EMERGENCY MEDICINE

A Comprehensive Review

Edited by

Thomas Clarke Kravis, M.D.

Chairman, Department of Emergency Care and
Medical Director, Ambulatory Care
Mercy Hospital and Medical Center;
Director, Emergency Care and Training Institute
San Diego, California

Carmen Germaine Warner, R.N., M.S.N., F.A.A.N.

Associate Professor, California State University System
Consultant, Community Health Systems and Emergency Medical Care
Coordinating Editor, Topics in Emergency Medicine
Leucadia, California

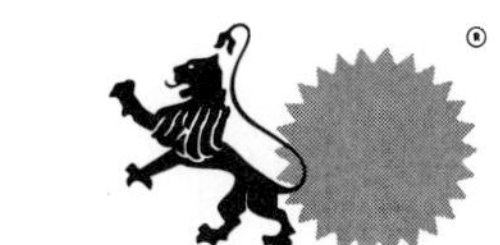

AN ASPEN PUBLICATION®
Aspen Systems Corporation
Rockville, Maryland
London
1983

Library of Congress Cataloging in Publication Data
Main entry under title:

Emergency medicine.

Includes bibliographical references and index.
1. Emergency medicine.   I. Kravis, Thomas
Clarke.   II. Warner, Carmen Germaine, 1941–
RC86.7.E585 1982   616'.025   82-11505
ISBN 0-89443-365-2

Publisher: John Marozsan
Editorial Director: N. Darlene Como
Managing Editor: Margot Raphael
Assistant Editor: Ruth Judy
Printing and Manufacturing: Debbie Collins

Library of Congress Catalog Card Number: 82-11505
ISBN: 0-89443-365-2

Printed in the United States of America

1 2 3 4 5

*To
Mavourneen,
Maureen,
Geraldine,
and Robert Oscar Peterson;
to the Sisters of Mercy,
friends, colleagues,
and other dedicated health care professionals
at Mercy Hospital and Medical Center.*

T.C.K.

*To my mother, Dorothy Loreen Warner,
and to my loving family,
John, Ryan Christopher, and Tracy Janée Robbins,
who encourage and support me in whatever I do.*

C.G.W.

Consultants

JOHN A. AALBERS, M.D.
Neurology, San Diego, California

SAM ASSAM, M.D.
San Diego, California

PAUL AUERBACH, M.D.
Associate Professor, San Francisco General
Hospital, San Francisco, California

G. RICHARD BRAEN, M.D.
Director of Emergency Services, Associate
Professor of Emergency and Internal Medicine,
University of Kentucky Medical Center, Lexington,
Kentucky

ALBERT B. BUTLER, M.D.
Department of Neurological Surgery, University of
Virginia School of Medicine, Charlottesville,
Virginia

DAVID L. CHADWICK, M.D.
Medical Director, Children's Hospital and Health
Center, San Diego, California

ARKY R. CIANCUTTI, M.D.
Natural Learning Center, Inc., Mendocino,
California

JACK L. CLAUSEN, M.D.
Department of Medicine, University of California,
San Diego, California

ROGER CORNELL, M.D.
Scripps Clinic and Research Foundation, La Jolla,
California

DONALD J. DALESSIO, M.D.
Chairman, Department of Medicine; Head,
Division of Neurology, Scripps Clinic and Research
Foundation, La Jolla, California

ARTHUR DAWSON, M.D.
Division of Chest Medicine, Scripps Clinic Medical
Group, Inc., La Jolla, California

HUGH A. FRANK, M.D.
Clinical Professor, Director, Regional Burn
Treatment Center, University of California, San
Diego, California

GORDON R. FREEMAN, M.D., F.A.C.S.
Private Practice, Otolaryngology, Dyersburg,
Tennessee

RICHARD FRIEDMAN, M.D.
Cardiologist, San Diego, California

JERALD GLASSMAN, M.D.
  Director, Pacemaker Center, Mercy Hospital and
  Medical Center, San Diego, California

PATRICIA S. GORMAN, R.N., M.I.C.N.
  Paramedic Coordinator, Mercy Hospital and
  Medical Center, San Diego, California

LELAND B. HOUSMAN, M.D., F.A.C.C.
  Cardiac Surgery Medical Group of San Diego, San
  Diego, California

RICHARD L. JUDD, PH.D.
  Professor of Emergency Medical Services, Central
  Connecticut College, New Britain, Connecticut

MARGO MCCAFFERY, R.N., M.S., F.A.A.N.
  Consultant in the Nursing Care of People with
  Pain, Santa Monica, California

THOMAS F. MCGEE, PH.D.
  Director, Mental Health, Mercy Hospital and
  Medical Center, San Diego, California

NINA MERRILL, R.N.
  Director, Life Flight of Southern California, Long
  Beach, California

RODRIGO A. MUÑOZ, M.D.
  Private Practice, Psychiatry, San Diego, California

DOUGLAS PAY, M.D.
  Assistant Clinical Professor of Dermatology,
  University of California, San Diego, California

GAIL PISARCIK, R.N., M.S., C.S.
  Psychiatric Nurse Clinical Specialist, Emergency
  Ward, Massachusetts General Hospital, Boston,
  Massachusetts

RANDOLPH A. READ, M.D.
  General and Forensic Psychiatry, San Diego,
  California

SUSAN J. REHM, L.C.S.W.
  Director, Social Work Services, San Diego,
  California

GORDON SPROUL, M.D.
  Cardiovascular Surgeon, San Diego, California

RICHARD L. STENNES, M.D.
  Diplomate, American Board of Emergency
  Medicine; Assistant Clinical Professor, Emergency
  Medicine, University of California, Los Angeles,
  California

RONALD R. STEWART, M.D.
  Assistant Professor of Medicine, University of
  Pittsburgh; Medical Director, Emergency Medical
  Services, City of Pittsburgh, Pittsburgh,
  Pennsylvania

DAVID K. SUBIN, M.D.
  Orthopedic Surgery, San Diego, California

MARK H. SUSSELMAN, M.D.
  Vice Chairman, Department of Emergency Care,
  Mercy Hospital and Medical Center, San Diego,
  California

LAWRENCE C. THUM, M.D.
  Medical Director, Department of Psychiatry,
  Mercy Hospital and Medical Center, San Diego,
  California

RICK TIMMS, M.D.
  Pulmonary Division, Scripps Clinic and Research
  Foundation, La Jolla, California

DONALD D. TRUNKEY, M.D.
  Chief of Surgery, San Francisco General Hospital,
  University of California, San Francisco, California

RICHARD ULEVITCH, PH.D.
  Department of Immunopathology, Scripps Clinic
  and Research Foundation, La Jolla, California

GAIL WALRAVEN, R.N., M.S.
  Consultant in Health Care Management and
  Emergency Medical Services, San Diego, California

DICK WILKIN
  Paramedic Coordinator, General Manager,
  Administrator, Hartsons Ambulance Service, City
  of San Diego, San Diego, California

JOHN J. WILLEMS, M.D., F.A.C.O.G.
  Assistant Professor, Department of Reproductive
  Medicine, University of California, San Diego,
  California

Contributors

Editors

THOMAS CLARKE KRAVIS, M.D.
Chairman, Department of Emergency Care, and
Medical Director, Ambulatory Care, Mercy
Hospital and Medical Center; Director, Emergency
Care and Training Institute, San Diego, California

CARMEN GERMAINE WARNER, R.N., M.S.N.,
F.A.A.N.
Associate Professor, California State University
System; Consultant, Community Health Systems
and Emergency Medical Care; Coordinating
Editor, Topics in Emergency Medicine, Leucadia,
California

JAMES W. ALLEN, M.D.
Emergency Services, Inc., Mt. Carmel Hospitals,
Columbus, Ohio

TODD D. BAILEY, JR., M.D., PH.D.
Clinical Instructor of Emergency Medicine, UCLA
School of Medicine, Los Angeles, California

GLEN S. BARTLETT, M.D., PH.D.
Elizabethtown Hospital for Children and Youth,
Elizabethtown, Pennsylvania; The Harrisburg
Hospital and Polyclinic Hospital, Harrisburg,
Pennsylvania

G. RICHARD BRAEN, M.D.
Associate Professor of Emergency Medicine and
Internal Medicine, Department of Emergency
Medicine, University of Kentucky, Lexington,
Kentucky

BARRY E. BRENNER, M.D., PH.D.
Assistant Director, Emergency Medicine Center,
UCLA Hospitals, Los Angeles, California

JAMES CABRAL, M.D.
Vitreo-retinal Surgeon, San Diego, California

MICHAEL L. CALLAHAM, M.D.
Associate Chief, Emergency Medicine, Highland
General Hospital, Oakland, California; Clinical
Assistant Professor of Medicine, UCSF, San
Francisco, California

STEPHEN V. CANTRILL, M.D.
Attending Staff Physician, Emergency Medical
Services, Denver General Hospital, Denver,
Colorado

WILLIAM D. CLARK, M.D.
Assistant Professor of Medicine, Harvard Medical School; Medical Director, Cambridge and Somerville Alcoholism Intervention Center of CASPAR, Inc., Cambridge, Massachusetts

MARY ANN COOPER, M.D.
Associate Professor and Director of Graduate Medical Education, University of Louisville, Louisville, Kentucky

DAVIS CRACROFT, M.D.
Mercy Hospital and Medical Center, San Diego, California

CARL DAVID CUCCO, M.D.
Senior Resident, Department of Obstetrics and Gynecology, Chicago Lying-in Hospital, University of Chicago, Chicago, Illinois

STEWART E. DADMUN, M.D., F.A.C.P.
Clinical Professor of Medicine, UCSD School of Medicine, San Diego, California

JOSEPH M. DOLPHIN
Chief Executive Officer and Chairman of the Board of Medevac, Inc., San Diego, California

DAVID J. DULA, M.D.
Associate, Department of Emergency Medicine, Geisinger Medical Center, Danville, Pennsylvania

FRANK E. EHRLICH, M.D.
Chairman, Department of Emergency Medicine, Conemaugh Valley Memorial Hospital, Johnstown, Pennsylvania

RICHARD T. ELLISON III, M.D.
Division of Infectious Disease, University of Colorado School of Medicine, Denver, Colorado

JACEK B. FRANASZEK, M.D.
Associate Director, Department of Emergency Medicine, Rhode Island Hospital; Associate Professor of Surgery (Emergency Medicine), Brown University, Providence, Rhode Island

RICHARD G. FRIEDMAN, M.D.
Diplomate, American Board of Internal Medicine; Diplomate, Subspecialty of Cardiovascular Diseases; Clinical Instructor of Medicine, UCSD; Mercy Hospital, San Diego, California

E. JOHN GALLAGHER, M.D.
Director, Emergency Medicine Service, Bronx Municipal Hospital Center, Albert Einstein College of Medicine, Bronx, New York

GORDON GENTA, M.D.
Chief Resident in Otolaryngology, University of Colorado Health Sciences Center, Denver, Colorado

JOEL M. GEIDERMAN, M.D.
Attending Physician and Research Coordinator, and Department of Emergency Medicine; Clinical Instructor, Emergency Medicine Center, UCLA Hospitals, Los Angeles, California

EMANUEL K. GORDON, M.D.
Attending Emergency Physician, Department of Emergency Medicine, Cedars-Sinai Medical Center; Clinical Assistant Professor of Medicine, UCLA School of Medicine, Los Angeles, California

STEPHEN P. GORMICAN, M.D.
Department of Emergency Medicine, Scripps Memorial Hospital, La Jolla, California

SHIRLEY A. GRAVES, M.D.
Associate Professor of Anesthesiology and Pediatrics, University of Florida College of Medicine; Medical Director of Pediatric Intensive Care Unit, Shands Hospital, Gainesville, Florida

B. KEN GRAY, M.D.
Director, Department of Emergency and Ambulatory Medicine, William Beaumont Hospital, Royal Oak, Michigan

STEPHEN HAMBURGER, M.D., F.A.C.P.
Associate Professor of Medicine and Vice Chairman, Department of Medicine, University of Missouri, School of Medicine, Kansas City, Missouri

BOB HEILIG, R.N., J.D.
Consultant, EMS Systems Design, Newport Beach, California

GEORGE L. HIGGINS III, M.D.
Department of Emergency Medicine, Maine Medical Center, Portland, Maine

GREGG T. HUSK, M.D.
Emergency Services, Jacobi Hospital, Bronx, New York

THEODORE L. JACKSON, M.D., F.A.C.S.
Director, Emergency Services, Martin Luther King Hospital; Associate Professor of Surgery, Charles R. Drew Postgraduate Medical School, Los Angeles, California

LESTER B. JACOBSON, M.D., F.A.C.C., F.A.C.P.
Director, Cardiovascular Education and Teaching, The Permanente Medical Group, Kaiser Foundation Hospital; Associate Clinical Professor of Medicine, UCSF, San Francisco, California

JOHN A. JANE, M.D., PH.D.
Department of Neurosurgery, University of Virginia, Charlottesville, Virginia

ROBERT C. JORDEN, M.D.
Staff Physician, Emergency Department, and Educational Coordinator, Emergency Medicine Residency, Denver General Hospital; Denver, Colorado

JOHN P. KELLY, D.M.D., M.D.
Harvard School of Dental Medicine; Oral and Maxillofacial Surgery, Massachusetts General Hospital, Boston, Massachusetts

MORRIS D. KERSTEIN, M.D.
Department of Surgery, Tulane Medical School, New Orleans, Louisiana

ERIC P. KINDWALL, M.D.
Assistant Adjunct Professor of Pharmacology, Division of Environmental Medicine, Medical College of Wisconsin; Director, Department of Hyperbaric Medicine, St. Luke's Hospital; Chairman, Wisconsin State Code Committee for Work in Compressed Air, Milwaukee, Wisconsin

RONALD L. KROME, M.D., F.A.C.S.
Chief, Emergency Medicine, Detroit Receiving Hospital and University Health Center; Chief, Section of Emergency Medicine and Professor of Surgery, Wayne State University School of Medicine, Detroit, Michigan

KEN KULIG, M.D.
Rocky Mountain Poison Center, Denver General Hospital, Denver, Colorado

GERALD S. LEVEY, M.D.
Professor and Chairman, Department of Medicine, University of Pittsburgh School of Medicine, Pittsburgh, Pennsylvania

LUKE K. LICALZI, M.D.
Department of Surgery, Yale University School of Medicine, New Haven, Connecticut

STUART J. MENN, M.D.
Clinical Assistant Professor of Medicine, UCSD School of Medicine; Scripps Clinic Medical Group, San Diego, California

Y. E. MILLER, M.D.
University of Colorado Medical Center, Denver, Colorado

JOHN A. MITAS II, M.D., F.A.C.P.
Naval Regional Medical Center; UCSD School of Medicine, San Diego, California

ATEF H. MOAWAD, M.D.
Professor, Department of Obstetrics and Gynecology and Chief of Obstetrics, Chicago Lying-in Hospital, University of Chicago, Chicago, Illinois

JAMES O. PAGE, J.D.
Executive Director, ACT (Advanced Coronary Treatment) Foundation; Publisher and Editor-in-Chief, *JEMS* (*Journal of Emergency Medical Services*); Basking Ridge, New Jersey

MERRILL-LYNN PAGE, R.N., M.N., C.S.
Massachusetts General Hospital; Boston-North Shore Associates, P.C., Boston, Massachusetts

PAUL M. PARIS, M.D.
Assistant Professor of Medicine and Program Director, Affiliated Residency in Emergency Medicine, University of Pittsburgh, Pittsburgh, Pennsylvania

ROBERTA PETERSON, M.S.S.W.
Pacific Asian and Latino Training Center, Union of Pan Asian Communities, San Diego, California

REBECCA W. RIMEL, R.N., B.S.N., N.P.
Department of Neurosurgery, University of Virginia Medical Center, Charlottesville, Virginia

DAVID ROSE, M.D.
Director, Critical Care, Mercy Hospital and Medical Center, San Diego, California; University of California, Irvine, California

MARK ALLEN ROSEN, M.D.
UCLA Medical Center, Los Angeles, California

DAVID RUSH, PHARM. D.
Associate Professor, Schools of Medicine and Pharmacy, University of Missouri, Kansas City, Missouri

NEAL W. SALOMON, M.D.
Northwest Surgical Associates, Portland, Oregon

JEFFREY A. SANDLER, M.D.
Endocrinologist, Mercy Hospital and Scripps Clinic Medical Group, San Diego, California

CLARICE A. SCHULTZ, R.N., B.S.N.
Instructor, Continuing Education Department, Nursing Division, Joliet Junior College, Joliet, Illinois

KENNETH E. SCHULTZ, M.D.
Director, Department of Emergency Medicine; Consultant, Emergency Medicine Services Associates, Harrisburg, Pennsylvania

CHARLES H. SCOGGIN, M.D.
Division of Pulmonary Sciences, University of Colorado Health Sciences Center, Denver, Colorado

BARBARA SECORD-PLETZ, R.N., M.I.C.N.
EMS Consultant, San Francisco, California

MARK ALLEN SHAFFER, M.D.
Assistant Professor, Department of Emergency Medicine, University of Chicago Hospitals and Clinics; Project Medical Director, Chicago South Mobile Intensive Care System, Chicago, Illinois

DANIEL SHINE, M.D.
Assistant Attending Physician, Montefiore Hospital and Medical Center; Assistant Professor of Community Health and Medicine, Albert Einstein College of Medicine; Medical Director, Montefiore Methadone Maintenance Treatment Program; Bronx, New York

ROBERT R. SIMON, M.D.
Assistant Professor, Emergency Medicine; Assistant Residency Director, Emergency Medicine Center, UCLA Hospitals, Los Angeles, California

GEORGE L. STERNBACH, M.D.
Deputy Medical Director, Emergency Services, Stanford University Medical Center, Stanford, California

CAROLYN M. STEWART, PHARM. D.
Staff Pharmacist, Mission Bay Hospital, San Diego, California

JAMES P. STEWART, PHARM. D.
Director of Pharmacy Services, Mercy Hospital and Medical Center, San Diego, California

RUTH I. STOLL, B.S.N. ED., M.S.N.
Doctoral Candidate at The Catholic University of America, Washington, D.C.

JOHN B. SULLIVAN, JR., M.D.
Assistant Professor, University of Colorado; Associate Director, Rocky Mountain Poison Center, Denver, Colorado

R. M. TATE, M.D.
University of Colorado Medical Center, Denver, Colorado

JUNE D. THOMPSON, R.N., M.S.
Assistant Professor, University of Texas School of Nursing, Houston, Texas

DORRIS E. TINKER, PH.D.
Assistant Professor of Pediatrics, Pennsylvania State University College of Medicine, Milton S. Hershey Medical Center, Hershey, Pennsylvania

GEORGE W. TYSON, M.D.
Assistant Professor of Neurosurgery, University of North Carolina, Chapel Hill, North Carolina

PETER VAKTOR, M.D.
Staff Physician, Department of Emergency Medicine, Royal Victoria Hospital; Lecturer, Department of Surgery, McGill University Faculty of Medicine, Montreal, Quebec, Canada

ALEXANDER D. VARGAS, M.D., F.A.C.S.
Assistant Professor of Surgery/Urology, LAC-USC Medical School, Los Angeles, California

GARY W. WILLIAMS, M.D., PH.D.
Scripps Clinic Medical Group, La Jolla, California

MIKE WILLIAMS, M.P.A.
Consultant, EMS Systems Design, Irvine, California

BEVERLEY C. YIP, B.S., M.S.W.
Executive Director, Union of Pan Asian Communties, San Diego, California

STEPHEN H. ZINNER, M.D.
Professor of Medicine and Head, Division of Infectious Diseases, Brown University, Roger Williams General Hospital, Providence, Rhode Island

Table of Contents

PART I

Section I
ORGANIZATION AND DELIVERY OF EMERGENCY MEDICAL CARE

Section II
SHOCK AND TRAUMA

Section III
METABOLIC AND ENDOCRINE EMERGENCIES

Section IV
GENERAL EMERGENCIES

Section V
PEDIATRIC EMERGENCIES

Section VI
ENVIRONMENTAL EMERGENCIES

Section VII
PSYCHIATRIC EMERGENCIES

Section VIII
SOCIAL AND BEHAVIORAL CONSIDERATIONS

PART II

Section IX
ALTERATIONS OF CENTRAL NERVOUS SYSTEM FUNCTIONS

Section X
ALTERATIONS OF CIRCULATORY SYSTEM FUNCTIONS

Section XI
ALTERATIONS OF RESPIRATORY SYSTEM FUNCTIONS

Section XII
ALTERATIONS OF URINARY AND REPRODUCTIVE SYSTEM FUNCTIONS

Section XIII
HEAD AND NECK EMERGENCIES

Section XIV
PRACTICAL APPLICATIONS OF EMERGENCY CARE

Foreword

The geometric rise in the number of patient visits to emergency departments over the past two decades made it clear that a new medical specialty had to be defined. Improvements in transportation and communications, the mobility among the people of the United States, the public's view of the hospital as a resource to be used for emergency medical needs, and the acknowledgment by leaders in the field of medicine that there was no planned response to medical and surgical emergencies has provided the substrate for the growth of emergency medicine as a distinct discipline. The recognition of emergency medicine as the newest medical specialty is fundamentally a response to unprecedented social, technological, and medical developments.

The character of the practice of emergency medicine is understandably unique. With rare exception, emergency departments accept any patient who seeks medical care. The emergency department is considered a critical care unit, but it is the only such unit to which patients admit themselves—before a physician has determined whether the patients' medical need requires admission. Furthermore, emergency medicine is a time-related specialty. Even if the problem is not a life- or limb-threatening condition, it must be handled expeditiously.

More than any other specialty, emergency medicine requires a team approach. Nursing staff commonly manage prehospital patient care, make triage decisions, apply standing orders, and make initial diagnostic decisions. The teamwork concept also extends emergency care into the community by means of specialized communications, transportation, and the emergency physicians' delegation of responsibility to those specially trained and skilled as paramedical personnel.

Emergency medicine is service-oriented, both to the patient and to the individual practitioner in the medical community. It deals with problem identification, palliation of symptoms, the reduction of patient anxiety, the referral of patients to appropriate physicians, and, in collaboration with physicians who will provide continuing care, the initiation of diagnostic testing and/or treatment of the patient.

The clinical practice of emergency medicine includes patients of all age groups with medical problems ranging from child abuse to cardiopulmonary failure, and from trauma to toxication. It is almost a certainty that more ambulatory patients with social, environmental, behavioral, cardiac, toxic, and trauma emergencies are initially treated by emergency physicians than by any other specialty group. Systematic planning with the collaboration of other medical specialists in providing for the secondary and tertiary needs of these patients is but another unique aspect of emergency care.

In the future, supplies and equipment that heretofore have been adapted and borrowed from other patient care settings will be developed especially for emergency medicine. This will result in further adaptations of critical care techniques as it becomes possible to use them in the prehospital arena. Research within emergency medicine, an essential hallmark of a specialty, will also evolve, further defining new diagnostic and treatment modalities for the future. A comprehensive review of emergency medicine should take into account the evolutionary process that requires subsequent adaptations in the clinical approach to patient care problems. This text, therefore, addresses the current clinical approach to problems seen in the emergency department; as such, it provides the most comprehensive and important codification to date of emergency medicine as it will be practiced in the 1980s.

B. Ken Gray, M.D.
Director, Department
 of Emergency and
 Ambulatory Medicine
William Beaumont Hospital
Royal Oak, Michigan
August 1982

Foreword

The emergency department mirrors the needs of health care consumers. It is far more than a reception and treatment center for the critically ill and injured. The center and the type of patients seen indicate the quality of life and health in the community.

Over the past 30 years, the emergency department has been catapulted into a busy primary, episodic, and emergency health care center. While the explosion is partly due to the sophisticated prehospital Emergency Medical Service (EMS) system by which patients who have suffered major physiologic deficits can be resuscitated and stabilized before they reach the hospital, it is mostly due to those individuals who visit the emergency department with minor, primary care type complaints. In 1954, 9.7 million persons visited the emergency department, or 5.9 visits for every 100 persons. In 1980, that figure had jumped to 83.5 million visits, or 38.2 for every 100 persons.

Alvin Toffler in *Future Shock* states that the present-day world is characterized by changes and stressors on every front. We have turned our country into a high-speed rat race, and our emergency departments are the best indicators of how that race is being run. Consumers using emergency services are experiencing maladaptation. Regardless of the factor that precipitated the problem, assistance is needed. The emergency center must be prepared to meet individual needs, whether they require advanced physiologic technologies and interventions, or simply self-care instructions.

As emergency health care providers, we must assess the needs of consumers and develop methodologies to meet those needs. Efforts to prevent disease and injury must include primary techniques, such as community education and accident prevention programs; secondary techniques, such as immediate physiologic and psychological care; and tertiary techniques, such as self-care instruction. If we are to produce harmony from the mounting dissonance among consumer needs, consumer expectations, and current health care delivery modes, we must recognize the contributions of our various disciplines and build on the strengths of each.

Together, the emergency care team can have a potentially dynamic impact on the health care needs of consumers. This text, written by an interdisciplinary team, is a text of emergency care. Rather than presume that total care is dictated by any single discipline, the authors have emphasized an interdisciplinary and interdependent approach to emergency care.

The field of emergency care has experienced both periods of growth and periods of stability during the past decade. We are now challenged to go on to the next level of emergency care delivery systems. We must stretch to understand consumer needs and the complex intervening sociological variables. We must study together and conduct research to advance our knowledge of physiologic processes and appropriate intervention techniques. We must work to improve and expand the emergency care delivery systems. We are working together, and we will succeed.

June D. Thompson, R.N., M.S.
Past President
Emergency Department Nurses
Association
Houston, Texas
August 1982

Foreword

Emergency medicine as a specialty is a relatively new concept, but the use of paramedics to provide prehospital emergency care is an even more recent development. Because of the many lives that paramedics have saved, however, the public now expects this service just as they expect police and fire protection.

The idea of paramedics as we know them today was first introduced in Ireland in the early 1960s. Their primary purpose was originally the resuscitation of patients who had suffered cardiac arrests. About ten years later, the first paramedic program in the United States was implemented in Miami Beach, Florida. Subsequently, paramedic programs have been established in numerous cities throughout the United States, and paramedics have become providers of advanced life support to victims of all serious medical and surgical emergencies. The current status of paramedics evolved from their raison d'etre—to provide advanced life support during the first few critical moments of the emergency. This concept allows paramedics to stabilize a patient's condition prior to transport, thus saving precious minutes that often mean the difference between life and death.

The comprehensive level of care that paramedics render in the prehospital environment has, in essence, extended the capabilities of today's sophisticated hospital emergency departments to serve the community when and where they are needed: at home, in the street, at work, at play—wherever and whenever a medical emergency may occur. This delivery of high-quality emergency medical care is truly a team effort, requiring a well-coordinated Emergency Medical Service (EMS) system. The importance of this teamwork to the effectiveness of any EMS system is difficult to overstate. If an individual element of the team fails to perform adequately, then the efforts of the entire system can be greatly diminished. Expert field treatment will do the patient little good if the hospital treatment is inadequate.

Thus, there is a certain "interdependency" among the EMS team members: the citizen bystander whose role is to alert the EMS system and render immediate aid until trained personnel arrive; the first responder, usually someone from the local fire or police department, whose function is to provide basic life support to the sick and injured until the paramedics arrive; the paramedics whose function is to act as the eyes, ears, and hands of the emergency department personnel; and the specially trained nurses and physicians who direct the paramedics in advanced care techniques, as well as receive and treat the patients brought to the hospital.

The underlying theme of this text is the interdependency of the emergency medical team members' skill and expertise. Recognition of this important insight can enhance the effectiveness of the individual, as well as of the emergency care team as a whole. The delivery of effective prehospital emergency medical care is dependent not only on good teamwork, but also on the mutual understanding of all team members' roles and the basis for their actions. It is in this capacity that this text will have significant value for paramedical personnel: it will allow them an in-depth understanding of the job performed by the emergency department nurses and physicians they work with daily. In addition, the sophisticated technology and rapid advances in emergency medicine require that all medical personnel frequently update their skills and expertise to remain competent. This text is an indispensable learning tool for medical professionals to keep abreast of the current state of the art.

Joseph M. Dolphin
Chief Executive Officer
and Chairman of the Board
of Medevac, Inc.
San Diego, California
August 1982

Preface

This comprehensive review of emergency medicine was conceived, designed, and developed for the purpose of enriching the quality of medical care provided to emergency patients. Although the emergency department was originally intended to provide initial care and treatment only to patients with acute illnesses or injuries, a variety of complex social and economic factors have caused people to seek medical attention at emergency departments for problems that are not always acute. The health care risks of patients who enter the emergency medical system will be significantly reduced if efficient and rapid triage, proper assessment, and appropriate intervention are accomplished when indicated. As increasing numbers of patients choose emergency departments for their care, new components of emergency medical systems have been introduced, and emergency medicine has emerged as a separate board specialty. Thus, one of the goals of this text is to provide an in-depth knowledge of a variety of different conditions so that emergency care personnel can quickly, accurately, and effectively distinguish between an urgent and a nonurgent problem.

Systems of emergency care have matured, and a trend toward sophisticated patient assessment and skilled intervention in the prehospital care setting has developed. It has also become increasingly clear that the high quality of care provided, as measured by patient morbidity and mortality rates, is determined not only by the knowledge and skills of the emergency department physician but also by the capabilities of the other integral members of the health care team, such as the emergency department nurse, the emergency medical technician, the paramedic, and the social worker. Each member of this multidisciplinary team in turn acknowledges the importance of the other essential components of the system, such as dispatch, land and air transportation, prehospital care communication, in-hospital services (e.g., laboratory tests and computerized axial tomography), and in-house specialists (e.g., the trauma surgeon), as well as the efficient management of the emergency department.

Because the editors are aware that each member of the emergency care team shares in the responsibility for the quality of care provided, representative team members were invited to participate in the preparation of this text. Among the contributing authors are practicing emergency physicians, emergency department nurses, medical educators, psychologists, surgeons, orthopedists, cardiologists, directors of emergency medicine training programs, paramedics, and social workers.

Thus, a second goal of this text is to provide the knowledge and skills required of this multidisciplined health care professional team.

This text has been divided into two parts. The first part commences with a section on emergency medical care systems and their relationship to prehospital care management; the remaining seven sections deal with both the urgent and nonurgent medical conditions that may affect multiorgan systems. The second part has been divided into sections concerning various medical emergencies involving different anatomical or physiological areas. The editors have presented pictorial representations of the anatomic areas under discussion within each section introduction. Throughout the text, each author has attempted, where possible, to follow the same general format: (1) the definition of the disease or process; (2) etiology; (3) pathology; (4) pathophysiology and clinical correlates, particularly the mechanism of injury or illness; (5) diagnosis; and (6) differential diagnosis.

Finally, the treatment of the various conditions discussed has been outlined to include the prehospital phase, the emergency department phase (including relevant diagnostic and therapeutic procedures), the indications for admission, and the suggested management of patients who can be discharged for continued ambulatory care. An atlas concisely illustrating some of the therapeutic and diagnostic procedures commonly utilized in the emergency department is provided in Chapter 71. For easy reference, every drug mentioned in the text, with its generic and trade names, dosage forms, uses, adult and pediatric dosages, contraindications, precautions, adverse reactions, and drug interactions, has been outlined in Chapter 72.

Thomas Clarke Kravis, M.D.
Carmen Germaine Warner, R.N.,
M.S.N., F.A.A.N.
August 1982

Acknowledgments

It is our pleasure to offer a warm and sincere thank you to the many competent, dedicated professionals who have participated in the design, development, and production of *Emergency Medicine: A Comprehensive Review*. To the contributors, who have adjusted their busy work schedules in order to adhere to rigid timetables, rewrite and revise manuscripts, and respond to numerous letters of inquiry, we extend our sincere gratitude for their exceptionally outstanding work. This indeed is a tribute to the authors who have made this book a reality.

The quality and comprehensiveness of the book has been enhanced by the comments of the many health care professionals who participated in the review and evaluation process. The consultants, whose names appear on page v, deserve recognition for their comments and recommendations.

Complementing the efforts of the health care professionals are the talents of several committed individuals whose energies have greatly benefited and influenced the design of this book. First of all, we would like to acknowledge B. Wallace Hood, Jr., former editorial director at Aspen Systems Corporation, who proposed the idea for this book. N. Darlene Como, currently the editorial director at Aspen Systems Corporation, continued the development of the project and, through her support, creativity, and special friendship, provided the much appreciated encouragement and motivation that has kept the project on schedule. Margot Raphael, managing editor at Aspen Systems Corporation, along with Ruth Judy, her assistant, and Debbie Collins, production specialist, has provided the top quality expertise and special attention that have resulted in an incredibly rapid production time without the sacrifice of excellence. Finally, we wish to recognize Gail Martin for her outstanding job as copy editor on the manuscript and Ann Beranek for her proofreading skill.

The illustrative design in this book has contributed significantly to its high quality. John W. Brown and Mary Zilinsky have displayed their unique talents for innovative design through the superb graphics that complement each chapter.

No editor has ever realized the dream of a scholarly endeavor such as this book without the encouragement, faithfulness, and loyalty of a professional secretary. Pat Summers, who for years has been a special friend and support system to Ms. Warner, and Catherine Serrato, who has proved to be of irreplaceable value to Dr. Kravis, are two remarkable and committed women. Their indefatigable strength has enabled us to maintain our enthusiasm and momentum during the development of this book.

Finally, we are grateful to you, the emergency care clinician, who has assisted in the development of an emergency medicine specialty through your desire for knowledge and quest for quality care. By your application of the material in this book, each of you will influence the continued growth and the ongoing search for excellence in emergency health care to which we are all committed.

Organization and Delivery of Emergency Medical Care

One of the goals of emergency care personnel is to distinguish quickly and accurately the urgent from the nonurgent condition. There is no better term than the French word *triage* to describe this process, defined as "the sorting of and allocation of treatment to patients . . . according to a system of priorities designed to maximize the number of survivors."* While the process, as explained in "Triage" (Chapter 1), usually begins in the prehospital care setting, the process changes according to the number of patients, the mechanism or degree of illness or injury, the availability of specialized care centers (Chapter 2), the level of sophistication of prehospital emergency care personnel (Chapter 3), and the time required for transport. Triage is continued in the emergency department as the nurse and physician evaluate the condition of each patient, and the principle is even employed in establishing priorities of care in an individual patient.

In "Emergency Systems: An Approach for Trauma Care" (Chapter 2), the author presents the unique problems encountered in the care of the trauma patient with multiple severe injuries and explores the various approaches available. While a plan for the development of a trauma center at a particular hospital is presented, it is recognized that this formula may not be effective in dealing with emergencies in all geographical areas or in all medical specialties.

In contrast to the *systems* approach, the *medical* approach to the patient with shock and trauma is reviewed in Section II, as well as in "Chest Trauma" (Chapter 61), "Genitourinary Emergencies" (Chapter 62), and "Head and Neck Emergencies" (Section XIII).

In "Prehospital Emergency Care and Transportation" (Chapter 3), the author provides an approach to patient assessment and care, emphasizes communications, describes the various vehicles and equipment utilized, and reviews some of the training, knowledge, and skills required by paramedics. An important but often neglected component of the emergency medical system is the care required while a patient is transported by air, and this is addressed in "Critical Care Air Transport" (Chapter 4). Another topic that is germane to the practicing emergency department physician, nurse, and paramedic is "Emergency Care and the Law" (Chapter 5), which is written by a practicing paramedic-lawyer.

---

* *Webster's New Collegiate Dictionary.* Springfield, Mass.: G.C. Merriam Co., 1981.

1. Triage

STEPHEN P. GORMICAN, M.D.

Emergencies are diverse and episodic. The goal of triage is to place the right patient at the right level of care at the right time. Optimal utilization of resources is the responsibility of emergency physicians from the earliest prehospital phase to final emergency department disposition.

Prehospital triage decisions include when to transport, when to treat in the field, when to bypass the nearest medical facility, and how to manage multiple patients simultaneously. Whether or not individual emergency physicians are involved in the planning and control of the emergency medical services (EMS) system, they must be familiar with their role in the system and the resources at their disposal and be ready to intervene in the event that they are needed.

In-hospital or emergency department triage is performed at the time a patient is first seen at the hospital. The actual categories used, the qualifications of the person performing triage, the extent of the triage examination, the use of protocols, and whether laboratory tests and radiographs are ordered at the time of triage vary from hospital to hospital. Of critical importance is that emergency physicians are responsible for the process and the results of triage while on duty and should ensure that the triage system operating at their hospital is optimally meeting the patients' needs.

In this chapter triage will be discussed first as it pertains to prehospital care and then as it pertains to emergency department care.

PREHOSPITAL TRIAGE

Prehospital triage can be divided into those decisions that affect a single patient and those that affect multiple patients.

Single Patient Field Triage

Triage decisions involving one patient include access triage, dispatch triage, whether or not to transport, whether to treat in the field or transport, and where to transport.

Access Triage

When to call an ambulance or paramedic service is a triage decision made by the public. Those involved with the EMS system should educate the public not to underutilize or overutilize the EMS system. Any repetitive inappropriate uses by a patient should be addressed by the emergency physician when the patient arrives in the ED, and whatever secondary gain the patient derives from this behavior should be identified and minimized. Taking a unit out of service for a patient who does not require access through this route weakens the EMS system's ability to respond to genuine emergencies elsewhere.

Dispatch Triage

If an EMS system has both EMT-I and EMT-P (paramedic) units, there is a critical triage decision made at the time of dispatch. The dispatcher must be able to identify those conditions when a paramedic unit should be sent immediately rather than waiting for a first responder assessment. Dispatch protocols should be written or reviewed by the local emergency physicians, taking into account the number of units available and the likelihood of simultaneous dispatch.

When to Transport

In general, each patient should be transported whenever an ambulance is called. Even when transport appears to be unnecessary, it would seem unwise for an EMT-I or paramedic to make that decision without having the patient assessed by a physician. If the patient feels that transport is not needed, a signed release form should be obtained. If the patient feels that transport is needed, there could be some legal hazard in denying transport regardless of the medical condition. (See Chapter 5.)

When an ambulance transport is medically indicated but the patient refuses, every effort should be made to convince that patient to go to the emergency department. If the patient persists in refusing transport, a release form must be signed. Those who are mentally incompetent, or a danger to themselves or others, should be taken into custody either by the paramedics, if this is allowed by state law, or by the police.

Field Treatment or Transport

The advantages of field medical treatment should be balanced by the disadvantages of delayed transport. The amount of time the paramedics spend in the field depends on the distance from the hospital, the duration of the specific field treatment, and the specific disorder being treated.

Transit times should always be taken into consideration. Treatment modalities that may be appropriate for a patient with a 20-minute estimated time of arrival may not be appropriate for the patient who has a transport time of 1 minute.

Obviously, fast, high-yield procedures are preferable over slow, low-yield procedures. Clearing an airway, controlling arterial bleeding, and administering epinephrine for acute systemic anaphylaxis are examples of the former. Elaborate wound dressings and extensive histories and physical examinations are examples of the latter. However, the value of any field treatment should be assessed in conjunction with a specific disorder.

At one end of the spectrum is the patient with severe multiple trauma. Trauma victims in hemorrhagic shock require definitive treatment by a qualified trauma surgeon in the operating room. They usually cannot be stabilized in the field, and everything should be done to minimize the accident-to-surgery time. The neck should be immobilized, the patient placed on an antishock garment (inflated, if appropriate), and transport begun with intravenous lines started en route. Occasionally it may be necessary to start an intravenous line at the scene of the accident, but any significant delay or extensive examination at the scene is to be avoided. Patients with nontraumatic cardiac emergencies are an example of the type of medical condition that is at the other end of the spectrum and frequently these patients can and should be stabilized in the field. If a patient is having a myocardial infarction, the time it takes to administer oxygen, connect an electrocardiographic monitor, start an intravenous line, and give morphine and/or lidocaine when indicated is usually worth the delay at the scene. (See Chapter 49.)

Where to Transport

Centers or specialized care facilities can often offer better care for certain critical patients. The Emergency Medical Services System Act of 1973 has identified the following critical categories: burn, neonatal, behavioral, spinal cord injuries, poisoning, cardiac, and trauma.

The multiple trauma category has raised the most controversy, and is discussed at length in Chapter 2. Centers for burn, neonatal, behavioral, and spinal cord injuries have evolved in many communities. Patients in those categories are often assessed and stabilized at the nearest medical facility first and are, therefore, more commonly involved in interhospital transfer rather than direct prehospital transport to the center. Poison centers are often telephone consultant services rather than treatment centers, and cardiac patients are often appropriately treated at the nearest facility that has cardiac care capability.

With regionalization of trauma care, major trauma victims usually bypass nearer facilities and are transported directly to a trauma center. The triage system that identifies those patients must be sensitive enough to select patients who do in fact need a trauma center, and still be specific enough to ensure that minor trauma is not inappropriately diverted to the center. Efforts to establish objective criteria for this task have led to various numerical scales. One of the simplest is the CRAMS scale. The acronym CRAMS represents each of the five categories measured: *c*irculation, *r*espiration, *a*bdomen, *m*otor, and *s*peech. It is numerically similar to the Apgar score and easy to memorize (Exhibit 1–1). A somewhat more involved scale is Champion's Trauma Score (Exhibit 1–2). Although the number of patients in the CRAMS scale study was small, an initial com-

Exhibit 1–1 CRAMS Scale

Circulation	Normal capillary refill and BP > 100......2
	Delayed capillary refill or BP 85 to 100......1
	No capillary refill or BP < 85 0
Respiration	Normal......2
	Abnormal (labored or shallow)......1
	Absent 0
Abdomen	Abdomen and thorax nontender 2
	Abdomen or thorax tender 1
	Abdomen rigid, flail chest, or penetrating wounds to abdomen or thorax......0
Motor	Normal......2
	Responds only to pain (other than decerebrate)......1
	No response (or decerebrate) 0
Speech	Normal......2
	Confused 1
	No intelligible words......0

Note: Score ≤8 = major trauma; score ≥9 = minor trauma.
Source: Gormican S: CRAMS scale: Field triage of trauma victims. *Ann Emerg Med* 11(3):132–135, 1982.

parison of the two scales seemed to indicate that the CRAMS scale was more sensitive in identifying those patients who need to go directly to the operating room for general surgery or neurosurgery.[1] Data collected since that study has statistically confirmed that trend, and a larger study is currently under way.

Although some form of objective criteria should be used as a starting point, the triage decision of the base station physician or medical authority involved should include factors such as mechanism of injury, age, underlying medical condition, increase in field time that might result from bypassing the nearest facility, and capabilities of the bypassed hospital. Patient preference should be considered when there is more than one trauma center in the area and the above factors are equal.

Multiple Patient Field Triage

Multiple patient field triage may involve care for two patients or for the many victims of a full-scale national disaster. The principles of single patient field triage also apply to multiple patient triage. Additionally, any time an EMS system is stressed beyond normal functioning, a reallocation of resources must take place. In a three-victim accident, this can involve simply dispatching a second transport unit and possibly activating a move-up system for the area left uncovered. As the number of casualties increases, additional facets of a plan should be phased in as needed, including full activation of the county and/or the state disaster plan.[2,3] All emergency physicians must be familiar with the plan to handle multiple casualties in the EMS system in which they

practice and should have no reluctance to activate the plan when indicated. Underreaction may result in poor patient care, while overreaction merely results in unplanned disaster drills. If the plan cannot be appropriately activated for seven to ten victims, it should probably be rewritten. While the specifics of the disaster plan depend on local resources, it should include establishing medical command, performing scene triage, determining the degree of field treatment, and establishing appropriate lines of communication.

Medical Command

The medical command is generally assumed by the most senior medical person at the scene who is familiar with the plan. This will likely be an EMT-I or paramedic initially, but command may be transferred to an emergency physician if the severity of the incident warrants a physician at the scene. The involvement in patient care of this person will vary depending on the number of victims. For example, if there are 10 victims, he or she may be totally involved in patient care; if there are 20, only assistance with triage may be practical; and if there are 50, the medical commander will likely be totally involved in mobilizing resources and coordinating activities of a triage officer, treatment officer, transportation officer, and communication officer. Before getting involved in any patient care, the senior medical person at the scene should step back and get an overview of the situation in order to make sure that resources are appropriately mobilized and utilized. This

Exhibit 1–2 Champion's Trauma Score

	RATE	POINTS	SCORE
A. *Respiratory:* Number of respirations in 15 seconds; multiply by four	10–24	4	
	25–35	3	
	>35	2	
	<10	1	
	0	0	A. _______
B. *Respiratory Effort:*	Normal	1	
	Shallow or Retractive	0	B. _______
Shallow—markedly decreased chest movement or air exchange *Retractive*—use of accessory muscles or intercostal muscle retraction			
C. *Systolic Blood Pressure:* *Systolic cuff pressure*; either arm—auscultate or palpate	>90	4	
	70–90	3	
	50–69	2	
	<50	1	
No carotid pulse	0	0	C. _______
D. *Capillary Refill:* *Normal*—forehead or lip mucosa color refill in 2 seconds	Normal	2	
	Delayed	1	
	None	0	D. _______
Delayed—more than 2 seconds capillary refill *None*—no capillary refill			

E. *Glasgow Coma Scale:*

1. *Eye Opening*

			Total GCS Points	Score
Spontaneous	___4		14–15	5
To voice	___3		11–13	4
To pain	___2		8–10	3
None	___1		5– 7	2
			3– 4	1 ___ E. _______

2. *Verbal Response*

Oriented	___5
Confused	___4
Inappropriate words	___3
Incomprehensible words	___2
None	___1

3. *Motor Response*

Obeys command	___6
Purposeful movement (pain)	___5
Withdraw (pain)	___4
Flexion (pain)	___3
Extension (pain)	___2
None	___1

Total GCS Points (1 + 2 + 3)   ______________

Trauma Score _______
(Total points A + B + C + D + E)

Source: Champion H et al: The Trauma Score. *Critical Care Medicine* 9(9):672–676, 1981. © 1981 The Williams & Wilkins Co., Baltimore, Maryland.

individual's most important function is to take command and bring order out of chaos.

Scene Triage

Scene triage should be performed by those designated by the medical commander. They will likely be paramedics and perhaps physicians if the severity of the incident warrants. The purpose of field triage is to separate those victims who need immediate transport or treatment from those who can wait. The means of identifying the victims and the categories used should be simple. One method is to write on the forehead of each patient an *I* for immediate, *U* for urgent, *N* for nonurgent, and *X* for unsalvageable. Another method is to use color-coded tags. The important fact is that the method chosen must be consistently used and familiar to everyone involved.

Treatment should generally be delayed until triage is complete. Fast, high-yield procedures such as clearing an airway or compressing a bleeding artery may be appropriate, but it is only after triage is complete that treatment priorities can be accurately established. It would be unfortunate to spend time reducing a fractured tibia when inserting an oral airway in another patient would be life-saving. Also, it is imperative that the medical commander know the results of triage as early as possible to activate whatever part of the plan is necessary.

Once triage is complete, it is helpful to separate physically those needing immediate and urgent care from those whose care can wait. Those needing immediate care should be moved to an ambulance loading/treatment area, and those with nonurgent disorders should be directed to a holding area or bus loading area at the opposite end of the field.

Field Treatment

A determination of the degree of field treatment should be made by the medical commander as soon as triage is complete. This will depend on the number of injured, the time it will take to transport them, the time it will take to move personnel and supplies to the field, and the capabilities of the area hospitals.

The person in charge of transportation should obtain an early estimate of the time to evacuate the patients needing immediate and urgent care. If the number of victims is large, it may be necessary to ask the police to commandeer vans or trucks. In general, efforts should be directed at moving seriously injured patients to hospitals where such treatment is best administered. However, since some delay is anticipated at the ambulance loading/treatment area, the medical commander should direct available medical personnel to that area to begin

treatment. If long delays are anticipated, additional medical personnel should be summoned to the scene. Predesignated physician/nurse teams with appropriate prepackaged supplies should be put on early standby and activated when needed.

If the number of victims will likely overwhelm local hospital disaster capability, it would be wise to set up a temporary field treatment facility for the patients with nonurgent disorders. This can be done at the scene or perhaps at some predesignated school auditorium. Supply and personnel coordination of a first aid station should be done with the local American Red Cross or relief agency.

Smooth management of multiple casualties requires a written plan that is flexible enough to be phased in as needed and a medical commander with common sense.

EMERGENCY DEPARTMENT TRIAGE

Until recently, the first person a patient encountered when entering the emergency department was the registration clerk.[4] The registration clerk, with little or no formal training in triage, would often decide whether the patient needed to be seen immediately or should register and wait. Since even low-volume emergency departments are occasionally confronted with delays of 2 or more hours, it is obvious that some triage system is necessary to avoid having a seriously ill patient wait while patients with relatively minor problems are being seen. The sophistication of the triage system used depends on the needs of the particular emergency department.[5]

Triage Categories

Triage may be divided into categories according to severity, medical specialty, and location.

The number of severity categories can vary from two to five or more. Dividing patients into those that need immediate care, urgent care, or nonurgent care is probably sufficient for most emergency departments. If the triage system allows for those needing nonurgent care to be sent to an outpatient clinic, an additional semiurgent or nonurgent emergency department category may be desirable. It would be unwise to have a formal or even an informal category of no care needed. Despite the desire to save the patient's time and money, triage personnel should be aware of their lack of protection in assuming that responsibility. Even if a physician makes that determination, to do so without a documented chart is legally hazardous.

An institution's need to triage patients into medical specialty categories such as surgical, pediatric, and psychiatric will generally be obvious and depend on the size, design, and staffing of the particular emergency department.

Location categories can include an outpatient clinic or private physician's office. However, prior to sending a patient to a private physician's office, approval should be obtained from both the private physician and the emergency physician, and all cases should have emergency department documentation. Also, in order to triage to the proper location, there should be some feedback on flow and space availability within the emergency department.

The sophistication and formalization of triage categories will depend to some extent on yearly patient census. If there is usually a brief waiting room time, all that may be necessary is to have the triage nurse obtain a brief history and determine whether the patient is well enough to register (nonurgent), needs to be seen next (urgent), or needs to be seen immediately. Very busy emergency departments with average waits of 2 or more hours will need a more elaborate system.

Triage Personnel

Once an emergency department determines the exact type of triage system to be used, the qualifications of the triage person will usually be clear. While any intelligent person could probably be trained, an experienced emergency department nurse in this position will make the process easier.[6,7] The cost of using such a highly trained individual will generally be preferable to the cost and effort of training less-qualified people and the potential legal liability in using them. Although there has been some favorable response to using paramedical personnel,[8-10] the standard of care is evolving to the point where primary evaluation is expected to be done by a nurse. One advantage of choosing nurses is the ability to rotate other emergency department nurses into the triage nurse position.[7] This helps increase scheduling flexibility, prevent burnout, and more efficiently utilize the position as the workload expands or contracts. Also, as this concept of emergency department triage is becoming more formalized, training and orientation programs for triage nurses are being described.[5,7]

Although the emergency physician should be available for consultation, utilizing physicians for triage has not been effective for various reasons and has been discontinued in the few places it was instituted.[7-9]

Triage Examination

The triage history and examination can be very brief or extensive. This should depend on the severity of the problem and the time between presentation and eval-

uation. A problem requiring immediate physician intervention such as a gunshot wound to the chest does not need an extensive triage examination. The same is true for someone at the other end of the severity scale. For example, a healthy appearing teenager with a sprained ankle could generally wait for the emergency department nurse to take vital signs and obtain a medication/allergy history.

The time interval between patient presentation and nurse evaluation should probably be less than 15 minutes. If the patient census is low for available staffing and the patient will likely see the emergency department nurse in less than 15 minutes, a very brief triage examination would be reasonable. If the waiting time is expected to be longer, a more thorough examination should be done. In addition to the history of the presenting complaint and physical examination of the system in question, vital signs should be taken since they have proved screening ability.[7,8,11] However, if the patient census is high for available staffing and there is a delay of greater than 15 minutes before even seeing the triage nurse, it may be necessary to shorten the triage examination.[5] The extent of the examination should be tailored to a particular hospital's patient census and staff and should have some flexibility at times of high patient load.

Triage Protocols

Written protocols should be a part of any triage system. They can be as simple as general statements on triage or as elaborate as having a specific algorithm for each presenting complaint. An algorithm is a question that branches into either another question or final statement, depending on a yes or no answer. The degree of independent medical decison making is a function of the expertise of the person utilizing the algorithm. If someone without prior medical knowledge is trained as a triage technician, it may well be appropriate to have all decisions derived from strictly followed algorithms. On the other hand, if emergency department nurses were to use detailed algorithms, the triage examination may be prolonged without any improvement in results and lack of challenge can lead to boredom and job dissatisfaction. If some detail is desirable, protocols or algorithms should be written by the nurses and physicians in the department.[12] Available algorithms[5,12-14] could be used as a resource, but writing one's own not only ensures tailored results and better staff reception but also is an educational process in itself.

If the goal of triage is expanded from simply sorting patients to regulating flow, it may be efficient for the triage nurse to order tests such as a complete blood cell count, urinalysis, or distal extremity radiograph. Whether this is subject to protocol would depend on perceived problems and extent of ordering. A large number of diagnostic tests such as a cardiac panel or trauma panel should probably be under protocol when initiated by a nurse.[5]

Triage Evaluation

Before evaluating individual performance, the triage system should be evaluated to ensure that it meets the intended goals without being overly complex. If the goals are to speed the flow of patients, improve public relations, and keep seriously ill patients out of the waiting room, then each of those areas should be monitored. If the average time per patient visit is decreasing, fewer patient complaints are received, staff morale has improved, and the quality of patient care has improved, then the system is a good one.

To evaluate individual patients, one could study either process or outcome. Process criteria could include seeing each patient within 15 minutes, completing the examinations in 5 minutes, or proper documentation of vital signs. Outcome criteria would address problems such as incorrect triage. Obviously it is safer to overtriage questionable cases, and any pressure to correctly triage should be weighed against the danger of undertriage.

REFERENCES

1. Gormican S: CRAMS scale: Field triage of trauma victims. *Ann Emerg Med* 11:132–135, 1982.
2. Holloway R, et al: The EMS system and disaster planning: Some observations. *J Am Coll Emerg Physicians* 7:60–61, 1978.
3. Melton R, et al: Revising the rural hospital disaster plan: A role for the EMS system in managing the multiple casualty incident. *Ann Emerg Med* 10:39–44, 1981.
4. Graves H: ACEP surveys hospital triage systems. *J Am Coll Emerg Physicians* 1:31–33, 1972.
5. Rund D, Rausch T: *Triage.* St Louis, C. V. Mosby Co, 1981.
6. Mills J, et al: Effectiveness of nurse triage in the emergency department of an urban county hospital. *J Am Coll Emerg Physicians* 5:877–882, 1976.
7. Estrada E: Triage systems. *Nurs Clin North Am* 16:13–24, 1981.
8. Rosen P, et al: A method of triage within an emergency department. *J Am Coll Emerg Physicians* 3:85–86, 1974.
9. DeAngelis C, et al: The effectiveness of various health personnel as triage agents. *Commun Health* 2:268–277, 1977.
10. Wilson F, et al: Algorithm-directed triage of pediatric patients. *JAMA* 243:1528–1531, 1980.
11. Goddard J: Triage and vital signs, letter to the editor. *J Am Coll Emerg Physicians* 6:224–225, 1977.
12. Podgorny G: Evaluation of an EMS algorithm system. *Ann Emerg Med* 9:534–536, 1980.
13. Wolcott B: Basic decisions in emergency department cases: A logical approach. *J Am Coll Emerg Physicians* 7:149–151, 1978.
14. Looney G, et al: Research algorithms for emergency medicine. *Ann Emerg Med* 9:12–17, 1980.

2. Emergency Systems: An Approach for Trauma Care

MIKE WILLIAMS, M.P.A.
BOB HEILIG, R.N., J.D.

Considerable debate has arisen in the past 10 years concerning the capability of the existing emergency medical care systems to provide care for critically injured patients. Even as early as 1966, when the National Research Council initially raised doubts about the care of critically injured patients in the United States, it was clear that trauma care was, in the words of the Council, "the most neglected disease of modern society."[1] With the recognition of this problem, a growing demand for adequate care for trauma victims has been emerging across the United States. Federal funding initiatives and media exposure have added tremendous momentum to the campaign for improved trauma care, particularly in the area of developing trauma centers.

Numerous deficiencies have been cited in the current system for the in-hospital treatment of major trauma victims.[2–8] Most experts agree that the continued practice of transporting major trauma patients to the nearest hospital, rather than to a more qualified designated hospital capable of surgical care for the most complex injuries, will mean unnecessary major trauma patient mortality. While at the surface the premise appears reasonable, the possibility of altering existing referral patterns has been threatening to the hospital administrators and physicians alike. Much of the apprehension is due to lack of clear understanding of the commitment and strategies necessary to implement trauma centers.

This chapter will discuss regionalization of trauma care as one example of a systems approach to emergency medicine.

Criteria for an individual hospital's involvement as a trauma center are also considered. An objective review process for prospective applicants is outlined and specific preparatory actions are recommended. Finally, a critical look is taken at the designation process, giving specific suggestions for applicant hospitals on writing their proposals, hosting the on-site survey, and reacting to the competitive and political influences of the designation process.

HISTORY AND DEVELOPMENT OF TRAUMA CENTERS

During the past 40 years, it has been the U.S. military that has made most of the advances in the care of seriously injured trauma victims. Trauma patient mortality was significantly reduced during World War II, and even further reductions occurred during the Korean and Vietnam conflicts. Most experts believe the military approach—the immediate attention to injuries by paramedical personnel, rapid transport by helicopters that bypassed local aid stations for trauma centers (or MASH units)—has been the single most important reason for the reduction in trauma mortality.

In 1961, a pioneering two-bed clinical shock-trauma unit at the University of Maryland was established under a grant from the United States Army to study the pathophysiological and immunobacteriologic response to shock in humans. The first civilian trauma unit was established in 1966 at Cook County Hospital in Chicago. In that same year, the Maryland Shock-Trauma Unit extended its research program to include biochemical investigations of the critically injured patient. In 1971, a statewide system of trauma centers was implemented in the state of Illinois. Three levels of trauma centers were identified, and hospitals participating across the state were designated accordingly. In 1974, San Francisco General Hospital, with federal and Johnson & Johnson Foundation funding, initiated a countywide system of care for trauma victims in the entire city and county of San Francisco.

Since that time, trauma center development has been growing at an increasing rate, largely because of public media pressure and funding made available through the federal emergency medical service (EMS) grants. With these incentives and with pressures from health systems agencies, it is expected that the trauma center issue will be addressed in nearly every urban, suburban, and rural area of the United States in the near future.

TRAUMA CENTER SYSTEM MODELS

Orange County, California: Suburban/Urban Model

Approximately two million people live in Orange County, California, a 780-square-mile area nestled between Los Angeles and San Diego Counties. The county is economically middle or upper class and well endowed with health care resources. There are 38 licensed hospitals, and 28 of them have 24-hour physician-staffed emergency departments. Early planning for trauma center development was initiated by the county's Office of Emergency Medical Services under direction of the local government. Technical advice was provided by a surgeon trained at the San Francisco Trauma Center. A paper was published in 1978 comparing trauma deaths in Orange County with those in San Francisco.[7] The study found that 73 percent of the non-CNS (central nervous system) deaths and 28 percent of CNS deaths were potentially preventable in Orange County, while only one death in San Francisco was judged preventable. The study indicated that the deaths in Orange County occurred in younger patients, in those with lower injury severity scores, and during the normal acute treatment phase. In San Francisco the deaths occurred in older patients, in those with higher injury scores, and days, even weeks later as a result of chronic complications. This study suggested that the single trauma center system in San Francisco was far superior to the system in Orange County that transported patients to the closest emergency department.

The publication of these results touched off a furor in the medical community and widespread media interest. Eventually a repeat study was done by the coun-

ty's EMS office in conjunction with the county medical society. This report's findings supported the earlier results. The county EMS office then began working with the medical society and hospital council to develop "trauma service hospital" criteria. After numerous drafts, committee meetings, hearings, protests, and confrontations, a jointly endorsed trauma service hospital plan was approved by the board of supervisors. The trauma center approved criteria closely resemble the published American College of Surgeons standards.[9]

The trauma service hospital plan adopted called for four to six hospitals to be designated as trauma centers based on regional needs and estimates of trauma volumes. An objective out-of-county expert physician panel was selected to make the recommendations. On June 7, 1980, five trauma service hospitals went into operation, three and one-half years after the planning had begun. Four hospitals began operations as level II community trauma centers, and one, the University Medical Center, began as a level I trauma center. Since then, two further studies have documented the clinical success of these centers.[10,11]

The Illinois System: Statewide Model

The Illinois trauma program, initiated in 1971, features a three-echelon system of designated trauma centers: local, areawide, and regional. Each level has specific functional capabilities for the care of the trauma patient. The Illinois program utilizes a combined total of 50 small community hospitals and large medical centers in the three tiers. The three-tiered functional and commitment breakdown is as follows:

Local Trauma Centers

Local trauma centers provide basic resuscitation and life support to trauma victims and are required to provide physician coverage 24 hours a day. In these local trauma centers a trauma nurse and an emergency physician are on duty at all times to provide initial care for the critically injured patient.

Areawide Trauma Centers

The areawide trauma centers have been established across the state in mid-sized community hospitals (approximately 500 beds) and in communities over 50,000 in population. These areawide centers are required to provide 24-hour staffing by highly competent medical and allied health care personnel who are able to perform resuscitative and definitive care for all injured patients. All services such as operating rooms, intensive care unit (ICU), laboratory, blood bank, resuscitation equipment, and radiology facilities including arteriography and nuclear medicine must be available on a 24-hour basis. The designated trauma director must be experienced in the initial care, triage, and priority determinations for victims of severe trauma. Specialty consultants are available 24 hours per day on call. The centers transfer the most critically injured patients to a designated regional center.

Regional Trauma Centers

The regional trauma centers are located in communities with established or developing university health education complexes or affiliations. They provide sophisticated treatment and educational support and coordination for the statewide program. They are also the designated facility for professional education, paraprofessional training, regional transportation, communication systems, data control, and epidemiological and clinical study efforts.

Special Regional Centers

Patients with unique clinical problems are selectively transported to special regional centers as rapidly and efficiently as possible. At present there are three such specialized units in the Illinois system: Midwest Regional Spinal Cord Center, Children's Memorial Hospital Trauma Center, and the Central Nervous System Trauma Study Center, University of Chicago. Other burn centers are located in Rock Island, Springfield, and St. Louis.

Baltimore, Maryland System: Urban Model

Baltimore's trauma network features an echelon system of care especially designed for an urban area with numerous hospitals of similar capability in caring for trauma. The network identifies four staffing requirements at a slightly higher level than required for the level I facility described by the American College of Surgeons. These centers receive the most critical trauma cases from within Baltimore, each having a distinct service area for patient triage. Additionally, each areawide center has been designated for specialty referral responsibilities as follows:

Areawide Trauma Centers

- Maryland Institute of Emergency Medical Service (MIEMS)
  - adult trauma—outside the city of Baltimore (via state police helicopter)
  - hyperbaric center
  - CNS-spinal cord center
- Sinai Hospital
  - adult trauma center
  - neonatal center

- University of Maryland
  - adult trauma center
- Baltimore City Hospital
  - adult trauma center
  - burn center
  - neonatal center
- Johns Hopkins Hospital
  - pediatric trauma center
  - neonatal center
  - eye injury center

Specialty Referral Centers

- St. Agnes Hospital
  - neonatal
- Union Memorial Hospital
  - hand center and limb replantations

ASSESSING HOSPITAL INTEREST AND INVOLVEMENT

Rationale for Involvement

At the hospitals that decide to apply for designation as trauma centers, there are generally three main reasons for that decision: (1) the clinical rationale, (2) the have and have-not theory, and (3) advantages for the hospital.

Clinical Rationale

It is generally agreed that not all hospitals can be all things to all people. A consensus has been reached on regionalizing care for such patient categories as premature newborns, burn patients, and open-heart surgery patients. Each of these patient categories has been regionalized based on the understanding that it was impossible for all hospitals to provide the necessary specialty staff, equipment, and support resources to treat the very specialized needs of these few patients. Additionally, the actual numbers of these patients in regions have been so limited that physician, nurse, and paraprofessional skills could not be properly maintained at all of the hospitals. Physicians and support staff in high-volume burn centers, neonatal centers, and open-heart surgery centers are better trained and equipped to treat these patients. The same rationale has now been applied to services for critically injured trauma victims.

The Haves and the Have-Nots

During the past five years federal and quasi-federal governmental organizations have been emphasizing regionalization as a means of improving the effectiveness and efficiency of the health care system. Regionalization has been the basis for health systems agency plans to provide more cost-effective health care across the United States.

The health systems agency planning and approval powers now provide the best example of the have and the have-not influence. Physicians or hospital administrators must place themselves in the shoes of the health systems agency policymakers, imagining themselves on a certificate of need (CON) approval committee (keeping in mind that the health systems agency committees are required to have a 51 percent consumer majority). Two requests to approve one new CT scanner are before the committee and two hospitals are competing: hospital A and hospital B. The administrators or physicians must imagine themselves as a committee member who is a parent of three children. Hospital A is a 214-bed, general practice hospital with a limited obstetric service, limited open-heart surgery program, and a small oncology unit. Hospital B is a 200-bed, general practice hospital with a larger obstetric service, a moderate open-heart surgery program, and a small oncology unit. However, hospital B has recently been designated as a regional trauma center and provides care to 500 multiply injured victims per year, 40 percent of whom have an associated head injury. Which hospital could make better use of this expansion? Would the same committee approve a trauma center designation for a low-volume obstetric hospital (what about a pregnant trauma victim?) or approve new pediatric beds for a non-trauma center rather than for a trauma center? (Trauma is the leading cause of death for children.) The permutations are endless, but in each case the committee member's decision will be influenced by the trauma center status of hospital B.

Even though health systems agencies may not endure in their present form, it must be recognized that their powers have been duplicated at various state and local governmental levels. The implications of this trend cannot be ignored by administrators.

Advantages for the Hospital

Hospitals have identified the following benefits resulting from their decision to become trauma centers.

Financial:

- The average length of stay for trauma patients in a hospital is usually considerably longer than that of the average patient. (The average trauma patient stays 15 days in the hospital.) The length of stay in an intensive care unit (ICU) is usually 4 to 6 days.

- Trauma patients utilize high-profit centers within the hospital (i.e., laboratory, radiology, respiratory therapy, pharmacy).

- Utilization of other services improves–particularly those services that may previously have been underutilized on the afternoon and evening shifts. (Normally 60 percent of serious trauma occurs between 9:00 P.M. and 3:00 A.M.)

- The projected trauma patient insurance mix tends to be better than that of the average emergency patient.

- In areas with trauma centers, the system has tolerated an overtriage of patients (12 percent in Orange County, 25 percent in Baltimore), thus affecting more than just the existing trauma volume at non-trauma centers.

- Depending on the patient mix, applicant hospitals have often projected a gross annual profit margin of between 4 and 18 percent.

Certificate of Need:

- Many hospitals believe that the trauma center designation is but one of a limited number of regional designations being handed out by government organizations, with each designation enhancing the chances for obtaining the additional designations.

- Because of the increased utilization of medical/surgical beds, ICU beds, the CT scanner, and ancillary services, trauma centers will better be able to justify expanded services.

- A trauma center is better able to fit the profile of the successful CON applicant because of its participation in a program that has a proven record of reducing unnecessary duplication of services and personnel and providing optimal utilization of resources.

Image/Prestige:

- Trauma centers have the potential to increase other services as a result of the trauma center designation. (An Orange County trauma center has experienced a 12 percent increase in emergency department volume since designation and has further experienced a significant increase in elective surgeries.)

- The trauma center designation has excellent potential for image enhancement that will have positive effects in every area, including nurse recruitment, attracting other physicians to join the staff, obtaining research grants, fund raising activities, and developing human interest stories.

- The trauma team concept will have a carry-over effect on other functions within the hospital, thus improving interdisciplinary cooperation and optimizing team efforts.

Objective Review of a Hospital's Capability as a Trauma Center

The decision to apply for trauma center designation must be based on a careful assessment of a variety of objective and subjective factors. There are seven specific considerations.

1. *ability to develop full institutional commitment of administrative staff, medical staff, and the hospital board of directors.* It is rare that such a commitment is solidly in place early in the hospital's deliberations, but a mechanism must be available to develop such a commitment should the hospital decide to proceed.
2. *surgical leadership.* Specific surgical leadership (e.g., trauma director, trauma surgeon panel) must be available or be capable of being developed.
3. *clinical support capability.* The specific surgeon and anesthesiologist support plus a full array of medical staff specialists (e.g., neurosurgeons, orthopedists, thoracic surgeons), 24-hour clinical support services (radiology, including specialized procedures; laboratory; respiratory therapy), and clinical philosophies (operational and treatment protocols) must be in place or have the capacity to be developed.
4. *capacity and depth of coverage.* Trauma resuscitation beds (in the emergency department), ICU beds, medical/surgical beds, operating rooms, and staffing capability, particularly in support services, must be available in sufficient quantities and depth to match the expected patient demands on the system. It is particularly important to consider the impact of scheduling for different periods of demand.
5. *financial means.* The specific fiscal capability must exist within the hospital to staff and equip the trauma center.
6. *equipment.* The basic equipment needed to treat trauma patients should be objectively assessed and in place to meet all foreseeable patient demands.
7. *geographic considerations affecting potential volume and patient access.* A review of the potential volume of trauma patients should be made to ensure the trauma team's ability to maintain clinical

skills and to provide for fiscal viability of the programs. Both areas should be assessed based on the expected demands on the system.

It is of paramount importance that these factors be objectively assessed, preferably with the help of unbiased outsiders. In-house reviews are seldom rigorous enough, and may even place the hospital in a competitive *disadvantage* because of the false sense of security an in-house review provides.

Preparatory Actions Prior to Official Designation

The most commonly asked question among the policy makers of potential trauma centers is: "Just how much do we have to be doing before designation?" The answer is: it depends on the level of competition and what the designee's expectations are. As a general rule, applicant hospitals should be striving to meet or exceed the standards for a trauma center as early as possible. The rationale for this is simple: what better way is there to prove total hospital commitment than to meet the trauma center standards before one is required to. Furthermore, an early commitment to meet the trauma center criteria is also a mechanism to develop an important track record. If a particular selection committee is to designate one of two hospitals, and one hospital states it will meet the criteria and make additional commitments *after* designation and the other hospital states it has been operating as a trauma center for six months prior to review, the latter hospital will have the competitive edge.

Another reason for early adoption of the trauma center criteria is to test the system. There are numerous variations permitted within any approved set of criteria that must be acted on based on actual experience. Furthermore, the hospital may consider proposing exceptions to specific items within the criteria and will want to test these exceptions first. The final and best reason is that no two trauma centers in the United States are alike. There are numerous protocols and policies to be adopted and implemented, and when it comes time to propose opening the door as a trauma center, one will be able to confidently state that this trauma center's machinery is finely tuned and the protocols and policies are field tested. The first step prior to designation is, therefore, to make a commitment for meeting as many of the trauma center criteria as possible, as early as possible.

The next step for preparing for trauma center designation is to develop a workable plan of action or strategies and to stick to it. This plan must identify the management arm of the trauma center (e.g., trauma director, trauma committee), ensure correction of known deficiencies, develop the medical framework for the center (treatment and operational protocols), address evaluation and quality assurance needs of the center (e.g., trauma registry, morbidity and mortality conferences), and then review support commitments (e.g., public education and prevention campaigns, nurse trauma training programs, advanced trauma life support classes). After adopting a well-organized strategy it is important to stick to that plan and not to be distracted by reports of what the competition is doing. Practical experience has shown that reacting to the competitor's efforts will often lead to a disorganized and fragmented program.

IMPLEMENTING THE TRAUMA CENTER

The Priorities

The first task in implementing a trauma center is to establish a set of priorities. An individual hospital will quickly become overwhelmed with the multifaceted implementation requirements of developing the trauma center unless such a priority plan is in place.

- Establish the trauma management structure, designating a trauma director and a trauma nurse coordinator and organizing a hospital trauma committee. This first-priority attention is justified because many unforeseen implementational problems that must be dealt with will be more effectively and expeditiously handled with this management structure in place. Additionally, a committed trauma director will often implement independent program enhancements that could not have been planned nor foreseen by the hospital's administrative staff.

- Establish the medical framework for the trauma center through written operational and treatment protocols. The planning for this medical framework should be led by the trauma director, with coordination and direction by the trauma committee.

- Establish in-hospital trauma support programs such as:
    - data collection and evaluation efforts
    - trauma team training programs
    - trauma grand rounds and morbidity and mortality conferences
    - advanced trauma life support training classes
    - psychological/social program development
    - research programs
- Establish external hospital support programs such as:
    - public awareness and prevention campaigns
    - fund raising activities
    - regional trauma advisory committees

- liaison/affiliation with other trauma centers or tertiary facilities (e.g., burn center, spinal cord center)
- government liaison
- community hospital affiliations
- trauma recovery group

Establishment of the Trauma Management Team

Of key importance to the success of an application or continuing designation of a trauma center is the soundness of the trauma management team. In an optimum program, the trauma management team will ensure medical credibility, help establish and maintain medical staff commitment, oversee all trauma center operations, and act as a source of support and advocacy for internal hospital policy matters.

Trauma Director

The leader of the management team is the trauma director. This general or thoracic surgeon or trained traumatologist has overall responsibility for program planning, implementation, operations, evaluation, and out-of-hospital liaison and coordination. In addition, the trauma director establishes and implements all trauma operational and treatment protocols and has supervisory responsibility for trauma victims in the acute and early definitive-care periods of their hospital stay. The trauma director also has overall responsibility for training of trauma team members and for trauma research within the trauma center. Additional responsibilities of the trauma director are listed in Exhibit 2–1.

Who is selected for the trauma director position and how that selection is made are matters entirely dictated by the applicant hospital. There are so many factors affecting that decision (e.g., attractiveness of the area for recruitment, potential volume of the trauma center, private practice opportunities, and availability of in-house talent) that a general approach cannot be identified. One should recognize, however, that a trauma director who is completely new to the hospital, even if a recognized expert, will have difficulty developing internal hospital medical staff commitment, while a trauma director selected from within the hospital should have better results developing medical staff support but may have trouble being documented as a trauma expert. Some trauma centers have developed a blend of the two approaches, with some going so far as to appoint a trauma director from within the hospital and also to appoint a full-time trauma chief who is a recent graduate of a residency program with recognized expertise in trauma care. The leader of the program must have strong

Exhibit 2–1 Trauma Director Job Description

Qualifications:	Experienced board certified general or thoracic surgeon or traumatologist with demonstrated clinical, administrative, and leadership competencies.
Responsibilities:	Plan, develop, implement, and direct the trauma center program to meet the needs of critically injured patients.
Duties:	• Coordinate the trauma service plan and review the performance of care for trauma patients. • Assist the trauma committee in establishing quality assurance programs and audits of trauma cases. • Assist the trauma committee with the development of policies and procedures for a multidisciplinary team approach to care of the trauma patient. • Establish rapport and coordinate efforts with emergency department, surgery, intensive care unit, laboratory, pharmacy, radiology, respiratory therapy, and other appropriate areas of services. • Recruit and assume responsibility for qualified trauma surgical physician coverage. • Chair the trauma committee and regional trauma advisory committee and maintain liaison with area hospitals. • Supervise the development of training for all trauma team members. • Assist in the development/monitoring of appropriate prehospital triage criteria. • Develop/implement trauma operational protocols. • Maintain liaison with other regional trauma centers. • Assume responsibility for accuracy and validity of the trauma statistics. • Develop written transfer agreements as appropriate to include secondary critical care transport mechanisms. • Conduct and coordinate research on trauma. • Organize and conduct grand rounds, morbidity and mortality conferences, and medical audits on trauma patients. • Act as liaison with regional disaster planning efforts.

Source: EMS Systems Design, Irvine, California.

leadership ability and must be able to look beyond the sphere of the typical community hospital program, and must be capable of representing the hospital well.

Trauma Committee

Because of the multidisciplinary and multifaceted nature of the issues associated with trauma center planning, development, and implementation, a working team should be organized under the direction of the trauma director to oversee this effort. This interdepartmental committee will plan the implementation of trauma center standards, particularly the development and approval of the trauma operational and treatment protocols. The committee should include representatives from the following individuals or departments.

- trauma director
- trauma nurse coordinator
- emergency department physician director
- emergency department nurse supervisor
- neurosurgery
- radiology
- laboratory
- respiratory therapy
- ICU (nursing)
- operating room (nursing)
- psychological/social service
- rehabilitation
- administration
- other representation based on individual hospital needs.

Trauma Nurse Coordinator

The planning and ultimate designation as a trauma center will carry with it a significant staff workload. A tremendous amount of in-hospital coordination will be necessary to simply meet the trauma center standards. The basic framework aspects of implementing the trauma center will be the same whether the volume predicted will be 200 or 1,000 patients per year. It is important to recognize that this is another pivotal position for affecting the hospital's designation chances, particularly in measuring hospital commitment. The hospital, then, should clearly plan out minimum qualifications, recruitment requirements, and intended time to be allocated (full-time or part-time) to the trauma center issue. A sample job description is shown in Exhibit 2–2.

The actual recruitment pattern will vary from hospital to hospital, but it is sufficient to say that currently there is not a large cadre of trained, experienced trauma nurse coordinators in the United States. Most hospitals will be looking for more locally available talent who have similar program experience, with the background and interest in trauma, and with the developed leadership, communicative, and assertiveness skills so necessary for this program.

Development of Trauma Protocols

Experience across the nation has influenced the development of trauma protocols to ensure predictable

Exhibit 2–2 Trauma Nurse Coordinator Job Description

Qualifications:	Licensed registered nurse with certified emergency nurse (CEN) or certified critical care registered nurse (CCRN) certification. This nurse will have demonstrated abilities as follows: • strong critical care–emergency department background • leadership qualities • good communication skills • guided assertiveness • goal orientation • educational program coordination
Responsibilities:	Responsible for overall staff education, patient care problem identification, and staff activity coordination with the trauma director.
Duties:	• Assess areas of education and performance skills requiring development and establish the priorities with individual trauma team members. • Staff and coordinate the trauma committee and regional trauma advisory committee meetings. • Maintain the trauma registry, including gathering statistics and data. • Assist staff members in the maintenance of advanced trauma life support specialty certifications. • Identify patient education needs for incorporation in community service projects and regional education programs. • Participate in establishing and coordinating the trauma treatment and operation protocols and policies. • Maintain communication with prehospital personnel and hospital; coordinate trauma matters. • Coordinate liaison of support services. • Coordinate public education/prevention programs.

Source: EMS Systems Design, Irvine, California.

success with the trauma system in general and with individual patients as well. The term *protocol* for physicians often suggests a loss of freedom. Protocols, or guidelines, if properly produced, merely ensure care for each patient consistent with the broad patterns professionals can agree on. Physicians and other health care professionals continue to respond to individual trauma patients and exercise individual clinical options within the broad parameters agreed on in the protocols.

Three specific categories of protocols should be developed in any trauma care system. They are:

- triage protocols: a predetermined schematic for prehospital distribution

- operational protocols: a delineation of each health care provider's role
- treatment protocols: step-by-step descriptions for each patient's specific clinical problem

The triage protocols must be addressed by the entire region's providers and health care planners, and are covered in detail in Chapter 1. Operational protocols and treatment protocols are of interest to individual hospitals for purposes of planning a trauma center.

Operational Protocols

The purpose of the trauma center operational protocols is to define the following:

- the trauma team
- how the trauma team is initiated
- who responds
- what resources and responsibilities are required
- how team members effect communication
- when to effect communication
- when to initiate specific responsibilities
- who relates to whom

The basic reason for these protocols is that they help identify system expectations and specific responsibilities for individuals within the trauma center. The specific individual responsibilities are now conceptualized as a team responsibility, with the trauma surgeon as the team captain. Trauma team members thus begin to understand their role as it relates to the whole team and how the team must work together effectively if there is to be an optimally functioning trauma center. Operational protocols should be developed for each member of the trauma team and trauma support team. Such membership should include:

Trauma Team

- trauma surgeon
- anesthesiologist
- emergency physician
- physician specialists
- trauma nurses A and B
- nurse recorder/assistant
- laboratory technologist
- radiology technologist
- respiratory therapist

Trauma Support Team

- operating room nurse
- ICU nurse
- psychological/social services
- recovery nurse

- hospital security
- nursing house supervisor
- clinical pharmacist

An example of a trauma operational protocol is shown in Exhibit 2–3.

Trauma Treatment Protocols

The purpose of trauma treatment protocols is to define standards or guidelines for the treatment of seriously injured trauma patients. The protocols (or clinical algorithms) provide a uniform, highly specific set of guidelines for the management of trauma; and since they are specific in detail, these protocols should represent tested and validated standards. The protocols may then offer medical-legal protection for the trauma team members. Experience in other trauma centers has shown that trauma treatment protocols also offer the following benefits:

- enhance conformity with defined, optimal standards of care
- facilitate evaluation
- form the basis for professional and paraprofessional training programs
- enhance the coordinated and integrated trauma team response

Protocols should be developed for each category of traumatic injury and at each phase of delivery (e.g., prehospital, hospital resuscitation, ICU, rehabilitation). An example of one such protocol or clinical algorithm may be found in Figure 2–1.

Implementing Trauma Programs

Once substantial progress has been made on developing the trauma management team and the trauma protocols then various other trauma programs may be implemented. These programs do not substitute for the basic clinical standards for trauma centers (i.e., American College of Surgeons' standards) or for various local medical standards that may be developed. These programs merely enhance these standards and provide for a better framework for actually operating a trauma center. Such programs not only help identify the hospital's commitment to the program but also indicate the hospital's depth of thinking on the issue of improved trauma care. The programs are broken down into internal hospital support programs and external hospital support programs.

Exhibit 2–3 Trauma Operational Protocol

Role:	Laboratory technologist
How Notified:	By voice or page of a trauma patient code
Response:	On notification, the designated trauma laboratory technologist shall respond immediately to the trauma resuscitation room where he/she will be under the direction of the trauma surgeon. On arrival, the technologist *super stat* shall obtain 50 cc blood, return to the laboratory and perform tests according to the trauma protocol. Results of the hemoglobin and hematocrit shall be immediately reported back by telephone with follow-up hard copy. The trauma battery of laboratory tests shall routinely include as a minimum: • complete blood cell count • type and cross match (6 units) • blood gases (may be performed by respiratory therapist) • sequential multiple analyzer 12 • prothrombin/partial thromboplastin time • blood urea nitrogen • urinalysis • blood alcohol • platelet count • amylase determination All tests are to be handled on a basis with results immediately reported as available.
Additional Personnel:	All additional laboratory personnel needed will be notified by the trauma laboratory technician or at his/her request by the switchboard operators.
Evaluation:	This operational protocol shall be reviewed at least bimonthly.

Source: EMS Systems Design, Irvine, California.

Internal Hospital Support Programs

Advanced Trauma Life Support Training. To the extent possible, the applicant hospital should train and certify as many emergency department physicians, trauma surgeons, and anesthesiologists as possible in the American College of Surgeons' advanced trauma life support course. This is a 2-day course covering the manual and cognitive skills for the emergency resuscitation of trauma patients. The strength in this course is really the exposure and practice of the priority pattern that has proved optimal for trauma patient resuscitation. Additionally, through individual physician certification, the course

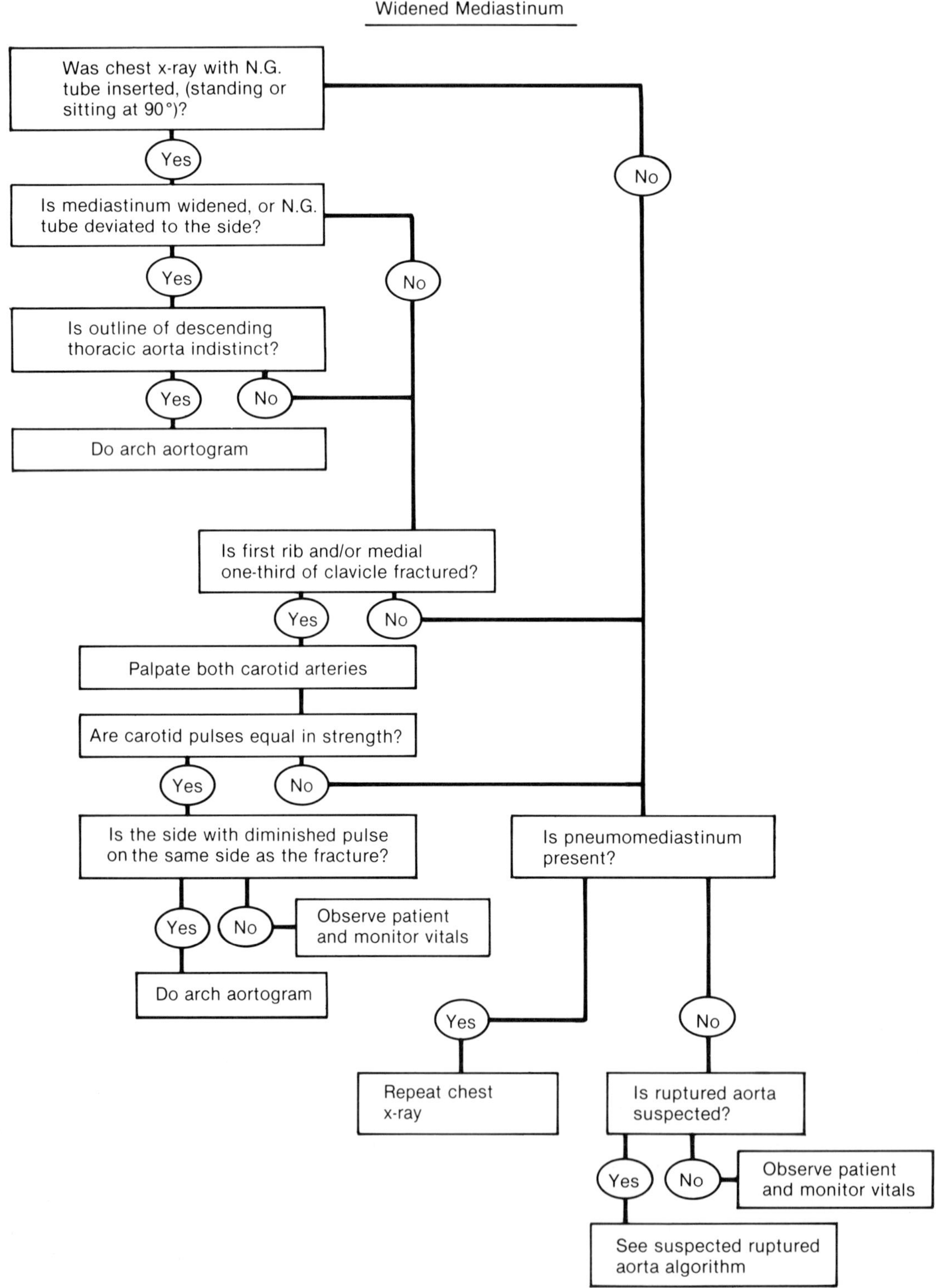

Figure 2–1 Trauma Treatment Algorithm. *Source:* Fountain Valley Community Trauma Center, Fountain Valley California, November 1980.

can help quantify trauma physician skills. Most applicant trauma centers should aim to provide their own advanced trauma life support training in-house for their own trauma center purpose as well as for satellite referral hospitals. Experience has shown that by training the staffs of satellite hospitals, the trauma center will improve its referral patterns. Future course schedules may be obtained by contacting the American College of Surgeons' national office in Lincoln, Nebraska, or the college's state coordinator.

Evaluation Program. Applicant hospitals should be taking steps to establish a comprehensive trauma evaluation program. A largely used data-base format is that of the trauma registry. The registry should provide a data bank of information on the prehospital, hospital, and follow-up care of trauma patients at the trauma center. (See Exhibit 2–4.) The registry data base should also include a retrospective review of all multisystem trauma patients treated at the hospital during the 12 months preceding designation. All trauma system-related data should be recorded, including: type of injury, location of accident, treatment time frames (e.g., time in emergency department, time to operating room, time of surgeon's response, length of stay, rehabilitation days). This retrospective view will indicate to the designating body the sincere interest of the applicant hospital in examining and evaluating its own track record.

Psychotraumatology Programs. Trauma center care should emphasize care of the total needs of trauma patients from clinical care, rehabilitation, and follow-up. Most current care focuses on the physical injuries of trauma patients and largely ignores the harmful emotional consequences of trauma. The psychotraumatology program for trauma centers should largely be a collaborative effort between psychological/social workers and the physician and nursing staffs. Trauma victims, some of whom would not survive under a less optimal system, must be taught to cope with changes in their body image, fears of dependency, and inabilities to perform former jobs. Additionally, families of trauma victims must be taught to cope with role changes of the victim within their own family structure. Finally, trauma centers must plan programs to recognize and treat staff burn-out and other associated problems as a result of the stressful trauma center environment. Program planning should be coordinated through the hospital's department of social work.

Trauma Nurse Training. An additional training program should be developed for all hospital nurses who will have responsibilities for treating trauma patients. In addition to the essentials of pathophysiology and the mandatory clinical skills, there should be "hands-on" training for nurses with equipment needed in a high-volume trauma center environment. Such skills training could be organized into several "skill days" or "equipment fairs" for this purpose.

External Hospital Support Programs

Tertiary Services. It is reasonable to assume that most applicant hospitals, when designated as trauma centers, will be unable to treat *all* trauma victims owing to special patient needs (e.g., burns, spinal injuries, limb replantation). Specific written transfer agreements should be developed with hospitals offering these services. A draft transfer agreement is shown in Exhibit 2–5.[12]

Community Hospital Affiliations. A significant advantage may be obtained during this application process if applicant hospitals are able to show other external hospital health care support for their designation. This support could come in several forms, including paramedic, physician, and other community hospital endorsements. Whenever possible, applicants should develop formal or informal support with other community hospitals, and in particular, specific endorsement on the applicant hospital's trauma center designation.

Public Education and Prevention. The nature of the cause of trauma lends itself to prevention campaigns and public awareness programs. Trauma, the leading cause of death for people under 40 years of age, is totally preventable. The establishment of a trauma public education and prevention program demonstrates that the applicant hospital has an interest in addressing the total problem of trauma care: prevention, and clinical treatment.

Regional Trauma Advisory Committee. In order to be fully effective in its region, the applicant trauma center must have the full participation and integration of other prehospital (police, fire, ambulance, and paramedic) and hospital participants in the area being served. A degree of suspicion and distrust will exist initially between the designated trauma center and the unsuccessful applicants or nondesignated hospitals. For these reasons, it is crucial that a regional trauma advisory committee be established. The designated trauma center would then utilize the regional trauma advisory committee as a forum for communication with other providers in the region served. By establishing a cooperative open communication system, problems in operational procedures will be avoided; and those problems occur-

Exhibit 2–4 County of Orange, Emergency Medical Services, Trauma Patient Registry

I. PREHOSPITAL PHASE

TRAUMA PATIENT REGISTRY #: _______________________

A. <u>PATIENT AND INCIDENT IDENTIFICATION DATA</u>

Age of patient _____________

Patient's sex: 1. Male
                2. Female

MICN Log #: _______________________

Medic Unit #: _____________   Time Medics
                                Arr. Scene _____________

Time Medics   Total Transport
Left Scene _____________   Time _____________

Incident Location:

____

Number   Street

____

                   City

Census Tract: ☐☐☐☐   ☐☐

INCIDENT TYPE:

01. Auto/Auto   07. Assault/Stabbing
02. Auto/Pedestrian   08. Assault/Other
03. Auto/Other   09. Fall
04. Motorcycle vs. _________   10. Fire
05. Bicycle vs. _________   11. Other: _________
06. Assault/Gunshot wound   12. Unknown

IF AUTOMOBILE ACCIDENT, WAS VICTIM:

1. Driver
2. Passenger, front seat
3. Passenger, back seat
4. Other: _______________________
5. Not applicable
6. Unknown

IF MOTORCYCLE ACCIDENT, WAS VICTIM:

1. Driver wearing helmet
2. Driver, no helmet
3. Driver, unknown whether wearing helmet
4. Passenger wearing helmet
5. Passenger, no helmet
6. Passenger, unknown whether wearing helmet
7. Other: _______________________
8. Not applicable
9. Unknown

Glasgow Coma Scale _______________________

Extrication Time _______________________

B. <u>PATIENT STATUS—PREHOSPITAL</u>

Vital signs: Pulse: _________ Resp: _________

Blood Pressure: _________ / _________

Traumatic injuries:
(Circle all that apply)   Estimated
                          blood loss:

1. Head/Neck Injury   _______________________
2. Chest Injury
3. Abdomen Injury
4. Extremity Injury
5. Other:

____

Level of consciousness: (Circle all that apply)	Pupils Right	Left	
		01	P.E.R.L.
1. Conscious	02	08	Pinpoint
2. Lethargic	03	09	Midposition
3. Confused	04	10	Dilated
4. Combative	05	11	Fixed
5. Unconscious	06	12	Respond
6. Uncon. Previously	07	13	Sluggish

C. <u>TREATMENT RECEIVED—PREHOSPITAL</u>

IV Fluids _________ cc   Airway:
# of lines _____   1. Nasal   4. Crico
                           2. Oral   5. Other:
                           3. EOA   _______________

TYPE OF TREATMENT: (Circle "#" if received)

01. Assisted ventilation   08. Cardiac Compression
02. Oxygen   09. Transmitted Telemetry
03. McSwain Dart   10. Backboard
04. MAST Suit Placed   11. C-Collar
05. MAST Suit Inflated   12. Sandbags
06. SST (Skeletal   13. Needlethoracentesis
    stabilization transport)   14. Other: _____________
07. Drugs _____________

D. <u>DISPOSITION—PREHOSPITAL</u>

Patient arrested in field:
1. Yes
2. No

If *Yes*, enter time of arrest: _______________
(24 hour clock)   hr   min

TRAUMA PATIENT DESIGNATED BY:
1. Base Station Hospital
2. Receiving Center
3. Trauma Center

<u>COMMENTS:</u>

Exhibit 2–4 continued

II. EMERGENCY DEPARTMENT PHASE

A. Patient and incident identification data

Trauma patient registry #: ________________________
    TC   PT#

Complete if patient transferred to TC:

Date admitted to E.D.: ________________________
    MO   DAY   YR

Time admitted to E.D.: ________________________
    HR   MIN

Trauma Center Admission data:

Date admitted to TC: ________________________
    MO   DAY   YR

Time admitted to TC: ________________________
    HR   MIN

Mode of Admission:
1. Paramedics (medic unit or ambulance)
2. Private ambulance (no medics in attendance)
3. Inter-facility transfer/ALS
4. Inter-facility transfer/BLS
5. Other: ________________________

If TRANSFER, state where from:

____

Reason for transfer: ________________________

If BURN PATIENT: Degree ______ BSA: ______%

              Degree ______ BSA: ______%

B. Treatment received—emergency department

Vital signs: Pulse ________   Resp ________

Temp: ________ __ C. GCS # ________

Blood Pressure ________ / ________

Crystalloids:	Blood:
Total number	Type:
of lines	1. Whole
functioning in	2. Products
ED: ______	Volume:
Volume:	
	________________cc
________________cc	Time of admin.:
	________________
	HR MIN

Airway:
1. Nasal	5. ET Tube	Chest Tube:
2. Oral	6. Trach	1. Single
3. EOA	7. Other:	2. Double
4. Crico	________________	3. None

Type of Treatment: (Circle "#" if received)
01. Cardiac Monitor	08. CPR
02. Assisted Ventilation	09. Foley
03. Oxygen	10. Nasogastric Tube
04. CVP	11. Autotransfusion
05. Pericardiocentesis	12. Thoracentesis
06. Paracentesis	13. Arterial line
07. Thoracotomy	14. Swan-Ganz

C. Laboratory and Radiology Orders

Laboratory (Ordered):	Radiology (Ordered)
01. Type and Cross	01. Chest Film
02. CB	02. Skull Film
03. Amylase	03. Abdominal Film
04. Urinalysis	04. IVP
05. Blood Gases	05. CT Scan
06. ECG	06. Angiogram ________
07. Alcohol/Toxicology	07. C-Spine
08. Coagulation	08. Extremity
09. Electrolytes	09. Pelvis
10. BUN/Sugar	10. Other: ________
11. Other: ________	

D. Consultations—Emergency Department

(USE 24 hour clock)	called:	arrived:
Trauma Surgery	________	________
Neurosurgery:	________	________
Thoracic Surgery:	________	________
Orthopedics:	________	________
Anesthesia:	________	________
________:		

E. Diagnosis at admission   *ICD.9.CM*

________________   ________   ________
________________   ________   ________
________________   ________   ________
________________   ________   ________
________________   ________   ________

F. Hospital Trauma Index
Enter highest index score recorded for each system:

System	Index
Respiratory	
Cardiovascular	
Nervous	
Abdominal	
Extremities	
Skin & Subcutaneous	
Complications	

G. Disposition—Emergency Department
(Circle all that apply)

1. Expired in ED	5. Transferred
2. Sent to OR	6. Discharged home
3. Admitted to ICU	7. Other:
4. Admitted to ward	________________

If patient was transferred:
where to: ________________

If patient expired, enter time
of death: ________________
    hr   min

Exhibit 2–4 continued

III. OPERATIVE CARE PHASE

TRAUMA PATIENT REGISTRY #: _________________

<u>Patient and incident identification date</u>

Date admitted to OR: _________________________________
          mo   day   yr

Time admitted to OR: _________________________________
          hr   min

Speciality of Surgical Assistant:
(First OR Surgery performed):

B. <u>Patient status—OR</u>

Vital signs: Pulse: _____________ Resp. _____________
Blood Pressure: _____________ / _____________

Crystalloids: Total number of lines functioning in OR:
Volume: _______________cc

Blood:
Type:
1. Whole
2. Products
Volume: _______________cc
Time of administration _______________
     hr   min

<u>Operations</u>

<u>Description</u> — Time — 24 hour clock — Date

ICD.9.CM   hr min   mo   day   yr

IV. ICU PHASE

A. <u>Patient and incident identification data</u>

_______________ days in ICU _______________ days on respirator

B. <u>Procedures</u> (Circle # of procedure if done in ICU)
1. Endotracheal intubation   4. Bronchoscopy
2. Arterial line   5. Swan-Ganz line
3. Tracheostomy   6. Other: _______________

C. <u>Complications</u>   mo   day   yr

1. Shock on admission
2. Cardiopulmonary arrest
3. Myocardial infarction
4. Pulmonary embolus
5. Gastrointestinal
   hemorrhage (stress)
6. Cardiac failure
7. Renal failure
8. Respiratory failure
9. Hepatic failure
10. Wound infection
11. Infection: _________(type)
12. Pulmonary infection
13. DIC
14. Other

Contact person: _______________________________

Phone #: _______________________________

V. FINAL DISPOSITION

A. <u>Patient and incident identification data</u>

Date of discharge: _______________________________
      mo   day   yr

# of days in hospital _______________
Disposition at discharge:
  If patient expired:
  date: _______________________________
      mo   day   yr

1. Disch. w/pre-injury capacity
2. Disch. w/handicap
3. Disch. to Convalescent Care
4. Death
5. Transferred   time: _______________
          hr   min
6. Other: _____________ ☐☐
  If tranferred, state
  where to:

Discharge diagnosis: *ICD.9.CM*

Autopsy: Coroner's Case   Coroners
1. Yes   1. Yes
2. No   2. No

B. *Financial data*   Source payments
Total treatment charge:
1. Medicare
2. Medicaid
3. 3rd Party
4. HMO
5. Cash
6. Other

Exhibit 2–4 continued

HOSPITAL TRAUMA INDEX

TRAUMA REGISTRY #: _____________
TC   PT#

Circle index score and
condition of final impression

SYSTEM	Initial Impression	INJURY	Class	INDEX
RESPIRATORY	NO INJURY		no injury	0
	chest discomfort—minimal findings		minor	1
	simple rib or sternal fracture (fx) chest wall contusion with pleuritic pain		moderate	2
	1st or multi-rib fx, hemothorax, pneumothorax		major	3
	open chest wounds, flail chest, tension pneumothorax normal (nl) blood pressure (bp), simple lac diaphragm		severe	4
	acute resp. failure (cyanosis), aspiration, tension pneumo. c + bp, bilateral flair, lac(s) diaphragm		critical	5
CARDIOVASCULAR	NO INJURY		no injury	0
	<10% (<500cc) blood volume (bv) loss, no change in skin perfusion		minor	1
	10–20% bv loss (500–1000cc), ↓ skin perfusion, urine normal (+300cc/hr), myocard, cont., bp normal		moderate	2
	20–30% bv loss (1000–1500cc), ↓ skin perfusion, urine (>30cc), tamponade, bp 80		major	3
	30–40% bv loss (1500–2000cc) ↓ skin perfusion, urine (<10cc), tamponade, conscious, bp <80		severe	4
	40–50% bv loss, restless, agitated, coma, cardiac contusion arrythmia, bp not obtainable		critical	5
	50% + bv loss, coma, cardiac arrest, no vital signs		fatal	6
NERVOUS SYSTEM	NO INJURY		no injury	0
	head trauma, c̄ or s̄ scalp lactns., no loss consciousness (coma), no fracture (fx)		minor	1
	head trauma c̄ brief coma (15′), skull fx, cervical pain c̄ minimal fndgs, one facial fx		moderate	2
	cerebral injury c̄ coma (+15′), depressed skull fx c̄ neuro fndgs, multi facial fxs		major	3
	cerebral injury c̄ coma (+60′) or neuro fndgs, cervical fx c̄ major neuro fndgs, i.e., paraplegia		severe	4
	cerebral injury c̄ coma c̄ no response to stimuli up to 24 hrs, cervical fx c̄ quadriplegia		critical	5
	cerebral injury c̄ no resp. to stimuli and c̄ dilated fixed pupil(s)		fatal	6
ABDOMINAL	NO INJURY		no injury	0
	mild abdominal wall, flank or back pain and tenderness s̄ peritoneal signs		minor	1
	acute flank, back or abdominal discomfort and tenderness, fx of a rib 7–12		moderate	2
	one of: minor liver, sm bowel, spleen, kidney, body pancr, mesentery, ureter, urethra, fxs 7–12 rib		major	3
	2 major: rupture, liver, bladder, head pancr, duodenum, colon, mesentery (large)		severe	4
	2 severe: crush liver, major vascular inclu.: thor and abdom aorta, cavae iliacs, hepatic veins		critical	5
EXTREMITIES	NO INJURY		no injury	0
	minor sprains & fx(s)—no long bones		minor	1
	simple fx(s): humerus, clavicle, radius, ulna tibia, fibula, single nerve		moderate	2
	fx(s) multiple moderate, cpd moderate, femur (simple), pelvic (stable), dislocation major, major nerve		major	3
	fx(s) two major, cpd femur, limb crush or amputation, unstable pelvic fx		severe	4
	fx(s) two severe, multiple major		critical	5

Exhibit 2–4 continued

SKIN AND SUBCUTANEOUS			
	NO INJURY	no injury	0
	<5% burn, abrasions, contusions, lacerations	minor	1
	5–15% burn, extensive contusions, avulsions, 3–6″ extensive lacerations (total 12″)	moderate	2
	15–30% burn, avulsions 12″–20″ laceration	major	3
	30–45% burn, avulsions entire leg, thigh or arm	severe	4
	45–60% burn (3rd degree)	critical	5
	60% + burn (3rd degree)	fatal	6

COMPLICATIONS

COMPLICATIONS			
	NO SIGNIFICANT COMPLICATIONS	none	0
	subq. wound infection, atelectasis, cystitis superficial thrombophlebitis, temp. <38.5° (101°F)	minor	1
	major wound infection, atelectasis, pyelonephritis, septic or deep thrombophlebitis, temp >38.5	moderate	2
	i.p. abscess, pneumonia, anuria or oliguria c̄ ↑ BUN (no dialysis), jaundice, <6u gi bleed, rds <1 day	major	3
	septicemia, empyema, peritonitis, pulm embolis (nl bp), renal failure (dialysis <1 wk), >6u bleed, <3d rds	severe	4
	septicemia c ↓ bp, pulm emb c̄ ↓ bp, renal failure 7–40d, gi bleed >12u. resp arrest >3d rds c̄ vent	critical	5
	pulm emb c̄ card arrest, cardiac arrest, renal failure >6 wks, coma >6 wks, >30d c̄ vent or >80% 02 >7d	fatal	6

DEFINITIONS: minor = trivial injury
moderate = minimal injury, short hospitalization anticipated
major = major injury, not immediately life-threatening
severe = life-threatening but survival probable
critical = survival uncertain
fatal = survival unlikely

ABBREVIATIONS:

bp — blood pressure	fx — fracture	s̄ — without	↓ — decreased
bv — blood volume	i.p. — intraperitoneal	sgns — signs	> — greater than
cpd — compound	lac–lactns — lacerations	u — units	< — less than
c̄ — with	mult — multiple	vent — ventilator	
d — days	nl — normal	wnd — wound	
fndgs — findings	rds — resp. distress synd.	↑ — increased	

Source: Orange County Office of Emergency Medical Services, Santa Ana, California.

ring will be resolved quickly. This committee will also act as a forum for other trauma centers to share data collected by the trauma registry. Suggested membership includes:

- trauma director
- trauma nurse coordinator
- regional or county EMS official
- emergency department physician from the trauma center and all non-trauma center hospitals of the region served
- emergency department nurse from all other non-trauma center hospitals in the region served
- fire department
- police department
- surgeons from all area hospitals
- land and air ambulance
- other individuals as needs may dictate.

The regional trauma advisory committee will additionally serve as the coordinating and planning arm for:

- regional trauma training
- regional trauma registry data collection and dissemination
- trauma prevention campaigns
- trauma awareness days
- case reviews and morbidity/mortality conferences

Exhibit 2–5 Referring Hospital Transfer Agreement

Agreement On Transfer Of Patients With
Certain Trauma Patient Conditions

TO: ____ Hospital

We, the undersigned, representing _____________________________ Hospital, as the referring hospital, request that _______________________________ Hospital, as the receiving hospital, enter into this transfer agreement with our hospital and our physicians to provide emergency care for patients with specific categories of critical conditions, when transfer of such patients is requested by a physician from the referring hospital and accepted by a physician of the receiving hospital staff. The specific categories are:

This transfer agreement reflects the emergency patient point-of-entry guidelines developed in Rhode Island to meet requirements of the Emergency Medical Services Systems Act of 1973 (P.L. 93–154) and the Emergency Medical Service amendments of 1976 (P.L. 94–573).

This agreement shall not be construed to create contract or other rights enforceable by members of the general public. This agreement will remain in force until superseded or modified by mutual agreement of the transferring and receiving hospital, with concurrence of the Department of Health. However, this agreement is also subject to termination by any party hereto in the event of cancellation or material adverse change in the malpractice liability insurance coverage of any other party hereto.

The undersigned undertake no responsibility for the transport of patients between hospitals or between the scene of any emergency and any hospital. In any case in which the carriage of a patient is deemed appropriate the obligation of any hospital or physician hereunder shall be limited to the taking of reasonable steps to arrange for such transport as is made available by the municipality or municipalities in which a patient or a referring hospital is located.

REQUESTED BY:

_______________________________	_______________________________
Chairman of Hospital Board	President of Medical Staff
_______________________________	_______________________________
Chief Executive Officer	Date

Source: Boyd D, et al: *Trauma Systems Development Manual For Emergency Medical Service Systems' Medical Directors and Clinical Consultants of Regional Trauma Centers.* Department of Health and Human Resources, 1979.

- regional trauma protocols
- coordination of helicopter services for trauma patients
- tertiary transport issues.

Trauma Recovery Group.   Many patients who previously would not have survived are surviving in a trauma center environment. These trauma patients undergo significant coping stresses as a result of body image changes, changes in family role, and career changes. A trauma recovery support group concept will assist these new survivors with coping problems subsequent to hospital care and rehabilitation. The recovery group may also be used to assist currently hospitalized victims to adjust and cope with their environment.

The Designation Process

What To Expect

Once the trauma system has been conceptualized within a community, a plan of action developed, and a specific criteria for trauma centers approved, the process for designation will begin. It is possible in urban/suburban areas that several hospitals will either meet the criteria or exceed it. In rural areas it is conceivable that no hospital will meet the criteria and that the designating body will be required to go to adjoining regions to obtain the necessary hospital resources. In either case a selection process will be initiated and the level of competition will be commensurate with the numbers and levels of applying facilities. An applicant hospital should insist, in the planning process, on a fair, objective, and medically based designation process.

It is impossible to predict the exact format and makeup of a selection process owing to the multiple variables and needs of individual communities. Most fair and objective reviews will include the following steps:

- request for proposal
- screening of proposals by staff to ensure proposals meet minimum standards
- review of proposals by an objective selection committee of trauma experts
- on-site visits by the selection committee
- selection committee recommendations
- an appeal process
- designations implemented

The most impartial selection committee would probably be a committee composed of trauma clinical experts from outside the region to be served, which has the *total authority* to make the designations based simply on medical capabilities and commitments of the applicant hospitals as they relate to the defined regional trauma center criteria.

Responding to the Request for Proposal

Applicant hospitals should keep in mind that responding to the trauma center request for proposal is not like writing a certificate of need application. The applicant hospital must define who will be reviewing the applications and what that reviewer's interest will be. A health systems agency staff person's interests and perceptions (i.e., cost containment, occupancy levels, and optimal resource utilization) will be quite different from the trauma surgeon reviewer (e.g., medical staff commitment, clinical protocols). Additionally, the application must be perceived as in two stages: the written proposal and the on-site survey. The proposal must be carefully written so as to state accurately the hospital's commitment. Many hours could be spent by the selection committee scrutinizing and discussing the written application to prepare the committee members for the on-site survey. When the comparison is made by the selection committees of the written application and the on-site survey, they should correspond to each other.

The following components should be reflected in a written response to a request for proposal:

- a basic description of the region's trauma problem, indirectly describing the applicant hospital's understanding of regional needs
- a conceptual overview of how the applicant hospital

will address the problems or how the system will work

- a description of how the applicant hospital meets the criteria, indicating in the case of exceptions how these exceptions enhance the total patient approach
- a description of how the applicant exceeds the criteria and why the applicant should be selected
- selected information based on the reviewers' orientations (e.g., clinical protocols for the trauma surgeon, utilization rates, and bed/day costs for health systems agency staff)

Sufficient time should be permitted for hospital staff input prior to submission to ensure their endorsement of the entire application and of specific components therein.

The On-Site Survey

Probably 60 percent of the applicant hospital's score will be assessed during the on-site survey. This is largely due to the lasting impressions (both positive and negative) that are left when the selection committee meets with the actual people who will operate the trauma center. If there is a need to ensure a good written proposal, it is doubly important to ensure an excellent on-site survey. It is possible for an applicant hospital to have a superior written application but to lose the designation during the on-site visit because of a lack of knowledge of key staff or a disagreement among hospital staff as to the extent of hospital commitment.

On-site surveys should be carefully rehearsed and practiced. Many hospital medical and nursing staff will not be familiar with the competitive on-site survey process, and their lack of familiarity with the process may make a poor impression on the survey team.

The on-site survey is usually a verification of commitments made in the proposal, and undoubtedly the surveyors will want to talk to those specific people making the commitments, such as the board of directors, medical staff, and administrative staff members. A thorough review of equipment, drugs, and medications is usually undertaken. This step will be a test of how thorough the hospital's own assessment has been. There is nothing more embarrassing than a survey team finding an expired drug, a thoracotomy tray without the required rib spreaders, or a nurse who does not know how to set up an autotransfuser. Finally, the survey team undoubtedly will want to look at the physical plant and a tour should be conducted from the *trauma patient's perspective*. The easiest points to score are those regarding drugs, equipment, and physical plant. The hardest points to win are those associated with a functional understanding of the trauma center commitments and those points associated with the personal commitment of individual trauma team members.

Competition and Its Impact

The level of competition in a trauma center designation process will depend on the number of competent facilities that apply. It is clear that if there were a selection system that kept hospitals from aggressively competing against each other, that system would probably be preferred. The associated long-term bitterness that exists with a highly competitive process is often difficult if not impossible to remove even years after the designation. From a regional standpoint, competition may be helpful because applicant hospitals are often willing to make more commitments under a competitive system. The key to a successful application process is to develop a blend of competition and commitment to preclude long-term hostility but to ensure that hospitals make commitments they are reasonably and permanently able to keep.

In any competitive trauma center process, it is not sufficient to state that the applicant hospital will meet the criteria, it is important to exceed the criteria in every aspect possible. Nor in such an environment is it sufficient to state that the applicant hospital will begin its commitments on the day of designation. The hospital must be meeting and exceeding trauma center standards as early as possible to provide that necessary track record and total hospital commitment. Additionally, the competitive environment often does not end with designation. The designated facility will often be required to defend the designation years after the formal title of trauma center is bestowed.

Community Politics

If a designation process were totally fair, objective, and medically based, community politics would not play a part in the designation process for trauma centers. The reality in most communities, however, is that politics does play a part and its actual impact and direction is not usually known until it is too late to counteract its effects. While it is not usually desirable to have a heavy "arm-twisting" political campaign prior to trauma center designation, it is important to maintain enough visibility that political policy makers, who may have an impact on the designations, know the level of commitment developing at the applicant hospital. Additionally, if the hospital makes a decision to apply for trauma center designation and believes in the need for it, the hospital should then be visible in its support for a trauma center system in the planning phases, even if there is some opposition. This support should also be voiced to the political policy makers. Political policy makers should also be reinforced (either in writing or by telephone) if they take any steps to improve trauma care. As an example, a board of supervisors or commissioners agreeing to fund a new ambulance or to fund a trauma study should quickly be formally recognized by the hospital as having taken a positive step toward improving trauma care in the community.

SUMMARY

Trauma center development will not occur in every community, and not all individual hospitals should develop such a service or make a decision to apply for such a designation. However, the conceptual framework of developing a trauma center (e.g., team development, objective assessments) may be applied to many other programs; and the proposed logical, organized implementation model can be applied to all hospitals. Fortunately, the trauma center issue forces individual hospitals to take an inventory of hospital priorities, medical staff commitments, and future hospital directions for the potential benefit of the critically injured patient. Such an inventory cannot help but be of tremendous help in improving trauma care.

REFERENCES

1. *Accidental Death and Disability: The Neglected Disease of Modern Society*. Washington, DC, National Academy of Services of the National Research Council, Committee on Trauma and Committee on Shock, September 1966.
2. Van Wagoner FH: Died in hospital: A three-year study of deaths following trauma. *J Trauma* 1:401–408, 1961.
3. Frey CF, Huelke DF, Gikas PW: Resuscitation and survival in motor vehicle accidents. *J Trauma* 9:292–307, 1969.
4. Gertner HR, Baker SP, Rutherford RB, et al: Evaluation of management of vehicular fatalities secondary to abdominal injury. *J Trauma* 12:425–431, 1972.
5. Moylan JA, Detmer DE, Rose J, et al: Evaluation of the quality of hospital care for major trauma. *J Trauma* 16:517–523, 1976.
6. Detmer DE, Moylan JA, Rose J, et al: Regional categorization and quality of care in major trauma. *J Trauma* 17:592–599, 1977.
7. West JG, Trunkey DD, Lim RC: Systems of trauma care: A study of two counties. *Arch Surg* 114:455–460, 1979.
8. Trunkey DD: Bay area trauma care. *San Francisco Medicine* 55:22–25, 1982.
9. Optimal Hospital Resources for Care of the Seriously Injured. Bulletin of the American College of Surgeons, February 1980.
10. West JG, Cazzaniga A, Cales R: The impact of regionalization. *San Francisco Medicine*, submitted for publication.
11. Cales R: A follow-up study of Orange County Trauma System. *San Francisco Medicine* submitted for publication.
12. Boyd D, Cowley RA, Edlich R, et al: *Trauma Systems Development Manual For Emergency Medical Services Systems Medical Directors and Clinical Consultants of Regional Trauma Centers*. Department of Health and Human Services (formerly Department of Health, Education and Welfare) contract #232–78–0170, 1979.

3. Prehospital Emergency Care and Transportation

BARBARA SECORD-PLETZ, R.N., M.I.C.N.

Prehospital care (PHC) incorporates all emergency rescue, medical, and transportation services provided to ill or injured patients outside the hospital. It has become an outreach of hospital-based emergency care into the community. Ultimate responsibility for each PHC system's medical quality rests with its emergency physicians. Over the past 15 years PHC has evolved from a "scoop-and-run" transport service, staffed by minimally trained attendants, to integrated emergency medical services systems (EMSS). Many systems deliver advanced life support to the patient at the emergency scene and during transport:

The year is 1965:

2:00 A.M. A 50-year-old man, previously in good health, awakens with crushing substernal chest pain and shortness of breath. His frightened wife is unsure how to summon assistance.

2:07 A.M. She consults the telephone directory. There is no medical emergency number listed. She checks the yellow pages and finds seven different ambulance companies listed.

2:09 A.M. She calls one and is informed that they do not offer a 24-hour service.

2:11 A.M. She reaches a second company, whose ambulances are momentarily unavailable but will respond as soon as possible.

2:21 A.M. The ambulance still has not arrived. She calls again and is told one is on the way.

2:23 A.M. Returning to the bedroom she finds her husband cyanotic, not breathing, and unresponsive. She helplessly waits.

2:29 A.M. The ambulance crew arrives. They load the patient into the ambulance and speed toward the closest hospital with red lights flashing and sirens screaming. The patient attendant attempts cardiopulmonary resuscitation in the rear of the lurching vehicle.

2:35 A.M. The ambulance arrives at the emergency room. The physician must be called in from home and the nurse on duty is reluctant to institute definitive medical care.

2:43 A.M. The physician arrives and carries out a heroic resuscitative effort that proves futile.

3:15 A.M. The patient is pronounced dead.

The year is 1980:

2:00 A.M. A 50-year-old man, previously in good health, awakens with crushing substernal chest pain and shortness of breath.

2:01 A.M. His wife dials 911 (the city's well-publicized emergency telephone number). The medical dispatcher obtains the vital information: location, telephone number, and the patient's chief complaint.

2:02 A.M. The dispatcher activates the closest fire station and the appropriate advanced life support mobile unit "code 3" (with red lights and siren).

2:04 A.M. Trained fire department personnel arrive, administer oxygen, assess the patient, and obtain vital signs.

2:06 A.M. The advanced life support mobile unit arrives. The two-member paramedic team quickly evaluates the patient's condition. The patient is ashen, profusely diaphoretic, in moderately severe respiratory distress, and has rales in his lungs. The cardiac monitor reveals frequent multifocal premature ventricular contractions.

2:10 A.M. Radio communication with the base hospital is established, and a patient report is relayed. The base hospital physician orders an intravenous line (dextrose 5%/water), morphine, oxygen, and lidocaine.

2:13 A.M. The paramedics start the intravenous line and administer the medications.

2:16 A.M. While the patient is being prepared for transport the base is informed that the premature ventricular contractions have been abolished and the patient appears stable. The base physician requests "code 2" transport (no red lights or siren) to the closest emergency department.

2:18 A.M. The base hospital physician notifies the receiving hospital and relays a complete patient report.

2:23 A.M. In transit the paramedics report that the patient's pain and shortness of breath have decreased and his color has improved.

2:25 A.M. The ambulance arrives at the emergency department. The patient is cared for expeditiously by the hospital staff.

2:45 A.M. The patient has been transferred to the coronary care unit and is resting comfortably.

Although these outcomes are not necessarily en-sured, a comparison of these two scenarios illustrates the changes that have taken place in PHC. Prehospital care now fits into an organized health care system that is rapidly accessible to the consumer. The providers are well trained and under physician medical control.

An effective PHC system requires coordination and cooperation among many agencies and categories of personnel. Many resources are necessary to bring care to the patient: system access, dispatch, biomedical communications, PHC providers, medical control personnel, public safety agencies, hospital facilities, and consumer education programs. One weak link within the system can render it ineffectual, despite the excellence of its other parts.

PHC differs from emergency department care significantly. The setting is "uncontrolled." Noise levels, scene confusion, and inconvenient and insufficient work space are frequent problems. Factors such as freeway traffic or a hostile crowd can endanger the patient and/or the care providers; there may be fewer personnel available or qualified to assist. Finally, the body of medical knowledge and the scope of PHC provider practice are much more limited than their hospital counterparts.

The scope of PHC may be basic life support, advanced life support, or limited advanced life support. The overall quality of patient care is probably more dependent on the smooth operation of the total system and effective medical control rather than on the scope of provider practice.

THE EMERGENCY MEDICAL SERVICES SYSTEM (EMSS) ACT

The federal EMSS Act was enacted in 1973. It outlines 15 separate EMS components, identifies 7 critical patient categories (trauma, burns, spinal cord injuries, poisoning, cardiac, neonatal, behavioral), and provides a national EMSS framework. Funding for programs was made available. The EMSS components include the following:

1. *manpower.* Sufficient manpower is a necessity. Major categories for personnel are medical control personnel, instructor-trainers, PHC providers, public safety and rescue workers, dispatchers, and staff for system administration and coordination.

2. *training.* National standards for provider training were published by the Department of Transportation in 1972 and 1975. Programs for the hospital-based team members are also necessary. Dispatcher training relative to telephone triage and medical information gathering is recommended.

3. *communications.* An effective communications system is critical. There must be a communications framework connecting the communications center, mobile units, and hospitals. Public safety agencies must also be linked to the communications center.

4. *transportation.* Transportation within an EMS system will include "scene" to hospital transport and interfacility transfers.

5. *facilities.* Receiving facilities must be designated and meet specified standards to guarantee optimal emergency care to the consumer. Receiving facility determination is based on the general nature and severity of the emergency condition and the location of facilities.

6. *critical care facilities.* Specialized and critical care must be available and accessible to patients in the seven identified critical categories.

7. *public safety agencies.* The cooperation and participation of law enforcement and fire safety personnel are often required. "First-in" responder, extrication, and scene safety are examples of how their skills and expertise are utilized.

8. *consumer participation.* Health care consumers work together with medical providers, agencies, and administrators in system planning and development.

9. *access to care.* System access is of utmost importance. Short response times for "first-in" and "second-in" responders are crucial. A single, standard, simple, and well-publicized telephone number makes system access easiest. The three digit "911" is optimal but is not universally operational.

10. *patient transfer.* Interfacility transfer of emergency patients is sometimes necessary so that the patient may receive specialized care. Transfer guidelines and protocols are an EMSS responsibility. These include establishing transfer criteria and clearly defining medical responsibility for the patient during transport. The medical expertise of the transport team must be appropriate for the patient's condition.[1]

11. *coordinated record keeping.* Standard record keeping is important for medical-legal reasons, patient care continuity, and system evaluation and to obtain relevant data for scientific analysis.

12. *public information and education.* Consumer education is necessary for a PHC system to be maximally effective. The media can assist by publicizing information relative to system access and the available services. The benefit of training large numbers of the lay public in cardiopulmonary resuscitation is becoming increasingly evident.

13. *review and evaluation.* All aspects of the PHC system (e.g., quality of patient care, system operations, cost effectiveness, provider competencies, and medical control) need ongoing evaluation.

14. *disaster plan.* Disaster planning takes place on the federal, state, and local levels. It is complex and requires the expertise and cooperation of a host of agencies and individuals. Frequent disaster drills are necessary to familiarize thoroughly all involved personnel with their roles and to identify and correct imperfections in the plan.

15. *mutual aid agreements.* Mutual aid agreements are formal agreements between agencies to provide assistance within another's response area when necessary. These agreements exist between PHC provider, fire safety, and law enforcement agencies.

SYSTEM DESIGN

Prehospital care systems are designed to meet the area's needs and to utilize the available resources most effectively. Physicians and nurses with emergency care experience must play a major role in designing the EMS systems. The design must ensure quality patient care through easy access, optimal PHC provider response times, an adequate communications network, sufficient medical control, and system evaluation. Cost effectiveness of the system is also a primary concern.

Local geographic features need to be considered. Some communications equipment will not function if the terrain is hilly or mountainous. Air transport may not be feasible in adverse weather.

Response times within the system are critical. Ambulance placement and "first-in responder" times must be carefully planned. Basic life support should be able to be initiated within 4 minutes. Central dispatching can decrease response times. Some urban areas have computer-assisted central dispatch.

Areas of low population density have some special needs. Specialized treatment centers will be further utilized by making air transport of patients to them advantageous. (See Chapter 4.) Provider response times are often too prolonged for patients to receive life-sustaining care within the necessary time frame. Some rural areas have attempted to solve this by establishing quick-response squads. These are volunteers trained in basic life support who are telephone dispatched and proceed to the scene carrying emergency equipment in their private vehicles.[2]

The administrative framework for PHC systems can be local, regional, statewide, or a combination of these.

Enabling legislation for the providers will be on the state level. It is very important that physicians work closely with other system planners in all phases of system design, implementation, and evaluation.

The scope of PHC practice is determined by a careful analysis of the area's needs, response times, transport times to emergency departments, available funding, and other resources. In some areas only basic life support is deemed feasible. Others may provide advanced life support capability to all prehospital patients. One expert estimates that a population base of 50,000 is needed to supply the necessary financial resources and clinical workload to support an advanced life support system.[3] An integrated approach utilizing both advanced and basic life support providers within the same response area is sometimes used. This requires expert dispatcher medical judgment.

Patient transportation is usually by land ambulance. Several types of ambulances are available: modular carry-all, van, and hearse design. Several selection criteria are recommended. The vehicle must be maneuverable and provide a reasonably comfortable ride. The patient compartment should be spacious enough to carry two patients and sufficient personnel, equipment, and supplies. Adequate head room is necessary to allow personnel to perform critical patient care functions.

In systems using air transport services, either helicopter or fixed-wing aircraft may be used. Air transport should be considered for interfacility transport of critical patients if the distance to the receiving hospital is great. Certain geographic areas can benefit from air transport services that respond to the emergency scene on request from field care providers.[4] The flight team's medical personnel will require specialized training in the unique aspects of flight medicine.

Selection of Provider Agencies

Selection of the PHC provider agencies will be based on several factors. Which agency can potentially provide the best quality of care? Which service will be most cost effective, on both the short and long term? Which agencies want to provide the service and what is their motivation?

There are four basic types of provider agencies: public providers (fire departments, police departments, health departments), private-commercial services, hospital-based programs, and volunteer services. Each type of agency has specific positive and negative attributes. A system may utilize more than one type of provider agency. Advanced life support may be provided by firefighter paramedics while transportation is by private ambulance. "First-in response" (basic life support) may be by the fire department while "second-in response" (advanced life support) is by a commercial service. In some systems provider agencies may differ from zone to zone.

Public Agencies

Firefighters are the advanced life support provider in many systems. They have traditionally responded to medical emergencies, are experts in rescue, and are not fully utilized on a 24-hour basis. The firefighter-paramedic functions in a dual role, thus increasing cost effectiveness. Fire departments have a strong administrative hierarchy, which may view the department's medical responsibilities as secondary to its fire-suppression role. This hierarchy is frequently resistant to medical control. The firefighter-paramedic usually has a limited paramedical career because the department's career ladder is channeled into firefighting rather than paramedicine.

A few systems have PHC providers based within the Public Health Department (San Francisco, Boston, and New York). These may have the advantage of being dedicated solely to medical care.[2] Some public service agencies do not have an established billing system for PHC services. The cost of the service is usually borne by the taxpayer rather than by a fee-for-service.

Private-Commercial Agencies

Privately owned ambulance companies are the traditional emergency transportation provider. Presently all systems utilize them for nonemergency transportation of patients and in some systems they are also the designated PHC provider. There is currently wide variation between these agencies in the quality of service they provide. With responsible company management and well designed performance contracts they can provide an excellent service. Cost of the service may be at least partially borne by user fees.

Hospital-Based Providers

In some areas, PHC providers are based at and employed by the hospital. The providers work in the emergency department between ambulance calls, utilizing them cost effectively while improving their skills. The providers clearly see themselves as part of the hospital team; therefore, medical control and cooperation is enhanced. Hospitals are not necessarily well distributed geographically, and response times to patients may not be optimal. There may be undue competition between hospitals to offer a PHC service, and hospitals are not generally well prepared to operate a fleet of ambulances.

Volunteer Services

Volunteer services are common in rural areas. These providers are highly motivated and the cost to the consumer is minimal. However, funding is unstable and staffing is unreliable. Maintenance of provider skills can be a problem and interface with the hospital-based team members too infrequent.

Cost Factors

The cost of the PHC system and who pays for it are important. Quality EMS systems are expensive to implement and maintain. Program planning must include an efficient administrative framework. Careful analysis of program costs and the elimination of unnecessary spending is necessary. In general the more sophisticated the program, the more it will cost. System planners and the consumers decide what level of service they wish to purchase, weighing the potential benefits against the cost.

Expenditures will include both "start up" costs and the expense of ongoing maintenance of the system. The initial expenses are very significant and include equipment procurement, biomedical communications, administrative costs, PHC provider training, and programs for medical control personnel. Provider training costs will be according to the program length and complexity and will also depend on the student's status with the provider agency. Trainees for private providers commonly pay for their own education. Costs to the consumers for training of public providers include program tuition, student salaries, and overtime pay for interim coverage.

Costs for system maintenance include provider salaries, equipment repair and replacement, medical supplies, and system administration. Training costs will accrue for continuing education programs and for primary training of personnel as necessary for attrition.

Specific methods of paying for the system vary. The system may operate entirely on a tax base or may charge a fee-for-service to the user. Often a combined approach of tax subsidy and user fees is employed. User fees are not a dependable method of total funding because collection rates are notoriously low.[2]

Rational system design is the key. There is no single ideal system that will be practical for all areas. System planners must consider the area's unique features and design accordingly, while utilizing the basic principles of EMS systems.

PATIENT ASSESSMENT AND CARE

The PHC approach to patient assessment and care is streamlined because of the time factors, the narrow knowledge base of the care givers, and the limited therapeutic modalities available in the field. This streamlined approach includes rapid patient assessment, prevention of further injury, patient stabilization, and transport.

The scope of "stabilization" will depend on the level of care available. For example, in a basic life support system, stabilization of a cardiac arrest victim consists of cardiopulmonary resuscitation and use of airway adjuncts. In an advanced life support system, stabilization of a cardiac arrest victim includes cardiopulmonary resuscitation, airway adjuncts, intubation, intravenous therapy, drug administration, and electrical countershock.

Patient assessment is the most complex and important skill that PHC providers perform. It must be performed very rapidly in critical situations. Emergency scenes are often loud and confusing and produce a good deal of stress in PHC personnel. Therefore, it is crucial that the providers be expert in assessment, have an organized approach, and be able to remain calm and efficient. The parameters for patient examination will focus on only those findings that directly affect the PHC care plan for the patient. Unnecessary and time-consuming parameters, such as evaluation of Babinski reflex, are specifically not included.

It is imperative that the providers be expert in their observation and communications skills. These skills are stressed within their primary and continuing education programs. Trainees need the opportunity to perform assessment on a wide variety of patients in a supervised setting.

Recognition of abnormal findings and life-threatening conditions is stressed, not diagnosis. For example, in a multiple trauma situation it is mandatory that the PHC provider recognize hypovolemic shock. The fact that the shock state is the result of a ruptured spleen is not of great significance until the patient reaches the hospital.

The patient history is abbreviated to include only the most relevant information. Providers are taught to ask certain questions based on the patient's chief complaint. For example, a patient complaining of chest pain would be asked: When did the pain start? Have you ever had this pain before? What were you doing when the pain began? On a scale from one to ten, how would you rank the severity of your pain? Describe what the pain feels like. Where is the pain; can you point to it? Does it go anywhere else? Do you feel short of breath? Are you under a doctor's care for any problems? Do you take any medications?

The physical examination is divided into three phases: (1) the overview, (2) the primary survey, and (3) the secondary survey. The overview includes the information that is immediately perceived on the provider's arrival. Is the patient unconscious or in obviously severe distress? What was the mechanism of injury? Does the scene environment pose a threat to the patient or to the providers?

The primary survey is frequently referred to as the "ABCs" (airway, breathing, circulation, spine and central nervous system). The airway is evaluated for patency. The rate of respirations and adequacy of tidal volume are determined. Pulse rate, quality, and regularity are evaluated. Blood pressure is taken. External hemorrhage, if present, is controlled. The skin color, moistness, and temperature are evaluated. If appropriate, cardiac rhythm is observed. The patient's level of consciousness is evaluated. The providers treat all life-threatening problems observed within the primary survey before proceeding to the more complete secondary survey.

The secondary survey takes approximately 2 minutes to complete, and it will be tailored somewhat for the specific patient situation. It consists of a complete but very basic head to toe examination.

Emergency field treatment is initiated in a carefully prioritized sequence that corresponds to the performance steps of the patient examination: (1) airway, (2) breathing, (3) circulation, (4) other. For example, take the case of a middle-aged female pedestrian who has been struck by a car. Witnesses state that the vehicle was traveling at a high rate of speed at impact. The patient appears critically injured. The closest hospital is 15 minutes away. The sequence of physical examination is shown in Table 3–1.

There are some key principles to adhere to when directing or providing prehospital treatment. Observing correct priorities in providing treatment is the first and foremost rule: treat those conditions that are most life-threatening first. Further injury should be prevented by instituting appropriate protection, such as immobilization of the cervical spine in a patient with a head injury. If possible, try to stabilize the patient prior to transport; some quick maneuvers such as antishock trousers can buy the patient valuable time.

Risk-benefit ratios to the patient must always be considered when contemplating medical intervention at the emergency scene. The potential benefit of the contemplated intervention must outweigh the risks relative to delayed arrival at the hospital. Decisions are based on the plan of care that will offer the patient the most potential benefit at the least risk.

THE PREHOSPITAL CARE TEAM

Prehospital care delivery depends on the coordinated expertise and cooperation of many people. It is a team effort of the highest order. All team members need specialized education and training to prepare them for their specific function. For the system to function smoothly, roles and responsibilities must be clearly identified and there must be open and frequent communication between the team members. The team members are "first-in responders," prehospital medical

---

TABLE 3–1   Example of Physical Examination Sequence

Assessment Step	Abnormal Finding(s)	Action	Result
Airway	Snoring	Perform and maintain jaw thrust while manually immobilizing cervical spine.	Snoring relieved
Breathing	Shallow at 8/minute	Assist with bag-valve-mask at 20/minute and supply supplemental oxygen.	Chest expansion equal Breath sounds equal
Circulation	Pulse: 140/minute, thready Blood pressure: 60/40 Skin: pale, cool and profusely diaphoretic	Inflate antishock trousers.	Blood pressure: 80/60 Pulse: 130/minute
Central Nervous System	Unconscious Hematoma on forehead	Immobilize spine using long backboard. Begin code 3 transport. Start intravenous lines with Ringers' lactate enroute.	
Secondary Survey	Multiple abrasions over right side of body Deformity right forearm	Splint right upper extremity.	

care providers, medical control personnel, receiving hospital personnel, members of public safety agencies, dispatchers, EMS administrators, PHC educators, and the lay public.

The Field Team

Until 1972 there were no accepted standards for PHC providers. In 1966 the National Academy of Sciences–National Research Council reported: "There are no generally accepted standards for competence or training of ambulance attendants."[5] Today there are defined categories and training standards for these individuals.

Currently, nomenclature for PHC providers is not nationally standardized but efforts to correct this situation are underway.[6]

Emergency Medical Technician—Ambulance (EMT-I)

The EMT-I is the first level of PHC provider. EMT-A, EMT-Basic, or EMT-1A are other titles for this category. The EMT-I is able to recognize acutely life-threatening conditions and render advanced first aid and basic life support. PHC systems offering basic life support alone will utilize the EMT-I as their sole provider. Advanced life support systems use the EMT-I as "first-in responder," to transport nonemergency patients, and to assist the advanced life support providers.

Current training programs for EMT-Is range in length from 81 to 150 hours.[7] The Department of Transportation published a national EMT-I curriculum in 1972 and revised it in 1977. This curriculum has had a significant impact on improving the overall quality of PHC nationwide.

The national training standard requires a minimum of 81 hours of training, including a 10-hour in-hospital experience. Additionally, the document recommends student participation on actual ambulance transport calls. Equipment categories in which the EMT-I is expected to be proficient are:

- stretchers
- airways (adjuncts, suctioning, oxygen)
- resuscitation techniques and devices
- splints (including backboards)
- dressings and bandages
- stethoscopes and sphygmomanometers.

Subject areas within the curriculum are identified by medical conditions: airway problems, cardiac arrest, external and internal bleeding, shock, injuries to all body parts, fractures, dislocations, sprains, poisoning, heart attack, stroke, diabetes, acute abdomen, communicable diseases, abnormal behaviors, alcohol and drug abuse, the unconscious state, emergency childbirth, burns, emergency conditions caused by hot and cold environmental conditions, and water hazards.[8]

A common misconception is that EMT-Is do not require as much medical control as advanced life support PHC providers. Frequently PHC systems do not provide tight medical control for EMT-Is, because they do not function as physician extenders. Medical control is necessary in all PHC systems, regardless of the scope of provider practice.

Emergency Medical Technician—Paramedic (EMT-P)

The EMT-P is a physician extender who renders advanced life support in the prehospital setting. The EMT-P is under medical control by voice communication and/or adherence to the system's patient care protocols. This provider may also be called EMT-2, EMT-3, mobile intensive care paramedic (MICP), or simply paramedic. In some systems an EMT-2 is actually an intermediate provider.

Training standards for the EMT-P have been identified. The programs are not currently standardized in course content, testing mechanisms, or course length. In the mid 1970s EMT-P training programs ranged in length from 60 to 2,000 hours.[9] In 1977, the Department of Transportation published an EMT-P curriculum that has become the national standard. It consists of 15 separate modules and requires both classroom instruction and clinical experience. Actual training hours are not specified, although the document states that many professionals estimate that the training can be provided and competencies achieved with 500 to 800 hours of training. Identified subject areas for the modules are:

1. the EMT-P role and responsibilities
2. human systems and patient assessment
3. shock and fluid therapy
4. general pharmacology
5. respiratory system
6. cardiovascular system
7. central nervous system
8. soft tissue injuries
9. musculoskeletal system
10. medical emergencies
11. obstetric/gynecologic emergencies
12. pediatrics and neonatal transport
13. emergency care of the emotionally disturbed
14. extrication/rescue techniques
15. telemetry and communications.

EMT-P skills include all EMT-I skills and the following (*optional skill):[10]

- peripheral intravenous insertion
- antishock trousers
- external jugular, internal jugular, and subclavian line insertion*
- drug administration (intravenous, subcutaneous, intramuscular, oral)
- use of nebulizers
- endotracheal intubation
- esophageal obturator airway*
- thoracic decompression*
- positive-end expiratory pressure*
- cricothyroidotomy*
- transtracheal jet insufflation*
- arrhythmia recognition
- ECG monitoring
- defibrillation
- cardioversion*
- rotating tourniquets*
- intracardiac injection*
- nasogastric tube insertion*
- urinary catheterization*
- extrication/rescue techniques
- communications.

State legislation and the system medical control authority will determine those skills to be included in actual practice. There is a trend away from being extremely explicit in statutory law because this practice makes it difficult to adjust for advances in the state of the art. Authorizing the very advanced skills, which are rarely performed, is controversial. Competency levels are not well maintained in seldom-used skills.[11,12] Many of the advanced skills require significant technical expertise, and many can result in fatal complications. Potential risk-benefit ratios must be carefully scrutinized before authorizing the EMT-P to perform a highly sophisticated skill.

A process for accreditation of EMT-P training programs was begun in 1979 under the auspices of the American Medical Association (Department of Allied Health Evaluation—Division of Educational Standards and Evaluation) in collaboration with the National Association of Emergency Medical Technicians, National Registry of EMTs, American College of Emergency Physicians, American College of Surgeons, American Psychiatric Association, and the American Society of Anesthesiology. The accreditation criteria include program sponsorship, curriculum design and content, teaching methods, program administration, medical control, and physician participation.[13]

Limited Advanced Life Support Categories

Some systems utilize an intermediate provider who is capable of rendering limited advanced life support. The training for these individuals consists of portions of the EMT-P curriculum. Some are called EMT-2, others are designated by that portion of the curriculum they have completed (e.g., EMT-Trauma, EMT-Cardiac). These providers are often utilized in rural areas where the need for prehospital medical intervention is real but an EMT-P program is not believed to be feasible.

"First-in Responder"

The "first-in responder" is usually the local fire department owing to geographic distribution, availability, and its traditional role in EMS. As "first-in" they assess the patient and situation, initiate basic life support, and assist the "second-in responders." "First-in responders" should be trained to the EMT-I level. In reality, the "first-on scene" is frequently the lay public, and thus the necessity for citizen cardiopulmonary resuscitation and first aid is obvious.

Dispatchers

All emergency calls are received and screened by a dispatcher. Many systems have central dispatching with one emergency telephone number for both medical and nonmedical assistance. The dispatcher gathers the pertinent information from the caller, interprets it, and notifies the appropriate responders. The dispatcher continually coordinates the movement of mobile units within the system. Dispatchers need specific medical training in order to perform triage effectively. It is recommended that they have EMT-I training.

Public Safety Agencies

Public safety agencies, law enforcement, and fire safety play a vital role in PHC. In many systems these agencies are also the designated medical care provider. Fire personnel are responsible for extrication and rescue operations. Law enforcement personnel are sometimes needed for traffic and crowd control and provision of protection. Public safety personnel need specific training programs to prepare them for their roles in PHC to facilitate cooperation and enhance teamwork.

Citizens

The lay public plays an important role in PHC. They must know how to recognize emergency situations, summon assistance, and provide first aid until the rescuers arrive. Citizen training in cardiopulmonary resuscitation is essential if the program is to be of maximum benefit to the victim of cardiac arrest. Studies show a significant improvement in patient outcomes when cardiopulmonary resuscitation is rapidly instituted. Seattle has conducted a massive citizen cardiopulmonary resuscitation program and estimates that over one-third of its population is trained, which may explain its high success rate in prehospital resuscitation.[14]

The Hospital-Based Team

A base hospital gives medical direction to PHC providers and maintains overall medical control of its assigned mobile units. The base hospital is also responsible for the ongoing continuing education of the prehospital team within the system's framework. Ideally, each mobile unit is assigned to a specific base hospital. This clearly defines medical control responsibility, enhances the team concept, and allows for easier system monitoring. The practice of permitting the mobile units to contact numerous base hospitals weakens medical control and encourages provider autonomy. The number of base hospitals in a region should be based on paramedic call volume. Each base hospital needs a large enough volume for its staff to maintain their expertise and enthusiasm.

A common misconception is that only base hospitals receive patients who have received advanced life support in the field. Although the base hospital directs field care and designates the receiving facility, the patients may be transported to non–base hospitals or satellite hospitals. The base hospital notifies the receiving hospital of the patient's impending arrival and provides a patient profile and description of the PHC rendered. Good communication between receiving and base hospitals is vital.

The Physician

The physician is the leader of the PHC team. Advanced life support providers are physician extenders and, therefore, function under the physician's medical license. Physician responsibilities include providing medical direction to field personnel via voice communication and patient care protocols, monitoring patient care standards, setting policy on medical matters, and actively participating in the educational programs for all PHC team members.

Base hospital physicians should be experienced and proficient practitioners of emergency medicine. An understanding of EMS systems, provider capabilities and limitations, field procedures, and biomedical communications is also necessary. Physician PHC educational programs are becoming available. Physician "ride along" with ambulance crews is an excellent way to gain insight into the unique aspects of field medicine, to evaluate provider competencies, and to foster mutual respect and understanding between the physician and the physician extenders.

Each base hospital needs a designated physician advisor for PHC activities. This individual is responsible for the overall medical control within the base hospital framework. Additionally, the system also needs a physician medical director who has overall medical responsibility for the total system.

The Mobile Intensive Care Nurse (MICN)

In California and North Carolina, advanced life support providers can receive medical direction from certified MICNs. These registered nurses receive specialized education and training in PHC and in principles of emergency medicine. In some areas registered nurses also act as PHC providers.

The MICN was first defined in law in California's Wedworth-Townsend Act as "a registered nurse who has been certified by a county health officer as qualified in the provision of emergency cardiac care and noncardiac care and the issuance of emergency instruction to mobile intensive care paramedics."[15] In California, there is slight variation between counties but generally the MICN is experienced in emergency and critical care nursing, is certified by the American Heart Association in advanced cardiac life support, has completed a formal MICN educational program, and has successfully passed the county's written and performance examinations. Certification criteria in North Carolina are similar, but the certification process is administered by the State Office of Emergency Medical Services and the Board of Medical Examiners.[16]

These nurses fulfill a vital role in the systems utilizing them. They direct field care, coordinate base hospital activities, and assist in educational programs for the PHC team. The scope of MICN practice is considerably broader than that of many other critical care nurses who initiate similar medical interventions in that the MICN gives medical orders that another individual will carry out. It is recommended that physicians must be immediately available for consultation to the MICN, since the physician has the ultimate medical-legal responsibility for the patient.[17] (See Chapter 5.)

MEDICAL CONTROL

Medical control of the PHC system must rest with physicians; they are the most medically qualified, and advanced life support providers practice under the physician's license. Medical control includes setting standards, determining policy relative to medical matters, directing PHC by voice communication and protocols, and evaluating the system and the levels of patient care. Lack of strong physician medical control and active physician participation in the system results in a poor care standard, provider autonomy, and ultimately a nonsystem. Medical control is provided prospectively in system planning and protocol design, immediately by voice direction, and retrospectively through system evaluation.[18]

Prospective Medical Control

Prospective medical control is vital to quality EMS systems. Physician participation begins in system design, long before the system is implemented. Physicians must assume a leadership role in determining the scope of provider practice, base hospital selection criteria, methods for immediate and retrospective medical control, patient care protocols, and the system's medical policies.

Policies will be needed for management of certain situations. Examples of these include transport and transfer protocols, pronouncement of death, criteria for mandatory base hospital contact, and patient refusal of treatment and/or transport. Establishing policies before they are needed will help avoid decisions that are detrimental to the patient and that are medically and legally unsound.

Prospective medical control also includes establishing criteria for PHC team members and evaluating their competencies before they are permitted to function. These team members include all PHC providers, MICNs, and base hospital physicians.

Immediate Medical Control

There are basically two methods of immediate medical control: (1) voice communication and (2) "standing orders" or written protocols. Both methods have benefits and pitfalls.

Voice communication seems more desirable because each patient's care is handled individually, decreasing the margin for error. The quality of medical direction is dependent on who answers the paramedic radio; therefore, the first pitfall is allowing individuals who are not well qualified to answer the radio and give medical directions. This can be prevented by establishing appropriate criteria and ensuring compliance. Some systems utilize a paramedic to direct field care.[3] This does not seem medically prudent nor does it enhance physician medical control of the system. The other major pitfall is inability to provide advanced life support in critical situations when radio equipment malfunctions.

The "standing orders" approach can be used only if the protocols are very well designed and the providers are extremely competent. This method has the advantage of standardizing treatment within the system. Care can be rendered rapidly without the delay for radiocommunication. Problems associated with a "standing orders" system are increasing the margin for provider error and increased provider autonomy.

Many EMS systems are now using a combined approach. With this approach the patient care protocols are considered as guidelines for treatment when medical direction is by voice communication. If radio contact cannot be established or maintained, the providers can follow the protocols as specified. These systems also permit the providers to initiate life-saving medical intervention prior to base hospital contact as a standard practice. The protocol shown in Figure 3–1 is an example of this approach.

Retrospective Medical Control

Medical control is also maintained retrospectively by ongoing evaluation. This will include both structured mechanisms and informal processes. Evaluation tools should be designed to adequately monitor standards of patient care, provider competencies, quality of medical direction, and the operational aspects of the system. The evaluation process includes determining the expected standard and then measuring actual compliance to the standard. Deficiencies are identified and methods to correct them are developed and implemented.

Mechanisms to achieve retrospective medical control include immediate critique of calls with the team members involved, formal case review as part of the continuing education program, observation of field care by "ride along" with emergency crews, incident reporting initiated by any team member alerting the medical control authority to deficiencies, and surveillance of prehospital medical records.

Accurate and standardized record keeping is necessary for continuity of patient care, for medical-legal reasons, and so that retrospective medical control can take place. The field providers complete a PHC record containing patient information and detailing care delivered. The form needs to be standardized within the system and should lend itself to retrieval of meaningful data. A copy will be included in the patient's medical record at the receiving hospital, and copies will be forwarded to the medical control authority.

In advanced life support systems in which immediate medical control is maintained by voice direction, the physician or MICN directing care will complete a standard written record and communications will be tape recorded. The tape recording and the base hospital record are considered part of the patient's medical record

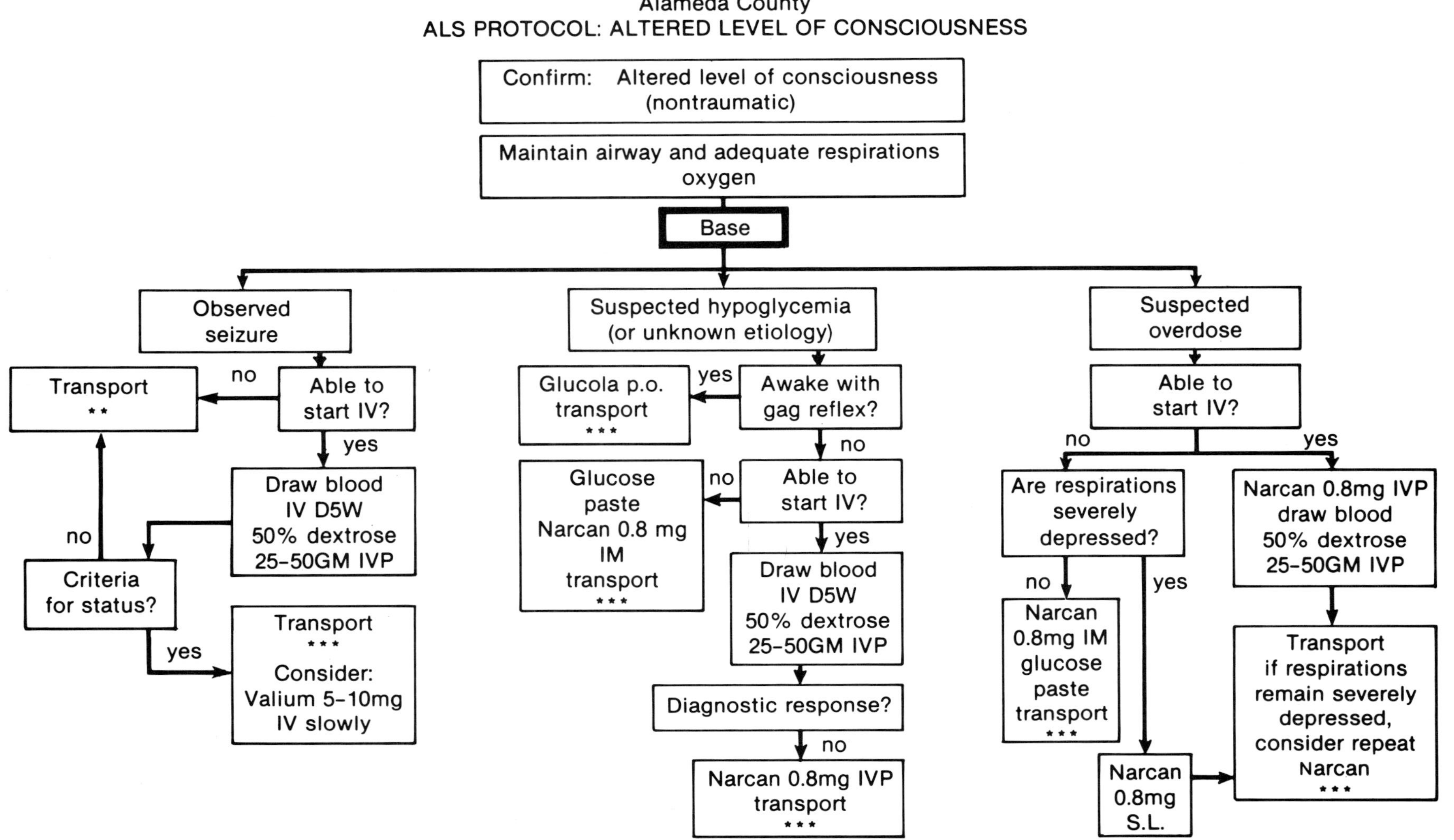

Treatment below *** not authorized without base station approval.
Note: In some medical communities base station authorization is required for the initiation of any treatment.

Figure 3–1   Advanced Life Support Protocol: Altered Level of Consciousness.

and are subject to all standard medical-legal requirements.

The tape recordings and written records are reviewed by the individual(s) responsible for monitoring patient care. Deviations from the established standard are identified and evaluated by the medical control authority, with input from the team members involved.

Formal retrospective audits are also necessary and include evaluation of patient care for selected patient groups and patient outcome data. Active participation by receiving hospitals in this process is essential.

Effective retrospective medical control is largely dependent on good communication between the PHC team members. Clear mechanisms must be established for alerting the medical control authority to problems and ensuring correction of deficiencies.

BIOMEDICAL COMMUNICATIONS

Biomedical communications are an integral part of all PHC systems. They tie the system together, permitting it to function. Biomedical communications within a PHC system have three major components: (1) a communications center that coordinates all radio communications, receives and screens calls, and dispatches responders; (2) mobile equipment that permits field personnel to communicate with the center, each other, and with hospitals; and (3) hospital equipment permitting the hospitals to communicate with the center, field units, and with each other.

All radio communications are subject to regulations of the Federal Communications Commission (FCC). The commission designates frequencies, establishes transmitter licensing criteria, and regulates equipment use and configuration. FCC rules applicable to PHC communications can be located in FCC Part 90—Private Land Mobile Radio Services, subpart C—Special Emergency Radio Service.[19] FCC regulations require that communicators identify themselves with each transmission by their designated call sign and specifically forbid the use of profane language.

Many factors will influence EMS radio system design. Terrain and the size of the area to be served are important considerations. The expected volume of radio traffic will also determine configuration of the system to some extent.

There are three basic modes of radio operation.

1. simplex. This mode allows for only one-way communication at a time. Only one frequency is used. The receiving unit cannot interrupt until transmission is completed.
2. duplex. This mode utilizes two radio frequencies, one for transmitting and one to receive, allowing

communicators to transmit and receive simultaneously.
3. multiplex. This mode is similar to duplex. It has the additional capability of being able to transmit from two sources simultaneously (the patient's ECG and the EMT-P's voice).[19]

Field Radio Equipment

Field radio equipment includes an antenna, an ambulance radio, a public address system, a vehicular repeater, and a portable radio. Portable radio equipment used in advanced life support systems typically consists of a transceiver (combination transmitter-receiver), ECG telemetry (transceiver and cardiac monitor), and a telephone coupler (see Figure 3–2).

The portable radio looks like a suitcase and weighs about 25 pounds. It has a handset with a "push-to-talk" feature. Many portable radios can operate in a "hands-free" mode in which base hospital transmissions are audible from the transceiver and the providers can communicate to the base hospital by speaking toward the transceiver instead of into the handset. The patient's ECG is transmitted to the base hospital by connecting the cardiac monitor to the transceiver and switching to the ECG telemetry mode.

The telephone coupler offers an alternative method for biomedical communications utilizing "land lines" (telephone lines) instead of radio frequencies. This method is used when there is radio interference or if all radio frequencies are in use. The provider attaches a telephone receiver to the telephone coupler and connects it to the transceiver. The provider then dials the base hospital's "dedicated land line," and communications are carried out in the standard fashion.

Base Hospital Equipment

The base station console is usually located in the hospital's emergency department. Its location should be outside of the department's traffic pattern, and it should allow for privacy in communications. It will be equipped with an audible alarm to alert the base hospital staff to incoming calls.

The console's components include a transceiver, hand set, oscilloscope, strip chart recorder, and tape recorder. The radio operator speaks into the handset as one would a telephone receiver. There is a "push-to-talk" button, making it necessary to depress the button in order to transmit. The radio communications are tape recorded. When the tape recording is played back on the base station console, the ECG transmissions will be displayed on the oscilloscope.

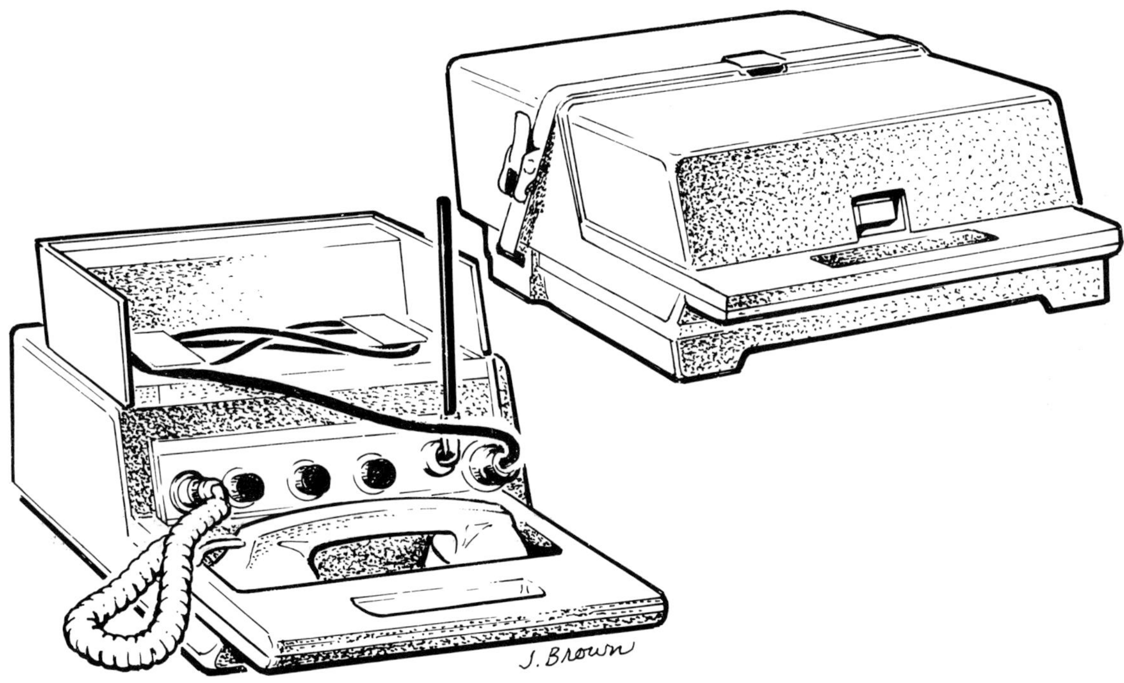

Figure 3–2　Biomedical Communications and Telemetry System.

General Principles of Biomedical Communications

Brevity is important in biomedical communications because radio traffic is congested and PHC time frames are short. When transmitting one needs to speak slowly and enunciate carefully. Radio transmissions have more inherent interference than do telephone communications, and the noisy emergency scenes make it difficult for the providers to hear the base hospital. Instructions need to be stated very clearly and specifically. The providers will repeat all orders they receive for base hospital confirmation.

Radio jargon should be minimal. Number codes and other common radio terms are not well understood by medical personnel. Plain, succinct, well-enunciated English suffices. Because private citizens are able to listen to EMS communications with scanning devices, it is recommended that the patient's name not be used so that patient confidentiality can be protected.

Radio interference is a common problem and can be caused by a variety of factors: equipment malfunction, jammed airways, hilly terrain, buildings, weather disturbances, and even cloudy skies. When communications are "broken" or otherwise inaudible, both communicators should troubleshoot their equipment. If clear communications cannot be restored, the communications center may be able to correct the problem or the providers may be able to utilize the "dedicated land line" alternative.

Another problem is overlapping of communications in areas with congested radio traffic. There are no absolute barriers to radio signals, and there are a very limited number of EMS frequencies. This can result in a transmission to be received by a mobile unit or base hospital for which it was not intended. This situation can result in an error with potentially catastrophic consequences—inappropriate medical therapy. This is yet another reason that the communicators must identify themselves and the intended receiver with each transmission.

Simultaneous emergency calls to one base hospital are sometimes unavoidable. If this occurs, the base hospital will inform the mobile units involved. The calls will be prioritized according to their urgency. It may be possible for one of the units to contact an alternative base hospital. If the calls must be directed simultaneously it is important that the base hospital radio operator be very organized and be very specific in mobile unit identity with each transmission.

Biomedical communications follow a standardized format. The format is prioritized to convey the most critical information first. The sequence is designed to help the provider supply an organized patient profile and complete information. The provider must communicate in such a way that the base hospital radio operator will receive an accurate mental picture of the patient. The concept of the paramedic being the physician's eyes, ears, and hands at the emergency scene is an accurate one.

An example format for initial communications about an acutely ill patient is shown in Table 3–2.

SUMMARY

PHC has undergone tremendous growth during the past decade. It has evolved from a "scoop and run" level of service to an integrated systems construct, with care delivered by well-trained paraprofessionals under the medical control of emergency physicians. No longer is it seen as an autonomous entity responsible only to the ambulance owner or the fire chief.

In the 1980s has come the realization that EMS systems are not without some serious problems. In an age of government cost containment, EMS systems represent a substantial expense for an intangible reward. Some systems have suffered from internal conflicts, "turf wars," and poor medical control.[20,21] There are still many areas in which PHC currently resembles the 1965 scenario presented at the beginning of this chapter. Sophisticated PHC has received a good deal of media attention, and consumers have come to expect PHC that is consistent with the media's portrayal. PHC is expensive to implement and to maintain. There is a

---

TABLE 3–2   Example of Format for Biomedical Communications

Content	Mobile Unit	Base Hospital
Contact established	Community Hospital, this is Medic 4. How do you copy?	
		Medic 4, this is Community Hospital. We copy you loud and clear. Proceed with your transmission.
Location	We are at a private residence	
Patient profile	with a 70-year-old female, weighing approximately 200 pounds.	
Level of distress	She is in severe distress,	
Chief complaint	complaining of shortness of breath	
History of chief complaint	that awakened her 30 minutes ago. She says she has never had this before.	
Mental status	She seems alert but is unable to talk very well because of her shortness of breath. She seems very anxious and is restless.	
Respiratory status	She is sitting in high Fowler's position and is leaning forward. Her respiratory rate is 32. She is coughing nonproductively. Breath sounds are equal, and she has rales bilaterally on chest auscultation. We started oxygen at 8 liters per minute.	
Circulatory status	Her pulse is 120 and irregular. Blood pressure is 160/100. Her skin color is dusky, and she is diaphoretic.	
ECG findings	We read atrial fibrillation and occasional PVC's on the monitor. We are preparing to send you a rhythm strip.	
Past medical history	We are unable to obtain much of a history due to her difficulty speaking. She says she has no allergies and takes no medications. We will give you the rest of her physical exam after we send you a rhythm strip.	
Estimated time of arrival to receiving hospital (ETA)	Our ETA to City Hospital is about 15 minutes, including loading time. We're awaiting your orders, Community.	
Initial orders		Medic 4, this is Community. We copy atrial fibrillation and occasional PVCs. Start an IV D5W to keep open. Get back to me with her physical exam when you can.
Confirm orders	Community, this is Medic 4. We copy an IV D5W to keep open.	
		That is correct, Medic 4.

need to justify the expense by more documentation of its benefit to patient outcomes.

Provider burnout is occurring at a rapid rate and is an expensive problem. As providers burn out, replacement personnel must be trained, and training is costly. There are numerous reasons cited for the burnout syndrome: lack of a career ladder,[22] few rewards, frustration with the system's hierarchy, inability to effect change within the system, sleep deprivation, frequent encounters with difficult patients, high stress levels, frequent exposure to death and dying, and few avenues for "letting off steam" and receiving emotional support.[23,24]

As PHC systems have proliferated across the nation, sound foundations in system design have not always been well constructed. Often the system components were not well in place, adequately planned for, or linked together. Without all 15 EMSS components, care will be less than ideal.

Some EMS professionals are questioning the rationale of establishing the most sophisticated advanced life support systems in highly urbanized areas where transport times are short. Perhaps where the service is most needed, yet least available, is in the rural setting.

Lack of both adequate physician participation and effective medical control have been cited as critical problems in some systems.[20,25] As these systems developed the void has been filled by bureaucrats and agency administrators.[7] The result is poor (or no) medical control, provider autonomy, a nonsystem, and frustration for the entire PHC team. Physicians are becoming aware of this problem and are attempting to regain medical control. Effecting medical control is time and energy consuming. It is hoped that physician interest and enthusiasm will not wane once the situation improves.

REFERENCES

1. Gough AR, Secord B, Behrens B: Emergency patient transfers: The medico-legal considerations. *Emergency* 12(7):49–52, 1980.
2. Cayton, GC: Prehospital care systems for advanced coronary life support. *Top Emerg Med* 1(4):9–18, 1980.
3. Rosen, P: Prehospital care: An integrated concept of emergency medicine. *Top Emerg Med* 1(4):19–26, 1980.
4. Cleveland HC: An air emergency service: The extension of the emergency department. *Top Emerg Med* 1(4):47–54, 1980.
5. Page JO: *The Paramedics: An Illustrated History of Paramedics in their First Decade in the U.S.A.* Morristown, N.J., Backdraft Publications, 1979, pp 4–7.
6. Vance M: EMT-paramedic defined. *Ann Emerg Med* 9(2):110, 1980.
7. Stewart RD: Prehospital care: Education, evaluation and medical control. *Top Emerg Med* 1(4):67–82, 1980.
8. *Basic Training Course/Emergency Medical Technician.* Washington, DC, US Department of Transportation, 1977.
9. Weigel AM: Tracking the trends in EMT-P training. *J Emerg Med Serv* 5(1):37–40, 1980.
10. *Emergency Medical Technician-Paramedic.* Washington, DC, US Department of Transportation, 1977, pp 59–69.
11. Latman NS, Wooley K: Knowledge and skill retention of emergency care attendants, EMT-A's and EMT-P's. *Ann Emerg Med* 9:183–189, 1980.
12. McSwain NE, Skelton MB: A study of cognitive and technical skills deterioration among trained paramedics. *J Am Coll Emerg Physicians* 6:436–438, 1976.
13. Essentials and guidelines of an accredited educational program for the EMT-P, special report. *EMT J* 4(1):22–26, 1980.
14. McElroy C: Citizen CPR: The role of the lay person in prehospital care. *Top Emerg Med* 1(4):37–45, 1980.
15. California Health and Safety Code, Section 1481.
16. Cummings PH: North Carolina's mobile intensive care nurse. *J Emerg Med Serv* 6(5):35–37, 1981.
17. Secord: The MICN: New critical care professional. *Crit Care Update*, December 1977, pp 16–18.
18. McSwain NE: Medical control: What is it? *J Am Coll Emerg Physicians* 7:114–116, 1978.
19. Felt H: A primer on radio communications. *J Emerg Med Serv* 5(4):23, 1980.
20. Page JO: A message from the coroner. *J Emerg Med Serv* 5(6):54, 1980.
21. Criley JM: Interview. *STAT* 1(1):52–56, 1979.
22. McSwain NE, Skelton MB: Burn out: Real or imagined? *Top Emerg Med* 1(4):93–97, 1980.
23. Graham K: Done in, fed up, burned out: Too much attrition in EMS. *J Emerg Med Serv*, January 1981, pp 24–29.
24. Graham NK: How to avoid a short career. *J Emerg Med Serv*, February 1981, pp 25–31.
25. Hurtado F: Letter to Robert White, Director, Department of Health Services, Los Angeles. *STAT* 1(1):57, 1979.

4. Critical Care Air Transport

MARY ANN COOPER, M.D.

During the late 1960s and early 1970s multiple civilian- and government-funded helicopter projects were originated to see if the successful military experience in air medical evacuation could be applied to the civilian sector. These included Project HELP in Philadelphia,[1] Project Flatiron in Alabama,[2] Operation Sky-Aid in Nebraska,[3,4] AMES in Arizona,[5] HASTE in Minneapolis–St. Paul,[3,6] CARE-SOM in Mississippi,[7] and others in Texas, Michigan, Pennsylvania, and California.[3] The Department of Transportation projects unanimously found that helicopter service to rural areas was feasible but that service to urban systems was impractical owing to limited landing space and to the ready availability of trained ground units. Helicopter services were found to be approximately five times more expensive than conventional ground units, although these costs could be decreased somewhat if the vehicles were employed for multiple other government uses.[3]

The military assistance to safety and traffic (MAST) system was begun in 1969 at Fort Sam Houston in San Antonio as a further experiment by the Department of Transportation to study the feasibility of military helicopters and crews augmenting existing emergency medical services (EMS).[8] It has expanded throughout the country and in its first 10 years flew more than 15,000 missions and transported nearly 16,000 patients.[9] While access to the MAST system is often limited, particularly when reserve units are all that are available, it will probably continue to be a major source of air transport in many rural areas.

In 1969 the Maryland State Police and University of Maryland Center for the Study of Trauma initiated a system utilizing paramedics and four helicopters situated throughout the state. When not carrying patients, the system conducts other civil duties such as crime investigation and traffic control.[10]

In 1972 Loma Linda University in California[11] and St. Anthony's Hospital in Denver[12,13] began air transport emergency service, joined a short time later by Hermann Hospital in Houston. By 1981 there were nearly 35 hospital-based air transport systems in the United States.

The hospital-based system seems to be the "Cadillac" of air emergency transport. Most programs deliver highly trained medical personnel and advanced equipment to the patient, operating as an extension of the hospital and more as a flying emergency department than as only a fast expensive ambulance.

From military and civilian experience it has been concluded that in rural areas where sophisticated medical care is not available air transport is the transport of choice for the critically injured provided an *appropriately trained caretaker who can handle the care of the patient and any complications is aboard.*

Each program of air medical transport has a different structure depending, for example, on type of vehicle used, management structure, emphasis on emergent versus nonemergent transfers, staffing, or financing. This chapter will deal with the differences between aircraft, with air ambulance standards, and with the most common types of management structure. Staffing, training, equipment, financing, marketing, and the other considerations in such a system also will be discussed.

TYPE OF AIRCRAFT

While many varieties of aircraft may be used, they can be divided into two broad classes: (1) fixed wing (airplanes) and (2) rotor wing (helicopters).

Fixed wing aircraft generally have the advantage of more room, more efficient fuel consumption, longer range, and greater speed, depending on the craft chosen.[14] They are about one-third to one-half as expensive to maintain and operate as helicopters, especially over long distances. Fixed-wing aircraft also are more readily available in pressurized models and may be quieter for their occupants. However, they have one major disadvantage: they must land at airfields.

Helicopters, particularly those that are now commonly used for civilian air ambulances, can land in areas as small as 60 to 100 feet in diameter. Newer types of helicopters have very reasonable maintenance times compared with their military ancestors. They are highly maneuverable, can land on an interstate highway or a hospital parking lot, and may be based at a hospital. Multiple transports of the patient and a medical team from referring hospital to EMS vehicle to airplane to EMS vehicle to receiving hospital are thus eliminated. Response time to the patient is also minimized. In the case of an engine failure, rotorcraft will autorotate and can be guided to a safe landing instead of gliding into the ground as an airplane does. Within a 150-mile radius helicopters are very cost and fuel efficient and are limited only by the availability of Jet A fuel for longer flights.

Ideally the craft and landing areas should be based at a hospital. However, if transport from a hospital to an aircraft or vice versa is necessary, a fully equipped EMS vehicle or similarly outfitted unit is mandatory in order to provide continuity of high level care, protection from the weather, and adequate lighting for patient care at night.

The ideal aircraft for medical transport would be totally safe, have a minimum of routine maintenance and no unscheduled maintenance, and have good range capabilities while still being very fast, smooth, quiet, and fuel efficient. It would have enough room to comfortably accommodate two or three attendants plus all their equipment and would provide good access and easy loading of two patients. It could be landed anywhere.

Unfortunately, there is no aircraft that is ideal for patient transport. Some of the characteristics that must be considered when choosing an aircraft are listed below:

- speed
- range
- lift and power
- fuel consumption
- maintenance
- parts availability
- safety record
- cost
- noise level
- smoothness of ride
- pressurization
- climate control
- communications system
- one vs. two engines
- patient loading and access
- work space
- convenience of oxygen, suction, and electrical outlets
- storage space
- room for one or two patients
- room for one to three attendants
- lighting

So many modifications are being made so rapidly on aircraft used by the health industry that it would be impractical to discuss in this chapter the individual craft that are currently available. Decisions as to how the program will be structured must be made, and then the craft best suited to the program can be chosen.

The best way to obtain information is to talk to the major vendors, to other program administrators, and to the pilots in the programs, realizing that each group will have its own biases. After studying the aircraft, the administrators must decide how much they can afford.

AIR AMBULANCE STANDARDS

Air ambulance systems vary from simple transport vehicles with no caretakers (air taxis) to highly sophisticated, custom-designed flying medical intensive care units with highly trained personnel. The advanced units may be fully outfitted with all the equipment available in any emergency unit, short of a heart-lung bypass pump or an x-ray machine. There is a great deal of variation of quality.[15] Attempts to develop standards for air ambulances by the Federal Aviation Administration (FAA) a number of years ago were aborted by intensive lobbying from pilots and aircraft organizations.[16]

The Department of Transportation and the American Medical Association have developed Guidelines for Air Ambulances,[17] although there are no statutes requiring compliance by the industry. The American Society for Hospital-Based Emergency Air Medical Systems

(ASHBEAMS) and the Committee on Trauma of the American College of Surgeons in cooperation with the American College of Emergency Physicians are presently attempting to develop health industry standards. Under these standards the public could trust that any service using the designation of "air ambulance" would meet certain criteria for staffing, equipment, and quality of care as opposed to the "air taxi."

AIR AMBULANCE OPERATORS

Currently, most air ambulance system operators can be divided into four groups: (1) private entrepreneur, (2) public agency, (3) military units, and (4) hospital operated.

The private entrepreneur is usually based at a local airport. For a fee an aircraft can be rented for transportation purposes. Any special equipment or medical personnel may or may not be supplied, and these private aircraft tend to fall in the "air taxi" classification.[16] It usually takes several hours' to several days' notice in order to arrange the charter, depending on the availability of a vehicle. These services rarely operate 24 hours a day and seldom can be considered emergency vehicles. This type of service is usually accessible to the public but may on occasion have agreements with hospitals to provide transport services for their personnel, as for transport of organs or blood products.

Several states (including Illinois and Maryland) and municipalities have services operated by public agencies such as the police, state highway patrol, fire-rescue service, or other para-military organization. While these programs are successful in some areas, many more have failed to serve as adequate emergency vehicles because of lack of trained medical personnel, unavailability of craft for medical transports owing to being on civil missions such as crime or traffic control assignments, and equipment modifications that are unsuitable for acute and critical patient transport. While sharing the high cost of aircraft between several functions may seem to be a logical solution, the shared system too often turns into a many-headed monster serving none of its masters well.

The military has sponsored many programs through the Coast Guard, Army, Army Reserve Units, and others like the MAST program that have saved the lives of many civilians and transported hundreds of organs and other body tissues when needed for medical emergencies.[14] The purposes of the MAST units in order of importance are to (1) provide continued training to military pilots, (2) provide support to military maneuvers, and (3) assist in emergency transport of civilians. By regulation, the first two priorities must override the third so that often MAST units may be unavailable

when needed, particularly when operated by reserve units that are only active on weekends. Medical caretakers may include a physician but more commonly involve only medics. While medics of the Vietnam era were often excellent, many new recruits who are assigned to the MAST unit are untrained but are still allowed to care for patients while training to a level analogous to the basic civilian emergency medical technician (EMT) level.[8] The helicopters used by the military are the UH-I ("Huey") and the newer Blackhawk. They are both made for multiple victim transport, are very large, use a tremendous amount of fuel, have high vibration levels, and are very noisy and much less maneuverable than the newer civilian models.

Since 1972 several hospitals have chosen to invest in air transport systems. Some market particular areas of specialization, whether it be their trauma center, neonatal unit, or some other area of expertise.[18] While some few programs provide transportation only, the vast majority supply advanced medical teams and sophisticated life-support equipment, as well as speed of response and smoothness of transport rather than just fast, expensive ambulance service. These systems are flying emergency and intensive care units, delivering a fully equipped medical team to support the patient.

All of these air ambulance operation styles will be discussed in this chapter. However, the hospital-based system provides the ideal in patient care and most items will be addressed to this type of system.

HEALTH CARE SYSTEM INTERFACES AND DISASTER RESPONSE

Medical air transport systems may interact with the rest of the health care system in a number of ways. The most common nonemergent medical transports are those used by the military to move hundreds of casualties from battlefield hospitals to larger facilities.[14] Chartered air taxis and air ambulances now commonly transport patients, filing flight plans and being scheduled from several hours to several days in advance.

The hospital-based programs that have been started in the past 10 years almost always respond immediately to an unscheduled patient situation, whether it be a scene run or an interhospital transfer. The helicopter system in Pensacola, Florida, is the only one that acts as a first responder. The program at both Hermann Hospital in Houston and Saint Anthony's Hospital in Denver frequently back up ground units responding to trauma or medical calls within the metropolitan area, landing on interstate highways and crowded parking lots.

Most programs choose not to compete with local ground EMS units.[16] They serve as back-up units when the EMTs may feel that more expert or specialized care is necessary than they can provide.

In rural areas, the rescue squads are often made up of volunteers who are reluctant to leave their community uncovered while they transport a critical patient to a distant medical center. A helicopter or other air ambulance that is properly staffed and equipped can provide the patient with a smoother ride, more rapid transport, and more advanced medical care[8,19] while the community squad is free to remain in service locally.

Some rural hospitals present their utilization of medical center helicopter services to their own communities as a demonstration of (1) their concern for increased cost effectiveness (in not attempting to duplicate services[20]) and (2) their medical expertise (as part of the "medical center team" that utilizes the helicopter).

A tornado, flood, or similar disaster may make victims inaccessible by road or ground vehicle. A helicopter can be used to deliver medical personnel and supplies that can be used to set up a field hospital or field triage system and later serve as an evacuation unit for patients. It is wise for any program to have a disaster plan, which should also include stockpiling and organization of "disaster packs" such as backpacks containing airways, splinting materials, and intravenous solutions to stabilize up to four victims apiece.

FEASIBILITY

Air EMS systems are very expensive to operate and should not be started lightly or unadvisedly, particularly with the current emphasis on health cost containment. Unless the service will be providing a level of medical care that is superior to what is already available by ground or unless it is solving some very rare and unusual problems of terrain, weather, or distance for an area, there is no reason to expend the large amount of money and resources necessary to make such a hospital-based helicopter system work effectively.

There are several conditions that must be met by any organization that wants to operate a system:[21–24]

- The medical team on the aircraft must have enough trained personnel to provide resuscitation and stabilization as well as patient support during transport.
- There must be a sufficient number of intensive care beds available to accept the patients at the receiving hospital.
- There must be a level of medical care at the receiving hospital that is superior to that already available to the patient locally.
- The physicians and staff at the receiving hospital must be willing to accept the responsibility for providing the support that these patients require, regardless of the time of day. Depending on the type of patient sought by the hospital, this may mean 24-hour in-house availability, for example, of a trauma team, a burn team, neonatal intensive care, cardiology, high-risk pregnancy management, an implantation team, medical intensivists, and neurosurgeons. Ancillary services such as blood bank, laboratories, or operating room teams may need to be increased in order to handle the patients.
- The population of the area served must be adequate to supply enough patients to make the program cost effective.
- The administration must be supportive, with funds for greater medical resources as well as for training, marketing, a communications center, and other support functions.
- The hospital must meet all the local zoning ordinances and have a landing site that is close enough to the emergency unit to avoid secondary ground transfer.
- Unless the service is supported by grants, benefactors, or the state, appropriate reimbursement mechanisms must be negotiated so that favorable cash flow and cost feasibility of the service may be continued.

Standards for hospitals implementing such a service are available through ASHBEAMS.

PERSONNEL

There is considerable variation among different programs in personnel requirements for the aircraft medical crew and administrative support team. It is still possible to hire an aircraft for transport of a critical patient with no medical personnel available to care for the patient. With increased public awareness and with the setting of standards for the industry it is hoped that the public will soon be assured that an air ambulance is not merely an air taxi with yellow pages advertising.

Emergency Medical Technicians: Level I

A few hospital-based helicopter services use EMT-Is. While EMTs are certainly of great value at the scene of an automobile accident, particularly when extrication is required, in most states these personnel are not trained to monitor the heart rhythm, adjust intravenous lines, or administer drugs of any kind and are prohibited from doing so.[19] To give this level of personnel the responsibility of caring for a critical patient transfer seems as inappropriate for air transport as it does for ground transport.[19] While many rural ground units may not have highly trained personnel available, an air service that purports to provide medical care should provide care during transfer that is on the level being supplied by the referring hospital.

Some hospital-based services that utilize only one caretaker sometimes elect to incorporate one of the ground squad EMTs into the flight team in order to provide extra help during transport as well as to provide continuity of care, especially when details of the accident scene and extrication may be helpful to the medical center team. This kind of teamwork also provides excellent ongoing liaison, training, and follow-up between the referring ground squads and hospital-based medical team. The disadvantage is that the EMT must be returned home by some means, which may be inconvenient and expensive if long distances are involved.

Emergency Medical Technicians: Paramedics

Some systems, including the Maryland system,[10] use paramedics for transport. Extensive training (up to 1,500 hours) is given in some instances, and EMT-Ps can be very good for scene runs. However, for interhospital transfers of cardiac and medical patients, neonates, and high-risk pregnancies it does not appear that paramedics are the best choice nor the most experienced for these areas requiring special expertise and training. It depends on the philosophy of the program as to what level of sophistication the medical care will be acceptable. The hospital that uses paramedics must determine that the paramedic practice act in their state does not prohibit paramedics from practicing within a hospital, since the aircraft is usually seen as an extension of the emergency unit for legal purposes.

Nurses

Almost all hospital-based programs use nurses either alone, in pairs, or in combination with physicians,[25,26] paramedics, or respiratory therapists. The nurses usually have extensive experience in critical care prior to becoming flight nurses, and almost all have had extra training in advanced cardiac life support, airway management and intubation, immobilization techniques, and central venous lines insertion. Some are trained to insert chest tubes, can do cricothyreotomies, and have other advanced skills.[21,27,28]

Again, the hospital and nurses must be aware of the nurse practice act within the states where they operate so that there is no question of the nurse "practicing medicine without a license." Certification as a nurse practitioner, nurse clinician, or paramedic may be necessary in order to circumvent these problems. The flight nurses organization through ASHBEAMS is attempting to establish certain guidelines for training and level of practice.

Flight nurses often provide an excellent level of care, particularly during transport when the vast majority of tasks required by a stabilized patient are nursing skills that many physicians are not accustomed to thinking of routinely. While some administrators feel that nurses can be less threatening to the local rural physician in the emergency or coronary care unit than a flight physician, others feel that the nurse who is more capable at resuscitation and stabilization than the local physician is more likely to be threatening as she or he takes over the case. In some programs nurses fly singly; others feel that nurses in pairs are better, particularly when extremely critical patients or multiple patients are involved.

Physicians

Physicians may fly as part of the team either on all flights or only on special flights as specified by their protocol (e.g., neonatal care, high-risk pregnancies, or at the request of the referring physician).[25,26] To be useful, the physician must be trained in the skills that are needed for the care of the patient. To send an intern or inexperienced resident is no better than sending an EMT-I and is not profitable for either the patient or for the physician as a training experience. Inexperienced physicians may be a particular hindrance at the accident scene, where they tend to attempt definitive rather than stabilizing procedures.

The well-trained and coordinated physician/nurse team can definitively treat the patient and do whatever procedures are necessary, particularly for the interhospital transports, including pacemaker insertion, complicated deliveries, and neonatal resuscitations. The service can then be truly marketed as a "flying emergency room," "flying trauma team," or "flying neonatal intensive care unit." For senior emergency, surgery, pediatrics, or other residents or fellows, being a member of an air EMS team can be a tremendous learning experience.

Medical Director

It is essential that any hospital-based or advanced medical air transport systems have a medical director who is responsible for quality control of the patient care on the flights and the relationship with both referring and receiving physicians.[23] The physician, unless the service is limited to neonates or some other particular subspecialty, should be experienced in all aspects of emergency care, particularly trauma and medical emergencies since these make up the vast majority of the transport (trauma, 60 percent; medicine, about 30 percent for most general programs). The medical director alone is responsible for the quality of the medical care delivered and must be involved in the training of the personnel, chart and run review, periodic evaluations of the staff, and establishment of medical protocols. The medical director is also the most visible focus of contact for referring physicians and agencies, the administration, the staff, and the news media and is responsible for letters of follow-up to the referring physician in order to ensure maintenance of the referral pattern and continued use of the program.

Dispatchers

Some programs use local EMS dispatch centers, but most have a separate team of dispatchers that handle not only the dispatch of the flight but also data collection from the referring source, coordination of the receiving team (notification of blood bank, CT scan team, intensive care unit, operating room, or special consultants), and care and guidance of the patient's family members to the receiving hospital.[21] The dispatchers may be trained as paramedics or EMT-Is or be chosen from the emergency unit clerks who are already familiar with emergency department operations. Depending on the sophistication of the communications system, several weeks to months of orientation and apprenticeship may be necessary before the dispatcher learns the complete system.

Administrator

When a hospital-based program is being initiated it is essential to have an administrator to handle contacts with the news media and referring hospitals, the certificate of need application, construction of the helipad, negotiations with third-party payers for reimbursement, and whatever other duties may be involved in setting up the program and doing the initial marketing. Even after the program is underway there is a need for ongoing marketing. Many of the day-to-day demands of ordering drugs, supplies, and equipment and scheduling staff may be handled either by the administrator, the head flight nurse, or by a manager assigned to these tasks. It is essential that the administrators and medical directors work very closely and well together, each handling their own spheres of expertise.

Pilots

Most hospital-based programs arrange for pilots through their leasing agreement with one of the major vendors or with their local fixed-base operator.[20,29] While the FAA in the past has partially exempted hospital pilots from the normal requirements for rest and time off, it is unlikely that this exemption will continue as more programs come into existence and those currently operating get busier.

Most programs in the past have operated with two pilots per craft even while covering 24 hours a day, 7 days a week. The FAA is beginning to require a minimum of three pilots in each program, depending on the volume of flight and number of flight hours.

Most companies, for helicopter programs, require a minimum of 3000 hours rotor wing time, including at least 500 hours night flying. While instrument flying is seldom used, most companies require instrument flight rating licenses for the extra experience that this gives the pilot in marginal weather conditions. If there are any other special demands of the region (e.g., mountains), then time and special training to handle these should also be required.

The pilot is responsible for the craft and the safety of the entire crew and the patient. The pilot alone makes the decision, based on weather and other considerations, as to whether any mission flies. Safety of the medical team should always be the top concern, even when an individual patient may suffer from lack of transport.[30]

The hospital pilot is a special breed of pilot, who must endure the boredom of long hours at the hospital while being ready to cope with the demands of the job at a moment's notice. The pilot must also act as a public relations representative for the hospital.[29] Some programs train pilots as EMT-Is or paramedics, but others feel that the pilot should be responsible only for flying the plane while others care for the patients.

Mechanic

Expert maintenance is essential to the availability and safety of the craft and for the program's success.[29] Most leasing companies supply an on-site dedicated mechanic who is on 24-hour call and who is experienced in maintenance of the particular craft used. This includes all the routine and scheduled maintenance as well as assisting with the major checks and overhauls mandated by the FAA for certain numbers of flight hours and any unscheduled maintenance.

FACTORS AFFECTING FLIGHTS

There are several important factors that will affect the accessibility and use of an air emergency transport system: weather, maintenance, response time, range, and fuel availability.

Weather is much less of a problem in air emergency transport than the general public believes. Most programs find that between 5 and 10 percent of their flights are missed as a result of bad weather. The most common weather problems are ground fog and gusty wind conditions. Some programs have special weather and climate conditions, ranging from blizzards to difficulty with lift over deserts and in high altitudes. Helicopter programs should all operate by stringent FAA visual flight rating standards. Airplanes, if properly equipped and flying to equipped landing sites, may operate by instrument flight rating standards. Both types of programs should plan for any conceivable deterioration in weather conditions that could occur during the flight. The pilot is the absolute arbiter of any decisions about weather conditions. The safety of the crew and patient must be of more concern than whether a flight can be made in marginal circumstances.

A firm contract must be written for the amount of permissible scheduled and unscheduled maintenance time and should include substantial penalties for the company that does not provide either acceptable service or a back-up craft properly configured for hospital work.

Response time may not be a crucial factor for non-emergency transfers. However, for scene runs, disaster response, and interhospital transport of unstable patients, it is critical. Many hospital-based programs boast lift-off times within 5 to 10 minutes of receipt of call. Other programs whose medical teams must be transported to the airport, be called in from home, or utilize the MAST may have dispatch times ranging from 30 minutes to several hours.

The range of the craft, special fuel availability, and need for a landing field can all limit the availability of the system to the health system user.

COMMUNICATIONS

Communications in an air transport system can be divided into two areas: (1) in-house and (2) interagency.[26,31]

When a call is received and the decision to dispatch has been made, there must be an excellent and foolproof way of paging the flight team (pilot, nurse, physician) and any other personnel involved secondarily (medical director, administrator, security, mechanic) that may, by protocol, need notification. Most programs use voice pagers that may be combined with a call-back system for verification of receipt of call by the members of the flight team.

The system may usually be accessed by dedicated land telephone lines or WATS lines and by radio network. The system should be able to communicate easily and directly with the EMS system, police, hospitals, civil defense authorities, and airports. Most systems limit access to dispatch to these parties. Some systems, however, also allow private citizens access to the system, particularly in areas where isolated farm or traffic accidents can occur. For those systems that deal only in interhospital transports, some type of call-back arrangement to the facility for verification of the call is sometimes used to cut down on bogus calls. Few, if any, programs use telemetry during transport at this time since the medical team should be trained to recognize and treat arrhythmias without need for verification by the base hospital.

MEDICAL EQUIPMENT

The emergency medical aircraft must be equipped to handle almost any emergency. Because of the small space available and weight limitations, particularly with helicopters, the equipment and supplies must be kept to a minimum and must be carefully chosen.[14,17,23,30] Since less than 10 percent of the time are two patients transported and even more rarely are mass casualties treated, supplies may be limited to that necessary to care for one, and at most two, patients.

Many programs have kits made up for different uses, including trauma, medical emergencies, pediatric/neonatal care, and obstetrical care. Depending on the problem, kits that are called for can be loaded for the transport. Often, supplies and drugs are available at the referring hospital or from paramedic squads on the scene for replenishing the kits for transport in case they are used up in the resuscitation/stabilization phase.

The standards recommended by ASHBEAMS for hospital-based emergency air medical services are listed below.[23] The aircraft utilized by a hospital-based emergency air medical service should at a minimum:

- be able to carry at least one patient and one medical attendant, with space for an additional attendant if indicated by the patient's medical condition
- carry the patient inside the cabin of the aircraft and allow access to the patient by medical attendants
- have radio communications with hospitals and public safety vehicles
- be equipped with at least the following:
  medical oxygen
  suction
  airway management equipment, including endotracheal intubation equipment
  cardiac monitor/defibrillator
  splinting and bandaging equipment
  all medications necessary for emergency cardiac, traumatic, and other patient conditions, as approved by the service medical director
  medical antishock trousers

- be equipped with survival gear appropriate to the environment (e.g., winter survival gear for cold environments or life raft for over-water operations)
- have adequate interior lighting for patient care arranged in such a manner so as not to interfere with the pilot's vision
- meet all necessary FAA safety requirements.

In addition many programs carry Bird pressure-cycled or volume ventilators that help to free the attendant to do other duties, especially during long transports. A respiratory therapist familiar with pressure, volume, and oxygen concentration changes with altitudes should be consulted to determine the appropriate settings, test and maintain the equipment, and instruct the flight crew in its use.

Because intravenous fluid flow changes markedly and is unpredictable with changes in altitude, most programs use Holter pumps to deliver fluids. Glass intravenous fluid bottles should never be used because of the high risk of breakage and because flow rates are less easily controlled. With plastic bags, blood pressure cuffs or blood pumps may be used to direct the flow, particularly since cabin space is often inadequate to let gravity make good flow possible.

Antishock trousers are commonly used. The Hare traction splint is too long to be used in most helicopters. However, the Klippel splint is easily accommodated. Immobilization of the cervical spine can be accomplished with the Philadelphia collar, sand bags, and tape. Cervical traction should ideally be done with a pneumatic traction device applied to the tongs rather than by hanging weights, which can be dangerous to both the patient and crew when unexpected turbulence is encountered.

Pleurovacs may sometimes be used successfully, but most programs find the Heimlich valve adequate for management of simple pneumothoraces. The Life-Pak 5 is the most commonly used monitor/defibrillator owing to its easy portability, low weight, and easily visible oscilloscope. The Doppler sphygmomanometer is used by many programs to monitor both pulse and blood pressure since they are audible in most aircraft.

Leather or other secure restraint devices are essential, particularly for patients with head injuries, overdoses, or psychiatric problems.

PATIENT CARE

Stabilization and Resuscitation

Any patient to be transported by air must be stabilized as much as possible prior to transport.[14,17,23,30,32] Intubation, chest tube insertion, and other procedures are difficult, if not impossible, in most aircraft owing to inadequacies of lighting, space, or patient configuration. A patient should not be transported in full cardiopulmonary arrest but should be resuscitated prior to loading, unless there are very strong overriding social, political, or medical considerations in the transport.

A pneumothorax must be treated, particularly if the patient is to be placed on a ventilator. Gas expands with altitude so that a pneumothorax will cause more respiratory compromise at higher altitudes.

At least two good intravenous lines should be established prior to transport and be large bore in the case of trauma. In the case of any type of shock, antishock trousers should be laid on the stretcher under the patient so that they may be inflated during flight if necessary; they are nearly impossible to put on after transport has begun. The pressure of any air splinting devices must be monitored before, during, and after flight to avoid overinflation and tourniquetlike action. Casts should be bivalved prior to transport.

Transport

Most, if not all, patients should be securely restrained prior to flight, both for their protection as well as for that of the crew. Restraints are mandatory for patients with head injuries, overdoses, or psychiatric disorders and in any other patient who might become excited or combative. Many programs routinely restrain all patients.

Oxygen should be used on any patient with respiratory compromise or anemia since atmospheric oxygen pressure decreases with altitude. It should certainly be used in all multiple trauma patients, patients with high-risk pregnancies, and cardiac patients. A nomogram for calculating arterial oxygen with changes in altitude is shown in Figure 4–1. The altitude limits recommended for patients by the American College of Chest Physicians are shown in Table 4–1.

Dysbarisms are those conditions aggravated by changes in atmospheric pressure. They include pneumothoraces, bowel obstructions, intracranial air (i.e., post-trauma or post-pneumoencephalography), and any other conditions in which trapped air will expand because of the increase in altitude causing attendant decreases in barometric pressure and expansion of gases. Vitreous and other intraocular tissues may expand and be extruded in the case of penetrating eye injuries.

Motion sickness may occur in some patients. Pre-transport nasogastric intubation with evacuation of stomach contents may help decrease the incidence of vomiting and aspiration. Occasionally sedation with an antiemetic is wise as long as the medication does not cloud another clinical condition.

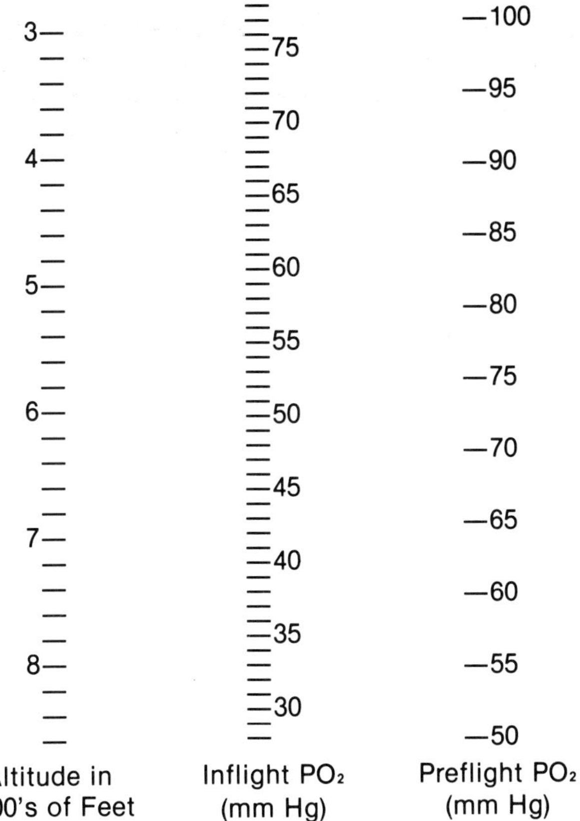

Figure 4–1 Nomogram for Predicting Inflight Arterial Oxygen Tension from Cabin Altitude and Preflight Arterial Oxygen Tension. (*Source:* Henry JN, Kremis LJ, Cutting RT: Hypoxemia during aeromedical evacuation. *Surg Gynecol Obstet* 136:49–53, 1973. Reprinted with permission of *Surgery, Gynecology & Obstetrics.*)

TABLE 4–1 Altitude Limits for Patients with Cardiorespiratory Diseases (without Supplemental O_2)

Limit (feet)	Problem
10,000	Any suspected or symptomatic cardiorespiratory disease
8,000	More than mildly symptomatic
	Marked ventilatory restriction
6,000	Recent myocardial infarction (8 to 24 weeks)
	Angina pectoris
	Sickle cell disease
	Alveolar block with cyanosis
	Patients with any one of the following:
	clinical cyanosis
	cor pulmonale
	respiratory acidosis
4,000	Severe cardiac disease with cyanosis or recent decompensation
	Patients with any two of the following:
	clinical cyanosis
	cor pulmonale
	respiratory acidosis
2,000	Cardiac patients in failure
	Myocardial infarction (8 weeks)
	Patients with all three of the following:
	clinical cyanosis
	cor pulmonale
	respiratory acidosis

Source: American College of Chest Physicians, Committee on Physiologic Therapy, Section on Aviation Medicine: Air travel in cardiorespiratory disease. *Dis Chest* 37: 579–588, 1969. (Reprinted with permission.)

The blood pressure can be palpated but cannot be audibly evaluated in most aircraft. A Doppler sphygmomanometer with the output wired into the caretaker's headphones can be placed over a pulse point prior to transport so that both pulse and blood pressure can be monitored during flight. Any digital automatic blood pressure read-out device should be flight tested since some are inaccurate at high altitudes.

None of the commercially available portable suction devices are acceptable for in-flight use. Most programs have wall suction mounted in the aircraft cabin near their oxygen outlets and use portable suction only at the scene or prior to loading in the aircraft.

If the patient has a cardiac arrest in the air, a judgment must be made whether to do cardiopulmonary resuscitation in the air or whether the helicopter should be landed and resuscitation carried out on the ground. The decision may depend on how far from a receiving hospital the craft is. Defibrillation, while it has been performed in the air, is probably more safely done on the ground, particularly for the crew, who may find it difficult to free themselves from all the metal stretcher supports and other structures in the craft.

Lighting at night, unless the patient compartment is completely separate from the pilot, should be with red or green lights so that the pilot's vision is not impaired. This, of course, makes patient assessment, particularly of patient color, difficult.

Helicopters and airplanes may seem cramped. However, since the attendant will never need to leave the patient's side, proper design and engineering of oxygen outlets, suction devices, and storage space for monitors, supplies, and drugs, and patient and caretaker configuration will make most aircraft as easy as possible to work in.

FINANCING

Both the costs and the revenue from a hospital-based emergency air medical system are substantial.

Aircraft Cost

With the rapid inflation and big interest costs in the early 1980s, several creative alternatives have been proposed for financing the original cost:[33]

Fixed-Based Operator (FBO)

Some programs have sought to decrease cost by using a local aircraft operator. A few of these have been very successful in their operation. However, others have found that while this type of contract ostensibly saves substantial sums, in reality the program may have problems in the following areas.

- *Expertise*—especially important to new programs, this includes advice in marketing, changing referral patterns, staff training, and communications system design.
- *Quality of pilots*—This may be low because of lack of sufficient flying experience, lack of familiarity with hospital operations, or high pilot turnover owing to poor pay scales or lack of job satisfaction.
- *Quality maintenance*—There may be delays in returning a vehicle to service or inadequacies in ensuring the safety and reliability of the operation. A back-up craft to continue the program in the event of an unexpected aircraft failure may not be available.

The advantages of having a local operator are that they are generally concerned with the community and the program and they are available and responsive to the needs of the hospital.

Lease from Vendor

The most common arrangement is a lease type of contract in which the craft, pilots, mechanic, and maintenance and repair for a year are leased from a major vendor. Many helicopter companies have found that the hospital market can be a stabilizing factor on their cash flow, smoothing out the profits and losses of their highly seasonal markets of forestry, seismic, and heavy construction. Thus, many companies with little experience are scrambling for contracts with hospitals. The track record and reputation of any company should be checked thoroughly prior to contract agreements or all of the problems mentioned with the fixed-based operator contracts can occur. Generally there is an additional charge per hour of flight time in addition to the base contract price, which will vary with the craft chosen.

Lease-Maintain, Lease-Purchase, and Other Alternatives

One solution to the high interest rates is the purchase of a craft by the hospital at an institutional interest rate or by financing with a bond issue. This saves money both by avoiding the higher interest and by reaping the tax benefits of depreciation and investment tax credits, for example. An agreement may then be made with a vendor to supply pilots, a mechanic to do all repairs and maintenance, and, in some cases, managerial and consulting services on marketing and implementation. This can save as much as one-third of the cost of the straight lease arrangement.

The vendor may agree to make payments on the craft in a lease-purchase agreement. The contract can be written so that there are still buy-out options should either the vendor or the hospital decide to cancel the service contract.

Of course, donation of aircraft by a benefactor, government agency, charity, or other granting institution can decrease the total cost to the hospital. The 1980s and 1990s should see multiple other creative financing alternatives for those institutions that want a program badly enough.

Other Program Costs

Other costs that must be considered are listed below:

- aircraft lease package:
  pilots
  maintenance
  mechanic
  aircraft
  flight hour charge
- staffing:
  medical director
  administrator or program manager
  physicians (none or one per flight)
  nurses (one or two per flight)
  dispatchers
  extra security
  other personnel or consultants
- helicopter support
  ground vs. rooftop helipad
  security precautions
  fuel
  maintenance area
  pilots quarters
  communications system
- medical equipment
  stretchers
  suction
  defibrillator/monitor

Doppler sphygmomanometer
ventilator
Holter pump
splints, medical antishock trousers
medical supplies and drugs
- insurance
liability
health and life
business
- training of staff
- marketing costs

Staffing decisions, as well as factors such as whether the helipad is at ground level or rooftop, can substantially change the cost of the program. Particularly during the first year the total cost for the non–aircraft areas approaches that of the aircraft lease, although it can decrease somewhat after that.

Revenue

Flight Charges

Air emergency transport and interhospital transfer of patients can be very profitable for the hospital, not only from the direct and indirect patient revenues but also from the standpoint of increased bed utilization.[26] Most programs do not try to recover the total cost of the program from flight charges since each flight costs $1000 to $1500, depending on the mileage. The administrators feel that either their referrals would be decreased or that third-party payers would be reluctant to reimburse the charges if the price were so high. The charges of these programs usually approximate ground ambulance charges, although clearly a superior level of care is being provided by the medical team on the aircraft.

Some programs, however, recover the entire program cost through flight charges. Their rationale includes the extra service and level of medical care plus the fact that they do *not* want to be seen as competitive with the ground units for patient transports.[24]

Inpatient Charges

Most hospitals realize that the benefit of a helicopter air transport program is in increased bed utilization at their institution by critical patients with large billings ($13,000 to $16,000 per patient), and long stays (16 to 22 days). Referral patterns are also inevitably changed for the area. An air transport system that is properly run and properly marketed can increase a hospital's prestige, improving its profits and changing the patient mix, attracting more and better physician staff, and providing more teaching cases for institutions affiliated with a medical school or other training program.

MARKETING

Proper marketing of an air medical transport system is essential if it is to be a financial success.[24,26,27,29] This is a particularly important factor for hospital-based programs.

Part of the initial marketing includes the certificate of need application. Other features of the marketing package must include in-house marketing (physicians, administrators, all supporting personnel), marketing to health users (hospitals, local and rural, referring physicians, EMS systems, and other public agencies such as sheriffs, highway patrol, and civil defense), and media exposure.

Unless the in-house personnel support the program the system will not be a success. The in-house personnel are the best public relations representatives to the public, both locally and to the referring communities. The physicians must be ready and willing to accept the additional critical patients that such a system will transport. The administrators must be farsighted enough to support the system with funding and good will prior to seeing the results of increased patient revenues and bed utilization.

Unless the system and method of accessing it is known to the referring medical personnel, hospitals, and other health care professionals, few referrals will be made. Some programs do several weeks of marketing flights to acquaint referring parties with the program prior to implementation of the system. It is essential to maintain excellent ongoing relationships with these organizations in order to maintain and increase referrals.

Letters of follow-up, return flights, and outreach education projects are all frequently used to maintain contact. Because of its newsworthiness the media will be constantly monitoring the program so that it pays to have good relations with them. Any problems must be dealt with openly and honestly. If the media has realistic expectations and a good understanding of the program, coverage that could otherwise be extremely damaging or derogatory can be favorably modified.

SUMMARY

Air medical transport can vary from uncontrolled and unstandardized air taxi services to highly sophisticated hospital-based medical helicopter services that offer both the advantages of speed and high quality medical care to the patient. Studies have shown a decrease in the mortality and morbidity of patients who are stabilized and transported by skilled personnel. A properly constructed air medical system can complement the already existing EMS system.

Hospitals have provided this service for a number of reasons:

- Critical patients transferred to an institution where they can receive definitive care have a decreased morbidity and mortality.
- The helicopter is an "image changer." It is a highly visible sign that a hospital is committed to patient care and adds to the hospital's prestige as a medical center.
- It will change patient mix, increase bed utilization and revenue, and change referral patterns.
- It increases the number and quality of seriously ill or injured patients, who may be utilized in the training of medical personnel.
- "Outreach" education programs and general improvement in the level of care in a region can be affected.

Many factors are necessary to make a program successful. The four most important components are (1) medical expertise and support at the base hospital, (2) a good communications system, (3) aircraft maintenance, and (4) marketing, both initially and ongoing.

REFERENCES

1. Myers RN, Angelides AP, Haupt GJ: A civilian aeromedical lifesaving plan, HELP. *Penn Med J* 68:51–53, 1965.
2. United States Army: *Army Flight Surgeon's Manual*, special text ST-1-105–8. Fort Reecher, Ala, Army Aeromedical Center, 1970.
3. United States National Highway Traffic Safety Administration: *Helicopters in Emergency Medical Service/NHTSA Experience to Date.* Washington, DC, 1972.
4. Cline RE: The air medical evacuation system concept. *US Army Aviation Digest*, July 1971, pp 22–25.
5. Arizona State University: *Air Medical Evacuation System (AMES)*, pp 1–207.
6. Hoffman R: Here come the helicopter ambulances. *Flying*, December 1970, pp 73–77.
7. Flexer M: What potential for helicopters in EMS? *Hospitals* 49(4):60–63, 1975.
8. Craig KC: MAST. *Emergency* 12(8):38–40, 1980.
9. United States MAST Interagency Executive Group: *MAST Missions Report.* Washington, DC, November 30, 1978.
10. Cowley AR, Hudson F, Scanlan E, Gill W et al: An economical and proved helicopter program for transporting the emergency critically ill and injured patient in Maryland. *J Trauma* 13:1029–1038, 1973.
11. This medevac program pays off in lives. *Emerg Med Serv*, September/October 1975, pp 67–70.
12. Cleveland HC: An air emergency service: The extension of the emergency department. *J Emerg Med Serv*, pp 47–54.
13. Flight for life. *Emerg Med Serv*, May/June 1975, pp 40–43.
14. Lam DM: *Aeromedical Evacuation: A Handbook for Physicians.* US Army 28–2038–4, August 1980.
15. United States Federal Aviation Administration: Letter from James Bowman, Alpha Aviation, Dallas, Texas, regulatory docket No. 17045. Washington, DC, 1977–1979.
16. Boyd K: Hospitals and helicopters: The ups and downs of care from the air. *J Emerg Med Serv* 5(9): 26–32, 1980.
17. United States Department of Transportation: Air ambulance guidelines, HS 805–703, February 1981.
18. Eastepp MS: One mission of mercy. *Emergency*, July 1978, p 10.
19. Gough AR, Secord B, Behrens BA: Emergency patient transfers: The medico-legal considerations. *Emergency* 12(7):49–52, 1980.
20. Farrell DF: Helicopters: Maximum mobility. *Emergency* 13(7):56–61, 1981.
21. Tye J: The role of a hospital-based emergency helicopter service in a rural state. *Emerg Med Serv* 9(4):17–23, 1980.
22. Tye J: In pursuit of excellence. Address given to the organizational meeting of ASHBEAMS, December 12, 1980.
23. Proposed ASHBEAMS Standards, 1980.
24. Cooper MA: A hospital-based helicopter service: Will it fly. *Am Emerg Med* 9:451–455, 1980.
25. Cordell WM: Lifetime: A physician-staffed, helicopter-mediated emergency service in Indiana. *J Ind State Med Assoc*, October 1980, pp 660–663.
26. Grider G: Air ambulances: What took so long? *Emergency* 12(8):52–56, 1980.
27. Farrell DF: Response from the Rockies: An air ambulance industry blossoms. *Emergency* 12(8):41–44, 1980.
28. McCombs CM: Air ambulance services: New horizons for emergency nursing. *J Emerg Nurs* 4(4):21–23, 1978.
29. Toler D: Taking your helicopter to the hospital. *Rotor Wing Int*, July 1980, pp 42–46.
30. Yancy RT: Stabilizing a critical patient for helicopter transport. *Emerg Med Serv*, 10(5): 72–76, 1981.
31. Brockway F: Helicopter to hospital communication. *Emergency* 12(8):61–62, 1980.
32. Welch BR: Some considerations before using the aerial ambulance. *J Am Coll Emerg Physicians* 6(5):155–157, 1977.
33. Stenstrud RL: Hospital-based air ambulance service extends emergency care. *Hosp Prog*, May 1980, pp 72–76.

5. Emergency Care and the Law

JAMES O. PAGE, J.D.

Among the many branches or divisions of the law, that which most concerns or interests the provider of emergency care seems to be the law of torts. A term derived from the Latin word meaning *to twist, torquere*, a tort is defined today as a private or civil wrong or injury. In the United States, this field of jurisprudence is most often referred to as the law of negligence.

The concept of civil remedies for civil wrongs can be traced to the early English law. In the feudal society that evolved from the Norman conquest of England, the question of court jurisdiction over conflicts and grievances was a source of contention between the king and nobles who sought to protect their own prerogatives of governance. Growing from this environment was a highly formalized system of procedure that continues to influence the processes of law in modern times.

Originally, trespasses, or wrongs that were subject to legal redress, were quasi-criminal. If the defendant were found guilty, not only were damages awarded to the successful plaintiff, but also the defendant was imprisoned until release was purchased by payment of a fine.[1] This criminal aspect of unintentional injury or damage to another was abolished by statute in 1697, leaving such matters to exclusively civil remedies.[2] Over the centuries, the common law distinctions between criminal acts and tortious acts have been the subject of protracted judicial debate. Gradually, the differences were clarified in legal opinions, and precedents that continue to serve as the substance of the common law were formed. With codification of the law through stat-utes, coupled with the enlightening though massive body of legal opinions, a rational and reasonably predictable system of civil law has been established.

The idea that the current system of civil law is rational and reasonable may be questioned by many who serve in the modern field of health care. This perception may be, in large part, the fault of those who practice and administer the law. Scientific knowledge has multiplied several times in recent decades, but the processes of the law have tended to retain a deliberate pace reflective of their heritage. Although the outcomes of civil law actions are just and fair in the preponderance of cases, they are often explained to the public in either imponderable legal esoterica or startling headlines that obscure the true substance. The resulting misperceptions tend to be exacerbated by unfounded rumor and relatively uninformed opinion.

In efforts to resolve disputes resulting from alleged negligence, U.S. courts have written volumes to describe negligence itself. Basically, negligence constitutes an omission to do something that a "reasonable" person would do, or it constitutes something done that a "reasonable" person would not do. In either case, negligence subjects other members of society to unreasonable risks of harm. When such harm does occur, an innocent member of society is personally injured, is wrongfully killed, or suffers some other form of loss to loved one or property. Any society that permits negligence to occur without penalty to the negligent party or remedy to the injured party must be deemed uncivilized in the mind of most U.S. citizens. To the extent the civil law of negligence penalizes the culpable by exacting compensation for injuries or damages caused, it probably discourages negligent behavior. To the extent the civil law of negligence compensates injured persons for their negligently inflicted injuries or damages, it provides the only rational form of justice to persons who otherwise would be uninjured.

In a free society, access to the processes of the civil law must be free and open. As with most aspects of liberty, however, this system provides many opportunities for abuse and indiscretion. It has been widely reported that health care providers have been victims of an abusive and indiscreet use of civil law in recent years. Although some would argue that this problem has been overstated, its impact on the attitudes, performances, and practices of health care providers has been both profound and expensive.

THE PERSPECTIVE OF THE PATIENT

Volumes of case reports detail instances in which it was alleged that a health care provider was less than reasonable in caring for a patient. Most providers yearn for practical guidance, but such guidance does not appear readily in the detail, dictum, and tedium of the case reports. Nonetheless, there lurks between the lines of those thousands of cases a common message that is far too simple to warrant judicial authorship—if the health care provider invariably cares for the patient as that provider would wish to be cared for as a patient, the demands and commandments of the civil law of negligence are satisfied.

In the emergency care setting, both before and after admission to the hospital, abandonment of patients has been a frequent cause of medical-legal confrontation. The abandoned patient, particularly one who has not been admitted to the hospital, tends to be socially or physically deviant. Apparently, it is difficult for health care providers to identify personally with the patient who is intoxicated, destitute, incontinent, or belligerent. In virtually every case in which it was held that the patient had been abandoned, however, had the patient been cared for by the provider as that provider would wish to be cared for in similar circumstances, the patient would not have been abandoned.

Another medical-legal confrontation may arise from resuscitation efforts if, for example, a patient suffers cardiac arrest and there is no attempt at resuscitation or the effort to resuscitate the patient is notably insufficient or inexpert.[3] In most cases that have resulted in litigation, the patient was neither elderly nor suffering from otherwise terminal illness. Obviously, health care providers responsible for such a patient, if similarly stricken, would wish for the attending medical personnel to be both expert and aggressive in their attempts at resuscitation.

Though litigation on the issue has been rare, failure to transfer a critical patient to a higher level of care may be another practical example of negligence. If a facility does not have the resources to meet a particular patient's critical care needs and the patient is not transferred to a more sophisticated level of care, the result is most often fatal. If in the position of the patient, the physician who has the opportunity to arrange for and initiate the transfer would obviously desire such action and would have little interest in the political or financial considerations that might stand in the way of transfer.

ELEMENTS OF THE LAW OF NEGLIGENCE

It is difficult to imagine an emergency medical problem or question that cannot be satisfactorily resolved from a medical-legal point of view by thinking through the provider-as-patient interposition. In order to understand *why* the processes of the civil law of negligence are likely to concur with such a resolution, it is necessary to examine the elements of history that have shaped the civil law over centuries and contributed to the creation and maintenance of a reasonably civilized society.

The case of *Weaver v. Ward,* which was brought before the King's Bench in the early seventeenth century,[4] is the earliest known case in which it was clearly recognized that a defendant might not be liable for a purely accidental injury that occurred entirely without his fault. At that time in the history of the civil law, however, the burden rested upon the defendant to prove his freedom from all fault. Although it was agreed that the injury inflicted by Ward upon Weaver was purely accidental and occurred through no fault of Ward's, he nonetheless was found guilty in that he failed to prove sufficiently his freedom from fault.

In modern times, the burden of proof rests upon the plaintiff, that is, the party who initiates an action under the civil law of negligence must prove that all the elements of negligence were present in the alleged incident or situation.[5] Very simply stated, the plaintiff must allege and prove that the defendant owed a duty to the plaintiff and, further, that the defendant breached that duty. The plaintiff must also allege and prove that a discernible injury, loss, or other form of damage was suffered and that there was a cause-and-effect link between the breach of duty and the injury, loss, or damage suffered.

Duty

It is possible to deal with most of the questions that arise in a typical negligence case in terms of the element of duty. In such cases, the term *duty* is often defined as an obligation, recognized by the law, to conform to a particular standard of conduct toward another. Whether such a duty to another exists at all may be an issue; if it does, the extent or limits of that duty may be an issue.

Since the early 1960s, medical-legal folklore has been rich with stories of lawsuits filed against physicians who have attempted to aid injured motorists.[6] Though factually without basis, such oft-repeated accounts seem to have generated apprehension among professionals who may provide health care to injured or stricken strangers.[7] It may be revolting to our moral senses, but it can be said that the law does not command affirmative action on behalf of a stranger in peril.[5] This rule, like so many in the law of negligence, has its roots in English common law. Largely because of the difficulties in setting workable standards for unselfish service to fellow citizens, the courts have avoided the temptation to impose a duty on the health care provider who encounters an injured or ill stranger outside the normal health care setting to render aid to that stranger.

Nonetheless, health care providers routinely do render assistance to ill or injured strangers at roadside, on ski slopes, and elsewhere. Although they had no initial duty, their affirmative action constitutes an automatic assumption of duty to the victim or patient. That duty, simply stated, is to care for the person as the rescuer would wish to be cared for in the same circumstances. In more conventional legal terms, the duty is to perform as a reasonable and prudent person of like training and experience would perform under the same or similar circumstances.

Breach of Duty

The process of litigation in the law of negligence nearly always involves both issues of law and issues of fact. Issues of law are reserved for decision by the court (judge), while issues of fact are the province of the jury. The distinction between legal issues and factual issues is seldom clear-cut. A general rule of thumb is that, if persons of reasonable intelligence might differ as to the conclusion to be drawn, the issue must be left to the jury. Otherwise, the issue is for the court to decide.

Whether or not a particular defendant has breached a duty to the plaintiff is most often an issue of fact, left to the jury for decision. For example, an unsuccessful effort by a health care provider to insert an adjunctive ventilation device in a patient may raise an issue of fact if it can be shown that the provider failed to participate in regular continuing education concerning the use of this procedure and device. The jury would be instructed to consider the actions of the defendant, measure them against the duty of care owed to the patient, and determine whether the defendant breached that duty. As in all elements of the law of negligence, the burden of proof rests with the plaintiff. Would a reasonable and prudent health care provider who had failed to maintain skills in such a technique attempt to use it? If the health care provider were in the position of the patient, how would the provider wish to be cared for, and by whom?

Damage

The plaintiff's burden of proof extends to a showing of actual loss or damage. Alleged violation of a technical right cannot result in an award for the plaintiff unless there is proof of actual loss or damage. Thus, negligence, in and of itself, cannot produce a verdict for the plaintiff; that negligence must have produced actual injury, damage, or loss to another person or persons.

Many of the hypothetical questions and concerns of health care providers in regard to the law of negligence involve this issue and cannot be answered without additional information or hypothetical conclusions. For example, questions may be raised about the liability of a physician or nurse who is notoriously unskilled at certain medical or surgical procedures. The lack of skill, in and of itself, will not produce a verdict for the plaintiff without proof that actual damage occurred as a result of that negligence. Thus, with sufficient luck and close scrutiny and assistance by aides and colleagues, the unskilled provider may escape liability despite shockingly negligent performance. Similarly, a certain act or omission will bring about liability only if that act or omission caused actual damage or loss.

Causation

Finally, the plaintiff's burden of proof requires a clear showing of a reasonably close causal connection between the breach of duty and the actual damage or loss. For example, in cases of cardiac and respiratory arrest, if an inexpert effort at resuscitation by the health care provider fails to revive the pulseless, nonbreathing patient, was the death caused by the preexisting condition of cardiac and respiratory arrest, or was it caused by the inexpert effort at resuscitation? If the resuscitative effort had been a textbook performance, would there have been a reasonable certainty of recovery?

In cases involving preexisting injury or illness, the plaintiff's burden of proof of a causal connection tends to be onerous, which may explain the relatively small number of cases involving alleged inexpert resuscitative efforts. The issue of causation has frequent application to another disastrous emergency medical incident, however—the spinal cord injury. When paralysis follows such an injury and litigation against a health care provider results, the plaintiff must prove that the actions or omissions of the provider have a causal connection to the damage suffered by the injured person. In most such cases, it is difficult for the plaintiff to counter the probability that the damage was caused by the precedent traumatic event, such as an automobile collision.

DEFENSES

One defense that may be raised by a defendant to prevent an adverse verdict and judgment is based on the theory of contributory negligence. More aptly described as "contributory fault," this theory commands that individuals comport themselves with the same degree of caution and prudence that they command of a defendant. If it is shown that a plaintiff's own conduct failed to meet the standard of the reasonable person of ordinary prudence under like circumstances, and if that conduct has been a substantial factor in causing the plaintiff's injury, the plaintiff's legal action may be barred by a device known as a "directed verdict."

Coincidental with growing judicial dislike for the doctrine of contributory negligence as a complete bar to a lawsuit, there has been increasing statutory activity with regard to the alternative concept of "comparative negligence." In those states in which this concept has been adopted, courts attempt to apportion monetary awards according to the percentage of fault of each of the parties.

The defense of assumption of risk may apply in three types of situations. It may apply when the plaintiff, in advance, expressly consented to relieve the defendant of an obligation of conduct toward the plaintiff and to accept the known risk of injury arising from defendant's acts or omissions. It may apply when the plaintiff, with knowledge of the risk, voluntarily enters into some relation with the defendant that will necessarily involve that risk, therefore actually or impliedly accepting the risk. Finally, it may apply when the plaintiff, already aware of a risk created by the negligence of the plaintiff, voluntarily encounters it.

In recent years, most often in response to the demands of organized groups of health care providers, state legislatures have enacted statutes that purport to protect certain classes of providers from civil liability. Commonly and inappropriately called "good Samaritan laws," these statutes constitute a form of defense that, if utilized, must be asserted by the defendant.[6,7] In essence, most of these statutory enactments seek to create for the described class of providers a form of immunity from liability.

Early in U.S. legal history, certain immunities from liability were established. For example, entities of government, charities, and judges were made immune from liability for reasons of public policy. At present, charitable immunity is all but ended, and governmental immunity survives in only a minority of jurisdictions. Many reasons have been advanced to explain this judicial and legislative trend, among them the fact that insurance is readily available to protect many previously immune entities from the hardship of judgments. At the same time, in little more than a decade, every state has enacted at least one statute that purports to make various classes of emergency care providers immune from liability for their ordinary negligence.

Legal scholars have been perplexed by this development, in part because many of the statutes are poorly composed; inconsistent; replete with contradictory language, undefined terms, and ambiguous requirements; and, in many cases, relatively ineffective. The immunity afforded by some of these enactments would leave injured persons without a remedy. It has been suggested that, under certain circumstances, an immunity statute singling out a specific group or class without evidence of a pressing social need would violate the equal protection provisions of the Fourteenth Amendment to the U.S. Constitution. Another criticism of the new wave of liability immunity statutes is that this presumed protection against liability may decrease the interest of health care providers in skill maintenance and continuing education.

The lack of need for such protections may be the most damning aspect of their development and existence. In virtually every state in which legislatures were persuaded to enact such immunity provisions, the supportive testimony included unfounded reports of litigation and liability involving providers of emergency medical care. Such testimony simply was untrue. There was no factual basis for the drastic reconstruction of the time-tested civil law of negligence. Litigation against the protected classes or groups was rare, and instances of liability, judgments, and awards against the protected classes or groups were rare to nonexistent. These facts lead the serious legal scholar to conclude that the recent liability immunity statutes are little more than a political placebo and of questionable value as a defense to litigation based on alleged negligence.

WITH AND WITHOUT PRECEDENT

Despite a virtual flood of legislative enactments during the past three decades, the U.S. legal system continues to rest on its common law foundations. That foundation is constructed around the principle of *stare decisis,* a Latin term meaning "to abide by or adhere to decided cases." Thus, when an appellate court renders a decision, it establishes a precedent. In subsequent cases based on similar facts, the precedent guides the courts in deciding those subsequent cases. Although the courts are free to depart from precedents when they conclude that earlier decisions are unreasonable or inconsistent with altered social conditions, the basic principle of the common law makes the course of the law reasonably predictable.

In certain fields, such as those involving common carriers or retail merchants, the casebooks are filled with reports of litigated cases and the resulting appellate court decisions. Analyzing the law's impact on given situations in those fields is largely a matter of research. In the field of emergency care, particularly outpatient care, however, there have been few instances of litigation and a minuscule number of appellate court decisions. Those who seek predictability in this field are obliged to examine the legal history of analogous fields, disciplines, and situations and even then can only speculate on the probable resolution of legal controversies that concern emergency medical care.

In the late 1960s, an innovative approach to the delivery of medical care began to appear in the United States.[8] Today, the concept is universal in U.S. urban centers. It involves training nonphysician personnel to deliver sophisticated advanced life support services in out-of-hospital settings. Under this concept, nonphysician personnel are guided or directed in their activities by written protocols or by radio or telephone communication. There is no body of legal precedents that concern this concept. On the other hand, it is not difficult to recognize the similarities between this situation and an agency relationship. The field provider, commonly known as a paramedic, is often employed by a public safety agency but controlled, directed, and guided in patient care by a physician who has no formal relationship with that public safety agency. In the end, who would be responsible for any negligent actions or omissions of the paramedic?

With some imagination, an analogy can be drawn between these medical personnel and nineteenth century farmers. When Farmer Brown prepared to harvest a crop, he might find that he needed to borrow several of Farmer Jones' farmhands to help with the harvest. If, while helping Farmer Brown, one of Jones' employees was negligent and caused injury or death to a third person, who would be liable ultimately? Then and now, the law would hold Brown responsible for injuries or damages caused by the negligence of Jones' employee during the period of the borrowing. Based on both public policy and logic, the "rule of the borrowed servant" has been stated as follows: "A servant directed or permitted by his master to perform services for another may become the servant of such other in performing the services. He may become the other's servant as to some acts and not as to others. . . ."[9] Another source has described the rule as follows: "When one person puts his servant at the disposal and under the control of another for the performance of a particular service for the latter, the servant, in respect of his acts in that service, is to be dealt with as the servant of the latter and not of the former."[10]

Control appears to be the essence of the rule of the borrowed servant. Farmer Brown would be responsible for the negligence of Jones' farmhand because Brown had control over the farmhand at the time the negligent injury or damage occurred. The public policy behind this conclusion presumes that those who know they will be held responsible for the acts or omissions of a borrowed employee will put forth special efforts to control that employee and prevent injury or damage to others. The conclusion is logical; between the two farmers, for example, Jones had the least opportunity to control his loaned servant and thus to prevent any negligence that caused injury or damage to the third party.

The rule can be applied to modern out-of-hospital advanced life support programs by placing the medical director of the program in the role of Farmer Brown and the primary employer of the paramedics, such as the fire chief, the private ambulance company owner, or the municipal ambulance service director, in the role of Jones. The paramedic would stand in the role of the borrowed employee. As the use of these programs has spread in the United States, there has been a tendency to assume that the personnel of the public safety or ambulance service (the farmhands) communicate with the program's medical director (Farmer Brown) only during medical incidents. This perception has been shown to be faulty on both medical and legal bases. The most serious defect is the universal lack of medical control in these types of systems.

At first glance, maintaining a degree of isolation or distance between physicians and paramedics employed by another agency or organization may seem to offer a degree of legal safety to the physician. In reality, the isolation or distance creates a vacuum of medical leadership and control, and it allows public service officials and administrators to set medical policy and control paramedic performances in patient care. It heightens the possibility of negligent performances by paramedics, thus increasing the possibility of litigation initiated by injured or damaged persons. Furthermore, in search of "deep pockets," the plaintiffs may seek out and involve the distant physician as a defendant.

Just as the early law sought to encourage Farmer Brown to control Jones' servant during the period of borrowing, modern law would expect the medical director to assert sufficient control over the paramedics to ensure reasonable and prudent behavior and performance, thus reducing or eliminating the possibility of negligence and injury or damage to patients. While the opportunity to control the patient care activities of paramedic personnel may be appealing to physicians, the prospect of being responsible for the consequences of their negligence may appear forbidding. The national experience between 1967 and 1980 should alleviate such concern, however. Approximately 20 million patients were seen, treated, attended to, and transported by paramedics during this 13-year period, but there is no record that any appellate court during that time determined the liability of paramedics or their medical directors for alleged negligence. It is estimated that 50 lawsuits were filed against paramedics, paramedic provider services, hospitals serving as the medical control base for paramedics, or the medical directors of out-of-hospital advanced life support programs. By using a conservative estimate of the numbers of patients seen during a duty shift and the average number of duty shifts worked by a paramedic team, it can be calculated that the average paramedic team generates litigation once in every 400,000 patient contacts. The average paramedic team would have to work for more than 600 years to encounter 400,000 patients.

There has been no formal study of the legal impact of out-of-hospital advanced life support programs. The foregoing information is based on periodic inquiry and ongoing investigation, with voluntary cooperation of many state and local emergency medical services organizations.[11] In that effort, it has been noted that there has been no litigation involving those systems that have embraced the borrowed servant doctrine and have given physicians a full measure of control over the patient care performances of paramedic personnel.

ISSUES OF CONSENT

In those instances of litigation that have been investigated and reviewed, abandonment of patients appears to be the most common allegation. In nearly every such case reviewed, it was alleged that paramedic personnel had assessed the patient's condition and, without consultation with their medical control facility, had concluded that the patient required no medical care.[12–16] Most often, litigation alleging wrongful death resulted from death of the patient. Interviews with personnel involved in several of these cases disclose that the patient may have been abusive or belligerent, may have been uncooperative, or may have refused care. In some of these cases, there was apparently some concern over the right of the patient to refuse care and the possible liability of providers who force care or transportation upon an unwilling patient.

These situations raise the issue of consent to care, which may occur in two forms, express or implied. Express consent is given through the actions, words, or written authorization of the patient; implied consent is deemed to exist whenever the patient is unconscious or otherwise unable to make a rational decision.

At the core of all consent issues in medical care is the established legal right of individuals to control their own body. This right includes the rational individual's right to refuse all medical care, even when the refusal may jeopardize the individual's life. There are no reliable guidelines for determining the rationality of the refusing patient, however. Particularly in the out-of-hospital setting, this can leave the provider with an emotional, possibly life-threatening, dilemma: to treat the individual in the face of refusal, thus taking the risk of legal action, or to conclude that the refusing individual is rational and discontinue efforts to provide care, thus taking the risk of legal action.

The legal history of modern out-of-hospital emergency care may be helpful in analyzing this dilemma. In more than a decade, there has been no reported litigation as a result of care allegedly rendered against the wishes of the patient in such a setting. It is common knowledge that nearly all paramedic teams frequently confront individuals who refuse care; in many cases, treatment and transportation are provided against the individual's stated wishes. The apparent absence of legal action in the face of frequent events would suggest that the risk of a lawsuit for providing care to the refusing patient is minimal.

As mentioned earlier, alleged abandonment of patients appears to be the most common progenitor of legal action against out-of-hospital emergency care providers. When confronted by refusal in the form of anger, determination, hostility, or even threatened violence, providers tend to conclude that the individual does not want their services and to leave, oftentimes without compiling a report or record of the event. Should the event result in litigation, however, the individual (or survivors of the individual) might argue that the patient's behavior was not rational and that the providers should have asserted themselves, assuming consent from the patient's irrational behavior and providing care, despite the outward manifestations of refusal. It would appear reasonable and prudent to opt for care and transportation in the face of adamant refusal, at least in those cases in which there may be some potential for aggravation of the medical condition or threat to the life of the patient or others. In California and a few other jurisdictions, legislation has been enacted to provide a lawful procedure for taking into protective custody individuals who may be endangered by their apparently irrational refusal of care or who may endanger others if left in the home or public setting.[17] This type of statute may serve as a model to other jurisdictions that are trying to resolve a common medical-legal problem.

In the hospital setting, there is frequent reference to "informed consent." This relatively recent legal requirement imposes upon health care providers the duty to explain to patients the nature and seriousness of their medical problem, the nature of the proposed medical or surgical procedure, and the risks of treatment. The patient must also be given sufficient opportunity to ask questions and receive informative answers before consenting to the procedure or treatment. More than anything else, the informed consent requirement is a judicial reaction to aloofness on the part of health care providers. The requirement is viewed by the courts as a way to ensure that health care providers communicate fully with patients and provide those patients with sufficient information to make an informed judgment. Although it has not been applied by the courts to out-of-hospital situations, it is a potential requirement in certain situations.

PROSPECTIVE LEGAL DEVELOPMENTS

It has become a matter of public knowledge that there are wide variances in the capability of individual hospitals to care for certain classes of seriously ill patients. Some hospital officials have been less than candid concerning those variances, however, and their hospitals may accept patients who have life-threatening medical or surgical problems that are beyond the care capability of that hospital.[18] In addition, medical personnel in those hospitals may be reluctant to initiate transfers of such patients to a more appropriate level of care.

At the same time, in the out-of-hospital setting, there appears to be a tendency—sometimes because of an official policy or protocol—to allow the patient's preference to determine the hospital to which the patient will be transported. Even though the patient may be aware of variances in the capabilities of individual hospitals in the community, it may be unreasonable to expect the patient (or the patient's spouse or guardian) to know which of several hospitals is best equipped and staffed to care for that patient's specific medical or surgical needs at that particular time. The current environment of relative ignorance, misinformation, and proprietary interest is a veritable seedbed of potential errors with undesirable consequences. Thus, it is likely to produce litigation that will reach the appellate courts.

It would seem reasonable to expect that the courts will require informed consent in out-of-hospital settings; i.e., the courts may require ambulance personnel to explain to a patient, or the patient's spouse or guardian if the patient is incapable of making a decision, the relative care capabilities of the several hospitals that may be within reasonable time and distance. The ultimate decision of the patient or the patient's representative could then be based on accurate information, rather than irrelevant experience or the impact of a particular hospital's efforts in public relations.

Should the patient arrive at an inappropriate facility, it would seem reasonable for the law to require medical personnel in the emergency department to make an honest, good faith, common sense assessment of the patient's status in relation to services and facilities available in that hospital facility. Although the legally imposed requirement may include the obligation to initiate and coordinate a transfer of the patient to a more appropriate facility, appropriate care in anticipation of or pending a transfer would also be required. The medical personnel first seeing a patient whose life is threatened should not conclude that their responsibility ends with the decision to transfer the patient. Recently, training programs for advanced cardiac life support and advanced trauma life support have been widely utilized by emergency care personnel. Courts would probably conclude that the skills embraced by those training programs constitute the minimum level of care to which a patient is entitled when suffering from a critical coronary disorder or life-threatening traumatic injury.

Finally, the courts could be expected to find offensive a hospital's overstated representations of patient care capability. Particularly in the area of designated trauma centers that have sought publicity for their trauma care services in the community, the courts might impose a strict national standard of service, facilities, equipment, staffing, and availability. Failure of a specialized center to provide what a reasonable person might expect in such a facility might lead to a legal conclusion that there were misrepresentations and that these misrepresentations constituted a breach of duty. If it could be shown that such a breach was the causative link in an injury or death, it is conceivable that negligence could be found in a legal action against the particular facility.

CONCLUSIONS

The health care provider should recognize that the law of negligence can be a common sense process of civilization. Although health care providers tend to see this branch of the law as incomprehensible and complex, it can be explained in terms of basic concepts and requirements. In the end, it should be recognized that the courts may be compelled to serve as the advocate of the patient in a system that is often captured by a network of interests competing to the detriment of the patient.

Aside from the rich history of the law and its modern rules and requirements, the obvious key to legal safety for the health care provider is to obviate the need for legal intervention. This can most easily be accomplished by the mental exercise of provider-to-patient interposition. If providers confront each situation as if they were the patient, it is likely that the judgments made and the performances rendered will conform to the reasonable requirements of the law of negligence.

REFERENCES

1. Prosser WL, Smith YB: *Cases and Materials on Torts,* ed 3. San Francisco, The Foundation Press, 1962.
2. Statute of 5–6 William and Mary, c. 12.
3. McIntyre KM: *Status of Liability Risk of the Lay Rescuer for Out-of-Hospital Cardiopulmonary Resuscitation.* Dallas, American Heart Association, 1978.
4. Hobart 134, 1616.
5. Prosser WL: *Law of Torts,* ed 3. San Francisco, West Publishing Co, 1964.
6. Chayet NL: The myth of the good Samaritan suit. *Medical Opinion,* June 1973.
7. Warren DG (ed): *Health Law Bulletin,* No. 36. Chapel Hill, Institute of Government, University of North Carolina, December 1972.
8. Page JO: *The Paramedics.* Morristown, NJ, Backdraft Publications, 1979.
9. American Law Institute, *Restatement of Agency,* Section 227.
10. *Denton v. Yazoo and M. Valley R. Co.,* 284 U.S. 305, 52 S. Ct. 141, 142, 76 L.Ed. 310.
11. Study conducted by ACT Foundation, P.O. Box 911, Basking Ridge, NJ 07920.
12. *Will Edward Brantley v. City of Dallas (Texas),* Case No. 75–6824–D.
13. Claim filed against the County of Los Angeles, July 25, 1977, by Ambrocio Ceniceros.
14. *Mary Gonzalez v. City of Los Angeles, et al,* Case No. C 172069.
15. Claim filed against the County of Los Angeles, October 6, 1975, by Bertha M. Tenney.
16. *Deborah J. Gaff v. City of Jacksonville, et al,* U.S. District Court, Middle District of Florida, Jacksonville Division, Case No. 79–128–CIV–J–C.
17. California Welfare and Institutions Code, Sections 300, 305, 5150, 5170, and 5343.
18. Houtchens B: Major trauma in the rural mountain west. *JACEP* 6:8, 1977.

Shock and Trauma

The different mechanisms of injuries and illnesses that may lead to shock share a common pathway of injury at the cellular and biochemical level, and this is presented in a four-compartment model in "Shock" (Chapter 6). One of the major causes of shock is multiple trauma, and a general medical/surgical approach to patients with such injuries is discussed in "Major Trauma" (Chapter 7).

The discussion of major trauma should be considered in conjunction with "Organization and Delivery of Emergency Medical Care" (Section I), particularly the systems approach for trauma care (Chapter 2). For patients with major trauma and specific traumatic injuries, emergency care personnel are referred to "Alterations of Central Nervous System Function" (Section IX), "Head and Neck Injuries" (Section XIII), "Vascular Injuries" (Chapter 53), "Heart and Great Vessel Emergencies" (Chapter 54), "Airway Management" (Chapter 56), "Respiratory Failure" (Chapter 59), and "Chest Trauma" (Chapter 61). Finally, physicians caring for patients with multiple trauma and injuries of the urinary and reproductive organs are referred to "Genitourinary Emergencies" (Chapter 62).

In "Orthopedic Emergencies" (Chapter 8), those orthopedic emergencies that may be encountered in the patient with multiple trauma are discussed, as well as the more common isolated bone and joint conditions that may not necessarily lead to shock, but may markedly impair function and ultimately lead to disability if not recognized early and managed appropriately. In treating patients with isolated joint disease, the reader may also refer to "Acute Gout" (Chapter 19) and techniques of joint aspiration and injection discussed in Chapter 71. Additional discussions of bony injuries of the cervical spine are reviewed in "Cervical Spine Injuries" (Chapter 43).

The patient with shock caused by trauma or medical conditions may require transfusion therapy, and a discussion of blood components, autotransfusion, and bleeding disorders is contained in "Transfusion Therapy" (Chapter 9). Finally, a practical discussion of minor injuries commonly encountered in the emergency department is reviewed in "Minor Lacerations and Abrasions" (Chapter 10).

6. Shock

MARK ALLEN SHAFFER, M.D.
JACEK B. FRANASZEK, M.D.

"A rude unhinging of the machinery of life" and "a momentary pause in the act of death" are among the earliest definitions of shock, yet these statements seem to encompass the essence and grim connotation that the shock state implies. Crile and Lower, Henderson, Cannon, and Blalock were just some of the early researchers who set the groundwork for understanding and treating this enigmatic pathophysiologic entity. Today, despite the decades of efforts by physicians to arrive at accurate definitions that could simplify the recognition and management of the various shock states, considerable controversy remains concerning all aspects of shock states.

Shock, in a broad sense, is a syndrome, a myriad complex of symptoms with varying hemodynamic characteristics. It indicates changes in the many systems designed to supply oxygen and nutrients to the cellular structures.

When damage occurs at any level of this system, a series of events occurs that if left uncorrected will ultimately lead to changes that will affect the transport of oxygen and nutrients to the cells. It is incumbent upon the paramedic in the field and the emergency physician to recognize the signs and symptoms associated with the early changes that occur in all shock states, since the crippling long term damage to vital organs increases as time elapses.

If therapy is not instituted promptly and hypoperfusion and hypoxia persist, the cellular structures are forced to utilize other metabolic pathways to survive at the expense of energy production and efficiency.

The persistence of cellular anoxia and starvation disrupts intracellular organelles, injuring normal molecular and enzymatic processes. If left uncorrected, shock results in progressive deterioration that ultimately reaches the point of irreversibility and cellular death.

In the initial stages, the changes observed are attempts by the body to compensate and correct the deficiencies initiated by the insult to the system. If the early pattern of insufficient oxygen delivery or utilization at the cellular level persists, an energy crisis develops, and the cellular metabolism is activated in such a way as to generate end products that may aggravate the initial injurious event. Thus, vital structures (i.e., brain, heart, kidneys) undergo changes that create a vicious cycle thereby secondarily affecting the cardiocirculatory system.

Since most of the physiologic derangements that accompany shock result from poor tissue perfusion, which causes inadequate transport of oxygen and nutrients at the cellular level, it seems appropriate to define those factors affecting blood flow and tissue perfusion. A model may be designed to identify four functionally dependent entities that interact to maintain normal cardiocirculatory function, cellular oxygenation, and nutrition. The components of the model are

Acknowledgment: The authors wish to thank Anita Shaffer and Donna Wicinski for their help in the preparation of this manuscript.

1. heart, the "pump" that generates the power necessary to maintain circulation.
2. conductance, i.e., the resistance and capacitance systems. These are composed of (a) arteries and arterioles, the primary function of which is to conduct blood to the capillary bed and to regulate blood pressure by changes in their caliber; and (b) the venous capacitance bed, which consists of veins and venules that act as a reservoir for blood and regulate circulating blood volume by contracting or dilating, directly affecting the capacitance system by means of the precapillaries that bypass the capillary bed.
3. capillary bed, where there is active exchange of oxygen and nutrients. The flow is regulated by precapillary and postcapillary sphincter muscles.
4. blood, which is the "priming" solution of the pump and carrier of oxygen and nutrients.

This four-component model explains the various forms of shock. A diagrammatic representation may be constructed to show the changes that occur in each component in differing clinical situations (Fig. 6–1).

A number of myocardial factors affect pump function and cardiac output, which is the amount of blood ejected by the heart per unit of time. (See Chapter 49.) The cardiac output is the product of stroke volume times the heart rate:

$$\text{cardiac output} = \text{stroke volume} \times \text{heart rate}$$

Stroke volume is the amount of blood ejected by the left ventricle with each contraction; it is determined by the venous return, the myocardial contractility, the length of the myocardial muscle fibers at the beginning of contraction, and the peripheral vascular resistance. Ventricular performance and the stroke volume are thus directly influenced not only by the venous return, increasing with increasing venous return, but also by peripheral vascular resistance, decreasing with increasing resistance. Inadequate stroke volume may result in a narrowed pulse pressure (i.e., difference between systolic and diastolic blood pressure), while a large stroke volume is suggested by a widened pulse pressure.

BLOOD PRESSURE

Normal values for systemic blood pressure are variable. One individual may normally have a blood pressure of 90/60 mm Hg, yet this blood pressure may be inadequate in another individual who is suffering from acute volume loss. Alternatively, a blood pressure of 120/80 mm Hg, which is considered well within normal values, may fail to support circulation in an individual who is usually hypertensive.

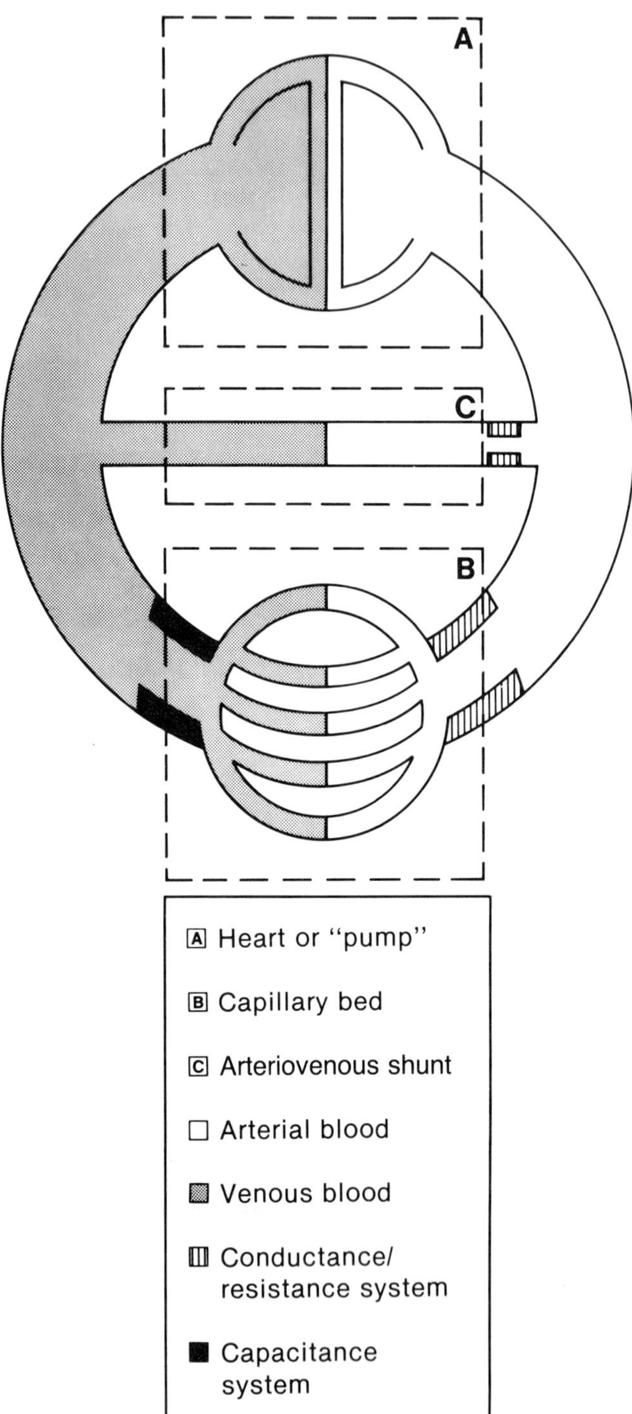

Figure 6–1   Model of Normal Circulatory System.

The size of the blood pressure cuff must be appropriate for the individual in order to obtain valid measurements. Intra-arterial blood pressure recordings are more accurate than cuff measurements in shock states. Thus, it is very important to obtain an adequate history and to correlate it with clinical findings. Low blood pressure is not considered indicative of shock unless it is accompanied by findings of decreased tissue perfusion (Fig. 6–2).

1. Preload refers to the length of myocardial fiber before contraction. With an increase of the ventricular size at the end of diastole, subsequent myocardial fiber shortening is greater and thus the extent of contraction is greater; this is called Starling's law. Preload is influenced by blood volume, venous tone, intrathoracic pressures, and intrapericardial pressures.

2. Contractility is the force of contraction of myocardial fibers, which is determined by force-generating processes at the contractile sites. The concentration of ionic calcium available to the heart's contractile proteins is one of the factors that determines the extent of myocardial fiber shortening and the velocity of myocardial contraction. Norepinephrine, as well as a number of other endogenous and exogenous agents (e.g., digoxin, isoproterenol, and calcium), exert a "positive" inotropic (force or strength of contraction) effect; i.e., they increase contractile effectiveness.

3. Afterload is defined as the wall tension that the left ventricle must generate in order to contract and to eject a given blood volume. Chamber size, shape, and thickness all contribute to ventricle wall tension. Increases in afterload result in decreases in stroke volume and cardiac output. Peripheral vasoconstriction, which raises arterial pressure and consequently afterload, depresses the extent of myocardial fiber shortening, thus depressing stroke volume. In a "failing" heart, the left ventricular end diastolic volume is increased, and the wall tension required to produce a contraction is greater than normal.

4. Heart rate is a function of the rhythmicity of the pacemaker cells of the heart. (See Chapter 50.) This intrinsic rhythmicity is increased by hyperthermia and hyperthyroidism, and decreased by hypothermia and hypothyroidism. Heart rate and rhythm may be adversely altered by ischemia of the pacemaker cells or surrounding tissues. Rate is also influenced by the extrinsic neural regulation mechanisms such as β-adrenergic stimulation (increasing heart rate) or parasympathetic stimulation (decreasing heart rate). Extrinsic humoral influences are mediated by circulating catecholamines and other substances.

Blood pressure is determined by the cardiac output and the peripheral vascular resistance. It is maintained relatively constant by an inverse relationship between the two modalities. Any increase or decrease in peripheral resistance is accompanied by a decrease or increase, respectively, in cardiac output:

Blood pressure = cardiac output × peripheral resistance.

An excessive increase in afterload, shunting of blood through arteriovenous communications, pooling of blood in the capillary system because of postcapillary sphincter resistance, loss of blood volume, puncture or damage to the myocardial muscle, or obstruction of the main flow of blood volume accounts for the majority of events that produce acute perfusion failure and clinical signs of shock. In Figure 6–3 shock states are classified according to the events that precipitate them. This categorization elaborates the abnormal mechanisms that trigger the ultimate damage pattern, disruption of cellular metabolism.

HYPOVOLEMIC SHOCK

Pathophysiology and Compensatory and Decompensatory Mechanisms

Shock caused by a decrease in the intravascular volume relative to the vascular capacity is hypovolemic

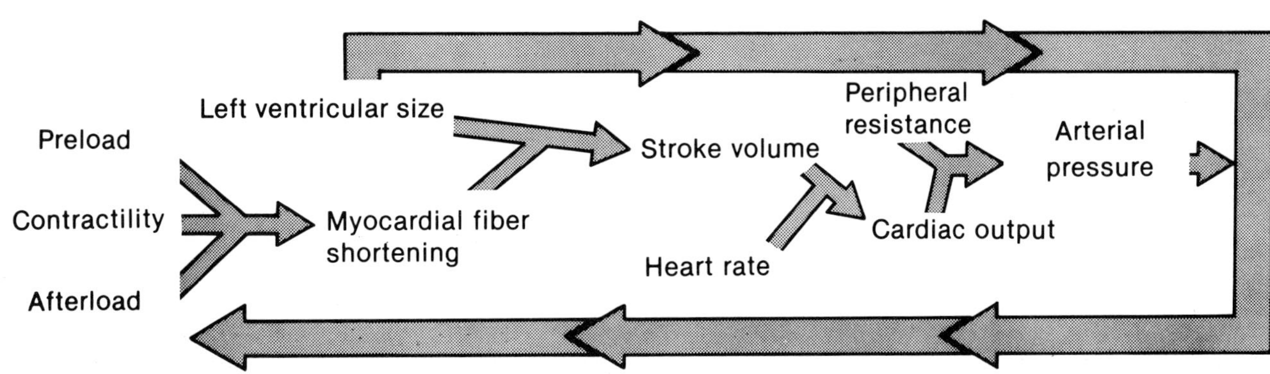

Figure 6–2 Interrelationship of Factors Supporting Hemodynamics.

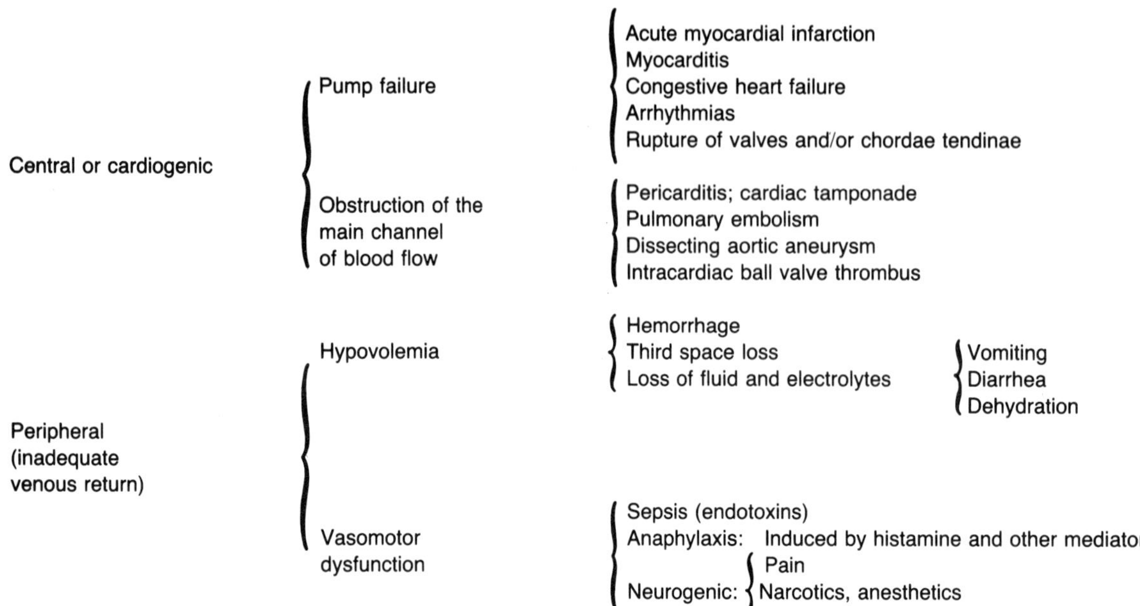

Figure 6–3 Etiologic Classification of Shock States.

shock. It is generally associated with a circulating blood volume deficit of at least 15 to 25 percent and is often accompanied by recruitment of large amounts of extravascular extracellular fluid. (See Figure 6–4a.) The clinical presentation may be characterized by altered mental status, ranging from restlessness and confusion to obtundation and coma; weakness, diaphoresis, tachycardia, hypotension, and tachypnea all reflect poor perfusion at the tissue level. Some of the manifestations may reflect a vigorous catecholamine response to the events that resulted in shock.

The initial response of the body to hypovolemia depends largely on the amount of intravascular volume lost. The rate at which it has been lost, the degree of associated injury, the patient's age, underlying systemic illnesses, and the ability of the cardiovascular system to adjust to the volume loss determine the clinical presentation. (See Figure 6–4b.) Compensatory mechanisms are initiated in several organ systems in an attempt to maintain adequate perfusion to the peripheral tissues.

Contraction of the capacitance system is the initial response. Intrinsic at first, it is mediated by the release of catecholamines as hypovolemia progresses. This mechanism is effective in maintaining adequate venous return until 10 to 15 percent of the volume is lost; metabolic and endocrine responses are minimal with this degree of volume loss. The physical signs and symptoms are transient and nonspecific at this stage. Narrowing of the pulse pressure, reflecting a decrease in stroke volume, is one of the earliest findings in these patients.

As hypovolemia progresses, hypotension and low stroke volume may stimulate baroreceptors and evoke an increase in circulating catecholamines via the vasomotor center's sympathetic discharge. Epinephrine and norepinephrine are released, and they act to increase the force, extent, and rate of myocardial contraction and to produce vasoconstriction at "nonvital" structures in an attempt to maintain perfusion pressure to the heart and brain (e.g., renal and mesenteric). Concomitantly, the signs and symptoms of adrenergic discharge are seen, i.e., tachycardia, restlessness, dry mouth, cool skin, diaphoresis, pallor, and mydriasis. Orthostatic hypotension (a fall in blood pressure and an increase in heart rate when the patient rises from the supine to the seated position) is a manifestation of hypovolemia. A pulse increase of greater than 30 beats/minute or symptoms of dizziness or syncope upon sitting are significant changes in orthostatic vital signs. Adrenergic responses are capable of counterbalancing acute volume losses of up to 30 percent. With severe volume loss of 45 percent of blood and more, several vascular, endocrine, and metabolic responses occur in an attempt to correct the underlying physiopathologic processes. Eventually, however, these responses may change from compensatory to decompensatory in effectiveness, causing a progressive deterioration in metabolic state that, if left uncorrected, leads to death (Table 6–1).

Fluid Resuscitation

While adrenergic responses are occurring after a moderate volume loss, extracellular fluid is redistributed into the intravascular compartment. Human studies have suggested that, after a loss of 10 to 20 percent of intravascular volume, plasma is transferred from the extracellular to the intravascular space at a rate of 50 to 90 ml/minute during the first two hours and averages 40 to 60 ml/hour for six to ten hours. It has been shown that plasma refill rates are considerably brisker in patients with profound volume depletion than in those with mild or moderate volume depletion. The hematocrit (normally 42 to 52 percent for a man and 37 to 47 percent for a woman) is a simple means of estimating red blood cell mass as compared with plasma volume. It may be used in instances of volume loss as a dynamic parameter that aids in determining plasma refill rates and the red blood cell mass. In a healthy 70-kg man, for example, the total blood volume is approximately 5,000 ml. Assuming his normal hematocrit is 45 percent, his red cell mass is 2250 ml (45 percent of 5,000 ml) and his plasma volume is 2750 ml. In the first few minutes after an initial depletion of red blood cells, as occurs in acute hemorrhage, these parameters remain constant; as plasma refill occurs, however, the red blood cell mass is diluted and hematocrit values drop. Plasma refill rates of nearly 1,000 ml/hour can follow severe acute blood loss. Thus, the body may compensate by increasing plasma volume. Additionally, fluid resuscitation with colloid or crystalloid continues to dilute red blood cell mass. At levels below 30 to 32 percent of the usual red blood cell mass, oxygen-carrying capacity is reduced, and hypoxemia may become manifest.

Cellular Metabolism

If the cell is to utilize energy and maintain its structural and functional integrity, it must be supplied with oxygen and nutrients. Most cellular activities are normally accomplished through metabolic pathways that require oxygen (aerobic metabolism). When the cell is forced to produce energy by means of anaerobic metabolic pathways (e.g., as a consequence of poor perfusion and hypoxia), it also produces increased amounts of lactic acid, amino acids, fatty acids, and phosphoric acids, resulting in metabolic acidosis. Acidosis has several deleterious effects. It damages intracellular organelles that contain lytic enzymes, releasing the enzymes and causing death of the cell. Also, when energy production is inadequate, the cell membrane pump does not function, resulting in cellular and mitochondrial edema. Furthermore, protein synthesis is hampered. In sum, all essential elements of the organism are injured.

Acidosis reduces myocardial contractility, depresses vascular response to catecholamines, and promotes intravascular coagulation. Acidemia promotes hypercoagulability, an effect that may be beneficial, for it tends to inhibit hemorrhage. Acidosis facilitates platelet ag-

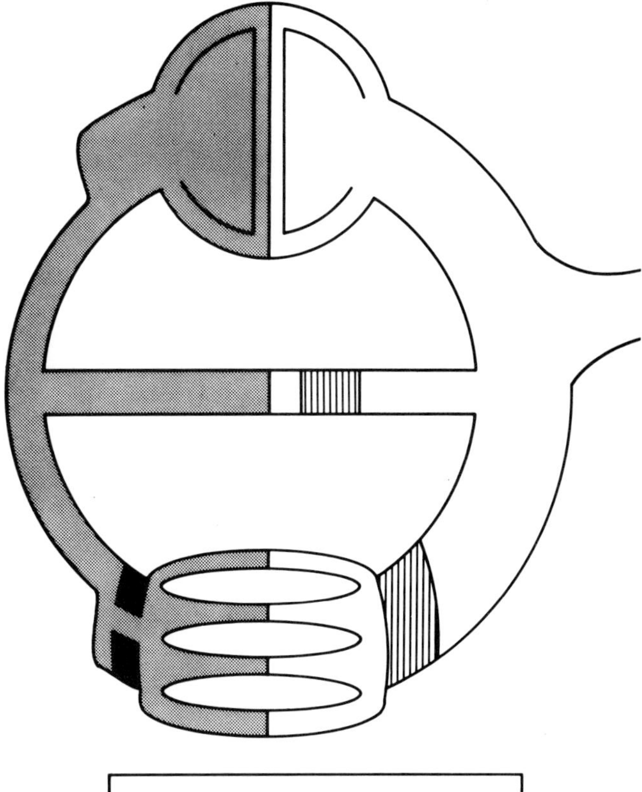

Figure 6–4*A* Hypovolemic Shock.

gregation, which may occlude small vessels. Blood may stagnate because of constriction by postcapillary sphincters in the face of acidosis and relaxation of precapillary sphincters, facilitating platelet aggregation and intravascular coagulation. All of these factors can precipitate a disorder known as disseminated intravascular coagulation. The development of microthrombi at capillary level may contribute greatly to irreversible injury and shock by inhibiting circulation to vital structures.

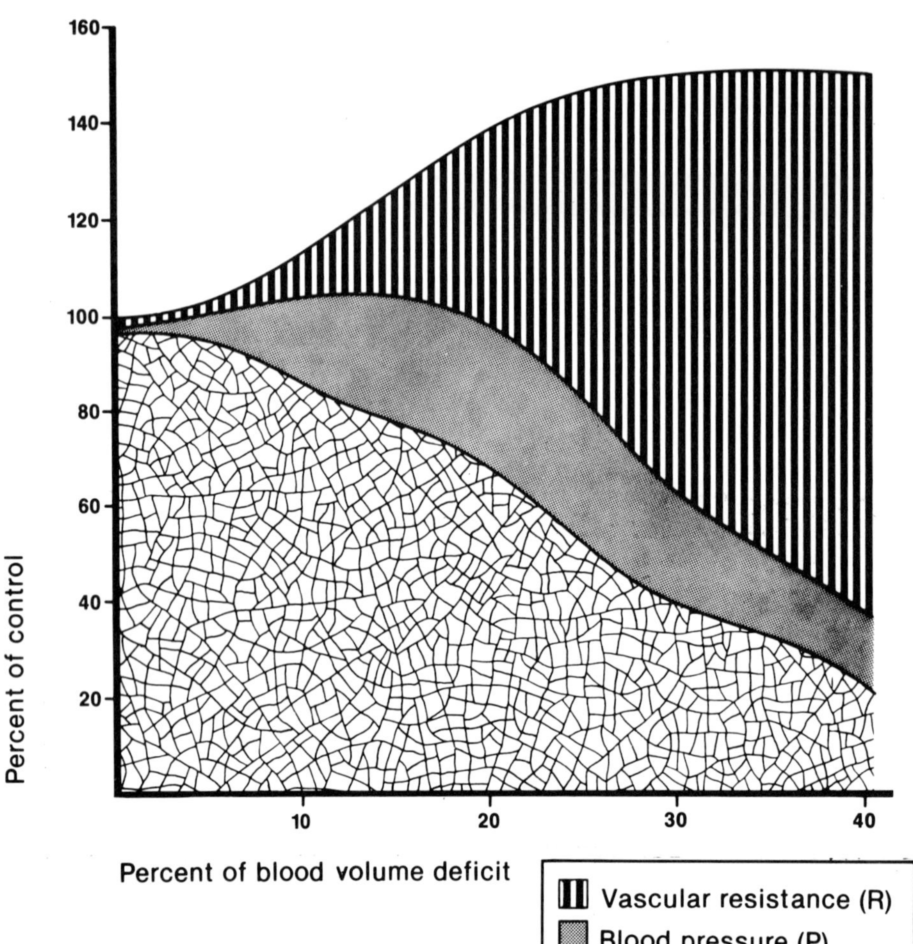

Figure 6–4*B* Changes in Vascular Resistance, Blood Pressure, and Cardiac Output with Increasing Blood Volume Deficits (P = QR). *Note:* Because of increasing vascular resistance, the blood pressure is usually maintained until the cardiac output falls about 25 to 33%.

TABLE 6–1   Changes Seen in Acute Hemorrhage

Degree of Volume Loss	Vascular Response	Endocrine Response	Signs and Symptomatology
Mild (0% to 20%)	Contraction of capacitance system	Minimal	Narrowing of pulse pressure Tachycardia Restlessness
	Recruitment of extravascular fluid		Diaphoresis
			Hypotension (90 to 100 mm Hg)
Moderate (20% to 30%)	Arteriolar constriction Narrowed pulse pressure Reduced cardiac output	Aldosterone Antidiuretic hormone Catecholamines	Diaphoresis Anxiety Decreased urine output Hypotension (approximately 60 mm Hg) Cool, clammy skin Obtundation
Severe (> 30%)	Hypotension Drastic reduction of cardiac output	Marked liberation of catecholamines	Dyspnea Coma Death

Anaerobic metabolism, as evidenced by increased serum and tissue lactate levels, may serve as a useful guideline in determining whether cellular perfusion is adequate during resuscitation and, to some extent, as a prognostic indicator; outcome is likely to be poor when high lactate levels persist. Furthermore, acidosis facilitates release of oxygen and uptake of carbon dioxide at the cellular level (owing to a shift of the oxygen hemoglobin dissociation curve to the right) and increases in the respiratory rate and cerebral blood flow. Persistent hypoperfusion of other tissues results in their decompensation.

Myocardial ischemia occurring as a result of conditions associated with a loss of volume may lead to a progressive decrease in coronary blood flow, or it may impair myocardial performance. However, adequate cardiac function can be maintained as long as venous return is sufficient; in fact, cardiac deterioration has been shown to occur only in very late stages of hypovolemia.

After prolonged ischemia to the kidneys, renal "shutdown" can occur and may become a permanent, devastating complication for long-term survivors. (See Chapter 63.) The reticuloendothelial system and the intestinal mucosa may be damaged during hypoperfusion of the hepatosplanchnic circulation, destroying barriers against bacterial invasion of the bloodstream. Consequently, sepsis may occur, and close monitoring of the patient for evidence of infection is essential.

Adult respiratory distress syndrome may develop from hypovolemia, hypotension-related damage to pulmonary vasculature, and changes in colloid osmotic pressure; it has become a major determinant in the prognosis of patients who survive the initial stages of shock.

Vasoactive Substances

The destruction of intracellular elements that follows prolonged hypotension and hypoperfusion liberates substances that have varied effects on the tone and integrity of the vasculature. Lysosomal enzymes and vasoactive substances are responsible for many of the decompensatory mechanisms found in late shock. Histamine, for example, is a vasodilator that not only affects arteriolar resistance but also increases capillary permeability; thus, it worsens hypovolemia, especially in the face of persistent venous sphincter tone that allows fluid to be sequestered in the capillary system and exuded into the interstitium. Serotonin, which is abundant in brain cells, intestinal cells, platelets, and mast cells, is felt to have an important role in coagulation and platelet aggregation following trauma. Lysosomal enzymes liberated from damaged cells are capable of converting active kinogens into kinins, which are plasma polypeptides with a potent vasoactive property. Bradykinin, for example, is a potent vasodilator. Another vasoactive polypeptide, myocardial depressant factor, may be produced by an ischemic pancreas; it affects splanchnic vasoconstriction and depresses myocardial contractility.

Hypoxia

In addition to responding to conditions that arise in the periphery because of hypoperfusion, acid, lysosomal enzymes, and vasoactive substances, the circulatory system is affected by hypoxia. Tissue hypoxia induces vasodilation at a local level, preferentially in organs requiring greater concentrations of oxygen; it stimulates chemoreceptor activity, which induces hyperventilation; it acts upon the vasomotor center, which produces peripheral vasoconstriction in an attempt to restore cerebral perfusion; and it also prevents appropriate autonomic circulatory adjustments.

Acid-Base Changes

One of the initial non specific responses to trauma, hypotension, or sepsis is alveolar hyperventilation. In the early stages of hypoperfusion, the expected arterial blood gas and pH determinants are pure respiratory alkalemia. The hypocapnia can further impair hemodynamics by inducing peripheral vasodilation. If hypoperfusion progresses to shock and cellular metabolism is altered, a metabolic acidosis ensues, first within the cell and then in the intravascular blood compartment as hydrogen ion moves out of the cell. By the time metabolic acidemia appears, the state of hypoperfusion is very advanced. Metabolic alkalemia can be produced by excessive intravenous sodium bicarbonate, nasogastric suctioning of gastric acid, excessive diuresis with loss of potassium, and steroids.

In severe shock, a respiratory acidosis due to impairment of gas exchange at the alveolocapillary level, combined with a metabolic acidosis due to acid accumulation resulting from abnormal metabolic processes, is a poor prognostic indicator. The morbidity and mortality are increased even when bicarbonate therapy is instituted. A further discussion of acid-base disturbances is found in Chapter 18.

SEPTIC SHOCK

A history of generalized or localized sepsis is often associated with septic shock. Shaking, chills, fever, vomiting, impaired mental status, and diarrhea may be present. The clinical syndrome covers a spectrum that ranges from bacteremia to frank septic shock. (See Figure 6–5.) In the early phases of sepsis, the patient is normovolemic and has a normally increased cardiac output, but is unable to utilize oxygen in the tissues because of arteriovenous shunting. In the late phases, the clinical picture is similar to that of hypovolemic shock.

Septic shock is characterized by poor tissue perfusion induced by vasodilation associated with bacteremia. It is usually caused by gram-negative enteric bacilli, such as *Escherichia coli, Proteus, Pseudomonas, Bacteroides,* and *Salmonella,* although it is occasionally produced by gram-positive cocci. Gram-negative septic shock occurs primarily in hospitalized patients with predisposing factors, such as diabetes, liver disease, and blood dyscrasias. Also, immunosuppression, childbirth, surgical interventions, and urinary, biliary, or gastrointestinal tract infections are associated with the development of septic shock.

As bacteria that have not been phagocytosed enter the bloodstream, endotoxins (from the cell membrane) and exotoxins (intracellular components of some bacteria) are released into the systemic circulation. These substances activate the coagulation, complement, fibrinolytic, and kinin systems. Each of these systems can destroy tissue if it is uncontrolled. For example, overactivation of the coagulation system can lead to disseminated intravascular coagulation. Activation of the complement system is a natural inflammatory response to bacterial invasion since it is required for bacterial phagocytosis and lysis; however, its severe "inflammatory" response to overwhelming bacteremia increases vascular permeability, leakage of fluid into the interstitium, and lysosomal release from white cells, producing some of the pathophysiologic changes of septic shock. Finally, activation of the kinin system creates vasoactive substances that increase vascular permeability and induce vasodilation, both of which tend to cause hypotension related to "hypovolemia."

The hemodynamic pattern during these reactions can be divided into a hyperdynamic stage at which peripheral resistance and vasodilation are initially decreased and cardiac output is increased to maintain blood pressure (also known as warm shock). If it is not recognized and the process continues uncorrected, there is a severe loss of plasma volume to the interstitial tissue through the damaged endothelium of the capillary system. This stage is followed by the hypodynamic stage, in which the circulatory response is similar to that of hypovolemic shock. An adrenergic response produces peripheral vasoconstriction and increases the heart rate. Cardiac output drops as a result of reduced preload and cellular hypoperfusion leads to anaerobic metabolism with all the consequences described previously in relation to the later stages of hypovolemic shock.

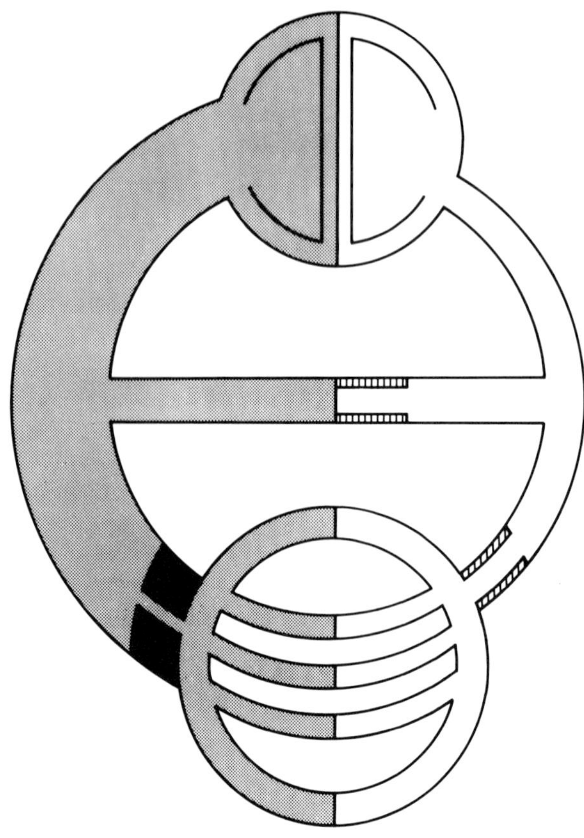

HEMODYNAMIC CHANGES
⬆ Cardiac output (early) Arterial vasodilation ⬆ Pulse pressure A-V shunting (early) ⬇ Cardiac output (late) Stagnation of blood in capacitance system Arterial vasoconstriction

SEPTIC SHOCK
CLINICAL FEATURES
Predisposing infection Hypotension ⬆ Temperature (early) Warm dry skin (early) Tachycardia Mental status changes Leukopenia, thrombocytopenia Leukocytosis Positive blood cultures

Figure 6–5 Septic Shock.

CARDIOGENIC SHOCK

The simplest definition of cardiogenic shock is a low arterial blood pressure (less than 90 mm Hg systolic) in the setting of acute myocardial infarction (Figure 6–6). The most common cause of cardiogenic shock—after acute myocardial infarction—is "pump failure." The hemodynamic abnormalities of pump failure secondary to myocardial infarction are due to paradoxical movement of the infarcted segment of myocardium. This leads to a reduction in stroke volume and consequently a fall in cardiac output and elevation of left ventricular pressure. When reduction in stroke volume and cardiac output are large enough, arterial blood pressure declines as does coronary blood flow. (See Chapters 49 and 50.) Cardiogenic shock is an advanced form of pump failure in which low cardiac output causes a functional deficit of tissue perfusion in one or more vital organs.

Since a history of prior myocardial infarction, age in excess of 65 years, and the physical findings of hypertension and congestive heart failure are associated with a poor prognosis, the emergency department physician must evaluate all of these factors when assessing a patient in cardiogenic shock. The following are the classic features of cardiogenic shock:

1. auscultatory systolic blood pressure less than 90 mm Hg
2. cool, moist skin
3. urine output less than 20 ml/hour
4. impaired state of consciousness
5. lactic acidemia
6. tachypnea

These findings are common to many different varieties of shock with widely varying therapeutic requirements; therefore, it is incumbent upon the emergency department physician to consider and eliminate noncardiac causes. Of primary importance in this regard is the correction of hypovolemia. Since even cardiogenic shock is often complicated by relative hypovolemia, a therapeutic trial of volume-expanding solutions or use of military antishock trousers (MAST) may be indicated in some cases. Anaphylactic, septic, and neurogenic causes of shock should be revealed by history and physical examination.

Many patients survive an acute myocardial infarction long enough to arrive at a hospital and then develop cardiogenic shock. This ongoing process, or period of deterioration, is termed the "preshock syndrome." Pathologic studies have demonstrated damaged cells at the fringes of a zone of infarction, and these damaged cells may or may not survive. The extent of pump failure is directly proportional to the mass of myocardium dis-

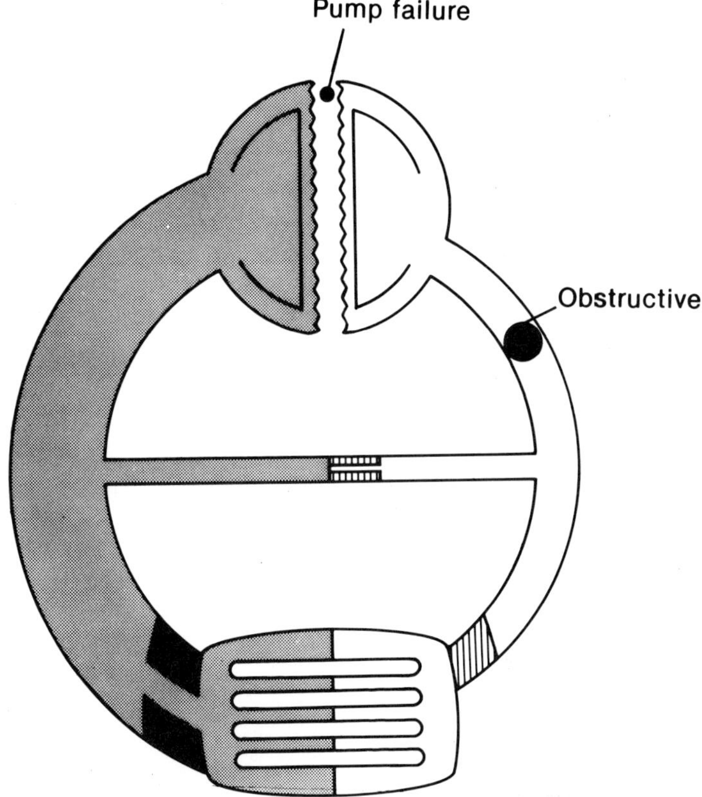

Figure 6–6 Cardiogenic Shock.

abled by ischemic injury; in cardiogenic shock more than 40 percent of the left ventricular myocardium is disabled. Most studies cite the incidence of cardiogenic shock among patients with acute myocardial infarction as 15 percent. Recently reported lower incidences may reflect a more aggressive approach in the treatment of preshock syndrome, including detection and treatment of congestive heart failure, dysrhythmias, fluid deficits, and metabolic abnormalities. Some therapy of the preshock syndrome may be accomplished in the prehospital care setting. Despite advances in therapy, the mortality rate has remained at 85 to 90 percent, once the shock syndrome has developed.

Hemodynamic subsets can be used to identify patients with a poor prognosis after myocardial infarction. With normal hemodynamics, the mortality rate is relatively low; however, it reaches 51 to 60 percent in the presence of pulmonary congestion and clinical evidence of hypoperfusion. As mentioned earlier, patients with cardiogenic shock, an extreme in which gross pulmonary congestion and hypoperfusion are involved, have a mortality rate approaching 90 percent. Survival rates with the intra-aortic balloon counterpulsation rarely exceed 17 percent. Emergency revascularization surgery and surgery to correct specific mechanical structural abnormalities, such as a post-myocardial infarction ventricular septal defect or mitral regurgitation, have been used with limited success. The intra-aortic balloon pump may be useful in stabilizing patients for surgery, but has a high complication rate, including arterial occlusion and local infection.

While acute myocardial infarction is the most common cause of cardiogenic shock, the syndrome may be precipitated by cardiac tamponade, pulmonary embolism, or acute cardiomyopathy, all of which produce similar hemodynamic results.

Cardiac Factors

Sympathetic activity is usually enhanced and parasympathetic activity diminished in response to lowered arterial blood pressure. This results in an increased heart rate in an attempt to compensate for reductions in stroke volume and maintain cardiac output. However, the increase in heart rate may increase the myocardial oxygen demand so that it is out of proportion to supply and worsen the ischemia. The endogenous sympathetic discharge may fail to produce adequate changes in myocardial performance because the ischemic myocardium may not respond properly to this stimulus. Lactic acidosis, a consequence of anaerobic metabolism, further impairs contractility. Moreover, cardiac performance may also be compromised by "myocardial depressant factor," a humoral substance accumulating in the blood in the presence of hypoperfusion.

An important determinant of stroke volume and, therefore, of cardiac output is preload. When volume is depleted, the fiber length decreases, reducing the force and extent of ventricular contraction and thus

decreasing stroke volume. In order to increase stroke volume, the heart must be given sufficient volume to increase diastolic fiber length to optimal levels (Frank Starling relationship). As diastolic fiber length increases, however, the pressure in the left ventricle increases also. In cardiogenic shock, the left ventricular filling pressure is markedly elevated, and an elevated left ventricular diastolic pressure may inhibit subendocardial perfusion and worsen ischemia, resulting in even more depressed left ventricular performance.

Another determinant of myocardial oxygen demand is left ventricular wall tension, which is influenced by outflow resistance (impedance), chamber geometry, and wall thickness. Increases in left ventricular wall tension during ejection, termed afterload, reduce stroke volume, while decreases in this tension generally increase it. These observations provide a rationale for vasodilators in therapy for cardiogenic shock with high filling pressures. Increases in left ventricular filling pressure induce elevated pulmonary interstitial pressures; when pulmonary wedge alveolar pressure exceeds 25 mm Hg, pulmonary edema develops. (See Chapter 48.)

Peripheral Vascular Factors

When cardiac output falls, arterial pressure falls; systemic vascular resistance reflex increases. While the arterial blood pressure may rise as a consequence, cardiac output may fall as a result of increased afterload. All too often, in cardiogenic shock, blood pressure is raised at the expense of worsening ischemia or regional underperfusion of some vascular beds.

ANAPHYLACTIC SHOCK

The rapidly developing allergic reaction that occurs when a previously sensitized individual is exposed to a specific antigen may progress to anaphylactic shock. The allergic reaction liberates histamine, a vasoactive substance, that opens capillaries and arterioles but has little effect on venular sphincters. In addition, capillary permeability is increased. Because of these changes, intravascular fluid passes into the interstitium, producing a relative hypovolemia that may be so marked as to result in shock. The vasodilation produces warm skin, and the increased permeability produces the edema so characteristic of this form of shock.

Atopic persons are predisposed to anaphylaxis. Parenterally administered drugs, especially penicillins and iodinated contrast media, are common offenders. Symptoms, which begin from a few minutes to an hour or so after exposure, are most commonly cutaneous and respiratory. Skin lesions range from urticaria to angioneurotic edema. Respiratory embarrassment may ensue, either because swelling of the tongue or larynx obstructs the upper airway, manifested by stridor, or because bronchospasm obstructs the lower airway, manifested by wheezing. If anoxia is severe, vascular collapse and cardiac dysfunction, such as dysrhythmia or cardiopulmonary arrest, may follow.

TREATMENT

Early recognition of shock and an evaluation of its possible cause are essential to the appropriate management of patients in shock. Therapy must be individualized to fit the needs of each patient. As there are common pathophysiologic manifestations to all forms of shock, however, certain general principles of therapy may be applied. Cellular anoxia and malnutrition are due to either ineffective circulating blood volume (e.g., hypovolemia or pump failure) or loss of tone of the reservoir system (e.g., sepsis or anaphylaxis). The goal of therapy is the correction of these derangements.

Field and emergency department management are probably the most important determinants of the eventual outcome of the patient with shock. What is done in the first hour after the initial insult directly determines morbidity and mortality; thus, all medical and paramedical personnel should take an aggressive, systematic approach (1) to stabilize and monitor the patient's condition, and (2) to recognize the etiologic factors in the shock state so that specific and definitive treatment can be instituted with dispatch. The important guidelines that should be followed once the diagnosis of shock has been made depend partly on the availability of advanced monitoring systems, regardless of the etiology.

The first priority is to assess the airway and ensure adequate ventilation. The delivery of high-flow oxygen is essential during the initial resuscitation. Once the airway has been cleared, assisted ventilation, if necessary, can be provided by a bag-valve-mask system. Use of the system is continued until the patient's condition has been stabilized and endotracheal intubation can be safely performed. In cases of traumatic shock, a suction apparatus is invaluable in clearing the airway and preventing aspiration. If the patient is conscious and alert, oxygen at high concentrations can be delivered by mask; however, the resuscitation team must closely monitor respiratory and mental status and be prepared to assist ventilation in cases of deterioration. The objective is to maintain an arterial PO_2 of at least 80 mm Hg.

Once proper oxygenation is ensured, a quick assessment of the overall condition of the patient is important to determine the next step. Under these circumstances, assessment and therapy are almost simultaneous. The initial evaluation includes

- measurement of blood pressure, pulse rate, respiratory rate and depth, and temperature
- inspection of external wounds for signs of hemorrhage
- assessment of mental status
- examination of the skin
- assessment of peripheral perfusion (cyanosis, capillary filling)
- determination of jugular venous pressure

If the patient is in shock and there is jugular venous distention, a cardiopulmonary cause, such as cardiac tamponade, pulmonary embolus, or myocardial infarction, can be assumed. If the neck veins are flat, hypovolemia should be assumed until proved otherwise.

At least two large-bore (16 gauge or larger) peripheral intravenous lines should be started. In case hypovolemic shock is evident, a balanced electrolyte solution, such as Ringer's lactate, or a normal saline solution is administered rapidly or over 20 to 40 minutes. This rapid volume administration serves as a therapeutic trial in evaluating preexisting or continuous blood loss. Markedly hypotensive patients may become normotensive with this regimen if blood loss is minimal. The MAST suit can also function as a quick reversible transfusion and may be very effective in correcting hypotension in both prehospital and hospital settings. If the fluid challenge elevates blood pressure and decreases pulse rate only temporarily, then a larger loss of blood volume is assumed to be present and other forms of intravascular volume expansion may be considered.

One main concern in the initial stages of resuscitation is the differentiation between pump failure and volume deficiency. This is important largely because the ensuing management depends on the relative contribution of these factors.

If inadequate cardiac function due to tension pneumothorax, cardiac tamponade, myocardial contusion, or pulmonary embolus is suspected, there is little the paramedic can do in the field to treat the underlying cause. In such cases, an initial fluid challenge of lactated Ringer's solution, use of a MAST suit in selected cases, monitoring, judicious use of inotropic and vasopressor medications, and rapid transport are the armamentarium that can be used as temporizing measures until the patient can receive definitive treatment at a medical facility. Other initial measures should include a neurologic assessment (mental status, pupillary response, motor response, and orientation), hemorrhage control by direct pressure or MAST suit, and splinting of fractures.

Adjuncts to Intravascular Volume Expansion: MAST Suit

The MAST suit, often known as the "G-suit" or "pneumatic suit," was first applied to medical practice by Crile in 1903 for control of hypotension occurring during surgical procedures of the head and neck. In studies conducted in Vietnam, Cutler and Daggett reported the effectiveness of the MAST suit for rapid stabilization of hypotension related to hemorrhage. Kaplan and associates reported successful civilian prehospital use of the MAST suit in hemorrhaging patients. The MAST suit has been used in a variety of prehospital emergencies (both traumatic and nontraumatic) with good results.

Because the beneficial effects of the MAST suit are varied, it can be used in several clinical settings. It has particular value in the resuscitation of patients in shock. It has been estimated that 750 to 1,000 ml whole blood are autotransfused from the pelvis and lower extremities once the MAST suit is applied, which diverts blood from nonvital structures into the heart-lung-brain circulation. Recent evidence suggests that the amount of blood transfused is actually considerably less and implies that increased peripheral vascular resistance is the mechanism of action for the MAST suit.

The MAST suit is most frequently used in the treatment of hypotension secondary to hemorrhage in the prehospital setting, emergency department, or intensive care unit. It is also commonly used in the management of (a) hemorrhage secondary to severe pelvic fracture and retroperitoneal hematoma, (b) hypotension induced by spinal anesthesia, (c) bleeding arising from hypocoagulation, (d) ruptured atherosclerotic abdominal aortic aneurysms, and (e) cardiogenic shock.

The MAST suit is a polyvinyl three-chambered trouser. It is wrapped around the patient's lower extremities and abdomen, one chamber for each lower extremity and a third chamber for the abdomen. The chambers are secured with Velcro fasteners. Each is independently connected to a foot-activated air pump that can be inflated to an internal pressure of 104 mm Hg; each has a pressure relief valve to prevent overinflation. The MAST suit is easy to apply and permits accessibility to the groin area. Its light chambers function both as volume replacers and as air splints.

An important characteristic of the MAST suit is its hemostatic effect. When applied, the external pressure decreases the wall tension of the injured vessel by reducing the difference between internal and external vessel pressure (transmural pressure). Laplace's law states that wall tension (T) varies directly according to the product of transmural pressure (P) and the radius of the lumen (R); i.e., $T = P \times R$. Because it is the wall tension that keeps the edges of lacerated vessels apart, reducing the transmural pressure, and thus the wall tension, narrows the separation. The MAST suit also decreases the vessel radius by compressing it, which reduces not only tension, but also flow. The reduction of both tension and flow through the injured vessel probably allows the patient's own clotting mechanism to act and to achieve hemostasis more readily.

It is clear that the physiologic effects of MAST suit application are varied. Blood pressure is increased and maintained by the autotransfusion of blood from the lower extremities and pelvis. Thus, the blood pressure rises appropriately, and the heart rate usually decreases, probably as a result of baroreceptor responses to increased aortic pressure and venous return. Carotid blood flow is increased; femoral blood flow, decreased. Vital capacity may be decreased (according to the results of a study done on eight volunteers).

Contraindications

There is no strong evidence to substantiate the theory that renal or pulmonary disease is a contraindication to MAST suit utilization. The MAST suit should be applied cautiously in patients with cerebral and pulmonary edema as acute MI, cardiogenic shock, and left ventricular heart failure may be aggravated. The suit has not been demonstrated to raise intracranial pressure in patients who are hypotensive because of hypovolemia. Although its use in patients with injuries or hemorrhage above the diaphragm is controversial, a recent review of patients with a variety of injuries failed to find any detrimental effects when the MAST suit was used in injuries above the diaphragm; indeed, good blood pressure augmentation and outcome were reported.

Complications

Acidosis, both metabolic and respiratory, is a phenomenon of MAST suit use reported in animal and clinical studies. Metabolic acidemia may occur if lactate is produced in ischemic extremities. There are no hard clinical data indicating that this occurs in humans, but respiratory acidemia due to restriction of diaphragmatic excursion and thoracic expansion and alveolar hypoventilation is theoretically possible. However, this problem was observed in a series of 25 patients on whom a MAST suit was used for variable periods of time; only those patients with head injuries were found to have impairment of alveolar ventilation with significant acid-base alterations. In this group of patients, prognosis was extremely poor.

Acidemia should be corrected as soon as possible, and the acid-base status should be closely monitored by means of arterial blood gas determinations. Alterations in renal function and respiratory function occurring with MAST use are difficult to evaluate, because it is not known if they are the consequence of application of the MAST suit or of hypotension and its attendant complications. Urinary output and pulmonary status must be closely monitored in patients who are treated with the MAST suit for prolonged periods of time.

Recommendations

Potential contraindications and complications of MAST use seem to be related to the magnitude of the inflation pressure. Ideally, pressure should be low enough to avoid problems, yet high enough to maintain hemostasis and permit proper immobilization of patients, especially for transportation. Pressures of 20 to 25 mm Hg seem adequate and fulfill these requirements.

Deleterious events all too commonly occur when the MAST suit is prematurely removed. If external pressure is removed without adequate fluid replacement, blood pressure may drop as much as 40 to 60 mm Hg. If the MAST suit is to be removed, it should be done cautiously over a 30-minute period; the deflation must be stopped if the blood pressure drops more than 5 mm Hg. One compartment at a time, beginning with the leg compartments, should be deflated. Should blood pressure drop, fluid must be infused to restore the blood pressure to its initial level before continuing deflation. In some instances the MAST suit should be removed in the operating room.

In summary, the MAST suit is a valuable adjunct in the prehospital and emergency department management of patients in shock. In the hands of experienced personnel, its use is associated with very low morbidity. The benefits outweigh the potential complications.

Trendelenburg Position

When a patient is in the recumbent position more than 50 percent of blood volume is located in the venous system; when intravascular volume is decreased, pooling occurs in the periphery. Theoretically, then, tilting a patient into the head-down position diverts this blood volume into the central circulation, thus increasing cardiac filling and augmenting stroke volume. The efficacy of this maneuver has been debated in the literature. Some authors propose that not only is it ineffective in improving the hemodynamic status of normotensive and hypotensive patients, but also it may be associated with untoward side-effects in pulmonary ventilation/perfusion, resulting in increased arteriovenous admixture and endotracheal tube displacement. Others support its use with hypotensive patients.

Data suggest that the Trendelenburg position improves hemodynamics in hypotension secondary to loss of vascular tone, but not in hypotension associated with hemorrhage and vasoconstriction. When the effects of the Trendelenburg position on systemic and pulmonary hemodynamics in critically ill, normotensive and hypotensive patients were studied, all subjects had Swan-Ganz catheters in place, and all important hemodynamic parameters were measured. The results failed to indicate that the Trendelenburg position has any significant beneficial hemodynamic effects. Its failure to increase central blood volume and mean arterial pressure in hypotensive patients is thought to be related to splanchnic pooling of blood. In some instances, a detrimental fall of mean arterial pressure was seen when the patient was in the Trendelenburg position. Considering the potential complications, the augmentation of intravascular volume seems to be better accomplished with the use of a MAST suit.

Selection of Fluid Therapy

After the initial fluid infusion, the advisability of further fluid replacement must be determined. Again, the basic indicator is the clinical condition of the patient. Once the patient is in the hospital, several monitoring parameters may be used. Urine output, differences in arterial and venous oxygen levels, colloid osmotic pressure, and measurement of left ventricular function such as pulmonary artery wedge pressure are among the most sensitive and useful parameters to evaluate intravascular volume and cardiac performance, and thus to gauge the necessity of further fluid replacement.

Types of Fluids

In hypoperfusion, the objectives of therapy are to replace lost blood, correct intravascular volume deficits, and identify the reason for the hypoperfusion. The mainstay of therapy for hemorrhagic shock is blood, properly typed and cross-matched, preferably fresh. (See Chapter 9.) There are complications associated with transfusing whole blood; for example, transfusion of large quantities of stored blood can increase the hemoglobin-oxygen affinity, resulting in poor oxygen release at the tissue level. The potential for severe allergic reactions, dysrhythmias (if the blood is cold), embolization of aggregates, hepatitis, and coagulation disorders is real, and the physician should consider these complications when selecting patients who require whole blood therapy. Blood banks currently separate whole blood into its component parts—the red cells, platelets, and plasma—thus limiting, to some extent, the risks and allowing a more selective use of blood substitutes. If blood replacement is needed urgently, type-specific (or Rh⁻, type O) blood can be utilized.

The objective of blood therapy is to maintain hemoglobin levels at 12.5 to 14 gm/dl or hematocrit at 30 to 32 percent. This level tends to maintain a better intravascular volume, and patients may have a lower incidence of respiratory failure. Below these levels, the oxygen-carrying capacity of the blood is reduced significantly, and the ensuing hypoxemia aggravates the clinical state. If the hemoglobin level is adequate, if red blood cell loss has been insignificant, or if whole blood is not readily available, further fluid therapy is carried out with blood substitutes. If multiple transfusions are required, fresh-frozen plasma replacement may be needed to restore clotting factors.

Physiologic Consideration

Starling's famous equation is a key to understanding the controversy surrounding the role of colloid and crystalloid solutions as volume replacements, and their contributing roles in the development of "shock" lung. The formula defines the factors regulating vascular fluid flux (Fig. 6–7):

$$FH_2O = K_c \times SA\,(P_c - P_i) + (OP_i - OP_c)$$

All these factors interplay to maintain fluid homeostasis. It can be seen that the extravascular fluid flux (FH_2O) is directly related to the intravascular hydrostatic pressure (P_c) and capillary permeability (K_c) and inversely

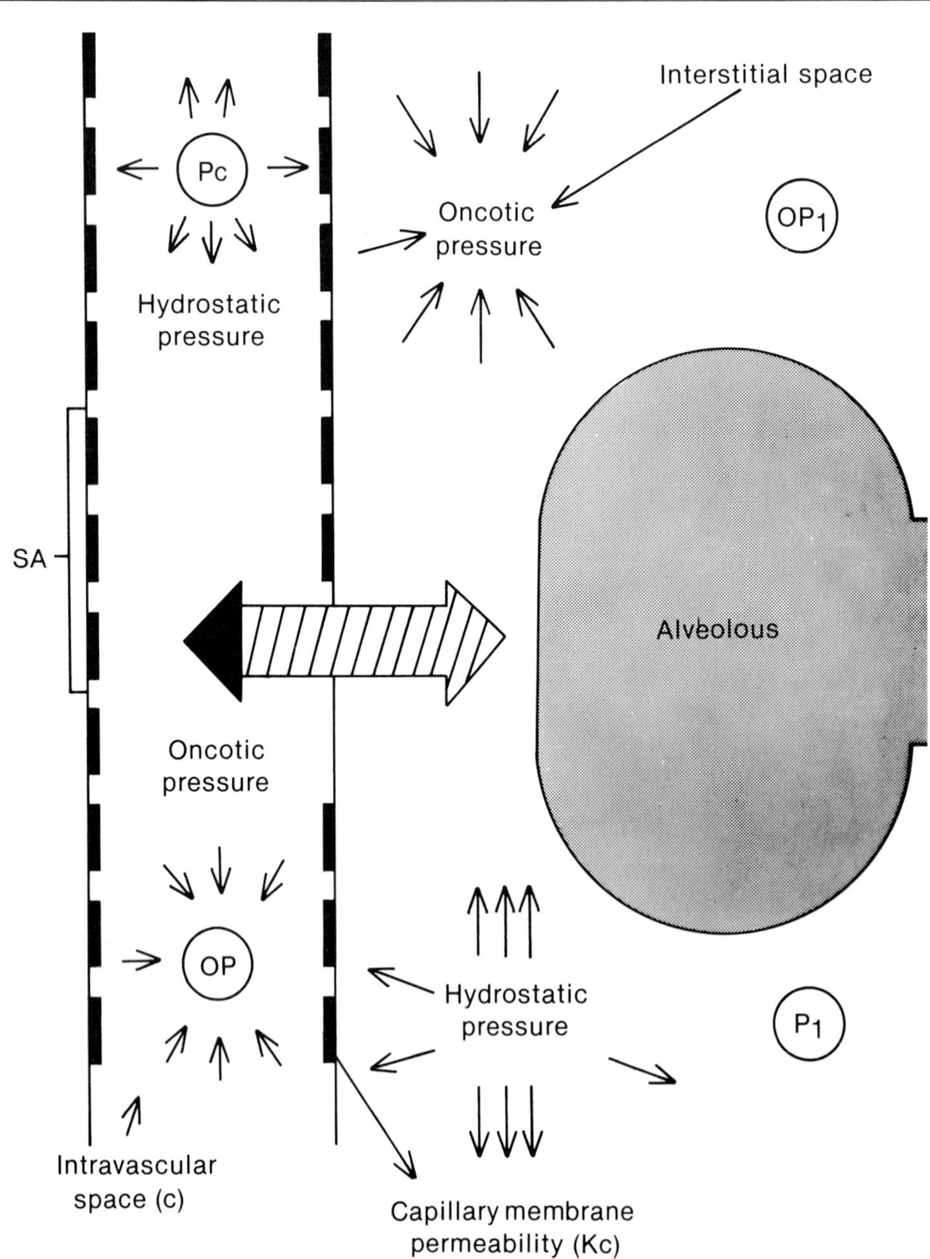

Figure 6–7   Vascular Fluid Flux.

related to the intravascular colloid oncotic pressure. Albumin, a circulating protein that maintains the colloid osmotic pressure, is the major determinant of the flux of fluids at capillary level. This information can be used to isolate two readily measurable parameters in the clinical setting: the intravascular colloid osmotic pressure and the pulmonary artery wedge pressure. Pulmonary edema can be associated with normal pulmonary artery wedge pressures. Reduction of the colloid osmotic pressure–pulmonary artery wedge pressure gradient, which is normally 10 to 20 mm Hg, is associated with the development of pulmonary edema and can be used as a prognostic indicator. In cardiogenic pulmonary edema, the reduction of this gradient is due to an elevation of pulmonary wedge pressure; in noncardiogenic pulmonary edema, it is due to severe reduction of colloid osmotic pressure. This was shown by studies of 17 patients with gradients of 13.6 mm Hg who developed noncardiogenic pulmonary edema. Furthermore, severe reduction of colloid osmotic pressure is a reliable prognostic indicator of mortality in 75 percent of cases.

Early correction of hypovolemia prevents renal and pulmonary complications. Shock lung, congestive atelectasis, and post-traumatic pulmonary insufficiency, are some of the terms used to define the pathologic findings associated with the common pulmonary complications of patients in shock. The cause of these complications varies.

Some authors suggest that resuscitation with crystalloid solutions is associated with fewer pulmonary complications, while others feel that resuscitation with colloid solutions results in less morbidity and mortality. Colloid proponents claim that crystalloids alone dilute plasma proteins, thereby reducing plasma colloid osmotic pressures, increasing hydrostatic pressure, and thus facilitating interstitial and intracellular fluid flux. When large amounts of balanced electrolyte solution are given, approximately 25 percent remains intravascular; the rest distributes itself within the interstitial spaces, promoting edema. Crystalloid proponents claim that albumin enters the interstitial pulmonary compartment, increasing the albumin pool and the interstitial colloid osmotic pressure, thus favoring fluid accumulation. A prospective clinical study, in which crystalloids were used in one group of patients and colloid was added to crystalloids in a second group, showed no significant difference in results; however, the cost of treatment with albumin was much greater.

The role of albumin in the development of interstitial edema during fluid infusion is unclear. In one study, not only was albumin found ineffective in preventing shock lung, but also pulmonary function was worse in patients receiving albumin than in those that did not. This is thought to be due to the "secondary effects" of albumin, such as impairment of myocardial performance, believed to be caused by a fall in the ratio of ionized to nonionized calcium; impairment of salt and water excretion, with subsequent elevation of central venous pressure and pulmonary wedge pressure; and interstitial entrapment of albumin within the lungs, which increases interstitial colloid osmotic pressure and extravascular fluid flux.

The quantity and quality of fluid therapy should be individualized, depending on a set of carefully obtained physiologic data. The causes of shock, shock lung, and pulmonary edema are so varied that no one therapeutic regimen can be recommended. Hence, the physician should take into consideration (1) the physiologic actions of each agent, (2) the pathophysiology of the disease entity, and (3) the specific aim of each therapeutic modality. Modern monitoring techniques are helpful in arriving at the proper balance of fluid replacement. Purified albumin solutions and pasteurized plasma (sold as 5 percent plasma protein factor) eliminate the risk that infections will be transmitted, but, like albumin, they are costly. Several artificial macromolecular polymers are available as plasma substitutes; they seem partially to correct the problem of rapid interstitial distribution that is seen with crystalloids, and they do not have the described disadvantages of albumin, including cost. However, they do have disadvantages of their own. With Dextran 70, for example, 70 percent remains in the circulation initially, and 30 percent is still present after 24 hours. Complications include a greater tendency for the patient to bleed because the dextran interferes with platelet function and increases blood viscosity. Furthermore, cross-matching of blood is difficult after dextrans have been used. Dextran 40, although it has a shorter half-life than Dextran 70, carries the same sorts of risks; in addition, it may precipitate renal failure. Both Dextrans 70 and 40 are allergenic; severe anaphylactoid reactions with shock and death have occurred. Hydroxyethyl starch has an intravascular persistence equal to or greater than that of Dextran 70. Like the dextrans, it increases bleeding times, but to a lesser degree. The advantage of hydroxyethyl starch is that it does not produce anaphylactoid reactions. It is considered a safe, effective colloidal solution for replacement of lost blood and for augmentation of blood volume. Recently developed fluorochemical blood substitutes need further study, but hold great promise as artificial blood replacements since they are capable of not only expanding blood volume but carrying oxygen as well.

Correction of Acid-Base Abnormalities

Most acid-base derangements can be corrected by adequate ventilation, oxygenation, and tissue perfusion. Maintaining the acid-base status as close to normal as possible improves both therapeutic response and physiologic recovery. When the acidemia creates a pH of less than 7.2, the bicarbonate dosage required to correct the deficit should be calculated by multiplying the base deficit times the approximate bicarbonate distribution space (considered to be 30 to 50 percent of body weight); only one-half the amount should be administered at one time at a rate of 3 to 5 mEq/minute. Overcorrection can lead to alkalemia and shift the oxyhemoglobin dissociation curve to the left, increasing hemoglobin affinity for oxygen and decreasing the availability of oxygen at the cellular level. (See Chapter 60.)

MONITORING THE PATIENT IN SHOCK

Urine Output

If there is no evidence of genitourinary trauma (e.g., pelvic fracture or hematuria), a Foley catheter should be inserted in the patient in shock. The flow of urine is a very useful and sensitive parameter of renal perfusion. Through mechanisms such as the aldosterone renin-angiotensin system and the release of antidiuretic hormone, the kidneys tend to compensate for hypovolemia by reabsorbing water and sodium; consequently, urine output falls. If a critically ill patient has an adequate circulating volume, changes in urine output, milliliter by milliliter and minute to minute, indicate the state of renal perfusion and help to determine the need for volume replacement. The usefulness of this parameter is limited in patients treated with diuretics, however.

Urinary electrolyte levels are used to determine replacement therapy. The urinary sodium concentration is useful in differentiating between a decreased urine output secondary to hypoperfusion (sodium level less than 20 mEq/liter) and that secondary to renal insufficiency (sodium level more than 40 mEq/liter). In the latter case, sodium is not reabsorbed and is lost in the urine. The urine/plasma creatinine ratio and the urine/plasma osmolality ratio are also used to make this distinction.

Intra-arterial Pressure

Because of discrepancies between central arterial pressures and cuff blood pressures, determination of intra-arterial pressure is required for proper blood pressure monitoring, particularly in those patients with hypotension and peripheral vasoconstriction (i.e., with cool upper extremities and thready brachial and radial pulses) because discrepancies are more common in these patients. This is accomplished by cannulating the radial, brachial, or femoral arteries and connecting the catheter to a pressure transducer and a continuous monitoring device. The catheter also permits frequent blood sampling for determinations of arterial blood gas levels, pH, electrolyte concentrations, glucose levels, and other values.

A new therapeutic approach to shock and volume resuscitation, introduced by Jelenko and co-workers, consists of a hypertonic albumin-containing fluid demand (HALFD) regimen. Mean arterial pressure, urine output, weight change, hematocrit, plasma and urinary sodium and potassium levels, and plasma and urinary volume are used as indicators for clinical administration of fluids. The objective is to maintain a normal mean arterial pressure, i.e., 60 to 110 mm Hg, and a urine volume of 30 to 50 ml/hour. In a prospective, randomized study of 19 burn patients treated with lactated Ringer's solution alone, hypertonic fluid alone, or the HALFD regimen, it was found that the HALFD group made better clinical progress, required the infusion of less fluid, gained less weight, and had less plasma leak. A fluorocarbon blood substitute has been used successfully to sustain life in blood-depleted experimental animals. This substance has also been used as a blood substitute in Jehovah's Witnesses who require additional intravascular oxygen-carrying capacity. The prospect of a shelf-stored plasma substitute with oxygen-carrying capability is an exciting development that awaits further clinical study.

Acid-Base Determinations

Frequent assessment of oxygenation and saturation of arterial blood as well as pH and PCO_2 is easily accomplished and provides invaluable information for the management of patients in shock.

Central Venous Pressure

There is a wide spectrum of opinion regarding central venous pressure monitoring. Some authors suggest there is little value in following the relationships between cardiocirculatory function and blood volume, while others find it helpful once certain preexisting factors (e.g., myocardial function) are taken into consideration.

It is our opinion that a central venous line should be established as soon as the patient arrives in the emergency department. Several approaches are possible. Physician skill, patient's body habitus, clinical circumstances, age, and any thoracic deformities should be considered in selecting one of the available internal jugular or subclavian techniques. (See Chapter 71.)

Common complications include pneumothorax, arterial puncture and laceration, air embolus, and sepsis; therefore, the physician must use meticulous, aseptic technique. Following insertion, a chest roentgenogram is mandatory to assess placement and detect any immediate complication.

Central venous pressure varies directly with circulating blood volume and inversely with vascular tone or right heart competence. This measurement is of particular value in patients who are in hemorrhagic shock but are otherwise healthy; in these patients, right atrial and left ventricular end diastolic pressures are closely related, even in the presence of controlled ventilation or positive end expiratory pressure (PEEP). Central venous pressure monitoring is not useful in patients with preexisting cardiocirculatory disease, since the relationship between the right atrial pressure and the left ventricular end diastolic pressure is variable and clinically misleading in these patients; however, a Swan-Ganz catheter gives accurate information as to left ventricular function. (See Chapter 71.)

Trends in central venous pressure measurements in response to infusion of fluid aliquots are more important than isolated readings. Assuming that right atrial pressure correlates well with left ventricular end diastolic pressure, the central venous pressure can be used to monitor right atrial and left ventricular function in relationship to circulating volume and vascular tone. At ten-minute intervals, 200 ml aliquots of volume-expanding fluids should be infused. If central venous pressure does not increase by more than 2 cm H_2O, the infusion is continued. If it increases by 2 to 5 cm H_2O, the challenge is interrupted briefly, and the patient's needs are reassessed; the challenge is stopped if the increase is more than 10 cm H_2O. Whatever formula is used in assessing response to volume challenge, it is the sequential changes in central venous pressure readings that are important.

Arterial-Central Venous Oxygen Difference

The measurement of oxygen consumption is a sensitive indicator of cellular metabolism. The oxygen consumption of patients in shock is decreased, owing to (a) limited oxygen transport because of a decrease in blood flow and a reduction of hemoglobin or (b) an inability of the cell to accept or utilize oxygen. Hemorrhagic or cardiogenic shock leads to the former; septic shock, the latter.

The calculation of arterial-mixed venous oxygen differences is easily performed by drawing arterial and central venous blood samples for PO_2 determination. The arterial-central venous oxygen content difference is calculated in volumes percent. The values may indicate trends in cardiac output:

$$C\ (A\text{-}V\overline{O})\ \text{difference}$$

$$= 1.34 \times Hb\ (aO_2 - V\overline{O}_2) + \frac{0.32}{100}\ (PaO_2 - PV\overline{O}_2)\ (\text{Vol \%})$$

where C is oxygen content and Hb is hemoglobin content. If the difference is greater than 6 volumes percent, it can be assumed that cardiac output is depressed. An arterial-mixed venous oxygen difference of less than 3 volume percent probably reflects a cardiac output that is abnormally high.

Under normal basal circumstances, oxygen consumption is about 145 ± 15 ml/minute/m^2 body surface. Oxygen consumption changes when the patient is hyperactive or hypotensive, for example. Yet, changes in the arterial-mixed venous oxygen difference, regardless of its initial value, provide information on the direction and degree of any change in the cardiac output. If oxygen consumption is assumed to be constant and the arterial-venous oxygen content difference is known, cardiac output can be calculated by substitution into the Fick principle:

$$Q = \frac{VO_2}{C(\text{a-}V)O_2 \times 10}$$

where Q is cardiac output and VO_2 is oxygen consumption. Cardiac outputs determined in this manner correlate well with measured outputs except at very low and very high ranges. Despite the inaccuracies introduced by the assumptions that oxygen consumption is constant and that right atrial oxygen content is equivalent to mixed venous oxygen content, the techniques allow an estimate of cardiac output to be made at the patient's bedside.

Swan-Ganz Catheter

Probably the most sensitive parameter of left ventricular function is pulmonary artery wedge pressure, which can be recorded easily with the Swan-Ganz catheter, a flow-directed, balloon-tipped pulmonary artery catheter that can be used to measure wedge pressure through a continuous electronic pressure monitor. This measurement is of particular value in patients with cardiogenic shock and severe sepsis, because there can be a great dichotomy between central venous pressure and pulmonary artery wedge pressure in these patients. A pulmonary artery wedge pressure greater than 17 mm Hg is correlated with pulmonary congestion; a pressure greater than 25 mm Hg, with pulmonary edema. With the Swan-Ganz catheter, cardiac output may be measured by the thermodilution method. The prognosis is poor when cardiogenic shock is associated with myocardial infarction and the cardiac output is less than 2.4 liters/minute/sq m.

Clinical trends are toward early placement of the Swan-Ganz catheter, perhaps even in the emergency department, in order to monitor fluid replacement therapy when the central venous pressure is not a clearly reliable indicator of left ventricular function. (See Chapter 71.)

SPECIFIC THERAPY

Fluid is the keystone to the management of shock, regardless of etiology (unless there are high left ventricular filling pressures). The initial objective is to replace volume, whether it be a few hundred milliliters or several liters. If the cardiocirculatory system cannot function properly when fluid therapy has been adequate, i.e., left ventricular filling pressure has been elevated to normal or even moderate levels, shock persists and other therapeutic modalities are necessary.

Inotropic and Vasopressor Agents

If patients remain in shock despite adequate fluid replacement, it may be necessary to administer medications that increase the cardiac output, elevate the perfusion pressure, or improve the tissue perfusion of the organism. Most inotropic drugs augment cardiac output by increasing the force and velocity of contraction, which also increases the oxygen demand of the already ischemic myocardium and may be ill-advised when acute myocardial infarction is associated with shock. Vasopressors are useful in raising arterial blood pressure to levels that ensure adequate coronary perfusion, but they may also enhance peripheral vasoconstriction, making tissue perfusion less adequate and increasing the workload of the heart. Therefore, pressors should be used very cautiously and transiently to maintain proper perfusion and vital circulation.

Levarterenol and metaraminol are commonly used vasoconstricting medications. While levarterenol does profoundly increase systemic vascular resistance, it produces a regional underperfusion. Isoproterenol significantly increases cardiac output by increasing contractility and heart rate, but both of these changes increase the myocardial oxygen demand. Clinical trials with isoproterenol have not demonstrated a reduction in the mortality rate for patients with cardiogenic shock; serious dysrhythmias are often associated with its utilization. Dopamine, while mimicking the vasoconstrictive effects of levarterenol at high doses, improves renal and mesenteric blood flow at low dosages; it also augments cardiac output. In general, total peripheral vascular resistance remains unaltered when dopamine is administered, and there is little or no increase in heart rate; blood pressure rises because of enhanced output. The drug may precipitate ventricular dysrhythmias, however.

Dobutamine, a more recently developed derivative of isoproterenol, may be superior to dopamine in augmenting cardiac output. It can be used in patients with cardiogenic shock, despite its lack of α-adrenergic effects.

The use of digitalis in patients with congestive heart failure and cardiogenic shock due to acute myocardial infarction is controversial. However, the drug seems to have beneficial hemodynamic effects in the presence of cardiogenic shock associated with cardiac failure and cardiomegaly.

The disadvantage of cardiac glycosides is that they produce a profound splanchnic vasoconstriction, aggravating preexisting ischemia and enhancing both the release of lysosomal enzyme and the formation of myocardial depressant factor. For this reason, although they improve myocardial performance, they are of questionable benefit in the absence of heart failure and cardiomegaly. (See Chapter 51.)

Vasodilators in Cardiogenic Shock

A reduction of left ventricular outflow impedance, resistance, and filling pressure may augment cardiac output by decreasing left ventricular workload and myocardial oxygen demand. In patients with acute myocardial infarction, best results are obtained when the left ventricular filling pressure is high and the blood pressure near normal. Among the most commonly used vasodilator drugs are sodium nitroprusside and nitroglycerin. In cardiogenic shock due to myocardial infarction, these medications often improve hemodynamic status, but long-term survival remains poor. Combination therapy, e.g., dopamine plus nitroprussides, might have a role in the therapy of cardiogenic shock, but control studies of alternative therapeutic regimens, including afterload reduction, are not yet available.

Corticosteroids

Many and varied actions have been attributed to corticosteroids, making them theoretically attractive for the correction of severe pathophysiologic derangements found in hemorrhagic, traumatic, and septic shock. In patients with shifts in the oxyhemoglobin dissociation curve following massive blood transfusion, corticosteroids restore p50 values to normal; this improves the availability of cellular oxygen, probably owing to restoration of pH within the red cell. In addition, corticosteroids stabilize lysosomal membranes, thus preventing the release of lysosomal enzymes that can damage intracellular organelles. Other theoretical actions include increased lactate metabolism, decreased systemic vascular resistance, and reduction of the size of an evolving myocardial infarction (although healing of the infarcted segment may be delayed).

Corticosteroids do have a role in the treatment of shock. In the best controlled study done to date, Shumer administered 30 mg/kg methyl prednisolone or 3 mg/kg dexamethasone to patients in septic shock and reduced the mortality rate to 10.4 percent in the treated group, compared with 38 percent in the control group. Despite some objections to the study, steroids appear to be strongly indicated in the treatment of septic shock, although not necessarily in the treatment of other types of shock.

The anti-inflammatory agent indomethacin has improved endotoxin shock survival in experimental animals. Naloxone also has been observed to reverse endotoxin shock in the animal model. Because septic shock consists largely of an uncontrolled inflammatory response initiated by the lipid A antigenic component of endotoxin, some interventions with antisera have been attempted; they have met with limited clinical success. Prolonged anaphylaxis with hypotension and/or bronchospasms should be treated with steroids, usually hydrocortisone sodium succinate (100 to 500 mg given intravenously). Obviously, shock in patients with adrenal insufficiency should be treated with corticosteroids.

Antibiotics

Patients in shock have a diminished resistance to infection because the increased permeability of the mucosa barrier of the intestine allows bacteria to enter the bloodstream. In addition, the reticuloendothelial system is depressed as a consequence of poor liver perfusion. Treatment with broad spectrum antibiotics should be started at any sign of systemic infection—after proper sampling of blood, urine, and sputum for culture and sensitivity tests. Once bacteriologic results return, the physician should choose the most specific, least toxic, and most likely to be effective treatment for the infecting agent. Side-effects, allergic reactions, and toxicity are of particular concern, since the condition of these patients is already compromised and fragile.

It must be remembered that, because of vasoconstriction and organ failure, distribution and half-life of drugs are often altered in patients who are in shock. Therefore, the route of administration and organ clearance of the antimicrobial are especially important considerations in drug selection. Particularly in the treatment of septic shock, it is incumbent on the emergency department physician to draw appropriate bacterial cultures from all sources before initiating therapy with antibiotics. Focal sites of infection should be sought vigorously. Every effort should be made to treat early in order to prevent bacteremia from progressing to generalized sepsis. Since symptoms can be subtle in the early phases of sepsis, particularly in the very young and very old, the physician should aggressively seek evidence of sepsis or any indication of a predisposition to infection, such as immunocompromise, underlying illness, recent instrumentation or surgery, intravenous drug abuse, or cytotoxic or steroid therapy. General supportive measures, including supplemental oxygen administration and volume expansion, should be initiated, and the search for metabolic and clotting abnormalities begun with standard laboratory tests. The chances for survival are better if cardiac output is maintained, but the mortality rate remains between 10 and 65 percent.

If the responsible organisms are not known, therapy with broad spectrum antibiotics is initiated. The first is usually an aminoglycoside, e.g., gentamicin, amikacin, or tobramycin, given in combination with a second antimicrobial. If anaerobic infection is suspected, the second drug is usually clindamycin, cefoxitin, or chloramphenicol. If *Pseudomonas* is suspected, carbenicillin is added to the regimen. A knowledge of whether the infection was acquired in the hospital and epidemiologic data about antibiotic sensitivities particular to the locale are invaluable management aids. Inotropic agents and pressors are indicated when intravenous fluid administration fails to maintain cardiac output and blood pressure adequately. (See Chapter 20.)

INTRA-AORTIC BALLOON COUNTERPULSATION

In order to use intra-aortic balloon counterpulsation, a catheter is threaded through the femoral artery into the thoracic aorta and a balloon located at the tip is inflated with 30 ml CO_2, using the R wave of the cardiogram for timing. The pump activates the balloon; the balloon is deflated prior to left ventricular systole, to lower outflow resistance, and then is reinflated at the onset of diastole after aortic valve closure, to augment ascending aortic and cerebral arterial pressures and diastolic coronary artery perfusion. With this technique, left ventricular wall tension is reduced, and stroke volume and coronary perfusion are improved. Initial improvements seen in patients with cardiogenic shock may not be supportable in the long term, however.

Another benefit of intra-aortic balloon counterpulsation is that it allows time for assessment of hemodynamic abnormalities and identification of potentially remediable surgical lesions, e.g., aneurysms, mitral regurgitation, rupture, and ventricular septal defects. Still, surgical intervention carries a high mortality rate.

The complication rate of intra-aortic balloon catheter insertion is as high as 26 percent. Complications include thrombosis, infection, and aortic dissection. Nevertheless, current trends in management are to use the intra-aortic balloon counterpulsation device earlier in the patient's clinical course. An external counterpulsation device is noninvasive and functions on the same principle, but its usefulness is minimal in profound cardiogenic shock.

THERAPY OF ANAPHYLAXIS

Hypotension associated with anaphylaxis should be treated by volume expansion with a balanced electrolyte solution. Administration of 0.3 to 0.5 ml aqueous epinephrine 1:1000, subcutaneously or intramuscularly, usually improves urticaria and bronchospasm. Profound peripheral vasoconstriction may necessitate slow intravenous administration of epinephrine in dosages of .1 to .5 cc of a 1:10,000 solution. Monitoring is necessary to detect cardiac dysrhythmia. Repetition of the dose, in 5 to 15 minutes, may be necessary. Local absorption of all antigen, e.g., bee sting, may be retarded by application of a tourniquet and local infiltration with epinephrine. Bronchospasm may be relieved by aminophylline. Oxygen should be administered and the airway maintained, by cricothyreotomy if necessary. Antihistamines (usually diphenhydramine hydrochloride 50 mg intramuscularly or intravenously) should be given early in the course. Pressors should be administered if hypotension persists despite the use of epinephrine and adequate volume replacement. Hemodynamic and electrocardiographic monitoring is essential.

BIBLIOGRAPHY

Alexander RS: Venomotor tone in hemorrhage and shock. *Circ Res* 3:181, 1955.

Alonso DR, et al: Pathophysiology of cardiogenic shock: Quantification of myocardial necrosis, clinical pathologic and electrocardiographic correlations. *Circulation* 45:588, 1973.

Bardet J, Masquet C, Kahn J, et al: Clinical and hemodynamic results of intraaortic balloon counterpulsatic and surgery for cardiogenic shock. *Am Heart J* 93:280–288, 1977.

Batalden DJ, Wickstrom PH, et al: Valve of the G-suit in patients with severe pelvic fracture. Controlling hemorrhage shock. *Arch Surg* 109:326, 1974.

Bates RJ, Beutler S, Resnekov L, et al: Cardiac rupture challenge in diagnosis and management. *Am J Cardiol* 40:429–437, 1977.

Bave AE, Chandry IH, Worth MA, et al: Cellular alterations with shock and ischemia. *Angiology* 25:31–42, 1974.

Blalock A: Experimental shock: The cause of the low blood pressure produced by muscle injury. *Arch Surg* 20:959, 1930.

Bland JHL, Laver MB, Lowenstein E: Vasodilator effect of commercial 5% plasma protein fraction solution. *JAMA* 224:1721–1724, 1973.

Bounous G, McArdle AH, Hampson LG, et al: The cessation of intestinal mucus production as a pathogenic factor in irreversible shock. *Surg Forum* 16:11, 1965.

Boutros AR, Olson L, et al: Comparison of hemodynamic pulmonary and renal effects of use in three types of fluids after major surgical procedures on the abdominal aorta. *Crit Care Med* 7:9, 1979.

Braunwald E: Control of myocardial oxygen consumption: Physiologic and clinical considerations. *Am J Cardiol* 27:588, 1970.

Braunwald E: Structure and function of the normal myocardium. *Br Heart J* 33(suppl):3–8, 1971.

Braunwald E: Regulation of circulation: I. *N Engl J Med* 290:1124–1129, 1974.

Braunwald E, Ross J Jr, Sonnenblick EH: *Mechanisms of Contraction of the Normal and Failing Heart.* Boston, Little Brown and Co, 1968.

Cannon WB: *Traumatic Shock.* New York, D Appleton and Co, 1923.

Carey CL, Lowery BD, Cloutier CT: *Hemorrhagic Shock. Current Problems in Surgery.* Chicago, Yearbook Medical Publishers, 1971.

Cervera AL, Moss G: Dilutional reexpansion with crystalloid after massive hemorrhage: Saline vs. balanced electrolyte solutions for maintenance of normal blood volume and arterial. *J Trauma* 15:498, 1975.

Christy JH: Treatment of gram negative shock. *Am J Med* 50:77, 1971.

Civetta JM, Nussenfeld SR: Prehospital use of military anti-shock trousers (MAST). *JACEP* 5:581, 1976.

Cloutier CT, Lowery BD, Carey LC: The effects of hemodilutional resuscitation on serum protein levels in humans in hemorrhagic shock. *J Trauma* 9:514, 1969.

Cohn JN: Blood pressure measurement in shock: Mechanisms of inaccuracy in auscultatory and palpatory methods. *JAMA* 199:972, 1967.

Cohn JN: Shock, in Hurst JW (ed): *The Heart.* New York, McGraw-Hill, 1978, pp 716–726.

Cope O, Litwin SQ: Contribution of the lymphatic system to the replenishment of plasma volume following hemorrhage. *Ann Surg* 156:655, 1962.

Coram AG, Ballantine TV, et al: The effect of crystalloid resuscitation in hemorrhagic shock on acid base balance: A comparison between normal saline and Ringer's lactate solutions. *Surg* 69:874–880, 1971.

Craham AJP, Douglas DM: Effect of the head down position on the circulation in hypotensive states. *Lancet* 2:941, 1949.

Crile GW: *Blood Pressure in Surgery in Experimental and Clinical Research.* Philadelphia, JB Lippincott Co, 1903, p 288.

Crile GW, Lower WE: *Anoci-Association.* Philadelphia, WB Saunders Co, 1914.

Crowell JW, Houston B: The effect of acidity on blood coagulation. *Am J Physiol* 201:379, 1961.

Crowell JW: Cardiac deterioration as the cause of irreversibility in shock, in Mills LC, Moyen JH (eds): *Shock and Hypotension. The 12th Hahnemann Symposium.* New York, Grune & Stratton, 1965.

Cutler BS, Daggett WM: Application of the G-suit to the control of hemorrhage in massive trauma. *Ann Surg* 173:511–514, 1971.

Cyres SM: The shock lung, in *The Organ in Shock. Proceedings of the Second Symposium on Recent Research Developments and Current Clinical Practice in Shock.* A Scope Publication, 1977, pp 24–32.

Dahn MS, Lucas CE: Negative inotropic effect of albumin resuscitation for shock. *Surgery* 86:235–241, 1979.

Da Luz PL, Weill MH, Shubin H: Current concepts on mechanisms and treatment of cardiogenic shock. *Am Heart J* 92:103–113, 1976.

Darling RC: Ruptured arteriosclerotic abdominal aortic aneurysms. *Am J Surg* 119:397–401, 1976.

Duncan GW, Sarnoff SJ, Rhode CM: Studies on the effects of posture in shock and injury. *Ann Surg* 120:24, 1968.

Du Point HL, Spink WW: Infections due to gram negative organisms: An analysis of 860 patients with bacteremia at the University of Minnesota Medical Center, 1958–1966. *Medicine* 48:307–332, 1969.

Espinoza MH, Updegrove JH: Clinical experience with the G-suit. *Ann Surg* 101:36–39, 1970.

Fletcher JR, Ramwell PW: *E coli* endotoxin shock in the baboon: Treatment with lidocaine or indomethacin. *Adv Prostaglandin Thromboxane Res* 3:183–192, 1978.

Geyer RF: Fluorocarbon-polyol artificial blood substitutes. *N Engl J Med* 289:1077–1082, 1973.

Grassford WD, Pandey N, Jensen CG, et al: Pulmonary changes in treated hemorrhagic shock. *Am J Surg* 124:738–743, 1972.

Gross SD: System of Surgery, 1850, cited by Mann FC. *Bull Johns Hopkins Hosp* 25:205, 1914.

Gunnar RM, Loeb HS, Winslow EJ, et al: Hemodynamic measurements in bacteremia and septic shock in man. *J Infect Dis* 128(suppl):5295–5298, 1973.

Guyton AC, Jones CE (eds): *Physiology Series One: Cardiovascular Physiology.* Baltimore, Butterworth and University Park Press, 1974.

Haller JA, Ward MJ, Cahill JI: Metabolic alterations in shock: The effect of controlled reduction of blood flow on oxidative metabolism and catecholamine response. *J Trauma* 7:727, 1967.

Hardaway RM: Syndromes of disseminated intravascular coagulation: With special reference to shock and hemorrhages. Springfield, Ill, Charles C Thomas, 1966.

Hardaway RM, James PM, et al: Intensive study of shock in man. *JAMA* 199:779–790, 1967.

Hartong JM, Dixon RS: Monitoring resuscitation of the injured patient. *JAMA* 237:242–244, 1977.

Hayes DF, Weiner MH, Rosenberg IK, et al: Effects of traumatic hypovolemic shock on renal function. *J Surg Res* 16:490, 1974.

Heinonen J, Takki S, Tammisto T: Effect of the Trendelenburg tilt and other procedures on the position of endotracheal tubes. *Lancet* 1:850, 1969.

Heistad DD, Abboud FM: Circulatory adjustments to hypoxia. *Circulation* 61:463–470, 1980.

Henderson Y: Acapnia and shock. *Am J Physiol* 24:66, 1909.

Holaday JW, Faden AI: Naloxone reversal of endotoxin hypotension suggests role of endophins in shock. *Nature* 275:450–451, 1978.

James PN, Myers RT: Central venous pressure monitoring: Misinterpretation, abuses, indications, and a new technique. *Ann Surg* 175:693–701, 1971.

Jelenko C III, Wheeler ML, et al: Shock and resuscitation II: Volume repletion with minimal edema using the "halfed" method. *JACEP* 7:326–333, 1978.

Jelenko C, Williams JB, et al: Studies in shock and resuscitation I: Use of a hypertonic albumin containing demand regiment (HALFD) in resuscitation. *Crit Care Med* 7:157–167, 1979.

Kaplan BC, Civetta JM, Nagel EL, et al: The military anti-shock trousers in civilian prehospital emergency care. *J Trauma* 13:843–848, 1973.

Knopp R, Dailey R: Central venous cannulation and pressure monitoring. *JACEP* 6:358–366, 1977.

Kuhn LA: Management of shock following acute myocardial infarction: I. Drug Therapy. *Am Heart J* 95:529–534, 1978.

Kuhn LA: Management of shock following acute myocardial infarction: II. Mechanical circulatory assistance. *Am Heart J* 95:789–795, 1978.

Lefer AM: Role of a myocardial depressant factor in the pathogenesis of hemorrhagic shock. *Fed Proc* 29:1836, 1970.

Lefer AM, Martin J: Relationship of plasma peptides to the depressant factors in hemorrhage. *Circ Res* 26:59, 1970.

Lefime AA: Results and complications of intra-aortic balloon pumping in surgical and medical patients. *Am J Cardiol* 40:416, 1977.

Lewis DG, McKenzie A, McNeil LF: The use of the G-Suit in the control of bleeding arising from hypocoagulation. *Ann R Coll Surg Engl* 52:53, 1973.

Libby P, Maroko PR, Bloor CM, et al: Reduction of experimental myocardial infarct size by corticosteroids administration. *J Clin Invest* 52:599–607, 1973.

Lister J, McNeill IF, Marshall VC, et al: Transcapillary refilling after hemorrhage in normal man. Basal rates and volumes; Effects of norepinephrine. *Ann Surg* 158:698–712, 1963.

Lowe RJ, Moss GS, et al: Crystalloid vs. colloid in the etiology of pulmonary failure after trauma—A randomized trial in man. *Crit Care Med* 7:107–112, 1979.

Lucas CE, Weaver DW, Higgins RP, et al: Effects of albumin versus non albumin resuscitation on plasma volume and renal excretory function. *J Trauma* 18:564–570, 1979.

Lucas CE, Ledgerwood AM, et al: Impaired pulmonary function after albumin resuscitation from shock. *J Trauma* 20:446–451, 1980.

Luz PL, Shubin H, Iveil MH, et al: Pulmonary edema related to changes in colloid osmotic and pulmonary artery wedge pressure in patients after acute myocardial infarction. *Circulation* 51:350–357, 1975.

McSwain NE: Pneumatic trousers and the management of shock. *J Trauma* 17:719–724, 1977.

Miller RD: Complications of massive blood transfusions. *Anesthesiology* 39:82–92, 1973.

Moore FD: *Metabolic Care of the Surgical Patient.* Philadelphia, WB Saunders Co, 1960.

Moore FD, Daher FD, et al: Hemorrhage in normal man. I. Distribution and dispersal of saline infusion following acute blood loss, clinical kinetics of blood volume support. *Ann Surg* 163:485–504, 1966.

Moss GS, Salletta JD: Traumatic shock in man. *N Engl J Med* 290:724–725, 1974.

Mudth ED: Mechanical and surgical interventions for the reduction of myocardial ischaemia. *Circulation* 53(1):176, 1976.

Mueller U, Ayres SM, Gregory JJ, et al: Hemodynamics coronary blood flow and myocardial metabolism in coronary shock: Response to L-norepinephrine and isoproterenol. *J Clin Invest* 49:1855–1902, 1970.

Mueller H, et al: Effects of isoproterenol, L-norepinephrine and intra-aortic counterpulsation on hemodynamics and myocardial metabolism in shock following acute myocardial infarction. *Circulation* 45:335, 1972.

Nishijima H, Weil MH, Shubin H, et al: Hemodynamic and metabolic studies on shock associated with gram negative bacteremia. *Medicine* 52:287–294, 1973.

O'Rourke MF, et al: Acute severe cardiac failure complicating myocardial infarction. *Br Heart J* 37:169, 1975.

Page DL, et al: Myocardial changes associated with cardiogenic shock. *N Engl J Med* 285:133, 1971.

Pelligra R, Sandbeig FC: Control of intractable abdominal bleeding by external counterpressure. *JAMA* 241:708, 1979.

Rackow EC, Fein IA, Leppo S: Colloid osmotic pressure as a prognostic indicator of pulmonary edema and mortality in the critically ill. *Chest* 72:709–713, 1977.

Ransom K, McSwain NE: Respiratory function following application of MAST trousers. *JACEP* 7:15–17, 1978.

Ratshin RA, et al: Hemodynamic evaluation of left ventricular function in shock complicating myocardial infarction. *Circulation* 45:127, 1972.

Reed JH Jr, Wood EH: Effect of body position on vertical distribution of pulmonary blood flow. *J Appl Physiol* 218:303, 1970.

Risk C, Rudo N, et al: Comparison of right atrial and pulmonary capillary wedge pressures. *Crit Care Med* 6:172–175, 1978.

Rutherford RB, Buerk CA: *The Pathophysiology of Trauma and Shock in the Management of Trauma,* ed 3, Philadelphia, WB Saunders Co, 1979, pp 38–79.

Salisbury PF, et al: Acute ischaemia of inner layers of ventricular wall. *Am Heart J* 66:650, 1963.

Sarnoff SJ, et al: Insufficient coronary flow and myocardial failure as a complicating factor in late hemorrhagic shock. *Am J Physiol* 176:439, 1954.

Scheidt S, et al: Intra-aortic balloon counterpulsation in cardiogenic shock. Report of a cooperative clinical trial. *N Engl J Med* 288:979, 1973.

Shenasky JH, Gillenwater JY: The renal hemodynamic and functional effects of external counterpressure. *Surg Gynecol Obstet* 134:253–258, 1972.

Shine KI (moderator): Aspects of the management of shock. *Ann Intern Med* 93:723–734, 1980.

Shires TG: Management of hypovolemic shock. *Bull NY Acad Med* 55:139–148, 1979.

Shoemaker WC: Pathophysiological basis of therapy for shock and trauma syndromes: Use of sequential cardiorespiratory measurements to describe natural histories and evaluate possible mechanisms. *Semin Drug Treat* 3:211–229, 1973.

Shoemaker WC, Carl JH: Critique of crystalloid vs. colloid therapy in shock and shock lung. *Crit Care Med* 7:117–124, 1979.

Shubin H, Weil WH: Bacterial shock. *JAMA* 235:421–424, 1976.

Shumer W: The microcirculatory and metabolic effects of dibenziline in oligemic shock. *Surg Gynecol Obstet* 123:787–791, 1966.

Shumer W, Sperlung R: Shock and its effect on the cell. *JAMA* 205:75–79, 1968.

Shumer W: Steroids in the treatment of clinical septic shock. *Ann Surg* 184:333–341, 1976.

Shumer W: Septic shock. *JAMA* 242:1906–1907, 1979.

Sibbald WJ, Patterson NA, Holliday RL, et al: The Trendelenburg position: Hemodynamic effects in hypotensive and normotensive patients. *Crit Care Med* 7:218–224, 1979.

Solen J, Muellen HA, Kennedy TJ: Clinical use of the G-suit. *JACEP* 5:609–611, 1976.

Starling EH: On the absorption of fluids from the connective tissue spaces. *J Physiol* 19:312, 1896.

Stein L, et al: Pulmonary edema during volume infusion. *Circulation* 52:483–489, 1975.

Swan HJC, et al: Catheterization of the heart in man with the use of a flow directed balloon tipped catheter. *N Engl J Med* 283:447, 1970.

Swank RL, Hissen W, Bergentz SF: 5-Hydroxytryptamine and aggregation of blood elements after trauma. *Surg Gynecol Obstet* 119:779, 1964.

Taylor J, Weil MH: Failure of the Trendelenburg position to improve circulation during clinical shock. *Ann Surg* 120:24, 1941.

Thompson WL: Rational use of albumin and plasma substitutes. *Johns Hopkins Med J* 136:220–225, 1975.

Triedman E, Grable E, Fine J: Central venous pressure and direct serial measurements as gauges in blood volume replacement. *Lancet* 2:609–614, 1966.

Trunkey DD, Sheldon GF, Collins JA: The treatment of shock, in Zuidema GD, Rutherford MD, Ballinger MD (eds): *The Management of Trauma.* Philadelphia, WB Saunders Co, 1979.

Valeri CR: Viability and function of preserved red cells. *N Engl J Med* 284:81, 1971.

Wagensteen SL, De Hall JD, Ludewig RM, et al: The detrimental effects of the G-suit in hemorrhagic shock. *Ann Surg* 170:187–192, 1969.

Walt AJ, Wilson RF: *The Treatment of Shock in Advances in Surgery.* Chicago, Yearbook Medical Publishers, 1975.

Wayne MA: The MAST suit in the treatment of cardiogenic shock. *JACEP* 7:3, 107, 1978.

Weber KT, et al: Left ventricular dysfunction following acute myocardial infarction. *Am J Med* 54:697, 1973.

Weedn RJ, Cook JH, McElreath RL, et al: Wet lung syndrome after crystalloid and colloid repletion. *Curr Top Surg Res* 2:335, 1975.

Wei JY, Hutchins GM, Bulkley BH: Papillary muscle rupture in fatal acute myocardial infarction. *Ann Intern Med* 90:149–153, 1979.

Weidner MG, Albrecht M, Clowes GH: Relationship of myocardial function to survival after oligemic hypotension. *Surgery* 55:73, 1964.

Weil MH, Shubin H, Carlson R: Treatment of circulatory shock. Use of sympathomimetic vasoactive agents. *JAMA* 231:1280–1286, 1975.

Wilson RF: Acid base abnormalities in clinical shock, in Schumer W, Nyhus LM (eds): *Treatment of Shock: Principles and Practice.* Philadelphia, Lea & Febiger, 1974, pp 37–52.

Wilson RF, Christensen C, Le Blanc LP: Oxygen consumption in critically ill surgical patients. *Ann Surg* 801–804, 1971.

Wilson RF, Gibson D: The use of arterial central venous oxygen differences to calculate cardiac output and oxygen consumption in critically ill surgical patients. *Surgery* 83:362–369, 1978.

Wilson RF, Saruer E, Birks R: Central venous pressure and blood volume determination in clinical shock. *Surg Gynecol Obstet* 132:631–636, 1971.

Young LS, Stevens P, Ingram J: Functional role of antibody against core glycolipid of enterobacteriaceae. *J Clin Invest* 56:250–261, 1975.

Ziegler EJ, McCutchan JA, Brande AL: Clinical trial of core glycolipid antibody in gram negative bacteremia. *Trans Assoc Am Physicians* 91:253–258, 1978.

7. Major Trauma

PETER VAKTOR, M.D.

Ever since the passage of the Emergency Medical Services (EMS) Act of 1973, great efforts have been made to provide comprehensive and optimal emergency medical care at the prehospital level. The development of training programs for paramedical personnel and the incorporation of these highly trained individuals into unified ambulance and emergency medical systems in the large urban centers have proved to be very successful. The reduction in morbidity and mortality resulting from these programs has been immeasurable. These new health professionals, the emergency medical technicians (EMTs) or paramedics, are providing basic and advanced life support not only for victims of acute cardiovascular events, but also for patients suffering from critical injuries. For the victim of major trauma, time is of the essence; delay jeopardizes not just future function, but life itself. EMS systems provide for rapid deployment of skilled paramedics to the scene of an accident, where evaluation, stabilization, and transport of the trauma victim is undertaken immediately. Such systems, currently operating in most areas of the United States, are certainly a far cry from the system used years ago when ambulance companies were mostly owned and operated by funeral parlors having an inherent conflict of interest. Today, it is common for the critically injured patient to arrive in the emergency department immediately and in same instances intubated and adequately ventilated, with an intravenous (IV) lifeline in place and musculoskeletal injuries properly immobilized.

The system for the prehospital management of the severely injured has been made the best possible; unfortunately, however, the same does not hold true for in-hospital care. The reason for this discrepancy is twofold: (1) unequal distribution of medical facilities capable of providing total continuing care for the multiple injured and (2) omissions in physician training in the management of the critically injured.

It is now widely recognized and accepted that the massively traumatized patient is best managed in a major trauma center, where specialized facilities and teams of physicians and surgeons trained in trauma care are immediately available. Therefore, certain hospital centers have been designated as regional trauma centers and are linked via rapid evacuation and transport facilities to the network of the EMS system. To maintain and refine both the in-hospital organization of resources and the expertise of the trauma team, a steady stream of patients is necessary. Efficiency and clinical skills are directly proportional to experience and decline rapidly when they remain dormant. Thus, the regional trauma centers, which are supplied with a constant flow of trauma victims, can become the ideals of trauma management. However, the reality is once again far from the ideal. (See Chapter 2.)

Serious accidents occur not only near urban university hospital centers, but also in rural, peripheral areas, where EMS systems and trauma centers are not as accessible as they are in urban areas. Small county and rural hospitals may lack both the facilities and the trained, experienced personnel to handle victims of major trauma. Emergency Departments in these hospitals have been staffed by general and family physicians working part-time; although competent, these physicians may lack the skills and judgment of the experienced traumatologist. The needs of the trauma victim are often beyond the resources in equipment, organization, and subspecialty consultation available to the rural hospital. The result is the often needless loss of hundreds of lives annually.

Trauma is the major cause of death in those under 40 years old and is one of the top three causes of death for all ages. In spite of this, there has been in the past an almost total lack of education and training in trauma management offered in medical schools and very little government funding for research and training programs. Basic research in traumatology is needed, and existing resources, knowledge, and skills must be reorganized into an effective unit, capable of managing the complex, shifting biologic parameters of the critically injured.

A great deal of interest has been focused on the development of emergency medicine over the last ten years, culminating in its acceptance as a distinct primary specialty in 1979. If a unique characterization could be applied to these new specialists, it would be their global knowledge in the art of resuscitation. This knowledge crosses the barriers of the various medical and surgical subspecialties and takes the whole complex of simultaneously interacting biological variables of the massively traumatized patient. The emergentologist, by virtue of training and experience, is most adept at rapid and accurate assessment of the patient's condition, resuscitation, determination of priorities, and delivery of primary care to the critically ill and injured. The three major causes of early death from massive trauma are (1) hemorrhage and resultant hypovolemia, (2) cardiorespiratory failure, and (3) central nervous system injury; if lives are to be saved, these must be averted by the rapid institution of resuscitative measures. Delayed or inadequate resuscitation invariably leads to late secondary organ failure from tissue anoxia and subsequent disability or death. It is only through decisive action and authoritative command of resources and personnel, interacting in a preestablished system of protocols, that care can be optimal. By controlling and directing the lines of communication between subspecialty areas, the emergentologist can also ensure continuity of care at secondary and tertiary levels.

As more and more emergentologists graduate from approved residency programs and as continuing medical education courses include more topics on trauma management, there should be a definite improvement in the primary care of the massively traumatized patient.

TRAUMA PREPAREDNESS

Whether it be in a major trauma center or a small, peripheral hospital, the principal common denominator for the successful management of the traumatized patient rests on preparedness.

Physical Resources

Trauma Room

The most appropriate place for the initial treatment of the trauma victim is the emergency department. Its strategic location and ease of access, because of its ambulance-receiving bay, make it ideal for this purpose. Inside the emergency department there should be a designated "crash" or trauma room reserved exclusively for the critically ill or injured. The location of such an area is important; not only does it have to be readily accessible from the ambulance-receiving area, but also it must facilitate subsequent transfer to either the operating room or intensive care unit. In addition, the trauma room should be located far enough away from the mainstream of emergency department activity to discourage the grandstand display of high drama that inevitably draws crowds of curious onlookers who may obstruct decisive judgment and action.

Recent literature[1] suggests that a considerable reduction in morbidity and mortality rates can be obtained by directly transferring major trauma victims to the operating room for both initial evaluation and definitive management. Such a system saves invaluable time and avoids excessive and repeated handling of the patient during transfer. Although useful for selected cases in major trauma centers, especially if the center can be notified beforehand of patient arrival, this procedure is not practical in most small urban and rural hospitals. Economic and staffing constraints do not allow smaller facilities to keep a fully staffed and equipped operating room in readiness exclusively for trauma victims. With a minimum of reorganization, however, a trauma room can be established in most emergency departments without incurring additional costs in either staffing or equipment.

Supplies and Equipment

The supplies and equipment that should be available in the trauma room naturally vary according to the number and types of trauma patients seen annually, the medical and surgical sophistication of the attending staff, and the budget of the emergency department. Through sound knowledge of the basic principles of trauma care and thoughtful organization, even minimally equipped trauma rooms can function effectively. Major trauma centers, owing to the large numbers and differing severity of trauma cases received, should have trauma rooms with the capabilities of operating theaters in which any type of surgery can be performed without delay.

The minimum requirement for successful resuscitation, aside from the skill and experience of the physician in charge, is equipment for cardiorespiratory monitoring and assistance. This should include portable or wall outlet suction units; oxygen supply; bag-valve mask; various sized oropharyngeal, nasopharyngeal, and endotracheal airways with accompanying laryngoscope and Magill forceps; and chest tube drainage sets. Useful, but not immediately essential on the premises is a respirator, preferably volume cycled, capable of delivering positive end expiratory pressure (PEEP). The presence of electrocardiographic monitoring and defibrillating equipment is an absolute necessity. Numerous IV administration sets, indwelling IV catheters, and central venous pressure lines should be immediately available for insertion. A generous supply of IV fluid, both crystalloids (Ringer's lactate and saline) and colloids (salt-poor albumin and plasma protein fraction-human [Plasmanate]) should be stored in the room. Sterile-packaged surgical trays, nasogastric suction tubes, peritoneal catheters, and Foley catheters are important diagnostic and therapeutic tools that should be instantly accessible. Numerous syringes; needles; blood-sampling tubes; sterile drapes, swabs, and bandages; and traction, splinting, and casting materials complete a small but effective trauma room, capable of managing most trauma cases.

As important as the actual equipment itself, is the attending staff's familiarity with both the functioning of each apparatus and its strategic location around the trauma room. Nothing is more disruptive or counterproductive during a resuscitation than needless, frantic searching for and fumbling with unfamiliar equipment. If there should be inflexibility in any area of resuscitation, it should be in the constant vigilance and maintenance of the trauma room according to daily established routines.

Radiology

As radiologic assessment is one of the most important tools available to the physician managing multiple trauma, some thought should be directed toward its accessibility. Most emergency departments have some form of radiology facility nearby, whether a completely autonomous branch of the radiology department is located in the emergency department or the main radiology department actually neighbors the emergency department. Although this arrangement greatly improves efficiency and patient comfort, compared with hospital centers where the radiology department is a considerable distance from the trauma room, it does not provide optimum care for the massively injured. When time is at a premium, patient handling must be reduced to a minimum, and constant surveillance of vital parameters is essential, any needless transport or breach of vigilance must be avoided. The ready availability of portable radiology equipment is the solution. Most of the radiologic examinations needed in the initial assessment of the critically injured patient are easily obtained with such an apparatus. Sophistication and efficiency can be increased by the addition of modifications to the examining table, e.g., a Potter-Bucky grid and cassette holders. However, the simplicity and ease of operation of portable radiologic equipment make it the ideal instrument for the trauma room.

The Trauma Team

As important, if not more so, than the physical resources available, are the medical personnel assigned to work in concert for the benefit of the massively injured.

Gill and Long, in their comprehensive and authoritative treatise on shock and trauma based on their many years of experience in the management of the severely traumatized at the Maryland Institute of Emergency Medical Services (MIEMS), advocated the "team approach" for the initial evaluation and resuscitation of the critically injured.[2] The team approach, which is an application of military experience to civilian practice, establishes a chain of command and ensures the coordination of action so important to optimal resuscitation. It can be used in small peripheral hospitals as well as at major trauma centers. At university hospitals, a multidisciplinary team could be composed of senior house officers and staff from the various subspecialties; they would be responsible to and guided by a single, preappointed chief of service. To ensure immediate availability, the team members on the trauma service would have no other clinical responsibility but trauma. This type of system would, or course, be feasible only in the larger teaching institutes, where a fair number of trauma patients are seen regularly. In the peripheral hospitals, the trauma team would be composed of available personnel with preassigned role functions. The team leader should have the most experience and should be immediately available when needed. When the team leader is the only physician involved, an effective trauma team can be formed by recruiting physician's assistants, nurses, and orderlies and assigning specific roles to them.

The trauma team must function as a single unit, with responsibility to but one leader who is capable of evaluating the complex parameters of the trauma victim and who can act authoritatively. It is imperative that each team member have a clear, precise preassigned job according to his or her level of competence and responsibility. Through the established system of priorities and protocols, each team member can function independently while the team leader concentrates on the total evaluation of the patient's condition and directs the whole process of resuscitation. The team leader, through consultation with other specialists, should also be able to ensure continuity of definitive care at secondary and tertiary levels. (See Chapter 2.)

THE GENERAL APPROACH TO THE INJURED PATIENT

Not all patients with multiple injuries arrive in the trauma room with critical, life-threatening pathology; obviously, trauma injuries vary in severity. However, in order to ensure effective and optimal trauma care, it is always wise to assume the worst and to initiate the resuscitation process to the fullest. A very common error—due to inexperience, insecurity, or the lack of a planned approach to trauma management—is to underestimate the extent and the life-threatening nature of injuries. A patient who initially appears stable may deteriorate rapidly and dramatically while the attending physicians concern themselves with an obvious, jagged, but superficial extremity laceration instead of the possibility of an occult critical injury. Only after the first priorities of resuscitation have been met, i.e., the adequacy of airway and respiration ensured, external hemorrhage controlled, and the force and volume of circulation restored, can attention be shifted to the secondary considerations of complete history, physical examination, and other diagnostic and therapeutic modalities. Rapid, early death due to massive trauma usually occurs as a result of either primary damage to the function of vital organs, e.g., lungs, heart, or central nervous system, or secondary failure of these structures as a result of diminished perfusion caused by hemorrhagic or hypovolemic shock. The main distinction between the trauma victim and the patient undergoing major elective surgery is the fact that vital organ functioning is not controlled during the traumatic event. It should, therefore, be the primary goal of the emergentologist to establish the same type of control over the vital physiologic parameters that is possible in the controlled setting of the operating room. Once this is under way, an organized, meticulous, etiologic investigation may be instituted.

THE FIRST PRIORITY

Rapid Overall Assessment

If it is possible, a forewarning of a trauma victim's arrival is extremely helpful, but the timing varies according to different EMS capabilities. The trauma team should be alerted, prepared, and positioned to receive the patient. As the multiply injured patient is being wheeled into the trauma room, the team captain makes a rapid overall primary survey of the patient's condition, focusing close attention on the most important vital parameters.

Airway

A quick verification of airway patency is first, and obviously obstructing foreign objects are removed. The presence of stridor, sternomastoid tug, crowing respiration, and intercostal retraction suggests airway obstruction and must be dealt with promptly. Any peripheral or central cyanosis is noted.

Breathing

The rate, depth, and rhythm of spontaneous respiration are noted. The chest is quickly examined for integrity, stability, and symmetry of expansion and air entry. Evidence of tracheal shift, dissymmetry of chest movement and air entry, and subcutaneous emphysema should alert the physician to the presence of a tension pneumothorax, and the chest should be prepared for tube drainage. Open, sucking chest wounds should be immediately occluded with an airtight dressing.

Circulation

Obvious, gross hemorrhage should be immediately arrested by means of direct pressure, pressure dressing, or hemostatic clamping when the source is identified. The pulse rate, rhythm, volume, and contour should be assessed as indicators of circulating volume and shock. Dissymmetric or varying pulses, or an absence of certain pulses, may indicate the existence of arterial occlusion, aortic rupture, or tamponade. Systolic and diastolic blood pressure measurements are obtained, and the pulse pressure is calculated. Pulsus paradoxus should be sought and noted. The state of perfusion can be easily assessed by looking at the color and temperature of the skin, lips, and nailbeds. Preparation for IV line insertion, if not already established, is begun.

Central Nervous System

Brief attention should be focused on the patient's state of consciousness, e.g., orientation, verbal and motor ability. The pupils can be quickly examined for equality of size, reactivity, and accommodation.

Initial Classification and Examination

After assessment of the vital signs, the patient can be classified, according to Gill and Long,[2] into the following three categories:

1. unstable: patients with grossly unstable vital signs, representing major cardiorespiratory and central nervous system failure.
2. potentially unstable: patients with moderately abnormal hemodynamic and ventilatory findings, but no immediate signs of deterioration. These are the patients who most often pose diagnostic problems and tend to suffer the consequences of physician underestimation of their injuries.
3. stable: patients with normal cardiorespiratory and central nervous system findings.

While the trauma team leader is performing the primary evaluation, the other team members are removing the patient's clothing. It is imperative that this be done expeditiously and completely. The patient must be stripped completely nude in order to ensure that no injuries are hidden by clothing. No time should be lost in trying to preserve a piece of clothing by gingerly removing it, anything not readily removable is cut away.

A very brief history can be obtained, meanwhile, from the ambulance attendants, police, paramedics, or others accompanying the patient as to the mechanism of injury, initial and subsequent condition during transport, and gross estimate of blood loss.

Owing to the expertise of the paramedics in the EMS systems, many trauma victims arrive at the emergency department with airways and IV lines already inserted, wounds bandaged, and fractures adequately immobilized. At this stage of the resuscitation, no attempt should be made to remove any previously applied bandages or dressings or to deflate pneumatic antishock garments, if they are in place, for doing so may precipitate massive hemorrhage and rapid decompensation of the patient. Correctly applied traction and splinting apparatus should also be left in place if the distal neurovascular function of the extremity involved is intact.

Attention is now directed to the immediate correction of vital organ dysfunction diagnosed during the rapid primary survey procedure.

Urgent Therapeutic Interventions

Airway

The management of airway obstruction naturally depends on the cause of the condition, but it must be rectified before any other resuscitative measure is undertaken. (See Chapter 56.)

Tongue. The most common cause of airway obstruction in the unconscious victim is occlusion of the posterior pharynx by the tongue. Because the usual techniques for relieving tongue obstruction, i.e., head tilt, jaw thrust, or triple airway maneuver, all involve mobilizing the head and neck to some degree, these prac-

tices are to be discouraged in the case of the trauma victim. At this stage of the resuscitation, especially with an unconscious victim, the possibility of cervical spine injury cannot be ruled out, and thoughtless action can lead to irreparable harm. A nasopharyngeal or oropharyngeal airway (Fig. 7–1) can be quickly and effectively inserted to relieve the obstruction, while preparations are made for endotracheal intubation. These airways are simple, safe, and often life-saving.

Foreign Bodies. With the availability of suction apparatus, the presence of blood, mucus, or vomitus in the oropharynx should pose no problem of management, as these can be cleared rapidly. However, broken teeth or pieces of dentures, solid particles of food, or other foreign objects may not be removable by suction; they may be impacted at the level of the epiglottis, or they may have slipped past the vocal cords to obstruct the trachea. These materials should be removed under direct vision, with the aid of either a laryngoscope and Magill forceps or a flexible fiberoptic bronchoscope, if available. No time should be lost, and there should be no hesitation whatsoever about performing a needle or a stab cricothyreotomy while preparations are under way to remove the obstruction. A needle cricothyreotomy (Fig. 7–2) is performed by first palpating the cricothyroid membrane beneath the inferior prominence of the thyroid cartilage and inserting a large-bore needle (14 gauge) through the skin and membrane beneath it into the trachea. A continuous flow of 100 percent oxygen should be administered through this needle, while another needle is inserted next to it to allow for expiration. However, a larger, more convenient airway can be created by means of a stab wound into the cricothyroid membrane and the insertion of an

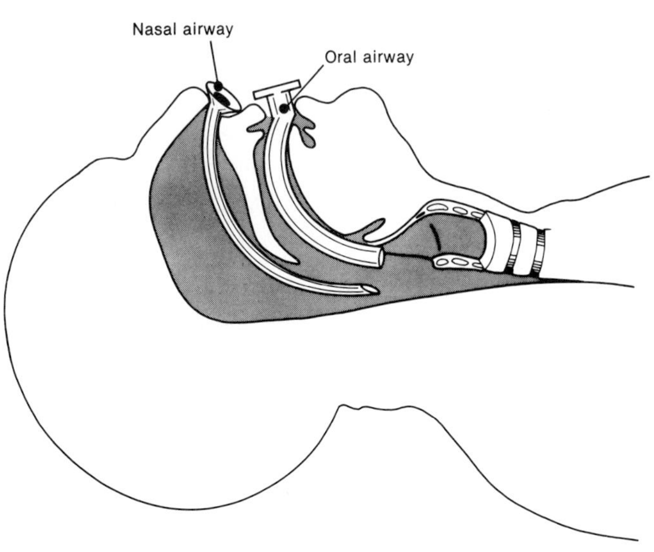

Figure 7–1 Nasal and Oral Airways.

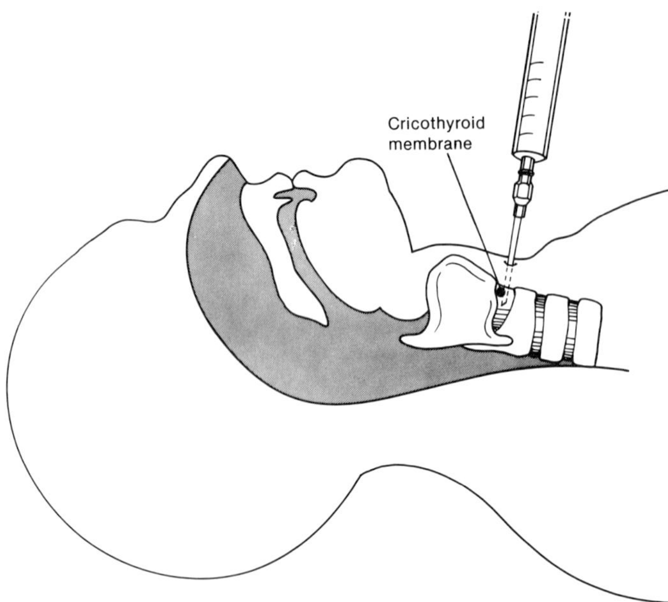

Figure 7–2 Needle Cricothyreotomy.

endotracheal tube through it into the trachea. This allows for both suctioning of the trachea and fiberoptic examination. A more permanent airway can be created when the patient's condition allows.

Structural Damage. Craniofacial trauma, e.g., a Le Fort III fracture, can result in the loss of the structural support of the upper airway, presenting a very real danger of airway obstruction. Fractures of the larynx and the trachea, diagnosed by the presence of cervical emphysema and palpable cartilage disruption, can lead to collapse of these structures and hence to traumatic asphyxia.[3] In these, as in other examples of obstruction, rapid access to the airway is imperative and can be accomplished via endotracheal intubation or cricothyreotomy.

All physicians who are involved in the care of the critically ill and injured should be thoroughly familiar with the technique of endotracheal intubation. It is not reserved solely for the care of patients in respiratory failure. Any trauma victim with a disturbed level of consciousness should be intubated, because stuporous and comatose patients are very prone to aspiration. Once the airway has been cleared of any obstruction it is essential to keep it clear. The endotracheal tube accomplishes this task most admirably.

Two routes of insertion are available: nasotracheal and endotracheal. Nasotracheal intubation, when performed "blind," is an especially useful technique when cervical injury has not been excluded. This technique can be rather difficult, however, even in the hands of experienced anesthesiologists. The flexible fiberoptic bronchoscope, on the other hand, can greatly facilitate

the placement of the endotracheal tube by this route.[4] Endotracheal intubation (Fig. 7–3) is readily performed with the aid of a laryngoscope, although it is necessary to mobilize the patient's head and neck. With the neck of the patient flexed and the head extended on the neck in the "sniffing" position, the mouth is opened with the right hand. Holding the laryngoscope in the left hand, the physician inserts the blade, following the curvature of the tongue posteriorly until the epiglottis is visualized. The tip of the blade is inserted into the vallecula, and the epiglottis elevated by lifting the laryngoscope upward, without rotation, to expose the vocal cords. The appropriate-sized endotracheal tube can then be passed into the trachea and its balloon inflated. Not only does the endotracheal tube protect the airway from aspiration or obstruction and facilitate bronchial suctioning, but also it allows the patient to be connected to a respirator for ventilatory support. Prophylactic ventilatory support to stave off respiratory depression is strongly urged for the patient with a depressed level of consciousness, hypotension, and chest injuries. (See Chapter 71.)

Respiration

With the airway secured, attention can be focused on the mechanics of respiratory function itself. As a baseline study, an arterial blood sample is immediately sent for blood gas determinations. The physician should not wait for the blood gas results to proceed with the course

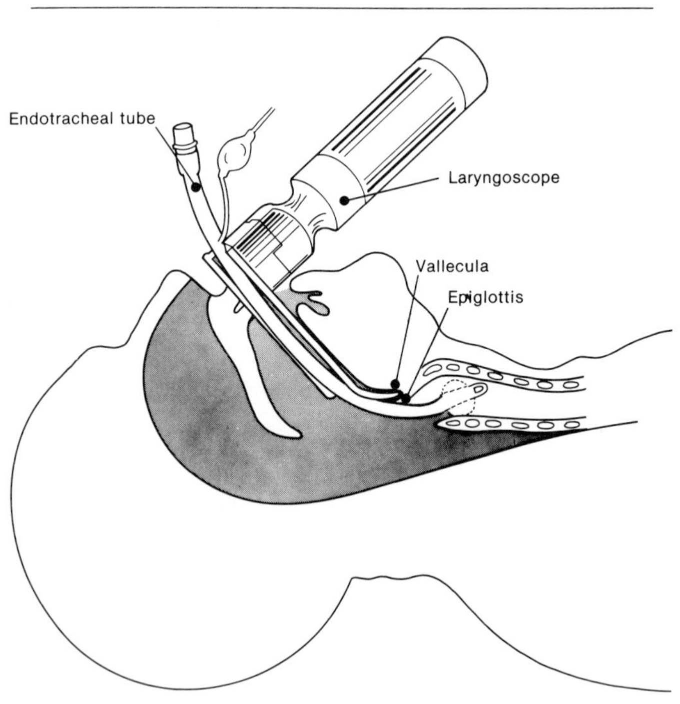

Figure 7–3 Endotracheal Intubation.

of action dictated by the clinical assessment, however. Blood gas values are most useful in the process of ongoing therapy, rather than as *the* diagnostic tool that determines when to initiate therapy.

The etiology of respiratory depression or inadequate ventilation in the trauma victim can often be divided roughly into two broad groups: central or peripheral.

Central Respiratory Depression. Central causes of respiratory depression are usually secondary to severe head trauma. Intracranial hemorrhage and/or cerebral contusion with edema can lead to transtentorial herniation and suppression of medullary centers. Increasing hypoxia and hypercapnia, owing to depressed respiration, further increase tissue anoxia and cerebral vasodilatation, which in turn perpetuates and augments cerebral edema. The management of centrally caused respiratory depression is, of course, immediate endotracheal intubation and ventilatory support to decrease arterial CO_2 tension and increase tissue oxygenation. Mannitol infusion is a temporizing measure to reduce cerebral edema until definitive treatment is possible. Another central cause of respiratory depression is spinal injury, which should be suspected whenever respiratory distress is associated with hypotension and bradycardia. Respiratory support is mandatory.

Peripheral Respiratory Depression. Ventilatory insufficiency from peripheral causes is due to trauma to the thoracic cage or its contents, that prevents adequate alveolar ventilation. This type of injury can be classified as either nonpenetrating (blunt) or penetrating. One of the most important considerations in the management of patients with chest trauma is the early and judicious use of the volume-cycled respirator. Whether they have experienced blunt or penetrating trauma to the chest, all patients benefit from maximal ventilation and oxygenation. It is far more prudent to ventilate the major trauma patient early than to hesitate and wait for the development of respiratory distress and shock. During the resuscitative process, the arterial PO_2 should be maintained above 80 mm Hg, if possible. This may require inspired oxygen concentrations of up to 100 percent. It is recommended that, whenever possible and indicated, PEEP be used, as this tends to reduce post-resuscitation complications of alveolar collapse, adult respiratory distress syndrome, and pneumonia.

Nonpenetrating injuries of the chest wall range from mild contusion to severely flailing segments of the thoracic cage. Morbidity and mortality result from either damage to the intrathoracic structures (e.g., lung or myocardial contusion, collapsed lung, or damage to the great vessels) or loss of integrity of the thoracic wall itself. When proper ventilatory mechanics cannot be maintained because of pain or unstable rib segments, the ensuing reduction in tidal volume (and, consequently, minute ventilation) makes respiratory distress

imminent, and respiratory support becomes a necessity. Of particular importance is the early recognition of fractures of the first and second ribs. Owing to their relatively protected location, any traumatic event that causes such fractures is assumed to be considerable and the patient's prognosis is guarded. The physician must search very thoroughly for other, underlying injuries, such as hemothorax, pneumothorax, transection of the aorta, or myocardial contusion, as the incidence of these associated complications is very high.[5]

Patients with respiratory distress, tracheal shift, asymmetric and reduced air entry, subcutaneous emphysema, tympanic percussion, and palpable, unstable rib segments should be treated for pneumothorax even before radiologic confirmation of the pneumothorax. Chest tube drainage should be instituted at once. If the diagnosis is in doubt, it is a simple and relatively complication-free procedure to place a thin (20 gauge) needle or Hemlich valve into the pleural space of the affected side, with a syringe, to check for free air. The procedure is at once diagnostic and therapeutic. Valuable time is often lost in awaiting roentgenograms to confirm the obvious, while the patient deteriorates with tension pneumothorax.

The trauma victim rarely has an isolated pneumothorax. Trauma to the chest nearly always involves some degree of hemorrhage; therefore, a hemothorax is to be expected as well. For this reason, it is advocated that chest tube thoracostomies be placed in the sixth intercostal space in the midaxillary line, as this placement facilitates the drainage of blood (Fig. 7–4). After skin preparation and local anesthetic infiltration (if required), a 2- or 3-cm incision is made parallel to the long axis of the rib. Using blunt and sharp dissection, the physician divides the serratus anterior and intercostal muscles, exposing the parietal pleura. After the pleura has been incised, the thoracostomy tube is placed in the thoracic cavity and sutured in place. The distal end of the tube is then placed under water seal drainage, with or without negative pressure. In the critically hypovolemic patient, chest tube drainage also allows for rapid autotransfusion of the blood collected in the pleural space.[6] (See Chapter 71)

Severe compression injuries of the chest can cause multiple rib fractures. Frequently, each rib has two or more fracture sites, resulting in an unstable, separated portion of the chest wall. This is known as traumatic flail chest. The paradoxical movement of the affected portion of the chest wall and, thus, the diagnosis are usually obvious. In order to reduce the large dead space inherent in this condition and increase the effectiveness of ventilation, the flailing segment must be stabilized. Sand bags are satisfactory initially; they reduce at least one component of the paradoxical movement. Definitive care (depending on the size of the flail) usually

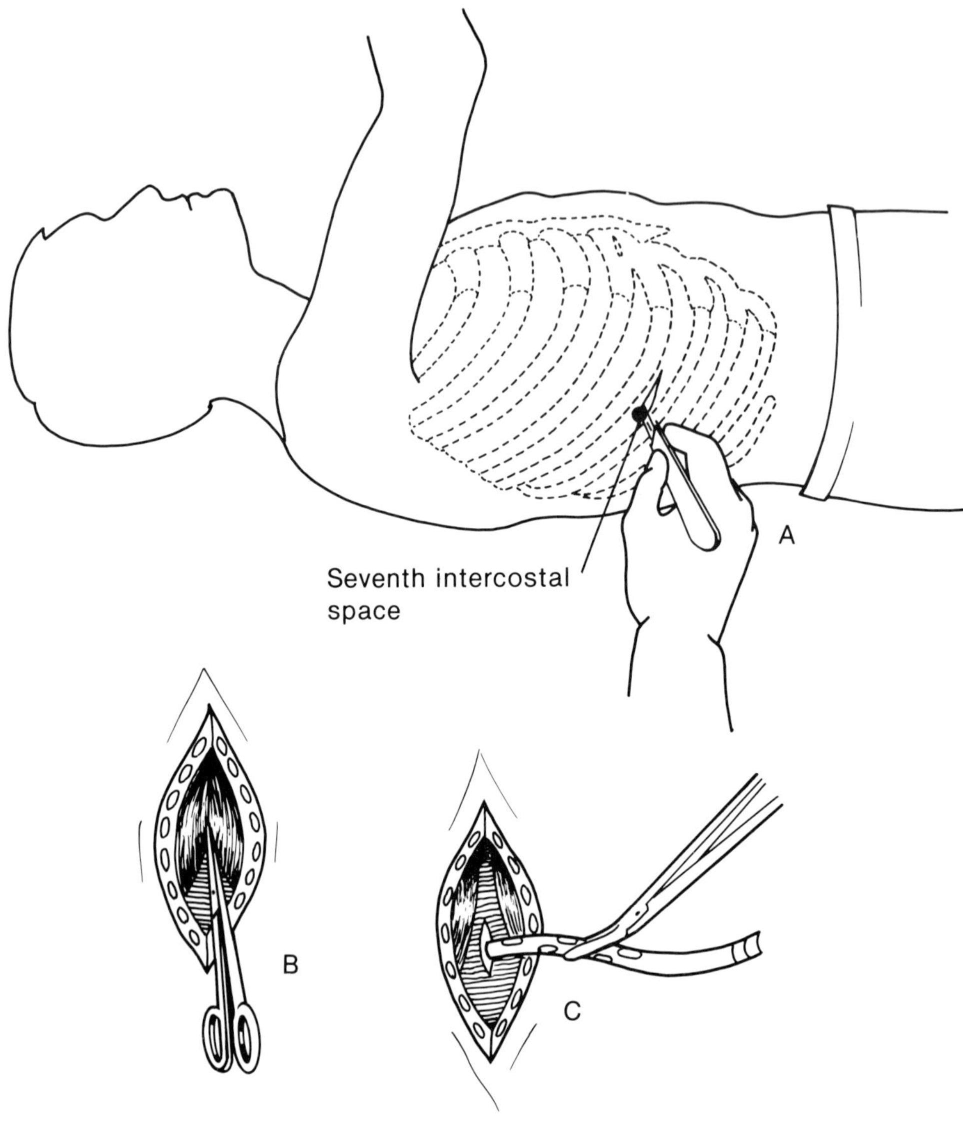

Figure 7–4 Tube Thoracostomy.

involves tracheostomy and respiratory support. Recently, intercostal nerve blocks for analgesia, with or without the use of external traction for stabilization, have been coming back into vogue since they do not have the complication rate characteristic of long-term respirator therapy. (See Chapter 61).

Fractures of the sternum are associated with trauma of great violence, and there is usually underlying mediastinal injury as well. These patients have severe cardiac contusions and hemopericardium. Flailing segments of the sternum generally involve both sides of the thorax, and severe respiratory distress can be expected. This is a surgical emergency that requires immediate attention.

Penetrating injuries of the chest wall can occur as a result of a low-velocity force (e.g., with a knife) or a high-velocity force (e.g., with a projectile). Usually, it is impossible to determine the extent of underlying organ damage by the external appearance of the wound; objects that penetrate the thoracic cavity are deflected by both bone and tissue planes, imparting their kinetic energies to the adjacent structures. For that reason, definitive treatment requires more extensive information about the injuring force than is usually available when life-saving action must be taken. Wounds of this type may require surgical exploration eventually, if not immediately. Defects in the chest wall, referred to as sucking chest wounds, may prevent the thoracic cavity from maintaining the pressures necessary for proper respiratory mechanics, and the resultant mediastinal shifts and ineffective to-and-fro movements of air make this a potentially lethal condition. Immediate management involves the rapid occlusion of these wounds with whatever is available, the only requirement being airtightness. If occlusion of the sucking wound creates a tension pneumothorax, the placement of a chest tube, as described previously, is indicated.

Circulation

Control of Hemorrhage. Control of the circulation involves bringing an immediate halt to any active hemorrhage and replacing lost intravascular volume. Any significant external hemorrhage should be stopped by any or all of the following methods: direct pressure, pressure dressings, tourniquets, ligature of bleeding vessels, or pneumatic trousers or splints. No time should be lost by trying to locate the exact source of the hemorrhage until the patient has been somewhat stabilized. It is enough at this stage to arrest the flow.

Pneumatic antishock garments have been in use for a number of years, and their importance at both the prehospital and the in-hospital level of care should not be underrated. Properly applied, they provide a rapid increase of intravascular volume in critical areas by decreasing blood flow to nonessential areas. Dramatic increases in blood pressure and augmentation of cerebral, myocardial, pulmonary, and renal perfusion[7] can be obtained. The tamponade effect of these pressure suits also decreases, if it does not actually arrest, active internal and external hemorrhage. As mentioned earlier, antishock garments previously applied by the paramedics should not be removed until adequate intravascular volume has been restored. Even then, the process of removal must be a carefully considered, slow, meticulous procedure with constant monitoring of vital parameters.

IV Catheter Insertion. Once external hemorrhage has been stopped and other measures have been initiated to stabilize the trauma patient's hemodynamic status, attention is focused on gaining access to the circulation, i.e., IV insertion for both fluid and drug administration. (Even though these various first-priority topics are discussed sequentially, with the team approach to trauma management, all of the life-saving measures are actually performed simultaneously.) The goal of IV catheter insertion is to make it possible to infuse massive volumes of fluids rapidly. Also, at the time of IV insertion, blood samples are withdrawn for a hemogram, determination of the coagulation times, biochemical studies, toxicology profiles, and typing and cross matching.

Although it is preferable to have access to the central circulation, physicians who are unfamiliar with the techniques of central venous catheterization should not hesitate to insert any other type of IV, be it a peripheral or a cut-down procedure. No one technique is favored above another; the criteria are speed of insertion and fluid flow capacity. There are also no rules about how many IVs should be started, although at least two (one on either side of the diaphragm) are recommended.[2] In practice, it is the patient's hemodynamic status and rate of response to volume infusion that determines the number and location of the IV lines.

Physicians who care for the critically injured should become familiar with at least one technique of central venous catheterization. (See Chapter 71.) The subclavian approach is one route that can be used in an emergency (Fig. 7–5). After skin preparation of the anterosuperior chest and administration of local anesthesia, the patient is placed in the Trendelenburg position to facilitate the filling and distention of the subclavian vein. One fingerbreadth below and lateral to the midclavicular point, a largebore needle on a syringe is introduced through the skin and passed just under the clavicle in the direction of the opposite shoulder. Once the vein is entered, as evidenced by the draw-back of blood in the syringe, a catheter is threaded through the needle into the superior vena cava. The needle is then withdrawn, and the catheter is sutured in place. Not only does this route allow the rapid infusion of large volumes of fluid, but also it permits measurement of the central venous pressure, which is a useful gauge of circulating volume.

A Foley catheter should be inserted at this stage to measure hourly urine output, which indicates the glomerular filtration rate and thus vital organ perfusion.

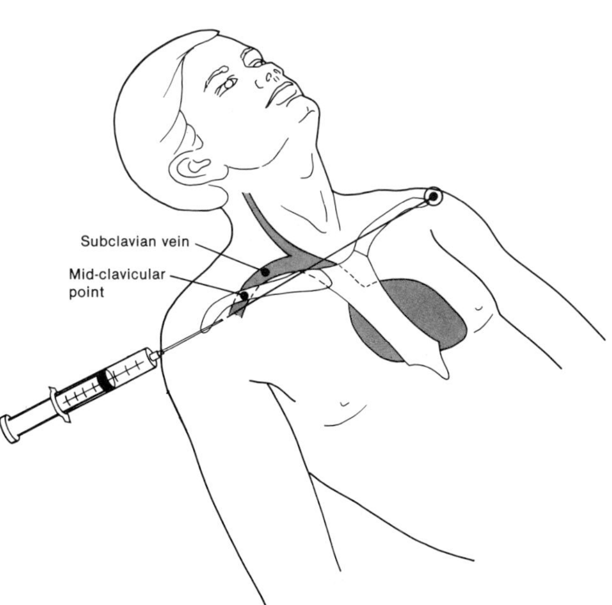

Figure 7–5 Subclavian Catheterization.

Fluid Resuscitation. The urgent fluid requirements of the multiple trauma patient include rapid expansion of intravascular volume and maintenance of sufficient hemoglobin for adequate oxygenation of tissues. It is obvious that the ideal fluid for replacement would be exactly what has been lost—fresh whole blood—but a controversy is raging about the composition of the initial resuscitation fluid when blood is unavailable. Colloid or crystalloid? It is an incontestable fact that colloids are better volume expanders, volume for volume, than crystalloids. They also match the fluid lost more closely and tend to stay in the intravascular compartment longer than crystalloids. On the other hand, crystalloid solutions have the advantages of immediate availability and low cost; therefore, crystalloids will probably continue as first-line resuscitative fluids in most minor and non-critical multiple trauma cases. Some centers, however, are turning to colloids, at least in part, for their resuscitative programs for the massively injured. Foremost among these is the MIEMS program.

In the MIEMS protocol, fluid resuscitation begins with the infusion of plasma protein fractions (Plasmanate) for blood pressure support. If the initial hematocrit of the patient is already low, i.e., less than 25 percent, then any further hemodilution will only worsen the already impaired oxygen-carrying capacity of the blood. Packed cells are infused as rapidly as possible; if necessary, uncross-matched type O Rh-negative blood is given. The rate of colloid and red cell infusion is coordinated to stabilize the blood pressure at a minimum of 90 to 100 mm Hg. Crystalloids in the form of Ringer's lactate or normal saline may be added to the resuscitation regimen once the patient's hemodynamic status has stabilized. The introduction of crystalloids at this stage is to improve urine output. This regimen for the immediate fluid management of the critically injured expands intravascular volume, restores oxygen transport capacity, and promotes renal function.[2,8]

The trauma victim's response to blood and fluid replacement is carefully monitored by continual assessment of blood pressure, pulse, oxygenation, level of consciousness, capillary refilling, urinary output, and central venous pressure. If the response of the patient is less than expected in view of the initial estimate of the extent of injury and volume of fluids infused, then occult blood loss with more extensive trauma must be suspected. A careful etiologic investigation should be undertaken.

THE SECOND PRIORITY

If, during the first phase of resuscitation, the trauma patient's cardiorespiratory status has been stabilized, attention may then be turned to a meticulous secondary survey of the patient's condition. This involves a thorough history of the traumatic event and a careful physical examination that is concentrated on hitherto unexamined areas, such as the central nervous system, the abdomen, the genitourinary tract, the musculoskeletal structures, and soft tissues. Monitoring and surveillance is continued, of course, and any trend toward instability is quickly noted and treated.

If the patient's initial status has not stabilized as expected after primary resuscitation, or if deterioration is detected in either the hemodynamic or neurologic status through the surveillance procedure, then certain urgent diagnostic procedures must be considered.

Hemodynamic Instability

Sometimes the cause of poor or deteriorating hemodynamic response is clear, as when major intrathoracic hemorrhage is indicated by a continual outpouring of blood through the thoracostomy tube. Although it is possible to tamponade such a hemorrhage by clamping the tube, this is a temporizing measure at best. The patient will certainly have to undergo surgical exploration of the wound for control of the source of hemorrhage. At other times, the reasons for continued or impending shock are not so evident. Two areas of investigation in these cases deserve special mention: pericardial tamponade and intra-abdominal injuries.

Pericardial Tamponade

In the presence of penetrating injuries of the chest or severe blunt trauma to the mediastinum, the physician should consider pericardial tamponade, especially if the patient is in shock but has no significant ventilatory impairment. At this point, either critical hypovolemia or pericardial tamponade may be suspected. Pericardial tamponade is confirmed, however, when shock persists and the central venous pressure is elevated or becomes so in response to IV infusion. It is important to have serial determinations of the central venous pressure as blood volume is being restored; otherwise, the elevation in central venous pressure may not be initially evident.[9] The classic triad of Beck (distended neck veins, low blood pressure, muffled heart sounds) and pulsus paradoxus are not reliable signs of pericardial tamponade in the trauma victim, owing to their nonspecificity and variability with time.

Once the diagnosis has been made, a substantial temporary improvement in the patient's hemodynamic status may be obtained by performing a pericardiocentesis and removing as little as 20 to 30 ml of blood (Fig. 7–6). Pericardiocentesis is performed following routine skin preparation under strict sterile technique. After local anesthetic infiltration, a 4-inch #18 spinal needle

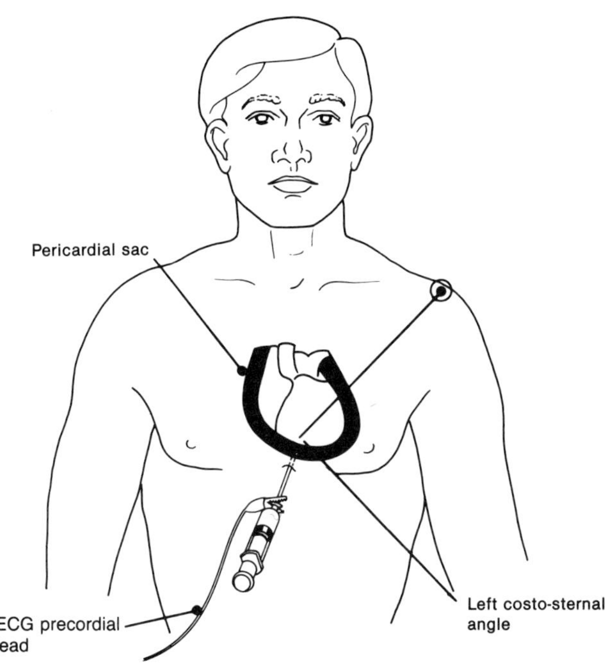

Figure 7–6 Pericardiocentesis.

is attached to the chest lead of an electrocardiogram (ECG) and introduced through the left costosternal angle in the direction of the left shoulder, at an angle of 45° to the chest wall. When the pericardium is entered, a "pop" is usually felt and blood can be withdrawn through a syringe. If an injury pattern begins to appear on the V lead of the ECG, then the needle tip is withdrawn slightly, as it is in contact with the myocardium. A catheter may also be introduced through the needle and left in place for continual drainage and pressure release. (See Chapter 71.)

Intra-abdominal Injuries

Like chest injuries, intra-abdominal injuries may be produced by either blunt or penetrating trauma. The main problem with all abdominal injuries is in arriving at the correct diagnosis soon enough to prevent extended morbidity or death (as in the actively bleeding, hypotensive patient). Two major types of life-threatening conditions may occur following either blunt or penetrating trauma: one immediate, i.e., severe hemorrhage, and the other delayed, i.e., rupture of the hollow viscus with subsequent chemical or bacterial peritonitis. Of the two, hemorrhage is the most critical. Penetrating abdominal injuries with concurrent, unexplained, persistent shock pose less of a diagnostic and therapeutic problem than do blunt injuries. The indication for emergency laparotomy in the former is well defined. The multiple trauma patient with blunt ab-

dominal injury, however, usually has equivocal and unreliable physical signs of intra-abdominal trauma. The patient may be unconscious or intoxicated; other conditions or injuries may mask abdominal injuries or prevent a proper evaluation of them. Although a careful, complete physical examination of the abdomen is needed, peritoneal lavage is an objective procedure that provides more accurate and faster information than the traditional examination in these cases (Fig. 7–7). Indications for emergency peritoneal lavage are (1) unexplained hypotension, (2) comatose or uncooperative, unreliable patient, or (3) equivocal physical findings. One important advantage of this test is that it can be performed at the bedside with local anesthesia and readily available equipment.

The bladder and stomach are decompressed by Foley and nasogastric tubes, respectively. If possible, an upright chest roentgenogram is taken to exclude preexisting intraperitoneal air. Once the abdomen is prepared and draped, a small amount of local anesthetic is infiltrated at a point between the superior and middle third of a line drawn between the umbilicus and the pubis; preexisting abdominal scars should be avoided. A small midline incision is made and the dissection

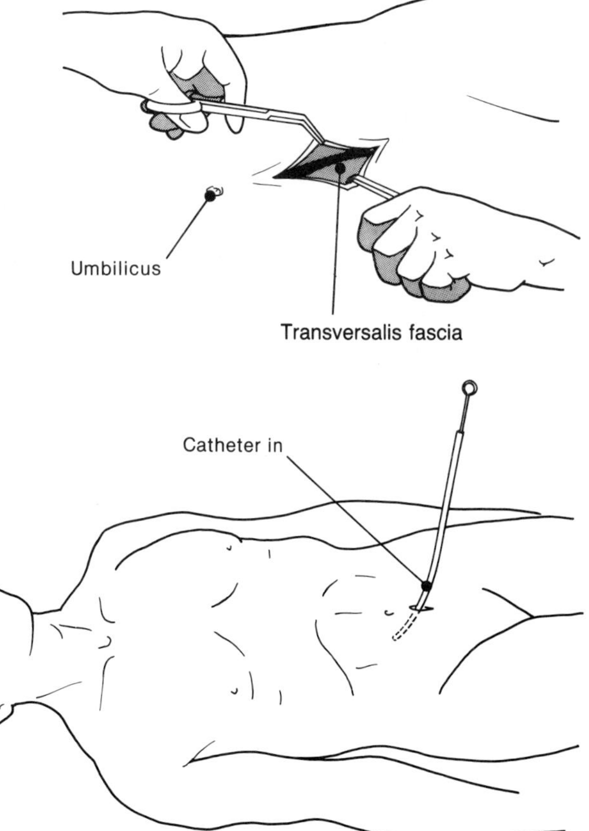

Figure 7–7 Peritoneal Lavage.

carried down to the peritoneum. After careful hemostasis, the peritoneum is opened and a catheter inserted into the abdominal cavity. If aspiration recovers gross blood, the lavage is considered positive and laparotomy is indicated. If there is no aspirate, then 1 liter normal saline is infused into the abdominal cavity and subsequently allowed to drain out. The lavage is positive if this fluid contains (1) more than 500 white blood cells/cu mm; (2) amylase greater than 100 Somogy units/100 ml; (3) more than 100,000 red blood cells/cu mm; or (4) bile, bacterial, or intestinal contents.[10] Usually, a positive lavage mandates laparotomy for further investigation. Until that can be accomplished, pneumatic trousers, as previously described, can provide a degree of tamponade to slow or control intra-abdominal hemorrhage. If the lavage is negative, then it can be assumed that the cause of the hemodynamic instability is not intra-abdominal injury.

An area not to be ignored when occult blood loss is being sought is the retroperitoneal space. It can collect several liters of blood without marked clinical manifestations. Bulging of the flank area, sometimes the only physical finding, and disappearance of the psoas shadows on plain roentgenograms of the abdomen suggest the diagnosis. Peritoneal lavage may be valuable in detecting this area of occult blood loss, for significant retroperitoneal hemorrhage has been associated with blood in the peritoneal cavity in spite of an intact peritoneum. In any event, the magnitude of trauma required to produce extensive retroperitoneal hemorrhage frequently results in intra-abdominal injuries detectable by peritoneal lavage. The high incidence of retroperitoneal hemorrhage as a result of pelvic fractures should be remembered when unexplained hypotension and pelvic fractures are concurrent.[11] The physician must deal not only with initial blood loss, which may exceed 2 liters, but also with continual hemorrhage from the pelvic venous plexus. (See Chapter 8.)

The most frequently overlooked sites of continual blood loss are closed tubular bone fractures. Because there is no laceration or visible bleeding, the significant amount of blood that may be sequestered in the soft tissues surrounding this area may be discounted. The failure to recognize this source of hemorrhage often leads to fluid loss underestimation and inadequate volume replacement.

Neurologic Instability

Only when all other possible sources of hemorrhage have been eliminated as the cause of a persistent hypotension can the possibility of central nervous system injury as the causative factor be investigated. Neurogenic shock can be seen in severe head trauma with brain stem involvement, as well as in spinal cord injuries. It is most important to document cervical spine injury early so that the patient will be handled appropriately. In a conscious, cooperative patient, the diagnosis of spinal injury is not problematic; pain, paralysis, and loss of sensation make it evident. In the comatose patient, however, it is somewhat more difficult, but bradycardia and hypotension without hypovolemia suggest it. Therefore, one of the few radiographs that is often mandatory early in the management of the trauma patient is a cervical roentgenogram that includes all seven vertebrae.

Patients with significant head injury should be monitored by repeated assessments of their level of consciousness and identification of focal neurologic signs. However, the majority of these patients are unconscious upon admission or have an assortment of injuries that make useful neurologic examination difficult, if not impossible. Often, the patient requires surgery for other critical injuries so that the prompt diagnosis of neurosurgically correctable lesions, such as an epidural or subdural hematoma, becomes imperative. A definitive diagnosis can best be accomplished with a computerized axial tomography (CT) scanner. If this is not readily available, or if the patent's condition precludes transport to a CT scanner, useful information may be obtained from a carotid angiogram, which can usually be done with portable equipment.

If the trauma patient's initial condition is neurologically stable, but the level of consciousness deteriorates or focal neurologic signs appear, the first response of the trauma team should be to exclude causes other than rising intracranial pressure. The prime causes to be investigated are ongoing ventilatory or circulatory insufficiency. When the deterioration in neurologic status has been found to be secondary to raised intracranial pressure, every attempt should be made to reduce it, even before confirmation of the exact etiology, i.e., intracranial hemorrhage or cerebral edema. If surgical decompression is required, any reduction in intracranial pressure that can be achieved while the patient is being prepared or transported is a valuable temporizing, time-saving procedure. If the cause of increased pressure is cerebral edema secondary to brain contusion, the definitive treatment is monitoring and controlled pressure reduction. This can begin in the emergency department. The modalities available for intracranial pressure reduction are

1. hyperventilation to obtain a reduction of the PCO_2 to 25 mm Hg.
2. hypothermia.
3. diuretics, e.g., mannitol or furosemide. Mannitol, in addition to being an osmotic diuretic, also increases cerebral blood flow. The dosage recom-

mended is 0.5 to 1 gm/kg infused over five minutes.[12] Some centers are beginning to use furosemide, in 40- to 80-mg boluses, in an attempt to circumvent the complications of fluid overload inherent with the use of mannitol.

4. dexamethasone. Although not an emergency drug, dexamethasone is believed to reduce mortality and morbidity in the severely brain injured. The recommended dosages are somewhat arbitrary, as there are no reliable dose-response data available. The Montreal Neurological Hospital advocates an initial 48 mg, followed by tapering dosages.

5. intraventricular drainage.

THE THIRD PRIORITY

Once the trauma team has resuscitated the patient and has begun treatment to correct any ongoing hemodynamic and neurologic instability, a careful review of the remaining body systems may be initiated. At this stage, a certain degree of flexibility in the planned approach to trauma care allows the physician to shift priorities according to circumstances.

Genitourinary System

A proper assessment of the urinary tract is almost totally dependent on radiologic examination. However, physical examination of the external genitourinary system, including the rectum, is still important. The presence of ecchymoses in the perineal or rectal areas could indicate urethral disruption. Since the insertion of a Foley catheter is recommended at the initial stages of resuscitation, early recognition of possible urethral injury is important. Catheterization of the urinary bladder not only monitors urinary output, but also provides information regarding the integrity of the urethra and bladder. If the Foley catheter does not pass into the bladder freely, it should not be forced. Gross blood obtained either on withdrawal of the catheter or through drainage from it could indicate urethral or bladder disruption. The presence of frank or microscopic hematuria may also signify injury in the urinary tract and requires thorough investigation.

Urethral injury may be determined by the retrograde injection of Renograffin into the urethra while radiographs are obtained. Similarly, the integrity of the bladder may be evaluated following Foley insertion and instillation of 250 ml Renograffin. The roentgenograms taken are then examined for urethral or bladder extravasation.

After the assessment of the lower genitourinary tract has been completed, the upper tract can be evaluated via the IV pyelogram. Information regarding renal function, as well as kidney and ureter integrity, can be obtained in this way. More sophisticated studes, i.e., renal angiography or renal scanning, can further elucidate any pathologic findings.

Special mention must be made of the association between fracture of the pelvic girdle and rupture of the urinary bladder, because it occurs so frequently.[13] If the bladder is full at the time of pelvic injury, it may rupture, either intraperitoneally or extraperitoneally. It is strongly recommended, therefore, that patients with pelvic fractures have a cystogram. (See Chapter 62.)

Musculoskeletal System

Injuries to the musculoskeletal system are usually fairly obvious clinically and easy to evaluate grossly. In spite of the striking nature of some of these injuries, the physician caring for the massively injured patient should not be deterred from the primary duties of resuscitation. In most instances, precise evaluation of musculoskeletal injuries can be delayed, but certain aspects of musculoskeletal injuries deserve early investigation.

The care of musculoskeletal injuries begins in the prehospital phase. Proper splinting and immobilization of fractures and dislocations en route to the hospital are absolute requirements if increased morbidity is to be avoided.

As discussed earlier, considerable blood loss can be concealed in and around fracture sites. This not only can seriously compromise circulation in the extremity, but also contributes to hypovolemia. The quantity of blood lost in this way must be calculated and restored to the circulation before radiologic examination or other investigations are undertaken.

Vascular deficiencies associated with musculoskeletal injuries have a high priority. Sites where capillary filling can be evaluated must be examined carefully and distal pulses should be checked thoroughly. Ultrasonic evaluation and selective angiography are useful and often indispensable adjuncts in determining vascular patency. It must be remembered that, many times, gentle manipulation or immobilization of a fracture or dislocation site can restore a pulse.

It is also important in musculoskeletal care to prevent additional contamination of open fracture sites. The skin surrounding the fracture site should be cleansed with surgical soap and the wound irrigated with sterile saline. The wound is then covered with a sterile occlusive dressing.

The basic tool for the evaluation of skeletal injuries, as it was for genitourinary trauma, is the roentgenogram. Once the clinical examination of skeletal injuries has been completed, radiologic examination is undertaken to confirm the extent of injury and plan for definitive treatment.

Very little has been mentioned earlier about radiologic examination of the massively traumatized patient because clinical evaluation is more important. The primary measures needed to stabilize a trauma victim depend almost entirely on clinical and procedural examination and cannot wait for roentgenograms. However, when it is time for radiologic efforts, they should be directed initially at the three major blind spots: the cervical spine, the chest, and the pelvis. The cervical spine examination consists of a lateral neck roentgenogram that demonstrates all seven vertebrae (most injuries involve the lower three vertebrae). An erect anteroposterior chest roentgenogram is taken after the cervical spine is determined to be normal. Specific attention is focused on widened mediastinal shadows, and aortography is performed if aortic rupture or dissecting aneurysm is suspected. A pelvic roentgenogram is obtained next, followed by other examinations as the situation warrants.[14] (See Chapter 8.)

Soft Tissue Injuries

With the exception of extensive burns, soft tissue injuries are low on the list of priorities. The usual management includes cleansing with surgical soap, irrigation, and application of a sterile occlusive dressing until more careful debridement and surgical repair can take place. This is adequate for most soft tissue wounds.

Thermal burns should be covered with saline-soaked sterile dressings until more definitive antibiotic and debridement therapy can be initiated. The top priority in major thermal burns (greater than 20 percent of the body surface area) is to replace plasma volume lost because of the increase in capillary permeability inherent in this condition. This loss is greatest in the first eight hours following injury.[15] Infection control is a secondary but equally important consideration in thermal burns. (See Chapters 10 and 21.)

Infection

The massively traumatized patient is especially prone to infection, not only because of the various types of injuries sustained, but also because of contaminants iatrogenically introduced through many invasive and therapeutic modalities. Supporting the immunologic defenses by providing adequate oxygenation, reducing shock, and preventing the post-traumatic catabolic metabolic state is the basis of infection control.

Cultures should be obtained from grossly contaminated wounds. Broad-spectrum antibiotic therapy should be commenced, especially in the presence of possible intestinal injuries. All patients with open wounds should receive tetanus immunization.

REFERENCES

1. Fischer RP, et al: Direct transfer to operating room improves care of trauma patients. *JAMA* 240:1731, 1978.
2. Gill W, Long W: *Shock Trauma Manual.* Baltimore, Williams & Wilkins Co, 1979.
3. Greene R, et al: Trauma of the larynx and trachea. *Radiol Clin North Am* 16:309, 1978.
4. Mulder DS, et al: The use of the fiberoptic bronchoscope to facilitate endotracheal intubation following head and neck trauma. *J Trauma* 15:638–640, 1975.
5. Wilson JM, et al: Severe chest trauma: Morbid implications of first and second rib fractures in 120 patients. *Arch Surg* 113–846, July 1978.
6. Symbas PN: Extra-operative autotranfusion from hemothorax. *Surgery* 84:722, 1978.
7. Raksom K, et al: Respiratory function following application of MAST trousers. *JACEP* 7:15, 1978.
8. Sohmer PR, et al: Transfusion therapy in trauma: A review of the principles and techniques used in the MIEMS Program. *Am Surg* 45:109, 1979.
9. Yao ST, et al: Haemodynamics and therapy of acute hemopericardium. *J Trauma* 13:36, 1973.
10. Fischer RP, et al: Diagnostic peritoneal lavage: 14 years and 2586 patients later. *Am J Surg* 136:1701, 1978.
11. Brownstein PW, et al: Concealed haemorrhage due to pelvic fracture. *J Trauma* 4:832, 1964.
12. Bruce DA, et al: Resuscitation from coma due to head injury. *Crit Care Med* 6:254, 1978.
13. Pokorny M, et al: Urologic injuries associated with pelvic trauma. *Urology* 121:455, 1979.
14. Ayella RJ: Radiology and the massive trauma victim. *Am Surg* 45:126, 1979.
15. Moncrief JA: Burns: Initial treatment. *JAMA* 242:179, 1979.

8. Orthopedic Emergencies

JAMES W. ALLEN, M.D.

Orthopedic emergencies constitute a very large part of the emergency department physician's daily practice. It is well known that vehicular accidents, industrial trauma, and the everyday hazards of living seem to supply the busy hospital emergency department with a steady stream of patients with orthopedic problems. Also, increased leisure time and a wide variety of recreational and sporting activities are contributing factors to the increase in orthopedic emergencies. It is imperative that the emergency department physician and emergency care personnel be skilled in the recognition, evaluation, and treatment of these problems.

PRIORITIES AND APPROACH TO DIAGNOSIS AND TREATMENT

Emergency department personnel must have established priorities and a systematic approach in dealing with all orthopedic emergencies. In the severely traumatized patient the establishment of airway, breathing, and circulation is, of course, of paramount concern. The need for immobilization of suspected cervical spine injuries until a more definitive judgment can be made is well known and recognized. Concern for possible intrathoracic or intra-abdominal injuries takes precedence over that for orthopedic injuries, unless there would be serious hemostatic or neurovascular compromise associated with the orthopedic injury.

An adequate history is essential, as is a complete, pertinent physical examination performed in a systematic manner. The patient should be viewed as a whole person with an injured part—not just as "a broken arm" or "a sprained ankle." The patient's age, sex, occupation, and style of living need to be considered and the nature of the problem, the usual course of events, and how it will likely affect the patient should be fully explained. The need for follow-up care should always be emphasized.

History

There are few medical specialties that lend themselves to deriving an accurate diagnosis more than orthopedics, because, for the most part, the injured or affected area is readily available to direct examination through inspection, palpation, and assessment of function. However, the importance of an accurate history cannot be overemphasized. From very minor injury to obvious severe trauma, a specific history and mechanism of injury can frequently yield the diagnosis before the physical examination is even attempted.

Included in the history should be the manner of presentation to the emergency department (e.g., by rescue squad, on a cart, by wheelchair, ambulatory, or with or without limp). A detailed account of the mechanism of injury can be truly enlightening. The patient's symptoms and disability produced by the injury are then recorded. Previous injury, symptoms, or disability is noteworthy.

Physical Examination

Physical examination requires the observation of the position and attitude of the affected part; the assessment of sensation and motor function, circulation, range of motion, swelling, apparent deformity, ecchymosis, discoloration, or loss of skin integrity; and, especially, the localization of tenderness (preferably the exact location of maximal tenderness). With care and experience this can be done with little or no additional harm or discomfort to the patient.

One of the common mistakes made in the emergency department is inadequate exposure of the patient and the affected part. For example, a patient with an injured knee who is sitting in a chair in the hallway cannot be adequately examined. The area to be examined must be fully visualized and inspected to ascertain the presence or absence of open wounds, abrasions, or signs such as discoloration, temperature changes, swelling, or other abnormalities that can be easily overlooked without proper patient preparation.

Use and Interpretation of Radiographs

Radiographs should be obtained when the signs and symptoms of the patient, or the mechanism of injury, lead the examiner to suspect skeletal damage. Bone or joint tenderness requires radiographic evaluation of the affected part. With few exceptions, radiographs will help to ascertain the integrity of bones and joints (and their relationships) but reveal little, if any, information concerning the soft tissues and supporting structures. Radiographs should be specific (e.g., navicular views instead of wrist or hand films when the clinical presentation reveals only point tenderness over the anatomical snuff box of the wrist; finger films "long," or "ring," for example, when the swelling, pain, and tenderness are primarily in the finger and not the hand). At least two views must be obtained, usually anteroposterior and lateral, but frequently oblique or tangential views are necessary. Inadequate or incomplete radiographs should never be accepted. Additional views can be ordered when indicated. Comparison views are also of benefit on occasion, especially in children.

Once radiographs are obtained, they must be interpreted properly. All too often radiographs are requested and then only briefly or cursorily evaluated. A systematic approach in reading radiographs will help prevent misreading or missing a diagnosis. An overview, at a distance from the film, can be very helpful in avoiding mistakes of "tunnel vision." The use of magnification and "bright lighting" is also helpful in resolving many questionable areas. When doubt or uncertainty remains, arrangements should be made for further radiographic evaluation and follow-up.

Terminology

Orthopedic injuries should be described accurately and specifically. The following terms are used:

- *fracture*—any disruption of a bone's structural integrity classified and described according to various criteria: open or closed; by location (e.g., middle third, metaphyseal, intra-articular, supracondylar, epiphyseal); by type (e.g., linear, spiral, oblique, transverse simple, comminuted); and by relationship of bone ends (e.g., alignment, angulation, displacement, impaction). There are also pathologic fractures, as a consequence of preexisting disease, and stress fractures, due to repeated loading or fatigue.
- *dislocation*—complete loss of apposition of the articulating bones of a joint
- *subluxation*—disruption of normal configuration of a joint but with some amount of apposition of bone ends remaining
- *contusion*—(bruise) direct trauma or blow to a specific body area without bone or ligamentous injury
- *sprain*—joint injury occurring as a result of applied force; classified in order of increasing severity as grade I, II, or III, signifying degree and extent of ligamentous damage
- *strain*—often applied to soft or supporting structures of the skeleton; usually affects muscle or tendon and is due to overuse, overload, or otherwise exceeding physiologic limits.

These terms will accurately describe almost all traumatic conditions or injuries. Terms such as *tendonitis, fasciitis, myositis, bursitis*, and *cellulitis* should be reserved for describing specific inflammatory conditions of a particular anatomical location or structure.

General Considerations of Patient Care

Attempts to arrive at a clear, concise, and accurate diagnosis as possible should be made, but if the diagnosis is in doubt, the patient should be told so and encouraged to get further evaluation and follow-up care. When a reasonably accurate diagnosis is made the physician can then be more specific in prescribing a course of treatment, outlining the limitations of activity, and anticipating a return of function.

The standard care of most orthopedic injuries in the first 24 to 28 hours remains rest, elevation, immobilization or limited use, application of ice, and administration of analgesics. It is helpful to think of all orthopedic injuries as a spectrum in which a lesser force may produce a contusion and a greater force a fracture; for example, a lesser stress may produce a first-degree sprain and a greater one, a second-degree sprain. This concept can then be expanded to include treatment, so that a contusion or first-degree sprain only requires immobilization for a few days, whereas a fracture or second-degree sprain may require three weeks or more of immobilization.

Individuals respond in different manners and with varying speed to bodily insults and injuries; therefore, it is not advisable to be dogmatic concerning projected healing time, disability, or duration or degree of pain and discomfort. Providing the patient with simple guidelines and an expected course of events is of considerable benefit, however.

In virtually all cases, the need for further evaluation and treatment should be stressed if the patient continues to experience symptoms of discomfort or disability past a reasonable time post injury. It is good emergency department practice to ensure that the patient at least have a physician or clinic to refer to even if the injury is minor. Patients should be adequately instructed, both verbally and in writing, on the care of their injuries before they leave the emergency department.

SPECIFIC ORTHOPEDIC INJURIES

The Multiple Trauma Patient

Vehicular accidents are the cause of the majority of multiple systemic injuries, but the principles of management remain true and constant whatever the etiology of multiple trauma. (See Chapter 7.)

The history, either from the patient, if possible, or from a reliable witness, can be most informative in giving a clue as to what injuries to suspect; for example, in a high-speed automobile accident the front seat passenger whose knee is thrust into the dashboard can sustain a fractured patella, knee ligament tears, fractured femur or tibia, or hip dislocation all by the same mechanism. More than one of these injuries can occur at the same time.

Once the airway is established, breathing is adequate, and circulation is maintained, a baseline evaluation of the neurologic status and examination of the chest and abdomen can be quickly performed. Any suspected cervical spine injury should be evaluated by portable, lateral, cross table, cervical spine radiographs, with the patient's neck adequately immobilized. This immobilization can usually be accomplished with sandbags or cervical collar in the awake, cooperative patient but may require manual restraint or traction by the physician or other experienced medical personnel in the mentally obtunded or uncooperative patient. The patient should be maintained in this position unless and until there is certainty that no significant cervical spine or cord injury exists. Potential cervical spine injury should be suspected in all patients with severe trauma, in patients with severe head injuries, especially when the patient is unconscious, and in the elderly population or those patients with degenerative disease of the cervical spine in which less than violent forces can produce neurologic pathology. (See Chapter 43.)

A routine should be established and followed for a thorough examination of extremity injuries. Even with a careful history, and especially without one, it is imperative to inspect and palpate all accessible areas, preferably leaving any obvious sites of injury until last. A good method is to proceed distal to proximal; inspecting and palpating in this manner avoids the potential for missing a fracture or significant soft tissue injury that could be overlooked by fixating on a more obvious injury. Pulses, skin color and integrity, sensation, and motor function are routinely and conscientiously noted in all cases. Obvious fractures or dislocations should be left immobilized until radiographs are obtained, unless there is evidence of neurovascular compromise. Any suspected areas of bone or joint tenderness should be investigated with radiographs.

Spine Injuries

All trauma victims with suspected spine injuries should be transported on a bed board and with the patients' neck immobilized by a cervical collar or, preferably, sandbags if indicated by the apparent severity of signs or symptoms. Immobilization is maintained until at least an initial evaluation and judgment is made by a physician in the emergency department.

Cervical Spine

The cervical spine is the most mobile portion of the entire spine and certainly the most frequently exposed and injured in vehicular accidents. Fortunately, the vast majority of cervical spine injuries are not life-threatening nor permanently disabling and represent varying degrees of muscle strain, due to the sudden, forceful flexion and extension of this very flexible area. Palpation will usually reveal specific areas of tenderness, although frequently this may be diffuse or ambiguous. The spinous processes of C2, C7, and T1 are the most prominent. If the patient is unresponsive or has real or suspected neurologic pathology or if the signs and symptoms dictate, a portable, lateral, cross table, cervical spine radiograph should be taken without moving the patient. Any neurologic abnormality is usually cause for strict immobilization and admission, regardless of radiographic findings.

Symptoms of severe occipital, neck, or extremity pain, numbness or tingling, or weakness or inability to use the extremities in a normal manner are all cause for concern and suggest cervical spine injury.

Dysphagia from pharyngeal edema or retropharyngeal hematoma is also a serious symptom in acute cervical spine injury. The lateral neck radiograph may verify forward displacement of the airway.

Signs of asymmetric or absent reflexes, demonstrable motor or sensory deficit, or loss of sphincter control also convey a high index of suspicion of cervical spine injury.

The careful placement of a nasogastric tube to avoid the threat of further neck motion from vomiting or the possibility of aspiration, is recommended in spinal cord injuries. A Foley catheter also should be inserted.

Negative neurologic and radiographic findings allow for most patients to be treated with varying degrees of rest, limited physical activity, heat to the neck, and analgesics or muscle relaxants used in an adjunctive role. Any symptoms or disability that persist for more than a week or 10 days mandates follow-up treatment. See Chapter 43 for a review of cervical spine injuries.

Thoracic Spine

The thoracic spine is infrequently injured, in contrast to the cervical and lumbar areas, mostly because of its relatively restricted motion. Two exceptions are severe torsional forces, which can cause vertebral injuries in healthy individuals, and minor trauma in older patients or in patients with metabolic abnormalities in which bone is resorbed. Because of bone demineralization in these patients, compression fractures can occur in the thoracic spine. Also, the physician must be aware that tumors, metastases, and abscesses may rarely be seen on thoracic spine radiographs, with or without symptomatology.

Lumbar Spine

The lumbar spine bears the workload of trunk and limbs to a large extent in many everyday endeavors, and thus it is not surprising that work-related low back injuries are observed frequently. There is hardly any activity from sedentary to the most strenuous from which the lower back is not susceptible to injury. Compressive forces, shearing forces, load forces, and many others are constantly acting on the flexible lower back.

Inquiries concerning previous low back problems or surgery, treatment modalities, and the existence of radicular symptoms are helpful in understanding the patient's presenting complaints. The initial mechanism of injury can be enlightening. It is useful to remember that the spinal cord terminates at the L1 to L2 level and that the cauda equina and nerve roots descend through the spinal canal to the levels where the specific nerve roots pass through the lumbar foramen to supply the lower extremities. Fractures at the levels T12 to L2 comprise over 50 percent of all vertebral body compression fractures. Fractures of the transverse processes can also occur (usually these are traction/avulsion injuries). The possibility of kidney injury must be considered in all significant lower back trauma, and a urinalysis should be obtained. (See Chapter 62.)

Lumbar radiographs are indicated in patients with acute, significant trauma, in patients with low back problems without previous radiographs, and in patients with previous back problems who present with a significantly different pattern of symptomatology or with newly acquired neurologic findings and no recent radiograph. In viewing spinal radiographs, the physician must note the general alignment, along with the transverse and spinous processes and degenerative or arthritic changes. On the anteroposterior view, abnormalities of the spinous or transverse processes may be the only clue to malalignment or discovery of a systemic or metabolic process, as illustrated by pedicle destruction in certain malignancies.

Most compression or transverse process fractures of the lumbar spine are stable and can be treated with bed rest and limited activity at home in the absence of complicating factors, such as associated neurologic deficit, severe ileus, or when the patient's age or home factors militate against it.

Pelvic Fractures

Most multiple trauma patients with severe injuries should have a pelvic radiograph, and most patients with pelvic fractures must provide a urine specimen for urinalysis to exclude urinary tract injuries, an exception being patients with traction injuries from muscle/tendon contraction, such as avulsion fractures of the ischial tuberosity. The severity of pelvic fractures may range from these avulsion fractures to a complete disruption of the pelvic ring, including diastasis of the symphysis or sacroiliac subluxations and their associated fractures. The insertion of a Foley catheter or an initial cystourethrogram is mandatory in patients with more severe pelvic injuries. Complications of pelvic fractures are: rupture of prostatomembranous portion of the urethra in males, intrapelvic or retroperitoneal hemorrhage, and bladder injuries.

Simple, uncomplicated pelvic fractures can be managed like compression fractures of the lumbar spine. Patients with more severe fractures, those with associated hematuria, or those in whom control of pain or home care represents a significant problem should be hospitalized.

Extremity Injuries

One of the true, absolute emergencies in the field of orthopedics is the extremity injury that disrupts or jeopardizes the blood supply and vitality of the part distal to the injury site. This is usually a severe fracture or dislocation and must be recognized and promptly treated if there is to be any hope for the survival and return of function of the involved part. Pulselessness, pallor, cyanosis, cold temperature (compared with opposite side), and decrease or lack of motor or sensory function are all findings of serious present or impending catastrophe, and immediate steps must be taken.

Careful attempts at distracting or applying traction to the above ends of a fracture or dislocation and restoring them to near normal anatomical position, and maintaining this position, may be all that is necessary to alleviate and control the problem. This must be done slowly and smoothly, without undue force, to prevent further injury or insult. If this does not accomplish the desired result and the fracture or dislocation is relatively stabilized in as desirable reduction as possible, no further manipulation should be attempted. Further evaluation and treatment should then be handled by a vascular surgeon as rapidly as possible if there is to be a reasonable chance to salvage the involved part. It is thus obvious why frequent neurovascular checks are necessary both before and after reduction of major fractures and dislocations.

Fractures and Dislocations of the Upper Extremity

Clavicle Fractures. Clavicle fractures are very common especially in the younger age-group. In displaced fractures, reduction is practically impossible to maintain by whatever means. Virtually all clavical fractures heal with satisfactory shoulder function, although there may be slight deformity or overabundant callus formation in a few instances.

Treatment with some form of clavicle strap and sling is all that is necessary for most clavicle fractures. This can vary from a few weeks in children to 5 or 6 weeks for adults.

Acromioclavicular Separations. Acromioclavicular separations usually result from a direct force on the point of the shoulder, resulting in local tenderness and swelling over the joint. There is usually some limitation of motion. These injuries are properly classified as grade I, II, or III separation since this is a joint injury, and the pathology is manifested by injury to both the acromioclavicular ligaments and the coracoclavicular ligaments. It is useful to obtain acromioclavicular joint radiographs with weights to differentiate grade I from grade II separations, although both of these types are treated conservatively with sling immobilization. In grade III injuries there is complete disruption of the ligaments, which is recognized by the prominent, superiorly protruding distal end of the clavicle. Surgical repair in grade III separations is the treatment in certain selected cases, at the discretion of the orthopedist, although the conservative approach will result in an essentially normal functional shoulder.

Shoulder Dislocations. Eighty-five to 90 percent of shoulder dislocations are anterior and occur as a result of abduction and external rotation forces. Pain and loss of motion are severe, and there is a loss of the normal rounded lateral contour of the shoulder. Before there is any attempt at replacing the humerus into the glenoid fossa, a neurovascular evaluation is done, pain medication is given, and a shoulder radiograph is obtained. Reduction is more easily accomplished with proper and sufficient sedation and muscle relaxation, whatever the method employed. The Kocher maneuver, in experienced hands, is generally safe, swift, and sure and consists of gentle downward traction on the arm with the elbow flexed about 90 degrees, slow and steady external rotation and abduction of the extremity, and then abduction with continued external rotations and, finally, internal rotation of the abducted arm. The Hippocrates technique (foot in axilla) and Stimson's technique (hanging weights) can also be employed. Caution should be employed in performing these maneuvers since fractures or neurologic or vascular injuries may occur.

In the rare case in which an atraumatic reduction cannot be accomplished, it may be necessary to give the patient a general anesthetic to accomplish the reduction. Once the shoulder is back in place, the neurovascular evaluation is repeated, a radiograph is taken to confirm the reduction and to ensure that no fracture has occurred. The extremity is immobilized in a sling, usually for 3 weeks, to allow for soft tissue healing. Recurrent shoulder dislocations should be referred to an orthopedic surgeon for consideration of operative repair.

The physician should be alert for subluxations of the glenohumeral joint when the patient complains of the shoulder "slipping out of joint" or "clicking" or "clunking," with residual shoulder aching or numbness or tingling of arm or forearm. Physical examination may reveal resistance to motion or apprehension when attempting external rotation as well as anterior shoulder tenderness; the radiograph will be negative.

Posterior dislocations should be mentioned, because, although rare, they are frequently missed. Physical and radiographic findings are more subtle, but pain and limitation of motion cannot be ignored.

Sternoclavicular Dislocations. Sternoclavicular sprains are much less common than acromioclavicular injuries but represent the same spectrum at the medial end of the clavicle. Posterior dislocation of the sternoclavicular joint (three degrees) requires prompt recognition and reduction since the posteriorly displaced clavicle can cause pressure on the trachea, esophagus, great vessels, and other vital mediastinal structures. The reduction can be accomplished by levering the clavicle from its retrosternal position with posterior pressure on both shoulders, with a fulcrum (e.g., sandbag, knee) in the interscapular area, or by direct pull anteriorly on the medial clavicle, with a towel clip, if necessary.

Scapula Fractures. Scapula fractures are usually nondisplaced and stable and are treated with sling immobilization until pain and discomfort recede.

Humerus Fractures. Eighty percent of proximal humerus fractures are nondisplaced or minimally displaced and require only Velpeau or sling and swathe type dressings or simply sling immobilization. The most common is probably the surgical neck fracture in the elderly, usually female patient. Early shoulder motion is a key goal in these patients. Fractures displaced greater than 1 cm, fragments blocking motion of a joint, fracture-dislocations, or less than anatomically aligned fractures in active younger patients may require operative treatment.

Humeral shaft fractures usually result from direct trauma and can be treated closed with a hanging arm cast, traction, sling and swathe, or by open methods (usually compression plating). It is important to note that the radial nerve is vulnerable in fractures of the distal third of the humerus.

Elbow Fractures and Dislocations. Before specific fractures and dislocations of the elbow region are discussed, the so-called fat pad sign should be mentioned. This is a radiographic finding of radiolucency posterior to the distal humerus as seen in the lateral view of the elbow and represents displacement upward of the normal fat pad by fluid or blood in the elbow joint. The significance of a positive fat pad sign lies in its correlation with subtle or occult fractures about the area of the elbow and in the fact that it may be the only radiographic abnormality. A patient with recent trauma, clinical findings of a potential fracture, and a positive fat pad sign should be treated as if the patient had a fracture (even if none is observed on the radiograph) and reevaluated in 7 to 10 days.

Supracondylar fractures are more common in children and usually result from a fall on an outstretched hand with the elbow in extension. The most common form is with the distal condylar fragment displaced posteriorly. It can be reduced by applying traction with the elbow in extension, reducing the fracture fragment, and carefully placing the elbow in flexion. Application of a plaster posterior sling will maintain reduction and allow for soft tissue swelling.

More frequent in adults, condylar fractures often require operative reduction. Restoration of function and motion of elbow is frequently more important than anatomical reduction.

Eighty to 90 percent of elbow dislocations are posterior, and reduction is accomplished by longitudinal traction and flexion of the elbow. It is important to flex and extend the elbow joint through a full range of motion following reduction to ensure complete reduction and verify that there is no mechanical block to motion and to ascertain if the joint is stable. The elbow is then immobilized in at least 90 degrees of flexion.

Olecranon Fractures. Treatment of nondisplaced olecranon fractures is simple immobilization, but displaced fractures, diagnosed by the inability to extend the elbow against gravity, involve disruption of the triceps mechanism and require open reduction and internal fixation.

Radial Head Fractures. Radial head fractures may not produce obvious signs or symptoms, and the patient may not seek medical attention until days after injury. Most fractures of the radial head or neck are caused by indirect trauma such as a fall on the outstretched hand. Pain elicited from passive pronation and supination of the forearm should make the examiner suspicious of a radial head fracture. Frequently only a positive fat pad sign will be seen on the radiograph. More severe radial head fractures may require primary or secondary excision of the radial head, but most can be treated by immobilization and plaster splint or cast, followed by relatively early motion.

Forearm Fractures. Shaft fractures of both the radius and ulna, in an adult, are generally displaced and frequently require operative treatment. The elbow and wrist joint must be included in the radiographic examination of all forearm fractures, especially in the case of fractures of only one of the forearm bones; this will help prevent the physician from missing the diagnosis in Monteggia fractures (fracture of the shaft of the ulna with dislocation of the radial head) and Galeazzi fractures (fracture of the distal third of the radius with dislocation of the proximal radioulnar joint). Associated injury at the elbow or wrist should not be excluded if there is any degree of displacement of a single bone fracture of the forearm. Nondisplaced forearm fractures can be treated with a long arm cast.

Wrist Fractures and Dislocations. Colles' fractures make up a large percentage of adult fractures; these are fractures of the distal radius (with or without fracture of the ulna) in association with dorsal displacement of the distal fragment (Fig. 8–1A). These fractures are frequently severely comminuted. Reduction can be accomplished by distraction, with or without hyperextension, then volar displacement of the distal fragment, volar flexion, and ulnar deviation.

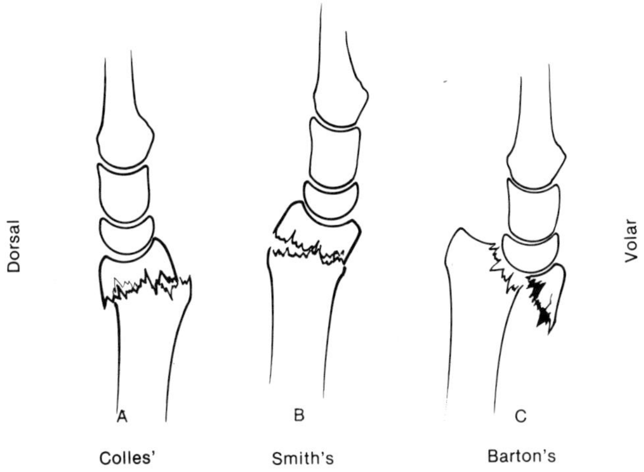

Figure 8–1   Fractures of Distal Forearm Bones. *A:* Colles'; *B:* Smith's; *C:* Barton's

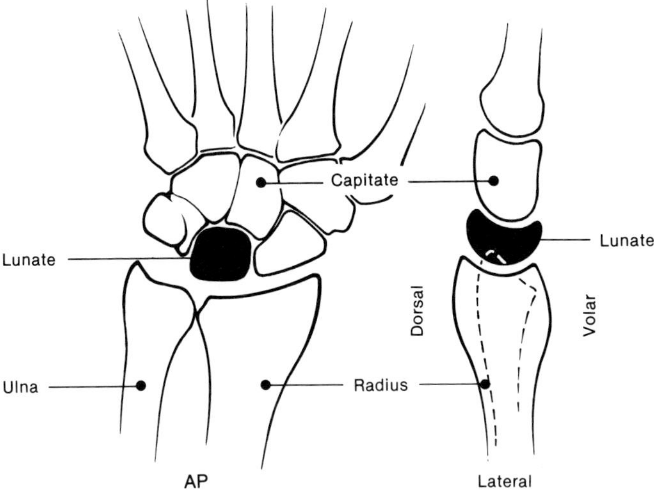

Figure 8–2   Normal Wrist, AP and Lateral View.

The opposite deformity, with volar displacement of the distal fragment of a distal radius fracture, is called a Smith's fracture (Fig. 8–1B) and tends to be more unstable than a Colles' fracture. Reduction of a Smith's fracture is by distraction, palmar flexion, and reduction of the distal fragment dorsally, with a cast applied with the wrist in neutral or slight flexion, not in dorsiflexion. Barton's fracture (Fig. 8–1C) is similar to Smith's fracture, but is usually more severe and may require open reduction and internal fixation. The normal bones of the wrist are shown in Figure 8–2.

Navicular fractures are diagnosed clinically by eliciting tenderness over the anatomical snuff box, just distal to the radial styloid. All patients with suggested navicular fractures because of localized tenderness, even when the radiograph is negative, should have their wrists

immobilized and rechecked in 2 to 3 weeks for tenderness or confirmatory radiographic findings at that time.

Dorsal chip or avulsion fractures of the carpal bones can be diagnosed by correlating the area of local tenderness on the back of the carpus with the presence of small chip fragments usually best seen on lateral radiographs. Lunate fractures and dislocations are fairly rare and frequently difficult to diagnose (Fig. 8–3).

Understanding the relationships on a wrist radiograph is the key to accurate diagnosis. In the lateral view, neutral position, the longitudinal axis of the long finger metacarpal, the capitate, the lunate, and the articulating face of the distal radius are all on the same horizontal line, and any distraction of this alignment represents a lunate or perilunate dislocation. In an anteroposterior view, these dislocations can be suspected by apparent shortening of the carpus with an overlap pattern. Closed reduction by traction and manipulation may be difficult, and open reduction may be necessary.

Perilunate dislocation may be seen either with or without a fracture of the scaphoid (Fig. 8–4). Although frequently overlooked on the initial radiograph, the diagnosis is made by the true lateral radiograph. The lunate and the radius are in the normal position but the capitate has dislocated dorsally around the lunate. Perilunate dislocation requires treatment by an orthopedic surgeon.

Metacarpal Fractures. Most fractures of the metacarpal shafts can be treated with cast or splint immobilization for 3 weeks. Fractures of the midshaft of phalanges and metacarpals may take longer. Fractures of the ring or small finger metacarpal neck with significant volar displacement (Boxer's fracture) should be reduced and a plaster splint applied. Fractures of the base of the middle metacarpals are frequently overlooked

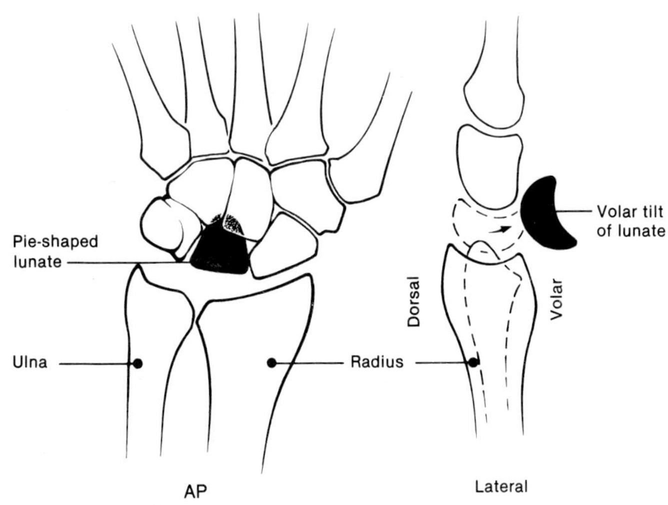

Figure 8–3   Lunate Dislocation AP and Lateral Views.

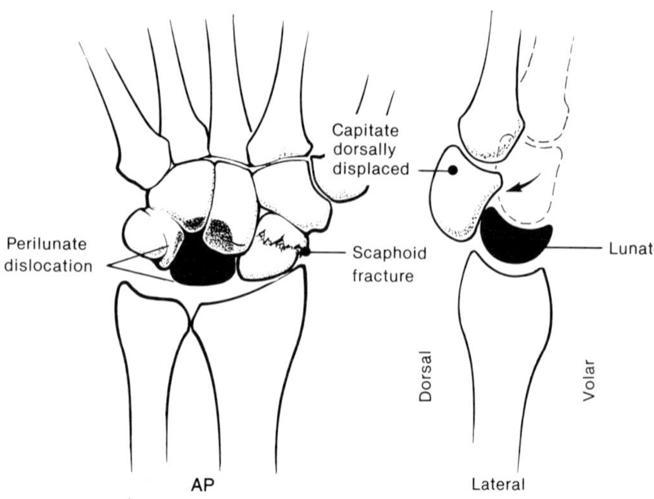

Figure 8–4　Perilunate Dislocation and Fracture of the Scaphoid.

on radiographs. The area of maximal tenderness must be examined carefully on the radiograph.

Phalangeal Fractures, Dislocations, and Ligamentous Injuries. Nondisplaced, nonarticular phalangeal fractures can be immobilized in position of function splints: 3 weeks for proximal phalanx, 2 weeks for middle phalanx, and 1 week for distal phalanx. Long oblique shaft or angulated fractures of the base of the phalanx need to be reduced and splinted with an adjacent, noninvolved digit—"buddy taping." Rotational deformities must be avoided in phalangeal fractures. Occasionally, open reduction or fixation may be necessary as in intra-articular fractures of the thumb metacarpal, the Bennett fracture, or the Rolando fracture.

The mallet finger, diagnosed by the volar displacement of the distal phalanx and inability to extend the distal interphalangeal joint, represents a disruption of the extensor tendon and may or may not have a dorsal chip avulsion fracture at the base of the distal phalanx on the lateral radiograph. Treatment is by splinting the distal joint in extension or mild hyperextension.

Dislocations occur at the metacarpophalangeal and the interphalangeal joints, most commonly at the proximal interphalangeal joints. A radiograph should be obtained first, and reduction should be accomplished with traction and gentle manipulation. The digit is splinted in position of function, and a second radiograph is obtained to confirm reduction and to rule out associated fracture.

Any finger joint with acute trauma, pain, tenderness, swelling, and limitation of motion deserves careful evaluation. Joint stability must be ascertained. Any joint instability represents significant damage to the collateral ligaments, volar plate, or both. Acute complete tears of the collateral ligaments should be operated on as in rupture of the ulnar collateral ligament of the

metacarpophalangeal joint of the thumb (gamekeeper's thumb). Joints with significant swelling or tenderness but that are stable should be immobilized in position of function and be reevaluated in a week.

Fractures and Dislocations of the Lower Extremity

Hip Dislocations and Fractures. The normal anatomy of the hip is shown in Figure 8–5. Considerable force is necessary to drive the femoral head from the acetabulum. Vehicular accidents are a common cause of hip dislocations. In anterior hip dislocations there is strong, forced abduction, resulting in an abducted and externally rotated lower extremity that can be flexed or extended. There is little, if any, shortening. Posterior dislocations result from a violent force applied against the flexed knee, as in a vehicular accident, with a resultant shortened, internally rotated, and abducted lower extremity with the hip in flexion. These injuries can occur with or without an associated fracture of the femoral head or acetabulum. Reduction must be accomplished quickly by exerting initial traction in the line of the femur with the pelvis stabilized by an assistant and by gentle manipulation following restoration of length. In central acetabular fracture-dislocation the femoral head is simply driven through the acetabulum.

Two broad categories serve to classify most hip fractures: the intracapsular or femoral neck fractures and the extracapsular or intertrochanteric fractures. The blood supply to the femoral head is somewhat tenuous and, therefore, relatively early treatment of femoral neck fractures is indicated if later vascular complications are to be avoided. Most femoral neck fractures are classified as stress, impacted, or displaced and can

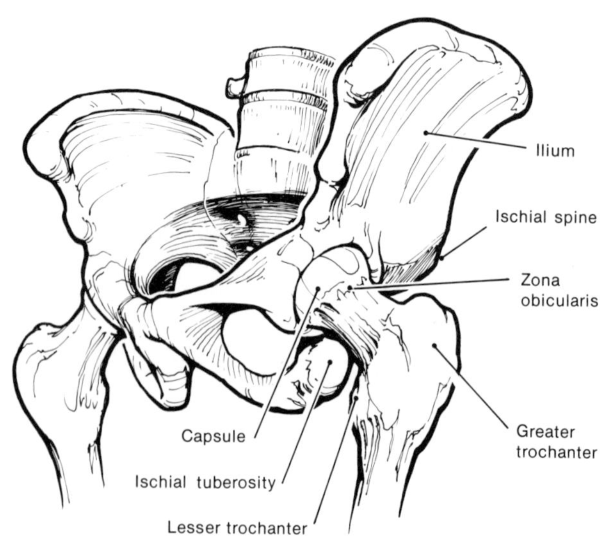

Figure 8–5　Normal Hip.

be described according to their radiographic appearance.

An intertrochanteric fracture presents as a shortened, externally rotated lower extremity (as some intracapsular fractures do). It may be stable, with an intact medial cortex, or unstable (e.g., the four-part intertrochanteric fracture involving both trochanters plus the medial cortex). Subtrochanteric fractures, just distal to the trochanters, represent another distinct entity.

Pelvic fractures may also be classified according to Type I (fracture of the pelvic bones with preservation of the pelvic ring); Type II (single fracture of the pelvic ring); or Type III (double fracture of the pelvic ring). See Figure 8–6.

Type IV fractures include displaced or undisplaced fractures of the acetabulum. Additional examples of fractures of the pelvis are shown in Figures 8–7, 8–8, 8–9, 8–10, and 8–11.

Femoral Shaft Fractures. The normal structures of the femur and tibia are shown in Figure 8–12. Fractures of the femur, below the trochanters and above the condyles, can be described in order of increasing severity as: (1) simple, including spiral or oblique fractures due to torque forces, (2) comminuted, often with a butterfly fragment, and (3) segmental owing to severe violence and with more marked soft tissue damage. Nerve injury is rare, but it is helpful to keep in mind that peroneal nerve disability can be avoided by preventing excessive traction in the treatment of the fracture. Diligence in anticipation, prevention, and prompt treatment of vascular complications is essential.

Supracondylar fractures require the expert care and handling of an orthopedist, since there is usually pronounced displacement due to the muscle pull and interactions of the quadriceps, hamstrings, and gastrocnemius, along with condyled and intra-articular fractures. These injuries can produce massive knee effusions and soft tissue swelling.

Patellar Fractures and Dislocations. It is helpful to describe the injured patella by the location of the fracture line in relation to the upper and lower pole, and especially by the presence or extent of comminution and displacement. (See Figure 8–13, A, B and C.) A direct blow is the usual mechanism, and the assessment and restoration of quadriceps function is the most important consideration.

Quadricep function can be disrupted by patellar fractures, patellar tendon rupture, quadricep tendon rupture, or tibial tubercle fracture. The ability to extend the leg against gravity is the hallmark of a functional quadriceps mechanism.

A common injury in teenage girls, patellar dislocations are a result of a direct blow or quadriceps contraction with the knee in flexion. A major force is not necessary for this injury. The patella dislocates laterally and is reduced by extension of the knee perhaps with a gentle medial push. This can easily be accomplished without sedation and may occur spontaneously if the patient extends the knee. Medial or lateral parapatellar tenderness and a positive patellar apprehension test, in which the patient reacts with fear and guarding when the patella is moved laterally toward dislocation, are presumptive evidence of a patellar dislocation having transpired.

Knee Dislocations and Fractures. Knee dislocation is rare, but it is an orthopedic emergency, since effects of the damage to the vascular structures of the popliteal fossa can be devastating. After reduction, surgical exploration and repair is mandatory because of the extensive disruption of the supporting structures necessary for knee stability and to ensure preservation of vascular continuity and function.

Condylar or tibial plateau fractures are usually from vertical compression and axial loading forces and torque. Hospitalization is usually necessary to ensure restoration of joint congruity and early knee motion.

Intra-articular fractures, including fractures of the tibial spine or intercondylar eminence, indicate probable alteration of cruciate ligament stability and possible cartilaginous injury. A rotatory component is one of the causative factors. In these injuries the knee will lack full extension and effusion will be present.

The proximal fibula is not involved in weight bearing. The salient features of fractures of the head or neck of the fibula are the potential for peroneal nerve injury, since it is vulnerable in this location; the need to search for associated fractures of the distal tibia or fibula; and the recognition of disruption of the proximal tibiofibular syndesmosis. A dislocation of the proximal tibiofibular joint may be diagnosed by inspection and palpation of the protruding fibular head.

Tibia Fractures. Simple and stable fractures of the long bones can usually be treated by closed reduction, if necessary, and casting. Goals of reduction are to correct alignment and rotation, minimize shortening and angulation, and reduce displacement as much as possible. Neurovascular complications occur most commonly in fractures of the proximal third of the tibia.

Any notable increase in pain, with acute tenderness over muscles of the anterior compartment or weakness or paralysis of these muscles, or sensory loss in the distribution of the common peroneal nerve should alert one to the likelihood of an anterior compartment syndrome. This can occur up to 24 to 48 hours after a tibial shaft fracture or trauma to the leg.

Fibula Fractures. Fibular fractures may be at the same or different level as the tibial fracture and may be treated simultaneously. More complicated tibial shaft fractures may be treated by open reduction or means other than casting, but consideration for hospital admission for all

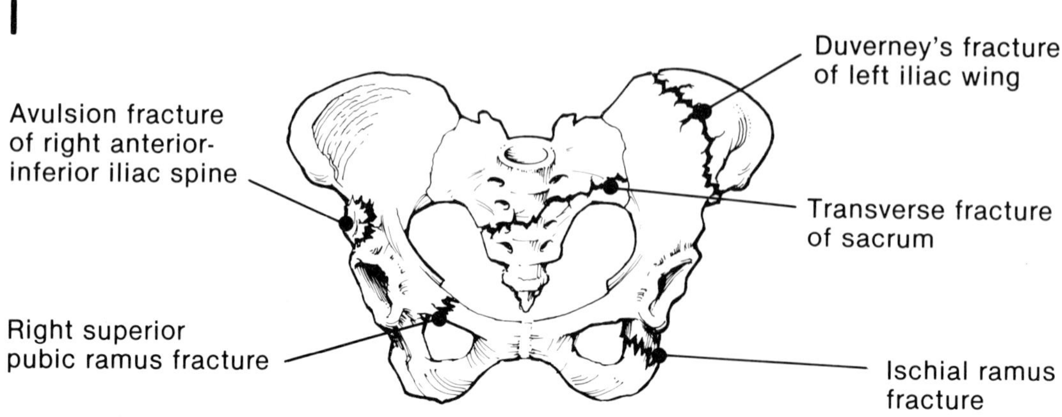

Type I: Fracture of individual bones without break in pelvic ring. (five examples shown)

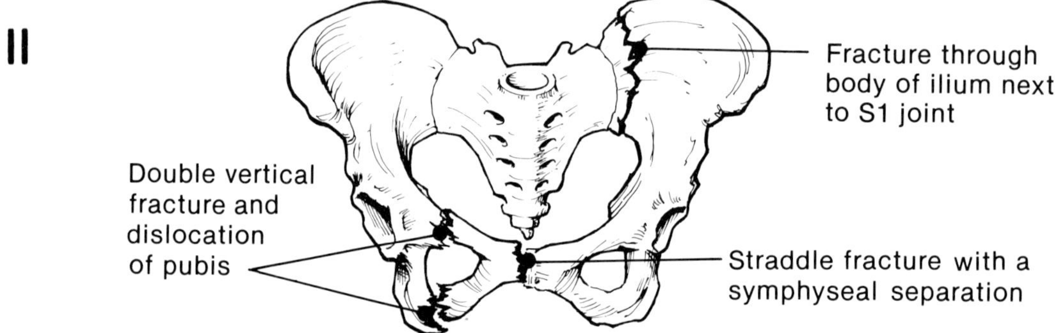

Type II: Three examples of single breaks in the pelvic ring.

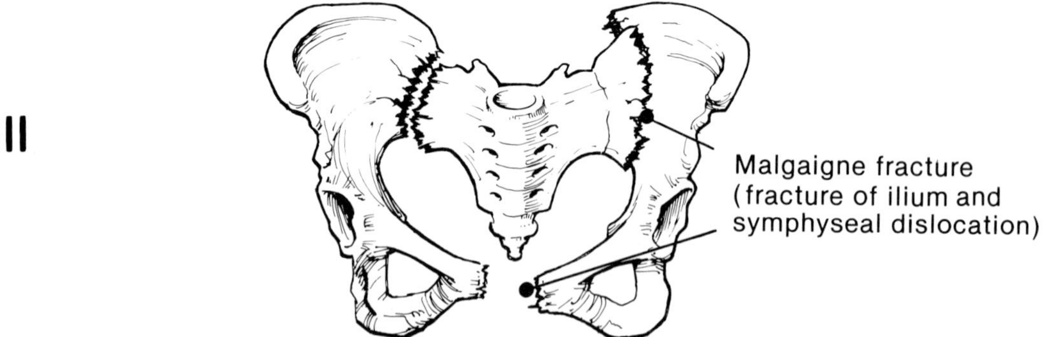

Type III: Double break in pelvic ring.

Figure 8–6 Pelvic Fractures, Type I, II, III.

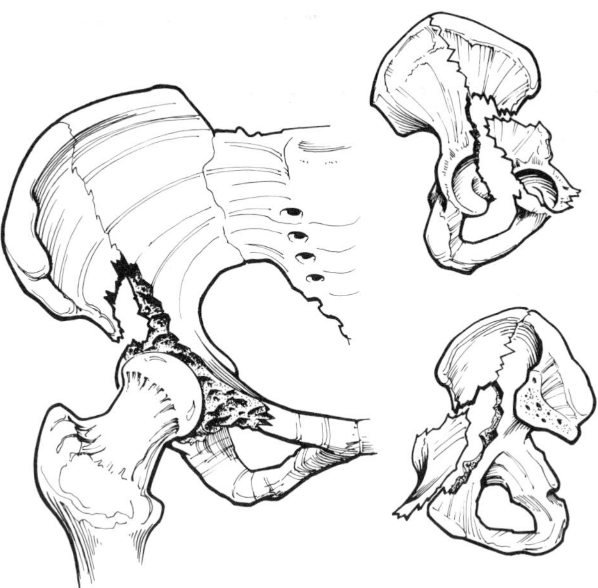

Figure 8–7 Iliopubic Fracture.

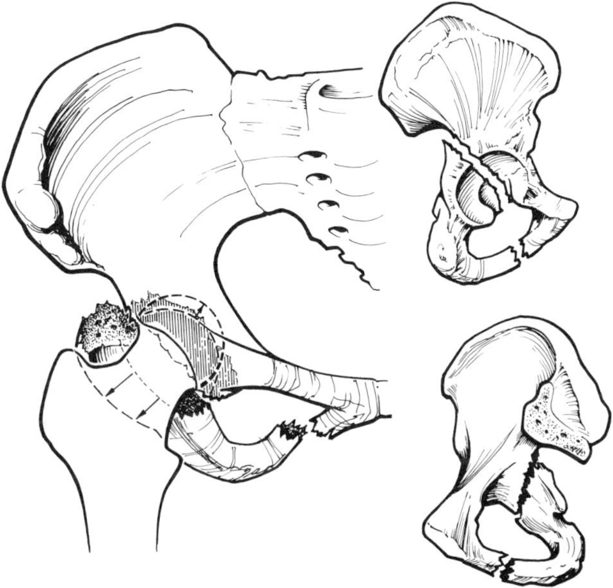

Figure 8–8 Ilioischial Fracture.

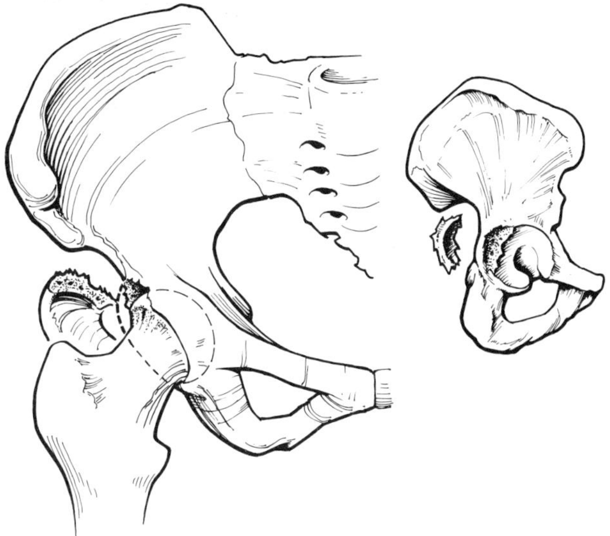

Figure 8–9 Fracture of the Posterior Lip.

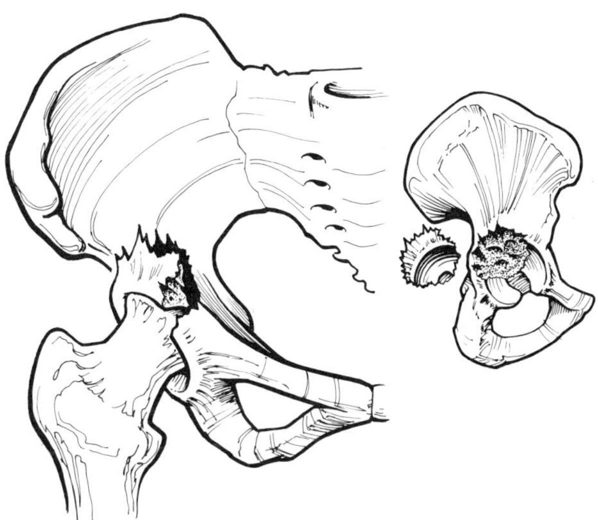

Figure 8–10 Posterior Superior Rim Fracture.

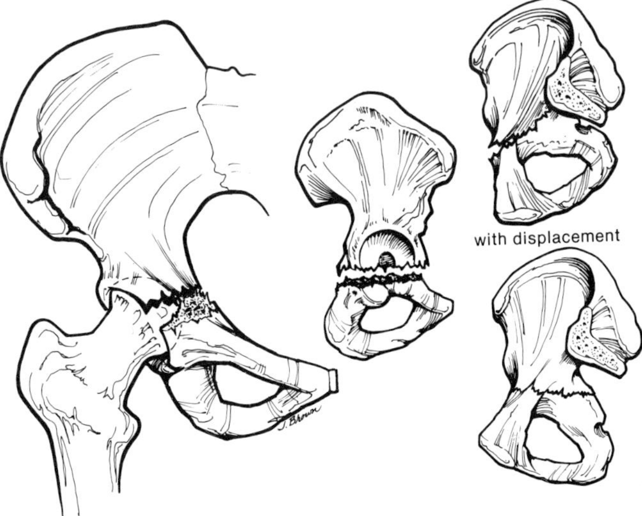

Figure 8–11 Transverse Fracture With and Without Displacement.

patients with fractures of the tibia should be entertained, especially in adults, since control of pain, swelling and patient compliance can be a major problem in outpatient treatment.

Ankle Fractures and Dislocations. If the ankle joint is viewed as a ring stabilized by three bones (the tibia, fibula, and talus) and their supporting ligaments (the deltoid medially, the lateral collateral ligaments as seen in Figure 8–14, and the tibiofibular syndesmosis), then accurate diagnosis and appropriate treatment is greatly facilitated. All of the appropriate areas should be examined for swelling, pain, and tenderness. Laterally,

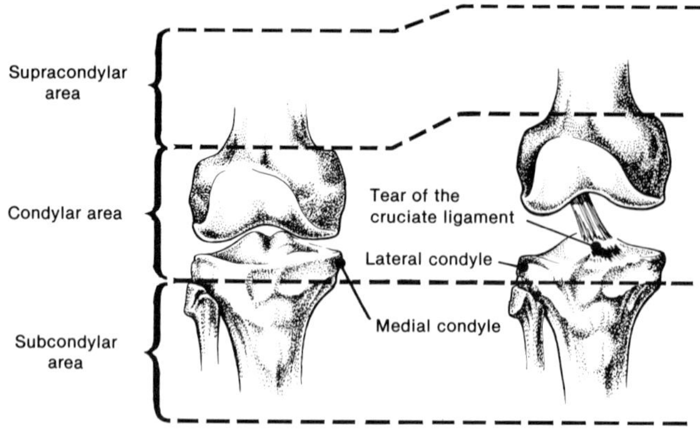

Figure 8–12   The Supracondylar and Condylar Areas of the Femur, and the Medial and Subcondylar Areas of the Tibia.

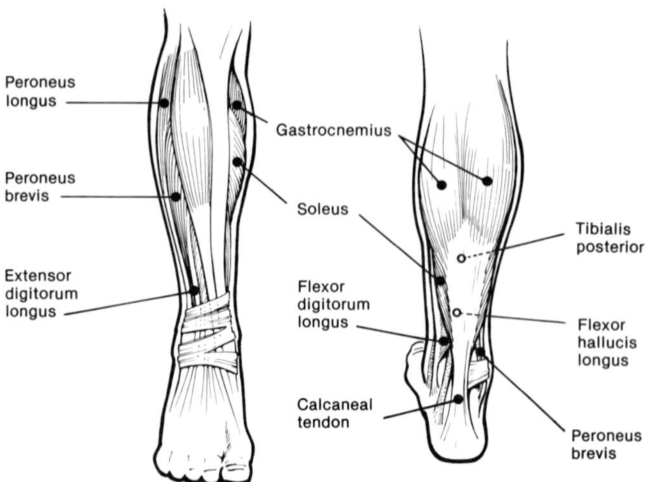

Figure 8–15   Posterior and Anterior Views of Ankle and Heel.

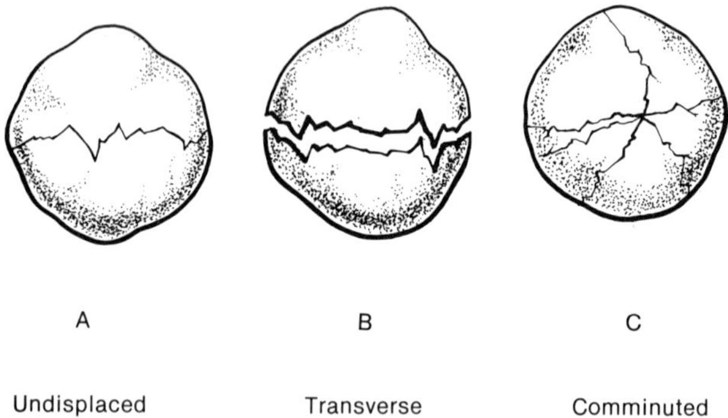

Figure 8–13   Types of Patellar Fractures (A, B, C).

the specific components of the lateral collateral ligament, namely, the anterior talofibular ligament, the calcaneofibular ligament, and the posterior talofibular ligament can be palpated. These ligaments are ruptured in order of frequency as listed above. A disruption of the ankle mortise occurs when there is a break in this osseous-ligamentous ring; a single break leaves a stable ankle whereas more than one break, such as a fibular fracture and a deltoid ligament tear, results in an unstable ankle. Views that can be utilized in evaluating injuries of the ankle are shown in Figure 8–15.

The important radiographic findings to be identified in ankle injuries are talar tilt, mortise incongruity, wid-

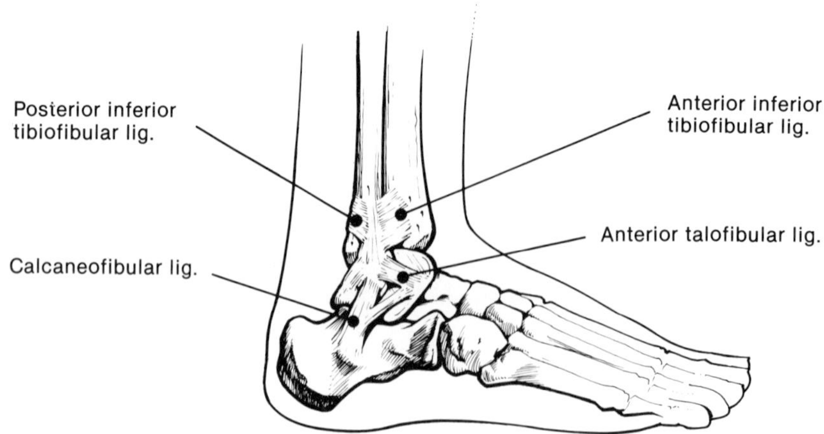

Figure 8–14   Lateral Ligaments of the Ankle.

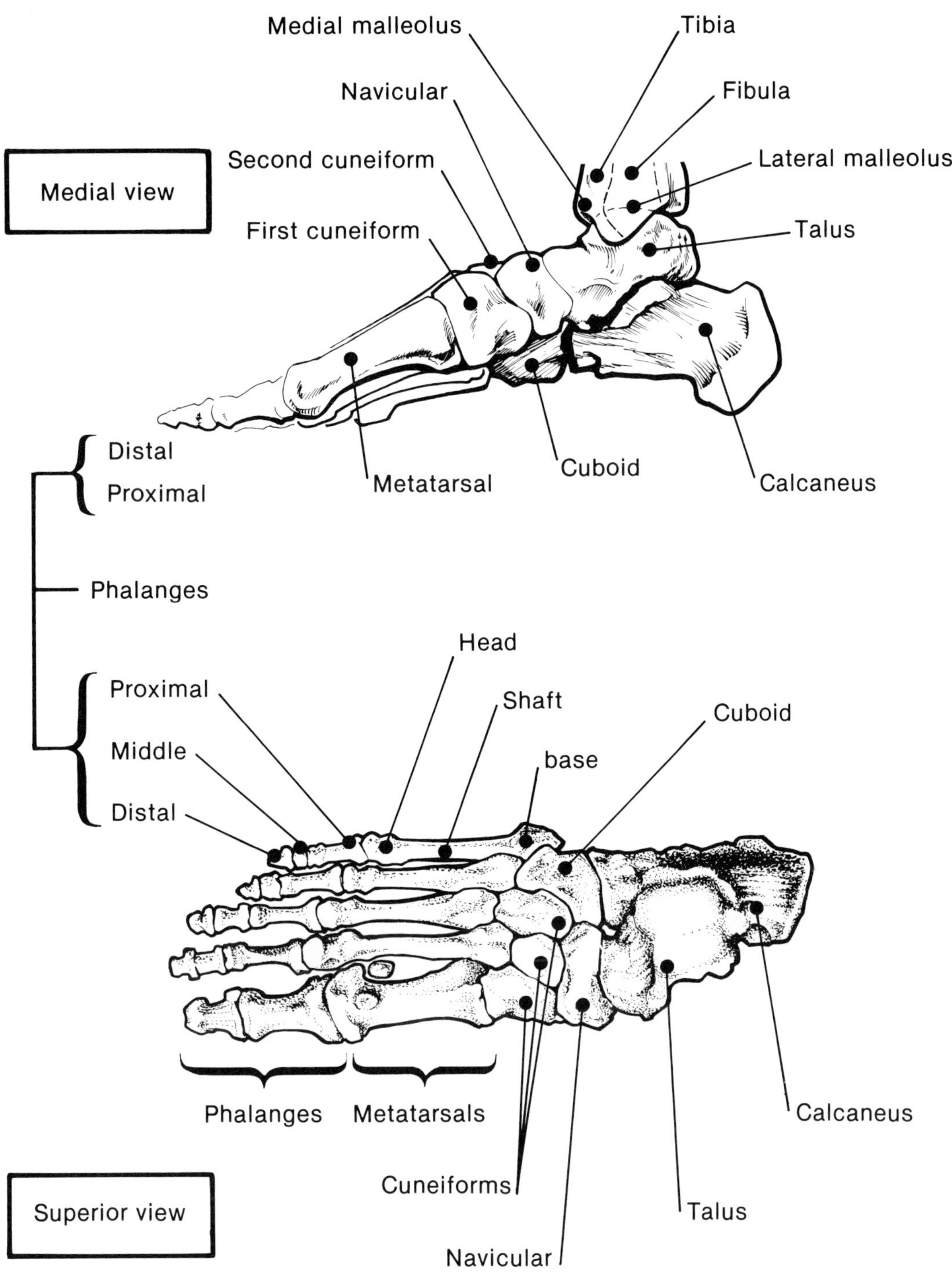

Figure 8–16 Bones of the Foot.

ening of the normal osseous relationships, displacement of fibular fracture, and avulsion fractures from the tip of the fibula or tibia or from the talus or calcaneus. All of these indicate significant ligamentous injury. All three radiographic views should be carefully inspected, because nondisplaced fibular fractures and fractures of the posterior malleolus of the tibia frequently are visible only on the lateral view; also small nondisplaced fractures of the distal articulating surface of the tibia or the

talus may defy detection if they are not meticulously searched for.

Treatment of stable ankle fractures and ligamentous injuries is conservative and includes immobilization, rest, application of ice, and elevation. Unstable injuries usually require reduction. What is considered to be a satisfactory reduction, and the methods employed in achieving such, may be somewhat controversial and may vary according to the nature of the injury and the inclinations of the attending orthopedist. This in no way lessens the vigilance of the physician in detecting and categorizing these injuries.

Foot Fractures and Dislocations. The normal anatomy of the foot is shown in Figure 8–16. Most talar fractures result from a forceful hyperextension of the foot impinging the talus against the anterior edge of the tibia. Usually, a cast is sufficient treatment, but severe or comminuted fractures may require open reduction or even secondary arthrodesis since the blood supply of the talus is somewhat tenuous and accounts for many of the difficulties in treatment.

Subtalar dislocation is a displacement, either laterally or medially, of the distal foot in relation to the talus, and may be recognized by tenting of the skin and ability to palpate the talus at the site of the deformity. Rapid reduction, with adequate muscular relaxation, is mandatory. Complete dislocation of the talus is rare.

A patient who falls from a height, even only a few feet, may suffer a fracture of the calcaneus. (See Figs. 8–17, 8–18, 8–19, and 8–20.) This mechanism can also produce compression fracture of the dorsolumbar spine. Thorough radiographic views (lateral, axial, and dorsoplantar) should be obtained. Posterolateral or posteromedial tenderness with compression is a more rewarding clinical sign than plantar tenderness when a fracture of the calcaneus exists.

Initial treatment of calcaneal fractures is with a compressive dressing (there is often much swelling and ecchymosis), rest, application of ice, elevation and strict non–weight bearing. Because of pain and swelling, hospitalization is frequently required. Definitive treatment is varied and controversial with no superior methods available to give consistent, satisfactory results.

The navicular, cuboid, and three cuneiforms comprise the midfoot. Fractures and dislocations of this area are somewhat less common than those of the hindfoot or forefoot, probably because it is the most rigid portion of the foot. Avulsion fractures are probably the most common, and immobilization with early weight bearing is the normal treatment of these injuries. Figure 8–21 demonstrates an axial view of the foot.

The metatarsals and the phalanges are often fractured. Fractures of the base of the fifth metatarsal are frequently encountered and are treated, as are most other types of metatarsal fractures, with immobilization and early weight bearing as tolerated. An orthopedic shoe is a useful adjunct in the treatment of these, and many other, foot injuries.

Toe fractures are treated by reduction, with restoration of alignment, if necessary, and taping to the adjacent toe, similar to the "buddy taping" employed in finger injuries. Care should be taken to pad the interdigital areas properly. Dislocations of the phalanges of the toe or even the metatarsal phalangeal joints are not

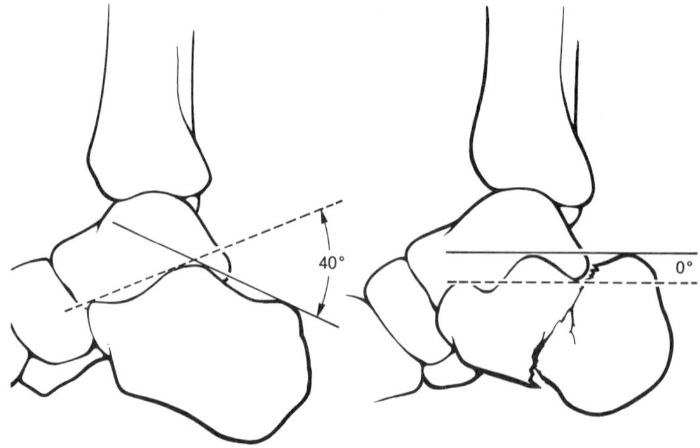

Figure 8–17 The Tuber Joint Angle of Zero Noting a Fracture of the Calcaneus.

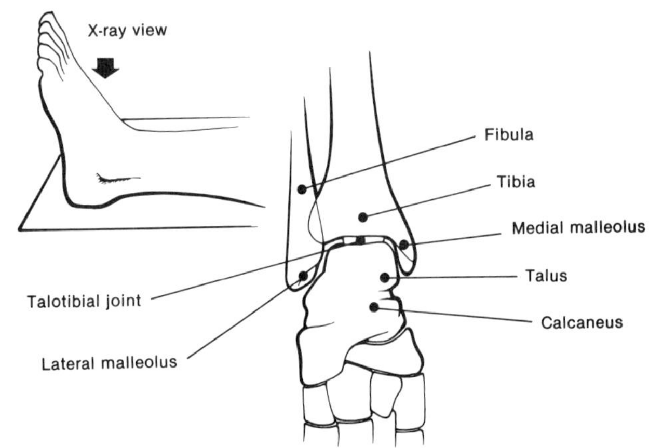

Figure 8–18 Anteroposterior View of the Calcaneus.

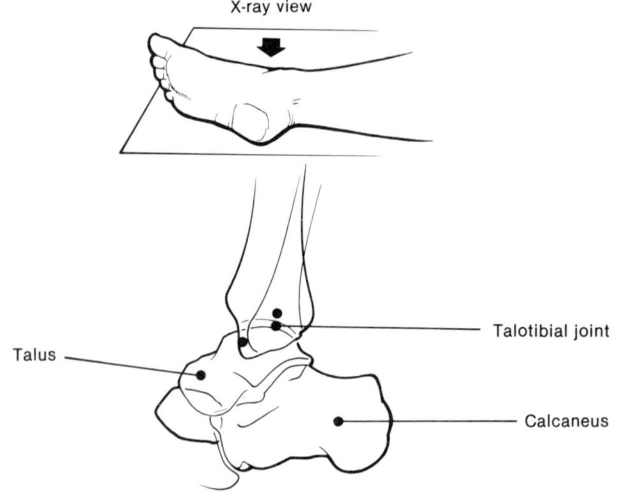

Figure 8–19 Lateral View of the Calcaneus.

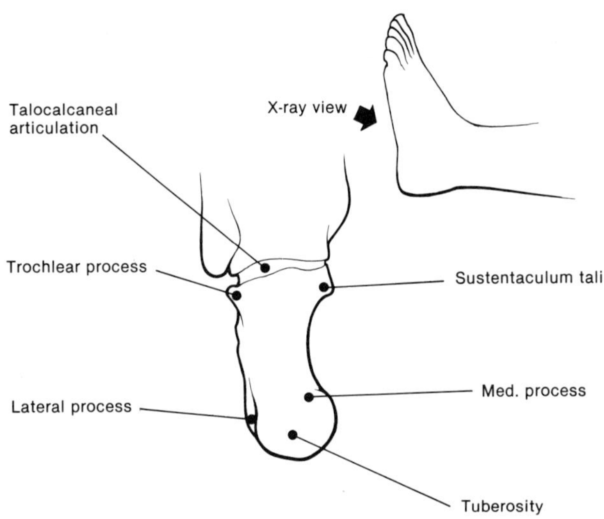

Figure 8–20   Axial View of the Calcaneus.

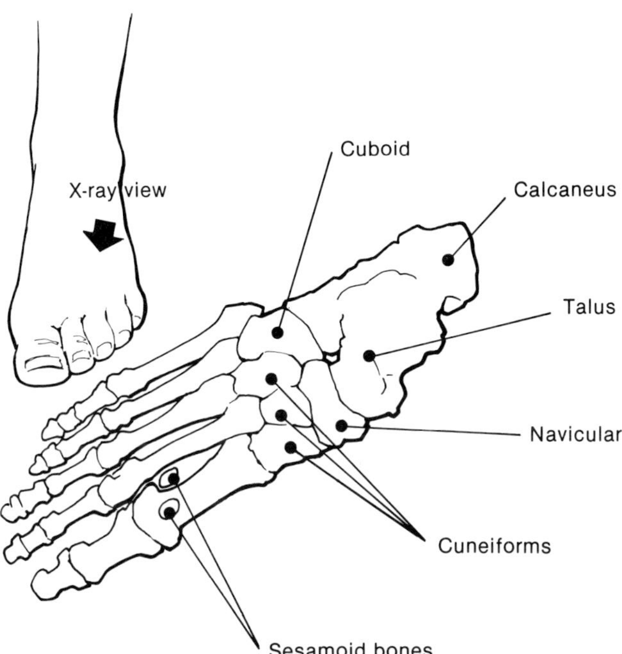

Figure 8–21   Axial View of the Midtarsal Bones of the Foot.

uncommon and are treated similar to toe fractures, after satisfactory reduction.

Pediatric Orthopedic Emergencies

Certain injuries and conditions that are unique to the pediatric age-group may present as orthopedic emergencies.

Torus Fractures

Torus fractures, simply representing a "buckling" of the cortex, are common, quite stable, and easily treated with a plaster splint or cast. However, the radiographic findings may be very subtle and overlooked. The patient may present with minimal or mild clinical findings but with well-localized tenderness.

Greenstick Fractures

An incomplete long bone fracture with one cortex essentially intact is called a greenstick fracture. There may be considerable clinical deformity, and proper reduction, with appropriate anesthesia, usually requires completion of the fracture by breaking the intact cortex. The forearm is a common site for this injury, with either one or both bones involved, and a long arm cast is necessary following satisfactory reduction.

Epiphyseal Injuries

The Salter-Harris classification of epiphyseal fractures is useful and should be employed. Point tenderness over an epiphysis may be treated as a Salter I fracture when the radiograph is negative. This is common at the wrist. Salter II fractures may be recognized by the presence of the Thurston-Holland sign on the radiograph; in this sign a triangular fragment of metaphyseal bone may be the only evidence that an epiphyseal injury has occurred. Most epiphyseal fractures require accurate reduction if subsequent growth deformities are to be avoided.

Elbow injuries in children can be difficult to diagnose because of the various growth centers that appear at different ages. Comparison views may be helpful, but in case of doubt, when no fracture or dislocation is evident but clinical findings dictate, immobilization and later reevaluation is the proper course of initial management. This is especially true in the patient with a positive fat pad sign.

Another epiphyseal condition that may confront the emergency physician is epiphysitis, such as Osgood-Schlatter's disease, which is actually an apophysitis of the patellar tubercle of the tibia. This condition is self-limiting, of a less acute nature, tends to be recurrent, and is exacerbated by activity and relieved by rest. The patient will complain of pain and swelling. Symptomatic treatment is indicated.

Pulled Elbow

Also referred to as subluxation of the radial head or nursemaid's elbow, this entity is commonly seen in the emergency department in children up to 4 or 5 years of age. A history of pulling or jerking a child by the wrist may not be revealed, but the patient typically resists active or passive motion of the extremity and will hold the arm comfortably at the side if left alone. Diagnosis and treatment is by rotating the forearm into complete supination with the thumb of the examiner's opposite hand on the radial head. A definite click will usually be felt; the child is left alone for a few minutes and then begins to actively use the arm. No immobilization or aftertreatment is needed and radiographs need not be obtained, except when the diagnosis is in doubt.

Hip Disorders

Transient synovitis of the hip in the younger child who appears healthy but will not walk or walks with a limp and has pain and restriction on passive motion of the involved side is a self-limiting condition treated with bed rest and observation until symptoms subside, usually within a few days. Radiographic studies will usually be normal but may show some evidence of capsular distention.

Hip joint infection is another matter since aggressive management is indicated. Differentiation is by more severe pain and irritability, with the extremity held in a fixed, flexed, abducted, and externally rotated position. The child is febrile and may appear toxic; laboratory findings indicate infection. Any questionable case should receive immediate orthopedic consultation.

Two other hip conditions, in which radiographs will be helpful, are infrequently seen in emergency practice. They are Legg-Perthes disease, or avascular necrosis of the femoral head, which presents much the same as transient synovitis; and slipped capital femoral epiphysis, which occurs in the prepubescent or adolescent age-group and is characterized by a loss of internal rotation on physical examination. Radiographs will confirm the diagnosis in these two conditions.

Soft Tissue Injuries

Together, these conditions comprise the vast majority of the problems that prompt the patient to seek emergency assistance. Unlike fractures and dislocations, the diagnosis of these conditions depends not so much on radiographic results and interpretation but on the clinical and diagnostic acumen of the examiner.

Back Disorders

Owing to the frequency with which lower back problems are encountered in the emergency department, it is important to be able to interpret findings of the back examination. The patient's general attitude (comfort or agony or appropriate behavior and response) is noted. Virtually all organic lower back syndromes are characterized by aggravation of symptoms with movement and relief with rest. Inspection may reveal a list in which the patient bends to lean away from the side of pain and discomfort, frequently in an attempt to relieve pressure on the sciatic nerve. Similarly, the patient with an acute disk syndrome may hold the affected leg in a flexed position to alleviate pressure on the nerve root. Loss of lumbar lordosis and paravertebral muscle spasm (asymmetry or obvious tightening of unilateral or bilateral paralumbar muscles) can also be visualized if present. Range of motion may be decreased and should be documented. Palpation of the spinous processes, paravertebral muscles, and sciatic notches should be performed, and areas producing tenderness or radicular symptoms should be noted.

Neurologic examination is probably the most important aspect of the examination. Motor examination is done by testing the toe and foot flexors (S1) and extensors (L5) and knee extension (quadriceps, L4). Atrophy of the quadriceps or anterior or lateral compartments of the leg is rarely seen but may verify significant motor deficit. Sensory changes may be documented on the posterolateral aspect of the leg and foot (S1) or on the anteromedial aspect of the leg and foot (L5). Reflex changes may include diminished or absent Achilles reflex (S1) or knee jerk (L4).

The straight leg raising test is useful in determining whether there is involvement of the sciatic nerve, usually caused by compression of a herniated lumbar disk. The patient is supine on the table, and the hip is flexed with the knee extended. If this maneuver produces radicular leg pain in the affected extremity, it is considered to be a positive contralateral straight leg raising test and is very suggestive of a herniated disk.

To confirm these findings and to help distinguish malingerers, several variations of this theme are available. Lasègue's test is positive when the radicular pain is reproduced by extending the knee after both the hip and knee are flexed to 90 degrees. Also, extending the knee with the patient sitting (hip flexed at 90 degrees) should reproduce the pain or force the patient to attempt to extend the hip.

The utilization of muscle relaxants may be helpful adjuncts to rest, physical therapy, ice or heat, and other modalities in the treatment of acute, painful, musculoskeletal conditions. Some of the more common muscle relaxants and their features are listed in Table 8–1.

Other muscle relaxants of value include carisoprodol (Soma), chlorzoxazone (Paraflex), and orphenadrine citrate (Norflex), used alone or in combination as Soma Compound, Parafon Forte, and Norgesic. Equagesic (meprobamate and ethoheptazine citrate with aspirin) is yet another popular combination drug employed to alleviate musculoskeletal discomfort. It should be pointed out that none of these medications directly acts on tense skeletal muscles to provide relaxation. It should also be emphasized that, if the patient's musculoskeletal discomfort is caused by pain, then analgesic medication,

TABLE 8–1   Common Muscle Relaxants

Generic Name	Brand Name	Dosage and Administration	Advantages	Disadvantages
Diazepam	Valium	IV: 5 to 10 mg, slowly IM: 5 to 10 mg PO: 2 to 10 mg three or four times daily	Good muscle relaxation; also reduces anxiety, tension	Dependency, abuse
Methacarbamol	Robaxin Robaxisal	IV: 1,000 mg, slowly IM: 1,000 mg PO: 500 mg four times daily PO: 750 mg three or four times daily	Especially effective if given IV for acute spasm	Dizziness, gastrointestinal disturbances
Cyclobenzaprine	Flexeril	PO: 10 mg three times daily	Effective, better tolerated, and less abused than methacarbamol or diazepam	Drowsiness, atropine-like effects

such as meperidine, codeine, propoxyphene (Darvon), zomepirac (Zomax), or, frequently, aspirin or acetaminophen, is indicated.

Knee Disorders

When radiographic findings rule out osseous pathology in knee problems, the diagnosis may still be unconfirmed. With proper evaluation, the physician should be able to arrive at a reasonably accurate diagnosis in almost all cases. The history, of course, can be extremely revealing, and the physical findings can be confirmatory. The crucial differentiation in knee injuries is in the detection of presence or absence of stability. The knee ligaments function as dynamic stabilizers and when the various stress forces are applied against them they are capable of producing a wide spectrum of insult and injury. Figure 8–22 shows the normal ligaments of the knee.

In the knee the term *sprain* should be reserved for those injuries that produce no demonstrable instability; accordingly, the severity of pain, swelling, tenderness, and loss of function can be classified as mild (first degree), moderate (second degree), or severe (third degree). A ligamentous injury producing any degree of instability is a rupture, by definition. Ruptures can be classified also as mild (first degree), moderate (second degree), or severe (third degree) by the amount of instability present and demonstrable. The differentiation between sprain and rupture is important because the former is treated conservatively while the latter may require surgical repair.

Instability is tested for by stressing the individual ligaments, with help of local or general anesthesia, when necessary. The uninvolved knee should be tested first since knee ligamentous laxity is variable in different individuals. The medial and lateral collateral ligaments and the anterior and posterior cruciate ligaments are all tested, and their stability is recorded. With the knee flexed, the examiner's hands are placed behind the leg and the tibia is drawn toward the examiner. A positive sign (excessive mobility) suggests a tear in the anterior cruciate ligament. See Figure 8–23. If the examination is inadequate, inconclusive, or equivocal, but instability is suspected, a stress test with radiography may help confirm the diagnosis. Proper relaxation is essential and usually requires some degree of analgesia or anesthesia. All questionable cases of ligament instability deserve an early orthopedic evaluation.

If bone and ligamentous pathology has been ruled out, the possibility of intra-articular pathology may still exist. The diagnosis of a meniscus tear is usually more difficult to define in the emergency setting and, fortunately, less critical in the proper care of the patient. The following features may serve to alert one to the probability of intra-articular pathology: previous knee problems; recurring knee symptoms with minor or no trauma; history of "clicking," "popping," "locking," "giving way," "catching," or "slipping"; slowly developing effusion (6 to 24 hours); localized joint line tenderness (usually medial); and lack of full extension. These patients should have the knee aspirated, if indicated, immobilized, and referred to an orthopedist for more definitive evaluation and treatment.

Contusion

Bruising of skin and underlying tissues caused by a direct blow is managed by initial rest, cold compresses, and pressure dressings or temporary splinting, followed by limited activity, heat, and protection of the area.

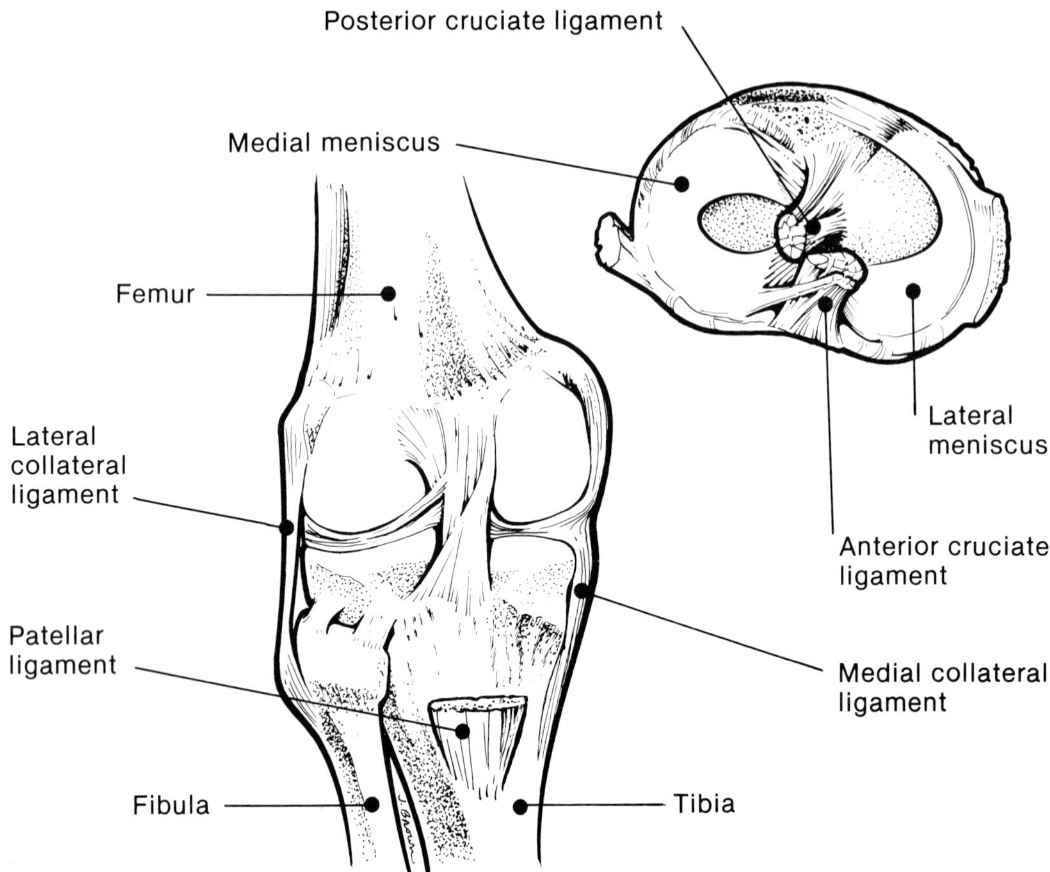

Figure 8–22 Ligaments of the Knee.

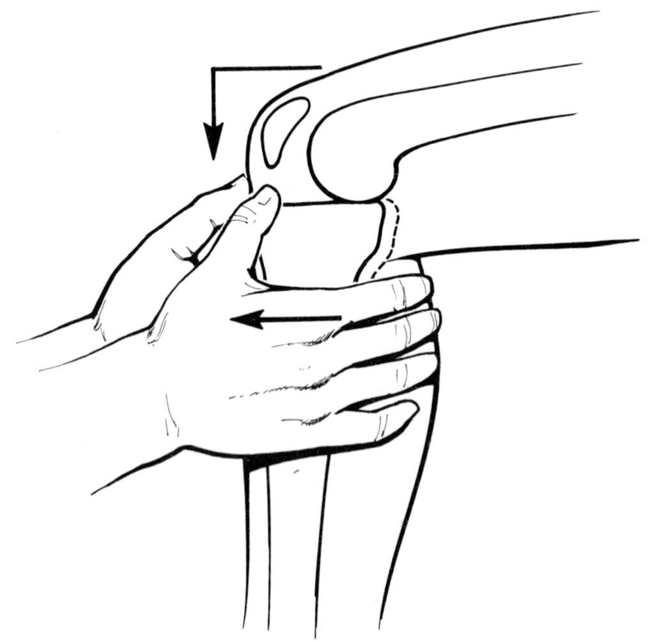

Figure 8–23 Anterior Drawer Sign.

Hematoma

A hematoma is a collection of pooled blood in a localized area that is not an anatomically closed space (e.g., joint). Deep-seated hematomas may be difficult to recognize. Treatment is rest. Cold compresses and pressure dressings are usually indicated. Aspiration, under sterile conditions, should only be done when there is sufficient quantity of readily accessible, aspirable blood present; external compression with a pressure bandage is then applied, and early application of heat and protection against excessive motion help to prevent excessive scar formation or calcification.

Myositis Ossificans

Rarely encountered in the emergency department is a complication of contusion and hematoma in which inflammation and calcification of muscle is a late result of trauma. In late stages radiographic evidence of this condition will exist, but if the impending condition is anticipated or suspected, preventive measures can be taken to try to avoid this complication. Rest with heat and limited, painless motion are indicated, along with close, continuing orthopedic follow-up.

Abrasion

A scraping injury to the skin should be treated by initial, mechanical cleansing of the area, application of protective dressing to prevent further trauma, and avoidance of active overuse of the skin. Extensive or raw, weeping wounds are best treated with burn ointments and dressings and with close early follow-up care.

Lacerations

A laceration is a skin wound with relatively sharp, separated edges. Determination of any underlying injuries, including joint penetration, is imperative. Exploration, cleansing, debridement, trimming of tissues, if necessary, and closure should be done after adequate anesthesia to the area. Insertion of a drain, if needed, and anticipation of potential for infection are important considerations. A proper protective dressing is placed over the wound. (See Chapter 10.)

Puncture Wound

Skin and tissue disruption by a penetrating object requires much the same initial care as for lacerations. Vigilance must be exercised when the puncture wound occurs directly over or near a joint since intra-articular involvement will result in serious consequences if this diagnosis is missed.

Foreign Bodies

If the history of a foreign body penetration is not that of an acute injury or is nebulous; if the foreign body is minute in size or of relatively innocuous material; or is not easily visible, palpable, or assessable, a surgical exploration should probably not be entertained. Radiographs are frequently helpful, and the use of metal skin markers can aid in the localization of the object. Efforts should cease if the foreign body is not removed after a reasonable time, usually 10 or 15 minutes. The patient should be told this before the search is begun, and the explorer should rigidly adhere to this limitation in the interest of avoiding iatrogenic damage to the tissues and the risk of infection. The wound should be closed or covered and the patient referred to a consultant.

Removing a foreign body, usually a splinter, from beneath a nail is accomplished by means of a digital block, followed by notching the nail as much as necessary and then removing the foreign body.

Blisters

Blisters are caused by friction and irritation that results in separation of dermis from epidermis with exudate. The best treatment is prevention; if considerable fluid is present, careful aspiration and a protective dressing is indicated. The overlying skin should be left intact unless it is in such condition that it can no longer adequately serve as a protective device. Guidelines in the treatment of second-degree burns will serve one well in the treatment of both blisters and abrasions.

Infections

The skin and underlying tissues are frequently involved in inflammatory and infectious processes, from trauma or more indirect causes. Prompt, appropriate action is needed to prevent unnecessary morbidity, permanent damage to the affected part, or spread of the infectious process. Cultures should be obtained whenever possible and the appropriate antibiotic chosen.

Before discussing specific conditions of established or suspected infections, it would be well to mention the indications for initiation of antibiotic therapy in high-risk patients and situations. Antibiotics should be begun promptly and adequately in patients with open fractures, open joint wounds, or exposed tendon wounds. Also, in grossly contaminated wounds, many hand wounds, and open wounds in high-risk patients (e.g., diabetics), antibiotic coverage should be entertained. Intravenous or intramuscular cephalosporins or the appropriate penicillin should be administered initially in the emergency department, with parenteral use continued in hospitalized patients and oral doses prescribed for outpatients.

Wound Infections. Once infection is suspected, treatment should be instituted. The wound should be opened, with removal of sutures, and cultured. Antibiotic therapy is begun and early follow-up is recommended.

Cellulitis and Lymphangitis. Cellulitis and lymphangitis are recognized by a diffuse, red, tender, swollen area and by "red streaking," respectively, and usually are caused by a group A β-hemolytic *Streptococcus*. Treatment is rest and elevation of the affected part. Oral penicillin, or erythromycin as a second choice, is indicated.

Abscess. A localized collection of pus, an abscess presents with fluctuance in addition to the signs of cellulitis. Treatment is by incision and drainage. Usually, installation of some form of drain for 1 to 2 days is necessary. Since staphylococcal organisms are frequently responsible for these infections, this should help one to choose the appropriate antibiotic if the abscess is extensive or deep or significant cellulitis is present or if systemic signs and symptoms are manifest.

Paronychia. A paronychia is a collection of pus beneath the eponychial fold at the base of the nail and is treated by the surgical elevation of this fold or by linear incision parallel to the nail edge.

Felon. Characterized by severe pain, tension, swelling, and marked tenderness, the felon is an abscess within the fat pad of the pulp space of a fingertip. Incision and drainage by a single lateral or medial approach is preferred, although the direct approach through the volar pad is recommended by some. Hockey stick or fishmouth incisions are to be avoided.

Suppurative Flexor Tenosynovitis. Suppurative flexor tenosynovitis represents a true surgical emergency, in which necrosis of the flexor tendons can occur if this condition is left untreated or treated improperly. Hospitalization with early incision and drainage is required if the following signs are present: when there is a very tender, red swelling extending along the flexor tendon sheath; when the finger is held rigidly in a semiflexed position; and, most importantly, when passive extension of the finger elicits excruciating pain. Hospitalization should be considered in any patient who is suspected of having this condition or any other potentially serious hand infection.

Joint Infection. The degree of pain, heat, redness, and limitation of motion should alert the examiner to the possibility of a joint infection. Septic arthritis is usually caused by a penetrating wound, but gonococcal or hematogenous spread of other organisms must also be considered. The joint should be aspirated, if effusion is present, and the appropriate laboratory tests on the aspirate should be employed to help pinpoint the diagnosis. Septic arthritis requires immediate orthopedic consultation, and hospitalization and parenteral antibiotics are often necessary.

Osteomyelitis. Osteomyelitis is rarely encountered in emergency practice. It can be suspected by history and verified by radiographic findings, when present. Local physical signs of drainage, inflammation, pain, and tenderness may be present or detected from the history. The chronicity of symptoms should direct one toward this diagnosis.

Human and Animal Bites. Human and animal bites deserve mention because of the frequency and potential for infection. These wounds should be surgically cleansed, debrided, irrigated copiously, and left open if at all feasible. Antibiotics to cover staphylococcal organisms should probably be employed in all but trivial or the most superficial wounds. (See Chapter 28.)

Standard practice of a tetanus booster injection, if more than 5 years have elapsed since the patient received the last booster, should be provided. Passive immunity with injection of human tetanus antitoxin (Hyper-Tet), along with the active immunity of the tetanus toxoid injection, is indicated for the unimmunized patient or the patient with a tetanus-prone wound, such as a barnyard injury.

Vascular Disease

Because certain vascular conditions may mimic musculoskeletal disorders, the patient may seek emergency care for symptoms that suggest an orthopedic problem. Differentiating these conditions requires an awareness of this fact.

Thoracic or low back pain that is not relieved by rest or exacerbated by activity could be caused by a slowly dissecting aortic aneurysm. Abdominal examination may reveal a pulsatile mass or bruit or distal pulse irregularities. Radiographs may demonstrate enlargement or characteristic calcification of the aorta.

Extremity pain is an all too common symptom and could be caused by arterial insufficiency. Vague or poorly localized symptoms may be related by the patient, and comparison of the extremities may reveal color or temperature changes, poor capillary filling, or diminished peripheral pulses. Sudden extremity pain and discomfort in a patient with mitral stenosis or atrial fibrillation suggests the possibility of peripheral embolization.

Varicose veins, venous stasis and insufficiency, as well as congestive heart failure can all cause problems of swelling and discomfort in the extremities. Thrombophlebitis can usually be differentiated from other causes of leg pain and discomfort by a careful physical examination. (See Chapter 53.)

Tumors and Tumorlike Growths

Skin and Soft Tissue Tumors. Few of these skin and soft tissue disorders are true tumors, and most are easily recognized, such as sebaceous cysts, lipomas, hemangiomas, keloids, fibromas, inclusion cysts, and warts.

Ganglion. A ganglion is a synovial cyst, usually found on either the dorsal or volar aspect of the wrist. Often, the patient is unaware of its existence until trauma to the area calls attention to it. Most ganglia are asymptomatic and require only an explanation and reassurance to the patient. Nonemergent surgical excision is the treatment for the occasional persistently symptomatic ganglion. Aspiration or smashing the ganglion with a large book are measures that will reduce its size or make it go away temporarily and are not recommended.

Benign Bone Tumors and Tumorlike Conditions. Benign bone tumors and tumorlike conditions deserve mention because not infrequently a patient will present to the emergency department for pain or trauma and the radiographic finding of bone irregularity or abnormality will be discovered incidentally. Osteochondritis dissecans, bone cysts, enchondromas, and hypertrophic osteoarthropathy, as well as many other less common conditions, fall into this category. The two most commonly encountered are nonosteogenic fibroma and subperiosteal cortical defect, and these can be diagnosed by their characteristic appearance on the radiograph. In any case, when diagnostic doubt exists, this should be resolved by consultation with a radiologist or orthopedist.

Malignant and Metastatic Bone Tumors. It is rare, indeed, that the emergency physician will make the initial diagnosis of a primary malignant bone tumor, except in the case of pathologic fracture. Clinical suspicion and awareness, as well as a careful and thorough radiographic examination, is necessary for correct diagnosis.

Practically any tumor can metastasize to bone, but by far the most common are cancer of the breast in women and cancer of the prostate in men. Cancers of the thyroid, kidney, and lung also frequently metastasize to bone.

Multiple myeloma, exhibiting multiple, destructive foci primarily in flat bones, may be found in patients over the age of 40 and should be differentiated from Paget's disease, which affects the same age-group but is considered a benign bone lesion and is characterized radiographically by areas of osteolysis and excessive repair. Thus, not only will there be areas of radiolucency in Paget's disease but also increased opacity with coarse and prominent trabeculae. Flat and cylindrical bones are about equally affected in patients with Paget's disease.

Arthritis

The various arthritides constitute the largest and most important group of crippling diseases, from the standpoint of incidence and economic loss, in the world. From a practical standpoint, arthritis can be classified as infectious and secondary, which refers to the joint manifestations of a more generalized disease.

Rheumatoid arthritis is considered to be a sensitivity (or collagen disease) arthritis and most often is seen as an emergency only because of increased pain or disability. Symptomatic treatment, without excessively limiting activity, is indicated. Other collagen diseases, with common joint manifestations, are disseminated lupus erythematosus, erythema nodosa, rheumatic fever, and serum sickness. The arthritis in these conditions is apt to run a milder and limited course, without the chronic problems of rheumatoid arthritis.

Gout and pseudogout are both manifested by an inflammatory synovitis and differentiated by their characteristic crystals on synovial fluid analysis. In the acute phase, treatment with colchicine tablets is initiated. Other anti-inflammatory agents may also be effective. (See Chapter 19.)

Degenerative joint disease is a result of repeated trauma and stresses placed on a joint, a progressive and accumulative effect, with structural and functional deterioration of the joint. It is a disease of the middle aged and elderly. The symptoms are usually pain and stiffness, which are worse after inactivity. Radiographic evidence of degenerative joint disease is often an incidental finding. Relief of pain and referral of the patient is indicated.

The work-up in the emergency department of an inflamed joint should include radiographs of the joint; aspiration of the joint with analysis of the aspirate for cell types and crystals, as well as a culture and a Gram-stain; and laboratory tests, including complete blood cell count, erythrocyte sedimentation rate, uric acid, rheumatoid factor, or latex fixation tests. If the diagnosis is in doubt, treatment should be initiated with rest and immobilization of the extremity, aspirin or anti-inflammatory medication, and referral of the patient to an orthopedist or internist in 5 to 7 days.

Bursitis

An inflammatory reaction within a bursa, usually secondary to repetitious trauma, bursitis can occur in virtually any area of the body. The most commonly involved bursae are the olecranon, which is easily recognized by its position overlying the olecranon process of the elbow; prepatellar, which is directly overlying the patella; and trochanteric, which can be distinguished from other sources of hip area pain by careful palpation of the greater trochanter of the femur. (See Chapter 71 for sites of injections.)

Tendinitis

Tendinitis is an irritation and inflammation of the tendon and is usually more painful and disabling than bursitis. Bicipital tendinitis involves the origin of the long head of the biceps, with localized tenderness at the intertubercular groove. Tendinitis of the Achilles tendon is easily diagnosed by localized tenderness just proximal to its insertion in the calcaneus. To test for the integrity of the Achilles tendon, the "heel squeeze" test is employed. The examiner squeezes the heel and attempts to resist plantar flexion. The patient with an intact Achilles tendon should be able to overcome this resistance easily. If the patient is unable to plantarflex the foot, Achilles tendon rupture is likely. DeQuervain's tendinitis is caused by overuse or excessive strain of the wrist and thumb and is localized at or near the styloid process of the radius. This condition, as well as most of the other forms of tendinitis, can also include involvement of the tendon sheath, in which case swelling, crepitation, or a "gritty" sensation may be present.

Treatment of tendinitis is rest to the area with adequate immobilization, local heat, and oral analgesics. Injection with lidocaine (Xylocaine) and a corticosteroid is helpful, especially in cases of calcific tendinitis of the shoulder. This differs from the treatment of the various bursitic conditions in that aspiration of fluid, if possible, and a compressive dressing are ordinarily the only measures that are necessary.

Neurapraxia and Other Nerve Disorders

Trauma, direct pressure, and other compressive forces can cause symptoms of pain, swelling, and sensory disturbances at the site of, and along the distribution of, a nerve. In the upper extremity, the following are seen:

- Saturday night palsy. (So called because it most typically occurs in an inebriated patient who loses consciousness with one arm draped over a bench or chair.) A radial nerve paralysis is caused by prolonged pressure on the distal humerus, with resultant loss of finger and wrist extension and sensory loss over the dorsoradial aspect of the thumb web space. Complete recovery can eventually be anticipated, but passive exercises, proper splinting, and referral is indicated.
- ulnar palsy. The ulnar nerve is susceptible to injury at the elbow, where it passes beneath the medial epicondyle ("the crazy bone"). A direct blow to this area can cause immediate pain and a shocking sensation extending all the way to the hand, particularly in the ring and small fingers. Usually, this paresthesia is transient. If symptoms persist beyond the acute phase or if later sequelae develop, referral is necessary. Ulnar neurapraxia is less commonly a result of entrapment in Guyon's canal at the wrist.
- carpal tunnel syndrome. The most common carpal nerve disorder is caused by pressure on the medial nerve within the confines of the carpal tunnel on the volar aspect of the wrist. Pain and tingling sensations at the wrist and especially in the distribution of the medial nerve are reported, and gently tapping over the nerve at the wrist (Tinel's sign) can reproduce these symptoms. Prolonged wrist flexion (Phalen's test) can also elicit the unpleasant sensations of carpal tunnel syndrome. Symptoms are usually worse at night or early morning, and the patient may recount having to shake the hand to "wake it up." Rest with wrist immobilization is the

treatment if early diagnosis is made. Injection of the carpal tunnel is to be avoided. If this condition does not respond to conservative management, surgical treatment is highly successful.

In the upper extremity, neurapraxias of the axillary and long thoracic nerves are rarely encountered (if axillary nerve paralysis, secondary to shoulder dislocation, is not considered).

In the lower extremity, peripheral nerve syndromes are usually limited to the peroneal nerve. This nerve is vulnerable to contusion or compression where it passes across the neck of the fibula. The typical pain and shocking feeling, with subsequent tingling and numbness, will be felt on the lateral side of the leg and foot. Treatment and complications of this injury are very similar to that for ulnar nerve palsy at the elbow.

Other Soft Tissue Conditions of Specific Anatomical Areas

Neck. Torticollis or wryneck can occur in children or adults. The patient reports severe neck pain, without trauma, and will tend to hold the head and neck rigid or tilted to one side. Often the patient will awaken with the symptoms, or they may progress gradually during the day. It is difficult to elicit any predisposing or causative factors. Rest is the hallmark of treatment, with use of a cervical collar, if needed, plus application of moist heat, oral administration of analgesics and muscle relaxants. Results of neurologic examination in this condition are normal.

Shoulder. The shoulder is susceptible to not only acute trauma but also the ravages of chronic irritation and wear and tear; as a result, the patient with a painful shoulder frequently appears in the emergency department. Bicipital tendinitis has been discussed but probably more common is the less well defined entity of shoulder cuff pathology.

The fibrous capsule of the shoulder joint, the musculotendinous rotator cuff, the subacromial bursa, and even the overlying deltoid muscle are all subject to the degenerative changes that afflict this area. Precisely pinpointing the pathology to the supraspinatus tendon or to the subdeltoid bursa, for example, is usually not of prime concern for the emergency department physician, since the essential treatment remains rest, with sling support, application of local moist heat, and analgesics.

Areas of point tenderness, particularly when calcification is seen on the radiograph, may be injected with a corticosteroid preparation and lidocaine. All patients should be referred for further evaluation, especially if a tear of the rotator cuff is suspected.

Acute rupture of the long head of the biceps tendon is recognized by the history of a sudden sharp pain and the characteristic bunching of the biceps muscle belly in the arm. Orthopedic consultation is necessary since surgical treatment may be indicated.

Elbow. Lateral epicondylitis, or tennis elbow, is attributed to chronic strain, attrition, and degenerative changes of the annular ligament of the radius and of the aponeurotic attachment of the extensor muscles of the forearm at the lateral epicondyle. This condition is more common than medial epicondylitis and may give rise to aching pain and local tenderness, which is aggravated by the use of these muscles in wrist and hand motion. Local injection of corticosteroids and Xylocaine is effective, in addition to conservative measures of rest and moist heat.

Hand. Trigger finger or trigger thumb is a stenosing tenosynovitis of the flexor tendon sheath, causing a constriction or binding of the tendon, which tends to lock the finger in flexion and produces an unpleasant snapping sensation when the finger is extended. The patient will refer this discomfort to the interphalangeal joint of the thumb or to the proximal interphalangeal joint of the finger, often to the dorsal surface. However, the pathology is localized to the volar surface at the level of the metacarpal head of the involved digit, where a firm, tender nodule may be palpated. Treatment with lidocaine injection into this nodule followed by application of ice and administration of analgesics will relieve this condition, but the patient must be cautioned that triggering may recur and repeated injection may be necessary.

Dupuytren's contracture will rarely be encountered as an emergency but should be easily recognized by the longitudinal band of contracture of the palmar fascia involving the little ring or long fingers. The patient should be referred to a hand surgeon.

Treatment of subungual hematoma is by puncturing the nail and releasing the hematoma, affording great relief to the patient. A nail avulsed at its base should be removed, using digital block, if necessary. Skin and soft tissue injury to the distal finger may take various forms, and treatment must be individualized. Many of these wounds will heal quite well if simply left alone, protected, and allowed to heal by epithelialization. Extensive or complex wounds require consultation and referral to a hand surgeon.

Recognition is the key in the treatment of nerve and tendon injuries of the hand. Simple inspection and observation will frequently confirm the diagnosis in tendon injuries. Sensation and tendon function should be checked in all lacerations before the wound is anesthetized.

Sensory examination of the median nerve is best performed around the nail fold of the index or long finger, of the radial nerve at the dorsal web space of the thumb, and of the ulnar nerve at the distal small finger.

Motor function of the median nerve is sometimes difficult to assess accurately but is best evaluated in a cooperative patient by pad-to-pad opposition of the thumb to the other digits. Integrity of the motor branch of the radial nerve is tested by extension of wrist, fingers, and thumb at the metacarpophalangeal joints. The ulnar nerve motor innervation is tested by digital abduction and adduction or, more specifically, by observing and palpating the action of the first dorsal interosseous muscle along the radial border of the index fingers.

Assessment of flexor tendon function is accomplished with the hand on a flat surface, palm upward; the sublimi are tested individually by holding the other digits flat and asking the patient to lift the finger to the ceiling; the profundi are tested similarly, but with the examiner immobilizing the proximal interphalangeal joints to prevent sublimis action.

After adequate anesthesia, a thorough exploration of the wound must be carried out. In this manner, the possibility of missing a partial tendon is negated.

Extensor tendon injury should always be suspected in dorsal hand and finger lacerations since the tendon lies only a few millimeters beneath the skin. A thorough exploration, including having the patient flex and extend the digit while the wound is being clearly visualized is required because extensor lacerations may not be clinically detectable by attitude and position or by testing extensor motion against gravity.

Extensor tendon lacerations of the hand and fingers can often be repaired in the emergency department, followed by proper immobilization and referral. All flexor tendon lacerations and digital nerve injuries should be referred. The most important of the digital nerves are those of the thumb, the radial nerve of the index finger, and the ulnar digital nerve of the little finger. Digital nerve injuries beyond the distal interphalangeal joint are usually not repaired.

Hip and Thigh. Contusion, with hematoma, to the hip and thigh may be massive, with extensive ecchymosis and swelling. Rest, with ice application, is imperative, and early referral is recommended.

Rupture of a significant amount of fibers of one of the large muscle bellies of this area, usually the hamstrings, may result in a large, palpable mass or knot. This can be readily differentiated from a soft tissue tumor by careful history and physical examination.

Knee. Baker's cyst is a cystic swelling of the popliteal fossa that, in adults, suggests intra-articular disease of the knee. The cyst frequently communicates with the knee joint and sometimes can become quite large. Specific treatment is usually not necessary, but orthopedic referral is indicated.

Iliotibial band syndrome and popliteus tendinitis are two similar entities caused by strain, usually from jogging or running, which are manifested by pain of the lateral knee over the lateral femoral condyle. Treatment is conservative and symptomatic.

Leg. Shin splints is an overuse syndrome that is poorly understood and that causes pain and tenderness of the distal two-thirds of the leg, either medial to the tibia, the usual reference, or lateral to the tibia (also referred to as an anterior compartment syndrome). Stress fractures must be ruled out, and treatment is the same as in other overuse syndromes.

Plantaris tendon rupture and partial rupture of the gastrosoleus muscle cannot always be distinguished, since both produce a sudden sharp, deep, midcalf pain. The subsequent appearance of swelling and ecchymosis will implicate the gastrosoleus. The Achilles tendon remains intact. Treatment is symptomatic.

Ankle. Dislocation of the peroneal tendons may be acute or chronic. The patient may describe a snapping sensation at the lateral malleolus or the awareness of something slipping out of place. These dislocations reduce easily, but orthopedic referral for defining possible operative treatment is indicated.

Foot. Spurs and exostoses are commonly encountered as incidental findings on the radiograph but, if symptomatic, can be treated with protective pads, lifts, and orthotics. Surgical excision may be necessary if conservative measures fail.

Plantar fasciitis is similar to spurs and exostoses and involves an inflammatory reaction at the insertion of the plantar fascia into the calcaneus. The radiograph may sometimes reveal a prominent heel spur. Injection of corticosteroid in the tender area may be tried in addition to conservative measures.

Plantar arch strain and actual rupture of the plantar fascia due to attrition and overuse can also occur. In these conditions symptoms are located more directly under the longitudinal arch of the foot. Rupture of the plantar fascia does not require surgical treatment.

Morton's neuralgia or neuroma is a thickening of the plantar nerve at the level of the metatarsal heads, before it divides into its digital branches. This disorder most commonly occurs between the third and fourth metatarsal heads and can usually be distinguished from strain or metatarsalgia by its characteristic nervelike pain. There is often a shocking sensation, tingling, or numbness that radiates to the inner aspects of the third and fourth toes. The pain can be excruciating at times. Longitudinal arch supports or a metatarsal bar may relieve the

pressure on the nerve. If this is unsuccessful, surgical treatment can be quite effective.

An ingrown toenail usually affects the great toe and should be managed nonsurgically in the emergency department. Analgesics, antibiotics, hot packs and soaks, and avoidance of irritation comprise suitable treatment. Referral for definitive surgical excision should be arranged.

Painful corns and calluses are caused by friction and pressure. Prevention, usually by means of properly fitting shoes, should be stressed. Padding and protection of the affected area, along with a softening agent or judicious trimming, will help once the corn or callus is established.

Plantar warts should be distinguished from a callus. They can be extremely painful and disabling. Treatment remedies include cauterization, surgical excision, or even freezing with liquid nitrogen. The best recourse for the emergency department physician is to recommend application of salicylic acid to soften the wart and careful, periodic scraping of the lesion.

IMMOBILIZATION

The role of immobilization as an initial mainstay in the treatment of many emergent orthopedic situations has been discussed. There are numerous available splints, wraps, and other mechanisms of preventing undesired motion and ensuring that the injured part remains at rest.

Splints are available in many shapes, sizes, and materials. For example, in the treatment of mallet finger injuries, there is a preshaped, easily fitted, "stack" finger splint made of plastic; a short, padded, aluminum "mallet" splint; or a malleable, plastic, "baseball" splint, all of which serve the same purpose of maintaining the distal interphalangeal joint in a neutral, or, the preferred, hyperextended position.

Aluminum or plastic finger splints, both padded and unpadded varieties, are probably most commonly employed. These can be preformed or malleable and are useful in immobilizing digits in a position of function. Whenever a digit, or the entire hand, is immobilized, the physician should strive to maintain the position of function (i.e., flexion of the interphalangeal and metacarpophalangeal joints and extension at the wrist with the thumb web space open).

The individual splint can thus be utilized for fractures, sprains, "stoved" fingers, lacerations, or any other condition that requires immobilization. If the immobilization is maintained longer than a few days, the patient should be told to expect some degree of joint stiffness that will require time and active motion to overcome.

Metal splints are more commonly employed for temporary immobilization of the large joints and long bone injuries, such as Colles' splints, elbow splints, and short and long leg splints. They allow for patient comfort, access for reexamination, safe transport, and radiographic examination while awaiting definitive treatment.

Other forms of immobilization include Shantz dressings (alternative layers of Webril and Ace wrappings) and Robert Jones dressings (heavy padding with cotton and fluffs). These are useful in lower extremity injuries such as nondisplaced fractures and ankle and knee sprains. The knee can also be immobilized with a knee immobilizer, a comfortable, brace-type apparatus that is frequently used in nondisplaced patellar fractures. Of course, clavicle fractures are treated with a clavicle strap or figure-of-eight dressing, with a sling as an adjunct. The sling is also an ideal immobilizer for most shoulder injuries.

Although all these forms of immobilization are effective and fairly easy to apply, the use of plaster is frequently best. Plaster splints for fingers, hands, and the rest of the extremities can be molded to fit any situation and need. Plaster can be combined with metallic splints in digital injuries or with Shantz or Robert Jones dressings in both lower and upper extremities.

Plaster volar splints or plaster posterior splints are often the best initial treatment in many hand/wrist fractures or elbow fractures, respectively, when there is much soft tissue swelling. These splints are simple to prepare and apply. The appropriate length and thickness of plaster slabs is selected, placed inside the correct size of stockinette, wet, applied to the extremity, and wrapped with an Ace dressing. When a fracture requires reduction, the proper position is most securely maintained by application of a circular plaster cast.

BIBLIOGRAPHY

Aegerter E, Kirkpatrick J: *Orthopedic Diseases*, ed 4. Philadelphia, WB Saunders Co, 1975.

Boyes JH: *Bunnell's Surgery of the Hand*, ed 5. Philadelphia, JB Lippincott Co, 1970.

Brody D: *Running Injuries*. Ciba Clinical Symposia, 1980, vol 32, no. 4.

Cozen L: *Office Orthopedics*, ed 4. Springfield, Ill, Charles C Thomas, 1974.

De Palma A: *The Management of Fractures and Dislocations*, ed 2. Philadelphia, WB Saunders Co, 1970.

Giannestros NJ: *Foot Disorders, Medical and Surgical Management*, ed 2. Philadelphia, Lea & Febiger, 1973.

Gillis L: *Diagnosis in Orthopedics*. London, Butterworths, 1969.

Hollingshead H: *Anatomy for Surgeons*, ed 2. New York, Harper & Row, 1969, vol 3.

Moore DC: *Regional Block*, ed 4. Springfield, Ill, Charles C Thomas, 1967.

Newmeyer, W: *Primary Care of Hand Injuries*. Philadelphia, Lea & Febiger, 1979.

Nicholas JA: *Internal Derangement of the Knee: Diagnosis and Management. American Academy of Orthopedic Surgeons Symposium on Sports Medicine*. St Louis, CV Mosby Co, 1969, pp 152–161.

O'Donoghue DH: *Treatment of Injuries to Athletes*, ed 2. Philadelphia, WB Saunders Co, 1970.

Rockwood C, Green D: *Fractures*, ed 2. Philadelphia, JB Lippincott Co, 1975, vols 1 and 2.

Tachdjian MO: *Pediatric Orthopedics*. Philadelphia, WB Saunders Co, 1972, vols 1 and 2.

9. Transfusion Therapy

STEWART E. DADMUN, M.D., F.A.C.P.

Traditionally, emergency departments have used blood products to stabilize acutely ill patients until more definitive care can be given. In recent years, many hospital emergency departments have had the added responsibility for elective transfusion therapy. Outpatient elective transfusion can be both cost effective and time saving.

HYPOVOLEMIA

Whole Blood

Until recent years, the term *blood transfusion* was equated with the infusion of whole blood. Modern blood banking techniques, such as the separation of whole blood into component parts; the chronic scarcity of donated blood; and the decreased risks of component transfusion have changed old concepts and habits of transfusion.[1] Nonetheless, the rapid, life-threatening loss of whole blood is still best managed by replacement with whole blood. Massive whole blood transfusion carries with it certain risks that must be borne in mind, however.

Bleeding Tendencies

With time, banked blood gradually loses labile clotting activity.[2] Factors V and VIII decline by about 50 percent in the first two weeks of blood storage. The infusion of 1 or 2 units of single-donor fresh plasma with each 5 to 8 units of banked blood helps to replace these factors.

Periodic platelet counts during massive transfusion warn of impending thrombocytopenia. One-day-old banked blood is essentially platelet-free. The availability of platelet transfusions as well as fresh-frozen plasma has markedly decreased the need for fresh drawn whole blood for transfusion.

Hyperkalemia

As blood cells deteriorate in banked blood, potassium is released into the plasma. This may become a serious problem for massively transfused patients with renal impairment or crush injury. Frequent patient serum potassium determinations may be helpful, but observation of peaking of the T waves on the electrocardiogram (ECG) can be a more rapid way to learn of possible significant hyperkalemia. (See Chapter 15.)

Hypocalcemia

Donated blood is mixed with calcium-binding anticoagulant solutions. These are most commonly anticoagulant-citrate-dextrose (ACD) or citrate-phosphate-dextrose (CPD). Because these solutions are present in excess, they can bind the patient's calcium as well. Massive transfusions can lead to tetany and seizure for this reason. The ECG may provide a clue to hypocalcemia, i.e., prolongation of the QT interval. One ampule calcium gluconate with every 2 units of transfused blood after the first 6 units should prevent significant hypocalcemia when transfusions must be given at a rate that exceeds the body's capacity to metabolize citrate. (See Chapter 17.)

2,3-Diphosphoglyceric Acid Depletion

Because 2,3-diphosphoglyceric acid (DPG) assists the hemoglobin molecule in its role of giving up oxygen to the tissues, depletion of 2,3-DPG in banked blood may hinder one of the main purposes of transfusion. Fortunately, the patient's body restores 2,3-DPG to banked blood within a few hours of transfusion.[3] Care should be taken to avoid other conditions that tend to prevent the transmission of oxygen from hemoglobin, such as alkalosis as a result of excessive bicarbonate administration or hyperventilation as a consequence of mechanically assisted respiration.

Other Risks

Volume must be carefully monitored, particularly in patients with heart disease and in the elderly, to prevent volume overload. Hypothermia can result from the rapid infusion of refrigerated blood (see Blood Warmers).

Autotransfusion

In recent years, many trauma centers have been equipped to reinfuse the patient's uncontaminated lost blood. This has been particularly helpful in the stabilization of victims of penetrating chest trauma and gynecologic emergencies, such as a ruptured ectopic pregnancy.[4] Many methods have been used to remove blood from the pleural or peritoneal cavities, treat it to prevent coagulation, and return it to the patient. The Sorensen Autotransfusion Unit (Sorensen Research Company, Salt Lake City, Utah 84115) has been well tested. It is quite safe, and it is not difficult to use.[5] Autotransfusion avoids the risk of transfusion reactions, is fast, and does not deplete valuable blood bank reserves. Naturally, it should not be attempted if the blood is contaminated. Emergency department personnel should become thoroughly familiar with this technique before attempting it.

Plasma Expanders

Hypovolemia due to minor bleeding can often be more safely treated with plasma expanders than whole blood. Severe burns, sepsis, intra-abdominal catastrophies, such as pancreatitis, may also be better treated with plasma expanders than with whole blood.

Normal Serum Albumin and Plasma Protein Fraction

If they are treated in such a way as to remove all bacteria, to inactivate hepatitis virus, and to remove ABO blood group antibodies, both normal serum albumin and plasma protein fraction (PPF) are suitable for treatment of hypovolemic shock. Infusions of PPF greater than 10 ml/minute can produce hypotension and are therefore contraindicated when rapid infusion is necessary. Normal serum albumin does not produce this complication. Solutions of 25 percent albumin have an oncotic equivalent five times greater than that of normal plasma. A 20-ml dose of this solution draws 70 ml fluid from extravascular tissues into the circulation in 15 minutes, thereby increasing total blood volume, reducing hemoconcentration, and lowering whole blood viscosity. It can be very helpful for patients with burns or cerebral edema, and in exchange transfusion of infants to prevent kernicterus. Normal serum albumin is not effective for treatment of chronic hypoalbuminemic states.

Dextrans and Hydroxyethyl Starch

Among the substances that have been found to be safe, effective plasma volume expanders are the dextrans and hydroxyethyl starch. Dextran is available either in a low-molecular-weight class (dextran 40), or high-molecular-weight class (dextran 70). Dextran 40 molecules are small enough to pass through capillary walls, so the plasma volume-expanding effect of this solution is lost in two to six hours. Dextran 70 has larger molecules and a circulating half-life of six hours. Small plugs of dextran 40 become lodged in renal tubules when glomerular filtration pressure is low, which may lead to renal failure.[6] This does not occur with dextran 70. Both dextrans interfere with platelet function and are therefore risky in acute bleeding situations. In addition, both forms can cause anaphylactic reactions.

Hydroxyethyl starch, a colloid derived from a waxy starch, is available as a 6 percent solution in normal saline. Its advantages over the dextrans include a 24-hour plasma volume expansion time, less bleeding tendency, no anaphylactic reactions, and no long-term side-effects.[7] Extensive blood loss has been adequately managed with only these synthetic plasma expanders.[8]

Crystalloid Solutions

Both normal saline and Ringer's lactate have the disadvantage of very brief plasma expansion. Their use is well understood. Many patients who receive only 1 or 2 units of whole blood for volume expansion could have been adequately managed with crystalloid infusion.[9]

BLOOD COMPONENT REPLACEMENT THERAPY

Patients deserve to be treated with just what is needed, no more and no less. Such treatment improves results and decreases complications. Blood component therapy exemplifies this kind of treatment precision.[10]

Packed Red Blood Cells

By separating the red blood cells (RBCs) from the plasma, serious anemia can be corrected with only about one-half the volume required when whole blood is used, thereby minimizing the chance of precipitating heart failure. Electrolytes, acid, and citrate that might be harmful to patients with heart, kidney, or liver disease are largely removed with the plasma. Packed RBCs are indicated in symptomatically anemic patients who cannot be readily returned to safe levels of hemoglobin with replacement therapy, such as iron, folate, or vitamin B_{12}.[11] Combinations of crystalloids and packed RBCs can be given for submassive bleeding.[12] The number of units of packed RBCs needed to correct anemia can be calculated as follows:

$$\frac{\left(\begin{array}{c}\text{Blood volume}\\ \times\ \text{hematocrit}\end{array}\right) + \left(\begin{array}{c}\text{No. of units}\\ \text{transfused}\\ \times\ 200\ \text{ml}\end{array}\right) \times 100}{\text{Blood volume} + \left(\begin{array}{c}\text{No. of units}\\ \text{transfused}\\ \times\ 300\end{array}\right)} = \text{New hematocrit}$$

The usual volume of a unit of packed RBCs is 300 ml, with a 200 ml RBC mass. Blood volume is about 75 ml/kg for men and 67 ml/kg for women.

Occasionally, packed RBCs must be purified further. Removal of leukocytes can prevent the febrile reactions to white blood cells often seen in patients who have received multiple transfusions or who have had many pregnancies. Use of leukocyte-poor RBC concentrations may delay the onset of antileukocyte or antiplatelet antibody formation in patients suffering from leukemia or aplastic anemia, who may later require white blood cell or platelet replacement as well. Leukocyte-poor packed RBCs irradiated with 1,500 to 3,000 rads may prevent the graft versus host reaction sometimes seen in immunodeficient transfusion recipients. Washing packed RBCs can remove substances potentially harmful to patients with paroxysmal nocturnal hemoglobinuria or IgA deficiency.

Glyceralized frozen blood allows for the prolonged storage of autologous blood, rare blood types, or even common blood types that must be stockpiled longer than the usual 21-day lifespan of refrigerated banked blood. Deglyceralized and thawed frozen blood can be given for the same indications that packed RBCs or leukocyte-poor packed RBCs are given. The freezing and deglyceralization process greatly increases the expense of transfusion, however, and is therefore of very limited practical application at this time.[13]

Platelet Transfusion

A platelet "pack" separated from whole blood shortly after donation contains at least 5.5×10^{10} platelets and each unit will raise the platelet count about 7,000/μl in a 70-kg adult. Platelet packs are used to treat bleeding secondary to thrombocytopenia (fewer than 50,000/μl) or for prophylaxis in patients with leukemia or other conditions associated with megakaryocytic failure who have platelet counts lower than 20,000/μl. Conditions that cause a loss of platelets from the circulation, such as idiopathic thrombocytopenic purpura or disseminated intravascular coagulation, do not respond to platelet transfusion. Patients with antiplatelet isoantibodies as a result of multiple transfusions may have a markedly blunted response to random donor platelet transfusions. These patients may respond better to platelets obtained by platelet phoresis from an HLA-matched sibling. Six to eight units of platelets or one platelet phoresis collection (comparable to seven to ten platelet packs from random donors) are usually sufficient for prophylactic treatment of a patient with a platelet count lower than 20,000/μl. A similar transfusion can successfully prepare a patient with fewer platelets than 60,000/μl for surgery. The three- to four-day half-life of platelets requires that prophylactic transfusion be carried out approximately twice a week. The efficacy of platelet transfusion can be checked by a platelet count done about one hour after the infusion. Platelet packs are more effective when stored at room temperature than when stored in the refrigerator, but room temperature storage increases the risk of bacterial contamination. Cross matching is not necessary for platelet transfusion.[14]

White Blood Cell Transfusions

The technique of white blood cell transfusion is used only for hospital patients with agranulocytosis and sepsis who are unresponsive to maximum antibiotic treatment. Therefore, a discussion of this procedure is not applicable to the emergency department at this time.[15]

Plasma Component Therapy

Plasma separated from the formed elements of blood can be prepared in a variety of ways to restore volume or to replace deficient plasma factors.

Single-Donor Fresh-Frozen Plasma

Units of fresh-frozen plasma contain all the clotting factors, including labile factors V and VIII. Plasma that has not been frozen immediately or from which cryoprecipitate has been removed can be used for volume expansion or replacement of the stable factors II, VII, IX, or X. Kept at −18°C the labile factors are active for up to one year of storage. Patients who have prolonged prothrombin times due to advanced liver disease or who are undergoing coumarin treatment can be corrected with 5 to 10 ml/kg fresh-frozen plasma. Deficiency of fibrinogen or factor VIII (hemophilia A, von Willebrand's disease) is better treated with factor VIII concentrates because of the potential volume overload from fresh-frozen plasma. Factor IX deficiency (hemophilia B) is treated with a lyophilized concentrate of the stable clotting factors.[2] Factor IX concentrate and plasma obtained from several donors carry a high risk of hepatitis transmission; this risk is much less with single-donor fresh-frozen plasma. Fresh-frozen plasma can cause allergic reactions with chills, fever, and urticaria, however. It also contains the normal red cell isoantibodies and therefore must be compatible with the ABO grouping of recipient red cells.

Factor VIII Cryoprecipitated Antihemophiliac Factor

A plasma concentrate, cryoprecipitated antihemophiliac factor contains about 80 units factor VIII, 250 mg fibrinogen, 30 percent factor XIII, and 40 to 70 percent von Willebrand's factor.[16] Cryoprecipitate bags are thawed at 30° to 38°C prior to infusion. The material should be transfused within six hours of thawing and four hours of pooling. Compatibility between donor plasma and recipient red cells is preferable, but not essential. In hemophilia A, the number of cryoprecipitate bags needed may be calculated as follows:

$$\frac{\left(\begin{array}{c}\text{Desired}\\ \text{factor VIII}\\ \text{level (\%)}\end{array}\right) \times \left(\begin{array}{c}\text{Plasma}\\ \text{volume}\\ \text{(ml)}\end{array}\right)}{100 \times 80 \left(\begin{array}{c}\text{Average}\\ \text{units per}\\ \text{bag}\end{array}\right)} = \text{No. of bags needed}$$

In order to maintain an even blood level of factor VIII, the concentrate must be given about every 8 to 12 hours because of the 12-hour half-life of factor VIII. Lyophilized factor VIII concentrates can be used in much the same way. The manufacturer records the number of units on the vial. Factor VIII levels should be monitored about one hour after infusion of the concentrate. Patients with anti-factor VIII antibodies may require massive doses of factor VIII replacement. Hemophiliacs can do quite well through most surgery or trauma with factor VIII levels of about 30 percent.

Patients with von Willebrand's disease should be treated with either fresh-frozen plasma or cryoprecipitated plasma because lyophilized factor VIII concentrates do not contain the von Willebrand's factor. These patients rarely have spontaneous bleeding and can be adequately supported through trauma and surgery with one bag of cryoprecipitate per 10 kg body weight per day. One unit of fresh-frozen plasma is equivalent to one bag of cryoprecipitate and may be used as an alternative, but fresh-frozen plasma may cause volume overload. Von Willebrand's replacement therapy should be started the day before surgery and continued until healing occurs.

Fibrinogen deficiency can be adequately treated with plasma cryoprecipitate. Pooled commercial fibrinogen is no longer available because of the great danger that it would transmit hepatitis. Eight bags of cryoprecipitated antihemophiliac factor contain about 2 gm fibrinogen. Hyperfibrinogenemia can be a complication of antihemophiliac factor therapy for factor VIII deficiency.

Factor XIII deficiency is a rare disorder that can be treated prophylactically with cryoprecipitate one bag/ 10 kg body weight every two to three weeks.

Factor IX Complex

A lyophilized complex of stable factors II, VII, IX, and X that remain in plasma after the cryoprecipitate has been removed is called the factor IX complex. This product can be used to manage patients with factor IX deficiency (hemophilia B), coumarin drug overdose, and rare congenital deficiencies of factor II, VII, and X. There is a high risk of hepatitis transmission with this product. Mild bleeding risks are best controlled with single-donor plasma. Most hemophiliac B bleeding episodes can be managed with factor IX complex in a loading dose of 30 units/kg, followed by a maintenance dose of 10 units/kg every 12 hours. Preparation for major surgery or treatment of major trauma requires a doubling of the loading dose, although the maintenance does remains the same. Reversal of the prolonged prothrombin time caused by coumarin drug therapy should be treated with factor IX complex only in patients who must have normal hemostasis in less than the five or six hours required for vitamin K to be effective. Factor IX complex is contraindicated in patients with disseminated intravascular coagulation or liver disease.

Removal of Blood Components

Occasionally, it is necessary to remove blood components that are abnormal or in excess.

Plasmapheresis

It is possible to remove whole blood, discard the plasma, and return the red blood cells with another plasma expander.[17] There is a growing list of indications for this technique.[18] Many communities look to the emergency department to perform plasmapheresis on an outpatient basis. Therapeutic successes have been reported in patients with Waldenström's hyperglobulinemia, myeloma, cryoglobulinemia, immune complex disease, antibodies against factor VIII, anti-insulin antibodies, Goodpasture's syndrome, myasthenia gravis, and antibodies to Rh factors in pregnancy. It has been used with questionable benefit in patients with Guillain-Barré syndrome and multiple sclerosis. Up to 4 liters plasma can be removed in a single session. This plasma is replaced with iso-oncotic fluids (i.e., the plasma and serum albumin products already mentioned).

Cell Removal

The cell separators used for plasmapheresis can also be used to remove platelets when they are excessive in number (as in chronic myelogenous leukemia or polycythemia vera), abnormal red cells (as in hemoglobinopathies), or abnormal white cells (as in leukemia blasts, rheumatoid lymphs, Sézary cells), thereby greatly expanding the potential therapeutic use of this technique. Cell separators are now made as portable units and can be brought from a central location to an emergency department.

Blood and Blood Component Administration

Concomitant Use of Intravenous Solutions

Normal saline (0.9 percent) is the only safe intravenous solution to use with blood infusions. Five percent dextrose in water is hypotonic and causes hemolysis of formed blood elements in the transfusion apparatus. Ringer's solution and other solutions containing calcium may induce clotting of citrated blood in vitro. Medication should never be put in the transfusion unit or infused with blood. Packed RBCs may be diluted with normal saline, single-donor plasma, or fresh-frozen plasma.

Blood Transfusion Apparatus

Blood products should always be infused through a standard transfusion apparatus. This contains a filter that traps particles greater than 170 μ. Otherwise, these particles would be trapped in the pulmonary microvasculature, causing microemboli.

Blood Warmers

Transfusion of cold blood at a rate faster than 100 ml/minute for 30 minutes, or 50 ml/minute for greater than 60 minutes may lower body temperature to less than 30°C. This can cause serious cardiac arrhythmias and death.[19] Warming devices are designed to warm the blood in the tubing (not the bag); they should be such that infusions do not exceed 40°C because of the risk of red cell injury and hemolysis above this temperature. Blood warmers are indicated during multiple rapid transfusions, exchange transfusions in infants, and transfusions in patients with cold agglutinin disease.

Untoward Reactions to Transfusion

Transmission of Infectious Diseases

Hepatitis B transmission has been reduced to about 7 percent by the use of volunteer donors and hepatitis B virus testing. No test is currently available to detect the presence of non-A, non-B hepatitis.[20] Malaria, brucellosis, toxoplasmosis, syphilis, Epstein-Barr virus, cytomegalovirus, Colorado tick fever, and other infections have been transmitted from blood donor to recipient via transfusion. A unit of blood can be infected by bacteria if allowed to sit at room temperature more than four hours. Septicemia as a result of transfusing such blood is always dramatic and often fatal.

Hemolytic Transfusion Reaction

Fatal transfusion reactions are almost always due to clerical error, not a cross-matching error.[21] The importance of care in identifying the unit and patient cannot be overemphasized. Potential sources of error must be sought and guarded against by such methods as double-checking by two individuals, centralization of blood drawing for cross match, and delivery of units by a few trained and motivated individuals in the hospital. Careful and frequent monitoring of the patient's vital signs and appearance during the first half-hour of each unit infusion is very important. Reactions can be divided into three categories:

1. Mild pruritus and urticaria may be due to an allergic reaction to one or more of the blood components and can usually be well treated with antihistamines. Such reactions can often be prevented by giving packed RBCs instead of whole blood.
2. Anxiety, palpitation, mild dyspnea, headache, chills, fever, and urticaria may indicate a moderately severe reaction. The transfusion is stopped. The intravenous line is kept open with normal

saline. All tubing and blood is returned to the hospital blood bank, along with samples of the patient's blood and urine. Vital signs are watched carefully. The clinician is notified and may order antihistamines, antipyretics, corticosteroids, or epinephrine. Such reactions may be caused by plasma protein sensitization, particularly in patients with a congenital deficiency of IgA immunoglobulin. Leukocyte and platelet antigen sensitivity occurs in patients who have been transfused many times or have had many pregnancies. Leukocyte-poor blood should avoid this complication. The use of washed packed RBCs is necessary for IgA-deficient patients. Pyrogens in the transfusion apparatus are rarely seen since the advent of disposable equipment.

3. Life-threatening reactions may be heralded by anxiety, chest pain, fever, restlessness, tachycardia, red urine, and unexplained bleeding. The same sequence of procedures is followed as mentioned previously; however, therapy must be more aggressive to treat shock, maintain renal blood flow, and prevent the development of serious bleeding from disseminated intravascular coagulation.

Delayed transfusion reactions, though potentially serious, would presumably occur long after the patient has left the emergency department and will not be discussed here. The risk of transfusion reaction must always be borne in mind, but the incidence of such reactions can be minimized by the use of careful technique and the appropriate use of blood components or other plasma volume expanders.

REFERENCES

1. Greenwalt TJ, Polesky HF, Chaplin H, et al: *General Principles of Blood Transfusion.* American Medical Association Editorial Board, 1978.
2. Biggs R: *Human Blood Coagulation, Haemostasis and Thrombosis,* ed 2. London, Blackwell Scientific Publications, 1976, pp 365–398.
3. Beutler G, Wood L: The in vivo regeneration of red cell 2,3-diphosphoglyonic acid (DPG) after transfusion of stored blood. *J Lab Clin Med* 74:300, 1969.
4. Von Hippel A: Autotransfusion of major hemothorax in a simple county hospital. *Alaska Med* 17:62, 1975.
5. Von Koch L, Wilson DW, Mattox KL: A practical method of autotransfusion in the emergency center. *Am J Surg* 133:770, 1977.
6. Morgan TO, Little JM, Evans WA: Renal failure associated with low molecular weight dextran infusion, abstracted. *Transfusion* 8:305, 1968.
7. Lee WH, Cooper N, Weidner MG, et al: Clinical evaluation of a new plasma expander—Hydroxyethyl starch. *J Trauma* 8:381, 1968.
8. Golub S, Baily CP: Management of major surgical blood loss without transfusion. *JAMA* 198:1171, 1966.
9. Kiman A: Presently useful plasma volume expanders. *Anesthesiology* 27:417, 1966.
10. *Blood Component Therapy: A Physician's Handbook, ed 3.* Washington, DC, American Association of Blood Banks, 1981.
11. Mollison PL: *Blood Transfusions in Clinical Medicine,* ed 6. London, Blackwell Scientific Publications, 1979, p. 44.
12. Chaplin H Jr: Packed red blood cells. *N Engl J Med* 281:364–367, 1969.
13. Roberts SC: Cryopreserved red blood cells: A blood component, in Myhre BA (ed): *A Seminar on Blood Components.* Washington, DC, American Association of Blood Banks, 1977, pp 37–52.
14. Daly PA, Schiffer CA, et al: Platelet transfusion therapy. *JAMA* 243:435, 1980.
15. Higby DJ, Burnett D: Granulocyte transfusions: Current status. *Blood* 55:2–8, 1980.
16. Ness PM, Perkins HA: Cryoprecipitate as a reliable source of fibrinogen replacement. *JAMA* 241:1690, 1979.
17. Jones JV: Plasmapheresis: Current research and success. *Heart Lung* 9:671, 1980.
18. Waldenstrom JG: Plasmapheresis: Bloodletting revived and refined. *Acta Med Scand* 208:1, 1980.
19. Boyan CP, Howland WS: Cardiac arrest and temperature of bank blood. *JAMA* 183:58, 1963.
20. Aach RD, Kahn RA: Posttransfusion hepatitis: Current perspectives. *Ann Intern Med* 92:539, 1980.
21. Schmidt PJ: Transfusion mortality: With special reference to surgical and intensive care facilities. *J Fla Med Assoc* 67:151, 1980.

10. Minor Lacerations and Abrasions

DAVIS CRACROFT, M.D.

Essential in the emergency department treatment of any wound is the initial evaluation of the patient's condition. Attention should be directed to the patient's age, allergies, medications being taken (e.g., steroids, chemotherapeutic agents), tetanus immunization status, and coexisting illnesses (e.g., diabetes mellitus, coronary artery disease). Blood loss replacement, intravenous (IV) fluid administration, and the treatment of life-threatening medical problems always precede definitive care of any wound. A sterile, dry gauze pad applied with pressure provides adequate hemostasis, prevents further contamination, and allows attention to be directed to more urgent problems. Occasionally, a cavity must be packed firmly to control bleeding; on an extremely rare occasion, a tourniquet is necessary to control the hemorrhage. Under these circumstances, the tourniquet is intended only as a temporary measure to provide a bloodless surgical field, allowing the accurate placement of hemostats and preventing damage to vital structures associated with blind clamping. Once hemostasis is ensured, the tourniquet is removed and some blood flow is restored to the limb until arterial reconstruction can be performed. Only in the case of the severely shattered limb, when amputation is inevitable, should the tourniquet be left in place. It should then be placed as close to the injury as possible and the limb amputated, preferably above the tourniquet.

WOUND EVALUATION

After the patient has been stabilized and associated injuries or illnesses treated or ruled out, attention can be directed to the wound. Information on the history and mechanism of injury is critical to the subsequent management of the patient. The injury may be the consequence of a more serious underlying disease. For example, a scalp laceration may be secondary to a dysrhythmia-induced syncopal episode. Suspicious location or appearance of wounds in children should suggest child abuse and prompt appropriate physical and social investigation. The history given by the patient may be suspect because of drug or alcohol intoxication, head injury, fear of potential legal consequences, senility, toxic or metabolic encephalopathy, and it may be necessary to seek the history of injury from family, friends, paramedics, police, or bystanders at the scene. The clinician should attempt to establish the age of the wound, the nature of any contamination, the causative agent (e.g., knife, dog bite, high- or low-velocity missile, blunt object), and the possibility of foreign bodies in the wound or distant sites. This information, combined with the location of the wound and overall physical and mental condition of the patient, allows the physician to plan the treatment of the injury logically.

Age of the Wound

The length of time between injury and treatment and the type and degree of contamination are important considerations in deciding whether to leave a wound open or to proceed with primary closure. Any accidental open wound can be considered contaminated. If left untreated, all but the most superficial wounds become infected. The presence of dead or devitalized tissue, blood clot, foreign bodies, moisture, and warmth enhances and hastens the process. The study of open wounds during World War I revealed that bacterial colony counts doubled at 10 to 12 hours postinjury.[1] Subsequent studies, based primarily on the experience of individual surgeons, have reduced the time necessary for a wound to be considered infected.

According to one classification, any incised wound less than 6 hours old is suitable for closure; a wound (either incised or ragged) 6 to 12 hours old is suitable for delayed primary closure after three to five days; and any wound older than 12 hours should be allowed to heal by secondary intention with subsequent grafting or delayed closure.[2] Any arbitrary classification based on the age of the wound or any other single factor may serve as a rough guide, but it is impossible to develop simple rules for complex problems. Each wound should be assessed individually.

Contamination and Infection

Infection occurs when the number of organisms at a given site exceeds the ability of local tissue defenses to control them. For most pathogens, a concentration of 10^6 organisms per gram of tissue produces an infection. With a lower concentration of bacteria, the wound is merely contaminated, and local humoral and cellular defenses prevent infection. Any contaminated wound can be converted to a surgically clean wound by means of mechanical cleansing and meticulous debridement. Infected wounds, however, cannot be converted to clean wounds by any quick simple procedure. Contamination can be differentiated from infection by the cardinal signs of inflammation—calor, rubor, dolor, and tumor. These signs are associated with infection and are an absolute contraindication to closure, regardless of the length of time the wound has been open.[2]

The blood supply to the region of injury plays an important role in the natural defense against infection. Facial and scalp lacerations may be closed primarily after 24 hours in many instances, owing to the rich blood supply in these areas. Conversely, as a consequence of diminished venous and lymphatic return and poor arterial supply, there is a high risk that distal lower extremity lacerations will become infected even when treated shortly after injury. The effectiveness of the defense provided by the blood supply to the upper extremity, proximal lower extremity, abdomen, and thorax falls between these two extremes.

Contusional damage to tissue surrounding a traumatic laceration may compromise local defenses and render a relatively clean wound unsuitable for closure. Additionally, the size and shape of the wound, the general condition of the patient, and damage to adjacent structures must all be considered by the physician who is deciding whether to close a wound. If there is any doubt, the wound should be left open or surgical consultation should be requested. A primary closure delayed three to five days does not appreciably alter the time of healing and avoids the discomfort, disability, time, and expense of treating an infected closed wound.

Causative Agent

The causative agent of injury may dictate whether the wound should be closed primarily. All partial thickness abrasions, puncture wounds, most animal (including human) bites, and most stab wounds are best treated with cleansing, exploration, debridement, and open drainage. Low-velocity missiles, such as a knife, low-caliber pistol bullet, or blunt object, usually create a relatively weak penetrating force that decelerates along its track. Surrounding injury is usually limited, and the greatest need is to review the anatomy of the region involved and ascertain the damage through the track. The destructive forces radiating from a high-velocity missile produce shock waves that extend several centimeters along its track, shatter bone, disrupt viscera, tear muscles, cause contusions, and usually leave a large ragged exit wound. Clearly, the emergency treatment of such injuries is centered about resuscitation and prompt transfer to the operating room.

Foreign Body Contamination

If there is any suspicion of foreign body contamination in a wound or distant site, radiographic examination in two planes should precede exploration. Radiopaque objects can be located by roentgenogram and removed under fluoroscopy. After the patient has been given local anesthesia, small-gauge (22 to 25) needles are passed through various angles and planes until the object is touched or seen to move. A small cutdown is then performed along the path of the needle in contact with the object, and the foreign body is retrieved. Only the most superficial foreign body, i.e., one that is readily seen or palpated after the injection of a local anesthetic, can be retrieved without the aid of fluoroscopy. A search for the proverbial "needle in the haystack" without fluoroscopy usually leads to excessive tissue damage and is often unsuccessful. Multiple shotgun pellets and less radiopaque foreign bodies in soft tissue are best left in place. If the object is not sterile, a localized abscess forms within a few days, allowing accurate removal by simple incision and drainage. Obviously, in the case of deep intraocular, intra-articular, or visceral foreign bodies, appropriate surgical consultation should be sought.

ANESTHESIA

Premedication

In general, premedication is not indicated for procedures performed under local anesthesia in the emergency department; it only adds to the potential complications. Careful explanations and ample reassurance usually allay fear in all but the most recalcitrant patients. When necessary, narcotics provide alleviation of apprehension, analgesia, and often some degree of euphoria. The recommended dose is roughly one-half that of the inpatient dose; meperidine hydrochloride (Demerol) 0.7 to 1 mg/kg or morphine sulfate 0.1 mg/kg. For children, a combination of meperidine hydrochloride (Demerol), 25 mg/ml; promethazine hydrochloride (Phenergan), 8 mg/ml; and chlorpromazine hydrochloride (Thorazine), 5 mg/ml provides excellent sedation. The dose is 1 ml/10 kg to a maximum of 2 ml. With all premedications, the clinician should wait 30 to 45 minutes before attempting the procedure. Caution should be used with children under the age of two; a papoose board or other restraint is the safer alternative. For procedures in which the uncooperative patient may jeopardize the outcome, general anesthesia is necessary.

Local Anesthesia

Most minor soft tissue injuries are best repaired under local infiltrative anesthesia. Lidocaine (Xylocaine), because of its low toxicity, rapid diffusibility, topical activity, and chemical stability is the drug of choice.[3] Toxic reactions vary from local skin wheals to convulsions, respiratory difficulties, and cardiovascular collapse. Resuscitative drugs and equipment should be readily available whenever local anesthetics are used. True allergic reactions are rare; most adverse reactions are due to overdosage. The maximum safe dose of lidocaine is 7.5 mg/kg up to 500 mg (50 ml 1 percent solution). Procaine hydrochloride (Novocain) with a maximal dose of 1,000 mg (100 ml 1 percent solution) is a good alternative to lidocaine in allergic patients. Strict limitation of dosages to below toxic levels, combined with aspiration in areas of suspected vascularity, prevents reactions in all but the rare hypersensitive patient.[4]

The local infiltrative technique is merely an infiltrate-as-you-advance process. Most wounds are best infiltrated through the open tissue, using fine-gauge (25 to 27) needles and systematically injecting the intradermal, subcutaneous, intrafascial, and intramuscular layers. With the addition of epinephrine (1:200,000), vasoconstriction occurs and absorption is delayed. The clinician should wait about ten minutes for maximal vasoconstrictive effect. In wounds of the head and neck, the use of lidocaine with epinephrine is standard. Avoid epinephrine-containing solutions where end-arteries are present (digits) or vasoconstriction may further compromise a tenuous blood supply (nasal tip, penis, or ear lacerations and skin flaps). Furthermore, avoid unnecessary distension of tissue by injecting small amounts of local anesthetics. High pressure injections only injure tissue, distort anatomy, compromise blood supply, and add tension to the wound closure.

DEBRIDEMENT AND IRRIGATION

Once the decision has been made to close a wound and the area has been properly anesthetized, a technique for converting the contaminated wound to a surgically clean one must be selected. In areas with sufficient tissue, such as the face, trunk, or an extremity, complete excision is by far the simplest and most certain way of eliminating damaged and contaminated tissue. Where excision is not feasible, irrigation and debridement are necessary. Hydraulic cleansing with sterile saline solution under moderate pressure (30 to 40 cm H_2O) provides optimal irrigation for the removal of blood clots, loose debris, and foreign bodies. A closed disposable irrigation system, consisting of a syringe attached via IV tubing to a saline irrigant bottle, makes an ideal irrigation device. Povidone-iodine (Betadine) solution is toxic to both bacteria and normal tissue; therefore, excessive soaking of wounds or irrigation with Betadine may retard healing and lead to excessive scar formation or infection. If contaminants can not be removed with saline irrigation or detergents, they must be excised.

Debridement is intended to remove all devitalized tissue and foreign material without doing harm to vital structures. Meticulous and often tedious attention to the removal of all small, often firmly adherent foreign bodies is mandatory if infection and tattooing are to be avoided. Repetitive saline irrigation, sponging with a dry gauze pad, and removal of adherent contaminants with fine-tipped Adson's forceps is recommended. Adequate visualization of the contaminated area may require extension of the wound. Partial thickness abrasions and lacerations should be debrided vigorously by scrubbing under topical, local, or general anesthesia. It must be remembered, however, that overzealous scrubbing can convert a partial thickness abrasion into a full thickness defect that will need skin grafting.

Excision should be done by sharp dissection, preferably with a scalpel and fine-toothed forceps, although sharp scissors can be used for removal of dead muscle, fat, and fascia. As a general rule, viable tissue bleeds freely and nonviable tissue does not. In skin debridement, only a narrow margin need be excised. On the face and scalp, questionably viable tissue can often be spared debridement; the abundant blood supply increases its chance of survival. Similarly, the facial subcutaneous tissue should be excised sparingly to avoid loss of supporting tissue that would result in a depressed scar. Elsewhere, fat should be excised back to a healthy, yellow plane free of any blood stains. Loose, ragged fragments of fascia should be excised. When ischemic or dead, muscle tissue is ragged and cyanotic; living muscle contracts when cut or pinched, bleeds when cut, and has a glistening, reddish brown color. Excision of muscle must be radical to prevent clostridial or other bacterial growth.

Flap lacerations and avulsions often present a difficult problem in management. Especially with distal-based and contused flaps, viability is not always easy to determine. Color demarcation is one important consideration. A slightly dusky end of a flap without a clear demarcation usually survives; if there is a clear-cut color line between normal tissue and cyanotic tissue, the cyanotic area should be removed. Often a flap has a good arterial supply, blanching and refilling when pressure is applied to its base, but local edema may impair venous return. This may lead to necrosis within the first few days. When doubt exists, the best method is to defat the flap and apply it as a full thickness graft with fine sutures placed close to the wound edges.

HEMOSTASIS

With most routine lacerations, hemostasis can be accomplished initially with a pressure dressing of sterile gauze. Following injection of a local anesthetic and preparation for closure, most wounds resume bleeding as vasodilatation occurs and clots are removed. If bleeding does not follow debridement, the excision was inadequate. In most superficial lacerations hemostasis can be adequately obtained with simple closure of the wound. Should bleeding be evident postclosure, local pressure for five minutes or a temporary suture around the bleeding site is normally sufficient. If this does not control hemorrhage, the wound should be reopened and the bleeding vessel ligated. Deeper wounds may require electrocauterization or, most often, suture ligatures of absorbable (4-0 or 5-0) material to effect hemostasis.

The physician should not attempt to ligate bleeders in the vascular subcutaneous tissue of the scalp. Most scalp lacerations can be closed primarily with deep, snugly tied skin sutures to control bleeding.[5] In deep scalp lacerations, traction and eversion of the galea with hemostats effectively controls subcutaneous hemorrhage and allows exploration of the wound. In other areas, clamping of larger vessels may be necessary to visualize the wound adequately. The physician should never clamp a vessel blindly; when faced with persistent bleeding, the physician must seek assistance. The assistant can sponge the area frequently, retract the edges of the wound, and apply pressure over the involved feeding artery or vein. Any wound that is too extensive to permit a systematic, thorough approach to its exploration and closure should be closed in the operating room.

SUTURING

Selection of Suture

Suture is used to obliterate spaces, stop hemorrhage, and impart physical strength to a discontinuous surface. The physician should select the best artificial fiber (suture) to maintain the edges in close apposition until a natural fiber (collagen) is synthesized. All suture material invokes a foreign body reaction, but using the most appropriate, and finest gauge suture that will do the job lessens the chances of postoperative infection. There are many types of suture available, and the appropriate type can be chosen according to the tissue to be closed, the proposed time required for healing, and the potential for infection in the wound.

Absorbable sutures are made of various materials including catgut, collagen, polyglycolic acid (Dexon), and a copolymer of glycolic and lactic acids in a ratio of 90:10 (Vicryl). Catgut sutures are digested by proteolytic enzymes derived from inflammatory cells. Plain catgut incites a greater inflammatory reaction than chromic catgut, and the reaction may persist for a prolonged period if plain catgut is used in or near the skin surface. Polyglycolic acid (Dexon) and polyglactin 910 (Vicryl) are slowly hydrolyzed by water, and the principal reaction occurs with invasion of the interstices of the suture by macrophages. While plain catgut and chromic catgut are digested at a variable rate (two weeks to two years), the synthetic sutures disappear at a more predictable rate. Polyglactin 910 disappears after approximately 80 days and polyglycolic acid after 100 to 120 days; both suture types are much more rapidly absorbed in the presence of infection. Absorbable sutures lose strength more rapidly than they disappear. At 14 to 21 days, both polyglactin 910 and polyglycolic acid have lost nearly all their tensile strength. Compared with catgut, however, both synthetic sutures exhibit greater tensile strength and cause less inflammation at all stages of healing in normal, irradiated, and infected tissue.[6] The overall superior qualities of Dexon and Vicryl, combined with their handling ease, make them the logical choice over catgut in emergency department use.

Nonabsorbable sutures are made of silk, cotton, nylon, polyester (Dacron), polypropylene (Prolene), or steel. They are further classified as monofilament—nylon, steel, polypropylene—or multifilament (woven)—steel, nylon, silk, cotton, or polyester. Silk is classified as nonabsorbable, but it has been shown to lose all its tensile strength after one year and usually disappears after two years. The unfortunate fatalities that have resulted from the failure of silk suture lines used to insert heart valve prostheses during the early years of cardiac surgery bear testimony to the absorbable nature of silk. Nylon may swell and lose some of its strength after one year, but this is probably not clinically significant.[7]

All nonabsorbable sutures induce a cellular reaction. Silk and cotton produce the greatest reaction; nylon, polypropylene, and steel, the least reaction. Polyester is intermediate in its reactivity. Because of their construction, multifilament sutures have a greater potential for infection than do monofilament sutures. Bacteria and tissue fluids can penetrate the interstices of the multifilament suture, but inflammatory cells cannot; the bacteria can multiply and convert a contamination into an infection. Monofilament sutures, on the other hand, provide no place for bacteria to hide and therefore are recommended when the possibility of infection is high.

When other characteristics of suture material are equal, the handling qualities of the suture may dictate the one to choose. Most multifilament sutures are easier to handle than monofilament. Usually, they are more pliable, lie flatter when tied, and do not project stiffly above the skin when cut. The latter is particularly important when suture is used near the eye, as such a projection could be a potentially dangerous corneal irritant. Nylon is notorious for coming untied and requires more knots than silk or cotton to secure. The absolute tensile strength of any suture is insignificant if the knot is weakened. Wire requires two throws to secure; silk, cotton, and other nonabsorbable braided sutures require three. Catgut, polymeric absorbables (Dexon and Vicryl), and the monofilament nonabsorbables—nylon and polypropylene—require four. All knots should be squared.

Nonabsorbable sutures should be utilized in the closure of skin and fascia, as well as in the approximation of lacerated tendons. Absorbable sutures can be utilized to close the periosteum, muscle, and subcutaneous tissue, and to ligate blood vessels. As a rule, the emergency department physician needs to become familiar with only one or two types of absorbable and nonabsorbable suture. Table 10–1 provides a general guide to suture; Dexon, Vicryl, and nylon are presented as examples, but personal preferences may be substituted.

Suturing Technique

The various layers of a wound should be placed in close apposition so that a minimal amount of new connective tissue will be required to restore structural integrity. Probably the most important single determinant of the final width of a scar is the tension under which the skin is originally closed. As a rule, the final width of any scar is approximately the size of the defect remaining after the subcutaneous tissue has been approximated. Up until the fifth to sixth day postinjury, the injured tissue has little tensile strength, and the wound edges are held together by the adhesiveness of cells, globular proteins, and fibrin. The deposition of collagen, which gives the tissue strength, is not even demonstrable until the fifth day. Collagen synthesis continues during the first six weeks, the proliferative phase of wound healing, but the injured tissue does not gain maximal strength for several months to years. If closed under any tension, the weakened, vulnerable scar will gradually widen for the first few weeks. Ideally, to optimize strength and minimize the tendency for the wound edges to separate, sutures should be left in place for two to three months. However, any suture left in place for more than two weeks produces unsightly railroad track scars or stitch abscesses. To reconcile these two inconsistencies, a subcuticular buried suture should be employed. In wounds that must be closed under tension, the suture material should be nonabsorbable to maintain the tensile strength of the closure until collagen synthesis is complete. In areas where little tension is exerted along the suture line, such as in the closure of facial lacerations parallel to relaxed lines of tension (Fig. 10–1), an absorbable suture combined with external support can be utilized.

Often the face is the only area of the body requiring meticulous closure with subcuticular support. If infection, drainage, or hemorrhage is anticipated, or if local edema and tissue damage are present, loose approximation or open drainage is recommended. A widened scar is an acceptable alternative to devitalization and infection in a wound improperly closed.

There is no hard-and-fast rule dictating the exact number of sutures necessary to close a wound. The physician should use only enough sutures to approximate the wound edges adequately. The finest gauge suture that is stronger than the tissue to be closed should be used. A wound edge is more effectively controlled when the sutures are placed nearer to that edge, but strangulation and necrosis can occur if the sutures are placed too close or under excessive tension. In general, the suture tension should be just enough to approximate the edges and no more. When tied too tightly, wound edges are inverted, making the suture line appear very

TABLE 10–1   Wound Closure Guide

	Skin	*Subcutaneous Tissue and Muscle*	*Stitch*
Face	6-0 nylon 6-0 nylon	4-0, 5-0 Dexon, Vicryl 4-0 nylon (subcuticular)	Simple, running simple (skin only)
Scalp	4-0 nylon	3-0, 4-0 Dexon, Vicryl	Simple, running locking (blanket) Simple running
Trunk	4-0 nylon	3-0, 4-0 Dexon, Vicryl	Simple, vertical mattress, Running simple or running Vertical mattress
Extremities	4-0 nylon	4-0 Dexon, Vicryl	Simple, vertical mattress Running simple or mattress
Hands, feet	5-0, 4-0 nylon	5-0, 4-0 Dexon, Vicryl	Simple, vertical mattress
Mucous membranes		5-0, 4-0 Dexon, Vicryl	Inverted simple or horizontal

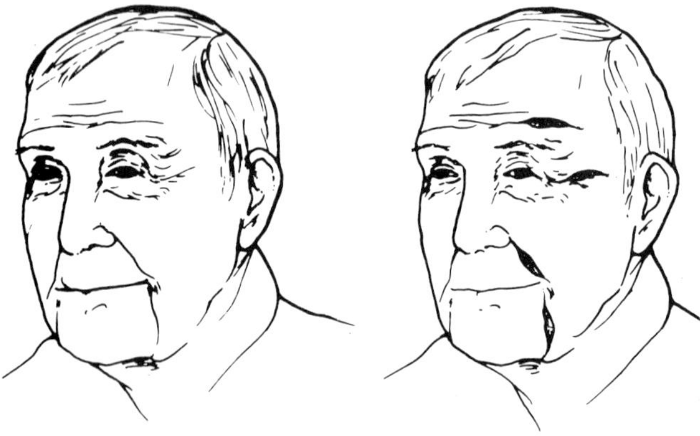

Figure 10–1   Relaxed Lines of Tension.

fine, but the rolled-under edges heal by secondary intention. To avoid wound edge inversion, a small probe or the tip of a forceps should be inserted along the entire length of the suture line at the end of the procedure. If the skin edges are not abutting, the sutures should be replaced. Excessive suture tension may also herniate subcutaneous tissue to the surface of the wound, producing a scalloped effect.

Several hours after closure, a wound should be watertight, unless drainage is excessive. Sutures may be removed from 2 to 14 days after closure if the epithelium has healed adequately. Cross-hatching inevitably occurs at 14 days and may occur sooner if the sutures are tied under excessive tension or infection supervenes. In debilitated patients or in patients with wounds of the distal lower extremity, it may be necessary to leave the stitches in place at least this long, however, in order to ensure wound healing. If there is some question about the removal of a suture, alternate sutures can be removed

and the wound rechecked in two days. A general guide to suture removal is provided in Figure 10–2.

The importance of using sharp, fine instruments in handling tissue should be stressed. An instrument tray for the closure of facial wounds in the emergency department should include diamond-tipped or smooth-tipped needle holders, skin hooks, fine mosquito hemostats, plain and toothed Adson's forceps, curved and straight iris scissors, #15 and #11 scalpels, curved Metzenbaum scissors, suture scissors, antiseptic solution, sterile gauze, and saline.

Types of Sutures

The Subcuticular Suture

In the closure of facial lacerations or anywhere where the final cosmetic result is important, subcuticular sutures should be used. They reduce tension on the skin edges and allow epidermal sutures to be removed early. Subcuticular stitches are placed after the underlying muscle fascia and subcutaneous tissue have been closed. Depending on the anticipated tension on the skin, either nonabsorbable (5-0 white silk or nylon) suture or absorbable (5-0 Vicryl or Dexon) should be used. Care should be taken to place the suture only in the dermis, as any perforation of the epidermis will lead to epithelial migration and the possible formation of an epithelial cyst or abscess. The skin edge is gently grasped and everted with fine-toothed Adson's forceps or skin hooks, and the lowest level of the dermis is approximated. The suture should be inverted with the knot cut close to avoid penetration of the overlying epidermis.

In straight or gently curved lacerations, the running subcuticular stitch may be used instead of interrupted

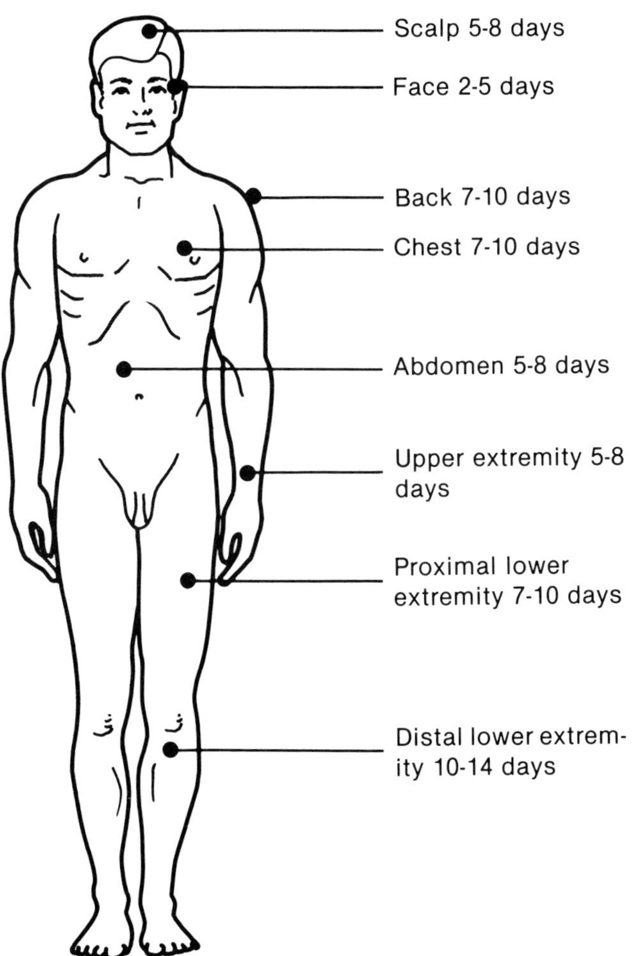

Figure 10–2 Guide to Suture Removal.

sutures. It prevents the occasional lumpy scar seen with simple interrupted subcuticular sutures and, with practice, can be placed with greater speed. The tensile strength of 4-0 nylon makes it ideal for a continuous intradermal suture. The needle is placed horizontally through the dermis, and small bites are taken alternatively on each side of the wound. If the laceration is long, it is wise to pass the suture through the skin every 6 to 8 cm to facilitate its removal. The physician should check the suture at the end of the procedure to make sure it slides back and forth easily. The suture can remain in place for two to three weeks. (See Fig. 10–3.)

The Simple Suture

Once the subcuticular layer has been approximated, the skin edges should be nearly touching. The simple epidermal suture is intended only to adjust the level of the two opposing edges and makes no contribution to the strength of the closure. The suture can be placed shallowly near the skin edge with 6-0 or 7-0 nylon or

silk. In three to four days it can be cut or, often, lifted off without being cut owing to the normal desquamating process of the skin.

In areas of the body where full thickness single-layer closure of the skin is desirable, the interrupted simple suture is the mainstay of cuticular sutures. The skin edge is readily everted by enclosing a greater amount of tissue at the bottom of the suture path than near the surface. The curved needle should enter the skin at a 90° angle, at least, with sufficient subcutaneous tissue included in the bite to aid eversion. Similarly, the exit angle of the needle should be at least 90° with an equal amount of subcutaneous tissue taken on the exit side of the wound. Often the needle should be regrasped after the first bite in the center of the wound to allow entry at the same level on the other side. This ensures proper skin edge alignment and obliteration of dead space (Fig. 10–4).

The simple or inverted simple suture is usually used in closure of subcutaneous fat, muscle, and fascia. It is important to take small tissue bites and to use as few sutures as possible in closing the subcutaneous tissue (see Fig. 10–5). The suture should be absorbable (4-0 or 5-0 Vicryl or Dexon) with inverted simple sutures used near the upper levels of the wound. Fascia should be approximated with 4-0 Prolene or nylon sutures as sutured fascia attains only 50 percent of its original strength in 50 days and may take one year to reach full strength.

Vertical Mattress Suture

Ideal for everting wound edges, the vertical mattress suture may be used anywhere except the face. It is especially useful in areas where the cut skin naturally inverts, such as on the dorsum of the hand, in web spaces, on the scrotum, at flexion creases, and for any laceration through atrophic skin. The vertical mattress suture is placed initially just like a simple suture, i.e., enclosing a larger rectangle of tissue in the base of the wound than near the surface. Instead of tying the knot at this stage, however, the needle is passed through the cuticular layer of skin on both sides of the laceration as near to the edge as possible. The knot is secured, everting and approximating the wound edges. Some physicians alternate vertical mattress and simple interrupted sutures. A running vertical mattress suture may also be utilized (Fig. 10–6, A). Also see Fig 10–6, B, C, and D for a demonstration of an interrupted vertical mattress.

Half-Buried Horizontal Mattress Suture

For approximating the point of a V-shaped laceration, the half-buried horizontal mattress suture is ideal.

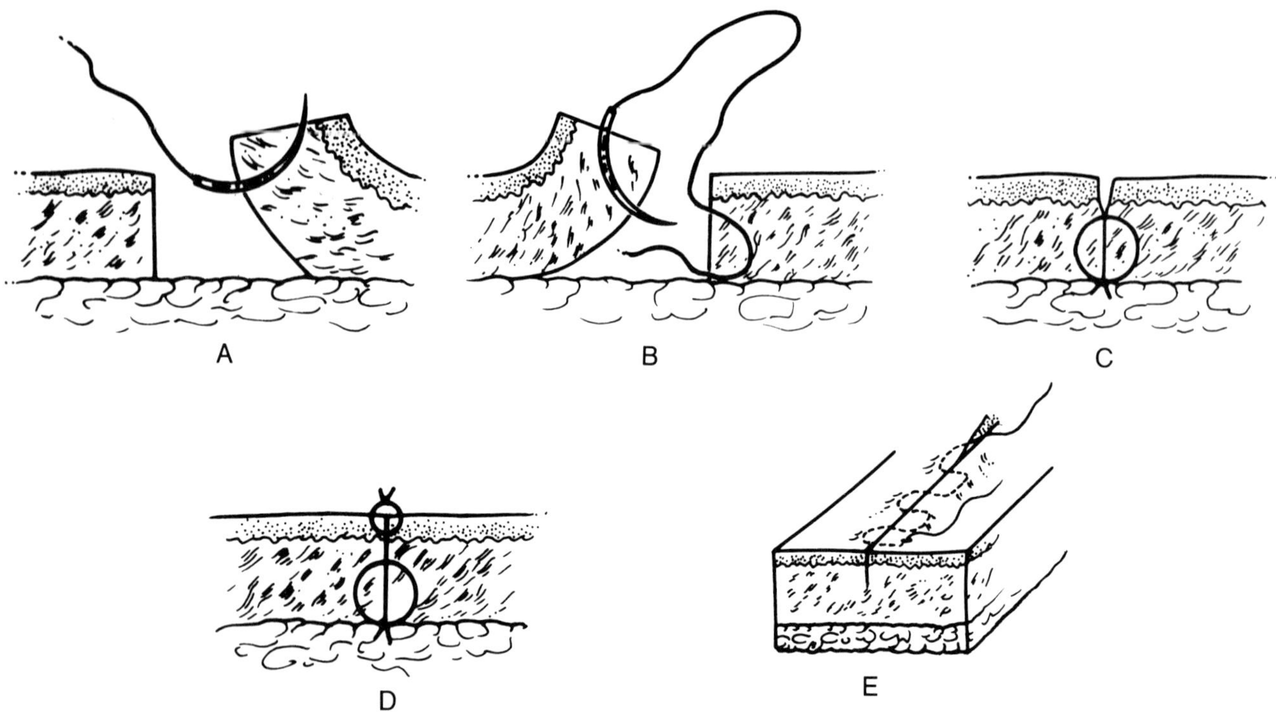

Figure 10–3 *A, B, C:* Subcuticular (Inverted) Stitch; *D:* Subcuticular and Cuticular Stitch; and *E:* Running Subcuticular Stitch.

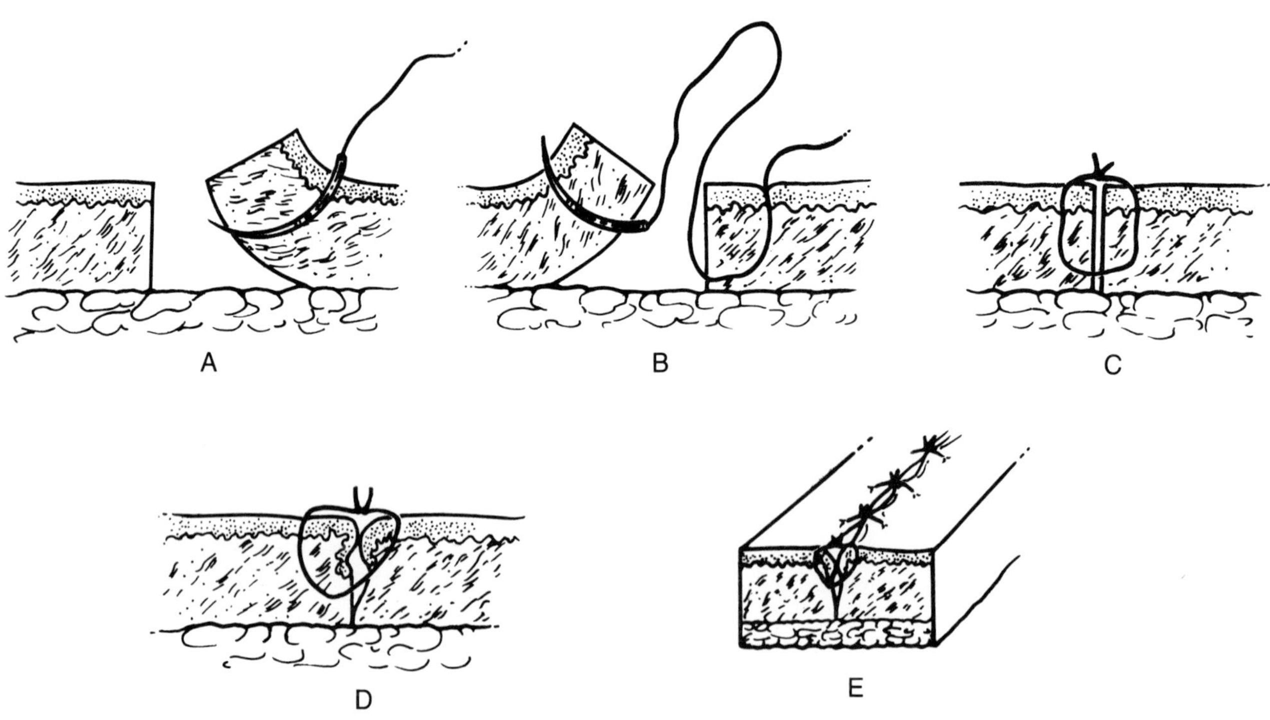

Figure 10–4 *A, B, C:* Properly Placed Simple Suture; *D:* Unequal Bites Produce Scars and Dead Space; and *E:* Bites Too Shallow and Tight Produce Scalloping.

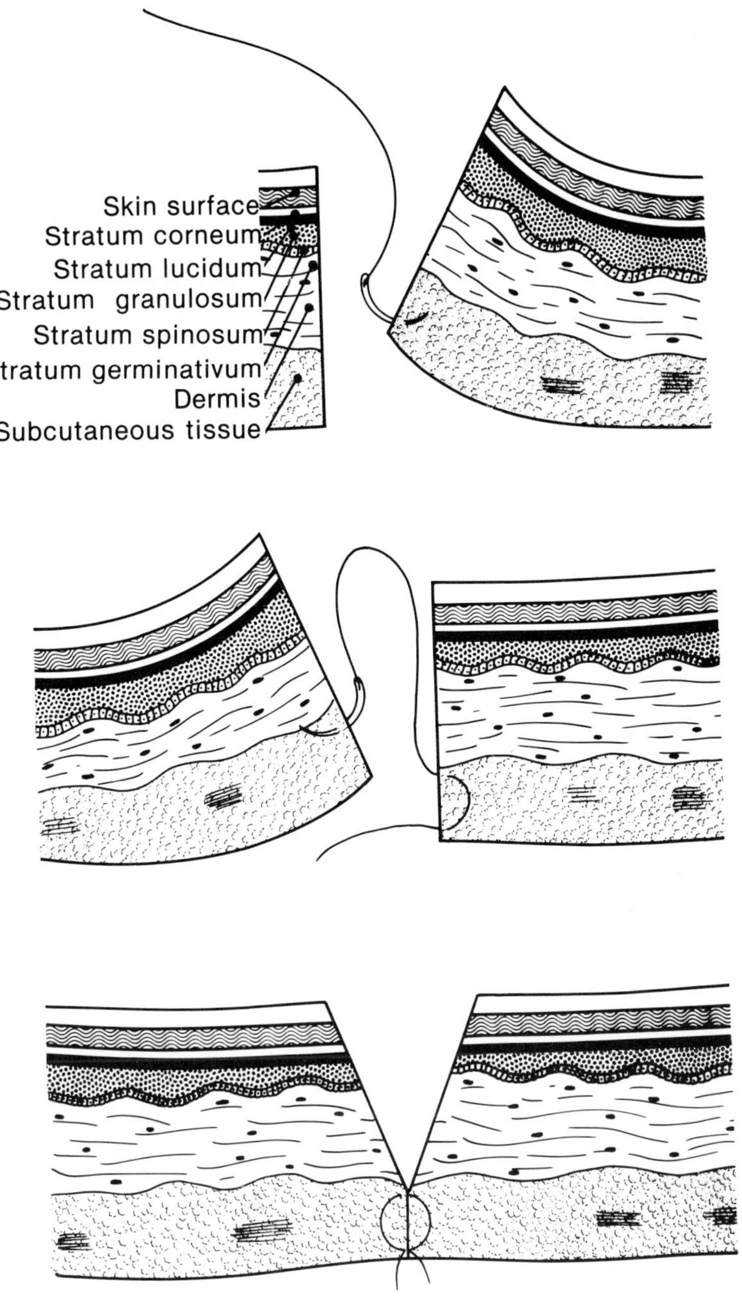

Figure 10–5   Inverted Simple Suture Placed in Subcutaneous Tissue.

Passing the buried portion of the suture through the lower portion of the dermis gives the stitch adequate strength and avoids necrosis of the delicate skin tip (Fig. 10–7).

Running and Running Locking (Blanket) Sutures

Running sutures are generally not used in the emergency department except in the closure of scalp lacerations or very long lacerations when the risk of infection is minimal. The final tension of a running suture is often difficult to adjust, and the suture line is lost if one knot unties or if a suture must be removed because of a localized infection. For these reasons, a running suture should never be used below the skin in wounds treated in the emergency department. In the scalp, however, tension can be maintained on the running suture and the wound rapidly closed. Each bite is taken as if a simple suture were being used, and the suture is usually advanced in the subcutaneous tissue (Fig. 10–8). Each bite may be locked, producing a blanket stitch. The abundant vascularity of the scalp ensures survival, even when the suture is tied under marked tension.

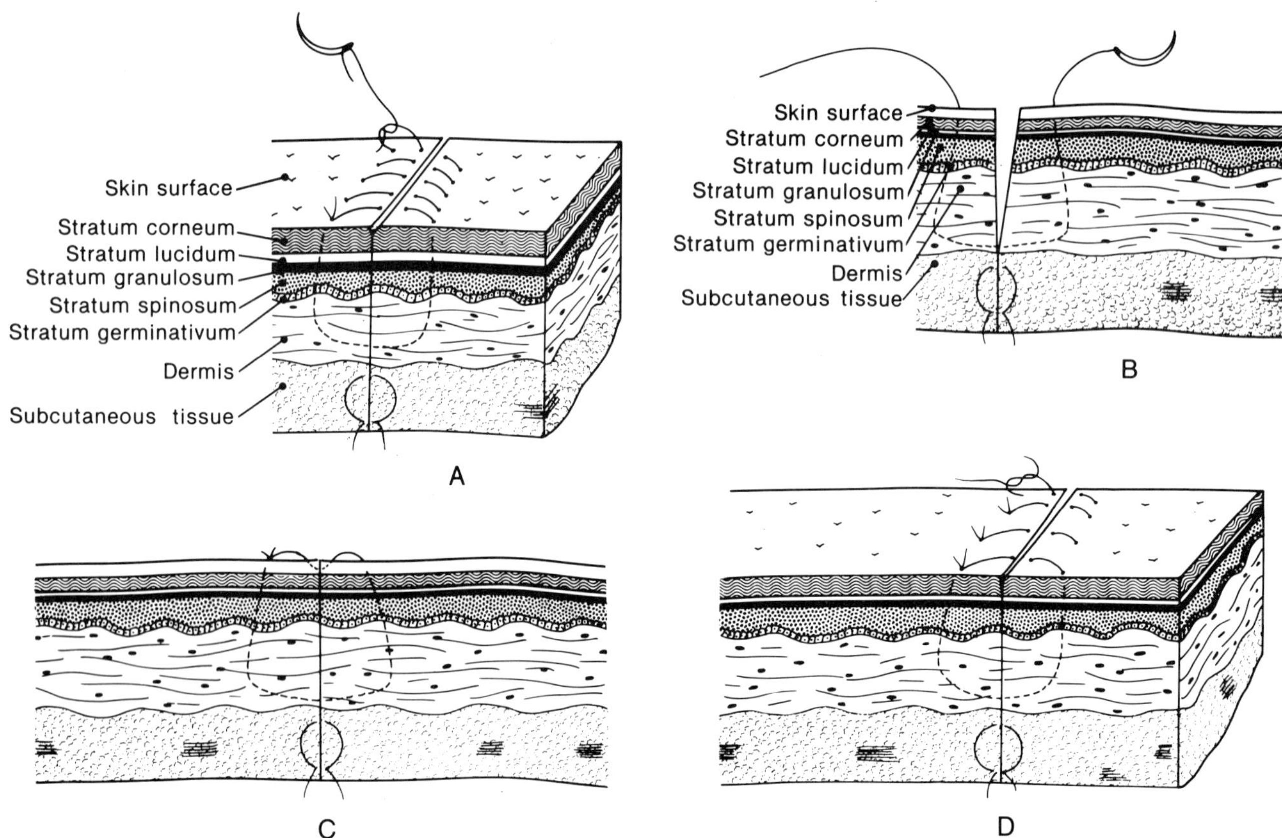

Figure 10–6 *A:* Running (Continuous) Vertical Mattress; *B, C, D:* Interrupted Vertical Mattress.

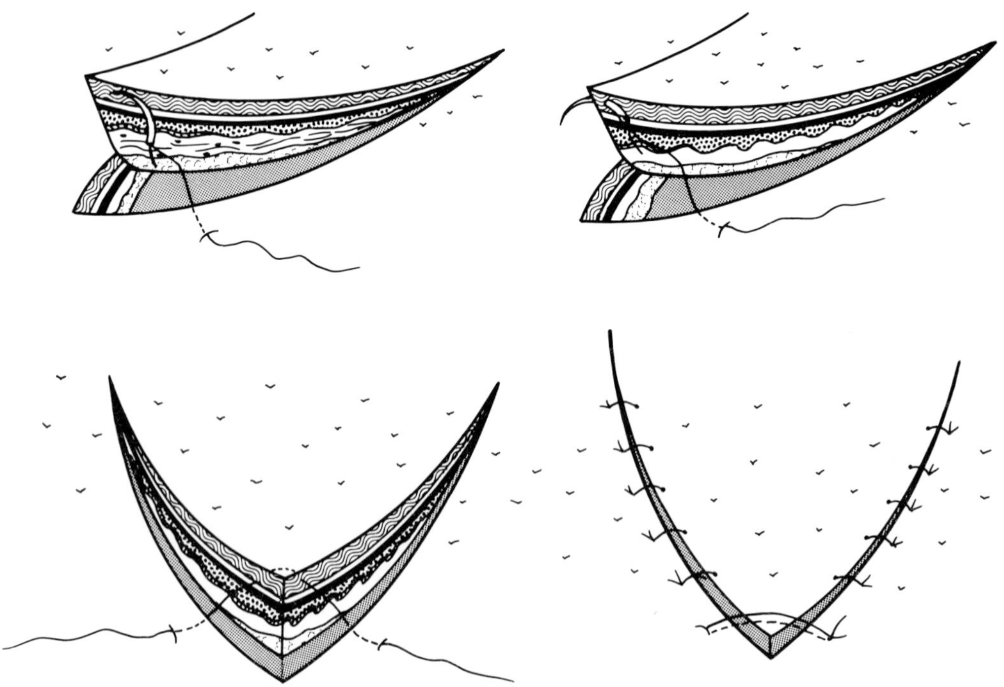

Figure 10–7 Method of Tip Closure; Half Buried Horizontal Mattress.

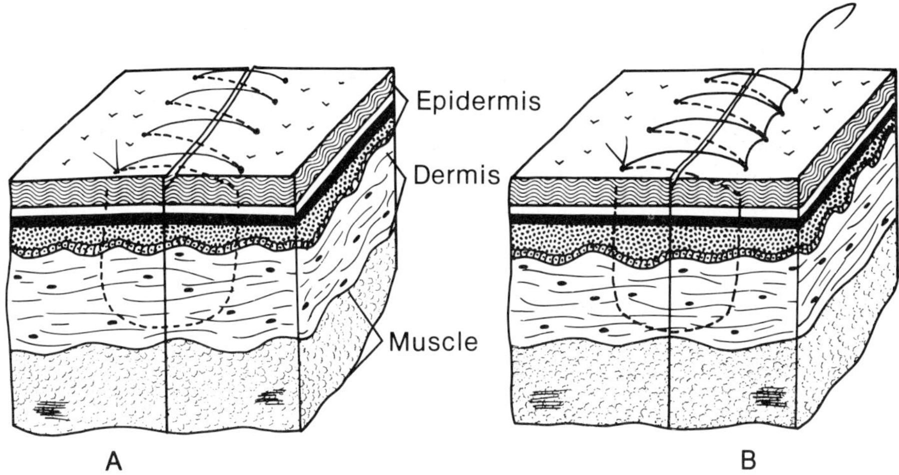

Figure 10–8   *A:* Running Simple Suture; *B:* Running Locking Suture.

TAPE CLOSURE OF LACERATIONS

Microporous surgical adhesive tape (Steri-strip), easily and quickly applied without anesthesia, can be useful in selected cases. The tape has a backing of viscous rayon fibers that are coated with an adhesive. Although pervious to perspiration, the tape does not permit the passage of blood or purulent material. Tape usually remains in place one to two weeks; if placed in areas of growing hair, however, it is pushed off in five to seven days. Tape is ineffective over areas in constant motion or over wrinkled, oily, or loose skin. Children and uncooperative patients often remove it, further limiting its usefulness.

Before tape is applied, the skin should be cleansed with soap and water and thoroughly dried; excess oily secretions can be removed with acetone or alcohol. The tape is applied perpendicular to the wound surface, one side first and then the other, bringing the edges together. Adhesives such as benzoin are contraindicated; they strengthen the adhesion initially, but after a few days they actually weaken it.[8]

Unfortunately, Steri-strips do not naturally evert skin edges. A meticulous subcuticular closure must precede their use on the face. Even then, cosmetic results are often inferior to those obtained by suturing. Their particular usefulness comes in the closure of finger burst lacerations and lower leg lacerations where local edema makes standard wound closure risky. In these cases, the use of Steri-strips makes it unnecessary to infiltrate anesthetic into an already edematous area, lessens the risk of marginal necrosis due to tight sutures, and allows prolonged coverage with a splint, cast, or bulky dressing.

All principles of wound closure with sutures apply equally to closure with Steri-strips. The tensile strength of adhesive strips is often greater than that of sutures, but the use of surgical tapes to close an infected or contaminated wound, or to approximate the edges of a puncture wound, is inviting disaster. Used alone or in conjunction with sutures, these tapes can be a valuable tool in delayed primary or secondary wound closure. In addition, by using tapes, the physician can avoid the troublesome bleeding encountered in tacking down skin grafts or approximating the avulsed, thin, atrophic skin frequently seen in steroid-dependent and elderly patients.

TYPES OF LACERATIONS

Scalp Lacerations

Laceration of the scalp is the most common head injury that requires surgical care in the emergency department. Nearly all scalp lacerations can be closed primarily; because of the rich vascularity of the scalp, there is little chance of subsequent infection.

The scalp is the thickest integument and functions as a protective layer for the cranium. It is composed of five distinct layers:

1. the thick (3 to 8 mm) skin
2. the dense and richly vascular subcutaneous layer
3. the epicranium, consisting of the paired occipitalis and frontalis muscles joined by the galea aponeurotica
4. the subepicranial layer (cavum subgalea) of loose areolar tissue that separates the galea from the pericranium
5. the pericranium or periosteum of the skull

There are five paired arteries from the external carotid system with many anastomoses throughout the subcutaneous layer. The veins of the scalp parallel the arterial supply. Unlike the arteries, however, the veins communicate intracranially by way of the diploid and emissary veins to the cavernous, superior sagittal, and lateral sinuses. Any extracranial scalp infection may thus precipitate sinus thrombophlebitis and meningitis.

Scalp lacerations should be thoroughly cleansed and shaved approximately 2 cm around the wound edges. Although shaving the area actually increases the chance of infection, it is necessary to keep hair from becoming entangled in the sutures. Shaving can be avoided in linear lacerations by using a soap solution to part and plaster the hair down along the sides of the laceration. The wound should be explored, thoroughly irrigated, and debrided of devitalized tissue. While an assistant applies local pressure on both sides of the wound, the physician can inspect it for foreign bodies or underlying skull fractures. If pressure fails to control hemorrhage, the galea should be grasped with a series of hemostats and everted over the wound edge to allow adequate visualization. Often, ground-in road dirt or other contaminants may be lodged in the cranium; these should be removed with a rongeur in order to avoid cranial osteomyelitis.

In most scalp lacerations, simple or running sutures of 3-0 or 4-0 Prolene or nylon effect hemostasis and provide adequate closure. In male patients with frontal or temporal lacerations, careful approximation is paramount as the naturally receding hairline may eventually uncover the scar. When a laceration extends across the galea, muscle pull may result in a gaping wound; separate closure of the galea with 3-0 or 4-0 absorbable suture is recommended in these cases. Irrigation or aspiration of blood clots is necessary to prevent infection. Skull roentgenograms should be obtained to rule out the presence of foreign bodies or associated fractures in all but the most superficial scalp injuries.

Scalp lacerations are often multiple, irregular, stellate, or trapdoor in nature. Simple debridement of only the tissue that is clearly devitalized and careful suturing of scalp flaps and irregular edges usually produce excellent results. In cases of extensive scalp laceration, or partial or total scalping injuries, prompt surgical consultation should be obtained. An avulsed scalp should be placed in iced saline and accompany the patient to the nearest center where microsurgical anastomosis can be performed.[9]

Facial Lacerations

In the management of a facial laceration, several factors work to the surgeon's advantage. The excellent arterial supply, lymphatic drainage, and venous drainage of the face almost guarantee success with primary closure, even in grossly contaminated wounds. Because of its innate elasticity, the skin can be undermined and mobilized to close lacerations with skin loss. Sutures can be removed early because facial skin heals rapidly. By handling the tissues delicately and accurately approximating the layers with little or no tension on the skin, the surgeon can almost always obtain a pleasing cosmetic result.

Many facial lacerations have a contusional component; the burst type injury damages skin edges, underlying muscle, and subcutaneous tissue. Closure without trimming the beveled skin edge results in a stepped scar. Whenever possible, it is best to trim the wound edges at right angles with a scalpel to ensure accurate everting apposition. Slight inward beveling of the edge also aids in eversion.

The subcutaneous tissue usually requires only minimal debridement; overzealous debridement produces a depressed scar with loss of facial contour. In small, ragged facial lacerations, the best technique includes wound excision, undermining, and closure without tension. Undermining is best accomplished by elevating the skin edge with skin hooks or Adson's forceps and sharply incising along the subdermal plane parallel to the skin surface with a #15 scalpel. Tension should be tested by grasping the two wound edges and apposing them; more undermining may be necessary if excessive tension is necessary to bring the edges together (Fig. 10–9). A subcuticular supporting suture should be utilized in nearly all facial lacerations. With more complex facial wounds, simplification with trimming to produce straight, gently curved, or sharply angled edges ideal for repair minimizes hypertrophic scar formation (Fig. 10–10).

When possible, wounds should be trimmed or mobilized to fit into or parallel to the lines of the patient's facial contour. However, all possible skin should be left in the vicinity of the lower eyelid, the nasal alae, and the angle of the mouth to avoid distortion of the surrounding structures. Similarly, only the nonviable edges of large ragged or stellate lacerations should be trimmed and the pieces of the jigsaw puzzle gently tacked back in place. Often, the results are cosmetically excellent; if not, ample skin remains for revision at a later time. The patient should be informed from the start of the possibility of revision but should be advised to wait at least six months before making any decision.

The Eyebrow

Because eyebrow hair grows very slowly and because it provides an accurate guide to approximation of cut edges, it should never be shaved. By gently grasping the wound edges with fine-tipped forceps and apposing

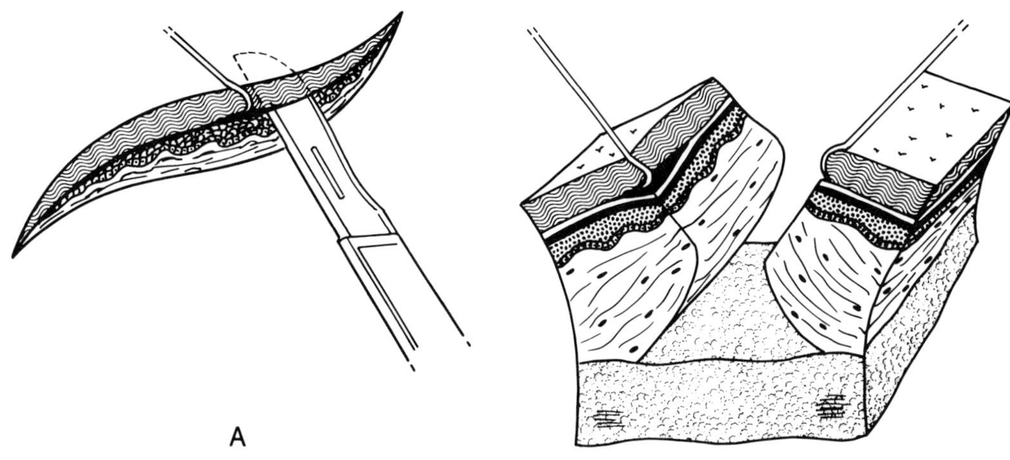

Figure 10–9   *A:* Method of Undermining Skin; *B:* Subdermal Plane Undermined.

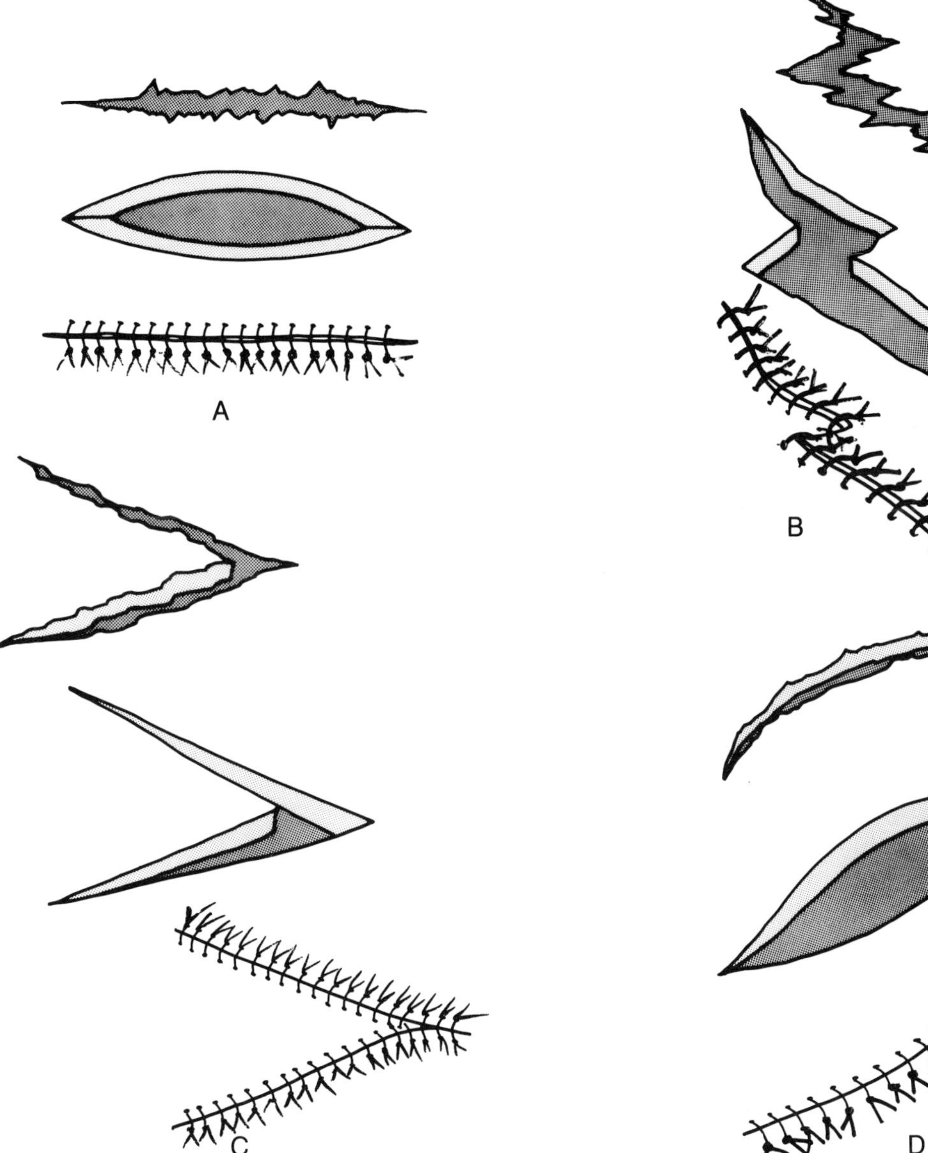

Figure 10–10   *A, B, C, D:* Simplification of Wounds by Excision.

them, the physician can determine the correct placement of sutures to avoid a discontinuity. Most eyebrow lacerations are burst type, and separate closures of muscle, subcuticular tissue, and skin are necessary.

The Eyelid

The location of an eyelid laceration determines the type of closure. If the laceration involves the inner one-sixth of the eyelid, the canaliculus is usually severed and must be repaired by a specialist using a stent. The key to successful repair of vertical lacerations involving the outer five-sixths of the lid margin is placement of the first suture through the gray line. This ensures alignment in the proper plane, and the remainder of the lid can be closed with absorbable suture (Dexon or Vicryl) for the tarsus and fine silk for the skin. The conjunctiva is adherent to the tarsal plate and does not require suturing. Knots should be tied facing the skin to avoid ocular irritation. Lacerations parallel to the lid margin can be closed as other facial lacerations are closed; they are not subject to the sideways pull of the orbicularis oculi muscle fibers. Occasionally, avulsion of thin eyelid skin creates small flaps of questionable viability. These usually survive if they are simply tacked into place.

The Cheek

When lacerations involve the cheek, injury to the facial nerve, parotid gland, or parotid duct is possible and should be ruled out before closure. Under ordinary circumstances, muscle paralysis on the involved side of the face indicates nerve injury. The parotid duct and buccal branch of the facial nerve course along a line from the tragus to the midportion of the upper lip (Fig. 10–10). Division of the nerve branches medial to the midpupillary line usually does not require nerve repair, as cross innervation and regeneration will reinnervate the appropriate muscle. If the injury is lateral to this point, however, nerve repair should be attempted in order to avoid permanent functional and cosmetic deformity. Severance of the temporal branch of the facial nerve, which is superficial and courses superiorly at a point halfway between the tragus and lateral canthus, causes particular disability, e.g., paralysis of the eyelid and potential exposure keratitis. Any suspected proximal nerve injury requires prompt surgical consultation.

Parotid duct injury may accompany injury to the buccal branch of the facial nerve. It is indicated by the leakage of clear fluid from the cut proximal end of the duct or blood at the orifice of Stensen's duct. Reanastomosis over a Silastic catheter or reimplantation of the proximal end into the buccal mucosa requires the skills of a specialist. Simple glandular lacerations need not be repaired; salivary fistulas are common and usually resolve spontaneously in approximately three weeks.[10]

The Nose

Simple lacerations or lacerations with small amounts of skin loss at the bridge of the nose can be readily closed. Alae lacerations should be closed in three layers: absorbable 5-0 suture for the mucosa and cartilage, 6-0 nylon or silk for the skin. The physician must be meticulous in obtaining hemostasis as an expanding alar hematoma can lead to extensive tissue necrosis. Nasal fractures are often associated with lacerations, and any septal hematomas should be incised and evacuated to prevent saddle back deformity. Full thickness skin losses at the tip of the nose usually require plastic surgical procedures.

The Ear

Full thickness ear lacerations should be closed in three layers: absorbable suture in interrupted stitches for the cartilage and 6-0 nylon or silk simple interrupted stitches for the two skin surfaces. An alternative method that can be used when cartilage must be trimmed to facilitate skin closure is a cutaneous-perichondrial suture. With 5-0 or 6-0 silk or nylon the skin and perichondrium are closed on both sides of the ear, thus apposing the cartilage without direct suturing. Flap type lacerations of the ear, often with small tenuous pedicles, are common. With careful handling and the use of fine, well-spaced tacking sutures, most of these flaps can be salvaged. Like nasal hematomas, ear hematomas should be evacuated before clot organization and fibrosis lead to the classic "cauliflower ear."

The Lips

Vertical lip lacerations are almost invariably untidy and require some degree of debridement or wedge excision before closure. Defects of up to one-third of the width of the lower lip and one-fourth of the upper lip can be closed by direct suturing after the laceration has been converted to a V or W. Proper alignment of the vermilion border is essential for a good cosmetic result. Three-layer closure of mucosa, muscle, and skin in lip lacerations and through-and-through tooth lacerations just below the lower lip is necessary to ensure adequate healing.

Leg and Foot Lacerations

Among the most difficult injuries to deal with in the emergency department are leg and foot lacerations. Without proper initial management, the patient may suffer discomfort and expense for several weeks. The classic example is the elderly or debilitated patient with a triangulated flap laceration over the tibia as a result of a fall against a curb or step. With the full body weight transmitted through the tibia, the injury results in real skin loss through crushing; widespread subcutaneous damage with edema invariably leads to secondary skin loss. The poor arterial supply, decreased venous return, and local edema, together with the patient's compromised ability to heal, render any closure liable to skin necrosis and cellulitis. If the flap is distally based, the blood supply and venous return are even more tenuous, and placing the leg in a dependent position inevitably leads to hematoma formation and flap necrosis.

Simple lacerations without skin loss can be closed primarily, provided the wound edges can be brought together without tension. Fine bites with 4-0 nylon suture widely placed without tension can be used. The wound should be dressed with sterile gauze and an encircling firm bandage from foot to knee. The lower leg and foot should be immobilized with a posterior plaster padded splint and elevated for the next week. Hospitalization may be required for some patients. If minimal tension is necessary to approximate the wound edges, the laceration should be closed with Steri-strips, combined with a pressure bandage. Immobilization and elevation are also necessary.

Even if there is a residual defect, either from the initial injury or subsequent debridement of nonviable tissue, primary closure under tension should never be considered. The triangulated flap can be tacked without tension to one side of the wound margin and checked for adequate capillary return, bleeding, and color. The remaining defect will require grafting that is best undertaken by a plastic surgeon. Likewise, when bone, tendon, or ligament is exposed or subcutaneous damage extends to these structures, hospitalization and plastic surgical care are necessary.

PRESSURE GUN INJURIES

Pressure (paint and grease) gun injuries can lead to profound and permanent disability if inappropriately treated. The small, seemingly innocuous entry wound belies the infiltration of often large amounts of grease or paint throughout the muscles, tendons, and fascial planes. On a rare occasion, the wound is tangential to the skin surface, and roentgenogram examination (if the paint is lead-based) reveals only superficial opacification. The wound can then be debrided or excised and closed. Unfortunately, most wounds are penetrating and require wide debridement in the operating room.[11]

BITES

Dog Bites

A common emergency problem, dog bites occur at a rate of 500 to 700 cases per 100,000 population, ac-

counting for 1 to 2 percent of all surgical cases.[12] (See Chapter 28.) More than 1 million dog bites occur annually, but controlled studies are few and treatment recommendations are often based on anecdotal information. Controversy still rages around the advisability of closing dog bite wounds primarily and the indications for antibiotic therapy.

Recent studies have shown wound debridement and irrigation of dog bite wounds to be the most important factors in preventing subsequent infection.[13] Large, deep lacerations and avulsion injuries were found to have insignificant infection rates when compared with puncture wounds and puncture lacerations, probably because the more extensive injuries received more intensive surgical toilet and were closed primarily. In puncture wounds, however, adequate mechanical cleansing and irrigation are impossible, and the infection rate was over 34 percent. A higher infection rate was also found in those patients over 50 years of age and those who delay treatment for 24 to 48 hours. Facial wounds have the lowest infection rate and should be closed or covered with grafts or transposition flaps. Hand lacerations consistently show the highest infection rates; generally, they should be debrided and left open for delayed closure. If tendon, bone, joint space, or large vessels are exposed or transected, appropriate consultation should be sought immediately. Puncture dog bite wounds are inflicted with a pressure of more than 400 psi and almost always have a severe contusional component. Their unacceptably high rate of infection suggests that extensive debridement or excision and delayed primary closure would be wise. If puncture wounds occur over joints, examination with the aid of a blood pressure cuff tourniquet is recommended (see Human Bites). Bulky dressings and immobilization, when practical, should be utilized in all but the most trivial of dog bite wounds.

Bacteriologic studies of normal canine flora reveal over 64 species.[14] Infected dog bite wounds reflect this wide array of pathogens, including *Staphylococcus aureus*, α-hemolytic streptococci, penicillin-resistant gram-negative rods, and anaerobic strains of *Bacteroides* species. Isolation of *Pasteurella multocida* varies from none to 50 percent of all infections in various studies. Overall, prophylactic penicillin reduced the wound infection rate by a factor of 2.5. While facial and scalp lacerations showed no difference in infection rates with or without penicillin, high-risk areas, such as the hand, were three times more likely to become infected without penicillin. Penicillin-resistant *S. aureus* is isolated in 10 to 15 percent of dog bites. The prophylactic value of a penicillinase-resistant penicillin or cephalosporin has not been investigated.

Initial wound cultures have shown a poor correlation with the subsequent development of infection; the infecting organism was predicted in only two-thirds of the initial cultures. The current recommendation is to treat all dog bite wounds with penicillin G and culture wounds only if infection supervenes. A cephalothin or penicillinase-resistant penicillin should then be started with appropriate local wound care.[15]

Cat Bites and Scratches

The nature of cat bite injuries is similar to that of dog bite injuries, except that the sharp, slender teeth of the cat often inflict deeper and initially less conspicuous damage. *Pasteurella multocida* is present in 50 to 80 percent of normal feline oral flora and accounts for more than 80 percent of all infections. It is unique in its ability to incite a severe inflammatory reaction within 24 hours of injury; most pathogens require 36 to 72 hours to produce clinical signs of infection. The organism may not be identified on culture unless the laboratory is aware of its possible presence. As with dog bites, *S. aureus*, anaerobes, gram-negative rods, diphtheroids, and streptococci may also be cultured from wounds.[16]

The initial treatment of cat bites and scratches should include cleansing, irrigation, debridement, excision of puncture wounds, dressing, and, when possible, immobilization. Facial lacerations may be closed primarily; in other areas, however, especially the hand, wounds should be left open. A seven- to ten-day course of oral penicillin or erythromycin is indicated. The patient should be seen again in 24 hours. If infection has supervened, hospitalization for IV antibiotics is indicated. The wound should be closely examined at both the initial and follow-up visits for tendon, bone, joint, or neurovascular injuries and appropriate consultation obtained.[17]

Human Bites

Inadequate treatment of human bites often leads to serious disabling sequelae. Human bites occur most often during altercations involving young individuals. They are also common in children, the mentally ill, and victims of sexual assault.[18] One of the most discouraging aspects of human bite wounds is the often long delay before the victim seeks treatment. In one study, the average length of time between injury and treatment was 2½ days; in many cases, it was several weeks.[19]

One of the most common wounds of this type seen in the emergency department is the clenched fist injury, which occurs when the patient's flexed metacarpophalangeal joints are impaled on another person's teeth. The skin stretched over the joint is lacerated, possibly accompanied by damage to the underlying extensor tendon and opening of the joint space. With the fingers extended, tendon and joint injury may go unnoticed.

Even with broad spectrum antibiotic coverage the patient with the clenched fist injury stands an almost 50 percent chance of developing suppurative tenosynovitis, septic arthritis, or osteomyelitis.[20]

The key to reducing the risk of complications associated with a clenched fist injury is prompt and aggressive treatment. The wound should be thoroughly inspected under regional block anesthesia after the arm has been elevated for five minutes and a blood pressure cuff has been applied at 250 mm Hg to ensure a bloodless examination. If the joint capsule has been violated, operating room debridement and hospitalization are indicated. If only a tendon laceration is found, the tendon should be approximated and the wound left open and splinted in extension for four weeks. Soft tissue injuries should be debrided and irrigated, a drain should be left in place, and the arm should be immobilized from finger tips to elbow. Movement is allowed at two weeks. The dressing and drain should be changed after 48 hours and dressing changes twice weekly thereafter. This regimen has significantly lessened the permanent disability resulting from such an injury.[21]

All human bite wounds, except those on the face, should be debrided and left open. Antibiotic coverage with a cephalothin is indicated for all but the most trivial of injuries. Group A streptococci, *S. aureus*, and *Eikenella corrodens* are the pathogens usually associated with human bite infections. Aerobic gram-negative rods and anaerobes (*Bacteroides* species) frequently are cultured, but their role in infection remains unclear. Isolated cases in which tetanus, gonorrhea, and syphilis were transmitted by human bites have been noted. *Eikenella corrodens* bacteria are present in a significant number of infected wounds; occasional strains are resistant to cephalothin but sensitive to penicillin. Therefore, penicillin G is a logical adjunct to cephalothin or penicillinase-resistant penicillin in the treatment of infected human bites.[22] Hospitalization is required for any patient with a human bite injury showing signs of cellulitis, lymphangitis, abscess formation, joint penetration. Severe, old, or facial wounds may also require specialized care.

DRESSINGS AND IMMOBILIZATION

All wounds should have a pressure dressing to help prevent local edema and hematoma formation, as well as to immobilize the wound edges and surrounding tissue. Mobility of any wound increases the chance of a cross-hatched scar and may lead to excessive scar formation. Patient comfort and the prevention of contamination are additional benefits of a properly dressed wound.

Facial dressings over convex surfaces, such as the forehead, malar region, or chin, are readily applied with strips of Elastoplast or adhesive tape placed over a fine gauze dressing (cocoon dressing). Where strapping is impossible, a collodion and fine mesh gauze dressing is a satisfactory alternative. Elevation of the head lessens edema. The patient should be advised against excessive talking or chewing postoperatively. The ear should be gently packed anteriorly and posteriorly with small gauze fluffs to prevent distortion or excessive pressure. Diagonal strips of Elastoplast or an encircling Kerlex bandage is used to exert firm, even pressure to the helix. Following nasal alae repairs, the ipsilateral nostril should be packed with petroleum gauze packing with an Elastoplast bandage exerting gentle counterpressure externally. After sutures are removed from facial lacerations, external support with strapping or Steri-strips should be continued for two weeks.

Scalp lacerations should be dressed with an encircling bandage of Kerlex under moderate pressure. The hemostatic bandage can be left in place for 24 hours, after which a loose, occlusive dressing is applied. Elastic bandages may lead to pressure necrosis and should not be used. Plastic spray dressings should be reserved for only the most superficial lacerations.

Splinting of extremity wounds is an important facet of total wound care; a properly applied splint hastens healing, reduces discomfort, and lessens scar formation. Abrasions, contusions, and lacerations all benefit from splinting. Simple finger lacerations at or near joint lines are best treated with immobilization of the entire digit. A forearm wound should be immobilized from the finger tips to the proximal forearm. The plaster splint should always be applied to the surface of the limb opposite the wound, and the limb should be splinted in the position of function whenever possible. A bulky, well-padded dressing with a splint is an ideal dressing for hand injuries. The finger tips should be left exposed to facilitate neurovascular evaluation. Prolonged immobilization always produces some degree of joint stiffness, and all splints should be removed as soon as the wound is adequately healed. A joint contracture is a poor trade off for a cosmetically acceptable scar. Splinting and elevation are essential in the treatment of most lower extremity injuries. Slings help decrease dependent edema in upper extremity injuries; when possible, the patient should elevate the arm on pillows.

ANTIBIOTICS AND WOUND INFECTIONS

Antibiotics are not indicated in the treatment of routine lacerations seen in the emergency department. They do not prevent infection in a wound improperly selected for closure or inadequately irrigated, debrided, or sutured. The risk of hypersensitivity reactions, especially with long-acting penicillins; the versatility of microorganisms in the selection of resistant strains; and the additional expense of antibiotic therapy render the indiscriminate use of antibiotics inadvisable. Emergency department studies have shown an infection rate of 6 percent in lacerations not treated with antibiotics.[23,24] There is no significant difference in the infection rate when prophylactic antibiotics (primarily depot penicillin) are used. In one study, Day noted a 23 percent infection rate for patients treated with antibiotics (depot penicillin or tetracycline wound irrigation) versus a 7 percent overall infection rate in the control group.[25]

When a distinction was made, studies showed that scalp and facial lacerations had the lowest infection rate (1 percent), while lacerations below the knee had an overall infection rate of 12 percent (6.5 to 17.5 percent). The overwhelmingly predominant organism cultured was penicillin-resistant *S. aureus*. No statistically significant differences were seen in the infection rate of ragged versus linear lacerations, wounds inflicted in different situations, or wounds caused by blunt versus sharp agents. Length of operating time and wound size were also not significant.[26] The inherent and often uncontrollable variables present in a busy emergency department render a well-controlled study extremely difficult, and more investigation is obviously necessary. Sound surgical judgment in deciding which wounds to close, meticulous debridement, and careful suturing appear at present to be the optimal tools in the prevention of infections.

Antibiotics are indicated in selected cases. For human bite wounds, a cephalosporin or penicillinase-resistant penicillin should be given for ten days. Penicillin is the drug of choice for dog and cat bites, with additional coverage with a cephalosporin or penicillinase-resistant penicillin if infection occurs. In patients without current active tetanus immunity, penicillin or tetracycline therapy should be instituted for severe, old (more than 24 hours), or neglected wounds. In open or closed wounds with signs of spreading cellulitis, lymphangitis, or suppuration, a penicillinase-resistant penicillin should be given, pending culture results. Sutures should be removed and local wound care initiated. Occasionally, prompt antibiotic therapy at early signs of inflammation in a closed wound will eliminate an impending infection. In such cases, close follow-up is mandatory, and sutures must be removed if the inflammation does not subside. In many instances of localized cellulitis and wound abscess formation, suture removal, wound debridement, and frequent dressing changes rapidly bring infection under control. Antibiotics, in such cases, should be held in reserve and used only if local measures fail.

Often the use of prophylactic antibiotic coverage is purely a clinical decision. In crush injuries and other wounds in which the blood supply has been imperiled, antibiotic coverage may prevent a low-grade infection that could lead to loss of valuable flap tips or skin edges. Where skin survival is essential, such as for cosmetic facial repairs or coverage of bone or tendon, many surgeons advocate antibiotic coverage. In every instance, however, proper wound cleansing, handling, and closure provide the optimal conditions for healing; no antibiotic can compensate for poor wound care.

REFERENCES

1. Peacock EE Jr, Van Winkle W Jr: *Wound Repair*. Philadelphia, WB Saunders, 1976, p 208.
2. Dudley HAF: *Emergency Surgery*, ed 10. Bristol: Wright, 1977, pp 47–57.
3. Goodman LS, Gilman A: *The Pharmacological Basis of Therapeutics*. London, The Macmillan Co, 1970, pp 371–390.
4. Moore DC: *Regional Block*. Springfield, IL, Charles C Thomas, 1965, pp 12–31.
5. Thompson RVS: *Primary Repair of Soft Tissue Injuries*. Melbourne, Melbourne University Press, 1969, pp 32–42.
6. Barham E, Butz GW, Angell JS: Comparison of wound strength in normal, irradiated and infected tissues closed with polyglycolic acid and chromic catgut sutures. *Surg Gynecol Obstet* 146:901–907, 1978.
7. Mach SD, Krizek TJ: Sutures and suturing: Current concepts. *J Oral Surg* 36:710–712, 1978.
8. Grabb WC, Smith JW: *Plastic Surgery*. Boston, Little, Brown and Company, 1979, pp 14–16.
9. Dingman RO, Johnson AJ: Surgery of the scalp. *Surg Clin North Am* 57(5):1011–1013, 1977.
10. Schultz RC, Oldham RJ: An overview of facial injuries. *Surg Clin North Am* 57(5):987–994, 1977.
11. Gaul JS Jr: Management of hand injuries. *Ann Emergency Med* 9(3):140, 1980.
12. Kizev KW: Epidemiological and clinical aspects of animal bite injuries. *JACEP* 8:134–141, 1979.
13. Thomson HG, Suitek EV: Small animal bites: The role of primary closure. *J Trauma* 13(1):22, 1973.
14. Bailie WE, Stowe EC, Schmitt AM: Aerobic bacterial flora of oral and nasal fluids of canines with reference to bacteria associated with bites. *J Clin Microbiol* 7(2):223–231, 1978.
15. Callaham ML: Prophylactic antibiotics in common dog bite wounds: A controlled study. *Ann Emergency Med* 9:410–414, 1980.
16. Goldstein EJC, Citron DM, Wield B, Blachmen U, Sutter VL, Miller TA, Finegold SM: Bacteriology of human and animal bite wounds. *J Clin Microbiol* 8(6):667–672, 1978.
17. Veitch JM, Omer GE: Case report: Treatment of cat bite injuries of the hand. *J Trauma* 19:201–202, 1979.
18. Weinstein RA, Stephen RJ, Morot A, Choukas NC: Human bites: Review of the literature and report of a case. *J Oral Surg* 31:792–794, 1973.
19. Guba AM, Milliken JB, Hoopes JE: The selection of antibiotics for human bites of the hand. *Plast Reconstr Surg* 56(5):538–540, 1975.
20. Farmer CB, Mann RJ: Human bite infections of the hand. *South Med J* 59:515–518, 1966.
21. Chuinard RC, D'Ambrosia RD: Human bite infections of the hand. *J Bone Joint Surg* 59A(3):416–418, 1977.
22. Goldstein EJC, Caffee HH, Price JE, Citronbaum DM, Miller TA, Finegold SM: Human bite infections. *Lancet.* 12:1290, 1977.
23. Gosnold JK: Infection rate of sutured wounds. *Practitioner* 218:584–585, 1977.
24. Hutton PAN, Jones BM, Law DJW: Depot penicillin as prophylaxis in accidental wounds. *Br J Surg* 65:549–550, 1978.
25. Day TK: Trial of prophylactic antibiotics in minor wounds requiring suture. *Lancet* 2:1174, 1975.
26. Rutherford WJ, Spence RAJ: Infection in wounds sutured in accident and emergency department. *Ann Emergency Med* 9(7):350–352, 1980.

Metabolic and Endocrine Emergencies

Various metabolic and endocrine emergencies may be encountered in the emergency department. In "Diabetic Emergencies" (Chapter 11), the author discusses the diagnosis of diabetes and considers the individualized treatment of the patient with insulin, the various components of intravenous fluid and electrolyte therapy required for adequate hydration, and the benefits of oral phosphate salt and alkali therapy. The recognition and treatment of less common but equally important and potentially life-threatening conditions, such as thyroid storm, myxedema coma, and adrenal disorders are discussed in "Thyroid Disorders" (Chapter 12) and "Adrenal Insufficiency" (Chapter 13), respectively.

"Electrolyte Abnormalities" (Chapter 14) is followed by detailed discussions on "Hyperkalemia and Hypokalemia" (Chapter 15), "Hypomagnesemia and Hypermagnesemia" (Chapter 16), and "Hypercalcemia" (Chapter 17). In "Acid-Base Disturbances" (Chapter 18), hydrogen ion concentration, acid-base physiology, and the various disturbances that may play a role in the metabolic disorders are discussed. Finally, the reader may wish to consider the discussion on the diagnosis and treatment of "Acute Gout" (Chapter 19) in conjunction with other conditions that involve the joint, as discussed in "Orthopedic Emergencies" (Chapter 8).

11. Diabetic Emergencies

STEPHEN HAMBURGER, M.D., F.A.C.P.
DAVID RUSH, Pharm.D.

DIABETIC KETOACIDOSIS

Diabetic ketoacidosis (DKA) is a medical emergency. Although the introduction of insulin into clinical medicine has lowered the morbidity and mortality rates of DKA tremendously, there is still an approximately 5 to 10 percent mortality in most medical centers.[1-3] In select subgroups of patients with DKA, such as the elderly, the mortality rate is significantly higher.[4] In recent years, interest in the treatment of DKA has focused mainly on the method of insulin administration.[5-8] Less dramatic, but possibly more important, has been the work involving the various components of fluid and electrolyte therapy: (1) the role of adequate hydration,[9] (2) the potential benefits of early use of phosphate salts,[10] and (3) the role of alkali therapy.[11]

The recent emphasis on the use of insulin in DKA has a potential negative impact; many physicians might assume that the treatment of DKA is standardized. This assumption could not be further from the truth—therapy of DKA must be individualized. As knowledge of the pathogenesis and the effect of the ketotic state on the host has evolved, awareness of the potential risk of DKA and its therapy has increased. There are few other conditions in which careful and continuous vigilance over the clinical and laboratory status of the patient is more important to the eventual outcome.

PATHOGENESIS

Diabetes mellitus is a complex syndrome. A component of this syndrome is a defect in intermediary metabolism resulting from the relative or absolute deficiency in insulin. DKA is the extreme clinical expression of this deficiency, which might be secondary to endogenous failure of insulin release (e.g., in the ketosis-prone diabetic), the exogenous administration of inadequate quantities of insulin in the known diabetic, or the antagonism of insulin by elevated circulating levels of anti-insulin hormones (glucagon, cortisol, growth hormone, and catecholamines) that might occur in numerous stressful conditions (Table 11–1). Whatever the reason, the normal balance between the anabolic hormone insulin and the catabolic anti-insulin hormones (growth hormone has both anabolic and catabolic functions) is shifted to the anti-insulin hormones, resulting in overproduction of glucose and ketone bodies.

TABLE 11–1   Metabolic Effects of the Anti-Insulin Hormones

	Insulin Release	Muscle Glucose Uptake	Gluconeogenesis	Lipolysis
Glucagon	↑	↓	↑	↑
Growth hormone	↑	↓		↑
Glucocorticoids	↑	↓	↑	↑

Source: Reprinted with permission from Family Practice Certification.

The hyperglycemia that is seen in most cases of DKA is a reflection of both overproduction and underutilization.[12] Circulating levels of insulin in these patients are usually quite low; thus, the insulin-dependent tissues, such as liver, muscle, and adipose tissue, which normally assimilate approximately 75 percent of a glucose load, are unable to use glucose.[13] In fact, the liver, which is normally a glucose-producing organ only during a fasting state, actively contributes to the hyperglycemia in DKA.[14] The increase in hepatic production of glucose is secondary to both glycogenolysis and gluconeogenesis. Both these glucose-producing mechanisms are primed by elevated levels of anti-insulin hormones, especially glucagon, cortisol, and catecholamines. Hyperglycemia results in an osmotic diuresis with loss of sodium, potassium, magnesium, chloride, and phosphorus. The urinary loss is usually hypo-osmolar to plasma. Clinically, the hyperglycemia is manifested as polydipsia and polyuria, leading to intravascular volume depletion.

Ketoacidosis is the end product of the accumulation of the ketone bodies: β-hydroxybutyric acid and acetoacetate. Another ketone body, acetone, is also formed; unlike β-hydroxybutyric acid and acetoacetate, however, acetone is neither an organic acid nor a hydrogen ion donor.[15] Because of the lack of insulin, there is an excessive lipolysis of triglycerides to free fatty acids and glycerol, as well as an excessive formation of β-hydroxybutyric acid, acetoacetate, and acetone. The free fatty acids are transported to the liver (glycerol is used for gluconeogenesis) where they are either oxidized to CO_2 or used in ketogenesis. In DKA, the oxidative capacity of the liver is overwhelmed; thus, ketogenesis is enhanced.

A working definition of DKA may be as follows: DKA is the state of relative or absolute insulin deficiency that results in an excess ketone concentration, a low arterial pH, and a low bicarbonate concentration. Hyperglycemia is *usually* present, and the results of a nitroprusside test are *usually* positive, although neither is a prerequisite to the diagnosis.[16,17] This definition of DKA takes into account the wide spectrum of severity of this illness.

DIAGNOSIS

Clinical Diagnosis

DKA is a common medical disorder that is seen not only in known diabetics, but also in previously unrecognized diabetics. Although the symptoms of DKA are variable, most can be explained by the defect in intermediary metabolism and the intravascular volume deficiency that causes poor tissue perfusion (Fig. 11–1).

Patients with DKA usually have increased urination and thirst secondary to the osmotic diuresis; increasing weakness and weight loss secondary to the catabolism of body fat and protein stores, anorexia, nausea, and vomiting; and variable mental symptomatology arising from the ketosis and intravascular volume depletion. In a known diabetic, these symptoms in increasing severity strongly suggest DKA; otherwise, the suspicion of DKA is a matter of clinical judgment. DKA should be very uncommon in the known, compliant diabetic, however, because the symptomatology of DKA is usually present for several days prior to severe clinical and metabolic decompensation and should be recognized by the patient. Furthermore, the patient who has had proper training in urinary testing for glucose and ketones will know when the test reflects a poor degree of control and will seek medical attention long before DKA develops.

Initial examination of the patient with DKA must include a meticulous search to determine the precipitating event (Exhibit 11–1). Patient noncompliance with the medical regimen or an infection is usually the underlying cause. A skin abscess, especially of the feet, is frequently overlooked. It is particularly important to seek an underlying condition in the elderly patient, for it is not uncommon for a diabetic to have a painless myocardial infarction with DKA.[18,19] The adequacy of the intravascular volume should be evaluated by measurement of blood pressure and pulse in both the supine and erect positions, if possible. Skin turgor and signs of tissue perfusion, such as central nervous system (CNS) symptomatology, urine output, and skin temperature, should be assessed.

The DKA patient with abdominal pain and tenderness presents a problem. Although the diabetic patient is certainly not exempt from surgical problems in the gastrointestinal tract, some DKA patients have a "pseudoappendicitis."[20] The serum amylase is elevated in a significant percentage of diabetic patients with DKA (as is the amylase/creatinine clearance ratio), but most of these patients do not have clinically significant pancreatitis.[21–23] Leukocytosis is common in uncomplicated DKA; therefore, this finding does not aid in the differential diagnosis. Since the abdominal signs and symptoms subside with treatment of the ketosis, it is of the utmost importance to correct the DKA as rapidly as possible in order to avoid unnecessary surgery. If, in spite of adequate treatment of the DKA, abdominal signs and symptoms persist, the possibility of a surgical condition should be strongly considered. Recent studies by Campbell and associates suggest that, in any DKA patient over the age of 40 years, abdominal pain is very likely to have an underlying precipitating cause. Also, it was found that abdominal pain in patients with a serum bicarbonate level greater than 10 mEq/liter is

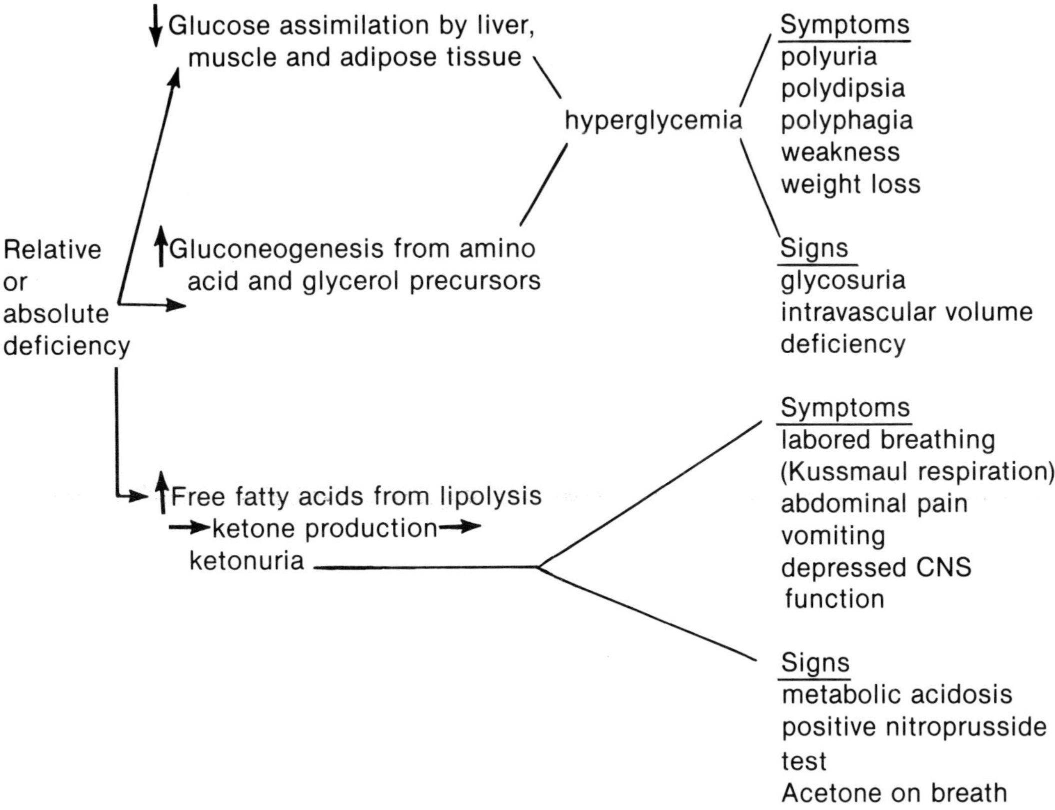

Figure 11–1 Pathophysiology of diabetic ketoacidosis.

very likely to be caused by an underlying condition. It must be stressed, however, that several of the conditions producing abdominal pain were of medical origin, such as pyelonephritis.[24]

Laboratory Diagnosis

Occasionally there is a significant delay in the laboratory reporting of biochemical determinations; however, any patient with a strongly positive reaction for ketones in undiluted serum, 4+ (2 percent) glycosuria, and a low arterial pH may be considered to have DKA and be treated as such. These tests may be done very rapidly in a semiquantitative fashion by means of nitroprusside tablets or reagent strips. Proper interpretation of the nitroprusside test is crucial and requires an understanding of the limitations of the test. It does not measure the level of β-hydroxybutyric acid, but it does reflect the concentration of acetoacetate and acetone.[25] Normally, the ratio of β-hydroxybutyric acid to acetoacetate (acetone is usually quantitatively much less significant) is 3:1. In DKA, the ratio might be greatly elevated, although both compounds are circulating at levels higher than normal.[26] If, as is often the case in DKA, tissue hypoxia leads to an increase in lactic acid, the β-hydroxybutyric acid/acetoacetate ratio is shifted further to favor β-hydroxybutyric acid. This is second-

ary to the increased level of NADH that results from tissue hypoxia. Thus, a patient may have a significant degree of ketoacidosis with only a weakly positive ketone test.[17] Then, too, a patient recovering from DKA may continue to have a strongly positive ketone test as the β-hydroxybutyric acid is converted to acetoacetate after the correction of the tissue hypoxia (Fig. 11–2).

The nitroprusside test is a poor indicator of the patient's response to therapy in DKA. This is true not only because the ketone equilibrium shifts as tissue hypoxia is relieved but also because the acetone that might have accumulated in the DKA patient is excreted so slowly. Acetone in high concentration might cause a positive nitroprusside test.[27] Thus, the patient might be fully recovered biochemically from DKA and yet have a positive ketone test if significant acetonemia remains.

Initial laboratory studies include a complete blood count; measurements of electrolytes, blood urea nitrogen (BUN), creatinine, magnesium, and blood glucose; urinalysis; and arterial blood gas and pH determinations. Interpretation of the serum sodium must take into account the "pseudohyponatremia" induced by hyperglycemia. Katz demonstrated that for every 100 mg glucose above 100 mg the percent serum sodium level is reduced by 1.6 mEq/ml.[28] Knowledge of this relationship is important in determining the water deficit in such a patient. An elevation in the serum triglyceride

Exhibit 11–1 Common Precipitating Factors of Diabetic Ketoacidosis

Failure of Endogenous Insulin
1. Previously undiagnosed diabetic
2. Viral infections of pancreas
3. Pancreatitis
4. Idiopathic/autoimmune

Failure of Exogenous Insulin
1. Change in diet or exercise
2. Patient noncompliance
   a. inadequate patient education
   b. poor vision
   c. wrong insulin concentration
   d. calibration/injection error
   e. mental deficiency
3. Inadequate dose or type prescribed
4. Insulin antibodies

Hormonal Antagonism of Insulin
1. Cushing's syndrome
2. Thyrotoxicosis
3. Pheochromocytoma
4. Acromegaly

Stress
1. Infection (e.g., pneumonia, abscess, urinary tract infection, gangrene)
2. Pregnancy
3. Myocardial infarction
4. Surgery
5. Trauma
6. Acute psychiatric illness

Source: Modified and reprinted with permission from Family Practice Certification.

level might also result in factitious hyponatremia.[29] A normal or increased serum osmolality, coupled with a low serum sodium level, suggests this possibility. An elevated uric acid level results primarily from decreased renal perfusion and competitive inhibition of uric acid secretion in the distal tubule of the kidney by the ketone bodies or lactic acid.[30,31] Test of kidney function might be misleading; the BUN, which is almost always high, might have a significant prerenal component in its increase, and the creatinine level might be spuriously elevated by the acetoacetate if the colorimetric method of determination is used.[32] The blood sugar level is invariably elevated, but a small percentage of patients with DKA have a normal glucose level.[16] Arterial blood gas determinations reflect a pure metabolic acidosis with a respiratory alkalosis as compensation in uncomplicated DKA. A superimposed lactic acidosis should be suspected if the nitroprusside test is weakly positive in the presence of significant acidemia and an elevated anion gap.* A baseline electrocardiogram (ECG) should always be obtained to diagnose a painless myocardial infarction. Appropriate Gram stains and cultures should be done to rule out an infection.

TREATMENT

The correction of DKA encompasses five areas:

1. diagnosis and treatment of the precipitating event(s)
2. replacement of fluid and electrolyte deficits
3. normalization of the intermediary metabolism
4. avoidance of complications
5. education of the patient to avoid recurrence

All patients with DKA should have a complete and up-to-date flowsheet (Fig. 11–3). This simple monitoring device allows the physician to see at a glance what therapy has previously been rendered and how the patient responded to the various modalities. If possible, central venous pressure lines and urinary catheters should be avoided so as to minimize the risk of a superimposed infection. In the unconscious patient, a patent airway must be established. Supplemental oxygen may be needed. Gastric aspiration benefits the patient with persistent vomiting or gastric atony. In the unconscious patient with an indwelling gastric tube, a cuffed endotracheal tube should be used to prevent an aspiration pneumonia.

Fluid Therapy

In all cases of DKA, it is crucial to replace the significant intravascular volume depletion as soon as possible. The average calculated loss of sodium is 8 mEq/kg body weight; that of water is approximately 75 ml/kg body weight.[34] The average patient with severe DKA requires approximately 4 to 6 liters normal and/or half normal saline during the first 12 to 24 hours of treatment.[35] The choice of normal or half normal saline is dictated by the status of intravascular volume and the serum osmolality. The intravascular volume, which is most easily corrected by normal saline, is measured by following the parameters of volume repletion, such as blood pressure, pulse, mentation, skin temperature, and urine output. During the repletion of the intravascular volume, the physician must continuously evaluate the patient's condition—not only for continued volume depletion but also for the development of signs and symp-

---

* Anion gap = $Na^+ - (Cl^- + HCO_3^-)$.
Normal anion gap = 12.4 ± 2 mEq/liter.[33]

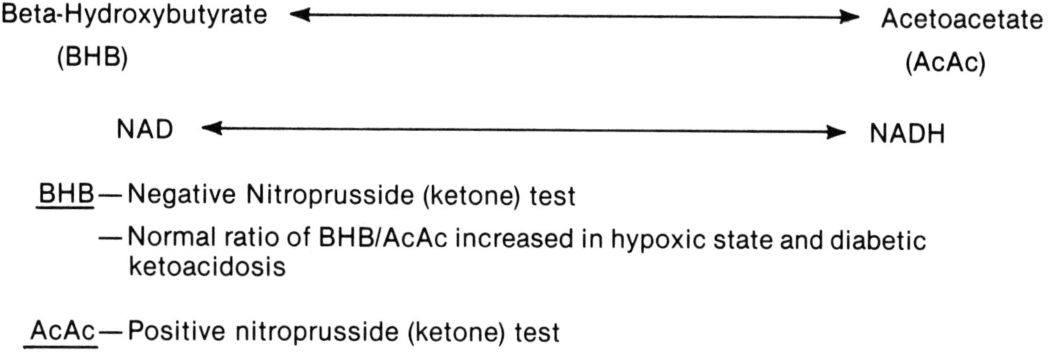

BHB — Negative Nitroprusside (ketone) test

— Normal ratio of BHB/AcAc increased in hypoxic state and diabetic ketoacidosis

AcAc — Positive nitroprusside (ketone) test

Acetone — Positive nitroprusside (ketone) test. Color intensity is much less than that of AcAc at equal concentration but if acetone concentration is greatly increased a positive nitroprusside test will result.

Figure 11–2   Interpretation of the Nitroprusside Test.
Key: BHBDH, β-hydroxybutyrate dehydrogenase; *NAD, NADH,* oxidized and reduced forms of pyridine nucleotide.

Clinical parameters	Laboratory parameters	Urine	Treatment parameters	
• Time • Blood pressure • Pulse • Urine output • Physical examination	Na, K, Cl, HCO$_3$, pH, glucose, BUN	• Glucose • Ketones	• Fluids (type, amount)	• Insulin (type, amount, and route of administration)

Figure 11–3   Flowsheet for Diabetic Ketoacidosis.

toms of sodium overload, such as congestive heart failure.

In the initial management of DKA, it is wise to determine the plasma osmolality (either by measurement or estimation*); this helps dictate early therapy and might warn of potential complications as the patient recovers. Most patients with DKA have some increase in plasma osmolality. This abnormality results mainly from loss of urine that is hypotonic to plasma. Studies have shown that the urinary output in DKA resembles half normal saline with 35 to 63 mEq/liter potassium.[35] With repletion of the intravascular volume by saline solutions and the reduction of the blood sugar level by insulin, much of the hyperosmolality is corrected. If the serum osmolality is still elevated, the use of hypotonic fluids such as half normal saline or free water by mouth lowers the osmolality to within normal range. It should be emphasized, however, that the rapid correction of the free water deficit has not been shown to be clinically beneficial and might be potentially harmful.[36]

Potassium

Studies that took place in the early 1950s have demonstrated that there is a significant loss of total body potassium in DKA.[37,38] Later studies confirmed these observations.[39–41] Causes of potassium depletion include the osmotic diuresis, acidemia with resultant intracellular buffering of hydrogen ions by potassium, and the catabolism of intracellular protein. Despite the *average* loss of approximately 6 mEq/kg[34] (some patients may lose as much as 10 mEq/kg), patients with DKA may have hypokalemia, normokalemia, or hyperkalemia. The mean admission concentration of potassium in a study by Beigelman was 5.3 mEq/liter (range 2.1 to 8.4), with 4 percent of the patients having an initial value less than 3.5 mEq/liter.[42] Initial hypokalemia signified a larger deficit of potassium, as those patients required a greater amount of parenteral administration of this cation for correction.

Aggressive therapy of DKA decreases the potassium level. This drop in potassium is secondary to rehydration and reuptake of potassium by cells under the influence of insulin therapy. If alkali therapy is begun to correct the acidosis, the decrease in potassium is more significant, owing to the intracellular shift of potassium; hence, additional exogenous potassium must be given to maintain a normal concentration. The study by Hockaday and Alberti showed the rapidity with which potassium is decreased after the start of therapy and the potential for significant hypokalemia without potassium

supplementation.[43] Their patients with DKA had an initial mean potassium of 4.4 mEq/liter, which decreased in one hour to 3.5 mEq/liter with little potassium supplementation. In light of this information, more aggressive potassium therapy was begun in the next group of patients. Five hours after therapy had begun, the mean potassium level was 4 mEq/liter (decreased from an initial mean of 4.4 mEq/liter), with an average of 87 mEq potassium being given to each patient. This drop in potassium was inversely related to the amount of exogenous potassium administered. Beigelman's study corroborated the fact that potassium levels drop rapidly with the initiation of treatment and further demonstrated the extreme range of potassium replacement needed to maintain a normal concentration (mean 170, range 0 to 620 mEq).[42]

Extreme hyperkalemia or hypokalemia is potentially lethal. (See Chapter 15.) In the absence of known hyperkalemia, ECG changes associated with hyperkalemia, or oliguria, it is recommended that potassium administration be initiated simultaneously with the initiation of other modalities of therapy. If the initial potassium level is found to be elevated, the administration of exogenous potassium should be stopped until the potassium level has decreased to the normal range. Potassium therapy should be individualized to maintain a normal serum concentration. Careful monitoring by frequent blood samples is essential. Serial ECGs to determine the prevailing serum potassium are not as useful as expected because many changes are nonspecific.[44]

Phosphorus

DKA is associated with total body phosphate depletion.[37,45] As with potassium, the serum level of phosphate can be normal or elevated in the patient with untreated DKA, in spite of the overall deficit.[46] In DKA, the possible deleterious effects of phosphate depletion include (a) decreased oxygenation of peripheral tissues, (b) depressed CNS function, (c) increased risk of infection, and (d) impaired carbohydrate utilization.

Decreased Oxygenation of Peripheral Tissues

Oxygen delivery at the cellular level is partially dependent on cardiac output and the arterial-venous oxygen difference. Phosphate depletion in DKA interferes with both of these mechanisms.

Cardiac Output. O'Connor and associates demonstrated that, in severely hypophosphatemic patients, the cardiac output (measured by thermodilution and cardiac stroke work) was impaired.[47] After the correction of the phosphate depletion, cardiac output improved significantly—possibly because of the repletion of intracellular adenosine triphosphate (ATP). Since many

---

* Estimated serum osmolality = $2(Na^+) + \dfrac{glucose}{18} + \dfrac{BUN}{2.8}$

patients with DKA already have a compromised myocardium and some of the complications in DKA might be related to cellular hypoxia, phosphate repletion seems warranted.

Arterial-Venous Oxygen Difference. Most of the interest in the treatment of DKA and the oxyhemoglobin curve (Fig. 11–4) has focused on 2,3-diphosphoglyceric acid (2,3-DPG) and the state of the arterial pH. 2,3-DPG levels are decreased in DKA by several mechanisms. Acidosis impairs the production of 2,3-DPG by inhibiting red cell glycolysis at the phosphofructokinase step.[48,49] Total body phosphate depletion is a factor in the low red cell 2,3-DPG. Travis has suggested that, in the presence of hyperglycemia with an increased conversion of glucose to sorbitol via the polyol pathway, production of 2,3-DPG is reduced.[50] Although the depletion of 2,3-DPG shifts the oxyhemoglobin association curve to the left, most *untreated* patients with DKA have a dissociation curve that approximates normal[51] because the acidosis shifts the curve to the right, compensating for the leftward shift. Clinically significant is the recovery of the 2,3-DPG during the treatment of DKA when phosphate is withheld. Although the pH may return to normal within 24 hours, the return of the 2,3-DPG to adequate levels may take as long as one week.[10] Thus, the protective effect of the acidosis on the oxyhemoglobin dissociation curve is lost rapidly, while the adverse effect of the depressed level of 2,3-DPG remains. This results in a potentially dangerous situation; i.e., the circulating hemoglobin has a high affinity for oxygen, and this may result in cellular hypoxia. The early administration of phosphate would

probably help in the recovery phase of 2,3-DPG. Studies in DKA patients who were given phosphate during early therapy have supported this contention.[52]

In regard to hyperalimentation, another clinical entity associated with hypophosphatemia, Travis has shown that supplemental phosphorus increases the red cell level of 2,3-DPG to the normal range more rapidly.[53]

Depressed CNS Function

CNS symptomatology is quite common in DKA. A depressed sensorium is the most frequent abnormality. Seizures and focal neurologic deficits are unusual in uncomplicated DKA.[54] If these neurologic findings are encountered in a patient with DKA, a secondary precipitating cause is usually present. The reason that seizures are uncommon in DKA may be related to the fact that concentrations of γ-amino butyric acid (GABA) are normal in the CNS of patients with DKA.[55] Although many causes have been proposed for this depressed sensorium, no one cause is probably at fault in the individual patient. Postulated factors in the pathogenesis of CNS depression in DKA include extracellular hyperosmolality,[56] hyperviscosity of the blood,[57] cellular hypoxia,[58] spinal fluid and presumably intracellular acidemia in the brain,[59] CNS utilization of the ketones[54] that occur in DKA, and a medical condition, such as a cerebrovascular accident or infection.

The role, if any, of phosphate depletion in the pathogenesis of CNS dysfunction is unclear. Droller and associates have shown that mental obtundation and seizures can occur in severely hypophosphatemic patients during hyperalimentation.[60] Travis and associates are in apparent agreement, but they found that many of the neurologic abnormalities could be prevented by adequate phosphorus supplementation during hyperalimentation.[53] Thus hypophosphatemia, possibly caused by impaired glucose utilization and/or depressed 2,3-DPG with resultant cellular hypoxia, seems to have a potential role in the CNS symptomatology of DKA.

Increased Risk of Infection

Although no defects in humoral antibodies or the complement system have been demonstrated in the diabetic patient, white cell function in patients with DKA or mildly uncontrolled diabetes is impaired.[61] This dysfunction affects not only chemotaxis, but also phagocytosis and microbiologic killing of ingested bacteria.[62,63] Therefore, the patient with DKA may be at an increased risk of infection, possibly related to phosphorus depletion. If true, the pathogenesis of this increased risk of infection seems related to a decreased level of intracellular ATP, with a resultant decrease in energy.

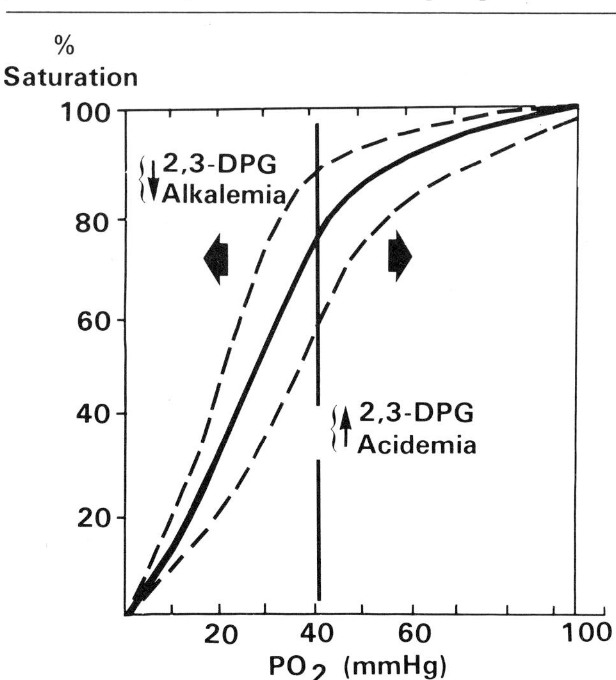

Figure 11–4 Oxyhemoglobin Dissociation Curve.

Impaired Carbohydrate Utilization

Several studies suggest that glucose utilization is improved following phosphorus administration. In his review of phosphorus depletion, Knochel showed that diabetic patients who received phosphorus had better glucose utilization.[64] In a more recent study Lichtman and associates showed that phosphorus depletion decreased the utilization of glucose by red blood cells.[65]

Phosphate Therapy

Phosphorus depletion in DKA is a clinical liability to the patient. Therefore, repletion of this deficit in the early therapy is logical, unless there are known contraindications to phosphate therapy, such as renal failure or a significant increase in plasma phosphorus. Intravenous preparations include potassium phosphate. If oral supplementation is possible, the patient should consume high-phosphate foods, e.g., dairy products, or solutions of sodium phosphate. Therapy must be carefully monitored—especially during intravenous therapy. Complications include hyperphosphatemia with possible metastatic calcifications, hyperkalemia due to the use of potassium phosphate salts, and hypocalcemia. Diarrhea occurs commonly during oral therapy with phosphates.

Magnesium

DKA is associated with a significant urinary excretion of magnesium.[66] As with potassium, the magnesium level might be normal or elevated initially, but it tends to drop with the administration of insulin and fluids. Clinical symptomatology of hypomagnesemia includes tetany, seizures, cardiac arrhythmias, and CNS depression. It is recommended that the serum magnesium level be determined as soon as possible in all patients with DKA. If low, magnesium should be administered. Intravenous magnesium supplementation is the preferred method of repletion in a severely magnesium-deficient patient. This is particularly true in the early therapy of DKA, as the uptake of magnesium after an intramuscular injection might be less than optimal until adequate hydration has been restored. In the presence of seizures or arrhythmias of uncertain etiology, magnesium therapy should be considered even if the initial magnesium level is within normal limits. Extreme caution must be used when magnesium is administered to patients with renal insufficiency, as these patients are prone to develop a toxic level. Both the blood level and the deep tendon reflexes, which tend to diminish as the magnesium concentration rises to toxic levels, should be checked frequently in these patients.

Alkali Therapy

The acidemic state in DKA results from the excess production and underutilization of the hydrogen ion–donating ketone bodies, β-hydroxybutyric acid and acetoacetate. The consequences of severe acidosis include cardiovascular collapse, respiratory depression, and CNS dysfunction. Although it would seem logical to treat all cases of DKA with alkali, this approach is invalid because (1) insulin can reverse the ketotic state and (2) alkali therapy has detrimental effects.

Lipolysis is inhibited by very low circulating levels of insulin, approximately 40 μU/ml in one study.[67] The metabolism of β-hydroxybutyric acid requires about 100 μU/ml in normal subjects.[68] Therefore, insulin levels readily achieved by current methods of therapy reverse the ketoacidotic state, usually within 24 hours. This fact is clinically documented thousands of times each year as DKA patients are returned to normal without resort to alkali therapy.

Potential adverse effects of alkali therapy include

- shift of the oxyhemoglobin dissociation curve to the left with resulting cellular hypoxia
- accentuation of the intracellular shift of potassium and phosphate
- accentuation of the "paradoxical" cerebrospinal fluid acidosis to levels associated with coma[69]
- sodium overload
- tetany secondary to hypocalcemia and/or hypomagnesemia
- induction of metabolic alkalosis

Weighing the benefits and risks of alkali therapy, it would appear wise to initiate alkali therapy only in those patients with a pH of approximately 7.0, significant cardiac arrhythmias in the acidemic state, or a compromised respiratory system. The latter may be suggested by an abnormal elevation of the PCO_2 according to the following formula in a primary metabolic acidosis:

$$\text{expected } PCO_2 = 1.54(HCO_5) + 8.34 \pm 1.1^{70}$$

In any case, the alkali therapy given should be estimated to give a final pH of approximately 7.20.[11]

The alkali therapy of choice is bicarbonate, not lactate, for two reasons:

1. Lactic acid usually makes a small contribution to the overall acidemic state in DKA.[71]
2. After high-dose insulin therapy, there is a small rise in lactate concentration during the early recovery phase of DKA.[72]

Close surveillance of the result of the bicarbonate therapy by arterial blood gas or venous pH determination is required.

Insulin Therapy

Much has changed in the therapy of DKA in recent years, particularly in regard to the route and amount of insulin administration. Since the highly quoted work by Root, as well as that of Black and Malins, during the 1940s, the supposed benefits of intensive, high-dose insulin therapy have been emphasized.[73,74] The occasional reports of "low"-dose insulin therapy (lower than generally used at the time but no where near current standards) during this era were largely ignored by practicing clinicians.[75]

This remarkable decrease in insulin dosage has been derived from elegant studies concerning the physiologic action of insulin in relation to carbohydrate and ketone metabolism in the normal person. It was found that low-dose insulin therapy of DKA results in circulating levels of insulin of approximately 100 μU/ml, which supports the rationale of high physiologic, not pharmacologic, concentrations of insulin for therapy.[76,77] This concentration of insulin has been readily achieved by several routes of administration, including intramuscular and intravenous (Table 11–2).

Intramuscular Administration

Studies by Binder have shown that intramuscularly administered insulin has a half-life of two hours.[78] By calculations and in actual practice, Alberti and associates have shown that an initial injection of 20 units insulin, followed by hourly injections of 10 units, results in an insulin concentration of approximately 100 μU/ml in less than three hours.[79] The intramuscular method of insulin administration in the treatment of DKA has worked quite well in several studies.[80,81] Advantages include a very predictable fall in the blood glucose level (approximately 80 to 100 mg/hour, assuming adequate hydration),[79–81] a decreased incidence of hypokalemia,[79] a decreased incidence of delayed hypoglycemia,[80] and a fall, not a rise, in the blood lactate level.[79] Although not yet documented, a smaller fall in serum phosphorus and magnesium levels, as well as a decreased incidence of cerebral edema, might be a consequence of low-dose insulin therapy of DKA. This regimen is also extremely convenient to administer. The recommended site of insulin injection is the deltoid muscle.[80] In the occasional patient who is adequately hydrated but does not respond to intramuscular insulin therapy (such a patient usually has an infection), a change to continuous infusion of intravenous insulin is recommended. If there is any doubt about the practicality of a continuous insulin infusion, the intramuscular route of insulin administration is the treatment of choice.

Intravenous Administration

Constant infusion of insulin is not new—only the dosage has changed. Since the work by Genuth,[82] who used a loading dose of 50 units regular insulin, followed by 50 units/hour, the dosage has plummeted to only 1 unit/hour in one study.[83] The goal of insulin therapy is to normalize the metabolic state of the patient; thus, circulating insulin concentrations of 100 to 200 μU/ml are probably adequate, if not excessive. This level is readily achieved by a constant infusion of regular insulin at a rate of 4 to 8 units/hour.[84,85] A loading dose is not necessary.

The advantages of a constant insulin infusion are similar to those of low-dose intramuscular therapy. Treatment should be continuous, since insulin administered intravenously has a half-life of only five minutes. Although a great advantage in preventing or in facilitating the recovery from hypoglycemia, the short half-life mandates constant surveillance of the intravenous apparatus. In the rush of the daily hospital routine, an accidental increase or decrease in the intravenous insulin infusion is all too possible.

It is well-known that insulin binds with glass and plastic—potentially up to 30 or 40 percent.[86,87] Thus, many centers recommend adding human albumin, a gelatin solution, or the patient's own blood to the insulin solution to prevent absorption.[88] The latter is preferred, since there is a risk of hepatitis with albumin and the gelatin solution is not available in the United States. Although of theoretical importance, the clinical significance of this absorption is questionable; several studies have shown excellent results with low-dose insulin therapy when no binding inhibitor was used.[6,89]

Despite the fact that the biologic action of insulin is longer than its immunologic half-life, bolus intravenous therapy is to be discouraged. The insulin levels fluctuate from initial pharmacologic levels to potentially suboptimal concentrations before the next dose is given.[90] Also, bolus therapy has been associated with rapid increases in anti-insulin hormones and lactate levels.[4]

As with other methods of insulin therapy in DKA, constant intravenous infusion is only part of the regimen. Total care of the patient is paramount. If the patient is not responding to the intravenous therapy in spite of adequate hydration, the insulin dosage should be doubled and an insulin-binding inhibitor added, if this has not been done already. As with intramuscular insulin therapy, patients with infections seem to respond more slowly.

TABLE 11–2   Methods for Low-Dose Insulin Therapy in Diabetic Ketoacidosis

	Subcutaneous	Intramuscular	Intravenous
Dose	1. 0.33 units regular insulin per kg as initial dose[a,b]	1. 0.22 units of regular insulin per kg as initial dose	1. 7 units of regular insulin per hour as continuous drip until plasma glucose reaches 250 mg/dl
	2. 7 units of regular insulin per hour thereafter until plasma glucose reaches 250 mg/dl	2. 0.1 units of regular insulin per kg hourly until plasma glucose reaches 250 mg/dl 3. Priming dose optional	2. Priming dose optional
Advantages[c]	1. Same as intramuscular	1. Predictable decrease in plasma glucose level (60–100 mg/dl/hour) 2. Possibly less incidence of hypokalemia 3. Possibly less incidence of hypoglycemia 4. Simplification of insulin therapy	1. Same as intramuscular
Disadvantages	1. Heavily dependent on intravascular volume replacement 2. Occasional nonresponder	1. Dependent on intravascular volume replacement 2. Occasional nonresponder	1. Dependent on intravascular volume replacement 2. Occasional nonresponder 3. Necessary to check infusion set frequently to ascertain that insulin delivery is correct

[a] If plasma glucose fails to decrease by 10 percent in the first hour, repeat initial dose each hour thereafter until a 10 percent decrease in plasma glucose is obtained.

[b] If there is no response in the plasma glucose after three doses, switch to intravenous insulin and search for an infection.

[c] In a patient with adequate replacement of intravascular volume and careful clinical and biochemical monitoring.

Source: Modified with permission from Missouri Medicine.

Complications of Insulin Therapy

Hypoglycemia. By any method of administration, insulin may induce hypoglycemia. With low-dose insulin therapy—because the drop in the blood glucose level is predictable—and with frequent monitoring of the blood sugar, this complication should be quite infrequent. When the blood sugar level approaches 250 mg/dl, exogenous glucose should be added either intravenously or, preferably, orally. As the exogenous sugar is added, insulin administration must be continued, but the dosage and route of administration should be reviewed. The correction of the acidosis tends to lag behind the normalization of the blood sugar, but this delay should be of little concern as long as the pH continues to improve.[91] In fact, this lag might be beneficial to the patient, because a correction of pH that is too rapid may result in significant complications.

Cerebral Edema. Fortunately, since it is frequently fatal, cerebral edema is very uncommon in DKA. This complication should be suspected in any patient whose clinical and biochemical improvement is followed by deterioration in cerebral function. Elevation of the intraocular or cerebrospinal fluid pressures (with or without papilledema) in such a patient strongly suggests cerebral edema. Although no treatment is of proved benefit, free water administration should be stopped and hypertonic saline or mannitol begun in hope of reversing the process.[92] It is hoped that early supplementation of exogenous sugar (at approximately 250 mg/dl) and less reliance on markedly hypotonic solutions to correct the increased serum osmolality will reduce this deadly complication.

Education of the Patient

The often quoted saying "an ounce of prevention is worth a pound of cure" certainly applies to DKA. A second episode of DKA in the same patient should be extremely uncommon. Education begins in the hospital. By the time of discharge, each diabetic patient should be thoroughly versed in proper diet, urine testing, drug therapy, and activity. This education is continued at each follow-up visit and should include the "sick day" management of diabetes mellitus. The following rules should be emphasized:

1. *Do not discontinue daily insulin injections.* Many diabetic patients are under the false impression

that, when they have an illness that causes a decrease in the intake of food, e.g., the flu or gastroenteritis, insulin is not needed. In reality, the insulin requirement usually increases, because the levels of anti-insulin hormones are elevated during an acute illness.

2. *Check urine fractional for sugar and ketones four times a day.* This should be done by many patients even when their condition is stable, but it is imperative during an acute illness. Double-voided urine specimens are preferred, as they usually reflect the prevailing blood glucose level more accurately.

3. *Know how to use regular insulin.* During an acute illness, a working knowledge of a rapid-acting insulin is essential. Injection of regular insulin at times determined by urine fractionals (approximately every six hours) helps prevent the illness from developing into overt DKA.

4. *Initiate a sick day diet.* Frequently, a normal diet cannot be tolerated during an acute illness. Substitution of a liquid or soft diet equal in calories to the food normally consumed is usually adequate. This diet must be adequate in sodium and potassium content as well. Substitutions of this type should be explained as part of the dietary education.

5. *Use common sense.* Close cooperation between patient and physician is essential. If this treatment regimen is not successful, admission to a hospital for more intensive treatment is advisable.

The success of the treatment of any disease must be measured by the decrease of morbidity and mortality that results from therapy versus the risk of treatment. There is no doubt that the treatment of DKA by the various modalities mentioned has considerably brightened the outlook of the patient with DKA. The risk of treatment has been reduced by the introduction of low-dose insulin therapy. Still, there is much to be achieved both in morbidity and mortality in DKA. Low-dose insulin therapy of DKA is not a panacea. Many deaths in DKA are associated with a major precipitating event; only in relation to hypoglycemia, hypokalemia, and possibly cerebral edema does low-dose insulin therapy have any impact. Future research will uncover other avoidable causes of morbidity and mortality in DKA. Until that time, and probably thereafter, the best therapy begins with a diligent physician dedicated to total patient management.

HYPEROSMOLAR HYPERGLYCEMIC NONKETOTIC COMA

In recent years, hyperosmolar hyperglycemic nonketotic coma (HHNK) has become a common complication of diabetes mellitus. Although HHNK was initially described nearly a century ago,[93] modern awareness of this syndrome is credited to the work of Sament and Swartz in 1957.[94] Since then, other reports have appeared.[95–97] Despite increased recognition of this syndrome, which is characterized by pronounced hyperglycemia, hyperosmolality, and dehydration in the absence of ketoacidosis, the mortality rate remains significantly higher than that of DKA, even in patients of comparable age.

PATHOGENESIS

The mechanism of HHNK has not been totally elucidated. Much interest in the pathogenesis of HHNK has focused on the lack of significant ketosis and the depressed sensorium.

Ketone bodies are normally produced by the liver in proportion to the circulating levels of free fatty acids, which act as substrate. Several reports have revealed that the levels of free fatty acids in HHNK are either normal or lower than those found in DKA, implying a defect in lipolysis.[98,99] Although the circulating levels of insulin have been found to be similar in patients with HHNK and DKA, the levels of growth hormone and cortisol, which are lipolytic hormones, have been found to be significantly lower in patients with HHNK than in patients with DKA. This suggests that, in some patients with HHNK, the low levels of free fatty acids and the lack of ketosis reflect a decrease in the activity of lipolytic hormones. Other mechanisms for the lack of ketosis in this syndrome have been postulated. For example, it has been suggested that severe dehydration might be antiketogenic, resulting in low plasma free fatty acid levels and ketone production.[100,101] In addition, in vitro studies have revealed that hyperosmolality inhibits both the release of pancreatic insulin to glucose and the production of free fatty acids from adipose tissue.[102]

Much of the work in the pathogenesis of the depressed sensorium in patients with HHNK has been done by Arieff and Carroll.[103] In a study of 40 patients with HHNK, they found that the depressed sensorium was highly correlated with the plasma osmolality. All stuporous or obtunded patients had a plasma osmolality of at least 350 mOsm/kg, while patients with a plasma osmolality of less than 350 mOsm/kg were alert. Sensorium did not correlate with the glucose concentration or the pH of either cerebrospinal fluid or plasma.

PATHOPHYSIOLOGY

Fundamental to the pathophysiology of HHNK is a relative lack of insulin and relative excess of anti-insulin hormones, such as growth hormone, cortisol, and glucagon (Fig. 11–5). The net result of the interaction of these hormones is the excessive production and the underutilization of glucose, which leads to a pronounced hyperglycemia. Osmotically active glucose is located only in the extracellular fluid. Total body water generally represents about 60 percent of body weight, with two-thirds of the water being intracellular and one-third being extracellular. As the plasma glucose level rises, water moves from the intracellular fluid to the extracellular fluid until osmotic equilibrium is achieved. Thus, pronounced hyperglycemia results in the loss of water from the intracellular fluid, producing intracellular dehydration and expanding the extracellular fluid. Both have diagnostic and therapeutic implications. When the plasma glucose level is elevated, the renal threshold for glucose reabsorption may be surpassed, resulting in glycosuria. Generally, the higher the glucose level, the greater the renal excretion of glucose. Glyosuria causes an osmotic diuresis by inhibiting the reabsorption of water, which increases the flow of urine.

In terms of electrolyte loss, the osmotic diuresis in patients with HHNK results in a urinary loss of sodium and potassium of approximately 50 mEq/liter each.[104] Thus, the osmotic diuresis produces a greater water loss than sodium loss, resulting in the hyperosmolar state and intracellular loss of water in most patients with HHNK. In addition, the loss of sodium leads to depletion of extracellular fluid volume. Other electrolytes, including magnesium and phosphate, have also been found to be depleted in patients with HHNK.

Much of the hyperglycemia in the HHNK patient probably results from decreased renal excretion of glucose rather than from overproduction or underutilization of glucose. As the extracellular fluid volume is depleted, the glomerular filtration rate decreases, which hampers the normal renal escape mechanism for glucose. Thus, a vicious cycle occurs: (1) the higher the plasma glucose level, the more pronounced the depletion of extracellular volume; (2) the glomerular filtration decreases; (3) less glucose is excreted in the urine; and (4) the plasma glucose becomes more elevated. A similar circumstance has been shown to occur in patients with DKA; as much as 80 percent of the hyperglycemia in DKA patients is secondary to impaired excretion of renal glucose.[105] In most instances, patients with HHNK have a more pronounced volume depletion and higher plasma glucose levels than do patients with DKA because of the longer duration of symptoms before therapy is given.

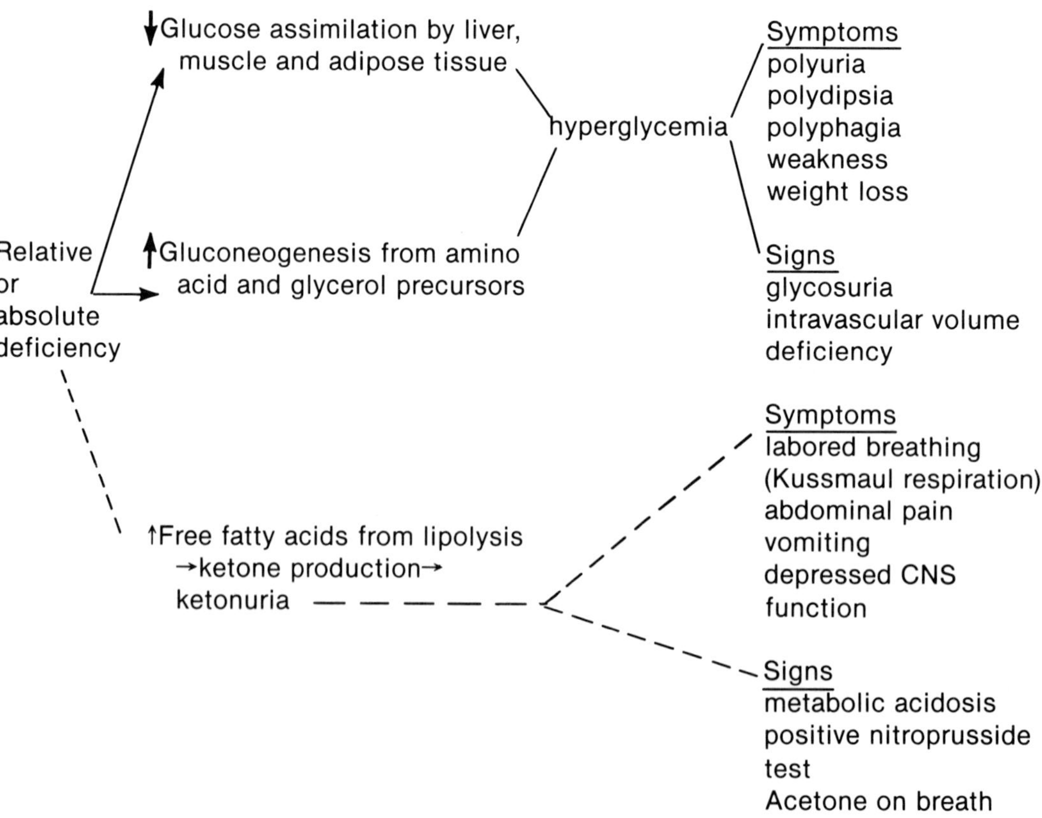

Figure 11–5 Pathophysiology of hyperosmolar hyperglycemic nonketoic coma (HHNK). In HHNK, the actions indicated by broken lines are suppressed.

DIAGNOSIS

Clinical Diagnosis

HHNK occurs mainly in the elderly; patients have an average age of 60 years, although one patient recorded was a nine-month-old child. The condition occurs with equal frequency in men and women. Prior to the onset of HHNK, many patients have no history of diabetes mellitus. Even those with diabetes have usually been well controlled with diet or hypoglycemic agents. Although symptoms usually develop over a few days to a week unless there is an acute precipitating cause, HHNK has occurred within several hours after peritoneal dialysis or major surgery. Symptoms, e.g., polyuria, polydipsia, and, occasionally, polyphagia, reflect the osmotic diuresis. Probably because ketosis (ketones are anorectic substances) and acidosis are insignificant, patients with HHNK generally have a longer history of illness than do patients with DKA.

Neurologic abnormalities are quite prevalent. As mentioned earlier, seizures are uncommon in uncomplicated DKA, but they are frequent in HHNK and occur in approximately 15 percent of patients. Localizing signs of a cerebrovascular accident, such as a positive Babinski sign, are also common and often resolve with successful therapy. In many instances, the admitting diagnosis is a cerebrovascular accident, which delays the recognition and management of the HHNK. Any comatose patient should have a screening test for glucose in blood and urine in order to prevent such a delay in the diagnosis of HHNK. In pure terms, all patients with HHNK are comatose; in reality, half are either obtunded or stuporous. A distinct minority is alert.

Physical examination usually reveals extensive evidence of extracellular fluid volume depletion. Relative or absolute hypotension and tachycardia are present in the majority of patients. Skin turgor is poor, but this sign is unreliable because most patients are elderly. Many individuals also have a precipitating illness:

- infection, particularly pneumonia
- cardiovascular disease
    myocardial infarction
    cerebrovascular accident
    gastrointestinal bleeding
- miscellaneous
    pancreatitis
    excessive carbohydrate intake
    surgery
    dialysis

In addition, the use of certain drugs has been associated with the onset of HHNK:

- diuretics, particularly thiazides, chlorthalidone, furosemide
- steroids
- propranolol
- immunosuppressive agents
- diphenylhydantoin (Dilantin)
- diazoxide

Hospital procedures, such as peritoneal dialysis, hemodialysis, hyperalimentation, and the administration of mannitol have also produced HHNK.

Laboratory Diagnosis

HHNK is easily diagnosed once the syndrome has been considered. No rigid criteria have been set, but a laboratory diagnosis may be defined as

1. glycosuria of 3+ or 4+ without ketonuria
2. extreme hyperglycemia, i.e., glucose usually greater than 600 mg/100 ml
3. negative or minimally positive nitroprusside test (Acetest), i.e., no greater than 2+ reaction when plasma is diluted 1:1 with water
4. serum osmolality greater than 350 mOsm/kg[105]

In addition, the serum sodium level is usually normal to elevated; the serum potassium level is normal to low; and the BUN, creatinine, and BUN/creatinine ratio (which is normally 10:1) are usually elevated.

In the absence of an osmometer, the approximate plasma osmolality may be calculated by using the following formula:

$$\text{Osmolality} = 2\,[\text{serum sodium}] + \frac{\text{blood glucose}}{18} + \frac{\text{BUN}}{2.8}$$

Normal osmolality is 285 to 300 mOsm. A low or low-normal plasma osmolality concomitant with extreme hyperglycemia may alter therapy. In any given series, the individual values for blood glucose and plasma osmolality vary widely. In the report by Arieff and Carroll, the mean blood glucose level was 1166 mg/dl (standard deviation $\pm$ 306), and the mean plasma osmolality was 384 mOsm/kg water (standard deviation $\pm$ 27).[105]

Initial studies should include a complete blood count; determinations of electrolytes, BUN, creatinine, and arterial blood gases; and urinalysis. Interpretation of these studies must take into account many of the same factors that must be considered with laboratory studies on DKA patients, e.g., "pscudohyponatremia" induced by hyperglycemia and factitious hyponatremia caused by an elevated triglyceride level. Many of the initial studies reflect the marked degree of dehydration. The hemoglobin and hematocrit are commonly elevated, but they return to normal with adequate fluid replacement. Many patients, successfully treated, will have residual impairment of kidney function. Like patients with DKA, those with HHNK have a total body depletion of potassium that is secondary to the osmotic losses in the urine and gastrointestinal tract. Unlike patients with DKA, who are usually acidemic, patients with HHNK are occasionally hyperkalemic. In the series by McCurdy, approximately 12 percent of patients with HHNK had initial hyperkalemia, whereas almost 30 percent had initial potassium levels below 4 mEq/liter.[96] In the series of patients studied by Arieff and Carroll, the mean initial values for BUN, creatinine, serum sodium, and potassium were 95 mg/dl, 5.6 mg/dl, 144 mEq/liter, and 5 mEq/liter, respectively.[105] The "normal" serum sodium in spite of extreme hyperglycemia demonstrates the tremendous loss of body water that occurs in patients with HHNK.

Metabolic acidosis is not infrequent in HHNK. In both the report by McCurdy and that by Arieff and Carroll, metabolic acidosis, as defined by a serum CO_2 level of less than 21 mEq/liter or an arterial pH of 7.35 or less, occurred in 40 to 60 percent of the patients.[96,105] Slight lactate elevations were frequent but did not account for the majority of cases of metabolic acidosis. Renal failure accounted for several. In a few patients, even though the nitroprusside test was not impressive, the level of acetoacetic acid (one of the prevalent hydrogen ion–donating ketone bodies in DKA) was slightly elevated, suggesting possible DKA. Interestingly, Sotos and associates have shown that pronounced hyperosmolality per se may cause metabolic acidosis in animals.[106] Thus, the cause for the metabolic acidosis is unknown in the majority of cases in HHNK; in most patients, it is probably multifactorial.

As with DKA, a baseline ECG should always be obtained to identify a painless myocardial infarction, and appropriate bacterial stains and cultures should be done to rule out an infection.

TREATMENT

The correction of HHNK encompasses four areas: (1) replacement of fluid and electrolyte deficits, (2) normalization of the intermediary metabolism, (3) prevention of complications, and (4) diagnosis and treatment of the precipitating event.

All patients with HHNK should have a complete and up-to-date flowsheet like that used in DKA (Fig. 11–3) to eliminate uncertainty about previous therapy and to indicate how the patient responds to various modalities. Catheters should be avoided if at all possible so as to minimize the risk of a superimposed infection. If required, a Swan-Ganz catheter is preferred to a central venous pressure line.

Fluid and Electrolyte Therapy

Fluid therapy in patients with HHNK is controversial. Some authors suggest fluid replacement with normal saline, while others prefer to use half normal saline providing the patient is not clinically hypotensive or oliguric.[34,107] In actuality, initial therapy is best determined by the clinical presentation of the individual patient. Whatever treatment is chosen, the patient's condition must be carefully monitored to determine progress and changes in fluid requirements.

Total body water loss in patients with HHNK has been estimated to average 24 percent, with approximately 50 mEq/liter each of sodium and potassium lost in the osmotic diuresis. Total body loss of sodium and potassium is similar to that in patients with DKA, i.e., an average of 8 mEq/kg and 6 mEq/kg, respectively. Thus, most patients with HHNK initially have marked clinical evidence of sodium depletion (relative or absolute hypotension, tachycardia, oliguria, and poor skin turgor) and require rapid and total correction of the sodium deficit. The amount of normal saline required varies among patients. The criteria mentioned earlier indicate the adequacy of sodium repletion. Since most individuals with HHNK are elderly, normal saline may not be innocuous, and hypertension with sodium overload must be carefully avoided.

In the face of clinical intravascular volume depletion, it may be advisable to withhold insulin early in the course of therapy. A few patients have no evidence of sodium depletion upon initial presentation, and, in these, cautious use of the half normal saline and insulin may be used. Careful and continuous monitoring of intravascular volume is necessary, however. Replacement with hypotonic fluids with simultaneous lowering of the plasma glucose by insulin has been shown to induce hypotension and oliguria because of the movement of water from the extracellular to the intracellular space.[108] Replacement of sodium deficit with normal saline instead of half normal saline results in a slower drop in the plasma osmolality.

The average loss of water is approximately 75 to 100 ml/kg of body weight or, as mentioned earlier, 24 percent of total body water. After the sodium deficit has been corrected, the free water deficit may be replaced.

The free water deficit may be calculated by the following formula:

$$\text{Water deficit} = 0.6 \times \text{body weight in kg} \left(1 - \frac{140}{\text{Plasma sodium}}\right)$$

Although this formula is based on several assumptions, it is adequate for the initiation of treatment. It is important to realize that the formula does not take into account the ongoing urinary and nonurinary losses of fluid and electrolytes. Generally, replacement of the water deficit is accomplished by 50 percent normal saline or 5 percent dextrose as the plasma glucose level approaches 250 mg/dl. As the patient becomes more alert, water may be taken by mouth. It must be remembered that too rapid correction of the water deficit may result in water intoxication with cerebral edema. Moreover, extreme caution is advisable in those patients with a low plasma osmolality because removal of the osmotic effect of glucose by insulin therapy or use of hypotonic fluids may also cause water intoxication.

Although total body potassium losses are probably higher in HHNK than in DKA, the mean initial potassium level in HHNK is lower. Thus, potassium replacement, with the chloride or phosphate salt, is generally indicated in the initial treatment. Contraindications to early potassium administration include ECG evidence of hyperkalemia, known hyperkalemia, or oliguria. The latter is a relative contraindication, since hydration and insulin-influenced cellular uptake of potassium cause a rapid drop in the potassium level. Careful monitoring of the potassium levels is required, as ECG evidence of hyperkalemia is nonspecific.

Normalization of the Intermediary Metabolism

As with DKA, there has been a shift to the use of low-dose insulin therapy in the treatment of HHNK. The main goal of insulin therapy in DKA is to reverse the ketotic state; the goal in HHNK is to return carbohydrate metabolism to normal. Hyperglycemia in HHNK reflects three conditions: (1) underexcretion of glucose by the kidney, (2) hepatic overproduction of glucose, and (3) peripheral underutilization of glucose. Studies have shown that circulating insulin levels of approximately 200 μU/ml are sufficient to inhibit gluconeogenesis and to produce almost maximal glucose uptake by adipose tissue and muscle.[109] This concentration of insulin may be achieved by intramuscular or intravenous administration. Bendezo and associates have shown satisfactory results in the treatment of HHNK with an intravenous loading dose of 5 to 10 units regular insulin, followed by a continuous infusion of 7 to 12 units/hour.[110] It must be emphasized that, no matter how the insulin is given, it is only part of the total management of the patient with HHNK.

REFERENCES

1. Beigelman PM: Severe diabetic ketoacidosis (diabetic "coma"). *Diabetes* 20:490–500, 1971.
2. Soler NG, Fitzgerald MG, Bennett MA, et al: Intensive care in the management of diabetic ketoacidosis. *Lancet* 1:951–954, 1973.
3. Alberti KGMM: Diabetic ketoacidosis: Aspects of management, in Ledingham JGG (ed): *Tenth Advanced Medicine Symposium.* New York, Pitman Publishing Corp, 1974, pp 68–82.
4. Alberti KGMM: Low-dose insulin in the treatment of diabetic ketoacidosis. *Arch Intern Med* 137:1367–1376, 1977.
5. Felig P: Insulin: Rates and route of delivery. *N Engl J Med* 291:1031–1032, 1974.
6. Page M, Alberti KGMM, Greenwood R, et al: Treatment of diabetic coma with continuous low-dose infusion of insulin. *Br Med J* 2:687–690, 1974.
7. Semple PF, White C, Manderson WG: Continuous intravenous infusion of small doses of insulin in treatment of diabetic ketoacidosis. *Br Med J* 2:694–698, 1974.
8. Kedson W, Casey J, Kraegen E, et al: Treatment of severe diabetes mellitus by insulin infusion. *Br Med J* 2:691–694, 1974.
9. Felig P: Diabetic ketoacidosis. *N Engl J Med* 290:1360–1363, 1974.
10. Ditzel J: Importance of plasma in organic phosphate on tissue oxygenation during recovery from diabetic ketoacidosis. *Horm Metab Res* 5:471–472, 1973.
11. Zimmet PZ, Taft P, Ennis GC, et al: Acid production in diabetic acidosis: A more rational approach to alkali replacement. *Br Med J* 3:610–612, 1970.
12. Felig P: Combating diabetic ketoacidosis and other hyperglycemic ketoacidotic syndromes. *Postgrad Med* 50:150–153, 1976.
13. Felig P, Wahren J, Handler R: Influence of oral glucose ingestion on splanchnic glucose and gluconeogenic substrate metabolism. *Diabetes* 24:468–475, 1975.
14. Nahren J, Felig P, Cerasi E, et al: Splanchnic and peripheral glucose and amino acid metabolism in diabetes mellitus. *J Clin Invest* 51:1870–1879, 1972.
15. McGarry JD, Foster DW: Regulation of ketogenesis and clinical aspects of the ketotic state. *Metabolism* 21:471–489, 1972.
16. Munro JF, Campbell IW, McCuish AC, et al: Euglycaemic diabetic ketoacidosis. *Br Med J* 2:578–580, 1973.
17. Marliss EB, Ohman JL, Aoki TT, et al: Altered redox state obscuring ketoacidosis in diabetic patients with lactic acidosis. *N Engl J Med* 283:978–980, 1970.
18. Faerman I, Faccio E, Milei J, et al: Autonomic neuropathy and painless myocardial infarction in diabetic patients: Histologic evidence of their relationship. *Diabetes* 26:1147–1158, 1977.
19. Soler NG, Bennett MA, Peneost BL, et al: Myocardial infarction in diabetes. *Q J Med* 44:125–132, 1975.
20. Beardwood UT Jr: Abdominal symptomatology of diabetic acidosis. *JAMA* 105:1168–1172, 1935.
21. Knight AH, Williams DN, Ellis G: Significance of hyperamylasaemia and abdominal pain in diabetic ketoacidosis. *Br Med J* 3:128–131, 1973.
22. Levine RI, Glauder FI, Berk JE: Enhancement of the amylase-creatinine clearance ratio in disorders other than acute pancreatitis. *N Engl J Med* 292:329–332, 1975.

23. Fridhandler L, Berk JE, Veda M: Isolation and measurement of pancreatic amylase in human serum and urine. *Clin Chem* 18:1493–1497, 1972.
24. Campbell IW, Duncan LJ, Innes JA, et al: Abdominal pain in diabetic metabolic decompensation: Clinical significance. *JAMA* 233:166–168, 1975.
25. Page LB, Culver PG (eds): *A Syllabus of Laboratory Examinations in Clinical Diagnosis: Critical Evaluation of Laboratory Procedures in the Study of the Patient*, rev ed. Cambridge, MA, Harvard University Press, 1960.
26. Stephens JM, Sulway MJ, Watkins PJ: Relationship of blood acetoacetate and 3-hydroxybutyrate in diabetes. *Diabetes* 20:485–489, 1971.
27. Sulway MJ, Malins JM: Acetone in diabetic ketoacidosis. *Lancet* 2:736–740, 1970.
28. Katz MA: Hyperglycemia-induced hyponatremia—Calculation of expected serum sodium depression. *N Engl J Med* 289:818–844, 1973.
29. Krumlovsky FA: Hyponatremia. *Ration Drug Ther* 9:1–6, 1975.
30. Padova J, Bandersky G: Hyperuricemia in diabetic ketoacidosis. *N Engl J Med* 267:530–534, 1962.
31. Goldfinger S, Klinenberg JR, Seegmiller JE: Renal retention of uric acid induced by infusion of β-hydroxybutyrate and acetoacetate. *N Engl J Med* 272:351–355, 1965.
32. Watkins PJ: The effect of ketone bodies on the determination of creatinine. *Clin Chem Acta* 18:191–196, 1967.
33. Murray T, Long W, Narins RG: Multiple myeloma and the anion gap. *N Engl J Med* 292:574–575, 1975.
34. Kleeman CR, Liberman B: Diabetic acidosis and coma, in Rand MM, Kleeman CR (eds): *Clinical Disorders of Fluid and Electrolyte Metabolism*, ed 2. New York, McGraw Hill, 1972, pp 971–994.
35. Winegrad AI, Clements RS: Diabetic ketoacidosis. *Med Clin North Am* 55:899–911, 1971.
36. Martin HH, Smith K, Wilson ML: The fluid and electrolyte therapy of severe diabetic acidosis and ketosis. A study of twenty-nine episodes (twenty-six patients). *Am J Med* 24:376–389, 1958.
37. Nabarro JDH, Spencer AG, Stower JM: Metabolic studies in severe diabetic ketosis. *Q J Med* 21:225–248, 1952.
38. Burnell JH, Villamil MF, Vyeno TB, et al: The effect in humans of extracellular pH changes on the relationship between serum potassium concentration and intracellular potassium. *J Clin Invest* 35:935–939, 1956.
39. Seftel HC, Kew MC: Early and intensive potassium replacement in diabetic acidosis. *Diabetes* 15:694–696, 1966.
40. Beigelman PM, Martin HE, Miller LV, et al: Severe diabetic ketoacidosis. *JAMA* 219:1082–1086, 1969.
41. Clementsen HJ: Potassium therapy: A break with tradition. *Lancet* 2:175–177, 1962.
42. Beigelman PM: Potassium in severe diabetic ketoacidosis. *Am J Med* 54:419–429, 1973.
43. Hockaday TDR, Alberti KGMM: Diabetic coma. *Clin Endocrinol Metab* 1:751–788, 1972.
44. Roberts KE, Magida MG: Electrocardiographic alterations produced by a decrease/increase in plasma pH, bicarbonate and sodium as compared with those produced by an increase/decrease potassium. *Circ Res* 1:206–213, 214–218, 1953.
45. Butler AM: Metabolic studies in diabetic coma. *Trans Assoc Am Physicians* 60:102–109, 1947.
46. Nabarro JDN, Spencer AG, Stowers JM: Metabolic studies in severe ketosis. *Q J Med* 21:225–243, 1952.
47. O'Connor LR, Wheeler WS, Bethune JE: Effect of hypophosphatemia on myocardial performance in man. *N Engl J Med* 297:901–903, 1977.
48. Rorth M: Dependence of oxyhaemoglobin dissociation and introerythrocytic 2,3-DPG on acid-base status of blood: I. In vitro studies on reduced and oxygenated blood. *Adv Exp Med Biol* 6:57–64, 1970.
49. Rapaport S: The regulation of glycolysis in mammalian erythrocyte. *Essays Biochem* 4:69–103, 1968.
50. Travis SF: Metabolic alterations in the human erythrocyte produced by increases in glucose concentration: The role of the polyol pathway. *J Clin Invest* 50:2104–2112, 1971.
51. Bellingham AJ, Detter JC, Lenfant C: Regulatory mechanisms of haemoglobin oxygen affinity in acidosis and alkalosis. *J Clin Invest* 50:700–706, 1971.
52. Stankl E, Ditzel J: The effect of red cell 2,3-DPG changes induced by diabetic ketoacidosis on parameters of the oxygen dissociation curve. *Man Adv Exp Med Biol* 75:89–95, 1976.
53. Travis SF, Sugerman AJ, Ruberg RL, et al: Alterations of red cell glycolytic intermediates and oxygen transport as a consequence of hypophosphatemia in patients receiving intravenous hyperalimentation. *N Engl J Med* 285:763–768, 1971.
54. Guisad OR, Arieff AI: Neurologic manifestations of diabetic comas: Correlation with biochemical alterations in the brain. *Metabolism* 24:665–679, 1975.
55. Flock EV, Tyce GM, Owen CA Jr: Glucose metabolism in brains of diabetic rats. *Endocrinology* 85:428–437, 1969.
56. Fulop M, Tannebaum H, Dreyer N: Ketotic hyperosmolar coma. *Lancet* 2:635–639, 1973.
57. Reubi FC: Glomerular filtration rate, renal blood flow and blood viscosity during and after diabetic coma. *Circ Res* 1:410–413, 1953.
58. Ditzel J: Impaired oxygen release caused by alterations of metabolism in the erythrocytes in diabetes. *Lancet* 1:721–723, 1972.
59. Posner JB, Plum F: Spinal fluid pH and neurologic symptoms in systemic acidosis. *N Engl J Med* 277:605–613, 1967.
60. Droller H, Siluis SE, Paragas PB: Paresthesia, weakness, seizures, and hypophosphatemia in patients receiving hyperalimentation. *Gastroenterology* 62:513–520, 1972.
61. Bagdade JD, Rout RK, Bulger RJ: Impaired leucocyte function in patients with poorly controlled diabetes. *Diabetes* 23:9–15, 1974.
62. Molenaar DM, Palumbo PJ, Wilson WR, et al: Leucocyte chemotaxis in diabetic patients and their non-diabetic first degree relative. *Diabetes* 25 (suppl 2):880–883, 1976.
63. Bagdade, JD: Infection in diabetes—Predisposing factors. *Postgrad Med* 59:160–164, 1976.
64. Knochel JP: The pathophysiology and clinical characteristics of severe hypophosphatemia. *Arch Intern Med* 137:203–220, 1977.
65. Lichtman MA, Miller DR, Cohen J, et al: Reduced red cell glycolysis, 2,3-diphosphoglycerate and adenosine triphosphate concentration and increased hemoglobin oxygen affinity caused by hypophosphatemia. *Ann Intern Med* 74:562–568, 1971.
66. Wacker WEC, Vallee BL: Magnesium metabolism. *N Engl J Med* 259:431–438, 475–482, 1958.
67. Zierler KL, Rabiosowitz D: Effect of very small concentrations of insulin on forearm metabolism. Persistence of its action on potassium and free fatty acids without its effect on glucose. *J Clin Invest* 43:950–962, 1964.
68. Sherwin RS, Hendler RG, Felig PF: Effect of diabetes mellitus and insulin on the turnover and metabolic response to ketones in man. *Diabetes* 25:776–784, 1976.
69. Ohman JC, Marliss EB, Aoke TT, et al: The cerebral spinal fluid in diabetic ketoacidosis. *N Engl J Med* 284:283–290, 1971.
70. Albert MS, Dell RB, Winters RW: Quantitative displacement of acid-base equilibrium in metabolic acidosis. *Ann Intern Med* 66:312–322, 1967.
71. Watkins PJ, Smith JS, Fitzgerald MG, et al: Lactic acidosis in diabetes. *Br Med J* 1:744–747, 1969.

72. Alberti KGMM, Hockaday TDR: Blood lactate and pyruvic acids in diabetic coma. *Diabetes* 21:350, 1972.

73. Root HF: The use of insulin and abuse of glucose in the treatment of diabetic coma. *JAMA* 127:557–564, 1945.

74. Black AB, Malins JM: Diabetic ketosis: A comparison of results of orthodox and intensive methods of treatment based on 170 consecutive cases. *Lancet* 1:56–59, 1949.

75. Shaw CE, Hurwitz GE, Schmukler M: A clinical and laboratory study of insulin dosage in diabetic acidosis: Comparison with small and large doses. *Diabetes* 11:23–30, 1962.

76. Menzel R, Aande E, Jutze E: Treatment of diabetic coma with low-dose injections of insulin. *Endocrinologie* 67:230–239, 1976.

77. Hannan TJ, Stahers GM: Constant low-dose infusion in severe diabetes mellitus. *Med J Aust* 1:11–13, 1976.

78. Binder C: *Absorption of Injected Insulin.* Copenhagen, Ejnar Munksgaaris Forlag, 1969.

79. Alberti KGMM, Hockaday TDR, Turner RC: Small doses of intramuscular insulin in the treatment of diabetic "coma." *Lancet* 2:515–522, 1973.

80. Kitabchi AE, Ayyagari V, Guerra SMO, et al: The efficacy of low-dose versus conventional therapy of insulin for treatment of diabetic ketoacidosis. *Ann Intern Med* 84:633–638, 1976.

81. Moseley J: Diabetic crises in children treated with small doses of intramuscular insulin. *Br Med J* 1:59–61, 1975.

82. Genuth SM: Constant intravenous insulin infusion in diabetic ketoacidosis. *JAMA* 223:1348–1351, 1973.

83. Piters K, Goodman J, Bessman A: Treatment of diabetic ketoacidosis with continuous low-dose intravenous insulin. *Diabetes* 24:396, 1975.

84. Malleson PN: Diabetic ketosis in children treated by adding low-dose insulin to rehydrating fluid. *Arch Dis Child* 51:373–376, 1976.

85. Martin MM, Martin ALD: Continuous low-dose insulin infusion vs. conventional intermittent subcutaneous injections in the treatment of diabetic ketoacidosis in children. *Diabetes* 25:376, 1976.

86. Weisenfeld S, Poldolsky S, Goldsmith L, et al: Absorption of insulin to infusion bottles and tubing. *Diabetes* 17:766–771, 1968.

87. Peterson L, Caldwell J, Hoffman J: Insulin absorpance to polyvinylchloride surfaces with implications for constant infusion therapy. *Diabetes* 25:72–74, 1976.

88. Sonksen PH, Ellis JP, Lowy C, et al: A quantitative evaluation of the relative efficiency of gelatine and albumin in preventing insulin absorption to glass. *Diabetologia* 1:208–210, 1965.

89. Herer D, Molitch M, Sperling M: Low-dose continuous insulin therapy for diabetic ketoacidosis: Prospective comparison with "conventional" insulin therapy. *Arch Intern Med* 137:1377–1380, 1977.

90. Clumeck N, DeTruyer A, Naeije R, et al: Treatment of diabetic coma with small intravenous boluses. *Br Med J* 2:394–396, 1976.

91. Soler NG, Fitzgerald MG, Wright AD, et al: Comparative study of different insulin regimens in management of diabetic ketoacidosis. *Lancet* 2:1221–1224, 1975.

92. Feig PV, McCurdy DK: The hypertonic state. *N Engl J Med* 297:1444–1454, 1977.

93. Dreshfeld J: The Bradshawe lecture on diabetic coma. *Br Med J* 2:358–360, 1886.

94. Sament S, Swartz MB: Severe diabetic stupor without ketosis. *S Afr Med J* 31:893–894, 1957.

95. Tyler FH: Hyperosmolar coma. *Am J Med* 45:485–487, 1968.

96. McCurdy DK: Hyperosmolar hyperglycemic non-ketotic diabetic coma. *Med Clin North Am* 54:683–699, 1970.

97. Miller EC: Diabetic emergencies. *Am Fam Physician* 18:115–121, 1978.

98. Gerich JE, Martin MM, Recant L: Clinical and metabolic characteristics of hyperosmolar nonketotic coma. *Diabetes* 20:228–237, 1971.

99. Joffe BI, Krut LH, Goldberg RB, et al: Pathogenesis of non-ketotic hyperosmolar diabetic coma. *Lancet* 1:1069–1071, 1975.

100. Passmore R, Johnson RE: The modification of post-exercise ketosis by environmental temperature and water balance. *Q J Exp Physiol* 43:352–358, 1958.

101. Gerich J, Penhos JC, Recant L: Metabolic consequence of hyperosmolarity. *Clin Res* 18:87, 1970.

102. Kuzuya T, Samols E, Williams RH: Stimulation by hyperosmolarity of glucose metabolism in rat adipose tissue and diaphragm in vitro. *J Biol Chem* 240:2277–2283, 1965.

103. Arieff AI, Carroll HJ: Cerebral edema and depression of sensorium in non-ketotic hyperosmolar coma. *Diabetes* 23:525–531, 1974.

104. Clements RS, Vourganti B: Fatal diabetic ketoacidosis: Major causes and approaches to their prevention. *Diabetes Care* 1:314–325, 1978.

105. Arieff AI, Carroll HJ: Nonketotic hyperosmolar coma with hyperglycemia: Clinical features, pathophysiology, renal function, acid-base balance, plasma-cerebrospinal fluid equilibria and the effects of therapy in 37 cases. *Medicine* 51:73–94, 1972.

106. Sotos JF, Dodge PR, Meara P, et al: Studies in experimental hypertonicity: II. Hypertonicity of body fluids as a cause of acidosis. *Pediatrics* 30:180–193, 1962.

107. Loeb JN: The hyperosmolar state. *N Engl J Med* 290:1184–1187, 1974.

108. Brown RH, Rossini AA, Callaway W, et al: Caveation fluid replacement in hyperglycemic, hyperosmolar, non-ketotic coma. *Diabetes Care* 1:305–307, 1978.

109. Christensen NJ, Orskou J: The relationship between endogenous serum insulin concentration and glucose uptake in the forearm muscle of non-diabetics. *J Clin Invest* 47:1262–1266, 1968.

110. Bendezo R, Wieland RG, Furst BH: Experience with low-dose insulin infusion in diabetic ketoacidosis and diabetic hyperosmolarity. *Arch Intern Med* 138:60–62, 1978.

12. Thyroid Disorders

GERALD S. LEVEY, M.D.

THYROID STORM

Hyperthyroidism is a readily recognized and treatable endocrine disease that is commonly encountered in the clinical practice of medicine. The clinical syndrome known as thyroid storm or thyroid crisis is one of the most dramatic and feared manifestations of hyperthyroidism. Thyroid storm occurs in a small percentage of hyperthyroid patients and accounts for much of the mortality associated with hyperthyroidism. Only prompt institution of appropriate therapy can prevent the dreaded sequelae of this syndrome. A number of excellent reviews have been written on this subject.[1-4]

The pathogenesis of thyroid storm is poorly understood. Such a crisis may occur in patients of either sex and at any age, although it is unusual in children. Thyroid storm almost always occurs in patients with preexistent hyperthyroidism due to diffuse toxic goiter that has been either untreated or inadequately treated before the onset of storm. While the extent of clinical symptoms is variable, thyroid crisis develops abruptly and is best characterized as a state of unregulated hypermetabolism with fever and tachycardia. Examination of patients with thyroid storm reveals excess sympathetic (adrenergic) activity, as well as evidence of chronically increased levels of thyroid hormone. A number of studies have demonstrated the importance of the interactions of both thyroid hormones and catecholamines as they affect the cardiovascular system, adipose tissue, and the central nervous system.[5-7] It is important to understand the role of both β-adrenergic stimulation and thyroid hormone in thyroid storm in order to institute effective treatment.

Precipitating Factors

While the pathophysiology of thyroid crisis is poorly understood, the clinical settings in which it arises are well-known. In general, there are two classes of precipitating factors in thyroid storm: surgical and medical. Surgical treatment of hyperthyroidism in a patient who has not been rendered euthyroid with antithyroid drugs prior to the operation may induce thyroid storm postoperatively. Operative procedures that do not involve the thyroid but are performed in untreated or inadequately treated hyperthyroid patients may also result in thyroid storm. In this instance, anesthesia per se or the general stress of the procedure may be responsible for the induction of storm.

The medical factors that place patients at risk for thyroid crisis include infection, trauma, diabetic ketoacidosis, pulmonary embolism, toxemia of pregnancy or labor, premature discontinuance of antithyroid drug therapy, and, rarely, radiation thyroiditis secondary to radioactive iodine therapy of hyperthyroidism. The manner in which these physiologic stresses induce thyroid storm is totally unclear. A variety of measurements, including measurements of serum thyroxine (T_4), serum tri-iodothyronine (T_3), and serum catecholamines, reveal no differences between patients with thyroid storm and those with uncomplicated hyperthyroidism.

Clinical Signs and Symptoms

Frequently thought to represent an exaggerated or decompensated state of ordinary hyperthyroidism, the signs and symptoms of thyroid storm are in some respects similar to those of uncomplicated thyrotoxicosis. The usual signs of hyperthyroidism include goiter; tachycardia; widened pulse pressure; warm, fine, moist skin; tremor; eye signs, e.g., lid lag, exophthalmos, ocular muscle palsies, and chemosis; and atrial fibrillation. The more frequent symptoms include nervousness, increased sweating, hypersensitivity to heat, palpitations, fatigue, weight loss, tachycardia, dyspnea, weakness, increased appetite, and frequent bowel movements.

Thyroid storm is characterized by more florid signs of thyrotoxicosis. The additional signs and symptoms include fever, which many consider to be the sine qua non for the diagnosis. The following may also be seen:

- extreme tachycardia
- restlessness, agitation
- emotional lability
- confusion
- psychosis
- diarrhea and vomiting
- jaundice
- hypotension
- coma

The patient may experience cardiovascular collapse and shock. The heart rate is usually increased out of proportion to the extent of the fever. Although the tachycardia is generally sinus in nature, it may be ectopic in origin, most commonly atrial fibrillation; rarely, heart block may be found, and the patient may be in congestive heart failure because of markedly hypertrophied heart muscle and the severity of the tachycardia. These patients are generally profusely diaphoretic; together with severe diarrhea and vomiting, this may produce marked electrolyte disturbances.

Diagnosis

The diagnosis of thyroid storm must be made promptly and is predicated on a careful clinical history and physical examination. Determination of serum T_4 and T_3 levels, and a measure of thyroxine binding globulin (T_3 resin uptake) are appropriate initial tests, but the results will not be known before therapy is initiated. If possible, a two-hour radioactive iodine (^{131}I) uptake is useful.

Laboratory tests are useful only in establishing the diagnosis of hyperthyroidism, since there is no specific laboratory test that indicates the presence of thyroid storm. The diagnosis of thyroid storm is considered more frequently than it is actually encountered. Patients with hyperthyroidism and intercurrent infections are particularly difficult to distinguish from patients with thyroid storm because both conditions are associated with fever, tachycardia, and diaphoresis. The treatment under these circumstances is the same, however.

Treatment

When thyroid storm is suspected, therapy should be initiated promptly. It is directed at decreasing the synthesis and release of thyroid hormones, blocking the increased adrenergic activity, treating congestive heart failure and electrolyte abnormalities, and reducing fever. The following treatment schedule is recommended:

1. propylthiouracil, 900 to 1200 mg/day by mouth or by gastric tube in three or four divided doses. Methimazole, 90 to 120 mg/day, may be used instead of propylthiouracil.
2. iodine, 30 drops potassium iodine daily by mouth in three or four divided doses or 1 or 2 gm sodium iodide/day by intravenous drip.
3. propranolol, 160 mg/day by mouth in four divided doses or 1 or 2 mg slowly intravenously every four hours under careful monitoring.
4. intravenous glucose solutions.
5. correction of dehydration and electrolyte imbalance.
6. cooling blanket for hyperthermia.
7. digitalis, if clinically indicated.
8. diagnosis and treatment of any underlying precipitating diseases (i.e., infection, diabetic ketoacidosis, or pulmonary embolism).
9. glucocorticoids, e.g., hydrocortisone, 100 to 300 mg/day intravenously or intramuscularly.
10. definitive therapy after control of the crisis, which consists of ablation of the thyroid gland with ^{131}I or surgical removal (subtotal thyroidectomy).

If an intercurrent illness is present, it must also be promptly treated.

Iodine

A critical therapeutic intervention involves iodine. In pharmacologic doses, it inhibits the release of T_3 and T_4 from the thyroid within a few hours of administration. Iodine also inhibits the organification of iodine, a transitory effect that lasts from a few days to a week. It is administered orally as Lugol's solution, 30 drops/

day in three or four divided doses, or is given as sodium iodide, 0.5 to 1 gm in 1 liter normal saline every 12 hours. If possible, antithyroid drugs should be administered prior to the initiation of iodine therapy in order to prevent any further incorporation of iodine into thyroid hormone. In practice, however, this is rarely possible in the treatment of thyroid storm.

Propylthiouracil and Methimazole (Tapazole)

The standard agents for the treatment of hyperthyroidism are propylthiouracil and methimazole. They decrease organification and impair the coupling of mono-iodotyrosines and di-iodotyrosines to T_4 and T_3. In addition, large doses of propylthiouracil (in excess of 800 mg/day) block the peripheral conversion of T_4 to T_3 in the liver. Therefore, propylthiouracil should be administered in amounts of 900 to 1200 mg/day. It may be given by mouth, or the tablets may be crushed and administered by nasogastric tube; parenteral preparations are not available. It requires about 24 hours of propylthiouracil therapy to decrease serum T_3 levels significantly; it is approximately five to seven days before serum T_4 levels decline. If methimazole is used, the doses are one-tenth those of propylthiouracil. Methimazole does not block the peripheral conversion of T_4 to T_3, however.

β-Adrenergic Blocking Drugs

Many of the signs and symptoms of hyperthyroidism are secondary to increased adrenergic activity. In the past several years, β-adrenergic blocking agents, notably propranolol, have replaced reserpine and guanethidine in the adjunctive treatment of hyperthyroidism. Thyroid storm is one of the major indications for propranolol, since it produces a very rapid decrease in heart rate (within two to three hours when given orally, in minutes when given intravenously). Propranolol occasionally results in rapid defervescence in thyroid storm. The drug is administered orally in a dosage of 40 to 160 mg daily in four divided doses. If given parenterally, patients should be titrated with 1 to 2 mg intravenously, which may be repeated every 4 hours, not exceeding 6 mg in 24 hours.

Propranolol and other β-adrenergic blocking agents are usually contraindicated in

- patients with chronic lung disease, such as asthma, emphysema, and bronchospasm
- patients with second-degree or greater heart block
- hyperthyroid patients with congestive heart failure
- patients with peripheral vascular disease
- diabetics receiving insulin or oral hypoglycemic agents
- patients receiving monoamine oxidase inhibitors
- pregnant women

The presence of any of these conditions should be considered in a plan of therapy. Heart failure is frequently related to the tachycardia. After congestive heart failure has been adequately treated with digitalis, the hyperthyroid patient may be cautiously titrated with propranolol under appropriate conditions of cardiac monitoring.

Plasmapheresis

Patients with thyroid storm sometimes fail to respond to the usual medical measures. Under these circumstances, plasmapheresis has been shown to be a useful adjunct to therapy.[8] The removal of large amounts of protein-bound thyroid hormone abruptly lowers the circulating T_4 and T_3. This measure is generally not used unless the patient's condition is deteriorating under medical management.

Other Measures

Dehydration and hyponatremia due to the fluid and electrolyte losses secondary to diaphoresis, vomiting, and diarrhea must be corrected. Glucose must be administered to prevent or correct hypoglycemia. A cooling blanket and, occasionally, ice packs may be required for the treatment of the underlying cause of the thyroid storm, such as intercurrent infection. It has been traditional to administer "stress" doses of adrenal steroids to patients with thyroid storm. Although a convincing rationale for such therapy has not been established, 300 to 400 mg hydrocortisone or its equivalent is generally given by continuous infusion each day.

Prognosis

The mortality of thyroid storm has been estimated at approximately 20 percent. The statistics are difficult to establish, however, since the incidence of thyroid storm is so low. It should also be noted that the mortality statistics that have been provided were calculated before the advent of β-adrenergic blocking drugs, such as propranolol, and before the development of plasmapheresis. These advances will probably lessen the mortality to some degree. Successful medical therapy generally produces improvement within 24 hours, and recovery occurs within a few days to a week. When the patient has recovered and is euthyroid, definitive therapy should be instituted either by ablation of the thyroid gland with ^{131}I or subtotal resection of the thyroid gland.

MYXEDEMA COMA

The end stage of improperly treated, neglected, or undiagnosed primary hypothyroidism is myxedema coma. This is a major medical emergency that requires prompt and effective treatment.[9,10] The underlying cause of the thyroid gland failure may be idiopathic, or it may be associated with autoimmune (Hashimoto's) thyroiditis, therapy (^{131}I) for hyperthyroidism or thyroid cancer, or thyroidectomy.

Precipitating Factors

There are a number of factors that predispose the hypothyroid patient to myxedema coma: exposure to cold, infection, trauma, and administration of central nervous system depressants, such as morphine, barbiturates, or general anesthesia. Coma is more common in elderly people with advanced coronary and systemic arteriosclerosis.

Clinical Signs

Patients with myxedema coma have many of the signs noted in uncomplicated hypothyroidism, i.e., dry skin, puffy appearance, coarse hair, cool skin, slow return of reflexes, carotenemia, periorbital swelling, facial puffiness, glossomegaly, and nonpitting edema. Myxedema coma is characterized by additional signs:

- hypothermia
- hypotension
- marked bradycardia
- hypoventilation with respiratory acidosis and carbon dioxide narcosis
- a variety of fluid and electrolyte abnormalities, such as decreased serum sodium level, increased serum lactate level, and inappropriate secretion of antidiuretic hormone
- hypoglycemia
- ileus

Hypothermia is considered by many to be the sine qua non for the diagnosis.

Diagnosis

The diagnosis of myxedema coma is based on the clinical picture; it requires a high index of suspicion and a careful history and physical examination. Uncomplicated hypothyroidism can be diagnosed by measuring the levels of serum T_4 and T_3, which are markedly decreased, and of serum thyroid-stimulating hormone (TSH), which is markedly elevated. These tests require

too much time to aid in the early management of myxedema coma, however. Thus, when this life-threatening medical emergency is seriously considered a possibility, therapy is initiated. Treatment can be altered later, depending on the results of the serum T_4, serum T_3, and serum TSH measurements. Serum levels of cortisol should also be determined, since these patients may have associated autoimmune adrenal failure.

Treatment

The patient's general medical condition, especially cardiovascular and pulmonary status, must be evaluated promptly and thyroid hormone replaced quickly by the intravenous administration of 500 µg L-thyroxine as a single loading dose, followed by 50 µg L-thyroxine on a daily basis intravenously. The large loading dose is necessary to saturate the unoccupied thyroid hormone binding sites on thyroxine. Intravenous therapy is required in this life-threatening situation because thyroid hormone is incompletely absorbed after oral administration. L-tri-iodothyronine is occasionally used because of its more rapid onset of action. However, commercial preparations of parenteral-tri-iodothyronine are not available, and the drug must be prepared fresh by the pharmacy immediately before use.

Adrenal corticosteroids are routinely administered to patients in myxedema coma; 100 mg hydrocortisone or its equivalent is administered intravenously by direct push, and a total of 300 to 400 mg hydrocortisone is administered in normal saline over the first 24 hours. Corticosteroids, 100 to 300 mg/day, should be continued until the result of the initial plasma cortisol determination is reported and adrenal status established. It is particularly important to administer corticosteroids if there is any suspicion of either adrenal cortical failure or pituitary insufficiency. Carbon dioxide narcosis must be treated promptly with mechanical ventilation, and any airway obstruction must be promptly relieved. Blood gases are monitored frequently. It should be emphasized that patients with hypothyroidism, particularly those in myxedema coma, metabolize drugs very slowly; therefore, narcotics and sedative drugs must be avoided entirely and the dosage of other drugs appropriately reduced. Hypoglycemia must be relieved by the intravenous administration of glucose. Electrolyte and water balance must be carefully monitored to prevent water intoxication, because patients with myxedema coma tend to retain water. Pressor amines may be administered cautiously to treat shock, although the effectiveness of pressor agents may be impaired until thyroid hormone is adequately replaced. Hypothermia is best treated by a covering blanket; the patient should not be actively warmed because of the risk of arrhythmias and peripheral vascular collapse. Other illnesses, such as intercurrent infections, that may have precipitated the myxedema coma must be diagnosed and treated vigorously and promptly.

Prognosis

The mortality rate for patients with inadequately treated myxedema coma is approximately 80 percent. Promptly treated myxedema is associated with a mortality rate of approximately 30 percent, one of the highest mortality rates of any medical emergency. Management must be prompt and effective, and all the physician's skills are required. Following recovery, the patient requires life-long treatment with thyroid hormone.

REFERENCES

1. Rosenberg IN: Thyroid storm. *N Engl J Med* 283:1052–1053, 1970.
2. Mackin JF, Canary JJ, Pittman CS: Thyroid storm and its management. *N Engl J Med* 291:1396–1398, 1974.
3. Ingbar SI: Thyroid storm in the thyroid, in Werner SC, Ingbar SH (eds): *The Thyroid*. Hagerstown, Md, Harper & Row, 1978, pp 800–804.
4. Levey GS: Beta adrenergic blocking drugs in the treatment of hyperthyroidism. *Hospital Formulary* 14:45–54, 1979.
5. Levey GS: Catecholamine sensitivity, thyroid hormone, and the heart. *Am J Med* 50:413–420, 1971.
6. Landsberg L: Catecholamines and hyperthyroidism. *Clin Endocrinol Metab* 3:697–718, 1977.
7. Levey GS: The heart and hyperthyroidism. *Med Clin North Am* 59:1193–1202, 1975.
8. Ashkar F, Katims RB, Smoak WM III, Gilson AJ: Thyroid storm treatment with blood exchange and plasmapheresis. *JAMA* 214:1275–1279, 1970.
9. Green WL: Guidelines for the treatment of myxedema. *Med Clin North Am* 52:431–450, 1968.
10. Werner SC: Myxedema coma, in Werner SC, Ingbar SH (eds): *The Thyroid*. Hagerstown, Md, Harper & Row, 1978, pp 971–973.

13. Adrenal Insufficiency

GEORGE L. HIGGINS III, M.D.

Adrenal insufficiency, in both its chronic and acute forms, often manifests itself in ways that bring the patient to the attention of the emergency medicine physician. Such manifestations range from subtle neuropsychiatric complaints to life-threatening complications. Unfortunately, in the busy and hectic atmosphere that exists in many of today's emergency departments, it is difficult at times to follow the superb example of clinical diagnosis set by Thomas Addison when he first described this disorder more than a century ago.[1] The responsibility, then, of the emergency medicine physician is to search for those clues in the history, physical examination, and laboratory data that allow the physician first to recognize and then to initiate therapy for this gratifyingly treatable disease.

ETIOLOGY

Autoimmune States

Autoimmune destruction of the adrenal glands is emerging as one of the more common causes of gland failure.[2] This recognition has come as developing technology has allowed identification of specific antibodies to specific adrenal gland antigens.[3] The glandular morphology reveals mononuclear inflammation, fibrosis, and atrophy. Numerous other disease entities that are presumed to have an autoimmune pathogenesis have been associated with this type of hypoadrenalism, e.g., chronic lymphocytic (Hashimoto's) thyroiditis,[4–6] silent thyrotoxic thyroiditis,[7] Graves' disease,[8] diabetes mellitus,[9–11] hypogonadism,[12–14] pernicious anemia,[15,16] vitiligo,[17] and hypoparathyroidism.[18,19] It is not uncommon for several of these disorders to develop sequentially in the same patient. Therefore, the presence of one of them should raise the possibility of the occult existence of another. Many of the previously so-called idiopathic forms of hypoadrenalism probably have an autoimmune basis.

Exogenous Steroid Administration

The frequent use of exogenous steroids in the treatment of various disorders and diseases has brought secondary adrenal insufficiency into prominence. In contrast to the primary type, secondary hypoadrenalism is not associated with hyperpigmentation, aldosterone deficiency,[20] or overproduction of cortisol precursors. Furthermore, the adrenal gland retains the capacity to respond to prolonged treatment with exogenous adrenocorticotropic hormone (ACTH). Most important, secondary hypoadrenalism is potentially a completely reversible disorder, although full recovery of adrenal responsiveness may take nine months or more. Prolonged administration of exogenous steroids is usually required for significant pituitary-adrenal suppression,[21,22] but short-term, high-dose steroid therapy can occasionally suppress adrenal function for a week or more.[23] Dexamethasone appears to have the most potent suppressive effect on ACTH secretion in humans.[24] Even very cautious steroid withdrawal not only can result in adrenal hypofunction but also may exacerbate the underlying disorder being treated.[25] In addition, maintenance doses of steroid occasionally become inadequate when stress is superimposed. It is important, then, to establish the possibility of exogenous steroid ingestion in the medical history.

It should be remembered, however, that the source of exogenous steroid may not always be obvious. Adrenocortical suppression has been found in workers who produce synthetic glucocorticoids, and it is recommended that these workers be screened periodically for adrenal responsiveness.[26] Topical corticosteroids used in the treatment of dermatologic disorders, such as psoriasis, have led to adrenal insufficiency,[27,28] as have inhaled steroids.[29–31] Switching from oral steroid to inhaled steroid therapy in the asthmatic patient may result in adrenal failure.[32] Maternal steroid therapy has caused adrenal gland suppression in the neonate.[33,34] Finally, to complicate matters further, there seems to be a true psychologic addiction to steroids. Withdrawing some patients from the drug leads to subjective signs and symptoms of adrenal insufficiency, although biochemically the hypothalamic-pituitary-adrenal axis remains intact and responsive.[35]

Sepsis

Fulminant bacterial infections can lead to or be complicated by absolute or relative hypoadrenalism. Like many other physiologically stressful situations, systemic bacterial infections are usually associated with elevated plasma cortisol levels.[36–39] Not only is adrenal hormonal secretion accelerated with septic stress, but supplemental ACTH administration during systemic infections can lead to additional hormonal production.

Careful prospective analysis of adrenal response to severe infections has revealed several patterns.[38–40] The highest baseline cortisol levels are usually seen in the most critically ill patients, many of whom succumb to their illness. A larger group of patients demonstrate higher than normal baseline levels and respond to synthetic ACTH administration with increased adrenocortical secretion. However, a significant minority of patients with severe infection have lower than expected baseline cortisol levels and fail to exhibit an appropriate increase in plasma cortisol levels following exogenous ACTH stimulation. Necropsy examination of the adrenal glands in such patients may reveal only cellular hyperplasia without hemorrhage or necrosis.

In the classic syndrome of fulminant meningococcemia, adrenal crisis has been well recognized; autopsy frequently reveals evidence of bilateral adrenal hemorrhage (the Waterhouse-Friderichsen syndrome).[41] The etiology of this hemorrhage has not yet been fully defined, but it has been ascribed to endotoxin-producing

thromboplastic activity as well as direct endothelial damage by the meningococi with subsequent thrombosis by the meningococci. Another postulated cause is that severe stress leads to rapid depletion of lipid hormone from the adrenal cells, causing tubular degeneration and, thus, predisposing the gland to hemorrhage.[42–44] In such cases, early steroid replacement can be life-saving.[45]

Hemorrhage

Adrenal gland hemorrhage can rapidly lead to adrenal crisis. Adrenal apoplexy, or idiopathic hemorrhagic infarction, is an uncommon but life-threatening development.[46–48] Hemorrhage is usually associated with physiologic stress caused by sepsis, burns, surgery, or trauma.[49] Since it has been demonstrated that marked adrenal stimulation can lead to tubular degeneration and necrosis, as well as increased vascularity, it has been hypothesized that such stress predisposes the adrenal gland to hemorrhagic events.[50] Flank or abdominal pain, a dropping hematocrit, and developing shock may be the initial manifestations of this syndrome. The presumptive diagnosis may be renal colic or a ruptured abdominal aortic aneurysm. Hemorrhage may be confined to the gland itself or the periadrenal tissues, but it can be massive. Signs and symptoms of adrenal insufficiency may be present. Radiographic procedures, including abdominal computerized axial tomography (CT) scanning, ultrasound, and angiography, are helpful in localizing the site of hemorrhage and ruling out an aneurysm. Once the diagnosis is established, immediate surgical intervention is indicated.

Anticoagulant-induced adrenal hemorrhage is a well-documented event. A review of over 4,000 autopsies revealed 30 cases of adrenal hemorrhage, 10 of which occurred in patients receiving anticoagulants in the treatment of thromboembolism or acute myocardial infarction.[51] In contrast to the fulminant course of adrenal hemorrhage associated with the Waterhouse-Friderichsen syndrome, which usually occurs in younger patients, anticoagulant-associated adrenal hemorrhage more often involves older patients (50 to 70 years of age). The primary medical disorders in these older patients tend to mask the signs and symptoms of hypoadrenalism, thus hindering diagnosis. Both heparin and coumarin compounds may be responsible for adrenal hemorrhage. Coagulation parameters are not always excessively prolonged, and there may be no evidence of generalized bleeding in these patients. Development of flank or abdominal pain, hypotension refractory to fluid management, anorexia, vomiting, mental status changes, and fever in patients on anticoagulation therapy should suggest adrenal hemorrhage.[52] Aggressive medical intervention, including corticosteroid replacement, can be life-saving.[53–55]

Anticoagulant-associated adrenal hemorrhage is often bilateral, but it may be unilateral. As it does in spontaneous adrenal hemorrhage, stress appears to play a role in this form. In the experimental animal, the administration of ACTH with anticoagulants increases the incidence of hemorrhagic complications significantly,[56] while hypophysectomized animals subjected to stress do not develop hemorrhages.

Neoplastic Disorders

Spontaneous and massive hemorrhage from intrinsic adrenal tumors, such as pheochromocytomas, can lead to adrenal insufficiency.[46] Less well understood is the role played in this syndrome by disease that has metastasized to the adrenal gland. Since the time of Addison, symptoms of terminal metastatic carcinomatosis have occasionally been attributed to adrenal gland replacement with tumor. Empiric treatment of weakness, fatigue, fever, anorexia, and orthostatic reactions with exogenous steroids in the terminally ill cancer patient has led to varying degrees of improvement. Response to this treatment obviously does not imply hypoadrenalism. Indeed, many cancer patients with symptoms resembling those of adrenal insufficiency are found to have elevated plasma cortisol levels and normal pituitary and adrenal glands at the time of autopsy.[57,58] Although some tumors demonstrate corticotropic activity with resultant hypercortisolemia, the stress of terminal carcinomatosis itself appears to be sufficient stimulation for elevated adrenal output.[57,59] Clinical response to administered steroids, then, may be independent of adrenal function, resulting instead from their nonspecific euphoretic effect or anti-inflammatory action. Even when disease that has metastasized to the adrenal glands (usually from lung or breast) leaves less than 20 percent of apparently normal tissue, adequate adrenal function and reserve remains.[60] It appears that, although adrenal insufficiency from metastatic disease does indeed occur and may even be the initial manifestation of malignancy,[61] it is a relatively uncommon event.

Surgical Procedures

Adrenal hemorrhage and necrosis may occur during certain abdominal operations that, because of anatomical proximity, result in direct trauma to the gland itself or embarrassment of its blood supply.[62] Operations of the stomach, lower esophagus, spleen, and kidneys appear to be especially prone to produce this complication.[63] In addition to disruption of the arterial supply of the gland, thrombosis or rupture of capsular and intra-adrenal veins can result in hemorrhage and necrosis. Destruction of one adrenal gland during or soon after the severe stress of a major operation may result in acute adrenal insufficiency.

Surgical procedures in areas of the body anatomically remote from the adrenal glands in patients without predisposing factors can also be complicated by postoperative adrenal hypofunction.[64–67] Hyperpigmentation is usually absent. Hypoglycemia, electrolyte abnormalities, and vomiting may be controlled by aggressive routine postoperative care; other manifestations of adrenal insufficiency, such as anorexia, abdominal pain, fever, and confusion, may be attributed to the stress of the operation. Recognition of adrenal insufficiency in these patients depends on a high index of suspicion when the postoperative course is complicated by bizarre, confusing, and apparently inappropriate symptoms. When the diagnosis is entertained, the pretreatment serum cortisol level should be determined and a therapeutic trial of steroid replacement promptly initiated to prevent death.

Granulomatous Disease

In Addison's time, granulomatous destruction of the gland by tuberculosis was the predominant cause of adrenal insufficiency. Over 70 percent of Addison's disease could be ascribed to tuberculosis in the early part of this century. The introduction of antitubercular chemotherapy and skin test screening programs has permitted earlier recognition and effective treatment of tuberculosis, dramatically reducing the incidence of adrenal insufficiency caused by this disease. A Danish study that reviewed 108 cases of Addison's disease identified tuberculosis as the primary cause in only 17 percent of the patients in the series.[68]

Tuberculous adrenal gland destruction in all age groups continues to be reported in the United States.[69–71] Often, active tuberculosis is also apparent in other organs, suggesting hematogenous spread. As might be expected, the symptoms and signs of adrenal insufficiency mimic those of active tuberculosis, making diagnosis difficult.[72] The combination of a suggestive chest roentgenogram, a positive tuberculin skin test result, adrenal gland calcifications (occurring in 5 to 10 percent of cases), and no serologic evidence of autoimmune adrenal gland destruction should cause the physician to suspect tuberculous involvement of the adrenal glands.[73]

There are other, less common causes of granulomatous adrenal gland destruction. Histoplasmosis is a recognized cause of adrenal insufficiency in the Ohio and Tennessee River valleys.[74,75] Disseminated North American blastomycosis frequently involves the adrenal gland and, rarely, can lead to adrenal crisis, suggesting that patients so infected should be screened for adrenal dysfunction.[76,77] Cryptococcosis and coccidioidomycosis have also been implicated in the etiology of adrenal insufficiency. Rarely, paracoccidioidomycosis (South American blastomycosis) can result in hypoadrenalism.[78]

Congenital Idiopathic Adrenal Hypoplasia

A relatively uncommon condition that affects newborns,[79] congenital idiopathic adrenal hypoplasia may not become manifest for several months.[80] There are both sporadic and familial cases,[81] and recessive and sex-linked inheritance occurs.[82–84] The association of anencephaly and adrenal insufficiency was noted as early as 1723 by Morgagni.

Secondary forms of adrenal hypoplasia in the very young have been ascribed to maternal Cushing's syndrome,[85] congenital adrenal cysts,[86] adrenal hemorrhage,[87,88] and steroid therapy during pregnancy.[33,34] The idiopathic type, however, is often associated with maternal pre-eclampsia, very low maternal estriol excretion[79,89] (the fetal adrenals produce the major portion of maternal urinary estriol precursors), and postterm pregnancy. The fetus is alive and radiographically normal. The living neonate may exhibit a salt-losing syndrome with dehydration, hyponatremia, hyperkalemia, acidosis, hypoglycemia, poor eating, failure to thrive, fever, vomiting, diarrhea, vascular collapse, and sudden infant death syndrome.[90] Autopsy findings include a normal pituitary and brain, no evidence of adrenal destruction, and diminished adrenal mass.[91] The mortality rate is high in these infants.

Other Causes

Adrenal insufficiency has been associated with systemic lupus erythematosus,[92] oral contraceptives,[93] bilateral adrenal venography,[94] hypopituitarism,[73,95] ACTH-releasing factor deficiency,[96] and isolated ACTH deficiency.[97]

Adrenomyeloneuropathy and adrenoleukodystrophy are rare, recessive sex-linked disorders that can lead to adrenal insufficiency, as well as to central and peripheral neurologic dysfunction (e.g., mental deterioration, sphincter disorders, objective sensory deficits, and spastic paraparesis). The neurologic deficits usually precede the endocrine manifestations. Long-chain cholesterol esters accumulate as cytoplasmic inclusions in brain, adrenal, and testes.[98–101]

SYMPTOMATOLOGY

Cutaneous

The diffuse hyperpigmentation of primary adrenal insufficiency, first described by Addison, is common (92 percent in patients[68]) and results from melanocyte stimulation by elevated levels of β-lipoprotein. ACTH is a weak melanocyte stimulant,[102] but some patients have a level high enough to produce hyperpigmentation. Diffuse hypermelanosis is by no means unique to primary hypoadrenalism, however; it can be found in association with endocrine and nonendocrine tumors, folate deficiency, cirrhosis, hemochromatosis, pernicious anemia, starvation, and many other disorders.[103] The hyperpigmentation of adrenal insufficiency has a predilection for extensor surfaces, pressure areas, palmar creases, scars from injuries that occurred after the onset of the adrenal disorder, mucous membranes, tongue, gingival margins, breast areola, scrotum, perineum, and the perivaginal and perianal areas.[73] Longitudinal banded pigmentation of fingernails has also been described.[104] An increased ability to tan or a longer lasting tan should raise the possibility of hypoadrenalism.[105] It must be remembered, however, that Addison's disease may exist without hyperpigmentation.[106,107]

An interesting case of Addison's disease associated with excessively salty sweat and ichthyosis has been reported.[108] Steroid replacement brought a dramatic decrease in the sodium and chloride, as well as an increase in the potassium content of the patient's sweat.

Vitiligo, yet another manifestation of autoimmune polyendocrine deficiency, has been associated with autoimmune primary adrenal insufficiency.[17] Cutaneous candidiasis appears to be more common in adrenal insufficient patients,[109] and abnormal calcification of the auricular and costochondral cartilages has been documented.[110]

Cardiovascular

Hypotension occurs in 88 percent of patients; postural dizziness, in 12 percent.[68] These findings reflect decreased intravascular volume, as well as diminished inotropy and cardiac output. Syncope may bring the patient to the physician's attention. Patients with severe adrenal insufficiency not uncommonly develop terminal vascular collapse and shock. The radiographic appearance of a small heart on chest roentgenogram should raise the possibility of hypoadrenalism.[111] Heart size in untreated, uncomplicated cases of Addison's disease is consistently reduced below normal, probably reflecting the cachectic and hypovolemic states of some of these patients. Steroid administration increases cardiac dimensions. Excessive therapy may lead to cardiomegaly.

Gastrointestinal

Gastrointestinal symptoms occur in 56 percent of patients.[68] Anorexia, weight loss, nausea, and vomiting are nearly universal.[112] Chronic diarrhea is not uncommon. Abdominal pain, at times severe, can result in "pseudoperitonitis" with signs of intra-abdominal catastrophe and may lead to unfruitful exploratory laparotomies.[113] Nearly all acute abdominal entities, including cholecystitis, pancreatitis, leaking abdominal aneurysm, ischemic or infarcted bowel, retroperitoneal hemorrhage, nephrolithiasis, perforated viscus, and cecal volvulus have been confused with acute adrenal crisis.[66] The exact mechanism of this pain syndrome has not been defined, but improvement with exogenous steroid therapy can be dramatic.

There is a decreased incidence of peptic ulcer disease in patients with adrenal insufficiency, possibly because of diminished gastric acid production.[114]

Neurologic

In addition to the full spectrum of mental status changes that manifest themselves during inadequate adrenal function (e.g., confusion, acute psychosis,[115] delirium, and coma), more unusual neurologic disorders have been observed. Adrenal insufficiency has been associated with the polyradiculoneuropathy of Guillain-Barré, with both disorders responding to steroid administration.[116] Morphological changes in the adrenal glands, including necrotizing inflammation and inclusion bodies, have been found at autopsy.[117,118]

The abrupt onset of "Addisonian encephalopathy" can be dramatic and confusing[119,120] and must be differentiated from other causes of metabolic encephalopathies. As noted previously, adrenoleukodystrophy and adrenomyeloneuropathy are rare disorders that can lead to adrenal hypofunction and rapidly progressive neurologic deterioration.

Miscellaneous

Adrenal deficiency may be associated with tachyarrhythmia;[121] delayed development of pubic hair;[122] chronic low back pain;[123] flexion contractures,[124] diffuse myalgias, and arthralgias;[125] more acute senses of taste, smell, and hearing;[126–128] and salt craving (in 15 to 20 percent of patients). One interesting case report involves a woman with undiagnosed adrenal insufficiency who noted that licorice ingestion abolished her lassitude, presumably owing to its mineralocorticoid effect.[129] The recent onset of asthma in a patient with weight loss or other constitutional signs should suggest hypoadrenalism.[130,131]

Laboratory Findings

Hyponatremia is common in adrenal insufficiency, occurring in 88 percent of patients in one study.[68] The degree of sodium depletion may at times be life-threatening. The etiology of this complication appears to be failure of aldosterone-directed renal sodium conservation, as well as poor handling of water loads.

Hyperkalemia, which occurs in 64 percent of patients, may become severe enough to produce cardiac arrhythmias and periodic paralysis.[132,133] Patients are also prone to potassium intoxication when given exogenous potassium. Both mineralocorticoid and glucocorticoid deficiencies play a role in the development of hyperkalemia. (See Chapter 15.)

Hypercalcemia, occurring in 6 percent of patients, can be treated successfully with corticosteroid administration. Hypercalcemic crisis has been reported as the initial manifestation of Addison's disease.[134,135] (See Chapter 17.)

Hypoglycemia, probably resulting from defective gluconeogenesis and lipolysis, is not uncommon[112] and is unmasked by fasting or excessive exercise. Patients with symptomatic hypoglycemia that has no obvious cause should be screened for adrenal insufficiency. It should be remembered that patients receiving insulin may develop insulin sensitivity as hypoadrenalism develops.

Decreased glomerular filtration rates can lead to elevated serum creatinine and blood urea nitrogen (BUN) determinations.

The findings or presence of eosinophilia should be investigated, although it is not invariably present. The eosinopenic effect of steroid administration can be explained by intravenous shift of eosinophils, as well as migration into tissues and diminished bone marrow production of these cells.[136]

Adrenal insufficiency can only be unequivocally diagnosed by biochemically demonstrating an absolute or relative adrenal hormone deficiency with abolished adrenal reserve. The combination of a low plasma cortisol level and an elevated plasma ACTH level confirms the diagnosis of primary adrenal deficiency. However, any of the previously described signs and symptoms may be missing in the patient with hypoadrenalism, and isolated serum and urinary steroid determinations may be in the normal range. It is not unusual, therefore, to establish the diagnosis by screening for adrenal gland unresponsiveness to exogenous ACTH or synthetic ACTH. A one-hour cosyntropin (synthetic ACTH) stimulation test has proved to be a safe, sensitive, and simple method.[137] It is also very helpful in determining when patients may be safely withdrawn from glucocorticoid therapy following a tapering schedule.[138] To prove that the adrenal insufficiency is primary or secondary to pituitary insufficiency or adrenal suppression usually requires a more prolonged ACTH stimulation with measurement of both plasma and urinary hormones. Other screening tests, such as the metyrapone test, are at times necessary to help establish the diagnosis.

Therapy

The emergency medicine physician routinely sees physiologically stressed patients. Conditions that can lead to acute adrenal insufficiency, such as systemic sepsis, acute myocardial infarction, trauma, burns, and gastroenteritis, are relatively commonplace in most emergency departments. Therefore, it is most important that physicians involved with emergency care consider adrenal crisis in patients who demonstrate the symptoms and signs that have been outlined. Patients being treated in the emergency department must be questioned about steroid usage, since augmentation of the daily dose of steroid is indicated in some patients treated as outpatients with certain disorders (e.g., pneumonia). Conditions that preclude the oral retention of medications (e.g., significant vomiting) might require a more liberal attitude toward hospitalization to ensure steroid administration. Obviously, a high index of suspicion is essential.

When the diagnosis of acute adrenal insufficiency is entertained, immediate treatment is mandatory. Blood should be drawn for cortisol, electrolyte, glucose, calcium, white blood count, hematocrit, BUN, and creatinine determinations. After a secure intravenous line has been established, hydrocortisone phosphate or hemisuccinate (100 mg intravenously over three to five minutes) is administered. The onset of action of this steroid is immediate, although it has a relatively short half-life (1½ hours). Over the first 24 hours, the total dosage of exogenous steroid should equal the amount that would be produced by normal adrenal glands subjected to severe stress—i.e., up to five times basal levels. Most patients require 100 to 300 mg during the first day, depending on body size. This can be given in the form of an intravenous bolus (e.g., 15 mg/kg every eight hours) or, more ideally, as a continuous drip (e.g., 100 mg in 1,000 ml 5 percent dextrose in normal saline to be infused at a rate of 10 to 15 mg/hour). Hydrocortisone in these doses has adequate mineralocorticoid activity; therefore, specific replacement is not usually indicated. If hypotension or electrolyte abnormalities persist, however, desoxycorticosterone acetate (2 to 3 mg in oil intramuscularly or fluorohydrocortisone 0.1 to 0.2 mg orally) may be required. Dexamethasone and prednisone lack a mineralocorticoid effect and probably should not be used in the management of adrenal crisis.

Most patients in adrenal crisis exhibit signs of significant dehydration, and an extracellular fluid volume deficit of 20 percent is not uncommon. Fluid therapy should be aggressive, especially in the presence of hypotension. One liter 5 percent dextrose in normal saline should be given over the first 30 minutes to one hour, and most patients require 3 to 4 liters the first day. Obviously, shock must be even more aggressively treated.

Patients with limited cardiac reserve require a more cautious approach. Placement of a central venous pressure or Swan-Ganz catheter can provide valuable monitoring information. If shock is severe, colloid solutions may be required; rarely, vasopressor agents are needed. The treatment of choice is fluid replacement. Persistent shock suggests sepsis or occult blood loss.

Hyponatremia is responsive to the measures that have been discussed. Hypertonic saline should be avoided, if at all possible. Hyperkalemia usually responds to the administration of glucose, steroid, and fluid. Should hyperkalemia be life-threatening, the traditional measures for rapidly lowering the serum potassium level should be used. It must be remembered, however, that such patients are sensitive to insulin and may be hypercalcemic. Hypercalcemia usually resolves with the measures described, and an effective calciuresis is established as the glomerular filtration rate improves.

A thorough search for the precipitating cause, especially infection, is mandatory. Appropriate cultures should be obtained and antibiotic therapy administered early when appropriate. Sedatives should be avoided and hypoglycemia corrected. Nonessential procedures should be postponed. If the patient fails to respond to this approach, other complications, such as sepsis, gastrointestinal bleeding, and panhypopituitarism, should be considered.

Once the life-threatening manifestations of the acute adrenal insufficiency have been controlled, the steroid dose is gradually tapered and a maintenance oral dose established, typically hydrocortisone (20 mg in the morning and 10 mg late afternoon) or the equivalent dose of prednisone (7.5 mg and 5 mg). At this time, the addition of a mineralocorticoid (e.g., fluorohydrocortisone, 0.1 to 0.2 mg daily) is often indicated.

REFERENCES

1. Addison T: *On the Constitutional and Local Effects of Disease of the Suprarenal Capsules.* London, Highly, 1855.
2. Nerup J: Addison's disease: Serological studies. *Acta Endocrinol* 76:142, 1974.
3. Nerup J et al: Antiadrenal cellular hypersensitivity in Addison's disease. *Clin Exp Immunol* 5:341, 1969.
4. Faber J et al: Subclinical hypothyroidism in Addison's disease. *Acta Endocrinol* 91:674, 1979.
5. McHardy-Young S et al: Serum TSH and thyroid antibody studies in Addison's disease. *Clin Endocrinol* 1:45, 1972.
6. Anderson P et al: Familial Schmidt's syndrome. *JAMA* 244:2068, 1980.
7. Parker M et al: Silent thyrotoxic thyroiditis in association with chronic adrenocortical insufficiency. *Arch Intern Med* 140:1108, 1980.
8. Gastineau C et al: Thyroid disorders in Addison's disease. *Mayo Clin Proc* 39:939, 1964.
9. Riley W et al: Adrenal autoantibodies and Addison's disease in insulin-dependent diabetes mellitus. *J Pediatr* 97:191, 1980.

10. Nelson R et al: Schmidt's syndrome in a child with diabetes mellitus. *Diabetes Care* 1:37, 1978.
11. Gharib H et al: Coexisting Addison's disease and diabetes mellitus: Report of 24 cases with review of the literature. *Mayo Clin Proc* 44:217, 1969.
12. Elder M et al: Gonadal autoantibodies in patients with hypogonadism and/or Addison's disease. *J Clin Endocrinol Metab* 52:1137, 1981.
13. Edmonds M et al: Autoimmune thyroiditis, adrenalitis, and oophoritis. *Am J Med* 54:782, 1973.
14. Appel G et al: The syndrome of multiple endocrine gland insufficiency. *Am J Med* 61:129, 1976.
15. Irvine W et al: Adrenocortical insufficiency. *Clin Endocrinol Metab* 1:549, 1972.
16. Strickland R: Pernicious anemia and polyendocrine deficiency. *Ann Intern Med* 70:1001, 1969.
17. Betterle C et al: Vitiligo and autoimmune polyendocrine deficiencies with autoantibodies to melanin-producing cells. *Arch Dermatol* 115:364, 1979.
18. Blizzard R et al: The incidence of adrenal and other antibodies in the sera of patients with idiopathic adrenal insufficiency. *Clin Exp Immunol* 2:19, 1967.
19. Fisher M et al: Candidiasis, vitiligo, Addison's disease and hypoparathyroidism. *Arch Dermatol* 102:110, 1970.
20. Liddle G et al: Dual mechanism regulating adrenocortical function in man. *Am J Med* 21:380, 1956.
21. Graber A et al: Natural history of pituitary adrenal recovery following long-term suppression with corticosteroids. *J Clin Endocrinol* 25:11, 1967.
22. Meakin J et al: Pituitary-adrenal function following long-term steroid therapy. *Am J Med* 29:459, 1960.
23. Spiegel R et al: Adrenal suppression after short-term corticosteroid therapy. *Lancet* 1:630, 1979.
24. Meikle A et al: Potency and duration of action of glucocorticoids: Effects of hydrocortisone, prednisone, and dexamethasone on human pituitary-adrenal function.. *Am J Med* 63:200, 1977.
25. Naik R et al: Serious renal transplant rejection and adrenal hypofunction after gradual withdrawal of prednisolone two years after transplantation. *Br Med J* 2:1337, 1980.
26. Newton RW et al: Adrenocortical suppression in workers manufacturing synthetic glucocorticoids. *Br Med J* 1:73, 1978.
27. Tan R: Pustular psoriasis with adrenal suppression following topical corticosteroids. *Proc R Soc Med* 67:719, 1974.
28. Carr R et al: Adrenocortical suppression with topical flumethasone. *Arch Dermatol* 96:269, 1967.
29. Harris D et al: The effect of intranasal beclomethasone dipropionate on adrenal function. *Clin Allergy* 4:291, 1974.
30. Michels M et al: Adrenal suppression and intranasally applied steroids. *Ann Allergy* 25:569, 1967.
31. Williams H: Beclomethasone dipropionate. *Ann Intern Med* 95:464, 1981.
32. Cayton R et al: Adrenal failure in bronchial asthma. *Br Med J* 2:547, 1973.
33. Bongiovanni A et al: Steroids during pregnancy and possible fetal consequences. *Fertil Steril* 11:181, 1960.
34. Grajwer L et al: Neonatal subclinical adrenal insufficiency: Result of maternal steroid therapy. *JAMA* 238:1279, 1977.
35. Dixon R et al: On the various forms of corticosteroid withdrawal syndrome. *Am J Med* 68:224, 1980.
36. Cornil A et al: Cortisol secretion during acute bacterial infections in man. *Acta Endocrinol* 58:1, 1968.
37. Melby J et al: Comparative studies on adrenal cortical function and cortisol metabolism in healthy adults and in patients with shock due to infections. *J Clin Invest* 37:1971, 1958.
38. Migeon C et al: Study of adrenal function in children with meningitis. *Pediatrics* 40:163, 1967.
39. Sibbald W et al: Variations in adrenocortical responsiveness during severe bacterial infections. *Ann Surg* 186:29, 1977.
40. Sandberg A et al: Metabolism of adrenal steroids in dying patients. *J Clin Endocrinol* 16:1001, 1956.
41. D'Agati V et al: The Waterhouse-Friderichsen syndrome. *N Engl J Med* 232:1, 1945.
42. Rick A: A peculiar type of adrenal cortical damage associated with acute infections and its possible relation to circulatory collapse. *Bull Johns Hopkins Hosp* 74:1, 1944.
43. Thomison J et al: Adrenal lesions in acute meningococcemia. *Arch Pathol* 63:527, 1957.
44. Levin J et al: Endotoxemia and adrenal hemorrhage. *J Exp Med* 121:247, 1965.
45. Bosworth D: Reversible adrenocortical insufficiency in fulminant meningococcemia. *Arch Intern Med* 139:823, 1979.
46. Lawson D et al: Massive retroperitoneal adrenal hemorrhage. *Surg Gynecol Obstet* 128:989, 1969.
47. Greendyke R: Adrenal hemorrhage. *Am J Clin Pathol* 43:210, 1965.
48. Batteri A et al: Adrenal hemorrhage and necrosis in the adult. *Acta Med Scand* 175:409, 1964.
49. Foley F et al: Adrenal hemorrhage and necrosis in seriously burned patients. *J Trauma* 7:863, 1967.
50. Wilbur O et al: A study of the role of adrenocorticotrophic hormone (ACTH) in the pathogenesis of tubular degeneration of the adrenals. *Bull Johns Hopkins Hosp* 93:321, 1953.
51. Amador E: Adrenal hemorrhage during anticoagulant therapy. *Ann Intern Med* 63:559, 1965.
52. Portnay G et al: Anticoagulant therapy and acute adrenal insufficiency. *Ann Intern Med* 81:115, 1974.
53. Harper J et al: Bilateral adrenal hemorrhage: A complication of anticoagulant therapy. Case report and review of the literature. *Am J Med* 32:984, 1962.
54. Klassen J et al: Survival after bilateral adrenal hemorrhage during heparin therapy. *Can Med Assoc J* 97:1162, 1967.
55. Danese C et al: Adrenal hemorrhage during anticoagulant therapy. *Ann Surg* 179:70, 1974.
56. Van Couwenberge G et al: Effect of ACTH with anticoagulants. *Can Med Assoc J* 79:536, 1958.
57. Cedermark B et al: Adrenal activity in patients with advanced carcinomas. *Surg Gynecol Obstet* 152:461, 1981.
58. Allot E et al: Increased adrenocortical activity associated with malignant disease. *Lancet* 2:278, 1960.
59. Bishop M et al: Adrenocortical activity in relation to prognosis. *Br J Cancer* 24:719, 1971.
60. Cedermark B et al: The clinical significance of metastases to the adrenal gland. *Surg Gynecol Obstet* 152:607, 1981.
61. Rosenthal F et al: Malignant disease presenting as Addison's disease. *Br Med J* 1:1591, 1978.
62. Fox B: Adrenal hemorrhage and necrosis resulting from abdominal operations. *Lancet* 1:600, 1969.
63. Henrich W et al: Adrenal insufficiency after unilateral radical nephrectomy. *Urology* 8:584, 1976.
64. Steer M et al: Recognition of adrenal insufficiency in the postoperative patient. *Am J Surg* 139:443, 1980.
65. Byyny R: Preventing adrenal insufficiency during surgery. *Postgrad Med* 67:219, 1980.
66. Alford W et al: Acute adrenal insufficiency following cardiac surgical procedures. *J Thorac Cardiovasc Surg* 78:489, 1979.
67. Hubay C et al: Occult adrenal insufficiency in surgical patients. *Ann Surg* 181:325, 1975.
68. Nerup J: Addison's disease: Clinical studies—A report of 108 cases. *Acta Endocrinol* 76:127, 1974.

69. Casten C et al: Tuberculosis, Addison's disease and thyrotoxicosis. *JAMA* 239:2014, 1978.

70. Morens D: Congenital tuberculosis and associated hypoadrenocorticism. *South Med J* 72:160, 1979.

71. Braedy J: Military tuberculosis presenting as adrenal failure. *Can Med Assoc J* 124:748, 1981.

72. Liddle G: Pathogenesis of glucocorticoid disorders. *Am J Med* 53:638, 1972.

73. Dillon R: *Handbook of Endocrinology*, ed 2. Philadelphia, Lea & Febiger, 1980.

74. Crispell K et al: Addison's disease associated with histoplasmosis. *Am J Med* 20:23, 1956.

75. Roofen R et al: Addison's disease due to *Histoplasma capsulatum*. *S Afr Med J* 47:1953, 1975.

76. Eberle D: Disseminated North American blastomycosis occurrence with clinical manifestations of adrenal insufficiency. *JAMA* 238:2629, 1977.

77. Chandler P: Addison's disease secondary to North American blastomycosis. *South Med J* 70:863, 1977.

78. Marsiglea I et al: Adrenal cortical insufficiency associated with paracoccidioidomycosis: Report of four patients. *J Clin Endocrinol Metab* 26:1109, 1966.

79. Colin R: Congenital idiopathic adrenal hypoplasia. *Obstet Gynecol* 41:655, 1973.

80. Tsung S et al: Sudden infant death and old adrenal hemorrhage. *JAMA* 241:2507, 1979.

81. Mitchell R: Congenital adrenal hypoplasia in siblings. *Lancet* 1:488, 1959.

82. McKusick V: *Mendelian Inheritance in Man*, ed 3. Baltimore, The Johns Hopkins Press, 1971, p 543.

83. Laverty C et al: Congenital idiopathic adrenal hypoplasia. *Obstet Gynecol* 41:655, 1973.

84. Wakefield M et al: X-linked congenital Addison's disease. *Arch Dis Child* 56:73, 1981.

85. Kreines K et al: Neonatal adrenal insufficiency associated with maternal Cushing's syndrome. *Pediatrics* 47:516, 1971.

86. Moore F et al: Adrenal cysts and adrenal insufficiency in an infant with fatal termination. *J Pediatr* 36:91, 1950.

87. Dickerman J et al: Adrenal hemorrhage in the newborn: The phenomenon of "enclosed" hemorrhage as a cause of neonatal jaundice and later adrenal calcifications. *Clin Pediatr* 16:314, 1977.

88. Stevenson J: Calcification of the adrenal glands in young children. *Arch Dis Child* 36:316, 1961.

89. Shackleton C et al: Deficient 3-Beta-hydroxy-5-ene steroid secretion by newborn infants. *J Clin Endocrinol Metab* 49:247, 1979.

90. Russell M et al: Sudden infant death due to congenital adrenal hypoplasia. *Arch Pathol Lab Med* 101:168, 1977.

91. Favara B et al: Idiopathic adrenal hypoplasia in children. *Am J Clin Pathol* 57:287, 1972.

92. Eichner H et al: SLE with adrenal insufficiency. *Am J Med* 55:700, 1973.

93. Das G et al: Adrenocortical insufficiency related to oral contraceptives. *JAMA* 207:2438, 1969.

94. Eagan R et al: Adrenal insufficiency following bilateral adrenal venography. *JAMA* 215:115, 1971.

95. Chakurakjian Z et al: Adrenocortical failure in panhypopituitarism. *J Clin Endocrinol Metab* 28:25, 1968.

96. Fehm H et al: Adrenal insufficiency secondary to hypothalamic CRF insufficiency with hyperpigmentation: A case report. *Horm Metab Res* 8:470, 1976.

97. Corrall R et al: Acute adrenal insufficiency due to isolated corticotrophin deficiency. *J R Soc Med* 72:530, 1979.

98. Toifl K et al: A combination of spastic paraparesis, polyneuropathy, and adrenocortical insufficiency: A childhood form of adrenomyeloneuropathy. *J Neurol* 225:47, 1981.

99. Davis L et al: Adrenoleukodystrophy and adrenomyeloneuropathy associated with partial adrenal insufficiency in three generations of a kindred. *Am J Med* 66:342, 1979.

100. Schaumburg H et al: Adrenomyeloneuropathy: A probable variant of adrenoleukodystrophy. *Neurology* 27:1114, 1977.

101. Menkes J et al: Adrenoleukodystrophy. *Neurology* 27:928, 1977.

102. Scott A et al: Adrenocorticotrophic and melanocyte-stimulating peptides in the human pituitary. *Biochem J* 139:593, 1974.

103. Greipp P: Hyperpigmentation syndromes. *Arch Intern Med* 138:346, 1978.

104. Bissell G et al: Longitudinal banded pigmentation of nails in primary adrenal insufficiency. *JAMA* 215:1666, 1971.

105. Strakosch C et al: Early diagnosis of Addison's disease: Pigmentation as sole symptom. *Aust NZ J Med* 8:189, 1978.

106. Goodwin T et al: Addison's disease without pigmentation. *Postgrad Med J* 49:305, 1973.

107. Hidden adrenocortical insufficiency, editorial. *Br Med J* 1:5, 1973.

108. Chan H et al: Salty sweat and ichthyosis in Addison's disease. *Br Med J* 1:145, 1977.

109. Blizzard R et al: Candidiasis studies pertaining to its association with endocrinopathies and pernicious anemia. *Pediatrics* 42:231, 1968.

110. Bedsole A: Calcified auricular cartilages in Addison's disease. *South Med J* 59:1268, 1966.

111. Jarvis J et al: Roentgenologic observations in Addison's disease: A review of 120 cases. *Radiology* 62:16, 1954.

112. Cohen E: *Adrenal Cortical Insufficiency, American College of Physicians Course in Clinical Endocrinology, Physiologic Basis for Current Diagnoses and Therapeutic Procedures*. Ann Arbor, Michigan, May 1971.

113. Turnipseed W et al: The acute abdomen in undiagnosed Addison's disease. *Wis Med J* 75:104, 1976.

114. Sparberg M: Addison's disease and peptic ulcer. *Gastroenterology* 53:450, 1967.

115. Harper M et al: Combined adrenal and thyroid deficiency presenting as an acute psychosis. *Med J Aust* 1:546, 1970.

116. Abbas D et al: Polyradiculopathy in Addison's disease. *Neurology* 27:494, 1977.

117. Spaar F et al: Adrenalitis inclusio-necroticans in Landry-Guillain-Barre syndrome. *Z Neurol* 193:195, 1968.

118. Sabin A et al: Visceral lesions in infectious polyneuritis. *Am J Pathol* 17:469, 1941.

119. Spinnler H et al: Unusual acute neurologic onset of Addison's disease. *Med J Aust* 1:280, 1979.

120. Kollmannsberger A et al: Addison's encephalopathy. *Electroencephalogr Clin Neurophysiol* 26:448, 1969.

121. Nora J: Tachyarrhythmia and hyperkalemia in adrenal insufficiency. *Chest* 71:686, 1977.

122. Hochberg Z: Delayed pubarche in adolescents with adrenal insufficiency. *Clin Pediatr* 19:827, 1980.

123. Sheridan P et al: Addison's disease presenting with chronic low backache. *Br Med J* 1:77, 1976.

124. Susac J et al: Flexion contracture in adrenal insufficiency. *Arch Phys Med Rehabil* 49:3, 1968.

125. Calabrese L et al: Musculoskeletal manifestations of Addison's disease. *Arthritis Rheum* 22:558, 1979.

126. Henkin R et al: Studies of olfactory threshold in normal man and in patients with adrenocortical insufficiency. *J Clin Invest* 45:1631, 1966.

127. Henkin R et al: Studies on auditory threshold in normal man and in patients with adrenocortical insufficiency. *J Clin Invest* 46:429, 1967.

128. Kosowicz J et al: The "taste" test in adrenal insufficiency. *J Clin Endocrinol Metab* 27:214, 1967.
129. Cotterill J et al: Self-medication with liquorice in a patient with Addison's disease. *Lancet* 1:294, 1973.
130. Green M et al: Bronchial asthma with Addison's disease. *Lancet* 1:1159, 1971.
131. Harris P et al: Bronchial asthma with Addison's disease. *Lancet* 1:1349, 1971.
132. Vilchez J et al: Hyperkalemic paralysis, neuropathy, and persistent motor neuron discharges at rest in Addison's disease. *J Neurol Neurosurg Psychiatry* 43:818, 1980.
133. Van Dellen R et al: Hyperkalemic paralysis in Addison's disease. *Mayo Clin Proc* 44:904, 1969.
134. Downie W: Hypercalcemic crisis as presentation of Addison's disease. *Br Med J* 1:145, 1977.
135. Siegler D: Idiopathic Addison's disease presenting with hypercalcemia. *Br Med J* 2:522, 1970.
136. Spry C: Eosinophilia in Addison's disease. *Yale J Biol Med* 49:411, 1976.
137. Speckart P et al: Screening for adrenocortical insufficiency with cosyntropin (synthetic ACTH). *Arch Intern Med* 128:761, 1971.
138. Byyny R: Withdrawal from glucocorticoid therapy. *N Engl J Med* 295:30, 1976.

14. Electrolyte Abnormalities

BARRY E. BRENNER, M.D., Ph.D.

Disorders of electrolytes pervade all areas of emergency medicine: surgery, medicine, pediatrics, and obstetrics and gynecology. Some electrolytic disorders may be life-threatening, even though there may be few symptoms or signs. These disorders may impair the function of critical organs, such as the brain or the heart. Abnormalities of electrolytes may be manifestations of an underlying disease process that is a major threat to the life of the patient; for example, mild lactic acidosis may signify sepsis.

Electrolytic disorders frequently require keen clinical judgment. The emergency physician may diagnose an electrolytic disorder tentatively and await laboratory test results only for confirmation. In an asymptomatic patient with a normal electrocardiogram (ECG), the laboratory may occasionally provide a startlingly abnormal result. It is important, however, to treat the patient, not the laboratory value. The treatment of electrolytic disorders may have serious side-effects, and the treatment must be based on symptoms, signs, and ECG findings rather than on the magnitude of any laboratory abnormality.

The rapidity of treatment should also depend on the clinical or ECG findings. As a general rule, one-half the electrolyte deficit should be corrected over a 6- to 12-hour period; then, the patient's condition should be reevaluated.

HYDRATION

The state of hydration of a given patient is dependent on the serum sodium concentration as well as the state of fluid hydration.

Fluid Physiology

A man has two physiologic components: a solid compartment, which makes up 40 percent of the total body weight, and a fluid compartment, which makes up 60 percent of the total body weight (Fig. 14–1). The fluid compartment, called the total body water (TBW), in a normal, lean 70-kg man is 42 liters. Two-thirds of the TBW is intracellular fluid; therefore, in a 70-kg man, the intracellular space contains 28 liters fluid. The extracellular space contains both the fluid in the interstitial space and the plasma volume. One-third of the TBW consists of extracellular fluid, which is 14 liters in a 70-kg man.

The interstitial fluid is the fluid that surrounds each cell and serves as the immediate medium for oxygen

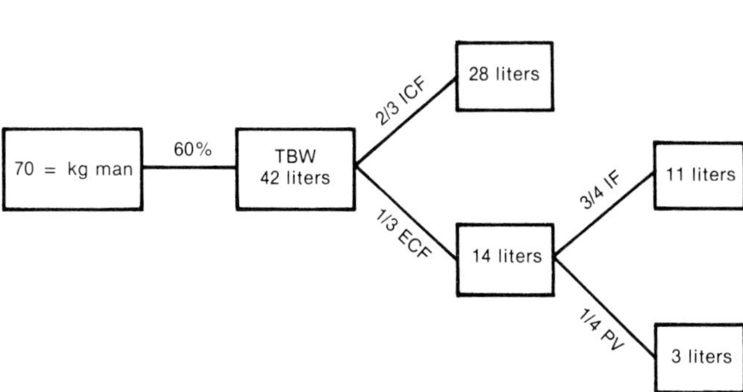

Figure 14–1 Fluid Compartments. *TBW*, total body water; *ICF*, intracellular fluid; *ECF*, extracellular fluid; *IF*, interstitial fluid; *PV*, plasma volume.

and nutrient delivery, as well as for the secretion and excretion of products. The interstitial fluid represents about 75 percent of the extracellular fluid. In a 70-kg man, interstitial fluid is 11 liters.

The plasma volume is the fluid that maintains the intravascular volume and is the fluid portion of blood. It is the supernatant fluid found after the centrifugation of blood in a capillary tube for a "routine" hematocrit. The plasma volume represents about 25 percent of the extracellular fluid; therefore, in a 70-kg man, it is 3 liters.

There is considerable variation in the apportioning of TBW. Variations from this 70-kg model occur because the water content of muscle is greater than that of fat. The more fat, the lower the percentage of TBW. Women have more fat than men; therefore, TBW in a woman is 50 to 55 percent of weight. Since the neonate has little fat, the TBW is 70 to 80 percent of the neonate's weight; the extracellular fluid is 40 percent of TBW.

Sodium Physiology

Sodium is a major extracellular cation in the body. Because it maintains extracellular volume by binding hydrogen in water, it plays an important role in metabolism. Sodium metabolism is clearly affected by the daily intake and excretion of sodium. With normal renal function, the daily intake of sodium is equal to the urinary output of sodium; i.e., the urinary sodium is 130 to 260 mEq/day, which is equivalent to the daily sodium intake. Clinically, it is important to remember that urinary electrolytes must be measured when the patient is not taking diuretics because these medications enhance sodium and potassium excretion, making the results difficult to interpret.

Some control mechanisms are involved in the maintenance of normal serum sodium. These mechanisms are thirst, antidiuretic hormone (ADH), and free water excretion.[1]

Thirst

Hypertonicity or an elevation of the plasma osmolarity causes thirst. As independent factors, a decrease in the extracellular fluid or an elevation in the level of plasma angiotensin also induces thirst. Therefore, hypovolemic patients may have increased thirst.

Antidiuretic Hormone

In order to understand the mechanism of action of ADH, it is necessary to understand renal physiology (Fig. 14–2). The plasma is passively filtered into the glomeruli. Sodium, bicarbonate, and small molecules,

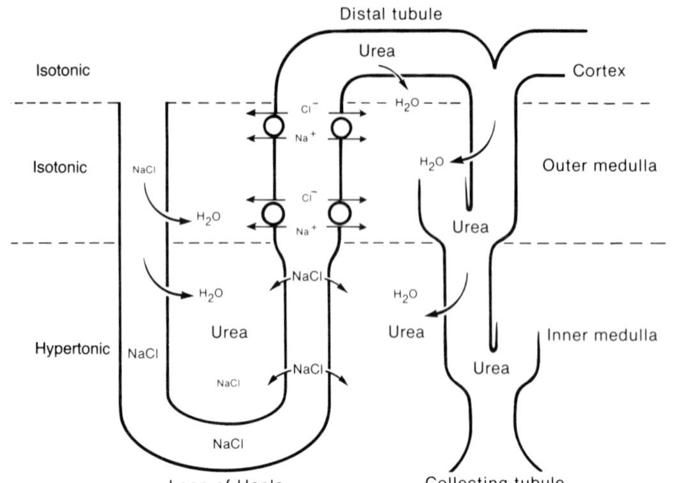

Figure 14–2   Renal Physiology.

along with water, are reabsorbed in the proximal tubule, which is located in the renal outer medulla. This filtrate is isotonic. Proceeding from the renal outer medulla, the filtrate descends through the descending limb of the loop of Henle, located in the inner medulla of the kidney. When the urine arrives in the ascending limb of Henle's loop, sodium is actively removed from the filtrate, leaving a hypotonic fluid. The medulla of the kidney is highly hypertonic, owing to the high concentration of urea that is maintained in the medullary interstitium of the kidney. The filtrate next proceeds to the distal tubule, located in the renal cortex. The urine is still hypotonic at this point. In the distal tubule, isotonic sodium and water reabsorption, as well as potassium and acid secretion, occur. These functions are controlled by the hormone aldosterone (see Potassium, Physiology later in this chapter). From the distal tubule, the urine enters the collecting tubule, which is located in the hypertonic medullary interstitium. Openings or "pores" in the cells of the collecting tubule permit equilibration between the hypotonic urine and hypertonic medullary interstitium, thereby causing an efflux of water from the hypotonic filtrate into the collecting tubule and the concentration of urine.[2,3] This pore size is regulated by ADH.

The mechanism of ADH action involves the second messenger, cyclic adenosine monophosphate (cAMP). ADH governs the water reabsorption at the collecting tubule and, in healthy individuals, is able to produce a maximum of 800 to 1,200 mOsm urine.[2–4] ADH secretion is normally increased during dehydration or hypovolemia.[5]

Free Water Excretion

The last control mechanism involved in the maintenance of a normal serum sodium is free water excretion.

A decrease in free water excretion means that less free water is being presented to the collecting tubule, either because of a decrease in the glomerular filtration rate or because of an increase in the proximal tubular reabsorption of water. Therefore, less free water can be conserved by the ADH mechanism, resulting in a loss of water.

HYPERNATREMIA AND FLUID DEFICIT

Pathophysiology

Since cell membranes are permeable to water, tonicity must be the same on both sides of a cell. Therefore, a decrease in TBW increases serum sodium concentration; conversely, an increase in TBW decreases serum sodium concentration.[6] For example, a 10 percent increase in serum sodium reflects a 10 percent deficit in TBW. In general, serum sodium is most highly influenced by TBW; therefore, the serum sodium is a poor indicator of sodium excess or deficit.[4]

In order to understand hypernatremia, it is necessary to understand the concept of hyperosmolarity or hypertonicity. The tonicity of the extracellular environment is influenced by sodium, glucose, and blood urea nitrogen (BUN). Sodium is maintained almost exclusively in the extracellular environment and is actively transported out of the intracellular space.[7] Owing to its high concentration extracellularly, sodium is the major osmotic agent. Glucose may enter the intracellular space but only at a slow, fixed rate and only when facilitated by a transport mechanism. BUN diffuses freely across cell membranes and is not affected by tonicity in vivo.[4] During in vitro measurements by freezing point depressions, BUN increases serum osmolarity.

The serum osmolarity can be calculated by the following equation[8,9]:

$$\text{Osmolarity} = 2 \times \text{Na} + \frac{\text{Glucose}}{18} + \frac{\text{BUN}}{2.8} \quad \text{(Equation 1)}$$

BUN is included in this equation so that the calculated osmolarity will agree with the measured osmolarity obtained from the laboratory; however, BUN does not affect osmolarity in vivo.[4] Hyperosmolarity is defined as a serum osmolarity greater than 350 mOsm.[10,11] Normal serum osmolarity is 270 to 300 mOsm.

Etiology

Hypernatremia and dehydration have many causes.[1,12–14] Patients in nursing homes are highly susceptible to dehydration for example, because they may not feed themselves adequately and may not be able to communicate with their caretakers when they are thirsty. Likewise, infants cannot communicate when they are thirsty, and the loss of even a small amount of water that is not replaced can rapidly result in dehydration in an infant.

Renal loss of more water than sodium also causes hypernatremia and dehydration. Patients whose renal losses of water are excessive have marked thirst, but, as long as they have access to water, they do not become dehydrated. This process occurs in diabetes insipidus. If patients with diabetes insipidus are not permitted access to water, they dehydrate quite rapidly. An osmotic diuresis, either drug-induced or due to the sudden release of urinary tract obstruction, also causes a significant renal loss of more water than sodium.[4] These patients may excrete as much as 1 to 2 liters urine every hour with a urine sodium more than 10 mEq/liter on a "spot" sample. If these patients do not have adequate fluid intake, usually by the intravenous (IV) route, severe dehydration rapidly ensues.

Gastrointestinal loss of more water than sodium because of nausea, vomiting, or diarrhea can lead to dehydration. During hot weather or fever, perspiring may cause a patient to lose more water than sodium and thus become dehydrated. Likewise, tachypnea, which may be associated with entities such as asthma, may result in dehydration.

Central neurologic lesions can decrease thirst. The hypothalamus is the area of the brain that controls thirst, and a lesion in the hypothalamus can eliminate thirst and predispose a patient to dehydration. Such lesions are rare, however. In patients with essential hypernatremia,[4,12] the mechanism maintaining a normal serum osmolarity or "osmostat" has been reset to a different level of serum sodium. Therefore, the body may vigorously maintain a serum sodium of 150 mEq/liter in the same fashion that most individuals maintain a serum sodium of 140 mEq/liter. A central hypernatremia has been associated with the presence of ectopic pinealomas located in the hypothalamus.[12]

Almost all cases of hypernatremia are due to a deficit in TBW, not to sodium excess.[4,12] It is most unusual for sodium excess to cause hypernatremia. Sodium excess, however, may result from excessive sodium bicarbonate administration during cardiopulmonary resuscitation, injection of hypotonic saline into a blood vessel by mistake during a saline abortion, administration of excessive amounts of hypertonic saline in the treatment of hyponatremia, the excessive ingestion of salt tablets or sea water, or, in infants, ingestion of cow's milk with a salt load that exceeds the ability of the infant to excrete sodium.[1,4,12,15]

Diabetes Insipidus: Central

ADH is produced by the paraventricular nucleus of the hypothalamus. Central diabetes insipidus results either from damage to the hypothalamus or, in the familial form, a defect in the ADH itself. Other causes of this condition include:

- trauma
- primary or metastatic carcinoma, such as carcinoma of the breast
- Hand-Schüller-Christian disease
- granulomas, as seen in tuberculosis, sarcoidosis, syphilis
- vascular conditions, such as aneurysm, Simmonds' syndrome, Sheehan's syndrome
- meningitis or encephalitis

The clinical manifestations of central diabetes insipidus include an abrupt onset, usually in patients 10 to 20 years old, with polyuria and polydipsia as major symptoms. The fluid intake and output are both usually 3 to 15 liters/day. Patients maintain a normal serum osmolarity, providing that they have access to water. Even if their intake decreases, however, their obligate production of urine continues because of the ADH deficiency. Therefore, patients with diabetes insipidus tend to develop dehydration. Most of the patients with central diabetes insipidus have only a partial deficit so that oral intake and renal output are only 3 to 5 liters/day.

Diabetes Insipidus: Nephrogenic

Congenital The congenital form of nephrogenic diabetes insipidus is rare. The clinical manifestations are fever, vomiting, dehydration, yet the presence of a markedly hypotonic urine.

Acquired The acquired form of nephrogenic diabetes insipidus is common. In the usual forms of nephrogenic diabetes insipidus, the oral intake balances renal output of 3 to 5 liters/day. The etiology of acquired nephrogenic diabetes insipidus includes the following:

- chronic renal failure. The diseased kidney may be unresponsive to ADH, but this does not tend to produce dehydration. Since the glomerular filtration rate (GFR) is less than 60 ml/minute, less compensatory polydipsia is needed to ensure adequate fluid intake in patients with chronic renal failure.
- starvation. When protein intake and urea excretion are diminished, less urea is provided to maintain the hypertonic medullary interstitium of the kidney. Therefore, the urine-concentrating mechanism of the hypertonic medullary interstitium is impaired, and the urine cannot be concentrated in the collecting tubule (see Antidiuretic Hormone).

- ethanol. Not only does ethanol directly inhibit the action of ADH on the collecting tubule, but also it inhibits ADH secretion by the hypothalamus, producing, in part, both a central and nephrogenic diabetes insipidus.
- hypercalcemia. A persistently elevated calcium level may produce nephrocalcinosis, which interferes with the ability of the kidneys to keep the medullary interstitium hypertonic and, therefore, impairs the action of ADH.
- hypokalemia. Hypokalemia impairs the renal ability to maintain the hypertonicity of the medullary interstitium. Patients with potassium values persistently less than 3 mEq/liter may develop an acquired nephrogenic diabetes insipidus and hypokalemic nephropathy (see Hypokalemia).
- sickle cell disease and sickle cell trait. Because they interfere with the vasa recta or the blood supply to the hypertonic renal medullary interstitium, sickle cell disease and sickle cell trait cause edema of the renal papilla.[16] Hence, they impair the urine-concentrating mechanisms of the kidneys.
- drugs. Several different drugs have been reported to cause a nephrogenic diabetes insipidus: most commonly lithium, demeclocycline, and amphotericin B.[17] In fact, lithium and demeclocycline have been used successfully in the treatment of excessive and inappropriate levels of ADH (syndrome of inappropriate ADH).

Clinical Manifestations

The clinical manifestations of dehydration vary with the severity. As the TBW deficit increases, there is a progressive increase in the symptomatology. One of the earliest manifestations of dehydration in children is the absence of tears when they cry; this reflects a 2 to 3 percent deficit in TBW. Next, sunken fontanelles appear, signifying a 3 to 5 percent deficit in TBW. Prominent in both adults and children who become dehydrated, dry mucous membranes mean a 4 to 8 percent deficit in TBW.[18–20] In adults with developed apocrine sweat glands, diminished axillary sweating is a reliable sign of a 4 to 8 percent TBW deficit. In adults, decreased skin turgor means at least a 6 to 10 percent deficit in TBW.[21] The most severe sign of dehydration is hypovolemia; orthostatic hypotension may be the earliest sign of hypovolemia, indicating at least a 10 to 15 percent deficit in TBW and a 20 to 25 percent deficit in the extracellular fluid.[22]

Mental aberrations, which occur in both adults and children with dehydration, are manifested as lethargy. In children less than two years of age, hypertonia, irritability, and seizures are seen when the sodium concentration exceeds 160 mEq/liter.[1,4,12,15] Also in children, minute cerebral vessels may rupture with dehydration, producing a xanthochromic cerebrospinal fluid with a high protein content. The rupture of these vessels is of no consequence.[23]

In dehydration, oliguria is defined as a urine output less than 10 ml/kg or less than 500 ml/day in adults. This oliguria reflects the physiologic response of ADH and aldosterone secretion to conserve water.[5,24] Adults or their family members may be able to report oliguria. It is important to ask parents of infants whether their child's diapers must be changed less often in order to document oliguria.

Diagnosis

Dehydration

The diagnosis of dehydration is aided by the clinical manifestations. The serum osmolarity should be more than 350 mOsm before it is classified as hyperosmolarity.[10,11] The serum sodium level should be elevated in dehydration, to more than 150 mEq/liter. If the actual level is more than 170 mEq/liter, however, the result of a laboratory determination will be artificially low.[25] This underestimation of the serum sodium is due to hyperviscosity and hyperosmolarity of the serum, which decreases the amount of serum that can be aspirated into the roller pump diluter. In addition, the standard curves for serum sodium are not linear when sodium values are greater than 170 mEq/liter.

To calculate the level of serum sodium, it is necessary only to use Equation 1. If the serum osmolarity, BUN, and glucose are known, then the serum sodium can be calculated. For example, a physician suspects that a patient's serum sodium level of 178 mEq/liter may be an underestimation of the serum sodium. The glucose is determined to be 180 mg/dl, the BUN is 56 mg/dl, and the serum osmolarity is determined to be 400 mOsm. Using Equation 1,

$$2 \times Na + \frac{180}{18} + \frac{56}{2.8} = 400 \text{ mOsm}$$

therefore,

$$Na = 185 \text{ mEq/liter}$$

With hypernatremia it is helpful to calculate the TBW deficit. In this calculation, it is assumed that the patient's condition is stable and that sodium excess is not the cause of the patient's hypernatremia. The TBW deficit may be used as an estimate of the amount of fluid that the patient will require to be hydrated.[4,6,15] To calculate the TBW, the physician must remember that the TBW represents 60 percent of a man's total body weight. The total body solute is calculated by multiplying the TBW by the serum osmolarity. For example, a 70-kg man has 42 liters TBW. This is multiplied by 400 mOsm in the dehydrated patient, resulting in 16,800 mOsm total body solute. In the calculation of the TBW deficit, a desired osmolarity of approximately 300 mOsm can be used. The total body solute is divided by the desired osmolarity; the expected TBW is subtracted from this result to arrive at the TBW deficit. In the above example, the total body solute, 16,800 mOsm, is divided by 300 mOsm. From this quotient, 56, the expected TBW, 42 liters, is subtracted, resulting in a 14-liter TBW deficit.

Diabetes Insipidus

If a dehydrated patient has a dilute urine, the physician should suspect diabetes insipidus. It is important to distinguish diabetes insipidus from psychogenic polydipsia. The onset of psychogenic polydipsia is vague rather than abrupt. Frequently, patients with psychogenic polydipsia have a history of psychiatric illness.[4] To distinguish central diabetes insipidus from incomplete diabetes insipidus, nephrogenic diabetes insipidus, and psychogenic polydipsia, a water deprivation test is performed (Table 14–1). In this test, the patient is deprived of water for 12 to 16 hours until there is a decrease in TBW of 3 to 5 percent or three consecutive urines are unchanged in osmolarity.[26] At this time, serum osmolarity and urine osmolarity are measured. Then, 5 units aqueous ADH are administered and the serum osmolarity and urine osmolarity are measured over the next one hour.

Treatment

Dehydration

The treatment of dehydration depends on the severity of the condition. If a patient is mildly symptomatic and has neither nausea nor vomiting, oral hydration may be possible. The maximum amount of oral hydration that may be considered is 2.5 to 3 liters/day.[15]

If the patient is mildly symptomatic and has more than a 5 percent deficit of TBW, or if the patient cannot tolerate oral hydration, then intravenous hydration is indicated. If hypotension or orthostatic hypotension is present, the TBW deficit is calculated and 1 to 2 liters normal saline administered over 48 hours. The baseline rate of fluid administration is equal to the rate of urine output, but the TBW deficit must be replaced by the administration of fluid above and beyond the amount excreted in the urine. The TBW deficit is replaced as 5 percent dextrose with one-half normal saline in

TABLE 14–1   Water Deprivation Test

Diagnosis	Initial Serum Osmolarity	Urine Osmolarity after Dehydration	Urine Osmolarity after Vasopressin
Normal	Normal, 275–300	Normal, 1,000	No response, 1,000
Complete diabetes insipidus	Normal	Dilute, 160	Excellent response, 400
Incomplete diabetes insipidus	Normal	Medium dilute, 440	Good response, 700
Nephrogenic diabetes insipidus	Normal	Dilute or medium dilute	No response
Psychogenic polydipsia	Dilute, 250–275	Isotonic, 300	Slight response, 370

Note: If patients with diabetes insipidus can drink, they have a normal serum osmolarity. Patients with psychogenic polydipsia cannot concentrate their urine secondary to their chronic hypotonicity, which "washes out" the countercurrent dilution mechanism of the interstitium of the medulla of the kidney.

adults.[1,4,15] In children, 5 percent dextrose with one-quarter normal saline is used.

It is important to treat dehydration over a prolonged period of time, such as 48 hours. The rapid administration of markedly hypotonic fluids, such as 5 percent dextrose, may cause hemolysis. Furthermore, rapid treatment of dehydration is associated with the development of cerebral edema and the subsequent marked deterioration in the mental status of the patient.[12] This cerebral edema may be due to the development of different osmotic gradients between the blood and the brain. To decrease these osmotic gradients and prevent cerebral edema, some physicians advocate normal saline for rehydration in patients without cardiac or renal disease; if the serum sodium level becomes more than 155 mEq/liter, a change to hypotonic fluids is recommended.[27]

During the hydration of children, mild hyperglycemia may develop. This hyperglycemia must not be treated with insulin, because rapid falls in glucose may alter the tonicity between the blood and the brain and predispose children to cerebral edema.[23]

During rehydration, it is important to avoid overhydration. A central venous pressure of 5 mm Hg or neck vein distention of 5 cm above the angle of Louis reflects adequate intravascular volume. Urine osmolarity and urine output are also useful determinations in avoiding overhydration. The physician must always be alert to the development of acute tubular necrosis with oliguria, which can develop secondary to the profound hypovolemia and decreased renal blood flow that occurs with severe dehydration.

Sodium Excess

Patients with sodium excess should be treated in the same manner as other patients with dehydration, except that normal saline is contraindicated. These patients should receive only one-quarter or one-half normal saline. Dialysis may be necessary to remove the excess saline in the presence of renal failure.[4]

Central Diabetes Insipidus

The treatment of central diabetes insipidus is beyond the scope of the emergency physician. These patients should be referred to the internist. A convenient and effective therapy for these patients has been developed. Deamino arginine vasopressin, a long-acting nasal spray with a half-life of 20 hours, has been highly effective as a single daily treatment in the patient with central diabetes insipidus.[1,4]

Nephrogenic Diabetes Insipidus

The treatment of congenital nephrogenic diabetes insipidus is the same as the treatment of any dehydration. These patients are treated with 5 percent dextrose with one-quarter normal saline. Interestingly, however, marked volume contraction with furosemide improves the patient's condition by increasing the proximal reabsorption of sodium and decreasing the delivery of sodium to the distal tubule.[4] Indomethacin has also been effective,[4] although the mechanism is unclear. In children with congenital nephrogenic diabetes insipidus, the combination of indomethacin and diuretics may decrease urine flow from 10 to 12 liters/day to 3 to 5 liters/day.

Prehospital and Nursing Care

Prehospital and nursing intervention should include the establishment of an IV catheter with normal saline or 5 percent dextrose with one-half normal saline infusion. If the dehydration is perceived to be severe, the nursing team should prepare the patient for admission. Any patient with dehydration so severe that it produces altered mental status, orthostatic hypotension, or hypotension requires prolonged therapy and should be admitted to the hospital.

HYPONATREMIA

Pathophysiology and General Etiology

The causes of hyponatremia may be divided into three categories according to the hydration status of the patient: edema, hypovolemia, and normovolemia.

Edema

Patients with hypervolemia have more water than sodium; the result is hyponatremia. This may occur in patients with nephrotic syndrome or in those with chronic renal failure who ingest excess water. The hypervolemia in congestive heart failure may diminish renal perfusion, causing a diminished sodium and water delivery to collecting ducts and thus decreasing free water excretion.[5,28,29] In addition, ADH secretion increases in an effort to compensate for the renal hypoperfusion, which in turn increases water retention.[5] In patients with chronic congestive heart failure or liver diseases, such as cirrhosis, metabolism of ADH is decreased, which also increases water retention.

Hypovolemia

Patients with hyponatremia and hypovolemia may be divided into two groups; those with renal salt-wasting and those with nonrenal salt losses.[29] Patients with hypovolemia and renal salt-wasting have a urine "spot" sodium of more than 40 mEq/liter in association with hypovolemia or orthostatic hypotension.[4] These patients may have hypopituitarism or Addison's disease; their high urine sodium and low serum sodium levels may be due to mineralocorticoid deficiency (see Hypokalemia).[1] In addition, a salt-losing nephropathy would produce severe renal salt losses and hyponatremia. Potent diuretics may produce salt-wasting and hyponatremia.[30]

Nonrenal salt losses occur with increased fluid retention secondary to compensatory and appropriate ADH secretion. In addition, free water excretion is decreased because of hypovolemia.[1,4] These nonrenal losses of fluid can result from gastrointestinal problems, such as diarrhea or vomiting, or retroperitoneal disease, such as pancreatitis.[1] Similarly, salt can be lost by profuse sweating during hot, humid weather; it is lost cutaneously in patients with severe burns.[1] Urine sodium is less than 10 mEq/liter on a spot sample in these patients, owing to the appropriate secretion of mineralocorticoids.[4]

Normovolemia

In the normovolemic patient, hyponatremia may result from several different causes. Hypothyroidism leads to hyponatremia, but the mechanism is unclear.[31] Sickle cell syndrome is a general phrase for a hyponatremia that occurs in patients who have a severe, usually chronic illness.[1,4,32] Both the existence of this disease and its pathophysiologic mechanism are controversial, however. It is postulated that sodium-potassium adenosine triphosphatase is not effective in a severe illness. Therefore, sodium enters the intracellular space and, owing to the ineffective sodium-potassium adenosine triphosphatase, is not actively transported out to the extracellular fluid.[7] Essential hyponatremia is similar to essential hypernatremia in that the pathophysiologic mechanism is that of a reset "osmostat" that maintains a lower serum osmolarity.[1,4] These patients are noted to have an increase in thirst. The existence of this entity is also controversial. Patients with psychogenic polydipsia drink 10 to 40 liters water per day. For this volume of fluid ingestion to produce hyponatremia a reset "osmostat" has been demonstrated. In contradistinction to diabetes insipidus, psychogenic polydipsia has a gradual onset.[33]

Pseudohyponatremia may develop secondary to hyperproteinemia or hyperglycemia. Patients with multiple myeloma or hyperlipemia may develop a pseudohyponatremia.[34] In the healthy patient, serum is 93 parts water and 7 parts solute (aqueous plus protein). The sodium is dissolved in the aqueous phase of serum at a concentration of 152 mEq/liter water. The sodium concentration reported from the laboratory is normally 140 mEq/liter serum, i.e., aqueous plus solid. In patients with hyperproteinemia, the relative proportion of water in serum may be decreased by an elevation of the solid phase (lipid or protein), producing a spurious decrease in the sodium concentration per liter of serum. Although the sodium concentration dissolved in the aqueous phase is unchanged, it shows 152 mEq/liter water.

In hyperglycemia, the serum sodium decreases 1.6 mEq/liter for each increase in glucose of 100 mg/dl.[35,36] Hyperglycemia produces hypertonicity in the extracellular fluid, and water transfers from the intracellular space to dilute the more hypertonic extracellular fluid. This increase in extracellular water decreases the concentration of sodium, producing hyponatremia. This reflects an actual hyponatremia in the extracellular fluid, but does not reflect a total body sodium deficit or TBW excess.

The syndrome of inappropriate ADH is a diagnosis of exclusion. It is based on the assumption that the patient has normal renal, adrenal, thyroid, and cardiac function. In addition, the patient must not have hypervolemia, which would make the ADH response appropriate and produce hyponatremia by mechanisms that have already been listed. The etiology of this syndrome includes the following[3,4,37]:

1. drugs. Carbamazepine and chlorpropamide increase ADH secretion. Both chlorpropamide and tolbutamide enhance the effect of ADH on the collecting duct. Amitriptyline hydrochloride, thioriadazine hydrochloride, narcotics, and barbiturates may also induce this syndrome by unclear mechanisms.
2. ectopic production. An inappropriate ADH response has been produced by various malignant tumors, ranging from carcinoma of the lung, pancreas, or prostate to lymphomas.
3. pulmonary disease. Many different pulmonary diseases may cause this syndrome. The most frequent pulmonary causes are pulmonary tuberculosis, pneumonia, and lung abscesses.
4. neurologic conditions. Since ADH is produced by the hypothalamus, it is not surprising that neurologic aberrations may cause increased secretion of this hormone. Patients with encephalitis, meningitis, brain tumors, cerebral aneurysms, or Guillain-Barré syndrome may develop the syndrome of inappropriate ADH.
5. miscellaneous factors. Various stress situations may induce an inappropriate ADH response. Presumably, this increased production of ADH is induced directly by the effect of stress on the hypothalamus. Acute intermittent porphyria, assisted ventilation, or emotional, physical, or surgical stresses are known to produce the syndrome.[38]

Clinical Manifestations

Only patients with a serum sodium level of less than 120 to 125 mEq/liter may have symptoms of hyponatremia.[1,4,39] The quicker the fall in the level of serum sodium, however, the higher the threshold for symptoms.[39] The symptoms of hyponatremia are altered mental status, headache, nausea and vomiting, asterixis, myoclonus, ataxia, and, in the most severe cases, seizures.

Diagnosis

The diagnosis of hyponatremia depends simply on the laboratory values. The presence of edema, congestive heart failure, or chronic renal failure suggests one set of diseases. The presence of hypovolemia with salt-wasting suggests a set of diseases different from those suggested by the presence of hypovolemia with non-renal salt losses. In patients with hyponatremia and normovolemia, the possibility of pseudohyponatremia due to hyperproteinemia or hyperglycemia must be considered. Hypothyroidism, sick cell syndrome, and essential hyponatremia are difficult to diagnose confidently in the emergency center. The syndrome of inappropriate ADH is a diagnosis of exclusion, as noted earlier. If the serum osmolarity is less than 270 mOsm, the urine osmolarity is more than 300 mOsm, and the urine sodium level is more than 40 mEq/liter on a spot sample, then the urine is inappropriately concentrated, despite a dilute serum, and the syndrome of inappropriate ADH is present.

Treatment

Nonsymptomatic Patients

The treatment of the nonsymptomatic patient with hyponatremia should in general be referred to the internist. The patient with hypervolemia or normovolemia requires fluid restriction to an intake of fluid that equals the insensible losses plus only one-third of the patient's urine output.[1,4] In patients with the syndrome of inappropriate ADH, if fluid restriction has been inadequate, the physician must use drugs that interfere with the action of ADH at the renal level. The drugs that have been used with success are lithium and demeclocycline.[40] Patients with hypovolemia and hyponatremia require the infusion of normal saline, which corrects both the volume deficit and the hyponatremia.[4]

Symptomatic Patients

If the patient is symptomatic, then urgent therapy is required. The water excess may be calculated in the same way as the water deficit. Patients with symptomatic hyponatremia should be treated with hypertonic saline.[41,42] Three percent saline may be administered over three to four hours to a volume of 500 ml. It is important to continue water restriction and administer furosemide, 1 mg/kg.[42] The physician must replace urine volume that is lost with an additional 3 percent saline. The aim of therapy is to remove one-half of the calculated water excess over the first three to four hours of treatment. The physician should check the urine electrolytes every hour, following the serum potassium and replacing as necessary. With these methods, most patients become asymptomatic in less than 12 hours. This vigorous treatment of hyponatremia is designed to achieve a serum sodium level of 120 mEq/liter. Efforts to raise the serum sodium level higher than this are unwarranted, for symptoms are unusual above 120 mEq/liter.

Prehospital and Nursing Care

The assessment of hyponatremia by the prehospital or nursing care team is nondiagnostic and nonspecific. The diagnosis is made in the laboratory. Once the diagnosis of hyponatremia has been made, nursing intervention should include establishment of an IV line and the preparation for a possible seizure in symptomatic patients.

All patients with symptomatic hyponatremia, e.g., altered mental status or seizures, or serum sodium levels lower than 125 mEq/liter should be admitted to the hospital.

POTASSIUM

Physiology

Potassium is found in abundance in the body. The normal adult has approximately 160 mEq/liter, nearly 98 percent of which is found inside the cells.[43] Potassium is also found in high concentrations in gastric secretions, bile, and pancreatic secretions. The serum or interstitial compartment contains 3.5 to 5.3 mEq/liter. Large fluctuations in intracellular potassium are well tolerated by the body, but even very small fluctuations in serum potassium can be life-threatening.

An average daily diet contains 40 to 100 mEq potassium. Although some is lost in feces, perspiration, or during vomiting, most is excreted by the kidney. Normal urine potassium is 40 to 80 mEq/day. Potassium excretion in the kidney varies with sodium retention.[43,44] This mechanism is under the influence of aldosterone, a hormone secreted by the adrenal gland.[5] Aldosterone causes reabsorption of sodium and a loss of potassium at the distal tubule. Potassium is lost in spite of a low serum level of potassium because the kidney cannot conserve it effectively. The amount of sodium and potassium exchanged depends on the amount of sodium delivered to the distal tubule and on the serum aldosterone level. A decrease in aldosterone secretion, as might be seen in adrenal insufficiency or Addison's disease, causes a decrease in sodium reabsorption, resulting in an increase in the amount of potassium retained by the tubules. An aldosterone antagonist, such as spironolactone, could increase the risk of hyperkalemia.

Aldosterone is under the influence of many feedback mechanisms (Fig. 14–3). Hypotension, standing, or low renal perfusion stimulate the kidney to secrete renin. Renin converts a liver protein, angiotensinogen, to angiotensin I, which is in turn converted to the potent hypertensive agent angiotensin II. Angiotensin II stimulates the zona glomerulosa to release increased amounts of aldosterone. High levels of aldosterone, high renal perfusion, or recumbency inhibits renin secretion by the kidney.[5,45]

The role of potassium parallels that of sodium in extracellular fluids, and its physiological action is almost solely related to its concentration in extracellular fluids. Potassium plays an important role in muscular con-

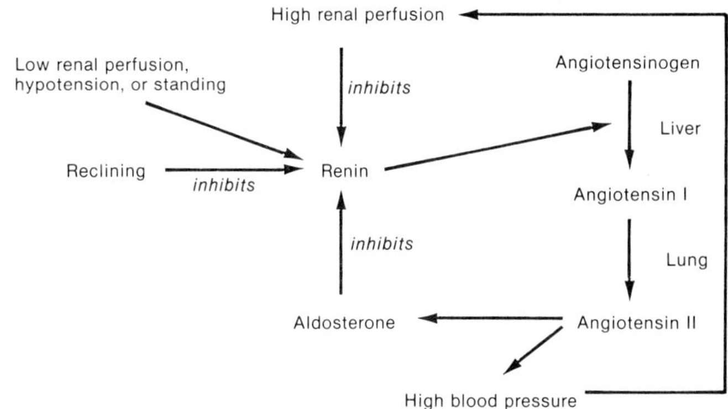

Figure 14–3 Model for Aldosterone, Renin-angiotensin Control Mechanisms. *Note:* Pointing arrows signify stimulation unless otherwise noted.

traction, conduction of nerve impulses, enzyme action, cell membrane function, and acid-base balance.

Acid-Base Balance

Body cells contain buffer systems that can either donate or accept hydrogen ions. Both hydrogen ions and potassium ions freely interchange across the cell membrane. In acidosis, the excess hydrogen ions in the serum migrate into the cells, displacing the potassium ions into the serum. Since the level of extracellular potassium is quite low compared with the intracellular levels, even a very small shift in potassium ions across the cell membrane can cause significant changes in the serum level. As a result, acidosis can cause hyperkalemia.[44]

Alkalosis can cause hypokalemia. The intracellular buffers dissociate to release hydrogen ions, which move out of the cell into the serum. To preserve electrical neutrality, potassium ions move into the cell, causing a decrease in the serum level.

An acid-base imbalance can mask a potassium imbalance. For example, a patient with a very low potassium level could appear to have an almost normal serum level if acidosis has caused potassium ions to move out of the cells into the serum.

The kidneys also influence the relationship of acid-base imbalances to potassium imbalances.[44–48] In acidotic states, the kidneys retain sodium ions instead of hydrogen ions,[49] and the excess hydrogen ions in the renal tubules prevent the normal renal excretion of potassium. In alkalotic states, the kidneys retain sodium and hydrogen ions, and excrete potassium ions into the renal tubules. By these mechanisms, hyperchloremic metabolic acidosis raises potassium 0.6 to 0.9 mEq/liter for each 0.1 decrease in serum pH.[50] However, in a metabolic acidosis with an elevated anion gap, a decrease in serum pH of 0.1 unit may not raise serum potassium at all (Fig. 14–4).[51,52]

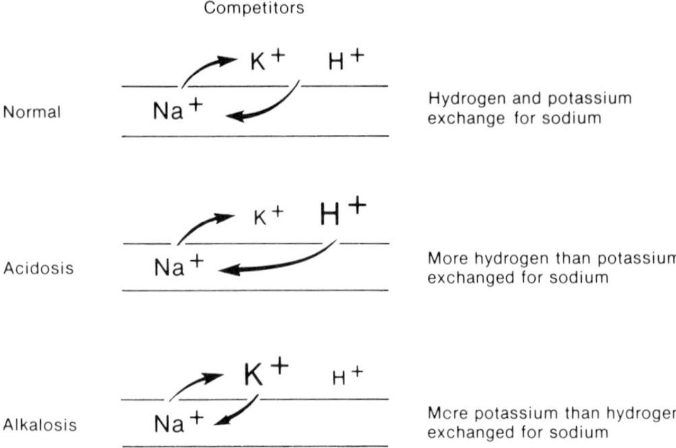

Figure 14–4   Effect of Alkalosis and Acidosis on Potassium-sodium Exchange.

Nerve Conduction and Muscle Contraction

The resting polarization of neurons and all types of muscle fibers (smooth, cardiac, and striated) is determined by the continual diffusion of potassium ions across the cell membrane. The magnitude or potential of the resting polarization is responsible for the duration and velocity of the subsequent action potentials (depolarization and repolarization).

Resting Membrane Potential. A nerve cell, to conduct an impulse, or a muscle cell, to contract and relax, must be polarized or "charged." A cell is polarized when ions of opposite charges are arranged on either side of the cell membrane. This ionic imbalance across the cell membrane creates an electrical "tension" or a potential; as long as the membrane remains undisturbed, the cell maintains itself in this state, referred to as the resting membrane potential. No current flows, since current flows only when negative and positive ions are in the same compartment, not separated by a membrane. The strength of the potential depends on the ionic imbalance across the cell membrane. In this resting state, sodium and potassium, both positively charged ions, establish an equilibrium across the cell membrane with more sodium ions outside and more potassium ions inside. Because the cell also contains negatively charged phosphate and protein molecules, the inside of the cell is more negative. Furthermore, in the resting state, the cell membrane is more permeable to potassium than to sodium; since the ratio of potassium ions inside the cell to those outside is 30:1, potassium can slowly leak out of the cell, causing the extracellular fluid to become less negative.[53,54] Normally, a cardiac muscle cell is polarized with an intracellular charge of -90 mV. During the resting potential phase, the cell is ready to receive a stimulus.

Action Potentials. A stimulus may be electrical (e.g., an impulse from the sinoatrial node), chemical (e.g.,

hypoxia), or mechanical (e.g., chamber dilation). This stimulus changes membrane permeability, which allows sodium to enter the cell. The sodium ions rush in, carrying their positive charges, and the inside of the cell becomes rapidly positive. Because polarity has been changed, the cell is said to be depolarized. Depolarization is an electrochemical event that precedes the mechanical event of contraction.

After depolarization, a series of further ionic movements, termed repolarization, takes place before the ionic balance is restored to the resting state (Fig. 14–5):

- During Phase 4, the cell is in the resting state with an inside negativity of -90 mV. The ionic "pumps" and membrane integrity maintain this resting membrane potential.
- Phase 0 represents the rapid depolarization of the cell. A stimulus causes a sudden change in cellular membrane permeability. Sodium rushes in, changing the polarity and producing the upstroke or first phase of the action potential or depolarization.
- Phase 1 is the initial phase of repolarization.
- During Phase 2, the process of repolarization decelerates, causing a plateau in the action potential. This plateau does not occur in skeletal muscles, but it is necessary in cardiac muscle to allow for a sustained contraction to expel all of the stroke volume from the ventricle. During this phase, calcium ions enter the cell.
- Phase 3 represents the last period of repolarization. Potassium ions enter the cell, and the resting membrane potential is restored.[53,54]

Pathophysiology

The magnitude of the resting membrane potential is dependent on the size of the potassium gradient across the membrane. The action potential (in Phase 0) is dependent on the strength of the resting membrane

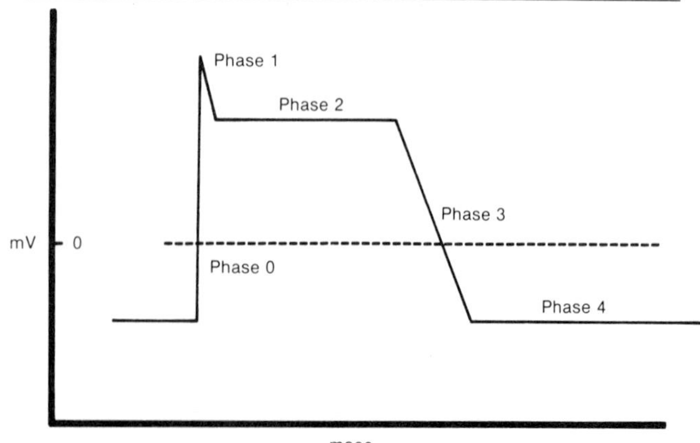

Figure 14–5   Action Potential.

potential, its amplitude (the degree of positive charge after depolarization), and the rate at which this amplitude is reached. These factors determine whether the rapid depolarization necessary to ensure adequate conduction velocity is possible. Contiguous muscle fibers are stimulated faster by a strong action potential and a steep rise in Phase 0.

If a rubber band were attached to the highest peak, stretched down to the point marked -90 mV, and suddenly released, it would snap upward to a point higher than the peak to which it was attached. Because the position was so high, it would take longer to descend. This analogy approximates events that occur in the presence of hypokalemia, which produces an increased electrical gradient across the membrane. A rubber band stretched only half the distance, however, not only would rise more slowly but also would be unable to rise as high. Because the rubber band did not ascend as high, it would take less time to descend. This analogy approximates thc events that occur when levels of potassium ions are elevated in the extracellular fluid and the gradient across the membrane is lessened.

Hypokalemia affects the action potential by increasing the potassium gradient across the cell membrane. The serum deficit facilitates the movement of potassium to the extracellular fluid. This increased negativity increases membrane excitability and interferes with the normal repolarization process. A potassium change from 4 to 2 mEq/liter causes the intracellular/extracellular potassium gradient to change from 30:1 to 60:1,[53,54] which increases the negativity of the resting membrane potential and, thus, increases the amplitude of the action potential. Therefore, in hypokalemia, slight to moderate increases in the amplitudes of P and QRS waves are seen on ECGs. The movement of potassium out of the cardiac cell, which occurs during Phase 3 of repolarization, involves a lower number of potassium molecules. The T wave of the ECG associated with hypokalemia, which is relatively small, reflects Phase 3 of the action potential, or the repolarization process. The fewer potassium molecules moving during Phase 3, the smaller the current generated and the smaller the T wave on the ECG. Owing to the increased magnitude of the action potential, Phase 3 is prolonged, resulting in a broad T wave.

U waves are positive deflections that are more than 1 mm in height and follow the position of the T waves on the ECG. U waves are characteristic of hypokalemia and are best seen in leads V_2 and V_3. They are secondary to repolarization of Purkinje fibers or to myocardial stretch potentials evoked during myocardial relaxation.

Hyperkalemia with a potassium change from 4 to 8 mEq/liter decreases the intracellular/extracellular potassium gradient from 30:1 to 15:1.[53,54] Such a change decreases both the negativity of the resting membrane

potential and the height of the action potential. Hyperkalemia, therefore, decreases the amplitude of the P and QRS waves. Advanced hyperkalemia decreases automaticity, increases atrioventricular conduction abnormalities, and produces asystole.[54] In hyperkalemia, the movement of potassium during Phase 3 involves a large number of potassium molecules; therefore, more current is generated and the amplitude of the T-wave height is increased, as is characteristic of hyperkalemia. Owing to the decreased magnitude of the action potential, Phase 3 is shortened, resulting in a peaked, short T wave. Hyponatremia and hypocalcemia increase membrane permeability to potassium and enhance the effects of hyperkalemia on the ECG and on the heart.[53]

HYPOKALEMIA

The causes of hypokalemia can be divided into two types: those associated with normotension and those associated with hypertension.

Normotensive Conditions

There are many causes of hypokalemia associated with normotension.

Poor Intake

Hypokalemia is common in cases of starvation. Despite inanition, there is an obligatory potassium loss of 5 to 15 mEq/day in the urine.[55] Ketones produced as a result of starvation serve as organic anions in the distal tubule. Their anionic charge produces an electrical gradient for cations, such as potassium,[56] causing the movement of potassium into the distal tubule and increasing potassium excretion.

Emesis

Another common cause of hypokalemia is emesis. The potassium concentration in gastric secretions is only 10 mEq/liter and therefore accounts for only minimal potassium loss during emesis.[43,44] During regurgitation, however, hydrochloric acid is lost from the stomach and a metabolic alkalosis develops. This alkalosis encourages the elimination of potassium by a renal mechanism.[44]

Diarrhea

Potassium concentration is greater than sodium concentration in diarrheal fluid, and diarrhea is a frequent cause of hypokalemia. The potassium loss with diarrhea varies with the volume and frequency of the stool. Villous adenoma in the colon may produce diarrhea and profound potassium depletion, and it should be considered in any patient with diarrhea and marked hypokalemia.[57] Some patients may abuse laxatives, causing diarrhea. Historically, these patients often deny laxative abuse, however. Their condition may simulate Bartter's syndrome, with high renin and low serum aldosterone levels that are unaffected by postural changes (Fig. 14–3).[58–60]

Bartter's Syndrome

Although there is a familial association with mental retardation, many patients with Bartter's syndrome have normal intelligence. There is an increased incidence in blacks. The histopathology demonstrates a hyperplasia in the cells located between the glomeruli and the macula densa; this is termed juxtaglomerular hyperplasia. These juxtaglomerular cells secrete renin.

A model of this syndrome was proposed by Bartter.[61] Although the model does not explain all the more recent findings, such as the role of prostaglandin E_2 in the pathogenesis of this syndrome,[62] it is still quite useful in understanding the different hormonal interactions in these patients. Bartter proposed that the mechanism for this syndrome is a hyporesponsiveness of the vasculature to angiotensin.[61] To compensate and maintain normotension, the juxtaglomerular cells produce excessive amounts of renin. High levels of angiotensin persist, however; these high levels of angiotensin stimulate aldosterone production, which causes hypokalemia. The hypokalemia in Bartter's syndrome impairs the renal ability to form urine (hyposthenuria) and, therefore, produces a nephrogenic diabetes insipidus. The severity of the hypokalemia in Bartter's syndrome usually varies from values of 1.5 to 2.5 mEq/liter.

Renal Tubular Acidosis

In Type I renal tubular acidosis, hydrogen ions cannot be secreted into the distal tubule. In Type II renal tubular acidosis, the kidney is unable to reabsorb bicarbonate in the proximal tubule.[63,64] Hypokalemia occurs because the net effect of renal tubular acidosis is to increase bicarbonate within the lumen of the distal tubule. Bicarbonate, with its negative charge, provides an electrical gradient for the migration of potassium to the lumen as well.[63,64]

Drugs

Carbenicillin and gentamicin both serve as nondiffusible anions within the distal tubule; therefore, they produce an electrical gradient that encourages the positively charged potassium ions to migrate into the distal tubule.[65] In addition, because each gram of carbenicillin contains 4.7 mEq sodium, carbenicillin increases the delivery of sodium to the distal tubule. This mechanism provides more sodium for exchange with potassium at the distal tubule by the normal physiologic mechanisms of aldosterone.

Amphotericin B may produce hypokalemia by causing a renal tubular acidosis.[66] This is a common finding in patients on amphotericin B.

Acetazolamide is an inhibitor of the enzyme carbonic anhydrase. Because of this inhibition, the urine is alkalinized, which produces an excess of bicarbonate within the renal tubule and an electrical gradient for the migration of potassium within the distal tubule.[67] Therefore, this alkalinization of the urine produces hypokalemia in the same way that renal tubular acidosis does.

Diuretic medications, such as mannitol, glycerol, furosemide, ethacrynic acid, and the thiazides increase delivery of sodium to the distal tubule so that more sodium is available for exchange with potassium.[43,44] This increased availability results in hypokalemia through the normal physiologic mechanisms of aldosterone. Similarly, other causes of diuresis, such as postobstructive diuresis, diabetic ketoacidosis, or the diuretic phase of acute tubular necrosis, may produce hypokalemia.

Acute Leukemia

In patients with acute leukemia, the chronic secretion of lysozyme may cause renal tubular damage.[68] This damage may result in renal potassium-wasting and explain the hypokalemia occasionally seen in these patients.

Transcellular Shifts

The sudden shift of potassium from the extracellular space to the intracellular space may result in hypokalemia on a serum sample. These transcellular shifts occur in several situations.

Alkalosis. Acute respiratory alkalosis, chronic metabolic alkalosis, and acute metabolic alkalosis all induce a renal loss of potassium. For reasons that are still unclear, hypokalemia does not occur in patients with chronic respiratory alkalosis.

Periodic Paralysis. The hypokalemic variety of periodic paralysis is inherited as an autosomal dominant trait. In these patients, there is no change in the urinary potassium excretion during periods of hypokalemia; therefore, the hypokalemia must be due to a shift of potassium from the extracellular fluid to the intracellular fluid. Adrenocorticotropic hormone (ACTH) induces attacks, but its effect is blocked by metyrapone, an agent that inhibits glucocorticoid synthesis by the adrenal cortex. The clinical manifestations of the hypokalemic form of periodic paralysis have an abrupt onset, usually within 10 to 20 minutes after various precipitating factors. Such factors include rest following exercise, high carbohydrate intake, infection, trauma, emotional stress, and ethanol ingestion. These manifestations last for approximately 24 hours.[43,44,69]

Insulin. In the therapy of patients with hyperglycemia, insulin encourages transport of glucose into the intracellular space.[70] Along with glucose, potassium is transported into the intracellular space, occasionally resulting in hypokalemia.

Trauma. In patients with marked trauma, hypokalemia seems to correlate with the degree of trauma.[71] The mechanism of this hypokalemia seems to involve a transcellular shift.

Heat Stroke

In patients with heat stroke, an acute respiratory alkalosis that may be due to exercise or to hyperventilation for heat dissipation is prominent. This acute respiratory alkalosis is responsible, in part, for the hypokalemia seen in patients with heat stroke. In addition, mucocutaneous fluid losses and hypovolemia may induce a physiologic aldosteronism that is a contributing factor to this hypokalemia,[72,73] since sweating results in an obligatory potassium loss under the control of aldosterone.[5]

Barium Poisoning

In barium poisoning, which may be induced by the ingestion of certain pesticides or depilatories, the patients have nausea, vomiting, and diarrhea. The severe hypokalemia that occurs is due to gastrointestinal losses.[74] It may be so severe that it produces arrhythmias or flaccid paralysis.

Vitamin B_{12} Therapy

During the therapy of pernicious anemia with vitamin B_{12}, there is a rapid formation of new platelets and erythrocytes. Formation of the new cells involves the formation of an intracellular space for each cell and the rapid uptake of potassium from the extracellular environment.[75] This mechanism is proposed to explain the occurrence of hypokalemia in association with vitamin B_{12} therapy.

Hypertensive Conditions

Hyperaldosteronism or Conn's Syndrome

Patients with inappropriately high levels of aldosterone usually have adrenal adenomas.[76–78] Occasionally, these patients may have adrenal hyperplasia. Patients with adrenal adenoma can not be distinguished from patients with adrenal hyperplasia by the serum aldo-

sterone level.[77] The striking feature of the high level of aldosterone in these conditions is that it is unresponsive to normal physiologic controls, e.g., it persists even when the patient is recumbent (Fig. 14–3).[77] This hyperaldosteronism continuously and primarily inhibits renin production, resulting in low plasma renin levels. This low renin production is also unresponsive to physiologic controls and persists despite volume contraction with diuretics or prolonged standing.

Cushing's Syndrome

The most common cause of Cushing's syndrome is adenoma of the adrenal cortex. Although unusual, carcinoma of the adrenal gland may also produce Cushing's syndrome. In addition, a pituitary adenoma that secretes excessive amounts of ACTH may induce bilateral adrenal hyperplasia. This cause of Cushing's syndrome is termed Cushing's disease.

The clinical manifestations of Cushing's syndrome are: truncal obesity, buccal fat pad, purple striae, ecchymosis, acne, hirsutism, and a buffalo hump.

Accelerated Hypertension

Hyperreninemia as a primary cause of accelerated hypertension results in increased serum aldosterone levels (Fig. 14–3), which, in turn, produces hypokalemia.[79] The clinical manifestations of accelerated hypertension are well described (see Chapter 52, Hypertensive Emergencies).

Renal Artery Stenosis

Renal artery hypoperfusion may induce hyperreninemia and therefore elevate angiotensin levels and serum aldosterone levels, which in turn produces hypokalemia (Fig. 14–3).[80] The salient clinical manifestations of renal artery stenosis are hypertension with an abdominal bruit.

Hemangiopericytoma or Robertson-Kihara Syndrome

A tumor of the juxtaglomerular cells may cause them to produce an excessive amount of renin.[43,44] The condition, called hemangiopericytoma or Robertson-Kihara syndrome, is characterized by hypertension, hyperreninemia, hyperaldosteronism, and hypokalemia.

Adrenogenital Syndrome

A disease in which there is a defect in the synthesis of adrenocorticoids is referred to as an adrenogenital syndrome. Many of these syndromes result in masculinization. A defect in hydrocortisone synthesis of the zona fasciculata of the adrenal cortex, owing to 11-

hydroxylase or 17-hydroxylase deficiency, may produce hypertension and hypokalemia in association with the adrenogenital syndrome.[43,44]

Because glucocorticoid levels are diminished in patients with these hydroxylase deficiencies, the pituitary gland secretes more ACTH to maintain adequate glucocorticoid levels. The glucocorticoid that substitutes for hydrocortisone is desoxycorticosterone. The elevated ACTH level also stimulates the zona glomerulosa of the adrenal cortex to synthesize aldosterone, thereby producing hypertension and hypokalemia.

The elevated ACTH levels and the blocked synthesis of hydrocortisone make it necessary for other glucocorticoid synthetic pathways to be utilized; this results in glucocorticoids with strong androgenic and masculinizing effects. Therefore, this syndrome often is seen in females who have had masculinized features from birth. A masculinized male patient may be less obvious. In addition, childhood hypertension suggests an adrenogenital syndrome.

Licorice Extract (Glycyrrhizic Acid)

Within licorice is a substance called glycyrrhizic acid that is biochemically similar to aldosterone and has many of the same clinical effects as aldosterone.[81] This substance is found in pipe tobacco and extracts for alcoholic beverages.[82] It can cause hypertension, hypokalemia, and laboratory evidence of hyperaldosteronism, i.e., a low plasma renin value unresponsive to provocative measures, but a low level of serum aldosterone.[81,82]

Clinical Manifestations

A low serum potassium level results in impaired neuromuscular function with profound weakness and cramping of skeletal muscle, leading to impaired ventilation or even rhabdomyolysis, and smooth muscle, producing distention and ileus.[43] In addition, hypokalemia may produce a nephrogenic diabetes insipidus and hyposthenuria (see Hypernatremia and Fluid Deficit), referred to as hypokalemic nephropathy.[44]

The ECG shows decreased amplitude and broadening of T waves, prominent U waves, sagging ST segments, and, at times, T-wave inversion in precordial leads and prolongation of the PR interval. The QT interval often appears prolonged because the T wave is difficult to discern from the U wave; however, it is actually of normal duration. This is referred to as pseudo–QT interval prolongation.[54] The best lead to measure the QT interval is aV_L, where the U waves are the smallest.[54]

Hypokalemia potentiates the toxicity of digitalized patients. Atrioventricular conduction defects, ventricular ectopic beats, tachycardias, ventricular fibrillation, or asystole also may occur. Hypokalemia decreases the effectiveness of vasoconstrictive pressors.[72] Myopathy may be severe enough to cause rhabdomyolysis and myoglobulinuria.[43]

Diagnosis

The method by which a potassium value is obtained may strongly affect the result. Hemolysis, which may occur during phlebotomy when the tourniquet remains too long on the arm, may profoundly elevate a serum potassium. In addition, agitation of a blood sample by passing it through a small-bore needle rapidly or by shaking the sample of blood in a glass tube may cause lysis of erythrocytes.

The serum should be rapidly separated from the cellular elements in the blood sample to obtain an accurate potassium value. If the blood components are not separated for prolonged periods of time, potassium will "leak" from the intracellular space into the serum, artificially raising potassium values. This effect is most prominent in patients with marked thrombocytosis or leukocytosis and produces a pseudohyperkalemia. Some patients have particularly "leaky" cells—a trait that is inherited on an autosomal dominant basis. These "leaky" cells are of no clinical concern, except that they routinely elevate the serum potassium unless blood samples have the cellular elements rapidly separated from the serum.

Hyperviscosity, as occurs in dehydration or Waldenström's macroglobulinemia, may artificially lower serum potassium by decreasing the amount of fluid that can be aspirated by the roller pump diluters of the automated blood analyzers.[25] It is recommended that, if a potassium abnormality is significant and important, a repeat value should be obtained by means of a different technique before intensive therapy for the abnormality is undertaken. The repeat value should be determined from an arterial blood sample that was obtained without a tourniquet on the arm during a phlebotomy.[83] In addition, rapid centrifugation of a plasma sample is preferable.

The ECG changes seen with hypokalemia may raise the index of suspicion for this abnormality even before the potassium value has been determined. The characteristic ECG changes are seen in 75 percent of patients with a potassium of less than 3 mEq/liter. Occasionally, the characteristic ECG changes of hypokalemia are seen in patients with a normal serum potassium but a depleted total body store of potassium.

Therapy

The following is a useful guide for the estimation of potassium deficits[6]:

1. In patients with potassium values of 3 to 3.5 mEq/liter, the associated deficit in total body potassium is 150 to 200 mEq.
2. Potassium values of 2.5 to 3 mEq/liter are associated with a total body potassium deficit of 300 mEq.
3. Potassium values of 2 to 2.5 mEq/liter are associated with a total body potassium deficit of 500 mEq.

Asymptomatic without Arrhythmias

In patients who are asymptomatic and do not have arrhythmias, one-half the potassium deficit can be replaced over 24 hours and the remainder replaced over the next 48 hours. It is important to account for any urinary losses of potassium that occur during this potassium replacement. In general, the physician should not replace potassium until an adequate urine output is ensured. In patients who have an asymptomatic hypokalemia without any arrhythmias, the oral route is preferable, provided an ileus is not present and the patient can ingest and absorb oral potassium. The effervescent solution of potassium Klorvess has been independently evaluated as the best tasting of the oral potassium preparations.[84] In addition, Klorvess is as inexpensive as potassium chloride solution. Potassium chloride salt found in Morton's salt substitute contains 27 mEq potassium chloride in each one-half teaspoon and is 15-fold cheaper than potassium chloride solution. Morton's salt substitute is an acceptable oral regimen for potassium chloride replacement.[85] If the etiology of hypokalemia is unclear, these patients should be referred to an internist.

Mildly to Moderately Symptomatic without Arrhythmias

The treatment of the patient with mildly to moderately symptomatic hypokalemia without arrhythmias requires more aggressive potassium replacement than the asymptomatic patient. One-half the deficit of serum potassium should be replaced over the first 12 hours of therapy, with the remainder of the deficit replaced over the next 24 hours. The physician should not replace potassium until adequate urine output is ensured, and all urine potassium lost during replacement must be considered. If possible, the oral route is preferable, and the recommendations for treatment of the asymptomatic hypokalemic patient can be followed. If oral therapy cannot be instituted, then IV therapy is indicated. During IV therapy ECG monitoring is desirable, since potassium is being administered more rapidly to these patients.

Patients with mildly to moderately symptomatic hypokalemia without arrhythmias should be admitted to the hospital if the etiology of the hypokalemia is unclear or if oral therapy is not possible, since prolonged therapy over a 36-hour period is indicated.

Severely Symptomatic with Arrhythmias

Patients with severe hypokalemia that causes impaired ventilation, rhabdomyolysis, or arrhythmias (e.g., ventricular tachycardia) require urgent treatment. One-half of the potassium deficit should be replaced over the first 6 hours and the remainder replaced over the next 24 hours. For this type of therapy, the IV route and ECG monitoring are essential. Potassium chloride at a rate of 40 mEq/hour or in solutions containing more than 40 mEq potassium should be administered only with ECG monitoring.[6] More than 60 mEq/hour should not be administered except under the most extraordinary circumstances. Potassium should not be administered through a central venous catheter because local hyperkalemia may result in myocardial arrhythmias, heart block, or asystole.[86]

All patients with hypokalemia that are severely symptomatic or manifest arrhythmias due to their hypokalemia should be admitted to the hospital.

Therapy of Specific Causes of Hypokalemia

The therapy of Bartter's syndrome is aided by the use of indomethacin.[62]

The therapy of periodic paralysis involves acetazolamide, which produces a metabolic acidosis and decreases the ability of potassium to enter the intracellular fluid. In addition, these patients are usually placed on spironolactone, which encourages the development of hyperkalemia because it is an aldosterone antagonist.[43,44,69]

Prehospital and Nursing Assessment and Intervention

The signs and symptoms of hypokalemia are only suggestive and are highly nonspecific. Only supportive therapy should be instituted before the serum potassium value is known. Clearly, an IV catheter should be placed in any patient with significant arrhythmias.

HYPERKALEMIA

Etiology

Hyperkalemia is one of the most serious electrolytic disturbances and can be immediately life-threatening. The emergency physician must be familiar with its etiology.

Pseudohyperkalemia

As mentioned earlier, potassium may "leak" into the serum of patients with thrombocytosis or leukocytosis if the serum is not rapidly removed from the cellular elements.[44] In fact, there is a familial disorder, inherited as an autosomal dominant trait, in which the erythrocytes "leak" potassium in vitro; however, these patients do not have a true elevated serum potassium,[87] and the condition is of no clinical concern.

Increased Exogenous Potassium Load

Patients with normal renal function can handle large amounts of exogenous potassium, but patients with renal failure may develop hyperkalemia with even small amounts of exogenous potassium. For example, whole blood more than ten days old contains potassium in amounts of 10 to 15 mEq/liter and may cause hyperkalemia if administered in large quantities.[88] Both potassium penicillin and oral or IV potassium may result in hyperkalemia in patients with any degree of renal failure.[6]

Increased Potassium Production

Tissue destruction may increase the amount of potassium released from the intracellular fluid.[44] This cellular damage occurs in patients with massive crush injury, burns, gangrene, and rhabdomyolysis. Destruction of tumors, such as lymphomas and leukemias, may also damage cells.

The administration of succinylcholine, a depolarizing muscle relaxant, produces muscle contraction and fasciculations that occur before paralysis. These extensive muscular reactions may also induce the release of additional potassium from the muscles and result in hyperkalemia.[89–91] These effects of succinylcholine may be prevented by pretreatment of the patient with diazepam before the administration of succinylcholine.

Transcellular Shifts

Shifting of potassium from the intracellular space to the extracellular space may be responsible for hyperkalemia.

Acute Digitalis Overdose. Digitalis inhibits the sodium-potassium adenosine triphosphate system, which maintains a normal sodium-potassium gradient in cells.[44] Through this inhibition, excessive amounts of potassium are permitted to remain in the extracellular space, resulting in hyperkalemia.

Periodic Paralysis. Patients with periodic paralysis are usually less than ten years of age. The onset of paralysis is abrupt, occurring over a period of 30 minutes; paralysis persists for less than 12 hours. These patients have an increased urinary potassium level, but a decreased urinary sodium level. This hyperkalemia is associated with hyponatremia and metabolic acidosis.[44]

Hyperosmolar Diuresis. The administration of hypertonic solutions, such as mannitol, may cause a diuresis. Potassium may shift from the intracellular space to the extracellular space,[92] resulting in hyperkalemia.

Acidosis. The mechanism by which acidosis causes hyperkalemia has been discussed (see Potassium, Physiology). Hyperkalemia in the presence of acidosis is much more prominent in hyperchloremic metabolic acidosis (as with administration of arginine hydrochloride) than in increased anion gap metabolic acidosis.

Decreased Renal Potassium Excretion. Patients with acute or chronic renal failure are unable to excrete potassium. Some patients have a selective renal defect in the excretion of potassium into the distal tubule and, therefore, develop hyperkalemia.

Aldosterone Antagonism or Deficit. Patients on potassium-sparing diuretics such as triamterene or the aldosterone antagonist, spironolactone, may develop hyperkalemia. Patients with hypoaldosteronism due to Addison's disease or hypopituitarism also may have hyperkalemia.[44]

Juxtaglomerular Hypoplasia

The juxtaglomerular apparatus produces renin (Fig. 14–3). Some patients have a juxtaglomerular hypoplasia and, therefore, have a hyporeninemic hypoaldosteronism.[93,94] Even when these patients stand or ingest diuretics, the hyporeninemia and the hypoaldosteronism persist. These patients usually have mild to moderate renal disease. This condition is associated with diabetes mellitus, gout, pseudogout, or hyperparathyroidism.[95] Although rare, some patients have a selective deficit in their aldosterone secretion; however, patients with this selective hypoaldosteronism have normal renin levels.[44,96]

Adrenogenital Syndrome

In the form of the adrenogenital syndrome with the 21-hydroxylase deficiency, patients do not synthesize aldosterone.[97] This deficit in the synthesis of aldosterone produces masculinization from birth, hyperkalemia, and salt-wasting at the renal level. These patients are normotensive, owing to the effect of other corticosteroids and angiotensin.

Miscellaneous

Heparin and acute barium poisoning may also cause hyperkalemia.

Clinical Manifestations

The ECG provides critical information to the emergency physician. The earliest manifestations of hyperkalemia with potassium values greater than 7 mEq/liter are prominent, tall, peaked T waves. Only 20 percent of patients with potassium values of 7 mEq/liter have such T waves.[98]

Potassium values of 8 to 10 mEq/liter produce prolonged PR and QRS intervals and decreased P-wave height. At these values, the ST segment may be elevated, superimposed upon the previously mentioned ECG abnormalities, a classic sine wave pattern of hyperkalemia occurs.[53,54] This pattern is frequently accompanied by bradycardia and sudden asystole, without intervening ventricular fibrillation.

Diagnosis

Hyperkalemia should be suspected in the emergency department even before laboratory values have been obtained. In addition, ECG monitoring of any patient with a potassium value of more than 6.5 mEq/liter should be initiated at once because hyperkalemia with ECG findings requires immediate therapy.

The differential diagnosis of hyperkalemia is based on the findings on the ECG. Tall, peaked T waves may be found congenitally or may occur early in patients with acute myocardial infarction. The broad QRS complex seen in patients with hyperkalemia must be distinguished from that caused by a left bundle branch block. In hyperkalemia, the left precordial leads show a wide S wave that is not found in patients with left bundle branch block. It is impossible to distinguish a slow, wide complex idioventricular rhythm of an agonal heart from the effects of hyperkalemia.[53]

Therapy

In patients with potassium values less than 7 mEq/liter and no ECG changes, it is important to reverse the underlying cause. If this is not possible, the emergency physician should administer sodium polystyrene sulfonate (Kayexalate) to maintain serum potassium values less than 5.5 mEq/liter. Kayexalate is a sodium-potassium cation resin that exchanges 2 mEq sodium for each mEq potassium. One mEq of the total body potassium store is removed per gram of Kayexalate.[6] The dose of Kayexalate, if administered orally, is 20 gm three times a day with 50 ml 20 percent mannitol. The mannitol is a cathartic and is added because Kayexalate is highly constipating. This dose of Kayexalate contains 120 mEq sodium/day.[44] These patients should be admitted to the hospital if the etiology of the hyperkalemia is unclear or the hyperkalemia proves difficult to reverse. In any case, they should be referred to an internist.

In patients with potassium values more than 7 mEq/liter and either no ECG changes or only tall, peaked T waves, it is also important to reverse the underlying cause. These patients should receive Kayexalate to remove potassium from the body. Dosage is the same as that just described.

In patients who are obtunded, Kayexalate can be administered as a 50-gm retention enema in 200 ml mannitol every one to two hours. Each dose so administered decreases the serum potassium 0.25 to 0.50 mEq. All patients in this category should be admitted to the hospital.

Severe Hyperkalemia

Patients with hyperkalemia and a broad QRS complex, a prolonged PR interval, or a decreased P-wave height in the appropriate clinical setting, for example, in the presence of renal disease, should receive treatment even before the potassium value returns from the laboratory. The institution of therapy must be immediate—these ECG findings represent a life-threatening emergency.

Calcium Gluconate. A first-line drug to be administered to patients with this severe hyperkalemia is calcium gluconate. It increases the permeability of the cell membrane to potassium and immediately reverses electrophysiologic manifestations of hyperkalemia. One to three ampules or 4 to 12 mEq of a 10 percent solution of calcium gluconate should be administered over 3 to 5 minutes.[44] The patient's ECG should be monitored. The effect of calcium gluconate has its onset within 1 to 5 minutes, but its duration of action is brief, only 30 minutes. More long-lasting therapy is needed.

Glucose-Insulin Infusion. An important second-line therapy for hyperkalemia is glucose-insulin infusion; it should be administered promptly. The dose is 1 unit insulin per 3 to 4 gm glucose. In a typical solution, 500 ml 10 percent dextrose in water is administered with 15 units regular insulin. This solution should be administered over 30 minutes, and the infusion slowed to maintain normokalemia. The onset of action is 30 minutes, and the duration is four to five hours.[6,44,99]

Sodium Bicarbonate. When the acid-base status of the patient is unknown or if the patient is alkalotic, 80 to 120 mEq sodium bicarbonate in 1 liter 5 percent dextrose and water should be administered over one to two hours. This therapy is effective within 20 to 40 minutes, and the duration of its action is four to five hours. When the acid-base status of the patient, however, shows metabolic acidosis, 80 to 120 mEq sodium bicarbonate may be administered over 2 to 3 minutes.[44]

Kayexalate. Either orally or by retention enema, Kayexalate should be administered in all patients with severe hyperkalemia. The administration of Kayexalate should not be delayed in the emergency department.

Dialysis. Hemodialysis or peritoneal dialysis is the treatment of choice for hyperkalemia in a patient with moderate to severe renal failure. These patients can not tolerate the high sodium load that is concomitantly administered with Kayexalate. In addition, any patient who does not respond appropriately to therapy with calcium gluconate, glucose-insulin infusion, sodium bicarbonate, and Kayexalate should be considered for immediate dialysis.

Specific Therapy

Patients with a renal potassium defect should receive diuretics, such as hydrochlorothiazide or furosemide (Lasix), which tend to induce a more normokalemic situation.

Patients with hyporeninemic hypoaldosteronism, selective hypoaldosteronism, or adrenogenital syndrome need mineralocorticoid replacement. The synthetic mineralocorticoid 9-α-fluorohydrocortisone or Florinef may be administered at a dose of 0.1 mg/day.

Prehospital and Nursing Assessment and Intervention

If the prehospital care team notes the ECG findings of hyperkalemia in the presence of hypotension, arrhythmias, electrical mechanical dissociation, or cardiac arrest, immediate therapy is required. Therapy with calcium gluconate, glucose-insulin, and sodium bicarbonate should be instituted as noted. If calcium gluconate is unavailable, calcium chloride may be substituted.

A nurse recognizing ECG manifestations of hyperkalemia should immediately establish an IV catheter and obtain a potassium value. The patient should have bedside ECG monitoring. Calcium chloride should be placed at the patient's bedside and the physician notified immediately.

CALCIUM

Physiology

The serum calcium level is affected by several different factors. Parathormone, a hormone secreted by the parathyroid gland, maintains serum calcium by stimulating osteoclastic activity that mobilizes the bony stores of calcium.[100] The renal mechanism involves the conversion of adenosine triphosphate (ATP) to cAMP, a second messenger that affects parathormone action and causes renal tubular excretion of phosphate and reabsorption of calcium and chloride. Parathormone also facilitates transport of calcium across the duodenal mucosa. Parathormone is controlled by feedback inhibition in which hypercalcemia suppresses parathormone secretion.

Vitamin D or calciferol, after absorption, is 25-hydroxylated in the liver and subsequently 1-hydroxylated in the kidney to form the active vitamin D, 1,25-hydroxylated calciferol. This active form increases calcium absorption from the gastrointestinal tract.[101]

Calcium is 50 percent protein-bound, mostly to albumin. Calcium values obtained from the laboratory reflect total calcium, that is, free plus protein-bound calcium.[100] This protein-bound calcium is in equilibrium with free calcium, and this balance is affected by the acid-base status of the patient. The free calcium is responsible for symptoms of either hypercalcemia or hypocalcemia. If albumin decreases 0.8 to 1 gm/dl, then total calcium diminishes 0.8 to 1 mg/dl, owing to the decrease in protein-bound calcium.[100] The free calcium, however, remains unchanged.

Alkalosis increases the electronegativity of proteins, so that more calcium is bound to the proteins and less calcium is free; therefore, symptoms of hypocalcemia may occur.[100] A respiratory condition such as respiratory alkalosis in association with hyperventilation may reduce the level of free calcium in the serum and produce symptoms identical to those of hypocalcemia. During alkalosis, total calcium (bound plus free) does not change; since the laboratory routinely measures only total calcium, this value is normal in the presence of alkalosis.

Acidosis decreases the electronegativity of proteins; therefore, less calcium is bound to proteins, and more calcium is free. Again, total calcium value remains unchanged.

Pathophysiology

Elevated levels of calcium stimulate the production of gastrin, which increases acid secretion and predisposes to peptic ulcer disease and pancreatitis.[100–104] Patients who have experienced prolonged periods of hypercalcemia may develop renal stones or nephrolithiasis or calcifications throughout the kidney, termed nephrocalcinosis, and renal failure.[105]

Hypercalcemia has marked effects on the ECG. It shortens the duration of Phase 2 of the action potential and causes a shortening of the ST segment on the ECG (see Potassium, Physiology).[106] In addition, calcium increases the duration of the ventricular ejection and causes a prolonged inotropic action.

Hypocalcemia has several important pathophysiological effects. A chronically low level of calcium in the serum and a high level of calcium in the lens results in cataracts.[100,107] Low levels of calcium, in addition, prevent troponin from inhibiting actin-myosin interaction; therefore, muscle contraction and even tetany may occur.[100,107]

The cardiac effects of hypocalcemia include a prolongation of the duration of Phase 2 of the action potential, thereby causing a prolonged ST segment on the ECG.[106] Hypocalcemia is the only cause of a prolonged ST segment. In addition, hypocalcemia shortens the duration of ventricular ejection.

HYPERCALCEMIA

Etiology

Carcinoma

The most common cause of hypercalcemia is carcinoma; in one series the incidence was 20 percent.[108–110] There are several mechanisms by which carcinoma produces hypercalcemia. Metastatic disease may induce bony destruction and thereby cause calcium release. Certain tumors may produce a parathormonelike substance that also causes the release of calcium. The mechanism of hypercalcemia in some tumors is unclear, but, in some manner, prostaglandin E_2 seems to be involved.[108,109,111–113] The cancers most often associated with hypercalcemia are those of lung, breast, and kidney, and multiple myeloma. The prognosis of patients with multiple myeloma and hypercalcemia is particularly poor.[114,115]

Hyperparathyroidism

The incidence of hyperparathyroidism is 2/100 cases of hypercalcemia. Hyperparathyroidism is frequently diagnosed in asymptomatic patients by means of automated chemistry tests.[116–118] In 80 percent of cases, the pathogenesis is an adenoma of the parathyroid. In 15 percent of the cases, it is diffuse hyperplasia of the parathyroid glands.[119]

With primary hyperparathyroidism, calcium values may be high or simply high-normal with an inappropriately high value of parathormone. Since parathormone increases the tubular reabsorption of chloride and enhances the secretion of phosphorus, a high chloride to phosphorus ratio, that is, more than 33:1, is maintained in 96 percent of cases.[120] The serum chloride is almost invariably more than 102 mEq/liter unless the patient has received diuretics; because diuretics enhance chloride secretion, the physician can not use this criterion in a patient on diuretics.[109] In addition, diuretics such as thiazide may increase the serum calcium level.[100] Since parathormone functions by a cAMP mechanism, the urinary cAMP value also is elevated in cases of primary hyperparathyroidism.

In hyperparathyroidism, there is prominent resorption of subperiosteal bone of the fingers and toes.[119] There is a central resorption of the vertebrae, resulting in alternating radiolucent and radiodense areas of the vertebrae. Owing to excess parathormone secretion, bony cysts may result from resorption of bone; this is called osteitis fibrosa cystica.[119] A late finding in hyperparathyroidism is resorption of the distal one-third of the clavicle.

Patients with suspected hyperparathyroidism should be referred to an internist.

Multiple Endocrine Adenopathies

Patients with a Type I multiple endocrine adenopathy, e.g., Wermer's syndrome, have adenomas in multiple endocrine organs.[100] Hypercalcemia is due to adenomas of the parathyroid. These patients may also have adenomas of the pituitary, adrenal cortex, pancreas, and, less commonly, the adrenal medulla and thyroid gland. Sipple's syndrome, a Type II multiple endocrine adenopathy, consists of adenomas of the parathyroid, explaining the hypercalcemia; adenomas of the adrenal medulla with pheochromocytoma; and medullary carcinoma of the thyroid.[100]

Sarcoidosis

Hypercalcemia may occur in association with sarcoidosis. In sarcoidosis there is increased gastrointestinal absorption of calcium and increased reabsorption of bone.[121,122]

Vitamin D

With excessive amounts of exogenous vitamin D (more than 150,000 IU/day), gastrointestinal absorption of calcium may be increased.[123,124] These patients are frequently health food faddists. Laboratory examination reveals an elevated serum phosphorus because the hypercalcemia suppresses parathormone levels.[100] These low parathormone levels, in turn, diminish tubular secretion of phosphorus.

Immobilization

During periods of immobilization, bony stores of calcium are mobilized in children and young adults, and hypercalcemia may occur.[100] Elderly patients with Paget's disease who are immobilized have increased osteoclastic activity that mobilizes their bony calcium stores, and they may also develop hypercalcemia.[100]

Renal Failure

Patients with chronic renal failure are unable to excrete calcium and therefore should be cautioned against excessive calcium intake. An increased calcium load in the presence of acute renal failure may result in hypercalcemia.[125,126] Calcium released during rhabdomyolysis, for example, may produce hypercalcemia because of the diminished ability of the kidney to excrete calcium. Classically, this occurs during the diuretic phase of acute tubular necrosis in patients with rhabdomyolysis.

Milk-Alkali Syndrome (Burnett's Syndrome)

Increased intake of calcium in the form of calcium carbonate antacids and milk in the treatment of peptic ulcer disease has been associated with severe hypercalcemia and nephrocalcinosis.[127] With the use of other treatments for peptic ulcer disease, this syndrome has markedly decreased in frequency.

Miscellaneous

Other conditions, such as hyperthyroidism (20 percent incidence), acromegaly, pheochromocytoma, and Addison's disease (endocrinopathies), are occasionally associated with hypercalcemia.[100,108,128,129]

Renal Transplant

During the first six months after surgery, renal transplant patients have a mild hypercalcemia.[130]

Thiazide Diuretics

Interference of thiazide diuretics with the renal excretion of calcium may lead to hypercalcemia.[100]

Idiopathic Hypercalcemia of Infancy

Patients with idiopathic hypercalcemia of infancy have enhanced vitamin D synthesis, which produces hypercalcemia. Some cases are associated with supravalvular aortic stenosis.[131]

Clinical Manifestations

The symptoms of mild hypercalcemia are subtle and difficult to discern. These symptoms are quite similar to typical functional complaints: malaise, weakness, anorexia, and arthralgia. In contrast, severe hypercalcemia results in nausea and vomiting, constipation and obstipation, polyuria, polydipsia, altered mental status, and hyporeflexia. In patients with prolonged hypercalcemia, calcium deposits in the lens or band keratopathy,

nephrocalcinosis, or nephrogenic diabetes insipidus may be present.[119,132,133]

Because hypercalcemia shortens Phase 2 of the action potential, a short ST segment may be noted on the ECG.[106] The interval, Q-aTc, defined as the time lapse from the beginning of the Q wave to the apex of the T wave measured in seconds divided by the square root of the R-R interval as measured in seconds,[134] is generally less than 0.29 seconds in hypercalcemia.

$$Q\text{-}aTc \ = \ \frac{Q\text{-}aT\ (sec)}{\sqrt{R\text{-}R}\ (sec)} \qquad \text{(Equation 2)}$$

Hypercalcemia markedly increases the sensitivity of the heart to digitalis and may induce digitalis toxicity. Therefore, in patients on digitalis, therapy with calcium-containing agents should be avoided.[135]

Diagnosis

Technical artifacts may affect serum calcium values. If the tourniquet is left around a vein for too long (two to three minutes), a transudate may exude from the intravascular space to the interstitial space, leaving a more highly concentrated sample of blood with a high concentration of protein-bound calcium to be assayed for serum calcium level. This may elevate the serum calcium level from 0.5 to 1.5 mg/dl.[136] In addition, erythrocytes may nonspecifically adsorb calcium to their surface and artifactually lower the serum calcium level.[136] Also, the cork stoppers supplied with some tubes of blood may cause a false hypercalcemia.[137]

It is recommended that, if the routine sample shows hypercalcemia, an arterial sample be obtained. An arterial sample is reliable[136] and can be obtained without a tourniquet. It is important not to use anticoagulants, however. For example, ethylenediamine tetra-acetic acid and oxalates may chelate calcium and falsely lower the serum calcium level. Also, only blood tubes with rubber stoppers should be used.

Treatment

Only patients with symptomatic hypercalcemia should be treated.[6,100,138] The initial treatment of all patients with hypercalcemia is to administer normal saline. A rate of at least 400 ml/hour for six hours to induce diuresis is recommended. It is important to try to maintain the urine output at a brisk pace, approximately 300 ml/hour and approximately 5 to 10 liters/day.[6] To increase the urine flow, some patients may need a potent diuretic, such as furosemide.[100] It must be recognized that many of these patients are dehydrated. Evaluation of intravascular volume by either neck vein distention or central venous pressure is desirable to maintain the appropriate level of hydration. During this rapid diuresis, it is also important to monitor serum potassium and magnesium that may be lost in the urine.[138]

If therapy with normal saline has been unsuccessful, the second-line therapy is mithramycin, an antibiotic, which blocks the resorption of bone and inhibits DNA-dependent RNA synthesis.[139,140] This drug is administered in doses of 25 to 50 μg/kg. The effect begins within one hour and peaks at two to three days.[139,140] The notable side-effects with this drug are nausea and vomiting.

Calcitonin, secreted by the thyroid gland, mobilizes calcium into bone.[141] In some medical centers it is actively used for the treatment of hypercalcemia, and there have been few side-effects. This drug has a rapid onset of action and is given intravenously at 4 units/kg with repeat doses at 12 to 24 hours. Approximately 20 to 25 percent of patients may not respond, and even in those that respond, resistance may develop. However, resistance may be avoidable with concomitant steroid administration.[142]

Ethylenediamine tetra-acetic acid and phosphate were formerly used in the therapy of hypercalcemia.[143] Normal saline, mithramycin, and calcitonin are less toxic and have replaced these drugs in the treatment of hypercalcemia.

Indomethacin inhibits prostaglandin E_2 and is especially effective in treatment of hypercalcemia associated with metastatic carcinoma. This drug is not effective for the management of acute hypercalcemia, however, because its effect is delayed several days.[144,145]

The mechanism by which corticosteroids inhibit hypercalcemia is not clear. They may inhibit vitamin D, which mediates calcium absorption. Corticosteroids inhibit hypercalcemia associated with vitamin D intoxication, multiple myeloma, sarcoidosis, carcinoma, and, very rarely, hyperparathyroidism.[146–150] Prednisone is given, 40 mg/day p.o. for seven to ten days. Corticosteroids do not control acute hypercalcemia, but they are useful for the differential diagnosis and treatment of chronic hypercalcemia.

Prehospital or Nursing Treatment or Assessment

Patients with hypercalcemia require no special prehospital or nursing assessment or intervention. Those with newly symptomatic hypercalcemia should be admitted to the hospital. All those with symptomatic hypercalcemia should be under the care of an internist.

HYPOCALCEMIA

Etiology

DiGeorge's Syndrome

Congenital absence of the third and fourth branchial pouches results in an absent thymus and absent T lymphocytes, as well as a congenitally absent parathyroid gland. This is called DiGeorge's syndrome. These patients have profound hypocalcemia.[151]

Hypoparathyroidism

The autosomal dominant form of idiopathic hypoparathyroidism is associated with candidiasis, hypogonadism, hypoadrenocorticism, and pernicious anemia.[152] The sex-linked variety of idiopathic hypoparathyroidism manifests itself early in life as neonatal tetany.[153–155]

Acquired hypoparathyroidism occurs commonly after thyroidectomies or parathyroidectomies.[155] Rarely, tumors of the neck, as in carcinoma, may infiltrate the parathyroid gland. Amyloid may infiltrate the parathyroid, resulting in hypoparathyroidism.[156,157] Medullary carcinoma of the thyroid may produce enough calcitonin to induce hypocalcemia, but this is unusual. Most cases of medullary carcinoma of the thyroid do not secrete enough active calcitonin to lower the serum calcium level.[142]

Hypomagnesemia

A low serum magnesium may cause hypocalcemia by inhibiting parathormone secretion and, thus, its action at the level of the renal tubules.[158–160]

Vitamin D Deficiency

Patients whose vitamin D intake or exposure to sunlight is inadequate may have vitamin D deficiency.[161,162] Since vitamin D is fat-soluble, patients with steatorrhea, e.g., those with malabsorption syndromes, may have vitamin D deficiency. Malabsorption is a relatively common cause of vitamin D deficiency and hypocalcemia. When vitamin D deficiency and hypocalcemia are prolonged, osteomalacia may result.

Pseudohypoparathyroidism

Patients with pseudohypoparathyroidism, an X-linked dominant trait, demonstrate a marked unresponsiveness to parathormone.[155,163] These patients have characteristic features: round face; short neck; short stature; squat appearance; short, stubby fingers; mental retardation; cataracts; short fourth metacarpal; thick calvaria, and calcifications in the basal ganglia.

Pseudo-pseudohypoparathyroidism is also an X-linked dominant trait. These patients have the somatic features of pseudohypoparathyroidism; however, they have no hypocalcemia.[155,163]

Acute Pancreatitis

In acute pancreatitis, release of parathormone is decreased. It was formerly believed that saponification of calcium by fats released by lipase during pancreatitis caused this hypocalcemia, but this is probably not the mechanism.[164] Serum calcium levels of less than 7 mg/dl correlate with a poor prognosis in hemorrhagic pancreatitis.[165]

Uremia

The mechanism of hypocalcemia in patients with uremia reflects a defect in the conversion of vitamin D into its active form by the kidney. (See Chapter 63.)

Diuresis

During diuresis, there is an obligatory calcium loss. Hypocalcemia may accompany the severe diuresis associated with an overdose of a diuretic.

Acute Renal Failure

Hypocalcemia may occasionally accompany acute renal failure.[100]

Massive Transfusion of Blood

During the massive transfusion of blood, citrate, which is used as an anticoagulant in blood, chelates calcium.[161] During massive transfusions, it is important to follow the patient for symptoms of hypocalcemia, prolongations of the QT interval, or low serum calcium values. Some physicians prefer to give 4 to 10 mEq calcium routinely for each 6 units of whole blood transfused.[100]

Clinical Manifestations

Acute hypocalcemia is manifested by paresthesias; altered mental status, especially surreal feelings; carpal or pedal spasm; irritability; Chvostek's sign, i.e., facial spasm, especially at the corner of the lip, caused by tapping along the facial nerve with reflex hammer (this test may be positive in 10 percent of healthy patients); and Trousseau's sign, i.e., severely painful carpal spasm induced by elevation of blood pressure cuff over the systolic pressure for three minutes. In severe cases, opisthotonus, tetany, and general or focal seizures may be seen.[100,161,166]

Patients with chronic hypocalcemia may also have a decrease in hair in the eyebrows, eyelashes, and pubic and axillary regions.[106,155,161] In addition, there is an increased predisposition for these patients to develop cataracts.[161]

Owing to the prolongation of Phase 2 of the action potential, there is a prolongation of the ST segment of the QT interval. As mentioned earlier, hypocalcemia is the only cause of QT interval prolongation due to elongation of the ST segment.[106] The QTc is the interval from the beginning of the QRS complex to the terminal part of the T wave measured in seconds divided by the square root of the R-R interval as measured in seconds.[167] This calculation is similar to that for the Q-aTC (see Equation 2).

$$QTc = \frac{QT\ (sec)}{\sqrt{R\text{-}R\ (sec)}} \qquad \text{(Equation 3)}$$

The QTc calculation takes into account the effect of heart rate on QT interval prolongation (Table 14–2).

Treatment[6,100,165,168]

In the treatment of hypocalcemia, parenteral medication is indicated only for the treatment of symptomatic hypocalcemia. For symptomatic patients, 10 ml 10 percent calcium gluconate (4 mEq/19 ml) should be administered at 2 mEq/minute. This drug should be administered at a much slower rate of infusion if the patient is receiving digoxin. The administration of calcium gluconate can be titrated to the patient's symptoms. However, it seems wise not to administer more than 50 mEq calcium gluconate without checking the serum calcium level, even in a symptomatic patient. In

TABLE 14–2   Effect of Heart Rate on QT Interval

Heart Rate	Lower Limit (sec)	Upper Limit (sec)
40	0.40	0.50
50	0.38	0.46
60	0.35	0.43
70	0.33	0.405
80	0.32	0.38
92.5	0.29	0.36
100	0.29	0.35
109	0.27	0.33
120	0.26	0.32
133	0.25	0.30
150	0.23	0.28

Note: These values vary ±0.02 seconds, depending on sex and age of the patient.

Source: Caty L: *Electrocardiography.* Philadelphia, Lea & Febiger, 1946.

such a patient, the persistent symptomatology may be due more to hypomagnesemia than to hypocalcemia.

Although calcium chloride contains more available calcium (14 mEq/10 ml), it causes massive tissue necrosis when infiltrated. Therefore, calcium gluconates are preferable in situations other than cardiac arrest, since they do not cause tissue necrosis.[169,170]

Another preparation, calcium gluceptate, is suitable for intramuscular use, although it is irritating to muscle.[170]

A patient with asymptomatic hypocalcemia may be treated with various preparations of calcium. Calcium gluconate (1 gm) or calcium lactate (300 mg) may be required in doses up to 8 gm/day orally.

Various vitamin D preparations have been useful in the treatment of hypocalcemia, the most effective of which is 1,25-hydroxycalciferol (calcitriol) which is the active form of vitamin D and is especially useful in the therapy of patients with uremia. The dosage is 0.2 µg/day, with increments of 0.25 µg/day to four-week intervals, depending on the clinical response.[171] Exposure to sunlight may induce calcitriol production and may be useful in refractory cases.[162]

If 1,25-hydroxycalciferol is unavailable, 50,000 to 100,000 units per day of dietary supplementation of calciferol may be tried.

Prehospital or Nursing Assessment and Intervention

Clinical manifestations such as altered mental status, Chvostek's or Trousseau's sign, muscle cramping or carpopedal spasm should lead the prehospital care team or nursing team to suspect hypocalcemia. Patients with suspected hypocalcemia should have an IV line, and blood should be obtained for calcium, magnesium, electrolytes, albumin, phosphate, and arterial blood gas studies. If an ST segment prolongation is seen on the ECG, calcium chloride should be available at the bedside.

Patients with newly symptomatic hypocalcemia should be admitted to the hospital. The condition of those with asymptomatic hypocalcemia should be evaluated by an internist, providing the albumin level is normal.

MAGNESIUM

Physiology

In a 70-kg man, there are 2,000 mEq magnesium. One-half of this magnesium resides in bone; one-third in muscle.[172–174] The serum concentration of magnesium remains remarkably constant, ranging from 1.5 to 2 mEq/liter. One-third of this is protein-bound.[172]

Magnesium plays an important role in many enzyme systems, especially in reactions involving ATP, because it stabilizes the highly negative charges of the triphosphates in such reactions.[173]

Pathophysiology

Although magnesium deprivation causes seizures in rodents, there has been no evidence to show that magnesium deprivation induces seizures in humans. The subject of magnesium-induced seizures is complicated by the fact that magnesium elevates the threshold for seizures.[172] Early investigators felt that hypomagnesemia, which is commonly found in alcoholic patients, was the cause of alcohol withdrawal seizures.[172]

Like potassium, magnesium metabolism is under the influence of aldosterone. Conditions that are frequently associated with hypokalemia are, therefore, frequently associated with hypomagnesemia. Similarly, hypermagnesemia tends to be found in patients with hypoaldosteronism.[172] There is also an obligatory loss of magnesium in the urine, a loss that increases with vigorous diuresis.[172,174]

HYPOMAGNESEMIA

Etiology

Ethanol Abuse

Ethanol inhibits the reabsorption of magnesium at the level of the proximal tubule. In addition, ethanol enhances the effect of aldosterone on the loss of magnesium at the renal level. Ethanol induces a diabetes insipidus, and the ensuing diuresis also increases the loss of magnesium in the urine.[175,176] For these reasons, hypomagnesemia is frequently found in patients who abuse alcohol.

Diabetic Ketoacidosis

Magnesium levels are usually elevated initially in diabetic ketoacidosis. This is due to the effect of acidosis on serum magnesium. During the vigorous diuresis that ensues during the first three to four hours of therapy for diabetic ketoacidosis, the magnesium level may fall precipitously—to dangerously low levels.[177,178]

Diuresis

Hypomagnesemia may occur in patients during periods of vigorous diuresis, such as diuretic overdose, or in patients on normal doses of diuretics but who have a predisposing cause for hypomagnesemia, such as alcohol abuse.[179]

Digitalis Preparations

Digitalis causes an increased renal excretion of magnesium. Hypomagnesemia in patients on digitalis may be responsible for digitalis toxicity, especially in patients refractory to the usual therapies.[180-184]

Malabsorption

In diarrheal fluid there is a large loss of magnesium. Patients with steatorrhea or malabsorptive syndrome may develop hypomagnesemia.[185-187] Hypomagnesemia also may occur in patients who abuse laxatives.

Hyperalimentation

During total parenteral nutrition, it is important for the physician to ensure that the patient is given an adequate supply of all the less common nutrients. Because of the obligatory magnesium loss in the urine, patients receiving hyperalimentation may develop hypomagnesemia without a continuous IV supply of magnesium.[188]

Renal-Wasting

There are several causes for renal-wasting of magnesium.[172-174] Hypercalcemia may cause diuresis and therefore result in an obligatory magnesium loss. Patients with renal tubular acidosis may have an excess of bicarbonate ion within the tubule that serves as a nondiffusible anion and therefore results in excess magnesium loss in the urine to maintain electrical neutrality. Occasionally, patients receiving gentamicin develop hypomagnesemia. Gentamicin within the renal tubule serves as a nondiffusible anion and, to preserve electrical neutrality, magnesium is lost in the kidneys. Patients with hyperthyroidism may have hypomagnesemia due to renal losses. Some patients have an obligatory magnesium loss in the renal tubules for which no reason has been found. In some patients with chronic renal failure, proximal tubular dysfunction may result in renal-wasting of magnesium.[172,173]

Acute Pancreatitis

Some patients with acute pancreatitis develop hypomagnesemia. This association may be due to the high frequency of alcohol abuse among patients with acute pancreatitis.[172] The presence of hypomagnesemia, however, seems to correlate with the presence of hypocalcemia.

Multiple Transfusions

The anticoagulants, such as citrate, that are administered during multiple transfusions, may bind magnesium and result in hypomagnesemia.[172]

Clinical Manifestations

The clinical manifestations of hypomagnesemia are anorexia, nausea, vomiting, and diarrhea; in severe cases, carpopedal spasm, tetany, Chvostek's and Trousseau's signs, tremors, hyperreflexia, and altered mental status may be seen.[189,190]

Studies on the ECG manifestations of hypomagnesemia have been complicated by the fact that many of the patients have other electrolytic abnormalities. In one study to evaluate the effect of hypomagnesemia alone on an ECG, it was noted that hypomagnesemia prolonged the QT interval and resulted in a low QRS complex, and a short, fixed PR interval.[191]

Diagnosis

It is not always necessary to determine the magnesium level when serum electrolytes or calcium are measured, but a magnesium level should be obtained in the presence of hypocalcemia or hypokalemia, during clinical manifestations suggestive of hypocalcemia, or in the presence of any of the conditions that may predispose to hypomagnesemia: digitalis intoxication, diabetic ketoacidosis, alcohol abuse, malabsorption, chronic renal failure, or vigorous diuresis. The value of the magnesium level should be used in a qualitative fashion; it should be considered only an indication of the presence or absence of hypomagnesemia. The absolute magnitude of the level of magnesium does not correlate with the severity of the symptoms or the severity of the deficiency. The clinical signs and symptoms determine if a low serum magnesium value reflects mild, moderate, or severe deficiency.

Not uncommonly, the magnesium level is normal, but the clinical manifestations suggest hypomagnesemia. In this instance, the physician should administer 1 gm magnesium sulfate IV and collect the urine for 24 hours. The excretion of less than 80 percent of the administered dose of magnesium sulfate over 24 hours indicates magnesium deficiency.[192,193]

Treatment

Patients who are asymptomatic with hypomagnesemia should receive 10 to 15 mEq/day orally (8.1 mEq magnesium = 1 gm). Oral absorption is erratic, however. The amount of magnesium that is absorbed orally depends on the magnitude of the deficit. In addition, many oral magnesium preparations are poorly tolerated.[6,173]

Several preparations contain magnesium and may be used for magnesium replacement: Maalox (1.2 gm/30 ml), Mylanta II (2.4 gm/30 ml), Milk of Magnesia (2.5 gm/30 ml).[172]

A patient with symptoms secondary to hypomagnesemia needs parenteral administration of magnesium. In these patients, the deficit is expected to be 1.5 mEq/kg or 100 mEq, or approximately 12 gm for a 70-kg man.[6,172,173] Even in the presence of an extreme magnesium deficit, the kidneys excrete more than 50 percent of an administered dose. Therefore, it is necessary to replace double the calculated magnesium deficit. In general, the physician should replace one-half the deficit, or 12 gm in a 70-kg man, during the first 24 hours, and the remainder of the deficit should be replaced over the next 48 to 72 hours.[6,172–174] Six grams of magnesium may be given continuously over 4 to 6 hours intravenously, but no more than 12 gm should be administered within 12 hours. Alternatively, 2 gm magnesium sulfate can be given intramuscularly every 2 to 4 hours.[194,195]

During the initial replacement of magnesium, the physician must monitor the patient's signs, symptoms, and reflexes in order to guide the rate of therapy; magnesium should be replaced at a slower rate once the patient becomes asymptomatic.

All patients with symptomatic hypomagnesemia should be admitted to the hospital.

HYPERMAGNESEMIA

Etiology

Hypermagnesemia is a rare entity that occurs only in certain clinical situations. Most patients with renal failure, for example, have a diminished ability to excrete potassium from the body. Continued intakes of magnesium, as with antacids, in these patients may result in severe hypermagnesemia.[196] In the treatment of eclampsia of pregnancy, magnesium is administered to elevate the seizure threshold. Some physicians may administer magnesium in excessive quantities in the treatment of alcohol withdrawal seizures. In both these instances, hypermagnesemia occasionally may ensue.[172,173]

Clinical Manifestations[172]

If the level of magnesium is less than 3 mEq/liter, the patient is asymptomatic. With values of magnesium of 3 to 9 mEq/liter, nausea, vomiting, hypotension, bradycardia, and confusion may be seen. At 5 to 6 mEq/liter, the deep tendon reflexes are diminished. At values of magnesium exceeding 10 mEq/liter, carbon dioxide narcosis, respiratory depression, paralysis, and hypotension may ensue.

On an ECG, hypermagnesemia may prolong the PR interval, increase the duration of the QRS interval, and occasionally cause heart block.[197]

Diagnosis

The diagnosis of hypermagnesemia is made by obtaining a magnesium level.

Therapy

Calcium neutralizes the effect of magnesium on a mEq/mEq basis. When patients are symptomatic with hypermagnesemia and serum levels are either known or suspected to be 5 to 8 mEq/liter, or when a patient is asymptomatic but the level is more than 8 mEq/liter, then 5 ml 10 percent calcium chloride can be administered IV over 30 seconds. If the patient is unimproved, calcium chloride may be repeated in 2 minutes. The effect is prompt.[172,198,199] Since calcium is such a rapid antidote of hypermagnesemia, calcium chloride should be at the bedside of all patients receiving parenteral magnesium therapy.

REFERENCES

1. Friedler RM, Koffler A, Kurokawa K: Hyponatremia and hypernatremia. *Clin Nephrol* 7:163, 1977.
2. Stein JH, Reineck HJ: Regulation of the excretion of sodium and other electrolytes by the collecting duct. *Kidney Int* 6:1, 1974.
3. Bartter F: The syndrome of inappropriate secretion of antidiuretic hormone (SIADH). *DM* 11:1, 1973.
4. Berl T, Anderson RJ, McDonald KM, Schrier RW: Clinical disorders of water metabolism. *Kidney Int* 10:117, 1976.
5. Robertson G, Athar S: The interaction of blood osmolality and blood volume in regulating plasma vasopression in man. *J Clin Endocrinol Metab* 42:613, 1976.
6. Lindeman RD, Papper S: Therapy of fluid and electrolyte disorders. *Ann Intern Med* 82:64, 1975.
7. Sweadner KJ, Goldin SM: Active transport of sodium and potassium ions: Mechanism, function and regulation, *N Engl J Med* 302:777, 1980.
8. Smithline N, Gardner KD Jr: Gaps—Anion and osmolal. *JAMA* 236:1594, 1976.
9. Glasser L, Sternglanz PD, Combic J, et al: Serum osmolarity and its applicability to drug overdose. *Am J Clin Pathol* 60:695, 1963.
10. Arieff AI, Carroll HJ: Non-ketotic hyperosmolar coma with hyperglycemia: Clinical features, pathophysiology, renal function, acid-base balance, plasma-cerebrospinal fluid equilibria and the effects of therapy in 37 cases. *Medicine* 51:73, 1972.
11. Sotos JR, Dodge PR, Meara P, et al: Studies in experimental hypertonicity: I. Pathogenesis of the clinical syndrome, biochemical abnormalities and cause of death. *Pediatrics* 26:925, 1960.
12. Arieff AI, Guisado R: Effects on the nervous system of hypernatremic and hyponatremic states. *Kidney Int* 10:104, 1976.
13. Zlerler KL: Hyperosmolarity in adults: A critical review. *J Chronic Dis* 7:1, 1958.
14. Harrington JT, Cohen JJ: Measurements of urinary electrolytes: Indications and limitations. *N Engl J Med* 293:1241, 1975.
15. Ross EJ, Christie SBM: Hypernatremia. *Medicine* 48:441, 1969.
16. Keitel HG, Thompson D, Itand HA: Hyposthenuria in sickle cell anemia: A reversible renal defect. *J Clin Invest* 35:998, 1956.

17. Singer I, Forrest N Jr: Drug-induced states of nephrogenic diabetes insipidus. *Kidney Int* 10:82, 1976.
18. Bruck E, Abal G, Aceto T: Pathogenesis and pathophysiology of hypertonic dehydration with diarrhea. *Am J Dis Child* 115:122, 1968.
19. Finberg L, Harrison HE: Hypernatremia in infants: An evaluation of the clinical and biochemical findings accompanying this state. *Pediatrics* 16:1, 1955.
20. Skinner AL, Moll FC: Hypernatremia accompanying infant diarrhea. *Am J Dis Child* 92:562, 1956.
21. Dorrington KL: Skin turgor: Do we understand the clinical sign? *Lancet* 1:264, 1981.
22. Knopp R, Claypool R, Leonardi D: Use of the tilt test in measuring acute blood loss. *Ann Emerg Med* 9:72, 1980.
23. Finberg L: Hypernatremic (hypertonic) dehydration in infants. *N Engl J Med* 298:196, 1973.
24. Chonko A, Bay W, Stzin J, Ferris T: The role of renin and aldosterone in the salt retention of edema. *Am J Med* 63:881, 1977.
25. Vader HL, Vink CLF: The influence of viscosity on dilution methods. Its problems in the determination of serum sodium. *Clin Chim Acta* 65:379, 1975.
26. Miller M, Dalakos T, Moses A, Fellerman H, Streeten D: Recognition of partial defects in antidiuretic hormone secretion. *Ann Intern Med* 73:721, 1970.
27. Alberti KGMM, Hockaday TDR: Diabetic coma: A reappraisal after five years. *Clin Endocrinol Metab* 6:421, 1977.
28. McDonald K, Miller P, Anderson R, Berl T, Schrier R: Hormonal control of renal water excretion. *Kidney Int* 10:38, 1976.
29. Epstein M, Pins D, Schneider N, Levinson R: Determinants of deranged sodium and water homeostasis in decompensated cirrhosis. *J Lab Clin Med* 87:822, 1976.
30. Fichman M, Vorherr H, Kleeman L, Telfer N: Diuretic-induced hyponatremia. *Ann Intern Med* 75:853, 1971.
31. Pettinger W, Talner L, Ferris T: Inappropriate secretion of antidiuretic hormone due to myxedema. *N Engl J Med* 272:362, 1965.
32. Sick cells and hyponatremia. *Lancet* 1:342, 1974.
33. Hariprasad M, Eisinger RP, Nadler IM, Padmanabhan CS, Nidus BD: Hyponatremia in psychogenic polydipsia. *Arch Intern Med* 140:1639, 1980.
34. Waugh WH: Utility of expressing serum sodium per unit of water in assessing hyponatremia. *Metabolism* 18:706, 1969.
35. Katz M: Hyperglycemia-induced hyponatremia—Calculation of expected serum sodium depression. *N Engl J Med* 289:843, 1973.
36. Moses AM, Miller M: Drug-induced dilutional hyponatremia. *N Engl J Med* 291:1234, 1974.
37. Bartter F, Schwartz W: The syndrome of inappropriate secretion of antidiuretic hormone. *Am J Med* 42:790, 1967.
38. Renzetti AD Jr, Kobayashi T, Bigler A, Mitchell M: Regional ventilation and perfusion in silicosis and in the alveolar-capillary block syndrome. *Am J Med* 49:5, 1970.
39. Arieff A, Llach F, Massry S: Neurological manifestations and morbidity of hyponatremia: Correlation with brain water and electrolytes. *Medicine* 55:121, 1976.
40. Forrest J, Cox M, Hong C, Morrison G, Bia M, Singer I: Superiority of demeclocycline over lithium in the treatment of chronic syndrome of inappropriate secretion of antidiuretic hormone. *N Engl J Med* 298:173, 1977.
41. Tallob L, Needle M: Hyponatremic syndromes. *Med Clin North Am* 57:1425, 1973.
42. Hantman D, Rossier B, Zohlman R, Schirer R: Rapid correction of hyponatremia in the syndrome of inappropriate secretion of antidiuretic hormone. An alternative treatment to hypertonic saline. *Ann Intern Med* 78:870, 1973.
43. Nardone D, McDonald W, Girard D: Mechanisms in hypokalemia: Clinical correlation. *Medicine* 57:435, 1978.
44. Kunau RT, Stein JH: Disorders of hypo- and hyperkalemia. *Clin Nephrol* 7:173, 1977.
45. Berliner RW: Renal mechanisms for potassium excretion. *Harvey Lect* 55:141, 1960.
46. Malnic G, DeMello G, Aires M, Giebisch G: Potassium transport across renal distal tubules during acid-base disturbances. *Am J Physiol* 221:1192, 1971.
47. Gennari FS, Cohen JJ: Role of the kidney in potassium homeostasis: Lessons from acid-base disturbances. *Kidney Int* 8:1, 1975.
48. Schultz R: Recent advances in the physiology and pathophysiology of potassium excretion. *Arch Intern Med* 131:885, 1973.
49. Burnell J, Villamil M, Uyeno B, Scribner B: The effect in humans of extracellular pH change on the relationship between serum potassium concentration and intracellular potassium. *J Clin Invest* 35:935, 1956.
50. Oster JR, Perez GO, Vaamonde CA: Relationship between blood pH and potassium and phosphorus during acute metabolic acidosis. *Am J Physiol* 235:345, 1978.
51. Orringer CE, Eustace JC, Sunsch CD, et al: Natural history of lactic acidosis after grand mal seizures: A model for the study of an anion gap acidosis not associated with hyperkalemia. *N Engl J Med* 297:746, 1977.
52. Fulop M: Serum potassium in lactic acidosis and ketoacidosis. *N Engl J Med* 300:1087, 1979.
53. Surawicz B: Relationship between electrocardiogram and electrolytes. *Am Heart J* 73:814, 1967.
54. Ettinger P, Regan T, Oldewurtel H: Hyperkalemia, cardiac conduction and the electrocardiogram: A review. *Am Heart J* 88:360, 1974.
55. Stoa KF, Knutsen KOH: Oestrogen excretion during cortisone therapy. *Acta Endocrinol* 25:209, 1957.
56. Sigler MH: The mechanism of the naturiesis of fasting. *J Clin Invest* 55:377, 1975.
57. Shields R: Absorption and secretion of electrolytes and water by the human colon, with particular reference to benign adenoma and papilloma. *Br J Surg* 53:893, 1966.
58. Gossain VV, Werk EE: Surreptitious laxation and hypokalemia. *Ann Intern Med* 76:671, 1972.
59. Larusso N, McGill D: Surreptitious laxative ingestion. Delayed recognition of a serious condition: A case report. *Mayo Clin Proc* 50:706, 1975.
60. Schwartz W, Reuman A: Metabolic and renal studies in chronic potassium depletion resulting from overuse of laxatives. *J Clin Invest* 32:258, 1953.
61. Bartter FC, Pronove P, Gill JR Jr, et al: Hyperplasia of the juxtaglomerular complex with hyperaldosteronism and hypokalemic alkalosis. *Am J Med* 33:811, 1962.
62. Gill J, Frolich J, Bowden R, Taylor A, Keisler H, Seyberth H, et al: Bartter's syndrome: A disorder characterized by high urinary prostaglandins and a dependence of hyperreninemia on prostaglandin synthesis. *Am J Med* 61:43, 1976.
63. Morris R Jr: Renal tubular acidosis. Mechanisms classification and implications. *N Engl J Med* 281:1405, 1969.
64. Narins RG, Goldberg M: Renal tubular acidosis: pathophysiology, diagnosis and treatment. *DM* 23:3, 1977.
65. Lipner H, Ruzany F, Dasgupta M, Lief D, Bank N: The behavior of carbenicillin as nonreabsorbable anion. *J Lab Clin Med* 86:183, 1975.
66. Douglas J, Healy J: Nephrotoxic effects of amphotericin B, including renal tubular acidosis. *Am J Med* 46:154, 1969.
67. Frazier H, Yager H: Drug therapy. The clinical use of diuretics. *N Engl J Med* 288:455, 1973.

68. Muggia F, Heinemann H, Farhangi M, Osserman E: Lysozymuria and renal tubular dysfunction in monocytic and myelomonocytic leukemia. *Am J Med* 47:351, 1969.

69. Forman BH: Hypokalemic periodic paralysis. *JAMA* 216:146, 1971.

70. Santeusanio F, Faloona G, Knochel JP, et al: Evidence for a role of endogenous insulin and glucagon in the regulation of potassium homeostasis. *J Lab Clin Med* 81:809, 1973.

71. Smith JS Jr: Hypokalemia in resuscitation from multiple trauma. *Surg Gynecol Obstet* 147:18, 1978.

72. Knochel J: Environmental heat illness. An eclectic review. *Arch Intern Med* 133:841, 1974.

73. Sprung CL, Portocarrero CJ, Fernaine AV, et al: The metabolic and respiratory alterations of heat stroke. *Arch Intern Med* 140:665, 1980.

74. Berning J: Hypokalemia of barium poisoning. *Lancet* 1:110, 1975.

75. Lawson DH, Murray RM, Parker JLW: Early mortality in the megaloblastic anemias. *Q J Med* 41:1, 1972.

76. Smithwick RH, Kinsey D, Whitelaw GP: Surgical treatment of hypertension-primary aldosteronism. *N Engl J Med* 266:160, 1962.

77. Vaughan NJA, Slater JDI, Lightman SL, et al: The diagnosis of primary hyperaldosteronism. *Lancet* 1:120, 1981.

78. Primary aldosteronism. *Lancet* 1:667, 1980.

79. Wrong O: Incidence of hypokalemia in severe hypertension. *Br Med J* 2:419, 1961.

80. Simon N, Franklin S, Bleiter K, Maxwell M: Clinical characteristics of renovascular hypertension. *JAMA* 220:1209, 1972.

81. Conn JW, Rovner DR, Cohen EL: Licorice-induced pseudoaldosteronism. Hypertension, hypokalemia, aldosteronopenia, and suppressed plasma renin activity. *JAMA* 205:492, 1968.

82. Blachley JD, Knochel JP: Tobacco chewer's hypokalemia: Licorice revisited. *N Engl J Med* 302:784, 1980.

83. Ward CF, Arkin DB, Venumof SL, Saidman LJ: Arterial versus venous potassium: Clinical implications. *Crit Care Med* 6:335, 1978.

84. Love DW, Foster TS, Bradley DL: Comparison of the taste and acceptance of three potassium chloride preparations. *Am J Hosp Pharm* 35:586, 1978.

85. Sopko JA, Freeman RM: Salt substitutes as a source of potassium. *JAMA* 238:608, 1977.

86. Surawicz B, Chlebus H, Mazzoleni A: Hemodynamic and electrocardiographic effects of hyperpotassemia. Differences in response to slow and rapid increases in concentration of plasma K. *Am Heart J* 73:647, 1967.

87. Stewart GW, Fyffe JA, Corrall RJM: Familial pseudohyperkalemia: A new syndrome. *Lancet* 2:175, 1979.

88. Bostic O, Duvernoy WFC: Hyperkalemic cardiac arrest during transfusion of stored blood. *J Electrocardiol* 5:407, 1972.

89. Roth F, Wuthrick H: The clinical importance of hyperkalemia following suxamethonium administration. *Br J Anaesth* 41:311, 1969.

90. Thomas ET: Circulatory collapse following succinylcholine: Report of a case. *Anesth Analg* 48:333, 1969.

91. Mazze R, Escue H, Houston J: Collapse following administration of succinylcholine to the traumatized patient. *Anesthesiology* 31:540, 1969.

92. Maroff DL, daSilva JA, Rosenbaum BJ: On the mechanism of hyperkalemia due to hyperosmotic expansion with saline or mannitol. *Clin Sci Mol Med* 41:383, 1971.

93. deLeiva A, Christlieb AR, Melby JC, Graham CA, et al: Big renin and biosynthetic defect of aldosterone in diabetes mellitus. *N Engl J Med* 295:639, 1976.

94. Szylman P, Better OS, Chaimowitz C, Rosler A: Role of hyperkalemia in the metabolic acidosis of isolated hypoaldosteronism. *N Engl J Med* 294:361, 1976.

95. Tan S, Burton M: Hyporeninemic hypoaldosteronism: An overlooked cause of hyperkalemia. *Arch Intern Med* 141:30, 1981.

96. Spitzer A, Edelmann C Jr, Goldberg L, Henneman P: Short stature, hyperkalemia and acidosis: A defect in renal transport of potassium. *Kidney Int* 3:251, 1973.

97. Iverson T: Congenital adrenocortical hyperplasia with disturbed electrolyte regulations: Dysadrenocorticism. *Pediatrics* 16:875, 1955.

98. Braun H, Surawicz B, Beuet S: T waves in hyperpotassemia. Their differentiation from simulating T waves in other conditions. *Am J Med Sci* 230:147, 1955.

99. Levinsky NG: Management of emergencies: VI. Hyperkalemia. *N Engl J Med* 274:1076, 1966.

100. Singer FR, Bethune JE, Massry SG: Hypercalcemia and hypocalcemia. *Clin Nephrol* 7:154, 1977.

101. Zerwekh JE: Vitamin D-dependent intestinal calcium absorption. *Gastroenterology* 76:404, 1979.

102. Ostrow JD, Blanchard G, Gray SJ: Peptic ulcer in primary hyperparathyroidism. *Am J Med* 29:769, 1960.

103. Barreras RF, Donaldson RM: Role of calcium in gastric hypersecretion, parathyroid adenoma and peptic ulcer. *N Engl J Med* 276:1122, 1967.

104. Cope O, Culver PS, Mixter CG, Nardi GL: Pancreatitis, a diagnostic clue to hyperparathyroidism. *Ann Surg* 145:857, 1957.

105. Parks J, Coe F, Favus M: Hyperparathyroidism in nephrolithiasis. *Arch Intern Med* 140:1479, 1980.

106. Bronsky D, Dubin A, Kushner DS, Waldstein SS: Calcium and the electrocardiogram. III. The relationship of the intervals of the electrocardiogram to the level of serum calcium. *Am J Cardiol* 7:840, 1961.

107. Juan D: Hypocalcemia: Differential diagnosis and mechanisms. *Arch Intern Med* 139:1166, 1979.

108. Muggia FM: Hypercalcemia associated with neoplastic disease. *Ann Intern Med* 73:281, 1970.

109. Lafferty FW: Pseudohyperparathyroidism. *Medicine* 45:247, 1966.

110. Fisken RA, Heath DA, Somers S: Hypercalcaemia in hospital patients: Clinical and diagnostic aspects. *Lancet* 1:202, 1981.

111. Stewart AF, Horst R, Deftos LJ, et al: Biochemical evaluation of patients with cancer-associated hypercalcemia: Evidence for humoral and non-humoral groups. *N Engl J Med* 303:1377, 1980.

112. Sherwood LM: The multiple causes of hypercalcemia in malignant disease. *N Engl J Med* 303:1412, 1980.

113. Skrabanek P, McPartlin J, Powell D: Tumor hypercalcemia and "ectopic hyperparathyroidism." *Medicine* 59:262, 1980.

114. Kyle RA: Multiple myeloma: A review of 869. *Mayo Clin Proc* 50:29, 1975.

115. Kapadia SB: Multiple myeloma: A clinicopathologic study of 62 consecutively autopsied cases. *Medicine* 59:323, 1980.

116. Boonstra CE, Jackson CE: Hyperparathyroidism detected by routine serum calcium analysis. Prevalence in a clinic population. *Ann Intern Med* 63:468, 1965.

117. Mundy GR, Cove DH, Fiskan R, et al: Primary hyperparathyroidism: Changes in the pattern of clinical presentation. *Lancet* 1:1317, 1980.

118. Heath H, Hodgson SF, Kennedy MA: Primary hyperparathyroidism: Incidence, morbidity, and potential economic impact in a community. *N Engl J Med* 302:189, 1980.

119. Mallette LE, Bilezikian JP, Heath DA, Aurbach GD: Primary hyperparathyroidism: Clinical and biochemical features. *Medicine* 53:127, 1974.

120. Palmer FJ, Nelson JC, Bacchus H: The chloride-phosphate ratio in hypercalcemia. *Ann Intern Med* 80:200, 1974.

121. Winnacker JL, Becker KL, Katz S: Endocrine aspects of sarcoidosis. *N Engl J Med* 278:427, 1968.
122. Cushard WG, Simon AB, Canterbury JM, Reiss E: Parathyroid function in sarcoidosis. *N Engl J Med* 286:395, 1972.
123. Chaplin H Jr, Clark LD, Ropes MW: Vitamin D intoxication. *Am J Med Sci* 221:369, 1951.
124. Paterson CR: Vitamin-D poisoning: Survey of causes in 21 patients with hypercalcaemia. *Lancet* 1:1164, 1980.
125. deTorrente A, Berl T, Chon P, Kawamoto E, Hertz P, Schrier R: Hypercalcemia of acute renal failure, clinical significance and pathogenesis. *Am J Med* 61:119, 1976.
126. Segal AJ, Miller M, Moses A: Hypercalcemia during the diuretic phase of acute renal failure. *Ann Intern Med* 68:1066, 1968.
127. Randall RE, Strauss ME, McNeely WF: The milk-alkali syndrome. *Arch Intern Med* 107:163, 1961.
128. Meier DA, Arnstein AR, Hamburger JI: Symptomatic thyrotoxic hypercalcemia. *Mich Med* 73:19, 1974.
129. Walser M, Robinson BHB, Duckett JW: The hypercalcemia of adrenal insufficiency. *J Clin Invest* 42:456, 1963.
130. Chatterjee SN, Friedler RM, Berne TV, et al: Persistent hypercalcemia after successful renal transplantation. *Nephron* 17:1, 1976.
131. Garcia RE, Friedman WF, Kaback MM, Rowe RD: Idiopathic hypercalcemia and supravalvular aortic stenosis: Documentation of a new syndrome. *N Engl J Med* 271:117, 1964.
132. David NJ, Verner JV, Engel FL: The diagnostic spectrum of hypercalcemia. *Am J Med* 33:88, 1962.
133. Goldsmith RS: Differential diagnosis of hypercalcemia. *N Engl J Med* 274:674, 1966.
134. Nierenberg DW, Ransil BJ: Q-aTc interval as a clinical indicator of hypercalcemia. *Am J Cardiol* 44:243, 1979.
135. Toda N, West TC: Modification by sodium and calcium of the cardiotoxicity induced by ouabain. *J Pharmacol Exp Ther* 154:239, 1965.
136. Dent CE: Some problems of hyperparathyroidism. *Br Med J* 2:1419, 1962.
137. Smith FE, Reinstein H, Braverman LE: Cork stoppers and hypercalcemia. *N Engl J Med* 272:787, 1965.
138. Aldinger KA, Samaan NA: Hypokalemia with hypercalcemia: Prevalence and significance in treatment. *Ann Intern Med* 87:571, 1977.
139. Perlia CP, Gubisch NJ, Walter J, Edelberg D, Dederick MM, Taylor SG: Mithramycin treatment of hypercalcemia. *Cancer* 25:389, 1970.
140. Smith IE, Powles TJ: Mithramycin for hypercalcaemia associated with myeloma and other malignancies. *Br Med J* 1:268, 1975.
141. Austin LA, Heath H: Calcitonin: Physiology and pathophysiology. *N Engl J Med* 304:269, 1981.
142. Wisneski LA, Croom WP, Silva OL, et al: Salmon calcitonin in hypercalcemia. *Clin Pharmacol Ther* 24:219, 1978.
143. Dudley HR, Ritchie AC, Schilling A, Baker WH: Pathologic changes associated with the use of sodium ethylene diamine tetra-acetate in the treatment of hypercalcemia. *N Engl J Med* 262:331, 1953.
144. Robertson RP, Baylink DJ, Marini JJ, Adkison HW: Elevated prostaglandins and suppressed parathyroid hormone associated with hypercalcemia and renal cell carcinoma. *J Clin Endocrinol Metab* 41:164, 1975.
145. Brereton HO, Halushka PV, Alexander RW, Mason DM, Keiser HR, deVita VT: Indomethacin-responsive hypercalcemia in a patient with renal-cell adenocarcinoma. *N Engl J Med* 291:83, 1974.
146. Ashkar FS, Miller R, Katims RB: Effect of corticosteroids on hypercalcemia of malignant disease. *Lancet* 1:41, 1971.
147. Deftos LJ: Medical management of the hypercalcemia of malignancy. *Annu Rev Med* 25:323, 1974.
148. Goldsmith RS: Treatment of hypercalcemia. *Med Clin North Am* 56:951, 1972.
149. Watson L, Moxham J, Fraser P: Hydrocortisone suppression test and discriminant analysis in differential diagnosis of hypercalcemia. *Lancet* 1:1320, 1980.
150. Binstock ML, Mundy GR: Effect of calcitonin and glucocorticoids in combination on the hypercalcemia of malignancy. *Ann Intern Med* 93:269, 1980.
151. DiGeorge AM: Congenital absence of the thymus and its immunologic consequences: Concurrence with congenital hypoparathyroidism. *Birth Defects* 4:116, 1968.
152. Graham K, Williams BO, Rowe MJ: Idiopathic hypoparathyroidism: A cause of fits in the elderly. *Br Med J* 1:1460, 1979.
153. Peden VH: True idiopathic hypoparathyroidism as a sex-linked recessive trait. *Am J Hum Genet* 12:323, 1960.
154. Richter PI, Chutorian AM: Familial hypoparathyroidism. Case reports and a review of the literature. *Neurology* 18:75, 1968.
155. Nusynowitz ML, Frame B, Kolb FO: The spectrum of the hypoparathyroid states: A classification based on physiologic principles. *Medicine* 55:105, 1976.
156. Horwitz C, Myers WP, Foote F Jr: Secondary malignant tumors of the parathyroid glands. Report of two cases with associated hypoparathyroidism. *Am J Med* 52:797, 1972.
157. Davis RH, Fourman P, Smith JWG: Prevalence of parathyroid insufficiency after thyroidectomy. *Lancet* 2:1432, 1961.
158. Anast CS, Motts JM, Kaplan SL, Burns TW: Evidence for parathyroid in magnesium deficiency. *Science* 177:606, 1972.
159. Reddy CR, Coburn JW, Hartenbower DL, et al: Studies on mechanism of hypocalcemia of magnesium depletion. *J Clin Invest* 52:3000, 1973.
160. Chase LR, Slatopolsky E: Secretion and metabolic efficacy of parathyroid hormone in patients with severe hypomagnesemia. *J Clin Endocrinol Metab* 38:363, 1974.
161. Juan D: Hypocalcemia: Differential diagnosis and mechanisms. *Arch Intern Med* 139:1166, 1979.
162. Holick MF, Vskokovic M, Henley JW: The photoproduction of 1,25-dihydroxyvitamin D_3 in skin: An approach to therapy of vitamin-D–resistant syndromes. *N Engl J Med* 303:349, 1980.
163. Farfel Z, Brickman AS, Kaslow HR, et al: Defect of receptor-cyclase coupling protein in pseudohypoparathyroidism. *N Engl J Med* 303:237, 1980.
164. Robertson GM Jr, Moore EW, Switz DM, Sizemore GW, Estep H: Inadequate parathyroid response in acute pancreatitis. *N Engl J Med* 294:512, 1976.
165. Edmondson HA, Berne CJ: Calcium changes in acute pancreatic necrosis. *Surg Gynecol Obstet* 79:240, 1944.
166. Blanchard BM: Focal hypocalcemic seizures 33 years after thyroidectomy. *Arch Intern Med* 110:382, 1962.
167. Howard E: Value of the Q-T interval. *Am Heart J* 59:789, 1960.
168. Avioli L: The therapeutic approach to hypoparathyroidism. *Am J Med* 57:34, 1974.
169. Pak CYC, Zisman E, Lotz M: Gluconate carrier in 47 Ca kinetic studies. *J Clin Endocrinol Metab* 27:433, 1967.
170. White RD, Goldsmith RS, Rodriguez R, et al: Plasma ionic calcium levels following injection of chloride, gluconate and gluceptate salts of calcium. *J Thorac Cardiovasc Surg* 71:609, 1976.
171. Calcitriol. *Med Lett Drugs Ther* 21:50, 1979.
172. Graber TW, Yee AS, Baker FJ: Magnesium: Physiology, clinical disorders and therapy. *Ann Emerg Med* 10:49, 1981.
173. Massry SG, Seelig MS: Hypomagnesemia and hypermagnesemia. *Clin Nephrol* 7:147, 1977.

174. Geiderman JM, Goodman SL, Cohen DB: Magnesium—The forgotten electrolyte. *J Am Coll Emerg Phys* 8:204, 1979.

175. Kalbfleisch JM, Lindeman RD, Ginn HE, Smith WO: Effects of ethanol administration on urinary excretion of magnesium and other electrolytes in alcoholic and normal subjects. *J Clin Invest* 42:1471, 1963.

176. Mendelson JH, Ogata M, Mello NK: Effects of alcohol ingestion and withdrawal on magnesium states of alcoholics: Clinical and experimental findings. *Ann NY Acad Sci* 162:918, 1969.

177. Martin HE, Wertman M: Serum potassium, magnesium and calcium levels in diabetic patients. *J Clin Invest* 26:217, 1947.

178. Martin HE, Smith K, Wilson ML: The fluid and electrolyte therapy of severe diabetic acidosis and ketosis. *Am J Med* 24:376, 1958.

179. Lim P, Jacob E: Magnesium deficiency in patients on long-term diuretic therapy for heart failure. *Br Med J* 3:620, 1972.

180. Iseri LT, Freed J, Bures AR: Magnesium deficiency and cardiac disorders. *Am J Med* 58:837, 1975.

181. Neff MS, Mendelssohn S, Kim KE, Banach S, Swartz L, Seller RH: Magnesium sulfate in digitalis toxicity. *Am J Cardiol* 29:377, 1972.

182. Seller RH, Cangiano J, Kim KE, Mendelssohn S, Brest AN, Swartz C: Digitalis toxicity and hypomagnesemia. *Am Heart J* 79:57, 1970.

183. Specter M, Schweizer E, Goldman R: Studies on magnesium's mechanism of action in digitalis-induced arrhythmias. *Circulation* 52:1001, 1975.

184. Burch GE, Giles TD: The importance of magnesium deficiency in cardiovascular disease. *Am Heart J* 94:649, 1977.

185. Balint JA, Hirschowitz BI: Hypomagnesemia with tetany in nontropical sprue. *N Engl J Med* 265:631, 1961.

186. Savage DCL, McAdam WAF: Convulsions due to hypomagnesaemia in an infant recovering from diarrhea. *Lancet* 2:234, 1967.

187. Fletcher RF, Henley AA, Sammons HG, Squire JR: A case of magnesium deficiency following massive intestinal resection. *Lancet* 1:522, 1960.

188. Flink EB, Stutzman FL, Anderson AR, Konig T, Fraser R: Magnesium deficiency after prolonged parenteral fluid administration and after chronic alcoholism complicated by delirium tremens. *J Lab Clin Med* 43:169, 1954.

189. Hanna S, Harrison M, MacIntyre I, Frazer R: The syndrome of magnesium deficiency in man. *Lancet* 2:172, 1960.

190. Shils ME: Experimental human magnesium depletion. *Medicine* 48:61, 1969.

191. Bajpai PC, Hasan M, Gupta AK, et al: Electrocardiographic changes in hypomagnesemia. *Indian Heart J* 24:271, 1972.

192. Fitzgerald MG, Fourman P: An experimental study of magnesium deficiency in man. *Clin Sci Mol Med* 15:635, 1956.

193. Fourman P, Morgan DB: Chronic magnesium deficiency. *Proc Nutr Soc* 21:34, 1962.

194. Pritchard JA: The use of the magnesium ion in the management of eclamptogenic toxemias. *Surg Gynecol Obstet* 100:131, 1955.

195. Flink EB: Therapy of magnesium deficiency. *Ann NY Acad Sci* 162:901, 1969.

196. Randall RE, Cohen MD, Spray CC Jr, Rossmeisl EC: Hypermagnesemia in renal failure. Etiology of topic manifestations. *Ann Intern Med* 61:73, 1964.

197. Berns AS, Kollmeyer KR: Magnesium-induced bradycardia. *Ann Intern Med* 85:760, 1976.

198. Massry SG: Pharmacology of magnesium. *Annu Rev Pharmacol Toxicol* 17:67, 1977.

199. Wacker WEC, Parisi AF: Magnesium metabolism. *N Engl J Med* 278:658 (part 1), 712 (part 2), 772 (part 3), 1968.

Appendix 14–A

TABLE 14–A1   Solutions

	Glucose (gm/liter)	Na (mEq/liter) NaCl Lactate		KCl (mEq/liter)	CaCl₂ (mEq/liter)	NH₄Cl	PO₄(gm/liter)
0.9% saline		154					
3% saline		513					
5% saline		856					
D₅W	50						
2% ammonium chloride						374	
1/6 molar ammonium chloride (0.9%)						167	
Ringer's lactate		103	27	4	4		
Sodium phosphate (pH 5.7)		400					93
Potassium phosphate (pH 6.6)				400			93

TABLE 14–A2   Common Ampules

	Volume (ml) in ampule	mEq in ampule (not concentration)
7.5% sodium bicarbonate	50	44
7.5% potassium chloride	20	20
14.9% potassium chloride	20	20
10.0% calcium gluconate	10	4
10.0% calcium chloride	10	14
26.8% ammonium chloride	20	100
25.0% magnesium sulfate	2	4
		Gram in Ampule
25.0% mannitol	50	12.5
50.0% glucose	50	25.0

TABLE 14–A3   Conversions

	mEq of anion or cation/gram of salt	Salt/mEq (mg)
CaCl₂ · 2H₂O	14	73
Ca gluconate · 1H₂O	4	224
KCl	13	75
KHCO₃	10	100
NaCl	17	58
NaHCO₃	12	84

15. Hyperkalemia and Hypokalemia

PAUL M. PARIS, M.D.

HYPOKALEMIA

An electrolyte disturbance seen relatively often in emergency medicine, hypokalemia may become life-threatening. Therefore, the emergency care physician must have a high index of suspicion and search for this condition even when its clinical manifestations are subtle.

ETIOLOGY

The causes of hypokalemia can be divided into four general groups: (1) decreased intake, (2) gastrointestinal losses, (3) renal losses, and (4) maldistribution.

Decreased Intake

It is unusual for clinically significant hypokalemia to result from decreased intake.[1,2,3] Potassium is present in almost all naturally occurring foods, including meats, vegetables, fruits, and juices.[2] The daily renal, gastrointestinal, and skin obligate losses of potassium are approximately 20 to 30 mEq/day.[3] Few diets contain less than this amount of potassium. In the rare circumstances in which less than 20 mEq/day potassium is consumed, mild hypokalemia may occur after several weeks, but other manifestations of malnutrition are usually more prominent.

Gastrointestinal Losses

All gastrointestinal secretions contain potassium[1,4] (Table 15–1). Any patient with fluid losses from the gastrointestinal tract should be considered a candidate for hypokalemia. Patients with vomiting, diarrhea, tube drainage, gastrointestinal fistulas, and villous adenomas should all be monitored for potassium loss. Hypokalemia may also result from laxative abuse or self-induced vomiting that may not be evident from the patient's history.

Renal Losses

The most common cause of significant hypokalemia is renal loss.[3,5,6] Several mechanisms cause increased urinary losses of potassium:

1. drug-induced
   a. potent saluretic agents
   b. osmotic diuretics

TABLE 15–1 Average Potassium Content of Gastrointestinal Fluids

Fluid	Potassium Content
Gastric	10 to 15 mEq/liter
Pancreatic	5 mEq/liter
Biliary	5 mEq/liter
Small bowel	5 mEq/liter
Diarrheal stool	25 mEq/liter or greater

c. carbonic anhydrase inhibitors
d. carbenicillin
e. sodium penicillin
f. licorice and extracts of licorice
2. mineralocorticoid activity
   a. Cushing's syndrome (adrenal neoplasm, pituitary neoplasm, ectopic adrenocorticotropic hormone [ACTH])
   b. primary aldosteronism
   c. Bartter's syndrome
   d. exogenous steroids
   e. edematous states (congestive heart failure, cirrhosis, nephrosis)
3. acid-base disturbances
   a. alkali loading
   b. renal tubular acidosis
   c. diabetic ketoacidosis
4. other
   a. magnesium deficiency
   b. leukemia

Almost all potassium that is filtered in the glomerulus of the kidney is reabsorbed in the proximal tubule and loop of Henle. Any potassium excreted in the urine has been secreted in the distal tubule and collecting duct. Factors that increase such secretion are (a) increased delivery of sodium to the distal tubule, (b) increased delivery of nonreabsorbable anions to the distal tubule, (c) alkalosis, and (d) increased urine flow rate. Loop diuretics, osmotic diuretics, and carbonic anhydrase inhibitors increase both urine flow rates and sodium delivery to the distal tubule, thus causing significant increases in kaliuresis.[1,2,3,7] Carbenicillin and sodium penicillin are nonreabsorbable anions that increase potassium secretions in the distal tubule.[1,8,9]

Certain chemicals with mineralocorticoid activity, such as licorice, increase distal tubule reabsorption of sodium, which is accompanied by the exchange of either potassium or hydrogen ion.

When an alkalosis is present, the distal tubular cell has a deficiency of intracellular hydrogen; therefore, most of the exchange of sodium is for potassium, which increases losses in the urine. Diabetic ketoacidosis causes significant potassium losses because of several factors. Glycosuria and ketonuria, for example, cause a tremendous osmotic diuresis and increase the delivery of nonreabsorbable anions to the distal tubule. Magnesium deficiency impairs the function of the renal tubular cells with subsequent potassium loss.[2] Edematous states (e.g., congestive heart failure, nephrosis, cirrhosis) increase the levels of aldosterone, owing to a decreased effective circulating volume. Aldosterone, like other mineralocorticoids, increases sodium exchange for potassium or hydrogen in the distal tubule. In acute myeloid leukemia, especially monocytic or myelomonocytic, increased loss of potassium in the urine is thought

to be due to the effect of lysozymes on the proximal tubule.[1] Bartter's syndrome is a rare, interesting disease in which hyperplasia of the renal juxtaglomerular apparatus results in overproduction of renin. In this syndrome, however, the renin does not cause hypertension, but increases aldosterone secretion, thus increasing potassium loss. Renal tubular abnormalities may also cause potassium loss. These tubular abnormalities may be mediated by prostaglandins, since many inhibitors of prostaglandins, such as indomethacin, are helpful in correcting the hypokalemia.[10]

Maldistribution

Normally, 2 percent of potassium is extracellular. In certain circumstances, potassium is shifted to the intracellular stores, leaving the serum hypokalemic.[1,3,4] With alkalosis, for example, potassium from extracellular stores is transported intracellularly in exchange for hydrogen ion. A rough estimate is that for each 0.1 change in pH there is a 0.6 mEq/liter change in the serum potassium level in the opposite direction.[1,3,4]

An unusual disorder caused by hypokalemia due to maldistribution is periodic paralysis. Patients with this disorder are subject to attacks of severe muscle weakness owing to the sudden intracellular shift of potassium. These shifts are frequently precipitated by carbohydrate loads in association with a lack of muscular activity, but the exact etiology is unknown.[11]

One action of insulin is to cause potassium to be transported intracellularly. With insulin therapy, therefore, care must always be taken to avoid precipitating hypokalemia. This is especialiy critical in the treatment of diabetic ketoacidosis, in which several other factors also predispose the patient to hypokalemia.[2,4]

In the early treatment of megaloblastic anemias with vitamin B_{12}, large amounts of potassium are transported into young red blood cells and platelets, which may lead to hypokalemia.[1]

CLINICAL MANIFESTATIONS

Hypokalemia has several manifestations, all of which depend on the severity and the duration of the hypokalemia. Losses greater than 5 to 10 percent of body potassium are usually symptomatic. The clinical effects of hypokalemia include[2,4,12]

- *skeletal and smooth muscle:* weakness, paralysis, rhabdomyolysis
- *cardiac:* electrocardiogram (ECG) abnormality, increased sensitivity to digoxin, increased premature atrial contractions and premature ventricular contractions

- *neurologic:* mental changes, decreased deep tendons reflexes
- *metabolic:* decreased release and sensitivity to insulin
- *gastrointestinal:* atony of the gastrointestinal tract
- *renal:* decreased concentrating ability, decreased glomerular filtration rate, increased ammonia production, decreased urinary acidification

Neuromuscular Effects

Frequently, the most prominent effect of hypokalemia is that on the neuromuscular system. When potassium is decreased in the extracellular space, the ratio of intracellular potassium to extracellular potassium increases. This change, in turn, increases the transmembrane potential, which widens the difference between the transmembrane potential and the resting potential, thereby impeding impulse conduction and muscular contraction. Skeletal muscle weakness is usually the first sign of this effect. Limb muscles are usually affected before trunk muscles. The classic pattern first involves the lower extremities, especially the quadriceps. The pattern of weakness may resemble ascending paralysis of primary neurologic origin (Guillain-Barré syndrome). Smooth muscle also becomes involved so that nausea, vomiting, constipation, paralytic ileus, and gastric distention are all possible. The muscle weakness may become severe enough to cause respiratory paralysis and death from respiratory failure.

When hypokalemia is severe, rhabdomyolysis may be induced by exercise; occasionally, it may occur even without muscular activity. Rhabdomyolysis frequently results in acute tubular necrosis secondary to myoglobinuria. This mechanism has even been implicated in cases of renal failure secondary to licorice ingestion.[13]

Cardiac Effects

Some of the most serious effects of hypokalemia are the cardiac changes, e.g., conduction disturbances, rhythm abnormalities, and possible decreases in contractility. The ECG changes that are seen with potassium depletion include[2,3,9,14]

- depression of ST segments
- decreased T-wave voltage and sometimes inversion
- increased U-wave voltage (with more severe changes)
- increased amplitude of P wave
- widening of the QRS complex
- prolongation of PR interval

The ECG changes of hypokalemia do not occur as reliably as those of hyperkalemia. Therefore, significant hypokalemia cannot be ruled out on the basis of an ECG. The most common arrhythmias seen with hypokalemia are premature atrial and premature ventricular contractions and disturbances in atrioventricular nodal conduction.[15] Severe hypokalemia may lead to the life-threatening ventricular rhythm of torsade de pointes. This rhythm is frequently fatal and is a variant of ventricular tachycardia with unique electrocardiographic features.[16] Digitalis causes a decrease in intracellular potassium and potentiates the cardiac manifestations of hypokalemia. Digitalis toxicity with hypokalemia is a life-threatening emergency. This association must be remembered because many patients taking digitalis preparations are also on diuretics, which predisposes them to hypokalemia. It is essential to monitor potassium levels in these patients. It must also be remembered that patients on diuretics frequently become deficient in magnesium, and replacement of the magnesium lost may be required to correct ventricular irritability seen with digitalis toxicity. There is some experimental evidence that hypokalemia decreases cardiac contractility and, therefore, may precipitate or exacerbate congestive heart failure.[3]

Renal Effects

Hypokalemia affects many aspects of renal function, including glomerular filtration rate, concentrating ability, ammonia production, urinary acidification, and bicarbonate and sodium reabsorption.[4,12,17,18] The renal abnormalities usually take weeks to develop. Because hypokalemia interferes with the kidney's responsiveness to antidiuretic hormone, the kidney's ability to concentrate urine is decreased, leading to polyuria and polydipsia. Hypokalemia induces an increase in the production of ammonia by renal tubular epithelial cells and diminishes the kidney's ability to acidify urine. Reabsorption of bicarbonate is increased, even in the face of alkalosis. Histologic changes associated with hypokalemia are seen in the renal tubular epithelial cells, but all functional and histologic abnormalities can be reversed with potassium replacement.

Metabolic Effects

Hypokalemia causes some interference in the release of insulin, and mild glucose intolerance is one of the signs of hypokalemia.[3] Since potassium is necessary for the synthesis of skeletal muscle and hepatic glycogen, this function is also impaired by hypokalemia.

DIAGNOSIS

The history usually suggests which patients are likely to have hypokalemia. Some patients, however, may have symptomatic hypokalemia without a history to suggest a cause. Patients can become hypokalemic from occult diuretic abuse, self-induced vomiting, or laxative abuse, but these patients frequently deny these practices. Therefore, it is necessary to determine the serum potassium level in patients with symptoms that suggest hypokalemia, even when there is no relevant history. In addition, hypokalemia may result from such entities as villous adenomas or Bartter's syndrome without a history to suggest these causes.

In patients with unexplained hypokalemia, it is frequently helpful to determine the urine potassium level. Patients with hypokalemia due to renal losses usually have a urine potassium level greater than 10 to 20 mEq/ liter. If the cause is extrarenal, a kidney is usually able to limit its potassium excretion to less than 10 to 20 mEq/liter.[2,3] Serum potassium determinations are extremely unreliable in estimating total body potassium deficits, but they are the easiest to obtain.

TREATMENT

Hypokalemia should be corrected as slowly as the clinical situation will permit. As mentioned previously, serum potassium determinations are very inaccurate, and it is impossible to predict precisely the amount of potassium that must be replaced.[2,3,19] The safest way to correct hypokalemia is via the gastrointestinal tract with oral supplements.[20] In life-threatening situations that involve severe muscle weakness or digitalis toxicity, or when oral preparations are not tolerated, intravenous potassium chloride must be used. When replacing significant quantities of potassium by the intravenous route, ECG monitoring is required to prevent the development of unrecognized transient hyperkalemia with its possible cardiotoxic effects.

Hypokalemia is frequently associated with alkalosis and a chloride deficit. When an alkalosis is present, bicarbonate acts as a nonreabsorbable anion in the distal tubule, leading to continued potassium losses in the urine unless chloride is replaced along with potassium. Therefore, potassium chloride should be used for replacement in this circumstance.[2,3] If no alkalosis is present, many compounds can be used, including potassium chloride, potassium acetate, potassium phosphate, or potassium bicarbonate.

All oral preparations of potassium chloride are irritating to the gastrointestinal tract and may cause ulcerations, especially if gastrointestinal motility is decreased. Even with enteric-coated tablets, ulcerations of the small bowel have been described. When intravenous replacement with potassium chloride is used, the rate should be limited to 20 mEq/hour, or a total of 200 to 250 mEq/day, unless losses continue at a rate

greater than this.[2,3,21,22] With peripheral intravenous administration, concentration should not exceed 40 mEq/ liter, owing to the risk of vein irritation. In severe life-threatening situations, potassium chloride can be administered via a central vein in a concentration of 60 mEq/liter, but continuous ECG monitoring is mandatory.

In patients with significant continuous losses of potassium, daily oral administration of potassium chloride may be necessary. The routine use of potassium chloride in all patients on diuretics does not seem to be justified, however. Several studies have shown that only a small minority of patients develop symptomatic hypokalemia on diuretic therapy. The Boston Collaborative Drug Surveillance Program in 1974 studied 4,921 patients on potassium chloride and found that 7 had died as a result of hyperkalemia and 21 others had developed life-threatening complications of hyperkalemia.[23] Eighty-six percent of the patients in this study were taking potassium chloride for prophylaxis rather than for any demonstrated hypokalemia. Patients on diuretic therapy should be monitored for the signs and symptoms of hypokalemia, but routine prophylactic potassium supplementation is not necessary in patients with a normal diet. The serum potassium level of patients on digitalis should be monitored more closely. Some patients benefit from the addition of potassium-sparing diuretics, such as spironolactone, triamterene, or amiloride hydrochloride; but, again, patients must be screened carefully for the development of hyperkalemia.[24,25]

Patients with diabetic ketoacidosis are a special group whose serum potassium levels must be extremely carefully monitored. Many of the deaths that occur in this disease are preventable consequences of hypokalemia. In diabetic ketoacidosis, there is a tremendous loss of potassium, owing to the osmotic diuresis and, occasionally, to vomiting. Initial serum potassium levels may be normal or even high. For each 0.1 decrease in pH, there is an approximate serum increase in potassium of 0.6 mEq/liter.[1,2,4] As the acidosis is corrected, the serum potassium level may decrease quite rapidly. Also, insulin causes a shift of potassium to the intracellular space. The combination of correcting the acidosis and using insulin therapy causes extremely precipitous drops in potassium levels, and serum levels should be monitored every 1 to 2 hours for the first 12 hours of therapy. Large doses of intravenous potassium supplementation must be anticipated in the treatment of this disease.

When hypokalemia is present, the magnesium level may also be decreased. Serum magnesium levels are notoriously unreliable indicators of body deficits. When hypokalemia is due to malabsorption or diuretic therapy, when losses of magnesium would be expected, it is frequently wise to add magnesium to the potassium supplement, especially if ventricular irritability is a problem. Hypocalcemia may also be associated with hypokalemia, especially in cases of malabsorption. If this is the case, the correction of either deficit without the simultaneous correction of the other will exacerbate the symptoms of the uncorrected deficit.[10,22]

HYPERKALEMIA

One of the most serious electrolyte abnormalities seen in emergency medicine is hyperkalemia. This term is usually applied when the plasma potassium level is greater than 5.5 mEq/liter. Severe hyperkalemia is life-threatening and represents a true medical emergency.

ETIOLOGY

The four main categories of hyperkalemia and differential diagnoses in each category are as follows:[4,7,18,23,26–29]

1. spurious
   a. lab error
   b. hemolysis in vitro
   c. pseudohyperkalemia secondary to thrombocytosis or leukocytosis
   d. poor venipuncture technique
2. excessive intake
   a. dietary
   b. intravenous infusions
   c. potassium salts
3. transcellular redistribution
   a. severe tissue trauma
   b. intravascular hemolysis
   c. acidosis
   d. insulin deficiency
   e. hyperkalemic periodic paralysis
   f. massive digitalis overdose
   g. administration of succinylcholine (especially in burn and trauma victims)
   h. rapid lysis of malignant cells
4. decreased potassium excretion
   a. acute renal failure
   b. chronic renal failure
   c. adrenal insufficiency
   d. potassium-sparing diuretics
   e. hyporeninemic hypoaldosteronism
   f. renal transplant

Spurious Hyperkalemia

Whenever hemolysis occurs before or after blood sampling, the serum potassium levels are elevated because intracellular potassium, which is present in a concentration of approximately 150 mEq/liter cell water has been released.[7,28] When markedly elevated platelet counts (greater than 500,000) or leukocyte counts (greater than 100,000) are present in the serum, potassium may be artificially elevated because potassium has been released in the clotting process.[7,28] When this is suspected, it can be confirmed by comparing simultaneously drawn serum potassium with a heparinized plasma potassium. Spurious hyperkalemia should be suspected when the potassium is elevated without any accompanying changes on ECG.

Excessive Intake

In individuals with normal renal function, the oral intake of potassium is rarely a cause of sustained hyperkalemia. The rapid administration of 50 mEq potassium can temporarily elevate potassium by 0.5 to 1 mEq/liter.[18] Individuals with any degree of renal impairment are candidates for significant hyperkalemia from oral and intravenous infusions. The potential sources of potassium include oral and intravenous potassium salts, potassium salts of penicillin (1.7 mEq/1 million units), salt substitutes, and banked blood. In Lawson's study of 16,048 patients receiving potassium supplements, approximately 4 percent developed hyperkalemia, and 7 died as a result of their hyperkalemia.[23] When patients are being treated for hypokalemia too rapidly, they may develop transient hyperkalemia prior to the intracellular equilibration of the potassium given.

Transcellular Redistribution

Ninety-eight percent of the body's potassium is intracellular. Owing to this high intracellular concentration of potassium, hyperkalemia may be produced by the release of intracellular potassium to the extracellular space. With severe tissue trauma, such as crush injuries or burns, massive amounts of potassium may be released. Hemolysis and the rapid lysis of malignant cells during drug therapy are other mechanisms of potassium release. During acidosis, hydrogen ions enter cells in exchange for potassium or sodium ions, with a resultant increase in the serum potassium level.[18,27–30] Insulin is very important in the intracellular transport of potassium, and hyperkalemia is one stimulus for insulin release.[31] In the presence of an insulin deficiency, the serum potassium level may be elevated because less potassium can be transported intracellularly. Massive digitalis overdoses block the sodium-potassium adenosinetriphosphatase (ATPase) pump in cell membranes that are responsible for maintaining the high intracellular concentration of potassium.[18,29] This action greatly elevates the serum potassium level, but it is seen only with massive doses of digitalis, not clinically therapeutic levels. Succinylcholine is a muscle relaxant that works by allowing potassium to leak out of cells, causing depolarization blockade of impulses.[18,28] Normally, the potassium level increases by only 0.5 mEq/liter or less, but significant potassium increases may occur in patients with burns, multiple trauma, or neuromuscular disease. If any of these states are present, succinylcholine is contraindicated owing to the risk of life-threatening cardiac toxicity.

Hyperkalemic periodic paralysis is a hereditary disease characterized by episodes of muscle weakness or paralysis due to sudden increases in serum potassium. Episodes are precipitated by small increases in dietary potassium or by exercise.[18,27-28] These patients have a diminished ability to transfer and maintain potassium intracellularly, but the exact nature of the defect is unknown. Attacks can be prevented by treatment with mineralocorticoids or acetazolamide. Success has also been reported with the use of salbutamol, a β-adrenergic agonist.

Decreased Excretion

Since greater than 90 percent of potassium excretion is mediated by the kidneys, major changes in the serum potassium level can occur if renal function is decreased.[18,29] The most severe condition is acute oliguric renal failure. In this condition, the potassium level may rise sharply, owing to the inability to excrete potassium. This may be exacerbated both by the acidosis that may develop and the increased potassium load that results from the catabolic state. With chronic renal failure, the ability to excrete potassium is frequently maintained because the surviving nephrons adapt, excreting four to five times their normal amount of potassium. Maintaining a normal potassium level in the presence of chronic renal failure is highly dependent upon urine volumes, however. Patients may be able to maintain potassium at normal levels until the potassium load is increased or potassium-sparing diuretics, such as spironolactone, triamterene, or amiloride, are used. These drugs work by different mechanisms, but all selectively block the aldosterone-mediated distal tubule reabsorption of sodium, therefore limiting the normal mechanism for potassium secretion. Because patients with decreased renal function are very sensitive to these drugs, they should be used with caution in these patients. Recently, a case of fatal hyperkalemia due to spironolactone in a patient with entirely normal renal function was reported.[32]

Patients with adrenal insufficiency have a decreased production of mineralocorticoid and, therefore, a decreased ability for distal tubular secretion of potassium.

In addition, patients with only mild degrees of renal insufficiency may have chronic hyperkalemia. These patients are reported to have decreased levels of renin and, thereby, decreased levels of aldosterone. Patients with this hyporeninemic hypoaldosteronism are frequently also diabetic, and many have a hyperchloremic metabolic acidosis.[18,27,29] Patients with renal transplants frequently have marked difficulty with the tubular mechanisms responsible for potassium excretion.[29,33]

CLINICAL MANIFESTATIONS

The major clinical manifestations of hyperkalemia include[4,18,27-29]

- cardiovascular: ECG changes, heart block, ventricular arrhythmias
- neuromuscular: paresthesias, weakness, flaccid paralysis
- gastrointestinal: nausea, vomiting, abdominal pain, ileus

All the manifestations of hyperkalemia can be attributed to the high extracellular potassium level on cell membranes. An increase in the ratio of extracellular to intracellular potassium decreases the resting membrane potential toward threshold levels with resultant delays in depolarization, hastening of repolarization, and decreased conduction velocity. Significant clinical abnormalities are not usually seen until the plasma potassium level exceeds the 6 to 6.5 mEq/liter level.

Cardiotoxicity

The most serious medical problem induced by hyperkalemia is cardiotoxicity. Cardiac tissue is very vulnerable to the effects of hyperkalemia. The ECG changes seen with hyperkalemia are relatively reliable; in fact, when hyperkalemia occurs without ECG changes, spurious hyperkalemia should be suspected. With increasing levels of potassium, the following changes are noted:[27-28,33-35]

1. peaking of T waves (with normal or slightly decreased Q-T interval)
2. PR lengthening with possible ST depression
3. disappearing P waves
4. increasing degrees of heart block
5. widening of the QRS complex
6. ventricular arrhythmias with possible sine wave pattern
7. ventricular fibrillation or standstill

The most reliable ECG change seen with hyperkalemia is the peaking of T waves, which can sometimes be distinguished from T-wave changes of ischemic heart disease by the lack of U waves and the lack of any T-wave axis changes in the horizontal plane. The presence of any ECG changes of hyperkalemia warrants immediate treatment, since the progression to fatal cardiotoxicity is unpredictable and frequently rapid. Hyponatremia, hypocalcemia, and acidosis all increase the cardiotoxicity of hyperkalemia and should be corrected if they exist.

Neuromuscular Effects

The first neuromuscular sign of hyperkalemia is usually the onset of paresthesias. This may be followed by weakness of several muscle groups in an ascending pattern. If hyperkalemia becomes severe, flaccid quadriplegia may occur. Cerebral and cranial nerve function is usually preserved, and respiratory muscle paralysis is very rare.

TREATMENT

Hyperkalemia is a life-threatening condition that deserves immediate medical attention. When ECG changes of hyperkalemia are seen, continuous ECG monitoring is mandatory until the hyperkalemia has been corrected. There are four general categories of treatment:

1. antagonism of membrane effects
   a. calcium (calcium gluconate or calcium chloride)
   b. sodium (if hyponatremia exists)
2. transfer of potassium intracellularly
   a. sodium bicarbonate
   b. glucose with or without insulin
3. removal of potassium from the body
   a. potassium exchange resins
   b. hemodialysis
   c. peritoneal dialysis
   d. loop diuretics
4. correction of underlying defects

The decision as to which modalities should be used in the treatment depends on the degree of potassium elevation and the associated medical conditions.[22,27–29,36,37]

Antagonism of Membrane Effects

When changes of hyperkalemia other than peak T waves are seen on the ECG, then immediate measures must be taken to prevent ventricular arrhythmias. The intravenous administration of calcium, either as calcium gluconate or calcium chloride, has the earliest action. Calcium decreases the membrane threshold potentials,

counteracting some of the effects of hyperkalemia on cell membranes. These actions are very rapid, but temporary; they are to be used only in conjunction with other measures. Calcium chloride or calcium gluconate may be administered intravenously as a 10 percent solution with 10 to 30 ml given over several minutes. Also, another 10 to 30 ml calcium can be added to a 1-liter bottle of a dextrose solution.

Hyponatremia exacerbates the membrane abnormalities induced by hyperkalemia. When a patient has any degree of hyponatremia, the administration of sodium frequently corrects some of the membrane effects of hyperkalemia. Care must be used to avoid fluid overload when sodium is administered as a hypertonic solution, however. The result of sodium use is not as reliable as that of calcium. An excellent way to add sodium is by means of sodium bicarbonate added to a dextrose solution, which combines the beneficial effects of sodium, bicarbonate, and dextrose.

Transfer of Potassium Intracellularly

An extremely useful strategy in the treatment of hyperkalemia is to increase the transfer of extracellular potassium to the intracellular space. When acidosis exists, it should be corrected immediately, since the serum potassium level increases approximately 0.6 mEq/liter for each 0.1 decrease in pH.[7,18,27–28] The bicarbonate ion increases the transfer of potassium to the intracellular space even when pH changes do not occur.[32] Fifty to 100 mEq/liter sodium bicarbonate can be administered over several minutes.

Insulin also facilitates the transfer of potassium intracellularly. In nondiabetics, administering glucose first as 50 ml 50 percent solution followed by 500 ml 10 percent dextrose enhances endogenous insulin secretion. It is frequently helpful to add 5 to 10 units regular insulin while administering this combination, being careful to avoid hypoglycemia. In patients with diabetes mellitus, insulin should be administered with the dextrose infusion. Approximately 1 unit regular insulin for each 3 gm glucose usually suffices, but serum glucose must be monitored.[27]

Removal of Potassium from the Body

Antagonizing the membrane effects of hyperkalemia and increasing the transport of potassium to the intracellular space are both temporary measures. The definitive treatment of hyperkalemia is to remove potassium from the body. The simplest technique to accomplish this is the administration of the cation exchange resin, sodium polystyrene sulfonate (Kayexalate). This resin can be administered orally or in a retention enema. For each gram of resin used, approximately 1 mEq potassium is removed.[18,28] When given orally, 20 to 30 gm Kayexalate can be added to an approximately equal amount of sorbitol. Sorbitol increases the amount of fluid entering the intestinal tract, thereby facilitating ion exchange. Retention enemas can be mixed by adding 50 to 100 gm Kayexalate to 200 ml water, and adding an appropriate amount of sorbitol. The enema must be retained for 30 to 45 minutes.

When extremely large amounts of potassium must be removed, hemodialysis and peritoneal dialysis can be considered. Hemodialysis is extremely effective—it can remove potassium at a rate of 25 to 50 mEq/hour. Peritoneal dialysis is less predictable and may not remove more than 10 to 15 mEq/hour. In patients who are nonoliguric with only minor elevations of serum potassium, the loop diuretics increase the renal excretion of potassium.

Correction of the Underlying Defect

Hyperkalemia is usually a short-term problem, but certain underlying medical conditions require continuing therapy. With hyperkalemic periodic paralysis, mineralocorticoids, acetazolamide, and salbutamol have all been shown to be effective at decreasing episodes of paralysis.[7,18,28] In chronic renal failure, potassium-sparing diuretics and large loads of potassium must be avoided. With adrenal insufficiency and with hyporeninemic hyperaldosteronism, chronic mineralocorticoid therapy is very effective at maintaining potassium within normal levels.

REFERENCES

1. Nardone DA, McDonald WJ, Girard DE: Mechanisms in hypokalemia: Clinical correlation. *Medicine* 57:435, 1978.
2. Rose BD (ed): *Hypokalemia: Clinical Physiology of Acid-Base and Electrolyte Disorders*. New York, McGraw-Hill, 1977, p 459.
3. Cohen J Jr, Madias NE: Acid-base disorders of respiratory origin, in Brenner BM, Stein JH (eds): *Acid-Base and Potassium Homeostasis*. New York, Churchill Livingstone, 1978, p 137.
4. Cohen JJ: Disorders of potassium balance. *Hosp Pract* 1:119, 1979.
5. Lowman DH, et al: Severe hypokalemia in hospitalized patients. *Arch Intern Med* 139:978, 1979.
6. Rose DB (ed): *Introduction to Disorders of Potassium Balance: Clinical Physiology of Acid-Base and Electrolyte Disorders*. New York, McGraw-Hill, 1977, p 448.
7. Kliger AS, Hayslett JP: Disorders of potassium balance, in Brenner BM, Stein JH (eds): *Acid-Base and Potassium Homeostasis*. New York, Churchill Livingstone, 1978, p 168.
8. Mohr JA, et al: Nafcillin-associated hypokalemia. *JAMA* 242:544, 1979.
9. Carlon GC: Drug associations in hypokalemia, letter to the editor. *Arch Intern Med* 140:989, 1980.
10. Bartter FC: Clinical problems of potassium metabolism. *Contrib Nephrol* 21:115, 1980.
11. Gastel B, Ehrlichman R (eds): Clinical conferences at the Johns Hopkins Hospital—Hypokalemic periodic paralysis. *Johns Hopkins Med J* 143:148, 1978.
12. Cronin RE, Knochel JP: The consequences of potassium deficiency in acid-base and potassium, in Brenner BM, Stein JH (eds): *Acid-Base and Potassium Homeostasis*. New York, Churchill Livingstone, 1978, p 205.
13. Laei F, et al: Licorice, snuff and hypokalemia, letter to the editor. *N Engl J Med* 303:463, 1980.
14. Schamroth L, Weiner S: A case of prolonged Q-T interval! *Heart Lung* 7:846, 1978.
15. Dychner T, Wester PO: Ventricular extrasystoles and intracellular electrolytes in hypokalemic patients before and after correction of the hypokalemia. *Acta Med Scand* 204:375, 1978.
16. Parrish C, et al: Les Torsades des Pointes. *Ann Emerg Med* 3:143, 1982.
17. Giebisch G, Malnic G, Berlinger RW: Renal transport and control of potassium excretion, in Brenner BM, Rector FL (eds): *The Kidney*, ed 2. Philadelphia, WB Saunders, 1981, p 908.
18. Cohen JJ, Gennari FJ, Harrington JT: Disorders of potassium balance, in Brenner BM, Rector FL (eds): *The Kidney*, ed 2. Philadelphia, WB Saunders, 1981.
19. Franklin JE Jr: Long-standing hypokalemia. *Hosp Pract* 9:153, 1979.
20. Ramsay LE, Ramsay MH: Rational potassium prescribing. *Practitioner* 219:529, 1977.
21. Zeluff GW, Suki WN, Jackson D: Hypokalemia—Cause and treatment. *Heart Lung* 7:854, 1978.
22. Levinsky N: Fluid and electrolytes, in Isselbacher KJ, Adams RD, Braunwald E, et al (eds): *Harrison's Principles of Internal Medicine*, ed 9. New York, McGraw-Hill, 1980, p 475.
23. Lawson DH: Adverse reactions to potassium chloride. *Q J Med* 171:433, 1974.
24. Ramsay LE, et al: Amiloride, spironolactone, and potassium chloride in thiazide-treated hypertensive patients. *Clin Pharmacol Ther* 4:533, 1980.
25. Pearce VR, et al: Total exchangeable potassium in response to amiloride. *Postgrad Med J* 54:533, 1978.
26. Lowenstein J: Hypokalemia and hyperkalemia. *Med Clin North Am* 57:1435, 1973.
27. Daniels GH: Metabolic and endocrine emergencies, in Wilkins EW Jr (ed): *MGH Textbook of Emergency Medicine*. Baltimore, Williams & Wilkins, 1981, p 264.
28. Falls WF: Hyperkalemia: Pathophysiology and management. *Virginia Medical* 107:184, 1980.
29. Rose BD (ed): *Hyperkalemia: Clinical Physiology of Acid-Base and Electrolyte Disorders*. New York, McGraw-Hill, 1977, p 482.
30. Hassan H, Gjessing J, Tomlin PJ: Hypercapnia and hyperkalaemia. *Anaesthesia* 34:897, 1979.
31. Cox M, Sterns RH, Singer I: The defense against hyperkalemia: The roles of insulin and aldosterone. *N Engl J Med* 299:525, 1978.
32. Wetli CV, Davis JH: Fatal hyperkalemia from accidental overdose of potassium chloride, letter to the editor. *JAMA* 240:1339, 1978.
33. Shapiro JB: Bifascicular block produced by hyperkalemia. *Cardiology* 64:303, 1979.
34. Schwartz AB: Potassium-related cardiac arrhythmias and their treatment. *Angiology* 29:194, 1978.
35. Burris AC, Chung EK: Pseudomyocardial infarction associated with acute bifascicular block due to hyperkalemia. *Cardiology* 65:115, 1980.
36. Levinsky NG: Management of emergencies: VI. Hyperkalemia. *N Engl J Med* 274:1076, 1966.
37. Fraley DS, Adler S: Correction of hyperkalemia by bicarbonate despite constant blood pH. *Kidney Int* 12:354, 1977.

16. Hypomagnesemia and Hypermagnesemia

JOEL M. GEIDERMAN, M.D.

Disorders of magnesium balance are now being recognized more frequently than they were in the past, owing largely to new techniques that allow rapid and accurate measurement of the cation. Both hypermagnesemia and hypomagnesemia may be life-threatening emergencies that require prompt medical treatment, or they may be less severe disturbances with subtle symptomatology.

MAGNESIUM HOMEOSTASIS

Magnesium is the fourth most abundant cation in the body and the second most plentiful intracellular element. An adult human body contains 21 to 28 gm, or about 2,000 mEq, magnesium. Approximately 50 percent of the total body magnesium is in bone; the other 50 percent is about equally divided between muscular and nonmuscular soft tissue.[1] Only about 1 percent of total body magnesium is extracellular. About 20 to 30 percent of serum magnesium is protein-bound; the remainder is in diffusible form, mainly as free ionized magnesium.[2] The normal serum magnesium concentration ranges between 1.6 and 2.1 mEq/liter.[3]

The level of magnesium in serum does not always accurately reflect total body magnesium stores, since the magnesium in the vascular space is only a fraction of the total body pool of the cation.[4] Serum and intracellular levels vary independently, and deficit or excess in one compartment may not indicate the level in the other. Skeletal muscle biopsy provides the most accu-

rate measurement of total body magnesium stores,[5] but it is not practical in the emergency setting. Measurement of serum magnesium must therefore suffice as the quickest, simplest, and most effective screening tool when magnesium depletion is suspected.[6]

An adult's average daily intake of magnesium is 20 to 40 mEq, much of which is contained in the chlorophyll portion of green vegetables.[1] Other sources include meats, grains, and seafood. The daily requirement of magnesium for the adult is approximately 5 mg/ kg body weight, or about 350 mg for a 70-kg person[7] (Table 16–1). This amount is contained in 3.5 gm magnesium sulfate.

Magnesium is absorbed primarily from the proximal small intestine; little is absorbed from the colon. Absorption begins within one hour of ingestion, continues at a steady rate for two to six hours, and has nearly ceased after 12 hours.[4] Under normal circumstances, 30 to 60 percent of orally ingested magnesium is absorbed. No apparent adaptation in absorption occurs in response to the body's need for the ion.

The kidneys are largely responsible for regulation of the serum magnesium concentration. Approximately 1,800 mg magnesium are filtered at the glomerule each day.[8] Since the diffusible fraction of magnesium is the moiety that is filtered, the filtered load is a function of both the serum concentration of diffusible magnesium and the glomerular filtration rate. Magnesium is actively reabsorbed along the entire nephron, but mainly in the proximal tubule. There seems to be a tubular

TABLE 16–1   Nutritional Requirements for Magnesium

Period of Life	Age (years)	Daily Amount of Magnesium (mg/day)
Infants	0–0.5	50
	0.5–1	70
Children	1–3	150
	4–6	200
	7–10	250
Males	11–14	350
	15–18	400
	19 and older	350
Females	11–14	300
	15 and older	300
	During pregnancy	300 + 150
	During lactation	300 + 150

Source: Food and Nutrition Board of National Academy of Sciences and National Research Council, 1980.

maximum for reabsorption (Tmax) beyond which all magnesium is excreted. Under normal circumstances, 3 to 5 percent of the filtered load is excreted in the urine.[2]

Many conditions can affect proximal tubular reabsorption of magnesium and result in variations in urinary excretion.[9] Factors that decrease tubular reabsorption include[10]

- extracellular fluid volume expansion (saline infusions)
- renal vasodilatation
- osmotic diuretics
- diuretics
- hypercalcemia
- alcohol ingestion
- high sodium intake
- growth hormone
- thyroid hormone
- calcitonin
- chronic mineralocorticoid excess
- phosphate depletion
- gentamicin
- tobramycin
- carbenicillin

Renal handling of magnesium is closely associated with that of sodium; in general, those agents that produce natriuresis produce magnesiuria as well.

The major factors that increase tubular reabsorption of magnesium are parathyroid hormone and hypomagnesemia.[2]

BIOCHEMICAL ASPECTS

Magnesium activates an array of enzyme systems that are vital to intracellular metabolism. Most prominent among these enzymes are those that hydrolyze and transfer phosphate groups, which are important in the synthesis of adenosine triphosphate (ATP).[4,11] ATP is necessary for glucose utilization; for synthesis of protein, nucleic acids, nucleoproteins, nucleotides, coenzymes, and carbohydrates; for muscle contraction; and for maintenance of the sodium-potassium pump.[4,7] Magnesium also stabilizes ribosomes and thereby facilitates polypeptide formation. Interference with magnesium balance can therefore affect all of these functions.

HYPOMAGNESEMIA

Clinical Manifestations

The predominant clinical manifestations of hypomagnesemia are gastrointestinal and neurologic, involving both the central and peripheral nervous systems:[1,2,3]

- anorexia
- nausea, vomiting, diarrhea
- fasciculations
- gross tremor
- athetoid movements
- tetany
- convulsions
- stupor, coma
- mental aberrations
- confusion
- hallucinations
- supraventricular arrhythmias
- ventricular arrhythmias

Magnesium has a curarelike effect at the neuromuscular junction, presumably because it interferes with the release of acetylcholine at the motor neuron terminal.[11] Thus, hypomagnesemia leads to hyperexcitability as a result of the accumulation of acetylcholine at the neuromuscular junction.[12]

Tetany caused by hypomagnesemia is clinically indistinguishable from tetany caused by any other condition.[13] In the past, the existence of tetany in humans as a result of hypomagnesemia alone, in the absence of other measurable serum electrolyte or acid-base disturbances, has been controversial. However, the magnesium deficiency tetany syndrome is now a recognized clinical entity. The diagnosis of human tetany is based on facial muscle and carpopedal spasm, convulsions, and, occasionally, laryngeal stridor.[13] Latent tetany may be elicited as Chvostek's and Trousseau's signs.

Supraventricular tachycardia, ventricular tachycardia, and paroxysmal ventricular fibrillation have all been reported in association with hypomagnesemia.[14,15] Nonspecific changes on the electrocardiogram (ECG), such as prolonged PR interval, ST depression, and inverted or peaked T waves, also occur.[15] The explanation for the cardiac arrhythmias seen with magnesium deficiency remains speculative. Since magnesium deficiency is almost always associated with imbalance of other electrolytes, it is difficult to be certain which electrolyte abnormality is responsible for the ECG changes.

Etiology of Hypomagnesemia

Hypomagnesemia may result from poor intake or a defect in absorption or excretion. The following conditions are associated with hypomagnescmia:

1. decreased intake
   a. protein-calorie malnutrition
   b. starvation
   c. prolonged intravenous therapy without added magnesium
   d. liquid protein diet
2. decreased intestinal absorption
   a. malabsorption syndromes, including nontropical sprue, celiac disease, and tropical sprue
   b. massive surgical resection of small intestine
   c. neonatal hypomagnesemia with selective malabsorption of magnesium
3. excessive losses of body fluids
   a. prolonged nasogastric suction
   b. excessive uses of purgatives
   c. intestinal and biliary fistulas
   d. severe diarrhea, as in ulcerative colitis and infantile gastroenteritis
   e. rarely, prolonged lactation
   f. cancer of the colon
4. excessive urinary losses
   a. diuretic therapy
   b. diuretic phase of acute renal failure
   c. chronic alcoholism
   d. primary and secondary aldosteronism
   e. hypercalcemic states, e.g., malignancy, hyperparathyroidism, and vitamin D excess
   f. renal tubular acidosis
   g. diabetes, especially during and following treatment of acidosis
   h. hyperthyroidism
   i. idiopathic renal magnesium wasting
   j. chronic renal failure with renal magnesium wasting
   k. gentamicin, tobramycin, and carbenicillin therapy
   l. alcoholic cirrhosis
   m. glomerulonephritis
   n. pyelonephritis
   o. familial and sporadic renal magnesium wasting
   p. cisplatin therapy
5. miscellaneous
   a. idiopathic hypomagnesemia
   b. acute pancreatitis
   c. porphyria with inappropriate secretion of antidiuretic hormone
   d. multiple transfusions or exchange transfusions with citrated blood
   e. malignant osteolytic disease
   f. cardiopulmonary bypass
   g. infant born of hypomagnesemic mother
   h. hypoparathyroidism

Alcoholism is the most common cause of hypomagnesemia.[10] A variety of factors, including decreased dietary intake, vomiting, diarrhea, hyperhidrosis, and increased urinary excretion, contribute to the hypomagnesemia.[15,16] Magnesium diuresis results from ethanol's interference with tubular reabsorption of the ion. In patients with alcoholic cirrhosis and ascites, hypomagnesemia may be caused by secondary hyperaldosteronism, which prevents distal tubular reabsorption.[17]

Because magnesium levels fall precipitously soon after the withdrawal of alcohol, the neurologic manifestations of hypomagnesemia may be seen at this time. This must be differentiated from delirium tremens, which may occur simultaneously.[15,16,18] While hypomagnesemia is common in severe alcoholism and may be symptomatic in some patients, it clearly is not the cause of delirium tremens.[13] The latter may develop and progress, despite vigorous magnesium replacement and normal serum magnesium levels. Each of these closely related symptom complexes must be considered separately.

Malabsorption syndromes, especially those associated with steatorrhea, may also result in hypomagnesemia.[5] This may be secondary to the excretion of large amounts of magnesium soaps. Steatorrheic hypomagnesemia has been reported in patients with nontropical sprue, following abdominal irradiation, and after extensive small bowel resection. It also may occur after jejunoileal bypass for morbid obesity.[4,19,20]

Patients who are maintained on magnesium-free parenteral fluids for long periods of time are at risk of developing magnesium deficiency.[21] This should be considered in a patient who comes to the emergency department after a recent long hospitalization. Another group of patients predisposed to hypomagnesemia secondary to reduced dietary intake are those on liquid protein diets for obesity.[22]

Diabetes is also associated with hypomagnesemia.[21,23] With glycosuria, there is a threefold increase in urinary magnesium excretion, resulting in depletion.[23] In the initial phases of diabetic ketoacidosis, serum magnesium levels may be normal or slightly elevated owing to the acidosis and dehydration.[24] However, fluid and insulin therapy not only lead to large urinary losses of magnesium but also facilitate the movement of the ion intracellularly. This may produce severe hypomagnesemia, resulting in fatal arrhythmias.[25] It is therefore recommended that magnesium be added to replacement fluids and that serum levels of the ion be monitored during treatment.

The other condition commonly seen in the emergency department that may be associated with hypomagnesemia is congestive heart failure.[22] (See Chapter 51.) Several factors may lead to magnesium depletion in these patients. Markedly congested splanchnic vessels may lead to malabsorption of the ion in the gut. Secondary hyperaldosteronism contributes to the hypomagnesemia[26] by preventing reabsorption at the distal convoluted tubule. Cardiac glycosides are known to reduce renal absorption of magnesium also. This can have catastrophic consequences, since hypomagnesemia has been shown to predispose patients taking digitalis to arrhythmias.[15,27] Serum magnesium and potassium levels should be checked in all patients with suspected digitalis-induced arrhythmias, and magnesium should be administered if serum concentrations are low. This has been shown effective in abolishing a number of arrhythmias.

Finally, thiazide diuretics and furosemide, commonly used in congestive heart failure, both increase renal magnesium clearance.[26,28] Some have suggested routine measurement of serum magnesium in all patients on diuretics and digitalis.

Treatment of Magnesium Deficiency

While asymptomatic magnesium-depleted patients may warrant treatment, only symptomatic hypomagnesemia should be treated in the emergency department.[6] Occult magnesium deficiency can be detected in skeletal muscle,[26] but only the magnesium in the intravascular space can be rapidly measured by the emergency physician. Some patients may require treatment on an empirical basis, before magnesium depletion has been demonstrated. This may be especially true in smaller hospitals that do not have the facilities to provide rapid measurements. Renal function must be shown to be adequate before therapy is begun, however. Azotemia does not exclude therapy but necessitates modification of dosage.[29]

Convulsive seizures due to magnesium deficiency represent a true medical emergency and require immediate, vigorous treatment. The loading dose for such a patient is 4 gm (33 mEq) magnesium given as a 10 to 20 percent solution of magnesium sulfate[30] over five to ten minutes, followed by either continuous intravenous or intramuscular administration. Intravenous magnesium sulfate should never be given as the 50 percent solution. A 20-ml dose of 20 percent solution (4 gm) can be made by mixing 8 ml 50 percent magnesium sulfate solution and 12 ml sterile distilled water. Each magnesium sulfate molecule, with a molecular weight of 246, contains 8.1 mEq/gm. Each magnesium chloride molecule, with a molecular weight of 203, contains 9.75 mEq/gm.

Serious arrhythmias occur frequently in the alcohol withdrawal syndrome. They require urgent treatment, since sudden death of patients with the alcohol withdrawal syndrome is probably related to tachyarrhythmias. In case of ventricular tachycardia or ventricular fibrillation in alcohol withdrawal, 2 gm (16.3 mEq) magnesium sulfate as a 10 to 20 percent solution should be given intravenously over five to ten minutes, followed by continuous intravenous infusion.[30]

Magnesium-depleted patients usually require 1 to 2 mEq/kg for parenteral replacement, and restitution of magnesium stores must take place over a three- to four-day period. Thus, magnesium-depleted patients usually require hospitalization, although treatment can be started in the emergency department as outlined in Table 16–2.

It has been shown that plasma levels of magnesium will not exceed 6.5 mEq/liter as long as the rate of administration of magnesium salt does not exceed 100 mEq/12 hours. Further, it has been shown that patients can normally excrete from 40 to 60 gm of magnesium sulfate every 24 hours.[30] Thus, complications should not occur when the recommended regimen is employed in normal individuals. However, kidney function must be evaluated before treatment is begun. In azotemic patients, therapy must be modified and carefully monitored.[7]

There does not appear to be any therapeutic advantage of the intravenous route over the intramuscular route, except when treating convulsions and arrhythmias. If any intravenous solution is being given already, magnesium should be added to it; otherwise, the intramuscular route is indicated.

HYPERMAGNESEMIA

Clinical Manifestations

Hypermagnesemia affects mainly the nervous and cardiovascular systems.[2] Deep tendon reflexes are usu-

TABLE 16–2   Suggested Dosage Schedule for Treatment of Magnesium Depletion

Route	Day	Dosage
Intramuscular (50 percent magnesium sulfate solution)	1	2 gm (16.3 mEq) q2° × 3 doses, then 1 gm (8.1 mEq) q4° × 4 doses
	2	1 gm (8.1 mEq) q4° × 6 doses
	3–5	1 gm (8.1 mEq) q6°
Intravenous (< 20 percent magnesium sulfate solution only)	1	6 gm (49 mEq) in 1,000 ml desired intravenous solution to be infused over 3 hours, then 5 gm (41 mEq) in each of two 1-liter solutions to be infused over the day
	2–5	6 gm (49 mEq) distributed equally in the total fluids of the day

Source: Information from Flink EB: Therapy of magnesium deficiency. *Ann NY Acad Sci* 162:901–905, 1969.

ally lost when the serum magnesium level reaches 6 mEq/liter, and the patient may be sedated. Muscle paralysis, respiratory depression, narcosis, and hypotension may occur,[3] as the serum concentration approaches 10 mEq/liter. ECG changes include lengthening of the PR interval, progressing to complete heart block, widening of the QRS complex, and transient rise in heart rate followed by bradycardia.[2,10] Asystolic arrest may occur if the level reaches 14 to 15 mEq/liter.

Etiology

Hypermagnesemia, less common than hypomagnesemia, may develop in a number of conditions (Exhibit 16–1).[10] The most common cause is severe renal failure,[3] especially when exogenous sources are not restricted. The other major cause is iatrogenic; hypermagnesemia may develop during therapy of the toxemic patient.

Therapy

Symptomatic patients with serum magnesium levels of greater than 5 mEq/liter and those with levels of 8 mEq/liter, regardless of whether they have symptoms, should be treated.[10] Treatment is 5 ml 10 percent calcium chloride solution by slow intravenous push. This may be repeated if symptoms do not subside within two minutes, thereafter as dictated by the clinical setting.[10] Peritoneal dialysis or hemodialysis should be considered for persistently high levels.

Exhibit 16–1 Clinical Settings of Hypermagnesemia

Common

    Acute renal failure
    Chronic renal failure with exogenous
       magnesium intake
    Toxemia therapy

Less Common

    Chronic renal failure without exogenous intake
    Rectal administration of magnesium-containing
       solutions

Uncommon or Producing Only Smooth Elevations of Magnesium

    Parasitosis with exogenous magnesium intake
    Lithium therapy
    Hypothyroidism
    Certain neoplasms with skeletal involvement
    Viral hepatitis
    Hyperparathyroidism with renal disease
    Pituitary dwarfism
    Milk-alkali syndrome
    Perforated viscus with exogenous magnesium
       intake
    Acute diabetic ketoacidosis
    Addison's disease

Source: Modified and reprinted with permission from Graber TW, Yee AS, Baker FJ: Magnesium: Physiology, clinical disorders, and therapy. *Ann Emerg Med* 10:49–57, 1981.

REFERENCES

1. Wacker WEC, Parisi AF: Magnesium metabolism. *N Engl J Med* 278:656–661, 712–716, 1968.
2. Massry SG, Seelig MS: Hypomagnesemia and hypermagnesemia. *Clin Nephrol* 7:147–153, 1977.
3. Fishman RA: Neurological aspects of magnesium metabolism. *Arch Neurol* 12:562–569, 1965.
4. Swenson SA, Lewis JW, Sebby KR: Magnesium metabolism in man with special reference to jejunoileal bypass for obesity. *Am J Surg* 127:250–255, 1974.
5. Booth CC, Babouris N, Hanna S, et al: Incidence of hypomagnesemia in intestinal malabsorption. *Br Med J* 2:141–144, 1963.
6. Geiderman JM, Goodman SL, Cohen DB: Magnesium—The forgotten electrolyte. *JACEP* 8:204–208, 1979.
7. Flink EB: Nutritional aspects of magnesium metabolism (nutrition in medicine). *West J Med* 133:304–312, 1980.
8. Heaton FW: The kidney and magnesium homeostasis. *Ann NY Acad Sci* 162:901–905, 1969.
9. Massry SG: Pharmacology of magnesium. *Ann Rev Pharmacol Toxicol* 17:67–82, 1977.
10. Graber TW, Yee AS, Baker FJ: Magnesium: Physiology, clinical disorders, and therapy. *Ann Emerg Med* 10:49–57, 1981.
11. Wacker WEC, Vallee BL: Magnesium metabolism. *N Engl J Med* 259:431–438, 1958.
12. Hamed IA, Lindeman RD: Dysphagia and vertical nystagmus in magnesium deficiency. *Ann Emerg Med* 89:222–223, 1978.
13. Vallee BL, Wacker WEC, Ulmer DD: The magnesium-deficiency tetany syndrome in man. *N Engl J Med* 262:155–160, 1960.
14. Iseri LT, Freed J, Bures AR: Magnesium deficiency and cardiac disorders. *Am J Med* 58:837–844, 1975.
15. Burch GE, Giles TD: The importance of magnesium deficiency in cardiovascular disease. *Am Heart J* 94:649–656, 1977.
16. Sullivan JF, Wolpert PW, Williams R, et al: Serum magnesium in chronic alcoholism. *Ann NY Acad Sci* 162:947–962, 1969.
17. Kalbfleish JM, Linderman RD, Ginn HE, et al: Effects of ethanol administration on urinary excretion of magnesium and other electrolytes in alcoholic and normal subjects. *J Clin Invest* 42:1471–1475, 1963.
18. Fankushen D, Raskin D, Dimich A, et al: Significance of hypomagnesemia in alcoholic patients. *Am J Med* 37:802–812, 1964.
19. Lipner A: Symptomatic magnesium deficiency after small intestinal bypass for obesity. *Br Med J* 1:148, 1977.
20. Houston BD, Turner T: Severe electrolyte abnormalities in a pregnant patient with a jejunoileal bypass. *Arch Intern Med* 138:1712–1713, 1978.
21. Jackson CE, Meier DW: Routine serum magnesium analysis. *Ann Intern Med* 69:743–747, 1968.
22. Fouty RA: Liquid protein diet, magnesium deficiency, and cardiac arrest, correspondence. *JAMA* 240:2632–2633, 1978.
23. Martin HE, Smith K, Wilson ML: The fluid and electrolyte therapy of severe diabetic acidosis and ketosis. *Am J Med* 24:376–389, 1958.
24. Martin HE: Clinical magnesium deficiency. *Ann NY Acad Sci* 162:891–899, 1969.
25. McMullen JK: Asystole and hypomagnesemia during recovery from diabetic ketoacidosis. *Br Med J* 1:690, 1977.
26. Calcium, magnesium and diuretics, editorial. *Br Med J* 1:170–171, 1975.
27. Ghani MF, Smith JR: The effectiveness of magnesium chloride in the treatment of ventricular tachyarrhythmias due to digitalis intoxication. *Am Heart J* 88(5):621–626, 1974.
29. Flink EB: Correspondence. *Arch Intern Med* 138:825, 1978.
30. Flink EB: Therapy of magnesium deficiency. *Ann NY Acad Sci* 162:901–905, 1969.

17. Hypercalcemia

EMANUEL K. GORDON, M.D.

Hypercalcemic crisis is a syndrome encountered in a minority of patients with hypercalcemia. A common condition, hypercalcemia occurs in up to 6 percent of asymptomatic patients who undergo routine screening.[1,2] Only a small proportion of hypercalcemic patients who become symptomatic develop the hypercalcemic crisis syndrome, a true medical emergency. Hypercalcemic crisis may be defined as hypercalcemia that causes the abrupt onset of severe symptoms, most commonly a comatose or semicomatose state, protracted nausea and vomiting accompanied by polyuria that markedly depletes intravascular volume, profound weakness, and deteriorating renal function.

The subgroup of hypercalcemic patients who develop hypercalcemic crisis is not determined simply by the absolute level of the serum calcium concentration. Factors such as the rapidity with which the serum calcium concentration rises, the underlying etiology of hypercalcemia, and variations in individual tolerance to the effects of hypercalcemia all seem to influence the development of hypercalcemic crisis. The syndrome may occur in a patient with an underlying malignancy who has a serum calcium concentration of 12 mg/dl, while an individual with chronic hypercalcemia can be virtually asymptomatic with a serum calcium concentration of 15 mg/dl.

The diagnosis of hypercalcemic crisis is based on the clinical symptoms and the demonstration of an elevated serum calcium concentration. The initial therapy of hypercalcemic crisis should be instituted immediately after the diagnosis is made. Therapy is similar for all patients with hypercalcemic crisis syndrome, no matter what the cause.

DIAGNOSIS OF HYPERCALCEMIC CRISIS

Even though hypercalcemia can produce symptoms referable to nearly every organ system in the body (Fig. 17–1), the diagnosis of hypercalcemic crisis is easily made by determining the serum calcium concentration. It is recommended that a serum calcium level be determined on every patient who comes to the emergency department with a disordered level of consciousness unless the cause is obvious.[3] A delirious or confused patient with a history of renal calculi, cancer, recent immobilization, or a combination of these should alert the physician to check the serum calcium concentration. Seizures are rarely seen in hypercalcemic crisis.[4] Unexplained gastrointestinal symptoms, weakness with hypotonia, and polyuric dehydration may also be initial clues to hypercalcemic crisis. In fact, serum calcium levels should be obtained in all emergency department patients with symptoms of uncertain origin that may be manifestations of hypercalcemic crisis. Once the serum calcium concentration has been determined, the diagnosis of hypercalcemic crisis is usually self-evident.

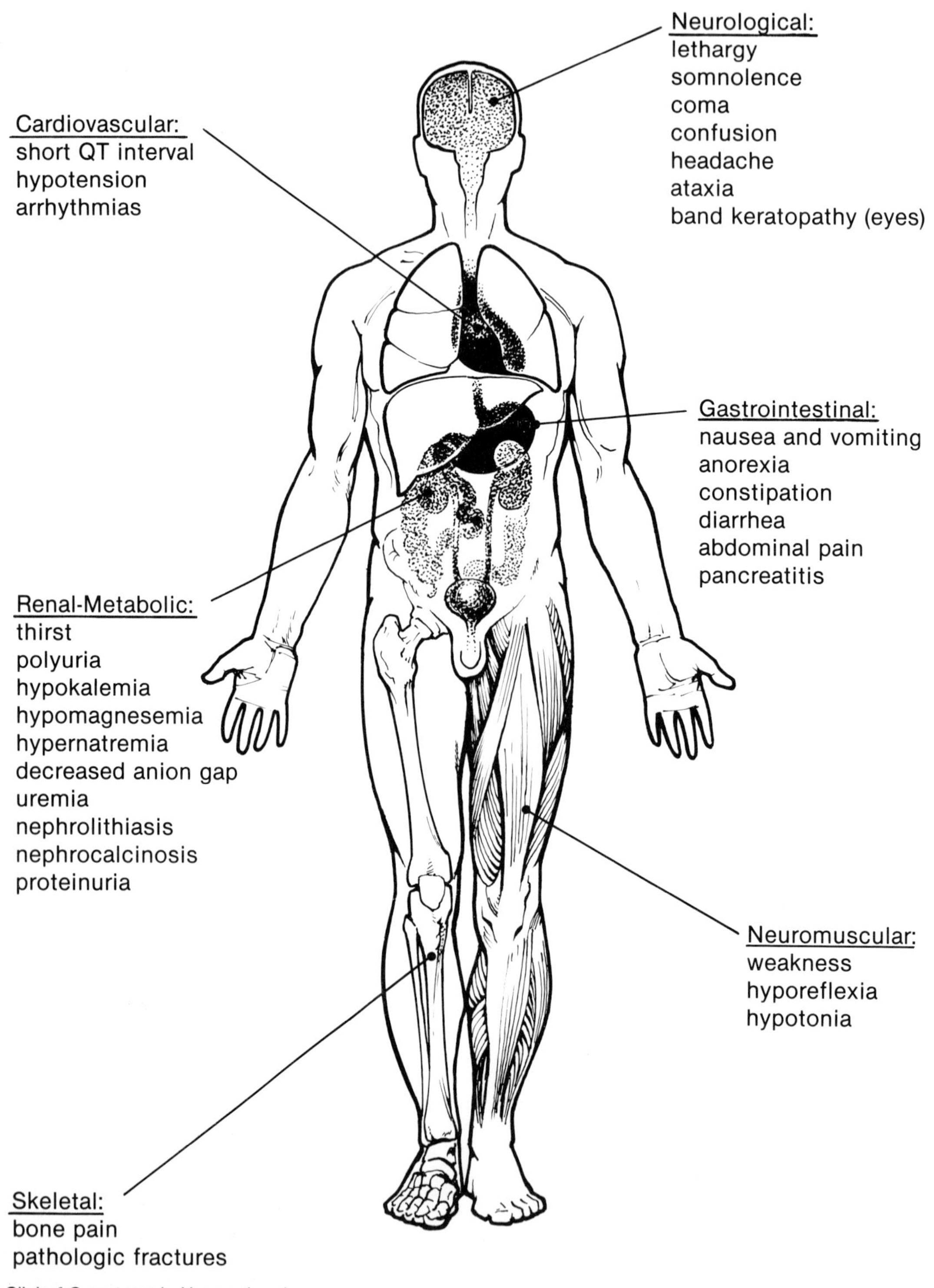

Figure 17–1 Clinical Symptoms in Hypercalcemia.

Interpretation of Serum Calcium Concentration

The normal range of serum calcium concentration is generally stated to be 8.9 to 10.3 mg/dl when determined by the EDTA titration method or 9.1 to 10.5 mg/dl when measured by atomic absorption flame spectrophotometry. This is roughly equivalent to 4.6 to 5.8 mEq/liter. Each laboratory should establish its own standard, depending on the technique used.[5]

The total serum calcium concentration measured on routine testing consists of the sum of the ionized and nonionized calcium present in the serum. It is the ionized calcium fraction that is responsible for the clinical disturbances in hypercalcemic crisis. In normal circumstances, the total serum calcium concentration is composed of 47 percent ionized calcium, 40 percent protein-bound calcium (primarily bound to albumin), and 13 percent calcium in a complex with various ions, e.g., citrate. A useful approximation is that one-half of the measured total serum calcium is ionized under normal circumstances.

Three circumstances may alter the relationship of ionized calcium to calcium that is bound or in a complex:

1. abnormalities in serum protein concentration
2. abnormal serum pH, i.e., systemic alkalosis or acidosis
3. elevations in soluble ligands that form complexes with calcium ions

A change in the serum albumin concentration of 1 gm/dl results in a corresponding change in the total serum calcium concentration of 0.8 mg/dl *in the same direction.* Thus, if the serum protein concentration is elevated, the fraction of protein-bound calcium is increased and the proportion of ionized calcium declines. This relationship may be significant when interpreting the total serum calcium concentration. For example, a hypoproteinemic cancer patient may have a low serum albumin concentration that normally leads to an appreciable decrease in total serum calcium concentration. With the decrease in serum albumin concentration, the fraction of ionized calcium increases. Therefore, a normal or slightly elevated total serum calcium level in this patient may actually represent a significantly elevated ionized calcium level. Conversely, a patient with multiple myeloma may have an elevated concentration of abnormal γ-globulin that binds calcium, raising the total serum calcium concentration. This situation may lead to a diagnosis of severe hypercalcemia, which would be in error, since the fraction of ionized calcium is decreased with hypergammaglobulinemia.[6]

It is important to remember that a tourniquet applied for unnecessary lengths of time can raise the concentration of calcium in the venous blood sample taken from that area. This phenomenon is due to the fact that the serum protein concentration of the blood rises as a result of the transudation of protein-free fluid from the capillaries. A tourniquet applied for three minutes has been shown to increase the measured total serum calcium concentration by 10 percent.[7] Therefore, it is important that the blood drawn for determination of the serum calcium concentration be obtained immediately after the tourniquet is applied.

Alkalosis leads to a decrease in ionized calcium and an increase in protein-bound calcium. Although the total serum calcium concentration may not be changed with alkalosis, the concentration of ionized calcium drops 1.6 mg/dl for each rise of 1 in the pH of the blood. This is the reason for symptoms of hypocalcemia (e.g., tetany) in cases of severe acute respiratory alkalosis, such as the hyperventilation syndrome. The assumption that 50 percent of the total serum calcium is ionized should therefore be modified in a patient with severe systemic pH abnormalities.

Abnormal elevations in the concentration of soluble ligands that form complexes with calcium may also make the 50 percent ionized calcium assumption invalid. This occurs with acute uremia and with elevations of citrate, sulfate, and phosphate levels in the serum.

In the absence of the conditions described, the assumption that the measured total serum calcium concentration reflects the physiologically active ionized serum calcium level is a valid and useful method of evaluating the magnitude of hypercalcemia. Direct measurement of ionized serum calcium is rarely available to the emergency department physician on an immediate basis.

An additional rapid diagnostic tool that can indirectly suggest hypercalcemia is the electrocardiogram (ECG). The earliest and most common finding on the ECG associated with hypercalcemia is shortening of the QT interval. This finding is not specific for hypercalcemia, but a rapid rhythm strip demonstrating a short QT interval should increase the suspicion of hypercalcemic crisis in a patient with appropriate symptoms. This information may be obtained while the results of the serum calcium concentration are pending.

CALCIUM HOMEOSTATIC MECHANISMS

Hypercalcemic crisis occurs when homeostatic control of calcium metabolism is severely impaired. Hypercalcemia always results from an increased calcium influx into the circulation, with or without impaired removal of calcium from the circulation; hypercalcemic crisis never results only from impaired removal of calcium from the circulation. Three sources contribute to the influx of calcium into the serum:

1. osteoclastic resorption of mineral from bone stores
2. gastrointestinal absorption of calcium
3. tubular reabsorption of calcium from the glomerular filtrate

The skeletal system contains over 95 percent of the total body calcium. Most hypercalcemic crises involve a relative increase of bone resorption over bone formation, which releases excess calcium into the blood. Bone resorption may be increased by hormonal agents that stimulate osteoclastic bone resorption or by skeletal osteolytic lesions that liberate calcium into the vascular space. The hormonal agents that increase calcium influx into the blood include parathormone, parathormonelike agents produced by malignancies, and neoplastic production of prostaglandins of the E series (PGE), which have been shown to augment bone resorption in tissue culture.[8]

Increased gastrointestinal absorption of calcium can also be mediated through hormonal mechanisms. The most potent stimulus of gastrointestinal calcium absorption is 1,25-dihydroxyvitamin D. By this means, hypervitaminosis D in faddists who consume enormous quantities of vitamin D is a rare cause of hypercalcemia. Increased gastrointestinal absorption can also result from increased calcium load in the intestine under certain circumstances, such as the milk-alkali syndrome.

Increased tubular reabsorption of calcium in the kidney is stimulated by parathormone, as well as by thiazide diuretics. By itself, increased tubular reabsorption of calcium is rarely a cause of significant hypercalcemia, but it is frequently a factor when combined with increased calcium influx from bone or gastrointestinal absorption.

The essential facts to remember in hormonal control of calcium homeostasis are that parathormone is the major hormone regulating bone resorption and renal reabsorption of calcium, and that vitamin D exerts its major effect on gastrointestinal absorption.

INITIAL THERAPY OF HYPERCALCEMIC CRISIS

It is essential to initiate therapy for hypercalcemic crisis immediately upon diagnosis. The order of priorities in managing hypercalcemic crisis is as follows:

1. Institute general supportive measures to prevent further elevation in serum calcium. Correct life-threatening hypovolemia and associated electrolyte abnormalities.
2. Lower serum calcium concentration by nonspecific methods that decrease calcium influx from bone, renal tubules, and gastrointestinal tract. Initiate therapy to stimulate calcium egress from the vascular space to bone and urine.
3. Determine the cause of the hypercalcemia and initiate specific measures to correct the primary disorder.

General Supportive Measures

A flowsheet, similar to that used in patients with diabetic ketoacidosis, is helpful in the initial therapy of hypercalcemic crisis. A suggested format appears in Figure 17–2.

Correcting Hypovolemia

Patients in hypercalcemic crisis have a marked intravascular volume depletion. Nausea, vomiting, and polyuria have usually been present for some time before the patient seeks treatment in the emergency department. Therefore, the most important initial therapeutic measure is to administer intravascular fluids, normal saline in most cases, to restore the markedly depleted extracellular fluid volume to an adequate level. The usual infusion rate is 1 to 2 liters normal saline during the first two hours of therapy (Table 17–1). To determine the amount of saline infusion required for volume replacement, insertion of a central line to monitor central venous or pulmonary wedge pressure is recommended; this is mandatory when patients are elderly or when renal function may be inadequate.[9] Urine output should be carefully monitored.

Correcting Electrolyte Abnormalities

Hypokalemia is the electrolyte abnormality most frequently associated with hypercalcemic crisis. Hypomagnesemia is also common in these patients. Correction of hypokalemia and hypomagnesemia should be instituted with the restoration of intravascular volume.

In the case of a patient in hypercalcemic crisis who takes a digitalis preparation, correction of hypokalemia and continuous monitoring are of extreme importance. Because calcium and digitalis are synergistic in their effects on the myocardium, such a patient may exhibit signs of digitalis toxicity as a result of hypercalcemia alone. Hypokalemia introduces an additional risk factor for digitalis toxicity. Any digitalized patient in hypercalcemic crisis should have continuous ECG monitoring until the hypercalcemia and hypokalemia have been corrected. Additional doses of digitalis should be withheld until the hypercalcemic crisis has resolved.

Withholding Medications That May Cause Hypercalcemia

In addition to digitalis, medications that may elevate the serum calcium level should be withheld from the patient in hypercalcemic crisis. The most common drug of this type is a thiazide diuretic. Pharmacologic agents that should also be discontinued during the initial therapy of hypercalcemic crisis include

- androgens and estrogens (especially tamoxifen) in patients with breast cancer
- vitamin D
- vitamin A

Time	Pulse	Vital Signs Blood Pressure	Central Venous Pressure (cmH₂O)/Pulmonary Wedge Pressure (mmHg)	Serum Calcium Level mg/%	Serum Potassium Level mEq/L	Serum BUN Creatinine	Intravenous Infusion Rate	Cumulative Total	Urine Output Per Hour	Cumulative Total	Medications	Remarks
00:00	110	90/60	1cmH₂O/4mmHg	16.5	2.5	28/1.2	Normal Saline + 40mEqKCl + 10mgMgSO₄ @ 1,500cc/hr	—	40cc	—	—	ECG monitoring: shortened QT interval noted.
01:00	90	110/60	1cmH₂O/6mmHg	16.0	2.9	24/1.1	Normal Saline + 40mEqKCl + 10mgMgSO₄ @ 1,000cc/hr	1,500	90cc	130cc	—	Furosemide is not given until ECF volume has been significantly restored as measured by rise in CVP or PWP.
02:00	90	120/70	3cmH₂O/7mmHg	15.8	3.2	23/1.1	Normal Saline + 30mEqKCl + 10mgMgSO₄ @ 1,000cc/hr	2,500	380cc	510cc	Furosemide 100mg IV at 02:00	
03:00	84	120/70	5cmH₂O/7mmHg	15.1	3.4	21/1.0	D₅W + 30mEqKCl + 10mgMgSO₄ @ 1,000cc/hr	3,500	400cc	910cc	Furosemide 100mg IV at 03:00	Substitute D₅W for normal saline every fourth liter intravenous fluid.
04:00	80	120/74	6cmH₂O/7mmHg	14.4	3.7	19/1.0	Normal Saline + 20mEqKCl @ 1,000cc/hr	4,500	580cc	1,490cc	Furosemide 100mg IV at 04:00	Goal of maintaining urine output at greater than 500cc/hr is achieved. Continue saline loading with diuresis until serum calcium falls below 12mg/%.

Figure 17–2 Flowsheet for Initial Therapy of Hypercalcemic Crisis.

- lithium
- calcium-containing antacids

Encouraging Mobilization

Immobilization increases the release of calcium into the extracellular fluid from bone. Although it may be impossible to mobilize a patient in hypercalcemic crisis initially, routine turning of the patient and specialized physical therapy regimens are helpful in reducing this source of calcium influx until adequate mobilization is possible.

Reduction of Serum Calcium Concentration

After general supportive measures have been initiated, therapeutic maneuvers to lower the serum calcium

TABLE 17–1   Schedule for Initial Therapy in Hypercalcemic Crisis*

Hour	Intravenous Normal Saline	Potassium Chloride (mEq)/liter	Magnesium (mEq)/liter	Furosemide (mg)
1	500 ml or more**			
2	500 ml or more**	10	5–10	
3	1 liter	20	10–20	100–200
4	Equivalent to urinary loss by volume	20	10–20	100–200
5	Equivalent to urinary loss by volume, replacement fluid D₅W	20	10–20	
6	Equivalent to urinary loss by volume	20	10–20	100–200

* In patients with normal renal function and without congestive heart failure.
** Volume of infusion sufficient to restore extracellular fluid volume as monitored by central venous or pulmonary wedge pressure.
Source: Adapted and reprinted with permission from Zawada ET, Lee DL, Kleeman CR: Management of hypercalcemia. *Postgrad Med* 66:105, 1979.

level should be begun. The most rapid methods involve urinary calcium excretion.

Increasing Caluresis

Sodium and calcium reabsorption in the kidney are closely correlated. Therefore, therapeutic interventions to increase urinary sodium excretion also increase urinary calcium excretion. The generally accepted method of increasing caluresis in hypercalcemic crisis is a combination of intravenous saline infusion and a loop diuretic, either furosemide (Lasix) or ethacrynic acid (Edecrin). A suggested schedule for the first six hours of combined saline and furosemide therapy is shown in Table 17–1. This schedule assumes normal renal function. During the initial two hours, saline infusion without furosemide is used to restore the extracellular volume deficit as described earlier. Once this has been accomplished, 1 to 2 liters of saline are "loaded" intravenously followed by furosemide (100 to 200 mg) given intravenously. The furosemide doses are repeated at one- to two-hour intervals with the goal of maintaining urine output at 500 ml/hour or more. Urine output is replaced on a volume-to-volume basis with intravenous fluid. After each 3 liters normal saline have been infused, 1 liter 5 percent dextrose in water should be alternated with the saline in replacing urine volume.

Potassium (20 to 40 mEq/liter) and magnesium (10 to 20 mEq/liter) are added to replace initial losses. Additional replacement therapy of potassium is guided by repeated serum potassium determinations.

Caluresis by combined saline and furosemide administration decreases the serum calcium level rapidly. With careful monitoring to detect fluid overload and oliguria, this method is safe and without side-effects. In the patient with renal insufficiency, renal failure, or congestive heart failure, however, it should not be attempted in the aggressive manner described. In these patients, either peritoneal dialysis or hemodialysis is the treatment of choice to remove calcium rapidly from the extracellular fluid.[10]

In the past, chelating or binding agents have been used to increase caluresis. They filter soluble complexes with calcium that are poorly reabsorbed by the renal tubule and thereby increase caluresis. These agents (e.g., edetate, sodium sulfate, and sodium citrate) all have serious side-effects, including renal tubular damage, renal failure, hypotension, hypernatremia, and potassium and magnesium depletion. They should not be used in the emergency treatment of hypercalcemic crisis unless all safer modalities fail and dialysis is unavailable.

Reducing the Movement of Calcium out of Bone

Three medications can be useful in decreasing the efflux of calcium from bone into the extracellular fluid: mithramycin, calcitonin, and corticosteroids.

Mithramycin is an antibiotic that has been found to be a potent antineoplastic agent. It was observed that serum calcium levels in patients treated with mithramycin for malignancies markedly decreased. This hypocalcemic effect has been used to treat patients in hypercalcemic crisis from both malignant and nonmalignant causes. Mithramycin inhibits ribonucleic acid (RNA) synthesis directed by deoxyribonucleic acid (DNA), which is thought to result in osteoclastic refractoriness to parathormone, thus decreasing bone calcium mobilization. The hypocalcemic effect of one dose of mithramycin can be as large as a drop of 7 mg/dl in the serum calcium concentration.[11]

The usual dosage is 25 μg/kg given intravenously over 3 to 8 hours. Reductions in serum calcium levels appear about 12 hours after administration, and the hypocalcemic effect peaks at 36 hours. The hypocalcemic effect of mithramycin may last for two weeks after a single administration of the drug. Mithramycin, in the usual dosage, frequently causes nausea and vomiting as side-effects. Severe side-effects are rare at this dose, although renal impairment, hepatic damage, and hemorrhagic disorders with thrombocytopenia have been reported.

Calcitonin is a polypeptide hormone secreted by the parafollicular cells of the thyroid gland in mammals. Its hypocalcemic action stems from its inhibition of bone resorption by osteoclasts. The calcitonin preparation available to clinicians (Calcimar) is derived from salmon.

Calcitonin is not as potent a hypocalcemic agent as mithramycin, but it has a lower incidence of side-effects, the only common ones being nausea and vomiting. The usual decrement in serum calcium concentration with calcitonin therapy is 1 to 2 mg/dl.[11] The onset of action is more rapid than that of mithramycin, occurring within two hours. Its hypocalcemic effect may persist up to 24 hours. The potency of calcitonin preparations is assessed by plasma calcium concentration lowering in rats and is measured in British Medical Research Council (MRC) units. The usual dose is 4 MRC units/kg, given subcutaneously or intramuscularly every 12 hours.

Corticosteroids have also been used in the treatment of hypercalcemic crisis. The efficacy of steroids is ill-defined, however, and the mechanism of action remains unclear. Glucocorticoids may lower serum calcium levels by inhibiting osteoclast precursor cells,[7] by inhibiting tumor growth and thus decreasing the efflux of skeletal calcium into the extracellular fluid,[12] or by inhibiting the synthesis of prostaglandins that stimulate bone resorption.[7] Glucocorticoids may also inhibit gastrointestinal calcium absorption and increase urinary calcium excretion. All of the postulated mechanisms are of little net effect in the treatment of hypercalcemic crisis. The hypocalcemic effect of glucocorticoids may take up to one week to manifest itself. If given, the recommended dosage is 80 mg prednisone daily.

Recent studies have demonstrated that PGE inhibitors, such as indomethacin and aspirin, cause a decrease in serum calcium levels in hypercalcemic cancer patients who have a clear elevation of circulating PGE.[13] This is an experimental method of therapy at present and is probably of use only in a clearly defined subset of cancer patients with hypercalcemic crisis.

Stimulating Movement of Calcium from the Extracellular Fluid into Bone

The administration of inorganic phosphates is an effective method of increasing movement of calcium from the extracellular space into bone. Inorganic phosphates stimulate osteoblastic activity, resulting in a shift of calcium and phosphorus into the skeletal system. This phenomenon is associated with

1. a decrease in the serum calcium concentration
2. a reduction in urinary calcium excretion
3. decreased rate of bone resorption

The hypocalcemic effect of inorganic phosphate given intravenously is extremely rapid, beginning within minutes. However, this method of therapy has a high incidence of serious side-effects, such as extraskeletal precipitation of calcium, hypotension, renal failure, and hypocalcemia. For this reason, intravenous phosphate is not recommended for therapy of hypercalcemic crisis unless safer methods, e.g., saline infusion combined with furosemide, fail to improve the patient's condition and the rapid reduction of serum calcium concentration would clearly be life-saving. In these rare circumstances, intravenous phosphorus (In-Phos, Hyper-Phos-K) in a dose of 1.5 gm (50mM) is infused intravenously over six to eight hours. Only one dose should be given.

Oral phosphate therapy is safer but is slow in onset of action (greater than 24 hours) and has no value in the initial therapy of hypercalcemic crisis.

Decreasing Intestinal Calcium Absorption

In the initial therapy of hypercalcemic crisis, very little can be gained by techniques that decrease gastrointestinal calcium absorption. Discontinuance of any calcium-containing foods or medications and vitamin D preparations should be routine, however.

Etiology of Hypercalcemic Crisis

The primary responsibility of the emergency department physician is to recognize hypercalcemic crisis and initiate therapy for the syndrome, regardless of its cause. The underlying condition responsible for the hypercalcemic crisis becomes clear in the majority of patients during the initial hours of therapy. Treatment of the underlying disorder does not play a significant part in the initial therapy of hypercalcemic crisis, but it is necessary for prolonged correction of the hypercalcemic state.

The list of causes of hypercalcemia is long:

1. neoplasms
   a. skeletal metastases
   b. increased production of parathormone or parathormonelike factors
   c. PGE production
   d. production of osteoclast-activating factor
2. hyperparathyroidism
   a. primary
   b. secondary
3. pharmacologic agents
   a. thiazides
   b. vitamin D toxicity
   c. vitamin A toxicity
   d. calcium (including massive transfusions)
   e. lithium
   f. androgen and estrogen therapy (especially in breast cancer)
4. hyperthyroidism
5. hypothyroidism
6. acromegaly
7. adrenal insufficiency
8. pheochromocytoma
9. milk-alkali syndrome
10. granulomatous disease
    a. sarcoidosis
    b. tuberculosis
    c. histoplasmosis
    d. coccidioidomycosis
11. renal failure
12. renal transplantation
13. phosphorus-depletion syndrome
14. immobilization
15. idiopathic infantile hypercalcemia

On the basis of the initial history, initial laboratory results, and knowledge of the frequency of various causes of hypercalcemic crisis, however, the underlying disorder responsible for the development of the syndrome is usually apparent to the emergency department physician.

One important axiom should be emphasized in the etiologic diagnosis of hypercalcemic crisis. Conditions leading to hypercalcemia coexist in patients who develop hypercalcemic crisis with a much higher incidence than would be expected by chance. Therefore, the physician should seek multiple causes or coexistent diseases that may combine to precipitate the hypercalcemic crisis syndrome.

The most common underlying disorder in patients with hypercalcemic crisis is malignancy. The overall incidence of hypercalcemia in malignant disease is 10 to 20 percent. The most common types of cancer underlying the development of hypercalcemic crisis are shown in Table 17–2; they account for over 90 percent of malignancy-associated cases.

In a patient with known malignancy, initiation of antineoplastic therapy can precipitate hypercalcemic crisis; the most frequent cause in breast cancer patients is tamoxifen. Immobilization, common in patients with malignancies, is a potential precipitating factor.

Primary hyperparathyroidism, although the most common cause of hypercalcemia in the general population, is less likely than malignancy to produce the rapid elevations and high levels of serum calcium concentrations (greater than 14 mg/dl) that usually characterize hypercalcemic crisis. Carcinoma of the parathyroid gland and acute hyperparathyroid crisis can, however, lead to the syndrome. Historical and laboratory evidence suggesting hyperparathyroidism as the cause of hypercalcemic crisis include the following:

- long history of hypercalcemia
- ureteral calculi
- hypophosphatemia
- hypochloremic acidosis
- a ratio of serum chloride to phosphate of greater than 33

A serum parathormone level is necessary to confirm the indirect evidence suggesting hyperparathyroidism.

The history obtained on arrival of the patient is important in diagnosing pharmacologic causes of hypercalcemia. The most common agents precipitating hypercalcemic crisis (usually in combination with another hypercalcemic disorder) are thiazide diuretics. Large amounts of vitamin D, vitamin A, or calcium containing antacids can result in hypercalcemia, as can lithium.

A chest roentgenogram, skeletal series, and, once the patient is adequately hydrated, an intravenous pyelogram, are helpful in detecting a malignant cause. The chest roentgenogram may also suggest sarcoidosis as an underlying cause. Rouleaux formation seen on the complete blood cell count suggests multiple myeloma.

TABLE 17–2   Malignancies that Commonly Underlie Hypercalcemia

Type of Malignancy	Incidence of Hypercalcemia (%)	Comments
Breast cancer	25–40	Most common cause: usually due to bone metastases
Lung cancer	10–15	Frequent in epidermoid and anaplastic cell types
Renal cell carcinoma	13	
Multiple myeloma	70	

REFERENCES

1. Prunell DC, Smith LH, Scholtz, DA, et al: Primary hyperparathyroidism: A prospective clinical study. *Am J Med* 50:670–678, 1971.
2. Christensson T, Hellström K, Wengle B, et al: Prevalence of hypercalcemia in health screening in Stockholm. *Acta Med Scand* 200:131–137, 1976.
3. Daniels GH: Calcium emergencies, in Wilkins EW (ed): *MGH Textbook of Emergency Medicine*. Baltimore, Williams & Wilkins Co, 1978.
4. Plum F, Posner JB: *The Diagnosis of Stupor and Coma*, ed 3. Philadelphia, FA Davis Co, 1980.
5. Yendt ER, Gagne RJ: Detection of primary hyperparathyroidism with special reference to its occurrence in hypercalcemic females with normal or borderline serum calcium. *Can Med Assoc J* 98:331–336, 1968.
6. Lindgärde F, ZeHervoll O: Hypercalcemia and normal ionized Ca^{++} in a case of myelomatosis. *Ann Intern Med* 78:396–399, 1973.
7. Lee DB, Zwada ET, Kleeman CR: The pathophysiology and clinical aspects of hypercalcemic disorders. *West J Med* 129:278–320, 1978.
8. Robertson RP: Prostaglandins and hypercalcemia of cancer. *Med Clin North Am* 65:845, 1981.
9. Zwada ET, Lee DB, Kleeman CR: Management of hypercalcemia. *Postgrad Med* 66:105, 1979.
10. Strauch BS, Ball MF: Hemodialysis in the treatment of severe hypercalcemia. *JAMA* 235:1347–1348, 1976.
11. Pak CYC: Pathogenesis and management of hypercalcemic states, in Isselbacher KJ, et al (eds): *Harrison's Principles of Internal Medicine,* ed 9. Update 1. New York, McGraw-Hill, 1981.
12. Deftos LJ, Neer R: Medical management of the hypercalcemia of malignancy. *Annu Rev Med* 25:323–331, 1974.
13. Robertson RP: Prostaglandins and hypercalcemia of cancer. *Med Clin North Am* 65:845–853, 1981.

18. Acid-Base Disturbances

BARRY E. BRENNER, M.D., Ph.D.

In 1923, Bronsted and Lowry independently defined an acid as a chemical that can donate a proton.[1] A base was defined as a chemical that would accept a proton. This concept of an acid and a base has been useful in the understanding of metabolic disturbances.

DISSOCIATION

The acid HA may dissociate into the anion (A^-) and a hydrogen ion (H^+). Henderson demonstrated that the rate of the reaction, K, is directly proportional to the concentration of the reactants (see Equations 1 and 2).[2]

$$K = \frac{(H^+)\,(A^-)}{(HA)} \qquad \text{(Equation 1)}$$

$$(H^+) = K\,\frac{(HA)}{(A^-)} \qquad \text{(Equation 2)}$$

In 1909, Sorenson proposed the concept of pH so that the numbers used to express hydrogen ion concentration would be conveniently small.[3] pH was defined as the negative log of the hydrogen ion concentration (see Equation 3).

$$pH = -\log (H^+) \qquad \text{(Equation 3)}$$

The hydrogen ion concentration in the normal metabolic situation was found to be 40×10^{-9} Eq/liter or 40 nEq/liter; therefore, the pH in the normal metabolic situation was 7.4. It was found that the normal pH ranged from 7.36 to 7.44.

Another useful formula is the modification of the Henderson equation (Equation 2) known as the Henderson-Hasselbalch equation.[4] By taking the negative logarithm of Equation 3, one can derive the following formula:

$$pH = -\log K + \log \frac{(A^-)}{(HA)} \qquad \text{(Equation 4)}$$

The $-\log K$ was defined as the pK. Rewriting this equation results in the formula:

$$pH = pK + \log \frac{(A^-)}{(HA)} \qquad \text{(Equation 5)}$$

From this Henderson-Hasselbalch equation (Equation 5), it can be seen that, when the salt (A^-) and the acid (HA) are of equal concentrations, the pH is equal to the pK.

OTHER METHODS OF EXPRESSING HYDROGEN ION CONCENTRATION

In addition to pH, there are other convenient methods for expressing the hydrogen ion concentration. As noted earlier, the hydrogen ion concentration can be expressed in units of 10^{-9} Eq/liter. Another method of expressing hydrogen ion concentration, therefore, is in nanoequivalents/liter, or nEq/liter. There are three methods for converting pH to hydrogen ion concentration and vice versa.[5]

Method 1

There is a linear relationship between pH and hydrogen ion concentration from pH 7.1 to 7.5. Each 0.01 unit pH change is equivalent to a change of 1 nEq/liter in hydrogen ion concentration. Therefore, for each 0.1 unit of pH, there would be a change in hydrogen concentration of 10 nEq/liter. For example, a pH of 7.5 is 0.1 pH units away from normal metabolic pH of 7.4 or 40 nEq/liter. Hence, a pH of 7.5 would result in a hydrogen ion concentration of 30 nEq/liter. It is important to note that Method 1 is only to be used for pHs ranging from 7.1 to 7.5.

Method 2

The second method is of value for pHs ranging from 6.8 to 7.7. To obtain a hydrogen ion concentration corresponding to each 0.1 pH unit decrement, sequentially multiply nEq/liter by 1.25. For example, given a pH of 7.2, one would multiply 40 nEq/liter by 1.25, resulting in 50 nEq, which corresponds to a pH of 7.3. To arrive at the number of nEq of hydrogen ions at pH of 7.2, the 50 nEq is again multiplied by 1.25, resulting in 62.5 nEq/liter, corresponding to a pH of 7.2. To obtain the hydrogen ion concentration corresponding to each 0.1 pH unit increment, it is necessary to multiply sequentially nEq/liter by 0.8. For example, to find the hydrogen ion concentration corresponding to a pH of 7.6, one multiplies 40 nEq/liter by 0.8, resulting in 32 nEq/liter, which corresponds to a pH of 7.5. To find the pH corresponding to 7.6, it is necessary to multiply the 32 nEq/liter again by 0.8, resulting in 25.6 nEq/liter, which is equivalent to a pH of 7.6.

Method 3

In order to use Method 3, it is important to remember that pH is based on a logarithmic scale and that the antilog of 0.3 is 2. Therefore, when the pH changes 0.3 units, the corresponding hydrogen ion concentration either doubles or halves. For example, when pH rises from 7.4 to 7.7 and then to 8, the hydrogen ion con-

centration falls from 40 to 20 and then to 10 nEq/liter, respectively.

HYDROGEN ION CONCENTRATION VS. pH

Commonly pH is used; however, the hydrogen ion concentration may have several advantages over the pH when used with the following equation:[6]

$$(H^+) = 24 \times \frac{PCO_2}{(HCO_3)} \qquad \text{(Equation 6)}$$

This equation is a derivation of the Henderson-Hasselbalch equation (see Equation 5). The PCO_2 and the bicarbonate in this equation are readily obtained by determining blood gas levels. The bicarbonate reflects the metabolic component of acid-base disturbances, and the PCO_2 represents the respiratory component of acid-base disturbances. If any two of these three parameters are known, the third parameter can be calculated. Therefore, the physician obtains an arterial blood gas level and can immediately double-check the laboratory results. All that is needed is the interconversion of pH to the hydrogen ion concentration by any of the three methods described. It is important to double-check the results of the laboratory because only the pH and the PCO_2 are determined directly. The bicarbonate level is determined from a nomogram, which is occasionally misread in the laboratory. Such an error can be rapidly detected by using this formula.

ACID-BASE PHYSIOLOGY

Acidosis represents processes that cause acid to accumulate; alkalosis reflects processes that cause base to accumulate.[7,8] Neither acidosis nor alkalosis necessarily cause pH to be altered out of the normal range. However, both acidosis and alkalosis cause pH changes to the low side or high side of normal, respectively. For example, alkalosis may increase pH from 7.40 to 7.44, and acidosis may decrease pH from 7.40 to 7.36.

Several terms are important in the understanding of acid-base physiology. The term *acidemia* indicates that the pH is less than 7.35; the term *alkalemia*, that the pH is more than 7.45.[7,8]

The anion gap is pivotal to understanding acid-base disturbances. To maintain electrical neutrality, positive charges (cations) must equal negative charges (anions); if they do not, there is a "gap." Normally, there are unmeasured negative charges within the body, two-thirds of which are proteins. Sulfates and phosphates constitute the other one-third. The cations and anions normally measured are sodium, chloride, and bicarbonate. The anion gap is calculated according to the following equation:[9]

$$Na - (Cl^- + HCO_3^-) = anion\ gap \qquad (Equation\ 7)$$

Normal values for the anion gap are 8 to 16 mEq/liter.[10]

METABOLIC ACIDOSIS

Compensation

In an attempt to maintain body pH within the normal range, despite the addition of acid, the respiratory center in the medulla compensates for metabolic acidosis by inducing hyperventilation. This profound hyperventilation decreases PCO_2 and causes a more normal pH in the presence of acidosis. This compensatory response is slow to occur, however, and may take 12 to 24 hours to be maximal after the onset of acidosis.[11] The slow response may be due to the slow diffusion of hydrogen ions through the blood-brain barrier. In addition, ketoacids that are commonly involved in metabolic acidosis do not cross the blood-brain barrier.

The degree of hyperventilation is directly proportional to the severity of the metabolic acidosis, although lactic acidosis seems to result in more hyperventilation than other acidoses because it directly affects the chemoreceptors of the brain.[5] Provided that the patient is in steady state and has had the metabolic acidosis for 12 to 24 hours, one of the following four methods could be used to calculate the expected response of hyperventilation, i.e., expected PCO_2, for a given degree of metabolic acidosis, i.e., bicarbonate level.[5]

1. The expected PCO_2 can be calculated by the following formula:

$$PCO_2 = 1.5\ (HCO_3) + 8 \pm 2 \qquad (Equation\ 8)$$

   The PCO_2 should be within 2 units of the value calculated by this method. For example, a bicarbonate of 10 should produce a significant respiratory compensation, i.e., a PCO_2 of 23.
2. The PCO_2 is expected to decrease 1 to 1.3 mm Hg for each 1-mEq fall in bicarbonate. For example, if bicarbonate drops from 25 mEq/liter to 10 mEq/liter, the PCO_2 would be calculated to decrease from 40 mm Hg to between 20.5 and 24 mm Hg.
3. The PCO_2 approximates the last two digits of the arterial pH. For example, an arterial pH of 7.19 produces a respiratory compensation that results in a PCO_2 of approximately 19 mm Hg.
4. For every 10-mEq increase or decrease in bicarbonate level, the pH decreases or increases, respectively, 0.15 units, providing the PCO_2 is unchanged. For example, given a pH of 7.4, a PCO_2 of 40, and a bicarbonate value of 24 mEq/liter, a sudden decrease in the bicarbonate to 14 mEq/liter produces a pH of 7.25, provided that the PCO_2 has not changed.

Except for the last, these methods for analyzing acid-base disturbances are valid only if the patient is in steady state and the metabolic acidosis has been present for at least 12 to 24 hours. If the degree of compensation is not proportional to the severity of the metabolic acidosis as determined by these methods, then it can be assumed that the patient has a primary respiratory disturbance or the patient's condition is not stable.

In the analysis of acid-base disturbances, the physician must be constantly aware of the possibility of errors in the laboratory values. For example, the patient's temperature has marked effects on pH, PCO_2, and PO_2 (Table 18-1).[12] Also, too much heparin in a blood gas syringe lowers PCO_2 without affecting pH or PO_2.[13] This causes the calculated bicarbonate level to be low and leads to an interpretation that the patient has a compensated metabolic acidosis.

Normal Anion Gap

The diagnostic approach to metabolic acidosis is greatly simplified when viewed in terms of the anion gap. For example, a normal (hyperchloremic) or high anion gap suggests specific diagnostic possibilities.

The addition of strong acids to body fluids converts bicarbonate to carbonic acid, which is subsequently degraded to water and carbon dioxide. The latter is then lost in the lungs. This loss of bicarbonate not only is acidifying, but also represents the loss of anions that were counterbalancing positive charges of sodium.[9] Thus, an anionic moiety is needed to replace the negative charge lost with the bicarbonate. In hyperchloremic

---

TABLE 18–1   Effect of Temperature on Blood Gases

	Increase 1°C	Decrease 1°C
pH	Decrease 0.015	Increase 0.015
PCO_2	Increase 4.4*	Decrease 4.4*
PO_2	Increase 7.2*	Decrease 7.2*

* Percent change from value at 37°C.
Source: Reprinted with permission from Reuler JB: Hypothermia: Pathophysiology, clinical settings, and management. *Ann Intern Med* 89:519, 1978.

metabolic acidosis, each mEq bicarbonate lost is replaced with chloride, often from the intracellular space. However, if an unmeasured anion replaces bicarbonate, then the anion gap continues to appear increased.[9] Patients who have been vomiting or receiving exogenous bicarbonate have a normal pH and a normal bicarbonate, but the anion gap remains elevated. The normal anion gap is 8 to 16 mEq/liter.

The etiology of metabolic acidosis associated with a normal anion gap includes the following:[9]

- diarrhea. Hyperchloremic metabolic acidosis is most commonly caused by the loss of bicarbonate in diarrheal fluid.
- pancreatic fistula. Bicarbonate is lost from alkalotic pancreatic secretions in the presence of pancreatic fistula.
- ureteroenterostomy. A urinary diversion procedure from ureter to sigmoid ileum, a ureteroenterostomy induces urea-splitting organisms to grow and function in the urine, where they produce ammonia and, most important, ammonium ion. The ion is systemically absorbed, causing the metabolic acidosis as well as an increase in the blood urea nitrogen (BUN)/creatinine ratio.
- acetazolamide (Diamox). Metabolic acidosis can also be caused by acetazolamide, a carbonic anhydrase inhibitor. The drug causes hydrochloric acid to be reabsorbed and bicarbonate to be excreted in the urine, resulting in alkalinization of the urine.
- mafenide acetate (Sulfamylon). The antibiotic mafenide acetate, useful in burn patients, converts to p-carboxybenzene sulfonamide, a carbonic anhydrase inhibitor.[14] The degree of acidosis is highest in the second to fourth hours after its application in the burned patient. Also, the degree of acidosis correlates directly with the amount of partial thickness burn.[14] Acidosis is particularly severe if the patient is in renal failure and cannot excrete this carbonic anhydrase inhibitor.
- cholestyramine. Daily oral ingestion of 32 gm cholestyramine, which binds bile salts, causes bicarbonate to decrease by 3 to 4 mEq after 1 to 2 months. The acidosis is secondary to the high chloride content in cholestyramine.[15]
- excessive acidifying agents. The use of excessive acidifying agents, such as ammonium chloride, may cause hyperchloremic metabolic acidosis.
- rapid intravenous hydration. Sodium and chloride increase during intravenous hydration without a commensurate increase in bicarbonate; hypoaldosteronism is induced by the volume expansion.[16] This may explain why hyperchloremic metabolic acidosis persists approximately eight hours after treatment of diabetic ketoacidosis, even though the

anion gap is decreased. Dilution of the anion gap may also have a role in this situation.[17] The development of a renal tubular acidosis Type II, administration of potassium chloride, and the loss of urinary ketones that would have been metabolized to bicarbonate also may explain the decrease in the anion gap and the presence of hyperchloremic metabolic acidosis in the therapy of diabetic ketoacidosis.[5,18]

- hyperalimentation. During hyperalimentation of infants, more cationic than anionic amino acids are administered. Metabolism of cationic amino acids causes increased generation of hydrogen ions and metabolic acidosis.[19]
- posthypocapnia. Chronic respiratory alkalosis decreases the bicarbonate by no more than 3 to 4 mEq/liter.[20] Sudden relief of the respiratory alkalosis, therefore, leaves a mild metabolic acidosis.
- early renal failure. In obstructive uropathies or other forms of early renal failure, a renal tubular acidosis may occur.[21]
- renal tubular acidosis. In Type I renal tubular acidosis, hydrogen ions cannot be secreted at the distal tubule; in Type II, bicarbonate cannot be reabsorbed at the proximal tubule (Tables 18–2 and 18–3).[22–25] In patients with a metabolic acidosis and a urine pH greater than 6, the physician should suspect renal tubular acidosis or laboratory error.

Increased Anion Gap

Uremia

Metabolic acidosis is not seen with chronic renal failure unless the glomerular filtration rate is less than 20 ml/minute and the BUN and the serum creatinine exceed 40 and 4, respectively. Fortuitously, the renal excretion of phosphates and sulfates parallels that of acid excretion. The increased anion gap associated with uremia is due to retained sulfates and phosphates, whereas acidosis is due to the inability to excrete acid. It is unusual for the anion gap to be more than 20 to 25 mEq/liter in uremia uncomplicated by a second metabolic acidosis.

Lactic Acidosis

The etiology of lactic acidosis includes shock, anemia, hypoxia, metabolic poisons, heat stroke, glycogenoses, malignancies, phenformin, and idiopathic causes.[26–30] An elevated lactate level (more than 5 mEq/liter) is the major finding of this covert but serious illness, which may be one of the earliest indications of sepsis. In lactic acidosis, profound degrees of acidosis can develop in a

TABLE 18–2   Distinction Between Proximal and Distal Renal Tubular Acidosis

	Type I *Distal Renal Tubular Acidosis*	*Type II* *Proximal Renal Tubular Acidosis*
Renal stones or nephrocalcinosis	Common	Rare
Phosphoglycosuria	Rare	Common
Serum bicarbonate	Less than 15	More than 15
Potassium	Low	Low
Urinary pH		
Random	Inappropriately alkaline	Inappropriately alkaline
First A.M. void	Never less than 6	Commonly less than 6
Post–acid load	More than 5.3	Less than 5.3
Ease of bicarbonate replacement	2–3 mEq/kg/day (sensitive)	More than 3–5 mEq/kg/day (resistant)

Source: Reproduced with permission from Narins RG, Goldberg M: Renal tubular acidosis: Pathophysiology, diagnosis, and treatment. *DM* 23:1, 1977.

matter of minutes, while most other acidoses, including diabetic ketoacidosis, develop much more slowly. After seizures, pH may be as low as 6.9, but it is rapidly restored to normal, usually in less than one hour.[31] During the reparative phase of lactic acidosis, the lactate is fully metabolized to bicarbonate, which returns the anion gap to normal. The physician can minimize the risk of an "alkaline overshoot" by anticipating this conversion and limiting the replacement of bicarbonate to maintain a pH of 7.2.[9] During reasonable respiratory compensation for metabolic acidosis, serum pH may be more than 7.2, but serum bicarbonate should be maintained at more than 10 mEq/liter. A lower bicarbonate level may induce arrhythmias and increase the incidence of ventricular fibrillation independent of pH.[32]

Lactic acidosis may be distinguished from ketoacidosis without directly measuring serum lactate. The phosphorus/creatinine ratio varies from 4.4 to 4.7 in lactic acidosis, whereas the ratio ranges from 1.7 to 2.3 in ketoacidosis.[33] These different ratios are due to hyperphosphatemia in lactic acidosis and a spurious elevation in serum creatinine in ketoacidosis.[34]

Ketoacidosis

When the mobilization of free fatty acids from adipose tissue is greatly increased, as it is with insulin deficiency, for example, the oxidative capacity of the liver is overwhelmed, free fatty acids combine, and ketogenesis dominates. Ketones are measured in urine by the nitroprusside reaction (Acetest), which measures *only* acetoacetate; in ketoacidosis, however, the concentration of another ketone, β-OH-butyrate, is in equilibrium at a three-fold higher concentration with acetoacetate so that the result of the urine Acetest is occasionally only weakly positive. Therefore a patient may have ketoacidosis due to a preponderance of β-OH-butyrate but only a weakly positive or negative urine Acetest. Hypoxia may increase the amount of reduced nicotine adenine dinucleotide (NADH) and drive the ratio of these two ketones toward even more β-OH-butyrate. When the ketoacidosis begins to resolve, the ratio shifts toward acetoacetate, paradoxically causing increased ketonuria in a patient who is improving.[5]

Isopropyl alcohol also is metabolized to acetone, causing a positive nitroprusside reaction.[35]

TABLE 18–3   Causes of Renal Tubular Acidosis

TYPE I

Hereditary elliptocytosis	States associated with edema
Chronic hydronephrosis	Lithium
Hyperthyroidism	Amphotericin
Hyperparathyroidism	Conn's syndrome
Vitamin D intoxication	Wilson's degeneration
Hyperglobulinemic states	Renal transplantation
(carcinoma)	Medullary sponge kidney
Amyloid	

TYPE II

Tyrosinemia or cystinosis	Carcinoma
Hereditary fructose intolerance	Heavy metal poisoning
Galactosemia	Carbonic anhydrase inhibitors
Glycogen storage disease	Out-dated tetracycline (not a problem unless saved from the 1960s)
(Type 1)	
Myeloma	
Nephrotic syndrome	Hyperparathyroidism
Amyloid	Renal transplantation

Source: Reproduced with permission from Narins RG, Goldberg M: Renal tubular acidosis: Pathophysiology, diagnosis, and treatment. *DM* 23:1, 1977.

Alcoholic ketoacidosis. The pathogenesis of alcoholic ketoacidosis is not fully clear, but it is related to increased lipolysis, an elevation in the plasma cortisol level, and a deficiency in growth hormone and insulin. The patients have a history of abdominal pain, protracted vomiting, and starvation for two to three days.[36,37] They may have low-grade temperature, i.e., less than 38.3°C, with epigastric tenderness; otherwise, physical examination is normal. The arterial pH may range from 7.0 to 7.6 (alkalosis secondary to severe vomiting), and the anion gap varies from 18 to 25 mEq/liter as average values. Hyperglycemia is seen, although it is generally less than 275 mg/dl, and 10 percent of patients have negative urine and serum nitroprusside reactions. When the urine nitroprusside reaction is negative, an increased β-OH-butyrate level is diagnostic. Hyperamylasemia may occasionally occur; hyperuricemia is common.

The treatment of choice is 5 percent dextrose water infused at a rate of 125 to 150 ml/hour, which resolves the syndrome in 12 hours. The use of normal saline alone may distort initial laboratory values, and the syndrome may persist even at 24 hours.[38] Glucose infusion restores the ability of the mitochondria to convert reduced nicotine adenine dinucleotide (NADH) to its oxidized form (NAD$^+$) and thereby to oxidize ketones. During therapy, phosphate should be replaced, for the level may fall from 7 to 1 mg/dl during the first 6 hours of therapy.[38] Also, the physician must follow the potassium level. Bicarbonate therapy is rarely needed in this syndrome. Insulin should never be used.

Diabetic Ketoacidosis. The therapy of diabetic ketoacidosis involves treatment of hyperglycemia, acidosis, dehydration (usually 10 percent of body weight), and treatment of potassium deficit, once adequate urine output is established. Initially, patients may have hyperkalemia, despite the total body potassium deficit.

Too rapid treatment of dehydration or hyperglycemia may lead to cerebral edema within 4 to 16 hours after the initiation of therapy.[39-42] The exogenous administration of bicarbonate may reduce cerebrospinal fluid pH, even though the serum bicarbonate is rising, because it also reduces the stimulus to hyperventilate.[43] However, this cerebrospinal fluid acidosis has not been a problem and remains more of theoretical interest.[44]

Treatment with insulin usually lowers the glucose level at a rate of 75 mg/dl each hour. The rate is quite constant in a given individual, but this decline occurs only half as fast if an infection is present.[45] Continuous intravenous administration of insulin may be preferred, since absorption by other routes is irregular in the presence of acidosis and dehydration. Furthermore, hypokalemia and hypoglycemia may occur less frequently during the administration of low-dose, intravenous insulin, and the

fall in glucose and serum acetone levels during the first two hours of therapy may be more rapid.[46,47]

Continuous intravenous infusion of regular insulin (5 to 10 U/hour after 0.33 unit/kg priming dose) is an excellent treatment for diabetic ketoacidosis. If 100 ml solution containing regular insulin (50 U/100 ml) is first run through the tubing, then there is no loss of insulin during initial infusions because of adherence to the plastic tubing or microscopic cracks in glassware. Once glucose values fall to less than 300 mg/dl, the regular insulin infusion should be stopped and glucose added to the solution used to hydrate the patient.[44] The physician should always check carefully for precipitating causes of diabetic ketoacidosis, such as infection, pancreatitis, or myocardial infarction.[48] During therapy of diabetic ketoacidosis it is important to replace magnesium and phosphorus (2.5 mg/kg over six hours) for levels of phosphorus less than 1 mg/dl.[49] (See Chapter 11.)

Paraldehyde Intoxication

There have been few cases of paraldehyde intoxication described in the literature. The typical history is one of abdominal pain and central nervous system depression in an alcoholic.[9] A garlic odor on the breath and leukocytosis of 24,000 to 65,000 are characteristic. All patients have survived.

Methanol Intoxication

Methanol is readily available in wood alcohol and paint thinner so that intoxication is inexpensive. The drug is easily absorbed through the skin, respiratory tract, and gastrointestinal tract. Pathologically, the concentration of methyl alcohol is highest per gram of tissue in the eye.[50] Methyl alcohol is oxidized at one-fifth the rate at which ethanol is oxidized; hence, it has a long persistence in the body.[50,51] It is metabolized to formic acid, which is an uncoupling agent and, like aspirin, causes an increase in the concentration of other organic anions and an increase in the anion gap.[52] Variations in individual responses to methyl alcohol are extreme. There is normally a latent period of 24 to 48 hours between ingestion and onset of symptoms, although symptoms may appear in less than 12 hours.

All patients who are frankly acidotic when first seen have visual impairment, and at least 50 percent with transiently normal bicarbonate have visual difficulties.[50] The most frequent complaint is blurred or indistinct vision. Headache is present in 62 percent.[50] Patients may have moderate to severe systemic hypertension. Nausea and vomiting are prominent in 52 percent of patients.[50] The abdominal pain is particularly violent, epigastric, and colicky; the abdomen is strikingly rigid and exquisitely tender, but rebound is not noted. Amylase was over 300 Somogyi units in 66 percent of patients, and pancreatic necrosis was regularly found at autopsy.[50] Only 25 percent had true Kussmaul breathing.[50] Patients have dilated pupils and papillitis. It is important to remember that these patients appear intoxicated. Chronic methanol abusers frequently develop an ophthalmic tolerance and do not become blind. The treatment is to keep the pH more than 7.2, maintain ethyl alcohol level at 100 mg/dl, and perform early hemodialysis.[53–55] For treatment protocol with alcohol see ethylene glycol intoxication.

Ethylene Glycol Intoxication

Ethylene glycol, which is contained in antifreeze, is a poor man's alcohol. It has a warm and sweet taste and may be the chosen agent for suicide. Ethylene glycol is nontoxic per se; however, its metabolites are aldehydes that are cytotoxic and oxalates that produce extensive renal damage.[56] High concentrations of oxalic acid, an uncoupling agent, result in the accumulation of organic anions that are responsible for the acidosis and increased anion gap.[9] These patients appear to be drunk, but there is no smell of ethanol on their breath. Central nervous system manifestations occur 30 minutes to 12 hours after ingestion; other symptoms include low-grade fever, nystagmus, ophthalmoplegias, papilledema, and cerebrospinal fluid findings consistent with a meningoencephalitis.[56] Moderate leukocytosis occurs. Hypocalcemia results from chelation of the calcium ion by oxalate. Profuse oxalate and, occasionally, hippurate crystalluria is noted.[56,57] Extreme ethylene glycol poisoning is associated with pulmonary edema, bronchopneumonia, and congestive heart failure. At 24 to 72 hours, the patient develops acute tubular necrosis, although normal renal function usually returns.[56] Early diagnosis and treatment reduce the mortality.[58] The estimated lethal dose is 100 ml, but one patient was saved after a 2-liter ingestion.[58]

Treatment includes thiamine and pyridoxine, which are cofactors needed in the degradation of ethylene glycol to less toxic metabolites. Osmotic diuresis increases renal clearance of ethylene glycol and reduces interstitial edema and renal cortical edema. Like methanol, ethylene glycol is a competitive inhibitor of alcohol dehydrogenase, reducing the half-life of ethylene glycol of three hours.[56,59] Ethanol should be started if ingestion occurred within four to six hours, keeping an ethanol level of 100 mg/dl using 0.1 ml/kg/hour of 100 percent ethanol as a 5 percent solution in 5 percent dextrose water preceded by a 1 ml/kg loading dose administered over 20 minutes.[56,59] Early hemodialysis is life-saving and is the procedure of choice. Ethanol infusion is a temporizing measure until hemodialysis can be instituted.

Osmolar Gap

The final diagnosis of ethylene glycol or methanol intoxication depends on toxicologic analysis, but these tests are difficult to obtain rapidly. Determinations of the serum osmolarity and osmolar gap are rapid screening tests for some circulating toxins, such as methanol and ethylene glycol.[57,60,61] At the concentration present in plasma, the osmotic coefficient of sodium chloride is $1.85 \times (Na^+)$. Doubling the factor (Na^+) in the formula does not overestimate the plasma osmolarity, since other cationic constituents of the plasma (potassium, calcium, and magnesium) are excluded from the calculation.

$$2 \times Na^+ + \frac{Glucose}{18} + \frac{BUN}{2.8} = \text{Calculated serum osmolarity}$$

(Equation 9)

The limit by which the measured osmolarity may exceed the calculated value is 10 mOsm. If the calculated value exceeds the measured value, either the laboratory made a mistake or there is an arithmetic mistake. If the measured value exceeds the calculated value, there are two possibilities: (1) if the measured serum osmolarity is normal but the calculated value is low, the free water content is decreased, or (2) if the measured and calculated osmolarities are elevated, there is an unmeasured osmole (Table 18-4) and osmolar gap.

Salicylate Intoxication

Aspirin solution is absorbed in less than 30 minutes. Addition of small amounts of antacids to aspirin solution increases the rate of absorption. Peak levels with tablets may take as long as 2 hours. Aspirin inhibits gastric emptying, and plasma salicylate levels may continue to rise for as long as 24 hours.[62]

The pathophysiology of salicylate toxicity involves two basic underlying mechanisms: (1) salicyclic acid directly stimulates the respiratory center of the brain, producing the predominant respiratory alkalosis, and (2) salicylate inhibits oxidative phosphorylation, as does thyroxine.[62,63] Uncoupling of oxidative phosphorylation from electron transport increases heat production, producing fever, tissue glycolysis, and peripheral demand for glucose because adenosine triphosphate is not being generated. This increased peripheral demand for glucose results in the mobilization of fats to free fatty acids and ketones. In addition, glycogen stores are mobilized initially, producing hyperglycemia; the subsequent depletion of the body stores of glucose results in hypoglycemia.[62] Hypoglycemia occurs much more frequently

TABLE 18–4   Toxic Substances Contributing 1 mOsm/kg Water to the Serum at Their Lethal Levels

Substance	Molecular Weight	Lethal Level (mg/dl)	mOsm/kg Water
Ethanol	46	350	80
Ethyl ether	26	180	70
Isopropanol	60	340 (toxic)	60
Methanol	32	80	27
Acetone	58	55	10
Trichloroethane	133	100	9
Paraldehyde	132	50	4
Ethylene glycol	62	21	4
Chloroform	119	39	3
Salicylate	180	50	3
Chloral hydrate	165	25	2
Ethchlorvynol	144	15	1

Source: Reproduced with permission from Glasser L, Sternglanz PD, Combic J, et al: Serum osmolarity and its applicability to drug overdose. *Am J Clin Pathol* 60:695, 1963.

in children than in adults. It is also more commonly reported in chronic salicylate intoxication.

Although metabolic acidosis is commonly associated with salicylate intoxication in children, it is rare in adults; only 10 percent of patients with a low pH had a metabolic acidosis, 30 percent had a respiratory alkalosis, and 57 percent had a combined respiratory alkalosis and a metabolic acidosis with the respiratory alkalosis being the overriding event.[64] Because it is an uncoupling agent, salicylate stimulates net organic acid production and causes a minor elevation in the anion gap.

The signs and symptoms of salicylate intoxication are secondary to all the laboratory value abnormalities that have been described. Other symptoms may be tinnitus, which is common, nausea, vomiting, and sensorineural hearing loss.[65] Anderson and associates studied 73 consecutive cases of adults with salicylate intoxication.[62] Twenty of these patients were older (mean age 53 years), had no psychiatric or suicidal history, and denied aspirin use, although they were taking aspirin for medical conditions. Diagnosis was frequently delayed up to 72 hours. Laboratory evaluation showed a mixed respiratory alkalosis and an anion gap type metabolic acidosis. In this study, the signs and symptoms noted were tachypnea and neurologic abnormalities, e.g., confusion, agitation, hyperactivity, slurred speech, hallucinations, generalized seizures, focal seizures (rare), and coma. The severity of the central nervous system manifestations correlated with the brain salicylate level. Cardiac dysfunction occurred as congestive heart failure or sudden death.

Some of the laboratory abnormalities are predictable from the pathogenesis, e.g., glucose aberrations, acid-base disturbances, and enhanced ketone formation. The severity of the acidosis varies inversely with age. Severe acidosis may be delayed in onset 12 to 24 hours following ingestion of excessive salicylate. Owing to increased insensible fluid losses from fever, increased renal losses due to a greater solute load, and organic aciduria, dehydration is in the order of 2 to 3 liters/sq m body surface area in moderate intoxications and 4 to 6 liters/sq m in severe intoxications. Respiratory alkalosis occurs initially and may persist throughout the intoxication. This acute respiratory alkalosis (unlike chronic respiratory alkalosis), together with nausea, vomiting, and dehydration (extracellular fluid contraction), encourages the development of an alkalosis and the renal excretion of potassium. Hypernatremia and hypokalemia are common findings. Occasionally, hyponatremia may occur secondary to inappropriate antidiuretic hormone secretion induced by aspirin. Salicylate intoxication also has hemostatic effects, e.g., decreased synthesis of prothrombin, decreased factor VII, and decreased aggregation of platelets.[63] With very high salicylate levels, hepatotoxicity has been described.[66] Neurogenic (i.e., noncardiogenic) pulmonary edema has also been described.[67] Owing to inappropriate antidiuretic hormone secretion and/or excessive administration of fluids during forced diuresis, cardiogenic pulmonary edema may ensue in the elderly. (See also Chapter 24.)

Treatment

In the treatment of metabolic acidosis, it is important to determine the base deficit.[68,69] The base deficit can be calculated as follows:

$$\text{Desired plasma bicarbonate} - \text{Actual plasma bicarbonate} = \text{Deficit of bicarbonate/liter}$$

Total body water = 60 percent total body weight

$$\text{Total body bicarbonate deficit} = \text{Total body water} \times \text{Deficit of bicarbonate/liter} \qquad (\text{Equation } 10)$$

For example, if a bicarbonate level of 18 mEq/liter is desired in a 50-kg patient in metabolic acidosis with a bicarbonate level of 12 mEq/liter, the bicarbonate deficit is $18 - 12$ or 6 mEq/liter. Total body water is 0.6×50 kg or 30 liters. Total body bicarbonate deficit is 30 liters $\times$ 6 mEq/liter or 180 mEq. One-half the initial deficit should be replaced over 5 to 10 minutes and the remainder of the deficit replaced according to the clinical condition of the patient. The proportion of bicarbonate passing into the intracellular space increases with bicarbonate values less than 5 mEq/liter. If bicarbonate values are this low, use total body water as 100 percent of total body weight.[70] To alkalinize urine orally, give 4 gm bicarbonate orally and then 1 to 2 gm orally every four hours.

Vasodilator therapy may help in severe idiopathic lactic acidosis.[71] Some success has been reported with nitroprusside. Tris-hydroxy-aminomethane (THAM) is an interesting buffer and an alternative to bicarbonate. Although THAM regularly depresses ventilation and therefore increases hypoxemia, it has the unusual property of lowering PCO_2 at the same time it raises the bicarbonate level. To reduce the PCO_2 by 25 percent for two hours, however, requires 500 mM THAM. This drug is useful in a ventilated patient who still has an increased PCO_2, such as a patient in cardiac arrest. In addition, THAM contains no sodium, which may make it the drug of choice in patients with cirrhosis, congestive heart failure, or nephrotic syndrome.[72] THAM is 0.3 M isotonic, with a pH of 10.6 and must be used within one hour of reconstitution. It catalyzes the following reaction:

$$(CH_2OH)_3 - C - NH_2 + H^+ \rightleftharpoons (CH_2OH)_3 - C - NH_3^+ \qquad (\text{Reaction 1})$$

Seventy-five percent of THAM is in ionized form at pH 7.4. The ionized form penetrates the cell and titrates the intracellular space. Since this removes H^+ without affecting bicarbonate level, PCO_2 is decreased because of a shift in equilibrium toward bicarbonate generation by the following reaction:

$$H^+ + HCO_3^- \rightleftharpoons H_2CO_3 \rightleftharpoons CO_2 + H_2O \qquad (\text{Reaction 2})$$

The decrease in PCO_2 may cause hypoventilation. THAM should be given according to the following formula:

$$\text{0.3 M solution THAM (ml)} = \text{kg body weight} \times \text{base deficit (mEq/liter)}$$

over one hour. In cardiac arrest, 100 to 300 ml may be administered via a large-bore intravenous catheter. This solution can occasionally cause hypoglycemia, prolonged prothrombin time, or hyperkalemia. Fifty to 75 percent of THAM is excreted from the body in 24 hours.[73]

All patients with an acute metabolic acidosis should be hospitalized except patients with chronic seizure disorders who have had a seizure within one hour.

ELEVATION OF THE ANION GAP WITHOUT ACIDOSIS

If more water is lost than salt, then the concentration of the remaining electrolytes increases.[9] If the loss is 20 percent of total body water, then electrolytes would be expected to increase by 20 percent and so would the unmeasured anions; however, a 20 percent increase in the anion gap, e.g., from 10 to 12 is trivial.

If lactate metabolism is slowed in shock or hypoxia, administration of lactated Ringer's solution has been shown to elevate the anion gap. In addition, each unit of whole blood contains 17 mEq citrate/liter.[74] This citrate is usually converted to bicarbonate; however, in shock or hypoxia, it is retained, elevating the anion gap.

Carbenicillin at 30 gm/day and penicillin at 50,000 to 100,000 U/day serve as unmeasured anions and elevate the anion gap.[75,76]

The accumulated organic anion in chronic hypocapnia may be lactate, which elevates the anion gap by 3 to 4 mEq/liter.[77]

Removal of chloride elevates the anion gap by 3 to 5 mEq/liter. It is believed that dehydration increases the concentration of unmeasured anions and alkalosis (pH 7.60), thus increasing the electronegativity of the serum proteins that constitute two-thirds of unmeasured anions in the normal anion gap.[78,79]

LOW ANION GAP

In contrast to dehydration, which increases the anion gap, dilution of the extracellular fluid decreases the anion gap.[9]

The replacement of the unmeasured anion albumin with the measured anion chloride in salt-retaining hypoalbuminemic states, such as a cirrhosis or nephrotic syndrome, causes a fall in the anion gap.[9] It is important to remember that albumin is responsible for most of the normal anion gap. The average anion gap in patients with nephrotic syndrome is 2 mEq/liter less than expected.

The combination of a spuriously lower than expected serum sodium level plus a high serum chloride level causes a low anion gap in patients with hypernatremia.[9] Hyperviscosity also results in an underestimation of the sodium level and causes a decreased anion gap by the same mechanism as hypernatremia.

The reaction of bromide with the automated analysis reagents is greater than that of chloride, causing a falsely elevated chloride level. A negative anion gap is a clue to this diagnosis. Nervine has bromide in the amount of 25 mEq/liter (200 mg/dl) and is the agent usually associated with toxicity. Symptoms and signs involve psychiatric and neurologic aberrations along with an acneiform eruption.[80,81]

The displacement of serum water by protein causes an artifactual decrease in the serum sodium concentration and, therefore, a decrease in the anion gap. In 76 patients with myeloma, the mean anion gap 9.2 ± 0.4. In fact, one-third of the patients had an anion gap less than 6 mEq/liter. Other causes of increased globulins, e.g., sarcoidosis, did not decrease the anion gap.[82]

The anion gap is affected on an mEq-by-mEq basis with hypercalcemia; therefore, only life-threatening hypercalcemia affects the anion gap.[9] Therapeutic levels of the cation lithium rarely exceed 3 mEq/liter, which hardly affects the anion gap. However, suicide attempts with lithium may be quite effective in lowering the anion gap.[9]

METABOLIC ALKALOSIS

Despite a widely diverse collection of clinical situations, hypokalemia or extracellular fluid depletion is nearly always associated with a metabolic alkalosis. For the most part, either acid or potassium is lost in the kidney or the intestinal tract, generating a metabolic alkalosis.[68,83]

Metabolic alkalosis can be rapidly life-threatening. An increase in the serum bicarbonate level of only 15 to 20 mEq/liter may cause marked alkalemia, because the compensatory respiratory response is a modest hypoventilation (PCO_2 of 50 to 55 mm Hg at most).[84,85] The following formula helps to predict the PCO_2 for a given value of bicarbonate:

$$PCO_2 = 0.9(HCO_3^-) + 9 \qquad \text{(Equation 11)}$$

A normal or lower than normal PCO_2 in the presence of a high bicarbonate level implies a respiratory alkalosis along with a metabolic acidosis.

Metabolic alkalosis can be divided into two groups: (1) that caused by gastric- or diuretic-induced chloride loss with subsequent replacement by the selective proximal reabsorption of bicarbonate in the renal tubules and (2) that caused by direct renal bicarbonate reabsorption without a chloride deficit. In group 1, the "spot" urine chloride is quite low, often less than 10 mEq/liter; in group 2, the urine chloride varies with the diet as usual (60 to 100 mEq/liter).[86]

Group 1

Gastric Loss

Chloride may be lost secondary to nasogastric suction or vomiting with reabsorption of bicarbonate.[68,83] The alkalosis stimulates a renal loss of potassium. Hypovolemia results in a low urine sodium level (i.e., less than 10 mEq/liter), whereas normovolemia is associated with a normal value for urine sodium (i.e., dependent on intake, but greater than 40 mEq/liter).

Contraction Alkalosis and Diuretic-Induced Metabolic Alkalosis

Enhanced excretion of sodium and chloride without the proportional loss of bicarbonate may result in contraction alkalosis and diuretic-induced metabolic alkalosis.[16] Acid excretion is brought on by the potassium depletion, as well as by a volume contraction induced by the physiologic response of aldosterone.

Relief of Chronic Hypercapnia

The abrupt reduction of carbon dioxide levels in patients with chronic hypercapnia may cause a sudden, severe metabolic alkalosis. For example, a patient with chronic obstructive pulmonary disease may have a pH of 7.37, PCO_2 of 58, and HCO_3 of 40; when placed on a ventilator, this patient develops a pH of 7.67, PCO_2 of 40, and HCO_3 of 40. If the reduction in PCO_2 is gradual (over two to three days), the excess bicarbonate is gradually excreted. If these patients are on a low salt diet or are treated with diuretics, however, proximal reabsorption of bicarbonate is enhanced, and the metabolic alkalosis that previously was compensating for a respiratory acidosis becomes primary. This primary metabolic alkalosis may develop even without diuretics; all that is needed is contraction of the arterial volume, e.g., congestive heart failure.[87]

Fasting Patients during Initial Feedings

Some patients who have been fasting are initially somewhat hypovolemic. Therefore, excess aldosterone has been secreted. With the addition of glucose, there is an increase in the proximal reabsorption of bicarbonate.

Hypoparathyroidism

Parathormone increases the renal absorption of chloride and enhances the renal loss of bicarbonate. Hypoparathyroidism causes a chloride deficit and a secondary reabsorption of bicarbonate.[68,83]

Hypercalcemia

Suppression of parathormone secretion in association with hypercalcemia causes a chloride deficit and a secondary reabsorption of bicarbonate. Hyperparathyroidism can be distinguished from all other causes of hypercalcemia, therefore, by the serum chloride level. A serum chloride level of greater than 102 mEq/liter should occur in hyperparathyroidism, presuming the patient is not on diuretics.[68,83] (See Chapter 17.)

Excess Bicarbonate Load

The oral intake of 140 gm bicarbonate every day for three weeks produces a metabolic alkalosis with bicarbonate levels ranging from 33 to 36 mEq/liter.[68,83] In renal failure, smaller doses of bicarbonate may produce a metabolic alkalosis because of the inability of the kidney to excrete this excess bicarbonate.

Congenital Alkalosis with Diarrhea

Although this syndrome is initially seen in infancy, children with congenital alkalosis with diarrhea survive into adulthood.[88] These patients have a defect in the chloride-bicarbonate pump in the ileum and are unable to transport chloride against an electrochemical gradient; this defect causes a loss of chloride and acid in the stool.

Group 2

All the causes of hypokalemia secondary to renal losses are included in Group 2 metabolic alkaloses.

Diagnosis

Symptoms of metabolic alkalosis may be tetany secondary to hypocalcemia (low free serum calcium), hyperirritability, convulsions, altered mental status, and respiratory depression.[68,83] Electrocardiogram (ECG) changes resemble those of hypokalemia. Hepatic failure is worsened by alkalosis secondary to an increase in the ratio of ammoniate ammonium ions in the presence of alkalosis, causing increased ammonia levels in the blood that may cross the blood-brain barrier and worsen hepatic encephalopathy.

The appropriate value to use as the bicarbonate level is controversial and varies between institutions. As an arterial blood gas determination, the calculated bicarbonate level depends on the reliability of the pH and the PCO_2; theoretically, small errors in these measured values could distort the resulting serum bicarbonate level.[89] The venous serum total carbon dioxide should be 2 to 3 mEq/liter higher than the calculated bicarbonate obtained from the arterial blood gas determi-

nation, since the total carbon dioxide obtained on a venous sample of blood measures the dissolved carbon dioxide, carbonic acid, and bicarbonate. The dissolved carbon dioxide and carbonic acid are usually no more than 2 to 3 mEq/liter, a value that must be subtracted when using the total carbon dioxide to calculate the anion gap. Although a measured value, the total carbon dioxide is unreliable and frequently results in two different values on the same sample. It is probably prudent to use the calculated arterial bicarbonate value as the "true" bicarbonate level.

Treatment

When considering therapy for severe metabolic alkalosis, the physician must remember that sodium chloride and potassium chloride infusions can usually correct alkalosis by suppressing renal acid excretion and enhancing the renal excretion of bicarbonate. However, these corrective mechanisms are slow and cannot be relied on for patients with extreme alkalosis, defined as a pH more than 7.6 with symptoms or more than 7.8 without symptoms. Nasogastric drainage should be stopped, if possible, and exogenous bicarbonate therapy discontinued. Patients in Group 1 respond to sodium chloride and potassium chloride replacement in three to four days, whereas patients in Group 2 are chloride-resistant but usually respond to spironolactone, an aldosterone antagonist.

In patients who retain sodium chloride (e.g., those with congestive heart failure or cirrhosis), arterial hypovolemia causes a secondary hyperaldosteronism with increased bicarbonate reabsorption. Volume expansion would obviously be detrimental in these cases. Spironolactone or acetazolamide (carbonic anhydrase inhibitor) may be given to increase the renal excretion of bicarbonate.

In the presence of extreme alkalosis or hepatic encephalopathy, the use of direct acidifying agents is justified:

1. Arginine hydrochloride supplies hydrochloride during its metabolism. It is the compound that is tolerated best parenterally. If commercial arginine is unavailable, a solution can be prepared from the powder with 50 mEq/100 ml.
2. Ammonium chloride contains H^+ in a concentration of 167 mEq/liter, and is well tolerated.
3. Lysine hydrochloride is an alternative to NH_4Cl.
4. Dilute hydrochloric acid can be used. This acid must be given through a central catheter. This method is the best treatment in patients with hepatic encephalopathy because no additional sources of ammonia, such as amino acids, are being supplied. Administration of acid should not prevent

therapy with volume expanders and potassium chloride, if needed, since these patients frequently require 4 to 5 liters fluid (isotonic saline) and 500 to 600 mEq potassium chloride for correction of their metabolic alkalosis. To prepare the solutions, 100 ml 1N hydrochloric acid is added to 900 ml normal saline or 5 percent dextrose and water, resulting in 0.1N hydrochloric acid containing 100 mEq H^+ per liter and a hypotonic 200 mOsm/liter solution. Alternatively, 200 ml 1N hydrochloric acid can be added to 800 ml normal saline or 5 percent dextrose and water, resulting in 0.2N hydrochloric acid with 200 mEq H^+ per liter and a hypertonic 400 mOsm/liter solution.[90–92]

5. Hemodialysis against low chloride and high acetate solution is well suited for uremic patients with severe metabolic alkalosis.

To calculate the amount of acid necessary to treat a metabolic alkalosis, the volume of distribution of bicarbonate must be known. The volume of distribution of bicarbonate is one-half the total body weight.[68,83] This volume is then multiplied by the desired decrement in bicarbonate, resulting in the base excess. In general, the physician should try to obtain a reduction in bicarbonate of 10 mEq/liter over 12 to 24 hours. For example, a 70-kg man with a severe metabolic alkalosis has a bicarbonate level of 50 mEq/liter, and a decrease in the bicarbonate level to 40 mEq/liter is desired. The volume of distribution is one-half of 70 kg, or 35 liters. Multiplying the volume of distribution (35 liters) by the desired decrement (10 liters) results in 350 mEq acid needed to decrease serum bicarbonate by 10 mEq/liter. This neutralization could be achieved with 0.2N hydrochloric acid in normal saline administered at a rate of 200 ml/hour. Faster decrements in bicarbonate can be achieved if the clinical situation warrants.

RESPIRATORY ACIDOSIS

Pathophysiology

Carbon dioxide is an end product of metabolism. The level of carbon dioxide reflects the balance between production at the cellular level and excretion by the lungs. Although carbon dioxide is produced at a relatively constant rate, the rate at which it is excreted varies with the efficiency of breathing. If alveolar ventilation is increased, the carbon dioxide level in the blood, or PCO_2, decreases.[93] Conversely, if alveolar ventilation is decreased, arterial PCO_2 increases.

Acute respiratory acidosis is uncompensated. There is no renal retention of bicarbonate.[94] For every 10 mm Hg increase in PCO_2, the hydrogen ion concentration increases 8 nEq/liter or decreases 0.08 pH units.[5,95] For example, if a patient with a PCO_2 of 40 mm Hg, a pH of 7.40, and a hydrogen ion concentration of 40 nEq/liter develops acute respiratory failure so that the PCO_2 becomes 60 mm Hg, the hydrogen ion concentration increases 16 nEq/liter or 56 nEq/liter and pH decreases 0.16 units to a pH of 7.24.

In acute respiratory acidosis, the elevation of PCO_2 increases the serum bicarbonate by a small amount owing to an equilibrium shift in the reaction catalyzed by carbonic anhydrase (see Reaction 2).[5] It is not a compensation for respiratory acidosis by the kidneys. Because of the shift in equilibrium, for every 10-mm Hg increment in PCO_2, bicarbonate increases 1 mEq/liter.

After 6 to 12 hours of acute respiratory acidosis, the renal synthesis and retention of bicarbonate is stimulated, and the patient is in chronic respiratory acidosis.[5,96] With the increased retention of bicarbonate, electrical neutrality is maintained by renal secretion of chloride. The renal compensation for respiratory acidosis is not complete, however. The pH remains in the low normal range from 7.36 to 7.39, provided that the PCO_2 is less than 60 mm Hg. When the PCO_2 is more than 60 mm Hg, only 15 percent of patients are able to compensate and maintain their pH within the normal range. Most of these patients have an arterial pH less than 7.36.[97] If the PCO_2 is more than 70 mm Hg, only 1 percent of patients have a pH within the normal range; the remainder have a pH less than 7.35.[97]

The hydrogen ion concentration in chronic respiratory acidosis does not vary as much as it does with acute respiratory acidosis because of the buffering capacity of the elevated bicarbonate values in chronic respiratory acidosis. In chronic respiratory acidosis, for each 10-mm Hg increase in PCO_2 there is a 3 nEq/liter increase in hydrogen ion concentration or a 0.03-unit decrease in pH.[5] For example, if the PCO_2 of a patient with a pH of 7.40, a hydrogen ion concentration of 40 nEq/liter, and a PCO_2 of 50 mm Hg is increased from 50 to 60 mm Hg, the hydrogen ion concentration is increased from 40 to 43 nEq/liter and the pH is decreased from 7.40 to 7.37.

Etiology, Diagnosis, and Treatment

For the etiology, diagnosis, and treatment of respiratory acidosis, see Chapter 59.

RESPIRATORY ALKALOSIS

Mechanism

Respiratory alkalosis develops when ventilation is increased to the point that carbon dioxide excretion exceeds carbon dioxide production.

Acute Respiratory Alkalosis

During acute respiratory alkalosis, a nonrenal compensation occurs secondary to the carbonic anhydrase reaction (see Reaction 2). In this reaction, the decreased level of carbon dioxide shifts the equilibrium so that bicarbonate is consumed, bringing the pH closer to normal and, therefore, functioning as a buffer. To maintain electrical neutrality, lost bicarbonate is replaced by chloride, which results in mild hyperchloremia. For every 10-mm Hg decrease of PCO_2, the bicarbonate level decreases 2 mEq,[98] the hydrogen ion concentration decreases 8 nEq/liter, and the pH increases by 0.08 units.[5] For example, if a patient with a pH of 7.40 and a PCO_2 of 40 mm Hg develops an acute respiratory alkalosis that decreases the PCO_2 to 20 mm Hg, the hydrogen ion concentration decreases 16 nEq/liter to 24 nEq/liter and the pH increases 0.16 units to 7.56.

Chronic Respiratory Alkalosis

By definition, chronic respiratory alkalosis is an acute respiratory alkalosis that has persisted for at least 12 to 24 hours and is being compensated for by the renal excretion of bicarbonate. As in all other acid-base abnormalities, the compensated pH is in the high normal range, i.e., 7.40 to 7.45. This persistence in a high normal range lasts for 7 to 9 days. After two weeks, however, the pH returns to a completely normal value without any superimposed metabolic acidosis.[5] Chronic respiratory alkalosis is unique among the acid-base disturbances in that it is the only one in which a completely normal pH is expected.[5] The serum bicarbonate level can be predicted in a chronic respiratory alkalosis. For every 10-mm Hg decrease in PCO_2, the serum bicarbonate level should fall 5 mEq/liter.[5,99] For example, if a patient with a pH of 7.4, a PCO_2 of 40 mm Hg, and a bicarbonate level of 25 develops a chronic respiratory alkalosis and a new PCO_2 of 20 mm Hg, the pH will be 7.4 and the expected serum bicarbonate level is 15 mEq/liter after two weeks.

Etiology of Respiratory Alkalosis

Hyperventilation Syndrome

Anxiety or stress may cause patients to develop the hyperventilation syndrome. They are usually totally unaware that they are breathing rapidly. Some patients, however, do not have tachypnea but simply increase the depth of inspiration without increasing the rate.

Central Neurogenic Hyperventilation

Massive brain injury may affect the medullary centers that inhibit respiration. Because these centers control the rate and depth of respiration, hyperventilation may follow such an injury. Central neurogenic hyperventilation is seen in patients with brain tumors, massive cerebrovascular accidents, encephalitis, or meningitis.

Respiratory Stimulants

Several entities stimulate the respiratory centers in the medulla. Progesterone secreted during pregnancy is responsible for the chronic respiratory alkalosis seen in pregnancy. During pregnancy, the PCO_2 usually is approximately 30 mm Hg, and the patient has a normal pH.[100] In fact, progesterone has been successfully used in the treatment of acute respiratory failure in patients with chronic obstructive pulmonary disease as well as in patients with pickwickian syndrome.[101,102] Adrenergic stimulation also may increase the respiratory rate. Excessive catecholamines, as may be seen in pheochromocytoma, may cause respiratory alkalosis. In a similar fashion, patients with analeptic overdose, e.g., with amphetamines or cocaine, also develop respiratory alkalosis.

Hepatic Insufficiency

The mechanism is unclear, but patients with marked liver disease frequently have respiratory alkalosis.

Restrictive Pulmonary Disease

Patients whose chest wall motion is restricted may complain of dyspnea. Although not associated with hypoxemia, this dyspnea and hyperventilation results in respiratory alkalosis. It has been postulated that restriction in chest wall motion stimulates the J receptors in the bronchi, which in turn enhance breathing. This mechanism may explain the dyspnea seen in nonhypoxemic patients with tumors of the lung, pneumothorax, pleural effusions, or pneumonia.

Pulmonary Hypoxemia

Chemoreceptors in the carotid body stimulate respiration in response to hypoxemia.[103] In normal individuals, there is a highly varied response to hypoxemia. Some patients develop a profound respiratory alkalosis in response to hypoxemia, while other patients do not hyperventilate at all in response to hypoxemia.[104] It is well known that patients with chronic obstructive pulmonary disease may have a blunted response to hypoxemia[105]; it is less well known that normal patients may also have a blunted response to hypoxemia and hyperventilate less than expected.[104] (See Chapter 57.)

Tissue Hypoxia

The pathophysiologic mechanisms behind tissue hypoxemia usually involve uncoupling. Uncoupling implies that oxidative phosphorylation has been uncoupled from electron transport in the mitochondria. Therefore, despite an abundant supply of oxygen, adenosine triphosphatase is not being generated. This is perceived by the body as hypoxemia, and hyperventilation ensues. This mechanism explains the respiratory alkalosis found during fever, gram-negative sepsis, hyperthyroidism, and salicylate intoxication. (See Chapter 6.)

Another pathophysiologic mechanism of tissue hypoxemia is impaired delivery of oxygen to the tissues. For example, carbon monoxide may occasionally produce respiratory alkalosis in association with a normal PO_2.[106] Carbon monoxide not only shifts the oxygen-hemoglobin dissociation curve to the left, which deprives tissues of oxygen, but also binds strongly to hemoglobin. Both these processes impair the ability of hemoglobin to release oxygen. Therefore, the patient may hyperventilate. Another cause of impaired oxygen delivery is methemoglobinemia, which may be congenital or acquired. The acquired form of methemoglobinemia can result in tissue hypoxemia secondary to impaired oxygen delivery and, subsequently, respiratory alkalosis.[107] These patients are quite dyspneic, with a normal PO_2 and a dark brown arterial blood gas rather than the normally red arterial blood sample.

Clinical Manifestations

During respiratory alkalosis, the ratio of charges between the cationic and anionic proteins is altered so that more anionic proteins are present. This results simply from the change in pH. The increased anionic proteins bind more free calcium, producing symptoms of hypocalcemia; the serum calcium is unaltered, however, since serum calcium measures both free and bound calcium. Therefore, the symptoms of respiratory alkalosis mimic those of hypocalcemia. Any other manifestations of acute respiratory alkalosis reflect the underlying etiology.

Treatment

The only treatment of respiratory alkalosis is treatment for the underlying condition. Respiratory alkalosis is highly refractory to any other forms of therapy.

REFERENCES

1. Van Slyke DD: Some points of acid-base history in physiology and medicine. *Ann NY Acad Sci* 133:5, 1966.
2. Henderson LJ: Theory of neutrality regulation in animal organism. *Am J Physiol* 21:427, 1908.
3. Sorenson SPL: Enzymestudien. II. Mitteilung. Uber die Messung und die Bedeutung der Wasserstaffionen-Konzentration bei enzymatischen Prozessin. *Biochem Z* 21:131, 1909.
4. Hasselbalch KA: Die Berechnung der Wasserstaffzahl des Blutes aus der Freien und gebundenen Kohlensaure desselben und die Sauerstaffbindung des Blutes als Funktion der Wasserstaffzahl. *Biochem Z* 78:112, 1916.
5. Narins RG, Emmett M: Simple and mixed acid-base disorders: A practical approach. *Medicine* 59:161, 1980.
6. Kassirer JP, Bleich, HL: Rapid estimation of plasma carbon dioxide from pH and total carbon dioxide content. *N Engl J Med* 272:1067, 1965.
7. Morgan HG: Acid-base balance in blood. *Br J Anaesth* 41:196, 1969.
8. Kaufman HE, Rosen SW: Clinical acid-base regulation—The Bronsted schema. *Surg Gynecol Obstet* 103:101, 1956.
9. Emmett M, Narins RG: Clinical use of the anion gap. *Medicine* 56:38, 1977.
10. Witte DL, Rodgers JL, Barrett DA: The anion gap: Its use in quality control. *Clin Chem* 22:643, 1976.
11. Pierce NF, Fedson DS, Brigham DE, et al: The ventilatory response to acute base deficit in humans: Time course during development and correction of metabolic acidosis. *Ann Intern Med* 72:633, 1970.
12. Reuler JB: Hypothermia: Pathophysiology, clinical settings and management. *Ann Intern Med* 89:519, 1978.
13. Goodwin NM, Schreiber MT: Effects of anticoagulants on acid-base and blood gas estimations. *Crit Care Med* 7:473, 1979.
14. Asch MJ: Acid-base effects of topical mafenide acetate in the burned patient. *N Engl J Med* 284:1281, 1971.
15. Runeberg L, Miettinen TA, Nikkila EA: Effect of cholestyramine on mineral excretion in man. *Acta Med Scand* 192:71, 1972.
16. Garella S, Chang BS, Kahn SF: Dilution acidosis and contraction alkalosis: Review of a concept. *Kidney Int* 8:279, 1975.
17. Oh MS, Carroll HJ, Goldstein DH, Fein IA: Hyperchloremic acidosis during the recovery phase of diabetic ketosis. *Ann Intern Med* 89:925, 1978.
18. Giammarco R, Goldstein M, Halpern M, Stinebaugh B: Renal tubular acidosis during therapy for diabetic ketoacidosis. *Can Med Assoc J* 112:465, 1975.
19. Heird WC, Dell RB, Driscoll JM, Grebin B, Winters RW: Metabolic acidosis resulting from intravenous alimentation mixtures containing synthetic amino acids. *N Engl J Med* 287:943, 1972.
20. Gennari FJ, Goldstein MB, Schwartz WB: The nature of the renal adaptation of chronic hypocapnia. *J Clin Invest* 51:1722, 1972.
21. Batlle DC, Aruda JAL, Kurtzman NA: Hyperkalemic distal renal tubular acidosis associated with obstructive uropathy. *N Engl J Med* 304:373, 1981.
22. Narins RG, Goldberg M: Renal tubular acidosis: Pathophysiology, diagnosis and treatment. *DM* 23:1, 1977.
23. Sebastian A, Morris RC Jr: Renal tubular acidosis. *Clin Nephrol* 7:216, 1977.
24. Morris RC Jr: Renal tubular acidosis. *N Engl J Med* 304:418, 1981.
25. Gennari FJ, Cohen JJ: Renal tubular acidosis. *Annu Rev Med* 29:521, 1978.
26. Ritz E, Heidland A: Lactic acidosis. *Clin Nephrol* 7:231, 1977.
27. Kreisberg RA: Lactate, homeostasis and lactic acidosis. *Ann Intern Med* 92:227, 1980.
28. Fraley DS, Adler S, Bruns FJ, et al: Stimulation of lactate production by administration of bicarbonate in a patient with a solid neoplasm and lactic acidosis. *N Engl J Med* 303:1100, 1980.
29. Nadiminti Y, Wang JC, Chou S-Y, et al: Lactic acidosis associated with Hodgkin's disease: Response to chemotherapy. *N Engl J Med* 303:15, 1980.
30. Sprung CL, Portocarrero CJ, Fernaine AV, et al: The metabolic and respiratory alterations of heat stroke. *Arch Intern Med* 140:665, 1980.

31. Orringer CE, Eustace JL, Wunsch CD, Gardner LB: Natural history of lactic acidosis after grand-mal seizures: A model for the study of an anion-gap acidosis not associated with hyperkalemia. *N Engl J Med* 297:796, 1977.

32. Gerst PH, Fleming WH, Malm JR: Increased susceptibility of the heart to ventricular fibrillation during metabolic acidosis. *Circ Res* 19:63, 1966.

33. O'Connor LR, Klein KL, Bethune JE: Hyperphosphatemia in lactic acidosis. *N Engl J Med* 297:707, 1977.

34. Molitch ME, Rodman E, Hirsch CA, et al: Spurious serum creatinine elevations in ketoacidosis. *Ann Intern Med* 93:280, 1980.

35. Grant DH: Pharmacology of isopropyl alcohol, a synopsis of available data. *J Lab Clin Med* 8:382, 1923.

36. Cooperman MT, Davidoff F, Spark R, Pallotta J: Clinical studies of alcoholic ketoacidosis. *Diabetes* 23:433, 1974.

37. Fulop M, Hoberman HD: Alcoholic ketosis. *Diabetes* 24:785, 1975.

38. Miller PD, Heinig RE, Waterhouse C: Treatment of alcoholic acidosis: The role of dextrose and phosphorus. *Arch Intern Med* 138:67, 1978.

39. Young E, Bradley RF: Cerebral edema with irreversible coma in severe diabetic ketoacidosis. *N Engl J Med* 276:665, 1967.

40. Metzger AL, Rubenstein AH: Reversible cerebral edema complicating diabetic ketoacidosis. *Br Med J* 3:746, 1970.

41. Kitabchi AE, Young R, Sacks H, et al: Diabetic ketoacidosis: Reappraisal of therapeutic approach. *Annu Rev Med* 30:339, 1979.

42. Alberti KGMM, Hockaday TDR: Diabetic coma: A reappraisal after five years. *Clin Endocrinol Metab* 6:421, 1977.

43. Ohman JL, Marliss EB, Aoki TT, Munichoodappa CS, Khanna VV, Kozak GP: The cerebrospinal fluid in diabetic ketoacidosis. *N Engl J Med* 284:283, 1971.

44. Kreisberg RA: Diabetic ketoacidosis: New concepts and trends in pathogenesis and treatment. *Ann Intern Med* 88:681, 1978.

45. Soler NG, Fitzgerald MG, Wright AD, Malins JM: Comparative study of different insulin regimens in management of diabetic ketoacidosis. *Lancet* 2:1221, 1975.

46. Kitabchi AE, Ayyagari Y, Guerra SM: The efficacy of low-dose versus conventional therapy of insulin for treatment of diabetic ketoacidosis. *Ann Intern Med* 84:633, 1976.

47. Fisher JN, Shahshahani MN, Kitabchi AE: Diabetic ketoacidosis: Low dose insulin therapy by various routes. *N Engl J Med* 297:238, 1977.

48. Knight AH, Williams DN, Ellis G, Goldberg DM: Significance of hyperamylasemia and abdominal pain in diabetic ketoacidosis. *Br Med J* 3:128, 1973.

49. Lentz RD, Brown DM, Kjellstrand OM: Treatment of severe hypophosphatemia. *Ann Intern Med* 89:941, 1978.

50. Bennett IL Jr, Cary FH, Mitchell GL, et al: Acute methyl alcohol poisoning: A review based on experiences in an outbreak of 323 cases. *Medicine* 32:431, 1953.

51. Erlanson P, Hagstam K-E, Liljenberg B, et al: Severe methanol intoxication. *Acta Med Scand* 177:393, 1965.

52. McMartin KE, Ambre JJ, Tephly TR: Methanol poisoning in human subjects: Role for formic acid accumulation in the metabolic acidosis. *Am J Med* 68:414, 1980.

53. Keyvan-Larijarni H, Tannenberg AM: Methanol intoxication: Comparison of peritoneal dialysis and hemodialysis treatment. *Arch Intern Med* 134:293, 1974.

54. McCoy HG, Cippole RJ, Ehlers SM, et al: Severe methanol poisoning: Application of a pharmacokinetic model for ethanol therapy and hemodialysis. *Am J Med* 67:804, 1979.

55. Gonda A, Gault H, Churchill D, et al: Hemodialysis for methanol intoxication. *Am J Med* 64:749, 1978.

56. Parry MF, Wallach R: Ethylene glycol poisoning. *Am J Med* 57:143, 1974.

57. Cadnapaphornchai P, Taher S, Bhathena D, et al: Ethylene glycol poisoning: Diagnosis based on high osmolal and anion gaps and crystalluria. *Ann Emerg Med* 10:94, 1981.

58. Stokes JB, Averon F: Prevention of organ damage in massive ethylene glycol ingestion. *JAMA* 243:2065, 1980.

59. Wacker WEC, Haynes H, Druyan R, et al: Treatment of ethylene glycol poisoning with ethyl alcohol. *JAMA* 194:173, 1965.

60. Smithline N, Gardner KD Jr: Gaps—Anion and osmolal. *JAMA* 236:1594, 1976.

61. Glasser L, Sternglanz PD, Combic J, et al: Serum osmolarity and its applicability to drug overdose. *Am J Clin Pathol* 60:695, 1963.

62. Anderson RJ, Potts DE, Gabow PA, Rumack BH, Schrier RW: Unrecognized adult salicylate intoxication. *Ann Intern Med* 85:745, 1976.

63. Temple AR: Pathophysiology of aspirin overdosage toxicity with implications for management. *Pediatrics* 62:873, 1978.

64. Gabow PA, Potts DE, Schrier RW, Anderson RJ: The acid-base abnormalities of adult salicylate intoxication. *Clin Res* 24:126A, 1976.

65. Myers EN, Bernstein JM, Fostiropolous G: Salicylate ototoxicity: A clinical study. *N Engl J Med* 273:587, 1965.

66. Zimmerman HJ: Aspirin-induced hepatic injury. *Ann Intern Med* 80:103, 1974.

67. Hrnicek G, Skelton J, Miller WC: Pulmonary edema and salicylate intoxication. *JAMA* 230:866, 1974.

68. Arruda JAL, Kurtzman NA: Metabolic acidosis and alkalosis. *Clin Nephrol* 7:201, 1977.

69. Lindeman RD, Papper S: Therapy of fluid and electrolyte disorders. *Ann Intern Med* 82:64, 1975.

70. Garella GD, Serafino AL, Dana CL, Chazan JA: Severity of metabolic acidosis as a determinant of bicarbonate requirements. *N Engl J Med* 289:121, 1973.

71. Taradash MR, Jacobson LB: Vasodilator therapy of idiopathic lactic acidosis. *N Engl J Med* 293:468, 1975.

72. Bleich HL, Schwartz WB: Tris buffer (THAM): An appraisal of its physiologic effects and clinical usefulness. *N Engl J Med* 274:782, 1966.

73. THAM. American Hospital Formulary Service 40:8, 1979.

74. Litwin MS, Smith LL, Moore FD: Metabolic alkalosis following massive transfusion. *Surgery* 45:805, 1959.

75. Lipner HI, Ruzany F, Dasgupta M, Lief PD, Bank N: The behavior of carbenicillin as a nonreabsorbable anion. *J Lab Clin Med* 86:183, 1975.

76. Brunner FD, Frick PG: Hypokalaemia, metabolic acidosis, and hypernatraemia due to "massive" sodium penicillin therapy. *Br Med J* 4:550, 1968.

77. Eldridge F, Salzer J: Effect of respiratory alkalosis on blood lactate and pyruvate in humans. *J Appl Physiol* 22:461, 1967.

78. Kassirer JP, Schwartz WB: The selective depletion of hydrochloric acid: Factors in the genesis of persistent gastric alkalosis. *Am J Med* 40:10, 1966.

79. Madias NE, Ayus JC, Adrogue HJ: Increased anion gap in metabolic alkalosis: The role of plasma-protein equivalency. *N Engl J Med* 300:1421, 1979.

80. Blume RS, MacLowry JD, Wolf SM: Limitations of chloride determination in the diagnosis of bromism. *N Engl J Med* 279:593, 1968.

81. Driscoll JL, Martin HF: Detection of brominism by an automated chloride method. *Clin Chem* 12:314, 1966.

82. Murray T, Long W, Narins R: Multiple myeloma and the anion gap. *N Engl J Med* 292:574, 1975.

83. Coe FL: Metabolic alkalosis. *JAMA* 238:2288, 1977.

84. Elkinton JR: Clinical disorders of acid-base regulation. A survey of seventeen years' diagnostic experience. *Med Clin North Am* 50:1325, 1966.

85. Fulop M: Hypercapnia in metabolic alkalosis. *NY State J Med* 76:19, 1976.

86. Harrington JT, Cohen JJ: Measurement of urinary electrolytes—Indications and limitations. *N Engl J Med* 293:1241, 1975.

87. Bear R, Goldstein M, Phillipson E, Ho M, et al: Effect of metabolic alkalosis on respiratory function in patients with chronic obstructive lung disease. *Can Med Assoc J* 117:900, 1977.

88. Bieberdorf FA, Gorden P, Fordtran JS: Pathogenesis of congenital alkalosis with diarrhea: Implications for the physiology of normal ileal electrolyte absorption and secretion. *J Clin Invest* 51:1958, 1972.

89. Schwartz WB, Relman AS: A critique of the parameters used in the evaluation of acid-base disorders: "Whole-blood buffer base" and "standard bicarbonate" compared with blood pH and plasma bicarbonate concentration. *N Engl J Med* 268:1382, 1963.

90. Wagner CW, Nesbit RR Jr, Mansberger AR: The use of intravenous hydrochloric acid in the treatment of thirty-four patients with metabolic alkalosis. *Am Surg* 46:140, 1980.

91. Frick PG, Senning A: The treatment of severe metabolic alkalosis with intravenous N/10 or N/5 hydrochloric acid. *German Medical Monthly* 9:242, 1964.

92. Williams DB, Lyons JH Jr: Treatment of severe metabolic alkalosis with intravenous infusion of hydrochloric acid. *Surg Gynecol Obstet* 150:315, 1980.

93. Pontoppidan H, Geffin B, Lowenstein E: Acute respiratory failure in the adult. *N Engl J Med* 287:743, 1972.

94. Goldring RM, Heinemann HO: Bicarbonate and the regulation of ventilation. *Am J Med* 57:361, 1974.

95. Martinez-Maldonado M, Sanchez-Montserrat R: Respiratory acidosis and alkalosis. *Clin Nephrol* 7:191, 1977.

96. MacDonald FM: Respiratory acidosis. *Arch Intern Med* 116:689, 1965.

97. Van Ypersele de Strihou C, Brasseur CL, DeConnick J: The "carbon dioxide response curve" for chronic hypercapnia in man. *N Engl J Med* 275:117, 1966.

98. Arbus GS, Herbert LA, Levesque PR, et al: Characterization and clinical application of the "significance band" for acute respiratory alkalosis. *N Engl J Med* 280:117, 1969.

99. Gennari FJ, Goldstein MB, Schwartz WB: The nature of the renal adaptation to chronic hypocapnia. *J Clin Invest* 51:1722, 1972.

100. Weinberger SE, Weiss ST, Cohen WR, et al: Pregnancy and the lung. *Am Rev Respir Dis* 121:559, 1980.

101. Sutton FD, Zwillich CW, Creagh E, et al: Progesterone for outpatient treatment of pickwickian syndrome. *Ann Intern Med* 83:476, 1975.

102. Morrison DA, Goldman AL: Oral progesterone therapy in COPD. *Am Rev Respir Dis* 119:154, 1978.

103. Lugliani R, Whipp BJ, Seard C, et al: Effect of bilateral carotid body resection on ventilatory control of rest and during exercise in man. *N Engl J Med* 285:1105, 1977.

104. Hirschman CA, McCullough RE, Weil JV: Normal values for hypoxic and hypercapnic ventilatory drives in man. *J Appl Physiol* 38:1095, 1975.

105. Flenley DC, Franklin DH, Miller JS: The hypoxic drive to breathing in chronic bronchitis and emphysema. *Clin Sci* 38:503, 1970.

106. Myers RAM, Linberg SE, Cowley RA: Carbon monoxide poisoning: The injury and its treatment. *Ann Emerg Med* 8:479, 1979.

107. Green ED, Zimmerman RC, Ghurabi WH, et al: Phenazopyridine hydrochloride toxicity: A cause of drug-induced methemoglobinemia. *Ann Emerg Med* 8:426, 1979.

19. Acute Gout

GARY W. WILLIAMS, M.D., Ph.D.

The term *gout* is used to represent a heterogeneous group of disease entities that occur exclusively in humans. They are characterized by hyperuricemia, single or multiple episodes of acute gouty arthritis, periods between attacks, and chronic tophaceous gout. The underlying abnormality in this metabolic disease is hyperuricemia, i.e., a sustained elevation of the serum urate above its solubility limit of approximately 7 to 7.5 mg/dl.

Asymptomatic hyperuricemia affects approximately 5 percent of the adult male population and may be present for life without additional features of gout. As the level of serum urate rises, however, the incidence of acute gouty arthritis increases. The Framingham study demonstrated that for men with an average age of 44 years, a serum urate level of 9 mg/dl was associated with a 90 percent risk of gouty arthritis within 14 years.[1] The factors contributing to hyperuricemia in the adult include increased production of uric acid due to an accelerated rate of purine synthesis, as well as decreased renal and intestinal excretion. Excessive consumption of purines is less important. Consequently, a rational classification of hyperuricemia involves three categories: (1) overproduction, (2) underexcretion, and (3) a combination of overproduction and underexcretion.

The diagnosis of hyperuricemia ideally is based on two separate measurements of serum urate, each following a 12-hour fast in a normally hydrated individual. Measuring the uric acid in a 24-hour urine specimen distinguishes overproduction from underexcretion. A value greater than 800 mg/24 hours indicates hyperuricosuria and suggests that the patient's hyperuricemia is due to overproduction of uric acid. If the 24-hour urinary uric acid excretion is normal, then underexcretion plays some role in the hyperuricemia, even though overproduction may also be present. These determinations are important in planning therapy and in assessing the risk of uric acid nephrolithiasis. It should be emphasized that the presence of hyperuricemia with a normal urinary uric acid excretion does not mandate therapy.

ACUTE GOUTY ARTHRITIS

Patients with acute gouty arthritis, which is frequently a nocturnal event, may seek medical care in the emergency department with complaints of severe monoarticular arthritis. Virtually any joint may be involved, with intense pain, swelling, heat, and redness. Occasionally multiple joints are involved in a single attack (polyarticular gout). The diagnosis can be made with absolute certainty only by the demonstration of needle-shaped, negatively birefringent crystals within polymorphonuclear leukocytes in synovial fluid. The failure to demonstrate such crystals suggests an acute monoarticular arthritis, and the leading diagnostic possibility is infection until proved otherwise. Therefore, synovial fluid should be removed from the affected joint whenever possible and appropriate cultures done if synovial fluid analysis does not demonstrate crystals. The emergency department physician should be familiar with the use of the polarizing microscope if technicians are not available on a full-time basis to perform synovial fluid analysis.

If it is not possible to obtain synovial fluid, a classic clinical history of gouty arthritis, the presence of hyperuricemia, and the demonstration of an appropriate response to colchicine or other anti-inflammatory agents suggest the diagnosis of monosodium urate gout. It should be emphasized, however, that crystals such as calcium pyrophosphate may produce a similar clinical picture (pseudogout) and may respond to colchicine. Furthermore, infectious arthritis may also improve somewhat with anti-inflammatory agents, leading to unnecessary and perhaps deleterious delay in the identification of an infecting organism and the initiation of appropriate antimicrobial therapy.

Hyperuricemia is also associated with specific enzyme or metabolic defects, as well as with so-called secondary forms of gout that result from increased purine biosynthesis. Finally, it should be kept in mind that increased nucleic acid turnover due to psoriasis or malignancy, as well as reduced renal function, may lead to hyperuricemia and may require therapy apart from that necessary to control the acute attack. Once the diagnosis has been made and aggravating factors or disease processes identified, prompt therapy should be instituted.

Colchicine administered orally or intravenously is an effective agent in the management of acute gouty arthritis. As indicated earlier, a response to such therapy does not firmly establish a diagnosis of acute gouty arthritis because pseudogout, calcific tendinitis due to hydroxyapatite, sarcoid arthritis, rheumatoid arthritis, and familial Mediterranean fever are also reported to respond to colchicine. If therapy is instituted within a few hours of the onset of joint symptoms, a similar interval may be expected before an improvement in symptoms. If, however, treatment is delayed for 12 hours or longer, an additional 12 to 48 hours may be required before improvement begins. If administered orally, 1 mg of colchicine should be given, followed by 0.5 mg every two to three hours until joint pain lessens or the patient shows signs of a toxic reaction. The major disadvantage of oral colchicine is that it may cause nausea, cramping abdominal pain, diarrhea, or vomiting before it relieves the arthritis. For this reason, many favor the use of intravenous colchicine, indomethacin, or phenylbutazone.

Intravenous colchicine is administered at an initial dose of 2 to 3 mg in 20 ml normal saline over 30 minutes. An additional 1 mg may be administered every six hours to a maximal dose of 4 to 5 mg. Oral colchicine should not be administered concomitantly. Local extravasation may cause painful inflammation and even necrosis of the surrounding tissue. The drug is contraindicated in patients who are neutropenic, since bone marrow suppression may be the first evidence of toxicity.

Indomethacin is also an effective agent in the treatment of acute gout when given at initial doses of 50 to 75 mg, followed by 25 to 50 mg every six hours. No more than 200 mg should be administered within the first 24 hours, however. At this point, the dosage may be decreased, although the drug should be continued for 2 to 3 days following resolution of symptoms to prevent a relapse. Like colchicine, indomethacin has significant gastrointestinal and central nervous system side-effects, particularly in elderly patients, which limit its usefulness. For patients with peptic ulcer disease, inflammatory bowel disease, or a previous history of intolerance to the medication, the physician should consider other forms of therapy.

Phenylbutazone, a powerful anti-inflammatory agent, is also effective in the treatment of acute gouty arthritis. An initial dose of 200 to 400 mg may be followed by 100 to 200 mg, three to four times daily. After 24 hours, a dosage of 100 mg four times a day is generally adequate. Rarely, phenylbutazone is associated with the development of serious bone marrow suppression. Even short-term therapy with this agent has led to bone marrow suppression on several occasions, and many physicians feel that its use is not justified in a disease for which many other agents are available. Virtually all of the nonsteroidal anti-inflammatory agents currently on the market have been tested in acute gout and may be used with good results at maximum doses.

Local injection of corticosteroids into an involved joint or bursa may limit the attack, but neither parenteral steroids nor adrenocorticotropic hormone (ACTH) is recommended because of the tendency for rebound attacks and somewhat inconsistent responses.

In terms of safety and efficacy, indomethacin is the drug of choice in patients who have documented gout. If the diagnosis cannot be substantiated by synovial fluid analysis, intravenous or oral colchicine may provide some diagnostic help.

It is important to arrange appropriate follow-up for all patients with a documented or presumed diagnosis of acute gouty arthritis. An assessment of serum urate, an appropriate history to exclude renal disease or renal stone formation, and measurements of renal function are helpful in subsequent decisions regarding long-term prophylaxis. The decision to place the patient on medications to decrease production of uric acid or to increase urate excretion depends on the cause of the patient's hyperuricemia. It is seldom possible to assess these factors accurately in the emergency department, however.

It may be possible to modify complicating factors, such as dehydration, obesity, improper diet, or excessive use of alcohol, without exposing the patient to long-term, expensive, and potentially toxic agents. It should be emphasized that some patients never have a second attack of gout; in others, the interval between attacks is as long as five years. Such patients generally have only minimally elevated serum urate values and often have normal 24-hour urinary uric acid excretions. In such patients, it is appropriate to try to alter the predisposing factors and to follow them until they have a second attack. In patients with more marked elevations of serum uric acid (greater than 9 mg/dl) or in those with elevated uric acid excretions, antihyperuricemic therapy should be considered. Such therapy should be individualized; it is *not* appropriate to treat every patient with an agent that inhibits uric acid production. The use of an agent that increases uric acid excretion is contraindicated in patients with hyperuricemia because it predisposes such patients to the development of uric acid nephrolithiasis or uric acid nephropathy.

HOSPITALIZATION

The primary consideration in a decision on immediate hospitalization must be the possibility of acute renal failure due to uric acid nephrolithiasis or nephropathy caused by excessively high serum uric acid levels. Although this is most commonly seen in patients with leukemia or lymphoma on ablative chemotherapy protocols, it has also been reported following epileptic seizures, strenuous exercise in poorly conditioned individuals, and episodes of gout in which patients have dramatically increased purine synthesis and high serum uric acid levels. Exercise and seizure activity appear to increase uric aciduria because of the associated acidosis and acid urines. In patients who are not anuric, the uric acid/creatinine ratio is typically greater than 1.

Proper therapy is necessary to prevent renal failure; it consists of adequate hydration, the use of allopurinol, and the maintenance of an alkaline urine.

Hospitalization is also recommended when infectious arthritis is suspected. It should be emphasized that acute gouty arthritis can occur concomitantly with an infection. If the clinical picture is consistent with infection, hospitalization, appropriate cultures, and careful observation are warranted.

LONG-TERM MANAGEMENT

Antihyperuricemic therapy should not be instituted during an acute attack of gouty arthritis, but should be delayed until the attack has resolved. Medications for lowering the serum uric acid include (1) xanthine oxidase inhibitors, of which allopurinol is the prototype, and (2) uricosuric agents, including probenecid and sul-

finpyrazone. In patients with hyperuricuria (a 24-hour urinary excretion of 800 mg uric acid or more), allopurinol is the drug of choice and should be administered at an initial dose of 4 mg/kg/day. This approximates 300 mg/day in the average adult and should be given as a single morning dose. Side-effects include gastrointestinal intolerance, as well as skin rash, leukopenia, and hepatic inflammation. Unfortunately, more serious side-effects, such as exfoliative dermatitis, toxic epidermal necrolysis, and vasculitis have been reported and are perhaps more frequent in patients with renal insufficiency. Occasionally, patients on allopurinol have developed xanthine stones because of the excessive excretion of hypoxanthine and xanthine. The initiation of allopurinol therapy has also been associated with acute attacks of gout, presumably due to rapid fluctuations in serum urate. Colchicine (0.5 or 0.6 mg twice a day) p.o. should be administered for several days prior to the institution of therapy with allopurinol. It may be necessary to continue the colchicine for several months after initiation of allopurinol, and in some patients one or two tablets of colchicine may be necessary indefinitely to prevent recurrence of attacks.

The specific indications for allopurinol in gout include renal insufficiency, a history of uric acid nephrolithiasis, documented uric acid overproduction with hyperuricuria, and chronic tophaceous gout. In some patients with tophi, a combination of a xanthine oxidase inhibitor and a uricosuric agent may reduce the total body urate load more rapidly.

URICOSURIC AGENTS

Probenecid and sulfinpyrazone may be used to correct underexcretion of uric acid. Probenecid should be initiated at 250 or 500 mg p.o. daily with adequate fluid intake to maintain a urinary output of 2 liters/day. Therapy may be increased gradually over four to six weeks to 1 gm in divided doses twice a day, if necessary. Side-effects include skin rash, as well as hepatic and renal dysfunction. Sulfinpyrazone may be administered at a dose of 100 mg daily and increased over two to four weeks to 200 or 300 mg p.o. daily, if needed. Side-effects include bone marrow depression, liver inflammation, and renal damage. The concomitant use of aspirin with either of these drugs may nullify their beneficial effect.

Acute gouty arthritis, although not itself a life-threatening condition, may be associated with significant renal complications that require hospitalization and aggressive therapy. The diagnosis of acute arthritis should be verified and therapy instituted promptly with the safest agent available for the individual patient based on the reasons for the hyperuricemia and the risk/benefit ratio of the proposed therapy.

REFERENCE

1. Hall AP, Barry PE, Dawber MR, McNamara PM: Epidemiology of gout and hyperuricemia: A long-term population study. *Am J Med* 42:27, 1967.

RECOMMENDED READING

Kelley WD: Gout and related disorders of purine metabolism, in Kelly WN, Harris ED, Ruddy S, Sledge DB (eds): *Textbook of Rheumatology*, ed 1. Philadelphia, WB Saunders, 1981, Vol. 2.

Wyngaarden JB, Holmes EW: Clinical gout and the pathogenesis of hyperuricemia, in McCarty DJ (ed): *Arthritis and Allied Conditions*, ed 9. Philadelphia, Lea & Febiger, 1979.

SECTION IV
General Emergencies

"Infectious Disease Emergencies" (Chapter 20) was written in great detail to cover not only minor nonurgent infectious processes, such as the "common cold" and pharyngitis, but also the potentially life-threatening illnesses, such as bacterial meningitis.

"Burns" (Chapter 21) contains a discussion of both minor and major burns, their prehospital care, and indications for transfer of these patients to specialized centers. Characteristic photographs of isolated skin disorders, as well as those that may manifest systemic diseases, seen in the emergency department are accompanied by a detailed text in "Dermatologic Emergencies" (Chapter 22).

"Gastrointestinal Emergencies" (Chapter 23) covers not only the common complaints of nausea, vomiting, diarrhea, and abdominal pain, but also gastrointestinal conditions that require definitive immediate surgical care.

In association with "Poisoning and Drug Overdose" (Chapter 24), the reader also may wish to refer to "Substance Abuse" (Chapter 35), "Alcohol Abuse" (Chapter 36), and "Depression, Anxiety, and Suicide" (Chapter 37). Since the symptoms of a patient who ingests an overdose of a drug may range from a paucity of signs and symptoms to coma, the reader may wish to refer to "Coma" (Chapter 45) and "Alterations of Central Nervous System Functions" (Section IX).

20. Infectious Disease Emergencies

RICHARD T. ELLISON III, M.D.
STEPHEN H. ZINNER, M.D.

Because an increasing number of patients are using the emergency department for walk-in medical care, the emergency department physician must have a ready approach to the diagnosis and treatment of common infectious diseases. With the exception of meningitis or septicemia from any source, few of these infections are bona fide emergencies, but prompt recognition and appropriate therapy are required to prevent the spread of infection and the development of potentially life-threatening disease.

Physicians must elicit the history pertinent to the patient's presenting complaint. Certain epidemiological clues are essential in the evaluation of bites, skin and soft tissue infections, respiratory infections, gastrointestinal infections, and genitourinary illness. The well-informed physician is able to obtain relevant data quickly.

Once the site of the presumed infection has been localized, the etiologic agent must be sought promptly and aggressively. The emergency department should have a simple mechanism to provide for the immediate preparation and reading of diagnostic material, such as Gram stains of sputum, pus, or cerebrospinal fluid; wet mounts of vaginal secretion or urine for the evaluation of trichomoniasis or yeast infection; routine urinalyses; and blood counts. Suitable cultures (e.g., of pus, blood, or urine) must be performed, and the emergency physician must have a follow-up system to link the patient with the appropriate culture report. Careful instructions must be given to the patient if therapy is to be based on the results of this culture. A system for data retrieval and patient recall is essential, since emergency department physicians may be the patient's only source of medical care. The responsibility of these physicians includes referral for follow-up visits when indicated, such as in the treatment of gonorrhea, urinary tract infections, and other infections that do not necessarily require hospitalization.

In life-threatening infections such as meningitis, the diagnosis must be made and specific appropriate therapy initiated in the emergency department with a minimum of delay. The physician must obtain spinal fluid for diagnostic studies and begin antibiotic therapy immediately. Rapid diagnostic tests such as countercurrent immunoelectrophoresis may be available and can provide rapid feedback to the physician.

Since many infections seen in the emergency department are self-limited, the presence of fever itself does not warrant a therapeutic course of antibiotics. It is imperative, however, that patients whose condition is initially evaluated in an emergency department have access to further medical care if the diagnosis and the proper therapeutic plan is not immediately apparent.

RESPIRATORY TRACT INFECTIONS

Common Cold

Acute upper respiratory infection is the most common illness in the United States. Children under one year of age have more than six "colds" each year, and most individuals average more than two per year until the fourth decade. The etiology of upper respiratory infection is almost exclusively viral, although Group A β-hemolytic streptococci may cause the illness in very young children. Rhinoviruses are responsible for 25 to 40 percent of upper respiratory infections; coronaviruses, parainfluenza viruses, adenoviruses, influenza virus, and respiratory syncytial viruses account for the remaining cases in which a pathogen can be identified. However, the pathogen may not be identifiable in 30 to 40 percent of adults and up to 70 percent of children.

Pathogenesis

Over 100 antigenically distinct viruses circulate among young children, who are the main reservoir for the respiratory viruses. While humoral immunity develops after exposure to a given viral strain, exposure to a new strain usually establishes clinical illness. Viral infections induce the secretion of large quantities of protein from the nasal mucosa. In rhinovirus infections, virus particles are shed in the secretions, beginning the day after infection, reaching a peak concentration two to four days into the clinical illness, and possibly continuing through the seventh day of illness. Infection is most often transmitted by hand-to-hand contact after contamination of hands with nasal secretions.

Diagnosis

After a 48- to 72-hour incubation period, a self-limited illness develops with rhinorrhea, nasal obstruction, and a scratchy or sore throat. Nonproductive cough, headache, malaise, myalgias, and loss of smell and taste are less common symptoms. Initially, the rhinorrhea is thin and watery, but it evolves to a mucopurulent discharge over several days. Low-grade fever may occur in children, but this is uncommon in adults. The symptoms are most prominent in the first two to four days of illness, and they may persist for as long as one week. Some patients may have persistent symptoms for up to six weeks. Examination shows a boggy nasal mucosa and obviously increased nasal secretions. Conjunctivitis and pharyngeal erythema may develop with adenovirus infections.

Differential Diagnosis

The typical syndrome is easily recognized, but a specific etiologic diagnosis usually cannot be made. Although allergic or vasomotor rhinitis can simulate an upper respiratory infection, they can be excluded by a careful history. It is important to rule out associated bacterial infections of the sinuses, the middle ear, or the lower respiratory tree. In patients with any atypical presentation, additional diagnostic studies should be performed (e.g., a throat culture), especially in febrile children under six years of age.

Treatment

Antibiotics have no role in the treatment of the common cold. Symptomatic therapy consists of oral or intranasal sympathomimetic decongestants, saline gargles, or oral analgesics. Codeine-containing cough suppressants are rarely necessary. A petrolatum-based ointment may be effective in preventing irritation of the nares by the nasal secretions. To limit the spread of infection, all patients should be instructed to wash their hands frequently.

Pharyngitis

One of the most frequent complaints brought to the emergency department physician is pharyngitis or sore throat. While most episodes of pharyngitis are self-limited, rheumatic fever may develop from unrecognized or untreated streptococcal infection. The management of this problem should be considered both from the individual and public health perspectives.

Etiology

Acute pharyngitis is caused predominantly by viral agents, e.g., rhinovirus, coronavirus, and adenovirus; by bacterial agents, e.g., Group A β-hemolytic *Streptococcus pyogenes*; and by *Mycoplasma pneumoniae*. The following are other infectious and noninfectious causes that must be considered:

I. Infection
   A. Localized pharyngitis
     1. Viral
       Rhinovirus
       Coronavirus
       Adenovirus
       Herpes simplex virus (Type 1 and 2)
       Parainfluenza
       Influenza virus
       Coxsackievirus A
     2. Bacterial
       Group A β-hemolytic *Streptococcus pyogenes*
       Mixed anaerobes
       Neisseria gonorrhoeae
       Corynebacterium diphtheriae
       Treponema pallidum
       Mycoplasma pneumoniae
       *Hemophilus influenzae**
       *Neisseria meningitidis**
       *Staphylococcus aureus**

---

* Rare proved cause of pharyngitis.

     3. Fungal
          Candida species
  B. Contiguous infections
     1. Epiglottitis
     2. Retropharyngeal abscess
     3. Peritonsillar abscess
  C. Systemic infection
     1. Viral
          Rubeola
          Rubella
          Epstein-Barr virus
          Cytomegalovirus
          Poliomyelitis
          Varicella zoster
          Viral hepatitis
     2. Bacterial
          Hemophilus pertussis
     3. Parasitic
          Toxoplasma gondii
 II. Trauma
  A. Heat
  B. Chemical injury, e.g., with paraquat
  C. Endotracheal intubation
III. Inhalation
  A. Smoke
  B. Industrial exposures
 IV. Dehydration
  V. Subacute thyroiditis

A specific etiology eludes definition in 30 to 40 percent of patients, however.

Pathogenesis

Adenovirus, coxsackievirus A, and herpes simplex virus directly invade the pharyngeal mucosa and produce local inflammation. Other viruses, such as rhinovirus, induce pharyngeal inflammation secondary to nasopharyngeal infection. Group A β-hemolytic streptococci invade the pharyngeal mucosa and produce inflammation by release of extracellular toxins and proteases such as streptolysin, hemolysin, DNAase, and hyaluronidase. The pharynx may be colonized with Group A β-hemolytic streptococci in 15 to 20 percent of individuals with no symptoms of disease. Actual infection by these organisms appears to be mediated by changes in the adherence of bacteria to the pharyngeal membrane mucosa.

Diagnosis

Acute pharyngitis is seen as a sore throat accompanied by fever and erythema of the pharynx. The erythema, which is related to vascular congestion, may extend to the soft palate and uvula. Frequently a patchy white or yellow exudate appears on the tonsils, and the anterior cervical lymph nodes may be enlarged and tender. This presentation can be seen with either viral or bacterial pharyngitis, and no single element or combination of clinical signs reliably indicates the etiologic agent. Occasionally, additional findings may suggest a specific pathogen. For example, the relative occurrence of streptococcal, mycoplasmal, and viral pharyngitis changes with the age of the patient. Streptococcal pharyngitis is most common in children under 12 years of age. Mycoplasmal disease is more common in the second decade, and viral disease is more frequent in older individuals. There is considerable overlap, however. A prior history of rheumatic fever is associated with an increased likelihood of both streptococcal pharyngitis and recurrent rheumatic fever. Coryza is seen occasionally in children with streptococcal infection, but coryza in adults is usually indicative of viral infection. A recent history of sexual contact increases the likelihood of gonococcal, syphilitic, or herpes simplex Type 2 pharyngitis.

Petechiae of the soft palate are associated with viral pharyngitis. Vesicles on the tonsillar pillars and soft palate occur with herpes simplex and coxsackievirus infections (herpangina). The presence of gingivitis and fetid breath suggests a mixed anaerobic infection, usually referred to as Vincent's angina. An ulcer on the soft palate or pharyngeal wall may indicate a syphilitic chancre. Any suggestion of stridor should prompt a search for epiglottitis.

Unilateral swelling of the pharyngeal wall is not a feature of uncomplicated pharyngitis and may represent a peritonsillar abscess or peripharyngeal infection. Membrane or pseudomembrane structures may develop in the pharynx in diphtheria, candidiasis, herpes simplex virus infection, Vincent's angina, and paraquat poisoning. Follicular conjunctivitis is present in 30 to 50 percent of patients with adenoviral pharyngitis. Posterior cervical adenopathy associated with pharyngitis is seen primarily in infectious mononucleosis. A scarlatiniform rash (involving an erythematous, fine, sandpaper-textured eruption on the trunk and extremities), circumoral pallor, and strawberry tongue are seen predominantly with streptococcal pharyngitis, although they may occur secondary to localized staphylococcal infection.

As there are no diagnostically distinguishing characteristics of streptococcal pharyngitis, a throat culture should be performed on all patients with pharyngitis. In a child under six years of age, streptococcal pharyngeal infection may appear only as an acute febrile illness in which the child's temperature rises above 38.3°C. Throat cultures should be performed on these patients also.

For optimal results, a sterile cotton or Dacron swab is used to brush the mucosa of both tonsillar pillars and the posterior pharyngeal wall. The swabs should be streaked on blood agar within 15 minutes. Unless special pathogens such as gonococci or *Corynebacterium diphtheriae* are suspected, the cultures should be used only to identify Group A β-hemolytic streptococci. Isolation of other bacteria is neither clinically nor economically useful.

A positive throat culture for Group A β-hemolytic streptococci does not definitely confirm the diagnosis of streptococcal pharyngitis. An acute rise in serum antibody titers to streptococci-associated proteins, such as streptolysin O, hyaluronidase, or DNAase, is confirmatory; however, this determination requires serial titrations over 10 to 14 days. All patients with clinical pharyngitis and a positive throat culture for β-hemolytic streptococci should be presumed to have a streptococcal infection.

Treatment

Pharyngitis itself is self-limited, and early antibiotic therapy shortens the duration of illness only minimally. Antibiotic treatment of streptococcal pharyngitis is directed to the prevention of acute rheumatic fever. If penicillin therapy is initiated within the first ten days after the development of pharyngitis, the risk of secondary acute rheumatic fever is significantly decreased. Antibiotic treatment also decreases the incidence of other complications of streptococcal pharyngitis and aids in limiting epidemics of streptococcal disease, but these effects are not related to the early timing of therapy.

Antibiotic therapy need not be initiated immediately in all patients with pharyngitis. In most patients, it is permissible to wait for the results of the throat culture. The success of this approach depends on adequate follow-up for all patients with throat cultures positive for Group A β-hemolytic streptococci; antibiotics can be prescribed immediately if follow-up cannot be ensured. Prompt antibiotic therapy is warranted in patients with a scarlatiniform rash or a past history of rheumatic fever and a high risk of recurrence.

Penicillin remains the drug of choice for treatment of streptococcal pharyngitis. For adequate therapy significant pharyngeal levels of penicillin must be maintained for ten days. This can be achieved with either penicillin V potassium (250 mg by mouth four times a day for ten days) or 1 intramuscular injection of 1.2 million units benzathine penicillin. The latter route is preferred for poorly compliant patients. For penicillin-allergic patients, erythromycin (250 mg by mouth four times a day for ten days) may be used (30 to 40 mg/kg/day erythromycin ethylsuccinate for a child).

Therapy for gonococcal pharyngitis should be initiated with either 4.8 million units intramuscular aqueous procaine penicillin plus 1 gm probenecid taken orally or 9.5 gm tetracycline taken orally over four days in divided doses. Trimethoprim-sulfamethoxazole (9 tablets in a single daily dose for three days) may be effective, especially against penicillinase-producing strains of gonococci. Ampicillin and spectinomycin have not been proved adequate therapy.

Any patient with suspected diphtheria should be immediately hospitalized. Initial therapy requires antibiotic treatment with either penicillin or erythromycin and the immediate use of diphtheria antitoxin.

Follow-up and referral should be arranged for all patients with pharyngitis whose symptoms persist for more than ten days because uncomplicated pharyngitis usually resolves in this time period.

Sinusitis

Acute sinusitis is an inflammation of the accessory nasal sinuses secondary to bacterial infection. *Hemophilus influenzae*, *Diplococcus pneumoniae*, and Group A β-hemolytic *Streptococcus* are the predominating pathogens in adults and children; together, they account for 65 percent of documented infections. *Staphylococcus aureus* and gram-negative rods are occasionally responsible for sinusitis, and mixed anaerobic bacteria have been isolated from about 10 percent of infected maxillary sinuses, a condition that may be secondary to dental abscesses.

Clinically, chronic sinusitis is considered a persistent or recurrent mucopurulent nasal discharge from a sinus with associated roentgenographic abnormality. Bacterial pathogens may be present, as they are in acute sinusitis, but this may represent simply colonization of the sinus with nasal flora.

Normally, the sinuses are lined with ciliated columnar epithelium that is covered with mucus produced by goblet cells. This mucus blanket is the primary defense against infection, since it has an intrinsic antibacterial effect mediated by IgA and lysozyme. In addition, a synchronized, rhythmic movement of the cilia on the epithelial surface continuously moves mucus out of the sinus. This mucociliary clearance mechanism removes particulate matter that might enter the sinuses and become trapped in the mucus. (See Chapter 67.)

Pathogenesis

When the host defenses are overcome, the result is acute purulent sinusitis. Viral upper respiratory infection is the most common factor predisposing patients to acute sinusitis. This infection produces edema of the nasal mucosa and increases the viscosity of the overlying mucus, resulting in obstruction of the sinus ostia. Consequently, mucus stasis develops within the sinus, which may then become infected secondarily. Nasal polyps, septal deviation, surgery, or nasal packing can similarly induce sinusitis by ostial obstruction. Acute sinusitis also may develop from contiguous spread of infection from a dental abscess, from infected soft tissues, or from fractures or osteomyelitis of surrounding bone.

Persistent purulent sinusitis, recurrent episodes of acute sinusitis, and/or local trauma may lead to gross and histological changes in the sinus anatomy that predispose a patient to chronic sinusitis. The epithelium becomes richer in stratified squamous epithelial cells, and the cilia may disappear. Goblet cell hyperplasia may develop, leading to edema and excessive mucus production that results in chronic mucus stasis and sinusitis. Rarely, congenital abnormalities of the mucociliary clearance mechanism may lead to chronic sinusitis. In cystic fibrosis, mucus is abnormally viscous and is not cleared readily. Mucus stasis secondary to impaired ciliary action also may occur in Kartagener's syndrome.

Diagnosis

Clinically, acute sinusitis is associated with fever and chills, purulent nasal discharge, and nasal obstruction. There may be tenderness over the involved sinus and a dull, asymmetric pain that changes with a change in position. The pain is localized to the forehead over the eyebrow in frontal sinusitis and to the superior lateral portion of the nose adjacent to the medical canthi in ethmoidal sinusitis. In maxillary sinusitis, tenderness is usually localized to the face over the sinus, but it may be referred to the upper teeth. Sphenoidal sinusitis produces symptoms over the mastoid prominence, the sphenoid processes, and the occipital skull.

Transillumination may be helpful in the diagnosis of maxillary sinusitis. With the room darkened, an intense, well-shielded light source is held against the patient's skin just below the orbital ridge, and the hard palate is observed through the mouth for the transmission of light. Complete opacity of the sinus is diagnostic of an abnormal sinus. Partial or dull light transmission is not diagnostically helpful, however. Roentgenographic evaluation of the sinuses should be performed to confirm sinusitis when the diagnosis is not clear. Sinusitis is suggested by an air-fluid level, complete opacification, or marked mucosal thickening of the sinus wall to greater than 5 mm.

Precise bacteriologic diagnosis of acute sinusitis can be obtained only by direct sinus puncture. Bacteria found by nasal swab cultures do not always correlate with infecting organisms within the sinus. Although lavage via catheter into the sinus ostia often yields infecting organisms, these cultures are usually contaminated with nasal flora. Gram-stain and aerobic and anaerobic cultures of material recovered by direct sinus puncture usually establishes the diagnosis, but this technique should be reserved for immunocompromised hosts and patients with persistent acute sinusitis unresponsive to initial therapy.

Differential Diagnosis

The major differential diagnosis in acute sinusitis is a prolonged common cold. A viral upper respiratory tract infection may simulate the clinical presentation of sinusitis, and roentgenograms are useful to determine the diagnosis. Cancer, tuberculosis, mucormycosis, aspergillosis, syphilis, and Wegener's granulomatosis should be considered in the differential diagnosis of chronic sinusitis.

Treatment

Acute sinusitis is treated with antibiotics effective against both *S. pneumoniae* and *H. influenzae*. At present, ampicillin (500 mg every six hours) or amoxicillin (500 mg every six to eight hours) p.o. is effective. In the penicillin-allergic patient, tetracycline, erythromycin, or trimethoprim-sulfamethoxazole can be used. Although not specifically indicated for sinusitis, cefaclor (250 to 500 mg every eight hours by mouth or 20 mg/kg in three divided doses in children) might be useful against ampicillin-resistant *H. influenzae*. Treatment should be continued for ten days. Decongestants may promote drainage, and mild analgesics may relieve pain.

Adequate follow-up must be provided to ensure clinical resolution. The complications of poorly treated or untreated sinusitis are severe, e.g., osteomyelitis, meningitis, brain abscess, orbital cellulitis, and cavernous sinus thrombosis. Patients with persistent acute sinusitis should be referred for direct sinus puncture.

The optimal therapy for chronic sinusitis has not been defined. A complete evaluation by an otolaryngologist is often useful, and surgical drainage might be beneficial.

Otitis

Otitis Externa

Sometimes called "swimmer's ear," otitis externa is an inflammation of the external auditory canal that may be produced by infection, trauma, seborrheic dermatitis, or sensitization to medications. Infection is most commonly caused by *Pseudomonas aeruginosa*, although *Streptococcus pyogenes*, *Staphylococcus aureus*, *Proteus* species, and *Candida* may be isolated. The squamous epithelium of the auditory canal is delicate and may be irritated by the retention of excess moisture.

Subsequent inflammation may be exacerbated by scratching with cotton swabs or other objects.

The patient complains of pain and tenderness of the affected ear. The pain may increase with movement of the jaw, and the patient may not be able to sleep on the involved side. Usually, there is no history of an upper respiratory tract infection and no fever. The external canal is tender and erythematous, and it may be completely obstructed by edema and cerumenous exudate. The tympanic membrane has normal landmarks and movement when it can be visualized.

The initial therapeutic approach is to remove any irritant and to prevent further exposure to irritants. The ear canal should be irrigated carefully. Although no controlled studies have been performed, a five- to seven-day course of topical antimicrobial agents may be useful. If such therapy is deemed appropriate, a cotton wick should be inserted down the length of the canal to ensure adequate penetration of the medication and to discourage continued self-trauma. Prolonged therapy with topical bacitracin, neomycin, polymyxin B, or chloramphenicol should be avoided, because these agents may induce sensitization and contact dermatitis. Topical 2 percent acetic acid solution also inhibits the growth of most pathogenic bacteria, and this can be used to treat uncomplicated otitis externa.

Erysipelas and cellulitis are occasional complications of otitis externa. Malignant otitis externa, a deep soft tissue infection, may develop if the infecting organism invades the junction of the cartilaginous and osseous external auditory canals; in such a case, *Pseudomonas aeruginosa* is usually found alone or with other pathogens. This is seen predominantly in elderly diabetic patients. These patients have persistent pain and may have facial nerve paralysis. They should be hospitalized for intravenous therapy and may require surgical drainage.

Otitis Media

Although otitis media is one of the most common illnesses in the pediatric population, ambiguities in its definition have obscured understanding of the disease. This discussion focuses on acute otitis media, defined as inflammation of the middle ear associated with the acute accumulation of the middle ear effusion. Chronic otitis media requires continued evaluation and should be referred to a specialist.

Otitis media may be produced by infection, allergy, or anatomical abnormalities. Bacteria are isolated from approximately 90 percent of specimens obtained by needle aspiration of the middle ear in children with acute otitis media. *Streptococcus pneumoniae* and nontypable *H. influenzae* are found in up to 60 percent of cases. *Branhamella catarrhalis*, *S. aureus*, Group A β-hemolytic streptococci, and anaerobic bacteria produce the remaining infections. In infants less than six weeks of age, the percentage of infections caused by gramnegative bacilli and *S. aureus* may be higher, but the predominant pathogens remain *H. influenzae*, *S. pneumoniae*, and *B. catarrhalis*. Viruses and *Mycoplasma* play only a minimal role in acute otitis media.

The pathogenesis of otitis media is related to abnormalities in the ventilation of the middle ear. The eustachian tube is obstructed by anatomical changes or edema of the nasal mucosa due to allergy or viral infection, and this isolates the middle ear as a closed space. Oxygen and carbon dioxide are absorbed through the middle ear mucosa, and negative pressure develops in the middle ear. Because of the negative pressure, fluid crosses the mucosa into the middle ear space, and bacteria migrate up the eustachian tube to infect the effusion. An immune response to bacterial pathogens develops in the middle ear, elevating the levels of specific immunoglobulins in the effusion. Increased concentrations of these antibodies help to clear bacteria from the middle ear and to localize the infection by their activation of histamine and slow-releasing substance of anaphylaxis. Additional edema is produced, fluid transudation continues, and obstruction of the eustachian tube occurs intermittently. Recurrent otitis media may result.

The diagnosis of otitis media should be suspected strongly in any patient with a febrile illness and otalgia; however, only 50 percent of children may have symptoms relating to the ear. Instead, a child may have gastrointestinal complaints or may show increased irritability. The peak frequency of otitis media occurs between one and two years of age. Infection recurs in 40 to 50 percent of patients.

Pneumatic otoscopy is the simplest technique to identify otitis media. It is relatively precise, but not definitive. The full tympanic membrane should be visualized, and its appearance, landmarks, the presence of a light reflex, and motion should be evaluated. With the pneumatic otoscope, gentle pressure changes in the external auditory canal cause the tympanic membrane to move. The normal membrane has a rapid fluttering movement; absent or sluggish movement indicates an effusion. When tympanic membrane motion is normal, the presence of erythema alone is not indicative of otitis media.

Tympanometry can be used to determine if middle ear fluid is present by measuring the acoustic compliance of the tympanic membrane. The external auditory canal is occluded, and a standard sound signal is reflected by the tympanic membrane as various air pressures are applied to the external canal. The normal drum has a peak in acoustic compliance at normal atmospheric pressure. In otitis media, the middle ear effusion dampens the membrane, and compliance is reduced. This technique does not require complete clearance of the external auditory canal and can be performed even if the entire tympanic membrane is not visualized.

Tympanocentesis, aspiration of the middle ear, is the only definitive study for otitis media. It is a relatively difficult procedure in an uncooperative patient, however, and should be reserved for those cases in which a pathogen must be isolated. Nasopharyngeal cultures have been proposed as a method of determining the etiologic agent in otitis media, but their usefulness is limited by high rates of false-positive and false-negative results. This technique is helpful only in determining the presence of resistant bacterial strains.

Therapy of otitis media is based on the use of antimicrobial agents active against both *H. influenzae* and *D. pneumoniae*. Many antibiotic regimens adequately treat these pathogens. Ampicillin (50 to 70 mg/kg/day) or amoxicillin (40 mg/kg/day) has been preferred because each is able to penetrate into the middle ear. With the increasing incidence of *H. influenzae* strains resistant to these agents, other antibiotics have been evaluated. Penicillin plus sulfonamides (100 to 150 mg/kg/day), erythromycin plus sulfonamides (50 mg/kg/day), trimethoprim 8 mg/kg/day, with sulfamethoxazole, 40 mg/kg/day, or cefaclor (40 mg/kg/day) is usually effective against the organisms responsible for otitis media. The latter three regimens should be useful against most strains of ampicillin-resistant *H. influenzae*. Although no controlled studies have been performed to determine the duration of therapy required, otitis media should be treated empirically for seven to ten days. Decongestants and antihistamines have been used frequently, but controlled clinical trials have not demonstrated any therapeutic effect. Surgical drainage by myringotomy should be considered in the immunocompromised patient, but this is not helpful in the treatment of the normal host.

In most patients, symptoms resolve within 72 hours, but middle ear effusion may persist for up to six months. This may predispose patients to more frequent recurrence and, possibly, to chronic otitis media. Consequently, all patients with otitis media should be seen in follow-up within two weeks or sooner if they remain symptomatic after three or four days of therapy. Patients with persistent effusion should be referred for continued evaluation of their condition.

Oral-Facial Infections

Oral Ulcerative and Vesicular Infections

The most common lesions of the oral mucosa are aphthous ulcers or "canker sores," the etiology of which is unknown. They are recurrent, painful, 1- to 3-mm vesicular lesions that appear singly or in clusters on the buccal mucosa, gingiva, and hard and soft palate. The vesicles ulcerate, leaving a clean white or gray crater. They occur more frequently in periods of stress and during menses and resolve spontaneously in several days. At present, there is no effective therapy, but saline mouthwashes or topical anesthetic ointments may provide symptomatic relief.

Herpes simplex viruses, Types 1 and 2, may produce a gingivostomatitis with vesicular ulcerating lesions on the gingiva, buccal mucosa, lips, tongue, and palate. In the initial infection, there is a 2- to 12-day incubation period; this is followed by fever, pharyngeal irritation, and the diffuse involvement of the oral mucosa with multiple vesicles on erythematous bases. Cervical lymphadenopathy is typical. Infrequently, halitosis and extension of the vesicular lesions onto the lips and cheeks may be seen. Patients normally have a gradual recovery over 7 to 10 days, although their clinical appearance may be unchanged during much of this period. The diagnosis can be confirmed if multinucleated giant cells are found in material scraped from the base of a fresh ulcer or aspirated from a vesicle and stained with methylene blue.

Following the patient's recovery from the initial infection, gingivostomatitis may recur through reactivation of viral organisms that remain in the trigeminal ganglion. Such a recurrence is characterized by a brief syndrome of pain or tingling, followed by the appearance of vesicular lesions that rapidly ulcerate and crust. The mucosal involvement is much less severe than that of the initial infection, and associated adenopathy and systemic toxicity are absent. Lesions may recur as often as several times a month or as infrequently as once or twice a year.

At present, there is no effective therapy for primary or recurrent gingivostomatitis caused by herpes simplex viruses. Patients may be treated symptomatically with saline mouthwash and topical anesthetics. They should be followed for bacterial superinfection and for possible dehydration with severe primary herpes simplex virus infections.

Several other pathogens may also produce oral lesions. Group A coxsackieviruses cause two syndromes with oral ulcerations, both of which occur primarily, but not exclusively, in children. Herpangina is a febrile illness that occurs predominantly in summer or autumn epidemics. It is manifested by fever, malaise, pharyngitis, and multiple discrete vesicles on the tonsils, anterior pillars, soft palate, and uvula. It is self-limited and resolves in five to seven days. Hand-foot-and-mouth disease, a variant of herpangina with a similar seasonal incidence, is associated with tender, painful vesicles on the palms and soles, as well as in the oral cavity. Compared with those in herpangina, the vesicles are small in number, and they may occur anywhere in the oral cavity. This is also a self-limited illness that resolves in approximately seven days.

Acute necrotizing ulcerative gingivitis is a synergistic anaerobic infection of the periodontal gingiva in patients with poor oral hygiene. It occurs in young adults as an acute febrile illness with bleeding and ulceration of the gingiva, pseudomembrane formation of the interdental papillae, foul breath, and cervical adenopathy. It is mediated by the endogenous fusobacteria and spirochetes of the oral flora and is rare in edentulous patients. The treatment of choice is oral penicillin and hydrogen peroxide mouthwashes.

Thrush is an infection of the buccal or gingival mucosa with *Candida* species. Although it is usually seen in immunocompromised patients or those on broad spectrum antibiotics, it can occur in diabetics and, rarely, in completely normal hosts. It is characterized by grayish white plaques with an erythematous base on the buccal mucosa, gingiva, and tongue, and by budding yeast forms. The first step in therapy is to stop antibiotics when possible. Then, nystatin may be given as a 4 to 6 ml oral suspension of 100,000 u/ml four times a day to be swished around the oral cavity, or as tablets or suppositories.

Oral lesions may be seen as manifestations of several systemic illnesses. Varicella can result in oral vesiculation with its characteristic exanthem. Syphilis not only can involve the mouth with a primary chancre, but also may produce oral lesions during its secondary and tertiary stages. One-third of patients with secondary syphilis have nonpainful, symmetric, silvery mucosal ulcerations in the oral cavity. These mucosal lesions occur concurrently with the exanthem of secondary syphilis and are highly infectious. Two noninfectious processes that must be considered with oral mucosal ulcerations are erythema multiforme and pemphigus vulgaris.

Deep Space Infections

Infections of the oropharynx may extend into the deep fascial spaces of the head and neck, producing maxillary space infections, peripharyngeal abscesses, retropharyngeal abscesses, and submandibular space infections. The natural history of each of these infections is determined by the anatomy of the involved space.

Infection of the canine space anterior to the maxilla can occur secondary to abscesses of the maxillary incisor and canine teeth. As with all infections of dental origin, the infection is due to mixed aerobic and anaerobic bacteria from the mouth, with *Bacteroides* species, *Peptostreptococcus* species, and *Streptococcus* species predominating. Swelling of the upper lip and soft tissues anterior to the maxilla is dramatic. The infection can

spread to the infratemporal space, to the maxillary bone and sinus, and into the orbit.

The peripharyngeal space, or pharyngomaxillary space, is a cone-shaped potential space bordered medially by the pharyngeal wall, laterally by the medial pterygoid muscles of the mandible and the parotid gland, and superiorly by the base of the skull. The carotid sheath passes through this space and may be involved in any infection of this space. Because of its location, this space can become infected in association with suppurative pharyngitis, a molar tooth abscess, mastoiditis, or suppurative parotitis. The usual pathogens are mixed aerobic and anaerobic bacteria, although suppurative parotitis is usually due to *Staphylococcus aureus.* Clinically, the patient is febrile and may have sore throat, dysphagia, hoarseness, marked facial pain, trismus, medial displacement of the pharyngeal wall, and swelling and induration of the soft tissue below the angle of the jaw. Typically, only a few of these findings are present in an individual patient, and the presentation can be very subtle. Complications from this infection arise either from spread to the retropharyngeal space or from involvement of the carotid sheath, which can cause septic carotid arteritis and septic jugular thrombophlebitis.

The retropharyngeal space lies directly posterior to the posterior pharyngeal wall and anterior to the prevertebral fascia of the cervical and thoracic spine; it extends from the base of the skull to the superior mediastinum. Infection in this space can arise from direct trauma to the posterior pharyngeal wall or contiguous spread of infecting organisms that have caused pharyngitis, peripharyngeal abscess, or vertebral osteomyelitis. It is usually caused by the same pathogens as peripharyngeal abscesses. Patients are febrile and complain of dysphagia. Laryngeal edema and bulging of the posterior pharyngeal wall may develop, resulting in upper airway obstruction that resembles epiglottitis. Bilateral cervical adenopathy is common. Upper airway obstruction and secondary suppurative mediastinitis are major complications.

The submandibular space lies below the floor of the mouth and extends posteriorly to the hyoid bone. Direct trauma or the erosion of the mandible by a dental abscess permits both aerobic and anaerobic organisms to enter the submandibular space and produces an infection known as Ludwig's angina. This space has very loose connective tissue, and, once it has been invaded, cellulitis rapidly involves the entire space without typical abscess formation. The patient is febrile and has severe dysphagia. There is submental induration and tenderness, and the entire floor of the mouth is elevated. The upper airway can be rapidly compromised as the tongue moves superiorly and posteriorly.

Since peripharyngeal, retropharyngeal, and submandibular infections can obstruct the larynx, the first priority when such an infection is suspected is to protect the airway. This may require immediate endotracheal intubation or tracheotomy. If this is not required, a lateral roentgenogram of the neck with soft tissue technique should be performed to evaluate the airway and to exclude epiglottitis.

With the airway controlled, therapy for the deep space infections requires surgical drainage and parenteral antibiotic therapy directed against a mixed anaerobic flora. Penicillin G (8 to 12 million units/day administered intravenously in six divided doses) remains the initial therapy of choice. Clindamycin or metronidazole is appropriate in patients with penicillin allergy. Occasionally, *S. aureus* must be considered in parotitis or vertebral osteomyelitis. In these instances, a semisynthetic penicillinase-resistant penicillin, such as nafcillin or oxacillin, should be used in high doses (2 gm administered intravenously every four hours). (See Chapter 70.)

Pneumonia

Acute pneumonia, both as a common community-acquired illness and a major nosocomial infection, is a leading cause of morbidity and mortality. Relatively few organisms are responsible for most cases of community-acquired pulmonary infection:

I. Viral
    Children: Respiratory syncytial virus
                   Parainfluenza virus
                   Influenza A virus

    Adults: Influenza A virus
                   Parainfluenza virus
                   Adenovirus
                   Varicella
                   Rhinovirus
                   Measles
II. Bacterial
    Pneumococcus *(S. pneumoniae)*
    Bacillis anthracis
    Enterobacteriaceae: *Klebsiella pneumoniae*
                             Escherichia coli
                             Enterobacter species
                             Citrobacter species
    Staphylococcus aureus
    Hemophilus influenzae
    Mixed anaerobic species
    Legionella pneumophila
    Legionella species
    Neisseria meningitidis
    Streptococcus pyogenes
    Streptococcus viridans
    Francisella tularensis

III. Mycoplasmal
    Mycoplasma pneumoniae
IV. Chlamydial
    Infants: *Chlamydia trachomatis*
    Adults: *Chlamydia psittaci*
V. Rickettsial
    Coxiella burnetii (Q fever)
VI. Fungal
    Histoplasma capsulatum
    Coccidioides immitis
    Aspergillus species

In young children, the predominant pathogens are respiratory syncytial and parainfluenza viruses; *M. pneumoniae, S. pneumoniae* (pneumococcus), *H. influenzae,* and *Chlamydia trachomatis* are less frequent causative agents in this age group. In adolescents and adults, *S. pneumoniae* and *M. pneumoniae* are the most frequent causes of pneumonia acquired outside the hospital. Pneumococci are implicated in at least 60 percent of patients who require hospitalization for pneumonia. *Staphylococcus aureus,* mixed anaerobic bacteria, and gram-negative bacilli, including *Klebsiella pneumoniae,* also are significant pathogens in the adult. *Hemophilus influenzae* is now recognized as a cause of adult pulmonary parenchymal infection. *Legionella pneumophila* may produce 1 to 2 percent of the cases of community-acquired pneumonia. Except for influenza virus strains that produce epidemic pneumonia in winter months, virus-mediated pneumonia is rare in the adult.

Patients who acquire pneumonia while they are in the hospital also may be infected with pneumococci, but infection with staphylococci and gram-negative rods is more common.

Pathogenesis

Primary pulmonary infections occur when infectious secretions or inhalation of aerosolized infectious particles introduce pathogenic organisms into the alveolar spaces. Secondary pneumonias may arise from hematogenous dissemination of microorganisms from other infected sites or by contiguous spread from adjacent infectious processes. The primary host defenses against pulmonary infection consist of mechanisms to prevent colonization of the lower tracheobronchial tree. For example, the gag reflex limits the aspiration of secretions, and the nasal turbinates and oropharynx act as filters to remove most inhaled particles greater than 10 μm in diameter. Materials that do reach the lower respiratory tree usually are trapped in the mucous lining of the tracheobronchial tree. This mucous layer transports aspirated particles up the trachea by the action of the ciliated epithelial cells. Microorganisms that are not cleared may be destroyed through opsonization by secretory immunoglobulins and subsequent phagocytosis by alveolar macrophages and polymorphonuclear leukocytes.

Infections generally develop because of an impairment in host defenses rather than because of contact with particularly virulent organisms; the latter may be the case with organisms such as *Mycobacterium tuberculosis* or pathogenic fungi, however. Most individuals aspirate small amounts of pharyngeal secretions during sleep, but possibility of aspiration is greatly increased when the gag reflex is blunted by sedatives, ethanol ingestion, heavy smoking, or advanced age. Alcohol, tobacco, and viral infection may impair mucociliary transport. In congestive heart failure increased intraalveolar fluid hinders the clearance of bacteria by alveolar macrophages.

Diagnosis

Community-acquired pneumonia occurs as acute lobar pneumonia or bronchopneumonia, atypical generalized pneumonia, or aspiration pneumonia. Acute lobar pneumonia, of which pneumococcal pneumonia is the prototype, usually develops in middle-aged or elderly patients during the winter or early spring, frequently following an upper respiratory tract viral infection. These infections are often associated with underlying illnesses, such as diabetes, chronic obstructive pulmonary disease, or congestive heart failure.

Lobar pneumonia begins with the abrupt onset of high fever and shaking chills, accompanied by a cough that produces yellow-green to rusty, possibly blood-streaked, sputum. Pleuritic chest pain over the involved lung is common; tachypnea and tachycardia are present. Physical examination reveals percussion dullness, increased tactile and vocal fremitus, and bronchovesicular breath sounds with crepitant inspiratory rales over the involved lung segments. The chest roentgenogram usually reveals dense lobar consolidation in one or more lobes, although it may show patchy localized infiltrates. Pleural effusions may occur late in the course of pneumococcal pneumonia. Significant early effusions should suggest empyema or pneumonia due to bacteria other than pneumococci. The peripheral white blood cell count is elevated to 15,000 to 30,000/cu mm with a predominance of neutrophils and a shift to immature forms. Arterial blood gas determinations may show a significant hypoxemia and an increased alveolar-arterial gradient. Levels of hepatic enzymes may be elevated.

Atypical pneumonia is usually seen in young adult or adolescent patients and does not have a particular seasonal predominance. The prodrome consists of three to four days of malaise, myalgias, coryza, and headache with a low-grade fever (less than 39°C) and a cough

that is initially nonproductive. Pleuritic chest pain early in the course is less common than it is in lobar pneumonia. Physical examination may reveal some localized crackles, but other chest findings are not impressive. Chest roentgenogram reveals diffuse, patchy infiltrates often out of proportion to the physical findings. Lower lobe involvement is common and may be unilateral or bilateral. Pleural effusions are unusual, and the white blood cell count is normal or only mildly elevated, often with a relative lymphocytosis.

Aspiration pneumonia is associated with an abnormal gag reflex and occurs most commonly in alcoholics or patients who have vomited heavily. The findings depend on the type of material aspirated. Aspiration of toxic secretions, such as gastric acid, may cause an immediate and intense chemical pneumonitis with acute dyspnea, bronchospasm, and the production of frothy sputum. Patients may be hypotensive, and diffuse inspiratory crackles are present on auscultation. Roentgenograms show mottled densities in the lower lobes, which may progress to diffuse infiltrates. Arterial blood gas measurements demonstrate severe hypoxia with normal or low pCO_2. Aspiration of solid particulate matter may cause acute respiratory distress, beginning immediately after the aspiration if the particle obstructs the trachea or a major bronchus. Aspiration of particles small enough to reach a peripheral airway produces cough, atelectasis, and recurrent localized infection. After the aspiration of oropharyngeal secretions, fever, chills, anorexia, weight loss, and a cough productive of copious, foul-smelling, and foul-tasting sputum develops gradually over an 8- to 14-day period. Physical examination reveals dullness to percussion, increased breath sounds, and bronchovesicular respirations. This process is usually localized to gravitationally dependent lobes. If aspiration took place while the patient was in the supine position, the superior segments of the lower lobes and the posterior segments of the upper lobes are involved; if the patient was in the upright position, the basal segments of the lower lobes are usually involved. Pleural effusions may occur. The peripheral white blood count is usually elevated.

Examination of the lower respiratory tract secretions is important in determining the etiology of pneumonia. Samples of sputum can be obtained by expectoration, transtracheal aspiration, flexible fiberoptic bronchoscopy, or lung puncture. Examination of expectorated sputum is the simplest, safest, and most economical technique, but its usefulness is limited because the patient may be unable to produce an appropriate specimen and because this sample may be contaminated with oropharyngeal flora. The sputum specimens should be observed for amount, purulence, color, and odor. A representative portion of mucopurulent material is selected for microscopic examination by Gram stain. The presence of columnar epithelial cells and polymorphonuclear leukocytes associated with a predominant bacterial flora intracellularly and extracellularly is indicative of lower respiratory tract infection with this predominant organism. Alternatively, the presence of large squamous epithelial cells and multiple bacterial forms indicates significant sample contamination with oral secretions. This type of specimen is unreliable for definitive diagnosis.

At best, the Gram-stained sputum smear permits putative identification of the offending organisms. The presence of contaminating normal mouth flora confounds the definitive identification of the pathogenic organism by culture. Nonetheless, a good correlation between culture and Gram-stain reading may provide a rough indication of the etiology of an episode of pneumonia. For a more definitive diagnosis in patients with an uninterpretable expectorated sputum Gram stain, with hospital-acquired pneumonia that developed during antibiotic therapy, additional diagnostic studies should be performed.

Transtracheal aspiration by means of a flexible catheter passed through the cricothyroid membrane to the trachea avoids specimen contamination with oral secretions. A pillow is placed under the patient's shoulders to hyperextend the neck. The cricothyroid membrane, between the cricoid and thyroid cartilage, is identified, prepared with an antibacterial solution, draped, and locally anesthetized. A large-bore indwelling intravenous catheter needle is inserted through the cricothyroid membrane into the trachea. The flexible catheter within the needle is advanced quickly, and the needle is withdrawn, leaving the catheter in place. A sterile syringe is connected to the catheter, and a sputum sample is aspirated. If a sample cannot be obtained in this way, 3 to 5 ml nonbacteriostatic sterile saline is injected into the trachea to induce coughing and produce a suitable specimen. The catheter is removed and firm pressure applied to the puncture site. A Gram stain and aerobic and anaerobic cultures should be performed on the specimen.

Significant complications, including subcutaneous emphysema, local bleeding, and rarely, death, may follow transtracheal aspiration. The risk of these complications can be reduced by strict attention to technique and careful patient selection. Minimal morbidity has occurred when (1) the patient is cooperative, (2) the normal cricothyroid membrane is easily identifiable, (3) the results of coagulation studies are normal, (4) arterial pO_2 of at least 70 mm Hg can be maintained with supplemental oxygen, and (5) the procedure is performed by an experienced physician.

It may be possible to obtain a good sputum sample by fiberoptic flexible bronchoscopy with a distally occluded telescoping cannula system, but such a procedure is rarely required in the emergency department. Bronchoscopy and transtracheal aspiration are difficult in young children. If an accurate etiologic diagnosis must be obtained to guide therapy, a direct lung puncture of the involved lung can be performed with little risk of morbidity. This procedure can also be utilized in the adult patient with pleura-based infection, but this is associated with a slightly higher risk of complications.

Any pleural effusion associated with a pneumonic process should be aspirated for diagnosis and therapy. Blood cultures should be performed on all patients, even though the results are positive in only 30 to 40 percent of patients with bacterial pneumonia. Additional diagnostic studies can be helpful in selected clinical situations. In approximately 50 percent of patients with mycoplasmal pneumonia, cold hemagglutinin titers rise in the first seven to ten days of illness and may remain elevated for several weeks. Occasionally, these titers are elevated in infection caused by adenoviruses, Epstein-Barr virus, rubella, influenza, and psittacosis. Fluorescent antibody techniques may be applied to smears of sputum or pleural fluid for the identification of *L. pneumophila* in Legionnaire's disease, and pneumococcal polysaccharides may be detected in the urine or, occasionally, in the serum by countercurrent immunoelectrophoresis in patients with pneumococcal pneumonia and bacteremia.

Differential Diagnosis of Pneumonia

Pulmonary embolism, atelectasis of a pulmonary segment, congestive heart failure, neoplastic disease, hypersensitivity pneumonitis, collagen and vascular diseases, sarcoidosis, and lipoid pneumonia are differential diagnostic considerations in the evaluation of a pulmonary infiltrate. Although the clinical presentation may indicate an infectious process, the precise diagnosis may be difficult and require additional studies. Pulmonary infarction may be associated with fever and a wedge-shaped pulmonary density on roentgenogram. Pulmonary angiography, if it is performed early, establishes the diagnosis. In congestive heart failure, a chest roentgenogram may show a pleural effusion that changes position with a properly performed lateral decubitis radiography and an infiltrate that may clear rapidly following diuretic therapy.

The major pathogen in acute lobar pneumonia is *S. pneumoniae*. Staphylococci, *H. influenzae*, mixed anaerobic bacteria, and *K. pneumoniae* also produce this syndrome. Evidence of necrotizing pneumonia is suggestive of staphylococcal or mixed anaerobic infection. Staphylococcal or streptococcal pneumonia may be more frequent following influenzal pneumonia, but pneumococcal disease also may occur in this setting.

Atypical pneumonia is most frequently due to *Mycoplasma pneumoniae*. It can be associated with myringitis, upper respiratory tract symptoms, myalgias, migratory arthralgias, and gastrointestinal symptoms; rarely, it is associated with meningoencephalitis, transverse myelopathy, and ascending paralysis. A carefully obtained history can aid in evaluating possible causes of atypical pneumonia. For example, a recent visit to the San Joaquin Valley in California or other parts of the southwestern United States increases the likelihood of coccidioidomycosis. Histoplasmosis is endemic in the Ohio River Valley. Exposure to an animal or bird increases the likelihood of psittacosis, tularemia, plague, brucellosis, and Q fever.

Legionnaire's disease may initially resemble atypical pneumonia, but the patient's condition may deteriorate with the development of headache, altered sensorium, and diarrhea—often with laboratory findings of hyponatremia, hypophosphatemia, and liver enzyme elevations. Specific direct fluorescent antibody tests on expectorated sputum or pleural fluid may reveal the presence of *L. pneumophila*.

Treatment

The management of patients with pneumonia depends on the clinical setting. Adults with uncomplicated, presumed pneumococcal or mycoplasmal pneumonia and no underlying disease can be managed outside the hospital, providing they can be followed closely. Most other patients should be hospitalized. Pneumococcal pneumonia is treated effectively with procaine penicillin (300,000 to 600,000 units intramuscularly twice a day for seven to ten days) or phenoxymethyl penicillin V (250 mg orally four times a day). Penicillin-allergic patients should receive erythromycin (500 mg orally every eight hours). If pneumococcal bacteremia or empyema is present, patients should be hospitalized and treated with aqueous penicillin G (5 to 10 million units/day intravenously in six divided doses).

Mycoplasmal pneumonia is treated with erythromycin (500 mg orally every six to eight hours) or tetracycline (250 mg orally four times a day for seven to ten days). Penicillin is not effective.

Aspiration pneumonia can be managed initially with aqueous penicillin G (8 to 12 million units intravenously for seven to ten days, including at least five afebrile days at the end of the course). Clindamycin (160 mg intravenously every six hours) is an alternative in the penicillin-allergic patient.

Pneumonia due to other pathogens, such as *S. aureus, K pneumoniae, P. aeruginosa,* or other gram-negative rods, should be treated in the hospital with agents selected by in vitro susceptibility testing.

GASTROINTESTINAL INFECTIONS

Acute Gastroenteritis

In acute gastroenteritis, diarrhea (an increase in the frequency or fluidity of bowel movements in relation to a patient's usual routine) occurs both with and without nausea, vomiting, and abdominal cramping.

Etiology

Gastroenteritis is caused by a diverse group of infectious and noninfectious agents. Viral agents can produce epidemics of explosive nausea, vomiting, and diarrhea in both children and adults, and viruses are the major cause of sporadic diarrhea in children under two years of age. Bacterial agents, including *Escherichia coli, Vibrio cholerae, Shigella* species, *Salmonella* species, *Clostridium* species, *Campylobacter fetus*, and *Yersinia enterocolitica* produce varied illnesses, ranging from profuse watery diarrhea to severe dysentery with rectal pain and bloody, purulent stools. The protozoa *Giardia lamblia* and *Entamoeba histolytica* produce watery diarrhea and dysenteric syndromes, respectively.

Drug ingestion is a frequent cause of noninfectious acute diarrhea. Many cholinergic agents, antacids, broad spectrum antibiotics, and antimetabolites produce diarrhea. Acute psychological stress may be responsible for diarrhea that usually occurs in the morning. Toxin or allergen ingestion can cause severe, but usually self-limited, gastroenteritis. Diverticulitis, fecal impaction, radiation proctitis, ischemic colitis, and inflammatory bowel disease, such as Crohn's disease, may first be seen as acute diarrheal illnesses.

Pathophysiology

Oral ingestion is the major route of infection in acute gastroenteritis, although there are several host defenses against such an event. The acid environment of the stomach is the first host defense, and over 99.9 percent of all coliform bacteria ingested are killed by the usual gastric pH of 4. In addition, normal intestinal motility helps to clear pathogenic microorganisms, thus decreasing the time they have available to establish infection. Intraluminal antibodies, either those secreted from plasma cells in the lamina propria of the bowel wall or serum immunoglobulins that migrate through the mucosal capillaries, also help to clear pathogens. The preexisting enteric flora of the normal small and large bowel limits colonization with pathogens. The effectiveness of these defenses against specific bacteria is quite variable. An inoculum of 10^5 to 10^8 organisms is required to establish enteritis with *Salmonella* or *Escherichia coli,* but the ingestion of only 10 to 50 *Shigella dysenteriae* produces disease.

Infectious diarrhea may be mediated by toxin formation or by invasion of the intestinal wall (Table 20–1).

Enterotoxins induce diarrhea by stimulating the small bowel mucosa to produce intestinal secretions at a rate that surpasses the reabsorptive ability of the gut, resulting in a profuse, watery diarrhea with isotonic fluid loss. Most of the enterotoxin-associated pathogens do not invade the intestinal mucosa. The prototype of the enterotoxin-mediated diarrheas is cholera, in which toxin induces cyclic adenosine monophosphate (cAMP) activity by stimulating adenyl cyclase. Enterotoxigenic *E. coli*, one of the major causes of traveler's diarrhea, produces a similar toxin.

Bacterial cytotoxins cause necrosis of the intestinal mucosa and induce an intense polymorphonuclear inflammatory response. The colon is the major site of involvement. The cytotoxin produces a dysenteric syndrome with abdominal cramping and small amounts of bloody or purulent stool. Antibiotic-induced pseudomembranous colitis due to the toxin of *Clostridium difficile* and much of the disease caused by *Shigella* and *Clostridium perfringens* are examples of disease mediated by cytotoxins.

Neurotoxins can induce upper gastrointestinal cramping, nausea, vomiting, and hyperperistalsis. Unlike enterotoxins and cytotoxins, which are produced within the intestinal lumen by ingested bacteria, neurotoxins are ingested preformed; disease develops without an established infection. A most common neurotoxin is that of *Staphylococcus aureus*, which produces acute gastroenteritis two to seven hours after ingestion of contaminated food.

Bacterial invasion of the intestinal epithelium, which occurs primarily in the colon and distal small bowel, produces an inflammatory response and a dysenteric syndrome. *Shigella*, enteroinvasive *E. coli* strains, and *Entamoeba histolytica* are the major pathogens in this category. The lamina propria of the large and small bowel is invaded by *Salmonella*, *Yersinia enterocolitica*, and *Campylobacter fetus*. Diarrhea produced by these organisms is usually watery and is probably mediated both by enterotoxins and by alteration in the intestinal wall due to bacterial invasion. Bacteremia and systemic febrile illness may accompany this syndrome.

The pathogenesis of gastroenteritis caused by other well-defined pathogens remains controversial. Viral agents, rotavirus, and the Norwalk agent infect the mucosa of the proximal small bowel, induce watery diarrhea, and alter the motor function of the upper gastrointestinal tract. *Giardia lamblia* colonizes primarily the proximal small bowel; and produces noninflammatory watery diarrhea.

Diagnosis

The acute gastroenteritides can be divided into several distinct clinical syndromes, according to the age of the patient, geography, the possibility of a food source, and the characteristics of the stool. For example, children between four months and two years of age develop water diarrhea from rotavirus infection, but this agent is unusual in other age groups. Travel provides exposure to "exotic" pathogens that may cause diarrhea. Recent food ingestion and similar illness in dining companions suggest a food poisoning syndrome.

The state of the patient's hydration is the major criterion of the severity of illness. Examination of the abdomen may indicate severe distention and high-pitched bowel sounds, suggesting intermittent partial bowel obstruction. Severe tenderness and peritoneal irritation may occur from either a diffuse process, such as toxic megacolon, or a localized process, such as diverticulitis.

Stool should always be examined for both occult blood and fecal leukocytes. The latter test can be performed quickly by mixing two drops of Löffler's methylene blue with a fleck of mucus or stool on the surface of a glass slide. After a cover slip has been placed over it, the material is allowed to incubate for two to three minutes

TABLE 20–1   Pathogenic Mechanisms of Infectious Gastroenteritis

Mechanism	Action	Agent
Toxin production	Enterotoxic	*Vibrio cholerae* *Escherichia coli* *Clostridium perfringens* *Bacillus cereus* *Shigella dysenteriae*
	Cytotoxic	*Clostridium difficile* *Clostridium perfringens* *Shigella dysenteriae*
	Neurotoxic	*Staphylococcus aureus* *Bacillus cereus* *Clostridium botulinum*
Invasion of the intestinal wall	Intraepithelial	*Shigella dysenteriae* *Escherichia coli* *Vibrio parahaemolyticus* *Campylobacter fetus* *Entamoeba histolytica* *Neisseria gonorrhoeae*
	Submucosal	*Salmonella* species *Yersinia enterocolitica* *Campylobacter fetus*
Undefined		Viral (e.g., Norwalk agent, rotavirus) *Giardia lamblia*

to provide good nuclear staining. The presence of sheets of polymorphonuclear cells indicates an inflammatory diarrhea, while the absence of white blood cells indicates a watery diarrhea syndrome. Occasionally, a small number of white blood cells is seen, e.g., 10 to 15 white blood cells per high-powered field. This indicates a low-grade inflammatory diarrhea or disease caused by those agents that invade the lamina propria, i.e., *Salmonella* species, *Campylobacter fetus*, or *Yersinia enterocolitica*.

Acute Watery Diarrhea

Sporadic, spontaneous, noninflammatory diarrhea is the second leading cause of illness, following upper respiratory tract infections. It occurs in infants from 6 months to 2 years of age after they have been weaned. Usually, there is a two- to three-day illness with frequent watery brown diarrhea, occasional vomiting, and a low-grade fever. The usual etiologic agents are the rotaviruses and, outside the United States, enterotoxigenic *Escherichia coli*. While gastroenteritis is so ubiquitous that every child has several episodes in the first two years of life, it may be the first indication of serious systemic infection in patients in this age group.

In older children and adults, the watery diarrhea syndrome can be produced by any of the enterotoxigenic bacteria, by bacteria that invade the lamina propria (i.e., *Salmonella, Campylobacter,* and *Yersinia*), by *G. lamblia*, and by viral agents (e.g., the Norwalk agent). Typically, there is anorexia, malaise, mild abdominal cramping, and progressive diarrhea. Depending on the volume produced, stool can vary in appearance from semiformed tan or brown to thin yellow and rice-watery. The volume of stool varies with the etiologic agent; the enterotoxin-producing bacteria cause the most profuse diarrhea. If adequate hydration is maintained, these patients usually are not toxic and the disease resolves spontaneously in three to five days.

Acute, noninflammatory diarrhea is particularly common in individuals who travel. This traveler's diarrhea usually develops as an explosive, watery diarrhea 5 to 15 days after arrival in the new environment. Enterotoxigenic *E. coli* is responsible for 75 percent of the cases worldwide, but other agents should be considered after travel to certain locales. For example, typhoid fever and cholera may occur after travel to endemic areas. *Giardia* has produced water-borne epidemics in Russian and southeast Asian cities and among hikers in many of the Rocky Mountain and eastern states.

Stool cultures and stool examination for ova and parasites should be performed in patients with prolonged or profuse diarrhea. If *Campylobacter* or *Yersinia* is suspected, the microbiologist should be informed because these pathogens require special growth conditions. When *Salmonella* or *Campylobacter* is likely, blood cultures should be obtained, as these organisms may cause bacteremia.

Dysenteric Gastroenteritis

Bloody or mucous diarrhea with severe abdominal cramping pain, tenesmus, rectal pain, and systemic toxicity may be seen in infections with the pathogens that invade the mucosal epithelium, such as *Shigella*, enteroinvasive *E. coli*, *Entamoeba histolytica*, *Vibrio parahaemolyticus*, and *Neisseria gonorrhoeae*. While this presentation is not specific for any given organism, *Shigella* is likely to produce these symptoms in children six months to six years of age, and outbreaks often occur in day care centers or institutions. *Campylobacter fetus* causes this syndrome in individuals exposed to animals, while *Vibrio parahaemolyticus* may be the causative agent if the patient has been in contact with salt water or seafood. *Gonococcal or chlamydial proctitis* is seen in patients who practice anal sexual activity.

Dysentery is also produced by cytotoxin-producing bacteria, particularly *Clostridium difficile*. This anaerobic bacteria has recently been implicated in antibiotic-associated pseudomembranous colitis, although it also may mediate some cases of watery diarrhea that occur after antibiotic therapy. While severe pseudomembranous colitis has been associated with clindamycin, it can occur after the use of almost any antibiotic; it may also occur spontaneously.

Additional studies that should be performed on all patients with a dysenteric syndrome include stool culture and stool examination for ova and parasites, as well as for *C. difficile* cytotoxin. In adolescents and adults, a sigmoidoscopic examination should be performed to evaluate the extent of inflammation and to determine whether idiopathic inflammatory bowel disease is present.

Food Poisoning

Several distinct gastroenteritic syndromes arise after the consumption of contaminated food. These syndromes are most readily distinguished by the duration of the incubation period. Food-related illness is especially likely if two or more individuals develop gastrointestinal or neurologic symptoms within 72 hours of sharing a meal.

Severe nausea, vomiting, abdominal cramping, and watery diarrhea occur within one to six hours after ingestion of preformed toxin from *Staphylococcus* or *Bacillus cereus*. The toxin forms in prepared food that has been stored improperly. *Bacillus cereus* has been associated with fried rice in particular. Disease induced by either bacteria usually resolves in less than 24 hours.

The major differential diagnosis is heavy metal poisoning with copper, tin, zinc, or cadmium.

Abdominal cramping and watery diarrhea that begin 8 to 16 hours after food ingestion can develop secondary to toxins produced by *Clostridium perfringens* or *B. cereus*. Vomiting is unusual, and the illness usually resolves spontaneously in 24 hours. One food-borne outbreak of diarrhea caused by *Giardia* has been described. Food-borne gastroenteritis developing 16 to 72 hours after a meal is usually related to *Salmonella*, *Shigella*, *V. parahaemolyticus*, enteroinvasive and enterotoxigenic *Escherichia coli*, and *Y. enterocolitica*. The simultaneous development of weakness or paralysis and gastroenteritis strongly suggests *Clostridium botulinum* toxin ingestion.

Treatment of Gastroenteritis

Initial treatment of any patient with gastroenteritis is directed at maintaining adequate hydration. Although fluid loss is minimal in most patients, the loss is so great in some patients that hospitalization is necessary for parenteral fluid replacement. In these patients, intravenous therapy should be initiated with normal saline solution because the lost fluid is isotonic. Serum electrolyte levels should be monitored because metabolic acidosis can develop from ongoing bicarbonate loss in the stool; properly diluted sodium bicarbonate is appropriate replacement fluid if acidosis develops. Fluid can be replaced orally in patients who are not severely dehydrated.

In the late 1960s, studies with cholera victims in Bangladesh demonstrated that patients could be effectively rehydrated with oral glucose-electrolyte solutions. The rationale for this therapy is based on the mechanisms for sodium transport in the gut. Normally, sodium is absorbed from the intestinal lumen by several active mechanisms, one that transports sodium alone and others that transport sodium coupled with glucose or neutral amino acids. Once sodium is transported, chloride and water follow passively. In patients with cholera and other enterotoxin-mediated diarrhea, only the transport of sodium is blocked. Coupled sodium transport continues and compensates effectively for the other impaired transport mechanism. The glucose-electrolyte solution must be isotonic and must contain replacement potassium and bicarbonate as well as sodium chloride. Two appropriate regimens from WHO and the Center for Disease Control are shown in Exhibit 20–1. Although these regimens were designed for treatment of cholera, they are effective for any diarrhea if the small intestinal mucosa is intact. While glucose is preferred, sucrose can be substituted if glucose is not available. This therapy does not decrease the stool volume; in fact, the volume will probably increase, as not all the oral fluids will be absorbed. Adequate volume can be maintained by matching the stool fluid losses with oral therapy, however.

Several agents have been marketed for the symptomatic treatment of diarrhea. They include agents that absorb toxins and water, such as kaolin, pectin, and psyllium hydrophilic mucilloid; and agents that decrease intestinal motility, such as paregoric, diphenoxylate hydrochloride, and loperamide hydrochloride. While both classes of drugs decrease stool fluidity and frequency, they do not decrease the intestinal fluid loss. Furthermore, agents that inhibit intestinal motility are contraindicated in dysenteric syndromes, as they have been demonstrated to prolong the duration of illness with *Salmonella* and *Shigella* infections and, rarely, may induce toxic megacolon.

Recent evidence demonstrates that bismuth subsalicylate (30 to 60 ml every 30 minutes for eight doses) decreases the fluid loss associated with enterotoxin-mediated diarrhea.

Antibiotic therapy is not indicated in patients with enterotoxigenic *E. coli*; antibiotic use increases the number of asymptomatic carriers of many diarrhea pathogens. Gastroenteritis caused by *Salmonella* is usually a self-limited illness, and antibiotics prolong the period of bacterial shedding. Antibiotic therapy is indicated for selected pathogens, however. *Shigella* dysentery is treated with trimethoprim-sulfamethoxazole (160/800 mg orally every 12 hours for five days; 10/50 mg/kg/day orally in two doses for children) or with tetracycline (2.5 gm orally as a single dose in adults). For ampicillin-sensitive organisms, amoxicillin or ampicillin may be given (100 mg/kg/day orally or intravenously in four doses for five days).

Erythromycin (500 mg orally every six hours for 5 days; 40 mg/kg/day orally in four doses for 5 days in children) is the initial treatment for *Campylobacter fetus* gastroenteritis. *Giardia lamblia* enteritis should be treated with either quinacrine hydrochloride (100 mg orally three times a day for 5 days; 6 to 7 mg/kg/day orally three times a day for 5 days for children) or metronidazole (250 mg orally three times a day for 10 days; 15 mg/kg/day orally three times a day for children). Symptomatic intestinal amebiasis should be treated with metronidazole (750 mg orally three times a day for 10 days; 30 to 50 mg/kg/day orally for children) plus di-iodohydroxyquin (650 mg orally three times a day for 20 days). Patients with pseudomembranous colitis due to *Clostridia difficile* are best treated with vancomycin (125 mg orally every six hours for 7 to 10 days).

All patients with dysenteric syndromes should be hospitalized or followed very closely as outpatients for the duration of the illness.

Exhibit 20–1 Oral Therapy of Diarrhea

Regimen A

3.5 gm NaCl	(Na 90 mEq/liter)
2.5 gm NaHCO$_3$	(HCO$_3$ 30 mEq/liter)
1.5 gm KCl	(K 20 mEq/liter)
20 gm glucose	(Glucose 110 mM/liter)
1 liter boiled water	

Regimen B

Prepare one glass of each of the following:

Glass 1		Glass 2	
Apple or other fruit juice (rich in potassium)	8 oz.	Tap water (boiled or carbonated if purity unknown)	8 oz.
Honey or corn syrup	½ tsp.	Baking soda	¼ tsp.
Table salt	1 pinch		

Drink alternately from each glass. Supplement with carbonated beverages, water (boiled if necessary), or tea, as desired.

INFECTIONS OF THE URINARY TRACT

Urethritis in Men

Urethritis with symptomatic urethral irritation and a urethral discharge is primarily a sexually transmitted disease that occurs in men. Classically, this disease has been associated with *N. gonorrhoeae*, but nongonococcal infection accounts for at least 40 percent of the cases of urethritis and is especially predominant in higher socioeconomic classes. *Chlamydia trachomatis* can be established as the causative pathogen in approximately 40 to 50 percent of patients with nongonococcal urethritis. *Ureaplasma urealyticum* also has been implicated strongly as a pathogen in this syndrome. *Trichomonas vaginalis* and herpes simplex virus appear to cause nongonococcal urethritis occasionally, but they are responsible for less than 5 percent of cases. Reiter's syndrome, associated with uveitis, conjunctivitis, circinate balanitis, oral mucosal ulcerations, and asymmetric arthritis, may be responsible for 1 to 2 percent of these cases. An etiology cannot be identified in almost 50 percent of these patients, however.

Pathophysiology

Both gonococcal and chlamydial urethritis are predominantly localized infections. Gonococcal infection is acquired by intimate contact of mucosal surface with the organism. The bacteria adhere to the epithelial surface and then penetrate to the subepithelial connective tissue, where they induce an intense inflammatory response and cause epithelial sloughing. Although untreated infection usually resolves spontaneously within six months, periurethral abscesses, urethral strictures, epididymitis, prostatitis, and disseminated gonococcal infection may develop as complications.

Chlamydia trachomatis is an obligate intracellular microorganism that infects columnar epithelial cells. Urethral infection results from contact with a cervix infected with *C. trachomatis*. While the infection is localized to the epithelial surface, it may extend along the urethra and produce acute epididymitis.

Diagnosis

The predominant symptom of urethritis is a urethral discharge, which may be purulent, mucoid, or watery and is manifested by staining of underwear or bedclothes. Occasionally, this is the only symptom. Urethral irritation is usually present with dysuria, frequency, urgency, a sensation of pressure in the groin, and continuous mild urethral pain or pruritis.

Physical examination should be performed two hours or more after the patient has last urinated to permit the accumulation of scant discharges that may have been cleared by the urinary stream. If there is no spontaneous discharge, manual stripping of the penis from the base to the meatus may express fluid from the urethra. Unless the patient is sexually aroused or has just urinated, the presence of any urethral fluid is abnormal and is considered a discharge.

Examination of the urethral secretions is essential in diagnosing urethritis and should include a Gram stain and culture for *N. gonorrhoeae*. With careful uniform swabbing of a 2 × 1 sq cm area on a glass slide, the Gram stain provides both diagnostic and etiologic information. On microscopic examination, an average of more than four neutrophils per high-powered field is a sensitive indicator of urethritis. Gonococcal urethritis is further characterized by the presence of intracellular gram-negative diplococci in association with the polymorphonuclear exudate. Although the exudate in nongonococcal urethritis is seen without intracellular bacteria, mixed extracellular coliform and coccobacillary forms may be present. The presence of extracellular gram-negative diplococcal organisms without intracellular organisms is suggestive but not diagnostic of gonococcal infection. All exudates should be cultured for *N. gonorrhoeae*, and rectal and pharyngeal swabs should be performed as required by the sexual history.

The urethral culture is taken with a urethral swab and plated immediately on Thayer-Martin agar or a specific gonococcal transport media. *Chlamydia trachomatis* and *U. urealyticum* cannot be cultured currently in all routine diagnostic laboratories.

Differential Diagnosis

Gonococcal urethritis in men has a short incubation period of two to seven days and is associated with significant dysuria and purulent exudate, although it may be asymptomatic at first. Nongonococcal urethritis has a more prolonged incubation period of one to three weeks. In many patients, a watery or mucoid discharge is the only symptom. Dysuria is more frequently mild or "itchy." Gonococcal urethritis is much more likely than nongonococcal urethritis to be associated with a spontaneous urethral discharge on examination. Because of the nonspecificity of the clinical presentations, microscopic examination and culture should be used to confirm the diagnosis in all patients.

The differential diagnosis of urethritis includes prostatitis, cystitis, and epididymitis, but they should be readily distinguished on clinical presentation. Hematuria and hemospermia are not seen with urethritis and suggest disease of kidneys, bladder, or prostate.

Treatment

Several drug treatment regimens for uncomplicated gonococcal infections have been recommended by the Center for Disease Control because no single therapy can be applied, optimally, to all patients. The recommendations are

- aqueous procaine penicillin G, 4.8 million units injected intramuscularly in two divided doses at separate sites, with 1 gm probenecid by mouth, or
- tetracycline hydrochloride, 0.5 gm by mouth four times a day for five days (total dose 10 gm), or
- ampicillin, 3.5 gm with 1 gm probenecid by mouth, or
- amoxicillin, 3 gm with 1 gm probenecid by mouth

The first two regimens appear to be slightly more efficacious. The use of aqueous procaine penicillin G is limited by penicillin allergy, pain from the injections, and, rarely, procaine reactions. Tetracycline should be utilized only when completion of the regimen is assured; if there is any question of patient compliance, a single-dose regimen is preferred. In patients who are allergic to penicillin, tetracycline or spectinomycin hydrochloride (1 gm in one IM injection) can be utilized. If concurrent anorectal gonococcal infection is suspected, aqueous procaine penicillin should be used. Gonococcal infection with a known penicillinase-producing strain should be treated with spectinomycin. Some of the new β-lactamase–resistant cephalosporins may also be useful.

The initial therapy of nongonococcal urethritis must be directed at both *C. trachomatis* and *U. urealyticum*, since the precise etiology is not usually established. Although both microorganisms are susceptible to tetracycline and erythromycin, tetracycline (500 mg by mouth four times a day for 7 to 10 days) may be preferred, as it is also effective against gonorrhea and syphilis. If tetracycline therapy has been ineffective or is contraindicated, erythromycin (500 mg by mouth four times a day for 14 days) is recommended.

The sexual partners of patients with urethritis must be examined and treated also, because both gonococcal and nongonococcal urethritis are sexually transmitted diseases. Failure to eradicate infection in both partners leads to recurrences.

Serologic studies for syphilis should be done in all patients with urethritis. All the regimens recommended for gonorrhea, except spectinomycin, are also adequate therapy for incubating seronegative syphilis.

Follow-up

All patients with urethritis must be reexamined in 7 to 14 days. A repeat culture for *N. gonorrhoeae* should be performed and should be negative to confirm cure. Following gonococcal urethritis, a small percentage of patients develop recurrent urethral symptoms associated with a mucoid discharge. At least 70 percent of these cases are due to a *Chlamydia* infection that probably occurred simultaneously with the initial *N. gonorrhoeae* infection. These patients usually have been treated with penicillin or ampicillin and respond to tetracycline therapy.

It is particularly important to arrange follow-up for patients with nongonococcal urethritis. Although over 80 percent of initial chlamydial infections are completely eradicated by tetracycline, patients with nonchlamydial, nongonococcal urethritis have a lower response rate. These patients may have infections with *U. urealyticum* strains resistant to tetracycline or urethritis due to *Trichomonas* or herpes simplex. The first 10 ml freshly voided urine should be examined by wet mount for *Trichomonas*; if positive, metronidazole (2 gm as a single dose, or 1 gm twice daily as total therapy, or 250 mg three times a day for seven days) should be given. If *Trichomonas* is not present and compliance with previous therapy was adequate, treatment with erythromycin should be initiated and further follow-up arranged.

Urinary Tract Infections

Infection of the urinary tract is a frequent cause of emergency department visits. Cystitis and pyelonephritis are primarily infections in women, and the incidence of these infections increases with age. Older men may develop urinary tract infection in association with prostatic hypertrophy and urethral instrumentation. Prostatitis is a disease of men that can be either acute or chronic. The urethral syndrome, which consists of symptomatic urethral irritation without evidence of cystitis or vaginitis, has been delineated recently as a distinct entity in women of childbearing age. While the clinical manifestations of urinary tract infections may be shared, the etiology and pathophysiology varies with the specific site involved.

The terms *cystitis* and *pyelonephritis* are clinical descriptions of acute symptomatic urinary tract infection caused usually by *E. coli* or other bacteria, such as *Klebsiella, Proteus* species, *Pseudomonas aeruginosa, Serratia marcescens, Enterobacter* species, and enterococci (e.g., *Streptococcus faecalis*). The first episodes of bacterial infection of the urinary tract are due to *E. coli*, which is very sensitive to most antibiotics, but recurrent episodes may be caused by other, more resistant organisms.

Bacteria can ascend the urethra and enter the bladder. Urinary tract infection in women results from colonization of the vaginal introitus by organisms that migrate from the fecal reservoir. Small bacterial inocula may be cleared by normal voiding. Factors that facilitate bacterial migration up the urethra, such as urethral catheterization, or those that prevent complete voiding, such as neurogenic bladder, pregnancy, urethral stricture, and benign prostatic hypertrophy allow bacteria to multiply within the bladder. Failure of local antibacterial defense mechanisms of the bladder mucosa results in the establishment of infection.

Infection may extend to the kidney, owing to reflux of urine from the bladder into the ureter. Bladder infection itself may cause a relative incompetence of the ureterovesical valve that permits such a reflux to the upper tract. Bacterial infection in the upper urinary tract (kidneys and collecting system) may occur without symptoms, or it may produce the signs and symptoms typical of acute pyelonephritis. Gram-negative bacteria may inhibit normal ureteric peristalsis, and this inhi-

bition facilitates the rapid ascent of bacteria to the renal pelvis and renal parenchyma. Infection usually begins in the renal medullary tubules and spreads cortically, inciting an inflammatory response. Microabscesses may develop in acute bacterial pyelonephritis.

Diagnosis

The clinical manifestations of bacterial urinary tract infections are urinary frequency, burning on micturition, pressure sensation over the bladder, urinary urgency, and pyuria and hematuria. Fever greater than 38.5°C, back pain at the costovertebral angles, rigors, nausea, and vomiting are associated with acute pyelonephritis. Patients may have upper tract bacterial infection without specific signs if their infection is clinically limited to the lower urinary tract. At present, there are no reliable, universally available techniques for localizing infection to the upper or lower urinary tract, but a test for antibody-coated bacteria may be useful.

The hallmark of acute urinary tract infection is the presence of a single bacterial species at counts equal to or greater than 100,000/ml urine. Because the urine sample must be uncontaminated with periurethral flora, the urethral orifice and periurethral area should be cleansed carefully with dilute green soap solution, and the patient should collect a urine sample while retracting the foreskin or labia. Although midstream specimens have been recommended, it is very difficult for women to obtain an adequate sample with this technique. Alternatively, an appropriate sample may be obtained by bladder catheterization or by suprapubic bladder aspiration. Either of these techniques can introduce bacteria into the bladder, however. In general, the urine should be obtained with the patient standing over a wide-mouthed collecting jar.

The sample should be either refrigerated immediately or transferred to culture media in a quantitative fashion within 30 minutes of collection, as bacteria will continue to multiply in a sample at room temperature. Failure to transport and culture the sample promptly results in artificially high colony counts, usually with multiple bacterial species. Patients may have true bacterial infection even when their bacterial count is below 100,000/ml if they produce large amounts of urine, diluting the colony count. Similarly, low urine pH and small doses of antibiotics may inhibit bacterial multiplication. Persistent low level bladder colonization (with colony counts of 10^3 to 10^4/ml) may be found in some patients with the urethral syndrome. Bacteriuria (colony count equal to or greater than 100,000/ml) may be present in the absence of symptoms; the presence of the same organism in three specimens taken over a three- to four-week period confirms the diagnosis of urinary tract infection.

In the symptomatic patient, a single positive urine culture is sufficient.

Microscopic examination of the urine is useful to determine rapidly the presence of bacteriuria. A mixture of one drop each of noncentrifuged urine and methylene blue or other bacterial dye is placed under a cover slip and examined. The presence of one bacterium per high-powered field on at least five fields is consistent with bacterial colony counts of at least 100,000/ml.

Urinalysis can be used to determine whether a large number of neutrophils and, often, microscopic hematuria are present. White blood cell casts are suggestive of renal tubular infection (pyelonephritis). The white blood cell count frequently reveals a polymorphonuclear leukocytosis in patients with acute pyelonephritis.

The localization of the level of infection within the urinary tract is difficult in the emergency department. There is no reliable diagnostic procedure, although ureteral catheterization and bladder catheterization with wash-out cultures have been used in specific studies. A search for antibody-coated bacteria in voided urine may reveal renal infection in women. The presence of antibody-coated bacteria correlates with upper tract infection in 62 to 95 percent of women patients studied. Men with prostate infections also have antibody-coated bacteria in the urine. This technique is not readily available in the emergency department, however.

The differential diagnosis of acute urinary infection includes vaginitis and the urethral syndrome in women, prostatitis in men, and renal stone disease in both sexes. Vaginal infections are even more common than urinary tract infections, and they may cause dysuria as well as vaginal discharge or irritation. A pelvic examination should be performed if these symptoms are present. Vaginitis and bacterial urinary tract infections may occur simultaneously in the same patient.

Treatment

Antimicrobial therapy is effective treatment for bacterial infections in the urinary tract. Antibacterial therapy can be instituted based on the clinical signs and symptoms or on the demonstration of bacteria in the urine. Cultures should be obtained and appropriate arrangements made for follow-up visits.

There is no clearly identified drug of choice; patients can be started on antibacterial therapy with any of the agents shown in Table 20–2. The optimal duration of therapy of uncomplicated urinary tract infection is not clear. Conventional therapy involves treatment for 10 to 14 days. Recently, single-dose therapy (such as amoxicillin 3 gm by mouth) has been shown to be as effective as conventional therapy in patients whose infection has been localized to the lower urinary tract. Since recurrent episodes of urinary tract infection can

be caused by new or reinfecting strains, careful follow-up of treated patients is essential. Patients may develop asymptomatic bacteriuria before a symptomatic episode recurs. In general, urine culture should be repeated within one to three weeks after therapy and again at 3, 6, and 12 months.

In patients with high fever, hypotension, or shaking chills, gram-negative rod bacteremia secondary to urinary tract infection should be suspected. These patients should be admitted to the hospital, blood and urine cultures should be obtained, and the patients should be treated with parenteral antibiotic therapy.

Patients with recurrent urinary tract infections are frequently infected with organisms that are resistant to many antibiotics. These patients should have a urine culture repeated 24 hours after empirical therapy has been initiated so that the adequacy of treatment can be ascertained. Antibiotics must act quickly, as they are rapidly excreted into the urine; therefore, the bacteriologic response to a treatment regimen is clear within 24 hours. If the antibiotic is appropriate for the infecting organism, the infection should be cleared within 24 hours. Should this not be the case, the addition of other antibiotics would be appropriate at that time. Patients with a history of recurrent urinary infections usually benefit from long-term suppressive therapy with trimethoprim-sulfamethoxazole or nitrofurantoin. Small doses of these agents can be taken as infrequently as two to three times a week and/or after intercourse in patients whose recurrent infections are related to sexual activity.

The Urethral Syndrome in Women

Also known as the dysuria-frequency syndrome or (in the past) nonbacteriuric urethritis, the urethral syndrome is responsible for up to 40 to 50 percent of episodes of dysuria and increased urinary frequency in women. In most of these women, low urinary counts (10^2 to 10^4/ml) of gram-negative rods or *Staphylococcus saprophyticus* are present; *C. trachomatis* is the second most commonly seen organism. No underlying cause can be defined in about one-third of patients. Frequently, women with chlamydial urethral syndrome have recently changed sexual partners, and the infection is probably transmitted sexually.

Diagnosis

The urethral syndrome is considered when vaginitis and typical acute urinary tract infection have been excluded in symptomatic women with dysuria, frequency, and urgency. The presence of low bacterial count cystitis or chlamydial urethritis can be determined by microscopic examination of the urine. Both of these conditions are associated with pyuria, more than eight white

TABLE 20–2 Antibacterial Therapy for Urinary Tract Infection

Drug	Adults	Children
Sulfisoxazole	1 gm orally 4 times a day	150 mg/kg/24 hours orally given in 4 divided doses
Ampicillin or amoxicillin	500 mg to 1 gm orally 4 times a day	100 mg/kg/24 hours orally given in 4 divided doses in children less than 20 kg
Cephalexin or cephradine	250 to 500 mg orally 4 times a day	25 to 50 mg/kg/24 hours orally given in 4 divided doses
Nitrofurantoin	50 to 100 mg orally 3 or 4 times a day	5 to 7 mg/kg/24 hours orally given in 4 divided doses
Trimethoprim-sulfamethoxazole	2 tablets orally twice a day	8 to 40 mg/kg/24 hours orally given in 2 divided doses
Tetracycline	250 to 500 mg orally 4 times a day	Not used in children under 8 years old

blood cells per high-powered field, which is absent in patients with the urethral syndrome without definable cause.

Treatment

Tetracycline or sulfonamides should be effective therapy for most women with urethral syndrome due to gram-negative bacteria and chlamydia. Doxycycline (100 mg orally twice a day for ten days) has been studied and shown to be effective in clinical trials. Urinary analgesics such as phenazopyridine hydrochloride may be helpful for these patients who complain of dysuria in the absence of pyuria.

Prostatitis

Acute bacterial prostatitis is caused by *E. coli*, other gram-negative bacteria, or, occasionally, *N. gonorrhoeae*. Infection is probably caused by reflux of bacteria from the urethra to the prostate. The normal prostate secretes an antibacterial zinc salt, but this secretion may be reduced in patients with bacterial prostatitis.

Diagnosis

Acute bacterial prostatitis has an abrupt onset with fever, chills, dysuria, frequency, and perineal and low back pain. Variable degrees of bladder outlet obstruction may occur. The physical examination reveals an enlarged, exquisitely tender prostate. Prostatic massage should be avoided to minimize the risk of bacteremia. Urinalysis reveals pyuria and bacteriuria, and a polymorphonuclear leukocytosis is found in peripheral blood.

Treatment

Hospitalization is required for patients who have severe infections or marked bladder outlet obstruction. Appropriate cultures of urine and blood should be obtained, and treatment with parenteral antibiotics should be started immediately. An aminoglycoside (gentamicin, tobramycin, or amikacin) with or without a broad spectrum penicillin or cephalosporin is reasonable, pending culture results. Trimethoprim-sulfamethoxazole in its new intravenous formulation also might be useful. Suprapubic bladder drainage should be performed if urinary retention is marked.

Outpatient management is acceptable in less severely ill patients. Few antibiotics other than trimethoprim and erythromycin penetrate well into prostate tissue. Trimethoprim or trimethoprim-sulfamethoxazole (160 mg/800 mg orally twice a day) is adequate therapy for bacterial prostatitis caused by sensitive organisms. Therapy should be continued for up to 30 days, and arrangements should be made for urologic follow-up.

CENTRAL NERVOUS SYSTEM INFECTIONS

Acute meningitis refers to inflammation of the subarachnoid space and the cerebrospinal fluid (CSF). Patients with aseptic meningitis have a mononuclear pleocytosis secondary to a variety of possible causes; patients with purulent meningitis have a pyogenic response to bacterial infection. Often an overwhelming infection, purulent meningitis is a true medical emergency and requires immediate antibiotic treatment in the emergency department.

Purulent Meningitis

Hemophilus influenzae, Neisseria meningitidis, and *S. pneumoniae* together account for 80 percent of all cases of purulent meningitis. No pathogen can be isolated in about 10 percent of patients with a classic clinical presentation of meningitis and CSF findings consistent with bacterial infection. The diagnosis is particularly obscured in patients who have received prior antibiotic treatment. Gram-negative bacilli are of major importance in meningitis in the elderly, in patients who have sustained head trauma or who have had neurosurgical procedures, and in neonates. Group B *Streptococcus* is also an important cause of meningitis in the neonate. *Staphylococcus aureus* and *Listeria monocytogenes* are infrequent meningeal pathogens. The former may cause meningitis secondary to contiguous infected foci; the latter may cause meningitis in immunocompromised patients. The relative frequency of *H. influenzae*, *N. meningitidis*, and *S. pneumoniae* in meningitis is related to age. *Hemophilus influenzae* is the predominant pathogen in patients from one month to 4 years of age and is uncommon after the age of 10. *Neisseria meningitidis* is the primary causal agent in patients 5 to 30 years of age, but it may be seen at any age. *Streptococcus pneumoniae* is the most frequent cause of meningitis in patients over 30 years of age.

Pathogenesis

The subarachnoid space is well protected from microbial invasion. It is surrounded by bone, ligaments, and three distinct membranes. CSF lacks intrinsic cellular and humoral immunity, however, and is thus particularly vulnerable to infection when bacteria are introduced. The subarachnoid space may be seeded by contiguous spread of infection from otitis media, mastoiditis, sinusitis, or osteomyelitis; or by direct invasion through CSF leaks due to trauma, surgery, or neuroectodermal defects. Seeding may also occur secondary to bacteremia. Several bacteria, particularly *N. meningitidis*, have intrinsic cellular properties that allow them to invade the subarachnoid space.

Vascular permeability of the choroid plexus, ependyma, and pia mater is increased by inflammation in the subarachnoid space, which also increases the protein content and cellularity of the CSF. Because active transport of glucose into the CSF is decreased, glucose concentration falls. CSF lactate concentration increases owing to increased anaerobic metabolism. Without prompt therapy, a thick purulent exudate forms and obstructs the normal CSF flow, occluding the vascular structures that pass through the subarachnoid space. Inflammation and edema of the underlying brain may produce cranial nerve palsies, seizures, stupor, coma, and death.

Diagnosis

Most patients with meningitis have fever, severe headache, and stiff neck. Other symptoms may be present, including nausea, vomiting, photophobia, and mental aberration. Many patients have had an antecedent upper respiratory tract infection or otitis media. Clinically, the meningeal irritation is reflected in nuchal rigidity, Kernig's sign (pain in the hamstring and paraspinal muscles when the knee is extended with the hip flexed), and Brudzinski's sign (flexion of the knees and hips when the neck is flexed). Patients may progress from lethargy to coma, and isolated cranial nerve palsies may occur. Papilledema is unusual; if present, a brain abscess or encephalitis should be considered. Meningitis in the infant is associated with bulging of the fontanelle.

The clinical presentation is variable and depends on the patient's age. Very young and very elderly patients may not have the usual signs of meningeal irritation. In these patients, the signs of meningitis may be very subtle, e.g., lethargy, increased irritability, and gastrointestinal disturbances with or without fever. Rapid, overwhelming infection is seen in about 10 percent of patients with purulent meningitis, and the rate of early mortality is significant.

The diagnosis is confirmed by examination of the CSF. Examination should include cell count and differential count, determination of glucose and protein concentrations, and Gram-stained smear of the sediment and culture. Meningitis is confirmed by the presence of spinal fluid pleocytosis with more than five neutrophils or ten leukocytes per cubic millimeter. A Gram stain indicates the etiology and guides the initial therapy of bacterial meningitis. A white blood cell count over 1,200/cu mm with a protein concentration greater than 150 mg/dl or a glucose concentration less than 30 mg/dl strongly suggests purulent meningitis, even if the Gram stain is negative.

Countercurrent immunoelectrophoresis, latex agglutination tests, and gas-liquid chromatography are useful and rapid techniques to identify bacterial antigens in the CSF. Countercurrent immunoelectrophoresis also can be performed on urine, since pneumococcal capsular polysaccharides may be detected in urine of infected patients.

Differential Diagnosis

The diagnosis is usually clear in overwhelming meningitis. However, aseptic meningitis, partially treated bacterial meningitis, viral encephalitis, brain abscess, epidural or subdural abscess, and vertebral osteomyelitis should be considered in patients with a more subtle presentation. Elderly patients frequently lose nuchal flexibility as a result of osteoarthritis, and nuchal rigidity may occur in these patients without true meningeal irritation. Patients with aseptic meningitis, partially treated bacterial meningitis, and viral encephalitis usually have a lymphocytic CSF pleocytosis. Localizing neurologic signs are often present with parameningeal abscesses, and vertebral osteomyelitis often produces point tenderness over the infected bone. Subacute bacterial endocarditis may result in embolic meningitis, and this usually produces a low-grade mixed pleocytosis. Bacteria may be seen on smear and are usually cultured from the CSF.

Treatment

Antimicrobial therapy should be initiated as soon as possible to limit morbidity and mortality in patients with fulminating meningitis (those whose total disease duration is less than 24 hours). A brief examination to exclude focal neurologic deficits or papilledema should be performed and a lumbar puncture obtained immediately. Blood cultures should also be obtained promptly. Empirical antibiotic therapy based on the age and condition of the patient must be instituted. Since the predominant pathogens in patients over eight years of age are *S. pneumoniae* and *N. meningitidis*, penicillin (50,000 units/kg intravenously every four hours, roughly 4 gm in adults) should be started in the emergency department. Penicillin (4 gm intravenously every four hours) should continue for ten days. Chloramphenicol (25 mg/kg intravenously every six hours) should be used in penicillin-allergic patients. In children between six weeks and eight years, chloramphenicol (25 mg/kg intravenously every six hours) plus ampicillin (50 mg/kg intravenously every four hours) or moxalactam (100 mg/kg intravenously, then 50 mg/kg every six to eight hours) plus ampicillin should be started because of the increased likelihood of *H. influenzae*.

In infants younger than two months of age, the major pathogens are Group B *Streptococcus* and gram-negative rods. Combined therapy with ampicillin (100 mg/kg intravenously every eight hours) plus an aminoglycoside such as gentamicin (2.5 mg/kg intravenously every twelve hours) is required. The initial therapy of fulminating meningitis in patients who are immunocompromised, who have experienced trauma, or who develop meningitis in the hospital should be directed against *Staphylococcus aureus* and gram-negative rods. Therapy with chloramphenicol (25 to 50 mg/kg intravenously every six hours), gentamicin (1.5 mg/kg intravenously every eight hours), and nafcillin (25 mg/kg intravenously every six hours) should be started in these patients, pending culture results. Cefoxitin and moxalactam are also useful in meningitis due to gram-negative bacilli.

Lumbar puncture is contraindicated in patients with focal findings consistent with a mass lesion. If the focal deficit suggests an intracranial or upper motor neuron lesion, then brain abscess, subdural empyema, or encephalitis become major considerations. These patients should receive chloramphenicol (25 to 50 mg/kg intravenously every six hours) and penicillin G (4 million units intravenously every four hours). Computerized axial tomography (CT) scans or sodium pertechnate brain scans should be performed. Lumbar puncture should be performed with extreme care in patients with spinal cord deficits to minimize the risk of introducing pathogens into the subarachnoid space. If an epidural abscess is suspected, immediate neurosurgical consultation should be obtained for surgical drainage.

Antibiotic therapy can be withheld until the results of lumbar puncture are known in patients whose symptoms are subacute. If the Gram stain and other studies are consistent with purulent meningitis, antibiotic therapy should be given as outlined. If the CSF findings are indeterminate and the patient's condition permits a delay in treatment, antibiotic therapy can be withheld and the lumbar puncture repeated in 8 to 12 hours. An increase in polymorphonuclear cells is suggestive of bacterial meningitis, and antibiotics should be given. Initial antibiotic therapy can be modified, if necessary, when the etiologic diagnosis is obtained by culture or bacterial antigen study. Crystalline penicillin G remains the agent of choice for pneumococcal, meningococcal, and listerial meningitis. When strains of *H. influenzae* are sensitive, ampicillin is the agent of choice. Chloramphenicol or moxalactam is appropriate for ampicillin-resistant strains. Staphylococcal meningitis requires large doses of semisynthetic penicillinase-resistant penicillins, such as nafcillin or oxacillin (2 to 3 gm intravenously every four hours).

The optimal therapy for gram-negative bacillary meningitis has not been determined. Chloramphenicol may be useful because it penetrates into CSF. Systemic intrathecal and intraventricular aminoglycosides are often used in adults, but intraventricular aminoglycosides are not helpful in neonates with meningitis. Moxalactam and other new experimental β-lactam agents may be proved useful in the future treatment of gram-negative rod meningitis. A repeat lumbar puncture should be performed 24 to 36 hours after antibiotic therapy is initiated to confirm sterilization of the CSF. Antibiotic therapy should be continued for at least ten days or for five afebrile days.

Prevention

Antibiotic prophylaxis with rifampin (600 mg orally every 12 hours in adults, 5 mg/kg in children under one year, and 10 mg/kg for older children in four divided doses) is appropriate for direct contacts of patients with meningococcal meningitis. Casual contacts, such as with fellow workers, schoolmates, or health care workers, do not require prophylaxis.

Aseptic Meningitis

Associated with meningeal irritation and a mononuclear cellular response, aseptic meningitis is usually due to enterovirus infection. Other agents may cause this syndrome, e.g., mumps, herpes simplex Types 1 and 2, varicella zoster, cytomegalovirus, adenovirus, measles, Epstein-Barr virus, hepatitis virus, poliomyelitis, and the encephalitis viruses. Meningeal irritation with mononuclear pleocytosis may be present in partially treated bacterial meningitis, parameningeal bacterial infections, tuberculosis, amebiasis, leptospirosis, syphilis, and fungal meningitis. Noninfectious causes include systemic lupus erythematosus, carcinomatosis, chemical injury from intrathecal medication, Behçet's syndrome, and Mollaret's syndrome.

Diagnosis

Aseptic meningitis is usually associated with signs of meningeal irritation (nuchal rigidity, headache, Kernig's and Brudzinski's signs) and fever after a short prodromal illness. A lumbar puncture should be performed immediately. The CSF examination reveals a normal glucose concentration, a protein concentration ranging from 50 to 200 mg/dl, and a white blood cell count of 50 to 1,000. Neutrophils predominate very early in the course, but mononuclear cells increase significantly after six to eight hours.

Other studies may reveal the specific etiology. An acid-fast smear obtained by means of the drop-on-drop technique may be positive in tuberculous meningitis, but usually the diagnosis must await cultural confirmation. India ink preparations and cryptococcal antigen determinations are useful in cryptococcal meningitis. If the clinical presentation suggests carcinomatosis, cytocentrifugation of CSF facilitates identification of neoplastic cells. Special studies for bacterial antigens should be obtained if partially treated bacterial meningitis is likely.

If the CSF examination is nonspecific, it should be repeated in 8 to 12 hours. Most patients with aseptic meningitis develop a lymphocytic cellular response in this length of time.

Treatment

The appropriate treatment of aseptic meningitis is determined by the clinical setting and, ultimately, by the proved etiology. These patients should be observed closely and most often require hospitalization for several days. In certain circumstances, for example, when there is a summer epidemic of viral meningitis, mildly ill patients do not require hospitalization. Antibiotics are not indicated unless a bacterial process is suspected. Partially treated bacterial meningitis requires full antibiotic therapy as outlined previously.

Infectious Mononucleosis

An acute febrile illness, mononucleosis produces pharyngitis, lymphadenopathy, and splenomegaly. It is associated with hematologic abnormalities, including absolute and relative lymphocytosis (greater than 50 percent of white blood cells) with many atypical lymphocytes. The causative pathogen is the Epstein-Barr virus (EBV) in over 90 percent of cases. The term *infectious mononucleosis* usually applies to these cases. Cytomegalovirus may cause the syndrome in 5 to 7 percent of cases. *Toxoplasma* can also cause this syndrome, but fewer than 1 percent of patients with mononucleosis actually have toxoplasmosis.

Pathogenesis

All three infecting agents produce systemic infection that involves lymph nodes, spleen, and liver. The central nervous system, the cardiovascular and respiratory systems, the kidney, and bone marrow are less frequently involved. The hematologic abnormalities associated with EBV infection may be mediated by viral infection of B lymphocytes and secondary proliferation of T lymphocytes, leading to the formation of atypical lymphocytes. The spread of this infection is mediated by prolonged, low-level excretion of EBV in salivary excretions. Cytomegalovirus mononucleosis is spread by low-level, close, person-to-person contact; it can also be transmitted by transfusion. Toxoplasmosis follows the ingestion of uncooked, infected meat or contact with infected cats or cat feces.

Diagnosis

Mononucleosis is most common in patients 15 to 25 years old, although it may occur at any age. The illness begins with a prodrome of fatigue, malaise, headache, and myalgias with the subsequent development of fever (38.3°C to 39.5°C). A severe exudative pharyngitis is prominent in infectious mononucleosis, but is less common with cytomegalovirus or *Toxoplasma* infections. Tender peripheral lymphadenopathy, involving particularly the anterior or posterior cervical nodes, is present in over 80 percent of patients infected with EBV or *Toxoplasma*, but is less common with cytomegalovirus.

Other early manifestations of the mononucleosis syndrome include an evanescent erythematous skin rash, periorbital edema, and palatal petechiae. Neurologic complications, such as encephalitis, cerebellar ataxia, cranial nerve palsies, transverse myelitis, or Guillain-Barré syndrome, may occur, although they are found in less than 1 percent of cases. Other rare manifestations of mononucleosis include myocarditis, pericarditis, hemolytic anemia, interstitial pneumonia, monoarticular arthritis, and splenic rupture, especially after vigorous palpation.

The atypical lymphocytes seen in the peripheral blood smear are large cells with vacuolated cytoplasm and horseshoe-shaped or oval nuclei that contain dense, irregular chromatin. Initially, mild agranulocytosis may be present, but leukocytosis develops in the second to third week of illness. Uncommonly, a leukemoid reaction is seen. Mild hepatic abnormalities are present in over 80 percent of patients with mononucleosis syndromes. While clinical hepatitis is rare, the levels of serum glutamic-oxaloacetic transaminase (SGOT), lactic dihydrogenase (LDH), alkaline phosphatase, and bilirubin are usually elevated and are useful in confirming the diagnosis.

With EBV infection, the production of immunoglobulins, including IgM heterophil antibodies, is characteristically increased. While several different heterophil antibodies are produced, a distinct elevation of the Paul-Bunnell heterophil antibody is found in infectious mononucleosis, and this has been used as a marker for the disease. Rapid slide tests (e.g., Monospot) utilizing formalinized horse or sheep erythrocytes are available to detect the presence of this heterophil antibody.

Antibody titers begin to rise with the onset of clinical illness and may remain elevated for as long as one year. The results of a heterophil test are positive in 85 percent of patients with EBV mononucleosis, although the titer elevation may not become significant for 6 to 12 weeks in some patients. Serologic studies for EBV-specific antibodies are available in research laboratories but they are difficult to perform and not available routinely.

Neither cytomegalovirus nor *Toxoplasma* infection induces heterophil antibodies. Cytomegalovirus mononucleosis is documented by a four-fold rise in serum antibody titer from the time of acute illness to the convalescent period. Complement-fixing antibodies or an immunofluorescent IgM assay may be used to determine the presence of antibodies. Toxoplasmosis is documented by serology or by specific lymph node pathology.

Differential Diagnosis

The initial evaluation, which includes a complete blood count and heterophil antibody study, usually establishes the diagnosis of mononucleosis in patients with EBV infection. Patients with the typical hematologic picture and a negative result on a heterophil antibody test up to six weeks after illness may have a cytomegalovirus or *Toxoplasma* infection. Adenovirus, rubella, the hepatitis viruses, and Group A streptococci may produce clinical illnesses that simulate mononucleosis.

Treatment

There is no specific therapy for EBV or cytomegalovirus mononucleosis. Both are self-limited illnesses that begin to resolve in two to three weeks, although fatigue may persist for several months. Symptomatic therapy should be offered, and patients should be advised against vigorous activity or contact sports until the splenomegaly recedes. Prolonged bed rest is not indicated. Short-term oral steroid therapy with 40 to 60 mg prednisone daily decreases the duration of fever and symptomatic illness. Its use is not necessary in most cases, but it should be considered (a) if severe pharyngitis threatens the airway or limits nutrition, or (b) if pericarditis, myocarditis, hemolytic anemia, thrombocytopenia, or neurologic complications develop. Because occasional patients have simultaneous streptococcal pharyngitis and infectious mononucleosis, throat cultures should be obtained routinely in patients with severe pharyngeal disease. The use of ampicillin in these patients is associated with a prominent erythematous papular eruption.

Mild cases of toxoplasmosis do not require therapy. Severe disease, especially in immunodeficient patients, can be treated with pyrimethamine and sulfadiazine, but this therapy requires close supervision.

SKIN AND SOFT TISSUE INFECTIONS

Cutaneous Abscesses

Either trauma or obstruction of the eccrine or exocrine glands in the skin can lead to cutaneous abscesses. Rarely, such abscesses may arise from hematogenous spread of infection from a distant focus. They are limited to the dermis, but deeper structures in the hand may be infected owing to the close spatial relations of potential and actual spaces. Infection is usually caused by resident skin flora and varies slightly with the anatomical location. Hand infections are primarily caused by *S. aureus*, which is also responsible for most infections on the head, neck, thorax, and extremities; however, some infections in these areas are due to mixed anaerobic and aerobic organisms. In perineal abscesses (including inguinal, buttock, pilonidal, and anorectal abscesses), the predominant pathogens are those comprising the anaerobic fecal flora, although *S. aureus* is occasionally isolated. The fecal aerobic gram-negative bacilli are found less commonly.

Diagnosis and Differential Diagnosis

A cutaneous abscess generally occurs as a painful, tender, warm, erythematous mass. Fluctuance is a particularly helpful diagnostic clue, but may be absent. The abscess may be accompanied by spreading cellulitis or lymphangitic streaking. A peripheral leukocytosis with a shift to immature polymorphonuclear leukocytes may be seen with large abscesses, although not with smaller lesions. The aspiration of pus is definitive, and Gram stain and culture of the aspirate determines the etiology.

A few lesions may mimic pyogenic abscesses. Sterile abscesses can develop in parenteral drug abusers owing to talc and other "cutting" materials. Acute relapsing panniculitis is associated with multiple subcutaneous nodules of fat necrosis on the abdomen and extremities. Erythema nodosum may produce similar lesions, primarily on the lower extremities. Herpetic whitlow may resemble staphylococcal paronychial infection. Localized arterial aneurysms may be seen as fluctuant masses, but they should be readily distinguished by their prominent pulsation.

Treatment

Systemic antibiotics do not always reach the center of an abscess cavity in adequate concentration, and the bacterial and phagocytic breakdown products within the abscess inhibit many antimicrobial agents. Consequently, surgical drainage is essential in the treatment of any abscess. The involved site should be scrubbed with organic iodine solution, the area anesthetized, and the abscess cavity incised. Purulent materials should be collected for culture in a syringe, and the cavity should be probed to break up any loculated pus. After irrigation with saline solution, the cavity should be loosely packed with a gauze wick. In most instances, cutaneous abscesses can be treated on an outpatient basis, but infections at several body sites require special attention and, often, hospitalization.

Hand infections are of particular concern. Infections on the palmar surface may be complicated by suppurative tenosynovitis or arthritis. Hospitalization is warranted if exploration of an abscess cavity suggests that infection has penetrated deep into the hand. Infection of the distal phalanges around the nail bed (paronychia) or in the deep pulp (felon) may induce compartmental syndromes. The dense fascial layers within the finger limit swelling, and infection below fascial planes may result in pressure necrosis. If deep space infection is suspected, adequate surgical drainage of the deep compartments must be ensured and careful follow-up maintained for at least 48 hours.

Anorectal abscesses involve the anal glands. They are usually limited to the perianal region, although extension to the ischiorectal fossa or the supralevator space may occur. Any anorectal abscess should be carefully explored; general or spinal anesthesia should be considered for adequate evaluation.

With uncomplicated cutaneous abscesses, supplemental antibiotics are usually not required after drainage unless the patient's defenses are compromised, cellulitis is marked, or infection appears to be systemic. In these instances, presumptive antibiotics should be prescribed, based on Gram-stain results and the anatomical location. When *S. aureus* is suspected, treatment with a penicillinase-resistant penicillin (such as cloxacillin (250 to 500 mg orally every six hours) or oxacillin (500 to 1000 mg orally or intravenously every six hours), or a cephalosporin should be instituted. Clindamycin, erythromycin, and trimethoprim-sulfamethoxazole have variable activity against *S. aureus*. Vancomycin (500 mg intravenously every six hours) is an alternative for the patient who is allergic to penicillin and cephalosporin. Hospitalization is usually necessary for these patients.

Small, superficial anorectal abscesses may respond to surgical drainage alone. Deeper infections require therapy directed toward anaerobic organisms with agents such as clindamycin, chloramphenicol, cefoxitin, carbenicillin, or metronidazole.

Erysipeloid

Erysipelothrix rhusiopathiae is a small, gram-positive pleomorphic rod found as a commensal in fish, marine animals, birds, and wild and domestic animals. It produces a self-limited infection in humans when infected organic material comes into contact with a break in the skin. The localized infection, known as erysipeloid, is seen in individuals with occupational exposure, for example, fishermen, fish workers, veterinarians, laboratory workers, meat packers, butchers, abattoir workers, poultry workers, and farmers.

Diagnosis

The infection usually develops at a site of trauma on the hands. After a one- to four-day incubation period, painful swollen erythematous or violaceous cellulitis develops at the contact site, and it slowly progresses to involve the entire hand. Systemic toxicity is unusual, and the disease usually resolves spontaneously without treatment in several weeks. Rarely, *E. rhusiopathiae* may invade the bloodstream and produce endocarditis or septicemia associated with arthritis and diffuse cutaneous involvement. Diagnosis may be confirmed by culture from the skin lesion, but it is often difficult to isolate the organism. The diagnosis must rest on clinical grounds alone in most cases.

Treatment

While the infection is usually self-limited, treatment is warranted to prevent systemic disease. *Erysipelothrix rhusiopathiae* is very sensitive to penicillin, and penicillin V (250 mg orally four times a day for five to seven days) is appropriate. Erythromycin, cephalosporins, and tetracyclines have in vitro activity against the organism and may be used in the penicillin-allergic patient.

Herpetic Whitlow

Herpes simplex viruses Types 1 and 2 may produce localized cutaneous infection. Three to seven days after direct contact with active oral or genital herpetic lesions, painful paresthesias and vesicles develop on the skin, most often on the finger near the nail bed. The vesicles may coalesce and become turbid, mimicking bacterial infection. Regional lymphadenopathy, low-grade fever, and malaise may accompany the initial infection. Complete healing occurs in 14 to 28 days, but, as with oral and genital lesions, frequent recurrences at the infection site are common. (See Chapter 22.)

Currently, there is no effective therapy for herpetic whitlow. Incision of the lesions should be avoided, as it may lead to extension of the herpetic infection or bacterial superinfection. Health care workers should avoid self-infection by wearing gloves during oral and genital examinations.

Septic Arthritis

A relatively common but serious infection, septic arthritis requires immediate therapy to prevent irreversible joint injury. At present, *Neisseria gonorrhoeae* is the most frequent cause of infectious arthritis in patients who are sexually active. In children and the elderly, *S. aureus* is the most common infecting organism, although *H. influenzae* is almost as frequent in children under five years of age who have septic arthritis. *Streptococcus pyogenes* and gram-negative bacilli are not uncommon at any age and *Pseudomonas aeruginosa* is particularly frequent in users of intravenous drugs. Other bacteria, such as *S. pneumoniae*, *Brucella* species, *Neisseria meningitidis*, and anaerobic gram-negative rods, may also cause septic arthritis. Viruses, fungi, and mycobacteria may produce arthritis, but they are not usually associated with acute, purulent, destructive disease.

Pathogenesis

Septic arthritis develops from hematogenous or contiguous spread of infection, or from direct invasion of the synovium and joint space by the infecting organism. In gonococcal infection, the arthritis is a manifestation of disseminated gonococcal infection, and hematogenous spread may have occurred as a complication of symptomatic or asymptomatic anogenital or pharyngeal infection. The characteristics of gonococci that produce disseminated disease differ from those of other gonococci, e.g., the former have an increased resistance to serum bactericidal activity and an increased sensitivity to penicillin. Parenteral drug use, prior joint disease, chronic illness, and trauma are predisposing factors to infectious arthritis with any pathogen.

Diagnosis

Septic arthritis is first seen as a painful, tender, swollen, erythematous and warm joint with associated fever. Concurrent extra-articular infection or sepsis may occur. Synovial effusion is not always obvious, and all of the major findings can be found in as few as 10 percent of cases. In infants, the initial complaint is commonly limited to an unwillingness to move the affected joint. Septic arthritis is most common in the knee, wrist, shoulder, elbow, hip, and ankle joints, although parenteral drug abusers appear to have a predilection for sternoclavicular joint infection. Most cases of nongonococcal arthritis involve a single joint, but gonococcal arthritis may have an asymmetric polyarticular distribution. Routine laboratory studies usually demonstrate a leukocytosis; however, 20 to 40 percent of patients have a total peripheral white blood count less than 10,000/cu mm. The erythrocyte sedimentation rate is usually elevated.

Arthrocentesis should be performed on any joint believed to be infected. The synovial fluid is examined by cell count and differential count, glucose determination, Gram stain, culture, and inspection of the mucin clot. In septic arthritis, the synovial fluid leukocyte count is typically 100,000 to 130,000/cu mm with more than 85 percent polymorphonuclear leukocytes. Glucose concentration is usually less than 40 mg/dl. The mucin clot is characteristically poor, and the Gram stain is positive in approximately 65 percent of cases. Additional diagnostic studies on the synovial fluid include lactic acid determination (greater than 100 mg/dl in nongonococcal septic arthritis and less than 75 mg/dl in gonococcal and nonseptic arthritis) and countercurrent immunoelectrophoresis for bacterial antigens. The blood cultures are positive in approximately one-third to one-half of patients with septic arthritis. With gonococcal arthritis, the pathogen frequently is isolated from a primary anogenital or pharyngeal site as well as from the urethra. Radiologic studies may demonstrate distention of the joint capsule or coexistent osteomyelitis.

Differential Diagnosis

Crystalline-induced synovitis, osteoarthritis, rheumatoid arthritis, Reiter's syndrome, and acute rheumatic fever may resemble suppurative arthritis. Gout and pseudogout may occur simultaneously with septic arthritis. In patients with rheumatoid arthritis, superimposed infection may be seen as a sudden asymmetric flare in joint symptoms. Arthrocentesis is critical to confirm the diagnosis.

Several clinical characteristics can be used to distinguish gonococcal from nongonococcal septic arthritis. Gonococcal arthritis arises in healthy, sexually active individuals. It occurs three times more frequently in women than in men, and 70 percent of the cases in women develop during menstruation, pregnancy, or the postpartum period. Sixty percent of patients have two or more joints involved. The wrists and hands are frequently infected in gonococcal arthritis; in contrast, the lower extremity joints are more commonly involved in other types of septic arthritis. Patients with gonococcal arthritis may have concurrent tenosynovitis in the hands, wrists, or ankles; in addition, diffuse, widely scattered skin lesions are present in 30 to 50 percent of patients. These lesions are painful papules and vesiculopapules that are located primarily on the distal extremities.

Nongonococcal septic arthritis is slightly more common in men. Most patients have a concurrent extra-articular infection or an underlying predisposing factor. The knee and hip are the most frequently involved joints.

Treatment

Therapy for septic arthritis depends on the pathogen involved, the joint infected, and the presence of prosthetic devices. Gonococcal arthritis is quite responsive to therapy and may be managed with antibiotics alone. In patients with gram-negative diplococci on synovial fluid Gram stain and presumed gonococcal arthritis, one of the following is considered appropriate therapy:

- aqueous penicillin G (10 million units/day intravenously in six divided doses) until improvement occurs, followed by ampicillin (0.5 gm four times a day) to complete seven days of antibiotic treatment
- ampicillin (3.5 gm) or amoxicillin (3.0 gm orally) with probenicid (1 gm orally), followed by ampicillin (0.5 gm) or amoxicillin (0.5 gm orally four times a day) for seven days
- tetracycline (0.5 gm orally four times a day) for seven days
- spectinomycin (2 gm intramuscularly twice a day) for three days
- erythromycin (0.5 gm orally four times a day) for seven days

Tetracycline should not be used in pregnant women because of risks to both mother and fetus. In patients with penicillinase-producing gonococci, spectinomycin is preferred. Cefoxitin and other second- or third-generation cephalosporins are additional alternatives for gonococcal infection.

Patients with gonococcal tenosynovitis, disseminated gonococcal dermatitis, or minimal synovial effusions can be managed as outpatients with daily follow-up. Patients with significant synovial effusion should be hospitalized and undergo repeat arthrocentesis if effusion reaccumulates. Intra-articular antibiotic administration is contraindicated, as it may produce an inflammatory response. Anti-inflammatory agents should be avoided because they may mask progression of the disease.

Nongonococcal arthritis is more destructive than gonococcal arthritis; therefore, all patients with nongonococcal arthritis require initial parenteral antibiotic therapy. In staphylococcal arthritis, therapy should be started with a penicillinase-resistant penicillin (12 gm/day intravenously in six divided doses). In penicillin-allergic patients, vancomycin (500 mg intravenously every six hours) is appropriate. If gram-negative bacilli are found on the Gram stain, initial therapy must be directed at *Pseudomonas aeruginosa*, which is frequently the pathogen, especially in parenteral drug abusers. A combination of an antipseudomonal semisynthetic penicillin and an aminoglycoside should be administered, for example, ticarcillin (250 to 300 mg/kg/day in four divided doses) plus tobramycin (3 to 4.5 mg/kg/day in three divided doses). If the Gram stain is negative but the clinical presentation suggests septic arthritis, the healthy, sexually active young adult should be treated initially for gonococcal arthritis. Other adult patients and older children should receive initial therapy directed against *Staphylococcus* plus an aminoglycoside for presumed gram-negative infection, pending culture results. Children under two years of age should receive treatment for *S. aureus* and *H. influenzae* with a penicillinase-resistant penicillin (200 mg/kg/day in six doses) and chloramphenicol (100 mg/kg/day in four doses). Cefamandole and other new cephalosporins may prove acceptable alternatives.

In addition to antibiotic therapy, nongonococcal septic arthritis requires drainage of synovial effusions to avoid joint damage. If the synovial fluid is neither loculated nor thick, daily or twice daily needle aspirations may provide better results than surgical drainage, except for hip infections (and shoulder infections in neonates). Aspiration should be continued until effusion resolves completely. The response to therapy can be monitored with cell counts and cultures of the serial aspirates. A good therapeutic response can be expected if synovial fluid leukocyte counts decrease and the synovial fluid is sterilized within four days. Complete joint immobility is not necessary, but weight-bearing should be avoided. The joint should be kept in the functional position as much as possible and passive range of motion exercises used to prevent contractures.

Septic Bursitis

One-third of patients with inflammation of the olecranon or prepatellar bursae have septic bursitis. *Staphylococcus aureus* is the causal pathogen in over 90 percent of the cases, but, rarely, Group A β-hemolytic streptococci, *Sporothrix schenckii*, or atypical mycobacteria may be isolated. Infection usually occurs in young or middle-aged men engaged in manual labor who have sustained trauma locally or distal to the involved bursa. Previous bursal disease is a predisposing factor. The major clinical features are tenderness, warmth, and distention of the involved bursa associated with erythema and cellulitis of the overlying skin. Fever develops in approximately 40 percent of patients.

Bursal fluid analysis can distinguish septic from nonseptic bursitis. Gram stain of the fluid yields organisms in 65 to 100 percent of infected cases, and the white blood cell count is usually greater than 1,000 cu mm, with a predominance of neutrophils. In noninfectious bursitis, the white blood cell count is less than 1,000 cu mm, with predominantly mononuclear cells. The bursal fluid glucose level is almost always less than 50 percent of the corresponding serum level with a septic bursitis and nearly the same as the serum level in other forms of bursitis.

The major differential diagnoses are traumatic, gouty, or rheumatoid bursitis. Septic bursitis should be suspected if the patient is febrile or has severe bursal tenderness. Needle aspiration should be performed in all cases of bursitis at these locations. As gouty and septic bursitis can occur simultaneously, all fluid should be examined for crystals as well as organisms. (See Chapter 71 for techniques of aspirating joints.)

Treatment should be initiated with a semisynthetic penicillinase-resistant penicillin, pending culture results. Adequate antibiotic levels can be achieved in bursal fluid with oxacillin (500 mg orally four times a day) or a corresponding dosage of cloxacillin or dicloxacillin. The time required to sterilize the bursal space increases with the duration of the untreated bursal infection; therefore, the length of therapy must be individualized. Repeat needle aspirations of the bursa achieve effective drainage and permit monitoring of the therapeutic response. Continuing therapy for five days after the bursa has been sterilized is effective and results in few complications.

Sporotrichosis

Sporothrix schenckii is a dimorphic fungus that is found in soil, wet or rotting wood, hay, and sphagnum moss. It can cause a local lymphocutaneous infection in humans after inoculation through a break in the skin and is an occupational risk for gardeners, nursery workers, and forestry workers. Children may develop infection after playing in infected soil or hay. Very rarely, an indolent pulmonary infection may develop after inhalation of the organism.

The initial presentation of cutaneous sporotrichosis is a subcutaneous nodule that develops from one week to six months after primary inoculation. The nodule gradually darkens and ulcerates through the skin, leaving a slowly healing dark chancre. Secondary ulcerating nodules can develop along the lymphatics draining the primary site, or a lymphatic cord may be formed. The patient is not febrile and has associated symptoms in less than 1 percent of cases. Disseminated illness may develop.

The diagnosis of sporotrichosis is confirmed by culturing the fungus from skin scrapings or lesion aspirates. Serologic tests are available but are not usually needed with cutaneous infection. The differential diagnosis should include other fungal diseases, such as coccidioidomycosis or blastomycosis, tularemia, leprosy, anthrax, and tuberculosis.

Cutaneous sporotrichosis is treated initially with saturated solution of potassium iodide. A 1 mg/ml solution is given orally as 8 to 12 ml/day in three doses, which should be continued for three weeks after the lesions have healed. Nonresponsive lesions should be referred to a dermatologist. (See Chapter 22.)

BIBLIOGRAPHY

Common Cold

Gwaltney JM, Moskalski PB, Hendley JO: Hand-to-hand transmission of rhinovirus colds. *Ann Intern Med* 88:463–467, 1978.

Monto AS, Ullman BM: Acute respiratory illness in an American community. The Tecumseh study. *JAMA* 277:164–169, 1974.

West S, Brandon B, Stolley P, Rumrill R: A review of antihistamines and the common cold. *Pediatrics* 56:100–107. 1975.

Pharyngitis

Glezen WP, Clyde WA, Senior RJ, et al: Group A streptococci, mycoplasmas and viruses associated with pharyngitis. *JAMA* 202:455–460, 1967.

Honikman LM, Masser BF: Guidelines for the selective use of throat cultures in the diagnosis of streptococcal respiratory infection. *Pediatrics* 48:573–581, 1971.

Kaplan EL, Bisno A, Derrick W, et al: American Heart Association Committee Report: Prevention of rheumatic fever. *Circulation* 55:51–54, 1977.

Komaroff AL: A management strategy for sore throat. *JAMA* 239:1429–1432, 1978.

Peter G, Smith AL: Group A streptococcal infections of the skin and pharynx. *N Engl J Med* 297:311–317, 365–370, 1977.

Stephens DS, Walker DM, Schaffner W, et al: Pseudodiphtheria: Prominent pharyngeal membrane associated with fatal paraquat ingestion. *Ann Intern Med* 94:202–204, 1981.

Wanamaker LW: Perplexity and precision in the diagnosis of streptococcal pharyngitis. *Am J Dis Child* 124:352–358, 1972.

Sinusitis

Carenfelt C, Lundberg C, Nord CE, Wretlind B: Bacteriology of maxillary sinusitis in relation to quality of the retained secretion. *Acta Otolaryngol* 86:298–302, 1978.

Chilton LA, Skipper BE: Antihistamines and alpha-adrenergic agents in treatment of otitis media. *South Med J* 72:953–955, 1979.

Evans FO, Sydnor JS, Moore WEC, Moore GR, et al: Sinusitis of the maxillary antrum. *N Eng J Med* 293:735–739, 1975.

Hamory BH, Sande MA, Sydnor A, Seale DL, Gwaltney JM: Etiology and antimicrobial therapy of acute maxillary sinusitis. *Infect Dis* 139:197–202, 1979.

Karma P, Jokiph L, Sipila P, Luotonen J, Jokiph AMM: Bacteria in chronic maxillary sinusitis. *Arch Otolaryngol* 105:386–390, 1979.

McLinn SE: Cefaclor in treatment of otitis media and pharyngitis in children. *Am J Dis Child* 134:560–563, 1980.

Morgan PR, Morrison WV: Complications of frontal and ethmoid sinusitis. *Laryngoscope* 80:661–666, 1980.

Schwartz R, Rodriguez WJ, Mann R, Khan W, Ross S: The nasopharyngeal culture in acute otitis media: A reappraisal of its usefulness. *JAMA* 241:2170–2173, 1979.

Shurin PA, Pelton SI, Donner A, Finkelstein J, Klein JO: Trimethoprim-sulfamethoxazole compared with ampicillin in the treatment of acute otitis media. *J Pediatr* 96:1081–1087, 1980.

Shurin PA, Pelton SI, Donner A, Klein JO: Persistence of middle-ear effusion after acute otitis media in children. *N Engl J Med* 300:1121–1123, 1979.

Shurin PA , Pelton SI, Finkelstein J: Tympanometry in the diagnosis of middle ear effusion. *N Engl J Med* 196:412–417, 1977.

Wald ER, Milmoe GJ, Bowen A, Ledesma-Medina J, Salamon N, Bluestone DC: Acute maxillary sinusitis in children. *N Engl J Med* 304:749–754, 1981.

Otitis

Brook I: Otitis media in children: A prospective study of aerobic and anaerobic bacteriology. *Laryngoscope* 89:992–997, 1979.

Giebink GS, Quie PG: Otitis media: The spectrum of middle ear inflammation. *Annu Rev Med* 29:285–306, 1978.

Halsted C, Lepow ML, Balassanian N, Emmerich J, Wolinsky E: Otitis media: Clinical observations, microbiology and evaluation of therapy. *Am J Dis Child* 115:542–551, 1968.

Sell SH, Wilson DA, Stamm JM, Chazen EM: Treatment of otitis media caused by *Hemophilus influenzae*: Evaluation of three antimicrobial regimens. *South Med J* 71:1493–1497, 1978.

Shurin PA, Howie VM, Pelton SI, Ploussard JH, Klein JO: Bacterial etiology of otitis media during the first six weeks of life. *J Pediatr* 92:893–896, 1978.

Wolinsky E: Otitis media: Clinical observations, microbiology and evaluation of therapy. *Am J Dis Child* 115:542–551, 1968.

Zaky DA, Bentley DW, Lowy K, Betts RF, Douglas RG: Malignant external otitis: A severe form of otitis in diabetic patients. *Am J Med* 61:298–302, 1976.

Orofacial Infections

Chow AW, Roser SM, Brady FA: Orofacial odontogenic infections. *Ann Intern Med* 88:392–492, 1978.

Miller GD, Tindall JP: Hand-foot-and-mouth disease. *JAMA* 203:107–110, 1968.

Spruance SL, Overall JC, Kern ER, Kaueger GG, Pliam V, Miller W: The natural history of recurrent herpes simplex labialis: Implications for antiviral therapy. *N Engl J Med* 297:69–75, 1977.

Pneumonia

Bartlett JG, Gorbach SL: The triple threat of aspiration pneumonia. *Chest* 68:560–566, 1975.

Kirby BD, Snyder KM, Meyer RD, Finegold SM: Legionnaire's disease: Clinical features of 24 cases. *Ann Intern Med* 89:297–309, 1978.

Murray HW, Masur H, Senterfit LB, Roberts RB: The protean manifestations of mycoplasma pneumoniae infection in adults. *Am J Med* 58:239–242, 1975.

Pratter MR, Irwin RS: Transtracheal aspiration: Guidelines for safety. *Chest* 76:518–520, 1979.

Sullivan RJ Jr, Dowdle WR, Marine WM, Hierholzer JC: Adult pneumonia in a general hospital: Etiology and host risk factors. *Arch Intern Med* 129:935–942, 1972.

Gastroenteritis

Horowitz MA: Specific diagnosis of food borne disease. *Gastroenterology* 73:375–381, 1977.

Plorde JJ: Current management of infectious diarrhea. *Drug Therapy* August 1979, pp 53–64.

Plotkin GR, Kluge RM, Waldman RM: Gastroenteritis: Etiology, pathophysiology and clinical manifestations. *Medicine* 58:95–114, 1979.

Urinary Tract Infections

Braude AI: Current concepts of pyelonephritis. *Medicine* 52:257–264, 1973.

Komaroff AL, Pass TM, McCue JO, Cohen AB, Hendricks TM, et al: Management strategies for urinary and vaginal infections. *Arch Intern Med* 138:1069–1073, 1978.

Meares EM Jr: Prostatitis and related diseases. DM 26:7–39, 1980.

Rubin RH, Fang LST, Jones SR, Munford RS, Slepack JM, et al: Single-dose amoxicillin therapy for urinary tract infection. *JAMA* 244:561–564, 1980.

Stamm WE, Running K, McKevitt M, Counts GW, Turck M, Holmes KK: Treatment of the acute urethal syndrome. *N Engl J Med* 304:956–958, 1981.

Stamm WE, Wagner KF, Amsel R, Alexander ER, Turck, M, et al.: Causes of the acute urethral syndrome in women. *N Engl J Med* 303:409–415, 1980.

Turck M: Urinary tract infections. *Hosp Pract* 15:49–58, 1980.

Urethritis

Center for Disease Control Recommended Treatment Schedules: Gonorrhea. MMWR 28:13–16, 21, 1979.

Jacobs NF, Kraus SJ: Gonococcal and nongonococcal urethritis in men: Clinical and laboratory differentiation. *Ann Intern Med* 82:7–12, 1975.

Medical Letter: Treatment of urinary tract infections. August 7, 1981.

Smith JW, Jones SR, Reed WP, Tice AD, Deupree RH, Kaiser B: Recurrent urinary tract infections in men. *Ann Intern Med* 91:544–548, 1979.

Swartz SL, Kraus SJ, Herrmann KL, Stargel MD, Brown WJ, Allen SD: Diagnosis and etiology of nongonococcal urethritis. *J Infect Dis* 138:445–454, 1972.

Infectious Mononucleosis

Evans A: Infectious mononucleosis and related syndromes. *Am J Med Sci* 276:325–339, 1978.

Ginsburg CM, Henle W, Henle G, Horwitz CA: Infectious mononucleosis in children: Evaluation of Epstein-Barr virus–specific serologic data. *JAMA* 237:781–785, 1977.

Horwitz CA, Henle W, Henle G, Polesky M, Balfour HH, et al: Heterophile negative infectious mononucleosis-like illnesses: Laboratory confirmation of 43 cases. *Am J Med* 63:947–957, 1977.

Meningitis

Feigin RD, Shackelford PG: Value of repeat lumbar puncture in the differential diagnosis of meningitis. *N Engl J Med* 289:571–574, 1979.

Geisler PJ, Nelson KE, Levin S, Reddi KT, Mose VK: Community acquired purulent meningitis: A review of 1316 cases during the antibiotic era, 1954–1976. *Rev Infect Dis* 1:725–745, 1980.

Karandanis D, Shulman JA: Recent survey of infectious meningitis in adults: Review of laboratory findings in bacterial, tuberculosis and aseptic meningitis. *South Med J* 69:449–457, 1976.

McCracken GH Jr, Mize SG, Threlked N: Intraventricular gentamicin therapy in Gram-negative bacillary meningitis of infancy: Report of the second neonatal meningitis cooperative study group. *Lancet* 1:789–791, 1980.

Singer JI, Maur PR, Riley JP, Burger Smith P: Management of central nervous system infections during an epidemic of enteroviral aseptic meningitis. *J Pediatr* 96:559–563, 1980.

Septic Arthritis

Goldenberg DL, Cohen AS: Acute infectious arthritis: A review of patients with nongonococcal joint infections (with emphasis on therapy and prognosis). *Am J Med* 60:369–377, 1976.

Holmes KK, Counts GW, Beaty HN: Disseminated gonococcal infection. *Ann Intern Med* 74:879–993. 1973.

Masi AI, Eisenstein BJ: Disseminated gonococcal infection (DGI) and gonococcal arthritis (GCA): II. Clinical manifestations, diagnosis, complications, treatment and prevention. *Semin Arthritis Rheum* 10:173–197, 1981.

Rosenthal J, Bole GG, Robinson WD: Acute nongonococcal infectious arthritis: Evaluation of risk factors, therapy, and outcome. *Arthritis Rheum* 23:889–897, 1980.

Septic Bursitis

Ho G Jr., Tice AD : Comparison of nonseptic and bursitis: Further observations on the treatment of septic bursitis. *Arch Intern Med* 139:1269–1273, 1979.

Ho G Jr, Tice AD, Kaplan SR: Septic bursitis in the prepatellar and olecranon bursae: An analysis of 25 cases. *Ann Intern Med* 89:21–27, 1978.

21. Burns

G. RICHARD BRAEN, M.D.

In the United States over 2 million people per year suffer thermal burns. A great majority of these burns are minor in nature, while 3 to 5 percent may be life-threatening. Most minor burns heal spontaneously, but inappropriate treatment may delay healing, lead to infection, or cause complications.

PATHOPHYSIOLOGY OF THERMAL INJURIES

The skin is the largest organ of the body. Its thickness varies from 1 to 3 mm, being thicker on the dorsal and extensor aspects of the body. It not only is a waterproof barrier for the body, but also aids in temperature regulation.

The skin is composed of two layers, the epidermis and the dermis. The epidermis comprises the outer layer of the skin and is further divided into five sublayers. From superficial to deep, these layers include (1) the stratum corneum, (2) stratum lucidum (present only in thick areas, such as the palms of the hands and soles of the feet), (3) stratum granulosum, (4) stratum spinosum, and (5) the stratum germinativum.

The stratum corneum forms the vapor barrier of the body because of its keratin and lipid content. When this layer is damaged, fluid loss may be extensive. The stratum germinativum is the layer from which new epidermal cells are produced. Portions of the stratum germinativum are also found around some of the epidermal appendages that lie in the dermis, e.g., hair follicles, sebaceous glands, and sweat glands. If the entire epidermis is damaged, but some of the epidermal appendages within the dermis remain intact, the stratum germinativum that surrounds these appendages may regenerate a new epidermis.

The dermis contains fibrous connective tissue and blood vessels that support the epidermis and supply it with nutrients. In addition to hair follicles, sebaceous glands, and sweat glands, the dermis contains peripheral nerve fibers that form a plexus near the lipodermal junction. Superficial burns are more painful than deeper burns because these pain-transmitting nerve fibers, which lie deep in the dermis, are irritated in superficial burns rather than being destroyed as they are in a deeper burn.

Beneath the dermis lies a layer of subcutaneous tissue that contains areolar and adipose tissue. The subcutaneous tissue also contains collagen fibers that bind and support the more superficial layers.

The water, lipid content, and vascularity of these various layers influence heat conductivity and subsequent depth of the burn. The greater the water content, the greater the heat conduction, and the more rapidly damage occurs. In highly vascular areas, however, heat can be transferred away from the burn site by blood flow, and this heat dissipation may decrease the depth of burn in such an area.

The water loss from burned skin may be considerable, ranging from 5 to 15 times normal. In conjunction with the evaporation of water, a considerable amount of body heat may be lost, and hypothermia may develop. In order to maintain the body's core temperature, metabolic and caloric demands are increased.[1]

The chance of localized and subsequent systemic infection increases greatly following a burn of the skin. In deeper burns, the skin undergoes coagulation necrosis, which provides an excellent growth medium for bacteria. Since blood vessels within a deeper burn may be destroyed and normal host defense mechanisms, such as white blood cell migration into the wound, may be altered, the natural defense against infection is decreased. Essentially, the immune response of the host decreases in proportion to the extent and depth of the burn.[2]

Almost immediately following a burn injury, the vascularity of the skin in the involved area changes. Three concentric areas of vascular change may be identified on the surface of the skin at the damaged site. The center area, which is called the *zone of coagulation* (seen particularly in deeper burns), is the area of greatest destruction.[3] Within this area, thermal coagulation and irreversible cellular death occur. Also within this area, all blood vessels and capillaries become occluded. As the intensity of the heat or length of exposure increases, this zone of coagulation extends more deeply into the skin, producing a full-thickness destruction.[4]

Surrounding the zone of coagulation is a *zone of stasis* that involves the vasculature of the dermis. Initially, it appears red and blanches on pressure. Within a few minutes, there is an abnormal aggregation of formed blood elements within this area, causing thrombosis. There is also vasoconstriction, which further decreases blood flow to the burned area. Some blood vessels in this zone remain patent, even though the overall blood supply is reduced, and circulation can be restored in these areas with appropriate treatment. Exposure of the wound to drying, further trauma, infection, or improper care may cause irreversible damage to this zone, however, converting it to a zone of coagulation with subsequent necrosis that could result in a full-thickness injury. This is preventable by appropriate treatment.

Surrounding the zone of stasis is a small *zone of hyperemia*, which is the area least affected by the burn. In this area, vascular integrity is maintained, and cellular death is minimal. This zone can be recognized by the bright red color that blanches on pressure. Almost all wounds have this zone of hyperemia at their margins.

Burn Shock

Shock following major thermal injuries is a common but preventable occurrence. Burn shock is due to changes in circulating blood volume and to cardiovascular changes. Circulating blood volume may decrease because of an extravasation of fluid and plasma into the burned area. In addition, there is an initial shunting of water and electrolytes into skeletal muscles throughout the body, even in areas not involved directly by the burn. This shift of sodium and water from the general circulation may play the greatest role in the development of shock during the first 1 to 2 hours following the thermal injury. Within a few more hours of the injury, however, the flow reverses, and sodium and water begin to move back into the intravascular compartment. By 20 to 24 hours following the burn, the fluid shift has largely stabilized.

Along with the fluid shifts, the cardiac output may fall to 30 to 50 percent of normal when the burn injury is extensive. This may be due in part to a circulating myocardial depressant factor that is created by the burn wound; this factor may directly decrease myocardial contractility, leading to a reduced cardiac output.[5] As the burn wound size and depth increases, the myocardial depression becomes greater, although there is wide variation among patients. (See Chapter 6.)

Other Pathophysiologic Considerations

Immediately following the burn injury, there may be an acute erythrocyte hemolysis because of direct heat damage to the red cells. Up to 15 percent of the total red blood cell mass may be lost in major burns. In addition to this direct damage to red blood cells, there may be a microangiopathic hemolytic anemia. During this time, both the patient's red blood cells and transfused blood cells have a shortened half-life. Platelets and leukocytes may also have shortened half-lives. This condition may last for up to two weeks after the burn episode.[6]

The kidneys may be damaged indirectly by the burn. Acute tubular necrosis may develop secondary to burn shock. Myoglobinuria may be a cause of renal failure. Fortunately, with adequate fluid resuscitation, acute renal failure due to hypovolemia is uncommon.

An acute adynamic ileus and gastric dilatation may develop after a major burn injury. As burn shock is corrected, the ileus and dilatation diminish. There may be a small amount of coffee ground gastric material aspirated from the stomach of the patient, which is probably due to a self-limited episode of hemorrhagic gastritis. Later, Curling's ulcers, accompanied by massive gastrointestinal bleeding, may develop in the burn patient.

PREHOSPITAL EVALUATION AND CARE

The prehospital care of burn injuries is concerned with (1) home care of a minor burn, possibly supplemented by telephone advice from a nurse or physician, and (2) initial assessment and care of a major burn by an emergency medical technician (EMT), followed by transport of the victim.

Most minor burn injuries occur at home, and it is common for emergency departments to be contacted by a patient or family member for advice on treatment. There are a few rules of general first aid that may be given. First, separate the victim from the cause of the burn; for example, any smoldering clothing should be removed. Next, the burn wound should be covered with a clean cloth (e.g., towels, handkerchiefs, sheets) soaked in cool water. This helps to stop the burning process and possibly minimizes the depth of injury by dissipating the heat. It also makes the patient feel more comfortable because it decreases the air currents over the wound.

Chemical burns may also mandate first aid measures. The injury to the skin is directly proportional to the duration of exposure and to the concentration of the offending substance. Any clothing that is soaked by the burning chemical should be immediately removed. (Those helping the victim must themselves avoid coming in contact with the agent.) Dry, powdered chemicals that may cause burning should be brushed off as much as possible. Specific neutralizing antidotes are not recommended, and the treatment of choice is *copious* irrigation with cool tap water.

Victims who consult emergency departments by telephone should be advised to avoid home remedies, such as butter, grease, or over-the-counter ointments. Some of these home remedies may promote bacterial growth on the burn wound, while others are difficult to remove for later wound evaluation. All patients who report burns should be encouraged to see a physician as soon after the burn as possible, since most burn victims are unable to judge the depth and severity of their own wounds.

EMTs and other ambulance personnel frequently are called to transport a burn victim from the scene of the injury. The EMT must initiate the proper care to decrease the morbidity and mortality of these patients. While the patient is removed from the source of heat, the airway, breathing, and circulation should be evaluated. There are 6,000 to 10,000 deaths annually from major burns, and half of these victims die at the scene of the burn, not uncommonly because of a simple problem such as an airway obstruction.[7]

After the airway, breathing, and circulation have been ensured and the burning process has been halted, the EMT may proceed to other treatment. The burn should be covered with clean sheets or sterile gauze dressings moistened with normal saline solution. This not only helps to arrest the burning process, but also may relieve some of the pain. Instead of saline moistened dressings, a dry, clean sheet may be used to cover a patient in

whom the burning process has been stopped and who feels relatively comfortable.

Some burn victims also require nasal oxygen (5 to 10 liters/minute). In addition to their burn, these patients may suffer from carbon monoxide-hemoglobin binding. This is particularly common when the patient has lost consciousness or has been burned in an enclosed space.

If the transportation time to the hospital will be short, no further treatment is necessary. However, if the anticipated transportation time is over one-half hour and the EMT or paramedic has the skill, an intravenous line with normal saline or lactated Ringer's solution may be started. During transport, the airway should be frequently reevaluated, particularly in patients with suspected respiratory burns.

EMERGENCY DEPARTMENT CARE OF THERMAL INJURIES

Initial Evaluation and Treatment

In the emergency department, initial evaluation of the burned patient's condition must include another assessment of the airway, breathing, and circulation, as well as an examination for other injuries that may have been sustained during the accident. For example, a patient burned in an automobile accident may have a cervical spine injury.

Since a major contributor to morbidity and mortality is burn wound infection, care should be taken from the onset of treatment to minimize contamination of the burn wound. Important steps include keeping the number of people dealing with the burned patient at a minimum; the use of sterile drapes; the use of surgical caps, masks, gowns, and gloves; and the use of sterile technique when starting intravenous lines.

The most immediate threat to the life of the burned patient is airway damage from an inhalation injury.[8] These injuries occasionally result from direct flame damage, but they more commonly result from superheated gases, steam, smoke, or toxic fumes that produce airway edema, changes in the physiologic properties of pulmonary surfactant, increased exudation in the upper and lower airways, deposition of carbonaceous material in the lungs, atelectasis, traumatic pneumonitis, and other types of damage to the airway and lung tissue.[9]

The diagnosis of an inhalation injury may be based on the history and physical findings. The history is important for the diagnosis, since many of these injuries occur when the victim is burned in an enclosed or confined space, such as an automobile. Physical findings (Fig. 21–1) suggestive of an inhalation injury include burns of the face, lips, tongue, or mucous membranes;

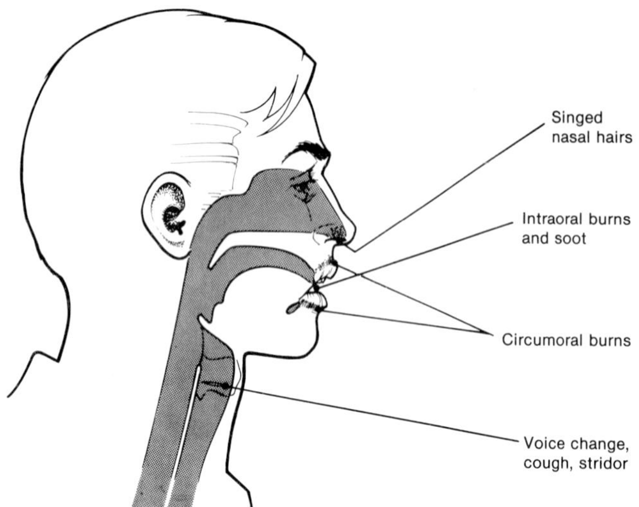

Figure 21–1 Physical Findings Suggestive of Inhalation Injury. *Source:* Adapted with permission from Marion Laboratories, Inc.

singed facial hairs; singed nasal hairs; hoarseness; wheezing; stridor; cough, particularly if it produces a carbonaceous material; or hemoptysis. The finding of stridor is particularly significant because it occurs when there is at least a 70 percent occlusion of the airway, an ominous sign.

The great majority of patients with inhalation injuries have associated burns of the face or neck, although the presence of head or neck burns does not necessarily indicate an inhalation injury. When these burns are present, a very careful evaluation of the patient's pulmonary status is necessary. Serial chest roentgenograms, arterial blood gases, possibly a diagnostic bronchoscopy, and serial pulmonary function studies are also needed. It is extremely important to consider the possibility of a pulmonary burn because this type of injury may lead to a significant reduction in the oxygen transfer potential of the lung with subsequent respiratory dysfunction and death.[10,11]

Circumferential burns of the chest may decrease respiratory excursions if significant edema and a constricting eschar develop. Such circumferential burns of the chest may require incision for release of the bandlike constriction. In addition, respiratory function may be altered by carboxyhemoglobinemia, which decreases the amount of oxygen that can be carried by the hemoglobin molecule, or by methemoglobinemia (due to inhaled chemicals) or a postburn hemolytic anemia, which also decreases the oxygen-carrying capacity of the blood. These factors working in concert may severely limit the transfer of oxygen to the tissues. Once the airway has been ensured, all major burn patients should be started on high-flow oxygen. An exception may occur with some patients having chronic obstructive lung disease, how-

ever, because carbon dioxide retention may become a problem in these patients.

If a respiratory burn is suspected, the initial step in treatment is the administration of humidified oxygen at a concentration of 40 to 100 percent with a flow rate of approximately 10 liters/minute. The use of humidified oxygen helps to keep the airway moist, inhibiting the inspissation of material that could produce atelectatic areas within the lung. The use of 100 percent oxygen is also important if carboxyhemoglobinemia is suspected. The half-life of carboxyhemoglobin is approximately 200 minutes in room air, but diminishes to approximately 40 to 50 minutes when 100 percent oxygen is given. When chronic obstructive lung disease is suspected in a burn patient, oxygen must be used cautiously to prevent the retention of carbon dioxide and subsequent carbon dioxide narcosis with respiratory depression. Initial blood gas determinations should be obtained as soon as possible, and the patient could be started on a 24 or 28 percent concentration of oxygen via Venturi mask. After 15 minutes, arterial blood gas levels should be measured again. If carbon dioxide has not been retained at that time, a higher concentration of oxygen may be used, followed by another blood gas determination in 15 minutes. When the patient begins to retain carbon dioxide, a lower concentration should be chosen for maintenance oxygen therapy.[10]

Particular attention should be given to the circulatory competence in burned patients. Minor burns generally do *not* require intravenous fluid therapy. If intravenous fluid therapy is necessary, the patient should probably be hospitalized. With extensive burns, intravenous fluid therapy should be initiated as soon as possible. The solution of choice for the initial resuscitation is Ringer's lactate through a peripheral vein cannulated with a large-bore catheter. Some experts in burn care feel that central venous lines are unnecessary and should be avoided in the management of major burns, except when no other intravenous route can be established. On the other hand, experts in the transport of burn victims feel that a central venous line is easier to maintain in the cramped quarters of a helicopter or ambulance and therefore prefer the use of central venous lines.

The physician may choose to begin intravenous fluids before the exact fluid requirement has been calculated. In this case, if an adult's burn wound is less than 30 percent of the body surface, an initial rate of 500 ml/hour may be chosen. Patients with greater than 30 percent body surface area burn should receive fluids at an initial rate of approximately 1 liter/hour.

Following the primary evaluation, the percent of the body surface burned is estimated. This estimation of percentage is used in calculating the amount of fluid to be given. There are several methods of evaluating burn wound size, such as the "rule of nines," the use of a Lund and Browder chart,[12] and the "rule of palms."

Under the rule of nines, the adult body surface is divided into 11 areas, each equal to 9 percent or multiples thereof (Fig. 21–2). The genitalia are assigned the final 1 percent. An adult patient with a burn of the entire left arm, the entire right arm, the anterior chest and abdomen, and the genitalia would have a 37 percent burn (9 percent + 9 percent + 18 percent + 1 percent), according to the rule of nines. The estimation of the body surface area in children is slightly different; during the first year of life, each leg accounts for 13 percent, while the head accounts for 18 percent. Until adolescence, these percentages of body surface in children change by a small amount each year.

The Lund and Browder method is more accurate than the rule of nines. With a Lund and Browder chart (Fig. 21–3), the patient noted in the previous paragraph would have a 9½ percent burn (right arm), 9½ percent burn (left arm), 13 percent burn (anterior chest and abdo-

men), and a 1 percent burn (genitalia), totaling 33 percent body surface area burn.

A very simple method of estimating burns is the rule of palms, by which the examiner compares the palm of the burn victim's hand with the size of the burn wound. Since the palm of the victim's hand approximates 1 percent, the examiner can compare the size of the burn with the number of "palms" to estimate the size of the burn. This is more useful for small burns than for large burns.

There are many formulas that can be used to calculate the fluid necessary for the resuscitation of burn victims. The lactated Ringer's formula is currently the most popular. According to this formula, the only intravenous fluid given during the first 24 hours is lactated Ringer's solution. The basic formula is as follows:

$$\text{Percent body surface area burn} \times \text{kg body weight} \times 4 \text{ ml}$$
$$= \text{Amount for the first 24 hours}$$

One-half of this total is given in the first 8 hours *following the burn*, and one-quarter of the total is given in the subsequent two 8-hour periods. The first 8 hours after the burn begins with the time of the burn and not with the time that the patient arrives in the emergency department. If 2 hours have elapsed from the time of the burn until the arrival of the patient, then one-half of the total 24-hour fluid requirement should be given within the next 6 hours. According to this formula, an 80-kg man with 50 percent body surface area burn would require 16 liters fluid during the first 24 hours of therapy; 8 liters would be given during the first 8 hours, 4 liters from the 9th through the 16th hours, and 4 liters from the 17th through the 24th hours.

To monitor the success of fluid resuscitation, urine output should be monitored in all extensively burned victims. The results of adequate fluid resuscitation include a urine production of 50 to 75 ml/hour in the adult, a slowing of the pulse, a stable blood pressure, a return to normal cerebration, and bowel sounds without an ileus. If these parameters neither stabilize nor improve within the first two hours of fluid resuscitation, the burn size should be recalculated and fluid administration altered accordingly. In addition, a careful search for hidden injuries that may have altered the fluid requirements should be made.

Two types of patients commonly demonstrate a reduced response to fluid resuscitation: those with massive burns and those with a decreased myocardial reserve, such as the elderly. The circulating myocardial depressant factor of burn shock, which directly depresses myocardial contractility and cardiac output, may be present. The failure of the cardiac output to respond to fluid therapy is manifested by a low blood pressure

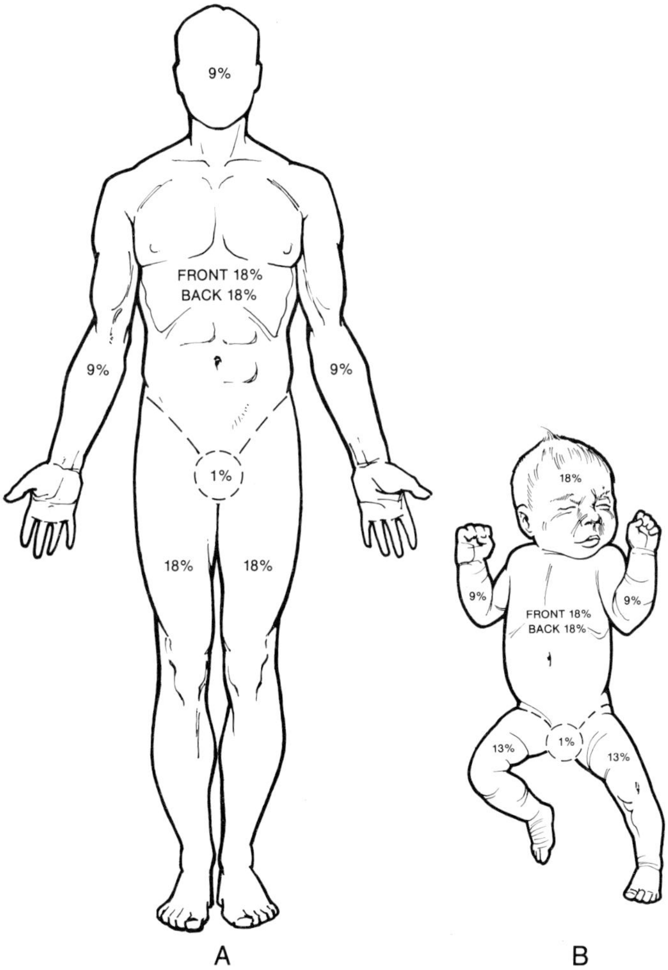

Figure 21–2 Rule of Nines. *A.* Adult. *B.* Adaptation for children. *Source:* Adapted with permission from Marion Laboratories, Inc.

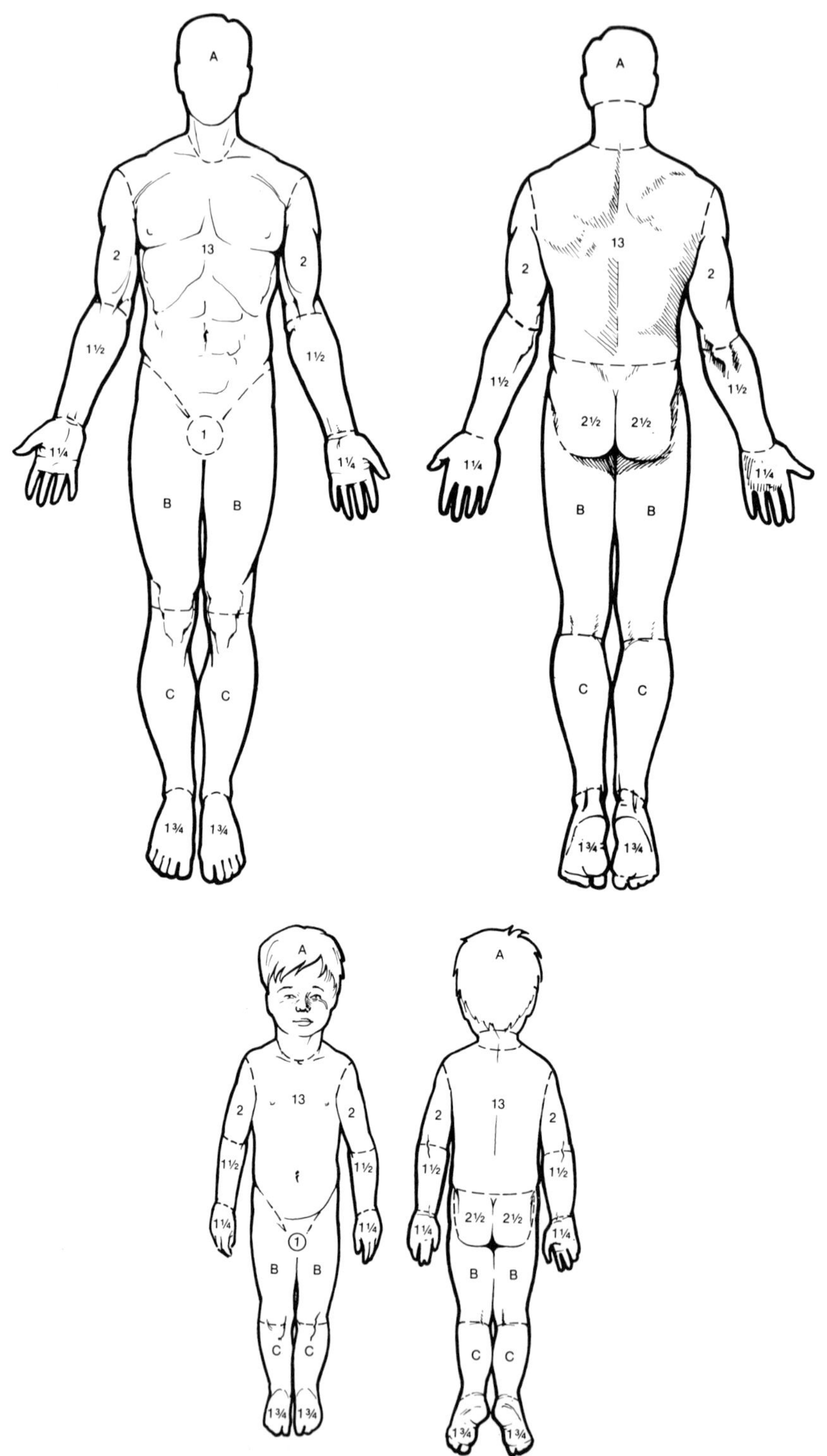

Figure 21–3 Lund and Browder Charts. *Source:* Adapted with permission from Marion Laboratories, Inc.

and elevated central venous pressure (possibly indicated by distended neck veins).

A nasogastric tube should be inserted for seriously burned patients, because it is common for them to develop gastric dilatation, gastric atony, and vomiting. The administration of antacids through the nasogastric tube may help reduce gastric irrigation and the devel-

opment of Curling's ulcers.[13,14] Cimetidine, which inhibits the action of histamine at the histamine (H_2) receptors of the parietal cells of the stomach, is being used in some centers to reduce the incidence of gastritis and ulcer formation in postburn patients. Cimetidine is rapidly absorbed following oral administration. Its half-life is approximately two hours when the patient has normal renal function, but the half-life is prolonged during renal impairment. The drug can also be given intramuscularly or intravenously. In an adult, the oral, intramuscular, and intravenous dosage is 300 mg every six hours. Clinical experience with cimetidine in pregnancy, during lactation, and in childhood is limited, and its use is not, therefore, recommended in these situations.

Laboratory Studies

Early in the resuscitation of a major burn victim, emergency care personnel should obtain baseline laboratory determinations on which further treatment can be based. These laboratory studies should include a complete blood count with differential blood cell count; measurements of serum electrolytes, glucose, blood urea nitrogen (BUN), creatinine, and arterial carboxyhemoglobin; arterial blood gas determinations, blood typing, and clotting studies. Patients may be under the influence of alcohol or drugs, and blood ethanol and drug screening should be considered. A baseline urinalysis should be obtained; if myoglobinuria is suspected, urinary myoglobin levels should be determined.

Precautions during Early Burn Treatment

There are a few precautions that the emergency personnel should take during the early burn treatment. First, burn victims frequently have associated traumatic injuries that must be treated before the burn wound is treated. For example, patients may have been involved in an automobile accident or an explosion in association with burns, or they may have jumped or fallen from buildings in attempts to flee a fire. Particular attention should be paid to the possibility of skull or cervical spine injuries.

Second, major burn victims should not be cooled excessively. Packing a patient in ice may initially relieve some of the pain of the burn, but this cooling may lead to hypothermia. Core body temperatures below 90°F (32.2°C) have been reported in burn patients who have been excessively cooled. Hypothermia not only increases the morbidity and mortality of burn patients, but also could freeze tissues, changing partial-thickness burns into full-thickness burns.

Third, narcotics should be avoided during the first few minutes of resuscitation until shock has been corrected and circulation restored. In addition, narcotics should be avoided if surgical consultation for abdominal trauma or neurosurgical consultation for head trauma is to be obtained.

Estimation of the Depth of the Burn

During the emergency phases of the care of major burn victims, it may be impossible to determine the depth of all areas of a burn because the depth of many burns is not clear until debridement has been performed. What may initially appear to be a partial-thickness burn may develop into a full-thickness burn during subsequent days.

First-degree burns, or superficial partial-thickness burns, involve only the most superficial layers of the skin (Fig. 21–4). The key diagnostic feature of the superficial burn is its erythematous, unblistered nature. Second-degree burns, or deeper partial thickness burns, involve the entire epidermis and parts of the dermis. Blisters form in this type of burn. Third-degree burns, or full-thickness burns, involve the epidermis, dermis, and subcutaneous tissues. Characteristically, the skin appears to be pearly white or charred, and the burn is *insensitive to pin prick.*

The American Burn Association further classifies burns into three categories: (1) major burn injuries, (2) moderate uncomplicated burn injuries, and (3) minor burn injuries. These distinctions have been made because the size and depth are not the only factors in the determination of the magnitude or severity of the injury.

Major burn injuries include

1. second-degree burns over more than 25 percent of the body surface area in adults and 20 percent in children
2. all third-degree burns involving 10 percent or more of body surface area
3. all burns that involve the hand, face, eyes, ears, feet, or perineum
4. all inhalation injuries
5. electrical burns
6. burn injuries complicated by fractures or other major trauma

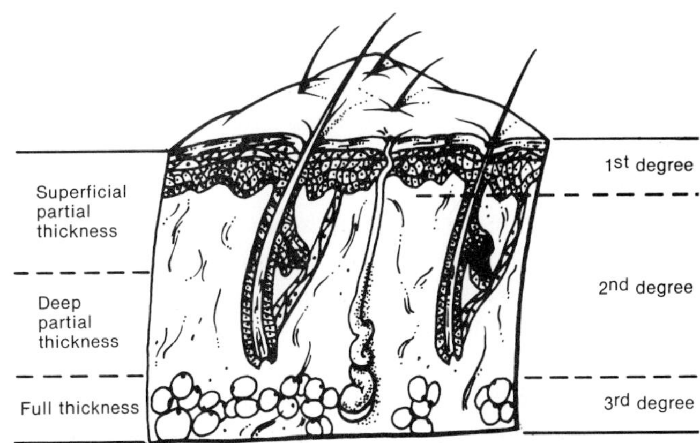

Figure 21–4   Depth of Burns. *Source:* Adapted with permission from Marion Laboratories, Inc.

7. all burns in poor-risk patients, such as those with cardiovascular disease, chronic obstructive pulmonary disease, chronic renal disease, hepatic disease, alcoholism, insulin-dependent diabetes, cerebrovascular accidents with residuals, head injuries associated with a loss of consciousness, severe psychiatric disabilities, and enclosed space injuries.

In addition, patients with sickle cell disease may develop a sickle cell crisis following a major burn. Almost all of these patients should be transferred to a burn center for care.

Moderate uncomplicated burn injuries include (1) second-degree burns of 15 to 20 percent of the body surface area in adults and 10 to 20 percent in children, and (2) third-degree burns of 2 to 10 percent of the body surface area if they do not involve the eyes, ears, face, hands, feet, or perineum. These patients should be cared for by a physician specifically trained in burn management.

Minor burn injuries include second-degree burns of less than 15 percent of the body surface area in adults and 10 percent in children, as well as third-degree burns of 2 percent or less if they do not involve the eyes, ears, face, hands, feet, or genitalia.

FURTHER MANAGEMENT OF THE BURN VICTIM

Drug Administration

The parenteral use of cimetidine and narcotics has been discussed earlier. The administration of penicillin and tetanus toxoid for prophylaxis should also be considered in many major burn victims, even though the use of prophylactic penicillin is controversial.

The first invaders of burn wounds are gram-positive organisms, particularly *Streptococcus*. The drug of choice for prophylaxis is aqueous penicillin G at a dosage of 1.2 to 2 million units for an adult and 0.6 to 1.2 million units for children. This is given by intravenous drip over 30 minutes in three to four divided doses each 24 hours. When the patient is allergic to penicillin, a substitute antibiotic, such as erythromycin, may be considered.

All burn patients should have up-to-date tetanus prophylaxis. In the previously unimmunized patient, 250 units human immunoglobulin should be given intramuscularly in one extremity, and 0.5 ml tetanus toxoid should be given intramuscularly in another extremity. The patient who has been adequately immunized previously should receive 0.5 ml tetanus toxoid intramuscularly.

Management of the Burn Wound

After all pieces of burned clothing, foreign bodies, and loose skin have been removed from the burn and after the initial life-saving resuscitative steps have been taken, care can be directed toward the burn wound itself. The burn wound may be washed gently with an antiseptic solution, with the exception of hexachlorophene-containing solutions in children; it has been reported that hexachlorophene is absorbed and causes an encephalopathy in isolated cases. After the skin has been cleansed with an antiseptic solution, a topical agent may be applied to the burn.

Over the past century many agents have been used for the topical therapy of burns. In the 1800s, carbolic oil was the agent most widely used, but early in the 1900s sodium bicarbonate paste was applied, followed by a solution of picric acid. In approximately 1910, the use of ammonium acetate was widespread, but it was replaced in 1918 by the application of warmed paraffin wax. During the Depression, tannic acid was the agent of choice.

Interest in thermal burns increased after World War II, mainly because of a fear of an atomic disaster. During that postwar period, extensive research was devoted to new topical agents and silver nitrate solution was introduced (1965), followed by mafenide acetate (1966), and silver sulfadiazine (1968). Numerous other compounds have been introduced for the care of major burn wounds, but they have not been as popular as these three.

Silver nitrate is effective on those burns in which an infection is not established. Some disadvantages of silver nitrate, however, have made this agent unpopular. For example, application is painful for the patient, and it leaves a dark stain on almost anything with which it comes in contact.

Mafenide acetate (Sulfamylon) penetrates burn wounds and eschars well, and it has an excellent antibacterial activity in infected wounds. There are, however, several disadvantages to the use of mafenide acetate: pain on application, maceration of the wound when used under a dressing, short duration of antibacterial potency, and the development of metabolic acidosis. Both mafenide acetate and its metabolite are excreted through the kidneys, and impaired renal function increases the risk of metabolic acidosis.

Silver sulfadiazine (Silvadene) is painless on application to burn wounds and does not inhibit carbonic anhydrase. The antibacterial potency of silver sulfadiazine is longer than that of mafenide acetate when used with a dressing. Local and systemic toxicity of silver sulfadiazine is very uncommon. Unlike mafenide acetate, however, silver sulfadiazine does not penetrate well into an eschar and should not be used in extensively infected burn wounds.

Minor burn wounds should be cleansed and debrided; then a number of methods can be used in the treatment of these minor burns. The burn can be treated in an open or closed fashion, with or without topical agents. Factors to be considered include the area of the body to be dressed, the depth and extent of the burn, the age and type of patient, the home or work situation, the patient's ability to care for the wound, and the availability of health care personnel to help in the home.[15]

Some clinicians treat minor burn wounds in selected areas, such as the head and neck, in an open fashion to allow exposure of the burned area to the air. Such exposure theoretically minimizes bacterial growth because moisture is decreased. As an alternative, burns in these areas can be treated with a topical antibacterial agent, but without a dressing. The antibacterial agent would be applied directly to the wound with a sterile tongue blade or a sterile-gloved hand. The dressing should be applied thickly enough to cover the wound completely. The agent is applied twice daily or as necessary if rubbed off. Before each reapplication, dried topical agent and exudate should be removed.

Closed dressings may be used for both outpatient and inpatient treatment. Closed dressings permit ambulatory management of small wounds, allow the patient to wear clothing over the burn, and may be used with or without topical therapy.

Burn dressings consist of a combination of layered materials, the innermost being a nonadherent, porous mesh gauze impregnated with a non–petroleum based, water-soluble lubricant. This mesh should be fine enough to prevent the ingrowth of new epithelium, but not so fine that the dressing becomes impermeable to exudation from the wound. Over the fine mesh layer is a layer of bulky, fluffed, coarse mesh gauze that absorbs any exudate and protects the wound from minor trauma. Securing this bulky layer in place is an outer layer of flexible semielastic coarse mesh bandage wrapped to apply a light, even pressure.

Closed, dry dressings are favored by many clinicians who view antibiotic agents as unnecessary for minor burns. Burns that cover less than 1 to 2 percent of the body surface area generally heal quite satisfactorily if simply enclosed in a dressing such as Xeroform or Adaptic and changed every three to five days.

Follow-up care for patients with minor burns treated in the emergency department is essential. Timing of the follow-up care depends on the extent and depth of the injury, the frequency with which the dressing must be changed, and the personal preference of the physician. When dressings that incorporate antibacterial agents are used, the first dressing should be changed at the end of 24 hours. When nonadherent, fine-meshed, po-

rous gauze is used, care should be taken to avoid simply pulling off this gauze during the dressing change because the underlying crust may adhere to the gauze. This crust is important because it protects the maturing wound, which is undergoing new epithelial growth.

Patients with newly healed burns should be cautioned against exposing that healed burn to the sun. These tissues are very sensitive to sunburning, and the application of a sun screen agent may be necessary. The patient may also notice itching and irritation of the newly healed burn wound; this can be relieved by the use of a mild lanolin cream (e.g., Alpha Keri or Nivea).

SPECIAL SITUATIONS

Myoglobinuria

Electrical and thermal burns occasionally cause myoglobinuria, which may be manifested by a brownish urine. Particularly in a patient who has a decreased urine output, myoglobinuria may damage the renal tubules. Myoglobinuria may be suspected rather than hemoglobinuria when the levels of serum muscle enzymes are greatly increased (especially that of creatine phosphokinase). Myoglobin may be positively identified in the urine by spectrophotometry or electrophoresis on gel or cellulose acetate. Treatment includes diluting the urine by increasing fluid therapy, using an osmotic diuretic such as intravenous mannitol at the rate of 25 gm/hour, or alkalizing the urine with IV sodium bicarbonate.

Escharotomy

Occasionally, escharotomies are performed in an emergency department. They may be needed in circumferential burns of extremities or chest wall burns when a constricting eschar and edema decrease respiratory excursions. The indications for an escharotomy in a burned extremity include peripheral cyanosis, decreased pulse strength, and a changing neurologic status. The most sensitive of these is a changing neurologic status, for example, the progressive loss of light touch or pin prick sensation of the hand in a burned arm. Early elevation and regular exercise of a burned extremity may decrease the need for an escharotomy. When edema develops beneath the constricting eschar, the interstitial pressure may rise to a point above that of the venous pressure, which could lead to ischemia and necrosis of otherwise uninjured tissues.

Transfer of Burn Patients

Many hospitals are unable to provide the total care that a patient with a major burn requires. In these cases,

Burn transfer checklist

TIME OF _______ AM

DATE_____________________CALL _______ PM

REFERRING DOCTOR_____________________

REFERRING HOSPITAL _____________________

PHONE #_____________________

CLOSED SPACE	YES	NO
ENDOTRACHEAL TUBE	YES	NO
VENTILATOR	YES	NO
IV LINES	YES	NO

(size & site) _____________________

CONSCIOUS NOW	YES	NO
DIABETES	YES	NO
HEART DISEASE	YES	NO

Type _____________________

ALLERGIES?   YES   NO

To what? _____________________

ASSOCIATED INJURIES: (Fracture, abdominal or chest injury, head trauma, etc) _____________________

_____________________ _____

THERAPY GIVEN THUS FAR

IV's ___________ cc Normal Saline

___________ cc Ringer's

___________ cc D₅W

Foley ___________ cc urine total

___________ cc urine last hour

IF PATIENT IS ACCEPTED SUGGEST:

1. M.D. accompany (if needed but must come with patient with endotracheal tube)
2. IV Morphine for sedation if needed
3. NG tube for burns over 30% or if drunk or intubated—DON'T CLAMP TUBE.
4. IV fluids—Ringer's fast enough to produce urine output
5. NO topical cream, antibiotics, IM meds of any kind. Debridement of burn wound to be discussed.
6. Escharotomy if needed
7. Does family know about transfer?

Widespread availability of this form for simultaneous use by both referring and receiving physicians will make telephone communication more precise.

PATIENT NAME _____________________

AGE _______ DATE & TIME OF BURN _____________________

TYPE OF BURN: FLAME   SCALD

ELECTRICAL   CHEMICAL   RADIATION

LAB RESULTS: Na_______, K_______, Cl_______,

CO₂_______, BUN_______, Sugar_______,

pH_______, PO₂_______, PCO₂_______

Is there blood in urine? _____________________

Chest x-ray _____________________

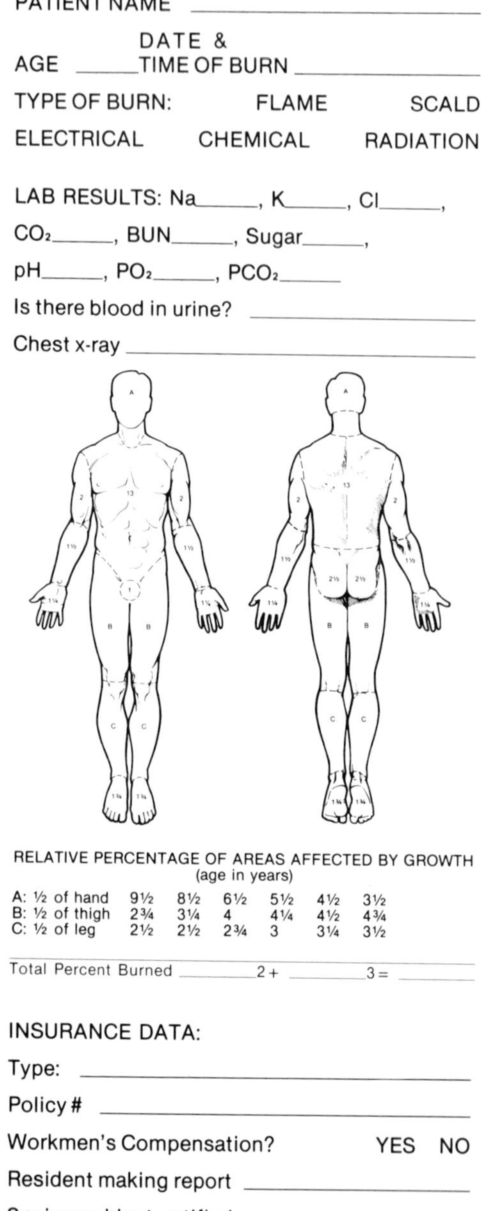

INSURANCE DATA:

Type: _____________________

Policy # _____________________

Workmen's Compensation?   YES   NO

Resident making report _____________________

Senior resident notified _____________________

Attending notified _____________________

Accept patient _____________________

Refer to _____________________

Adapted from *JAMA* 238:489-492, 1977.

Figure 21–5   Burn Transfer Checklist. *Source*: Reprinted with permission from Marion Laboratories, Inc.

transfer may be necessary. The patient should not be transferred, however, until fluid resuscitation is adequate, the airway has been ensured, and there are signs of reversal of burn shock. Even for local transfers, both telephone contact with a receiving physician and the use of a burn transfer checklist are essential.[16] Telephone contact with a receiving physician and hospital should include the following:

- patient's name and age
- extent of burn
- pertinent medical information
- fluid therapy started
- topical burn care initiated
- use of escharotomy
- adequacy of airway
- sedatives and analgesics used
- systemic antibiotics administered
- tetanus immunization given

In addition, the referring physician should outline a precise transfer plan to the receiving hospital, including the expected time of departure and the expected time of arrival, information on all aspects of air and ground transfer (e.g., ground ambulance to airplane to ground ambulance), and who will accompany the patient. The burn transfer checklist (Fig. 21–5) should accompany the patient along with any other pertinent medical records from the transferring institution.

CONCLUSION

Burns are not simply injuries to the skin. Many other organ systems can be involved, making this type of injury a challenge to emergency care personnel. In addition, the treatment of a burn brings out almost all of the evaluative skills that are necessary for a practicing emergency care professional. Appropriate emergency care can mean the difference between early recovery or even death.

REFERENCES

1. Artz CP: What's new in burns. *Med Times* 104:128–141, 1976.
2. Baxter CR: Pathophysiology and treatment of burns and cold injury, in Hardy JD (ed): *Rhoads Textbook of Surgery, Principles & Practice*, ed 5. Philadelphia, JB Lippincott Co, 1977.
3. Noble HG, Robson MC, Krizek TJ: Dermal ischemia in the burn wound. *J Surg Res* 23:117–125, 1977.
4. Zawacki, BE: Reversal of capillary stasis and prevention of necrosis in burns. *Ann Surg* 180:98–102, 1974.
5. Baxter CR, et al: Serum myocardial depressant factors of burn shock. *Surg Forum* 17:1–2, 1966.
6. Lloyd JA: Thermal trauma: Therapeutic achievements and investigative horizons. *Surg Clin North Am* 57:121–138, 1977.
7. Artz CP, Moncrief JA, Pruitt BA: *Burns: A Team Approach*, ed 1. Philadelphia, WB Saunders Co, 1979.
8. Moylan JA, Chan CK: Inhalation injury—An increasing problem. *Ann Surg* 188:34–37, 1978.
9. Jelenko C, Garrison AF, McKinley JC: Respiratory problems complicating burn injury. *Postgrad Med* 58:97–102, 1975.
10. Boutros AR, et al: Algorithm for management of pulmonary complications in burn patients. *Crit Care Med* 5:89–92, 1977.
11. Diamond AW, Piggott RW, Townsend PLC: Immediate care of burns. *Anesthesia* 30:791–802, 1975.
12. Lund CC, Browder NC: The estimation of areas of burns. *Surg Gynecol Obstet* 79:352–358, 1944.
13. Baxter CR, Marvin JA, Curreri PW: Early management of thermal burns. *Postgrad Med* 55:131–139, 1974.
14. Boswick JA: Burns. *Surg Clin N Am* 58, 1978.
15. Wagner MM: Emergency care of the burned patient. *Am J Nurs* 77:1788–1791, 1977.
16. Stein JM, Stein ED: Safe transfer of civilian burns casualties. *JAMA* 238:489–492, 1977.

22. Dermatologic Emergencies

GEORGE L. STERNBACH, M.D.

Skin conditions frequently induce patients to seek treatment in the emergency department because of the accompanying pruritus or the unaesthetic appearance of the skin lesions. Although common skin lesions are usually not indicative of serious illness, the possibility that a dermatosis may be a marker of infection or systemic illness should always be considered.

ACANTHOSIS NIGRICANS

The association of acanthosis nigricans with internal malignancy is well known, despite the fact that most cases are benign.[1] These benign cases may be familial, or they may be related to endocrine disease or obesity. *Malignant acanthosis nigricans* is the term used to designate that form associated with neoplastic disease. This term may be misleading, since acanthosis nigricans is only a marker of the underlying disease and is never infiltrated with malignant cells.

The lesion appears as a hyperpigmented, verrucous, velvetlike hyperplasia and hypertrophy of the skin, with accompanying accentuation of the skin markings. The chief sites of involvement are the body folds—especially the axillae, antecubital fossae, neck, and groin.

More than 90 percent of cases of malignant acanthosis nigricans are associated with intra-abdominal malignancies, about two-thirds of which are adenocarcinomas of the stomach.[2] Carcinomas of the breast and lung make up the majority of the remaining cases.[3] Regardless of the tumor type, acanthosis nigricans is associated with tumors that usually are highly malignant and metastasize early.[2] The mechanism by which this dermatosis develops in internal malignant disease is unknown.

ATOPIC DERMATITIS

The cutaneous manifestation of atopy, atopic dermatitis is associated with allergic diseases such as asthma and allergic rhinitis. Patients with atopic dermatitis are known to display both humoral and cell-mediated abnormalities of immunity.[4] Although the skin condition is chronic, patients frequently seek treatment of exacerbation at the emergency department.

Skin lesions appear as inflammatory macules or papules with indefinite borders. The skin is typically dry and scaly, but lesions in the acute phase may be vesicular, weeping, or oozing. The distribution of lesions varies with the age of the patient. Infants may have inflammatory, exudative plaques on the cheeks and in the diaper area. Older children have lesions in the antecubital and popliteal flexion areas. In adults, areas of involvement include the hands, feet, forearms, groin, and scalp.

Intense pruritus is the hallmark of atopic dermatitis, and low itching thresholds have been demonstrated in patients with this disorder.[4] Itching may be focal or generalized. It is worse during the winter and may be triggered by increased body temperature and emotional stress. Excoriations may be a prominent part of the clinical picture, and secondary bacterial infection of excoriated lesions is common. Repeated scratching and rubbing produces lichenification, a feature of chronic atopic dermatitis that consists of hyperpigmentation, thickening of the skin, and accentuation of skin furrows.

Exudative areas should be treated by application of wet dressings to reduce itching and crusting. Two to three layers of gauze soaked in Burow's solution should be applied for five minutes four times a day. Administration of antihistamines not only reduces pruritus, but also has useful sedative and soporific effects. Topical corticosteroids are the cornerstone of therapy, and should be prescribed in ointment form since this form is an effective lubricant for dry skin. Small amounts should be applied to involved areas three to six times daily.

BACTERIAL INFECTIONS

For a discussion of infectious disease emergencies, see Chapter 20.

Erythrasma

An infection caused by *Corynebacterium minutissimum*, erythrasma appears as dry, brown, scaly plaques with sharp margins, frequently localized to the groin. It is more commonly seen in diabetic patients. A coral red fluorescence under Wood's light is characteristic. Erythromycin (250 mg four times a day) is the treatment of choice.[5]

Gonococcal Dermatitis

The most common presentation of disseminated gonococcal disease is the arthritis-dermatitis syndrome.[6] It affects approximately 1 to 2 percent of patients with gonorrhea and is seen primarily in women.[7] Fever and migratory polyarthralgias frequently precede or accompany skin lesions. The lesions are often multiple and have a predilection for the distal periarticular regions. They begin as erythematous or hemorrhagic papules that may resemble the lesions of meningococcemia. Lesions evolve into pustules and vesicles with an erythematous halo. They are tender and may have a gray necrotic or hemorrhagic center. They usually heal with crust formation within several days, although recurrent crops of lesions may continue to appear for some time.[6,7]

Gram stain occasionally reveals the organisms within the lesions, but culture is usually negative. Immunofluorescent antibody staining of pustular fluid may be a more reliable diagnostic technique.[8] This has been thought to indicate that the lesions are the result of hematogenous dissemination of nonviable gonococci.[6]

Current therapeutic recommendations call for treatment with ampicillin, amoxicillin, tetracycline, spectinomycin, erythromycin, or penicillin. Ampicillin may be given as 3.5 gm orally, accompanied by 1 gm probenecid, followed by 0.5 gm ampicillin orally four times a day for seven days. The amoxicillin schedule is similar, calling for 3 gm orally with 1.0 gm probenecid, followed by 0.5 gm amoxicillin orally four times a day for seven days. Tetracycline may be administered orally as 0.5 gm four times a day for seven days. Tetracycline is not recommended for treatment of complicated infection, however, and should not be given to pregnant women.

Spectinomycin is administered intramuscularly, 2 gm twice a day for three days. Erythromycin is taken orally, 0.5 gm four times a day for seven days. Aqueous crystalline penicillin G is given intravenously, 10 million units/day until the patient's condition improves, followed by ampicillin, 0.5 gm four times a day for a total of seven days of antibiotic treatment.

Hospitalization is recommended for patients whose diagnosis is uncertain or for those who have purulent septic arthritis, meningitis, or endocarditis.[9]

Meningococcemia

The severity of meningococcemia varies from a mild febrile illness to a fulminant infection capable of producing death within hours. The onset is usually sudden, with the development of fever, chills, myalgias, and arthralgias. A rash appears in approximately three-quarters of cases; initially, it consists of nonpruritic, macular, erythematous lesions on the trunk or extremities. The lesions may be 2 to 15 mm in diameter, and they blanch on pressure. Petechiae may be present, and these occasionally coalesce to form large intracutaneous hemorrhages. The latter are seen in the Waterhouse-Friderichsen syndrome, which occurs in 10 percent of cases.

Meningococci can be recovered from blood and cerebrospinal fluid, as well as from fresh skin lesions. Immediate culture and treatment is imperative. Penicillin G is the drug of choice. Adults with meningococcemia or meningococcal meningitis should receive 24 million units daily in divided intravenous boluses. Children require 250,000 units/kg daily. Chloramphenicol can be administered as an alternative drug to patients with penicillin allergy.

Pyoderma

Most bacterial infection of the skin and subcutaneous tissue is caused by streptococci or staphylococci. Patients predisposed to pyoderma are those with various other skin diseases, obesity, diabetes, chronic granulomatous disease, dysglobulinemia, leukemia, and those receiving corticosteroids or immunosuppressive chemotherapeutic agents. Common skin infections include impetigo, the staphylococcal scalded skin syndrome, cutaneous abscess, and cellulitis.

Impetigo

Although impetigo, a pustular eruption, occurs at all ages, it is most commonly seen in preschool-age children. Group A *Streptococcus* is the primary pathogen. Poor health and hygiene, malnutrition, and various antecedent dermatoses—scabies, varicella, contact dermatitis, atopic dermatitis—predispose patients to impetigo.

Lesions are found most often on the face and upper extremities. They begin as 1- to 2-mm vesicles with erythematous margins. These break, leaving a red erosion covered with a golden yellow crust. Regional lymphadenopathy is frequently present. Impetigo may be pruritic, but it is not painful as a rule. The infection is very contagious among infants and young children, less so in older children and adults. Postpyodermal acute glomerulonephritis is a recognized complication.

Bullous impetigo, caused by Group 2 *Staphylococcus*, is less common than the streptococcal form. It is seen primarily in infants and young children. The initial skin lesions are thin-walled, 1- to 2-cm bullae. These persist longer than the vesicles of streptococcal impetigo and leave a thin serous crust when they rupture. Regional lymphadenopathy occurs rarely.

Impetigo should be treated with systemic antibiotics; topical treatment alone is not effective. Although systemic treatment shortens healing time of skin lesions and reduces the number of recurrences, there is no evidence that systemic antibiotics prevent the development of acute glomerulonephritis.[10] Treatment of choice is intramuscular benzathine penicillin: 40,000 units/kg for children under six years old; 1.2 million units for older children and adults. Alternatively, phenoxymethyl penicillin (penicillin V) may be given orally, 25 mg/kg daily or 250 to 500 mg four times a day for ten days. Penicillin-allergic patients may be treated with erythromycin, 250 to 500 mg four times a day.

Bullous impetigo may be treated with cloxacillin, dicloxacillin, or erythromycin. Topical therapy, useful as an adjunct, should consist of soaking in warm water three to four times daily to remove crusts, followed by the application of povidone-iodine (Betadine) or topical antibiotic ointment.

Staphylococcal Scalded Skin Syndrome

Although it generally occurs in children younger than six years of age, staphylococcal scalded skin syndrome has infrequently been described in adults.[11] It is also caused by infection with Group 2 exotoxin-producing staphylococci. The illness begins with erythema and a crusting lesion around the mouth. The erythema then spreads down the body, and bulla formation and desquamation follow. Mucous membranes are involved to a minor extent, if at all. After desquamation, the lesions tend to dry up quickly; clinical resolution occurs in three to seven days. Although this syndrome resembles toxic epidermal necrolysis in some respects, these two entities can be distinguished both clinically and histologically (see Toxic Epidermal Necrolysis).

Since most Group 2 toxin-producing organisms are penicillin-resistant, treatment has been with penicillinase-resistant penicillins—methicillin or dicloxacillin—although it is recognized that most patients recover completely without any antimicrobial treatment.[12]

Cutaneous Abscess

Folliculitis, furuncles, and carbuncles can be distinguished from each other by their size and the extent of involvement of deeper tissue layers. *Staphylococcus* is the usual infecting organism, although other infecting flora may be present simultaneously.[13] Folliculitis is an infection of hair follicles. The skin surrounding the follicle is not involved, and there is little erythema or pain. A furuncle, or boil, may develop from folliculitis as a result of infection of the dermal glands. This lesion begins with swelling and erythema that progresses as the center of the furuncle liquefies. The overlying skin becomes tense and very tender, and there may be significant surrounding induration or cellulitis.

Hidradenitis suppurativa is a disorder of apocrine sweat glands. It is associated with recurrent abscess formation in the axilla and groin. These abscesses should be incised and drained as indicated. The condition tends to be recurrent and may be extremely resistant to therapy. Antistaphylococcal antibiotics are useful if administered early and for a prolonged course.[10] Many cases do not respond, however, and local excision and skin grafting of the involved area may eventually be required. A carbuncle is a large abscess that develops in the thick, inelastic skin of the back of the neck, back, or thighs. Carbuncles produce severe pain and fever. Septicemia may accompany the lesions.

Superficial folliculitis should be treated with local cleansing and application of topical antibiotics. Furuncles and carbuncles should be treated by the local application of heat and they should be incised and drained when they point. Antibiotics need not be administered if incision and drainage is performed unless cellulitis or septicemia is present.

Cellulitis

An infection of subcutaneous tissue, cellulitis is manifested by erythema, swelling, and local tenderness. The margins of the infection are not elevated or sharply defined. Chills and fever may be present. The causative organism may be *Staphylococcus* or Group A *Streptococcus*. Treatment should include the application of moist heat and administration of antibiotics. If an extremity is involved, it should be immobilized and elevated. Severe or extensive cases may require hospitalization for parenteral administration of penicillin or nafcillin.

Erysipelas is a streptococcal cellulitis that affects the skin and subcutaneous tissue, most frequently on the face. The involved area is red, indurated, and edematous; its borders are elevated and sharply demarcated. Fever, chills, and systemic toxicity may be present. Treatment should consist of daily injections of procaine penicillin G (600,000 units) or oral phenoxymethyl penicillin (250 to 500 mg four times a day for ten days). Rapid improvement is the rule, but patients who are elderly or suffer from severe chronic illness may require hospitalization.

The appearance of cellulitis in very young children suggests infection with *Hemophilus influenzae*. Patients infected with this organism are usually six months to two years of age. The infection typically involves the face, causing a bluish or purple red discoloration, accompanied by marked temperature elevation.[14] Blood cultures are positive for *H. influenzae*. Treatment with ampicillin (50 mg/kg/day) or chloramphenicol (50 mg/kg/day) typically results in defervescence and rapid recovery within 24 hours.[15]

Scarlet Fever

Infection with Group A hemolytic streptococcal organisms causes scarlet fever. The illness has an abrupt onset with fever, chills, malaise, and sore throat. This is followed within 12 to 48 hours by the appearance of a distinctive rash, i.e., a generalized papular eruption overlying a hyperemic base. The eruption begins on the chest and spreads rapidly, occasionally involving the entire body within 24 hours. Classically, it spares the perioral area. The skin has a rough "sandpaper" texture owing to the multitude of pinhead-sized papules. The pharynx is infected, and erythematous or petechial lesions may be seen on the palate. Following resolution of symptoms, desquamation of the involved areas occurs. This desquamation is as characteristic of the disease as is the eruption.

Complications include streptococcal infection of lymph nodes, the middle ear, and the respiratory tract. Rheumatic fever and acute glomerulonephritis may be late complications. Treatment is aimed at providing adequate antistreptococcal blood levels for at least ten days, and penicillin is the drug of choice. In children younger than ten years, benzathine penicillin (600,000 units) and aqueous procaine penicillin (600,000 units) should be injected intramuscularly. In older children and adults, the dosage of benzathine penicillin is 900,000 units. In patients allergic to penicillin, erythromycin (250 mg four times a day) may be given orally for ten days.

CONTACT DERMATITIS

Contact dermatitis is an inflammatory reaction of the skin to chemical, physical, or biologic agents that act as irritants or allergic sensitizers. Irritant contact dermatitis is the more common form, with caustics, detergents, and industrial solvents being prominent causes.[16] Allergic contact dermatitis is a form of delayed hypersensitivity mediated by lymphocytes that have been sensitized by contact of the allergen to the skin. Clothing, jewelry, soaps, cosmetics, plants, and medications contain allergens that frequently cause allergic contact dermatitis. The most common allergens are listed in Table 22–1.[17]

The primary lesions of contact dermatitis are papules, vesicles, or bullae on an erythematous bed. Of the allergens, *Rhus* plants are the most likely to cause bullous eruptions. Oozing, crusting, scaling, and fissuring may be found. Lichenification is seen in chronic lesions. The distribution of the eruption depends on the specific contactant, but mucous membranes are usually not involved. A history of exposure and an appropriate distribution of the lesions are the most significant indications of the diagnosis. If there is doubt, the patient should be referred for allergic patch testing.

The first step in treatment is to avoid the irritant or allergen. Oozing or vesiculated lesions should be treated

TABLE 22–1   Common Allergens Causing Contact Dermatitis

Source	Sensitizing Agent
Topical medications	Ethylenediamine
Topical antibiotics	Neomycin
Jewelry	Nickel
Hair and fur dyes	Paraphenylenediamine
Leather	Potassium dichromate
Topical and parenteral medications	Thimerosal
Rhus plants: poison ivy, oak, and sumac	Urushiol

with cool, wet compresses of Burow's solution, applied for five minutes three to four times daily. Topical corticosteroid lotions help to reduce inflammation and pruritus. In some instances—such as severe cases of *Rhus* contact dermatitis—a short course of systemic corticosteroids is necessary.[18] Prednisone, 30 to 50 mg daily, may be prescribed initially, with the dosage reduced over a one- or two-week period.

DIABETES MELLITUS

A number of skin conditions are associated with diabetes mellitus. The most characteristic is necrobiosis lipoidica diabeticorum, which occurs predominantly in women, usually in the third or fourth decade of life. It precedes the diagnosis of diabetes in about 15 percent of patients.[19] The typical lesion is an oval or round yellowish plaque with sharply demarcated borders and a shiny atrophic surface, localized to one or both shins. A telangiectatic pattern often develops within the lesions. Control of the diabetic condition has no effect on necrobiosis lipoidica diabeticorum. Its appearance and course are similar in well controlled and poorly controlled diabetics, as well as in nondiabetics, in whom it also may occur.[20]

Diabetic dermopathy is the most common skin lesion found in diabetics. It is a nonspecific sign, however, since it also appears in nondiabetics. The lesions are oval or round macules located in groups or in a linear pattern, usually on the anterior shins. They are also found on the forearms. They are atrophic and depressed; they may be dull red or hyperpigmented. The lesions of diabetic dermopathy likewise do not fade with control of the hyperglycemia.[21]

Localized pruritus is very common in diabetics. The vulva, perianal area, and legs are frequent sites of involvement. The cause of this itching is often either *Candida* infection or excessive dryness of the skin.[21]

DRUG ERUPTION

Drugs may cause virtually any type of dermatosis, so a rash in a patient taking medication always raises the possibility that the drug is involved. Reactions tend to appear within a week after the drug has been taken, although reactions to the semisynthetic penicillins frequently occur later than this. Skin lesions may appear after a drug has been discontinued if the drug or its metabolites persist in the system.

The most acute and potentially life-threatening allergic reaction is anaphylaxis. Diffuse erythema, pruritus, and urticaria are the skin manifestations of anaphylaxis; they may accompany hypotension, bronchospasm, and laryngeal edema. Any of these manifestations may be seen, isolated or in combination. Although an anaphylactic reaction most frequently follows parenteral drug administration, it may also be triggered by oral ingestion. Symptoms of dyspnea, substernal discomfort, nausea, vomiting, and hyperperistalsis typically develop within 5 to 30 minutes following administration of the drug.

Epinephrine is the drug of choice in treatment. It should be administered subcutaneously, 0.3 to 0.5 ml in a 1:1,000 solution, unless shock is present. In this case, it may be given intravenously, 1 to 2 ml in a 1:10,000 solution. Intravenous fluids should also be administered. Pressor agents such as levarterenol or dopamine should be considered if hypotension cannot be reversed by these measures. Diphenhydramine hydrochloride (Benadryl), 50 mg, may be administered intravenously or orally for therapy of urticaria, but this should be considered of secondary importance in the treatment.

Serum sickness is a systemic allergic reaction comprised of an urticarial or maculopapular rash accompanied by fever, myalgia, arthritis, edema, and lymphadenopathy. Although initially described as a reaction to horse serum, it is now found most frequently associated with drugs. There is a latent period of 5 to 14 days between the administration of the inducing drug and the onset of symptoms. The syndrome is usually self-limited, resolving within a week. When a long-acting penicillin or sulfonamide is involved, symptoms may appear as late as three weeks after termination of therapy and persist for a month.[22] Other medications that cause serum sickness include aspirin, barbiturates, digitalis, insulin, phenylbutazone, diphenylhydantoin.[23] Treatment for serum sickness is far less urgent than that for anaphylaxis. Allergic symptoms may be controlled by discontinuation of the drug and administration of corticosteroids or antihistamines.[24]

Drug eruptions have numerous forms. Skin lesions of urticaria, erythema multiforme, erythema nodosum, and toxic epidermal necrolysis may be drug-induced. In addition, drug eruptions may be exanthemic, eczematous, vasculitic, purpuric, photosensitive, and fixed.

Exanthemic drug eruptions are the most common type. Resembling the skin manifestations of various viral infections, they are usually widespread, symmetrical maculopapular eruptions. Severe cases may progress to exfoliative dermatitis. Drugs that commonly produce exanthemic reactions include barbiturates, chloral hydrate, insulin, isoniazid, meprobamate, penicillin, phenothiazines, phenylbutazone, quinine, quinidine, salicylates, sulfonamides, tetracycline, and thiazide diuretics.

Eczematous drug rashes resemble contact dermatitis but are generally more extensive. They begin as erythematous or papular eruptions that may become vesicular. Prior sensitization to a topical medication is common. Aminophylline, meprobamate, methyldopa, penicillin, phenothiazines, sulfonamides, and thiazides are common causes of this type of eruption.

Vasculitic lesions begin as erythematous papules or nodules, but they may ulcerate and become gangrenous. Chloramphenicol, quinidine, iodides, guanethidine, quinine, and other antimalarials may cause such lesions. Purpuric drug eruptions may be the result of bone marrow suppression or platelet destruction. In severe cases, inpatient management with systemic corticosteroid administration, platelet transfusion, plasmapheresis, or splenectomy may be necessary. Quinidine is a frequently implicated causative agent.

Photosensitive reactions result from excessive exposure to sunlight. Patients who are subject to photosensitive drug eruptions should utilize sun-screening agents during any prolonged ultraviolet light exposure. Anovulatory drugs and tetracyclines are well-known causes of photosensitive drug eruption.

Fixed drug eruptions are those that appear and recur at the same site following repeated exposures to a drug. The lesions are usually round or oval in shape and sharply marginated. They may be pigmented, erythematous, or violaceous; they may itch.

Treatment of drug eruptions should begin with discontinuation of the inciting agent. Pruritus may be controlled as needed by the application of drying antipruritic lotion (calamine) or lubricant (Eucerin with 0.25 percent menthol and 1 percent phenol). Cool compresses or tepid water baths with Aveeno or cornstarch may be useful. Diphenhydramine (Benadryl), 50 mg, or hydroxyzine (Atarax, Vistaril), 25 to 50 mg every six hours, is likely to be of benefit. If the condition is severe, systemic corticosteroid therapy—such as prednisone, 25 mg every six hours until improvement is noted—should be instituted. This is most likely to be necessary for severe erythema multiforme, drug-induced toxic epidermal necrolysis, or vasculitis.

ERYTHEMA MULTIFORME

An acute disease that is usually self-limiting, erythema multiforme is characterized by skin lesions that are erythematous or violaceous macules, papules, vesicles, or bullae in a symmetrical distribution (Fig. 22-1). This involves most frequently the soles and palms, the backs of the hands or feet, and the extensor surfaces of the extremities. Particularly characteristic is the presence of lesions on the soles and palms. The hallmark of erythema multiforme is the target lesion, which may be a papule surrounded by a zone of normal skin or a vesicle surrounded by a halo of erythema. This lesion is frequently found on the hands or wrists.

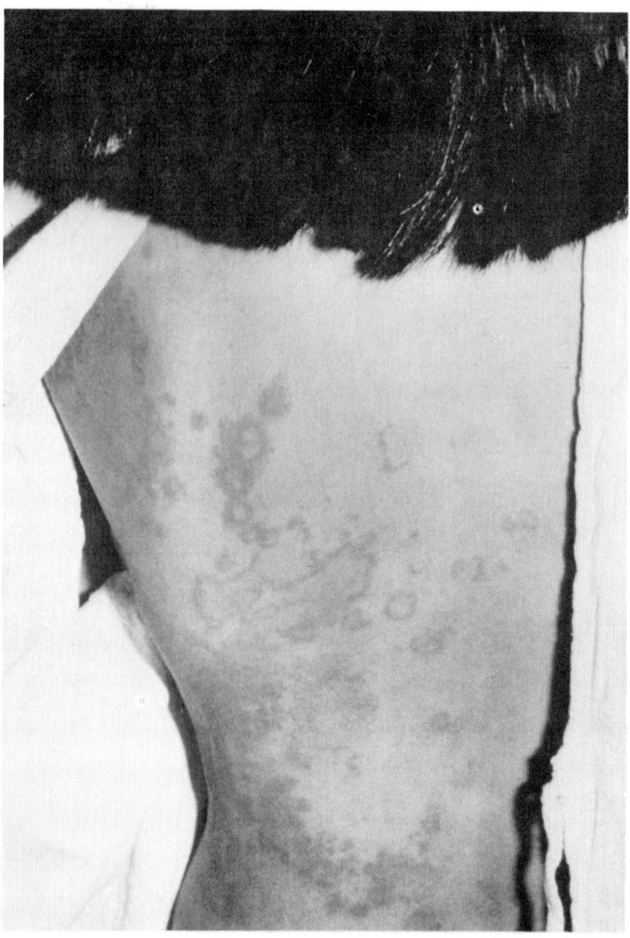

Figure 22–1 Erythema multiforme.

The Stevens-Johnson syndrome is a severe form of erythema multiforme that is occasionally fatal. It is characterized by bullae, mucous membrane lesions, and multisystem involvement. The patient may be acutely ill, with chills, headache, fever, malaise, tachycardia, and tachypnea, in addition to the skin lesions.

Erythema multiforme has a variety of precipitating causes:

- collagen-vascular disease
    - dermatomyositis
    - periarteritis nodosa
    - rheumatoid arthritis
    - systemic lupus erythematosus
- drugs
- infectious disease
    - fungal infection—systemic and dermatologic
    - hepatitis
    - herpes simplex
    - influenza A
    - streptococcal infection
    - tuberculosis

- malignancy
  - Hodgkin's lymphoma
  - leukemias
- pregnancy

The most common of these are exposure to drugs and herpes simplex infection. Drug-induced erythema multiforme is frequently caused by barbiturates, halogens, penicillin, phenolphthalein, phenothiazines, phenylbutazone, quinine, quinidine, salicylates, and sulfonamides. The long-acting sulfonamides in particular have been linked to the Stevens-Johnson syndrome. In about half of all cases, no provocative factor can be identified.

Treatment should begin with a search for an underlying cause. Severity of the condition varies; mild forms resolve spontaneously over a few weeks, while severe cases may require hospitalization. Treatment for severe cases consists of intravenous hydration and systemic corticosteroid therapy. Bullous lesions should be treated with application of wet compresses soaked in 0.25 percent silver nitrate solution several times per day.

ERYTHEMA NODOSUM

Patients with erythema nodosum have painful erythematous or violet nodules that represent an inflammatory reaction of the dermis and adipose tissue. The nodules occur most frequently over the anterior tibiae, but may also be seen on the arms or body (Fig. 22-2). Women are affected more frequently than men by a 3:1 ratio.[25]

A number of conditions produce erythema nodosum; e.g., tuberculosis, sarcoidosis, coccidioidomycosis, histoplasmosis, ulcerative colitis, regional enteritis, and streptococcal infections. Erythema nodosum has also been found in association with leukemia, Hodgkin's disease, and metastatic carcinoma.[26] As in erythema multiforme, many cases are idiopathic. The relationship of drugs to erythema nodosum has already been noted; oral contraceptive agents are the leading cause of drug-induced cases.[27]

Erythema nodosum is a self-limiting process that usually resolves in three to eight weeks.[27] When an underlying condition can be identified, this should be treated. Bed rest, elastic stockings, and elevation of the legs reduce pain and edema. Aspirin, 600 mg every four hours, may also afford some relief. Very symptomatic patients may be treated with potassium iodide, 360 to 900 mg orally daily for three to four weeks.

FUNGAL INFECTION

The dermatophytoses are superficial fungal infections of the skin that are characterized by scaling, pruritic

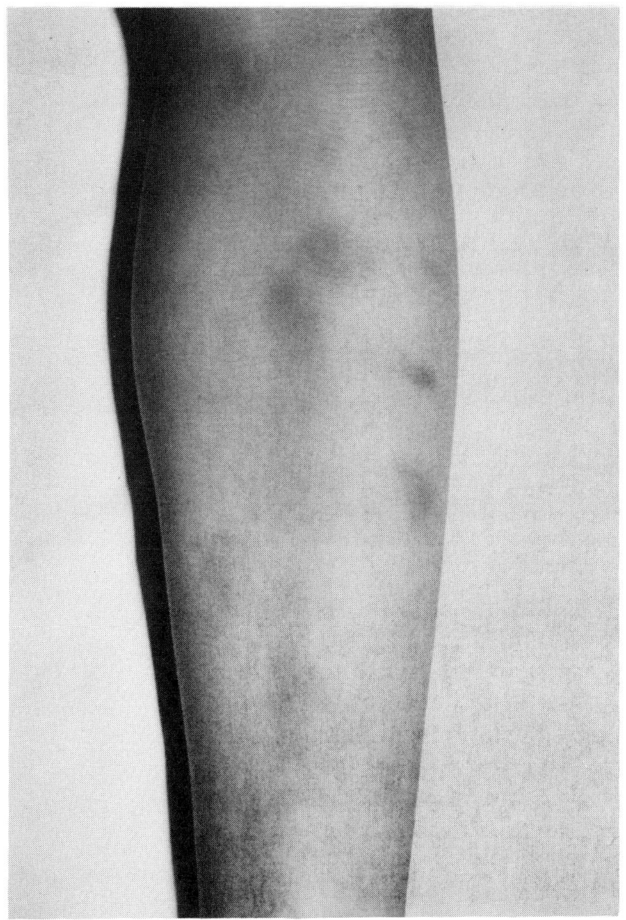

Figure 22–2 Erythema Nodosum.

lesions. Since dermatophytes generally grow best in hot, moist areas and grow only in the keratin layer of the skin, they are most often found in the areas where keratin tends to accumulate, e.g., in the body folds, between the toes, in the groin, and in the axillary and inframammary areas. With the exception of tinea capitis, the dermatophyte infections are not markedly contagious.[28]

Infection of the scalp—tinea capitis—occurs primarily in children. It may cause hair loss, resulting in circular patches of partial baldness. Infected hairs may fluoresce green yellow under long-wave ultraviolet (Wood's) light, although not in all cases. The disease may be transmitted by close child-to-child contact, as well as by contact with household pets, hats, combs, barber's shears, and similar items.

Tinea corporis affects the trunk and extremities. It is classically a sharply marginated, annular lesion with raised or vesicular margins and central clearing (Fig. 22-3). Lesions may be single or multiple. Dermatophytosis of the groin—tinea cruris—is similar in appearance. The perineum, thighs, or buttocks may be in-

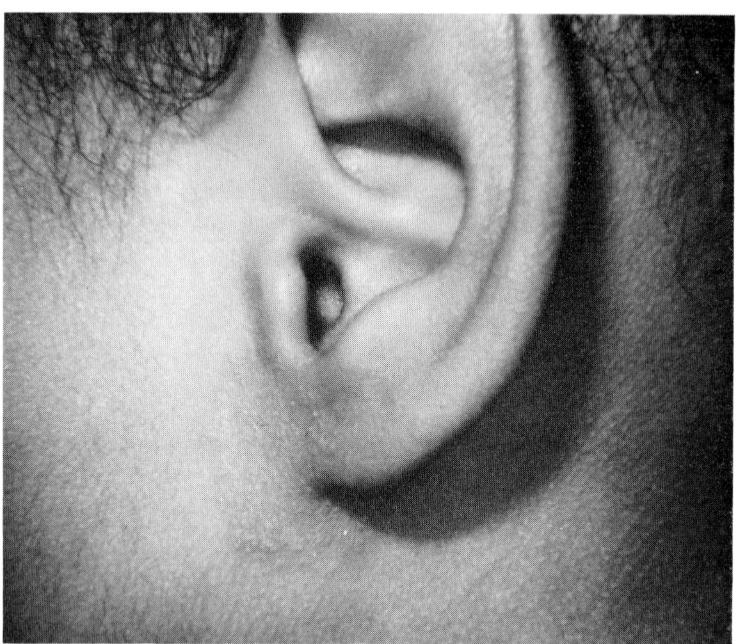

Figure 22–3   Tinea Corporis.

volved, but the scrotum is characteristically spared. It is often accompanied by involvement of the feet and toenails.[29]

Tinea pedis, or athlete's foot, is associated with scaling, maceration, vesiculation, and fissuring between the toes and on the plantar surface of the foot. In extensive cases, the entire sole may be involved. Nail involvement—tinea unguium—results in nails that are opaque, thickened, cracked, and crumbled; there are yellowish longitudinal streaks on the nails. The big toe is the digit most frequently involved.

An eruption thought to be a dermatophyte infection should be sampled and examined under the microscope in a potassium hydroxide preparation. The lesion should first be sponged with alcohol and allowed to dry. A specimen from the border of a lesion should be gently scraped onto a glass slide with a scalpel blade. The tops of vesicles or subungual debris can also be examined. A drop of 10 percent potassium hydroxide solution should then be applied and the specimen covered with a cover slip. The slide is heated over an alcohol lamp flame for a few minutes. The specimen should be examined for the characteristic long, thin, branching hyphae.

Infections of the body, groin, and extremities usually respond to topical measures alone. A number of effective topical antifungal agents are available, including clotrimazole (Lotrimin), haloprogin (Halotex), miconazole (MicaTin), and tolnaftate (Tinactin). The cream or solution of any of these should be applied two to three times a day; most superficial lesions heal in one to three weeks with this treatment. Acute inflammatory lesions with oozing or blisters should be additionally treated with wet compresses of Burow's solution.

Involvement of hyperkeratotic skin, such as on the palms and soles, may also require the use of a keratolytic agent, such as salicylic acid. Application of the gel form under an occlusive dressing overnight softens hyperkeratotic skin and leads to exfoliation. Keratolytic agents may, however, cause significant skin irritation.

Infections of the scalp and nails require additional treatment. Oral micronized griseofulvin, 5 to 10 mg/kg/day, should be given to patients with tinea capitis until lesions have cleared completely and scrapings are negative. This usually requires three to six weeks of therapy. There is also some evidence that alternate day or twice-a-week griseofulvin therapy may be as efficacious as daily administration.[30] Shaving or cutting the hair is not a necessary part of treatment.

Tinea unguium often poses a difficult therapeutic problem. Topical therapy of nails alone rarely results in a cure. Administration of griseofulvin, 0.5 to 1 gm/day for 6 to 12 months, is necessary. Headache, gastrointestinal discomfort, and photosensitization are common side-effects.

There are a number of predisposing factors to infection of the skin or mucous membranes by *Candida albicans*. These include infancy, old age, pregnancy, obesity, malnutrition, diabetes and other endocrine imbalances, malignancy, or other debilitating illness. Patients treated with corticosteroids, immunosuppressive agents, and antibiotics are also prone to such infection.

Oral thrush is the most frequent clinical expression of *Candida* infection.[31] It is most frequently due to inoculation of the infant's mouth during the passage through the maternal vaginal canal.[32] It appears as patches of white or grey friable material covering an erythematous base on the buccal mucosa, gingiva, tongue, palate, or tonsils. There may also be fissuring or crusting at the corners of the mouth.

Cutaneous candidiasis favors the moisture and maceration of the intertriginous areas. Lesions appear as moist, bright red plaques with scalloped borders, and small satellite vesicles or pustules are present just peripheral to the main body of the rash. Intertriginous lesions are prone to bacterial superinfection. Potassium hydroxide preparation reveals blastospores—oval budding yeast forms—or pseudohyphae, which have indentations at the septae.

Treatment of thrush involves painting the mouth with oral nystatin suspension—2 ml (100,000 units/ml) for infants, 4 to 6 ml for older children and adults—four times a day. Treatment should be continued for five to seven days after the lesions disappear. Gentian violet, 1 to 2 percent solution, is an alternate treatment.

Treatment of intertriginous lesions requires the removal of excessive moisture and prevention of maceration. Lesions should be exposed to circulating air from a fan several times a day. Inflammatory lesions should be soaked in or covered with compresses of cool water or Burow's solution. Nystatin dusting powder, lotion, cream, or ointment can then be applied. Clotrimazole and miconazole are also effective as topical agents.

PEDICULOSIS

The diagnosis of pediculosis pubis (crabs) is made by identifying louse eggs—nits—in the pubic hair or, occasionally, in other body hair. Nits, which are more commonly found than the adult lice form, appear as white dots attached to the bases of hair shafts. Adult forms look like blue or black grains. Patients complain of intense itching and scratching.

Treatment is the application of gamma benzene hexachloride (GBH—Kwell, Gamene) lotion or cream to the infested and adjacent hairy areas. A thin layer is applied following a warm bath or shower and left in place for 24 hours before being washed off. A second treatment may be administered in one week, although it is not usually necessary. GBH should not be applied to the face. Involvement of the eyelashes may be treated with the topical application of 0.5 percent physostigmine or petrolatum, applied twice a day for eight days.

Sexual partners should also be treated, but other uninfested household members need not be. Underclothing, pajamas, sheets, and pillowcases should be machine-washed and dried (hot cycle), laundered and ironed, or boiled. Pruritus that persists following a course of therapy may be due to irritation of the skin by GBH, sensitization, or anxiety.

Pediculosis capitis (head lice) is seen more frequently in small children than adults. Pruritus is the major symptom, although excoriation frequently results in secondary bacterial infection. Diagnosis is made by identification of nits cemented to hairs at the hair-scalp junction. Treatment consists of shampooing for four minutes with one tablespoon of GBH shampoo. The shampoo should be applied while the scalp is dry. Shampooing may be repeated in one week, if needed. Household contacts should be examined for involvement, but uninfested persons need not be treated. Clothing and linen should be washed as described earlier.

The organisms that cause pediculosis corporis (body lice) reside in the seams of clothing and bedding materials while they feed on the human host. Except in heavily infested individuals, the parasites are absent from the body itself. Erythematous macules or wheals may be present, along with intense pruritus. Treatment consists of laundering or boiling clothing and bed linen. If nits are found in the body hair, a treatment with GBH lotion may be used, but this is unnecessary in most cases.[33]

PEMPHIGUS VULGARIS

Although pemphigus vulgaris is an uncommon dermatologic disorder, it is an important one because it is potentially fatal. It is a bullous disease that is most common in the 40- to 60-year-old age group and affects men more often than women. The typical lesions are small flaccid bullae that break easily, forming superficial erosions and crusted ulcerations. Any area of the body may be involved, although mucous membrane lesions antedate cutaneous lesions by several months.[34] The most common site of these mucous membrane lesions is in the mouth, especially the gums and vermilion borders of the lips. Blisters may be extended or new bullae formed by firm tangential pressure of a finger on the intact epidermis; this is known as Nikolsky's sign and is characteristic of the condition.

The cause of pemphigus is unknown, although studies suggest an autoimmune mechanism.[10] The diagnosis may be confirmed by cytologic testing—Tzanck smear—or serum immunofluorescence. Once the diagnosis is made, treatment with oral glucocorticoids, initial dosage of 100 to 200 mg prednisone daily, should be instituted. Despite the condition's localization to the skin and mucous membranes, mortality in the presteroid era was 95 percent and continues to be substantial.[34] Most deaths relate to uncontrolled spread of the disease; secondary infection, dehydration, and thromboembolism may also contribute to mortality. Patients may also succumb to the side-effects of corticosteroids.

PITYRIASIS ROSEA

A benign skin eruption, pityriasis rosea is seen predominantly in children and young adults. The lesions are multiple oval pink or pigmented papules or plaques, 1 to 2 cm in diameter, appearing on the trunk and proximal extremities. Lesions may be scaly and are arranged parallel to the long axis of the ribs, forming a "Christmas tree distribution" on the trunk. In about one-half of cases, the generalized eruption is preceded by a week by a "herald patch." This is a larger lesion—2 to 6 cm in diameter—that resembles the smaller lesions in other respects (Fig. 22-4). The eruption is usually asymptomatic, although pruritus may be present.

Pityriasis rosea is a self-limited condition, usually resolving in 8 to 12 weeks. The etiology is unknown, although a viral etiology is suspected. Recurrences are rare. Treatment is usually unnecessary, except for symptomatic alleviation of pruritus.

ROCKY MOUNTAIN SPOTTED FEVER

Although originally described in the western United States, Rocky Mountain spotted fever occurs in other portions of North, South, and Central America. Most cases are currently reported from the southeastern United States. Rocky Mountain spotted fever is an acute infectious disease caused by *Rickettsia rickettsii*, an organism harbored by certain ticks.

Onset is usually abrupt, with headache, nausea, myalgias, chills, and a fever spiking to 104°F (40°C). Occasionally, the illness begins insidiously, with progressive anorexia, malaise, and fever. The rash usually develops on the second to fourth day of the illness. It consists of erythematous macules that blanch on pressure; they appear first on the wrists and ankles, then spread up the extremities to the trunk and face. This spread is rapid, occasionally occurring in a matter of hours. The presence of lesions on the palms and soles is particularly characteristic. Lesions may become petechial or hemorrhagic, capillary fragility may be increased, and splenomegaly may be present.

The Weil-Felix test is the best known serologic diagnostic test, but Weil-Felix agglutinins are not always present in Rocky Mountain spotted fever, and more specific immunofluorescent procedures have been developed.[35] Treatment should not await the result of such tests, but should begin as soon as the disease is diagnosed on clinical grounds.

Tetracycline is the antibiotic of choice. It should be given orally, 25 to 30 mg/kg daily in divided doses. If the patient is unable to take oral medications, tetracycline may be administered intravenously, with a 15 mg/kg loading dose followed by a maintenance dose of 15 mg/kg/day. Chloramphenicol may be used in patients allergic to tetracycline. Treatment should be continued until the patient is afebrile for 72 hours.

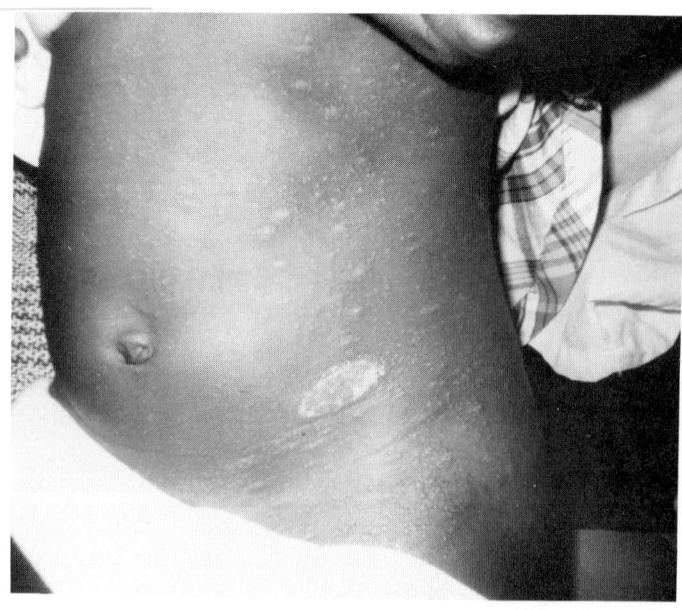

Figure 22–4 Pityriasis Rosea.

While deaths can occur in untreated cases, the response to treatment with antibiotics is uniformly favorable. The patient usually shows symptomatic improvement in 24 hours and is afebrile in three days. Administration of antibiotics should be continued for three days after defervescence.

ROSEOLA INFANTUM

High fever and a rash characterize roseola infantum, but there is a paucity of other physical findings. Ninety-five percent of cases are seen in children six months to three years old. The fever typically has an abrupt onset and rapid rise to 103°F (39.5°C) to 106°F (41°C). Fever is present consistently or intermittently for three to four days, then drops precipitously to normal.

The rash appears when the fever subsides. Lesions are discrete pink to rose-colored macules or maculopapules 2 to 3 mm in diameter; they blanch on pressure and rarely coalesce. The trunk is involved initially, with eruption typically spreading to the neck and extremities. The rash clears over one to two days without desquamation.

Despite the presence of a high fever, the infant may not appear particularly ill. Other physical findings are entirely nonspecific. The etiology of roseola is unknown, and there are no diagnostic tests. The prognosis is uniformly excellent, the most common complication being the occurrence of febrile convulsions.

SCABIES

Epidemics of scabies, a mite infestation characterized by severe itching, occur in 15-year cycles, with a 15-year gap between the end of one epidemic and the beginning of the next. The most recent epidemic period began around 1964.[36]

Areas of the body most commonly involved are the interdigital web spaces, the flexion areas of the wrists, the axillae, buttocks, lower back, penis, scrotum, and breasts. Infestation tends to be more generalized in infants and children than in adults. Typical lesions are reddish papules or vesicles surrounded by an erythematous border and scratch marks. Impetigenization of lesions is common. Close personal contact is involved in transmission of scabies, and multiple family members are likely to become infested. The infestation is also transmitted venereally.

Among effective treatment agents are GBH (Kwell, Gamene) and crotamiton (Eurax) lotion and cream. Patients who do not respond to the former may respond to the latter.[37] Following a warm bath or shower, the scabicide is applied to the entire body, except the face

and scalp, even though lesions may be localized. It should be left in place for 12 to 24 hours and then washed off during another bath. Children younger than five years should be treated with GBH for four hours only; alternatively, crotamiton may be used for these patients. A second treatment course may be applied in one week.

All family members and sexual contacts should be treated. In addition, intimate articles of clothing, sheets, and pillowcases should be washed and dried by machine (hot cycle), laundered and ironed, or boiled.[33] It may take several weeks following therapy for signs and symptoms to abate. Hypersensitivity or anxiety may prolong symptoms long after the mites have been destroyed.

SYPHILIS

The causative organism of syphilis is the spirochete *Treponema pallidum*. The primary lesion appears 10 to 90 days after exposure, remains for 3 to 12 weeks, and heals spontaneously. Six weeks to six months following exposure, the disease enters the secondary stage, which may include a variety of mucocutaneous lesions. These lesions also heal spontaneously in two to six weeks, when the disease enters the latent phase. Either a prolonged latent phase or tertiary syphilis follows. Twenty-five percent of untreated patients have at least one relapse of mucocutaneous lesions during the latent phase.[38] Such lesions are often located in the oral cavity or anogenital region.

The chancre is the principal manifestation of primary syphilis. Although they may be multiple, chancres usually appear as single lesions at the site of spirochete inoculation, generally the mucous membranes of the mouth or genitalia. The chancre begins as a papule and characteristically develops into an ulcer about 1 cm in diameter, with a clean base and raised borders. Painless unless secondarily infected, it may be accompanied by nontender regional lymphadenopathy.

There are a number of cutaneous manifestations of secondary syphilis. Lesions may be erythematous or pink macules or papules, usually with a symmetrical, generalized distribution. Pigmented macules and papules classically appear on the palms and soles. Lesions may be scaly, but are rarely pruritic. Papular, annular, and circinate lesions are more common in nonwhites (Fig. 22-5). Generalized lymphadenopathy and malaise accompany the skin lesions. Irregular, patchy alopecia may be seen. Moist, flat, verrucous condylomata lata may appear in the genital area. These lesions are highly contagious.

The diagnosis of primary syphilis is made principally by identification of spirochetes on darkfield microscopy. If darkfield examination is negative, another ex-

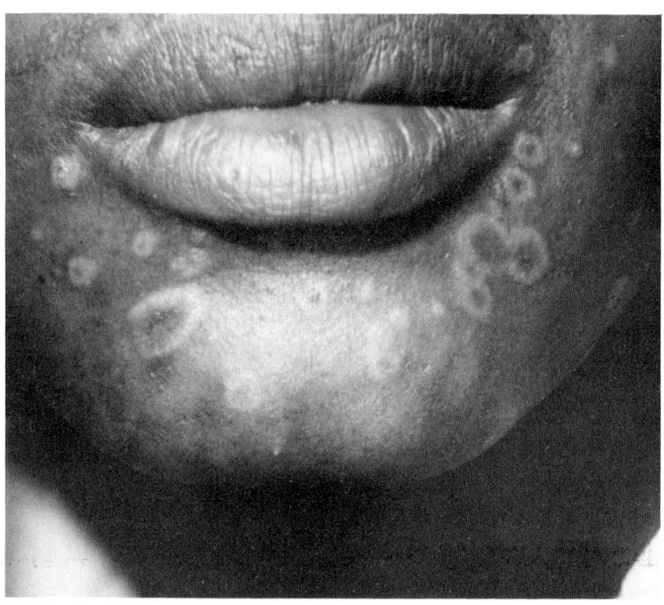

Figure 22–5   Secondary Syphilis.

amination is indicated in 24 hours.[38] The result of the Venereal Disease Research Laboratory (VDRL) test, the most commonly used diagnostic serologic test, is positive in about three-quarters of patients with primary syphilis, but it tends to be negative in the very early stage.[38] The result of the VDRL test is invariably positive in secondary syphilis, usually in titers of 1:16 or greater. Darkfield examination of moist lesions may also be positive.

The most specific and sensitive serologic test is the Fluorescent Treponemal Antibody Absorption (FTA-ABS) test. A biologic false-positive serologic reaction for syphilis is defined as a positive VDRL test result with a negative FTA-ABS test result. This is seen following vaccination or infections—especially mycoplasmal pneumonia, mononucleosis, hepatitis, measles, varicella, and malaria—and in pregnancy. Chronic biologic false-positive reactions, i.e., those lasting longer than six months, may occur with systemic lupus erythematosus, thyroiditis, lymphoma, or narcotic addiction; they may also be seen in the elderly. Most false-positive reactions are in low titer ranges of 1:1 to 1:4.[39]

Incubating syphilis—the stage prior to the appearance of primary lesions—may be treated with 4.8 million units procaine penicillin given intramuscularly along with 1 gm probenecid orally. Primary and secondary syphilis calls for treatment with benzathine penicillin G, 2.4 million units intramuscularly, or daily intramuscular injection of 600,000 units aqueous procaine penicillin G for 8 days. Patients allergic to penicillin may be treated either with oral tetracycline or erythromycin, both 500 mg four times a day for 15 days.

TOXIC EPIDERMAL NECROLYSIS

There are two forms of toxic epidermal necrolysis, both of which are characterized by the loosening of large sheets of epidermis from underlying layers of epidermis or dermis. One form is associated with *Staphylococcus aureus* (the staphylococcal scaled skin syndrome, see Bacterial Infections) infection and has an excellent prognosis, regardless of treatment. The other form may be associated with drugs, infection, or medical illness, or it may be idiopathic. This form carries a substantial risk of mortality. The two conditions are histologically distinguishable at skin biopsy.

The main feature of non–staphylococcal-induced toxic epidermal necrolysis is the separation of large sheets of epidermis from underlying dermis. The full thickness of epidermis is involved. In pigmented skin, the pigment is entirely removed when the skin desquamates. In contrast, substantial pigment remains in staphylococcal scalded skin syndrome. Toxic epidermal necrolysis usually appears first on the face, and mucous membrane involvement is the rule. Erythema usually precedes loosening of the epidermis.

Medications are an important cause of toxic epidermal necrolysis. Among those that have been implicated as inciting agents are the long-acting sulfa drugs, aspirin, penicillin, barbiturates, phenylbutazone, diphenylhydantoin, and allopurinol. Toxic epidermal necrolysis has followed vaccination and immunization against poliomyelitis, measles, smallpox, diphtheria, and tetanus. It has also been found in association with lymphoma.

The mechanism that results in toxic epidermal necrolysis is not known. Treatment includes fluid replacement and the administration of systemic corticosteroids. Prednisone, as much as 300 mg daily or its equivalent, has been used, but deaths occur despite high-dose steroid therapy.[40]

URTICARIA

Among the most common skin lesions seen in emergency medicine, urticaria appears as circumscribed, raised wheals that represent localized edema produced by transvascular fluid extravasation (Fig. 22-6). The wheals, or hives, may be slightly erythematous with central clearing. Urticaria is classified as acute or chronic, depending on whether its duration is greater than some arbitrary time limit, usually four to six weeks. Acute urticaria, which is seen in patients of both sexes, is more likely to have an allergic cause. Chronic urticaria is more common in women in their 40s and 50s, and it may persist for years.

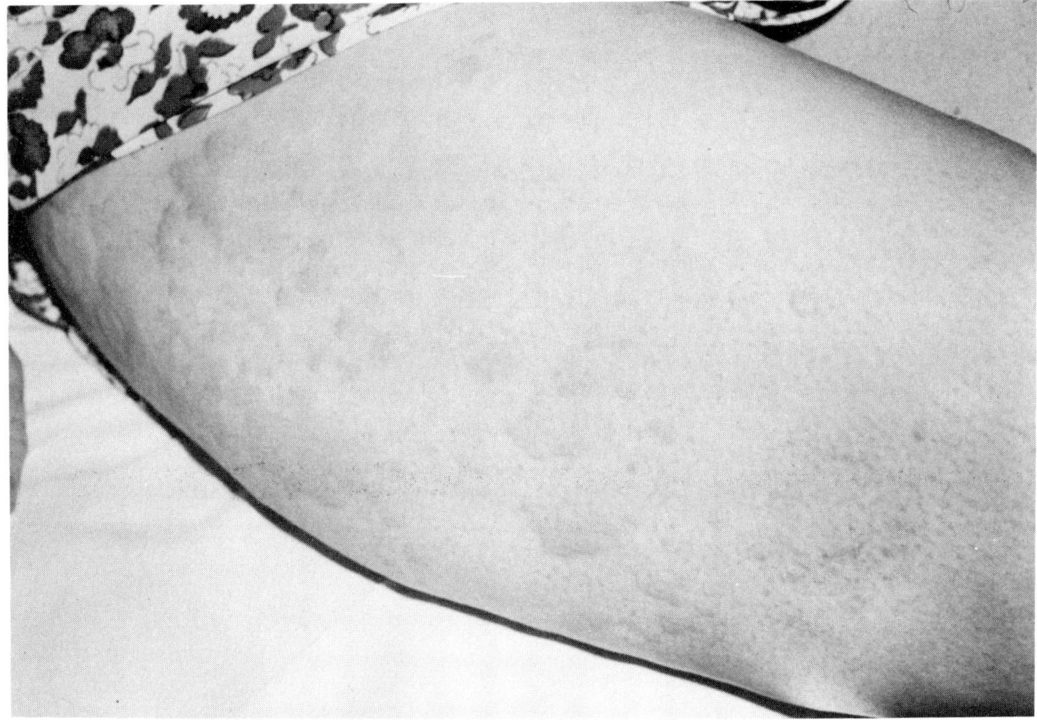

Figure 22–6 Urticaria.

Various mediators, including histamine, bradykinin, kallikrein, and acetylcholine, are thought to play a role in urticaria. Their release may be initiated by immunologic mechanisms, as in anaphylaxis and serum sickness, or by nonimmunologic degranulation of mast cells. The latter may be accomplished by a number of drugs and foods.

Substances that can cause urticaria by contact with the skin include foods, textiles, animal dander and saliva, plants, topical medications, chemicals, and cosmetics.[41] Although virtually any drug can cause urticaria, aspirin and penicillin most frequently produce this eruption.[23,42] Penicillin may be present in trace amounts in dairy products, as well as in medications. Drug-induced urticaria is not invariably allergic. Some drugs—notably the narcotics—may cause urticaria by the direct release of histamine.

A variety of food allergies may result in urticaria, such as sensitivity to fish, eggs, and nuts. In addition, foods such as lobster and strawberries are able to release histamine through a nonimmunologic mechanism. Hereditary forms of urticaria include familial cold urticaria and hereditary angioneurotic edema.

Infections are an uncommon cause of urticaria, although infection with *Candida*, the dermatophytes, bacteria, viruses, and parasites may trigger hives. Bacterial infections usually involve the respiratory or urinary tracts.

Viral infections that may produce urticaria include hepatitis, mononucleosis, and coxsackievirus infections.

Inhalation of pollens, mold, animal dander, dust, plant products, and aerosols may produce urticaria. Respiratory symptoms may accompany the dermatosis, and the pattern of occurrence may be seasonal. Stings and bites of insects, arthropods, and various marine animals may produce an urticarial eruption. (See Chapter 34.)

Urticaria is uncommonly associated with internal disease and malignancy. It is occasionally found in Hodgkin's disease, more rarely in leukemia and carcinoma. Systemic lupus erythematosus, hyperthyroidism, rheumatic fever, and juvenile rheumatoid arthritis are also occasionally associated with an urticarial eruption.

A number of physical agents produce urticaria. Dermatographia, i.e., when firm stroking of the skin produces an urticarial wheal within 30 minutes, is the most common form of physical urticaria. Pressure urticaria is distinct from dermatographia in that the onset of urticaria is delayed by four to eight hours after the application of physical pressure.

Cold urticaria may be either familial or acquired, although the latter is more common. Cold urticaria may also be associated with underlying illness, such as multiple myeloma, cryoglobulinemia, cryofibrinogenemia, syphilis, and connective tissue disease.[41]

Cholinergic urticaria is induced by exercise, heat, or emotional stress. It may be associated with pruritus, nausea, abdominal pain, and headache.[43] Wheals of cholinergic urticaria are characteristically small, 1 to 3 mm, and surrounded by extensive erythematous flares. Heat rarely induces hives. Solar urticaria, also uncommon, is confined to sun-exposed areas of skin and clears rapidly when light stimulus is removed. Extensive sun exposure may cause wheezing, dizziness, and syncope in the susceptible individual.[43]

Treatment of urticaria involves removal of the inciting factor, where applicable, and administration of antihistamines or other antipruritics. Diphenhydramine (Benadryl), 25 to 50 mg; hydroxyzine (Atarax, Vistaril), 25 to 50 mg; and chlorpheniramine maleate (Chlor-Trimeton), 2 to 8 mg, all provide symptomatic relief. When anaphylaxis accompanies urticaria, treatment of this life-threatening condition obviously takes precedence.

The most important diagnostic steps are a history of inciting factors and a physical examination to investigate the possibility of an underlying illness. An allergic work-up may be in order, especially for acute urticaria. In a significant number of patients with urticaria, however, the cause is not determined.

VIRAL INFECTIONS

Herpes Simplex

Two variants of herpes simplex virus (HSV) are known to cause human infection. These are designated HSV-1, which affects primarily nongenital sites, and HSV-2, which produces lesions in the genital area predominantly. HSV-2 is thought to be transmitted primarily by venereal contact.[44] Lesions found above the waist are usually caused by HSV-1, while those below the waist are generally caused by HSV-2.

The oral region is the most common site of HSV-1 infection, and children are affected more frequently than adults.[45] Initial lesions are small clusters of vesicles, but these are soon broken, leaving irregularly shaped, crusted erosions. Herpetic gingivostomatitis varies in severity from small areas of erosion to extensive ulceration of the mouth, tongue, and gums. Severe cases may be accompanied by fever and cervical lymphadenopathy. Infection may be severe enough to inhibit adequate food and fluid intake. Healing typically takes place in 7 to 14 days, unless the lesions are secondarily infected with streptococci or staphylococci.

The hallmark of herpesvirus infection is the presence of grouped vesicles on an erythematous base. The lesions are usually localized in a nondermatome distribution, although the skin distribution may become more generalized in patients with atopic dermatitis and other skin disease.[45] HSV infection in the immunocompro-

mised host is a potentially fatal infection, owing to its propensity for generalization and dissemination to the internal organs.[46]

HSV-2 infections in the male appear as either a single vesicle or multiple vesicles on the shaft or glans penis. Fever, malaise, and regional lymphadenopathy may also be present. A prodrome of local pain and hyperesthesia may precede the appearance of the cutaneous lesions. Erosion of vesicles after several days to form a crust that heals in 10 to 14 days is the rule. The infection is much more severe in the female. It may involve the introitus, cervix, or vagina; vesicles may be grouped or confluent. Herpetic cervicitis or vaginitis may be the cause of severe pelvic pain, dysuria, or vaginal discharge,[47] and hospitalization may be necessary to control pain. Although recurrences are common, symptoms tend to be less severe in subsequent episodes.

Several therapeutic modalities have been suggested for the treatment of cutaneous HSV infection, but no agents currently available have been found to be both benign and beneficial in controlled trials.[48–50] The most effective current therapy is the application of a drying solution that promotes crusting and speeds involution of the cutaneous lesions.[48] The application of 2 percent topical lidocaine jelly is of benefit in the symptomatic treatment of oral or female genital herpes. (See Chapter 20.)

Herpes Zoster

Infection with varicella-zoster (V-Z) virus causes herpes zoster, or shingles. Individuals who have previously been infected with chickenpox virus are affected exclusively. The patient typically develops pain in a dermatomal distribution prior to the appearance of the rash. This pain is of variable intensity and is sharp, dull, or burning in quality. It precedes the eruption by one to ten days. The rash consists of grouped vesicles on an erythematous base and involves one or several dermatomes. The thorax or abdomen is involved in the majority of cases. The appearance of herpes zoster in the trigeminal nerve dermatomes is also common.

The vesicles, which are initially clear, become cloudy and then progress to scab and crust formation. This process takes 10 to 12 days, and the crusts heal over the next two to three weeks. Unusual in children, herpes zoster has a peak incidence in the 50- to 70-year-old age group. The majority of cases occur in healthy individuals.[46] Although the association with Hodgkin's lymphoma and other malignancy is well-known, rarely does the appearance of the rash antedate the diagnosis of such disease.[46]

Herpes zoster may be transmitted from patients infected with chickenpox to susceptible individuals. It is generally believed, however, that most herpes zoster is caused by reactivation of V-Z virus present since the initial infection with chickenpox. During the latent period between the two illnesses, the virus is thought to reside in dorsal root ganglion cells.[51]

Herpes zoster has a very low mortality rate, rarely being life-threatening even when disseminated to the visceral organs as occurs occasionally in immunosuppressed patients.[52] Possible complications include central nervous system involvement, e.g., meningoencephalitis, myelitis, and peripheral neuropathy. Ocular complications occur in half of the cases that involve the ophthalmic division of the trigeminal nerve.[46] The severity of this varies from mild conjunctivitis to panophthalmitis that threatens the eye. Ophthalmologic consultation or follow-up should be sought in these cases. Postherpetic neuralgia, i.e., pain that persists after lesions have healed, is a troublesome complication. It occurs more frequently in elderly and immunosuppressed patients.[51] The pain may last for months and is often severe and resistant to standard analgesic medications.

Treatment is rarely necessary. Analgesics may be prescribed as needed. Burow's solution compresses, 1:20 to 1:40 diluted in water, may be applied to hasten the drying of lesions. Early systemic corticosteroid therapy may shorten the duration of postherpetic neuralgia, but it does not reduce the severity of pain or accelerate the rate of healing.[46] Some clinicians feel that systemic steroids, if not otherwise contraindicated, may reduce the incidence of postherpetic neuralgias.

Measles

A viral illness, measles is highly contagious. Following an incubation period of 10 to 11 days, fever and malaise develop. The fever usually escalates daily until it reaches around 105°F (40.5°C) on the fifth or sixth day of the illness. Cough, coryza, and conjunctivitis begin within 24 hours of the onset of symptoms.

The second day of the illness is marked by the appearance of the pathognomonic Koplik's spots on the buccal mucosa. Although these small, red spots with whitish centers are usually located opposite the molars, they may involve an extensive portion of the oropharynx. The cutaneous eruption begins on the third to fifth day of the illness. Maculopapular erythematous lesions appear on the forehead and upper neck initially, then spread to involve the face, trunk, arms, and finally the legs and feet. The rash begins to fade after three days, disappearing from the various sites in the same order. The fever subsides and Koplik's spots begin to disappear during this time.

Otitis media is the most common complication. Other common complications include encephalitis and pneumonitis. Encephalitis occurs in approximately 1/1,000 cases of measles and carries a 15 percent mortality. Measles pneumonia may also be life-threatening.

If bacterial invasion occurs in the presence of otitis media or pneumonia, antibiotics are indicated. Otherwise, treatment is supportive. Quarantine is of limited value, as others are usually exposed before the appearance of the rash and Koplik's spots render the diagnosis apparent. Measles is not contagious after the rash has been present for five days.

The illness can be modified or prevented by the administration of human immune serum globulin, which induces a passive immunity of about four weeks' duration. The dosage is 0.22 ml/kg as an intramuscular injection, which is administered within five days of exposure.

Rubella

The chief characteristics of rubella, or German measles, are fever, skin eruption, and generalized lymphadenopathy. The incubation period is typically 16 to 18 days. In children, the rash heralds the onset of the illness; in adults, a 1- to 5-day prodrome of headache, malaise, sore throat, coryza, and a low-grade fever antecedes the rash. These prodromal symptoms generally disappear within the first day following the appearance of the skin eruption. Reddish spots on the soft palate may be seen prior to the development of the rash.

The rash first appears on the face, then spreads to the neck, trunk, and extremities. Its appearance is that of pink to red maculopapules. Lesions on the face and trunk may coalesce, but those on the extremities typically do not. Mild pruritus may be present. The rash remains for one to five days, classically disappearing at the end of three. Clearing is occasionally accompanied by some desquamation.

Lymphadenopathy may be apparent from one day to one week before the rash appears. In general, the nodes most apparent in their enlargement are the suboccipital, postauricular, and posterior cervical groups. Tender adenopathy may be apparent several weeks after other signs and symptoms subside.

Major complications of rubella, e.g., encephalitis, arthritis, and thrombocytopenia, occur more frequently in older children and adults who contract the disease. The most severe complication is fetal damage. Twenty percent of children born to mothers infected during pregnancy have congenital anomalies. Maternal infection may be determined by comparing serum hemagglutination-inhibition antibody during the acute illness with that of two weeks later. A four-fold rise in titer is diagnostic of rubella infection.

Varicella

An infection caused by V-Z virus, varicella, or chickenpox, begins with low-grade fever, headache, and malaise, following an incubation period of 14 to 16 days. The exanthem coincides with these symptoms in children, follows them by 1 to 2 days in adults. The skin lesions progress from macules to papules to vesicles to the crusting stage very rapidly, sometimes within hours. The vesicles are usually 2 to 3 mm in diameter and surrounded by an erythematous border. Drying begins centrally, producing umbilication. The dried scabs fall off in 5 to 20 days.

Lesions are most highly concentrated on the trunk. Crops are also common in the scalp, face, and extremities. The hallmark of varicella is the appearance of skin lesions in various stages of development in a single region of the body. Extensive eruptions are often associated with high and prolonged fever.

The illness is self-limited, and treatment should be symptomatic only. Complications include encephalitis, pneumonia, and bacterial cellulitis. As the disease may be transmitted before the diagnosis is clinically evident, isolation of infected patients is futile. The illness is contagious until all vesicles are crusted and dried, so children should be kept at home until this stage is reached.

Other Viral Exanthems

An exanthem is a skin eruption that occurs as a symptom of a systemic disease. Enteroviruses, predominantly the coxsackievirus and echovirus groups, and adenoviruses are known to produce exanthems, and other viruses may do so as well. The exanthems of the coxsackievirus and echovirus have been the most thoroughly studied. Although most viral exanthems are maculopapular, other forms of rash are occasionally seen, e.g., erythematous, vesicular, and petechial eruptions. These are variable in the extent of involvement, are nonpruritic, and do not desquamate. Oropharyngeal lesions, enanthems, may accompany or precede the skin rash. Fever, meningitis, interstitial pneumonitis, or stomatitis may be part of the viral exanthem syndrome.[53]

REFERENCES

1. Sibrack LA: Cutaneous signs of internal malignant disease. *Primary Care* 5:263–280, 1978.
2. Safai B, Grant JM, Kurtz R, et al: Cutaneous manifestations of internal malignancies (I). Acanthosis nigricans. *Int J Dermatol* 17:312–315, 1978.
3. Rosenberg FW: Cutaneous manifestations of malignancy. *Cutis* 20:227–234, 1977.
4. Hanifin JM, Lobitz WC: Newer concepts of atopic dermatitis. *Arch Dermatol* 113:663–670, 1977.
5. Robins DN: Cutaneous groin lesions. *Primary Care* 5:215–232, 1978.
6. Bennett RM: Disseminated gonococcal infection: The problems of diagnosis and management. *J Reprod Med* 11:99–103, 1973.
7. Kraus SJ: Complications of gonococcal infection. *Med Clin North Am* 56:1115–1125, 1972.
8. Holmes KK, Wieser PJ, Pederson AHB: The gonococcal arthritis-dermatitis syndrome. *Ann Intern Med* 75:470–471, 1971.
9. *CDC-Recommended Treatment Schedules: Gonorrhea,* 27–29, 1979.
10. Causey WA: Staphylococcal and streptococcal infections of the skin. *Primary Care* 6:127–139, 1979.
11. Sturman SW, Malkinson FD: Staphylococcal scalded skin syndrome in an adult and a child. *Arch Dermatol* 112:1275–1279, 1976.
12. Pearson RW: Advances in the diagnosis and treatment of blistering diseases: A selective review, in Malkinson FD, Pearson RW (eds): *Yearbook of Dermatology.* Chicago, Year Book Medical Publishers, 1977, pp 7–52.
13. Meislin HW, Lerner SA, Graves MH, et al: Cutaneous abscesses: Anaerobic and aerobic bacteriology and outpatient management. *Ann Intern Med* 87:145–149, 1977.
14. Feingold M, Gellis SS: Cellulitis due to *Haemophilus influenzae* Type B. *N Engl J Med* 272:788–789, 1965.
15. Rapkin RH, Bautista G: *Hemophilus influenzae* cellulitis. *Am J Dis Child* 124:540–542, 1972.
16. Smith SZ: Contact dermatitis. *Primary Care* 5:653–659, 1978.
17. Farber EM, Abel EA: Contact dermatitis, in Rubenstein E, Federman DD (eds): *Scientific American Medicine.* New York, Scientific American Inc, 1980, pp 2 V 1–14.
18. Fisher AA: The notorious poison ivy family of anacardiaceae plants. *Cutis* 20:570–595, 1977.
19. Braverman IM: Cutaneous manifestations of diabetes mellitus. *Med Clin North Am* 55:1019–1029, 1971.
20. Stawiski MA, Voorhees JJ: Cutaneous signs of diabetes mellitus. *Cutis* 18:415–421, 1976.
21. Gouterman IH, Sibrack LA: Cutaneous manifestations of diabetes. *Cutis* 25:45–54, 1980.
22. Parker CW: Drug allergy, Part one. *N Engl J Med* 292:511–514, 1975.
23. Fisher AA: Drug eruptions in geriatric patients. *Cutis* 18:402–409, 1976.
24. Parker CW: Drug allergy, Part three. *N Engl J Med* 292:957–960, 1975.
25. Soderstrom RM, Krull EA: Erythema nodosum. *Cutis* 21:806–810, 1978.
26. Cormia FE, Domonkos AN: Cutaneous reactions to internal malignancy. *Med Clin North Am* 47:655–680, 1965.
27. Sibulkin D: Drug eruptions. *Primary Care* 5:233–248, 1978.
28. Mescon H, Moretti G: The treatment of cutaneous mycoses. *Med Clin North Am* 38:1301–1308, 1954.
29. Sutton RL Jr, Waisman M: Dermatoses due to fungi. *Cutis* 19:377–394, 1977.
30. Oskui J: Intermittent use of griseofulvin in tinea capitis. *Cutis* 21:689–692, 1978.
31. De Villez RL, Lewis CW: Candidiasis seminar. *Cutis* 19:69–83, 1977.
32. Greenspan JS: Oral mucous membrane disease. *Int J Dermatol* 17:31–41, 1978.
33. Orkin M, Epstein E Sr, Maibach HI: Treatment of today's scabies and pediculosis. *JAMA* 236:1136–1139, 1976.
34. Sanders SL, Nelson CT: Pemphigus and pemphigoid. *Med Clin North Am* 47:681–694, 1965.
35. Walker DH, Cain BG, Olmstead PM: Laboratory diagnosis of Rocky Mountain spotted fever by immunofluorescent demonstration of *Rickettsia rickettsii* in cutaneous lesions. *Am J Clin Pathol* 69:619–623, 1978.

36. Orkin M, Maibach HI: Scabies in children. *Pediatr Clin North Am* 25:371–386, 1978.

37. McRae ME: Scabies. *Cutis* 20:90–92, 1977.

38. Swartz MN: Syphilis, in Rubenstein E, Federman DD (eds): *Scientific American Medicine.* New York, Scientific American Inc, 1980, pp 7 VI 1–15.

39. Lee TJ, Sparling PF: Syphilis: An algorithm. *JAMA* 242:1187–1189, 1979.

40. Rosenthal AL, Binnick S, Panber P, et al: Drug induced toxic epidermal necrolysis in children. *Cutis* 24:437–440, 1979.

41. Monroe EW, Jones HE: Urticaria. *Arch Dermatol* 113:80–90, 1977.

42. Fellner MJ, Baer RL: Cutaneous reactions to drugs. *Med Clin North Am* 49:709–724, 1965.

43. Akers WA, Waverson DN: Diagnosis of chronic urticaria. *Int J Dermatol* 17:616–627, 1978.

44. Josey WE, Nahmias, AJ, Naib ZM: The epidemiology of type 2 (genital) herpes simplex virus infection. *Obstet Gynecol Surv* 27:295–302, 1972.

45. Olmstead CB: Genital herpes: The newest venereal disease. *Cutis* 20:113–127, 1977.

46. Miller LH: Herpes zoster in the elderly. *Cutis* 18:427–432, 1976.

47. Jarratt M, Smith R, Knox JM: Therapy of herpes simplex infection. *Int J Dermatol* 18:357–361, 1979.

48. Lopyan L, Young AW Jr, Menegus M: Generalized acute mucocutaneous herpes simplex type 2 with fatal outcome. *Arch Dermatol* 113:816–818, 1977.

49. Guinan ME, MacCalman J, Kern EA, et al: Topical ether and herpes simplex labialis. *JAMA* 243:1059–1061, 1980.

50. Taylor CA, Hendley JO, Greer KE, et al: Topical treatment of herpes labialis with chloroform. *Arch Dermatol* 113:1550–1552, 1977.

51. Dolin R, Reichman RC, Mazur MH, Whitley RJ: Herpes zoster-varicella infections in immunosuppressed patients. *Ann Intern Med* 89:375–388, 1978.

52. Gallagher JG, Merigan TC: Prolonged herpes-zoster infection associated with immunosuppressive therapy. *Ann Intern Med* 91:842–846, 1979.

53. Lerner AM, Klein JO, Cherry JD, et al: New viral exanthems. *N Engl J Med* 269:678–685, 736–740, 1963.

23. Gastrointestinal Emergencies

RONALD L. KROME, M.D., F.A.C.S.

This chapter deals with a variety of gastrointestinal (GI) emergencies, excluding trauma because it is dealt with separately.

THE ACUTE ABDOMEN

In distinguishing between the acute and nonacute abdomen, the first concern is conditions requiring immediate surgical intervention; then, those that require immediate medical therapy; and, finally, those that require careful and complete evaluation in an outpatient or hospital setting, but not immediate intervention.

The most likely diagnoses of sudden severe abdominal pain in patients who are over the age of 13 include acute appendicitis, diverticulitis, perforated peptic ulcer, acute cholecystitis, small bowel obstruction, and acute pancreatitis. In women, especially those in the young and reproductive years, acute salpingitis and ruptured ectopic pregnancies, as well as pyelonephritis should be considered in the differential diagnosis.

At least one author has suggested that misdiagnosis may occur in as many as 30 percent of those patients with abdominal pain, because the symptoms and signs do not fit into a classic pattern.[1] Therefore, a careful history and examination, indeed, repeated examinations when the diagnosis is in doubt, and a high index of suspicion of the less common causes of abdominal pain are important factors in the accurate diagnosis.

Generally, abdominal pain may arise in the abdomen itself or from an extra-abdominal location, as for example, in the chest. Pain of sudden onset generally represents an acute condition.

Intra-abdominal Pain

Intra-abdominal pain may be caused by peritoneal inflammation or irritation, obstruction of a hollow viscus, or vascular compromise of the small or large bowel.

Peritoneal Inflammation

Any infection or even stretching of the mucous membrane of the GI tract can permit leakage of normal bacterial inhabitants of the GI tract through the wall with the subsequent development of peritonitis, retroperitoneal infection, or hematogenous spread of organisms. Peritonitis is the inflammation of the peritoneum due to the action of any irritant, either bacterial or chemical. It may be produced by gastric juice, bowel contents, urine, blood, or pancreatic secretions.

Peritoneal inflammation is frequently accompanied by the transudation of large volumes of fluid. When all or a great deal of the peritoneal lining is involved, fluid loss may be sufficient to produce shock and electrolyte disorders.

Inflammation involving the peritoneal covering of the GI tract (visceral peritoneum) frequently results in paralytic ileus, with bowel distention, small or large, and fluid accumulation within the bowel lumen. Consequently, small and large bowel dilatation may accompany inflammation of a retroperitoneal, or even an intraperitoneal organ without perforation or obstruction. That is, a functional obstruction may occur as a result of a localized paralytic ileus resulting from inflammation.

These pathophysiologic changes account for the hypotension and electrolyte disorders seen in these patients, as well as the abdominal distention and decreased bowel sounds. In a roentgenogram, air fluid levels can also be seen, although usually without a stepladder effect. Therefore, the diagnosis of paralytic ileus (adynamic ileus) remains a clinical diagnosis.

Although extremely uncommon, primary peritonitis can occur, and is most frequently caused by *Pneumococcus, Streptococcus, Escherichia coli,* or *Myobacterium tuberculosis.* Secondary peritonitis is produced by a disease or injury of the abdominal or pelvic viscera, resulting in a crossing through the intestinal wall of the bacterial contents and causing infected or septic peritonitis.

Rigidity, involuntary contraction of the abdominal musculature, when it occurs is a sign of peritonitis. Guarding, that is the voluntary production of abdominal musculature "spasm," may result from any intraabdominal or extra-abdominal pain. In addition to rigidity and abdominal pain present with peritonitis, rebound tenderness, fever, vomiting, decreased or absent bowel sounds, and abdominal distention are frequently present. The quality of the pain varies with the nature of the irritant that is producing the peritonitis, but generally, it is constant and diffuse, only becoming localized when the peritonitis is localized. If the material is sterile, the pain may be acute and intense, but if highly acid, the pain may be initially minimal.

When peritonitis is localized as, for example, when there is inflammation surrounding a perforated duodenal ulcer, subsequent to pelvic inflammatory disease or an abscess of the appendix, rigidity is not generally present, but guarding is. There is generally point tenderness over the area of inflammation with rebound tenderness as well. Every female patient with intraabdominal pain must have a rectal and pelvic examination.

Mechanical Obstruction

Generally speaking, pain resulting from obstruction of the GI tract is intermittent and crampy in nature, and accompanied by abdominal tenderness with vomiting and abdominal distention. Obstipation or constipation, although generally present, may be absent, and in fact, the patient may have normal bowel movements or diarrhealike bowel movements, depending on the location of the obstruction.

The nature of the vomitus may give some indication of the level of obstruction, and indeed, the duration of obstruction. For example, feculent material in the nasogastric suction may be associated with longstanding lower small bowel obstruction. Most often, this is produced by gangrenous bowel. The presence of green bilious return in the nasogastric tube at least indicates that the pyloric canal is open, and the obstruction—functional or mechanical—is distal to the ligament of Treitz. Clear colorless fluid in large volumes occurs with gastric outlet obstruction.

The most common cause of mechanical bowel obstruction in the United States is adhesions as a result of previous abdominal surgery, and the second most common is an incarcerated inguinal hernia.

Although the abdominal distention may initially be localized and detectable only on abdominal radiologic examination, as it progresses, the distention becomes generalized and clinically apparent. The intermittently colicky pain of small bowel obstruction is often localized in the periumbilical area, while pain resulting from large bowel obstruction is usually referred to the hypogastric region. Pain location is not always helpful in determining the point of obstruction.

Rigidity is not present unless peritonitis is present. Guarding is frequently present, and bowel sounds may be hyper- or hypoactive, depending on the duration of the obstruction. Classical, mechanical bowel obstruction produces high-pitched rushes of bowel sounds, whereas in paralytic ileus, the bowel sounds are hypoactive. When the bowel sounds in mechanical obstruction change from hyperactive to hypoactive, the obstruction has been longstanding—an ominous sign.

Vascular Conditions

Perhaps the most catastrophic abdominal emergency is that involving vascular disorders. At times impingement of the patient's vascular supply to the bowel may present occult signs requiring a high index of suspicion to establish the diagnosis. Obviously, patients with bowel infarction have severe central abdominal pain, frequently colicky and intermittent, followed by progressive signs of toxicity with fever, leukocytosis, and hypotension ending in shock and death if surgical intervention is not rapid. Some patients present with much less obvious signs, e.g., abdominal back pain and loose mucoid bloody stools.

Hematemesis may also be present, and if the vascular problem persists, functional bowel obstruction will occur with an area of dead bowel through which peristalsis does not pass. In this case, the bowel sounds will be hyperperistaltic, and mucoid bloody loose stools may be present. Vomiting is often present, and may be feculent in nature.

Electrolyte disturbances, occult blood loss manifested by anemia, and guaiac-positive stools may be among the early manifestations. An elevated white blood cell count with a shift to the left is frequently present.

Elderly patients (over 60 or 65 years of age) may not manifest all of the clinical and laboratory signs noted above, and the diagnosis is especially difficult in them. Tachycardia, signs and symptoms of hypovolemia, mild to moderate abdominal pain, and Hematest-positive stools may be the only findings.

Aortic dissection produces abdominal pain. Generally, the pain originates in the chest or abdomen, and radiates through to the back, rather than around to the back. Depending on the length of dissection, focal neurologic signs or loss of pulses in an extremity may be present. Mesenteric or renal artery occlusion may accompany aortic dissection with anuria and signs of vascular impingement of the bowel also developing. If blood loss is sufficient, hypotension, tachycardia, shock, and death may result.

Rupture of an abdominal aortic aneurysm is most often characterized by sudden cardiovascular collapse, following a period of severe back pain. A leaking or expanding aortic aneurysm may produce abdominal or back pain with guarding. Abdominal distention may appear to be present because of retroperitoneal or intra-abdominal bleeding resulting from the aneurysm. Cross table lateral roentgenographic examination will show that the air fluid level of the small bowel is "floating" on a glassy-appearing abdomen. In these patients, if time allows, an abdominal or back bruit should be sought. (See also Chapter 54.)

Extra-abdominal Causes of Abdominal Pain

Abdominal pain can originate from the chest, pelvis, or abdominal wall itself. Pain localized solely to the abdomen is usually caused by intra-abdominal disease.

Referred Pain

In patients with upper abdominal pain, especially those with pain in the left or right upper quadrants, intrathoracic disease should be suspected. Not only can inferior wall myocardial infarction produce upper abdominal pain, but so too can pneumothorax, pneumonia, pulmonary infarction or embolism, pleural fusion, and even upper gastric or lower esophageal rupture.

Pelvic Disease

In women, especially young women, acute pelvic pain may be caused by a number of problems related to reproductive organs. Perhaps the most common cause of intra-abdominal pain from the pelvis is acute salpingitis, or salpingo-oophoritis, especially if it is unilateral. When unilateral salpingitis occurs, it is extremely difficult to distinguish from acute appendicitis.

Symptoms are a history of the onset of symptoms just after menses, vaginal discharge, and marked cervical tenderness on motion. However, cervical tenderness on motion may also be present with acute appendicitis, especially when the appendix falls into the pelvic area.

Ruptured ectopic pregnancy should always be considered as a cause of abdominal pain in women of reproductive age. It is classically associated with sudden abdominal pain, hypotension, tachycardia, or cardiovascular collapse. In this age-group vaginal bleeding, which may be limited to spotting, in the presence of an abdominal mass and tenderness should raise this suspicion. On bimanual examination, the uterus may be enlarged or an extrauterine mass is palpated. Culdocentesis may be diagnostic, but the presence of a negative cul-de-sac tap does not rule out an ectopic pregnancy. Ectopic pregnancies have been reported to occur even in women who have had tubal ligation, and therefore in young women with abdominal pain it is best to include a pregnancy test as part of the initial evaluation. (See Chapter 64.)

Other Causes

Metabolic Causes

Porphyria is classically described as producing severe abdominal pain, often of sufficient severity to mimic intestinal obstruction. However, these patients rarely exhibit rigidity or hypoactive bowel sounds.

Classically, patients with diabetic ketoacidosis and hyperlipemia also have abdominal pain of varying intensity. In those patients who have associated pancreatitis, of course, the pancreatitis itself may produce the abdominal pain.

Black widow spider bites and scorpion bites are among the insect bites that may produce abdominal pain. Patients with sickle cell disease who present in crisis frequently have abdominal pain. Bowel sounds are normal and rebound tenderness or rigidity generally absent. Guarding may, however, be present. At times it is extremely difficult to distinguish between an acute surgical abdomen and a painful crisis in a patient with known sickle cell disease. In fact splenic infarcts and cholelithiasis, both of which in their own right produce abdominal pain, occur with some frequency among these patients.

Neurogenic Causes

Some neurologic diseases produce abdominal pain by compression or irritation of the spinal nerves or roots. In these patients, however, the other findings that would indicate intra-abdominal disease are absent and there are other signs or symptoms associated with the primary disease process.

EVALUATION OF THE PATIENT

History

The first step in the evaluation is to characterize the pain. The onset of the pain and the mode of onset should be clearly identified; its character and quality, location, whether it shifts or radiates to any specific location, and what factors relieve or aggravate the pain are all part of the characterization. In addition, the presence of any symptoms that occur at the same time as the pain should also be elicited.

In some conditions onset of pain is typically acute and sudden. The classic example is a perforated duodenal ulcer when the patient may be able to tell virtually the exact time of onset. Other causes of acute sudden pain include ruptured aneurysms, acute pancreatitis, and ruptured ectopic pregnancy.

More slowly developing conditions are characterized by slowly intensifying pain. This most characteristically occurs in a mechanical bowel obstruction, when the pain increases in severity as the distention of the GI tract also increases.

The character of the pain, that is, the quality of the pain, may be helpful in determining the diagnosis. Colicky and intermittent pain generally indicates obstruction of a hollow viscus. The pain is produced by the distention, and is related to the peristalsis. Such crampy abdominal pain may result from obstruction of the biliary ducts, as for example, by a stone. The biliary ducts are hollow and peristalsis does occur. Similarly, obstruction of a ureter produces crampy intermittent pain initially and severe constant pain reflecting the degree of obstruction, as well as the duration.

When increased abdominal pressure or movement extenuate the pain, the abdominal pain is usually a result of peritoneal irritation or inflammation. Such maneuvers as having the patient cough or jump to elicit pain may be very helpful. If the peritonitis is localized, the pain will be localized; if it is generalized, the pain will also be generalized.

Frequently, patients with peritonitis lie in bed curled up, knees toward chest. This position relieves the tension on the parietal peritoneum and, therefore, minimizes peritoneal irritation and the pain. In fact, patients with pelvic inflammatory disease frequently walk "hunched" over to relieve the pain produced by the peritonitis. In addition, patients with acute pancreatitis will lie in bed in the knee-to-chest position for the same reason.

Pain may start in one location and gradually shift to another. Classically, the pain of appendicitis starts in the periumbilical region and as time progresses, moves to the right lower quadrant and to McBurney's point.

This sort of shifting pattern may also occur with intestinal obstruction, where it is at first localized and then becomes diffuse and generalized. The pain of ureteral obstruction may start in an upper quadrant and then move to a lower quadrant, eventually radiating into the scrotum or labia.

In some instances, where the disease entity involves an organ abutting the inferior aspect of the diaphragm, the pain generated may start in the shoulder or scapular areas ("referred"), and subsequently, become localized to an upper quadrant. The process occurs because of irritation of the underside of the diaphragm and the sensory innervation of the diaphragm. This can occur in acute hepatitis, acute cholecystitis, and acute splenic infarcts, among others. Ruptured ectopic pregnancies may also produce the same pain pattern, secondary to irritation of the diaphragm by the blood. Subdiaphragmatic abscesses also produce a similar pain pattern.

Localized pain, pain located in only one area of the abdomen, is frequently a result of local peritonitis or local peritoneal irritation, as may occur in acute pancreatitis, acute cholecystitis, or acute hepatitis. Pain originating from the intestinal tract is more diffuse in location, and does not generally become localized.

Some acute abdominal problems produce not only localized pain, but also a particular radiating pain. While the pain of acute cholecystitis is crampy, colicky, and localized to the right upper quadrant and radiates around to the back; that of acute pancreatitis, although generally localized to the hypogastrium or to both upper quadrants frequently penetrates straight through to the back. Classically, pain of ureteral stones radiates from the abdomen or flank into the scrotum or labia.

Other Aspects

Vomiting and the appearance of the vomitus are essential elements of the history. If the vomitus is clear and colorless, gastric outlet obstruction may be present. Blood in the vomitus, whether bright red, coffee-ground, or speckled flecks, indicates upper GI bleeding. Generally speaking, this signifies that the bleeding has occurred proximal to the ligament of Treitz. Hematemesis can occur in a wide variety of conditions.

Common causes include the Mallory-Weiss syndrome, gastritis, varices, and peptic ulcer disease. In addition, however, hematemesis may occur as a result of erosion of the mucosa, not only from carcinoma, but also from a gallstone eroding through the common duct into either the duodenum or the stomach. Generally, the latter is associated with only small amounts of bleeding. It is unusual for a perforated duodenal ulcer to produce significant upper GI bleeding. There may, however, be a small amount of bleeding at the initial onset of the perforation.

A history of hematemesis requires confirmation. Therefore, patients who have a history of hematemesis must be aspirated with a nasogastric tube, and the aspiration checked with guaiac or Hematest. If the return is clear, and the tube not otherwise indicated, it may be removed. If the gastric return is green, not only is the gastric outlet open, but so is the common bile duct. Intestinal obstruction, if present, must be distal to these two points. This can occur in both small and large bowel obstruction.

In longstanding small bowel obstruction, especially in low small bowel or longstanding large bowel obstruction, the patient may complain of feculent vomitus. That is, the vomitus appears as though it were liquid stool and even has the same odor. If confirmed, this should be considered an ominous sign; it is frequently present with dead or gangrenous bowel.

Another part of the history that deserves special attention is the patient's bowel movements. Most commonly, complete obstipation is associated with large bowel obstruction. Obstipation implies that the patient has had no bowel movements nor passed any flatus. It can occur with lower large bowel obstruction, especially mechanical bowel obstruction. However, it is not unusual, when a tumor is impinging on the bowel, for a patient to complain of diarrheal bowel movements, and indeed, in patients with mechanical small bowel obstruction, the patient may have frequent bouts of diarrhea. In some tumors, especially villous adenomas of the rectum, diarrhea with significant potassium loss is not unusual.

In summary it is possible, therefore, for patients with mechanical bowel obstructions to have one or several normal stools, and indeed, complain of diarrheal bowel movements. In patients with diverticulosis that becomes diverticulitis, a past history of intermittent episodes of constipation alternating with diarrhea is not unusual.

The stool should be examined and tested for the presence of blood. Any melena is generally associated with bleeding of the upper GI, that is, proximal to the ligament of Treitz. It is possible for even red blood in the stool to occur following massive GI bleeding. In fact, the most common cause of lower GI bleeding (blood in the stool) is upper GI bleeding.

Other causes of blood in the stool include, of course, anal diseases, such as hemorrhoids or fissures. Guaiac-positive stools can be detected when carcinoma of the common duct, or even common duct stones, have eroded into the GI tract producing some bleeding. Lower GI bleeding, therefore, must be confirmed by the presence of blood in the stool, and the absence of blood in the nasogastric return. This does not, of course, rule out bleeding from the small bowel, but does help localize the process.

Physical Examination

In addition to the general physical examination, special attention must be paid to several areas. Obviously, specific attention must be paid to the abdominal findings. The localization of tenderness and rebound tenderness already alluded to is very important. Local peritonitis will produce localized tenderness and localized rebound tenderness. This may occur in patients with appendicitis and salpingo-oophoritis. Rigidity, when present, indicates generalized peritonitis, and the next step is surgical exploration. Guarding occurs frequently in many patients with abdominal pain; it should be considered a nonspecific finding.

Bowel sounds should be auscultated for approximately 30 seconds in each quadrant of the abdomen. High-pitched rushes of bowel sounds of an intermittent nature may be associated with bowel obstruction. A quiet abdomen is generally considered to indicate paralytic ileus. However, a quiet abdomen, that is, one with diminished or absent bowel sounds, may occur when a bowel obstruction has been present for a prolonged period of time; it should be considered an ominous sign. The presence or absence of masses, tender or not, should be noted and recorded. A nasogastric tube should be inserted in virtually every patient suspected of having any significant GI emergency. This is done for several reasons:

- to detect gastric outlet obstruction (large volume of return),
- to assess the color of the vomitus and the presence or absence of blood, and
- in some cases to give therapy.

Patients with pancreatitis frequently get relief from their abdominal pain within minutes when the nasogastric tube is inserted. Patients with ileus and small bowel obstruction get some relief of their pain because the abdominal distention will be somewhat diminished by drainage of the upper GI tract.

In patients with upper GI bleeding, the nasogastric tube should generally be left in place, even if lavage returns are clear. In patients with pancreatitis, the nasogastric tube is therapeutic and should be left in place until such time as either the amylase returns to normal or the patient becomes asymptomatic and nontender.

Additionally, the rectal examination is a mandatory part of the physical examination of a patient with a GI problem. Not only is this necessary in order to obtain a stool specimen to check for blood, but it is also necessary to rule out large bowel obstructions related to tumors in the rectum. In addition, the examiner may be able to detect pelvic abscesses, either related to an appendiceal abscess or to pelvic inflammatory disease. Finally, some additional assessment of the presence or absence of abdominal masses may be possible during the rectal examination.

Pelvic examination is indicated in most women with abdominal pain and possible GI emergencies. In sexually active women, pelvic examination may pinpoint the problem to pelvic inflammatory disease. In addition, such conditions as ovarian cysts and ectopic pregnancies cannot be diagnosed adequately without a complete pelvic examination. Not only should a bimanual examination be done, but also a speculum examination. Some assessment of the cervix including the presence or absence of bleeding and the color of the cervix should be made prior to the bimanual examination. At the same time, if and when pelvic inflammatory disease is entertained in the diagnosis, not only should routine cultures be obtained, but cultures for gonorrhea. Even when pelvic inflammatory disease is not the prime diagnosis, in women who are in the sexually active age-group, the pelvic examination is an integral part of establishing the diagnosis and the etiology of the abdominal pain. Therefore, in all women (but especially in this age-group), a pelvic examination is a mandatory part of the physical examination for abdominal pain not related to trauma.

Other less common signs include the presence or absence of pain or tenderness when the hip is flexed and the knee pointed externally (the psoas sign). The presence or absence of any discoloration of the abdomen, asterixis, or pedal edema, which may be indicative of congestive heart failure, should also be sought.

Laboratory Examination

Virtually every patient who presents with any significant GI problem or abdominal pain should have a complete blood count. It is not unusual to detect unsuspected anemia in patients with large bowel obstruction, especially when a tumor is present on the right side of the colon. In addition, an elevated white count with a shift to the left should lead to suspicion of an inflammatory process. The absence of this, however, does not rule out abscesses—whether appendiceal or diverticular—or more esoteric causes of abdominal pain, such as lymphomas and leukemias.

Young black patients should generally have a reticulocyte count and a sickle cell test. Commonly, however, most adult patients who have sickle cell disease are aware of their disease and their problems, and generally give this information as a part of their history.

Elderly patients, especially with gangrenous bowel, may not show anything other than a very slight anemia, and the white count may be within normal limits, without a shift to the left. The presence of dead bowel in the elderly is difficult to diagnose, and a high index of suspicion must be maintained.

Electrolytes should be assayed, not routinely, but in virtually any patient who has a significant history of either vomiting or diarrhea. Electrolyte disturbances must be corrected in the emergency department, even when surgery is indicated as part of the resuscitation and stabilization. Blood urea nitrogen (BUN) and creatinine assays do give some indication of the patient's general renal function. Uremia may produce abdominal pain, and in the elderly patient especially or in patients with a past history of renal disease, BUN and creatinine are part of the general evaluation of the patient. The use of the BUN to assess the patient's state of hydration is not reliable; other means, including the physical diagnosis, are much more accurate.

Liver studies, including enzymes, alkaline phosphatase, and bilirubin may be indicated only in those patients in whom liver or gallbladder disease is considered a possibility. Patients with pancreatitis may have associated changes in the bilirubin and the alkaline phosphatase. Edema of the head of the pancreas from pancreatitis producing a functional obstruction of the common bowel duct may lead to an elevated bilirubin and an elevated alkaline phosphatase.

In addition, patients with sickle cell crisis frequently have elevated bilirubin and anemia. The bilirubin is related to the hemolytic crisis that occurs in this disease process. The finding of an elevated bilirubin in a patient with severe abdominal pain, unless the patient is known to have sickle cell disease, can frequently lead to a difficult differential diagnosis. The reticulocyte count will also be elevated during the hemolytic crisis.

Amylase

The serum amylase level is fraught with difficulty in interpretation and diagnosis when it is either the sole abnormal finding or is elevated in a patient known to be an alcohol abuser. Pancreatitis, the disease most commonly associated with elevated amylase, can occur in nonalcoholics as well. When it does occur in nonalcoholics, it is related to biliary disease, and in addition to the elevated amylase, elevated bilirubin and elevated serum alkaline phosphatase will be detected. However, to further compound the problem, patients who have pancreatitis with significant edema of the pancreatic head may also have elevated bilirubin and alkaline phosphatase. A normal serum amylase level may be found in patients with active pancreatitis, although this most likely occurs in patients who have chronic pancreatitis and an activation of their problem. In addition to pancreatitis, serum amylase may be elevated in acute cholecystitis, perforated viscuses, mesenteric thrombosis, and high large bowel obstruction. Penetrating ulcers that burrow into the head of the pancreas also elevate the serum amylase.

Recent evidence from Donald Weaver suggests that in patients with abdominal pain there may be a minimal elevation that does not have as its source the pancreas (personal communication). Some studies indicate that salivary amylase may be elevated in alcoholics (personal communication with David Bowman), and this finding in addition to the combination of acute alcoholism, abdominal pain, and minimally elevated serum amylase may be difficult to interpret. Urinary excretion of amylase is significantly higher in patients with pancreatitis and in patients with other sources of amylasemia. Serum lipase studies may be done in the emergency department but have limited usefulness in acute conditions. Patients with hyperlipidemia may also have elevated serum amylase.

Urinalysis

Urinalysis is frequently helpful in the differential diagnosis of the patient with an acute abdominal problem. Although classically pyuria and hematuria indicate urologic sources of the patient's abdominal pain, appendiceal abscesses and even retrocecal appendicitis may produce microscopic hematuria and pyuria. Pelvic abscess, regardless of the source, frequently irritates the bladder, producing dysuria, frequency, and urgency, as well as hematuria and pyuria.

In addition, the genitourinary tract may indeed be the source of the patient's abdominal problem. Abdominal pain radiating into the groin, and associated with microscopic or gross hematuria, is the classic finding in renal calculi.

Peritoneal Lavage

Although classically peritoneal lavage has been used to establish the diagnosis of visceral injury caused by blunt abdominal trauma, its use has been expanded. In a patient with acute onset of abdominal pain in whom the physician has difficulty distinguishing between a nonoperative and operative cause, peritoneal lavage may be of some benefit. (See the anatomical representation of the procedure in Figure 23–1.) Obviously, the same contraindications apply to the nontrauma patient as to the trauma patient.

The finding of elevated amylase in the peritoneal lavage fluid, white cells, bowel contents, and even stool can assist in establishing the source of the patient's ab-

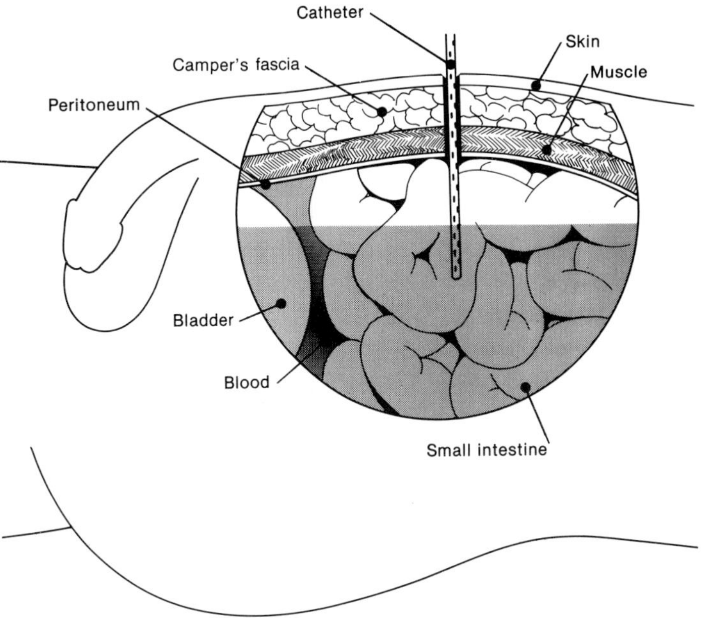

Figure 23–1   Peritoneal Lavage.

dominal problem. However this should not be considered a routine study for all patients with acute abdominal pain, because ileus or bowel distention as a result of mechanical obstruction may be present. In this circumstance, peritoneal lavage may lead to perforation of the large or small bowel. However, with care and using the open method of peritoneal lavage, inspecting and lifting the peritoneum prior to entering it, it is possible to do this study with relative ease. The effluent should be sent to the laboratory for examination, and a sample should be Gram-stained for bacteria. (See Chapter 71.)

X-rays

Each hospital has its own routine "acute abdomen series," but when roentgenograms are indicated in such a patient they should include a chest roentgenogram in the upright position. Free air under the diaphragm can be best seen when the patient is in this position. A flat and upright abdominal film should be obtained to detect air-fluid levels in the small and large bowel, to look for calcifications, and to look for a sentinel loop. Although most frequently the sentinel loop is described as occurring in association with pancreatitis, it can occur over or adjacent to any inflammatory process. For example, a sentinel loop can be detected over a kidney when pyelonephritis is present.

Air in the biliary system, which may appear as a series of small bubbles in the liver or right upper quadrant, should also be sought. Common duct stones that erode through the small bowel, or carcinoma involving the large or small bowel that erodes through into the biliary system or into the liver may produce biliary tract air. Retroperitoneal air is also an abnormal finding and should be sought on these films. This may occur with any retroperitoneal perforation of a hollow viscus.

One should also look carefully for foreign bodies in the abdomen. Some patients will not admit to ingesting foreign bodies; others will. Foreign bodies, of course, can be the source of perforation of a viscus.

Even in patients with an elevated amylase, a careful scrutiny of the abdominal film should be conducted to look for free air. A perforated duodenal ulcer which, obviously, can produce free air is associated with elevated serum amylase. Decubitus films are helpful in localizing fluid. A cross-table lateral view should be taken if an abdominal aortic aneurysm is suspected. In this case, the small bowel will be pushed anteriorly. Calcification in the wall of the aorta may also be detected.

Fluid in the chest roentgenogram, especially on the left, can occur with pancreatitis and subphrenic abscesses. Intra-abdominal abscesses may also be detected by looking for extraintestinal air-fluid levels, and multiple small "bubbles" grouped together.

In patients with sickle cell crisis, calcifications, either in the right upper quadrant (cholelithiasis) or the left upper quadrant (calcified splenic infarcts) may be found.

Other Special Studies

Radioactive Imaging

Radioactive imaging of the liver or spleen may be helpful in diagnosing splenic infarcts or hepatic abscesses; either may produce abdominal pain. In addition, liver and lung scans may enable one to establish the diagnosis of a subphrenic or subhepatic abscess since a "cold space" will appear on the image. Abscesses appear as a cold area in whatever organ is scanned.

Ultrasonography

Ultrasonography has gained increasing acceptance in the emergency department in the evaluation of the patient with abdominal pain. Ultrasonography can detect biliary stones and other calcifications in the abdomen, and pancreatic pseudocysts and pancreatic enlargement. Finally, ultrasonography is sometimes helpful in diagnosing an abdominal aortic aneurysm. Pelvic ultrasonography is useful in detecting ectopic pregnancies.

CT Scanning

The use of CT scanning has broadened beyond diagnosing intracerebral lesions, and without question will find ever-increasing acceptance in diagnosing abdominal problems. Recent studies indicate that in some circumstances, CT scanning of the abdomen may enable the detection of masses, including cystic structures, abscesses, retroperitoneal bleeding, contusions, or bleeding in the spleen, liver, or kidney, and aortic aneurysm.

Gastroscopy

The flexible gastroscope, although restricted to specialists other than emergency physicians, frequently enables establishment of the source of upper GI bleeding early in the management of the patient. Emergency physicians should be aware of this technique because its early use may be extremely helpful, and because more and more it is becoming the primary diagnostic tool in patients with upper GI complaints.

CONCLUSION

All too often physicians provide symptomatic relief for the patient without having a clear sense of diagnosis. Virtually every patient given Demerol and a tranquilizer will feel better. But nowhere is such an act so dangerous as in abdominal pain. Pain should only be relieved when the physician feels comfortable with the diagnosis, and when further consultation is not required.

The nasogastric tube will give many patients symptomatic relief and will allow time for further diagnostic evaluation. Repeated observation of the patient with repetition of the physical examination, preferably by the same observer, and the laboratory studies helps a great deal.

No examination of a patient with abdominal complaints is complete without the rectal or pelvic examination, and perhaps, even the nasogastric tube.

REFERENCE

1. Nase HW: The diagnosis of appendicitis. *Am Surg* 46:504, 1980.

BIBLIOGRAPHY

Berk JR, et al: Does hyperamylasemia in the drunken alcoholic signify pancreatitis? *Am J Gastroenterol* 7(6):557, 1979.

Blumhagen JD, et al: Ultrasound in the diagnosis of hypertrophic perforic stenosis. *J Clin Ultrasound* 9(6):289, 1981.

Daffner R: Computed tomography in the diagnosis of intra-abdominal abscesses. *Am Surg* 189:29, 1979.

Davis S, et al: The plain radiograph in acute pancreatitis. *Clin Radiol* 31:87, 1980.

Dixon AK, et al: Computed tomography in patients with an abdominal mass: Effective and efficient? *Lancet* 1(8231):1199, 1981.

DuPriest TW, et al: Open diagnostic lavage in blunt trauma victims. *Surg Gynecol Obstet* 148(6):392, 1979.

Freitas JE, et al: Rapid evaluation of acute abdominal pain by hepatobiliary scanning. *JAMA* 244:1585, 1980.

Gonez A, et al: Acute appendicitis during pregnancy. *Am J Surg* 137(2):180, 1979.

Kudsk KH, et al: Acute surgical illness in patient with sickle cell anemia. *Am J Surg* 142(1):113, 1981.

Lazrus HM, et al: A technique for peritoneal lavage without risk or complication. *Surg Gynecol Obstet* 149:889, 1979.

Levitt M: Extrapancreatic origin of chronic unexplained hyperamylasemia. *N Engl J Med* 302:670, 1980.

Miller RE, et al: Detection of pneumo-peritoneum: Optimum body position and respiratory phase. *Am J Roent* 135:487, 1980.

Nase, HW: The diagnosis of appendicitis. *Am Surg* 46:504, 1980.

Pederson F: Ultrasonic scanning in suspected ectopic pregnancy. *Br J Radiol* 53:1, 1980.

Philbrick TH, et al: Abdominal ultrasound in patients with acute right upper quadrant pain. *Gastrointest Radiol* 6(3):251, 1981.

Piironiken O, et al: The use of ultrasonography in the diagnosis of ectopic pregnancy. *Clin Radiol* 32(3):331, 1981.

Powers DN: Ectopic pregnancy: A five-year experience. *South Med J* 73:1012, 1980.

Smith GW, et al: Oral cholecystography in assessment of acute abdominal pain. *Arch Surg* 115:642, 1980.

Solomon AR: The value of the amylase/creatinine clearance ratio in the diagnosis of acute pancreatitis. *CRC Crit Rev Clin Lab Sci* 9:367, 1978.

Stone, KS, et al: Ultrasound as the initial diagnostic study in patients with suspected gallstones. *Am Surg* 46:444, 1980.

Vine HS, et al: Ultrasound evaluation of pelvic pain. *JAMA* 244:2540, 1980.

Warshaw AL, et al: Inhibition of serum and urine amylase activity in pancreatitis with hyperlipidemia. *Ann Surg* 182:72, 1975.

Wolk LA, et al: Computerized tomography in the diagnosis of abdominal aortic aneurysms. *Surg Gynecol Obstet* 153(2):299, 1981.

24. Poisoning and Drug Overdose

JOHN B. SULLIVAN, JR., M.D.

The condition of a patient who has ingested an overdose of a drug should receive special pharmacologic, toxicologic, and clinical evaluation, since the manifestations of such an overdose range from a paucity of signs and symptoms to coma and complete cardiorespiratory arrest. Not all poisons or drug overdoses result in immediate symptomatology. The patient may initially be asymptomatic, but serious morbidity may develop over a period of hours or days. Physiologic antagonists are available for a select number of toxic agents; however, basic and advanced critical care are imperative to the management of the patient with a poisoning or a drug overdose. The emergency department physician should understand the clinical toxicology and pharmacology of a drug in overdose, the changing absorptive process, the possible changing kinetic process, and the effect of patient age and disease on drug metabolism.

PREHOSPITAL MANAGEMENT

Basic prehospital care of a poisoned patient does not differ from the care rendered any seriously ill patient. Emergency care personnel should attempt to ascertain what substance was ingested, how much was ingested, and when it was ingested. They should search the area of initial contact with the patient for evidence of an empty container or drug prescription. Supportive prehospital care consists of the following:

- airway management. Intubation should be considered if the patient is comatose, experiences seizures, or has a depressed gag reflex. The airway should be protected at all times, and the aspiration of vomitus or secretions should be prevented.
- intravenous lines. Poisoned patients may be hypotensive because of vasodilation, peripheral pooling of intravascular volume, or myocardial depression. Intravenous administration of crystalloid fluids may be indicated to correct hypotension. Administration of other drugs may also be necessary.
- naloxone, glucose, and oxygen. The intravenous administration of naloxone (two ampules of 0.4 mg each) with glucose and supplementary oxygen by mask or nasal cannula is not harmful to any comatose patient if the diagnosis is not yet established. Hypoglycemia may be present, or a narcotic may be involved in the overdose.
- basic and advanced life support. Cardiopulmonary resuscitation of a poisoned patient is generally the same as that of any other critically ill patient.

EMERGENCY DEPARTMENT MANAGEMENT

The evaluation of the poisoned patient's condition in the emergency department should begin with a baseline history and physical examination. Historical information concerning the poison or drug may be difficult to obtain, however, owing to coma, seizures, cardiopulmonary arrest, or delirium. The history supplied by a friend or family member may not be accurate. A depressed patient who has attempted suicide with a drug may also be reluctant to reveal the substance ingested. The physical examination may provide the only data base in a comatose patient when a history is not available. If the patient is not comatose and can supply information, the emergency department physician should try to ascertain what was ingested, when it was ingested, and how much was ingested. Also, it is useful to know if any type of first aid treatment was administered by friends or family, for example, an outdated antidote.

The emergency department physician must first determine if the patient's life is in immediate danger and if advanced critical care is required. It is also imperative that the physician, in the initial and subsequent evaluations, rule out any associated illness or injury. An acute abdomen, neck injury, or intracranial injury is easily overlooked in a comatose poisoned patient or in a patient assumed to be poisoned.

Good supportive care is the foundation for proper management of any poisoned patient, and the physician should always provide this basic care instead of hurriedly searching for an antidote.

Airway Management

The poisoned patient who is deeply comatose, is having seizures, or has a depressed gag reflex has an unprotected airway. Endotracheal intubation, either by the oropharyngeal or nasotracheal route, is necessary in these patients. If the patient cannot be intubated, then correct positioning of the head to prevent aspiration or airway occlusion by the tongue is important. Intubation may be required to protect the airway during orogastric lavage, and the endotracheal tube cuff should always be properly inflated. Tracheal intubation may also be necessary to provide ventilatory assistance. Possible complications to tracheal intubation should be anticipated, however.[1] A poisoned patient may be supported on a respirator until a drug is metabolized and eliminated from the body. (See Chapter 56.)

Fluid Resuscitation of Hypotensive Patients with a Drug Overdose

Hypotension secondary to a drug overdose may result from[2,3]

1. peripheral pooling of vascular volume and vasodilation because of a drug-induced effect on the vascular tone, either directly or through central nervous system action

2. myocardial depression through drug effects on contractility, heart rate, stroke volume, and peripheral resistance
3. direct injury to the vascular endothelium
4. direct caustic effect of the drug on the gastrointestinal tract, producing necrosis and hemorrhage

Fluid resuscitation of shock following a drug overdose should be initiated with a crystalloid. The rapid administration of a crystalloid such as Ringer's lactate or normal saline usually brings about some correction of hypotension, although the administration of large volumes of crystalloid solutions can precipitate noncardiogenic pulmonary edema[4-7] and worsen cerebral edema.[8,9] An adult should be given 250 to 500 ml crystalloid solution rapidly to begin restoration of intravascular volume. A child in shock should be given isotonic saline or Ringer's lactate intravenously (15 to 20 ml/kg over 30 minutes).[10] If large volumes of fluids are required, the addition of a vasopressor such as dopamine (Intropin) or norepinephrine (Levophed or Levarterenol) should be considered. The adult and pediatric dosage of dopamine is 5 to 10 μg/kg/minute by intravenous infusion. The adult dosage of norepinephrine is 0.1 to 0.2 μg/kg/minute by intravenous infusion; the pediatric dosage, 0.05 μg/kg/minute.[11] The infusion rate can be varied to titrate blood pressure.

Physical Examination and Neurologic Evaluation

Associated illnesses and injuries should be ruled out in the poisoned patient. Neurologic evaluation should include a determination of the level of consciousness, as well as an examination of pupillary reflexes, oculovestibular reflexes, and muscle-strength reflexes. The pattern of respiration should be noted with attention to the rate and depth. Funduscopic examination may provide some information as to the cause of coma. Naloxone, glucose, and oxygen should be administered. The depth of coma should be determined and any changes noted. (See Chapter 45.)

Cardiac Monitoring

Many drugs may be associated with cardiac dysrhythmias when taken in overdose. This is especially true with tricyclic antidepressants and phenothiazines. An electrocardiogram (ECG) should be obtained and the PR, QRS, and QT intervals noted.

Electrolyte and Acid-Base Determination

Serum electrolyte and arterial blood gas determinations are helpful in managing a poisoned patient. The presence of acidosis and electrolyte derangement may help determine the type of toxicity involved.

Advanced Life Support

The clinical status of a poisoned patient may deteriorate rapidly. Cardiorespiratory depression, pulmonary edema, deepening coma, seizures, and life-threatening dysrhythmias may occur and must be treated appropriately. The critical care of a poisoned patient is no different from that of any other critically ill patient. Advanced life support techniques should be applied when necessary.

Toxic Drug Screen

Drug screens are overused in emergency departments. The physician should attempt to ascertain from the history, physical examination, and clinical presentation the pharmacologic class of drugs that may have been ingested; any drug screen ordered should be to confirm the clinical suspicion. Also, the physician should be familiar with the various drugs that can be identified by laboratory screening. Communication with the toxicology laboratory concerning the clinical status of the patient and the drug or class of drugs that may be involved can facilitate rapid screening for the suspected drugs.

TOXICOLOGIC-PHARMACOLOGIC SYNDROMES OF POISONED PATIENTS

Various pharmacologic syndromes may occur in poisoned patients. Knowledge of the differential drug diagnoses can direct the physician to investigate certain classes of drugs or poisons that the patient may have ingested.

Coma, Depressed Reflexes, Hypotension

Many drugs can cause coma when taken in an overdose. Coma of various degrees associated with depressed muscular activity and depressed reflexes is characteristic of the sedative-hypnotic drugs, which include barbiturates, benzodiazepines, ethanol, chloral hydrate, glutethimide, and ethchlorvynol.[12–17] Other drugs associated with coma and flaccidity are narcotics, meprobamate, and valproic acid.[18–21] All these drugs can cause coma, respiratory depression, depressed muscle stretch reflexes, loss of oculogyric and oculocephalic reflexes, and hypotension. With the narcotics, however, miosis is generally present. Valproic acid is not known to cause hypotension in overdose. Clonidine hydro-

chloride overdose has been reported to result in coma, areflexia, and hypotension.[22,23]

Coma, Hyper-reflexia, Seizures, Hypertonicity, and Myoclonus

Certain drugs in overdose may be associated with a combination of coma, seizures, increased muscle tone, and myoclonic activity. This toxicologic syndrome is most commonly caused by the anticholinergics such as tricyclic antidepressants and phenothiazines.[24,25] Overdose with methaqualone, a sedative-hypnotic, can result in coma, hyper-reflexia, hypertonicity, and seizures.[26,27] Other drugs associated with this type of symptomatology are phencyclidine hydrochloride, strychnine, amphetamines, cocaine, phenytoin, haloperidol, and fluoroacetate.[28–36] Propoxyphene (Darvon) overdose may be associated with seizure activity, along with coma, miotic pupils, and pulmonary edema.[37] Propranolol or metoprolol overdose has been reported to be associated with seizure and coma, along with the cardiac manifestations of atrioventricular block and hypotension.[38,39]

Overdose with carbamazepine (Tegretol), a drug being employed more frequently as an anticonvulsant for grand mal seizure disorders, may result in coma, hyperreflexia, seizures, and myoclonic activity.[40] Patients with cyanide and carbon monoxide poisoning may manifest seizures, coma, and hypertonicity.[41–44] Isoniazid also produces coma and seizures in overdose.

Intense, prolonged seizure activity and myoclonus can result in rhabdomyolysis with possible acute renal failure secondary to myoglobinuria. Rhabdomyolysis has been associated with various drug overdoses[45,46] and is particularly noted with overdose of amphetamine, heroin, phencyclidine hydrochloride, or carbon monoxide.[45,47,48]

Coma, Pulmonary Edema, Hypotension

The syndrome of coma, pulmonary edema, and hypotension may be caused by drug overdoses with sedative-hypnotics, narcotics, or salicylates. Ethchlorvynol (Placidyl) has been reported to be associated with noncardiogenic pulmonary edema.[49,50] Sedative-hypnotic drugs may also be associated with respiratory distress and pulmonary edema secondary to shock and aspiration of gastric contents. Narcotics have long been known to be associated with pulmonary edema, hypotension, and coma.[51,52] An overdose of propoxyphene should be suspected in a comatose patient with pulmonary edema, seizures, and miotic pupils.[37,53] Salicylate toxicity is associated with noncardiogenic pulmonary edema,[54,55] and the mechanism is thought to be increased permeability of alveolar and capillary endothelial cells.[56] Insult to the lungs following shock with development of the respiratory distress syndrome can accompany any drug overdose that produces coma and hypotension.

Narcotic-Opiate Toxicologic Syndrome

All of the opiates and narcotic drugs may produce a similar toxicologic syndrome, i.e., a combination of coma, hypotension, areflexia, brodycardia, miosis, pulmonary edema, and seizures. Miosis may not always be present in overdoses with meperidine (Demerol).[57,58] Miosis may not be extreme in some cases, and clinical suspicion is important in making a diagnosis of narcotic toxicity. Bowel sounds may be decreased or absent, and reflexes may be depressed. Lomotil (diphenoxylate and atropine) poisoning may have some anticholinergic symptomatology along with the narcotic syndrome; furthermore, symptomatology may be delayed for 12 or more hours.[59] Treatment with the narcotic antagonist naloxone (Narcan) is warranted if narcotic or opiate toxicity is suspected.

Cardiac Dysrhythmias, Seizures, Coma

Many drugs in overdose are associated with cardiac dysrhythmias, seizures, and coma. The tricyclic antidepressants are probably the most commonly used drugs that cause cardiac dysrhythmias in overdose; they are also frequently associated with seizures.[3,24] Other poisons and drugs associated with cardiac dysrhythmias, seizures, and coma in overdose are theophylline, caffeine, arsenic, chloral hydrate, propranolol, cocaine, amphetamine, phencyclidine hydrochloride, fluoroacetate, clonidine, carbamazepine, phenothiazines, lead, digoxin, and lithium. Theophylline and caffeine are known to produce seizures and ventricular dysrhythmias in overdose, as well as gastrointestinal bleeding.[60–62] Arsenic has been associated with ventricular irritability, as has lead, which may also produce a myocarditis.[63,64] Chloral hydrate has produced both supraventricular and ventricular dysrhythmias in overdose.[65] Clonidine overdose can result in coma, seizures, and atrioventricular block of varying degrees.[66,67] Sodium fluoroacetate was previously used in rodenticide preparations, but it is now banned because of its toxic effects on humans. Symptomatology from fluoroacetate may consist of coma, seizures, nystagmus, and cardiac dysrhythmias ranging from ST segment and T wave changes to ventricular premature contractions.[32,68] Propranolol overdose may result in coma, seizures, and atrioventricular block.[69] Carbamazepine overdose has been reported to result in QRS and QT interval prolongation in at least one case, as well as coma and

seizures.[40] Cocaine, amphetamines, and phencyclidine hydrochloride are commonly abused drugs that may be associated with cardiac dysrhythmias and hypertension, as well as coma and seizures.[3]

Hypothermia and Hyperthermia

A patient who is comatose from a drug ingestion may become hypothermic through exposure to environmental ambient temperature and through loss of heat secondary to peripheral vasodilation and depression of central nervous system (CNS) thermoregulation. Because hypothermia may add to metabolic acidosis, hypoxemia, CNS depression, and cardiac dysrhythmias,[70,71] the temperature of a comatose patient should always be taken rectally to rule out complicating hypothermia. Drugs or poisons frequently associated with hypothermia are ethanol, barbiturates, other sedative-hypnotics, general anesthetics, phenothiazines, tricyclic antidepressants, and carbon monoxide.[72–75]

Hyperthermia may be present with salicylate, phenothiazine, tricyclic antidepressant, phencyclidine hydrochloride, cocaine, and amphetamine overdose.[25,28,73,76] Agents that uncouple oxidative phosphorylation, e.g., salicylates, pentachlorophenol, and dinitrophenol, may result in hyperthermia, tachycardia, and coma.[76,77] (See Chapters 29 and 30.)

Cyanosis

Many disease processes can produce cyanosis. The differential diagnosis of a cyanotic patient includes acute myocardial infarction, pulmonary thromboembolism, right-to-left arteriovenous shunts, impaired pulmonary function, and abnormal hemoglobins, either hereditary or acquired. Cyanosis is clinically evident when there are more than 5 gm reduced hemoglobin per 100 ml blood (33 percent reduced hemoglobin). At this point, the arterial blood is usually less than 80 percent saturated.[78]

Cyanosis is also clinically evident when there is 1.5 gm methemoglobin per 100 ml blood (approximately a 10 percent methemoglobinemia). Many drugs and chemicals can result in methemoglobinemia, and the most common etiologic agents are sulfonamides, nitrates, and nitrites.[79] Aromatic amino and nitro compounds, such as aniline, trinitrotoluene, nitrobenzene, nitrophenol, dinitrobenzene, and nitroaniline, are well absorbed through the skin and can result in methemoglobinemia and hepatotoxicity.[80] Other common causes of methemoglobinemia are azo dye compounds such as those used in urinary analgesics. Most of these products contain phenazopyridine hydrochloride.[81] Benzocaine is present in many proprietary compounds and can cause methemoglobinemia when ingested.[82] The diagnosis of methemoglobinemia should be considered in a patient who is cyanotic, does not respond to oxygen therapy, and has no other historical or cardiac reason for being cyanotic.

Sulfhemoglobinemia is another chemical cause of cyanosis that is again unresponsive to oxygen therapy. This is a rare disorder thought to be due to sulfur-containing drugs or to chronic constipation with absorption of sulfur compounds.[83] Sulfhemoglobinemia is not responsive to methylene blue therapy and lasts the life of red blood cells. As little as 0.5 gm sulfmethemoglobin per 100 ml blood can result in clinical cyanosis.[84]

Metabolic Acidosis

Anion gap metabolic acidosis may be caused by a toxic ingestion of salicylates, methanol, ethylene glycol, isoniazid, iron, ethanol, or paraldehyde.[76,85–89] Other common causes of metabolic acidosis, such as diabetic ketoacidosis and sepsis, should be ruled out. Phenformin ingestion is associated with a severe lactic acidosis, but it is uncommon now. Renal tubular acidosis without an anion gap has been associated with chronic sniffing abuse of toluene-containing products.[90] Toluene ingestion has also been reported to cause an anion gap metabolic acidosis.[91] Salicylates, methanol, and ethylene glycol are the most commonly ingested substances that cause an anion gap metabolic acidosis and should always be considered in a comatose, acidotic patient. Seizures may also occur with ingestion of these drugs; seizures almost always occur with isoniazid poisoning. (See Chapter 18.)

DISORDERS OF MOVEMENT

Both nontoxic ingestions and overdoses can cause movement disorders. Phenytoin is known to be associated with movement disorders in both therapeutic and toxic concentrations. Choreoathetosis and orofacial dyskinesias have been reported at therapeutic levels,[92] and choreoathetoid movements have been reported with ingestion of amounts in the toxic range.[93] Phenytoin toxicity is also associated with ataxia and nystagmus.[94] Phenothiazines and the butyrophenone haloperidol (Haldol) are known to cause extrapyramidal reactions. Tricyclic antidepressants in overdose have been associated with choreoathetoid movements.[95] Heavy metals such as lead, mercury, and arsenic can cause movement disorders of ataxia and choreiform motions through chronic toxicity.[63,96,97] Lithium toxicity is associated with ataxia and tremors.[98]

BEHAVIORAL DISORDERS

Drug-induced disorders of behavior include psychoses, delirium, paranoia, hallucinations, excitability, abusive and violent behavior, disorders of perception, extreme agitation, fatigue, and depression. Phencyclidine hydrochloride, cocaine, and amphetamines can produce a toxic psychosis indistinguishable from a true paranoid schizophrenia. Phencyclidine hydrochloride intoxication may be associated with paranoid and violent reactions, as well as agitation and hallucinations.[28,99] Chronic abuse of cocaine and amphetamines can result in depression, paranoia, hallucinations, perceptual difficulties, emotional lability, and irritability as well as a toxic psychosis.[100–102] Anticholinergic drugs such as antihistamines, tricyclic antidepressants, phenothiazines, atropine, scopolamine, and over-the-counter products can produce a syndrome of hallucinations, delirium, and agitation in overdose.[24,25,103,104] Chronic heavy metal poisoning with mercury, lead, or arsenic can produce a toxic psychosis and other behavioral disturbances.[63,96] Caffeine and theophylline toxicity may also produce an acute confusional state with hyperalert behavior. Phenytoin can also produce a confusional state in high therapeutic plasma levels, and in toxic plasma ranges can cause excitation, delirium, nystagmus, myoclonus, and, in rare cases, seizures.

GENERAL MANAGEMENT

The general approach to managing a patient with a poisoning or drug overdose can be summarized as (1) prevention of absorption, (2) enhancement of elimination, and (3) use of physiologic antagonists as necessary.

Prevention of Absorption

Skin and Ocular Decontamination

Contamination of the eyes by an alkaline, acidic, or irritating chemical should be managed immediately by flushing the eyes with tap water. A low pressure continuous stream should be applied to the exposed eye for a minimum of 20 minutes if an alkali is involved, for 10 minutes if an acid or hydrocarbon is involved. The eye should be irrigated for 20 minutes if the substance involved is unknown. Treatment in the emergency department is to continue the irrigation if flushing may have been inadequate and to examine the eyes for corneal injuries.

Gasoline and hydrocarbon solvents not only may cause burns of the skin, but also they may be absorbed dermally.[105] These substances should be removed by means of thorough detergent and water decontamination.

Organophosphate and carbamate insecticides are readily absorbed through clothes and skin. The decontamination procedure for these insecticides should be carried out away from the emergency facility to prevent contamination of medical personnel. The person performing the decontamination should wear a protective apron, gloves, and disposable shoe covers. The patient's clothes should be removed and placed in specially marked plastic bags. Two separate water-detergent washes should be performed. Studies have demonstrated that two separate washes removed up to 94 percent of skin contamination with an organophosphate six hours postexposure.[106,107] It is important to wash all parts of the body, including the hair and under the fingernails.

Induction of Emesis

The clinical condition of the patient and what was ingested determine the appropriateness of inducing emesis. It is contraindicated when the patient

- has ingested acid or alkali
- is unconscious
- is having seizures
- has a depressed or absent gag reflex

Many drugs can delay gastric emptying, and emesis may be effective in removing some amount of these drugs even hours after the overdose. Emesis should be induced with syrup of ipecac, which works by both local gastric irritant effects and CNS effects.[108] The adult dose is 30 ml; the pediatric dose is 15 ml. After the syrup of ipecac, water should be given to distend the stomach. The dose may be repeated once if vomiting does not occur in 15 to 20 minutes. Stimulation of the pharynx with a tongue blade may also help in inducing emesis.

The use of apomorphine to produce vomiting has no advantage over the use of syrup of ipecac. In fact, because apomorphine may also produce drowsiness and protracted vomiting, it should be avoided. Sodium chloride should not be used as an emetic because of the possibility that it will lead to a serious hypernatremia. Deaths have been reported.

Lavage

If a patient is becoming unconscious, is unconscious, has lost the gag reflex, or is having seizures, endotracheal or nasotracheal intubation followed by the insertion of a large orogastric tube is the preferred method of removing the remainder of the drug. A 28 French Ewald with multihole tip is the smallest bore orogastric tube that should be used. A 36 French Ewald that is

about 1 cm in diameter and has large holes is preferable. The usual size nasogastric tube of 16 or 18 French is completely worthless except for liquids. Tablets cannot be aspirated through it. The preferred lavage solution is saline. The patient should be in the left side, head down position. Lavage should continue until no solid material returns. Rarely can all the ingested substance be removed at this point, however.

Charcoal

Most drugs and chemicals are well absorbed by activated charcoal, which can be made up in water and administered orally or by nasogastric or orogastric tube after emesis or lavage has been completed. The universal antidote, consisting of burnt toast, magnesium oxide, and tannic acid, is not a replacement for activated charcoal. The universal antidote is worthless in poison management.

There are no known contraindications to the administration of activated charcoal. It should be remembered that activated charcoal also absorbs syrup of ipecac and these should not be given simultaneously. The dose of activated charcoal is usually 50 to 100 gm for an adult and 15 to 30 gm for children. The dose of charcoal may be repeated during the clinical course to ensure adequate absorption.

Cathartics

Another method by which drug absorption is prevented is through the use of cathartics to enhance gastric motility. The use of magnesium cathartics is contraindicated in renal failure. Oil-based cathartics should probably be avoided, owing to the potential for a lipoid pneumonia if aspiration occurs. The cathartic dose is 15 to 30 gm magnesium sulfate or magnesium citrate in all adults and 250 mg/kg in children. The use of cathartics helps to mobilize the activated charcoal through the gastrointestinal tract. The cathartic dose may need to be repeated to stimulate bowel action. An enema may also be helpful to stimulate bowel clearance.

Enhancement of Excretion

Enhancing the removal of a drug includes the techniques of forced diuresis, dialysis, or hemoperfusion.

Forced Diuresis

The excretion of some drugs can be facilitated by a neutral, alkaline, or an acid diuresis. Alkaline and acid diureses employ the principle of ion trapping. Drugs with a dissociable group carry a charge at a pH that is distant from the pKa. At a pH equal to the pKa, a drug is half-dissociated and half-undissociated. Promoting an alkaline urine to a pH of 7 or greater accelerates the renal elimination of salicylates and phenobarbital, since both of these drugs are weak acids.[109,110] An alkaline urine causes the drugs to remain ionized in the renal tubular lumen and thus not readily able to cross the tubular cell membrane. Forced diuresis is not helpful for drugs with large volumes of distribution, such as tricyclic antidepressants, phenothiazines, and digoxin. Cerebral edema and pulmonary edema may be exacerbated by forced diuresis, and caution is in order in these cases.

Alkaline diuresis is accomplished with bicarbonate (1 to 2 mEq/kg) administered intravenously. The addition of potassium chloride may be necessary to ensure that the urine becomes alkaline. Alkaline diuresis is useful in the treatment of salicylates and phenobarbital poisoning. The urine pH must be increased to 7.5 to achieve the maximum elimination effect.

Acid diuresis is accomplished with ammonium chloride (2 to 6 gm/day orally in adults and 75 mg/kg orally divided into four doses for children). The urine pH should be reduced to 4.5 or less. Acid diuresis has been reported for amphetamine and strychnine intoxication,[29,111] but its effectiveness is not established. Also, if rhabdomyolysis has occurred secondary to seizures or myoclonic activity, acid diuresis can precipitate myoglobinuric renal failure. Intense myoclonic activity and seizures can occur with PCP, amphetamines, and strychnine toxicity.

Neutral diuresis may be helpful in renal elimination of isoniazid.

Pharmacologic diuretics should be given, together with adequate fluids. Usual urine flow is 0.5 to 2 ml/kg/hour; with forced diuresis, urine flow should be 3 to 6 ml/kg/hour. Alkaline or acid diuresis should be chosen on the basis of the drug's pKa, protein-binding capacity, and volume of distribution so that ionized drug is trapped in the tubular lumen and not reabsorbed. Osmotic load is also important, and either type of diuretic may be employed. Reabsorption proximally occurs if inadequate osmotic load is not maintained in the tubule.

Dialysis

Hemodialysis or peritoneal dialysis can be useful in some poisonings. Dialysis is considered part of the supportive care of most poisoned patients—not a primary form of treatment. Dialysis may be considered if the patient's condition fits any of the following criteria:

1. coma or seizures that are caused by a dialyzable drug and cannot be treated by conservative means
2. acid-base and electrolyte disturbances that cannot be controlled
3. marked hyperosmolality that is not due to easily corrected fluid problems
4. marked hypothermia or hyperthermia
5. drug-induced hypotension that is uncontrollable and threatens renal or hepatic function
6. renal failure

More specifically, dialysis should be considered if the substance involved is

- ethylene glycol and acidosis cannot be controlled with an ethanol infusion or the patient is in renal failure
- methanol and acidosis cannot be controlled with an ethanol infusion and sodium bicarbonate or cerebral edema is present
- a heavy metal and chelation has occurred or the patient is in renal failure
- theophylline and seizures and arrhythmias cannot be controlled
- salicylate and pulmonary edema, acidemia, seizures, or cerebral edema is uncontrollable
- ethanol and the blood level is extremely high and respiratory depression has occurred

The dialyzability of a drug is dependent upon its physiochemical properties and its pharmacokinetic parameters.[112,113] The factors involved in the dialyzability of a drug can be summarized as follows:

1. molecular weight. Drugs with a lower molecular weight cross the dialyzing membrane more readily than drugs with a higher molecular weight.
2. solubility. Water-soluble drugs are dialyzed more easily than lipid-soluble drugs in an aqueous dialysate solution.
3. plasma protein binding. Only free drug is available for removal. Drugs with a high degree of protein binding are poorly dialyzed.
4. distribution phase. For drugs having a long tissue-to-plasma redistribution phase, extracorporeal methods of removal will be less successful.
5. apparent volume of distribution. Drugs with large volumes of distribution are highly tissue bound, and very little of the drug is actually present in the vascular compartment. Thus, less is available for removal by dialysis.
6. elimination half-life. The half-life of a drug in an overdose situation may change as a result of the change in elimination kinetics. A drug's half-life may be shorter or longer in an overdose than in a therapeutic situation.
7. dialysis clearance relative to total body clearance. The overall clearance must be increased in order to shorten the elimination half-life of the drug.

Even if the overall clearance with dialysis is greater than total body clearance, dialysis may not remove a significantly larger fraction of the drug during a reasonable period.

8. metabolites. The same considerations of dialyzability must be given to metabolites as well as the parent compound. Many metabolites are pharmacologically and toxicologically active.

Hemoperfusion

The use of hemoperfusion as an extracorporeal technique to remove ingested drugs is increasing in the management of overdoses.[114,115] The technique involves passing the patient's venous blood over a fixed adsorbent bed that consists of either coated activated charcoal or amberlite resin. The fixed bed provides a solid surface area with a continuous porous phase so that the blood can penetrate the pores and be exposed to a large surface area. Hemoperfusion has a few advantages over hemodialysis. It is particularly useful for drugs with a high degree of protein binding, since both protein-bound and non–protein-bound drug is removed. Charcoal-based hemoperfusion beds can remove both polar and nonpolar drugs, as well as their metabolites. The amberlite adsorbent, however, removes nonpolar drugs and metabolites better than it removes polar drugs.

The limiting factors of hemoperfusion are the affinity of the drug for the adsorbent material, the rate of blood flow through the adsorbent bed, the volume of distribution of the drug, and the redistribution of the drug back into the vascular compartment following termination of the procedure. A drug with a slow redistribution from tissue to plasma can result in rebound levels after hemoperfusion. Hemoperfusion is best used for drugs that have a low intrinsic clearance and a small volume of distribution. Drugs such as tricyclic antidepressants, phenothiazines, ethchlorvynol and digoxin do not have an effective total body burden clearance. Hemoperfusion can significantly decrease the total body burden of theophylline, salicylates, and phenobarbital. The patient must be heparinized, however, and there is a substantial decrease in platelet count up to one-half the prehemoperfusion value. The platelet count usually returns to normal within one to two days following the procedure. There may also be a loss of plasma protein and calcium.

Specific Poisons and their Physiologic Antagonists

Some physiologic antagonists reverse the symptomatology of certain poisons and drug overdoses. It is important to be aware of the pathophysiology of the specific toxic agent involved.

Oxygen

The agent employed in carbon monoxide poisoning is oxygen. Carbon monoxide is produced by incomplete combustion of organic products. Automobile exhaust fumes account for approximately 60 percent of carbon monoxide emitted per year into the atmosphere. Other causes of carbon monoxide poisoning are fires, industrial processes, gas and water heaters, and methylene chloride exposure. Tobacco smokers may have carboxyhemoglobin levels between 5 and 20 percent.[116] There is also an endogenous carbon monoxide production that results in a carboxyhemoglobin level of 0.4 percent secondary to heme catabolism.[117]

Carbon monoxide has an affinity for hemoglobin 200 times that of oxygen. It also has an affinity for other heme-containing proteins, such as cytochrome oxidase, peroxidases, P-450 cytochrome oxidase, and myoglobin. The effect of carbon monoxide on the oxyhemoglobin dissociation curve is a shift to the left, which inhibits the release of oxygen to tissues.[117] The pathophysiology of carbon monoxide is tissue hypoxia and interference with cellular respiration.

Several factors are involved in carbon monoxide poisoning: (1) the concentration of carbon monoxide in the environment, which need not be very high since carbon monoxide has a great affinity for hemoglobin; (2) alveolar ventilation; (3) preexisting cardiovascular disease and anemia; (4) duration of exposure; (5) cardiac output; (6) physical activity of the person exposed.

The signs and symptoms of carbon monoxide poisoning vary according to the level of carboxyhemoglobin and the duration of exposure (Table 24–1). The absolute

TABLE 24–1 Signs and Symptoms of Acute Carbon Monoxide Poisoning

Level of Carboxyhemoglobin (%)	Signs and Symptoms
10–20	Headache, fatigue, dizziness
20–30	Headache, fatigue, nausea, vomiting, decreased motor ability
30–40	Syncope, increased respirations, tachycardia, confusion, obtundation
50–60	Coma, convulsions, Cheyne-Stokes respirations
60–70	Cardiorespiratory depression, bradycardia, pulmonary edema
70–80	Cardiovascular failure, death

carboxyhemoglobin concentration may not correlate with the signs and symptoms at all times since the level declines once exposure is terminated. A patient with a low level of carboxyhemoglobin may be comatose and having seizures because the level was very high during primary exposure. The half-life of carboxyhemoglobin is approximately six hours in 21 percent FIO_2 (room air). With 100 percent oxygen, the half-life is 30 to 60 minutes, and with 2 atmospheres oxygen (hyperbaric) the half-life is 15 minutes.[118] A person with carbon monoxide poisoning should be given 100 percent oxygen if a hyperbaric chamber is not available or while preparations are being made for hyperbaric therapy. One hundred percent oxygen therapy should continue until the carboxyhemoglobin concentration is less than 5 percent. Any patient who is symptomatic secondary to carbon monoxide poisoning should be observed for other signs of a toxic reaction, and a patient with a concentration greater than 20 percent should be admitted to the hospital.

When a patient is brought to the emergency department following a fire exposure, carbon monoxide poisoning should be considered. However, other toxic gases may also be produced in the combustion process, such as hydrogen cyanide and hydrochloric acid from burning plastic and foam products. The levels of arterial blood gases may be normal in carbon monoxide poisoning except for a decreased oxyhemoglobin saturation. In order to detect a decreased oxyhemoglobin saturation, direct measurement of the concentration by an oximeter is required.

The normal solubility of oxygen in blood is 0.3 ml/ 100 ml blood at a PaO_2 of 100 mm Hg (FIO_2 of 21 percent). With 100 percent oxygen there is a six- to seven-fold increase in the amount of dissolved oxygen, up to 2 ml/100 ml blood. Breathing 100 percent oxygen should produce a PaO_2 of 673 mm Hg at sea level. Hyperbaric (2 atm) oxygen therapy dissolves 4.3 ml/100 ml blood. Thus, therapy with oxygen in carbon monoxide poisoning involves increasing the dissolved oxygen in the blood for delivery to tissues.[118] If patients do not improve despite 100 percent oxygen or hyperbaric oxygen therapy, the possibility of cerebral edema should be considered.

Carbon monoxide poisoning can result in myocardial ischemia and myocardial infarction with increased myocardial oxygen consumption. ST segment and T-wave changes can be seen in acute and chronic carbon monoxide poisoning. Neurologic sequelae can involve cerebral edema, seizures, cortical necrosis, cerebellar lesions, focal and disseminated cerebral atrophy, demyelination of white matter, and basal ganglia lesions. Neurologic lesions may thus result in personality changes, dementia, memory impairment, visual loss, and retardation.[119,120] The exposure of a pregnant woman to carbon monoxide may have severe CNS effects on the fetus.[121]

Most clinicians are not aware that methylene chloride is a source of carbon monoxide poisoning. Used as an industrial solvent and present in paint remover, methylene chloride can produce carbon monoxide poisoning if used in a poorly ventilated area because it is converted into carbon monoxide. Also, the half-life of carbon monoxide from methylene chloride exposure is twice that from other sources.[122] (See Chapter 60.)

Cyanide Kit

A cyanide kit is marketed by Lilly and Company and is the only treatment form for cyanide poisoning generally available in the United States. The cyanide kit should be in every emergency department and should be checked frequently for expiration. The kit contains an amyl nitrite ampule, a 3 percent sodium nitrite solution, and a 25 percent sodium thiosulfate solution. The drugs should be used sequentially. The amyl nitrite ampule should be crushed and the patient made to breathe it for 30 seconds of every 60 seconds until the sodium nitrite can be administered. The sodium nitrite is in an adult dosage form; if a child is being treated, the dose must be adjusted.

The goal of therapy is to produce a state of methemoglobinemia, since the cyanide ion has a great affinity for iron in the ferric (Fe^{3+}) state. The amyl nitrite produces a 5 percent methemoglobinemia. The 3 percent sodium nitrite solution is then administered intravenously. The adult dose is 300 mg or 10 ml; the pediatric dose is 10 mg/kg or 0.2 ml/kg, not to exceed 300 mg. If a child is given the adult dose of sodium nitrite, a fatal methemoglobinemia may be produced. The pediatric dosage regimen should be affixed to the kit so it will be readily seen. The 25 percent sodium thiosulfate solution is then administered intravenously. Packaged as a 50-ml volume (12.5 gm), it provides substrate for conversion of cyanide to thiocyanate. Sodium thiosulfate has a low toxicity and is well tolerated. Should symptoms recur, the sodium nitrite and sodium thiosulfate can be repeated but at half the dose previously administered.

Cobalt compounds, e.g., cobalt edetate and hydroxocobalamin, have been studied with regard to their use in the treatment of cyanide poisoning, but their effectiveness as compared to the nitrite-thiosulfate treatment remains to be seen. The treatment of hydrogen sulfide poisoning is the same as that for cyanide poisoning except the sodium thiosulfate is not administered.[123–125]

Atropine

The cholinergic effects of organophosphate and carbamate insecticides can be reversed by atropine, although the patient's condition will be refractory to the usual doses. An adult should be given 2 mg intravenously at a slow rate and then observed for a reversal of signs and symptoms. The pediatric starting dose is 0.05 mg/kg administered intravenously. The organophosphate and carbamates inhibit the acetylcholinesterase enzyme and thus allow acetylcholine to stimulate the cholinergic receptor sites continually. Atropine blocks the muscarinic effects of increased salivation, pulmonary secretions, bradycardia, bronchospasm, and diarrhea, but it does not block the nicotinic effects of skeletal muscle weakness and paralysis. The amount of atropine required may be tremendously large, sometimes approaching as much as 2 gm over a 24-hour period.[126–129]

The end point of treatment with atropine is to dry all secretions. Only when all secretions are dried is the patient fully atropinized. At this point, the patient's heart rate is most likely to be increased and pupils dilated; however, if the pulmonary secretions or oropharyngeal secretions are still present, the patient has not been given enough atropine. A patient who has been fully atropinized may also suffer a respiratory arrest secondary to skeletal muscle paralysis, owing to the fact that the nicotinic receptors have not been blocked. The airway of the patient should be protected at all times, and the physicians should be prepared to intubate the patient and support respiration during the course of the treatment. A patient may even succumb to a respiratory arrest late in the course of treatment.

Pralidoxime (2-PAM, Protopam Chloride)

An acetylcholinesterase regenerator, 2-PAM is useful in organophosphate poisonings in which the red blood cell-cholinesterase level is depressed below 50 percent of normal. 2-PAM should be given early in the course of treatment and may not be beneficial more than 24 hours postexposure. However, atropine should always be given first and 2-PAM administered after atropinization is complete.[130]

Naloxone (Narcan)

Naloxone, a pure narcotic antagonist with no agonist properties, effectively reverses the CNS and cardiorespiratory effects of narcotic overdoses. Naloxone may be administered intravenously, subcutaneously, or intramuscularly. Because the half-life of naloxone is approximately 60 minutes,[131] the dose may need to be repeated as the antagonistic effect disappears. Naloxone, unlike nalorphine (Nalline), is devoid of respiratory depressant effects. The usual adult dose of naloxone is 0.4 to 0.8 mg, and the usual pediatric dose is 0.01 mg/kg. However, larger doses of naloxone may be required in narcotic overdoses involving methadone, propoxyphene, or pentazocine. Ten times the usually recommended dose may be necessary as an intravenous bolus to reverse the narcotic effects of propoxyphene. Narcotic toxicity may not be reversed until five to ten ampules (2 to 4 mg) are administered as an intravenous bolus. An adequate naloxone trial for any narcotic overdose should be at least 2 mg intravenously.[132–134] Relatively large doses of naloxone have been administered without adverse effects or addictive potential.[135]

Methylene Blue

A nonenzymatic catalyst, methylene blue is used to treat methemoglobinemia caused by nitrates, nitrites, and other nitro compounds. Methemoglobin is the oxidized form of hemoglobin with the iron in the ferric (Fe^{3+}) state. Since methemoglobin in unavailable for oxygen transport and release to tissues, the oxyhemoglobin dissociation curve shifts to the left.[79] An endogenous physiologic methemoglobinemia usually does not exceed 2 percent because the erythrocyte expends energy to keep hemoglobin in the reduced state. This function is normally performed by methemoglobin reductase enzymes that are NADH-dependent. This system is activated by electron transport carriers such as methylene blue. If the normal methemoglobinemia exists, then the methemoglobin reductase-NADPH system increases its activity about 60-fold. The addition of the nonenzymatic electron carrier methylene blue increases the activity rate of the methemoglobin reductase-NADPH system ten-fold above the rate at which methemoglobin stimulates it.[79]

Methylene blue is oxidized in the enzymatic process as it reduces the methemoglobin to hemoglobin. The secondary methemoglobin reductase system requires an intact pentose phosphate shunt and normal glucose metabolism to provide NADPH as a cofactor. The congenital absence of glucose-6-phosphate dehydrogenase results in an absence of NADPH. Individuals with this condition do not respond to methylene blue and develop a hemolytic process when exposed to oxidant agents. Persons with a deficiency or absence of methemoglobin reductase are also more likely to develop methemoglobinemia from oxidant drugs.

The clinical presentation of a patient with methemoglobinemia depends on the percent of hemoglobin oxidized to the ferric state. Cyanosis, dyspnea, lethargy, coma, seizures, hypotension, bradycardia, and cardiac arrest may occur. At low levels of methemoglobinemia, below 30 percent, mild symptomatology of headache, cyanosis, and lethargy may occur. As the methemoglobin level increases above 50 to 70 percent, the symptomatology may progress to coma, hypotension, bradycardia, and seizures with cyanosis. Levels greater than

70 percent may result in death.[81] Cyanosis develops when the level of methemoglobin is greater than 1.5 gm/100 ml blood or about 10 percent methemoglobinemia. The cyanosis is also unresponsive to oxygen therapy. A simple test can be performed at the patient's bedside to determine if a significant methemoglobin level should be investigated. If a drop of the patient's blood on a piece of blotter paper appears darker than a normal control, methemoglobinemia should be suspected.

Treatment of methemoglobinemia is with high-flow oxygen and methylene blue. The dose of methylene blue is 0.1 to 0.2 ml/kg intravenously of a 1 percent solution.[79–81] Caution is in order since large doses of methylene blue can also cause a methemoglobinemia; therefore, only one repeat dose should be administered if the patient with a severe case of poisoning has not improved. Also, if a patient does not respond to methylene blue therapy, the possibility of a glucose-6-phosphate dehydrogenase deficiency should be considered.

Physostigmine

In order to reverse both the peripheral and central effects of anticholinergic drug overdose, physostigmine is employed. Physostigmine is a reversible inhibitor of acetylcholinesterase and reverses the anticholinergic syndrome of tricyclic antidepressants, antihistamines, atropine, and other drugs with anticholinergic effects in overdose.[136–138] The adverse effects of physostigmine are bradycardia, increased tracheobronchial secretions, decreased atrioventricular conduction, and seizures. The half-life of physostigmine is estimated to be 20 to 30 minutes. Physostigmine is available as an injectable in 1 mg/ml ampules. The adult dose is 1 to 2 mg slowly administered intravenously. The pediatric dose is 0.5 mg administered intravenously at a slow rate.

The effective dose can be repeated in 20 minutes if needed. However, the dose should be repeated only if the symptomatology is serious enough to warrant continued drug treatment. No maximum dose of physostigmine has been established, but a conservative approach to physostigmine administration is indicated in order to avoid seizures and other adverse effects.

PHARMACOKINETICS AND DRUG OVERDOSES

A basic understanding of drug pharmacology and pharmacokinetics is necessary if the clinical course of a patient with an overdose is to be understood. Pharmacokinetics involves the basic processes of drug absorption, distribution, biotransformation, and elimination from the body. A drug ingested in an overdose may act much differently pharmacokinetically than a drug taken in therapeutic amounts.

Drug Absorption

The various routes of drug administration include intravenous, intramuscular, rectal, subcutaneous, dermal, ocular, sublingual, and inhalation; however, the oral route is the most commonly employed, with the gastrointestinal tract forming the absorptive barrier to entrance into the vascular compartment. After entering the vascular compartment, a drug is distributed to various tissue receptor sites. Various factors affect the absorption of a drug from the gastrointestinal tract and thus the distribution of the drug to the receptor sites in tissues.[139–141]

Absorptive Process

Two barriers affect absorption of a drug through the gastrointestinal tract: the columnar epithelium of intestinal villi and the endothelium of the capillary wall. Because the capillary endothelium is relatively porous, the intestinal villi epithelium is the main biologic barrier to drug absorption. Absorption may be by passive diffusion or by active transport. The integrity of the villi epithelium is very important for drug absorption, and any pathologic state that disrupts this integrity may affect absorption, either increasing it (as in massive iron poisoning), or decreasing it by causing diarrhea and loss of absorptive area.

Fasting State

The absence of food in the stomach increases the absorption of most drugs. Drugs may combine with food particles, which can retard or inhibit absorption.

Gastric Juices and Digestive Enzymes

Some drugs may be destroyed, precipitated, or altered by gastric juices and enzymes present in the stomach.

Drug Dissolution

A drug must be dissolved before it can be absorbed; therefore, the dissolution rate of a drug influences absorption. A drug with a slow dissolution rate has a slow absorptive rate. The dissolution rate of a drug depends on its solubility, the pH of the gastrointestinal juices, food content of the stomach, and the salt or crystalline form of the drug.

Gastrointestinal Surface Area and Motility

The large surface area of the intestinal villi and the rate of emptying of gastric contents are the two most important factors in drug absorption.[140] The absorptive capacity of the small intestines is much greater than that of the stomach; if gastric emptying into the intestines is rapid, drug absorption is not delayed. Any factor that decreases gastric emptying, e.g., drugs such as anticholinergics and narcotics, also delays drug absorption.[142] Once the drug is in the small intestines, the large absorptive area compensates for other factors that may affect the absorption.

The motility of the small intestine also influences the absorption of a drug. Decreased intestinal motility increases the contact time with the epithelial surface and, thus, absorption of a drug. Increased intestinal motility decreases surface contact time and delays or decreases absorption. Since the absorptive area of the small intestine is greater in the duodenum and proximal area, absorption would be thought to be expedited here. However, since the motility of the proximal small intestines is greater than that of the distal small intestines, a drug may actually be absorbed in the distal segment because the contact time with the epithelial area there is longer.

pH Influence on Drug Absorption

The influence of gastric pH on the absorption of a drug is not clinically significant. A nonionized drug penetrates a biologic membrane much more rapidly than an ionized drug; however, the large absorptive area of the small intestines more than compensates for pH effect.

First Pass Elimination

The venous blood from the intestinal villi goes directly into the liver via the portal system. A drug may be metabolized by the liver at this point to a great extent before it reaches the general circulation.

Drug Distribution

Following an intravenous dose of a drug, there is a biphasic decline in drug concentration over time (Fig. 24–1). The decline in the drug concentration is represented by a distribution phase (alpha) as the drug is distributed from the blood into tissue sites and a slower drug elimination phase (beta). The drug in the vascular compartment is bound to some extent to plasma proteins, and an equilibration is reached between protein-bound drug and free drug. The free drug interacts with drug receptors at the tissue distribution sites to produce pharmacologic or toxicologic activity.

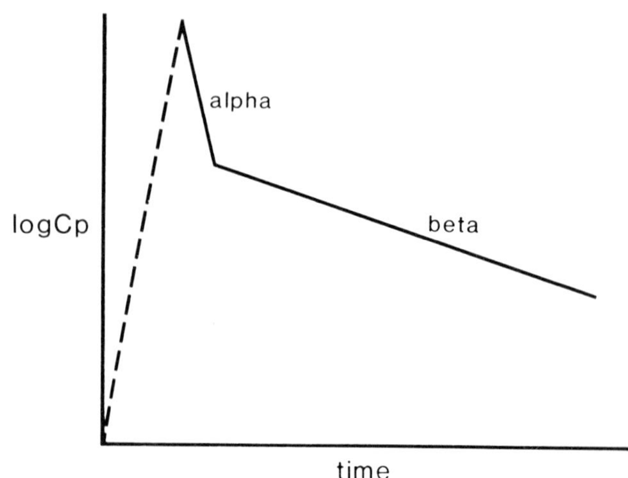

Figure 24–1   Biphasic Decline in Drug Concentration Over Time.

The distribution of a drug into the vascular space, body water space, and tissue sites is a pharmacologic concept termed the *apparent volume of distribution.* This is not a real volume, but a concept that describes the characteristics of the drug, e.g., its lipid or water solubility and the extent of its plasma protein binding and tissue binding. A drug that is confined chiefly to the vascular and body water space with relatively low tissue binding has a low volume of distribution; a lipid-soluble drug with a high degree of tissue binding has a large volume of distribution. The volume of distribution is also affected by plasma protein binding. A decrease in protein-bound drug provides more free drug to diffuse into tissue sites. Increased binding to plasma protein tends to decrease the volume of distribution. Volume of distribution is given in units of liters/kg.

A large volume of distribution would be greater than 1 liter/kg. The volume of distribution (Vd) is related to the plasma concentration (Cp) and administered drug dose (D) by the following equation (in a simplified one-compartment model):

$$Vd = \frac{D}{Cp}$$

where Vd = liter/kg × body weight in kg
D = mg
Cp = mg/liter (μg/ml)

The volume of distribution can be determined for a drug by administering a known dose intravenously, determining several plasma levels, and extrapolating back to what the concentration would have been at time zero ($Cp0$) once equilibration has occurred, and then entering these values into the equation. The drug concentration at time zero is the assumed concentration if instantaneous distribution had occurred. This is based on a one-compartment model, i.e., the distribution and elimination of the drug from the central plasma compartment. This is a relatively simple model to use. In reality, several different compartments, representing various tissue distribution and elimination sites, may be involved. The one-compartment model (Fig. 24–2) is useful for gaining a basic understanding of drug distribution and elimination, however.

The volume of distribution can be used to calculate either the amount of certain drugs in the body when plasma concentration is known or to calculate a loading dose needed to obtain a specific plasma concentration. (A partial listing of volumes of distribution is given in Table 24–2.) For example, using a known volume of distribution (Vd) to calculate the loading dose (D) required (in a one-compartment model), to obtain a theophylline blood level of 15 μg/ml in a 70-kg adult results in the following calculation:

$$Vd = 450 \text{ ml/kg for theophylline in an adult}$$

$$450 \text{ ml/kg} = \frac{D}{15 \text{ μg/ml}}$$

$$(450 \text{ ml/kg}) \times (70 \text{ kg}) = 31.5 \text{ liters}$$

$$15 \text{ μg/ml} = 15 \text{ mg/liter}$$

$$31.5 \text{ liters} = \frac{D}{15 \text{ mg/liter}}$$

$$(31.5 \text{ liters}) (15 \text{ mg/liter}) = 473 \text{ mg}$$

$$D = 473 \text{ mg}$$

Since aminophylline is 80 percent theophylline, the adjusted dose of aminophylline in a 70-kg adult would be 591 mg administered slowly over 30 minutes intravenously to achieve a 15 μg/ml therapeutic level.

The volume of distribution can also be useful when a patient is subtherapeutic on either theophylline or phenytoin and the level needs to be increased. In order

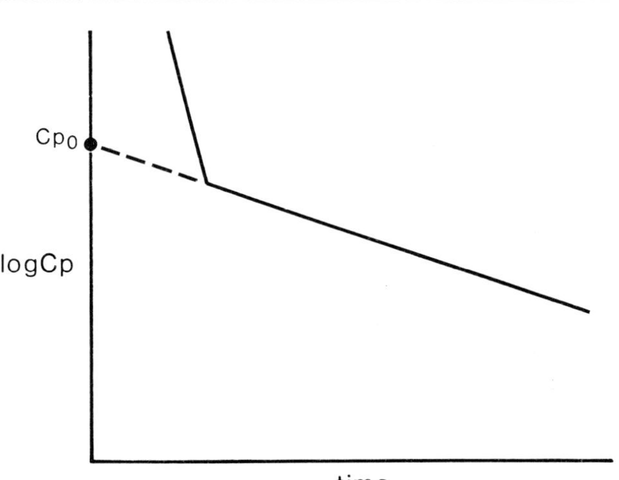

Figure 24–2 The One-Compartment Model.

TABLE 24–2   Volumes of Distribution (Vd = liters/kg)

Drug	Older Children	Adults
Acetaminophen	1–1.2	1–1.2
Digoxin	15	7.5
Furosemide	0.20	0.25
Phenobarbital	0.75	0.75
Phenytoin	0.75	0.60–0.80
Salicylates	0.3–0.6*	0.3–0.6*
Theophylline	0.45	0.45
Ethanol	0.60	0.60

* Vd of salicylate changes in an overdose from 0.30 to 0.60 liters/kg.

Source: Modified and reprinted with permission from Silver H, Peterson R, Rumack B: Drug therapy, in Kempe H, Silver H, O'Brien D (eds): *Current Pediatric Diagnosis and Treatment*, ed 7. Los Altos, CA, Lange Medical Publications, 1982, p 1015.

to raise a phenytoin plasma level from 5 ng/ml to 15 ng/ml, an increment of 10 ng/ml, the following calculation can be made:

$$Vd = 600 \text{ ml/kg for phenytoin}$$

$$600 \text{ ml/kg} = \frac{D}{10 \text{ ng/ml}}$$

$$(600 \text{ ml/kg}) (10 \text{ ng/ml}) = D = 6000 \text{ ng/kg} = 6 \text{ mg/kg}$$

Therefore, to raise a phenytoin blood level 10 ng/ml, 6 mg/kg can be administered intravenously.

Biotransformation

Elimination of a drug includes biotransformation into pharmacologically active or inactive metabolites. Polar drugs and metabolites are primarily excreted by the kidneys, whereas nonpolar drugs are first metabolized by the liver to more polar compounds. Biotransformation of a drug taken in overdose may be very important clinically. For example, amitriptyline, imipramine, and doxepin are tertiary amines and are metabolized to their respective secondary amines nortriptyline, desipramine, and nordoxepin. Both the parent compounds and metabolites are further hydroxylated. All of these are toxicologically active and influence the clinical course of a tricyclic antidepressant overdose.

Drug Elimination and Clearance

Following distribution, elimination begins. Elimination is through the central compartment. The elimination phase of drug metabolism may follow one of two pharmacokinetic processes or a combination of two processes: (1) first order elimination kinetics and (2) zero order elimination kinetics.

Most drugs are eliminated by a first order process, i.e., the amount of drug metabolized per unit of time is a constant fraction of the total drug present and does not vary with the plasma concentration of the drug. Most drugs are eliminated in this manner. In contrast, a constant amount of drug is metabolized per unit of time with zero order elimination. The metabolic mechanism for the drug elimination is saturated and cannot proceed faster than its maximal rate of metabolism.

The time required for one-half of a drug to be eliminated from the body is termed the drug half-life. Since most drugs are eliminated by a first order process, it can be predicted that 97 percent of a drug will be removed from the body in five half-lives. Thus, if a patient has a theophylline level of 40 μg/ml with a half-life of four hours, then the patient will have a level of 20 μg/ml in four hours and 10 μg/ml in eight hours. Detailed reviews of clinical pharmacokinetics are available elsewhere.[143,144]

Understanding the two processes can be clinically useful in certain overdose instances. For example, phenytoin elimination is normally a first order process at levels below 20 μg/ml and the drug has a half-life of 22 hours. In an overdose, however, the elimination process changes from first order to zero order as the plasma level rises above 20 ng/ml. Thus, owing to the saturation of the hydroxylation process that is the major metabolic route of phenytoin, the patient with a phenytoin overdose may require several days to eliminate the drug. Knowing this will help the clinician predict the course of a patient with such an overdose.

Pharmacokinetic Considerations in the Neonate and Elderly

Patients in the extremes of age groups present special pharmacokinetic problems that must be considered in both therapeutic and overdose situations. The neonate and premature infant generally have a larger volume of distribution because of an increase in the extracellular fluid and the decreased ability of fetal plasma proteins to bind drugs. The premature infant has much less protein-binding ability than the neonate. Adult values for plasma protein may not be attained until the infant is over one year of age.[145] Free fatty acids and bilirubin are also increased in neonates, which would tend to displace some drugs from protein-binding sites. Highly protein-bound drugs, such as salicylates and phenytoin, can displace bilirubin from binding sites, leading to possible hyperbilirubinemia. Salicylate plasma protein binding is decreased in the neonate, and the volume of distribution is approximately 600 ml/kg, twice the adult

value.[145,146] Premature infants and neonates also have a relative hypoxemia and a lower blood pH that can lead to increased tissue concentrations of salicylates.[145]

The volume of distribution of phenytoin in the neonate is twice that of the adult.[147,148] The level of non–protein-bound phenobarbital is 60 percent in the neonate versus 50 percent in the adult.[149] Tricyclic antidepressants are generally greater than 90 percent protein-bound in plasma; however, increased free levels in the neonate can certainly result in increased toxic reactions. In general, the increased volume of distribution of drugs and the decreased plasma protein binding can result in a higher plasma/tissue ratio of the drug than would be expected in an older child or adult, leading to possible toxicity.

The premature infant and neonate also have a decreased ability to biotransform drugs through hydroxylation and a decreased plasma esterase activity.[145] However, the ability to N-demethylate is present.

Renal function is reduced in the newborn; adult functional levels are not reached until 6 to 12 months of age.[150] The renal functions of glomerular filtration and tubular secretion do not mature at the same rate. The development of tubular secretory capacity lags behind the development of glomerular filtration capacity so that the premature infant has difficulty handling some drugs even though glomerular filtration is possible. Furosemide (Lasix), for example, is a drug that depends on both glomerular filtration and active tubular transport.[151] The ability of a premature infant to secrete furosemide actively is much different from that of the full-term infant. Furosemide half-life in the premature infant may be prolonged up to 20 hours, whereas in the full-term infant the half-life may be only 7 hours. In the healthy adult, it is 30 minutes.[152]

In general, the elderly have difficulty handling some drugs, mainly because of decreased cardiac output with decreased renal blood flow and decreased hepatic clearance.[153] Absorption of drugs from the gastrointestinal tract is not significantly altered in the elderly, although it may be in the neonate because the neonate has irregular peristalsis and prolonged gastric emptying. Also, the premature infant has a relative achlorhydria compared with the full-term infant. The gastric pH of a neonate is 6 to 8, but reaches adult values by one year of age.[145] The elderly do not have drastic changes in drug volumes of distribution; however, some decrease in plasma protein binding can occur.

Theophylline is a commonly used drug that has different kinetics in the different age groups. In the premature infant, it has a prolonged elimination half-life, owing to a decreased elimination rate and an increased volume of distribution up to 690 ml/kg.[150] Elderly patients may also have a decreased theophylline elimination; the drug may have a prolonged half-life owing to a decrease in hepatic and renal blood flow secondary to congestive heart failure or decreased cardiac output associated with aging.

The disposition of drugs in the newborn and elderly must be a real concern to the physician in order to manage an intoxication properly or to prevent an iatrogenic complication.

COMMON DRUG OVERDOSES

Theophylline

The therapeutic range for theophylline is 10 to 20 μg/ml,[154] and levels above 20 μg/ml can produce a toxic reaction. Overdose of theophylline-containing compounds can cause ventricular dysrhythmias, focal and generalized seizures, hallucinations, tremors, hyperreflexia, hyperpnea, tachypnea, hyperthermia, gastrointestinal hemorrhage, coma, hypotension, tachycardia, and cardiovascular collapse.[60,61,155] Theophylline-induced seizures may be refractory to conventional anticonvulsant therapy; ventricular ectopy may also be difficult to control. Theophylline overdose may result in certain metabolic effects, such as lipolysis and a lactic acidosis.[156-158] There is increasing evidence that theophylline in high overdose concentrations may be eliminated by mixed first and zero order kinetic processes.[159] Prolonged theophylline half-lives with toxic plasma concentrations have also been reported.[160]

Toxic reactions to theophylline may occur secondary to decreased clearance in patients with pulmonary edema, liver disease, and congestive heart failure.[161] These patients require the same theophylline loading dose as other patients, but the maintenance doses should be decreased to avoid toxicity.

Some patients may tolerate very high theophylline levels with a paucity of signs and symptoms.[162] Therefore, if a toxic reaction to theophylline is suspected, the level should be determined as soon as possible. Such a toxic reaction may also be seen as an acute surgical abdomen with gastrointestinal bleeding.

The treatment for a toxic reaction to theophylline is mainly supportive. However, if seizures and dysrhythmias occur, conventional antiarrhythmic and anticonvulsive therapy should be employed and hemodialysis should probably be considered. A patient may be treated with cardiac monitoring and electrolyte replacement as long as the theophylline half-life is following a first order elimination process and seizures and dysrhythmias are controlled. Theophylline half-life in an adult is usually four to seven hours. Should the half-life be prolonged significantly, then hemodialysis should be considered. Hemoperfusion has a greater clearance of theophylline as compared with hemodialysis, but may have more complications in a theophylline overdose, and can result in a substantial decrease in platelets and significantly increase the risk of hemorrhage in an already seriously ill patient.

Tricyclic Antidepressants

Commonly ingested in overdose, tricyclic antidepressants may result in a clinical spectrum ranging from lethargy, hyperreflexia, sinus tachycardia, and delirium to coma, seizures, respiratory depression, hypotension, ventricular ectopy, and cardiac arrest. The mechanisms of tricyclic activity are (1) direct anticholinergic effect, (2) direct myocardial depression, and (3) blockade of norepinephrine reuptake. Cardiotoxicity is common, with intraventricular conduction delay, premature ventricular contractions, ventricular tachycardia, and ventricular fibrillation.[163] Neurologic effects include seizures, myoclonus, choreoathetosis, loss of oculovestibular reflexes, loss of muscle stretch reflexes, and pupillary changes.[164] Tricyclics are highly lipophilic, are absorbed rapidly from the small intestines, and have a large volume of distribution, signifying extensive tissue binding. The parent compounds of tricyclic antidepressants have a half-life of 24 to 36 hours. The active metabolites may take much longer to be eliminated.[24] Total plasma levels of tricyclic antidepressants do not correlate with symptomatology and cannot be depended on to predict outcome.

Amitriptyline (Elavil), doxepin (Sinequan), and imipramine (Tofranil) are tertiary amines and are N-demethylated by the liver to the corresponding secondary amines nortriptyline, nordoxepin, and desipramine, which are pharmacologically and toxicologically active. These are further hydroxylated to toxic metabolites.

Treatment is mainly supportive, e.g., cardiac monitoring and pulmonary care. Intubation with respirator support may be required because of respiratory depression. Hypotension can be managed initially with crystalloid fluids and secondarily with a vasopressor. The vasopressor of choice is norepinephrine. Clinical reports in the literature support the use of sodium bicarbonate to prevent or reverse ventricular dysrhythmias.[165] Physostigmine has also been reported to reverse coma, seizures, delirium, myoclonus, and ventricular dysrhythmias.[95] However, conservative use of intravenous physostigmine is in order since the adverse effects are seizures, bradycardia, and increased tracheobronchial secretions. Lidocaine has been employed with success in reversing ventricular ectopy. Phenytoin has also been employed if ventricular dysrhythmias are refractory to other pharmacologic intervention. Propranolol is a last choice drug that may terminate ventricular tachycardia or ventricular fibrillation,[166] but it can also further depress an already compensated myocardium.

Physostigmine, propranolol, and sodium bicarbonate have been demonstrated to counter the effect of amitriptyline on the frequency of extrasystole threshold.[167] The mechanism of action of sodium bicarbonate was previously believed to be an increased protein binding of the tricyclics as the plasma pH became more alkaline and thus decreased the amount of active free drug;[168] however, further studies have demonstrated that plasma protein binding of tricyclic antidepressants does not change significantly over a pH range 7 to 7.6.[169] The mechanism of action of sodium bicarbonate remains unknown. The drugs of choice for reversing ventricular ectopy in tricyclic toxic reactions are

1. sodium bicarbonate in an intravenous infusion of 1 to 2 µg/kg to maintain a plasma pH of 7.4
2. lidocaine, 1 to 2 mg/kg administered intravenously followed by a maintenance infusion of 2 to 4 mg/minute
3. phenytoin in a loading dose of 1,000 µg over 20 to 30 minutes to achieve therapeutic levels of 10 to 20 µg/ml
4. physostigmine, 1 to 2 mg administered intravenously at a slow rate (in the event that none of the first three methods is effective).

Methanol and Ethylene Glycol

Aliphatic alcohols that cause severe metabolic acidosis with a large anion gap, both methanol and ethylene glycol are nontoxic in the parent compound, but are metabolized by alcohol dehydrogenase and aldehyde dehydrogenase to their respective acids and aldehydes—which are toxic. Both methanol and ethylene glycol are ingredients of antifreeze and deicers. Ethylene glycol is metabolized to glycoaldehyde by alcohol dehydrogenase and then to glycolic acid by aldehyde dehydrogenase. The glycolic acid is the major metabolite and together with lactic acid, is most likely responsible for the metabolic acidosis.[167] Other acids are formed in the metabolism of ethylene glycol, but they are rapidly metabolized. Less than 3 percent of ethylene glycol is actually converted to oxalic acid.[170,171] Ethylene glycol poisoning is diagnosed by findings of a marked anion gap, metabolic acidosis, hyperoxaluria, intoxication similar to ethanol intoxication, seizures, and coma.

Methanol is metabolized by alcohol dehydrogenase to formaldehyde, which is metabolized by aldehyde dehydrogenase to formic acid. Methanol by itself may cause gastrointestinal distress with epigastric pain, but does not seem to produce the intoxication syndrome as ethanol does. Optic nerve damage can occur with methanol poisoning and may result in blindness. The optic nerve damage is possibly due to the accumulation of formate in the choroid plexus and optic nerve tissue, which damages the mitochondria and inhibits cytochrome oxidase activity.[172,173] Another CNS aspect of methanol poisoning is putaminal infarction, which can be readily evaluated by computerized tomographic scanning.[174,175]

Treatment of both ethylene glycol poisoning and methanol poisoning is correction of the existing severe metabolic acidosis, prevention of further metabolism of the parent compounds, and consideration of hemodialysis. Ethanol can block the metabolism of both methanol and ethylene glycol by alcohol dehydrogenase. It has a greater affinity for the alcohol dehydrogenase enzyme and can be given in a loading dose of 1 ml/kg intravenously (diluted in normal saline or dextrose and water) of absolute ethanol to achieve a blood level of approximately 130 mg/dl. An ethanol level of 100 mg/dl completely saturates the alcohol dehydrogenase enzyme and blocks further methanol and ethylene glycol conversion to organic acids. Sodium bicarbonate is also administered to correct the existing acidosis. After the loading dose of ethanol is given and the blood ethanol level is documented to be at least 100 mg/dl, an ethanol maintenance infusion is begun. Ethanol is metabolized at a rate of 75 to 175 mg/kg/hour on the average.[176] Calculation of the maintenance infusion is based on the mean of 125 mg/kg/hour as follows:

$$\frac{(125\,\text{mg/kg/hour})\,(\text{kg wt of patient})}{790\,\text{mg/ml (density ETOH)}} = \frac{\text{ml/hour of absolute ETOH to}}{\text{maintain level at 100 mg/dl}}$$

The density of absolute ethanol is 790 mg/ml, and dividing by this gives the milliliters per hour of absolute ethanol required to maintain the desired 100 mg/dl ethanol level. Once the metabolism of ethylene glycol and methanol is blocked, the parent compounds are renally eliminated over a period of days. Hemodialysis should be considered for a patient with severe acidosis and electrolyte imbalance that cannot be controlled. Also, since the renal excretion of methanol and ethylene glycol may require up to five days once metabolism is blocked, hemodialysis morbidity can be weighed against the morbidity of ethanol therapy for several days in a critical care unit. Even if hemodialysis is performed, ethanol infusions should be maintained during the procedure. The infusion rate will have to be almost doubled because the ethanol will be dialyzed also. Hemodialysis is very effective at removing methanol, ethylene glycol, and ethanol.[177] (See also Chapter 18.)

Salicylates

Overdose with aspirin is a common cause of metabolic acidosis with an anion gap. Salicylates have numerous pharmacologic, toxicologic, and metabolic effects in overdose:

- direct stimulation of the CNS respiratory center with resulting hyperpnea and tachypnea
- uncoupling of oxidative phosphorylation
- interference with glucose metabolism
- interference with the Kreb's cycle
- increased lipolysis
- increased plasma amino acids
- fluid and electrolyte loss with total body potassium depletion
- decreased platelet adhesiveness
- decreased prothrombin formation
- decreased level of factor VII
- increased pyruvate and lactic acid with a severe metabolic acidosis.[178,179]

Interference with glucose metabolism most frequently results in hyperglycemia, although hypoglycemia can occur. Salicylates have also been demonstrated to produce a decrease in CNS glucose levels with a peripheral normoglycemia.[179,180] Adults usually develop a combined metabolic acidosis and respiratory alkalosis, whereas children and infants develop a profound metabolic acidosis. Hyperpyrexia can also occur as a result of the hypothalamic effect of salicylates and uncoupling of oxidative phosphorylation.

Coma, seizures, and pulmonary edema are signs of serious salicylate intoxication. Morbidity and mortality are related to the CNS salicylate concentration, cerebral edema, the severity of the metabolic disorder, and pulmonary edema. Noncardiogenic pulmonary edema as a result of salicylate toxicity is well recognized and is attributed to increased epithelial permeability in the alveolar-capillary membrane.[56] Fluid retention with hyponatremia has been noted in a few cases of salicylate overdose. The CNS concentration of salicylates may be the most important factor contributing to morbidity and mortality.[181] The CNS and other tissue concentrations of salicylates are directly related to the alkalemia or acidemia of the patient. At a blood pH of 7.4, more than 99 percent of the salicylate is in an ionized form (pKa equals 3); as acidemia supervenes, the amount of nonionized salicylate, and thus the amount available to cross biologic membranes, increases. As the pH of blood decreases from 7.4 to 7.2, the amount of nonionized salicylate that is available to enter the CNS doubles.[181]

The volume of distribution of salicylates increases with increasing plasma levels. The normal volume of distribution of salicylates ranges 150 to 300 ml/kg at therapeutic concentrations, but it is increased in overdoses and may be as high as 600 ml/kg.[182] This increase may be attributed to increased tissue binding in an overdose.

The elimination of salicylate is zero order at two metabolic pathways: formation of salicyluric acid and salicyl phenolic glucuronide metabolites. Thus, in an overdose, the elimination kinetics can change from first order to zero order. The metabolites of salicylate are excreted renally when they are formed.[182]

Salicylism can be divided into acute and chronic conditions. Both types are associated with dehydration, potassium depletion, and acidosis; however, in chronic salicylism, the hypokalemia and acidosis may be more profound. The salicylate blood level in chronic poisoning can be very low as opposed to a high level seen with an acute overdose. Chronic salicylism results from continued administration of aspirin that saturates the metabolic pathways. Usually, this occurs in a child who is already dehydrated from vomiting and diarrhea and is receiving salicylates for fever therapy. Treatment of salicylate poisoning is often delayed because it is not recognized until late in the clinical course when metabolic acidosis is a prominent feature. The clinical presentation can include lethargy, coma, vomiting, diarrhea, tachypnea, hyperpnea, pulmonary edema, seizures, and hyperthermia, as well as the electrolyte and metabolic derangements. Treatment is aimed at restoring depleted vascular volume and electrolytes, and correcting the metabolic acidosis. Alkaline diuresis has proved effective in increasing renal salicylate elimination by trapping anions in tubular lumen. However, before an alkaline urine can be achieved, total body potassium must be repleted.

The Done salicylate nomogram is useful in determining the severity of intoxication in acute overdose cases,[183] but the nomogram requires that a salicylate level be obtained no earlier than six hours postingestion. Therefore, the nomogram is not helpful with chronic salicylism. Hemodialysis may be indicated in salicylate poisoning if the patient is having seizures, has pulmonary edema, or has electrolyte abnormalities and an acid-base imbalance that cannot be controlled. (See Chapter 18.)

Acetaminophen

Commonly used as an aspirin substitute for analgesia, acetaminophen has become recognized as a cause of hepatotoxicity in overdose. Acetaminophen is a pharmacologically active metabolite of phenacetin. Its metabolism involves sulfate conjugation, glucuronide conjugation, and glutathione conjugation. Although the conjugation with glutathione involves only 3.8 percent of the metabolic pathway,[184] this is the pathway that determines whether or not hepatotoxicity will occur. Should glutathione reserves be depleted in a massive acute overdose, then a reactive intermediate is formed via this minor metabolic route. This active intermediate covalently binds to protein structures in hepatocytes, causing hepatocellular necrosis. Animal studies indicate that 70 to 80 percent of the intracellular glutathione stores must be depleted before hepatotoxicity occurs.[184]

The earliest symptoms of an acute overdose are gastrointestinal distress with some epigastric pain. Hepatocellular damage is usually manifested in 48 hours with rising levels of hepatic enzymes. Abnormalities of coagulation and renal failure may also occur. The levels of hepatic enzymes usually peak in four to five days and then return to normal.

Treatment involves the administration of N-acetylcysteine (Mucomyst), which acts as a glutathione surrogate to detoxify the active intermediate.[185] N-acetylcysteine is administered orally as a loading dose of 140 mg/kg and then given as a maintenance dose of 70 mg/kg every 4 hours for three days.[185] It should be administered within the first 24 hours following the overdose to be effective. A nomogram is available to aid in deciding the probability of hepatotoxicity in an acute overdose.[186] Death from acetaminophen-induced hepatotoxicity is usually due to a combination of hepatic encephalopathy and acute renal failure, but it can be prevented with the administration of N-acetylcysteine within 24 hours of the overdose and supportive care.

Anticonvulsants

The most common anticonvulsants encountered by the clinician in overdose are phenytoin (Dilantin), phenobarbital, primidone (Mysoline), carbamazepine (Tegretol), and valproic acid (Depakene). Each of these anticonvulsants has its own unique clinical toxicologic spectrum in an overdose.

Phenytoin

One drug that changes elimination kinetics from first order to zero order in overdose situations is phenytoin. The therapeutic range for phenytoin is 10 to 20 μg/ml. At these levels, phenytoin is eliminated by first order process, and the half-life is approximately 22 hours. The half-life may be much shorter in some situations, however. When phenytoin levels rise above 20 μg/ml, the enzymatic process that hydroxylates the phenyl ring and forms hydroxylphenylphenylhydantoin (HPPH), the major phenytoin metabolite, becomes saturated and thus the elimination of phenytoin becomes dependent on the maximal rate of an enzymatic process. Thus, a patient with a phenytoin overdose and high phenytoin plasma levels can be expected to have a prolonged elimination course, i.e., over days instead of the usual 22 hours half-life.

The change in phenytoin kinetics also has implications for therapeutic dosage. Due to the saturation proc-

ess, even small changes in phenytoin doses can lead to large changes in plasma levels of the drug.

Phenytoin has a systemic bioavailability of 80 to 95 percent after oral dosing.[187] It is a weak acid, poorly soluble in water, and slowly absorbed from the small intestines. Being a weak acid, phenytoin precipitates in the acid medium of the stomach. Thus, in an overdose, it would be expected to be slowly absorbed over a period of 6 to 12 hours, and the clinician may see slowly rising plasma levels for hours. Therefore it becomes important to clear the stomach and small intestines of a patient who has overdosed on phenytoin, even if it is 12 hours after the ingestion.

Phenytoin has a volume of distribution of approximately 600 ml/kg (body water space) and is about 90 percent bound to plasma albumin. It is displaced from albumin binding sites by hepatic disease, uremia, valproic acid, and salicylates.[188] Because it also readily crosses placental membranes, neonatal levels may be equal to maternal levels, a fact to be kept in mind in overdoses involving pregnant women.[188]

The clinical spectrum of phenytoin poisoning may range from nystagmus, slurred speech, and ataxia at lower levels to more pronounced cerebellar signs, confusion, choreoathetoid movement disorders, coma, and decerebrate rigidity at higher levels.[36,94] Treatment is mainly supportive, with monitoring of vital signs and plasma phenytoin levels. Hemodialysis is of no benefit. The clinician should be aware that plasma phenytoin levels in an overdose decline slowly over days and that the complete absorption of the drug from the gut may take hours.

Phenobarbital

The volume of distribution of phenobarbital is approximately 600 ml/kg, and the drug is 40 to 50 percent protein-bound. The plasma half-life of phenobarbital ranges from one to three days and is shorter in children than in adults. The metabolism of phenobarbital is by hepatic first order elimination. The therapeutic plasma level of phenobarbital is 20 to 30 μg/ml. Phenobarbital is also a potent inducer of hepatic enzymes. In an overdose, phenobarbital may cause a clinical spectrum ranging from lethargy, nystagmus, and increased muscular activity to deep coma, areflexia, hypotension, hypothermia, and cardiovascular collapse.[189,190] The treatment of phenobarbital intoxication is based on mainly supportive care and the use of urinary alkaline diuresis to increase excretion. There is a four-fold increase in the excretion of phenobarbital when the pH of the urine exceeds 7.5.[191] An alkaline diuresis should result in a fairly rapid recovery from coma in phenobarbital overdoses. The effect of an alkaline diuresis is considerably less when a short-acting barbiturate, such as secobarbital or pentobarbital, is ingested, however.[191] Should pulmonary edema be present, a diuresis would be relatively contraindicated. Hemodialysis can also effectively remove a phenobarbital body burden.

Primidone

An anticonvulsant that is chemically related to phenobarbital, primidone is converted to phenobarbital and phenylethylmalonamide by hepatic metabolism. The anticonvulsant effects of primidone are primarily due to phenobarbital. The parent compound, primidone, and the phenylethylmalonamide metabolite have weak anticonvulsant properties. Therapeutic plasma levels of phenobarbital are obtained with chronic administration of primidone. An overdose of primidone should be managed as if it were a phenobarbital overdose. Primidone itself can result in mild CNS depression and over a period of 12 to 24 hours following an acute overdose the phenobarbital levels should peak.

Carbamazepine

Now being more commonly employed as an anticonvulsant for grand mal seizures, carbamazepine is slowly absorbed from the small bowel over 12 hours.[192] The half-life of carbamazepine in an overdose has been reported to range from 10 to 29 hours.[40] Carbamazepine follows first order elimination, and the major metabolite is carbamazepine-10,11-epoxide, which has anticonvulsant properties of its own. The clinical spectrum of carbamazepine intoxication may include various degrees of coma, respiratory depression, nystagmus, ataxia, slurred speech, seizures, hyperreflexia, absent bowel sounds, myoclonus, depressed reflexes, atrioventricular conduction delay with prolongation of the QRS interval, and sinus tachycardia.[40] Cyclic coma has been described following acute overdoses.[40,193] Carbamazepine is similar in chemical structure to imipramine hydrochloride and has anticholinergic properties that delay gastric emptying. Supportive care is essential in the management of acute overdoses. The removal of any remaining drug from the gastrointestinal tract is important, since delayed absorption occurs with delayed gastric emptying. Carbamazepine is 75 percent protein-bound and has a volume of distribution ranging from 0.79 to 1.40 liter/kg.[194] There are no data presently available on hemodialysis and hemoperfusion in acute overdoses. Cardiac monitoring is important until the ECG is normal. Therapeutic levels of carbamazepine range 2 to 8 µg/ml, but intoxication is generally evident at levels greater than 10 µg/ml.

Valproic Acid

One of the newer anticonvulsants being used to manage seizure disorders is valproic acid, which is dipropylacetic acid, a fatty acid. Valproic acid has a small volume of distribution (100 to 400 ml/kg) and is greater than 90 percent protein-bound. It is absorbed from the gastrointestinal tract within 1 to 4 hours following ingestion.[195] The plasma half-life of valproic acid is 8 to 15 hours.[195] In neonates and young infants, the elimination half-life may be prolonged to 60 hours.[195] Valproic acid displaces phenytoin from plasma protein binding sites, lowers the total phenytoin plasma level,[196] and increases plasma levels of phenobarbital by interfering with elimination.[195,196] An overdose of valproic acid may cause deep coma.[196] Gastrointestinal irritation with vomiting may also occur. Hepatotoxicity associated with valproic acid has been reported only with therapeutic dosages,[197] which range from 50 to 100 µg/ml. Treatment is supportive.

Isoniazid

A drug that produces seizures and extreme metabolic acidosis with a large anion gap when ingested in an overdose, isoniazid is rapidly absorbed from the gastrointestinal tract; plasma levels peak in one to two hours. The volume of distribution of isoniazid is approximately 600 ml/kg, and the drug is only 15 percent bound to plasma proteins.[198] Isoniazid is acetylated by the liver to inactive metabolites. One of these metabolites is N-acetylhydrazine, which is thought to be responsible for isoniazid-induced hepatitis. Acetylation of isoniazid may be classified as slow or rapid, based on genetic phenotype; rapid acetylators have an autosomal dominant allele. Ingestion of a single large dose of isoniazid does not result in hepatotoxicity. The hepatitis is a result of chronic therapeutic doses. The half-life for isoniazid varies, depending on whether the patient is a rapid or slow acetylator. In rapid acetylators, the drug has a half-life of approximately one hour in slow acetylators, two to four hours.[198]

In an overdose, isoniazid may cause coma, convulsions, anion gap, metabolic acidosis, and hyperglycemia.[199] Owing to the rapid absorption of isoniazid, symptomatology usually occurs within an hour or less. The metabolic acidosis is due to lactic acidemia. The treatment of acute intoxication is based on controlling the seizure activity and correcting the lactic acidosis. The seizures may be difficult to control until the acidosis is also corrected. The mechanism of the seizures is unknown, but it may be an interference with pyridoxine action. Seizures can be adequately controlled with intravenous diazepam and sodium bicarbonate, even if pyridoxine is not administered. Most investigators, however, feel that large amounts of pyridoxine should be administered intravenously. Patients who ingest large amounts of isoniazid-pyridoxine combination tablets still have seizures and acidemia. Phenobarbital and/or diphenylhydantoin may be required to control seizures. Once the seizures have been terminated and the acidemia corrected, the isoniazid is usually rapidly eliminated, and the coma resolves within 24 hours or less. Isoniazid excretion can be enhanced by a forced neutral diuresis. Also, should the seizures and acidemia be difficult to control, hemodialysis may be beneficial in removing the isoniazid body burden.

An important point in therapy is that isoniazid interferes with diphenylhydantoin metabolism, resulting in diphenylhydantoin intoxication. Therefore, if diphenylhydantoin is employed to terminate seizures, the normal loading dose can be administered, but plasma levels must be monitored and maintenance doses either withheld or decreased.

OVER-THE-COUNTER DRUGS

Nonprescription drugs are commonly ingested in overdoses, sometimes accidentally by small children.[104,200] Most of these drugs contain various anticholinergic compounds, salicylates, acetaminophen, salicylamide, or phenacetin, and some small volume of ethanol.[200] These drugs are sold as cold preparations, sleep aids, or sedatives. Over-the-counter sleep aids contain methapyrilene hydrochloride or pyrilamine and in overdose may cause seizures, delirium, tachycardia, hypertension, and coma. Children are more susceptible than adults. The anticholinergic syndrome is common with toxic ingestions of the cold preparations and sleep aids. Cold preparations usually contain a form of antihistamine, such as chlorpheniramine maleate or phenylpropanolamine, together with an antipyretic in many cases. Preparations containing ethanol can result in seriously high blood ethanol levels if ingested by small children.

Management of over-the-counter ingestions is mainly supportive and is directed at controlling the severe symptomatology that can result from the anticholinergic drugs. The clinician should be aware of other ingredients in these preparations, such as caffeine, which can cause seizures, tachycardia, gastrointestinal bleeding, and cardiac dysrhythmias; acetaminophen, which may result in hepatocellular necrosis; salicylates, which may result in a metabolic acidosis; and ethanol, which can result in coma and hypoglycemia in children.

Tetracyclics

The tetracyclics are new antidepressant drugs that are being used in foreign countries. One tetracyclic, maprotiline (Ludiomil), is available in the United States. Mianserin (Norval, Organon, Bolvidon) is a tetracyclic that is currently being investigated in the United States.

Overdoses of these will be seen by clinicians. The clinical pharmacokinetics of the tetracyclics are similar to those of the tricyclics with large volumes of distribution and high plasma protein binding. Mianserin differs from the tricyclic antidepressants in clinical pharmacology, however. The tricyclics block the reuptake of norepinephrine and have central anticholinergic properties; mianserin has presynoptic α-adrenergic blocking effects, sedative effects, and very few central anticholinergic effects.[201] Mianserin is reported to be less cardiotoxic and less anticholinergic than the tricyclics in overdose situations.[202]

Benzodiazepines and Other Sedative-Hypnotics

The benzodiazepines include the commonly used drugs diazepam (Valium), chlordiazepoxide (Librium), oxazepam (Serax), lorazepam (Ativan), flurazepam (Dalmane), chlorazepate (Tranxene), and clonazepam (Clonopin). The benzodiazepines are commonly ingested in drug overdoses, most frequently diazepam and chlordiazepoxide. An overdose of a benzodiazepine alone does not cause serious intoxication,[203] but, in combination with other drugs, it may result in serious intoxication, including respiratory depression. The elimination half-lives for diazepam and chlordiazepoxide vary between 20 and 50 hours. Diazepam, chlordiazepoxide, flurazepam, and chlorazepate are long-acting benzodiazepines and have a common pharmacologically active intermediary metabolite—desmethyldiazepam.[204] Chlorazepate undergoes acid hydrolysis in the stomach to desmethyldiazepam, whereas the other long-acting benzodiazepines are demethylated by the liver to desmethyldiazepam. Oxazepam and lorazepam, short-acting benzodiazepines, are both metabolized by hepatic glucuronidation. Oxazepam and lorazepam are metabolites of desmethyldiazepam.[204]

Other sedative-hypnotics encountered in overdose are ethchlorvynol (Placidyl), glutethimide (Doriden), and chloral hydrate. Ethchlorvynol is rapidly absorbed in an overdose. It has a large volume of distribution, signifying a great deal of tissue binding. Clinically, ethchlorvynol overdose produces coma, usually prolonged, and respiratory depression. The half-life for ethchlorvynol is about 70 hours. Supportive care is the mainstay of treatment. Resin hemoperfusion has been advocated to treat serious overdoses,[205] but hemoperfusion techniques are limited by the large tissue distribution of ethchlorvynol plus its very slow redistribution back into plasma from tissue.[206] The benefit of hemoperfusion in ethchlorvynol intoxication remains questionable.

Glutethimide intoxication usually results in coma and respiratory depression. The drug is irregularly absorbed from the gastrointestinal tract, has a large volume of distribution, and a half-life of up to 40 hours in overdose.[207] Conservative management usually results in a good outcome.[208] Chloral hydrate intoxication results in coma, respiratory depression, and sometimes cardiac dysrhythmias.[65] Chloral hydrate is metabolized to trichloroethanol, the active metabolite, by alcohol dehydrogenase. The half-life of trichloroethanol has been calculated to be around 13 hours.[209] Hemodialysis appears to remove the trichloroethanol metabolite and may be beneficial in serious intoxication.[209]

Ethanol

The ingestion of ethanol in overdose can result in coma, respiratory depression, hyperosmolality, hypoglycemia, gastrointestinal bleeding, and metabolic acidosis.[86] Small children who ingest ethanol-containing products may experience seizures,[210] respiratory depression, and hypoglycemia. The chronic ingestion of ethanol is associated with many problems as a result of interference with carbohydrate, lipid, and protein metabolism.[86] Alcoholic ketoacidosis and lactic acidosis are commonly seen in the alcoholic population.[211] The management of ethanol ingestion in overdose includes providing respiratory support and correcting electrolyte problems and hypoglycemia. Ethanol can be removed by hemodialysis, if necessary. (See Chapter 36.)

Heavy Metals

The most common heavy metals involved in poisonings are lead, mercury, and arsenic, although zinc, copper, and cadmium may also result in poisoning. Heavy metals may be inorganic, organic, or elemental. Acute heavy metal poisoning usually results in immediate gastrointestinal distress with vomiting and diarrhea. Chronic heavy metal poisoning in general may result in CNS disturbances and toxic psychoses.

Mercury poisoning can be caused by elemental mercury vapors absorbed through the lung, resulting in cough, dyspnea, and lethargy. The most severe form of mercury poisoning is due to organic methylmercury, which is used as a fungicide. Methylmercury produces severe CNS disorders that are usually irreversible.[97] Organic mercurials are difficult to treat by chelation.

Lead poisoning results from chronic ingestion of lead in either the elemental or organic form. Various CNS, hematologic, renal, and metabolic problems result from lead poisoning. Tetraethyl lead poisoning from gasoline sniffing results in permanent cerebellar lesions.[96] The diagnosis of lead poisoning is best made from an elevated blood lead level, i.e., a level in excess of 40 ng/100 ml blood.

Arsenic may cause acute pulmonary problems when inhaled in dust. Cardiac dysrhythmias, seizures, neurologic sequelae, and hematologic abnormalities with thrombocytopenia, leukopenia, aplastic anemia, and marrow hypoplasia have been described following arsenic intoxication.[212,213] Acute leukemia following arsenic-induced aplastic anemia has also been described.[213]

The treatment of heavy metal poisoning is based on the use of chelator agents. The most commonly employed chelators are calcium disodium ethylenediaminetetraacetic acid ($CaNa_2EDTA$) for lead poisoning; dimercaprol (BAL, British antilewisite) for lead, arsenic, and mercury poisoning; and D-penicillamine for lead, mercury, arsenic, and copper poisoning.[214–216]

REFERENCES

1. Applebaum E, Bruce D: Complications of tracheal intubation, in *Tracheal Intubation*. Philadelphia, WB Saunders Co, 1976, pp 74–94.
2. Berne R, Levy M: Interplay of central and peripheral factors in the regulation of the circulation, in *Cardiovascular Physiology*. St. Louis, CV Mosby Co, 1972, pp 237–253.
3. Benowitz N, Rosenberg J, Becker C: Cardiopulmonary catastrophes in drug-overdose patients. *Med Clin North Am* 63:267–296, 1979.
4. Carrico C, Canizaro C, Shires T: Fluid resuscitation following injury: Rationale for the use of balanced salt solutions. *Crit Care Med* 4:46–54, 1976.
5. Stein L, Berand J, Morissette M, et al: Pulmonary edema during volume infusion. *Circulation* 52:483–489, 1975.
6. Rackow E, et al: Relationship of colloid osmotic pressure and pulmonary capillary pressure to pulmonary edema. *Cardiovasc Med* 3:407–412, 1978.
7. Rackow E, Fein A: Fulminant noncardiogenic pulmonary edema in the critically ill. *Crit Care Med* 6:360–363, 1978.
8. Shoemaker W: Comparison of the relative effectiveness of whole blood transfusions and various types of fluid therapy in resuscitation. *Crit Care Med* 4:71–78, 1976.
9. Skillman J: The role of albumin and oncotically active fluids in shock. *Crit Care Med* 4:55–61, 1976.
10. Burrington J: Emergencies and accidents, in Kempe C, Silver H, O'Brien D (eds): *Current Pediatric Diagnosis and Treatment*, ed 5. Los Altos, Calif, Lange Medical Publications, 1978.
11. Silver H, Peterson R, Rumack B: Drug therapy, in Kempe C, Silver H, O'Brien D (eds): *Current Pediatric Diagnosis and Treatment*, ed 6. Los Altos, Calif, Lange Medical Publications, 1980.
12. Long acting barbiturates, in Rumack BH (ed): *POISINDEX*. Englewood, Colo, Micromedex Publishers, 1980.
13. Greenblatt D, Allen M, Noel B: Acute overdosage with benzodiazepine derivatives. *Clin Pharmacol Ther* 21:497–514, 1977.
14. Lansky L: An unusual case of childhood chloral hydrate poisoning. *Am J Dis Child* 127:275–276, 1974.
15. Chazan J, Garella S: Glutethimide intoxication. *Arch Intern Med* 128:215–219, 1971.
16. Adelson L: Fatal intoxication with isopropyl alcohol (rubbing alcohol). *Am J Clin Pathol* 38:144–151, 1962.
17. Westerfield B, Blovin R: Ethchlorvynol intoxication. *South Med J* 70:1019–1020, 1977.

18. Maddock K, Bloomer H: Meprobamate overdosage. *JAMA* 201:999–1003, 1967.

19. Opiates and narcotics, in Rumack BH (ed): *POISINDEX*, Englewood, Colo, Micromedex Publishers, 1980.

20. Steiman G, Woerpel R, Sherard E: Treatment of accidental sodium valproate overdose with an opiate antagonist. *Ann Neurol* 6:274, 1979.

21. Browne T: Valproic acid. *N Engl J Med* 302:661–666, 1980.

22. Moore M, Phillipi P: Clonidine overdose. *Lancet* 2:694, 1976.

23. Saperia J: Clonidine overdose. *Br Med J* 4:580, 1975.

24. Biggs J, Spiker D, Petit J: Tricyclic antidepressant overdoses—Incidence of symptoms. *JAMA* 238:135–138, 1977.

25. Goldfrank L, Bresnitz E: Phenothiazines. *Hospital Physician* 15:42–53, 1979.

26. Matthew H, Proudfoot A, Brown S: Mandrax poisoning: Conservative management of 116 patients. *Br Med J* 2:101–102, 1968.

27. Brown S, Goenechea S: Methaqualone: Metabolic, kinetic and clinical pharmacologic observations. *Clin Pharmacol Ther* 14:314–324, 1973.

28. Aronow R, Done A: Phencyclidine overdose: An emerging concept of management. *JACEP* 7:56–59, 1978.

29. Teitelbaum D, Ott J: Acute strychnine intoxication. *Clin Toxicol* 3:267–273, 1970.

30. Gay G, Rappolt R, Inaba D: Cocaine. *Clin Toxicol* 8:149–178, 1975.

31. Haddad L: 1978: Cocaine in perspective. *JACEP* 8:374–376, 1979.

32. Reigart J, Brueggeman L, Keil J: Sodium fluoroacetate poisoning. *Am J Dis Child* 129:1224–1226, 1975.

33. Hart J, Wallace J: The adverse effects of amphetamines. *Clin Toxicol* 8:179–190, 1975.

34. Kalant H, Kalant O: Death in amphetamine users: Causes and rates. *Can Med Assoc J* 112:299–304, 1975.

35. Tenckhoff H, Sherrard D, Hickman R: Acute diphenylhydantoin intoxication. *Am J Dis Child* 116:422–425, 1968.

36. McLellan D, Swash M: Choreoathetosis and encephalopathy induced by phenytoin. *Br Med J* 2:204–205, 1974.

37. Lovejoy F, Mitchell A, Goldman P: The management of propoxyphene poisoning. *J Pediatr* 85:98–100, 1974.

38. Salzberg M, Gallagher E: Propranolol overdose. *Ann Emerg Med* 9:26–27, 1980.

39. Lagerfelt J, Matell G: Attempted suicide with 5.1 grams of propranolol. *Acta Med Scand* 199:517–518, 1976.

40. Sullivan J, Peterson RG, Rumack BH: Carbamazepine toxicity in acute overdose: Serial blood levels and clinical presentations. *Neurology* 31:621–624, 1981.

41. Stewart R: Cyanide poisoning. *Clin Toxicol* 7:561–564, 1974.

42. Mascarenhas B, Geller A, Goodman A: Cyanide poisoning, Medical Emergency. *NY State J Med* 69:1782–1784, 1969.

43. Gordon E: Carbon monoxide encephalopathy. *Br Med J* 1:1232, 1965.

44. Winter P, Miller J: Carbon monoxide poisoning. *JAMA* 236:1502–1504, 1976.

45. Grossman R, Hamilton R, Morse B: Nontraumatic rhabdomyolysis and acute renal failure. *N Engl J Med* 291:807–811, 1974.

46. Ralph D: Rhabdomyolysis and acute renal failure. *JACEP* 7:103–106, 1978.

47. Myers R, Linberg S, Cowley R: Carbon monoxide poisoning: The injury and its treatment. *JACEP* 8:479–484, 1979.

48. Finley J, VanBeek A, Glover J: Myonecrosis complicating carbon monoxide poisoning. *J Trauma* 17:536–539, 1977.

49. Teehan B, Maher J, Carey J: Acute ethchlorvynol (Placidyl®) intoxication. *Ann Intern Med* 72:875–882, 1970.

50. Burton W, Vender J, Shapiro B: Adult respiratory distress syndrome after Placidyl® abuse. *Crit Care Med* 8:48–49, 1980.

51. Duberstein J, Kaufman D: A clinical study of an epidemic of heroin intoxication and heroin induced pulmonary edema. *Am J Med* 51:704–714, 1971.

52. Katz S, Aberman A, Fraud V: Heroin pulmonary edema: Evidence of increased pulmonary capillary permeability. *Am Rev Respir Dis* 106:472–474, 1972.

53. Bogartz L, Miller W: Pulmonary edema associated with propoxyphene intoxication. *JAMA* 215:259–262, 1971.

54. Tweedale M: Salicylate and pulmonary edema. *Ann Intern Med* 81:710, 1974.

55. Bowers RE, Brigham K, Owen P: Salicylate pulmonary edema: The mechanism in sheep and review of the clinical literature. *Am Rev Respir Dis* 115:261–268, 1977.

56. Glauser F, Egan P, Miller J: The effect of salicylate infusion on the alveolar epithelial membrane in the isolated perfused lung. *Crit Care Med* 6:181–184, 1978.

57. Grant M (ed): *Toxicology of the Eye*, ed 2. Springfield, Ill, Charles C Thomas, 1974, p 800.

58. Jaffe J: Narcotic analgesics, in Goodman L, Gilman A (eds): *The Pharmacological Basis of Therapeutics*, ed 4. New York, Macmillan Co, 1970, p. 256.

59. Rumack B, Temple A: Lomotil poisoning. *Pediatrics* 53:495–500, 1974.

60. Vaucher Y, Lightner E, Walson P: Theophylline poisoning. *J Pediatr* 90:827–830, 1977.

61. Zwillich C, Sutton F, Neff T: Theophylline induced seizures in adults—Correlation with serum concentrations. *Ann Intern Med* 82:784–787, 1975.

62. Sullivan J: Caffeine poisoning in an infant. *J Pediatr* 90:1022–1023, 1977.

63. Petery J, Rennert O: Arsenic poisoning in childhood. *Clin Toxicol* 3:519–526, 1970.

64. Kline T: Myocardial changes in lead poisoning. *Am J Dis Child* 99:48–54, 1960.

65. Gustafson A, Svensson S, Ugaander L: Cardiac arrhythmias in chloral hydrate poisoning. *Acta Med Scand* 201:227–230, 1977.

66. MacFaul R, Miller G: Clonidine poisoning in children. *Lancet* 1:1266–1267, 1977.

67. Kibler L, Gazes P: Effect of clonidine on atrioventricular conduction. *JAMA* 238:1930–1932, 1977.

68. Harrisson J, Ambrus J, Ambrus C: Acute poisoning with sodium fluoroacetate. *JAMA* 149:1520–1523, 1952.

69. Salzberg M, Gallagher E: Propranolol overdose. *Ann Emerg Med* 9:26–27, 1980.

70. Reuler J: Hypothermia: Pathophysiology, clinical setting and management. *Ann Intern Med* 89:519–527, 1978.

71. Stine R: Accidental hypothermia. *Ann Emerg Med* 6:413–416, 1977.

72. Goldfrank L, Kirstein R: Emergency management of hypothermia. *Hospital Physician* 1:47–52, 1979.

73. Noble J, Matthew H: Acute poisoning by tricyclic antidepressants: Clinical features and management of 100 patients. *Clin Toxicol* 2:403–421, 1969.

74. Subin H, Weil M: Shock associated with barbiturate intoxication. *JAMA* 215:263–268, 1971.

75. Myers R, Linberg S, Crowley R: Carbon monoxide poisoning—The injury and its treatment. *JACEP* 8:479–484, 1979.

76. Temple A: Pathophysiology of aspirin overdosage toxicity with implications for management. *Pediatrics* (suppl)62(5)II:873–879, 1978.

77. Hamilton A, Hardy H: Pesticides, in *Industrial Toxicology*, ed 3. Littleton, Mass, Publishing Science Group Inc, 1974, pp. 353–369.

78. Comroe J: Manifestations of pulmonary disease, in *Physiology of Respiration*, Chicago, Ill, Year Book Medical Publishers, 1970.

79. Harris J, Rumack B, Peterson R: Methemoglobinemia resulting from absorption of nitrates. *JAMA* 242:2869–2871, 1979.

80. Hamilton A, Hardy H: Aromatic nitro and amino compounds, in *Industrial Toxicology,* ed 3. Littleton, Mass, Publishing Science Group Inc, 1974, pp 305–311.

81. Green E, Zimmerman R, Ghurabi W: Phenazopyridine hydrochloride toxicity: A cause of drug-induced methemoglobinemia. *Ann Emerg Med* 8:426–431, 1979.

82. Potter J, Hillman J: Benzocaine-induced methemoglobinemia. *Ann Emerg Med* 8:26–27, 1979.

83. Leavell B, Thorup O: Hemolytic anemia, in *Fundamentals of Clinical Hematology,* Philadelphia, WB Saunders Co, 1971.

84. Cartwright G: Methemoglobinemia and sulfhemoglobinemia, in *Harrison's Principles of Internal Medicine,* ed 6. New York, McGraw Hill, 1970.

85. Clay K, Murphy R: On the metabolic acidosis of ethylene glycol intoxication. *Toxicol Appl Pharmacol* 39:39–49, 1977.

86. Isselbacher K: Metabolic and hepatic effects of alcohol. *N Engl J Med* 296:612–616, 1977.

87. Terman D, Teitelbaum D: Isoniazid self poisoning. *Neurology* 20:299–303, 1970.

88. James J: Acute iron poisoning: Assessment of severity and prognosis. *J Pediatr* 77:117–119, 1970.

89. Kittel J: Paraldehyde toxicity. Hosp Pharmacy 8:263–265, 1973.

90. Taher S, Anderson R, McCartney R: Renal tubular acidosis associated with toluene sniffing. *N Engl J Med* 290:765–768, 1974.

91. Fischman C, Oster J: Toxic effects of toluene—A new cause of high anion gap metabolic acidosis. *JAMA* 241:1713–1715, 1979.

92. Rasmussen S, Kristensen M: Choreoathetosis during phenytoin treatment. *Acta Med Scand* 201:239–241, 1977.

93. Kooiker J, Sumi S: Movement disorder as a manifestation of diphenylhydantoin intoxication. *Neurology* 24:68–71, 1974.

94. Tenckhoff H, Sherrard D, Hickman R: Acute diphenylhydantoin intoxication. *Am J Dis Child* 116:422–425, 1968.

95. Burks J, Walker J, Rumack B: Tricyclic antidepressant poisoning—Reversal of coma, choreoathetosis and myoclonus with physostigmine. *JAMA* 230:1405–1406, 1974.

96. Browder A, Joselow M, Louria D: The problem of lead poisoning. *Medicine* 52:121–139, 1973.

97. Gerstner H, Huff J: Selected case histories and epidemiologic examples of human mercury poisoning. *Clin Toxicol* 11:131–150, 1977.

98. Saran B, Gaind R: Lithium. *Clin Toxicol* 6:257–269, 1973.

99. Burns R, Lerner S: Phencyclidine deaths. *JACEP* 7:135–141, 1978.

100. Haddad L: 1978—Cocaine in perspective. *JACEP* 8:374–376, 1979.

101. Gay G, Inaba D, Sheppard C: Cocaine—History, epidemiology, human pharmacology, and treatment. *Clin Toxicol* 8:149–178, 1975.

102. Hart J, Wallace J: The adverse effects of amphetamines. *Clin Toxicol* 8:179–190, 1975.

103. Reyes-Jacang A, Wenzl J: Antihistamine toxicity in children. *Clin Pediatr* 8:297–299, 1969.

104. Hooper R, Conner C, Rumack B: Acute poisoning from over-the-counter sleep preparations. *JACEP* 8:98–100, 1979.

105. Binns H, et al: Gasoline contact burns. *JACEP* 7:404–405, 1978.

106. Fredriksson T: Percutaneous absorption of parathian and paraoxon. *Arch Environ Health* 3:67–70, 1961.

107. Hayes W (ed): *Toxicology of Pesticides.* Baltimore, Williams & Wilkins Co, 1975, p 459.

108. Manno B, Mano J: Toxicology of ipecac—A review. *Clin Toxicol* 10:221–242, 1977.

109. Morgan A, Polak A: The excretion of salicylate in salicylate poisoning. *Clin Sci* 41:475–484, 1971.

110. Bloomer H: A critical evaluation of diuresis in the treatment of barbiturate intoxication. *J Lab Clin Med* 67:898–905, 1966.

111. Innes I, Nickerson M: Sympathomimetic drugs, in Goodman L, Gilman A (eds): *The Pharmacologic Basis of Therapeutics.* New York, Macmillan Co, 1975.

112. Gibson T, Nelson H: Drug kinetics and artificial kidneys. *Clin Pharmacokinet* 2:403–426, 1977.

113. Watonabe A: Pharmacokinetic aspects of the dialysis of drugs. *Drug Intell Clin Pharm* 2:407–417, 1977.

114. Pond S, Rosenburg J, Benowitz N: Pharmacokinetics of hemoperfusion for drug overdose. *Clin Pharmacokinet* 4:329–354, 1979.

115. Winchester J, Gelfand M, Knepshield J: Dialysis and hemoperfusion of poisons and drugs. *Trans Am Soc Artif Intern Organs* 23:762–842, 1977.

116. Jaffe L: Carbon monoxide in the environment—Sources, characteristics, and fate of atmospheric carbon monoxide. *Ann NY Acad Sci* 174:76–88, 1970.

117. Ayres S, Giannelli S, Mueller H: Myocardial and systemic responses to carboxyhemoglobin. *Ann NY Acad Sci* 175:268–293, 1970.

118. Winter P, Miller J: Carbon monoxide poisoning. *JAMA* 236:1502–1504, 1976.

119. Anderson R, Allensworth D, DeGroot W: Myocardial toxicity from carbon monoxide poisoning. *Ann Intern Med* 67:1172–1182, 1967.

120. Garland H, Pearce J: Neurological complications of carbon monoxide poisoning. *Q J Med* 36:445–455, 1967.

121. Ginsberg M, Myers R: Fetal brain injury after maternal carbon monoxide intoxication. *Neurology* 26:15–23, 1976.

122. Ratney R, Wegman D, Elkins H: In vivo conversion of methylene chloride to carbon monoxide. *Arch Environ Health* 28:223–226, 1974.

123. Stewart R: Cyanide poisoning. *Clin Toxicol* 7:561–564, 1974.

124. Cerami A, Allen A, Graziano J: Pharmacology of cyanate—General effects on experimental animals. *J Pharmacol Exp Ther* 185:653–666, 1973.

125. Evans L: Cobalt compounds as antidotes for hydrocyanic acid. *Br J Pharmacol* 23:455–475, 1964.

126. Milby T: Prevention and management of organophosphate poisoning. *JAMA* 216:2131–2133, 1971.

127. Namba T, Nolte C, Jackrel J: Poisoning due to organophosphate insecticides—Acute and chronic manifestations. *Am J Med* 50:475–492, 1971.

128. Richards A: Malathion poisoning successfully treated with large doses of atropine. *Can Med Assoc J* 91:82–83, 1964.

129. Organophosphates, in Rumack B (ed): *POISINDEX,* Englewood, Colo, Micromedex Publishers, 1980.

130. Quinby G: Further therapeutic experience with pralidoximes in organic phosphorus poisoning. *JAMA* 187:111–118, 1964.

131. Berkowitz B: The relationship of pharmacokinetics to pharmacological activity: Morphine, methadone, and naloxone. *Clin Pharmacokinet* 1:219–230, 1976.

132. Moore R, Rumack B, Conner C: Naloxone—Underdosage after narcotic poisoning. *Am J Dis Child* 134:156–158, 1980.

133. Sesso A, Rodzvilla J: Naloxone therapy in a seven month old with methadone poisoning. *Clin Pediatr* 14:388–389, 1975.

134. Lovejoy F, Mitchell A, Goldman P: The management of propoxyphene poisoning. *J Pediatr* 85:98–100, 1974.

135. Jasinski D, Martin W, Haertzen C: The human pharmacology and abuse potential of N-allylnoroxymorphone (naloxone). *J Pharmacol Exp Ther* 157:420–426, 1967.

136. Rumack B: Anticholinergic poisoning—Treatment with physostigmine, *Pediatrics* 52:449–551, 1973.

137. Lee J, Turndoff H, Poppers P: Physostigmine reversal of an-

tihistamine induced excitement and depression. *Anesthesiology* 43:683–684, 1975.

138. Nattel S, Bayne L, Ruedy J: Physostigmine in coma due to drug overdose. *Clin Pharmacol Ther* 25:96–102, 1979.

139. Schanker L: Drug absorption, in LaDu B, Mandel H, Way E (eds): *Fundamentals of Drug Metabolism and Drug Distribution.* Baltimore, Williams & Wilkins Co, 1971.

140. Levine R: Factors affecting gastrointestinal absorption of drugs. *Digestive Diseases* 15:171–188, 1970.

141. Rowland M: Drug administration and regimens, in Melmon K, Morrelli H (eds): *Clinical Pharmacology—Basic Principles in Therapeutics.* New York, Macmillan Co, 1972.

142. Nimmo W: Drugs, diseases and altered gastric emptying. *Clin Pharmacokinet* 1:189–203, 1976.

143. Hug C: Pharmacokinetics of drugs administered intravenously. *Anesth Analg* 57:704–723, 1978.

144. Curry S: *Drug Disposition and Pharmacokinetics.* London, Blackwell Scientific Publications, 1977.

145. Morselli P: Clinical pharmacokinetics in neonates. *Clin Pharmacokinet* 1:81–98, 1976.

146. Levy G: Clinical pharmacokinetics of aspirin. *Pediatrics* (suppl) 62:867–871, 1978.

147. Rane A: Urinary excretion of diphenylhydantoin metabolites in newborn infants. *J Pediatr* 85:543–545, 1974.

148. Rane A, Garle M, Borga O: Plasma disappearance of transplacentally transferred diphenylhydantoin in the newborn studied by mass fragmentography. *Clin Pharmacol Ther* 15:39–45, 1974.

149. Ehrnebo M, Agurell S, Jalling B: Age differences in drug binding by plasma proteins—Studies on human fetuses, neonates, and adults. *Eur J Clin Pharmacol* 3:189–193, 1971.

150. Rane A, Wilson J: Clinical pharmacokinetics in infants and children. *Clin Pharmacokinet* 1:2–24, 1976.

151. Peterson R: Pharmacologic considerations for the newborn and premature, in Aldrete J, Stanley T (eds): *Trends in Intravenous Anesthesia.* Chicago, Year Book Medical Publishers, 1980.

152. Peterson R, Simmons M, Rumack B: Pharmacology of furosemide in the premature newborn infant. *Pediatrics* 97:139–143, 1980.

153. Crooks J, O'Malley K, Stevenson I: Pharmacokinetics in the elderly. *Clin Pharmacokinet* 1:280–296, 1976.

154. Mitenko P, Ogilvie R: Rational intravenous doses of theophylline. *N Engl J Med* 289:600–603, 1973.

155. McDonald J, Turk J, Dietzler D: Theophylline toxicity. *Clin Chem* 24:1603–1608, 1978.

156. Arnman K, Carlstrom S, Thorell J: The effect of norepinephrine and theophylline on blood glucose, plasma free fatty acids, plasma glycerol and plasma insulin in normal subjects. *Acta Med Scand* 197:271–274, 1975.

157. Eldridge F, Salzer J: Effect of respiratory alkalosis on blood lactate and pyruvate in humans. *J Appl Physiol* 22:461–468, 1967.

158. Emmett M, Narrins R: Clinical use of the anion gap. *Medicine* 56:38–54, 1977.

159. Lesko L: Dose dependent elimination kinetics of theophylline. *Clin Pharmacokinet* 4:449–459, 1979.

160. Kadlec G, Jarboe C, Pollard S: Acute theophylline intoxication—Biphasic first order elimination kinetics in a child. *Ann Allergy* 41:337–339, 1978.

161. Diafsky K, Sitar D, Rangno R: Theophylline kinetics in acute pulmonary edema. *Clin Pharmacol Ther* 21:310–316, 1978.

162. Snodgrass W, Sawyer D, Conner C: Asymptomatic theophylline overdose. *Drug Intelligence and Clinical Pharmacy* 14:783, 1980.

163. Vohra J, Burrows G, Hurst D: The effect of toxic and therapeutic doses on tricyclic antidepressant drugs on intracardiac conduction. *Eur J Cardiol* 3:219–227, 1975.

164. Biggs J, Spiker D, Petit J: Tricyclic antidepressant overdose—Incidence of symptoms. *JAMA* 238:135–138, 1977.

165. Brown T: Tricyclic antidepressant overdosage—Experimental studies on the management of circulatory complications. *Clin Toxicol* 9:255–272, 1976.

166. Roberts R, Mueller S, Lauer R: Propranolol in the treatment of cardiac arrhythmias associated with amitriptyline intoxication. *J Pediatr* 82:65–67, 1973.

167. Tobis J, Aronow W: Effect of amitriptyline antidotes on repetitive extrasystole threshold. *Clin Pharmacol Ther* 27:602–606, 1980.

168. Brown T, Barker G, Dunlop M: The use of sodium bicarbonate in the treatment of tricyclic antidepressant induced arrhythmias. *Anesth Intens Care* 1:203–210, 1973.

169. Sullivan J, Peterson R, Rumack B: Amitriptyline plasma protein binding versus plasma pH. Presented at American Academy of Clinical Toxicology, Minneapolis, Minn, August 1980.

170. Clay K, Murphy R: On the metabolic acidosis of ethylene glycol intoxication. *Toxicol Appl Pharmacol* 39:39–49, 1977.

171. Parry M, Wallach R: Ethylene glycol poisoning. *Am J Med* 57:143–149, 1974.

172. Amat-Martin G, Tephly T, McMartin K: Methyl alcohol poisoning—Development of a model for ocular toxicity in methyl alcohol poisoning using the rhesus monkey. *Arch Ophthalmol* 95:1847–1850, 1977.

173. Hayreh M, Hayreh S, Baumbach G: Methyl alcohol poisoning—Ocular toxicity. *Arch Ophthalmol* 95:1851–1858, 1977.

174. McLean D, Jacobs H, Mielke B: Methanol poisoning—A clinical and pathological study. *Ann Neurol* 8:161–167, 1979.

175. Aquilonius S, Bergstrom K, Enoksson P: Cerebral computed tomography in methanol intoxication. *J Comput Assist Tomogr* 4:425–428, 1980.

176. Wagner J, Wilkinson P, Sedman A: Elimination of alcohol from human blood. *J Pharm Sci* 65:152–154, 1976.

177. Tobin M, Lianoa E: Hemodialysis for methanol intoxication. *J Dial* 3:97–106, 1979.

178. Brem J, Pereli E, Gopalan S: Salicylism, hyperventilation, and the central nervous system. *J Pediatr* 83:264–266, 1973.

179. Hill J: Salicylate intoxication. *N Engl J Med* 288:1110–1113, 1973.

180. Spector R, Lorenzo A: The transport and metabolism of salicylate in the central nervous system—In vivo studies. *J Pharmacol Exp Ther* 185:276–286, 1973.

181. Hill J: Experimental salicylate poisoning—Observations on the effects of altering blood pH on tissue and plasma salicylate concentrations. *Pediatrics* 47:658–665, 1971.

182. Levy G: Pharmacokinetics of salicylate elimination in man. *J Pharm Sci* 54:959–967, 1965.

183. Done A: Salicylate intoxication—Significance of measurements of salicylate in blood in cases of acute ingestion. *Pediatrics* 26:800–807, 1960.

184. Mitchell J, Thorgeirsson S, Potter W: Acetaminophen-induced hepatic injury—Protective role of glutathione in man and rationale for therapy. *Clin Pharmacol Ther* 16:676–684, 1974.

185. Rumack B, Peterson R: Acetaminophen overdose—Incidence, diagnosis and management in 416 patients. *Pediatrics* 62(suppl):898–903, 1978.

186. Rumack B, Matthew H: Acetaminophen poisoning and toxicity. *Pediatrics* 55:871–876, 1975.

187. Neuvonen P: Bioavailability of phenytoin: Clinical pharmacokinetic and therapeutic implications. *Clin Pharmacokinet* 4:91–103, 1979.

188. Richens A: Clinical pharmacokinetics of phenytoin. *Clin Pharmacokinet* 4:153–169, 1979.

189. Matthew H, Lawson A: Acute barbiturate poisoning—A review of two years experience. *Q J Med* 35:539–551, 1966.

190. Shubin H, Weil M: Shock associated with barbiturate intoxication. *JAMA* 215:263–268, 1971.

191. Bloomer H: A critical evaluation of diuresis in the treatment of barbiturate intoxication. *J Lab Clin Med* 67:898–905, 1966.

192. Kevey R, Pitlick W, Troupin A: Pharmacokinetics of carbamazepine in normal man. *Clin Pharmacol Ther* 17:657–668, 1975.

193. DeZeeuw R, Westenberg H, VanDerkleijn: An unusual case of carbamazepine poisoning with a near fatal relapse after two days. *Clin Toxicol* 14:263–269, 1979.

194. Rawlins M, Collste P, Bertilsson L: Distribution and elimination kinetics of carbamazepine. *Eur J Clin Pharmacol* 8:91–96, 1975.

195. Gugler Rand von Unruh G: Clinical pharmacokinetics of valproic acid. *Clin Pharmacokinet* 5:67–83, 1980.

196. Browne T: Valproic acid. *N Engl J Med* 302:661–666, 1980.

197. Suchy F, Balistreri W, Buchino J: Acute hepatic failure associated with the use of sodium valproate. *N Engl J Med* 300:962–966, 1979.

198. Weber W, Hein D: Clinical pharmacokinetics of isoniazid. *Clin Pharmacokinet* 4:401–422, 1979.

199. Hyatt H: Acute poisoning from overdose of isoniazid. *Am J Dis Child* 102:106–110, 1961.

200. Thornton W: Sleep aids and sedatives. *JACEP* 6:408–412, 1977.

201. Drugdex: Drug evaluation—Mianserin, in Conners C, Watanabe A, Rumack B (eds): *POISINDEX,* Englewood, Colo, Micromedex Publishers, 1981.

202. Crome P, Newman B: Poisoning with maprotaline and mianserin. *Br Med J* 2:260, 1977.

203. Greenblatt D, Allen M, Noel B: Acute overdosage with benzodiazepine derivatives. *Clin Pharmacol Ther* 21:497–514, 1977.

204. Greenblatt D, Shader R: Pharmacokinetic understanding of antianxiety drug therapy. *South Med J* 71:2–9, 1978.

205. Lynn R, Honig C, Jatlow P: Resin hemoperfusion for treatment of ethchlorvynol overdose. *Ann Intern Med* 91:549–553, 1979.

206. Benowitz N, Abolin C, Tozer T: Resin hemoperfusion in ethchlorvynol overdose. *Clin Pharmacol Ther* 27:236–242, 1980.

207. Maher J: Determinants of serum half-life of glutethimide in intoxicated patients. *J Pharmacol Exp Ther* 174:450–455, 1970.

208. Wright N, Roscue P: Acute glutethimide poisoning—Conservative management of 31 patients. *JAMA* 214:1704–1706, 1970.

209. Stalker N, Gambertoglio, Fukumitsu C: Acute massive chloral hydrate intoxication treated with hemodialysis—A clinical pharmacokinetic analysis. *J Clin Pharmacol* 12:136–142, 1978.

210. Cummins L: Hypoglycemia and convulsions in children following alcohol ingestion. *J Pediatr* 58:23–26, 1961.

211. Goldfrank L, Starke C: Metabolic acidosis in the alcoholic. *Hospital Physician* 4:34–38, 1979.

212. Peterson R, Rumack B: D-penicillamine therapy of acute arsenic poisoning. *J Pediatr* 91:661–666, 1977.

213. Kjeldsberg C, Ward H: Leukemia in arsenic poisoning. *Ann Intern Med* 77:935–937, 1972.

214. Oehme F: British antilewisite, the classic heavy metal antidote. *Clin Toxicol* 5:215–222, 1972.

215. Chisolm J: The use of chelating agents in the treatment of acute and chronic lead intoxication in childhood. *J Pediatr* 73:1–38, 1968.

216. Chisolm J: Poisoning from heavy metals (mercury, lead, and cadmium). *Pediatr Ann* 9:28–42, 1980.

SECTION V
Pediatric Emergencies

"Common Pediatric Emergencies" (Chapter 25) has been kept brief because many of the emergencies encountered in pediatric patients are discussed elsewhere in the text, for example, "Orthopedic Emergencies" (Chapter 8), "Minor Lacerations and Abrasions" (Chapter 10), "Diabetic Emergencies" (Chapter 11), "Acid-Base Disturbances" (Chapter 18), "Infectious Disease Emergencies" (Chapter 20), "Burns" (Chapter 21), "Dermatologic Emergencies" (Chapter 22), "Gastrointestinal Emergencies" (Chapter 23), "Poisoning and Drug Overdose" (Chapter 24), "Drowning and Near-Drowning" (Chapter 32), "Depression, Anxiety, and Suicide" (Chapter 37), "Cardiopulmonary Resuscitation" (Chapter 55), and "Obstructive Lung Diseases" (Chapter 57).

When reviewing "Child Abuse" (Chapter 26) and "Sexual Abuse" (Chapter 27) the reader is invited to refer to chapters elsewhere in the text that may also be of interest: "Rape and Sexual Assault" (Chapter 65) and "Social and Behavioral Considerations" (Section VIII).

25. Common Pediatric Emergencies

FRANK E. EHRLICH, M.D.

The majority of general hospital emergency departments primarily treat adults. When small children appear in one of these emergency departments, they usually create anxiety among the emergency personnel. It is therefore imperative that the staff prepare themselves for the arrival of these patients. It is likely that no patient is easier to treat in the emergency department, since there is generally no secondary gain involved. A child who appears sick is in fact a sick child. A playful, romping child has, more than likely, no significant acute illness.

"Children are not small adults." This statement is something that health professionals must be reminded of regularly. Pediatric patients have their own pathophysiology, which emergency physicians should become familiar with.

INITIAL ASSESSMENT

Any emergency department situation involving pediatric patients involves a triangular relationship bringing into play the patient, the patient's parents or guardian, and the emergency department personnel (Fig. 25–1). If this is managed thoughtfully, many problems in the initial assessment can be resolved.

The first corner of the triangle and the most important is the patient. Emergency department personnel realize that invariably they are dealing with a frightened patient. Hospitals and people in white uniforms often evoke memories of previous traumatic experiences. Even a

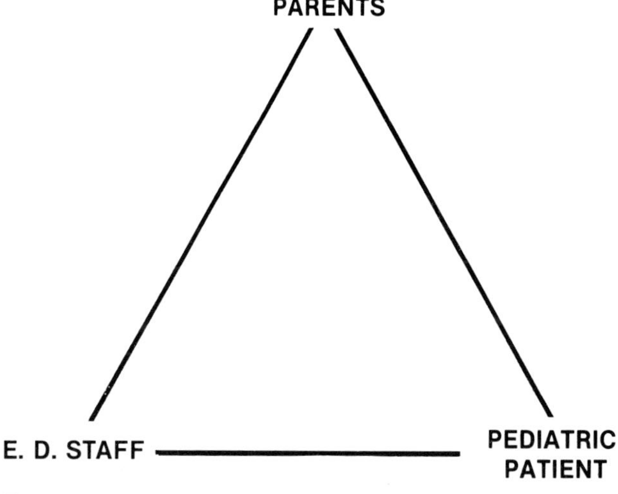

Figure 25–1 Triangular Relationship.

child who has never been in an emergency department can sense the similarity to a physician's office. It is therefore imperative that every effort be made to make the hospital experience as atraumatic as possible. It should be remembered that a child who has a bad experience today may be an unmanageable patient in the future.

Separating child from parents, in order to facilitate diagnostic procedures, often enhances their fear. A thoughtful and understanding staff can do much to alleviate this problem. On the other hand, efforts directed at convincing a small child to voluntarily submit to a painful procedure are largely wasted time and energy.

The effort to convince a 4-year-old to hold still for blood drawing may be productive, but if the child does not cooperate readily, the child should be properly restrained and the blood drawn. It is much better to do what is necessary in an understanding yet firm manner than to battle a screaming, frightened, unrestrained child.

Another important aspect of pediatric patients is that they live in a world of simple truths—to deceive, lie, or create distrust destroys all hope of dealing with them. Children should be given all the necessary information in terms they can deal with. As an example, telling a child that the needle used for drawing blood will not hurt or that an injection will not hurt creates distrust for any future efforts. A gentle, firm, honest, and reassuring approach with the child over 3 years of age often enables the physician to perform a complete initial assessment with minimal difficulty. Explaining procedures in detail to the patient under the age of 3 is usually a waste of time. It is better to tell the child what is going to happen, restrain the child properly, and then carry out the necessary procedures.

At the second corner of the triangle are the parents of the patient. It is absolutely essential for emergency personnel to remember that they are dealing not only with a patient but the parents of that patient as well. For most parents, their child's illness is a frightening experience. They feel helpless and may even sense failure over the situation. They may feel guilty because the child is ill or injured and wonder if it was something they could have prevented. All of this leads to an anxiety-laden experience. Their behavior may be totally different from when the illness involves one of them. Understanding this situation will lead to a better experience for all concerned.

Parents should be completely informed of the physician's impressions of the cause of the problem and what studies and treatment are planned. Just as no secrets should be kept from the patient, none should be kept from the parents either. A helpful and thoughtful word from the physicians and nurses will do much to alleviate anxiety.

The mother appearing in the emergency department at three o'clock in the morning with a child whose temperature is 101°F (38°C) and who has a runny nose, is herself in need of help. The child probably has nothing more than an upper respiratory infection, but the mother is telling the staff, "I am insecure and do not really understand what to do for my child." She is indirectly asking for help. The child will be helped as much by educating the mother as by a prescription for a decongestant.

The final corner in the triangle is the emergency department personnel. The arrival of a pediatric patient can create significant anxiety for the staff. First, personnel are often afraid of dealing with such small patients. They are unable to understand the child's pathophysiology, uneasy performing the necessary diagnostic procedures, and often uncertain as to the appropriate therapy. Finally, they are afraid of similar problems with their own children. It is imperative that emergency personnel deal with their anxieties in a constructive way and not allow them to interfere with relationships with parents and patients.

The staff must serve as the conductor, orchestrating the relationships surrounding a pediatric patient. It is interesting to talk with children and parents who have been treated in the emergency department of a pediatric hospital. In these institutions the staff are readily familiar with pediatric patients and have voluntarily chosen to work with them. The anxiety level among this staff is usually much lower. The experience in these emergency departments, for child and parent alike, is better when compared with that in a general hospital emergency department. Obviously, effort must be put forth to offset this problem.

History

Another point to remember is that for the vast majority of children the medical history comes primarily from the parents. Nevertheless, when taking a history always have the child in the room with the parents; talking with the parents away from the child usually arouses distrust on the part of the child. In addition, it is sometimes beneficial to ask questions directly of the child but in the presence of the parents. The child who understands the question will give a reliable answer. This same technique is helpful in completing the physical examination since the presence of a parent will help to alleviate fear and distrust.

The details of history-taking are quite similar to the adult patient. The one point that should be emphasized for the pediatric group is the time factor. In a small child, such as a 6-month-old infant, tremendous devastation can occur in a short period of time. Twenty-four hours of diarrhea in a 6-month-old can produce far more significant fluid loss than 24 hours of diarrhea in a 20-year-old.

Physical Examination

As for the physical examination the basic premise is that nothing should be done to frighten or startle the child and initiate fear and crying. Instruments should be room temperature; nothing is more frightening to a small infant or child than to have a cold instrument placed on the chest or abdomen. Likewise, the examiner's hands should be warm. Along these same lines it is imperative that the examiner have available pediatric-size instruments. This includes otoscope attachments, a pediatric stethoscope so that pulmonary and heart sounds can be adequately localized, and needles and syringes for drawing blood samples.

It is important that the blood pressure cuff be of the appropriate size. The correct size cuff covers approximately two-thirds of the upper arm. If the cuff is narrower, readings will be erroneously high and if the cuff is wider, erroneously low.

During this stage of the initial assessment the parent may hold the child. In particular, examination of the chest is aided by the parent's holding the child to the chest with the child's back turned to the examiner. The object, once again, is to maintain the child's sense of security. If for some reason the parents must leave the room, it is advisable to explain to the child why they are leaving and what will happen while the parents are away. It is often helpful to allow the child the opportunity of playing with some of the instruments and exploring them prior to using them on the patient.

It is important to realize that the sequence of the adult physical examination, which usually begins at the head and proceeds to the toes, is not appropriate for small children. It is easier for everyone if those areas which are most apt to produce crying are examined at the very end. Therefore a good beginning is listening to the chest, a procedure which is the least invasive and least obnoxious to the child and enables the child to stay in the parent's arms and be most secure. Then proceed to auscultation of the heart and anterior chest.

Then if the abdomen is not involved with the problem, examine that area, perhaps tickling the child and beginning some sort of play relationship.

In general, examining the ears, throat, and nose produces the child's most vivid response. Distracting the child by pretending to produce things from the child's ears may make it possible to carry out this part of the assessment without difficulty. However, if the child has an earache on one side, then that will certainly be the last area to examine. If the problem is external otitis, expect minimal cooperation from the child. When the physician examines the throat and ears of small children an assistant should restrain the child in order to make the procedure as atraumatic and rapid as possible.

It is important when examining a sick child to be as patient as possible. Haste will only result in pain, needless trauma, and fear. In turn this will result in the least amount of cooperation and produce a sequence that benefits no one.

Restraining the Child

A child can be restrained in three ways. The simplest method is to ask a staff assistant to hold the child in the proper position. Parents often shrink from using the force required to restrain their children. During the initial assessment, the parent may be allowed to hold the child's feet since this maintains contact between them. Another form of restraint entails the use of a commercially available device that consists of a board and Velcro straps. These are, in general, quite effective. They are especially useful when dealing with patients with lacerations. The third type of restraint involves "mummifying" the child in a bed sheet. This is probably the most inexpensive effective way to immobilize a small child for examination of the areas around the upper extremities and head.

RESUSCITATION AND LIFE-THREATENING EMERGENCIES

Cardiac arrest in a pediatric patient is fortunately a rare event. Nevertheless, the protocol for the Basic Cardiac Life Support program as outlined by the American Heart Association and supported by the American Academy of Pediatrics should be familiar to all staff members. (See Chapter 55.) It involves the basic ABC format, with particular attention to the variations of pediatric patients.

Infant Intubation

The child under the age of 2 years has an exceptionally soft and pliable trachea. Extension of the neck, done in the adult to clear the airway, should not be done in the small child as it may occlude the airway. Intubation of a small child can be disheartening in the hands of the inexperienced. It is a dangerous procedure unless there has been an opportunity for practice. The technique of infant intubation as practiced in the Advanced Cardiac Life Support program of the American Heart Association should be familiar to all emergency personnel, and maintaining such skills should be an integral component of each clinician's continuing education program.

A good rule of thumb for the correct size of endotracheal tube is that the tube that will fit in the child's external nares is the correct size for the child's trachea. The tube should be without a cuff and should be taped securely in place, preferably with some form of bite block in the mouth. This latter device is usually a taped gauze roll which fills the mouth and prevents any movement of the tube. Remember that in a 6-month-old child a 1- to 2-cm tube movement may move the tube from the subglottic area to the right main stem bronchus.

It is important to remember that the tidal volume of a small child is markedly less than that of an adult. There have been many documented cases of iatrogenic pneumothorax in infants because an overzealous staff member squeezed too much air into an intubated child's lungs with a respiratory assistance bag. An approximation for the tidal volume in children can be made using 8 cc/kg. Observing and listening to the chest are most beneficial when evaluating how much respiratory assistance is appropriate.

Cardiac Compression

The rules for cardiac compression as advocated by the American Heart Association's Basic Life Support program should be followed rigidly. These include location, rate, and depth of compression. Supporting the infant's thorax posteriorly is imperative since the infant's anatomy creates an open space behind the spine and, with their pliable thorax, effective compressions are difficult to achieve.

Drug Administration

Another important aspect in the resuscitation of a small child is expedient administration of drugs. It is probably impossible for active emergency department personnel, 90 to 95 percent of whose patients are adult, to remember the correct dosage for drugs used to resuscitate a critically ill child. Therefore, a pediatric drug dose chart (Exhibit 25–1) should be used. This is maintained on the resuscitation cart in a clear plastic envelope with an attached wax pencil.

While the patient is undergoing the initial steps in the resuscitation, for example, removal of clothes, attachment of electrodes, and initiation of an intravenous (IV) line, the nurse who will run the drug box either estimates (by a weight per year graph) or is told the child's weight. This number is placed in the upper right-hand corner of the drug dose chart. Then that number is multiplied by the numbers in the dose column and the answer is written on the clear plastic envelope over the final dose column. This usually takes a matter of seconds and by the time the first drug is requested, the nurse has fully completed the chart and is ready to hand out the correct dosage of each drug.

The concentrations on this chart are standard adult concentrations requiring no second drug box for pediatric patients. This type of chart can obviously be modified to suit the needs of any emergency department. It will allow the average general hospital emergency department to be better prepared for the arrival of a critically ill pediatric patient requiring resuscitation.

FLUID AND ELECTROLYTE REPLACEMENT

One of the most significant problems in the pediatric age-group involves the loss of fluids from such common causes as diarrhea and vomiting. Viral gastroenteritis in a 9-month-old child can cause significant dehydration in a very short period of time. It is therefore imperative to understand pediatric fluid and electrolyte replacement as well as maintenance requirements. Many formulas are available for these calculations. One of the most accurate, and one which can be used for the smallest of pediatric patients as well as the largest of adult patients, relates water requirements to calories burned and that in turn is a function of the patient's weight.

As can be seen in Table 25–1 appropriate maintenance fluid volumes can be determined for a patient in any weight bracket. An infant weighing up to 10 kg will require 100 cc/kg for maintenance fluid. A child between 10 and 20 kg requires for maintenance fluid 1,000 cc of water for the first 10 kg and 50 cc of water for each kilogram between 10 and 20. For a child or adult over 20 kg the maintenance fluid requirement is 1,500 cc of water for the first 20 kg and 20 cc of water for every kilogram over 20. Table 25–2 shows the calculations for maintenance fluid requirements in a 6.5-kg infant, a 17-kg child, and a 27-kg child, as well as for a 70-kg adult. The latter amount is the standard 2,500 cc/day volume, usually administered (100 cc/hour) as maintenance fluid to adults.

The electrolyte requirements for maintenance purposes are 3 mEq of sodium, 2 mEq of potassium, and 2 mEq of chloride for every 100 cc of water administered to the patient.

Dehydration occurs primarily in the extracellular fluid. The extracellular space occupies approximately 30 percent of the child's body mass. The interstitial space occupies approximately three-quarters of the extracellular volume and it is into this space that so-called third-space loss occurs. In the replacement of dehydration losses, if the patient has a significant volume depletion and is in shock, then every effort should be made to correct the vascular space deficit within two hours. The overall extracellular fluid-space deficit can then be corrected over the ensuing 24 hours. Fluid can be administered empirically at 10 to 15 cc/kg/hour up to a maximum rate of 20 to 30 cc/kg for prompt correction. This should, within the initial two hours, restore the blood pressure and other vital parameters so that the patient's primary problems can be treated and the overall dehydration corrected.

The general symptoms of dehydration are decrease in skin turgor, drying of the mucous membranes, tachycardia, hypotension, oliguria, and thirst if the deficit is greater than 2 percent of the body weight. It is extremely important when examining a possibly dehydrated child to question the mother as to the amount of urine in the diapers and the number of wet diapers during the previous 24 hours.

Exhibit 25–1 Pediatric Drug Dose Chart

Patient Weight (Kg)_____________

Drug	Dilution	Concentration	Dose	Final Dose
Epinephrine		1:10,000	0.1 ml/kg	EPI
Sodium bicarbonate		1 mEq/ml	1 ml/kg	NaHCO$_3$
Atropine		0.1 mg/ml	0.1 ml/kg	ATROP
Calcium chloride		10%	0.1 ml/kg	CaCl
Calcium gluconate		10%	0.3 ml/kg	CaGl
Lidocaine	2 gm in 100 cc D$_5$W	20 mg/ml	0.05 ml/kg	LIDO
Narcan		0.4 mg/ml	0.025 ml/kg	NARC
Dopamine	200 mg in 500 cc D$_5$W	400 μg/ml	5 μg/min/kg	DOPA
Isuprel	1 mg in 100 cc D$_5$W	10 μg/ml	6–24 cc/hr absolute dose	ISUP
Defibrillations	2 watt-sec/kg per shock; may double and repeat as needed			

Dehydration therapy is usually figured according to a clinical estimate of the amount of dehydration. If one is fortunate enough to have a recent weight for the child, then the actual amount of fluid loss can be determined by comparing weights. If this information is not available, then clinical expertise is required.

Dehydration can be graded as simple (5 percent), moderate (10 percent), or severe (15 percent). The child with 5 percent dehydration will present with a diminution of urine output, slight tachycardia, minimal loss of skin turgor, and dry mucous membranes. At the other extreme will be the child with severe or 15 percent dehydration. This child will be in shock, and will have significant tachycardia, hypotension, diminution of urine output to the point of oliguria, dry and coated mucous membranes, and essentially no skin turgor. If the patient is a small infant the fontanelles will be soft or sunken. The child with 10 percent or moderate dehydration is somewhere in the middle of these two extremes and it requires greater clinical acumen to make this evaluation.

The amount of fluid needed to replace an isotonic dehydration loss is shown in Table 25–3. A child with simple dehydration should receive 50 cc/kg of water in addition to maintenance requirements. The amount of electrolytes needed will be approximately 4 mEq/kg of sodium, 3 mEq/kg of potassium, and 3 mEq/kg of chloride if the loss is isotonic. For the child with 10 percent dehydration the volume replacement should be 100 cc/kg with the electrolytes as shown. This of course is in addition to maintenance fluid and electrolytes. Finally, the severely dehydrated child will require 150 cc/kg of fluid as well as 12 mEq of sodium, and 9 mEq each of potassium and chloride just to offset the dehydration. It is important to replace approximately half the calculated volume in eight hours and then a quarter over each of the succeeding eight-hour periods. These patients should be reevaluated frequently so that errors in the original evaluation can be corrected promptly.

Table 25–4 shows the calculations for fluid and electrolyte replacement in a 3-kg infant with a 10 percent clinical estimate of dehydration. The patient's serum sodium is 146, potassium 4.8, osmolarity 285, and pH 7.28. Based on the calculations for this patient, who appears to be in a state of isotonic dehydration, the concentration of replacement solution and the volumes over the ensuing eight-hour intervals can be determined.

TABLE 25–1   Maintenance Fluid Requirement

Weight	Daily Maintenance Fluid Requirement
0 – 10 kg	100 cc water/kg
10 – 20 kg	1,000 cc for first 10 kg + 50 cc water for each kg between 10 and 20 kg
Over 20 kg	1,500 cc for first 20 kg + 20 cc water for each kg over 20 kg

TABLE 25–2   Sample Maintenance Fluid Calculations

6.5-kg Infant	6.5 × 100 = 650 cc water/day
17.0-kg Child	10.0 kg × 100 = 1,000 cc 7.0 kg × 50 = 350 cc 1,350 cc water/day
27.0-kg Child	10.0 kg × 100 = 1,000 cc 10.0 kg × 50 = 500 cc 7.0 kg × 20 = 140 cc 1,640 cc water/day
70.0-kg Adult	10.0 kg × 100 = 1,000 cc 10.0 kg × 50 = 500 cc 50.0 kg × 20 = 1,000 cc 2,500 cc water/day

TABLE 25–3   Dehydration Requirements

% Dehydration	Fluid cc/kg	Electrolytes mEq/kg Na	K	Cl
Simple (5%)	50	4	3	3
Moderate (10%)	100	8	6	6
Severe (15%)	150	12	9	9

TABLE 25–4   Sample Calculation for Dehydrated Patient

	Water	Na	K	Cl
Maintenance	300 cc	9	6	6
Dehydration replacement	300 cc	24	18	18
Total	600 cc	33 mEq	24 mEq	24 mEq

33 mEq in 600 cc = x mEq in 1,000 cc

x = 55 mEq

∴ fluid of choice is about ⅓ NS

Consideration should be given as well to whether dehydration is isotonic, hypertonic, or hypotonic (Table 25–5). Alterations are required in the volume and electrolyte content of the fluid used for replacement if the dehydration is other than isotonic. Table 25–5 can be used with the results of the clinical exam and laboratory tests to determine the type of dehydration. This infor-

mation is most helpful in deciding the type of fluid to use for replacement and the rate at which that fluid should be replaced. It is of primary importance in the management of hypertonic dehydration, for example, that the solution used contain salt. If water were used as the replacement fluid, the patient's serum sodium would be lowered too rapidly and an intracerebral bleed might result.

Certain axioms should be kept in mind when managing fluid and electrolyte disorders in pediatric patients. The first has already been mentioned—replace half the deficit over eight hours and reevaluate the patient critically during that time. The second axiom is, never trust the laboratory. The third axiom is, replace all deficits at the same rate that they arose. A patient who is in a state of hypertonic dehydration after a four-day illness does not need to be totally corrected within the first 24 hours. The final axiom is an anonymous quotation, "Dying in balance is unnecessary."

Many formulas are available to help with ancillary fluid and electrolyte problems in the pediatric patient. For example, the formula for administering whole blood is 2 cc of whole blood for every percent hematocrit per kilogram body weight the patient's hematocrit should be raised. The formula for packed cells is similar except the number is 1.2 cc of packed cells for every percent hematocrit per kilogram body weight the hematocrit should be raised.

If bicarbonate will be used to help with acid-base problems, multiply the base deficit by the patient's body weight (kilograms) by 0.3 (which conforms to the distribution of bicarbonate in the extracellular space). This gives the total amount of bicarbonate needed in milliequivalents. Usually half of this can be given as an IV bolus and the rest can be delivered over four to six hours. In an emergency, administer 3 mEq of bicarbonate/kg as an IV push.

In patients with diarrhea, loss of bicarbonate exceeds loss of chloride and therefore acidosis results. In the case of vomiting with loss of gastric secretion, chloride loss exceeds bicarbonate loss and alkalosis results. The increased fluid loss in a patient with fever can be accommodated by increasing the maintenance requirement 12 percent for every centigrade degree rise in temperature.

PROBLEMS IN THE FIRST YEAR OF LIFE

Infants in this age-group are probably the most frightening patients to the staff of a general hospital emergency department. At the same time they are often the easiest to diagnose and treat. The majority of patients in this age-group are brought to the emergency de-

TABLE 25–5   Types of Dehydration

Type Dehydration	Type Loss	ECF Volume	ICF Volume	Serum Na	Osmolarity
Isotonic	Iso	↓	WNL	WNL	280 mOsm
Hypertonic	Hypo	↓	↓	> 150	> 280 mOsm
Hypotonic	Hyper	↓	↑	< 150	< 280 mOsm

partment for some form of infection. The presenting complaint is usually fever, a frightening experience for most parents when it involves their own children. Usually, they make some effort to control the fever and when that fails they bring the child immediately to the emergency department. If the child has additional symptoms such as diarrhea or vomiting or is tugging at an ear, then the diagnosis is simplified.

On the other hand, many children are brought to the emergency department with a complaint of fever and no localizing signs or symptoms. The physician must then do a thorough head-to-toe examination looking for the cause. Otitis media, urinary tract infections, and pharyngitis are often hidden causes for fever. If a cause is found treatment is rendered accordingly. If no cause is found then the laboratory should be used for assistance. A complete blood cell count (CBC), urinalysis, and chest roentgenogram should be done. Throat and blood cultures are done as indicated, as is a cerebrospinal fluid (CSF) evaluation.

The appropriate dosage for aspirin and acetaminophen products is based on the weight of the patient. The dose for aspirin used as an antipyretic is 30 to 60 mg/kg/day. This is given orally and divided into doses every four hours. Another good general rule to teach parents is to administer 1¼ grains of aspirin for every year of life. Since most of the pediatric aspirin tablet preparations come as 1¼-grain tablets, this is a simple system to use. The American Academy of Pediatrics recommends avoiding the use of aspirin in young children with flu or chicken pox, because of the risk of Reye's syndrome. The dose for acetaminophen, for infants under 1 year of age is 60 mg orally every four hours; for children under 3 years of age 120 mg every 4 hours orally; and for children over 3 years of age 120 to 240 mg every three or four hours orally. Parents should be advised that for children who are vomiting, both medications are available in suppository form. The dosage for aspirin and acetaminophen administered rectally is the same as the dosage orally. It is often helpful in the management of high fevers to use both medications, alternating them at two-hour intervals.

Fever in the first 3 months of life is a serious symptom and any temperature over 101°F (38°C) most likely warrants hospital admission and a complete work-up in terms of diagnostic studies, including lumbar puncture, cultures, chest roentgenogram, CBC, and urinalysis.

Respiratory Infections

In the case of a child under 1 year of age with an upper respiratory infection, management should include humidification and increased fluid intake and should not include the use of antibiotics, decongestants, or antihistamines.

Urinary Tract Infections

Urinary tract infections in children in this age-group are difficult to diagnose because of the lack of symptoms. Sterile urine for culture must be collected in order to make the diagnosis. Various commercial kits are available for strapping the child in order to collect a sample. If these do not work then a suprapubic tap is indicated. Once the diagnosis of a urinary tract infection is established, appropriate antibiotic therapy should be instituted and a diagnostic work-up of the urinary tract should be initiated by referral to a urologist.

Gastrointestinal (GI) Infections

Another form of infection common in this age-group involves the GI tract. Therapy entails replacement of fluid loss as discussed. An important consideration is that for the outpatient management of children with GI infections and fluid loss, the oral replacement fluid should be a simple electrolyte solution. The child should be fed small amounts of these liquids at frequent intervals and no attempt made to give large bolus volumes. Agents such as Kaopectate and Lomotil should be avoided in the management of diarrhea since they may prolong the problem. If any of these problems persists to such a degree that adequate oral intake cannot be given and the child seems to be worsening clinically, hospital admission for IV fluid replacement and a culture work-up is required.

Surgical Conditions

A few surgical conditions that occur in the first year of life can present as problems to the emergency department. Chronologically, the first of these is pyloric stenosis. This usually presents in a patient between 2 and 6 weeks of age. The infant is brought to the emergency department because of persistent projectile vomiting. The vomiting is usually worse later in the day than in the morning. The characteristic history and the palpable mass in the child's right upper quadrant lead to the definitive diagnosis. The treatment is, of course, surgery.

Another surgical problem is intussusception. These children are usually between 6 months and 1 year of age, and more often male than female. The patient usually presents with intermittent crampy abdominal pain. Often the parents describe the child as having "fits"—drawing up the legs and crying in apparent pain. There may be bloody diarrhea and emesis, depending on the degree of intestinal obstruction. Physical examination usually reveals a tender abdomen and on occasion a palpable mass on the right side of the abdomen. This can be a difficult diagnosis to make and requires a high index of suspicion. The treatment is to obtain the diagnostic (and often therapeutic) barium enema after a surgical consultation.

Inguinal hernias can present as a problem in this age-group. They are usually frightening to the parents and get far more attention than they deserve. If the hernia can be reduced, then the parents should be reassured and referred to their pediatrician for eventual surgical consultation. Efforts to reduce the hernia can be made but an overzealous effort to squeeze the hernia contents back into the abdominal cavity should be avoided. If the hernia cannot be reduced easily, then immediate surgical consultation is required.

SEIZURES

Febrile seizures are common in the pediatric population, and are associated with some form of febrile illness such as viral gastroenteritis or roseola. They usually occur between 6 months and 5 years of age. They are of short duration lasting generally less than ten minutes.

The important steps in management involve immediate supportive treatment. This consists of airway maintenance, oxygen, and initiating an IV line. Anticonvulsants are used when indicated, the most appropriate being diazepam. It can be given in a dose of 0.5 mg/kg up to a maximum dose of 5 mg in small children. The intramuscular (IM) route is by no means as effective as the rectal or IV route. If diazepam is given IV it should be administered slowly. Since it may be difficult to establish an IV in a small child, rectal administration of the standard IV diazepam preparation in the same dosage, via a small rubber catheter is recommended. The dosage should be titrated carefully,

since respiratory depression may occur with an overdose.

Once the seizure has been controlled then the fever should be evaluated and the child treated with appropriate medications. The central nervous system should be evaluated as a possible source of the convulsion. Whether these children should be placed on daily prophylactic therapy, whether they should be given prophylactic phenobarbital during febrile episodes, or whether they should be managed with neither is controversial. A careful review of the literature suggests that doing nothing is most likely the best management.

COMMON VIRAL INFECTIONS

It is imperative for the emergency physician in a general hospital to be adept at recognizing certain of the viral infections common to the pediatric population. These include rubeola, rubella, roseola, erythema infectiosum, varicella, and mumps. (See Chapter 20.)

Rubeola

Rubeola, or measles, has an incubation period of 10 to 12 days. The prodromal phase is characterized by a low-grade to moderate fever, a mild cough, and the general symptoms of an upper respiratory infection. This in turn is followed by the appearance of Koplik's spots which are pathognomonic of measles. These spots are grayish punctate lesions on the buccal mucosa opposite the lower molars. Next the rash of measles begins to appear, first as macules along the neck and face area. Then it becomes more maculopapular as the rash spreads over the upper body and arms, then to the torso and abdomen, and eventually the feet. The rash may take two to three days to reach the distal lower extremity. The rash may be confluent. Pruritus is unusual. Isolation should be continued for approximately one week after the rash starts. The rapid decline in the number of cases of measles throughout the United States only underscores the need for greater awareness on the part of the emergency physician as to the diagnosis.

Rubella

Rubella, or German measles, has an incubation period of two to three weeks. The prodromal period consists of mild catarrhal symptoms and often goes unnoticed. The characteristic physical finding in rubella is the posterior or retroauricular lymphadenopathy. These nodes are often quite large and tender. Few alternative diagnoses cause this finding in this age population. The rash of rubella varies from discrete maculopapular lesions to flushing with confluence of the maculopapular lesions particularly over the face. The rash usually lasts about three days. The photophobia (light sensitivity) present with measles is not present in German measles. Fever is usually low-grade, and pruritus is not generally a problem.

Roseola

Roseola, or exanthem subitum, is characterized by the sudden onset of four to five days of high-grade fever, often as high as 103° to 105°F (39° to 40°C). Febrile seizures are not uncommon when the fever is this high. There may be minimal symptoms of an upper respiratory infection. The most outstanding characteristic of roseola is the complete absence of any physical findings to explain the fever. This clinical characteristic is often used to support the diagnosis. The disease occurs most commonly in infants and young children. The fever usually falls precipitously around the fourth day and at about the same time a macular or maculopapular eruption appears over the trunk and then spreads to the arms, neck, and finally the face and legs. The rash usually lasts only 24 hours and then fades.

Erythema Infectiosum

Fifth disease, or erythema infectiosum, is characterized by a rash which seems to appear in two separate stages. The rash may be preceded by very nonspecific signs and symptoms of an upper respiratory infection, including sore throat and coryza. The first stage of the disease is characterized by erythematous, coalescent, maculopapular lesions overlying the cheeks—the so-called "slapped cheeks." The rest of the face is usually spared. The lesions resemble, at least superficially, early erysipelas. The facial rash generally lasts one to four days.

The second-stage rash, which begins about one day after the first, consists of an erythematous maculopapular eruption on the extensor surfaces of the arms, hands, and then shortly thereafter the thighs and buttocks. The trunk is usually spared. The rash spreads to the flexor surface of the arms as the extensor surface lesions begin to clear. The rash may take from one to two weeks to fade completely with the entire course of the disease lasting up to 24 days. A peculiar characteristic of the rash of fifth disease is its marked variation in intensity from moment to moment. There is often mild pruritus. These patients are usually afebrile particularly in the latter stages of the disease.

Varicella

Varicella, or chickenpox, has an incubation period of two to three weeks. The prodromal symptoms consist of a mild fever with malaise. Following this, the specific rash of chickenpox appears. It begins as small red papules that shortly thereafter develop into clear vesicles overlying an erythematous base. Subsequently the vesicle content becomes cloudy. The vesicles are broken easily and are coated with an eschar. Vesicle eruption continues for between two and five days. They spread from the trunk to the face and scalp, sparing the extremities. Pruritus is a predominant symptom of varicella. The fever may range from low-grade to as high as 105° F (40°C).

Mumps

Mumps has an incubation period of two to three weeks. Prodromal symptoms are rare but, if present, usually consist of mild myalgia in the neck area. The onset of the illness is characterized by pain and then swelling in the area of one or both parotid glands. These symptoms persist for one to three days and then over the ensuing week gradually subside. Bilateral swelling is much more common than unilateral. High fever is a rare complication of mumps. On occasion, the submandibular gland may be swollen as well or may even be the only gland involved with mumps.

ACUTE ABDOMEN

One of the most common problems for which children are brought to an emergency department is abdominal pain. It is absolutely essential that an emergency medicine physician be adept at discerning the nonsurgically from the surgically treatable causes. The emergency physician must be able to decide that a child most likely has appendicitis and will require surgery or has a viral mesenteric adenitis and can go home.

Appendicitis

The story of epigastric pain followed by nausea, anorexia, vomiting, malaise, and subsequent migration of the pain to the right lower quadrant is classical for appendicitis. The diagnosis of appendicitis in a child should be based on clinical findings and not laboratory tests. The physician must take a careful history of the nature, onset, and progression of the pain, and must elicit a history of the child's overall behavior during the time of the illness. A child who has been playing and jovial throughout the illness is much less likely to have appendicitis than one who has been lying around watching television or playing quietly in bed or on the couch. The critical part of this diagnosis is a careful abdominal examination and eliciting peritoneal signs along with localized right lower quadrant abdominal tenderness.

The standard technique for producing rebound tenderness is to push into the abdominal cavity and then sharply release the abdominal wall. This should *never* be done as part of the examination of children. It produces a pain over which the child has no control. It will assuredly destroy the examiner's rapport with the child. A far better technique for discovering the same information is to use the cough rebound sign. If in fact the peritoneum is irritated, the child will limit the excursion of the cough and protect the abdomen.

At this point the diagnosis of acute appendicitis should be entertained and, whether or not the white blood cell count is elevated, surgical consultation should be requested. Many children have had a gangrenous appendix removed while their WBC count was normal, and many children with a WBC count of 20,000 to 25,000 have been operated upon only to find a normal appendix. Although the majority of patients with acute appendicitis have a mildly to moderately elevated WBC count, emergency department physicians cannot allow themselves the luxury of using it as a basis for diagnosis. They should base their impressions on the physical examination and history, particularly if they intend to avoid the catastrophe of sending a patient out of the emergency department with acute appendicitis.

Once the diagnosis of acute appendicitis has been clinically ruled out, the child often can be managed as an outpatient. One exception involves the abdominal pain of sickle cell disease.

It is imperative that a child sent home with abdominal pain and instructions for outpatient management have a follow-up visit arranged for the next day.

COMMON PEDIATRIC TRAUMAS

A child can be traumatized in any area and the ability to manage these injuries is required of all emergency department physicians. This section covers some of the common forms of trauma. The battered child, pediatric orthopedic injuries, drowning, burns, or injuries to the genitourinary tract are discussed in other chapters.

Foreign Bodies

A common problem for which children are brought to the emergency department involves the ingestion of a foreign body. If the foreign body is in the tracheobronchial tree, immediate surgical consultation is required. This should be done only after the child's airway has been evaluated and secured. (See Chapter 57).

If the foreign body has been swallowed and is in the stomach then therapy will depend on the nature of the object. If it is a blunt object such as a coin, no further attention is necessary. These patients can be followed once a week with routine roentgenograms so as to follow the course of the foreign body. In addition, the parents should be instructed to check the bowel movements for the foreign body. If the child has swallowed a pointed or sharp object, the type and location of the object will determine the management.

Esophageal foreign bodies need immediate attention. In the child under the age of 4, coins can be removed from the esophagus without the use of the esophagoscope. This can be done with a Foley catheter. The technique involves placement of the Foley catheter in the esophagus. Inflation of the Foley balloon is done under the fluoroscope with radiopaque dye so that it is exactly the same size as the coin. This prevents any damage to the esophagus by the balloon. The child is then tipped head down and the Foley catheter withdrawn. The coin will fall out onto the table. The child is then observed overnight on a liquid diet and sent home after a repeat chest roentgenogram.

Foreign bodies in the ears and nose can pose a difficult problem. Many foreign bodies lodged in the nose can be extracted with fine forceps. If this does not work, then a small Foley catheter can usually be passed beyond the object, the balloon inflated, and the object and catheter withdrawn simultaneously.

Foreign bodies in the ear can be difficult to remove, and most of them should be referred directly to an otolaryngologist. They require a great deal of expertise in working through an otoscope with a head mirror, light, and delicate instruments. If the ear canal is irritated and bleeding initiated, the task of the otolaryngologist will only be more difficult and general anesthesia and an operating room may be needed. (See Chapter 67, Fig. 67–4.)

Another site for foreign body presentation is the vagina. Little girls whom you suspect of having vaginal foreign bodies should be examined with thought and patience and only in the presence of their mothers and a nurse. A good deal of explanation will be necessary, as well as reassurance and a gentle manner. The correct size instruments are an absolute prerequisite.

Lacerations

Lacerations around the head, eyes, ears, nose, and face are common in this age-group. The management of these injuries is the same for children as for adults. (See Chapter 10.)

One injury more common in children than adults involves lacerations of the tongue. This can be a difficult injury to treat, particularly at three in the morning with minimal assistance. Suturing such a laceration should be done only after conservative means to control the bleeding fail. Also, the minimum number of assistants is two and appropriate lighting and equipment must be available. The mouth should be held open, with the tongue outside the oral cavity, by means of some form of mouth gag or an assistant. This requires fine absorbable suture material as well as a great deal of suction and patience. Anything less is doomed to failure. If repair cannot be accomplished in the emergency department, the patient should be managed by the appropriate specialist and will more than likely require general anesthesia and an operating room.

Electric Burns

Another common injury involves burns around the mouth from contact with electrical current. Such injuries usually occur because the child bit into a plug or electrical cord and sustained an injury, most often in the corner of the mouth. This injury may look like a superficial burn initially and be covered with an eschar. The eschar in turn will slough around the fifth to the seventh day at which time significant bleeding may occur. All of these children should be admitted to the hospital if any tissue loss has taken place. They can be treated conservatively and appropriate surgical consultations obtained as needed. (See Chapter 21.)

MAJOR TRAUMA

The management of a child with major multisystem trauma resembles that of an adult with similar trauma. Attention to the ABCs of trauma resuscitation are paramount. The possibility of a fracture of the cervical spine must constantly be emphasized. The ability to gain airway control in a child with head and neck trauma requires a skilled intubationist or a skilled surgeon to perform a tracheostomy or cricothyroidotomy. A tracheostomy in a traumatized 3-year-old child, in the best of hands, is a difficult procedure. Cricothyroidotomy, while difficult, is certainly easier than a tracheostomy

and should be a skill in which the emergency physician maintains some degree of expertise.

Access to the circulation of a child via the various large peripheral veins is another skill required of an emergency physician. Venous cutdown at the saphenous vein in the ankle or groin or the basilic or cephalic veins in the upper extremity, and the percutaneous techniques of external jugular or subclavian puncture are procedures that may need to be performed rapidly in a small child.

The necessary steps for evaluation of injuries to the chest, abdomen, and head are similar in children and adults. One major difference is that peritoneal lavage should be a routine part of the management of the pediatric patient with an abdominal injury. Since the history is often difficult to obtain and may be of doubtful validity, peritoneal lavage provides a basis, but not a definitive one, for the initial diagnosis. That is, a positive lavage has meaning while a negative lavage does not. The administration of fluids and maintenance of adequate urine output, with appropriate monitoring of either wedge pressure or central venous pressure, are mandatory for the pediatric patient.

The basic format for trauma management outlined in the Advanced Trauma Life Support course of the American College of Surgeons should be familiar to every emergency department physician managing a traumatized pediatric patient. (See Chapters 6 and 7.)

BIBLIOGRAPHY

Gellis SS, Kagan M: *Current Pediatric Trauma*. Philadelphia, WB Saunders, 1964.

Irving G: Pediatric emergencies, in Schwartz GR (ed): *Principles and Practice in Emergency Medicine*. Philadelphia, WB Saunders, 1978.

Smith C: *The Critically Ill Child*, ed 2. Philadelphia, WB Saunders, 1977.

Vaughan VC, McKay RJ, Behran RE: *Nelson Text Book of Pediatrics*, ed 11. Philadelphia, WB Saunders, 1979.

American College of Emergency Physicians: *The Study Guide in Emergency Medicine*. November 1980.

26. Child Abuse

GLEN S. BARTLETT, M.D., Ph.D.

Child abuse may be defined as any act by a parent, guardian, or other person responsible for the well-being of a child that is physically or mentally injurious to that child. Four specific types of child abuse are recognized by law in most states: (1) physical abuse, (2) emotional or mental abuse, (3) neglect, and (4) sexual abuse, including incest.

Physical abuse is any act that produces a physical injury in the child. These injuries include multiple bruises, abrasions, and lacerations; burns; fractures; head, face, eye, ear, and mouth injuries; internal abdominal injuries; and genital injuries. *Mental abuse*, which is more difficult to define and recognize, includes constant belittling, repeated shouting at the child, abusive name calling, scapegoating, and similar verbal assaults on the child. *Neglect* may be physical, emotional, or medical and includes situations in which the parents or caretakers fail to provide adequate nourishment, physical care, or emotional support; circumstances in which the parents or guardians fail to provide adequate supervision or guidance to the point where the child's life may be potentially or actually endangered; and situations in which medical care is not sought for illness or injury. *Sexual abuse* is any illicit sexual act carried out by an adult on a child or a nonconsenting adolescent, including exposure; fondling; oral, anal, or genital intercourse, either attempted or completed; situations in which a child is forced to perform sexual acts on or with an adult; and exposure to or involvement in prostitution or pornography. Incest is intercourse between the child and an adolescent or adult family member, whether or not pregnancy results.

All of the acts that constitute forms of child abuse lead to serious social and psychological problems as well as medical problems. The more severe forms of abuse are symptomatic of family disorganization and poor social and psychological development on the part of the responsible adults. Physical abuse, including sexual abuse, while perhaps carried out by only one parent, is characteristically done with the knowledge and complicity of the other parent.

Each state has its own law or statute defining the specific forms of child abuse recognized in that state. Most states exclude from the definition of child abuse medical neglect cases where medical care is withheld for religious reasons. Nevertheless, there is ample precedent throughout the United States for court intervention when the child's life is at stake, as when courts order blood transfusions for children raised by parents who are Jehovah's Witnesses. Many states specifically absolve parents of responsibility for neglect of the child when that neglect results solely from socioeconomic factors, such as inadequate resources and inadequate housing.

The individual state laws vary considerably, but they have many characteristics in common, including a requirement for reporting cases of suspected abuse or neglect whenever individuals in the course of their professional activity have contact with such a child. The list of mandated reporters in all states includes physicians, nurses, and other health care personnel. In addition, each state law specifies the responsible agency to which reports of suspected abuse and neglect are to be made and defines the procedures for making such reports. Each physician and other health care provider coming in contact with children should be familiar with the child abuse laws within his or her own state.

ETIOLOGY

Many factors may be involved in cases of child abuse. Some relate to the child, some to the parents, and some to the family as a whole or to the situation in which the family finds itself.[1]

A detailed list of factors relating to the child is presented below:[1]

- an injury unexplained or inadequately explained by the history given
- evidence of repeated injuries
- injuries that are not mentioned in history
- characteristic radiographic changes to long bones
- evidence of sexual abuse or molestation
- evidence of dehydration and/or malnutrition without obvious cause
- evidence that child has been given inappropriate food, drink, and/or drugs
- evidence of overall poor care
- unusual fearfulness
- child was a premature infant, is a twin, has a physical defect, or has been a "difficult" child to care for
- child is seen as "different" or "bad" by the parents
- child "takes over" and tries to care for parents' needs.

While extensive, this list is not exclusive, and the presence of any one or even a small number of these factors in a given situation does not in itself constitute sufficient evidence for making the diagnosis of suspected child abuse. A common theme is that the child is seen by the parents either as a special child or as a child with characteristics that make him or her less than perfect. In this category are twins or children with many siblings, the long-awaited child, the unplanned or unwanted child, and the child that takes the place of a child who has died. Negative factors relating to the child include prematurity and the presence of any physical defect, mental retardation, or difficult behavior.

Factors relating to parents include characteristics of background and current behaviors:[1]

- presents a history that cannot or does not explain the injury

- presents contradictory or inconsistent history
- gives a history of repeated injury
- projects cause of injury onto a sibling or third party
- gives specific "eyewitness" history of abuse
- is reluctant to give information
- reveals inappropriate awareness of seriousness of situations (either overreaction or underreaction)
- continues to complain about irrelevant problems unrelated to the injury
- has delayed unduly in bringing child for care
- refuses consent for further diagnostic studies
- hospital "shops"
- cannot be located
- shows detachment from the child
- has unrealistic expectations of the child
- shows evidence of loss of physical or emotional control, or fear of losing such control
- has no one to "bail" her (him) out when "up tight" with the child
- has been reared in an atmosphere lacking a consistent parenting figure
- personally is misusing drugs or alcohol
- is psychotic or psychopathic.

It is often the case that the abusive parents were themselves abused as children or came from family environments in which physical striking out or abuse was common behavior. Some abusive parents come from disorganized families with inadequate parental role models.

A variety of family and situational factors may be present in cases of child abuse:

- continuous friction in the home
- marital discord
- broken home, divorce, and frequent remarriages
- recent or recurrent crises
- loss of support of relatives, friends, community
- recent or recurrent relocation of living quarters
- immature parents
- mental retardation of parents
- mentally ill parents
- excessive drinking or addiction to drugs
- overly severe control and discipline, physical or psychological
- failure to give constructive discipline for the child's proper development of good character, conduct, and habits
- criminal environment of parents; encouragement of delinquency in child
- incestuous sex relations
- promiscuity and prostitution
- harsh and improper language
- failure to give good adult example

- failure to inculcate value system in guidance and care of children (lack of moral training)
- failure to offer motivation and stimulation toward learning and receiving an education in keeping with child's ability and intelligence.

In general, these factors impose serious stresses on the family and/or represent acute crisis situations.

It should be noted that physical and mental abuse, neglect, and sexual abuse are seen at all levels of society and in families representing all educational, occupational, racial, and ethnic backgrounds. Nevertheless, within the context of the usual urban or public hospital emergency department practice, emergency care personnel are more likely to encounter abused children of lower socioeconomic status and minority group membership. Children from higher socioeconomic levels are more likely to appear in private physicians' offices or suburban private hospital emergency departments.

The investigation of a particular situation of abuse will often reveal that some combination of the above-mentioned child, parent, and situational factors is present, and that the family has recently experienced a crisis. In cases of sexual abuse, an unrelated crisis may precipitate a further investigation into the situation.

A typology of forms of sexual abuse is shown in Table 26-1. The dynamics of sexual abuse are even more complex than those of physical abuse,[2] and sexual abuse may be considered one of the most severe consequences of family disorganization.[3] The emergency care professional must have special training and skill in techniques for recognizing and interviewing child sexual abuse victims. A more thorough review of the subject of sexual abuse is presented in Chapters 27 and 65.

Studies have shown that as many as 10 percent of children coming to emergency departments with physical injuries have sustained these injuries as a result of physical abuse.[4] Beyond this there is a larger percentage of children who present with physical injuries sustained in situations where a parent has failed to protect a child against injury or has failed to provide adequate supervision of a child, or where the injury is the result of a parent's poor judgment in allowing or encouraging the child to carry out potentially dangerous activities. It is important to recognize the nature of these injuries and to offer help and guidance, but it may not be appropriate to report these cases as instances of abuse. Guidance on what constitutes child abuse can be obtained from the hospital's child abuse team or social service department, or from a responsible community agency.

PATHOLOGY, PATHOPHYSIOLOGY, AND CLINICAL CORRELATES

Physical Abuse

The physical signs of child abuse may be manifested in a variety of ways.[5,6] The skin may show bruises, abrasions, lacerations, grip marks, rope burns, cigarette burns, flame or liquid burns, and hot instrument brands.

Certain skin injuries are characteristic and diagnostic of child abuse in themselves, while others are not. Abusive injuries are more likely to be located over the cheeks, trunk, genitals, buttocks, and upper legs and are less likely to involve lacerations.[7] Many instruments that are used to strike children will leave characteristic marks. A severe hand slap will leave one or more irregular lines of petechiae, which represents the space between the fingers (Fig. 26-1). This can often be identified by placing the hand of the examiner over the area of petechiae and recognizing the anatomical matchup. A punch with a closed fist leaves a large bruise (Fig. 26-2).

A narrow instrument such as a belt, coat hanger, or electric wire will yield a double parallel line of petechiae or bruise marks (Fig. 26-3). When a coiled rope or wire

TABLE 26-1   Typology of Child Sexual Abuse and Incest

Not Involving Intercourse	*Involving Intercourse*
Indecent exposure	Anal or vaginal intercourse
"Carnal knowledge"	Sibling intercourse
Fondling of breast or genitalia	Statutory rape
Cunnilingus	Forcible rape
Fellatio	
Sodomy	
Pornography	

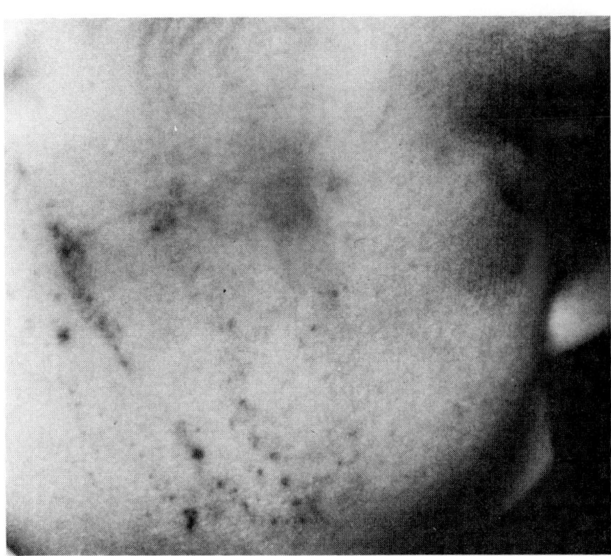

Figure 26–1 Hand Slap Markings on Face.

has been used, a characteristic loop-shaped bruise will reproduce the shape of the striking instrument (Fig. 26–4). A broad strap or belt will leave a solid bruise the shape of the striking instrument rather than the parallel line of bruises marking the edges, as seen with a narrow instrument. Marks such as these often present on multiple body surfaces or are so distributed over a single body surface that they could not have occurred accidentally.

When one finds multiple bruises on many body surfaces of a comatose child there is clear reason to suspect either intracranial injury in the form of subdural hematoma or intracerebral hemorrhage accompanying the skin injuries. When multiple bruises are present on the trunk of the young child, the abdomen must be carefully examined, since the young child does not protect the abdomen with muscle tightening and is at significant risk of sustaining intra-abdominal organ injury with little or no evidence of overlying skin injury. The abdominal findings may indicate free blood in the peritoneal cavity or a ruptured viscus.

Burns are among the most serious skin injuries found in situations of child abuse.[8,9] These burns may be hot water burns, hot grease burns, flame burns, or various forms of branding burns. Many of these burns will have

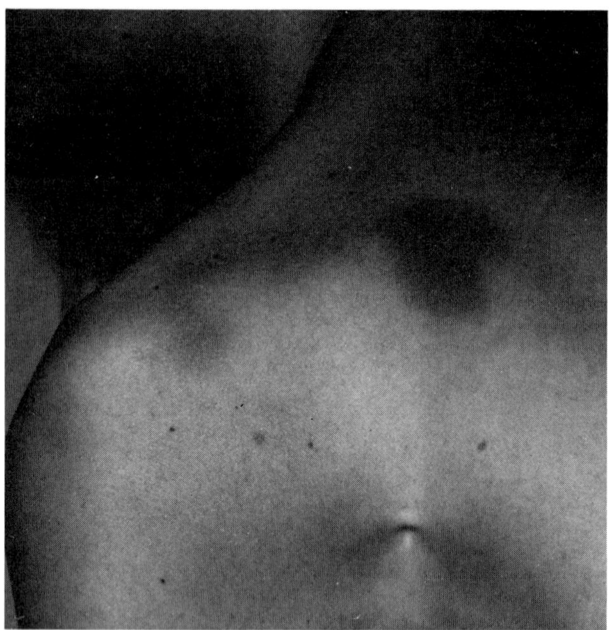

Figure 26–2 Punch Bruise on Shoulder from Blow with Fist.

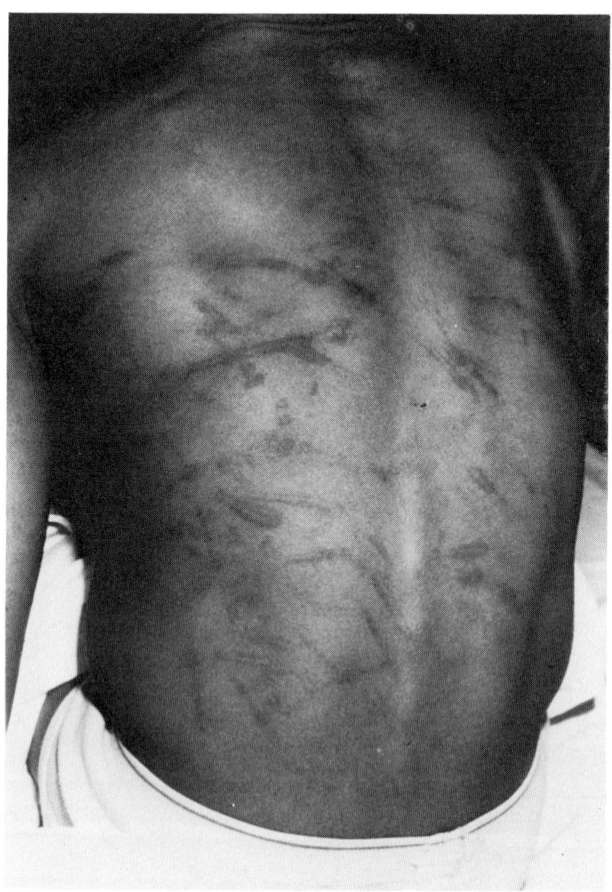

Figure 26–3 Multiple Bruises from Beating with a Narrow Belt.

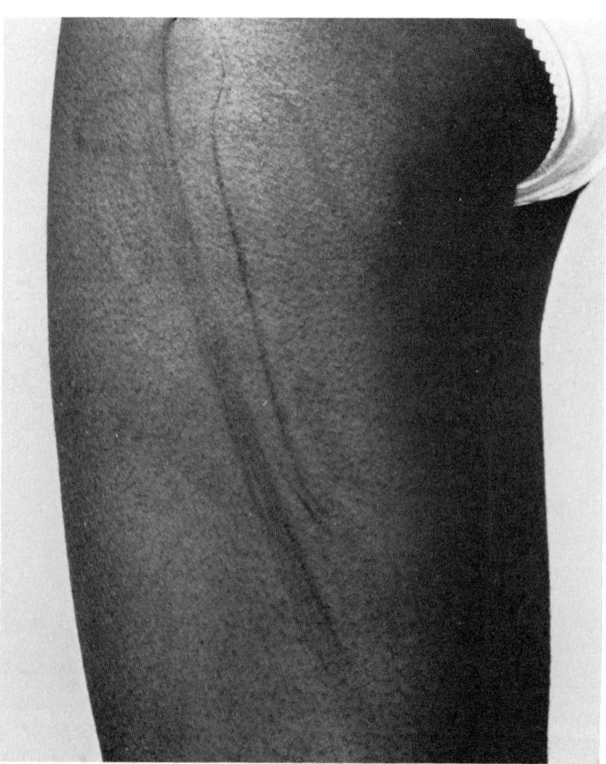

Figure 26–4 Bruise from Loop of 3-Wire Heavy-Duty Extension Cord.

been inflicted deliberately, such as the immersion scald burn that occurs as a misguided form of punishment (Fig. 26–5) or in an attempt to quiet a crying infant (Fig. 26–6). Immersion burns of this type are often seen on the genitalia, buttocks, or thighs of toddlers at the time of toilet training. Other burns, such as cigarette burns, may have been inflicted as a form of punishment or as a purely malicious act. A burn may also result from an accident in which a child has pulled over a hot coffee pot or frying pan. In such situations, the parent or caretaker may have used poor judgment in failing to protect the child from the hazard.

One or more fractures may be present in a child who has been a victim of child abuse.[10,11] These fractures may involve the skull, jaw, arms or legs, ribs, or spine. The presence of an extremity deformity or of a deep hematoma in the vicinity of a joint will provide a clue to skeletal injury. Certain fractures, such as the Salter type 2 or "bucket handle" fracture, which results from a twisting traction force applied to an extremity, are rarely seen in any situation other than child abuse (Fig. 26–7). Rib fractures are rarely seen in children except

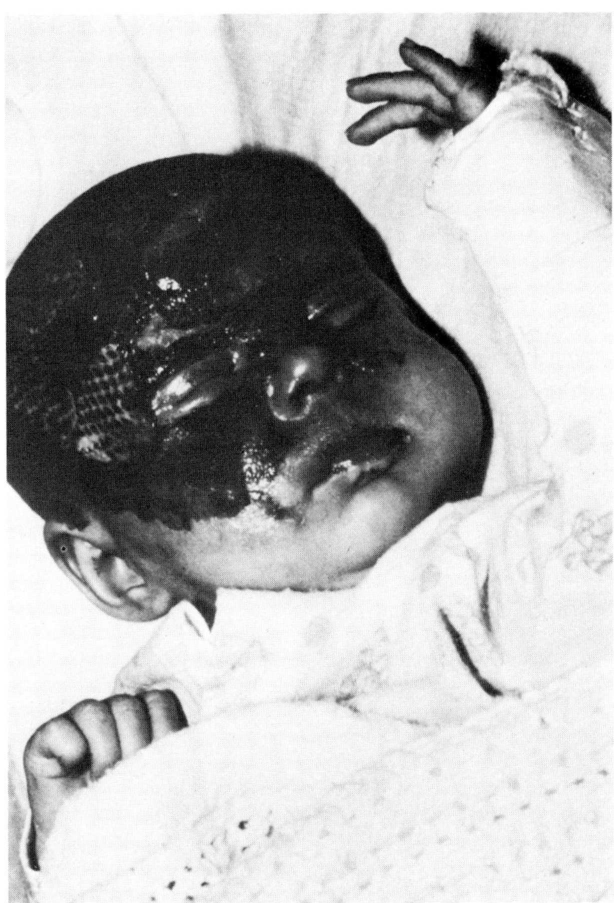

Figure 26–6   Immersion Burn of Face (After Grafting).

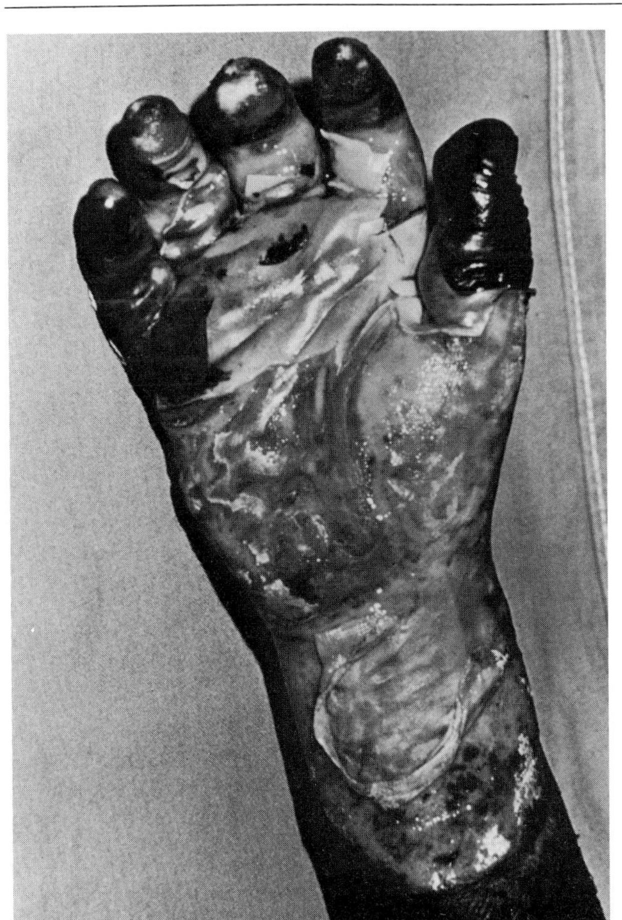

Figure 26–5   Immersion Burn of Hand Held in Boiling Water.

in severe accidental injury (e.g., vehicular accident) and are a strong indication of possible child abuse. It is not uncommon in obtaining radiographs of a site of suspected fracture to discover old healing (Fig. 26–8) or healed (Fig. 26–9) fractures or other fresh fractures that were not suspected. Such findings are a strong indication of child abuse.

Careful examination of eyes, ears, nose, and mouth are also indicated in cases of suspected abuse. Vigorous shaking of infants may produce subdural hematomas or retinal hemorrhage. Blows to the side of the head may lead to an acute traumatic rupture of the ear drum, and blows to the mouth may result in broken or dislodged teeth or other intraoral injuries.

Situations still occur in which a child arrives in an emergency department already dead as a consequence of inflicted injuries. In the absence of clear evidence that such a death occurred accidentally, or in a young infant as a result of the sudden infant death syndrome, child abuse must be suspected. A careful postmortem inspection and autopsy examination will usually substantiate or refute the suspicion of abuse.[12]

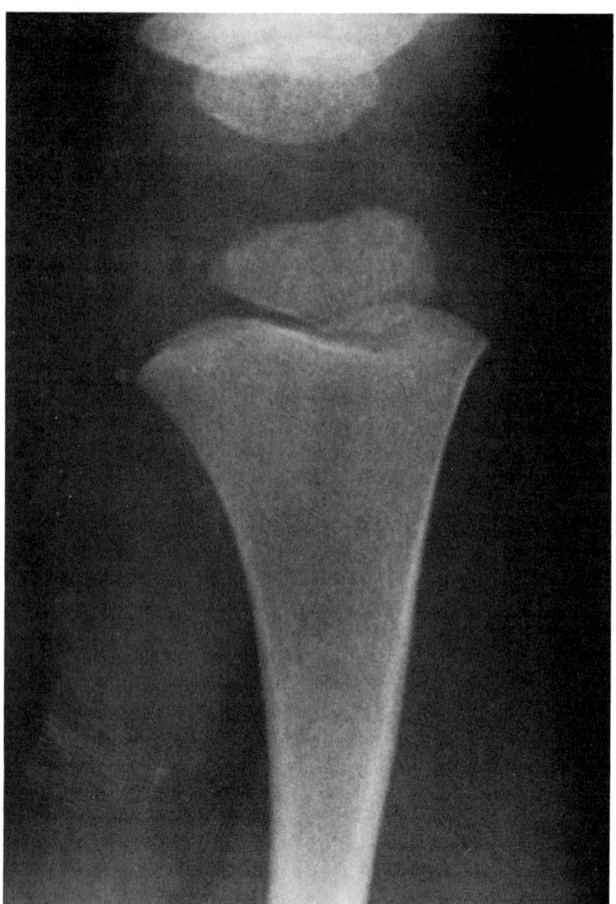

Figure 26–7   Bucket-Handle Fracture of Distal Femur.

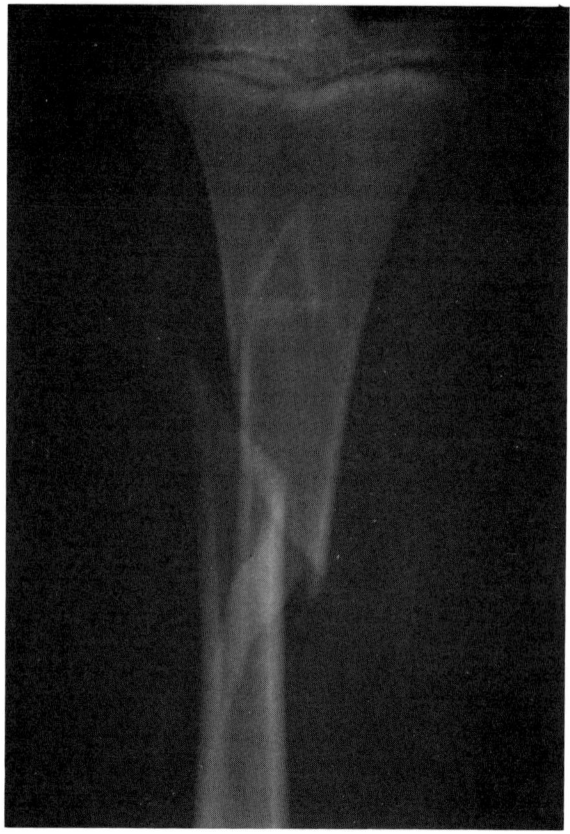

Figure 26–8   Metaphyseal Tear (New Fracture) and Subperiosteal New Bone Formation (Old Fracture) in Infant with Multiple Fractures and Skin Abrasions.

Mental Abuse

Mental abuse is far more difficult to recognize than physical abuse, and children are unlikely to come to the emergency department solely because of mental abuse. Nevertheless, if emergency care personnel observe patterns of parent-child interaction closely or inquire as to the usual mode in which the parent or parents relate to the child, a high index of suspicion may be generated. A parent who is being mentally or emotionally abusive to a child will typically make fun of the child, tease the child, belittle the child, or tend to ignore the child until the child misbehaves in some way and then the parent will lash out verbally at the child. Such parents also typically have derogatory nicknames for their child, such as "stinker" or "dummy." They may refer to their child as "bad" or "evil" or be able to describe only the negative characteristics of the child. Such a child is made to feel of little worth and typically behaves in such a way as to elicit further derogatory responses from the parent. Some of these children have poor self-images and are habitual misbehavers, since the only reaction they receive from a parent occurs when they misbehave. Others are exceptionally well behaved, apparently to avoid the wrath of a parent.

Many children who have been mentally abused are also victims of at least mild degrees of physical abuse. It is not uncommon for such children to be repeatedly hit or slapped, although perhaps never to the extent where a detectable injury is inflicted. The most serious consequences for the child occur when mental abuse is accompanied by some degree of physical abuse alternating with periods of emotional or physical neglect.

Neglect

The most common result of serious physical and emotional neglect is the condition referred to as *nonorganic failure to thrive*. Infants manifesting this condition typically show evidence of moderate to severe undernutrition characterized by failure to gain weight or loss of

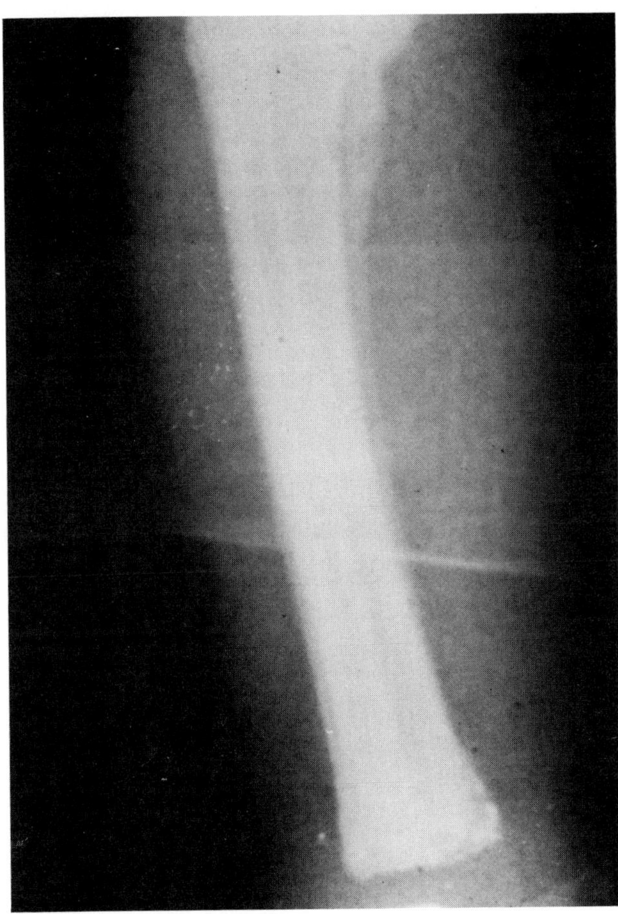

Figure 26–9   New Fracture and Fully-Healed Old Fracture in Same Bone in Child with Multiple Fractures.

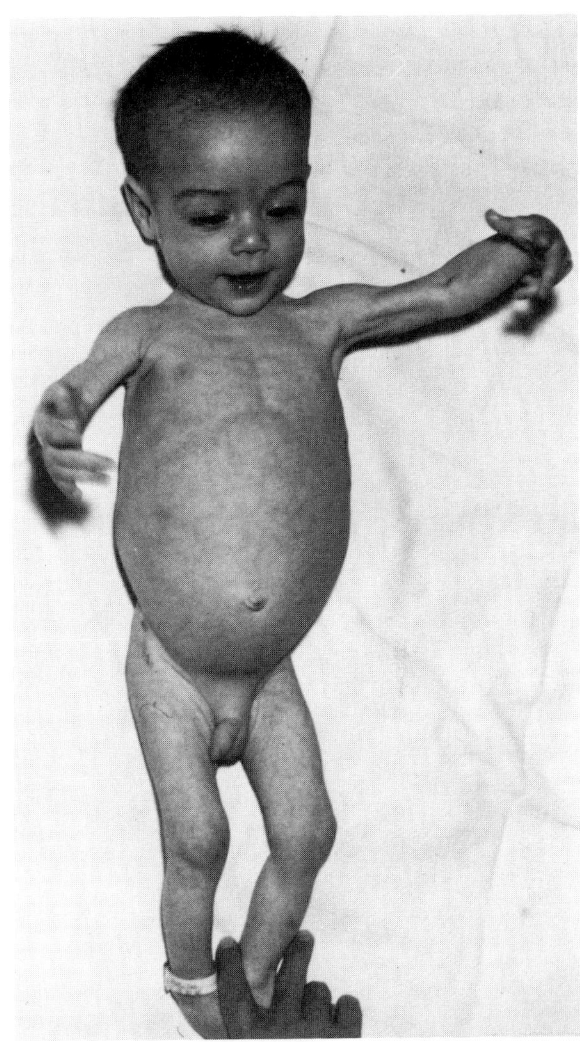

Figure 26–10   Infant with Nonorganic Failure to Thrive from Neglect and Undernutrition.

weight, failure to grow in length (in somewhat lesser degree), and, in severe cases, retardation of head circumference growth.[13] The infant who has failed to gain weight or who has lost weight will have little subcutaneous tissue; this will be most evident over the buttocks (Fig. 26–10). The infant with nonorganic failure to thrive resulting from frank neglect may have other evidence of physical neglect or injury (e.g., bruises, diaper rash). The infant with physical neglect in association with emotional neglect or other forms of emotional maltreatment may also manifest signs of withdrawal or avoidance behavior, depression, rumination, or bizarre behavior. A combination of these signs is sometimes referred to as *psychosocial dwarfism*.

Evidence of physical neglect in the older child is more difficult to evaluate, since with the slower rate of growth beyond infancy the consequences of inadequate nutrition are less evident. Also, as the child becomes a toddler, he or she is more self-reliant and can obtain food when it is available. In the older child, physical neglect is most evident in the dirty, poorly clothed child, particularly the underweight and anemic-looking child.[14]

One of the most serious consequences of neglect in the older child is the occurrence of serious accidental injuries. There is an overlap in the types of injuries seen in physical abuse and preventable accidental injuries. A review of 30 children hospitalized for intracranial bleeding demonstrated that approximately 60 percent of the children sustained injuries that were either definitely or apparently abusive or were a result of preventable accidents (Table 26–2). The children with preventable accidental injuries were much older than the abused children, but came from families sharing many of the social characteristics of the abused children. They sustained their injuries in circumstances of apparently inadequate supervision.[15] In another study involving 105 children, 35 percent of the serious fractures and 91 percent of the serious burns requiring hospitalization occurred in situations that could have been prevented through better parental supervision.[16] Once again, these children were older and had an increased number of abuse-related social and familial characteristics (Table 26–3).[16] Thus, when an older child has sustained a serious injury, attention should be directed to the circumstances in which the injury occurred and the degree of supervision that was provided to the child at the time of the injury.

Sexual Abuse

In most situations of sexual abuse, there will be very few physical findings (see Chapter 27). Many of the episodes of sexual abuse involve exposure, fondling, and the carrying out of acts by the child on the adult or other acts that will not produce physical findings in the child.[17] Even in the situation in which there have been alleged attempts at sexual intercourse, unless penetration of the preadolescent girl has been violent, there is usually no evidence of external injury. Since many acts of sexual abuse are discovered long after the act occurs, one cannot rely on physical findings as one might in a case of rape (see Chapter 65).

TABLE 26–2   Characteristics of 30 Children Hospitalized with Subdural Hematomas

Etiology	No. Patients (%)	Age at Hospitalization Mean (±1 SD)	Number of Abuse-Related Characteristics Mean (±1 SD)
Inflicted or preventable	18 (60)		
Nonaccidental injury (child abuse)	7 (23)	4.3 ± 1.9 mo.	8.7 ± 7.8
Probable nonaccidental injury (suspicious for abuse)	5 (17)	5.8 ± 3.6 mo.	3.4 ± 3.5
Preventable accidental injury (neglect)	6 (20)	50.5 ± 20.6 mo.	2.3 ± 2.1
Noninflicted or nonpreventable	12 (40)		
Nonpreventable accidental injury	4 (13)	63.0 ± 26.6 mo.	0.8 ± 0.6
Birth injury	8 (27)	22.4 ± 42.8 mo.	0.4 ± 0.6

Source: Data from Wenger A: Subdural hematomas in children: What proportion are caused by non-accidental injury? Project report, Pennsylvania State University College of Medicine, 1977.

TABLE 26–3   Characteristics of 105 Children Hospitalized with Major Fractures or Serious Burns

Etiology	No. Patients (%)	Age at Hospitalization Mean (±1 SD)	Number of Abuse-Related Characteristics Mean (±1 SD)
Fractures			
Nonaccidental injury (child abuse)	3 (4)	8.7 ± 4.9 mo.	6.3 ± 3.8
Preventable accidental injury (neglect)	14 (20)	31.5 ± 25.8 mo.	1.3 ± 1.7
Potentially preventable accidental injury (possible neglect)	11 (15)	85.6 ± 23.3 mo.	1.3 ± 1.7
Nonpreventable accidental injury	44 (61)	64.5 ± 28.2 mo.	0.3 ± 0.5
Total*	72 (100)		
Burns			
Nonaccidental injury (child abuse)	1 (3)	3.0 mo.	8.0
Preventable accidental injury (neglect)	26 (74)	38.0 ± 36.1 mo.	1.4 ± 2.0
Potentially preventable accidental injury (possible neglect)	6 (17)	34.8 ± 28.7 mo.	0.7 ± 1.2
Nonpreventable accidental injury	2 (6)	11.0 ± 1.6 mo.	0.0
Total*	35 (100)		

* Two children sustained both major fractures and serious burns.
Source: Data from Janesky C, Bartlett GS: Serious preventable injuries as a manifestation of child neglect. Paper presented at the Ambulatory Pediatric Association annual meeting, Atlanta, April 30, 1979.

When sexual abuse is suspected, the information can be elicited by a careful and sympathetic interview with the child and the parents.[3] In certain circumstances, a history may also be appropriately taken from another family member, such as an older brother or sister. Sexually abused children may be very frightened at the time they are interviewed and may exhibit either withdrawn or overly aggressive behavior. They may initially be reluctant to describe the events that have occurred. On the other hand, children who can describe and even demonstrate the types of sexual acts that they claim have been perpetrated on them can generally be assumed to be reporting these events accurately, since preadolescent children do not have the level of cognitive development or prior experiences to fabricate such stories. It is common for the child to be willing to describe the events only once and then refuse further discussion. Thus, it is important that a sensitive and skilled interviewer should conduct the initial interview.

General Findings

Numerous findings may be present in children who have sustained any form of child abuse.[1,18] There is often poor behavioral adjustment, evidenced by aggressive behavior or markedly withdrawn or inappropriately good behavior.[19] Poor school performance and truancy are quite common in children who are physically or emotionally abused at home. Adolescents may have a record of delinquency or running away. A runaway teenage girl has often experienced sexual or physical abuse at home. Adolescents who have attempted suicide should also be interviewed very carefully about the possibility of a predisposing episode of physical or sexual abuse.

Mental retardation and neurologic sequelae such as hemiplegia and seizure disorders may be a late outcome of physical abuse. The history must be obtained carefully, since children who are retarded or who have neurologic disorders are at increased risk of being physically abused.

Many of the behavioral consequences of physical or emotional abuse or sexual abuse may remain long after the child has been removed from the home or environment. Typically, these children and their families require long-term psychiatric counseling to attenuate the effects of the early abuse or neglect.

DIAGNOSIS

The diagnosis of apparent child abuse, like any other medical diagnosis, is based on obtaining an appropriate history, performing a physical examination, and obtaining supportive laboratory and radiographic studies. When abuse is suspected, it is particularly important that the personnel obtaining the history be as nonthreatening, nonjudgmental, and nonpunitive as possible. Many parents who have injured their children come to the emergency department in a state of extreme remorse. If emergency department personnel are supportive, the parents can be made sufficiently comfortable to describe the events as they occurred. On the other hand,

when the medical personnel are threatening and judgmental or take a punitive approach, the parent may refuse to talk and may attempt to remove the child from the emergency department.

In obtaining the history, a careful exploration of the circumstances surrounding the injury should be made. This is true of the apparent accidental injury as well as the apparent abusive injury. The parent should be allowed to reveal the history as he or she wishes to present it. A thorough physical examination must be carried out, with examination of all body surfaces. All physical findings should be described in detail and, when appropriate, diagrams or sketches should be drawn. An effort should be made to relate the physical findings to the history as obtained.

In cases of abuse there will often be inconsistencies in the histories given by the same person to different medical personnel, or histories given by different parties that are inconsistent with each other, a history that does not explain the physical findings, or a history that is clearly not credible (e.g., an infant too young to roll over who is said to have fallen out of a crib). An injury may be attributed to a third person, such as an older sibling or a baby sitter, or the parent may disclaim any knowledge of how a serious injury may have occurred. Occasionally a parent will describe the circumstances in which an injury was inflicted, either by the parent or by another person.

Further evaluation of the child should include all appropriate diagnostic studies that are required to investigate the evident injuries. When bruising is present or a parent reports that the child "bruises easily," a complete blood cell count and a clotting screen should be obtained. Radiographs of all apparent fracture sites are also necessary. When the child is 5 years of age or younger, a complete skeletal radiographic survey should be ordered, including at least a lateral skull radiograph, upper and lower extremity radiographs in their entirety, and rib radiographs. These radiographs should be studied for indications of recent fractures, for fractures of different ages, and for the presence of old healing fractures, as well as for any fractures that may be suspected on the basis of physical findings. Attention should be given to all aspects of these radiographs, because on abdominal radiographs one may occasionally find chips of paint, indicating ingestion of lead-containing paint (pica), or other foreign bodies in the stomach, intestine, urethra, vagina, or bladder.

In cases where there are visible physical findings, such as bruises, abrasions, or distorted limbs, or the child is comatose, photographs should be obtained as soon as possible without delaying necessary medical procedures. These photographs may be taken by a physician, a nurse, a hospital photographer, a representative of the appropriate social agency, or by the police, as permitted or required by the relevant state law. Procedures for obtaining such photographs as admissible evidence in court have been outlined.[20] (See Chapter 65.)

The behavior of the parents or responsible caretakers should also be observed very carefully, with particular attention to the way in which the adults relate to the child. These interaction patterns have been described in the section on mental abuse.

DIFFERENTIAL DIAGNOSIS

The differential diagnosis of physical abuse includes specific medical conditions that may produce similar skeletal or skin findings.[12] Other skeletal conditions that must be considered and that can be evaluated on the radiographs include metabolic bone disorders, bone tumors (including leukemia), and bone infections (osteomyelitis).[10,11] The child with multiple bruises may be suffering from bleeding disorders such as hemophilia in its several forms, Henoch-Schönlein vasculitis, thrombocytopenic purpura, and the acute onset of leukemia. Studying the child's prior health status, family history, and other results of the physical examination should clarify these possibilities.

If the child is unconscious and has petechiae or ecchymoses on multiple body surfaces, a temperature should be obtained and the optic fundi carefully examined. In fulminating infections such as septicemia and meningitis, particularly those due to *Neisseria meningitidis*, the child will either be febrile or will have a markedly depressed body temperature. Retinal hemorrhage frequently accompanies intracranial hemorrhage resulting from trauma to the head or vigorous shaking[21] and may be the only visible indicator of injury in unexplained coma.

In the child with multiple severe injuries, the history should be sufficient to differentiate the child who has been involved in a serious traumatic episode such as a vehicular accident.[15] In the case of burns, the differential diagnosis is between accidental and inflicted burns.[16] The child between the ages of 2 months and 2 years who is dead on arrival in the emergency department should be considered a possible victim of sudden infant death syndrome if there is no evidence of external physical injury or of overwhelming infection. Accidental strangulation or asphyxiation, such as may occur in highchair and crib accidents,[22] usually produces some external physical evidence to corroborate the history given by the parents.

The child presenting with evidence of serious failure to thrive should be hospitalized and carefully examined for organic causes for this condition, particularly if the child is a very young infant. The presence of characteristic behavior patterns will help to distinguish the nonorganic from the organic failure-to-thrive child[13] and the physically neglected child from the emotionally neglected and maltreated child. A detailed exploration of the family's social and economic situation is appropriate in the situation of failure to thrive.

The child presenting with a serious behavioral disturbance should have the primary behavioral disorders, including hyperactivity and acute psychological or psychiatric disturbances, considered in the differential diagnosis.

MANAGEMENT

Prehospital

Multiple injuries that may have resulted from child abuse require the same pattern of care as corresponding injuries from any other cause. The most important aspect of dealing with the child who may have sustained abusive injuries is that the child must be protected from further injury. If necessary, some person other than the parent should bring or accompany the child to the hospital.

Emergency Department

In the emergency department, the first concern is to provide appropriate medical care for any injury or illness that may be present. In the unconscious or severely injured child, this may need to take place prior to obtaining a detailed history of the apparent cause of the illness or injury.

If, after the history has been obtained and diagnostic studies have been ordered and reviewed, there is reason to suspect that child abuse may have occurred, the following additional procedures should be carried out. The parents should be informed that on the basis of the history and physical findings there is reason to suspect that an abusive injury may have occurred, that the physical findings in the child cannot be explained by the history as given, or that an episode of sexual abuse may have occurred. The emergency department personnel should further state that *as required by law* they must report these suspicions to the appropriate agency, but that this reporting in no way establishes that physical abuse, neglect, or sexual abuse has occurred. The parents should be allowed to react to these statements and have the option of rebuttal. The professional should not be talked out of the suspicion of abuse, neglect, or sexual abuse by any disclaimer of the parents. It is *not* the physician's responsibility to prove the existence of abuse; that is the responsibility of the appropriate social agency and the courts.

Immediate contact should be made by telephone with the local social agency responsible for handling cases of suspected abuse. Typically this will be a child welfare agency, child protective service, or children and youth agency, although in some states the report must be made to the police department or juvenile authorities. All states now have a central child abuse registry that must also be notified of suspected abuse. Specific arrangements should be made for the representative of the responsible agency to meet with the family *before* the family leaves the hospital.

The options available on completion of the assessment are listed below:

- admission to hospital
- admission to child care shelter
- referral to women-in-crisis shelter
- agency custody in foster care
- agency custody in home
- return to home with supervision
- return to home without supervision.

When it is not possible to ensure the safety of the child outside the hospital,[18] the child should be admitted, regardless of the nature or severity of the injuries. *No child should leave the hospital who does not have a safe place to go.*

When in doubt, admit the child. If necessary, emergency custody of the child may be obtained by contacting the local juvenile court judge with jurisdiction over the area of residence of the child to allow a protective admission. In general, utilization review criteria for cases of suspected child abuse allow a hospitalization for the duration of an emergency court order without further admission or length of stay justification, regardless of the nature of the injury.

Continued Ambulatory Care

Medical care and social service follow-up should be arranged prior to discharge from the emergency department. If the child is admitted to the hospital, the follow-up care should be arranged prior to discharge from the hospital, in conjunction with other aspects of social service follow-up as part of a comprehensive management plan. Follow-up medical care should include management of all identified medical, surgical, or psychiatric problems and, when possible, should involve a long-term follow-up health care resource. Continued social service or protective service follow-up will be required to help the family deal with the behaviors or social conditions that led to the abuse or neglect.

REFERENCES

1. Helfer RE., Kempe CH: The child's need for early recognition, immediate care and protection, in Kempe CH, Helfer RE (eds): *Helping the Battered Child and His Family*. Philadelphia, JB Lippincott, 1972, chap 5.
2. Summit R, Kryso J: Sexual abuse of children: A clinical spectrum. *Am J Orthopsychiatry* 48:237–251, 1978.
3. Burgess AW, Groth AN, Holmstrom LL, Sgroi SM: *Sexual Assault of Children and Adolescents*. Lexington, Mass, Lexington Books, 1978.
4. Holter JC, Friedman SB: Child abuse: Early case findings in the emergency department. *Pediatrics* 42:128–138, 1968.
5. Sussman SJ: Skin manifestations of the battered child syndrome. *J Pediatr* 72:99–101, 1968.
6. Kempe CH: Uncommon manifestations of the battered child syndrome. *Am J Dis Child* 129:1265, 1975.
7. Pascoe JM, Hildebrandt HM, Tarrier A, Murphy M: Patterns of skin injury in nonaccidental and accidental injury. *Pediatrics* 64:245–247, 1979.
8. Lung RJ, Miller SH, Davis TS, Graham WP III: Recognizing burn injuries as child abuse. *Am Fam Physician* 15:134–135, 1977.
9. Hight D, Bakalar HR, Lloyd JR: Inflicted burns in children. *JAMA* 242:517–520, 1979.
10. Silverman FN: Radiologic aspects of the battered child's syndrome, in Helfer RE, Kempe CH (eds): *The Battered Child*, ed 2. Chicago, University of Chicago Press, 1974.
11. Cameron IM, Roe LJ: *Atlas of the Battered Child Syndrome*. Edinburgh, Churchill Livingstone, 1975.
12. Weston JT: The pathology of child abuse, in Helfer RE, Kempe CH (eds): *The Battered Child*, ed 2. Chicago, University of Chicago Press, 1974.
13. Barbero GJ, Shakeen E: Environmental failure to thrive: A clinical view. *J Pediatr* 71:639–644, 1967.
14. Young LR: *Wednesday's Children*. New York, McGraw Hill, 1964.
15. Wenger A: Subdural hematomas in children: What proportion are caused by non-accidental injury? Unpublished project report, Pennsylvania State University College of Medicine, 1977.
16. Janesky C, Bartlett GS: Serious preventable injuries as a manifestation of child neglect. Paper presented at the Ambulatory Pediatric Association annual meeting, Atlanta, April 30, 1979.
17. National Center on Child Abuse and Neglect: *Child Sexual Abuse: Incest, Assault, and Sexual Exploitation*, publication No. (OHDS) 79–30166. Department of Health, Education and Welfare, 1978.
18. Friedman SB: The need for intensive follow-up of abused children, in Kempe CH, Helfer RE (eds): *Helping the Battered Child and His Family*. Philadelphia, JB Lippincott, 1972, chap 6.
19. Martin H: The child and his development, in Kempe CH, Helfer RE (eds): *Helping the Battered Child and His Family*. Philadelphia, JB Lippincott, 1972, chap 7.
20. Ford RJ, Smistek BS, Glass JT: Photography of suspected child abuse and maltreatment. *Biomed Communications* 3(4):12–17, 1975.
21. Caffey J: The whiplash shaken infant syndrome: Manual shaking by the extremities with whiplash-induced intracranial and intraocular bleedings, linked with residual permanent brain damage and mental retardation. *Pediatrics* 54:396–403, 1974.
22. Smialek JE, Smialek PZ, Spitz WU: Accidental bed deaths in infants due to unsafe sleeping situations. *Clin Pediatr* 16:1031–1036, 1977.

27. Sexual Abuse

DORRIS E. TINKER, Ph.D.

Sexual abuse of children is a component of child abuse. It is an involvement of children, without their consent, in fondling, vaginal or oral intercourse, fellatio, cunnilingus, and other adult sexual practices. Sexual abuse also includes using children for pornography, insisting that they view sexual intercourse repeatedly, and exposing them to sexual stimulation that is inconsistent with their chronological age and stage of development. The abuse is incestuous if the child is forced to participate in such activities by a family member (e.g., father, mother, stepfather, sister, brother, uncle, cousin, or grandfather). Incest is an indication of extreme family pathology.

ETIOLOGY

Like child abuse, sexual abuse knows no racial, ethnic, cultural, educational, or socioeconomic boundaries. Current thinking and research indicates that, for every reported case of sexual abuse, three cases go unreported.[1] In 1968, it was reported that 14 percent of child abuse cases were in reality cases of sexual abuse.[2] Many of the cases of sexual abuse that are seen in an emergency department are unrecognized, however. Improved diagnosis by physicians, more alertness in members of the community, and prompt attention from parents and family have resulted in the increased reporting of sexual abuse.

The physician, alone or as a member of a health care team, may be the first person to respond to a child who has been sexually abused. In a busy emergency department, the physician may choose *not* to pursue a thorough investigation because of time constraints, a lack of cooperation from parent or family, or personal discomfort with the situation. Ideally, one person should be designated to help sort out and identify the psychological and family problems that may result from and contribute to sexual abuse, as well as to help the child deal with the medical and judicial systems. If suspected cases of child sexual abuse are consistently referred to the same person, that individual develops an expertise in dealing with this problem. This designated person could be a representative of the local rape crisis center or county child protection agency.

Emergency department personnel must have a high index of suspicion about the child who frequents the emergency department with many vague, psychosomatic symptoms (e.g., headache, abdominal pain). This child may be trying to say that something is drastically wrong. The differential diagnosis should include sexual abuse.

In all emergency departments, it is common for a parent to bring in an adolescent girl and demand to have her "checked." The girl may have run away from home or stayed out all night, and the parent wants to know whether she has been sexually active. The presence or absence of a hymen and its relationship to virginity should be explained, and a referral to a mental health professional is indicated.

"Acute" Rape

The rape of a child is termed acute when the child is sexually attacked "out of the blue." The child may have been accosted on the way to school, followed home by an intruder who entered the house, attacked while baby-sitting for a neighbor, or raped under other, equally unpredictable circumstances.

Incest

Complaints of girls and boys involved in an incestuous relationship are increasing. It has been recognized that, in an isolated population of English origin, the medieval concept of *le droit de seigneur* (the right of the lord of the manor to have the first sexual contact with the vassal bride on her wedding night) has been distorted through the years and has become the right of fathers to have sexual contact with their daughters. The oldest girl in the family is the most vulnerable, but each succeeding female child becomes a potential target for the father's sexual abuse.

Characteristics of the incestuous family as described by the American Humane Association, Children's Division, include:[1]

- a home-centered family with limited outside contacts
- rigid, restrictive control by the father of the children's activities, particularly those of the daughters
- a history of alcoholism and physically abusive behavior on the part of the father
- the absence of extramarital relationships
- an early marriage of long duration and the absence of acting-out behavior by the children
- the "too good" children

These families guard against exposure. Often, the mother has been aware of the situation but has not responded to the daughter's plea for help, generally blaming the child for what has occurred. These adolescent girls report a history of sexual abuse by the father over a period of time and also indicate that their sisters have been sexually abused. Many girls impart this information for the first time in the emergency department.

In cases of incest, mothers frequently refuse to prosecute their husbands or partners because they fear loss of income, loss of companionship or lover, or severe physical retaliation to themselves or their other children, or because they need to preserve the integrity of the family. A safe place *must* be provided for the incest patient, even if it means admission to the hospital. Often,

a relative or neighbor can help for a short period of time.

Consenting Intercourse

The sequel of normal teen-age sexual experimentation may be acute rape or the cry of "rape." Girls who feel the need to confide in their parents about previous sexual activity sometimes accuse their sexual partner of rape in the hope that the onus may be removed from them and directed toward their partners. Professionals need to take a careful history from the girl, by herself, in order to sort out the data. The conflict between the patient's need for confidentiality and the parent's desire to know the facts creates a dilemma that must be handled with tact and understanding. The positive handling of this situation by an objective professional should facilitate communication between the child and parent.

Abuse by Friends and Neighbors

Children who have been sexually abused by a relative, friend of the family, or baby sitter tend to become confused, as do the parents. Parents have difficulty believing that a friend or neighbor could sexually abuse their child. These children feel guilty and often turn their feelings inward, thus laying the groundwork for future emotional problems. If managed appropriately, a one-time incident may leave few emotional scars. However, parents should be told to talk about the incident and to absolve the child from blame.

PARENTAL ATTITUDE

Parents reflect their feelings about their sexually abused children in their choice of words to describe these children (e.g., "dirty," "ruined," "damaged for life"). Parents need help in sorting out their feelings and reestablishing a nurturing relationship with their child. Because they feel guilty and fearful, they may become overprotective and restrictive. This overreaction is understandable, but it must be explored and dealt with over a period of time. If the sexual abuse occurs when the child is already feeling isolated, deprived, and helpless, the child may attach a particular significance to the event and, although feeling guilty and anxious, may seek further sexual attention and affection.

SPECIAL CONSIDERATIONS OF MENTALLY RETARDED CHILDREN

Of particular concern are those children who are mentally retarded. Parents often deny that their retarded child is physiologically mature enough to have the same sexual desires that the normal child experiences as part of the developmental process. They may not provide the education or protection that is necessarily a parental obligation. Some parents do not give their children, retarded or not, adequate explanations of developmental landmarks. For example, when menarche occurs, many parents say only, "You are now a woman . . . don't mess around . . . don't let boys touch you." Such ambiguous phrases are frightening, titillating, and vague, particularly for those children who are less intellectually capable.

GUIDELINES FOR EMERGENCY DEPARTMENT MANAGEMENT

Adult professionals must be prepared to cope with their feelings of disgust, disbelief, and anger when confronted with cases of sexual abuse or exploitation. Professional training includes techniques to deal effectively with crisis situations, and new techniques are taught as a part of continuing education. The emergency department staff must remember that each person has had different experiences, including sexual experiences. With this approach, it is hoped that a professional empathy and calmness can be maintained, and the crisis that often arises with a case of sexual abuse can be defused.

Privacy is essential, even in a busy, overwhelmed emergency department. In a case where the child has been attacked by a male, the presence of a female professional is strongly recommended, whether the patient is male or female, since the male professional may be perceived by the child as a second assailant. Whatever history may be considered necessary for legal protection of the child should be included in the emergency department chart notes, preferably in the patient's own words. It is helpful to the child and the family if feelings are put into descriptive words, such as "scary," "strange," or "worried."

Each medical procedure must be explained carefully before it is begun. It is very important to make the patient and the family feel that the staff are their advocates. An obstetrician/gynecologist is often called to perform the pelvic examination, and this physician serves as an "expert" in any subsequent hearing. The sustained cooperation among several clinical departments (i.e., pediatrics, child mental health, obstetrics/gynecology) not only aids the patient and family but also establishes an excellent model for students of all disciplines.

Assessment

Interview

Interviewing children who are victims of alleged sexual abuse is difficult for the professional, the child, and the family. Different children have different responses to crisis situations. Even though a child is not screaming or crying, a sexual assault may have occurred. The interviewer should be experienced in interviewing children and assessing their responses, because many children will tell their story only once. Again, the attitude of the professional is of the utmost importance.

The police should be permitted to interview the child only if a staff member is present, because a child may be very intimidated by the police. Since the child should not be prompted by the parent, a staff member should be present in order to make the child feel as comfortable as possible and to protect the child's rights.

Physical Examination

In dealing with children, a calm, empathic approach is essential. A complete medical history should be elicited, as always. Then, a complete physical examination can be conducted in the manner to which the child is accustomed, i.e., the examination should begin with the eyes, ears, and throat, and proceed caudad.

Genital examination should be initiated with an inspection of the perineum. Trauma should be recorded with appropriate diagrams. The condition of the hymenal ring and the diameter of the hymenal opening should be observed and recorded. If a pelvic examination is to be performed, consideration should be given to admitting a child under seven years of age to the hospital and performing the examination with the child under anesthesia. Professionals trained in the use of clinical hypnosis are often helpful when a pelvic examination must be performed on the older child or adolescent.

The child should be examined for bruises, burns, rope marks, wounds, erythema, edema, or dilation of the rectal sphincter. These should be noted in the chart. Clothing and undergarments should be retained. As previously noted, the medical history should be recorded in the child's own words. Diagnosis should be *suspected* sexual abuse.

If the physician suspects that sexual abuse has occurred, the following medical tests should be performed:

- cultures of pharynx, urethra (male), urethra and vagina (preadolescent female), endocervix (adolescent female), and rectum for gonorrhea.
- serologic test for syphilis.
- stool guaiac or anoscopy, if indicated.
- Woods' light screening of perineum for fluorescence. Record as + or − . If areas of skin fluoresce, swab with moistened saline and place in appropriate tube for acid phosphatase determination.

- wet mount. Record as + or − for sperm and whether motile or nonmotile.
- pregnancy test for postmenarche females.
- photographs, if indicated.

Treatment

The following medical treatment is recommended:

- tetanus prophylaxis for injuries. The guidelines of the Center for Disease Control and Public Health Service should be used.
- prophylaxis against venereal disease, if indicated: probenecid, 1 gm orally, plus ampicillin, 3.5 gm orally; or probenecid, 1 gm orally, followed in 20 minutes with procaine penicillin G, 4.8 million units intramuscularly. If the patient is penicillin-allergic, spectinomycin, 4 gm intramuscularly, or tetracycline, 500 mg four times a day for 4 days, may be substituted.

Many physicians use prophylactic treatment for all children who are victims of sexual abuse. I favor oral medication, since an intramuscular injection is painful and children may interpret an injection as punishment. Probenecid, 1 gm orally, followed in 20 minutes by amoxicillin, 50 mg/kg orally is recommended.[3]

The goals of the crisis management are the following:

- Give whatever medical care is necessary according to an established protocol.

- Establish a relationship with both the patient and the family.

- Explain to the child and the family that the child is neither "bad" nor to blame for the incident.

- Attempt to deal with the parent's anger and often expressed wish to punish the assailant and to help the family understand that it is the responsibility of the judicial system, not the physician or the family, to judge and punish.

- Encourage and facilitate verbal communication between the child and the family. If parents do not discuss the incident with their children, the children often feel that they have been involved in, and responsible for, something so terrible that their own parents cannot talk about it and do not initiate discussion with parents.

- Have the child and the family return within 24 to 48 hours for psychological follow-up. Unless the patient and the family are seen often within the first few weeks after the incident, the problems

cannot be assessed and managed. Follow-up medical care should include reculture for gonorrhea in five to seven days, repeat serologic test in six to eight weeks, and reevaluation of any medical problems that were found on initial evaluation. Psychological follow-up can often be accomplished by group therapy with skilled leaders. With this technique, more children and families can be helped in a given time period, and the patients can provide emotional support for each other.

Children appear to go through several stages after a sexual assault or when an incestuous relationship is uncovered:

- *Stage I:* an initial reaction of withdrawal, tremulousness, and crying or a pseudocalm with over-verbalization

- *Stage II:* anxiety and somatic complaints with excessive clinging to one parent (usually the mother), nightmares, enuresis, alterations in appetite, extreme fearfulness, hyperactivity, stomachache, headache, increased perineal sensation, academic problems, and, possibly, venereal disease and pregnancy

- *Stage III:* denial and suppression of the incident with a reluctance to discuss feelings with anyone

- *Stage IV:* placement of the incident in its proper perspective after appropriate therapy and indications that age-appropriate activity and development have been reestablished

Recently, I studied 95 cases of sexual abuse that were reported to the emergency department or pediatric clinic of the county hospital in a large metropolitan area over a 14-month period. The patients (families) reporting sexual abuse are grouped by age and sex in Table 27–1. The ratio of male to female is 1:8, with the highest incidence of abuse reported in the age group 14 to 17 years. Boys below the age of 4 years appear to be at less risk than girls, and the risk increases for both sexes

TABLE 27–1   Age and Sex of Victim

Age	Male	Female	Total	Percent
2–3		5	5	5.3
4–5	2	13	15	15.8
6–9	8	13	21	22.1
10–13		21	21	22.1
14–17	1	32	33	34.7
Total	11	84	95	100

as the age increases. Since no boys in the age groups 2 to 3 years and 10 to 13 years reported sexual abuse, it is hypothesized that either they cannot or do not tell their parent(s) about a sexual attack or the parent(s) are not as concerned about their sons' early sexual activity and do not report such attacks to the police or health care system. (Male homosexuality, involving young boys, is being increasingly reported, however.)

The study suggested that more children (Table 27–2) were seen in the emergency department during the hours of 5 P.M. to 8 A.M. than during daytime hours of 8 A.M. to 5 P.M. The investigation indicated that this more frequent use of the emergency department was not always because the incidents occurred during the evening and night but because the parents learned of the incident during the evening, the parents considered the incident an "emergency," or transportation to the hospital was available only after 5 P.M.

The fact that few patients were admitted is consistent with the philosophy of not separating families (particularly mothers and young children) in a crisis unless there is a medical need for hospitalization or there is no other safe place for a child or family.

In Table 27–3 it is indicated that 44 percent of the children in the study were from two-parent families, and 51 percent of the children were from a single-parent family with the mother as head of household.

As seen in Table 27–4, child sexual abuse generally involves a person who is known to the child. In only 20.1 percent of these cases was a stranger involved.

TABLE 27–2   Number of Patients Admitted in Emergency Department and Outpatient Clinic

	Seen (%)	Admitted (%)	Total (%)
Emergency department	55 (57.9)	3 (3.2)	58 (61.1)
Outpatient clinic	35 (36.8)	2 (2.1)	37 (38.9)
Total	90 (94.7)	5 (5.3)	95 (100)

TABLE 27–3   Composition of Family

	No. Patients	Percent
Two-parent family	42	44.2
Mother only	48	50.5
Father only	2	2.1
Other (relative, foster parents)	3	3.2

TABLE 27–4   Relationship of Assailant to Victim

	No. Patients	Percent
Family member	47	49.4
Acquaintance	29	30.5
Stranger (same sex)	4	4.2
Stranger (opposite sex)	15	15.9

RECOMMENDATIONS

All personnel must maintain an accepting and matter-of-fact attitude. Established medical and mental health protocols should be followed. The emergency department staff of each hospital are unique in their experiences and training. Each unit must assess its own strengths and form a team that can deal consistently and efficiently with problems of sexual abuse. It would be helpful to have, as a member of the team, a representative of the community agency legally responsible for emergency custody, child care, and child placement to help during possible court proceedings. The hospital attorney is often a useful member of the team.

Periodic review of cases and protocols not only keeps professionals up to date on the medical regimen but also provides follow-up on the outcome of cases.

REFERENCES

1. Brandt RS, Tisza V: The sexually misused child. *Am J Orthopsychiatry* 17:80–90, 1977.
2. Center for Disease Control: Gonorrhea: Recommended treatment schedules. *Arch Intern Med* 90:255–257, 1979.
3. Burgess G, et al: *Sexual Assault of Children and Adolescents.* New York, D. C. Heath & Co., 1978.

BIBLIOGRAPHY

Groth AN, Burgess A, Thale, B: Rape: Offender and victim. *Am J Psychiatry* 137:806–810, 1980.

Jaffe A, et al: Sexual abuse of children: An epidemiologic study. *Am J Dis Child* 129:689–692, 1975.

Kempe CH: Sexual abuse, another hidden pediatric problem: The 1977 C. Anderson Aldrich Lecture. *Pediatrics* 62:382–389, 1978.

Orr D, Prietto S: Emergency management of sexually abused children. *Am J Dis Child* 133:628–631, 1979.

Prince R, Barried D (eds): *Configurations: Biological and Cultural Factors in Sexuality and Family Life.* New York, D. C. Heath & Co., 1974.

Tinelli JA, et al: Sexual Abuse of Children: Clinical Findings and Implication for Management. *N Engl J Med* 302:319–323, 1980.

Environmental Emergencies

Common bites and stings inflicted by a human, dog, cat, snake, spider, and hymenoptera, as well as their epidemiology, are discussed in "Bites and Stings" (Chapter 28). The controversy regarding various treatment modalities is addressed, and an extensive reference list is provided for the reader who wishes to consult the original sources in the literature. Other approaches to bites are considered in "Minor Lacerations and Abrasions" (Chapter 10) and "Infectious Disease Emergencies" (Chapter 20).

The discussion of heat stroke, exhaustion and cramps in "Hyperthermia" (Chapter 29) might be considered with the processes reviewed in "Alterations of Central Nervous System Functions" (Section IX). "Hypothermia" (Chapter 30) may be read in association with "Cervical Spine Injuries" (Chapter 43), "Thyroid Disorders" (Chapter 12), "Alcohol Abuse" (Chapter 36), and "Poisoning and Drug Overdose" (Chapter 24).

The author of "Altitude-Related Emergencies" (Chapter 31) discusses the effect of high altitude on human physiology and the important systemic manifestations that may require emergency medical attention. The four major clinical manifestations of high altitude sickness are discussed: (1) acute mountain sickness, (2) high altitude pulmonary edema, (3) cerebral edema, and (4) chronic mountain sickness. The reader may wish to refer to "Dyspnea and Pulmonary Edema" (Chapter 48) and "Congestive Heart Failure" (Chapter 51) for discussion of pulmonary edema due to other causes.

A presentation on "Drowning and Near-Drowning" (Chapter 32) provides a clear definition of these processes and their pathophysiology. Because of the involvement of the respiratory system in this emergency, the reader may choose to read "Airway Management" (Chapter 56), "Obstructive Lung Diseases" (Chapter 57), and "Respiratory Failure" (Chapter 59). Successful resuscitation of patients with near-drowning, may also require an in-depth knowledge of the material covered in "Acid-Base Disturbances" (Chapter 18) and "Cardiopulmonary Resuscitation" (Chapter 55). "Diving Emergencies" (Chapter 33) includes a review of barotrauma, cerebral air embolism, and decompression sickness. "Dangerous Marine Organisms" (Chapter 34) virtually exhausts the list of common and exotic injuries that may result from encounters with dangerous marine organisms.

28. Bites and Stings

ROBERT C. JORDEN, M.D.

The vast number of animals capable of inflicting injury makes it impossible to cover all types of animal bites and stings in a single chapter. Therefore, this discussion has been limited to the more common of these injuries. First, only injuries caused by animals inhabiting the continental United States are included. Second, marine injuries are not included; the reader is referred to Chapter 34, "Dangerous Marine Organisms," and to Halstead's three-volume work *Poisonous and Venomous Marine Animals* for an extensive review of this specific subject. Likewise, large animal bites, e.g., those of bears, wolves, and cougars, as well as most insect bites, have been excluded.

DOG BITES

Epidemiology

Several studies have documented the fact that dog bites are truly becoming epidemic in the United States.[1-4] This problem seems to be more acute in large urban areas where there are great numbers of unsupervised dogs. The magnitude of the dog bite problem is difficult to ascertain, however, since the exact number of dogs is not known. Various estimates of the dog population have been published; the American Humane Society, for example, has estimated that there are 36 million dogs in the United States.[5]

The exact incidence of dog bites is also unknown. The Center for Disease Control in 1972 reported that animal bites ranked fourth among all reportable diseases in the 29 reporting states.[2] Of these bites, 84 percent were inflicted by dogs. A reasonable estimate of the number of dog bites is 500/100,000 population,[1] or a staggering 1.2 million bites per year.

Other interesting epidemiologic aspects of dog bites include the population most often bitten, location of bites, activity of the person being bitten, and the breed of dog most often involved. Children are by far the most frequently bitten segment of the population. In one large series, 40 percent of victims were under 10 years of age;[2] another series showed 60 percent of victims under 15;[3] and a third survey showed 52 percent were less than 20.[6] In most studies, approximately 60 percent of all victims are males.[2,3,6]

The anatomical location of the bites, as indicated in several studies, is most often the extremities. Data from several studies show that 63 to 74 percent of injuries occur on the extremities, the right arm being the most common site. Of the remainder, 10.6 to 21 percent occur on the head and neck, and 3 to 9 percent occur on the trunk.[2,4,6] An interesting point is that, in all series, young children were most often the victims of facial bites. These data are indicative of the young child's inherent curiosity and inexperience concerning animals.

The relationship between victim and dog varies. The dog is owned by the victim or the owner is known in 78 to 98 percent of cases; the dog is a stray in 3 to 25 percent.[4,6] The attack of the dog is also subject to analysis. The majority of attacks are either provoked by the victim's interaction with the dog (43 percent) or occur in sick or fighting animals (18 percent). The remaining 39 percent are unprovoked.[6]

The physical characteristics of the biting dog are also noteworthy. Most bites are inflicted by larger breeds, and a dog bite is likely to be more severe if inflicted by a larger dog. In recent years, there has been a trend toward owning larger, more aggressive breeds of dogs, primarily for self-protection and property protection. If this trend continues, the problem of dog bites may become even more serious. In one large study, 43.4 percent of the dogs were classified as large (50 pounds or more); 25.8 percent, medium (15 to 25 lbs); and 4.6 percent, small (less than 15 lbs).[4] In the remaining 26.2 percent, the size was not recorded. In another series, in which specific breeds were studied, the most frequently implicated breed was mixed (31 percent) and German Shepherd (28 percent). All other breeds accounted for the remaining 41 percent.[6]

The economic impact of dog bites is significant. The average cost for treatment of a dog bite, based on survey studies, ranges from $26 to $38.50.[2,7] The total annual cost then is $31.2 to $46.2 million for 1.2 million bites. This figure represents only medical expenses; it does not include work losses or damaged clothing and is therefore a conservative figure.

Nature of Injury

The type of wound incurred from a dog bite runs the gamut from contusion or superficial abrasion to fatal injuries.[8] In addition to the obvious superficial lacerations seen with dog bites, there may be contusions, crush injuries, deep puncture wounds, and tissue loss. All of these types of tissue damage must be considered in choosing proper treatment.

The majority of dog bites are not serious. In one series of over 9,000 bites, 6 percent did not puncture the skin, 55 percent showed skin punctures only, 32 percent showed a small skin tear, and 6 percent showed a laceration greater than 1 inch (2.5 cm). Less than 1 percent of these bites required plastic surgery.[2]

Complications

Infection is by far the most common complication of dog bites. The incidence of infection varies with each series reported, however. In some of these series, the patients were treated with prophylactic antibiotics, further confusing the issue. Generally, the infection rate ranges from 0.4 to 29 percent,[9–18] with a reasonable average of 5 to 6 percent. The only prospective study

in the literature shows an infection rate of 17 percent.[14] Regardless of the exact incidence, there does seem to be a predilection for infection.

The physician's problem is to identify the wounds that are likely to become infected and treat them accordingly. Callaham, in the detailed retrospective study of 106 dog bites, made several interesting observations, such as the fact that patient age may be a risk factor. Children under age 4 and adults over age 55 have a higher infection rate, particularly the latter group. Location of the wound is also an important risk factor. In Callaham's study, 28 percent of hand and arm bite wounds became infected in contrast to 4 percent of facial wounds, 12 percent of scalp wounds, and 15 to 16 percent overall.[12] The type of wound also has a bearing on the risk of infection. Obviously, a wound from a bite that does not penetrate the skin is not likely to become infected. On the other hand, a deep puncture wound to the hand may be very susceptible to infection. The reports vary, but puncture wounds are generally more likely to become infected than lacerations. One study showed a 48 and 29 percent infection rate for punctures versus lacerations.[17] Another study showed 22 and 13 percent infection rates, respectively.[12]

In the vast majority of cases, the only evidence of infection is a local cellulitis. In extremities, particularly the hand, deeper poorly vascularized tissues, such as tendons, are occasionally infected. Rarely, systemic infection occurs, which can lead to overwhelming sepsis and death. Several case reports of sepsis with *Pasteurella multocida* and other organisms attest to the potential for serious morbidity and death.[19–21]

Other forms of infection that have been reported after dog bites include osteomyelitis,[22,23] tenosynovitis, meningitis,[19] brain abscess,[24] and endocarditis.[25] Although these complications are rare, it is clear that thorough evaluation of dog bites and the judicious use of antibiotics are necessary.

Complications other than infection are uncommon. Probably the most important is disfigurement as a result of the bite. As mentioned earlier, however, data from one large survey indicate that less than 1 percent of all dog bites require the services of a plastic surgeon, which implies that few dog bites are seriously disfiguring. Psychological complications of dog bites no doubt occur, but their incidence and seriousness are unknown. No data are available to suggest how often tissue loss and subsequent loss of function occur. Dysfunction can also result from infection, particularly involving the hand. Fractures of underlying bones rarely occur, although there are case reports documenting depressed skull fractures as a result of dog bites.[24–26] For the most part, however, the main problems are infection and local tissue destruction. (Also see Chapter 10.)

Treatment

There is no treatment protocol that is ideal for all dog bite wounds. Furthermore, there is no unanimity among clinicians regarding the management of comparable wounds. Available data are not definitive. Treatment must be individualized to the particular patient and the particular wound. Treatment can be broken down into local care, surgical treatment, and infection prevention and control (Table 28–1). The protocol outlined in the following is a compilation based on data from the literature which is given as *an* approach (not *the* approach) to dog bites.

Skin Intact

Wounds with intact skin include abrasions and contusions. The protective barrier has been violated, yet there is no laceration per se. These wounds require the least amount of attention. Local care consists of cleansing the wound with an antiseptic soap. No surgical treatment is indicated, and prophylactic antibiotics, likewise, are not recommended. Infection control is limited to tetanus prevention, as follows:[27,28]

1. Patients who have had no tetanus toxoid, who have had only one dose, or who are uncertain of their immunization history, require
   a. an initial dose of diphtheria-tetanus (DT), 0.5 ml, injected intramuscularly for minor, clean wounds.
   b. tetanus immune globulin (TIG), 250 units subcutaneously, in addition to the DT for more extensive or dirty wounds. (If tetanus toxoid and TIG are given simultaneously, they should be given in separate arms.)
   c. a follow-up DT booster in four to six weeks.
2. Patients who have had two previous doses of tetanus toxoid require a DT booster, regardless of the extent or contamination of the wound. TIG is given for extensive or contaminated wounds only if they are more than 24 hours old.

3. Patients who are fully immunized, i.e., who have had three doses of DT, require
   a. no treatment for clean, minor wounds unless it has been more than ten years since their last tetanus booster.
   b. no treatment for extensive or dirty wounds unless it has been more than five years since their last tetanus booster.

Rabies precautions are also taken (Exhibit 28–1). *All subsequently described wounds also require tetanus prophylaxis and rabies precautions.*

Lacerations

Some lacerations are cosmetically important, and some are not. Generally, the former group consists of facial wounds. Cosmetically unimportant wounds are carefully cleansed with an antiseptic soap solution and irrigated thoroughly with saline. Irrigation has been shown to be effective in decreasing the incidence of wound infections. Once the wound has been thoroughly cleansed, devitalized tissue should be excised. The wound is left open and a nonadherent dressing applied. Large gaping wounds may be an exception, however. Even in a relatively unimportant cosmetic area, these injuries can be disfiguring. Although there are no data that address this point specifically, a delayed primary closure five days after the injury may be a reasonable compromise for such a wound.

Antibiotics are given prophylactically for five days. The patient is instructed to cleanse the wound twice a day with soap and water and to return for a wound check in two days, sooner if infection develops.

Facial wounds are cleansed in the same way and devitalized tissue debrided. Wound edges are also excised. The wound is then closed in a routine fashion, and the patient is started on antibiotics.

The literature is not clear on whether the incidence of wound infection is increased when a bite wound is sutured. There are studies to support both sides of the issue. However, it does not seem warranted to risk

---

TABLE 28–1 Management of Dog Bites

	Cleansing	Irrigation	Debridement	Antibiotics	Suturing	Tetanus and Rabies Precautions
Skin intact	Yes	No	No	No	No	Yes
Facial laceration	Yes	Yes	Yes	Yes	Yes	Yes
Nonfacial laceration	Yes	Yes	Yes	Yes	No	Yes
Puncture	Yes	No	Yes	Yes	No	Yes

Exhibit 28–1 Rabies Precautions and Prophylaxis

The following recommendations are only a guide. In applying them, take into account the animal species involved, the circumstances of the bite or other exposure, the vaccination status of the animal, and presence of rabies in the region. Local or state public health officials should be consulted if questions arise about the need for rabies prophylaxis.

	Animal species	Condition of animal at time of attack	Treatment of exposed person*
DOMESTIC	dog and cat	healthy and available for 10 days of observation	none, unless animal develops rabies†
		rabid or suspected rabid	RIG ‡ and HDCV §
		unknown (escaped)	consult public health officials. If treatment is indicated, give RIG ‡ and HDCV §
WILD	skunk, bat, fox, coyote, raccoon, bobcat, and other carnivores	regard as rabid unless proven negative by laboratory test ¶	RIG ‡ and HDCV §
OTHER	livestock, rodents, and lagomorphs (rabbits and hares)	Consider individually. Local and state public health officials should be consulted on questions about the need for rabies prophylaxis. Bites of squirrels, hamsters, guinea pigs, gerbils, chipmunks, rats, mice, other rodents, rabbits, and hares almost never call for antirabies prophylaxis.	

* All bites and wounds should immediately be thoroughly cleansed with soap and water. If antirabies treatment is indicated, both rabies immune globulin (RIG) and human diploid cell rabies vaccine (HDCV) should be given as soon as possible, regardless of the interval from exposure.

† During the usual holding period of 10 days, begin treatment with RIG and vaccine (preferably with HDCV) at first sign of rabies in a dog or cat that has bitten someone. The symptomatic animal should be killed immediately and tested.

‡ If RIG is not available, use antirabies serum, equine (ARS). Do not use more than the recommended dosage.

§ If HDCV is not available, use duck embryo vaccine (DEV). Local reactions to vaccines are common and do not contraindicate continuing treatment. Discontinue vaccine if fluorescent-antibody (FA) tests of the animal are negative.

¶ The animal should be killed and tested as soon as possible. Holding for observation is not recommended.

Source: Reprinted with permission from Rabies Prevention. *Morbidity Mortality Weekly Rep* 29:279, 1980.

possibly increasing the infection rate by closing wounds that are not of cosmetic concern and will heal if left open. The risk, if any, does seem warranted for wounds of the face. Not only are these injuries cosmetically important, but also the risk of facial infection is lower, given the excellent blood supply.

Puncture Wounds

Regardless of location, puncture wounds are handled in the same way. All wounds are thoroughly cleansed, and grossly devitalized tissue is excised. Wounds are not irrigated, since egress of fluid is not usually possible. All patients are placed on antibiotics and instructed to return if there are any signs of infection. An alternative approach is to excise the puncture wound completely and close the wound. It must be emphasized that many variations in treatment are possible, since the data on treatment are inconclusive. Until definitive data are available, treatment is not likely to be uniform.

The choice of antibiotics in the management of dog bites is also controversial. In a study of 50 dogs, 30 different species of bacteria were isolated from oral and nasal mucosa.[29] In that study, the following 11 species

or groups of bacteria were isolated from 50 percent or more of the dogs:

1. IIj
2. EF–4
3. *Pasteurella multocida*
4. *Staphylococcus aureus*
5. *Staphylococcus epidermidis*
6. group D streptococci
7. *Corynebacterium* species
8. enterobacteria
9. *Neisseria* species
10. *Moraxella* species
11. *Bacillus* species

The organisms designated by the alphanumeric code IIj and EF–4 had been previously identified by the Center for Disease Control. In this cited series, IIj and EF–4 were isolated in 90 and 94 percent, respectively, from the canine oral and/or nasal secretions. Both of those organisms are sensitive to the penicillins. Subsequent studies have not duplicated this high incidence of IIj and EF–4 in cultures of both infected and uninfected dog bite wounds, however.

Anaerobes are frequently present in dog bite wounds. In one series of 26 dog bites, 15 anaerobic organisms were isolated in ten patients.[15] Only six of the isolates were associated with clinical infections, and in no instance was the anaerobe the sole organism isolated. The most common isolate from all wounds was alpha-hemolytic streptococci,[12,25] but it was associated with only one clinical infection. *Staphylococcus aureus* was isolated in eight wounds, four of which were infected. *Staphylococcus aureus* and *Staphylococcus epidermidis* were the organisms most often associated with infection: four each.

Pasteurella multocida has frequently been implicated as the most common cause of dog bite wound infections. Some series cite a 50 percent incidence of *P. multocida* in infected wounds.[30] In Callaham's prospective, however, there were no clinical infections caused by *Pasteurella*.[14] In the series by Goldstein et al., this organism was isolated from eight wounds, two of which were infected.[15] In the study of the normal flora of 50 dogs, *P. multocida* was present in the oral mucosa in 30 of 50 dogs, in the nasal swab taken from 7 of the 50, and in both areas in 4 of 50.[29] In the same study, *S. aureus* was present in 21 of 50 oral and 30 of 50 nasal cultures. Again in Callaham's prospective study, no organism accounted for more than 15 percent of the infections. *Streptococcus*, gram-negative rods, *Pseudomonas* and *Staphylococcus aureus* accounted for approximately 10 percent each of the infections.[14] Thus, it appears that the importance of *Pasteurella multocida* in dog bite infections has been overemphasized.

Most of the commonly cultured pathogens are sensitive to penicillin, the exception being coagulase-positive *S. aureus*. Because there is a significant incidence of infections caused by this organism, antibiotic coverage against it seems reasonable. Although *P. multocida* is very sensitive to penicillin, some strains are resistant to the semisynthetic penicillins, such as dicloxacillin.[31] A logical choice for antibiotic prophylaxis therefore is a cephalosporin. Cephalosporins are effective against streptococci and staphylococci, as well as many gram-negative organisms.[32] Sensitivity studies also indicate that *P. multocida* is sensitive to most cephalosporins. For example, in adequate dosages, cephalexin (Keflex), 500 mg every six hours, readily provides minimal inhibitory concentrations.[31,33] Some of the newer cephalosporins have not been investigated with regard to *Pasteurella* sensitivities and therefore cannot yet be recommended.

The question of using prophylactic antibiotics for dog bite wounds is controversial. Although these wounds are significantly infection-prone, the effectiveness of prophylaxis in preventing infection remains to be proved. A large prospective study is needed to settle that question, as well as to determine which antibiotic should be used and whether wounds should be sutured. Until such a study is available, the conservative approach is to use prophylactic antibiotics and leave all but cosmetically important wounds open.

The treatment of established infections of dog bite wounds is less controversial. Infected wounds that have been closed should be opened and irrigated. Devitalized tissue should be excised. Initial antibiotic choice should be based on the Gram stain; it can be altered subsequently, depending on culture and sensitivity studies. Most often, the Gram stain shows a fixed flora; however, if there is an overgrowth of a single organism, antibiotics effective against that class of bacteria should be started (e.g., dicloxacillin for a staphylococci overgrowth). If several organisms are seen, a broader spectrum antibiotic should be started until culture results are available (a cephalosporin). Depending on the severity of the infection, the presence of systemic signs, and the location of the wound, the patient may require hospitalization and intravenous therapy with antibiotics.

CAT BITES

Cat bites are much less common than dog bites. In a 17-year survey of all animal bites in Maryland, dog bites accounted for 95 percent of the injuries; only 3 percent were cat bites.[6] Although recognized for many years as a potential cause for infection, little attention has been focused on cat bite or scratch injuries.

In many ways, cat bites are similar to dog bites. Tissues are disrupted and inoculated with bacteria, and infection is the most common complication of both types of injuries. A variety of organisms can be cultured from both cats' and dogs' oral and nasal mucosa, as well as from wounds inflicted by either animal. However, the pathophysiology of cat bites is quite different from that of dog bites. Cats are smaller animals and, therefore, do not produce the crush injury that dogs inflict. Feline teeth are sharper and smaller in diameter, and they tend to produce deep puncture wounds rather than the tearing injuries often seen with dog bites. The puncture wounds of cat bites, because they are deep, also have a tendency to involve superficial tendons and to penetrate joint spaces.[9,34,35]

Infection is much more commonly seen with cat bites than with dog bites. Two studies indicate a 30 percent infection rate for cat bites.[6,9] The infecting organisms vary and are often mixed. *Pasteurella multocida* is isolated from cats' oral or nasal mucosa 50 to 80 percent of the time,[35] but the incidence of *P. multocida* in infected cat bites is not well documented. It is known, however, that *P. multocida* is a more common cause of infection in cat bites than in dog bites. One series of

50 cat bites and scratches documented the finding of *P. multocida* in 80 percent of cultured wounds.[6] Of those patients with clinical infections in the same series, 27 percent of the infected wounds had *P. multocida* alone or in combination with other organisms. In another small series of 18 cat bites, 9 of 9 cultured wounds showed *P. multocida*.[36]

Cat scratches have a tendency to become infected even in the absence of bite wounds.[34] This is not true of canine injuries. Cats frequently groom their claws by licking them, and the saliva thus deposited on the claws is thought to be the source of the infecting bacteria. Again, *P. multocida* is a frequent offender.

The same treatment principles outlined for dog bites apply to cat bites. Wounds should be cleansed, irrigated, and debrided, when appropriate. Since cat bites usually consist only of small puncture wounds, little can be done to remove the bacterial inoculum. Prophylactic antibiotics are recommended for all cat bites that penetrate the skin. Less controversy surrounds this treatment for cat bites than for dog bites, since the incidence of infection is so much higher.

Not all clinicians agree on the choice of antibiotics. Because of a higher incidence of *Pasteurella*, many authors recommend penicillin.[34,35,37] At least one author documented the presence of multiple organisms, including penicillin-resistant *S. aureus*, as the infecting organisms in clinically infected wounds, however.[35] The same author also documented treatment failures with penicillin. For this reason, cephalosporins may be a better choice as the first-line drug in cat bite infection prophylaxis. A seven- to ten-day course of antibiotics (penicillin 500 mg or cephalexin 500 mg q.i.d) is therefore recommended as prophylaxis.

For wounds that are grossly infected, Gram stain and cultures should be obtained. Initial treatment should be instituted with a cephalosporin or penicillin, unless the Gram stain is characteristic of a particular organism.

The same precautions and prophylaxis against tetanus and rabies that were recommended for dog bites apply also to cat bites.

HUMAN BITES

There are two categories of human bites: true bites and fight bites. Like any other type of bite, a true bite is an occlusional injury that occurs when tissue is grasped between maxillary and mandibular teeth. Fight bite injuries occur when an assailant strikes another person in the mouth and sustains a hand laceration as a result of contact with the person's tooth. Human bites, regardless of etiology, occur most often on the hand.[38–40] This fact, probably more than any other, accounts for the higher morbidity rate of human bites. Studies that include human bites at sites other than the hand have shown that human bite wounds do not have any higher incidence of infection than other types of bite wounds.[41]

The exact incidence of human bites is unknown. The majority of injuries are never reported because medical attention is not sought. Human bites are not uncommon injuries, however. Since the first reported case in 1910,[42] there have been over 1,000 cases reported in the literature.

Nature of the Injury

The injury inflicted by the human bite is similar to that of dog bites. Deep puncture wounds are less likely, since humans do not have long fangs, but certainly crush injury, laceration, and tissue loss occur. Because the majority of bites occur on hands, there is a significant incidence of traumatic finger tip amputation. Hand bites often violate multiple tissue planes and damage tendons, bones, joint capsules, and articular cartilage.

Fight bites have a particular pathophysiology that is conducive to major infections. Typically, these lesions are sustained when the striking hand is in a clenched fist. In this position, the extensor tendon and its underlying bursa are pulled distally over the metacarpal-phalangeal joint, and it is this joint that usually impinges on the tooth. The result is a deep laceration that can disrupt superficial and deep fascia, the extensor tendon and its bursa, and the joint capsule. When the fingers are extended, the skin and tendon retract proximally, sealing off the contaminated wound inflicted to the deep tissues. These anatomical relationships set the stage for serious infections.[43]

Complications

The most serious complication of human bites is infection. Human bites are notorious for causing severe infections that lead to functional disability, amputation, sepsis, and even death.[36,38,39–41,44–53] The advent of antibiotics and a general increased awareness of the injury have significantly reduced the incidence of serious complications, however.

Several factors in human bites predispose to infection—hand anatomy, as discussed earlier, is one factor. Another is delay in seeking treatment.[22,25,26,43,46,49] Victims may not seek help because of embarrassment, the initial innocuous appearance of the wound, or their general socioeconomic class. Alcoholics, for example, generally do not take good care of themselves and are not likely to see a physician until an infection is well established. Several studies have documented a poor outcome when the injury is not attended to until 12 hours after it occurred. On the other hand, patients seen promptly and treated aggressively rarely develop long-term problems.

The virulence of the infecting bacteria is also very significant. The early data on human bite infections are sketchy. Most serious infections reportedly were due to fusiform bacilli and Vincent's spirochete in a synergistic type of infection.[38,39,44] More recent data indicate that mixed infections are frequent (25 to 89 percent) and that the most commonly found organisms are staphylococci[36,47,48,51] and streptococci (78 percent in one series, 68 percent in another).[36] In one series, 64 percent of all staphylococci were resistant to penicillin. Several series have documented the importance of *Staphylococcus aureus*. One study noted 100 percent of patients with *S. aureus* alone or in combination with other organisms had serious complications.[52]

The nature of the infections that develop from hand bites, in particular fight bites, has been well established by the work of Kanavel[54] and the study of Mason and Koch.[43] The latter authors injected barium into and around the metacarpal-phalangeal joints and documented radiographically how infection is likely to spread. They concluded that several weak points in the joint capsule result in a characteristic spread of infection. The sites of infection in hand bites in order of frequency are (1) the subcutaneous space of the dorsum of the hand, (2) the fascial space of the dorsum of the proximal phalanx, (3) the metacarpal-phalangeal joint, (4) the palmar fascial spaces, and (5) the flexor tendon sheaths.

Treatment

Given the potential for serious infection and long-term disability, the most important treatment principle is to recognize the injury and to take an aggressive approach. Any laceration over the metacarpal-phalangeal joints must be assumed to be a bite wound until proved otherwise. For various reasons, patients may not divulge the true nature of the injury.

Once identified as a bite wound, the next step is to determine the depth of the wound. The wound should be carefully explored to determine if deep tissues, i.e., tendon and joint capsule, have been violated. If the wound is less than 12 hours old, it should be carefully examined for signs of infection. Typically, the infected wound is inflamed and slightly swollen at the metacarpal-phalangeal joint. A thin grayish exudate, which is often foul-smelling, may be present. Passive motion is painful if the joint is infected. All of these findings indicate an acute infectious process.

Some physicians routinely debride all hand bites, regardless of the depth of penetration or the signs of infection.[47,50] Some also hospitalize all patients for intravenous administration of antibiotics. Others take a more conservative approach to the wounds,[36,48,49] surgically debriding the noninfected wound only if the joint has been penetrated or if devitalized tissue or foreign material is present. The patient with an infected wound is taken to the operating room for debridement if the joint is involved or if there is a localized collection of pus. It is unanimously agreed that human bites of the hand should never be sutured.

Nonsurgical management consists of cleansing and irrigating the wound, administering antibiotics, elevating the hand, and splinting the wound. The antibiotic chosen should be one that is effective against coagulase-positive *S. aureus*. Cultures and Gram stain should be performed, but antibiotic therapy should not be delayed for culture results. Cephalosporins are effective against staphylococci and streptococci, as well as many gram-negative organisms that are also frequently cultured. Therefore, a cephalosporin is a good choice for antibiotic coverage. Roentgenograms should be obtained to determine the presence of fractures, foreign bodies, or air in joints.

From the emergency physician's point of view, management must be in conjunction with the local hand surgeon. The decision to hospitalize the patient is dependent on the practice of the individual surgeon. Certainly, patients with grossly infected wounds should be admitted. Likewise, those with deep wounds in which tendons have been injured or the joint space has been violated should have at least a trip to the operating room for thorough debridement, if not admission. In addition, the reliability of the patient must be carefully considered. Patients' reliability is inversely proportional to the need for admission.

Aggressive surgical management and antibiotic therapy have markedly improved the outcome of human bite injuries of the hand. In the preantibiotic era, one of ten patients seen soon after injury came to amputation. In those patients seen after 12 hours, one in three required amputation, and another one in three had permanent stiffness of the affected digit.[44] More recent series show a marked improvement, although the number of people who require amputation, develop osteomyelitis, or have permanently stiff fingers is still significant.

The management of human bites in other areas of the body is as controversial as dog bite management. Generally, the recommendations for cleansing, irrigation, and debridement in human bites are the same as those for dog bites. Wound closure is recommended only for facial wounds. Prophylactic antibiotics are recommended and should include an antibiotic effective against staphylococci. Acceptable antibiotics include a cephalosporin (Keflex, 500 mg orally four times a day) or dicloxacillin (500 mg orally four times a day for seven to ten days). Tetanus prophylaxis is recommended, even though tetanus bacteria are rarely found in the human oral flora,[55] because the wound may be contaminated from other sources, particularly in view of the patient population likely to sustain a human bite.

Unusual infections can be transmitted via a human bite. These infections include syphilis,[56] tuberculosis,[57] actinomycosis,[58] and hepatitis.[59] Although rare, these infections do occur, and the emergency care physician should be aware of them.

SNAKE BITES

Each year in the United States, 45,000 people sustain snake bite injuries. Of this number, only about 8,000 bites are inflicted by poisonous snakes.[60] Unlike dog, cat, and human bites, in which the primary concern is tissue loss and infection, snake bites are important because of the local and systemic effects of the venom injected.

Taxonomy and Physiology

There are 2,500 to 3,000 species of snakes in the world, 375 of which are venomous.[60] These species are members of five families of poisonous snakes (Table 28-2). Each of the 50 states, except Alaska, Hawaii, and Maine, has at least one venomous species.[61] These species are members of two families, Crotalidae and Elapidae. The Crotalidae include the genera *Crotalus* (rattlesnakes), *Agkistrodon* (cotton mouth and copperhead),[62] and *Sistruris* (massasauga and pigmy rattlesnake). The Elapidae family includes two genera of coral snakes,[63] *Micruroides euryxanthus* (Sonoran) and *Micruris fulvius* (Eastern and Texas).

Poisonous snakes deliver their venom by way of their fangs. The pit vipers have two long, curved, canaliculated, retractable fangs located in the anterior maxilla. In their retracted, resting position, these teeth are tucked up into the mucosa of the upper jaw. In the striking position, the jaws are opened wide and the fangs projected forward so that they are perpendicular to the maxilla. The snake has control over the movement of the fangs, being able to retract or extend them at will. Each fang is hollow with an anterior opening near its distal tip. Venom is produced in a modified salivary gland that lies in the soft tissue of the maxilla just below the eye and is delivered to the sheath of each fang by a salivary duct. The sheath forms a pocket around the base of the fang and transmits the venom into the hollow fang. The actual release of venom is controlled by muscles surrounding the venom gland. The innervation of this musculature is separate from that of the biting musculature. Thus, the snake has the ability to control the amount of venom injected, independent of the biting process. In addition to the fangs, pit vipers also have two rows of smaller teeth in both the upper and lower jaws; occasionally, superficial bite wounds caused by these smaller teeth can be seen around the two fang marks. These teeth and the wounds they inflict are of no clinical significance.

The dentition of the coral snakes, the other group of poisonous snakes found in the United States, is different from that of the *Crotalus* species. The coral snakes also have bilateral maxillary fangs in addition to their smaller dentition, but their fangs are not as long as those of the pit vipers and they are fixed, not retractable. Their function, however, is the same as that of the fangs of the pit vipers—the delivery of venom into prey or adversaries.

Epidemiology

Snakes are generally quiet, nonaggressive creatures that rarely seek out adversaries. They bite humans only as a defensive measure. Bites occur most commonly in the natural environment, either when people accidentally stumble into the snake's habitat or when they deliberately disturb a snake. Snakes in captivity are responsible for a significant number of bites, however. These victims are usually herpetologists, zoo keepers, hobbyists, entertainers, or cultists.[60] Snake bites occur five times more commonly in males than in females because of a greater occupational and recreational exposure. Half of all snake bites occur in children or young adults, the highest incidence being in the 10- to 19-year-old age group. The vast majority of bites occur on the extremities (99 percent), with 65 percent occurring on the upper and 34 percent the lower extremity.[60]

Snakes are poikilothermic, i.e., their body temperature equilibrates with the environment; they are unable to regulate their own body temperature. At 8°C (46°F), snakes become motionless, and at 42°C (108°F) they survive only 10 to 12 minutes. Their optimal temperature range is 27°C to 32°C (81°F to 90°F).[61] Because of these temperature constraints, the snakes' activities

TABLE 28–2   Poisonous Snakes

Family	Examples
Crotalidae (pit vipers)	Rattlesnake,* copperhead,* cotton mouth*
Elapidae	Coral snakes,* cobras, mambas
Viperidae (true vipers)	Puff adder
Hydrophidae	Sea snakes
Colubridae	Boomslang

* Found in the continental United States.

and therefore snake bites are subject to seasonal as well as diurnal temperature fluctuations. The peak season for snake bites is the warmer months, March 15 to October 15; the peak time of day for bites is the evening.[60]

Because of their cardiac physiology, snakes do not oxygenate peripheral tissues well, which severely constrains their activity level. Snakes are thus slow-moving animals, with a maximum speed of 3 miles/hour. Nevertheless, the snake can strike with great speed (8 feet/second), and their otherwise slow movement should not lull anyone into a false sense of safety.[61]

Effects of Venom

Snake venoms are complex poisons consisting of enzymes, peptides, glycoproteins, and other substances.[60] Knowledge of the pharmacology of venoms and their component parts is far from complete, despite extensive research. In the past, venoms have been labeled and categorized as various toxins, i.e., neurotoxin, cardiotoxin, necrotoxin, and hemotoxin. This practice is an oversimplification of the total action of venoms and may lead to therapeutic errors.[64] Certainly, snake venoms do exhibit these toxic effects, but it is dangerous to assume a given species has a particular toxic effect to the exclusion of any other. Nevertheless, various clinical findings seen with snake bites can be related to certain venom components and their in vitro actions.

Local Necrosis

Generally a hallmark of pit viper envenomation, local necrosis is probably due to a number of venom constituents. Proteolytic enzymes, which are trypsinlike enzymes that digest tissue protein, have been found in all crotalid venoms that have been analyzed. Venoms with high concentrations of these enyzmes cause marked tissue destruction. Pit viper venom also contains a nonproteolytic enzyme that is directly myonecrotic and contributes to local necrosis. Collagenase, which digests collagen, and hyaluronidase, which decreases connective tissue viscosity and thus permits venom penetration, also contribute to tissue necrosis.[64]

Shock

There are several potential causes of shock after pit viper envenomation. Initial hypotension may be attributed to pulmonary and, to a lesser extent, splanchnic pooling of blood. This pooling is a transient phenomenon that gives way to hypovolemia as the cause of shock. Hypovolemia is secondary to transudation of fluid across endothelium that has been damaged, probably by polypeptides found in the venom. Overall then, fluid loss and sometimes hemorrhage into tissue is the primary cause of shock in pit viper envenomation.[60] Renal failure is possible from the effects of hypotension or the circulating hemoglobin and myoglobin. Vasodilation and myocardial depression may also play a role, but the latter is not well established in humans. (See Chapter 6.)

Coagulopathy and Hemorrhage

Coagulopathy can result from one of three mechanisms operative in snake venom poisoning: anticoagulation, defibrination, and procoagulant effect.[60] Venom's procoagulant effect results from the stimulation of the clotting mechanism in a number of places in the clotting cascade. Crotalid venom has been shown to affect Factors X, IX, V, and II.[60] In addition, venom contains a thrombinlike enzyme that converts fibrinogen to fibrin. As a result of this enzyme's activity, fibrinogen is consumed and a secondary fibrinolysis occurs. Fibrin split products are therefore increased; interestingly, however, platelets are not aggregated, and platelet function remains normal. The net result of this thrombinlike enzyme's activity is to deplete fibrinogen, resulting in a marked hypofibrinogenemia.[60]

Anticoagulant effects of various venoms are also well documented. Venom activity at several sites in the cascade inhibit normal clotting function.[60]

Some *Crotalus* species are also known for a direct fibrinolytic effect. The exact mechanism of action is not known, although activation of plasminogen has been eliminated as a possible mechanism.[60]

Hemorrhage secondary to coagulopathy does not generally occur unless there are hemorrhagic factors in the snake's venom, as there are in a number of *Crotalus* species. The hemorrhagic factors are nonproteolytic, nonenzymatic proteins that are toxic to the vascular wall. The damage to the endothelial lining leads to bleeding into the vessel wall and surrounding tissues, platelet aggregation, and red cell destruction. The result is significant hemolysis, hemorrhage, and thrombocytopenia.[65,66]

Neurotoxicity

Most *Crotalus* venom is only slightly neurotoxic; the venoms of the coral snake and the Mojave rattlers, however, are severely neurotoxic. The specific component of these venoms that is responsible for the neurotoxicity is not known, although it is thought to be a polypeptide. The mechanism of action is likewise unknown, but it is possibly a nondepolarizing blockade at the neuromuscular junction.[64] The net result is a severe neurotoxicity, causing a paralysis that leads to respiratory insufficiency.

Clinical Manifestations of Snake Bite

Snake bite produces a variety of clinical manifestations, depending on the size, age, and species of the biting snake; the amount of venom injected; and the individual's resistance. The pit vipers account for 98 percent of all venomous snake bites in the United States,[67–69] and the signs and symptoms of their bite can be divided into two broad categories; local effects and systemic effects. As stated earlier, local symptomatology is due to severe tissue necrosis. The bite wound typically consists of two fang marks that penetrate the skin. The depth of the wound is variable, but generally the deep fascial layers have not been penetrated. Pain and swelling at the site are almost immediate. The pain caused by the bite itself is probably due to the venom and usually is not severe. As edema progresses, pain becomes more severe. Swelling usually occurs within 5 minutes, although it may be delayed up to 15 minutes. If there is no swelling at 20 to 30 minutes after the bite, envenomation probably has not occurred.[60,67] Edema tends to progress very rapidly and may continue to spread for as long as 36 hours.

Ecchymosis is common in the area of the bite, as well as in contiguous areas.[70] This finding is variable, depending on the species of the biting snake. Vesiculation is also related to the snake species. Vesicles appear 8 to 36 hours after envenomation and may be filled with serous fluid or blood.[60] They rarely appear if antivenin has been administered promptly and in adequate amounts. The administration of adequate antivenin should also prevent the tissue necrosis that commonly resulted in gangrene and ultimately in amputation before the advent of antivenin.

Systemic symptoms, commonly seen in snake venom poisonings, usually indicate a serious envenomation. Nausea and vomiting are very common but may be due to the administration of narcotics. At least one author does not consider this symptom serious if it is the only systemic manifestation.[71] Weakness is a common symptom of severe envenomation.[60,61] Immediate, transient weakness following snake bite is probably more of an emotional response to the injury and is not significant; it should not be confused with more persistent weakness.

Numbness and tingling, particularly in the perioral and scalp areas, are frequently seen.[60,61] These symptoms also may occur in the fingers and toes or may involve the entire body. They occur early in the course of a bite and indicate significant envenomation.

The presence of a metallic, minty, or rubbery taste in the mouth is a common early symptom of envenomation by several of the crotalid species.[60] It, too, indicates significant envenomation. This is a symptom that must be elicited, however, since the patient may not spontaneously voice this complaint.

Neurologic manifestations of *Crotalus* envenomation may include muscle fasciculations, pinpoint pupils, focal paresis, and paralysis (rarely, diffuse paralysis). Convulsions occasionally follow *Crotalus* bites, but such convulsions are more likely to result from anoxia rather than a direct effect of the venom, since venom does not cross the blood-brain barrier.[72]

Hemorrhage can be a severe problem as a consequence of snake bites. Its presence indicates moderate to severe poisoning. Bleeding can occur in the form of melena, hematemesis, hemoptysis, hematuria, or epistaxis. The results of coagulation studies in such cases are abnormal, and platelet counts may be markedly depressed.

The signs and symptoms of Mojave rattlesnake envenomation differ from those of the typical pit viper envenomation. Mojave rattlesnake bites produce little local reaction, even when poisoning is serious. The venom of these snakes contains a potent neurotoxin that can result in paralysis with respiratory arrest.[60,65,67] These injuries should be aggressively treated with antivenin, despite a lack of significant local symptoms.[60]

The coral snake poisonings can also be deceptive, because local symptoms are lacking and systemic symptoms may be greatly delayed, even in severe poisonings. Apprehension, giddiness, dyspnea, nausea, salivation, vomiting, and weakness are early symptoms, although they may actually be delayed for several hours. Bulbar palsy, which is seen in four to seven hours, heralds the onset of a diffuse paralysis that follows in one to two hours. Once symptoms do occur, progression is rapid.[63,73] An aggressive use of antivenin in coral snake poisoning is therefore recommended.[74] Coral snake antivenin is effective only in treating the more serious bite of the Eastern coral snake.[67] The venom of the Sonoran variety is not neutralized by the antivenin, but these bites rarely result in serious envenomation.[74]

Management of Snake Bites

The treatment of snake bite victims can be divided into two phases, the first aid given at the scene and the definitive care given in the hospital. Snake bites are true medical emergencies and must be given the same attention that any other life-threatening emergency deserves. The first few hours in the course of a snake bite are crucial. Delays in treatment can result in serious morbidity and mortality. The importance of prompt assessment and treatment cannot be overemphasized.

First Aid Management

Recommendations for first aid measures vary in the literature. Some authors feel that no first aid is indicated; others recommend a number of measures. Generally, the importance of rapid transport to a medical facility is emphasized. A few simple measures are universally recommended—rest, reassurance, immobilization of the bitten part, observation for complications, and transportation to a definitive care facility.[60] More aggressive first aid may be indicated if signs of serious envenomation develop or if medical care is several hours away.[69,70,73]

Calm the Victim. The victim should be removed from the immediate vicinity of the snake and instructed to lie down and do as little physical activity as possible since such activity may facilitate the absorption of venom. The victim should be reassured as much as possible that the injury is not fatal and that effective medical treatment is available. An extremity that has been bitten should be kept immobile in a slightly dependent position.

Identify the Snake. An effort should be made to locate and retrieve the offending snake. If possible, the snake should be killed and brought to the hospital with the patient for identification. Extreme caution must be used in handling the snake, even after it has been killed. Reflex biting has been reported up to 45 minutes after decapitation.[67] The snake, in particular the head of the snake, should not be mutilated since this may make identification impossible.

Apply a Constricting Band. A loosely applied constricting band should be placed above the joint proximal to the bite or 2 to 4 in. (5 to 10 cm) proximal to the wound. The band should be tight enough to occlude superficial veins and lymphatics, but care must be taken not to occlude arterial flow. To be of any value, however, the band must be applied within 30 minutes of the bite. There is some controversy surrounding the periodic release of the band. Some experts feel the band should be released for 90 seconds every 10 to 15 minutes. Others oppose this practice, stating that it releases a bolus of venom into the circulation.[73,75] At any rate, the band should not be removed until after antivenin has been given. When the band is released, it should be done gradually to prevent delivery of a large bolus of venom. In treating coral snake poisonings, the constricting band is of little value.[60,76]

Incise and Suction the Wound. If done early, incision and suction of the snake bite wound has therapeutic value. It has been experimentally shown that prompt initiation of this technique can result in removal of 22 to 50 percent of radioisotope-labeled venom.[77] The procedure must be properly performed, however, or unnecessary tissue damage will result. The two fang marks should be incised in the direction of the strike. The incision should extend only $\frac{1}{8}$ to $\frac{1}{4}$ in. (3 to 6 mm) and should penetrate only the skin. Deeper incisions are not necessary and only risk damage to vital structures.[67]

Cruciate incisions or multiple incisions in the area of edema are disfiguring and do not improve the yield of extracted venom. Suction should be applied once the incisions have been made. Ideally, this should be done with suction cups supplied in snake bite kits. If the cups are not available, oral suction may be used, provided that the person applying the suction has no open oral sores. This practice is condemned by some authors, however, who claim it contaminates the wound.[78] Suction should be applied for one hour; beyond that time, no benefit can be derived. Beginning the suction more than 30 minutes after the bite is probably of little or no value.

Immobilize the Involved Area. The affected part should be splinted to prevent excess movement.

Do Not Apply Ice. Cryotherapy is mentioned only to be condemned. Although it was a popular form of therapy in the recent past, cryotherapy has been uniformly denounced as detrimental. The application of ice enhances tissue ischemia and ultimately causes additional tissue necrosis, possibly leading to amputation.

Some authors recommend the application of an ice pack as a temporary first aid measure to help ease the pain of the bite. However, even this practice is condemned by some.

Evacuate the Victim. The final step in first aid treatment of snake bites and by far the most important is evacuation of the victim. First aid care is by no means a substitute for definitive medical care. The latter care should be obtained as soon as possible; there should be no inordinate delays at the scene in order to accomplish first aid measures.

Emergency Department Management

The medical management of snake bites is multifaceted. It requires the simultaneous performance of several procedures. Therefore, just as it is for any patient who has a life-threatening or potentially life-threatening condition, a team approach is desirable. Despite the potential severity of these injuries, tissue loss is the exception, not the rule, and fatalities nationwide are less than 15/year.[60,79] The following is a step-by-step approach to the snake bite patient. The order in which these steps are accomplished depends on the needs of the individual patient and the availability of extra personnel. The goals of therapy are to prevent further venom absorption, neutralize what has been absorbed, remove unabsorbed venom, prevent and treat complications, and provide supportive care.

Obtain a Thorough History. The emergency physician must obtain a detailed history regarding the circumstances of the bite. Specific details about the time of injury, the activity of the patient when bitten, the number of bites, activity since the bite, and the first aid measures, if any, that were taken should be elicited. Inquiry about previous snake bites and allergies, particularly to horse serum, should be made. If the snake was not recovered, the victim must be asked to describe the snake in an attempt to determine species and size.

The physician must first allow the patient to relate the symptoms and then ask specific questions concerning numbness, tingling, lightheadedness, weakness, nausea, vomiting, or abnormal tastes. If local swelling is present, the physician should ask when it started and whether it is progressing.

Examine the Patient. Physical examination is conducted with emphasis on vital signs, neurologic function, and the wound itself. Serial measurements of limb circumference are made to determine the extent of swelling. Signs of envenomation are specifically sought. Depending on the urgency, one or two intravenous lines are established and blood obtained for a baseline complete blood cell count, electrolyte, measurements, coagulation profile, platelet count, and determinations of blood urea nitrogen (BUN), glucose, and arterial blood gas levels. In critically ill patients, central venous pressure lines or Swan-Ganz catheters may be helpful in guiding fluid therapy. It is also wise to obtain blood for typing and cross matching, even in the absence of bleeding, since later cross matching may be difficult because of the presence of venom. A baseline electrocardiogram (ECG) and chest roentgenogram are also obtained. Urine is analyzed for blood and/or hemoglobin.

Provide General Supportive Measures. The physician institutes supportive measures based on the vital signs and physical examination. Other general measures include wound cleansing, pain control, airway support (if needed), and infection and tetanus prophylaxis. Rabies precautions are not necessary, however. Wound cleansing with antiseptic soap solution is adequate local care. Pain may be controlled with oral medications in most instances. If pain is severe, however, systemic narcotics may be needed. Prevention of infection by administration of prophylactic antibiotics is generally recommended, even though there are no studies to support this practice.

In bacteriologic studies on snake venoms, a large variety of both aerobic and anaerobic organisms have been isolated.[80] In view of the amount of tissue necrosis and this degree of contamination, broad spectrum antibiotic prophylaxis seems warranted, at least until a prospective study indicates that it is not. Russell recommends broad spectrum antibiotics, but does not specify which one, for severe tissue involvement.[60,81] Cephalosporins once again seem like a logical choice.

Determine the Need for Antivenin. The cornerstone of treatment for snake bites is antivenin. It is effective against both systemic manifestations and local effects of venom. Its administration is not without risk, how-

ever; therefore, it should be given only when indicated. The need for antivenin is determined by the severity of the bite and the type of snake involved. The mere fact of a penetrating bite by a Mojave rattler or a coral snake is all that is required for the administration of antivenin. With other *Crotalus* species, the need for antivenin is determined by the patient's signs and symptoms.

It must first be determined whether the patient actually sustained a snake bite. If the patient has only superficial scratches with no evidence of fang marks, envenomation did not occur. If the patient has fang marks, envenomation *may* have occurred. About 10 percent of the time, envenomation does not occur despite a significant bite.[60] Envenomation must be determined by the presence of other signs and symptoms.

Two classifications of snake bites have been developed to determine the severity of the injury and the need for antivenin. The first classification, established by Wood, Hoback, and Green, was subsequently modified by Parish, as well as by McCollough and Gennaro.[74] There are five categories in this system, 0 through IV, corresponding to a nonpenetrating wound through minimal, moderate, severe, and very severe bites. Each category has certain signs and symptoms (Table 28–3). Antivenin is recommended for moderate and more serious bites. The second classification system is that recommended by Russell.[60] This schema uses only four categories: no envenomation, minimal, moderate, and severe envenomation (Table 28–4). Antivenin is given for envenomations classified as minimal, moderate, or severe. If the area of swelling is limited to the bite area and there are no systemic symptoms, antivenin is withheld.

TABLE 28–3 Classification of Severity of Crotalid Envenomation According to McCollough and Gennaro

Category	Signs
Grade 0	No envenomation
Grade I, minimal	Fang marks, minimal or no local swelling, moderate pain, no systemic signs
Grade II, moderate	More severe and widely distributed edema and pain; possibly local petechiae and ecchymoses; occasionally weakness, nausea and vomiting, and bloody oozing from fang marks
Grade III, severe	Signs of Grades I and II in rapid progression with immediate systemic signs and symptoms
Grade IV, very severe	Sudden pain and rapid swelling that may involve the trunk; ecchymoses and progressive edema; bleb formation; early systemic signs and symptoms; shock, bleeding from body orifices, convulsions, coma, renal failure

TABLE 28–4   Classification of Severity of Crotalid Envenomation According to Russell

Category	Signs
No envenomation	No local or systemic signs
Minimal	Local swelling, no systemic reactions
Moderate	Swelling progressing beyond the site of the bite and systemic signs and/or laboratory changes, e.g., a fall in hematocrit
Severe	Marked local reaction, severe systemic symptoms, and laboratory changes

Administer Antivenin. The administration of antivenin is by the intravenous route only. Intramuscular or local injections are ineffective.[60,67,74] Administration must always be preceded by skin or conjunctival testing to determine if the patient is allergic to horse serum.[82] The test is performed by the intradermal injection of 0.02 ml 1:10 dilution of the antivenin with saline. If there is no inflammatory reaction in 15 minutes, the test result is negative. In patients with a known allergy to horse serum, the conjunctival test is performed. A drop of 1:10 dilution of antivenin with saline is instilled in the eye. A positive test result consists of itching, slight edema, and dilation of conjunctival vessels. If positive, a drop of 1:1000 ml epinephrine diluted with saline should be instilled in the eye.

A positive result to the skin or conjunctival test is not a contraindication to the administration of antivenin. If a patient's life or limb is in danger, the antivenin should be administered in spite of a positive test result. A desensitization process for use in this situation is described in the antivenin package insert,[82] but this process is cumbersome and time-consuming. In a critically ill patient, it may be necessary to administer the antivenin by slow intravenous drip with a simultaneous epinephrine drip.[60] This procedure is obviously risky and should not be undertaken without proper emergency resuscitation equipment and personnel on hand. In general, even under ideal circumstances, antivenin should not be administered in anything but a critical care setting, be it the emergency department or the intensive care unit.

The exact manner of administration of the antivenin is variable. Some clinicians give it by intravenous push; others put the antivenin in 500 ml saline and drip it in over an hour. Additional vials of antivenin can be added to a second 500 ml fluid as needed.[60]

The antivenin for pit vipers that is available in the United States is produced by Wyeth Laboratories and is called Antivenin (Crotalidae) Polyvalent. It is produced by injecting a combination of four crotalid venoms (*Crotalus atrox*, *Crotalus adamanteus*, *Bothrops atrox*, and *Crotalus terrificus*) into horses.[82] The hyper-immune horse serum is then standardized by its ability to neutralize a standard venom injected intravenously into mice. Wyeth also manufactures an antivenin for the Eastern coral snake venom. This antivenin is administered in the same way as the crotalid antivenin.

The success of antivenin therapy depends not only on early administration but also on adequate amounts of antivenin. For coral snake poisoning it is easy to administer an adequate amount, since 3 to 6 vials neutralize the maximum envenomation.[60,74] For crotalids, however, the case is less clear-cut. The amount recommended is variable and frequently changes. Russell's current recommendations are shown in Table 28–5. It should be emphasized that the administration of one dose of antivenin does not preclude the administration of another. If signs and symptoms persist or worsen after the first dose, more antivenin is needed.

The optimal time for giving antivenin is in the first four hours after the snake bite. Beyond this time, the efficacy of the antivenin progressively lessens. However, some benefit might be derived from late administration. Russell has identified venom in serum of victims as long as 26 hours after the snake bite,[60] which implies that the administration of antivenin even this late may be of benefit.

Other than the immediate complications of anaphylaxis, the major drawback to the administration of antivenin is the development of serum sickness. This complication is very common, occurring in as many as 75 percent of patients who receive antivenin.[74] Russell reports a 100 percent incidence in patients who receive more than seven vials (70 ml) of the antivenin.[60,67] The physician must watch for the development of serum sickness. Typically, symptoms develop six days to three weeks after antivenin administration. Symptoms include malaise, fever, arthralgia, swollen joints, urticaria, lymphadenopathy, and, rarely, peripheral neuritis and meningism.[67] Steroid therapy should be initiated at the onset of symptoms and continued until symptoms subside; at this point, dosage of the steroids is tapered. Wingert and Wainschel use dexamethasone, 16 mg initially administered intramuscularly and then 8 to 16 mg every four to six hours. For less severe symptoms, pred-

TABLE 28–5   Dosage of Antivenin

Category of Snake Bite	No. of Vials
No envenomation	None
Minimal	3–5
Moderate	6–9
Severe	10–20 or more

nisone, 40 mg by mouth every four to six hours, can be given.[68]

The use of steroids in the management of snake venom poisoning has been advocated in the past.[83,84] One author in particular has used large doses of steroids with good results.[84] Controlled studies in animals, however, demonstrated no advantage to steroids and in fact, suggest a detrimental effect.[85] Based on available data, there is no place for steroids in the management of snake bites.

Snake Identification

It is important to identify the biting snake in order to determine if a snake is indeed venomous and, if venomous, the probable severity of its envenomation. The snakes of some species are more dangerous than others because of their size or the nature of their venom. For example, the Eastern diamondback is the largest of the domestic rattlesnakes, and its bite results in some of the most severe envenomations.

Snake identification can be carried out at two levels. The treating physician can make the distinction between venomous and nonvenomous snakes, while the herpetologist can make a very specific identification. Identification by an expert should always be sought ultimately, but such an expert may not be available for several hours. The initial identification by the nonexpert, treating physician is probably clinically more important.

Venomous snakes in the United States (pit vipers and coral snakes) can be easily distinguished from nonvenomous snakes by a few simple characteristics. Pit vipers (e.g., *Crotalus, Agkistrodon,* and *Sistrurus*) have the following characteristics (see Figure 28–1):[83]

- the pit, a heat-sensing device, described as a depression between the eye and nostril
- vertically elliptical pupils
- the rattle (a series of rings composed of keratin not seen in *Agkistrodon* species)
- large anterior retractile maxillary fangs
- a single row of subcaudal scutes

These characteristics are contrasted to those of nonvenomous snakes in Figure 28–2.

Coral snakes must also be distinguished from nonvenomous snakes that closely mimic them.[83] The key to coral snake identification is knowing the sequence of their circumferential bands. The following are characteristic of the coral snake:

- The head is always black.
- Red and black bands are separated by more narrow yellow or white bands.

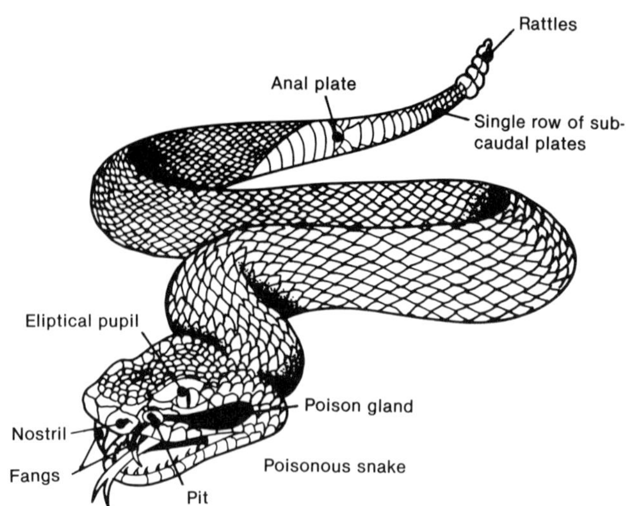

Figure 28–1 Poisonous Pit Vipers.

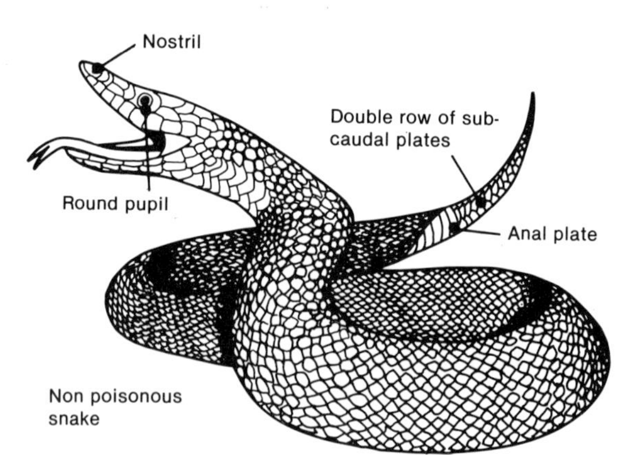

Figure 28–2 Nonpoisonous Snakes.

- Red bands are bordered on either side by yellow bands.

Coral snakes, in contrast to other venomous snakes, have round pupils and a double row of subcaudal plates.

Surgical Management

Some experts feel there is no place at all for surgery in snake bite therapy,[60] while others consider it the mainstay of therapy. Some use surgery as an adjunct to medical management, while others use surgery as the primary therapy, reserving antivenin as an adjunct only for very serious injuries.[86] As in most controversial areas of medicine, the correct therapy is not easily identified and may be between the two extreme positions.

Surgical management includes any or all of the following procedures: incision and suction, excisional therapy with or without extensive debridement, and fasciotomy. Incision and suction may have been performed as a first aid measure; if not, some clinicians feel that this procedure should be a routine part of definitive medical therapy. The procedure is recommended by some as a first step, even if two hours have elapsed since the injury was incurred.[74]

Excisional therapy is a popular form of treatment that has been practiced for many years. The exact technique of excision varies greatly among clinicians. Some recommend excising the skin and necrotic subcutaneous tissue only. The amount of tissue removed varies from an area of ¼ to 1 in. (approximately ½ to 2½ cm) distance from the fang marks.

Some experts take a more aggressive approach.[78,87] They advocate making a longitudinal incision into the affected tissue around the bite, excising necrotic tissue, and opening the deep fascia to inspect the underlying muscle. If necrotic, the muscle is also debrided. The majority of experts, however, are more conservative with fasciotomy and perform it only when vascular compromise is apparent.

The rationale for excisional therapy is based on Snyder's 1968 study involving radioisotope-labeled venom. He was able to demonstrate that 80 to 90 percent of the injected venom was present locally two hours after injection.[76] The proponents of this therapy feel that significant amounts of venom can be removed by excision, thus diminishing both the local and systemic toxic effects of the venom.

Those opposed to surgical management of snake bites, particularly Russell, feel that any surgical manipulation is unnecessary if antivenin is properly administered. Those in favor of surgery counter that the hazards of antivenin can be avoided by using excisional therapy and reserving antivenin for only the severe envenomations. Both groups argue strongly in support of their positions and cite good results from their respective protocols. The controversy is not readily resolved.

ARTHROPOD ENVENOMATION

All spiders are venomous, but they generally do not attack humans unless severely provoked. Except for the bites of a few species, spider bites do not cause serious problems. Most commonly, a local inflammatory reaction and a minor stinging pain at the time of the bite are the only symptoms. In the United States, the black widow (*Latrodectus mactans*) and the brown recluse (*Loxosceles reclusa*) are the two species that cause significant morbidity and mortality. In his ten-year survey from 1950 to 1959,[79] Parrish documented 65 deaths in the United States from spider bites. Two of these were by the brown recluse, the remaining 63 were attributed to the black widow.

Black Widow

The black widow spider is a small black spider with a characteristic red or yellow hourglass marking on the ventral surface of the abdomen. The body measures 6 mm in diameter, while its maximum leg span is 4 cm.[88] These spiders usually build their webs in wood piles, under rocks, or in outdoor structures, such as garages. Occasionally, however, they nest in houses; in such cases, victims often sustain bites while in bed or putting on clothing.[89] Geographically, the black widow is distributed throughout the continental United States.[88]

Venom

The venom of the black widow spider has not been specifically characterized. It may contain as many as 15 proteins and 5 nonproteins.[89] The venom appears to be mainly neurotoxic, with the primary site of action at the neuromuscular junctions. Although studies of the effects of black widow venom on isolated ganglia and neuroeffector junctions have been performed,[90–96] the venom's mechanism of action has not been precisely defined. Nevertheless, the black widow venom has been observed to cause an initial, massive release of neurotransmitter from the presynaptic membrane,[88,94] an initial increase in miniature end plate potentials,[95] an inhibition of presynaptic neurotransmitter reuptake,[93] and the inhibition of normal neurotransmission.

The role of calcium in the entire process is also unknown, although calcium seems to be required for the increased neurotransmitter release.[96] Black widow venom has been shown to increase intracellular calcium at the presynaptic nerve terminal, which results in mitochondrial swelling and clumping of neurotransmitter vesicles.[92] Exactly what this means in vivo is not clear.

Clinical Presentation

The clinical course of a person bitten by a black widow spider is usually benign. At the time of the bite, the patient feels an immediate stinging, sharp pain. This pain frequently causes the patient to kill and retrieve the spider, which is helpful diagnostically. After a few minutes, the pain becomes less severe and more dull in character. Usually, the next and most prominent symptom is muscle cramping. This symptom is delayed in onset, generally 15 minutes to 2 hours. The cramping can be local initially, but it usually becomes more generalized with time. If the upper extremity is involved, pleuritic chest pain may be severe, mimicking pulmonary embolism. Bites of the lower extremity tend to produce abdominal wall rigidity and pain, sometimes so severe that it simulates an acute abdomen. Other symptoms frequently elicited from victims of black widow spider bites include nausea, dizziness, headache, anxiety, and weakness.[88,89]

The signs of black widow spider bite generally complement the symptoms. Patients appear restless and in pain from their muscle cramps. Muscle spasms and fasciculations usually occur. The bite wound itself consists of two small puncture wounds surrounded by a small area of inflammation. There is no local necrosis. Other signs that may be seen include ptosis, edema, conjunctivitis, skin rash, pruritus, vomiting, and respiratory distress. Blood pressure may be elevated.

Victims with serious envenomations become weak, stuporous, and, sometimes, delirious. Seizures can occur, particularly in children. Shock and respiratory depression with their attendant symptomatology may develop. Death can occur.

Although the duration of symptoms is variable, the intensity of the symptoms usually peaks a few hours after the bite and then gradually diminishes. Symptoms are usually gone in 24 hours, but they may persist one to four days.[79]

The mortality rate associated with black widow bites is not known. Estimates of 4 to 5 percent[97] have been reported, but this seems exaggerated if one recalls that only 63 people died in a ten-year period from this spider's bite.[79] People generally recover completely from these bites.

Treatment

For most black widow spider bites, treatment is symptomatic. The most prominent symptom is muscle cramping, and therapy is aimed at relieving the pain of these cramps. Intravenous calcium gluconate has been used for many years for this purpose.[89] Although it is not a specific antidote and the physiologic basis for this treatment is not proved, anecdotal literature does support its use. As noted earlier, black widow venom increases nerve terminal intracellular calcium by allowing extracellular calcium to flow into the cells. Perhaps calcium gluconate replenishes this extracellular calcium, resulting in a cessation of tetanic contractions and fasciculations.

The calcium gluconate (10 ml in a 10 percent solution) can be administered in 50 to 100 ml fluid over 10 to 15 minutes. Exact guidelines for administration and the amount of calcium that should be given have not been established. Hypercalcemia can develop if treatment is overzealous.[98] (See Chapter 17.) It is advisable to give no more than two or three ampules over a two- to three-hour period and to monitor cardiac function during the infusion. If successful, pain relief is dramatic, usually occurring within minutes after administration.

Intravenous muscle relaxants have also been recommended.[89] Methocarbamol (Robaxin), given intra-venously over five minutes, may be very helpful in relieving symptoms. The dose is 1 gm (10 ml). The initial bolus can be supplemented with a drip of 500 to 1,000 mg in 250 ml of saline over one to two hours. If successful, therapy can be continued with oral Robaxin every six hours after the patient has been discharged. Intravenous diazepam (Valium) may be equally effective, but little is written on specific dosages.

Narcotics may be necessary to relieve the painful cramps induced by the black widow's bite. Meperidine hydrochloride (Demerol) or morphine may be given intramuscularly as needed every three to four hours. However, since the venom may cause respiratory depression, caution must be exercised in giving the narcotics. Antivenin is readily available in the United States[99] and may be needed to prevent serious secondary complications. Russell recommends that it be used in patients with hypertension or a history of hypertension and in patients less than 16 or more than 60 years of age.[89] The probable rationale for the age indications is the fact that most fatalities of black widow bites occur in these two age groups. Severe hypertension may be sustained, probably as a result of the action of the venom at the arteriolar neuromuscular junctions.

Antivenin must be administered with the same precautions required in the administration of snake bite antivenin. Skin testing is done prior to administration, and preparations must be made for the treatment of an anaphylactic reaction. The dose for adults and children is one vial (2.5 ml) of antivenin given intravenously in 10 to 50 ml saline over 15 minutes.[99] Relief of pain may be apparent in minutes, or it may take one to three hours. Like snake antivenin, spider antivenin is prepared from horse serum, and serum sickness is therefore a possible complication. The amount of antivenin given for spider bites is much smaller than that given for snake bites, however, and serum sickness is therefore less likely.

Admission to the hospital for black widow bites is usually not necessary. Patients who require antivenin as well as patients whose symptoms cannot be controlled by the measures outlined obviously should be hospitalized. Again, the elderly and the young should be observed as inpatients, even if antivenin is not given. The usual patient can be treated successfully by several hours of observation and symptomatic treatment in the emergency department, followed by oral administration of muscle relaxants and/or minor pain medications.

Brown Recluse

The other spider in the United States that can cause significant morbidity and, rarely, mortality is the brown recluse spider. This spider is light brown in color and has a characteristic dark brown, violin-shaped marking on the dorsum of its thorax. The spider is small in size, being 1 to 1.5 cm in length and 0.5 to 1 cm in width. As the name implies, this spider is not a social animal and tends to remain in dark areas, such as closets and basements.[88]

Epidemiology

The geographical distribution of the recluse spider in the United States is limited to the southeastern and South Central states, including Tennessee, Kentucky, Georgia, Alabama, Indiana, Illinois, Ohio, Iowa, Missouri, Kansas, Oklahoma, Arkansas, Mississippi, Louisiana, Texas, and South Carolina.[100] Other species of *Loxosceles* have been identified in Arizona, New Mexico, and southern California.[100] Isolated cases of recluse bites have been recorded from other states, possibly indicating an expanding range.

The incidence of recluse spider bites is not precisely known, but the fact that only two deaths were reported in the ten-year survey by Parish[79] suggests that the incidence is probably not high. According to Hufford's review, over 150 case reports are recorded in the literature, the first being in 1940.[100]

Venom

The venom of the brown recluse has been analyzed by several investigators, and the presence of esterase, protease, lipase, and hyaluronidase has been reported. The absence of phospholipase A, C, and D has also been reported. Geren and coworkers, utilizing thin layer gel filtration and Sephadex column chromatography, have been able to identify several venom components of varying toxicity. The same authors have shown no direct hemolysis of human red cells in vitro and no antigen-antibody activity in the venom.[101] The fact that hemolysis can occur after a brown recluse bite indicates either that these investigators did not have enough venom in their preparation or that the hemolysis occurs by an unexplained indirect process.

Clinical Presentation

The clinical manifestations of the brown recluse bite can be divided into common local effects and systemic effects. The local effects are referred to as necrotic arachnidism. Typically, the victim feels no pain or only a mild stinging sensation at the time of the bite. Local pain and a blue gray constrictive halo around the bite are usually the only manifestations in the first 8 hours after the bite.[100,102] After 12 to 18 hours, a bleb that is surrounded by a zone of erythema and edema develops. This area progresses to aseptic necrosis, dry gangrene, and eschar formation over the next five to seven days.

When the eschar separates, an open ulcer remains. The sequence of events leading to necrotic arachnidism is thought to be endothelial damage, fibrin formation, platelet thrombi, and leukocyte infiltration.[100]

Systemic symptoms from the *Loxosceles* bite include fever, chills, malaise, nausea, vomiting, and arthralgias. More serious problems, which are usually seen in children, include disseminated intravascular coagulation, convulsions, hemolysis, renal failure, and death.[100,102] As stated, the symptoms of the recluse spider bites range from local pain to death. The reason for this varied sensitivity is not known. Fortunately, the serious systemic complications are relatively uncommon.

Treatment

As the treatment for bites of the brown recluse spider has not been well established, it is controversial. Steroids have not been unequivocally proved effective, but most authors recommend their use. The exact dosage and type of steroid is not clearly defined, but pharmacologic doses are generally given. In addition to systemic steroids, intralesional injections of steroids have also been given in an attempt to halt local necrosis; however, the results of this treatment are not clear. Many of the patients with local necrosis eventually require surgical debridement and grafting. In fact, some authors recommend early excision and grafting as primary therapy.[103,104]

The treatment of systemic complications is entirely symptomatic. Hemolytic anemia is treated by transfusion as needed, and the secondary hemoglobinuria is treated by hydration and alkalinization.[102] Disseminated intravascular coagulation is also treated in the established fashion, i.e., with supportive care, replacement therapy, and, possibly, heparin.

Scorpions

Scorpionism in the United States is a problem limited to the Southwest, in particular, to Arizona. Although there are approximately 40 species of scorpions in the United States, only one, *Centruroides sculpturatus*, possesses a potentially lethal venom. This species is located primarily in Arizona, but it can also be found in parts of Texas, California, and northern Mexico.[105]

Scorpions are not aggressive creatures and generally sting humans only in self-defense. They do not envenomate by biting, as spiders do, but by stinging. Venom is produced in a specialized segment at the tail called a telson. A stinger located at the caudal end of the telson delivers the venom into the scorpion's adversary. Scorpion activity varies with temperature and tends to reach a peak in the cool of the evening. It is during this time that most scorpion stings occur.

Venom

Certain effects of scorpion venoms are species-specific and cannot be attributed to all scorpions. The *C. sculpturatus* venom is primarily neurotoxic. It contains four neurotoxins[106] that appear to act at neuronal synapses and neuromuscular junctions. Increased sodium permeability of the presynaptic neuron of neuronal synapses[107] and possibly increased calcium permeability of the presynaptic neuron at the neuromuscular junctions have been demonstrated (although the latter has not been shown with centruroid venom).[107] Increased calcium permeability leads to increased acetylcholine release at the neuromuscular junction and causes muscle twitching and fibrillation. The clinical significance of the findings is not known.

Clinical Presentation

The clinical manifestations of scorpionism include a great many symptoms, some of which are helpful diagnostically. Unlike the nonlethal sting of the *Vejovis spinigerus*, the *C. sculpturatus* sting produces no local signs of inflammation and swelling. In fact, the exact site of the sting cannot be determined in most instances, in spite of the fact that one of the most common symptoms is local pain with hyperesthesia.[89,105,108] Another common sign is extreme restlessness and agitation. This agitation is so severe that it may be mistaken for seizure activity.[105] In Rimsza's series, this sign was limited to those patients under ten years of age. Rimsza also noted roving eye movements, a sign that had not previously been reported, in 8 of her 24 patients.[105] Other signs of *C. sculpturatus* stings include tachycardia, hypertension, tachypnea, salivation, blurred vision, poor coordination, slurred speech, paresthesia, wheezing, vomiting, stridor, and dysphagia.[105] Respiratory depression is a less common symptom and may actually be a complication of oversedation.

Treatment

The treatment for stings of nonlethal scorpions is symptomatic and nonspecific.[89] The management of the *C. sculpturatus* sting is also largely symptomatic. In the past, heavy sedation with barbiturates has been recommended to control agitation, but there seems to be no advantage to this treatment and, in fact, it may result in respiratory depression. Measures to support ventilation and blood pressure should be taken as necessary. An antivenin derived from goats is available through the Arizona State University at Tempe, Arizona; it has not undergone adequate clinical investigation,[105] and its use is currently limited. It does, however, remain an option in cases of severe envenomation. Steroids are frequently used for scorpion stings, but are of no proved benefit.

The mortality statistics for *C. sculpturatus* stings are interesting. Stahnke reported that from 1929 to 1948 scorpions were responsible for more deaths in Arizona than any other venomous animal, including rattlesnakes.[108] More recent statistics, however, differ markedly. In the past ten years, there have been no reported deaths from scorpion stings in Arizona.[105] The improved survival is probably a reflection of more sophisticated supportive care and possibly more effective eradication programs.

The need for tetanus prophylaxis in spider and scorpion bites is not clear. Generally, routine tetanus prophylaxis is recommended.

HYMENOPTERA

The class hymenoptera contains many stinging insects, but only a few of these insects are associated with anaphylaxis, e.g., the honey bee, the yellow jacket, hornets, wasps, and fire ants.[109,110]

Unlike the previously discussed animals who inflict their injury by direct trauma, infection, or by injection of potent venoms, hymenoptera cause morbidity and mortality by inducing anaphylaxis. Although these creatures inject venom into their victims, only in cases of massive numbers of stings does the venom itself cause a serious problem. Rather, the reaction of sensitized patients to the injected venom is responsible for the serious morbidity and death that the hymenoptera sting can cause.

Epidemiology

The incidence of hymenoptera sting, though unknown, must be extremely high given the large number of hymenoptera and the number of people who have experienced their stings. The incidence of sting anaphylaxis, obviously, is much lower. It is estimated that approximately 0.4 percent of the population in the United States are at risk for serious reactions.[111] Most often, sensitive patients give a history of sting reactions that were initially small and progressed to extensive local reactions and, ultimately, to systemic reactions. There are, however, many exceptions to this typical pattern. Some individuals deny any previous stings or report only "normal reactions" prior to a serious systemic reaction. Others claim repeated systemic reactions with no evidence of progression or variation. Fifty percent of 2,606 sting allergy patients surveyed by the Insect Allergy Committee of the American Academy of Allergy reported no warning of their systemic reactions, based on previous stings.[112] This suggests that many people with sting allergy are unprotected simply because they are unaware that they have such an allergy.

Stings are likely to occur under a variety of circumstances. People who handle the insects, such as bee keepers and their families, are obviously at great risk. Accidental or intentional encroachment on hives or nests also provokes an attack and subsequent stings. Walking in meadows or going barefoot in clover patches can result in stings when the insects are disturbed. Other practices that attract the insects and therefore increase the chances of a sting are wearing brightly colored clothes or sweet-smelling fragrances, or eating sweets outdoors.[113]

Venoms

Like other venoms, hymenoptera venoms are complex poisons. Detailed analyses of all the important hymenoptera are not available, but analyses of the honey bee and wasp venoms, particularly the former, are well characterized.[114,115] Honey bee venom consists of three groups of pharmacologically and biochemically active ingredients: biogenic amines, nonenzymatic proteins and polypeptides, and enzymes. Biogenic amines, which include histamine, dopamine, and norepinephrine, account for about 1 percent of the venom. Their clinical effects are minimal and are obscured by the presence of other substances in the venom. The proteins and polypeptides include mellitin, apamin, mast cell degranulating peptide (MCD-peptide) and minimine.[115] Mellitin is the major component of bee venom (50 percent by weight) and probably accounts for the majority of its toxicity. It is a basic polypeptide with hydrophilic and hydrophobic terminals. Its main action is to alter cell permeability, which can result in hemolysis of red blood cells or the destruction of any other cells it contacts. Indirectly then, mellitin could destroy specific cells and release lysosomal enzymes. Clinically speaking, mellitin causes local pain and increases vascular permeability.[115]

Apamin is a neurotoxin, but its exact mechanism of action is unknown. The substance seems to affect the central more than the peripheral nervous system and has an excitatory effect.[115]

MCD-peptide, composed of 22 amino acids, comprises 1 to 2 percent of bee venom. The substance is very potent in its effect on mast cells, causing them to release histamine and other vasoactive substances.[115]

Minimine is a minor peptide found in bee venom; its effects are not well-known. It accounts for 3 percent of the venom volume.

Of the enzymes present in bee venom, those of known clinical importance include phospholipase A and possibly B, hyaluronidase, and acid phosphatase. The primary action of phospholipase A is the hydrolysis of phospholipids, particularly in membranes, resulting in cell destruction and the release of toxic reaction products such as lysolecithin, a hemolysin. Fortunately, not all phospholipids are susceptible to phospholipase A, which limits its toxicity.[115] Hyaluronidase is present in significant amounts in bee venom (2 to 3 percent by weight). It is not toxic, but it acts as a spreading factor, allowing the toxic components of the venom to disseminate.[115] Acid phosphatase does not produce serious toxic effects, but it is one of the major allergens of the venom.[116]

Wasp venom is similar to bee venom with some notable differences.[115] In addition to histamine, dopamine, and norepinephrine, wasp venom contains serotonin. Wasp venom does not contain any of the proteins and polypeptides of bee venom, but it does possess a kinin similar to bradykinin. Enzymes include hyaluronidase and phospholipase A and B.[116]

The clinical significance of the hymenoptera venom is minimal. In the usual case of one or a few stings, the venom is not systemically toxic. With great numbers of simultaneous stings, however, systemic toxicity is possible.

The most important allergens in bee venom are phospholipase A, hyaluronidase, acid phosphatase, mellitin, and allergen C–9.[116] Of these, phospholipase A is the most important.[117] Wasp allergens are antigen-5 (a protein of unknown function), phospholipase A, and hyaluronidase. Of these, antigen-5 is the most important.

Clinical Presentation

The signs and symptoms of hymenoptera sting vary from minimal local reactions to anaphylactic shock. The onset of symptoms may be immediate or delayed.

Local Reaction

The "normal" response to a sting is an immediate, sharp, burning pain that is accompanied in a few minutes by swelling and itching.[109] Part of the stinging apparatus may be retained in the victim, particularly if it is a honey bee sting, because the stinger of the honey bee is barbed and cannot be removed by the bee. The usual local reaction is minimal, involving a 2 sq in. area.[109]

Extensive local reactions may involve an entire extremity. Because the swelling is contiguous with the sting site and because there are no systemic manifestations, these reactions are classified as local. It is important to note these types of reactions, however, since they may indicate increasing sensitivity in the patient.

Such patients are at greater risk for systemic reactions with subsequent stings.[112]

Stings of certain body areas are problematic even if the reaction is local. Stings of the eye can be very damaging, particularly to the cornea and structures of the anterior chamber. Severe pain and photophobia, corneal clouding and edema, or iritis and hypopyon can occur.[118] Intraoral stings are also important, since airway-occluding edema may result.[119] (See Chapter 57.)

Systemic Reactions

An allergic response to a sting is indicated by a systemic reaction. These reactions vary in severity and symptomatology. Minimal systemic signs and symptoms may include diffuse pruritus, urticaria, swelling distant from the sting site, or flushing. More severe reactions are so labeled because of their location or because they interfere with vital functions.[112,120] For example, even with no other systemic manifestations, laryngeal edema is an immediate threat to life. Severe bronchospasm and bronchorrhea can severely compromise oxygenation. Profound hypotension, a frequent component of anaphylaxis, has obvious serious ramifications, including myocardial infarction, brain damage, and renal failure.

Delayed Reactions

Arbitrarily defined as reactions that begin more than 1 hour after injury, delayed reactions may also be local or systemic. Although most serious anaphylactic reactions occur within the first hour, a significant percentage of serious and fatal reactions are delayed even up to 48 hours. The mechanism for the delay is not well understood, but it is clinically well documented.[112]

Treatment

In the nonsensitive patient, the treatment of hymenoptera stings is nonspecific and symptomatic. In the sting-allergic patient, treatment can be divided into immediate care, prevention of subsequent stings, self-treatment, and hyposensitization.

Immediate treatment varies with the severity of the reaction, but the mainstay of therapy is epinephrine. Management of anaphylactic reactions consists of appropriate supportive care and administration of drugs to counteract the anaphylactic reaction (see Chapter 6, Shock). Supportive measures include airway management and blood pressure support with intravenous fluids and, occasionally, vasopressors. Specific drugs for counteracting anaphylactic reactions include epinephrine and theophylline, which inhibit the release of vasoactive substances; antihistamines, which counteract the peripheral effects of some of the vasoactive substances,

and steroids, whose role is unknown.[121] The route of administration and dosages of these agents vary with the severity of the reaction. It should be emphasized that, although steroids are helpful, they have no immediate beneficial effect. Their action is delayed for several hours, and therefore steroids should not be given as the sole treatment of anaphylaxis.

Prevention of subsequent stings in sensitized patients is a matter of common sense. Practices such as going barefoot, strolling in flower gardens, and wearing perfumes or brightly colored clothes outdoors should be avoided.

Self-treatment for sting allergy patients involves kits for emergency treatment. These kits consist of a syringe of 1:1,000 epinephrine, needles, antihistamine tablets, and a tourniquet. Allergic patients are taught how to administer the epinephrine. One other measure that might be considered self-treatment is wearing a Medic Alert tag. All patients with sting allergies should wear such tags to help ensure prompt treatment even if they are unconscious.

Hyposensitization is the most promising treatment for sting-allergic patients. Allergic reactions are mediated by IgE antibodies. (See Chapter 57.) In sensitized patients, production of these IgE antibodies has been stimulated by previous stings. On reexposure to the antigen, these antibodies mediate the anaphylaxis. The purpose of hyposensitization is to stimulate the production of IgG blocking antibodies.[122,123] This is accomplished by injecting a small dose of venom intradermally. This dose is gradually increased until it approximates the venom transmitted by two insect stings; this amount is then given as a maintenance dose every month for the rest of the patient's life. More than 95 percent of those treated by this technique can tolerate subsequent bee stings without developing anaphylaxis.[124]

For a number of years, allergists debated the relative effectiveness of hyposensitization with whole body extract versus venom.[125,126] The controversy now appears to be resolved—whole body extract has been shown to be ineffective and should no longer be given for hyposensitization.[110,124,126] Unfortunately, venom hyposensitization is very expensive. Furthermore, there remains a number of unanswered questions, e.g., which patients should undergo hyposensitization and what level of IgG antibody is protective.[124,127] It is hoped that these questions will be answered as experience with the technique grows, because, of all the biting and stinging creatures discussed, hymenoptera account for the most deaths in the United States, 29 to 100/year.[111,120,128,129]

REFERENCES

1. Beck AM: The public health implications of urban dogs. *Am J Public Health* 65:1315–1317, 1975.

2. Moore RM, Zehmer RB, Moulthrop JI, Parker RL: Surveillance of animal-bite cases in the United States, 1971–1972. *Arch Environ Health* 32:267–270, 1977.

3. Berzon DR, Farber RE, Gordon J, Kelly EB: Animal bites in a large city—A report on Baltimore, Maryland. *Am J Public Health* 62:422–426, 1972.

4. Harris D, Imperato PJ, Oken B: Dog bites—An unrecognized epidemic. *Bull NY Acad Med* 50:981–1000, 1974.

5. Animal Control Survey, April 1971—December 1971. The American Humane Association, 1972.

6. Kizer KW: Epidemiologic and clinical aspects of animal bite injuries. *JACEP* 8:134–141, 1979.

7. Berzon DR: Medical costs and other aspects of dog bites in Baltimore. *Public Health Rep* 89:377–381, 1974.

8. Winkler WG: Human deaths induced by dog bites, United States, 1974–75. *Public Health Rep* 92:425–429, 1977.

9. Douglas LG: Bite wounds. *Am Fam Physician* 11:93–99, 1975.

10. Graham WP, Calabretta AM, Miller SH: Dog bites. *Am Fam Physician* 15:132–137, 1977.

11. Schultz RC, McMaster WC: The treatment of dog bite injuries, especially those of the face. *Plast Reconstr Surg* 49:494–500, 1972.

12. Callaham ML: Treatment of common dog bites: Infection risk factors. *JACEP* 7:83–87, 1978.

13. Goldstein EJC, et al: Editorial—Animal bites. *JACEP* 7:417, 1976.

14. Callaham, M: Prophylactic antibiotics in common dog bite wounds: A controlled study. *Ann Emerg Med* 9:410–414, 1980.

15. Goldstein EJC, Citron DM, et al: Bacteriology of human and animal bite wounds. *J Clin Microbiol* 8:667–672, 1978.

16. Torphy DE, Ray CG: *Pasteurella multocida* in dog and cat bite infections. *Pediatrics* 43:295–297, 1969.

17. Thomson HG, Svitek V: Small animal bites: The role of primary closure. *J Trauma* 13:20–23, 1973.

18. Zook AG, et al: Successful treatment protocol for canine fang injuries. *J Trauma* 20:243–247, 1980.

19. Bobo RA, Newton EJ: A previously undescribed gram-negative bacillus causing septicemia and meningitis. *Am J Clin Pathol* 65:564–569, 1976.

20. Butler T, et al: Unidentified gram-negative rod infection. *Ann Intern Med* 85:1–5, 1977.

21. Findling JW, Pohlmann GP, Rose HD: Fulminant gram-negative bacillemia (DF-2) following a dog bite in an asplenic woman. *Am J Med* 68:154–156, 1980.

22. West M, Gibbs M, Hansman D: *Pasteurella multocida* infection after a dog bite. *Med J Aust* 1:585–586, 1976.

23. Szalay GC, Sommerstein A: Inoculation osteomyelitis secondary to animal bites. *Clin Pediatr* 11:687–689, 1972.

24. Klein DM, Cohen ME: *Pasteurella multocida* brain abscess following perforating cranial dog bite. *J Pediatr* 92:588–589, 1978.

25. Gump DW, Holden RA: Endocarditis caused by a new species of *Pasteurella*. *Ann Intern Med* 75:275–278, 1972.

26. O'Riordan WD, Hubbell DV: Compound depressed skull fracture. *JACEP* 5:123–124, 1976.

27. Diphtheria and tetanus toxoids and pertussis vaccine. *Morbidity Mortality Weekly Rep* 26:41, 1977.

28. Fraser DW: Preventing tetanus in patients with wounds, editorial. *Ann Intern Med* 84:95–97, 1976.

29. Bailie WE, Stowe EC, Schmitt AM: Aerobic bacterial flora of oral and nasal fluids of canines with reference to bacteria associated with bites. *J Clin Microbiol* 223–231, 1978.

30. Lee MLH, Buhr AJ: Dog-bites and local infection with *Pasteurella septica*. *Br Med J* 1(1):169–171, 1960.

31. Stevens DL, Higbee JW, Oberhofer TR, Everett ED: Antibiotic susceptibilities of human isolates of *Pasteurella multocida*. *Antimicrob Agents Chemother* 16:322–324, 1979.

32. Thompson RL: The cephalosporins. *Mayo Clin Proc* 52:625–630, 1977.

33. Rosenthal SL, Freundlich LF: In vitro sensitivity of *Pasteurella multocida*. *Health Lab Sci* 13:246, 1976.

34. Tindall JP, Harrison CM: *Pasteurella multocida* infections following animal injuries, especially cat bites. *Arch Dermatol* 105:412–416, 1972.

35. Veitch JM, Omer GE: Case report: Treatment of catbite injuries of the hand. *J Trauma* 19:201–202, 1979.

36. Peeples E, Boswick JA, Scott FA: Wounds of the hand contaminated by human or animal saliva. *J Trauma* 20:383–389, 1980.

37. Francis DP, Holmes MA, Grandon G: *Pasteurella multocida*. *JAMA* 233:42–45, 1975.

38. Boyce F: Human bites: An analysis of 99 (chiefly delayed & late) cases from Charity Hospital of Louisiana at New Orleans. *South Med J* 35:631, 1942.

39. Boyce F: Human bites: A study of a second series of 93 cases from the Charity Hospital of Louisiana at New Orleans. *Southern Surgeon* 14:690, 1948.

40. Butz R: Human bites, a series treated with antibiotics. *Am J Surg* 91:525, 1956.

41. Boland F: Morsus humanis. *JAMA* 116:127–131, 1941.

42. Hultzen JR: Partial gangrene of the left index finger. *JAMA* 55:857, 1910.

43. Mason M, Koch S: Human bite infections of the hand. *Surg Gynecol Obstet* 51:591, 1930.

44. Welch CE: Human bite infections of the hand. *N Engl J Med* 215:901, 1936.

45. Levin I, Longacre A: Antibacterial therapy in infections resulting from human bites. *JAMA* 147:815, 1951.

46. McMaster P: Human bite infections. *Am J Surg* 45:60, 1939.

47. Mann RJ, et al: Human bites of the hand: Twenty years of experience. *J Hand Surg* 2:97–104, 1977.

48. Chuinard RG, D'Ambrosia RD: Human bite infections of the hand. *J Bone Joint Surg* 59-A:416–418, 1977.

49. McConnell CM, Neale HW: Two-year review of hand infections at a municipal hospital. *Am Surg* 45:643–646, 1979.

50. Malinowski RW, et al: The management of human bite injuries of the hand. *J Trauma*, 19:655–659, 1979.

51. Guba AM, Mulliken JB, Hoopes JE: The selection of antibiotics for human bites of the hand. *Plast Reconstr Surg* 56:538–541, 1975.

52. Farmer C, Mann R: Human bite infections of the hand. *South Med J* 59:515, 1966.

53. Kock S: Acute rapidly spreading infections following trivial injuries of the hand. *Surg Gynecol Obstet* 59:277, 1934.

54. Kanavel AB: *Infections of the Hand*, ed 6. Philadelphia, Lea & Febiger, 1933.

55. Robinson IB, Loskin DM: Tetanus of oral origin. *Oral Surg* 10:831, 1957.

56. Owen HR: Chancre complicating laceration of the hand. *Ann Surg* 8:783, 1928.

57. Kankat CT: Direct innoculation of tuberculosis through bite on cheek by tuberculous patient. *Turk Tip Cemiy Meem* 12:168, 1946.

58. Robinson RH: Actinomycosis of the sub-cutaneous tissue of the forearm secondary to a human bite. *JAMA* 124:1049, 1944.

59. MacQuarrie MB, Forghani B, Wolochow DA: Hepatitis B transmitted by a human bite. *JAMA* 230:723–724, 1974.

60. Russell FE: *Snake Venom Poisoning*. Philadelphia, JB Lippincott, 1980.

61. Wingert WA, Wainschel J: Diagnosis and management of envenomation by poisonous snakes. *South Med J* 68:1015–1026, 1975.

62. Parrish HM, Carr CA: Bites by copperheads (*Ancistrodon contortrix*) in the United States. *JAMA* 201:107–112, 1967.

63. Parrish HM, Khan MS: Bites by coral snakes: Report of 11 representative cases. *Am J Med Sci* 77:561–568, 1967.

64. Jimenez-Porras JM: Biochemistry of snake venoms. *Clin Toxical* 3:389–431, 1970.

65. Clement JF, Pietrusko RG: Pit viper snakebite in the United States. *J Fam Pract* 6:269–279, 1978.

66. Hasiba Ute, Rosenbach LM, Rockwell D, Lewis JH: DIC-like syndrome after envenomation by the snake, *Crotalus horridus horridus. N Engl J Med* 292:505–507, 1975.

67. Strickland NE: Snake bites: A review. *J Arkansas Med Soc* 73:69–77, 1976.

68. Wingert WA, Wainschel J: A quick handbook on snake bites. *Med Times* 105:68–75, 1977.

69. Parrish HM, Hayes RH: Hospital management of pit viper venenations. *Clin Toxicol* 3:501–511, 1970.

70. Russell FE, et al: Snake venom poisoning in the United States. *JAMA* 233:341–344, 1975.

71. Sabback MS, Cunningham ER, Fitts CT: A study of the treatment of pit viper envenomization in 45 patients. *J Trauma* 14:569–573, 1977.

72. Rosenberg P: Pharmacology of phospholipase A-2 from snake venoms, in Lee CY (ed): *Handbook, Experimental Pharmacology, Snake Venoms.* New York, Springer-Verlag, 1979, pp 403–447.

73. Russell FE: First-aid for snake venom poisoning. *Toxicon* 4:285–289, 1976.

74. McCollough NC, Gennaro JF: Treatment of venomous snakebite in the United States. *Clin Toxicol* 3:483–500, 1970.

75. Watt CH: Poisonous snakebite treatment in the United States. *JAMA* 240:654–656, 1978.

76. Snyder CC, Pickins JE, Knowles RP, et al: A definitive study of snakebite. *J Florida Med Assoc* 55:330–337, 1968.

77. McCullough NC, Genarro JF: Evaluation of venomous snake bite in the southern United States from parallel clinical and laboratory investigation: Development of treatment. *J Fla Med Assoc* 49:959, 1963.

78. Glass TG: Early debridement in pit viper bites. *JAMA* 235:2513–2516, 1976.

79. Parrish HM: Analysis of 460 fatalities from venomous animals in the United States. *Am J Med Sci* 245:129–141, 1963.

80. Goldstein EJD, et al: Bacteriology of rattlesnake venom and implications for therapy. *J Infect Dis* 140:818–821, 1979.

81. Russell FE, Ruzic N, Gonzalez H: Effectiveness of Antivenin (Crotalidae) Polyvalent following injection of *Crotalus* venom. *Toxicon* 71:461–464, 1973.

82. Wyeth Antivenin (Crotalidae) Polyvalent, advertisement. Marietta, Pa, Wyeth Laboratories, 1977.

83. Minton SA: Identification of poisonous snakes. *Clin Toxicol* 3:347–362, 1970.

84. Glass TG: Early debridement in pit viper bite. *Surg Gynecol Obstet* 136:774–776, 1973.

85. Cunningham ER, et al: Snakebite: Role of corticosteroids as immediate therapy in an animal model. *Am Surg* 45:757–759, 1979.

86. Huang TT, et al: The use of excisional therapy in the management of snakebite. *Ann Surg* 179:598–607, 1974.

87. Henderson BM, Dujon EB: Snake bites in children. *J Pediatr Surg* 8:729–733, 1973.

88. Toewe, CH: Bug bites and stings. *Am Fam Physician* 21:90–95, 1980.

89. Russell FE: Venomous animal injuries. *Curr Probl Pediatr* 3:3–47, 1973.

90. D'Ajello V, Magni F, Bettini S: The effect of the venom of the black widow spider *Latrodectus mactans tredecimguttatus* on the giant neurones of *Periplaneta americana. Toxicon* 9:103–110, 1971.

91. Frontali N, et al: Purification from black widow spider venom of a protein factor causing the depletion of synaptic vesicles at neuromuscular junctions. *J Cell Biol* 68:462–479, 1976.

92. Smith JE, Clark AW, Kuster TA: Suppression by elevated calcium of black widow spider venom activity at frog neuromuscular junctions. *J Neurocytol* 6:519–539, 1977.

93. Rothlin RP, et al: Supersensitivity to norepinephrine induced in vitro by crude *Latrodectus mactans* venom in the rabbit ear artery. *Toxicon* 15:71–74, 1977.

94. Pumplin DW, McClure WO: The release of acetylcholine elicited by extracts of black widow spider glands: Studies using rat superior cervical ganglia and inhibitors of electrically stimulated release. *J Pharmacol Exp Ther* 201:312–319, 1977.

95. Pinto JEB, et al: Peripheral adrenergic effect of *Latrodectus mactans* venom. *Toxicon* 11:395–400, 1973.

96. Pardal JF, Granata AR, Barrio A: Influence of calcium on H-noradrenaline release by *Latrodectus antheratus* (black widow spider) venom gland extract in arterial tissues of the rat. *Toxicon* 17:455–465, 1979.

97. Breland OP: Bionomics and significance of some venomous arthropods. *Cutis* 19:749–757, 1977.

98. Black widow spider bite, in Rumack B (ed): *Poisindex.* Englewood, Colo., Micromedex, 1981.

99. Antivenin (*Latrodectus mactans*), MSD. advertisement, Merck Sharp & Dohme, West Point, Pa., 1975.

100. Hufford DC: The brown recluse spider and necrotic arachnidism: A current review. *J Arkansas Med Soc* 74:126–129, 1977.

101. Geren CR, et al: Composition and properties of extract of fiddleback (*Loxosceles reclusa*) spider venom apparatus. *Toxicon* 11:471–479, 1973.

102. Madrigal GC, et al: Toxicity from a bite of the brown spider. *Clin Pediatr* 11:641–644, 1972.

103. Auer AI: Surgery for necrotic bites of the brown spider. *Arch Surg* 108:612–618, 1974.

104. Hershey FB, Aulenbacher CE: Surgical treatment of brown spider bites. *Ann Surg* 170:300–308, 1969.

105. Rimsza ME, Zimmerman DR, Bergeson PS: Scorpion envenomation. *Pediatrics* 66:298–302, 1980.

106. Rabin DR, et al: Amino acid sequence of neurotoxin I from *Centruroides sculpturatus Ewing. Arch Biochem Biophys* 166:125–134, 1975.

107. Cahalan MD: Modification of sodium channel gating in frog myelinated nerve fibres by *Centruroides sculpturatus* scorpion venom. *J Physiol* 244:511–534, 1975.

108. Stahnke HL: The Arizona scorpion problem. *J Ariz Med Assoc* 7:23–29, 1950.

109. Itkin: Bee sting. *Am Fam Physician* 13:124–125, 1976.

110. Busse WW, et al: Immunotherapy in bee-sting anaphylaxis. *JAMA* 231:1154–1156, 1975.

111. Reisman RE; Stinging insect allergy. *J Allergy Clin Immunol* 64:3–4, 1979.

112. Insect Allergy Committee of the American Academy of Allergy: Insect-sting allergy. *JAMA* 193:109–114, 1965.

113. Frazier CA; The hazards of hymenoptera. *Am Fam Physician* 15:91–96, 1977.

114. Banks BEC, Hanson JM, Sinclair NM: The isolation and identification of noradrenaline and dopamine from the venom of the honey bee, *Apis mellifica. Toxicon* 14:117–125, 1976.

115. Habermann E: Bee and wasp venoms. *Science* 177:314–322, 1972.

116. Hoffman DR: Allergens in hymenoptera venom. V. Identification of some of the enzymes and demonstration of multiple allergens in yellow jacket venom. *Ann Allergy* 40:171–175, 1978.

117. Sobotka A, et al: Honeybee venom: Phospholipase A as the

major allergen, abstracted. *J Allergy Clin Immunol* 53:103–104, 1974.

118. Gilboa M, Gdal-on M, Zonis S: Bee and wasp stings of the eye. Retained intralenticular wasp sting: A case report. *Br J Ophthalmol* 61:662–664, 1977.

119. Mader CL: Intraoral hymenoptera sting. *JADA* 100:386–387, 1980.

120. Feingold BF: Allergic reactions to hymenoptera stings. *J Asthma Res* 9:55–70, 1971.

121. Kelly JF, Patterson R: Anaphylaxis. *JAMA* 227:1431–1436, 1974.

122. Lessof MH, Sobotka AK, Lichtenstein LM: Effects of passive antibody in bee venom anaphylaxis. *Johns Hopkins Med J* 142:1–7, 1978.

123. Muller U, Johansson SGO, Streit C: Hymenoptera sting hypersensitivity: IgE, IgG and haemagglutinating antibodies to bee venom constituents in relation to exposure and clinical reaction to bee stings. *Clin Allergy* 8:267–272, 1978.

124. Lichtenstein LM, Valentine MD, Sobotka AK: Insect allergy: The state of the art. *J Allergy Clin Immunol* 64:5–12, 1979.

125. Voss HE, Coleman M: Treatment of bee stings, editorial. *N Engl J Med* 291:16, 1974.

126. Lichtenstein LM, Valentine MD, Sobotka AK: A case for venom treatment in anaphylactic sensitivity to hymenoptera sting. *N Engl J Med* 290:1223–1227, 1974.

127. Yunginger JW: The sting—revisited, editorial. *J Allergy Clin Immunol* 64:1–2, 1979.

128. Gottlieb PM, et al: NIH consensus development conference on emergency treatment of insect sting allergy. *J Allergy Clin Immunol* 63:77–79, 1979.

129. Barnard JH: Studies of 400 hymenoptera sting deaths in the United States. *J Allergy Clin Immunol* 52:259–264, 1973.

29. Hyperthermia

MICHAEL L. CALLAHAM, M.D.

Heat illness is a spectrum of disease resulting from the physiologic toll of attempting to maintain normal body temperature in the face of a large internal or environmental heat load. The body's cooling mechanisms are usually well equipped to cope with the ordinary heat loads experienced every day in normal life. However, if heat load is great enough even the healthiest of persons may experience heat illness.

The spectrum of heat illness ranges from minor (and poorly understood) types such as heat edema and heat syncope to the most lethal form, frank heat stroke. These entities are discussed separately in this chapter.

HEAT STROKE

Heat stroke occurs when the body is unable to maintain temperature control, and body temperature rises to levels of 105.8°F (41°C) or higher, interfering with central nervous system, cardiovascular and cellular function. If the condition is not promptly reversed, permanent disability or death will occur.

Heat stroke occurs when the internal or external heat load exceeds the ability of the body's cooling mechanisms to dissipate it. The result is a net gain in total body heat, and thus a rise in temperature.

Pathology

Cellular metabolism increases 13 percent for each 1°C (1.8°F) rise in temperature; at 105°F (40.6°C) metab-olism is 50 percent above normal. As metabolism increases cellular needs outstrip oxygen supply, and at 107.6°F (42°C) oxidative phosphorylation becomes uncoupled. At about 113° to 114.8°F (45° to 46°C) direct cell breakdown begins. All organ systems are affected, and the underlying pathology is that of cell death, literally by cooking.

Pathophysiology and Clinical Correlates

The basic defect in heat stroke is cooling system failure. There is wide individual variation in ability to tolerate heat load, but all humans rely on circulation of blood (functioning as a coolant) from the hot inner core to the dilated vessels in the cooler skin where heat is lost to the atmosphere. The heat load can come from either the environment or from the body itself. Environmental heat load is created by

- ambient air temperatures higher than that of the body (saunas or even hot tubs);
- high humidity (which reduces the evaporation of sweat, and therefore, of cooling);
- high radiant heat loads (as in hot metal buildings, automobiles, or ship boiler rooms).

Increased endogenous heat load is created by:

- fever;
- hyperactivity from delirium tremens, seizures, psychosis;

- muscular exertion from work, athletics, or labor during childbirth (e.g., healthy marathon runners develop rectal temperatures of 104°F (40°C));
- malignant hyperthermia, a rare form of heat load caused by a genetic defect of cell membrane, triggered by exposure to anesthetic drugs.

The cardiovascular system and skin bear the brunt of dissipating this heat load. Skin vessels dilate increasing blood flow up to 20-fold as peripheral vascular resistance drops. This in effect creates a shunt of up to 4 liters per minute. To maintain normal blood pressure (BP), cardiac output must double or quadruple. This is accomplished partially by increased stroke volume, but mostly by increased rate. Despite this cooling, with sufficient heat load body temperature will rise, and eventually a point will be reached where cardiac output cannot meet cooling needs. At this point hypotension occurs.

There is a continuum from the normal physiologic response to heavy heat load (tachycardia, temperature elevation to 104°F (40°C), tachypnea, lactic acidosis with exertion, and lowered glomerular filtration rate) to actual heat stroke. Normally the body's cooling systems remain able to maintain body temperature at a stable, although somewhat elevated, level. In heat stroke, however, such control is lost and the temperature soars out of control, to levels of 107.6°F (42°C) or higher, where cell damage is virtually certain. The exact temperature varies among individuals; some have demonstrated true heat stroke at temperatures of only 105.8°F (41°C). In addition, cell and organ damage is a function of time and temperature, not temperature alone. Concomitant hypotension, acidosis, and dehydration also greatly increase the severity and irreversibility of heat damage.

Diagnosis

It is frequently stated that the diagnosis of heat stroke is made on the basis of body temperature (usually some absolute figure is given) and hot dry skin. Recent physiologic research proves neither of these beliefs true. The heat stroke victim has an elevated temperature (often 107.6°F (42°C) or higher) but there is considerable individual variation. In addition, even the simplest of initial cooling efforts by bystanders or prehospital health teams may have lowered the temperature several degrees. In addition, perfectly well athletes exercising in the heat have rectal temperatures to 104°F (40°C). Thus elevated temperature is suggestive, but not diagnostic of heat stroke.

Dry skin is also not a prerequisite. Many heat stroke victims present this way, particularly the elderly classic heat stroke (CHS) victim, who is often dehydrated from several days of illness and inability to obtain sufficient oral fluids. However, external heat stroke (EHS), usually seen in healthy young athletes, soldiers, and laborers, often presents with copious sweating still present.

The diagnosis of heat stroke, then, calls for a high index of suspicion. It is a diagnosis that must be made quickly, as time is critical in reversing it and preventing permanent disability or death. The CNS is the organ system that fails first in the heat stroke. Therefore, *the diagnosis of heat stroke must be suspected whenever alteration or loss of consciousness (including bizarre behavior) occurs under conditions of internal or external heat load.*

Typically, CNS dysfunction starts with irritability and poor judgment, then progresses to incoherence, confusion, delirium, seizures, and frank coma. Tremor, dystonia, decerebrate positioning, transient hemiplegia, and fixed and dilated pupils have all been reported, and all are potentially reversible with prompt cooling. (See Chapter 47.)

The following presenting symptoms are usually, but not invariably, present:

- Hot flushed skin, either with or without sweating.
- Tachycardia (to 180).
- Hypotension (representing high-output cardiac failure).
- Hyperventilation (to 60)—the resultant respiratory alkalosis can cause tetany.
- Vomiting and diarrhea are common.

Laboratory work-up of a suspected heat stroke patient is only done *after* cooling is initiated. It should include:

- Complete blood cell count (CBC)—(WBC often elevated to 30,000).
- Platelet count, prothrombin time, partial thromboplastin time, fibrin degradation products—all clotting factors are decreased in heat stroke, and disseminated intravascular coagulation (DIC) is seen as a late complication.
- Glucose.
- Blood gases; metabolic acidosis is very common and may be severe enough to need treatment.
- Electrolytes and blood urea nitrogen (BUN).

Although many lab tests are abnormal in heat stroke, none are diagnostic except SGOT, lactate dehydrogenase (LDH), and creatine phosphokinase (CPK), which are often spectacularly high on admission. Repeated normal serum enzymes essentially rule out heat stroke. In infections and other diseases, enzymes are elevated slightly if at all on admission, and fall promptly with treatment. In heat stroke, values rise for the next 7 to 14 days even with prompt treatment.

Differential Diagnosis

In most situations, differential diagnosis should be entertained *after* cooling has begun, not before. No harm will be done to patients with other causes of elevated temperature, and critical treatment will not be delayed (with disastrous results) in those who have heat stroke. Those with heat stroke will respond to cooling with lowered temperature and usually improved mental status and a return to normal blood pressure. If they do not, the differential is essentially that of febrile coma, particularly:

- Meningitis or encephalitis. The diagnosis is made by lumbar puncture, which is normal in heat stroke.
- Cerebral falciparum malaria is rare in nontropical areas. The peripheral blood smear confirms the diagnosis.

Other possibilities in the differential are diagnosed by history, initial blood work, and early clinical course; they include:

- Seizure disorders.
- Cerebrovascular accident (CVA).
- Thyroid storm. This is essentially a clinical diagnosis. The initial treatment, which fortunately includes modalities, such as cooling, used in heat stroke.
- Diabetic ketoacidosis.
- Severe heat exhaustion. There is a gray zone between this entity and heat stroke; heat exhaustion is also reported with temperatures to 41° to 42°C, hypotension, and confusion. Serum enzymes are normal. Initial treatment should be the same as for heat stroke.

Treatment

The mainstay of treatment is rapid *cooling*. In the field, patients' clothing should be removed, and they should be moved to a cool location and have any available aqueous liquids or ice splashed on them. Fanning and massaging (to prevent cold-induced vasoconstriction and thus decreased rate of cooling) are also helpful.

Once the patient arrives in the emergency department, this process is continued if the rectal temperature is 41°C or greater. (Most clinical thermometers register no higher than 42°C; a long steel thermistor is preferable as it has a higher range, gives continuous readings, and will not break during seizures.) Immersion in a tub of ice water, though controversial, is the quickest method, but impractical unless staff is experienced with it.

For the emergency department that does not treat heat stroke frequently, ice water soaks are more practical and almost as effective. The patient's clothing should quickly be removed, and the patient wetted down with a slurry of water and ice chips. A fan directed over the area will help maximize cooling. It is helpful to place sheets or towels on the patient and to wet them, because they absorb the liquid keeping it in contact with the patient's skin and preventing its running on the floor, which creates a safety hazard. The sheets or towels should be changed frequently and kept cold. The contact with the ice will cause reflex vasoconstriction in the skin, which will slow core cooling. To counteract this, body massage must be carried out continually during cooling to aid circulation.

Cooling by this method is rapid. When the temperature declines to 39°C, cooling is stopped to avoid overcooling, which may result in hypothermia. Rebound hyperthermia may occur three to six hours after cooling. Heat stroke patients have poor thermoregulatory control for months after the episode, and it may become permanent.

No scientific study or comparison of cooling methods in humans has been done. Although other methods have been used, they are not as effective as the icing method just described. Cold air inhaled by intermittent positive-pressure breathing (IPPB), cold intravenous (IV) solutions, and cold gastric lavage are all useful but contribute only a small fraction of the needed cooling. Ice water enemas are ineffective (since pelvic venous circulation is poor) and may cause water intoxication. Peritoneal lavage with dialysate solution at 6° to 10°C cooled dogs at 0.56°C per minute—five times more rapidly than an ice slush bath—and therefore increased survival rates.[1] This presumably was due to the immediate initial cooling of the core rather than the exterior. Its use has not been reported yet in humans.

Aspirin is ineffective in heat stroke; it acts by returning to normal the thermoregulatory set-point, which is elevated in fever. Heat stroke is a different phenomenon; the set-point remains normal, but the organism is physically incapable of eliminating enough heat to maintain it.

Simultaneous with cooling, the airway, arterial oxygen tension, IV fluids, dehydration, and hypotension must be addressed. The airway should be protected since coma, convulsion, and vomiting are common; this usually mandates endotracheal intubation. Although arterial oxygen saturation is usually normal, tissue oxygen needs are high, and oxygen enrichment may be helpful. An IV infusion should be started with normal saline (NS) or Ringer's lactate, or 5.5 percent dextrose in normal saline; no one fluid has demonstrated superiority over another.

Patients may or may not be dehydrated. If not hypotensive, aggressive fluid replacement should await evaluation of dehydration by serum sodium, hematocrit, and BUN.

Hypotension

This may simply represent high output failure, or true volume depletion. Hypotension usually responds to cooling, but it also increases the risk of renal failure, so that it should be remedied as soon as possible. This suggests that a central venous pressure (CVP) line or Swan-Ganz catheter should be placed, a fluid challenge of 250 to 500 cc be given over several minutes, and the patient's response carefully watched in terms of pulse, BP, and CVP or pulmonary wedge pressure. Fluid replacement can continue aggressively until BP is normal or CVP or pulmonary wedge pressure rise excessively. When this happens, fluid overload is a risk, particularly in view of the incidence of acute renal failure of 5 percent in CHS and 25 percent in EHS. In this manner, treatment is individualized, and only patients who really need large volumes of fluid will receive them.

Shivering

Violent shivering, leading to convulsions, often is seen as cooling proceeds. Such shivering generates heat and should be suppressed. Chlorpromazine is the drug usually recommended, in a dose of 25 to 50 mg IV. Chlorpromazine suppresses shivering and decreases metabolic oxygen consumption; it also dilates skin vessels and thus maximizes cooling. However, chlorpromazine also lowers the seizure threshold, and thus would seem to be contraindicated. No controlled studies of any kind in humans exist, but empirically the problem of increased seizures has not been noted. Controlled studies on this issue are needed.

Barbiturates also inhibit shivering and decrease oxygen demand, but some types can obscure the sensorium for long periods of time. Thiopental sodium has been used successfully, despite its theoretical anticonvulsant inferiority to phenobarbital. Diazepam reverses the seizures but does not decrease oxygen consumption. Phenytoin is reported to be ineffective.

Electrolyte Disorders

Serum potassium often is low, usually due to the hyperventilation and respiratory alkalosis seen in heat stroke. When this is the cause, the hypokalemia is transient. Serum potassium does not accurately reflect total body potassium, which may be low, particularly during the first few weeks of acclimatization. Hypokalemia in the presence of acidosis indicates a true deficit and the need for replacement. Much more serious is a high potassium level, most often seen in EHS, reflecting cell damage to muscles from exertion or seizures, and later, renal failure. Treatment is the same as for other causes of potassium abnormalities. Calcium occasionally is drastically decreased, especially in EHS patients with rhabdomyolysis. It usually is fruitless to treat this hypocalcemia, since any elevation of plasma levels will be transient because the calcium is rapidly deposited in injured muscle. A few days later, it will dissolve and may cause hypercalcemia if the patient is anuric. Glucose may be normal or quite low.

ECG Changes

Virtually any abnormalities may be seen, with non-specific ST- and T-wave changes most common. Myocardial infarction may be simulated, or actually precipitated. Arrhythmias and bundle branch blocks are also seen, and revert to normal with cooling.

Further Treatment

Any patient with heat stroke needs hospital admission, as major cellular injury has occurred. Late complications (occurring within six hours to three days of admission) should be anticipated, and include the following.

Acute Renal Failure

Some 5 percent of CHS and 25 percent of EHS patients develop renal failure. (See Chapter 63.) Hypotension probably contributes to its development; renal blood flow is compromised under even mild heat stress. Early fluid replacement to correct this decreased perfusion is vital. The use of mannitol and furosemide to maintain urine output is advocated by some, but is still controversial. Dialysis is needed for hyperkalemia and rising BUN. Abnormalities in all clotting factors in the direction of hypocoagulability are pronounced in heat stroke. In severe cases they may lead to a DIC syndrome. Treatment with heparin and epsilon-aminocaproic acid (EACA) is the same as for DIC coagulopathies caused by other illnesses. Initial studies are useful for baseline values. The more prolonged the prothrombin time early in the case, for example, the more severe the damage.

Rhabdomyolysis

Rhabdomyolysis may be seen in EHS, with muscle tenderness, myoglobinuria, and the danger of ischemic compartment syndromes. Patients with rhabdomyolysis have dangerously elevated levels of potassium, elevated uric acid, CPK up to 1 million, and plummeting calcium. There is a huge plasma leak into damaged tissues, and

10 to 12 liters of fluid may be needed the first day. Treatment consists of fluid replacement, calcium replacement if respiratory and CNS dysfunction dictate it, and efforts to prevent renal failure by diuresis with mannitol and furosemide.

Liver

Liver damage is virtually universal and is signaled in the second day by jaundice and falling prothrombin levels; the latter may need treatment with vitamin K.

CNS Sequelae

If the patient survives the first 24 hours, recovery may be complete or partial. The brain is most sensitive to irreversible damage; any of the CNS symptoms mentioned earlier may persist. Cerebellar defects are the most common. The other major sequela in survivors is an apparently permanent susceptibility to heat stroke in the future, combined with relatively unstable thermoregulatory control.

Prognosis

The duration of coma provides a rough guide to prognosis. If coma is present for more than ten hours, a fatal outcome is likely. Coma of less than three or four hours usually indicates a favorable outcome.

Also useful in the first 24 hours are SGOT levels. Less than 1,000 IU/liter indicates a good prognosis with serious brain, liver, and kidney damage unlikely; greater than 1,000 IU/liter indicates likely damage to all three organs and high mortality. The duration of the high temperature, rapidity of cooling, and preexisting disease and predisposing factor all help predict severity as well. A rectal temperature greater than 42.2°C on admission is also a poor prognostic sign.

HEAT EXHAUSTION

Presenting Symptoms

The symptoms of heat exhaustion are very vague and nonspecific. They include headache, giddiness, anorexia, nausea and vomiting, malaise, thirst, muscle cramps, irritability, and anxiety. There may be orthostatic blood pressure drops, tachycardia, and syncope; the patient may or may not be significantly dehydrated. Temperature is usually normal or only moderately elevated (to 38°C or so). There are no lab tests diagnostic of this condition, although BUN, hematocrit, and sodium may be increased if dehydration is severe.

Differential Diagnosis

From the nonspecificity of the symptoms, it is obvious that heat stroke is a diagnosis of exclusion. The typical patient is elderly and has one or several of the predisposing factors listed in Exhibit 29–1. They come to medical attention due to a flulike malaise. The diagnosis is made if other illness can be excluded, and a source of heat load (such as a heat wave or broken air-conditioning at home) can be identified.

Treatment

The treatment of heat stroke is as nonspecific as are the symptoms. It consists of rest in a cool place and rehydration. Dehydration is common, and is assessed by orthostatic changes in BP, rapid pulse, elevated serum sodium, hematocrit and BUN. The amount and type of fluid replacement depends on these findings. In mild

Exhibit 29–1 Predisposing Factors in Heat Stroke

Patient types
  Elderly
  Athletes and military recruits (particularly the
    unacclimatized)
  Individual sensitivity
  Previous episodes of heat stroke

Physiologic predispositions
  Dehydration (especially deliberate weight loss in
    athletes)
  Fever
  Hyperactivity from: seizures
                       delirium
                       psychosis
                       psychomimetic drugs
                       labor of childbirth
  Abnormalities of skin: burns
                          severe sunburn
                          cystic fibrosis
                          scleroderma
  Drugs: anticholinergics: tricyclic antidepressants
                            antihistamines
                            antispasmodics
                            phenothiazines
         alcohol
  Lack of acclimatization
  Fatigue, lack of sleep
  Heavy clothing
  Infection or reaction to immunization

Environmental
  High temperature
  High humidity
  High radiant heat load
  Hot mini-environments: enclosed vehicles in sun
                          deep mines
                          ship boiler rooms
                          saunas
                          hot tubs
                          hot springs

cases, oral 0.1 percent saline solution will suffice. In more serious cases, NS, D5.5NS, or 0.5NS may be used IV according to the patient's cardiovascular status. For example, a fit young soldier may receive 4 liters of fluid in six to eight hours. Patients should be well in 12 hours and can be discharged with no expected sequelae.

HEAT CRAMPS

Presenting Signs and Symptoms

Heat cramps—painful cramps in an otherwise well person—usually affect the most used muscles, such as shoulders and thighs, and often commence after the end of work. They usually occur in young, muscular athletes or laborers during hard work in hot weather. These individuals sweat copiously (more than unacclimatized persons), which helps keep them cool but also increases their losses of salt in the sweat. They drink large quantities of hypotonic fluids, usually water, and do not take any salt supplements. It is theorized that the cramps occur as a result of a falling serum sodium level, although this is unproved.

Differential Diagnosis

Heat cramps are most often confused with tetany from other causes. This can include the cramps of muscle exhaustion or hyperventilation. The history usually suffices to make the diagnosis, but arterial blood gases will help pinpoint hyperventilation in difficult cases. (It should be noted that moderate hyperventilation is a normal response to heat.) The patient with hyperventilation will still be hyperventilating when seen by the physician, whereas the person with heat cramps will not. Although hypocalcemia or one of the other myriad causes of tetany is usually mentioned in the differential diagnosis, it is extremely rare, and lab work to rule out such conditions is not justified in straightforward cases.

Treatment

The treatment of heat cramps is very simple. It consists of salt. This is most easily given orally as 0.1 percent saline solution (two 10-grain tablets or ¼ teaspoon salt in 1 quart of water). Plain salt tablets should not be swallowed whole since they cause gastrointestinal (GI) irritation, nausea, and vomiting. Alternately, NS solution can be given IV. The cramps quickly disappear with this treatment (if they have not done so with rest and a cool environment alone) and have no permanent effects.

OTHER SYNDROMES

This chapter focuses on three types of heat illness: heat stroke, heat exhaustion, and heat cramps. Although eight types of heat illness are listed in Exhibit 29–2, the last five types are not serious disorders and are discussed only briefly. They are reviewed in more detail elsewhere, but there is very little information about their diagnosis and treatment.[2,3]

Heat edema is a self-limited mild swelling and tightness of hands and feet (occasionally even appearing as pitting edema of the ankles) which appears in the first few days of exposure to a hot environment.

Heat tetany is the occurrence of carpopedal spasms during exposure to heat. Although the Chvostek sign may be positive, serum calcium is normal. Heat tetany probably is related to the hyperventilation seen universally in persons under heat load; it develops in those in whom the changes in pH and body temperature are the most rapid, rather than simply the greatest. Heat tetany may appear in persons suffering other heat syndromes such as heat exhaustion or heat stroke. It is self-limiting and resolves promptly on removal of the person from the hot environment.

Heat syncope is simply postural hypotension causing syncope in unacclimatized persons in the early days of heat exposure. Water and salt depletion do not contribute to it. It probably is related to the large shunt through dilated cutaneous vessels. Rest and the avoidance of sudden or prolonged standing are adequate treatment.

Prickly heat is an erythematous maculopapular rash that causes a prickly sensation. It occurs chiefly in unacclimatized persons in humid regions, where the skin constantly is kept wet from unevaporated sweat. The only treatment is to provide access to air conditioning to allow several hours a day of dry skin.

Anhidrotic heat exhaustion is a poorly understood syndrome of weakness, failure of normal sweating, and vasopressin-resistant polyuria which occurs after several months of heat acclimatization. It is preceded by prickly

Exhibit 29–2 Spectrum of Heat Illness

1. Failure of thermoregulation   Heat stroke

2. Thermoregulation maintained
   Heat exhaustion
     Water depletion
     Salt depletion
   Heat cramps
   Heat edema
   Heat tetany
   Heat syncope
   Prickly heat
   Anhidrotic heat exhaustion

heat in 80 percent of cases, often involves slightly elevated temperature, and may lead to heat stroke. Knochel has shown that a total-body potassium depletion of about 517 mEq (20 percent) occurs by the third week of acclimatization and has postulated this as the cause of this syndrome. Treatment involves rest in a cool environment and potassium supplements may be useful since serum potassium does not reflect the depletion of body stores.

PREVENTION

It never will be possible to prevent all heat illness, even in the disciplined military environment, due to the multiple risk factors. However, substantial decreases in incidence can be effected. The factors listed in Exhibit 29–1 should be avoided as much as possible.

Exertion should be timed to avoid sunlight exposure. Light clothing should be worn; it should minimize the amount of sun striking the body, but should otherwise permit maximal air flow over body surfaces. This is particularly pertinent in sports such as football and auto racing where heavy clothing may mandate cancellation at lower temperatures than shown in Exhibit 29–3.

Fluid intake is most critical. In the past, fluid restriction in sports has been the rule. Nothing could be more dangerous. Fluids should be encouraged before and during all heavy exertion, even when persons do not feel thirsty.

Dehydration is universal in persons working in the heat. Such persons are at least 3 percent dehydrated

and do not replace fluid lost by exertion regardless of availability of drinks. Sweat losses can be large, on the order of 1.5 liters/hour. Sodium and potassium also are lost by this route, but the loss of water is far more important than the loss of electrolytes. Additionally, work in the heat produces an almost immediate plasma volume decrease of 10 to 14 percent, because water shifts into muscle cells in response to the osmotic gradient created by the breakdown of glycogen during exercise.

Dehydration by itself has been shown to elevate the rectal temperatures of runners; in one study it was found that 5 percent dehydration elevates rectal temperature about 2.5°C by the end of the race.[4,5] Even 1 percent dehydration causes a decrement in work and hemodynamic performance. Wrestlers often lose weight deliberately to make weight classes. Match winners had much lower specific gravities of urine (less than 1.015) than did losers.[6] Dehydration, especially hypernatremic dehydration, long has been known to increase body temperature even at rest.

Before competition, 400 to 500 ml of fluids should be consumed, as well as a minimum of 200 to 300 ml at 20-minute intervals during exertion. Although athletes may feel they are receiving adequate fluid, studies show this is not the case.[7] Runners are unable to gauge their own fluid consumption accurately, and football players replace only 65 percent of measured weight loss after two hours of practice. In regular sports practice, daily weights should be taken; a weight loss of 3 percent indicates the need for increased fluid intake. A weight loss of 5 percent should cause cancellation of that individual's participation that day, and 7 percent may require prompt fluid replacement.

The choice of liquid used for fluid replacement is a matter of some debate. The goal is to maximize voluntary intake and gastric emptying, so that the fluid rapidly can enter the small bowel, where it is absorbed. Authorities differ as to whether plain water or electrolyte solutions are most beneficial to athletes. Gastric emptying is accelerated by large volumes (500 to 600 ml) at cold temperature (10° to 15.8°C). The ideal osmolality for rapid emptying is about 200 mOsm/liter or less. A typical solution contains 2.5 gm of glucose and 0.2 gm of sodium chloride per 100 ml of water. Several commercial solutions of this type are available. Solutions with higher osmolality drastically slow gastric emptying.

Full fluid restoration does not occur until six to eight hours after exertion, regardless of efforts to increase intake. There appears to be no need to replace electrolytes or glucose during exertion; only water is needed. After exertion, supplements of minerals may be needed, including iron and magnesium, which are lost in sweat. However, further studies of these losses are needed to

Exhibit 29–3 Wet-Bulb Globe Temperature and Recommended Activity Levels

°C	°F	Activity
15.6	60	No precautions.
19 to 21	66 to 70	No precautions as long as water, salt, and food are easily available.
22 to 24	71 to 75	Postpone sports practice, avoid hiking.
24	76	Lighter practice and work with rest breaks.
27	80	No hiking or sports.
28	82	Only necessary heavy exertion with caution.
30	85	Cancel all exertion for unacclimatized persons; avoid sun exposure even at rest.
31.5	88	Limited brief activity for acclimatized, fit personnel only.

Source: Adapted from Callaham M: *Emergency Management of Heat Illness.* Emergency Physician Monograph Series, American College of Emergency Physicians, 1979.

determine precise requirements. For practical purposes, cold water or weak electrolyte solutions are probably equally good initial replacements.

Salt supplements generally are not needed, since the body's ability to conserve sodium is great. Many natives of tropical areas maintain work in the heat on 3 to 5 gm of sodium a day or less, with no dietary salt supplements of any kind. The average western diet with no added salt contains 4 to 5 gm of sodium chloride; the average salted diet contains two to three times more. The salted diet is sufficient for most situations, particularly in the acclimatized person whose sodium conservation in sweat glands and kidneys is high. The large sodium supplements (10 to 20 gm/day) previously recommended not only are not needed, but are actually harmful. They slow acclimatization, paradoxically increase potassium loss, and worsen symptoms of heat exhaustion if given acutely.

The ingestion of salt tablets without fluid replacement increases the risk of hypernatremic dehydration and cardiovascular collapse. During acclimatization, a potassium deficit of 500 mEq develops by the second to third week (the time when most cases of heat stroke occur) due to inappropriate urinary secretion. Dietary sodium supplements actually worsen this deficit. Perhaps the only time salt supplements may be needed is in brief exposures to work in the heat in unacclimatized persons who sweat less but lose more sodium in their sweat than acclimatized persons. Even then, liberal salting of food usually will be adequate.

Potassium supplements have not been well studied in relation to heat illness. It is known that a potassium deficit occurs in persons who are not yet acclimatized and are not receiving a potassium supplement. There is no potassium deficit in the fully acclimatized person when dietary intake (70 to 100 mEq) is adequate to replace sweat losses. The issue needs to be studied further, but there seems to be no reason for supplementation.

Acclimatization is another means of preventing heat illness. This process takes several weeks; it can be accomplished partially by exertion in a cool environment, but can occur fully only with exertion in heat. Exercise should occur in graduated increases of one to two hours a day. Unacclimatized persons should take extra precautions, as should those with any of the predisposing risk factors previously discussed.

A wet-bulb globe temperature (WBGT) index is the most accurate measure of environmental heat stress. The WBGT measures three forms of heat load. A regular thermometer measures dry air temperature. A wet-bulb thermometer measures the effect of humidity on temperature. The globe thermometer measures the effect of radiant heat. Details for construction and measurement are available in Army, Navy, and Air Force Technical Bulletin No. 175.[8] Activity should then be based on the WBGT reading, as shown in Exhibit 29–3.

Since the WBGT is complex, and 70 percent of the resultant value is derived from the wet-bulb temperature, an economical and simple alternative is the construction of a sling psychrometer, which measures wet-bulb temperature (air passing over the wetted thermometer bulb cools the bulb in inverse proportion to humidity). Construction of such a device is described in Army, Navy, and Air Force Technical Bulletin No. 175.[8]

Public education is another important prophylactic measure. Athletes in particular should know that some of the unpleasant sensations experienced during exertion in the heat may be warnings of imminent collapse. The severity of heat stroke must be emphasized to the public, as must its simple but life-saving treatment. Organizers of athletic events have a responsibility to encourage and even demand adequate fluid intake before and during competition. Coaches, team physicians, school nurses, and others have a responsibility to be knowledgeable about the risk and symptoms of heat illness and to ensure that athletes observe basic precautions.

REFERENCES

1. Bynum GP, Patton J, Bowers W, et al: Peritoneal lavage cooling in an anesthetized dog heat stroke model. *Aviat Space Environ Med* 49(6): 779–784, 1978.
2. MacPherson RK, O'Brien JP: Effects of heat, in Hunter G, Swartzwelda JC, Clyde DF (eds): *Tropical Medicine*, ed 5. Philadelphia, WB Saunders Co, 1976.
3. Callaham M: Heat illness, in Rosen P, Dailey R, Braen R, et al (eds): *Advanced Textbook of Emergency Medicine*. New York, CV Mosby Co, in press.
4. Maron M, Wagner J, Horvath SM: Thermoregulatory responses during competitive marathon running. *J Appl Physiol* 42:909–914, 1977.
5. Wyndham CH: Heat stroke and hyperthermia in marathon runners. *Ann NY Acad Sci* 301:128, 1977.
6. Hursh L: Food and water restriction in the wrestler. *JAMA* 241:915–916, 1979.
7. American College of Sports Medicine, Position statement: Prevention of heat injury during distance running. *Med Sci Sports* F(1):VII, 1975.
8. Etiology, prevention, diagnosis, and treatment of adverse effects of heat. Department of Army, Navy, and Air Force Technical Bulletin No. 175, April 1969.

BIBLIOGRAPHY

Bartley JD: Heat stroke: Is total prevention possible? *Milit Med* 142:528, 1977.

Bynum GP, Randolf KB, Schuette WH, et al: Induced hyperthermia in sedated humans and the concept of critical thermal maximum. *Am J Physiol* 235:R228–R236, 1978.

Callaham M: *Emergency Management of Heat Illness*. Emergency Physician Monograph Series, American College of Emergency Physicians, 1979.

Costrini AM, Pitt HA, Gustafson AB, et al: Cardiovascular and metabolic manifestations of heat stroke and severe heat exhaustion. *Am J Med* 66:296, 1979.

Cowes GHA, O'Donnell TF: Heat stroke. *N Engl J Med* 291:564, 1974.

Dasler AR, Karas S, Bourman JS, et al: Adverse effects of supplementary sodium chloride on heat adaptation, abstracted. *Fed Proc* 32:336, 1973.

Ellis FP: Mortality and morbidity associated with heat exposure. *Int J Biometeorol* 6(suppl 2):36, 1976.

Ellis FP: Heat illness. *Trans R Soc Trop Med Hyg* 70:402–425, 1976.

Greenleaf, JE, Convertino VA, Stremel RW, et al: Plasma, Na, Ca, and volume shifts and thermoregulation during exercise in man. *J Appl Physiol* 43:1026–1032, 1977.

Heat stroke, medical staff conference, University of California at San Francisco. *West J Med* 121:305–312, 1974.

Hubbard RW, Matthew WR, Criss REL, et al: Role of physical effort in the etiology of rat heat stroke injury and mortality. *J Appl Physiol* 45:463–468, 1978.

Kew MC: Temperature regulation in heat stroke in man. *Isr J Med Sci* 12–759, 1976.

Kew MC, Bershas I, Sefteh H: The diagnostic and prognostic significance of the serum enzyme changes in heat stroke. *Trans R Soc Trop Med Hyg* 65:325, 1971.

Knochel JP: Dog day and siriasis: How to kill a football player. *JAMA* 233:513–515, 1975.

Knochel JP: Environmental heat illness: an eclectic review. *Arch Intern Med* 137:841–864, 1974.

Knochel JP, Dotin LN, Hamburger RJ: Potassium depletion during physical conditioning in a warm climate. *Clin Res* 16:388, 1968.

Ladell WSS: Disorders due to heat. *Trans R Soc Trop Med Hyg* 51:189–216, 1957.

O'Donnell T: The hemodynamic and metabolic alterations association with acute heat stress injury in marathon runner. *Ann NY Acad Sci* 301:262–269, 1977.

Rhabdomyolysis, medical staff conference, University of California at San Francisco. *West J Med* 125:298–304, 1976.

Ryan AF: Balancing heat stress, fluids and electrolytes. *Physician Sports Med* August:43–52, 1975.

Shapiro Y, Magazanik A, Udassin R, et al: Heat intolerance in former heat stroke patients. *Ann Intern Med* 90:913–916, 1979.

Shepard RJ, Kavanagh T: Fluid and mineral needs of middle-aged and postcoronary runners. *Physician Sports Med* May:90–102, 1978.

Shibolet S, Lancaster M, Danon Y: Heat stroke: A review. *Aviat Space Environ Med* 47(3):200–301, 1976.

Simon HB: Extreme pyrexia. *JAMA* 236:2419–2421, 1976.

30. Hypothermia

MICHAEL L. CALLAHAM, M.D.

ACCIDENTAL HYPOTHERMIA

The term accidental hypothermia is applied to a human body temperature of less than 35°C (95°F) when it occurs accidentally due to disease or exposure to a cool environment. It excludes all forms of therapeutic hypothermia, such as are used in cardiac surgery, and that induced by anesthesia.

Etiology

Ultimately, all accidental hypothermia is caused by the loss of body heat to the environment. Since the environmental temperature is usually less than that of the human body, this can happen under many circumstances. Often conditions are not severe environmentally, but certain of the patient's conditions predispose to heat loss in excess of heat production.

Many disease states predispose a person to such excess heat loss, and thus bring the patient to medical attention with the problem of hypothermia (Exhibit 30–1). Some mental diseases and CNS lesions are thought to affect the hypothalamic thermostat. Spinal cord transection causes loss of cutaneous vasomotor control, one of the body's major mechanisms of heat conservation. Myxedema is the most common endocrine disorder presenting with hypothermia, which is caused by decreasing heat production via a lowered metabolic rate. Alcohol depresses thermoregulation, reduces shivering, causes vasodilation and thereby loss of heat to the environment, and produces immobility and decreased sensory awareness. Barbiturates do the same in large doses, as do phenothiazines. Interestingly, alcohol and barbiturates also seem to exert a protective effect against hypoxia on the cells of the CNS, thus helping protect against some of the effects of hypothermic coma. A number of metabolic states, such as hypoglycemia, uremia, and sepsis, can produce hypothermia by means not fully understood. Burns, exfoliative skin disease, and large amounts of cold intravenous (IV) infusions (as in trauma resuscitation) cause excess heat loss despite normal or increased heat production.

The aged are prone to hypothermia even in the absence of disease; their ability to regulate body temperature declines, as does their awareness of cold. Surveys of elderly persons living at home have consistently found that about 10 to 20 percent of them have oral temperatures of 35°C (95°F) or lower. Neonates are also very susceptible due to their proportionately greater ratio of surface area to body mass, and less subcutaneous fat.

Finally, healthy and fit individuals can become hypothermic when inadequately protected from cold and wet weather. These conditions need not be extreme; a body temperature of 26.7°C (80°F) is fatal in the majority of cases, and yet this is the temperature of a warm summer day. Improper clothing is as significant as environmental temperature in causing hypothermia in campers and hikers. Wind chill is another very significant factor. Wetness is even more critical, since heat loss is increased fivefold by wet skin, and 25 times by immersion in cold water. For example, even the fittest person immersed in 2°C (35°F) water for one hour has a 99 percent expectancy of death. Movement in water increases heat loss, so that in most cases attempts at swimming ashore are not recommended unless the distance is only about 1 kilometer.

In air, exercise helps combat hypothermia by generating heat, but at the risk of eventual exhaustion. However, after a rest period it takes more exercise to regain lost heat than if no rest break is taken. In addition, one of the early symptoms of hypothermia is poor judgment and irrational behavior, which sometimes leads victims to take off their clothes due to an illusory sensation of heat.

Exhibit 30–1 Predisposing Factors in Hypothermia

Disease States
  CNS:
    CVA
    cerebral neoplasm
    basilar skull fracture
    Parkinsonism
    Wernicke's encephalopathy
    spinal injury (above T1)
    Shapiro's syndrome
  Mental disorders:
    schizophrenia
    paranoia
    senile dementia
    anorexia nervosa
  Endocrine:
    hypopituitarism
    hypothyroidism
    adrenal failure
  Drugs:
    alcohol
    barbiturates
    phenothiazines
  Metabolic:
    hypoglycemia
    uremia
    diabetes
    shock
    sepsis
    protein undernutrition
    trauma (including massive cold IV
      infusions and blood
      transfusions)
    extremes of age
  Skin:
    burns
    exfoliative dermatitis
    (erythroderma)
Exposure
  Wet and cold weather

Pathology

Specific pathologic changes are few. All cases develop fatty changes in myocardium, renal tubules, adrenals, and liver. Many organs demonstrate multiple infarcts, presumably due to shock, hypoxia, acidosis, and sludging of red cells. Pancreatitis seems to be particularly common. However, many victims are elderly and ill, making interpretation of such changes difficult.

Pathophysiology and Symptoms

Heat loss in humans is largely controlled by constriction of skin vessels, controlling blood flow and thus heat loss through the skin. This cutaneous heat loss occurs via radiation, convection, and conduction, and is greatly accelerated by wind and wetness, as previously described. Humans respond to this heat loss by vasoconstriction, and then, as body temperature begins to drop, by shivering. Shivering increases heat production fivefold by increasing muscular work, but also increases heat loss. It is generally thought to disappear clinically below about 33°C (91°F), but it is still seen on ECG at lower temperatures, and gross shivering has been reported as low as 29°C (84°F). At body temperatures of 33° to 38°C (91° to 100°F), the increased heat production can balance losses, but below 33°C (91°F) it cannot, and further body heat loss is inevitable unless the environment is changed.

As body temperature falls, metabolism drops by half for every 10°C (18°F) decrease. The initial manifestation is in the CNS, where cerebral blood flow drops 6 percent for every degree centigrade. Poor judgment and confusion begin to appear about 32°C (90°F). Reflexes diminish or become absent; pupils become fixed and dilated at 30°C (86°F). Coma occurs at about 28°C (82.4°F), and the EEG is flat at 20°C (68°F). Nonetheless, all these changes are reversible and the patient is not dead. In fact, the hypothermia itself, by decreasing metabolic rates and oxygen and nutrient demands, greatly increases tolerance to circulatory failure and shock.

The cardiovascular system reacts with bradycardia and hypotension, which are marked below about 25°C (77°F). The microcirculation suffers sludging of red cells and stagnation, with attendant hypoxia and acidosis, due to dehydration and the increased viscosity of the blood. Intravascular and CNS thromboembolism is common. Most important of all, myocardial irritability is increased below 30°C (86°F), and conduction is increasingly blocked. Arrhythmias are common below this critical temperature, and include atrial fibrillation, premature ventricular contractions, ventricular fibrillation, and conduction blocks. These are all very difficult to reverse—the traditional drugs are useless—until temperature is restored to 32°C (90°F) or above. Asystole occurs at about 15°C (59°F), and this or ventricular fibrillation is the usual specific cause of death in hypothermic patients.

Acidosis is universal. It is due to both alveolar hypoventilation as the respiratory rate slows, and the effects of tissue hypoxia from poor perfusion. The oxyhemoglobin curve shifts to the left, making less oxygen available to the tissues. (However, solubility of oxygen in plasma increases with lowered temperature.) Lactic acid production is increased, but hepatic metabolism is slowed and less able to deal with it. Hepatic metabolism of other metabolites, drugs, and toxins is also severely depressed, greatly increasing their half-life and toxicity.

Dehydration is also universal, as intravascular fluid moves into tissues. Cold depresses renal tubular function, with a resultant "cold diuresis" occurring with increased urine output and increased sodium and water losses. As the plasma volume is shifted from the vasoconstricted periphery of the body to the core organs, the body inappropriately interprets this as an excess fluid volume, and antidiuretic hormone secretion is suppressed, causing further fluid loss.

Respiration is depressed, and carbon dioxide retention may occur, with resultant respiratory acidosis. Copious bronchial secretions are a physiologic response to cold, and may cause aspiration. Respiratory tract infections such as pneumonia are a frequent complication in those who recover from the hypothermia.

Plasma glucose is often high, due to decreased uptake by cells and inhibition of pancreatic insulin production. This high extracellular fluid glucose draws water from cells and dilutes the extracellular fluid (ECF). Thus the administration of hypertonic dextrose during hypothermia is unwise, as it only worsens this problem. Hyperglycemia resolves spontaneously with return to normal temperatures. On the other hand, hypoglycemia itself can cause hypothermia, so that either hypo- or hyperglycemia may be found in the hypothermic patient.

Diagnosis

The diagnosis of hypothermia per se presents few problems. Patients with mild hypothermia (greater than 32°C or 90°F) may appear relatively normal, but will usually be detected by routine temperature taking. It is important not to dismiss a low reading automatically as being due to mouth breathing. Most clinical thermometers only register down to 94°F. Thus, such a reading requires the use of a special extended-range mercury or electronic thermometer, which every emergency department should possess. Once a low temperature is documented, the diagnosis is not in doubt, although the etiology remains to be identified.

Early recognition of hypothermia in the field by clinical symptoms is important. Fatigue, weakness, apathy, incoordination, and slowing of gait are common. Shivering, although an important sign, may not occur during heavy physical exertion, and disappears clinically at lower temperatures. Impaired judgment, hallucinations, and gross confusion eventually occur.

The severely hypothermic patient is unconscious, cold to the touch, stiff, and often has no palpable pulse or detectable blood pressure. Respiration is slow, and the patient may inhale as seldom as once or twice per minute. Pupils are fixed and dilated. The patient's hypothermia will be obvious to the touch, and is documented by a low-range thermometer. The main diagnostic dilemma is whether the patient is truly dead, as may erroneously be assumed. However, patients have been successfully resuscitated who showed no signs of life and had core temperatures as low as 17°C (63°F), without CNS sequelae. In addition, the length of time without signs of life does not have the same significance as in a euthermic patient. Cold protects the brain against hypoxia, and full recovery has been documented after more than 30 minutes' complete submersion in very cold water. Thus, no patient suspected of being hypothermic should be pronounced dead until body temperature is restored to at least 32°C (90°F) and there are still no signs of life.

The rectum is usually chosen as the location for monitoring the temperature, for reasons of convenience and familiarity. Core temperature, of course, is the critical temperature, since it is that of the heart with its temperature-sensitive arrhythmias. Oral and axillary temperatures do not at all reflect core temperature, and in fact rectal temperature does not accurately reflect changes in the core either. Esophageal temperature does, but is not a familiar procedure to most physicians, is affected by any warm intermittent positive pressure breathing (IPPB) treatments given, and may cause vagal stimulation and fatal arrhythmias. Thermistor monitoring of the tympanic membrane avoids the latter two disadvantages, but is even more unfamiliar and requires special equipment. For the time being, then, the rectal thermometer reigns supreme.

Although the thermometer makes the diagnosis, along with clinical state, other tests may be suggestive. The ECG shows any of the previously mentioned arrhythmias, particularly atrial fibrillation, as well as muscle tremor artifact in about two-thirds of patients, even in those without shivering. In addition, about 10 to 20 percent of patients whose temperature is under 25°C (77°F), show the pathognomonic J or Osborn wave (Figs. 30–1 and 30–2).

Laboratory values usually reflect dehydration, with an elevated hematocrit and blood urea nitrogen readings. Sodium and potassium may be normal or decreased due to urinary losses. Glucose is often high, but without ketones. Amylase may be elevated. Crea-

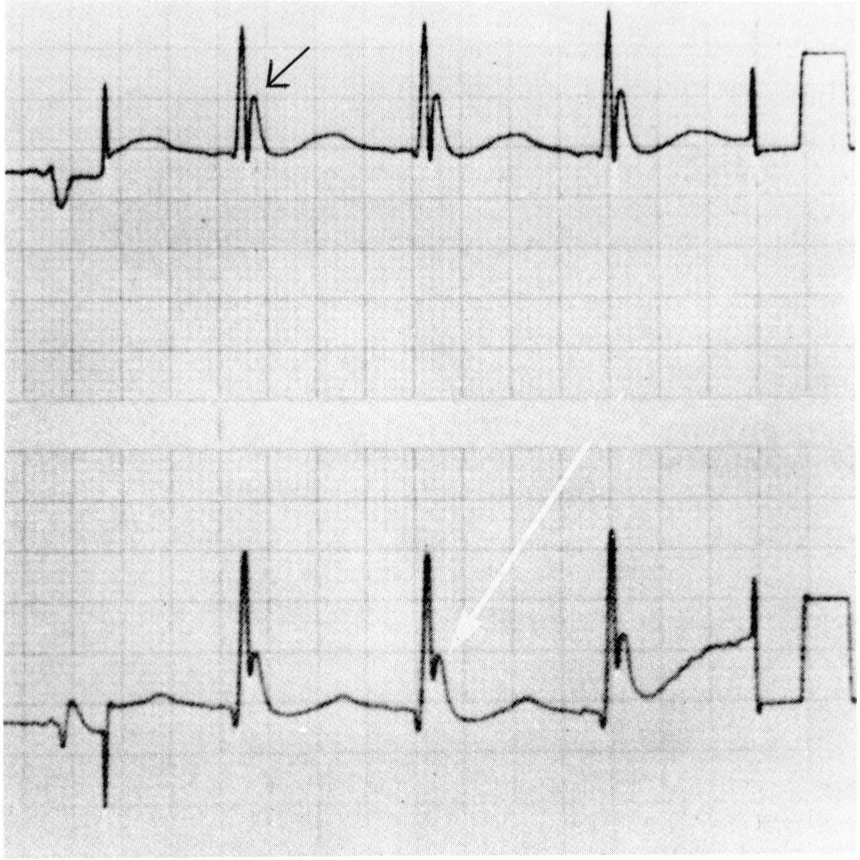

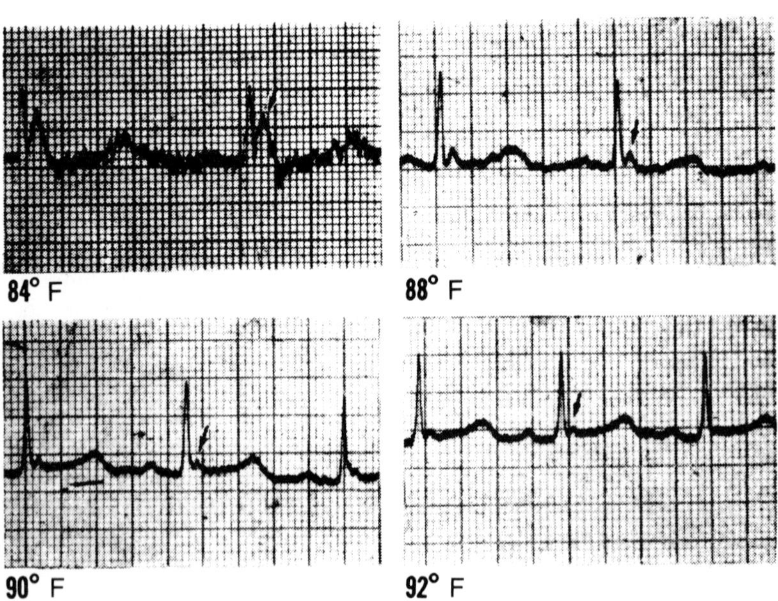

Figure 30–1   Prominent J or Osborn Waves in the ECG of a Patient with Hypothermia. Reproduced with permission from Reuler JB: Hypothermia: Pathophysiology, clinical setting and management. *Ann Intern Med* 89:519–527, 1978.

Figure 30–2   ECG of a Patient with Resolving Hypothermia, Demonstrating the Disappearance of J or Osborn Wave as Temperature Approaches Normal. Reproduced with permission from Johnson L: Accidental hypothermia: Peritoneal dialysis. *JACEP* 6(12):556–560, 1977.

tine phosphokinase (CPK), lactate dehydrogenase, and SGOT may be elevated in cases of severe exertion with hypothermia. Isoenzymes of CPK have been elevated to 27 percent without any evidence of myocardial infarction. Acidosis is commonly seen, and PO_2 is often low. However, it is important to remember that blood gases must be corrected for temperature; PO_2 drops for every degree centrigrade drop in temperature 7.2 percent, PCO_2 drops 4.4 percent, and pH increases 0.015 units. Lactate level is often elevated, reflecting acidosis; this should be suspected whenever the anion gap is greater than 15.

Other tests may be indicated in certain cases, and blood should be drawn for them early. They are not immediately useful in the emergency department, but may be later. These include thyroid function tests, serum cortisol or corticotropin levels, and blood cultures. Obviously the decision to obtain them will be based on the history; a healthy 20-year-old mountain climber caught in a snowstorm would not need them, whereas a 60-year-old invalid found comatose in bed probably would. A chest roentgenogram should also be obtained, looking for evidence of aspiration or infection.

Differential Diagnosis

There is no differential diagnosis of hypothermia per se, but only of its underlying and predisposing conditions. This particularly includes sepsis, hypothyroidism, hypoglycemia, and uremia. Routine lab work as described will detect these conditions.

Treatment

Prehospital

Care of hypothermic patients in the field largely consists of removing them to as warm and protected an environment as possible. This may be a sleeping bag, tent, or heated building. The patient is warmly dressed or covered with blankets; other persons may need to join them in a sleeping bag to speed up rewarming. Other than this, there is no active rewarming method that is safe and practical in the field. This includes inhalation of heated air or oxygen, which creates a risk of oral and tracheal burns and does little to accelerate reheating (see below). Rapid transportation to a hospital should be provided. If the patient is comatose and severely hypothermic, care should be taken to avoid airway suctioning, intubation, and other vagal maneuvers which could cause ventricular fibrillation. If there are no signs of life, cardiopulmonary resuscitation (CPR) should be started and not stopped until there is still no response at a body temperature of 32°C (90°F). Areas

of frostbite should be identified and treated as described in the section on that subject below.

Hospital Treatment

When the patient arrives in the emergency department, the respiratory support started in the field must be continued. An IV line is established, blood drawn for initial tests, and ECG and chest roentgenogram obtained. Frostbite is searched for and treated as described below. From this point on, treatment is controversial. The literature is not very extensive, and no large or controlled studies exist. The treating physician would do well to remember that no true consensus exists.

Clearly hypothermic patients need to be rewarmed. The problem is, how quickly and by what method? Mildly hypothermic patients (greater than 28° to 30°C or 82° to 86°F) can generally be rewarmed fairly slowly and by virtue of their own generated body heat. Warmly covered in a heated environment, they should spontaneously rewarm without problems. This is particularly so in young, previously healthy individuals who become hypothermic quickly due to exposure. When appropriate, this is the safest method, and the easiest to apply.

The patient who cannot spontaneously rewarm under these conditions at a rate of at least 1°C per hour has essentially failed a diagnostic test; it suggests the existence of one of the previously mentioned underlying disorders. A careful search for such disease must then begin. The coexistence of other disease is a significant poor prognostic factor, in contrast to the body temperature, vital signs, cardiac rhythm, and lab tests, which are not prognostic. While the search for other factors commences, active external rewarming can begin, using a rewarming blanket or other methods discussed below. The patient will of course need admission.

The severely hypothermic patient, particularly at the fibrillation-prone temperature of 28° to 30°C (82° to 86°F) and below, presents difficult problems in treatment. For one thing, any vagal stimulation, such as intubation, IV cardiac pacing, nasogastric tubes, esophageal cardiac leads, or even vigorous suctioning, can precipitate fibrillation. Thus good bag-valve-mask ventilation may in this case be much safer than intubation. Inappropriate CPR can also cause fibrillation, so this must be applied only when truly needed, and must then be continued until rewarming occurs—sometimes a matter of hours.

After-drop. The danger of "after-drop" or "rewarming collapse" is often mentioned in connection with rapid rewarming. The after-drop is an actual (but small, less than 1°C) drop in core temperature that occurs even after external rewarming has begun. German experimenters at Dachau in the 1940s were the first to postulate that this is due to cold, acidotic blood being released from the periphery as external heat causes dilation of cutaneous vessels.[1] This has been cited as the cause ever since, without any real documentation. The only study done,[2,3] carried out in pigs, showed that while there was an after-drop of esophageal, rectal, and gastric temperatures, central venous blood temperature showed no after-drop at all, and central venous blood warmed very rapidly. The after-drop itself is easily explained by the thermal properties of the body with its insulated inner core; this occurred in the same magnitude in pigs whose hearts were stopped. There is thus good reason to doubt the conventional explanation as well as the significance of after-drop.

Another postulated cause of rewarming collapse is that the severely hypothermic patient is dehydrated, and the peripheral vasodilation caused by external warming causes a further loss of volume. In some patients hyperkalemia from cell damage may contribute to this problem. Previously normal serum potassium may also drop once treatment is begun, for reasons not known. The blood released at the periphery is also acidotic, which is theorized to cause central venous pH to drop suddenly, although this has not been documented in the literature.

Arrhythmia. Despite the lack of knowledge regarding the causes of rewarming collapse, it does occur, and the ventricular fibrillation that usually accompanies it is the usual cause of death in patients who survive to be hospitalized. The cold heart is very prone to arrhythmia, and the fibrillation is intractable to the usual drugs and defibrillation until normal temperature is restored. Any sudden change in acid-base balance (including that induced by hyperventilation) triggers fibrillation at the critical temperature. In dogs, alkalosis induced by excessive bicarbonate treatment of acidosis also had this ill effect, whereas animals whose pH was kept stable remained in stable rhythms.[4] Since all the other organ systems of the body are actually protected by hypothermia and can survive long periods of hypoxia, the heart is the critical link. Much study remains to be done in this controversial area; present data only suggest that therapy be aimed at rapid rewarming (excessively slow rewarming increases the period of risk) without rocking the physiological boat. Preliminary studies[5,6] have shown that bretyllium is useful in both preventing and terminating the ventricular fibrillation of hypothermia.

Core rewarming. Core rewarming of severely hypothermic patients is recommended by most authors, because it is faster than external methods and at least theoretically avoids some of the risk of rewarming collapse. (This theoretical advantage is also poorly documented.) Cardiovascular bypass is a rapid and effective means of core rewarming which has the further advantage that effective cardiac rhythm is not needed. This is the method of choice where it is rapidly available and

emergency personnel are proficient in its use. It is, however, expensive and carries risks of its own.

In most hospitals bypass is not readily available, and other techniques must be used. Suggested methods include heated peritoneal dialysis, heated gastric lavage, heated mediastinal lavage through chest tubes or a thoracotomy, and heated IPPB. Peritoneal lavage is simple and available in most hospitals. It is carried out with isotonic dialysate with 1.5 percent dextrose, heated to 43°C (110°F). Using a single abdominal peritoneal dialysis catheter, about 4 liters/hour can be exchanged; placing two catheters with suction at the outflow can increase the rate to 12 liters/hour. At this rate body temperature can increase 6°C/hour. Dialysis is discontinued in favor of external rewarming once the temperature reaches 30°C (86°F). In addition to rapid core warming, dialysis helps ensure acid-base and potassium balance, as well as helps remove drugs such as barbiturates, glutethimide, and salicylates which may be present. Close monitoring of electrolyte and acid-base balance is mandatory, but this is the safest and most effective core rewarming technique for most hospitals. It is claimed that rewarming collapse and after-drop do not occur with this technique.

Heated gastric lavage operates on the same principle, but due to the rather limited surface area of the stomach, is not very effective. Heated IPPB suffers from the same drawback. Although the surface area of the lungs is huge, almost all the actual heat exchange takes place above the carina due to the mixing of inhaled and exhaled gases. Saturated air at 44°C (111°F) is used (higher temperatures can cause burns), but even at high respiratory rates the major benefit is to prevent the normal 10 percent body heat loss through respiration. However, some proponents have argued that since mediastinal temperature is raised more and sooner than other core temperatures by this method, the vulnerable heart receives more benefit than those core temperatures suggest. Rates of rewarming and degree of after-drop seem to be the same as for peripheral rewarming methods, however. In any event, although this is a useful, safe, and readily available treatment adjunct, it cannot be relied upon by itself. For prehospital care, the small amount of heat transferred and the difficulty of controlling inhaled temperature with portable apparatus have caused rescue teams to abandon it.

Lavage of the heart or mediastinum with warm saline or lactated Ringer's solution is a traditional method of resuscitation of the hypothermic arrest in surgery. If the chest is not already open, such lavage can be accomplished through dual chest tubes (usually placed on the left). The method has not been studied, but is safe and may be faster and more effective than peritoneal lavage. It should be considered in cases of resistant ventricular fibrillation.

Heated IV fluids (or blood in the trauma patient) do not contribute much to body heat, but help prevent further heat loss from cold solutions. This is particularly helpful in the stressed, often naked and uncovered trauma patient receiving 5 to 10 liters or more of IV fluids.

Peripheral rewarming of the severely hypothermic patient in a 40° to 42°C (104° to 108°F) water bath has previously been advocated, with arms and legs elevated out of the bath by slings to minimize peripheral vasodilation and after-drop. Aside from the physical difficulties of such a set-up, a patient needing such aggressive rewarming probably warrants core rewarming instead.

Supportive Treatment. Other than rewarming, treatment is supportive. Electrolyte abnormalities should be corrected. Vasopressors are not normally used, except when shock is unresponsive to fluids; it has been suggested that catecholamines are depleted in hypothermia. Steroids have no place in routine treatment and should be used only if adrenal insufficiency is suspected. In the patient who fails to show any spontaneous rewarming, hypothyroidism is a possibility, and 500 µg of levothyroxine should be given IV. Although respiratory infection is a common complication, antibiotics should not be given until signs of specific infection develop.

Summary. Patients with mild hypothermia (greater than 32°C or 90°F) are probably best treated with external or endogenous rewarming. Cardiovascular complications are rare, and thus aggressive treatment is not warranted. If temperature does not rise, hypothyroidism or other underlying disorder should be suspected. Such a patient, successfully rewarmed in the emergency department over several hours, can be discharged if there is no underlying disease and if the home situation is excellent.

Patients with a temperature less than 32°C who have a stable cardiovascular status should be rewarmed rapidly with blankets, heated IPPB, and perhaps peritoneal dialysis. Any unnecessary manipulations (especially endotracheal intubation or central venous catheterization) and sudden changes in acid-base balance (including hyperventilation and aggressive bicarbonate therapy) should be avoided. Watchful caution should be employed, and all these patients should be admitted, usually to the intensive care unit.

Patients with a temperature of less than 32°C who are in asystole or fibrillation need CPR and rapid core rewarming. Drugs and electrical countershock are generally useless. If necessary CPR should be continued for hours, since full recovery is possible and death can only be diagnosed by absence of vital signs at a temperature of 32°C or more. Bypass or mediastinal lavage (preferably by thoracotomy, with open-chest cardiac message) should be initiated as soon as possible; if this is not possible, peritoneal dialysis should be combined with heated IPPB and IV solutions.

LOCALIZED COLD INJURY

Chilblains

This entity is commonly seen in climates that are damp and cool for long periods of time. A localized nodule, probably representing a vasculitis, forms on the skin and superficial fatty tissue. These lesions are self-limiting and heal within a few days. Older people with poor circulation may develop ulcerated areas.

Frostnip

This term is given to early and mild frostbite. It is characterized by whitening and pain in the area involved.

Frostbite

Frostbite is the injury and death of localized areas of tissue (most often on the extremities) due to local cold and freezing. Cold conditions cause arteriolar vasoconstriction in the affected part; capillary circulation stops secondary to the increased viscosity and sludging of the blood. Eventually the tissues freeze. Ice crystals form within the extracellular space, creating physical damage, hypertonic ECF, and dehydration of cells. Tissue damage is irreversible; pathologic changes include necrosis, with later atrophy, inflammatory changes, and fibroblastic proliferation. The bones may show punched-out lesions near joints.

A number of factors predispose a person to frostbite. Any disorder of the peripheral circulation (such as arteriosclerosis) increases the risk, as does previous frostbite, which seems to permanently damage vasomotor stability. Lack of acclimatization to cold may also be a risk factor, as is race. Blacks suffered a disproportionate share of cold injuries in the Korean War. In addition, type of clothing and activity—particularly wetness and contact with metal, which accelerates heat loss greatly—contribute considerably to the occurrence of frostbite.

The diagnosis of frostbite is relatively simple, although there is as yet no accurate means of determining the true extent of damage on the initial assessment. The first symptoms (which are actually those of frostnip) are a burning pain and whitish discoloration of exposed parts, such as fingers or toes, face, nose, or earlobes. Later a feeling of warmth replaces the pain, and the skin becomes waxy and whitish. As the frostbite becomes deeper the appearance changes little, except that it is firm to the touch and lacks sensation, feeling numb or "heavy." This appearance, combined with a history of cold exposure, makes the diagnosis and excludes other ailments.

The treatment of frostbite in the field, as in the emergency department, is rapid rewarming. In the field this can be accomplished by holding the affected part in the axilla or crotch. Warming in warm water is desirable if the temperature of the bath can be controlled and the resultant pain treated. Great care must be taken to avoid worsening damage by excessive exposure of the numb part to a fire, radiator, or other such heat source. All friction (including the traditional rubbing with snow) must be avoided, as must all weight-bearing. If the leg is thawed or partially thawed, the patient must not walk on it but must be carried; a frostbitten arm must not be used. If this is impossible, it is better to leave it frozen until proper treatment can be assured. Alcohol should be avoided in the field due to its potentiation of hypothermia. Smoking is prohibited due to its deleterious vasoconstrictor effects, which further jeopardize blood supply.

In the emergency department, rewarming is done in a water bath kept at 40° to 42°C (104° to 110°F). Lower temperature of the bath increases tissue loss; higher may cause thermal burns. Socks or gloves that are frozen on are thawed with the extremity and then carefully removed. The bath is continued until the distal areas of the affected part flush and remain flushed even when removed from the bath. This may take an hour or more. Since it is often very painful, analgesia with morphine or meperidine may be required. Once thawed, the part is protected from any friction or pressure.

Blisters, varying in size, form in minutes to hours; their total absence is a very poor prognostic sign. As in thermal burns, debriding the blisters is controversial, but if punctured they pose an infection risk and should be removed. Systemic hypothermia should be suspected and thoroughly searched for in any victim of frostbite. Transient cyanosis is common in the thawed part, but persistent cyanosis or ischemia despite thawing may indicate a developing compartment syndrome (perhaps due to a fracture, soft tissue sprain, or associated injury). Fasciotomy may be needed if circulation is threatened.

Since depth of injury cannot be initially determined, all but frostnip patients should be hospitalized. Vigorous whirlpool baths in antiseptic solution, with active physical therapy, provide safe debridement and mobilization of joints. Antibiotics should be reserved for actual clinical infection. Tetanus prophylaxis must not be forgotten. The true extent of the damage may not be apparent for weeks, although arterial pulses, Doppler studies, and technetium-99 scans can help demarcate the injury.

As in accidental hypothermia, controversy abounds and few data exist regarding other treatment modalities. Early intra-arterial injection of 0.5 mg of reserpine provides a medical sympathectomy of the affected limb and increases blood flow, thus improving survival of marginal tissue and relieving pain. Phenoxybenzamine, starting at 10 mg/day and increasing to 60 mg/day if needed does the same thing by the oral route. Fasciotomy may be needed in severe tissue damage if compartment syndromes develop; low molecular weight dextran is advocated by a few. Surgical sympathectomy also has its advocates, but diathermy and hyperbaric oxygen are not recommended. There is little in the way of hard data to support any of these treatments, which appear to be largely a matter of personal experience and preference on the part of their advocates.

REFERENCES

1. Coniam SW: Accidental hypothermia. *Anesthesia* 34:250–256, 1979.
2. Golden F St C, Harvey GR: The mechanism of the after-drop following immersion hypothermia in pigs. *J Physiol* 272(1):26–27, 1977.
3. Marcus P: Treatment of acute accidental hypothermia: Proceedings of a symposium held at the RAF Institute of Aviation Medicine. *Aviat Space Environ Med* 50(8):834–843, 1979.
4. Southwick, FS, Dalglish PH: Recovery after prolonged asystolic cardiac arrest in profound hypothermia. *JAMA* 243:1250–1253, 1980.
5. Buckley JJ, Bosch OK, Bacaria MB: Prevention of ventricular fibrillation during hypothermia with bretyllium tosylate. *Anesth Analg* 50(4):507–593, 1971.
6. Dronen S, Nowak RM, Tomlanovich MC et al: Bretyllium tosylate and hypothermic ventricular fibrillation. *Ann Emerg Med* 9(6):335–336, 1980.

BIBLIOGRAPHY

Bangs C, Boswick J, Hamlet M, et al: When your patient suffers frostbite. *Patient Care*: 132–157, February 1977.

Carlson CJ, Milson B, Rapaport E: CPK MB isoenzyme in hypothermia: Case reports and experimental studies. *Am Heart J* 95(3):352–358, 1978.

Clements SD, Hurst JW: Diagnostic value of ECG abnormalities observed in subjects accidentally exposed to cold. *Am J Cardiol* 29:729–734, 1972.

Edwards RD: *Emergency Management of Accidental Hypothermia.* American College of Emergency Physicians Monograph Series, 1978. (A movie on the same topic is available for a nominal charge from Abbott Laboratories, prepared by the same author.)

Hayward JS, Steinman A: Accidental hypothermia: An experimental study of inhalation rewarming. *Aviat Space Environ Med* 46(10):1236–1240, 1975.

Jessen K, Hagelsten JO: Peritoneal dialysis in the treatment of profound accidental hypothermia. *Aviat Space Environ Med* 49(2):426–429, 1978.

Kyosola K: Clinical experiments in the management of cold injuries: A study of 110 cases. *J Trauma* 14:32–35, 1974.

Marcus P: Laboratory comparison of techniques for rewarming hypothermic casualties. *Aviat Space Environ Med* 49(5):692–697, 1978.

Marcus P: Treatment of acute accidental hypothermia: Proceedings of a symposium held at the RAF Institute of Aviation Medicine. *Aviat Space Environ Med* 50(8):834–843, 1979.

O'Keefe K: Accidental hypothermia: A review of 62 cases. *JACEP* 6:491–495, 1977.

Reuler JB: Hypothermia: Pathophysiology, clinical setting and management. *Ann Intern Med* 89:519–527, 1978.

31. Altitude-Related Emergencies

CHARLES H. SCOGGIN, M.D.
Y.E. MILLER, M.D.
R.M. TATE, M.D.

In the middle of the nineteenth century, all the dogs and cats in the high mountain region of McNulty's Gulch, in the mountain range that divides the Arkansas and Blue Rivers of Colorado, died within three months. The physician of the area at that time, Dr. Irving J. Pollok, attributed this unusual occurrence to high altitude ozone. He also ascribed the death of a 13-year-old child to the same cause.[1] While this 1860 report of high altitude–related illness remains somewhat mysterious, today it is understood that high altitude indeed affects human physiology and is responsible for important systemic manifestations that may require emergency medical attention. The term *high altitude–related illnesses* can be defined as those disorders that occur as a direct consequence of exposure to altitudes greater than 2,000 meters (approximately 7,200 feet).

It is particularly important to appreciate the severity and increasing frequency of high altitude–related illnesses. The increased mobility of populations throughout the world now makes it possible for unacclimatized sea level dwellers to reach high altitudes virtually within hours. The high altitude illnesses frequently affect young, otherwise healthy individuals; are rapid in onset; and are potentially fatal if not promptly recognized and treated.

ETIOLOGY OF ALTITUDE-RELATED ILLNESS

It is estimated that some 12 percent of the world's population, or 25 billion people, live in high mountains and valleys.[2] In addition, a vast number of people now visit places at high altitudes for recreational or occupational purposes. The most obvious impact of high altitude on normal persons is a decreased ability to perform muscular work. As measured on a treadmill, the ability to do maximum work at 3,000 meters is reduced some 20 percent from the ability to perform similar activity at sea level.[3] This reduced capacity for work means that more time and effort are required to perform a given task at high altitude than are required at sea level. For example, because of the approximate 25 percent reduction in work performance during an eight-hour shift at 3,400 meters, it took 25 percent longer to complete the Johnson-Eisenhower Tunnel through the Continental Divide in Central Colorado than it would have taken had the tunnel been constructed at sea level.[4] Similarly, this reduced work capacity can affect the endurance and peak performance of individuals caught in high altitude emergency situations.

PATHOPHYSIOLOGY OF HIGH ALTITUDE

With ascent to high altitude, there is an immediate decrease in the amount of oxygen available to breathe. This necessitates a series of acute and chronic physiologic responses, most of which are advantageous. Such adaptive responses affect respiration, pulmonary gas exchange, pulmonary circulation, the ability of hemoglobin to carry oxygen, the cardiovascular system, and the renal system.

Effect of High Altitude on Respiration

Probably the most critical initial response the body makes to high altitude is hyperventilation. This is reflected in the fact that the degree of ventilation is greater for every level of exercise at altitude than for an equivalent amount of exercise at sea level. Such a response is physiologically economical; that is, the increase in the amount of oxygen transported as a result of hyperventilation greatly outweighs the amount of oxygen consumed in the process of hyperventilation.

The ventilatory response to ascent to high altitude is mediated through a series of highly sensitive chemoreceptors located in the carotid bodies and brain stem. In response to the decrease in the arterial oxygen level at high altitude, these receptors stimulate the brain stem respiratory center to increase breathing. This is the expected response in normal individuals. However, individuals may have an aberrant chemosensitivity to hypoxia as a result of disease, drugs, or long-term residence at high altitude, or they may have a genetically low sensitivity to hypoxia. For instance, it has been noted that some individuals with chronic obstructive pulmonary disease have an attenuated ventilatory response to hypoxia, causing them to respond abnormally to an increase in altitude and, thus, to be susceptible to serious systemic hypoxemia. Certain classes of drugs, particularly the opiate, sedative, and hypnotic drugs, depress respiratory drives and may interfere with the normal ventilatory response to an ascent to high altitude. Finally, it has been noted that natives of areas at high altitudes have a blunted ventilatory response to hypoxia, possibly because of prolonged residence in these areas.[5] In this situation, it appears that the blunted sensitivity to hypoxemia may be adaptive.

The initial hyperventilation that occurs with ascent to high altitude may have a deleterious effect on another determinant of breathing—the ventilatory response to carbon dioxide. The initial stimulation to breathing produces arterial hypocapnia and respiratory alkalosis.[6,7] After 24 to 36 hours of residence at a particular altitude, most individuals undergo a spontaneous bicarbonate diuresis to compensate for this respiratory alkalosis. However, until the acclimatization takes place, respiratory alkalosis predominates, and the effect of alkalemia is to depress the ventilatory response to hypoxia.

During this period of respiratory alkalosis, most symptoms of acute mountain sickness occur. This is mirrored by such objective findings as arterial oxygen desaturation, particularly during sleep.[8] Reversal of alkalosis with drugs that induce a secretion of bicarbonate by the kidney, such as acetazolamide (Diamox) improves oxygenation.[8,9] The use of this drug has also been associated with an improvement in the symptoms of acute mountain sickness.

Pulmonary Gas Exchange at High Altitude

The gradient between the alveolar oxygen concentration and arterial oxygen concentration is increased in high altitude natives.[10] Furthermore, such activities as exercise, sleeping, and even lying down may increase this gradient even more. The increase is probably due to ventilation/perfusion mismatching within the lung, and it may explain the potential for hypoxemia in individuals residing at high altitude. Interestingly, the actual capacity of the lung to diffuse molecules such as carbon monoxide (a commonly used parameter of gas transport in pulmonary function tests) is increased in natives of high altitudes,[11] but it does not appear to change in sojourners to high altitude.

Effect of High Altitude on the Circulatory System

With ascent to high altitude, cardiac output decreases at rest in spite of the increase in heart rate that occurs. The mechanism for this decrease in cardiac output appears to be a reduction in the stroke volume of the heart.[12] The cardiac output remains subnormal for increasing levels of exercise as compared with that for similar activities at sea level. This, as well as the diminished supply of oxygen, limits an individual's capacity to perform strenuous work at high altitude.

Effect of High Altitude on the Blood

High altitude has at least two effects on the blood itself. As a chronic adaptive response, red cell mass increases.[13] This is mediated through hypoxic stimulation of erythropoietin production and is reflected in an elevation in the blood hematocrit. The increase in red blood cells serves to increase the oxygen-carrying capacity of the blood. Although this response requires a period of weeks to occur, it is of potential benefit to the person who wishes to become conditioned to high altitudes. This conditioning was the subject of intense study prior to the 1968 Olympic Games, which were held in Mexico City at an altitude of over 1,600 meters (1 mile). Training at a specific altitude appeared to improve performance at that altitude.[14] No advantage of high altitude training has been conclusively demonstrated in similar competition at sea level, however. Other factors that might explain a beneficial effect of training at high altitude include increased capillary density within the body, proliferation of intracellular mitochondria for energy transfer, and an increased level of cytochrome oxidase in muscle myoglobin.[15]

The second effect of high altitude on the blood is that it decreases the affinity of oxygen for hemoglobin,[16] which probably improves oxygen transfer at the tissue level. Whether or not this is of any clinical benefit is controversial. This rightward shift of the oxyhemoglobin dissociation curve is evidenced within weeks after ascent to high altitude. It is mediated through increased levels of 2,3-diphosphoglycerate (2,3-DPG). It is important to remember that certain persons with rare disorders characterized by poor binding of oxygen to hemoglobin or with disorders such as sickle cell anemia are susceptible at high altitudes to either poor oxygenation or sickling of red blood cells.

Effect of High Altitude on the Renal System

As mentioned earlier, the kidney usually spontaneously begins to excrete bicarbonate after 24 to 36 hours.[6] This expected adaptive phenomenon compensates for the respiratory alkalosis and usually brings about an improvement in the oxygenation of the blood as well as in the symptoms of persons who experience acute mountain sickness. This loss of bicarbonate is accompanied by the loss of fluid. In the typically dry environment of high altitude, the loss of fluid through the lungs may lead to volume depletion.

It is important to keep in mind that the adaptive response, i.e., hyperventilation and renal compensation, must recur with each incremental increase in altitude. The person who has become acclimatized at 2,745 meters (9,000 feet) will not necessarily adapt well to a further increase in altitude, even an increase as little as 305 meters (1,000 feet).

DIAGNOSIS AND TREATMENT OF HIGH ALTITUDE–RELATED ILLNESSES

The adaptive responses to high altitude generally benefit both the sojourner and resident. In some circumstances, however, the altitude-induced changes are not beneficial; rather, they produce medical syndromes that are now well associated with high altitude. In addition, because of the decreased availability of oxygen at high altitude, individuals with the following conditions should generally avoid high altitudes:

- chronic obstructive lung disease
- cyanotic congenital heart disease
- congestive heart failure requiring diuretic or vasodilator therapy
- sickle cell anemia
- pulmonary hypertension
- pregnancy (altitudes greater than 3,000 meters)

Four major clinical manifestations of high altitude illnesses have been recognized:[17] (1) acute mountain sickness, (2) cerebral edema, (3) high altitude pulmonary edema (HAPE), and (4) chronic mountain sickness. Although they can be considered distinct clinical entities, it is probably best to regard them as a spectrum of disease with many common overlapping presentations of variable severity.[18] Mechanisms of pathogenesis remain controversial and mainly speculative, but empiric methods of treatment have been developed. These disorders usually occur in otherwise healthy persons at altitudes greater than 2,300 meters (7,000 feet).

Acute Mountain Sickness

The clinical presentation of acute mountain sickness includes headache, nausea, vomiting, anorexia, insomnia, palpitations, dyspnea, irritability, poor concentration, and, occasionally, visual and gait disturbances.[7,19] Usually, acute mountain sickness occurs within the first 24 hours of rapid ascent to high altitude, and it may recur with each progressive elevation in altitude. It generally has both its onset and its peak during the first day after ascent. Rarely, the onset of symptoms may not be seen for three to four days after ascent to high altitude. As the individual remains at the high altitude, the symptoms usually abate over the next three- to five-day period.

Poor-quality sleep is often a bitter complaint of sojourners to high altitude.[8,9] Patients complain of frequent arousals; periodic breathing, i.e., apnea interspaced with hyperpnea; and a failure to feel refreshed upon arising in the morning. This poor-quality sleep may also be reflected in an inability to concentrate or mentate. As a consequence, individuals may be prone to make errors in judgment. This can result in injury or even death, for example, when members of a high altitude expedition with milder symptoms of irritability or problems with mentation do not recognize the more severe symptoms in companion climbers. Thus, it is important that all members of an expedition be aware of the possibility that errors in judgment will result from the effects of high altitude. Typically, affected individuals note nausea and loss of appetite as early symptoms. While lethargy may be noticeable, sleep is fitful and of poor quality. Headache is often prominent. Symptoms and findings may improve spontaneously with acclimatization; however, some individuals develop confusion and even coma.

Acute mountain sickness may well be more prevalent in younger individuals. Furthermore, the higher the altitude, the greater the likelihood of acute mountain sickness and the more severe its degree. Physical conditioning or prior exposure to altitude does not appear to decrease the risk of acute mountain sickness in any individual. Finally, acute mountain sickness tends to recur in individuals who have previously experienced it.

The treatment of acute mountain sickness includes

- bed rest
- oxygen, if available
- descent to low altitude if symptoms are severe or persist beyond 24 to 48 hours
- avoidance of sedation
- acetazolamide prophylaxis, which may be effective for altitudes up to 4,200 meters

The most definitive treatment for acute mountain sickness is the prompt evacuation of the affected individual to low altitude. In high altitude expeditions, logistic factors or weather conditions may prevent moving the victim, however. If this is the case, then oxygen should be administered at high-flow rates. The use of medications such as diuretics or corticosteroids is controversial. Probably little harm could be done by the empiric administration of corticosteroids, but the use of diuretics may induce appreciable systemic dehydration and complicate an already difficult situation.

Mild cases of acute mountain sickness are usually self-limited and can be treated with bed rest and oral intake of fluid. Headache is often a prominent symptom, but medications aimed at improving headache, such as aspirin and codeine, should be used only with caution. Codeine may further depress respiration and increase systemic hypoxemia. Anecdotal experience suggests that most individuals affected with severe headache will accept such risks in order to seek relief, however.

The use of acetazolamide has been reported in the mountaineering literature to be effective in preventing acute mountain sickness. This may result from the drug's effect in correcting the acute respiratory alkalosis that occurs with ascent to high altitude, as noted earlier.[20] Recently, objective evidence has been provided that this agent improves oxygenation at high altitudes,[8,9] particularly during sleep. This correlates with subjective improvement in symptoms. The usual recommendation is that individuals who regularly develop severe nausea, headache, or marked sleeping problems at high altitude take 125 to 250 mg acetazolamide prior to ascent. A single dose should also be administered following ascent. Contraindications to the use of acetazolamide include preexisting metabolic acidosis.

Slow ascent to high altitude also apparently lessens the severity of acute mountain sickness. The use of potent diuretics such as furosemide has been recommended by Indian investigators;[19] however, some recent studies have shown either no benefit or accentuation of symptomatology when this medication was used.[20]

Cerebral Edema

A small percentage of people who ascend to high altitude may develop manifestations of illness primarily expressed as central nervous system signs and symptoms.[18,21] Findings of lassitude, headache, mental dullness, and ataxia predominate. Physical examination may show papilledema and retinal hemorrhage. These individuals also may experience high altitude pulmonary edema. Focal neurologic defects vary; paresthesia, loss of sensation, decreased cerebellar function, and paralysis may occur.

Treatment is much the same as that for other causes of cerebral edema. Because of their possible beneficial effects on cerebral edema in general, potent corticosteroids (10.0 mg IV), e.g., dexamethasone, should be administered. The dosage of corticosteroid that should be given is somewhat controversial. In an acute case, it is probably best to err on the side of too much rather than too little. For that reason, an initial dose of 100 mg, administered intravenously, is recommended. Every effort should be made to evacuate the individual with cerebral edema to a lower altitude.

High Altitude Pulmonary Edema

A unique type of noncardiogenic pulmonary edema, HAPE occurs both in lowland residents who sojourn to high altitude and highland children and adolescents who return to high altitude after visiting a low altitude, even if the visit was only a brief one.[22] Such people develop accentuated hypoxemia upon return to high altitude when compared with healthy lowland residents of similar age. Another group of individuals who appear to be predisposed to high altitude pulmonary edema are those with unilateral pulmonary artery atresia.[23] The exact mechanism of its occurrence is unknown; however, youth appears to be particularly important.[24]

The characteristic symptoms of HAPE occur within 24 to 48 hours after ascent to high altitudes. Symptoms include cough, which may progress to hemoptysis and frothy sputum; weakness; and other symptoms that can be related to coexisting conditions, such as acute mountain sickness or cerebral edema. Physical examination shows the characteristic findings of pulmonary edema. Patients are cyanotic and dyspneic; they have crepitant rales upon auscultation of the chest, but notably do not have distention of the jugular vein or cardiac S_3 gallops. Low-grade fever may be present, but it does not necessarily indicate an infectious process. Laboratory findings are nonspecific, except for the characteristic finding of interstitial and alveolar infiltrates on chest roentgenogram without enlargement of the cardiac silhouettes.

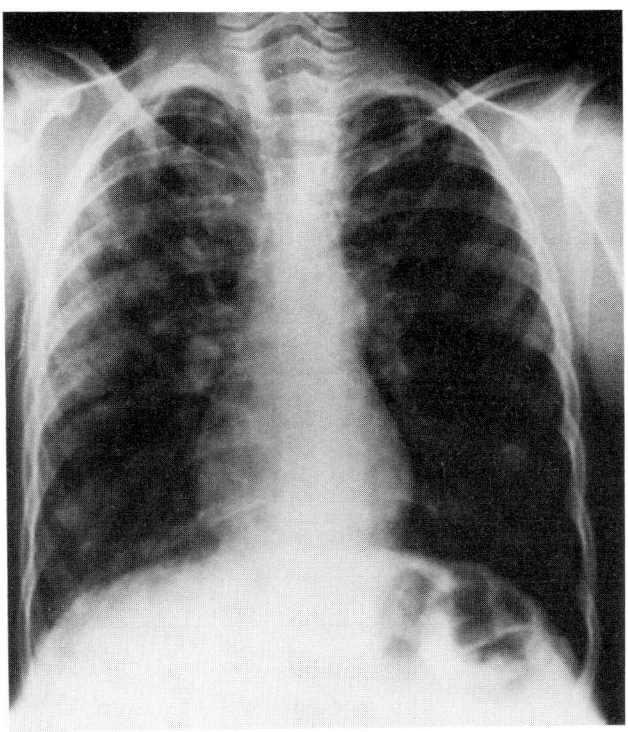

Figure 31–1   Typical Radiographic Appearance of High Altitude Pulmonary Edema. *Note:* Bilateral fluffy pulmonary alveolar infiltrates with normal-sized cardiac silhouette.

These patchy infiltrates tend to be more severe in the right midlung zone (Fig. 31–1). The electrocardiogram (ECG) typically shows sinus tachycardia and evidence of right ventricular strain. Pleural effusions are rare. Hemodynamic findings include an elevated pulmonary artery pressure in association with a normal pulmonary capillary wedge or left atrial pressure, indicating the absence of left ventricular failure.[25] Cardiac index is normal or slightly decreased. The administration of 100 percent oxygen typically fails to correct associated arterial hypoxemia completely because of a marked mismatching of perfusion of the lung with blood and ventilation of the lungs with air.

Death can occur as a result of HAPE. Typically, a protein-rich alveolar exudate is found within the lungs. Hyaline membrane formation and in situ thrombus and platelet aggregation to the capillaries of small pulmonary arteries have been described.[26]

It is important not to confuse HAPE with more common conditions. Individuals who rapidly ascend to high altitudes commonly complain of shortness of breath, and this does not necessarily mean that they have HAPE. It must be recalled that asthma may be precipitated by exercise, particularly in the cold, dry environment of high altitude.[27] If HAPE is suspected, the diagnosis should be confirmed by a chest roentgenogram if logistically possible.

There are many treatment modalities for HAPE:

- bed rest, shown to be effective for mild or moderate HAPE
- oxygen, if available
- avoidance of sedation
- evacuation of patients with severe symptoms to low altitude unless an adequate supply of oxygen is available
- if symptoms persist beyond 48 hours in spite of therapy or if patient worsens, evacuation to low altitude

A study from Peru has suggested that bed rest alone may relieve some episodes of HAPE.[28] This may be effective for the high altitude native who wishes to remain at high altitude; however, the treatment of choice remains evacuation to lower altitude. Other treatment modalities, e.g., diuretics, corticosteroids, intermittent positive pressure breathing, and morphine sulfate, have been proposed, but these are unproved. Furthermore, drugs such as morphine sulfate may depress respiration to a dangerous level. Digitalis, corticosteroids, and aminophylline have been advocated but are probably of no benefit. Of all the active treatment modalities, supplementary oxygen remains the only proved treatment. It should be administered at high flow rates of 4 to 10 liters/minute, since oxygen has not been shown to induce elevations of arterial carbon dioxide tension in HAPE as it does in chronic obstructive pulmonary disease. (See Chapter 57.)

Finally, suspected severe HAPE, necessitating mechanical ventilation and positive end expiratory pressure (PEEP), has been reported.[29] These cases appeared as severe respiratory failure, and the diagnosis of HAPE was made circumstantially. Thus, the spectrum of HAPE symptomatology, as well as the treatment necessary, may vary widely.

In summary, the individual who is suspected of having HAPE should be given oxygen immediately and, if possible, evacuated to a lower altitude. The one exception is the individual who is a native of high altitude and who experiences reascent HAPE. In this circumstance, oxygen therapy alone is usually sufficient to reverse HAPE.[24] These individuals can apparently remain at high altitude following recovery without consequence.

An important aspect of the management of HAPE is its prevention. It appears that individuals who have experienced one episode of HAPE are likely to have another under similar circumstances. Experience in high altitude populations in North America suggests that people tend to "outgrow" susceptibility to HAPE.[24] Acetazolamide prophylaxis has been advocated by the physicians at Leadville, Colorado, where the altitude is approximately 3,000 meters (10,200 feet), to prevent recurrence of HAPE in susceptible individuals. While controlled studies have not been performed, there is probably little danger in empirically administering acetazolamide, as it is administered for prophylaxis against acute mountain sickness, to individuals with a documented episode of HAPE.

Efforts directed at promoting acclimatization and minimizing physical exertion upon arrival may minimize the occurrence of HAPE.[30] For example, visitors to an altitude such as that found in Colorado should spend a day or two at 1,600 to 2,500 meters (5,000 to 8,000 feet) before ascending to a higher altitude. Furthermore, a day of rest following ascent to that altitude probably also decreases the likelihood of HAPE.

HAPE has occasionally been seen in individuals with congenital absence of one major pulmonary artery.[23] If an individual has documented HAPE that is unilateral in nature, a radionucleotide profusion lung scan should be performed to determine whether blood flow is uniform to both lungs. In individuals with unilateral pulmonary artery atresia, the image of only one lung is seen.

Chronic Mountain Sickness (Monge's Disease)

While a person with chronic mountain sickness is unlikely to be seen as an emergency, this condition is of interest because it again demonstrates the effect of high altitude on otherwise normal individuals. Chronic mountain sickness characteristically occurs in highland persons, usually males, and is associated with chronic lethargy, complaints of headache, and excessive elevation of the hematocrit (usually 55 percent or greater).[31] Pulmonary hypertension may or may not be present. The traditional treatment for chronic mountain sickness has been periodic phlebotomy to treat the excessive elevation of the hematocrit. It appears that this disorder is secondary to chronic hypoventilation, particularly during sleep, which stimulates the bone marrow to produce an excessive number of red blood cells.[8] Limited experience with respiratory stimulant drugs, e.g., medroxyprogesterone acetate (Provera), has suggested that such measures may improve both sleep-associated hypoxemia and the more general symptoms of chronic mountain sickness.[32] These agents have not been shown to be of benefit in normal individuals who rapidly ascend to high altitude, however.

Other High Altitude–Related Disorders

Other disorders of high altitude may be seen as medical emergencies. Isolated episodes of thrombosis have been reported at altitudes greater than 4,000 meters (12,000 feet). These include cerebral thrombosis as well as deep vein thrombosis with associated pulmonary thromboembolism. The exact mechanism of this thrombosis remains unknown. Inactivity and dehydration may be contributing factors. In addition, a "hypercoagulable" state may occur at high altitudes.[33] Treatment for such thrombosis includes adequate hydration, descent to low altitude, and anticoagulation therapy. Such anticoagulation therapy probably does not need to be continued beyond 14 days after its initiation, except in the individual who appears to be predisposed to thrombosis even at low altitude. (See Chapter 58.)

A second disorder that may occur at high altitude is retinal hemorrhage.[34,35] (See Chapter 66.) Hemorrhage appears to be mediated by increased retinal blood flow and perhaps hypoxic injury to retinal vessels. The exact incidence of retinal hemorrhage at high altitude is difficult to determine because spontaneous retinal hemorrhage may occur with strenuous exercise even at sea level. Retinal hemorrhage may or may not be associated with other manifestations of acute illness. It is often asymptomatic, but it may be associated with visual blurring and scotoma. Permanent visual impairment occurs only rarely. Measures used in the management of the other acute disorders of high altitude, primarily bed rest and evacuation, are also important for symptomatic retinal hemorrhage.

Exercise-induced asthma may also occur at high altitude. It is thought that this type of bronchospasm is precipitated by the flux of heat and water across the respiratory epithelium owing to breathing cold and dry air,[27] a circumstance almost synonymous with high altitude activity. In many patients, such asthma can be prevented by wearing a cold weather mask to prewarm air before it is inhaled. In addition, the inhalation of β-adrenergic aerosols prior to physical exertion may prevent exercise-induced asthma.[36] Symptoms usually consist of exertional chest tightness, dyspnea, and cough. β-adrenergic aerosols or subcutaneous injection of epinephrine or terbutaline often easily control such asthmatic attacks. Because the cholinergic nervous system is thought to play a prominent role in mediating exercise-induced asthma, inhalation of atropine (1 mg via nebulizer) may also be effective.

A disorder that may occur in black individuals who ascend to high altitude is red blood cell sickling.[37] Such a disorder should be considered in any black patient with chest pain, shortness of breath, joint pain, or abdominal pain. The sickling hemoglobinopathies most notable for producing this disorder include S–S hemoglobin, S–C hemoglobin, and S–β-thalassemia hemoglobin. S–C sickling due to high altitude may result in pulmonary or splenic infarction.[38] Sickle crises may generate fat emboli syndrome if sufficient bone marrow infarction occurs.[39] Treatment usually consists of oxygen, bed rest, and evacuation to low altitude.

A final disorder that has been associated with ascent to high altitude is high altitude flatus expulsion (HAFE).[40] Characterized by an increase in both volume and frequency of the passage of flatus, it arises from the expansion of intestinal gases as the barometric pressure decreases with ascent to high altitude. The possibility of colonic rupture has been reported.[41] Alteration in digestive processes may also contribute to the excessive production of flatus. To date, no definitive preventive measures have been described.

CONCLUSION

The common denominator for conditions associated with high altitude appears to be hypoxia. The cornerstone to treatment is correction of hypoxemia and evacuation to a lower altitude. Simple correction of hypoxemia may result in complete recovery and may allow the person to remain at high altitude. Simple awareness of such high altitude illnesses is extremely important for any physician taking care of patients in an emergency. The function of the physician is not only to care for patients already afflicted, but also to provide informed counseling to individuals who anticipate ascent to high altitude. It should be emphasized to these individuals that there is no "magic bullet" to prevent high altitude–related complications. Once they are recognized, reason dictates that the best treatment is to remove the affected individual from the environment that has induced the illness.

REFERENCES

1. Pollok IJ: Report on diseases peculiar to high altitudes. *Transactions of the Colorado Territorial Medical Society*, 1873, pp 26–30, 1873.
2. DeJong GF: The demography of high altitude populations (report to WHO/PAOH/IBP). Washington, DC, Pan-American Health Organization, 1968.
3. Reeves JT, Grover RF, Cohn JE: Regulation of ventilation during exercise at 10,200 feet in athletes born at low altitude. *J Appl Physiol* 22:346–431, 1967.
4. Grover RF: High altitude geoecology, in Webker PJ (ed): *AAAS Selected Symposium 12*. Boulder, Colo, Westview Press Inc, 1979, pp 127–138.
5. Sorenson SC, Severinghaus JW: Irreversible respiratory insensitivity to hypoxia in man born at high altitude. *J Appl Physiol* 25:217–222, 1968.
6. Lenfant C, Sullivan K: Adaptation to high altitude. *N Engl J Med* 284:1298–1309, 1971.
7. Hacket PH, Rennie D: The incidence, importance and prophylaxis of acute mountain sickness. *Lancet* 2:1149–1154, 1976.
8. Weil JV, Kryger MH, Scoggin CH: Sleep and breathing at high altitude, in Guilleminault C, Dement W (eds): *Sleep Apnea Syndromes*. New York, Alan R Liss Inc, 1978.
9. Sutton JR, Houston CS, Mansell AL, et al: Effect of acetazolamide on hypoxemia during sleep at high altitude. *N Engl J Med* 301:1331, 1979.
10. Kreuzer F, Tenney SM, Mithaefer JC, et al: Alveolar-arterial oxygen gradient in Andean natives at high altitude. *J Appl Physiol* 19:13–16, 1964.
11. DeGraff AC, Grover RF, Johnson RL, et al: Diffusing capacity of the lung in caucasians native to 3100m. *J Appl Physiol* 29:71–76, 1970.
12. Alexander JK, Hatley L, Modelski M, et al: Reduction of stroke volume during exercise in man following ascent to 3,100m altitude. *J Appl Physiol* 23:849–856, 1967.
13. Weil JV, Jamieson G, Brown DW, et al: The red cell mass-arterial oxygen relationship in normal man. *J Clin Invest* 47:1627–1639, 1968.
14. Buskirk ER, Kollias J, Picon-Reatique E, et al: Physiology and performance of track athletes at various altitudes in the United States and Peru, in Goddard RF (ed): *The Effects of Altitude on Physical Performance*. Albuquerque, Albuquerque Athletic Institute, 1967, pp 65–71.
15. Heath D, Williams DR: *Man at High Altitude*. London, Churchill-Livingston, 1977, pp 54–55.
16. Lenfant C, Torrance J, Englis E, et al: Effect of altitude on oxygen binding by hemoglobin and on organic phosphate levels. *J Clin Invest* 47:2652–2660, 1968.
17. Hultgren HN: High-altitude medical problems. *West J Med* 131:8–23, 1979.
18. Hackett PH, Rennie D: Rales, peripheral edema, retinal hemorrhage, and acute mountain sickness. *Am J Med* 67:214–218, 1979.
19. Singh I, Khanna PK, Scrivastava MC, et al: Acute mountain sickness. *N Engl J Med* 208:175–183, 1969.
20. Cain SM, Dunn JE: Low doses of acetazolamide to aid accommodation of men to altitude. *J Appl Physiol* 21:1195–1200, 1966.
21. Houston CS, Dickinson J: Cerebral form of high-altitude illness. *Lancet* 2:758–761, 1975.
22. Hyers TM, Scoggin CH, Will DH, et al: Accentuated hypoxemia at high altitude in subjects susceptible to high-altitude pulmonary edema. *J Appl Physiol* 46:41–46, 1979.
23. Hackett PH, Creagh CE, Grover RF, et al: High-altitude pulmonary edema in persons without the right pulmonary artery. *N Engl J Med* 302:1070–1073, 1980.
24. Scoggin CH, Hyers TM, Reeves JT, et al: High-altitude pulmonary edema in the children and young adults of Leadville, Colorado. *N Engl J Med* 297:1269–1272, 1977.
25. Hultgren HN, Lopez CE, Lundberg E, et al: Physiologic studies of pulmonary edema at high altitude. *Circulation* 29:393–408, 1964.
26. Heath D, Moosavi H, Smith P: Ultrastructure of high-altitude pulmonary oedema. *Thorax* 28:694–700, 1973.
27. McFadden ER, Ingram RH Jr: Exercise-induced asthma: Observations on the initiating stimulus. *N Engl J Med* 301:763–769, 1979.
28. Marticorena E, Hultgren HN: Evaluation of therapeutic methods of high altitude pulmonary edema. *Am J Cardiol* 43:307–312, 1979.

29. Simmerman GA, Crapo RO: Adult respiratory distress syndrome secondary to high altitude pulmonary edema. *West J Med* 133:335–337, 1980.

30. West JB, Lahiri S, Gill MB, et al: Arterial oxygen saturation during exercise at high altitude. *J Appl Physiol* 17:617–621, 1962.

31. Heath D, Williams DR: Monge's disease, in Heath D (ed): *Man at High Altitude*. New York, Churchill-Livingstone, 1977.

32. Kryger M, McCullough RE, Collins DD, et al: Treatment of excessive polycythemia of high altitude with respiratory stimulant drugs. *Am Rev Respir Dis* 117:455–464, 1978.

33. Singh I, Chohau I: Blood coagulation changes at high altitude predisposing to pulmonary hypertension. *Br Med J* 34:611–617, 1972.

34. Wiedman M: High-altitude retinal hemorrhages. *Arch Ophthalmol* 93:401–403, 1975.

35. Shults W, Swan KC: High-altitude retinopathy in mountain climbers. *Arch Ophthalmol* 93:404–408, 1975.

36. Anderson S, Seale JP, Ferris L, et al: An evaluation of pharmacotherapy for exercise-induced asthma. *J Allergy Clin Immunol* 64:612–624, 1979.

37. Bromber PA: Pulmonary aspects of sickle cell disease. *Arch Intern Med* 133:652–657, 1974.

38. Sears DA: The morbidity of sickle cell trait. *Am J Med* 64:1021–1036, 1978.

39. Chmel H, Bertles JF: Hemoglobin S–C disease in a pregnant woman with crisis and fat embolization syndrome. *Am J Med* 58:563–566, 1975.

40. Auerbach P, Miller YE: High altitude flatus expulsion (HAFE). *West J Med* 134:173–174, 1981.

41. Davis EY: HAFE in Nepal. *West J Med* 134:366, 1981.

32. Drowning and Near-Drowning

SHIRLEY A. GRAVES, M.D.

Drowning and near-drowning are marine emergencies that constitute leading causes of morbidity and mortality throughout the world. Over 7,000 deaths result from drowning each year in the United States alone. These figures may represent only a small part of the problem of aquatic near-disasters because no accurate statistics reflect the number of persons who near-drown. Modell has extrapolated data and has estimated that more than 1.2 million patients have been treated for near-drowning in the past 25 years.[1] Drowning implies a terminal event, death. The emergency medical team is concerned, however, with the survivor, the near-drowned patient.

DEFINITIONS

A decade ago, Modell defined the terms drowned and near-drowned[2] and, recently, revised these definitions.[3]

To drown, with or without aspiration, is to die while submerged in water. Approximately 10 percent of drowning victims do not aspirate water but die of respiratory obstruction and asphyxia while submerged.[4] Those who aspirate die from both the asphyxia and the effects of the aspirated water.

To near-drown, with or without aspiration, is to suffocate by submersion in water and to survive, at least temporarily. Approximately 12 percent of near-drowned persons do not aspirate and suffer only laryngospasm or breath holding, which prevents the aspiration of fluid.[5]

Delayed death may occur secondary to near-drowning after an initial apparently successful resuscitation. Delayed death may be the result of pulmonary injury, infection, or irreversible cerebral injury.

EPIDEMIOLOGY AND ETIOLOGY

Drowning is one of the leading causes of accidental death among young people; the highest incidence occurs during the second decade of life.[6] These victims are generally healthy. Approximately 65 percent cannot swim. The backyard swimming pool is a particular hazard for the child under 10 years of age.[7] Pearn reported an overall annual mortality of 3.1 drownings per 100,000 children from the city and county of Honolulu. The swimming pool fatality rate of 0.9 per 100,000 is low compared with other studies and may be related to more fencing of pools in Honolulu.[8]

The ability to swim is certainly desirable in the prevention of drowning; however, it is not the only factor. At least 35 percent of drowned victims can swim,[7] which indicates the importance of other factors, such as regard for safety rules, estimation of one's own ability, use of drugs and alcohol when engaging in aquatic activities, and physical illnesses, e.g., labyrinthitis or preexisting cardiac diseases.

The author thanks Dr. Jerome H. Modell for review of the manuscript and Ms. Lynn Carroll for editorial assistance.

Hyperventilation before underwater swimming has been documented by Craig to be a dangerous practice.[9,10] If an individual hyperventilates before underwater swimming, the PCO_2 in the blood is lowered sufficiently so that the individual can stay under water longer without feeling the urge to surface and take a breath. Unfortunately, during this time the PO_2 also decreases; the individual becomes hypoxemic and unconscious and drowns.

Immersion in cold water causes hypothermia. As body temperature falls the resultant disorientation and subsequent loss of consciousness can lead to submersion and drowning.[11] If the individual does not drown or near-drown because of the disorientation associated with hypothermia, arrhythmias and even death may occur from the hypothermic effects on the heart. Hypothermia does, of course, decrease oxygen consumption and cases are reported in the literature of complete recovery after prolonged submersion in cold water.[12] Also, when submerged in cold water, the individual may experience the diving reflex, whereby blood is shunted preferentially to the heart and brain.[13] (See Chapter 30.)

Many factors are involved in drowning and near-drowning. Prevention is the most valuable and life-saving measure; however, once the accident has occurred, it should be realized that no two near-drownings are identical and each case must be evaluated and treated individually.

PATHOLOGY

Autopsies of drowned persons reveal varied findings, depending on the amount and type of fluid aspirated, the length of submersion, the degree of hypoxia, the duration of survival, and the effects of therapy. The most extensive changes occur in the lungs and brain.[14]

Goose flesh, or cutis anserina, and water wrinkling of the palms of the hand and soles of the feet may appear. A pale or plasmalike watery foam may be present in the nose and mouth and may be mixed with mud, debris, or vomitus. This material may also appear in the lower airway.

Upon opening the pleura, the lungs frequently appear large, hyperexpanded, and irregularly congested with pink or red mottling. If the patient survives initially but dies later, the lungs may show hyaline material in the alveoli, pneumonia, and mechanical injuries such as barotrauma. Microscopic sections of the lung may show alveolar distention, hyaline precipitates, and intra-alveolar hemorrhage. (See Chapter 33.)

The changes in the brain vary with the degree and duration of cerebral anoxia. If death occurs within the first few hours or days, brain edema and perivascular hemorrhages may be the only gross changes. With severe anoxia, basal ganglia or midbrain cystic degenerations may appear after a week or two. All of these findings are secondary to anoxia and are not necessarily unique to drowning.

PATHOPHYSIOLOGY

Significant experimental and clinical data obtained since the 1940s have changed our understanding of the pathophysiology of drowning and near-drowning and, thus, have altered the approach to therapy. The evolution of the understanding of the pathophysiology can be divided into three phases: first, serum electrolyte concentrations and blood volume; second, pulmonary and acid-base changes; and third, neurologic damage and brain preservation.

In the 1940s and 1950s, clearly, the emphasis in treating the near-drowned patient was on the serum electrolyte concentrations and the blood volume changes that might have occurred.[15,16] However, in the 1960s, Modell and colleagues experimentally and clinically demonstrated that pulmonary insufficiency and acid-base changes were the primary pathophysiology in near-drowned patients.[5,17]

In the late 1970s, concern not only for survival after an anoxic insult but for survival with intact cerebral function led to considerable investigation. Although no controlled studies have been done in the area of near-drowning and brain preservation, techniques to preserve the brain have been advocated and used by some.[18–20]

Pulmonary, Blood Gas, and Acid-Base Alterations

The most important and immediate consequence of near-drowning is hypoxemia (Fig. 32–1).[5,17,21,22] Hypoxemia may occur whether or not the individual as-

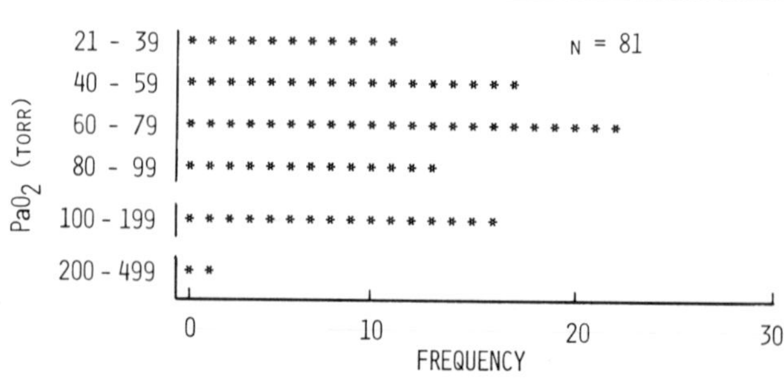

Figure 32–1 Values for PaO_2 on Admission to Hospital after Near-Drowning. FIO_2 ranged from 0.2 to 1.0. Each point represents one patient. *Source:* Modell JH, Graves SA, Ketover A: Clinical course of 91 consecutive near-drowning victims. *Chest* 70:232, 1976. Reprinted with permission.

pirates. As reported by Cot,[4] 10 percent of drowned humans did not actually aspirate fluid, but died secondary to upper airway obstruction. Similarly, 12 percent of near-drowned victims do not aspirate but suffer hypoxemia from breath holding and laryngospasm.[5] In near-drowning without aspiration, if effective ventilation and circulation can be restored before irreversible cerebral damage occurs, the victim should recover with little or no additional therapy. This situation has been simulated in the laboratory by using dogs anesthetized with barbiturates.[23] When the airway was occluded, the arterial oxygen tension (PaO_2) decreased from a normal control value to 40 torr at one minute and 4 torr at five minutes. The rise in the carbon dioxide tension ($PaCO_2$) was 3 to 6 torr per minute. Eighty percent of these animals could be successfully resuscitated if they were manually ventilated with room air five minutes after tracheal occlusion. Some of the animals required external cardiac massage in addition to the positive pressure ventilation.

If the victim aspirates fluid, then the pulmonary picture is substantially more complicated. Aspiration of even small quantities of water yields significant decreases in PaO_2.[17,22,24,25] If significant quantities (11 ml/kg) of fresh water or seawater are aspirated, profound hypoxemia occurs within one minute and persists for at least 72 hours in surviving animals. This initial hypoxemia is accompanied by hypercarbia and acidosis.[17,22] The hypercarbia is readily reversible once the victim breathes spontaneously or mechanical ventilation is instituted.[5,21] Just as the hypoxemia persists, so does the metabolic component of the acidosis.[5,26] Some investigators have been unable to always correlate PaO_2 or pH with survival, but these values do indicate the severity of the lesion.[5]

Hypoxia occurs after the aspiration of either fresh water or seawater; however, the mechanism in each case differs. Seawater is hypertonic (approximately three and one-half times more concentrated than plasma); therefore, fluid is drawn into the alveoli from the circulation in response to this hypertonicity. If 22 ml/kg of seawater is aspirated by dogs, approximately 33 ml/kg can be drained from the lungs by gravity. The result of seawater aspiration is fluid-filled but perfused alveoli.[25,27] Pulmonary surfactant after seawater aspiration has normal surface tension properties. After freshwater aspiration, fluid is absorbed across the alveolar surface into the circulation and no water can be drained from the airway by gravity.[24] Fresh water alters surface tension properties of the pulmonary surfactant,[28] which produces unstable alveoli and atelectasis. These poorly ventilated and atelectatic alveoli, in turn, produce ventilation/perfusion mismatching and intrapulmonary shunting (Fig. 32–2).[17] With both freshwater and seawater aspiration, pulmonary compliance decreases, dead

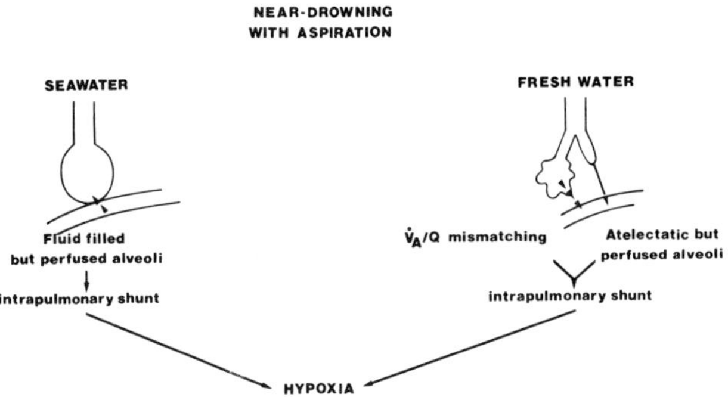

Figure 32–2   Effects of Seawater and Freshwater Aspiration. After seawater aspiration, fluid fills the alveoli, which produces intrapulmonary shunt. After freshwater aspiration, alteration of surfactant causes partially collapsed and completely atelectatic alveoli, which produces intrapulmonary shunt. Aspiration of either type of water causes hypoxia.

space to tidal volume ratio and airway resistance increase, and ventilation/perfusion mismatching and intrapulmonary shunting occur.[17,25,29–31] Pulmonary edema may occur secondary to either type of aspiration.

It has been demonstrated in the laboratory that the application of positive end-expiratory pressure (PEEP) or continuous positive airway pressure (CPAP) to the airway can significantly improve oxygenation and decrease intrapulmonary shunting after the aspiration of fresh water or seawater. Animals aspirating seawater improved significantly when they breathed spontaneously with CPAP or were mechanically ventilated with PEEP.[27] The animals aspirating fresh water, on the other hand, did not always improve significantly with CPAP alone, but some required positive pressure ventilation also.[32] Both PEEP and CPAP increase functional residual capacity (FRC), improve oxygenation and ventilation/perfusion, and reduce intrapulmonary shunt. Why does the animal aspirating fresh water often require positive pressure ventilation in addition to CPAP? One hypothesis is that, because the alteration of surfactant produces unstable alveoli and atelectasis, a high peak inspiratory pressure is necessary to open the alveoli and, once opened, CPAP is necessary to keep them inflated.

The near-drowned victim may suffer gastric distention, may vomit, and may aspirate gastric contents, which compounds the pulmonary injury of aspirating water. Gastric distention may also interfere with ventilation (Fig. 32–3). Neurogenic pulmonary edema may also complicate the primary injury.[33]

Although there may be acute and severe pulmonary insufficiency after near-drowning, those who survive the initial insult suffer no long-term alteration in pulmonary function.[34,35]

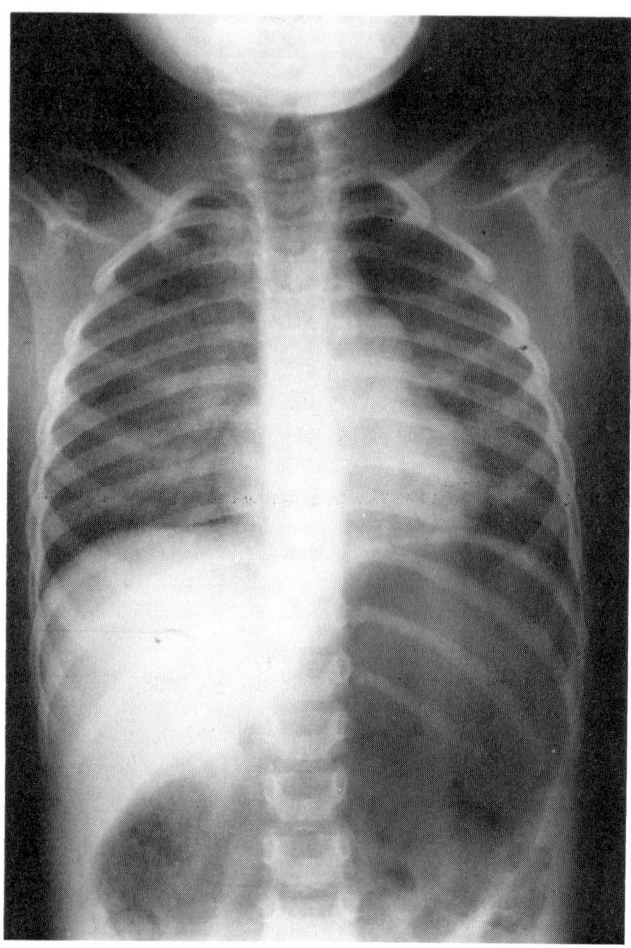

Figure 32–3 Chest Roentgenogram Postresuscitation of a Child. Note the massive gastric distention. This may predispose to vomiting and may also interfere with ventilation.

Serum Electrolyte and Blood Volume Changes

In the 1940s and 1950s, serum electrolyte and blood volume changes were thought to be the primary cause of morbidity and mortality after near-drowning. This phase of understanding the illness and approaching its therapy was based on investigations by Swann and colleagues who demonstrated significant serum electrolyte and blood volume changes after total immersion of dogs in either seawater or fresh water.[15,16] After total immersion in seawater, animals showed marked increases in serum electrolyte concentrations and in blood density and a decrease in blood volume. If the animals were immersed in fresh water until death, blood density and serum electrolyte concentrations decreased and blood volume increased. These animals frequently died of

ventricular fibrillation in contrast to animals submerged in seawater, none of which suffered ventricular fibrillation.

In the 1960s, Modell and colleagues investigated further the fluid and electrolyte changes after near-drowning and found that these changes depend both on the type and the volume of water aspirated and are transient.[22,24,25] Animals aspirating 22 ml/kg of either fresh or seawater showed no life-threatening changes in serum electrolytes. When 22 ml/kg of fresh water were aspirated, the serum sodium and serum chloride decreased 10 to 20 mEq/liter within three minutes but returned to normal within 30 minutes. Aspiration of the same quantity of seawater transiently raised these electrolytes 20 to 30 mEq/liter. In these animals, potassium concentrations rose acutely after the aspiration of either fresh water or seawater. These levels also were not life-threatening and returned to normal within 30 minutes. If 44 ml/kg of fresh water were aspirated, 80 percent of animals died of ventricular fibrillation. An analysis of blood from humans drowned in either fresh water or seawater demonstrated similar findings.[36] The 85 percent who did not have severe changes in serum electrolyte concentrations presumably died of anoxia and acidosis. On the basis of these data for both drowned and near-drowned animals and humans, survivors probably do not aspirate enough fluid to change electrolytes profoundly, but rather manifest transient electrolyte changes that revert to normal without specific therapy (Fig. 32–4).[5] The hypotonic fresh water is rapidly absorbed into the circulation after near-drowning;[24] however, in survivors, fluid is rapidly redistributed and hypervolemia is transient. After seawater aspiration, blood

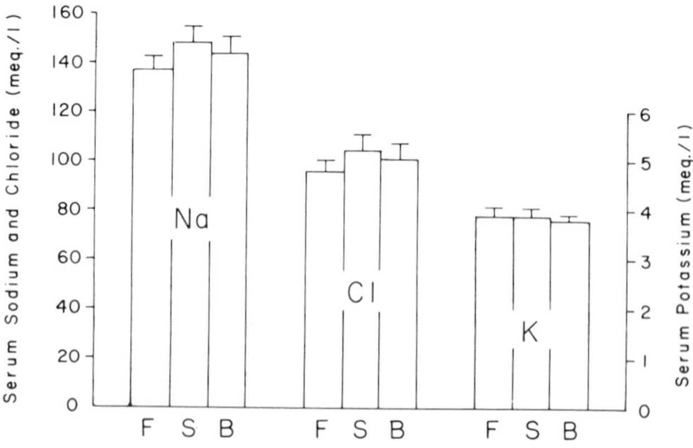

Figure 32–4 Serum Concentrations (Mean ± SD) of Sodium, Chloride, and Potassium in Patients Who Suffered Near-Drowning in Fresh (F), Sea (S), or Brackish (B) Water. *Source:* Modell JH, Graves SA, Ketover A: Clinical course of 91 consecutive near-drowning victims. *Chest* 70:234, 1976. Reprinted with permission.

volume decreases in proportion to the quantity of fluid aspirated.[25] Pulmonary edema can occur after freshwater or seawater aspiration and can produce hypovolemia, which may require replacement therapy.

Cardiovascular Changes

Most cardiovascular changes are related to hypoxia and acidosis, which accompany pulmonary insufficiency in the near-drowned victim. The usual situation is cardiovascular stability in the patient without any preexisting cardiovascular compromise. Numerous arrhythmias have been reported after near-drowning.[7,22,24,25,37–41] Ventricular fibrillation after total immersion in fresh water was identified by Swann and colleagues as a mechanism of death secondary to drowning,[15,16] however, aspiration of this quantity of water by humans is infrequent.[36] Central venous pressure (CVP) increases transiently after the aspiration of either fresh water or seawater;[24,25] if death occurs immediately after the aspiration of large quantities of fresh water, the elevation persists until death.[15,38,41] Otherwise, the CVP returns to normal after approximately an hour.[22,24] After seawater aspiration, fluid is lost into the lungs and the CVP rapidly decreases and approaches zero.[16]

Cardiac output (CO) transiently falls after the aspiration of fresh water. Controlled mechanical ventilation decreases CO, and this decrease may be accentuated by the application of PEEP.[32] In the dog, if the intravascular volume is augmented with crystalloid, this decrease in CO can be reversed. Contrary to this, inotropic stimulation of the myocardium with dopamine does not restore CO.[42] This effect of dopamine has not been evaluated in near-drowned humans.

Hypothermia may occur secondary to near-drowning and, if the body temperature is below 28°C, arrhythmias, including ventricular fibrillation, frequently occur.[11] (See Chapter 30.)

Hematologic Changes

Significant changes in hemoglobin and hematocrit rarely occur in the near-drowned victim.[5] This suggests that near-drowning victims do not aspirate large quantities of fluid. In a retrospective study of 86 consecutive near-drowned patients, hemoglobin and hematocrit values were normal and those of freshwater victims could not be differentiated from those of seawater victims (Fig. 32–5).

If large volumes of fresh water are aspirated and absorbed, hemolysis of red blood cells and hemoglobinemia can occur. Although the hemolysis of RBCs relates to the tonicity of this fluid, the hemolysis increases when combined with hypoxemia. After the IV

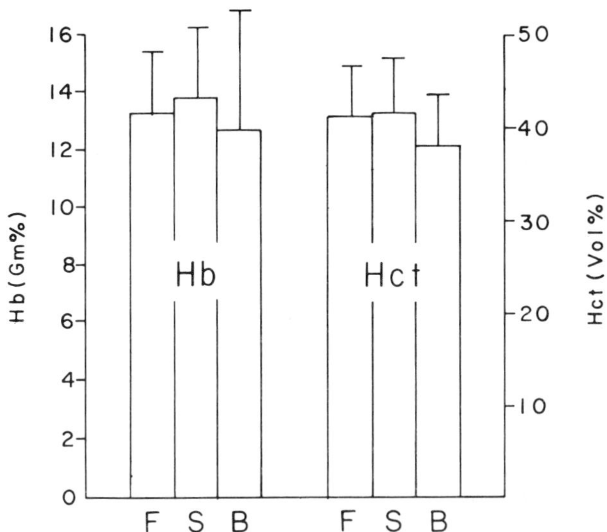

Figure 32–5   Hemoglobin (Hb) Levels and Hematocrit (Hct) Readings (Mean ± SD) in Patients Who Suffered Near-Drowning in Fresh (F), Sea (S), or Brackish (B) Water. *Source:* Modell JH, Graves SA, Ketover A: Clinical course of 91 consecutive near-drowning victims. *Chest* 70:234, 1976. Reprinted with permission.

injection of 44 ml/kg of fresh water into animals, plasma hemoglobin levels were not significantly elevated as long as the animals were not hypoxemic; if the airway was occluded and the same volume of water infused, plasma Hb concentration exceeded 100 mg/liter.[23] In near-drowned humans, the plasma Hb levels rarely exceed 10 mg/liter; although patients with higher levels have reportedly survived without specific therapy for the hemoglobinemia.

Disseminated intravascular coagulation as well as other coagulative disorders have been reported in the drowned victim. The etiology of these disorders is unknown but might be related to severe hypoxemia and acidosis, sepsis, shock, or hemolysis of the RBCs with the release of factors that disrupt the coagulative cascade.[43–45] This is a rare occurrence in a near-drowned patient with no complications.

Renal Function

If oxygenation and renal perfusion are maintained, renal failure is unusual in the near-drowned patient. This is not to say that such abnormalities cannot occur. There are numerous reports of abnormal findings such as albuminuria, hemoglobinuria, oliguria, anuria, and acute tubular necrosis.[46–50] Any biochemical effects of the absorbed water on the kidney are unknown; however, it seems likely that the abnormalities relate to acidosis, hypoxia, and compromised renal perfusion. Hemoglobinuria is not usually a problem in the near-drowned patient; however, it should be considered a potential problem deserving evaluation.

CNS Changes

Central nervous system compromise may be associated with near-drowning. The underlying cause has not been defined; but seems likely to be secondary to cerebral hypoxia. The reported incidence of neurologic dysfunction after near-drowning varies considerably, 0 to 30 percent of survivors.[5,19,51–53] The high incidence of brain damage reported has led some persons to recommend the consideration of significant neurologic damage before instituting hospital-based intensive care and life support.[53] These same fears lead others to pursue aggressive measures for cerebral resuscitation and brain preservation.[18–20]

Pearn and coworkers, attempting to define the best indicator of neurologic outcome, reviewed childhood drownings and near-drownings over a five-year period.[52] All children who were resuscitated survived without neurologic sequelae; 5 of the 104 children died. Based on these findings, the time until the first spontaneous gasp during rescue was the best indicator of neurologic sequelae. Most patients who survived made spontaneous respiratory efforts within two minutes after removal from the water. The authors concluded that no spontaneous gasps within an hour of rescue indicates that neurologic complications will occur.

More recently, to better define the patient at risk from neurologic deficit, two retrospective studies divided the victims of near-drowning into three groups classified according to neurologic status in the emergency department.[20,54] Patients in group one arrived at the hospital awake and alert, although they may have suffered cardiopulmonary arrest during the accident and may have required resuscitation on the scene; 100 percent survived normally.

Group two arrived at the hospital with a blunted level of consciousness. These patients were described as lethargic, combative, disoriented, semicomatose, and confused. One hundred percent in one study and 90 percent in the other survived without neurologic sequelae. Three patients died of pulmonary insufficiency and had no neurologic deficit beforehand. Therapy was directed at pulmonary and cardiac parameters for this group in both studies.

In the third group, comatose patients, one study included adults of whom 73 percent survived and were normal.[54] In both studies, approximately 44 percent of children survived with normal function. Patients from one institution received therapy directed primarily at pulmonary and cardiac resuscitation and, in some patients, hyperventilation and steroids.[54] In the other study, therapy was aimed at aggressive cerebral resuscitation including hyperventilation, hyperoxia, fluid restriction and diuresis, hypothermia, muscle paralysis, steroids, and barbiturate coma.[20] A well-controlled prospective study is needed to resolve many of the questions about the most important elements in producing normal survival of the comatose near-drowned patient.[55]

DIAGNOSIS AND DIFFERENTIAL DIAGNOSIS

Unlike many medical illnesses, the diagnosis of near-drowning is usually obvious from the history; however, the degree of injury to various organs requires thorough investigation and a complete knowledge of the pathophysiologic changes induced by near-drowning. Also important in assessing the victim is the recognition of associated problems.

Although near-drowning may appear to be the only accident, trauma to the head, neck, or other organs may have occurred if the patient fell or was diving into the water. Injuries such as fractures of the neck or back or intracranial hemorrhage must be considered. Whether or not the victim was imbibing alcohol or taking drugs at the time of the accident should be ascertained. It is important to know the patient's previous state of health. For example, an older patient may suffer a myocardial infarction while in the water and may aspirate terminally; a diabetic might suffer hypoglycemia, lose consciousness, and near-drown; or the epileptic patient might have a seizure, near-drown, and be postictal or have cerebral depression secondary to cerebral anoxia. As in all serious illnesses, a careful history and a complete physical examination are imperative to determine the extent of the physiologic damage the patient has sustained.

TREATMENT

Prehospital

The outcome of the near-drowned patient depends greatly on the quality of the resuscitation at the scene of the accident. The primary objective is to maintain oxygenation and acid-base balance. The ABCs of cardiopulmonary resuscitation recommended by the American Heart Association apply to the resuscitation of the near-drowned victim. Safar and coworkers have shown mouth-to-mouth or mouth-to-nose ventilation to be the most effective methods of ventilation in a situation such as near-drowning.[56] If the victim is apneic, hypoxia increases rapidly and the victim may be just a breath away from cardiac arrest. If the rescuer is experienced and a good swimmer, it may be possible to begin mouth-to-mouth ventilation while still in the water; however, the rescuers should not jeopardize themselves or delay resuscitation by attempting a technique in the water that exceeds their abilities.

If the victim remains apneic, mouth-to-mouth ventilation should be replaced with a positive pressure breathing device as soon as available. Hand-operated units are generally preferable to automatic pressure-cycled devices. In the face of decreased pulmonary compliance, pressure-cycled or pressure-limited devices may fail to deliver an adequate tidal volume. Supplemental oxygen should be supplied as soon as possible.

Heimlich recommended subdiaphragmatic compression to remove aspirated water from the lungs of the near-drowned victim.[57] This author does not recommend such a maneuver and thinks that it may even be hazardous because the fluid, swallowed water and gastric secretions, is probably extruded from the stomach. If the patient is apneic or without airway reflexes the gastric secretions could be aspirated and could further compound the pulmonary injury. Attempting to remove fresh water from the lungs is futile because it is so rapidly absorbed into the circulation. Seawater is hypertonic and, in animals resuscitated after the aspiration of large quantities of this type of water, gravitational drainage of the lungs did improve survival.[27] Based on this, if a seawater victim can be resuscitated in a slightly head-down position, some theoretical advantage might be gained; however, it is far more important that rapid and effective artificial ventilation be instituted to restore oxygenation.

If the victim has not aspirated and effective ventilation and oxygenation are restored before permanent circulatory or cerebral hypoxic changes occur, the prognosis for normal recovery is excellent. On the other hand, if water has been aspirated, then pulmonary insufficiency usually ensues and the problem is more complicated. In addition to ventilation, if the patient does not have an effective heartbeat, closed-chest cardiac massage should be instituted immediately.

Many communities have emergency medical personnel who can deliver sophisticated care at the scene. These paramedics and emergency medical technicians can easily replace mouth-to-mouth ventilation with bag-and-mask ventilation or, in some situations, endotracheal intubation. If the rescue personnel are skilled at endotracheal intubation, then the patient who is comatose or apneic or who cannot maintain ventilation should be intubated at the scene. However, it is far better to continue mouth-to-mouth or bag-and-mask positive pressure ventilation or to use an esophageal obturator airway if endotracheal intubation proves difficult or impossible or if the rescuers are not skilled in performing endotracheal intubation. A rescue team may also be able to establish an intravenous infusion and,

if telemeterized monitoring and radio contact is available between the physician and the team, additional drugs and therapy may be administered. These advanced life-support procedures should be performed according to established protocol and under the direction of a physician.

If the patient is breathing spontaneously at the time of rescue or begins to breathe after resuscitation, supplemental oxygen should be continued, preferably 100 percent oxygen through a nonrebreathing mask, and the patient should be transferred to a hospital for further evaluation.

Regardless of how well the patient looks during transport, oxygen should be continued. Respiratory and circulatory assistance should also be continued as dictated by the patient's condition.

If there is a history of diving or trauma or there are physical signs of trauma, cervical spine injury should be suspected and the patient should be treated as though this were the case. These patients should be placed in a cervical collar and a spine-board should be used for transportation.

Cardiopulmonary and Acid-Base Therapy

The near-drowned patient requires an uninterrupted continuum of care from the time of rescue through the emergency department and to the intensive care unit until vital body functions have stabilized (Fig. 32–6). On arrival at the emergency department, immediate assessment of ventilation and circulation is most important. The target organ is the lungs, making intensive evaluation for pulmonary insufficiency and treatment the immediate goal. For other organs to maintain normal function, oxygenation and oxygen delivery must be ensured. The level of ventilatory support required will vary from patient to patient. For example, the spontaneously breathing patient may require only supplemental oxygen whereas the apneic patient requires immediate endotracheal intubation. One hundred percent oxygen should be continued until arterial blood gas and pH values are determined. The fractional concentration of inspired oxygen (FIO_2), the ventilatory support, and the administration of sodium bicarbonate solution will be dictated by these values as well as by the physical assessment of the patient. If the patient is alert and has a PaO_2 of greater than 80 torr while breathing room air, aspiration probably did not occur and observation for 12 to 24 hours is all that is necessary if blood gas values and physical status do not deteriorate.

At the other end of the spectrum, the comatose or apneic patient should be intubated to protect the airway and to provide further ventilatory support. The patient who cannot maintain adequate oxygenation with an FIO_2 of less than 0.4 also requires more aggressive therapy.

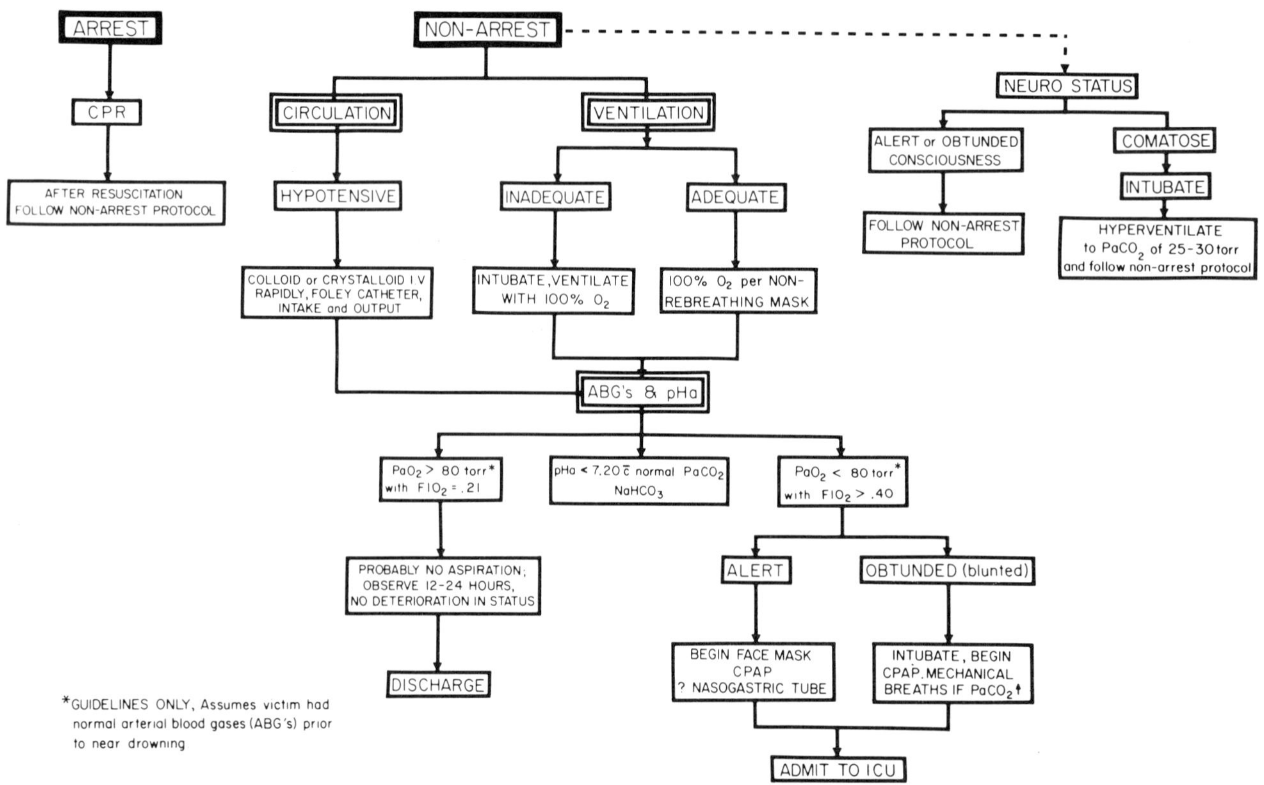

Figure 32–6 Guidelines for Treating the Near-Drowned Patient. See text for details.

Application of PEEP or CPAP to the airway improves ventilation/perfusion matching and oxygenation.[27,32,58] If the patient is alert and can adequately clear CO_2, CPAP may be applied by a special tight-fitting face mask. Most patients easily tolerate 10 to 12 torr of CPAP applied by this method. If levels greater than 12 torr are used or aerophagia is present, then a nasogastric tube should be inserted to prevent gastric distention. If oxygenation does not improve with this technique, if the patient cannot maintain adequate alveolar ventilation to clear CO_2, if respiration is labored, or if the patient is at high risk from vomiting, the patient should be intubated. Once the trachea is intubated, CPAP can be titrated to higher levels to improve oxygenation and mechanical ventilatory breaths can be added.

The degree of venous admixture after near-drowning varies. The exact amount of CPAP each patient will require must be individualized based on the therapeutic effect achieved. The optimal level of CPAP is when the greatest decrease in intrapulmonary shunting and improvement in ventilation/perfusion ratio are achieved

without adversely affecting CO.[59,60] In addition to CPAP, mechanical breaths will occasionally be necessary, not only to maintain $PaCO_2$ within a normal range, but also to improve PaO_2, particularly after freshwater aspiration.[32] If controlled ventilation is necessary, CO may be compromised.[32] The addition of PEEP or CPAP at high levels may decrease CO, particularly if hypovolemia is present. Cardiac output may be improved by augmenting intravascular volume with crystalloid, colloid, or, rarely, blood.[42] With spontaneous ventilation CPAP results in decreased intrapleural pressures and improved venous return, which also help to maintain a better CO. Once CPAP has been titrated to optimal levels and the beneficial effects on oxygenation realized, any interruptions in the expiratory positive airway pressure should be minimized; sudden discontinuation results in a decreased FRC and PaO_2 within seconds. The more severe the pulmonary insufficiency, the more pronounced are these changes and the more difficult it is to restore oxygenation to the previous level.[61] Unnecessary disconnections for suctioning and such should also be avoided.

Bronchospasm may occasionally occur after near-drowning and, if so, should be treated with a bronchodilating agent such as IV aminophylline. Pulmonary edema may accompany near-drowning with either fresh water or seawater and is best treated with CPAP as just described. Bronchoscopy is not indicated after near-drowning unless solid material has been aspirated.

Steroids should not be used to treat aspiration pneumonitis associated with near-drowning. Animals who have aspirated foodstuff[62] or acid[63-65] or have near-drowned in fresh water[66] show no significant improvement in PaO_2 or in survival with the addition of steroids to therapy. According to Wynne and colleagues steroids may actually prevent normal healing after pulmonary injury caused by aspiration of foodstuff.[62] Retrospective analysis of data from near-drowned humans also shows that survival did not improve with steroids.[5] The use of steroids to treat cerebral edema may be justified.[67,68]

Prophylactic antibiotics are also not recommended to treat aspiration pneumonitis after near-drowning unless clinical symptoms and cultures indicate an infection. Routine use of antibiotic prophylaxis may actually cause superinfection with resistant organisms. If the patient is intubated, tracheal secretions should be stained and cultured at once and then daily thereafter as those results may be of some value in deciding what antibiotic to use should signs and symptoms of a pulmonary infection occur.

Sodium bicarbonate is indicated to treat persistent metabolic acidosis in a near-drowned patient. The dose of bicarbonate to be administered should be based on determinations of arterial blood gas values and acid-base balance. The formula for calculating the dose of bicarbonate is: sodium bicarbonate (mEq) equals weight (kg) $\times$ base deficit (mEq/liter) $\times$ 0.20.

Fluid Therapy

Fluid resuscitation is rarely necessary after near-drowning unless pulmonary edema occurs and an excessive loss of fluid results. If hypovolemia does occur, resuscitation with crystalloid, such as lactated Ringer's solution, or colloid is indicated. Ordinarily, only maintenance fluids are required and, if the patient is comatose and has cerebral edema, fluids might actually have to be restricted after the initial resuscitation and evaluation. The patient's electrolyte changes are usually transient and require no specific therapy; however, if persistent imbalances do occur, they should be corrected. Most near-drowned patients do not aspirate a sufficient quantity of fluid to cause electrolyte changes that will be evident on arrival at the emergency department.[5]

Significant hemolysis of RBCs after near-drowning is extremely rare; however, if combined with profound hypoxia, clinically significant hemolysis may occur. If hemoglobinemia and hemoglobinuria occur, consideration should be given to the use of osmotic diuresis to increase urine flow and elimination of plasma Hb. Circulating blood volume must be adequate before the administration of an osmotic diuretic.

CNS Therapy

Although the immediate emphasis of therapy after near-drowning is directed at the lungs and the improvement of oxygenation and oxygen delivery, other organ systems may be affected, particularly if hypoxia has been sustained.[44] The final measure of successful therapy is survival without neurologic deficit. In the emergency department, a careful neurologic examination must be performed. If there is a history of falling or diving or signs of facial trauma, cervical spine injury and intracranial hemorrhage must be ruled out with roentgenography of the cervical spine, CT scan, or, occasionally, arteriography. A cervical collar should be placed on the patient until cervical injury is ruled out. If the patient is alert, then no specific therapy aimed at cerebral salvage is necessary. If the patient has a blunted level of consciousness, therapy aimed at cardiopulmonary resuscitation and improved oxygenation is all that is necessary and should result in survival of 90 to 100 percent of patients.[20,54]

The comatose patient is a more complicated problem. In addition to the guidelines outlined so far, therapy aimed at preserving the brain and decreasing cerebral edema must be considered. Hyperventilation to a $PaCO_2$ of approximately 25 to 30 torr will reduce cerebral blood flow and cerebral volume and, thereby, will reduce intracranial pressure (ICP).[69] This is unquestionably indicated if cerebral edema is present and should be started in the emergency department. Other therapy is more controversial. Although the data supporting beneficial effects are inconclusive, steroids have been advocated and are used frequently to treat cerebral edema.[67,68,70,71]

Conn and colleagues have recommended a more aggressive approach to the comatose, near-drowned patient regardless of the state of ICP.[19,20] They recommend high-dose barbiturate therapy, induced hypothermia (30°C), muscle paralysis, hyperventilation, diuresis with furosemide, steroids, and a PaO_2 of 150 torr or greater. High concentrations of inspired oxygen are used as necessary to produce this hyperoxia. There are no controlled prospective studies evaluating the ratio of risk to benefit of such therapy.

If cerebral edema and elevated ICP are present, therapy to reduce ICP below 20 torr is indicated. High-dose barbiturate therapy can decrease ICP by increasing cerebral vascular resistance, which decreases intracranial blood volume. This therapy should be used if ICP cannot be controlled with hyperventilation and with judicious use of drugs such as mannitol (0.25 gm/kg)[72] or furosemide (0.5 to 1 mg/kg). Weighing the potential risk versus the benefit of hypothermia and hyperoxia makes this therapy questionable. If ICP cannot be controlled or if the patient cannot be adequately oxygenated with aggressive pulmonary intervention, hypothermia may be justified. Even in the face of cerebral edema, a PaO_2 of approximately 100 torr should be adequate. Barbiturate therapy, hypothermia, and other aggressive measures for cerebral salvage are instituted in the intensive care unit. Given the present state of the art, patients ideally should be triaged to a unit with full-time staff to administer and monitor such therapy. A complete discussion of barbiturate therapy is beyond the scope of this text and the reader is referred to the bibliography for further information.[73–77]

Monitoring

All near-drowned patients must have vital signs (heart rate, blood pressure, respiratory rate, and temperature) monitored. If hypoxemia persists and any type of prolonged support is necessary, ECG and intake and output must also be monitored.

Most important is the analysis of arterial blood gases and pH. If multiple determinations are necessary, an arterial catheter facilitates the sampling of blood.

In addition to determinations of arterial blood gases and pH, Hb, Hct, and serum electrolytes should be determined. If the Hct is near normal and the plasma is free of Hb, it is unlikely that the patient has aspirated enough fluid to affect electrolyte concentrations. If hemolysis is present on inspection of the plasma, determination of plasma Hb is indicated. Chest and, also, if indicated, cervical spine roentgenograms should be obtained. Those patients requiring extensive cardiopulmonary resuscitation should also have baseline coagulation values determined—prothrombin time, partial thromboplastin time, and platelet counts—and a baseline renal metabolic profile performed.

Patients with cardiovascular instability need venous pressure monitoring. Central venous pressure reflects pressure proximal to the right atrium and has limited benefit during pulmonary insufficiency and when high levels of expiratory pressure are required. In these situations, a flow-directed thermistor-tipped pulmonary artery catheter is helpful in assessing pulmonary artery and pulmonary artery occlusion pressures, CO, intrapulmonary shunt, and arterial-venous content difference.[78–80] The ICP of patients who remain comatose after resuscitation should be monitored.[18,81]

In summary, therapy must be directed at rapid cardiopulmonary resuscitation as indicated by the victim's condition at the scene of the accident and must be continued uninterrupted until all vital functions are stabilized or death is confirmed. Fear of resuscitating a permanently neurologically damaged patient should not be a consideration as there are reports of intact survival after prolonged submersion.[12]

Ambulatory and Follow-Up Care

Patients whose PaO_2 is greater than 80 torr while breathing room air probably did not aspirate. If the patient is alert and, after in-hospital observation for 12 to 24 hours, has no deterioration of physical status or arterial blood gas values, such a patient may be discharged without further specific follow-up. Always advise the patient to return if any signs of respiratory distress, fever, or other related problems occur within 48 hours of release.

Patients who have minimal alteration of arterial blood gases that rapidly return to normal while being observed or treated in the intensive care unit should return to a physician familiar with their history after approximately a week, or sooner if problems occur.

Patients who require more prolonged and extensive therapy for respiratory insufficiency, cerebral damage, or damage to other organs require more extensive follow-up, the exact extent of which will depend on the severity of the injury and the residual deficits.

REFERENCES

1. Modell JH: Biology of drowning. *Annu Rev Med* 29:1–8, 1978.
2. Modell JH (ed): *The Pathophysiology and Treatment of Drowning and Near-Drowning*. Springfield, Ill: Charles C Thomas, 1971.
3. Modell JH: Drown versus near-drown: A discussion of definitions. *Crit Care Med* 9:351–352, 1981.
4. Cot C: *Les Asphyxies Accidentelles (Submersion, Electrocution, Intoxication Oxycarbonique). Etude Clinique, Therapeutique et Preventive*. Paris, Editions medicales N. Maloine, 1931.
5. Modell JH, Graves SA, Ketover A: Clinical course of 91 consecutive near-drowning victims. *Chest* 70:231–236, 1976.
6. Press E, Walker J, Crawford I: An interstate drowning study. *Am J Public Health* 58:2275–2289, 1968.
7. Webster DP: Pool drownings and their prevention. *Public Health Rep* 82:587–600, 1967.
8. Pearn JH, et al: Drowning and near-drowning involving children: A five year total population study from the city and county of Honolulu. *Am J Public Health* 69:450–454, 1979.
9. Craig AB Jr: Causes of loss of consciousness during underwater swimming. *J Appl Physiol* 16:583, 1961.
10. Craig AB Jr: Underwater swimming and loss of consciousness. *JAMA* 176:255–258, 1961.
11. Keatinge WR: *Survival in Cold Water: The Physiology and Treatment of Immersion Hypothermia and of Drowning*. Oxford, Blackwell Scientific, 1969, pp 5, 42.
12. Siebke H, Breivek H, Rod T, et al: Survival after 40 minutes' submersion without sequelae. *Lancet* 1:1275–1277, 1975.

13. Gordon BA: Drowning and the diving reflex in man. *Med J Aust* 2:583–587, 1972.
14. Davis JH: Autopsy findings in victims of drowning, in Modell JH (ed): *The Pathophysiology and Treatment of Drowning and Near-Drowning*. Springfield, Ill: Charles C Thomas, 1971, pp 74–82.
15. Swann HG, Brucer M: The cardiorespiratory and biochemical events during rapid anoxic death. VI. Fresh water and sea water drowning. *Tex Rep Biol Med* 7:604–618, 1949.
16. Swann HG, Brucer M, Moore C, et al: Fresh water and sea water drowning: A study of the terminal cardiac and biochemical events. *Tex Rep Biol Med* 5:423–437, 1947.
17. Modell JH, Moya F, Williams HD, et al: Changes in blood gases and A-aDO$_2$ during near-drowning. *Anesthesiology* 29:456–465, 1968.
18. Conn AW, Edmonds JF, Barker GA: Near-drowning in cold fresh water: Current treatment regimen. *Can Anaesth Soc* 25:259–265, 1978.
19. Conn AW, Edmonds JF, Barker GA: Cerebral resuscitation in near-drowning. *Pediatr Clin North Am* 26:691–701, 1979.
20. Conn AW, Montes JE, Barker GA, et al: Cerebral 'salvage' in near-drowning: Following neurological classification. *Can Anaesth Soc* 27:201–210, 1980.
21. Modell JH, et al: Blood gas and electrolyte changes in human near-drowning victims. *JAMA* 203:337–343, 1968.
22. Modell JH, Gaub M, Moya F, et al: Physiologic effects of near-drowning with chlorinated fresh water, distilled water, and isotonic sodium chloride. *Anesthesiology* 27:33–41, 1966.
23. Modell JH, Kuck EJ, Ruiz BC, et al: Effect of intravenous vs. aspirated distilled water on serum electrolytes and blood gas tensions. *J Appl Physiol* 32:579–584, 1972.
24. Modell JH, Moya F: Effects of volume of aspirated fluid during chlorinated fresh water drowning. *Anesthesiology* 27:662, 1966.
25. Modell JH, Moya F, Newby EJ, et al: The effects of fluid volume in seawater drowning. *Ann Intern Med* 67:68–80, 1967.
26. Hasan S, Avery WG, Fabian C, et al: Near-drowning in humans. A report of 36 patients. *Chest* 59:191–197, 1971.
27. Modell JH, Calderwood HW, Ruiz BC, et al: Effects of ventilatory patterns on arterial oxygenation after near-drowning in sea water. *Anesthesiology* 40:376–384, 1974.
28. Giammona ST, Modell JH: Drowning by total immersion: Effects on pulmonary surfactant of distilled water, isotonic saline and sea water. *Am J Dis Child* 114:612–616, 1967.
29. Colebatch HJH, Halmagyi DFJ: Lung mechanics and resuscitation after fluid aspiration. *J Appl Physiol* 16:684–696, 1961.
30. Colebatch HJH, Halmagyi DFJ: Reflex airway reaction to fluid aspiration. *J Appl Physiol* 17:787–794, 1962.
31. Colebatch HJH, Halmagyi DFJ: Reflex pulmonary hypertension of fresh water aspiration. *J Appl Physiol* 18:179–185, 1963.
32. Bergquist RE, Vogelhut MM, Modell JH, et al: Comparison of ventilatory patterns in the treatment of freshwater near-drowning in dogs. *Anesthesiology* 52:142–148, 1980.
33. Ducker TB, Simmons RL, Anderson RW: Increased intracranial pressure and pulmonary edema. III. The effect of increased intracranial pressure on the cardiovascular hemodynamics of chimpanzees. *J Neurosurg* 29:475–483, 1968.
34. Butt MP, Jalowayski A, Modell JH, et al: Pulmonary function after resuscitation from near-drowning. *Anesthesiology* 32:275–277, 1970.
35. Jenkinson SG, George RB: Serial pulmonary function studies in survivors of near drowning. *Chest* 77:777–780, 1980.
36. Modell JH, Davis JH: Electrolyte changes in human drowning victims. *Anesthesiology* 30:414–420, 1969.
37. Fainer DC: Near drowning in sea water and fresh water. *Ann Intern Med* 59:537–541, 1963.
38. Farthmann EH, Davidson AIG: Fresh water drowning at lowered body temperature: an experimental study. *Am J Surg* 109:410, 1965.
39. Lougheed DW, Janes JM, Hall GE: Physiological studies in experimental asphyxia and drowning. *Can Med Assoc* 40:423–428, 1939.
40. Redding JS, Pearson JW: Management of drowning victims. *GP* 29:100–104, June 1964.
41. Spitz WU, Blanke RV: Mechanism of death in freshwater drowning. I. An experimental approach to the problem. *Arch Pathol* 71:661–668, 1961.
42. Tabeling BB, Modell JH: Drowning and near-drowning: pathophysiology and treatment, in Tinker J, Rapin M (eds): *Care of the Critically Ill Patient*. Berlin, Springer-Verlag, in press.
43. Culpepper RM: Bleeding diathesis in freshwater drowning. *Ann Intern Med* 83:675, 1975.
44. Hoff BH: Multisystem failure: A review with special reference to drowning. *Crit Care Med* 7:310–320, 1979.
45. Ports RA, Deuel TF: Intravascular coagulation in freshwater submersion: Report of 3 cases. *Ann Intern Med* 87:60–61, 1977.
46. Fuller RH: The 1962 Wellcome Prize Essay. Drowning and the post-immersion syndrome. A clinicopathologic study. *Milit Med* 128:22–36, 1963.
47. King RB, Webster IW: A case of recovery from drowning and prolonged anoxia. *Med J Aust* 1:919–920, 1964.
48. Kvittingen TD, Naess A: Recovery from drowning in fresh water. *Brit Med J* 1:1315–1317, 1963.
49. Munroe WD: Hemoglobinuria from near-drowning. *J Pediatr* 64:57–62, 1964.
50. Rath CE: Drowning hemoglobinuria. *Blood* 8:1099–1104, 1953.
51. Pearn JH, Bart RD Jr., Yamaoka R: Neurologic sequelae after childhood near-drowning: A total population study from Hawaii. *Pediatr* 64:187–191, 1979.
52. Pearn JH, Nixon J, Wilkey I: Freshwater drowning and near-drowning accidents involving children: A five-year total population study. *Med J Aust* 2:942–946, 1975.
53. Peterson B: Morbidity of childhood near-drowning. *Pediatr* 59:364–370, 1962.
54. Modell JH, Graves SA, Kuck EJ: Near-drowning: Correlation of level of consciousness and survival. *Can Anaesth Soc J* 27:211–215, 1980.
55. Conn AW, Modell JH: Current neurological considerations in near-drowning. *Can Anaesth Soc J* 27:197, 1980.
56. Safar P, Escarraga LA, Elam JO: A comparison of the mouth-to-mouth and mouth-to-airway methods of artificial respiration with the chest-pressure arm-lift methods. *N Engl J Med* 258:671–677, 1958.
57. Heimlich HJ: The Heimlich maneuver: First treatment for drowning victims. *Emerg Med Serv* 10:58–61, 1981.
58. Ruiz BC, Calderwood HW, Modell JH, et al: Effect of ventilatory patterns on arterial oxygenation after near-drowning with fresh water. A comparative study in dogs. *Anesth Analg (Cleve)* 52:570–576, 1973.
59. Downs JB, Klein EF Jr, Modell JH: The effect of incremental PEEP on PaO$_2$ in patients with respiratory failure. *Anesth Analg (Cleve)* 52:210–214, 1973.
60. Downs JB, Modell JH: Patterns of respiratory support aimed at pathophysiologic conditions, in Hershey SG (ed): *ASA Refresher Courses in Anesthesiology*, Philadelphia, JB Lippincott, 1977, vol 5, pp 71–85.
61. Rose DM, Downs JB, Heenan TJ: Temporal responses of functional residual capacity and oxygen tension to changes in positive end-expiratory pressure. *Crit Care Med* 9:79–82, 1981.
62. Wynne JW, Reynolds JC, Hood CL, et al: Steroid therapy for pneumonitis induced in rabbits by aspiration of foodstuff. *Anesthesiology* 51:11–19, 1979.
63. Chapman RL Jr, Downs JB, Modell JH, et al: The ineffectiveness

of steroid therapy in treating aspiration of hydrochloric acid. *Arch Surg* 108:858–861, 1974.

64. Chapman RL Jr, Modell JH, Ruiz BC, et al: Effect of continuous positive-pressure ventilation and steroids on aspiration of hydrochloric acid (pH 1.8) in dogs. *Anesth Analg (Cleve)* 53:556–562, 1974.

65. Downs JB, Chapman RL Jr, Modell JH, et al: An evaluation of steroid therapy in aspiration pneumonitis. *Anesthesiology* 40:129–135, 1974.

66. Calderwood HW, Modell JH, Ruiz BC: The ineffectiveness of steroid therapy in treating fresh water near-drowning. *Anesthesiology* 43:642–650, 1975.

67. Faupel G, Reulen JH, Müller D, et al: Double-blind study on the effects of steroids on seven closed-head injuries. In Pappius HM, Feindel W (eds): *Dynamics of Brain Edema.* Berlin, Springer-Verlag, 1976, pp 337–343.

68. Gobiet W, Bock WJ, Liesegang J, et al: Treatment of acute cerebral edema with high dose dexamethasone, in Beks JW, Bosch DA, Brock M, et al (eds): *Intracranial Pressure III.* Berlin, Springer-Verlag, 1976, pp 231–235.

69. Severinghaus JW, Lassen HA: Step hypocapnia to separate arterial from tissue PCO₂ in the regulation of cerebral blood flow. *Circ Res* 20:272–278, 1967.

70. Fishman RA: Brain edema. *N Engl J Med* 293:706–711, 1975.

71. Gudeman SK, Miller JD, Becker DP: Failure of high dose steroid therapy to influence intracranial pressure in patients with severe head injury. *J Neurosurg* 51:301–306, 1979.

72. Marshall LF, Smith RW, Rauscher LA, et al: Mannitol dose requirements in brain-injured patients. *J Neurosurg* 48:169–172, 1978.

73. Marsh MI, Marshall LF, Shapiro HM: Neurosurgical intensive care. *Anesthesiology* 47:149–163, 1977.

74. Michenfelder JD: The interdependency of cerebral functional and metabolic effects following massive doses of thiopental in the dog. *Anesthesiology* 41:231–236, 1974.

75. Pierce EC Jr, Lambertson CJ, Deutsch MC, et al: Cerebral circulation and metabolism during thiopental anesthesia and hyperventilation in man. *J Clin Invest* 41:1664–1671, 1962.

76. Rockoff MA, Marshall LF, Shapiro HM: High-dose barbiturate therapy in humans: A clinical review of 60 patients. *Ann Neurol* 6:194–199, 1979.

77. Siesjo BK, Carlsson C, Hagerdal M, et al: Brain metabolism in the critically ill. *Crit Care Med* 4:283–294, 1976.

78. Colgan FJ, Mahoney PD: The effects of major surgery on cardiac output and shunting. *Anesthesiology* 31:221–231, 1969.

79. Gustafson I, Nordstrom L: Central venous PO₂ and open-heart surgery. *Acta Anaesth Scand (suppl 37)* 14:112–113, 1970.

80. Swan HJC, et al: Catheterization of the heart in man with use of flow-directed balloon-tipped catheter. *N Engl J Med* 283:447–451, 1970.

81. Mickell JJ, Reigel DH, Cook DR, et al: Intracranial pressure: Monitoring and normalization therapy in children. *Pediatr* 59:606–613, 1977.

33. Diving Emergencies

ERIC P. KINDWALL, M.D.

Any diver—whether using deep-sea dress supplied by a compressor on the surface or a self-contained underwater breathing apparatus (scuba) supplied by tanked air carried on the back—is subject to pressure-related accidents. Barotrauma associated with scuba use can produce sudden death in as little as 4 feet of water. Thus, severe diving accidents can occur in a relatively shallow swimming pool.

BAROTRAUMA

The word barotrauma is derived from the same Greek root as the word barometer and refers to any damage done to the body by a change in pressure. Barotrauma of the ears is most common. As the diver descends, the pressure in the middle ear must equalize through the eustachian tube. If it does not, the eardrum usually ruptures between 10 and 15 ft. Simple damage to the eardrum can be managed easily with decongestants to help open the passage to the middle ear and drain any blood from the middle ear. If the eardrum is broken, it usually heals within two weeks, but the patient should be cautioned not to dive before being reexamined. A ruptured eardrum contraindicates diving, since cold water entering the middle ear can cause sudden vertigo and incapacitation underwater.

Another consequence of barotrauma to the ear may be "round-window blow-out." In this case, the patient has usually tried to use Valsalva's maneuver vigorously to equalize middle ear pressure during descent. Symp-toms are tinnitus, deafness, and perhaps vertigo after returning to the surface. If 48 hours of complete bed rest with the head elevated fails to completely clear this, surgical exploration is mandatory.

Sinus squeeze is the next most common form of barotrauma experienced by scuba divers. The patient frequently complains of extreme frontal sinus pain and may spit out blood after surfacing. Maxillary and ethmoid pain are much less common. If the patient complains of pain at the occiput or vertex of the skull, the sinus most likely involved is the sphenoid, which refers pain to these areas. Treatment is again the use of simple decongestants.

Tooth pain is sometimes encountered by divers but if it is in the upper jaw it must be differentiated from maxillary sinus squeeze. It is sometimes difficult for the patient to differentiate the pain because pain can often result from an improperly or incompletely filled tooth which becomes symptomatic with compression or decompression. Treatment is for the dentist to revise the filling, being sure that there are no gas spaces.

Cerebral Air Embolism

Cerebral air embolism results from pulmonary barotrauma or overdistention of the lungs during ascent, usually with a closed glottis. This is sometimes termed burst lung.

The mechanism is as follows. While submerged in water, the diver is breathing air from the scuba tank at a pressure exactly equal to the pressure of the surrounding water. For example, at a depth of 4 ft, the pressure of the air in the diver's lungs equals that of the surrounding water which is 1.78 psi above normal atmospheric pressure at the surface. This corresponds to a pressure differential between the surface and the diver's alveoli of 92 mm Hg. If the diver then takes a deep breath and holds it while ascending 4 ft to the surface, the air within the lungs will expand, and the diver will arrive at the surface with a pressure within the lungs 92 mm Hg greater than the surrounding air pressure.

Animal experiments have shown that the pulmonary alveoli rupture at a transpulmonic pressure of 80 mm Hg. Once alveolar rupture occurs, the air can be forced medially to produce pneumomediastinum; laterally through the pleura to cause pneumothorax; or in the worst case, into the pulmonary capillaries themselves and thence to the pulmonary veins and the left heart. From the left ventricle the air is pumped directly into the brain via the carotids. As little as 0.5 ml of blood air foam delivered to the right anatomic area in the brain can cause death. The onset of symptoms is abrupt, usually within seconds of surfacing. If symptoms first appear longer than about 5 minutes after surfacing, the cause is usually not air embolism. Symptoms and signs of cerebral air embolism include sudden unconsciousness, hemiplegia with paralysis extending vertically from face to toes, a dilated pupil on the affected side, sudden numbness or weakness of an extremity or confusion, coma, and death. Sometimes, a white mottling of the tongue may appear due to an embolization of the arteries to the tongue; this is termed Liebermeister's sign. Thus, symptoms can vary from death within a minute or two to a strokelike syndrome or a weakness limited to one part of an extremity. Sometimes, the patient may have only a personality or mental change which the examining physician may not note but which can be recognized by querying the patient's companions.

Treatment is recompression in a hyperbaric chamber to a depth of 165 ft in order to compress the bubbles to one-sixth of their original volume and restore circulation. The patient must be referred to a chamber NO MATTER HOW FAR AWAY IT IS. Even hyperbaric treatment carried out a number of hours after the embolism will usually prove very effective.

Subcutaneous emphysema frequently accompanies cerebral embolism as air moves upward from the mediastinum. Crepitus below the angles of the jaw or anywhere in the neck in the absence of trauma is pathognomonic of burst lung. Always palpate the neck first when a diving casualty is brought to the emergency department. It is helpful to remember that if the accident occurred in less than 33 ft of water, decompression sickness can be ruled out. Anyone experiencing sudden neurologic dysfunction of any kind on surfacing from a dive, even in a shallow swimming pool, should be assumed to have air embolism until proved otherwise.

Immediate management of cerebral air embolism is placing the patient in steep Trendelenburg position and administering 100 percent oxygen by tight-fitting mask. In the head-down position, the increased hemostatic pressure in the brain dilates the blood vessels. Animal experiments have shown that air bubbles tend to pass through the capillary bed when local blood pressure is thus increased, and circulation may be partially restored. The purpose of the oxygen is to increase the gradient for nitrogen elimination from the bubbles in the circulation, not to oxygenate the patient per se. Thus, the mask should fit extremely tightly—tightly enough that it would permit the patient to breathe from it while lying supine underwater. The usual plastic masks in most emergency departments are totally inadequate. An anesthesia mask with attached 5-liter bag will suffice. A double-seal or nasal aviator's mask with a demand regulator is ideal.

The most common error made by a physician is to dismiss the symptoms because of the trivial depth or, if the patient is recovering or "nearly normal" when seen in the emergency department, to miss the diagnosis completely. *All* patients suffering from burst lung should be referred to a hyperbaric specialist. Many scuba divers' deaths are ascribed to drowning when in reality cerebral air embolism was the cause of death.

DECOMPRESSION SICKNESS

Decompression sickness, also termed the bends or Caisson disease, is caused by the evolution of nitrogen bubbles in the blood and tissues following ascent from a dive or other exposure to increased ambient pressure. Nitrogen from the air breathed during the dive is absorbed into the tissues where it causes no problem (aside from a narcotizing effect at depths in excess of 100 ft) while the dive is in progress. However, if the diver has been diving deeply or has remained a long time and then ascends too rapidly to the surface, nitrogen bubbles out of solution and causes difficulty.

The rule of thumb is that decompression sickness cannot occur at depths shallower than 33 ft in the usual sport diver. However in compressed air, tunnel workers who work seven- and eight-hour shifts at increased pressure, decompression sickness is a possibility if pressures are in the range of as little as 11 to 12 psi. This corresponds to a sea-water depth of 25 to 27 ft. According to Navy diving tables published in the *U.S. Navy Diving Manual,*[1] the diver can remain for up to 200 minutes at 40 ft without the necessity of taking decompression stops on the way back to the surface. However, the deeper the diver goes, the shorter the time before decompression becomes a requirement. Thus, the time limit for "no-decompression" diving is 100 minutes at 50 ft and 25 minutes at 100 ft. Descent time is included in the actual bottom time for purposes of decompression. Most sport scuba divers have copies of these tables.

A particular danger in sport scuba diving is that the diver may make more than one dive within a 12-hour period. This can cause difficulty as after the first dive, a certain amount of residual nitrogen remains in the body and, using tables developed by the Navy, this residual nitrogen time must be added to the total bottom time of the second dive. Because of the residual nitrogen which takes over 12 hours to leave the body, two or three no-decompression dives made during any 12-hour period might produce decompression sickness if this residual nitrogen is ignored. Since there is a great variation among individuals, the possibility of decompression sickness cannot be dismissed even in someone who has followed the tables exactly. A certain percentage of people approaching the limits of the decompression tables will suffer decompression sickness even if the tables are used properly. Increasing age, obesity, postalcoholic state, viral illness, dehydration, recent strain or sprain, and extreme hard work while under water can all contribute to an increased incidence of decompression sickness.

Diagnosis

Decompression sickness is divided into two types, type I being simple "pain only" bends. In this situation, pain is experienced in a muscle belly or near a joint and is typically described as being boring or like a toothache. Ninety percent of all patients with decompression sickness present with pain. To be classified as type I decompression sickness, there must be no symptom other than pain. The pain commonly appears in an extremity but may appear anywhere in the body. Abdominal pain should be viewed with some alarm as this may be referred from the spinal cord and in such case is not a simple type I case. Divers most commonly experience pain in the upper extremities whereas compressed-air tunnel workers more commonly experience pain in the legs.

Type II decompression sickness includes all cases in which serious symptoms appear. Pain is often present also. Twenty-five percent of all cases of decompression sickness present with neurologic symptoms, commonly associated with the middle third of the spinal cord. Thus, in decompression sickness the paralysis tends to be from T10 down and a paraplegia results. This contrasts with air embolism which often produces a hemiplegia. Sometimes, a type-II case may present with only a small patch of numbness on an extremity that may easily be missed by the examining physician. Symptoms include numbness, weakness, and loss of bladder and bowel control so that these patients often require a Foley catheter. *Any diver who complains of "pins and needles" anywhere in the body following a dive deeper than 33 ft should be considered to have spinal cord decompression sickness until proved otherwise.*

Another form of type-II decompression sickness is a vestibular disturbance often called the "staggers." The patient has true vertigo and nystagmus with vomiting made worse by any movement of the head. Vestibular decompression sickness must be treated within 45 minutes after the onset of symptoms if dramatic relief is to be achieved in the recompression chamber. If the patient is received later than this, recompression is still mandatory.

Another form of serious decompression sickness is known as "chokes." Here, some hours after the dive, nitrogen bubbles collect in the lungs and when more than one-third of the pulmonary capillaries are blocked, symptoms of asphyxiation may occur. Only about 2 percent of the cases involve chokes. In chokes, the patient breathes less and less deeply as time progresses, because taking a deep breath causes pain and paroxysms of coughing. Even in a heavy smoker, one puff from a cigarette will provoke a violent paroxysm of coughing and chokes. This is known as Behnke's sign.

In very severe cases of decompression sickness, usually after a long exposure underwater, decompression sickness shock may result. Here, the hematocrit may rise, since capillary permeability permits an outflow of plasma into the third space. In decompression sickness shock, massive fluid replacement with plasma or plasma substitutes is an absolute requirement in addition to recompression in the hyperbaric chamber.

Treatment

Recompression in a hyperbaric chamber as soon as possible after symptoms appear is the sine qua non of treatment in decompression sickness. If blockade of the vasculature draining the hips or shoulders is permitted to remain for more than six to twelve hours, aseptic necrosis or dysbaric osteonecrosis may result months or years later. Vascular blockade is painless and the patient might develop osteonecrosis of a hip even though the only complaint is muscle pain near the shoulder. Also, any diver who has for some reason missed taking required decompression according to standard tables following any dive is a candidate for later dysbaric osteonecrosis, *even if asymptomatic.* Thus all decompression sickness cases, no matter how mild or doubtful, must be referred to a treatment chamber. If the diagnosis is in doubt, a test of pressure or brief exposure to pressure in the chamber breathing oxygen can be carried out by hyperbaric personnel. It is wise to consult with experts in any diving-related accident.

Immediate Treatment Measures

While arranging transfer to a recompression facility however, there are a number of things the emergency physician can do to be of immediate help. Immediate hydration of the patient is of utmost importance. Forcing fluids either orally or intravenously (IV) to produce a urine output of 1 to 2 ml/kg or more is a necessity. Again it is emphasized that a urinary catheter must be placed if the patient is unable to urinate and becomes distended. Oral fluids can be forced at the rate of 1 liter/hour for the first one or two hours, or Ringer's lactate may be given IV. The use of plain dextrose 5% and water is discouraged as the glucose will be metabolized away leaving water which may worsen neural tissue edema. Evidence now shows that patients hydrated before arriving at the hyperbaric chamber fare much better than those who have not been so managed.

Aspirin has theoretical value as it appears to inhibit platelet aggregation even though there are no experimental data to demonstrate its prophylactic value. Two tablets taken orally will exert maximum effect in this regard in 30 minutes. Platelet aggregation seems to play a role in decompression sickness as well as sludging of all of the formed elements of the blood. However, once platelet aggregation is complete and the vessel blockade has been established, the theoretical value of aspirin is nil. Thus, it must be given immediately after symptoms appear.

Steroids can be given as they tend to stabilize membranes and endothelium and have an anti-edema effect which has been noted by neurosurgeons. For this reason the indication is usually serious decompression sickness affecting the brain and spinal cord. The recommended dosage appears to be 1 gm of a rapidly acting steroid such as hydrocortisone hemisuccinate given IV in a bolus with 4 mg decadron given concomitantly intramuscularly (IM). The latter drug is continued in 4-mg doses every six hours for two to three days.

Glycerol may be of value in treating spinal cord edema secondary to decompression sickness and has been used in this way with good effect. It is given orally, 0.8 ml/kg of body weight in a 50% solution of water, which may be flavored with lemonade to make it more palatable. It is superior to mannitol and urea in that it does not derange electrolyte balance and it exerts its maximal effect in one hour with a duration of effect of six hours. This is faster than all other agents. It does not cause rebound edema. The only major disadvantage of glycerin is that it is an unpalatable concoction which may induce nausea and thus may have to be given via nasogastric tube.

The use of narcotic analgesics or opiates is contraindicated unless there is some overriding necessity. Respiratory depression caused by morphine can exacerbate oxygen toxicity during later treatment in the hyperbaric chamber, and additionally, potent analgesics may mask symptoms and hinder evaluation of response to treatment.

Diazepam appears to be the drug of choice should the patient be convulsing. It may be administered IV in 10-mg doses as required. Barbiturates are not safe as they produce more respiratory depression, again with the increased liability of central nervous system (CNS) oxygen toxicity during treatment in the hyperbaric chamber.

If the patient is extremely restless requiring sedation during transportation or if agitation is so great that sedation is required to carry out treatment, diazepam is again the preferred drug. The IV route is best and the dosage is the same as indicated for convulsion suppression.

Oxygen should be given by tightly fitting mask, if available. As stated above, the purpose is not to oxygenate but to *denitrogenate* the patient.

While these immediate first aid measures are being carried out, arrangements must be made to transport the patient to a recompression chamber no matter how far away it is.

The National Oceanic and Atmospheric Administration, in conjunction with the National Institute of Occupational Safety and Health and the Department of Energy, has established a free emergency consultation and referral service for diving accidents occurring anywhere in North America or Hawaii. This service, the Diving Accident Network (DAN), knows the location and operational status of all recompression facilities as well as the best means of transportation to use. The service functions 24 hours a day, seven days a week, with headquarters at the F. G. Hall Laboratory, Duke University Medical Center in Durham, North Carolina. The United States has been divided into seven regions, each with its own coordinator. The telephone number of this consultation service, which will give access to any of the regions, is 919-684-8111. Collect calls will be accepted for real emergencies. Ask for the Diving Accident Network. The center will also be able to advise on other disorders that require treatment in a hyperbaric chamber, such as severe carbon monoxide poisoning, postsurgical air embolism, and gas gangrene.

REFERENCE

1. *U.S. Navy Diving Manual*, Navships 0994-001-9010, vol 1, Washington, D.C., Government Printing Office, 1973.

BIBLIOGRAPHY

Davis JC, Hunt TK (eds): *Hyperbaric Oxygen Therapy.* Bethesda, Md, Undersea Medical Society Inc, 1977.

Edmonds C, Lowry C, Pennefather J: *Diving and Subaquatic Medicine,* Mosman N.S.W., Australia, Diving Medical Centre, 1976.

Kindwall EP: Medical aspects of commercial diving and compressed air work, in Zenz C (ed): *Occupational Medicine,* Chicago, Year Book Medical Publishers, 1975, pp 361–421.

National Oceanic and Atmospheric Administration, Office of Marine Resources: *NOAA Diving Manual.* Washington, D.C., Government Printing Office, 1975.

Strauss RH (ed): *Diving Medicine,* New York, Grune & Stratton, 1976.

34. Dangerous Marine Organisms

KENNETH E. SCHULTZ, M.D.

The marine environment, in which our earliest ancestors were nurtured, has shaped the evolutionary development of the most beautiful, majestic, and—in many cases—deadly organisms on earth.

When one thinks of dangerous marine life, the usual initial reaction is, "Shark!" However, the majority of illnesses caused by marine life occur through direct contact with or ingestion of a variety of less obviously dangerous organisms. Sims quite accurately describes the broad spectrum of organisms and resultant illnesses.[1]

Dangerous marine life of the oceans ranges in size from minute viruses to large whales, and consists of micro-organisms, plants, and animals. *ANY* marine species which produces human injury or illness may be identified as a dangerous marine organism. Human beings are provided the opportunity to encounter dangerous marine organisms in the native habitat of these organisms while wading (e.g., stingray stings), swimming (e.g., Portuguese man-of-war stings), snorkeling (e.g., coral cuts), scuba diving (e.g., moray eel bites), boating (e.g., red tide-induced asthma), fishing (e.g., fish fin wounds), board surfing (e.g., shark bites), body surfing (e.g., lyngbya dermatitis), beachcombing (e.g., stings from dried-out jellyfish), marine spec-

imen collecting (e.g., palythoa intoxication), shellfish harvesting (e.g., sea urchin stings), sponge harvesting (e.g., sponge poisoning), and shell collecting (e.g., sea snake bites). The development of effective technology for maintaining saltwater aquaria has enabled dangerous sea creatures to be brought to public aquaria (where aquarium workers and researchers would be potential victims), private research aquaria (where researchers and aquarium workers would be at risk), and, importantly, home aquaria (where the unwary aquarium enthusiast would be at risk for injury or illness) . . . these aquaria being found scores to thousands of miles *inland* as well as in coastal areas. Home aquariums are sometimes stocked with living venomous "tropical fish" (such as the Lionfish *Pterois volitans*), cone shells, sea urchins, moray eels, surgeon-fish, and other noxious sea creatures. Aquaria also pose a threat of exotic marine bacterial infections, such as those attributed to *Mycobacterium marinum* and *Pseudomonas cepacia*, for the unprotected person dipping into or changing the aquarium water.

Dangerous marine organisms also affect persons in both coastal and inland areas through the human diet. There are fish and shellfish which, *in the absence of spoilage*, are toxic despite cooking or canning. These ingestion intoxications are endemic in certain areas of the world and include the not so esoteric poisonings such as ciguatera fish poisoning, paralytic shellfish poisoning (PSP), sardine

The author wishes to acknowledge the invaluable review of this manuscript by J.K. Sims, M.D., Chief, Emergency Medical Services Systems, Department of Health, State of Hawaii.

poisoning, pufferfish poisoning, and many others. Travel, scientific research programs, diving expeditions, and war campaigns have brought the unknowing into these endemic areas with resultant fish or shellfish poisoning upon the consumption of toxic species. Inadvertent importation of toxic fish and toxic shellfish has introduced the intoxicating species into the areas well away from the endemic source, although such occurrences are generally uncommon except in a few areas. Inland and coastal scombroid poisoning (by tuna, mahimahi, bonito, sardines, saury, et al.), by fresh, frozen, and canned fish and shellfish allergies occur worldwide in many ethnic groups and are presently felt to represent true allergic reactions and not a poisonous ingestion. Bacterial fish and shellfish poisoning will always remain a serious worldwide problem for fresh, frozen, and canned products whenever the prospect of spoilage is not eliminated. The human diet, then, is an example of the opportunity which living and nonliving marine organisms have to produce human illness and injury.

HISTORICAL PERSPECTIVE[2–5]

Historically, poisoning from ingestion of fish has been well recognized, and references to the dangers of eating certain marine organisms, specifically skates and rays, have been found in the writings of early Roman and Greek scholars. The biotoxicological syndrome of ciguatera fish poisoning is described in the *Odyssey* (800 B.C.). Alexander the Great (356–323 B.C.), during military campaigns, cautioned his legions to refrain from eating certain species of fish for fear of poisoning. Ch'en T'sang-chi, during the Tang Dynasty (618–907 A.D.), indicated in his writings the danger of eating yellowtail (amberjack), and for centuries yellowtail has been well known to cause human intoxication (i.e., ciguatera fish poisoning) after ingestion.

Peter Martyr of Anghera (1457–1526) is credited with the first published reference to ciguatera poisoning in the Americas. One of the earliest reported mass poisonings by ciguatera occurred during the voyage of Pedro Fernandez Quiros in the waters of the southern Pacific off the New Hebrides in 1606. The largest mass outbreak of ciguatera poisoning occurred during the British naval invasion of Mauritius, when the entire fleet of over 1,500 men succumbed after eating what appears to have been grouper (*Epinephelus fuscogutatus*).

Sauvages (1758–1770) is credited with the first report of oral intoxication from eating shark (*Squalus catulus*), and on July 23, 1774, one of the most noted outbreaks of ciguatera fish poisoning occurred on Captain James

Cook's ship *Resolution*. The crew became ill after ingesting snapper. One of the most fascinating accounts of ciguatera fish poisoning occurred on June 8, 1789, after the mutiny on the *Bounty* and the voyage of Captain Bligh. Several of his crew, after being cast adrift in a small lifeboat by the mutineers led by Fletcher Christian, became ill from eating a small dolphin (class Osteichthyes, family Coryphaenidae, genus (Coryphaena). This remarkable story is brilliantly outlined by Steinfield and Steinfield.[5]

Buniva in 1803 was the first to comment on the opiatelike effects from a poison found in ratfish (*Chimaeras*), and Chevallier and Duchene (1851) were the first to call attention to cyclostome (hagfishes and lampreys) poisoning. There have been numerous reports of fish poisoning in the 20th century, and from a historical perspective it becomes clear that there have been and will continue to be food-borne diseases caused by the ingestion of poisonous marine organisms.

TRAUMATIC LACERATIONS AND INJURIES

Shark[1,3,4,6–10]

The frightened cry of "shark" sends chills down the spine of most people, especially those in imminent danger. However, the actual incidence of shark attacks worldwide is less than 100 per year for which the fatality rate is approximately 35 percent. Of the 250 to 300 species of shark, only 27 species have been definitely implicated in attacks on humans.

Shark attacks seem to be seasonal, occurring with greater frequency in tropical waters where the temperature is above 68°F (20°C), and increasing during the late afternoon or evening hours when greater numbers of people are swimming and sharks are more likely to be feeding. Most attacks occur in waist-high water and are generally unprovoked. It is difficult to explain these unprovoked shark attacks, but they may be related to mistaken identity: a shark feeding on a fish may accidently bite a swimmer's leg. Furthermore, sharks seem to be territorial creatures and may perceive humans as invaders and a threat to their habitats. Unprovoked attacks may be precipitated by blood or commotion in the water, as occurs with spear fishing or near-drowning. Drowning victims whose bodies have never been recovered may indeed have been victims of a shark attack.

Provoked attacks certainly occur, usually as a consequence of the provocateur's foolhardiness. The divers who have been attacked have often been teasing, hitting, spearing, riding, and generally annoying the sharks that attack them. Instances of individuals being devoured alive have been documented, but there has been no significant evidence that sharks are true man-eaters that specifically prey on human beings.

The most notorious and frightening instances of shark attacks occurred in sea disasters during World War II. Specifically, on November 28, 1942, in the Indian Ocean south of Africa, the U.S.S. *Nova Scotia* was sunk and 1,000 men were reported killed by sharks. On July 3, 1945, after the sinking of the U.S.S. *Indianapolis*, only 370 men survived out of a crew of 1,200; the others died from exposure, drowning, and mass shark attack.

The most dangerous aspect of shark behavior is unpredictability. They may suddenly strike without warning, and have been known to attack one individual among a large group of swimmers. Even in the presence of blood and water turbulence, the shark develops "tunnel vision" and becomes oblivious to others splashing about in the bloody water.

Sharks range in size from about 6 inches (*Squaliolus laticautus*) to over 50 feet (the whale shark *Rhincodan typus*, a plankton eater). The largest of the carnivores is the great white shark *Carcharodon carcharias*, attaining lengths of over 20 feet and weights of over 1,000 pounds. There are both fresh- and saltwater sharks, the former being found in freshwater lakes of Nicaragua, Guatemala, and New Guinea.

The chief mechanism of injury inflicted by sharks is their dentition and the powerful force exerted by their jaws. Each jaw has several outer rows of sharp teeth (functional teeth) that are constantly being replaced by the inner rows of teeth (residual teeth). A second system that can inflict injury is their placoid teeth or dermal denticles, which form a sandpaperlike skin known as shagreen. A swimmer or diver brushing against this coarse integumentary layer can sustain severe abrasions or lacerations; this may incite the shark into a full-blown attack because of the victim's agitation and the presence of blood in the water.

Physiologically, sharks have an acute sense of smell, and are able to detect blood measured in parts per billion. Their hearing, combining inner ear labyrinthine structures with pressure-sensing devices along the length of their bodies (lateral lines) and specialized receptors (ampullae of Lorenzini), enables them to detect low-frequency sounds or vibrations miles away.

When all of the various sensory systems of sharks are taken into consideration, it becomes obvious that the shark is a highly integrated "computerized" sensory marvel possibly without equal either in the aquatic environment or on land.[9]

Of further interest is the fact that neither heart disease nor cancer has ever been detected in sharks. They are cannibalistic, yet repelled by dead sharks, are insensitive to pain, and are extremely difficult to kill.

Killer Whales[1,4,6,9,10]

The killer whale *Orcinus orca,* one of the largest dolphins, has become very familiar to the public as a result of the recent motion picture *Orca,* and various marine animal shows. The killer whale has been portrayed as the relentless man-killer and ferocious predator. However, there seems to be no factual justification for the former characterization. Although the killer whale can effectively devour a large sea lion, it is generally believed to be a case of mistaken identity if a person is attacked. Killer whales are generally found in packs of 40, feeding upon invertebrates as well as sea lions, seals, walrus, birds, and fish. Injuries to human beings can be severe as a consequence of bites or blunt trauma from the animal's use of its body, flippers, or tail.

Barracuda[1,3,4,6,8–11]

Of the approximately 20 species of barracuda, the most dangerous is the great barracuda *Sphyraena barracuda.* They are particularly awesome creatures, having large dangerous canine teeth, and attaining weights of over 100 pounds and lengths of 6 to 8 feet. Barracuda are generally very inquisitive yet seem to be quite timid when approached. Underwater they seem to be constantly observant and wary, and to exhibit an ever-present wolf-like smile. They are attracted to bright, shiny, colorful objects; the metallic reflection from a diver's watch or "sun flash" off a swimmer's bare foot can trigger a lightning-fast attack resulting in a significant laceration, usually consisting of two straight parellel cuts. Luckily, barracuda rarely strike twice.

Moray Eels[1,3,4,6,9,10,12,13]

Moray eels are similar to barracuda in that they present a very fierce countenance but generally wish to remain unmolested. Moray eels present a double threat to man: the unwary diver may sustain a nasty laceration or fall victim to serious poisoning after ingesting their flesh.

Of the family Muraenidae, approximately 34 species have been described.[12] Moray eels are generally distributed throughout the tropical waters of the world. The most common species in U.S. coastal waters are the green moray *Gymnothorax funibris* (Carribean Sea south to Brazil), the spotted moray *Gymnothorax moringa* (Gulf of Mexico to Brazil), the *Muraena insularum* (eastern Pacific Ocean), the *Muraena argus* (Gulf of California to Peru), and the *Gymnothorax mordax* (California coast).

Moray eels are rock and reef dwellers, often attaining lengths of 10 feet. Usually they can be seen with their heads protruding from a coral reef looking extremely forbidding while their jaws open and close rhythmically as water is flushed across their gills. The moray eel has a formidable set of sharp teeth pointing caudad, making it difficult to remove any object unlucky enough to be caught in its viselike grip. In most instances divers are injured when they reach before they look into coral crevices and holes in the reef. Rarely will a moray eel come out of its coral home to attack a diver. If provoked when swimming free, however, the moray can prove to be a very dangerous adversary. Many divers befriend local moray eels and routinely feed them pieces of meat or fish. The novice should refrain from such practices.

Grouper[1,3,4,6,9,10]

Groupers (family Serranidae) inhabit the tropical waters of the world. Some of the more than 30 species attain lengths of 10 to 12 feet and weights of 300 to 500 pounds. They are very inquisitive, pugnacious creatures, and by their size alone can be menacing. Injuries to humans can be as a consequence of bites from their crushing jaws or damage inflicted by fin contact, such as abrasions, lacerations, and puncture wounds. Most groupers encountered when diving or fishing weigh 2 to 30 pounds. Often after gaining familiarity with friendly divers, the smaller groupers can be petted and fed by hand. Beware, however, because when the food is gone the grouper often goes for ears, fingers, and thighs.

Treatment of Traumatic Lacerations[1,4,7,9,10,14,15]

The extent of the injury, obviously, depends upon the species of the attacker. Sharks, killer whales, sea lions, seals, and barracudas generally inflict greater damage than moray eels, groupers, crabs, lobsters, and annelid worms. All traumatic wounds are prone to infection. The marine environment (sea water, sea sediment, corals, marine life) contains many micro-organisms including a wide variety of bacteria, fungi, parasites, protozoa, and viruses. Thorough wound management with copious irrigation and appropriate debridement is paramount in the successful treatment of minor and extensive injuries. Primary closure of most injuries is desirable but wounds involving deeper structures or displaying contamination with foreign debris may require delayed primary closure or healing by secondary intention and granulation.

Most wounds require local anesthesia or systemic analgesics to permit adequate cleansing and should be treated as follows. All wounds should be thoroughly cleansed before primary closure is effected.

- Provide anesthesia and analgesia as needed.
- Cleanse with 3% hydrogen peroxide (external wounds only). Hydrogen peroxide is excellent for chemical debridement and can be very helpful in removing foreign matter, such as sand or minute pieces of coral, but it kills very few bacteria.
- Irrigate the wound copiously with normal saline.
- Remove all foreign matter, including sand, coral, and (in cases of shark bite) deciduous teeth that may be present in the wound.
- Debride all necrotic tissue.
- Irrigate again with normal saline.
- Take a soft tissue roentgenogram in order to evaluate the effectiveness of decontamination procedures.
- Make every effort to facilitate a primary closure, even if skin grafting is required.
- Provide antitetanus prophylaxis.
- Schedule postinjury checkups at 3 and 7 days.

The patient's tetanus immunization status must be ascertained and updated with a booster vaccination if necessary. Passive immunization with tetanus antitoxin must be given to those who have not been fully immunized, or when injuries are extensive or contaminated with significant debris and foreign matter.

Antibiotic ointment such as neosporin or bacitracin can be used although their efficacy is not supported by controlled clinical data. Withholding systemic antibiotics is appropriate in minor lacerations and abrasions, while obtaining initial wound cultures for aerobic and anaerobic organisms may prove helpful if subsequent infection develops. Broad-spectrum antibiotics (which are effective against penicillinase: producing staphylococci) should be used for deeper puncture wounds and lacerations or when subcutaneous tissue has been violated or exposed. One also must remember that with marine mammal (e.g., seals, sea lions) bites the possibility of rabies infection must be recognized, although the possibility is extremely remote.

Life-threatening wounds are those involving traumatic amputation, significant lacerations involving major vessels, evisceration, and extensive tissue and bone damage. As a consequence, profuse blood loss, hypotension, and shock may ensue. Sterile pressure dressings or clean cloths should be placed over the wounds, and if necessary tourniquets may be used (with appropriate safeguards), or antishock garments. At least two peripheral intravenous (IV) lines, using large-bore intracatheters and infusions of Ringer's lactate or normal saline, should be started. Plasma expanders or blood replacement may be necessary. Wounds of the extremities can be particularly dangerous because of major vessel tears and associated disruption of bone, tendon, and nerve compartments. For proper treatment, most life-threatening wounds require surgical intervention and the talents of several surgical subspecialists.

One must also keep in mind that any person sustaining a significant injury from the bite of a marine organism should also be evaluated for secondary complications of aspiration of sea water, near-drowning, dysbaric accidents, and decompression sickness, as appropriate. (See Chapters 32 and 33.)

Proper initial management of these traumatic injuries may not only save lives but may also decrease the length of hospitalization, prevent recurrent surgical procedures, and lower the incidence of future complications of infection, limitation of motion, and psychological stress.

MARINE ORGANISMS THAT STING

Marine organisms that sting may cause injury with chemical toxins or puncture wounds or both.

Stinging with Spicules

Sponges (Porifera)[1,2,6,9,16–18]

Of the approximately 4,000 known species of sponges only a dozen or so are toxic to humans. The fire sponge *Tedania ignis*, and *Fibulia nolitangere* inhabit the West Indies. The red moss sponge *Microciona prolifera* is found off the northeast coast of the United States from Cape Cod to South Carolina and causes dermatitis in oyster fishermen and divers. Another interesting dermatitis, known as sponge fishermen's disease, occurs in Mediterranean sponge divers; however, the term is a misnomer. This chemical dermatitis is thought to be caused by a sea anemone *Sagartia rosea*, which adheres to the base of the sponge, and not by a toxin originating in the sponge itself.

Structurally, sponges have minute spicules, composed of silica or calcium carbonate, which bear the chemical toxin. Subcritine, halitoxin (*Haliclonia* sp.), and okadaic acid are some of the sponge toxins. When handled, the spicules penetrate the skin, depositing their toxic substances.

Sponge poisoning precipitates a local chemical dermatitis characterized initially by erythema, swelling, and a painful stinging sensation, often followed by joint stiffness in the affected extremity, vesicle formation, and skin desquamation. The dermatitis often lasts several months. Generalized skin eruptions of erythema multiforme type, as well as anaphylactoid reactions, can be seen, although they are very rare.

Treatment consists of removing any remaining spicules with adhesive tape, soaking the affected area with a diluted solution of acetic acid (vinegar will suffice)

three or four times a day, and using analgesics. Updating tetanus immunization is also necessary. Antibiotics should only be used after definite signs of infection exist and given only after obtaining appropriate specimens or swabs for culture and sensitivity studies. Steroid ointments have not been shown to be effective and indeed may worsen the dermatitis. Anaphylactoid reactions and erythema multiforme should be treated in the usual manner according to their severity.

Stinging by Nematocysts[2,6,8–10,19–21]

Coelenterates (Coelenterata)[1,2,6,9–11,21–23]

Coelenterates are marine organisms comprising three classes: Hydrozoa (hydroids), Scyphozoa (jellyfish), and Anthozoa (sea anemones and sea corals).

Common to all coelenterates is their stinging apparatus or nematocyst. Thousands of nematocysts are found along the tentacles, protuberances, ridges, and oral epidermis of these organisms. The morphologic characteristics of nematocysts have been well documented by Weill.[23] Basically, the nematocyst consists of a pouch-like structure, the cnidoblast, within which rests the venom capsule opening at the operculum. The venom capsule contains a coiled "thread tube" through which the venom is ejected. In some coelenterates, a sensitive receptor, the cnidocil, is located at the tip of the cnidoblast and when touched, signals a sudden opening of the operculum. The coiled thread tube springs forth, inverting the venom sac and injecting toxin into the offending object.

Thus, the unwary prey—whether zooplankton swept by the currents into the waiting embrace of the sea coral (Anthozoa), a small fish darting for safety among the outstretched arms of the sea anemone (Anthozoa), a swimmer's torso embraced by the drifting tentacles of the Portuguese man-of-war (Hydrozoa), or the diver's hand caressed by the deadly, spindly fingers of the sea wasp (Schyphozoa)—becomes the unwitting victim of nature's ever-present intoxication.

The venoms of coelenterates vary in effect from that causing an annoying dermatitis (e.g., fire coral *Millipora alcicornis*), to inflicting a sting causing death within minutes (e.g., sea wasp *Chironex fleckeri*). In human beings, this variability in degree of toxicity depends upon the coelenterate species involved, its type of nematocyst and potency of its toxin, the dose injected, the extent of tissue exposure, and the victim's sensitivity to the venom.

Stinging Hydroids (Hydrozoa)

The class Hydrozoa contains approximately 2,700 species, which fall into three basic types:

Stinging Hydroids.[1,2,6,9,10] These hydroids grow in plumelike colonies (e.g., *Aglaophenia*) or mosslike colonies (stinging seaweed *Aglaophenia cupresina*) attaching to pilings, rocks, rafts, and shells, and are often mistaken for seaweed.

Hydroid Corals (*Millepora*).[1,2,6,8–10,21,24,25] These coral-like organisms live among true corals, having calcareous lime carbonate exoskeletons with thousands of pores within which communicate a network of tiny tentacles containing nematocysts. Colonies may attain beautiful shapes of varying sizes and are capable of inflicting a fiery sting when touched; thus, the term stinging fire coral.

Siphonophores.[1,2,6,8–10,21,26,27] These organisms are free-floating hydroids, such as the well-known Portuguese man-of-war (*Physalia*), having a balloonlike body (pneumatocele) within which is contained several gases: oxygen, nitrogen, carbon monoxide, and carbon dioxide. The pneumatocele, floating on the surface of the water, has numerous tentacles dangling from it which may reach lengths of over 30 feet. These tentacles contain thousands of toxic nematocysts. The Pacific Portuguese man-of-war (*P. utriculus*) has a smaller pneumatocele (3 to 5 inches) than the Atlantic Portuguese man-of-war (*P. physalis*) whose pneumatocele can attain sizes of 12 to 16 inches.

Symptoms of Hydroid Stings[1,2,6,8–10,21]

The stinging hydroids and hydroid corals generally are less toxic than the siphonophores (e.g., Portuguese man-of-war). Local reactions are common in all hydroid stings but siphonophores can cause significant systemic symptoms with fatal outcomes. Generally speaking, hydroids and hydroid corals produce local reactions, including a stinging, often burning sensation, followed by an urticarial wheal-and-flare reaction, erythema, and edema. These lesions may become hemorrhagic or vesicular, and desquamation of the skin can be severe. Siphonophores produce linear, multilinear, or serpiginous local reactions of edema, erythema, urticarial reactions, petechiae, pruritus, and excruciating pain. Systemic reactions include paresthesias, malaise, headache, abdominal cramps, nausea, vomiting, abdominal rigidity, fever, chills, respiratory distress (including wheezes, stridor, laryngospasm), weakness, pallor, cyanosis, anaphylaxis, cardiovascular collapse, hypotension, shock, and death from cessation of respiratory and cardiac function.

Jellyfish (Schyphozoa)[1,2,6,8,9–11,19,20,27–29]

Jellyfish are open sea creatures varying in size, shape, and color. They are free-swimming medusae, passively carried about by the currents and winds, but can move vertically by pulsations of their bell-shaped bodies. Approximately 200 species are known to be capable of envenomation by nematocysts. The cubomedusae comprise a group of marine organisms whose venom is among the most lethal in the marine environment. The sea wasp *Chironex fleckeri* or box jelly (*Chiropsalmus quadrigatus, Chirop. quadrumanus, Chrysaora quinquecirrha, Carybdea alata, Ca. rastoni*) are extremely toxic. *Chir. fleckeri* may indeed be the most lethal organism on earth, producing death almost instantaneously. The venom of *Chir. fleckeri* is a cardiotoxin, causing cessation of cardiac function. Of further interest is the jellyfish named lion's mane or sea blubber (*Cyanae capellata*), which can attain a diameter several feet across.

Symptoms after contact with jellyfish range from a localized painful stinging sensation to almost instantaneous death, as mentioned previously. The pain may be restricted to the specific area of envenomation or may radiate to other areas of the body, characterized as an excruciating shooting pain and, in cases of the sea wasp, may be so severe as to cause unconsciousness, with subsequent drowning as the cause of death. The local urticarial reaction may progress to vesiculation and necrosis involving the affected area. *Chir. fleckeri* produces a specific ladder-type tentacle mark that can be helpful in identifying the sting of this particular jellyfish. Severe systemic reactions consisting of muscle spasms and respiratory distress (from pulmonary edema or pulmonary failure) can be followed by prostration, hypotension, cardiovascular collapse, and death within an average of 15 minutes.

Sea Anemones and Sea Corals (Anthozoa)[1,2,6,9,10,21,30]

The class Anthozoa is subdivided into Alcyonaria (soft corals, sea fans, sea pens, and sea pansies) and Zoantharia (sea anemones and true corals). Sea anemones and true corals belong to the orders Actiniaria and Madreporaria, respectively. The approximately 1,000 species of sea anemones generally are sessile carnivores attaching to rocks, coral heads, and crevices of the marine environment. Morphologically, the sea anemone's tentacles are fingerlike projections, having on their surface the majority of the nematocysts. Sea anemones are very beautiful creatures, with their tentacles having variously colored tips (e.g., pink, green, and yellow). The toxin injected from nematocysts serves to incapacitate various invertebrates and fish which the creature preys upon. The sea anemone often lives in a symbiotic relationship with the clown fish, which seems to be immune to the sea anemone's venom.

The sea anemone's stings tend to be milder and more localized in their effects than the stings of hydroids and jellyfish. As with stinging hydroids, envenomation causes a painful burning sensation, usually followed by swelling, erythema, and a localized urticarial reaction. Lesions may undergo necrosis and eventually ulcerate, forming multiple abscesses with a purulent discharge. Desquamation of the skin may be severe and systemic reactions consisting of nausea, vomiting, abdominal discomfort, general malaise, fever, chills, and prostration may occur.

True corals are one of the primary constituents of the living reef and marine environment. The stony corals with their anemonelike polyps are carnivores that feed basically on zooplankton. Envenomation from corals is usually insignificant. The danger, however, is related to traumatic injury that may become infected if left untreated. Lacerations can ulcerate, resulting in a cellulitis, lymphangitis, and systemic infection. It is well known that coral cuts take a long time to heal. This may be the result of infection by micro-organisms, contamination by coral debris, or envenomation of small amounts of toxin.

Therapy for Nematocyst Stings[1,2,8–10,14,15,21,27]

Therapy for nematocyst stings consists of pain relief, prevention of envenomation, and treatment of systemic reactions. Morphine sulfate or other opiates may be needed for analgesia. Initial inactivation of nematocysts and prevention of continued discharge has been achieved by utilizing vinegar and/or unseasoned papain (meat tenderizer, applied as a paste). After neutralization with vinegar, removal of tentacles is mandatory, and drying agents such as flour, baking soda, diver's talc, sand, or towels can be used, but care must be taken not to touch the tentacles with the bare hands. Remove the tentacles with a clamp, pliers, comb, stick, or other tool.

Local therapy using topical and oral steroids and antihistamines has been effective in relieving symptoms and resolving urticarial skin reactions. Epinephrine may be needed for moderate to severe stings as well as anaphylactoid reactions followed by antihistamines such as diphenhydramine in doses of 1 mg/kg intramuscularly or intravenously. Intravenous injections of 5 to 10 cc of a 10% calcium gluconate solution have been effective in relieving muscle spasms. Systemic reactions involving anaphylaxis or neurologic, respiratory, or cardiovascular collapse require appropriate supportive care, including artificial ventilation, use of the MAST suit, IV fluids, epinephrine, high-dose steroids, antihistamines, critical care monitoring, and careful observation.

SPINE OR PUNCTURE INJURIES CAUSED BY INVERTEBRATES

Cone Shells[1,2,6,8–10,15,21,31,32]

Cone shells (phylum Mollusca, class Gastropoda, subclass Prosobranchia, order Archaeogastropoda, suborder Toxoglossa, family Conidae, genus *Conus*) consist of land, fresh-water, and marine snails and slugs comprising over 30,000 species. Inhabiting the tropical and subtropical areas of the world, cone shells are univalve mollusks. Cone shells puncture their prey, causing injury by envenomation through a minute harpoonlike tooth. The shells are very colorful and sought by divers, snorkelers, shell collectors, and aquarium enthusiasts, many of whom are unaware of these organisms' lethal natures.

The venom seems to be a multicomponent neurotoxin; its main component is a relatively heat-labile peptide, but quaternary ammonium compounds and amines may be present as well.

Symptoms consist of an initial burning, painful sensation, with local ischemia and cyanosis at the puncture site. However, excruciating pain, pruritus, nausea, and neurologic symptoms of paresthesias, weakness, incoordination, paralysis, dyplopia, dysphagia, dysphonia, aphonia, and coma predominate in the clinical picture. Death is caused by cardiovascular collapse.

Therapy for cone shell envenomation is directed at decreasing pain, preventing local absorption by incision and suction at the puncture site, placing a venoconstrictive tourniquet to limit systemic spread, applying hot water to the affected area to partially inactivate the toxin and to promote bleeding, and supportive care for neurologic and cardiovascular collapse. Respiratory failure (although rare) may occur secondary to muscular paralysis and mechanical ventilatory support may be required. Treatment of shock by the usual methods must be instituted when appropriate. Intravenous 10% calcium gluconate may be helpful in treating pruritus and muscle spasms. Antitetanus prophylaxis and follow-up wound care are also essential for proper management of these injuries.

Sea Urchins[1,2,6,8–10,14,21,33–37]

Sea urchins are of the phylum Echinodermata. They are free-living nocturnal feeders inhabiting crevices in the coral reef during the day. They can also be found motionless on sandy beaches and ocean bottoms, thereby endangering the unwary wader or swimmer.

Sea urchins have oval, egg-shaped bodies, and their internal organs are encased by a hard shell. Their bodies are covered by several types of venomous and nonvenomous spines that may inflict a painful puncture wound. Sea urchin spines are designated according to size (primary spines are long spindly spines; secondary spines are shorter blunt calcareous spines), and according to location (oral spines are located on the ventral surface, and aboral spines on the dorsal surface). Some species of sea urchins also have tiny venomous pincers called pedicellariae. Venomous sea urchins usually have either spines with venom glands or pedicellariae, but rarely both types of venom apparatus.

Most species of sea urchins have nonvenomous round-tipped spines. However, echinoids of the families Echinothuridae and Diadematidae have long sharp spines that are brittle and very dangerous. The more common sea urchins with toxic spines are the black sea urchin *Diadema antillarum* (West Indies), the white sea urchin *Lythechinus variegatus* (West Indies, North Carolina south to Brazil), and the white sea egg *Tripneustes ventricosus* (West Indies south to Brazil, and the west coast of Africa). Examples of those sea urchins that envenomate through pedicellariae are the sea urchin *Toxopneustes pileolus* (Indo-Pacific and Japan), the sea urchin *T. elegans* (Japanese waters), and the sea urchin *Asthenosoma ijimai* (southern Japan to the Moluccan Sea). Contact with sea urchins produces a danger to bathers, swimmers, and divers. Protective gloves, stockings, and flippers may prove inadequate to prevent puncture wounds. Individuals should refrain from handling sea urchins, particularly those with long slender spines and those short-spined urchins with pedicellariae.

Symptoms from sea urchin puncture wounds can be very painful and very difficult to treat. Spines often break off and disintegrate when attempts are made to remove them. Calcareous spines penetrating bone may have to be removed surgically in order to prevent chronic inflammation and infection. Foreign body granuloma may form about sea urchin spines, and pustules with draining sinuses can occur. Spines causing envenomation as well as puncture wounds often produce an aching burrowing type of pain, while pain from envenomation secondary to those urchins with pedicellariae is usually more radiating and severe. Redness, swelling, numbness, paralysis, aphonia, respiratory distress, and anaphylactoid reactions can also occur.

Treatment of sea urchin puncture wounds and envenomation consists of adequate cleansing of the affected area (vinegar soaks may be helpful in dissolving the thin spines, but not the thick calcium carbonate ones) and removal of deeply embedded shorter calcareous spines under local anesthesia. The latter is often necessary to prevent chronic inflammation, draining sinuses, and chronic arthritis. Soaking the affected area in hot water (45 to 50°C) will help to inactivate the heat-labile toxins of venomous urchins, and when necessary the accepted therapy for anaphylactoid symptoms should be instituted. Again, tetanus toxin immunization must be considered, and antibiotic therapy should be withheld until overt signs of infection develop. In addition, specimens should be obtained for proper culture and sensitivity studies.

Starfish, Sea Stars (Asteroidea)[1,2,6,9,10,14,21,38]

Starfish are free-living organisms comprising six families (Acanthasteridae, Asteriidae, Asterinidae, Astropectinidae, Echinasteridae, and Solasteridae). The only starfish known to be poisonous, the crown of thorns starfish *Acanthaster planci*, inhabits the Indo-Pacific region from Polynesia to the Red Sea. Starfish in general are star-shaped with a central body and five or more radiating arms. The ventral surface of starfish contains furrows along the arms, from which protrude tubelike structures (tube feet) that enable locomotion, digestion, and sexual function. The dorsal surface contains spines emanating from their hard, calcareous exoskeletons. Starfish have large mouths that can engulf fairly large organisms. *A. planci* has played a significant role in the destruction of the coral reefs of the Indo-Pacific. The production of its own venom may be in part the result of ingestion of hydroid coral nematocyst venom.

Wounds inflicted by *A. planci* can be very painful, as a result of both traumatic puncture and envenomation injuries. Pain, redness, swelling, nausea, vomiting, and neurologic symptoms of numbness and paralysis are seen. *A. planci* thorns contain a red-pink pigment which may stain the tissues, helping to identify injury caused by this venomous organism.

Treatment consists of analgesia, thorough wound cleansing, removal of spines under local anesthesia, immersion of the affected extremity in hot water, 40 to 50°C (to inactivate heat-labile toxins), and careful follow-up in order to detect delayed infections, granuloma formation, cellulitis, lymphangitis, and sepsis.

Bristle Worms (Annelida)[1,2,6,8,9]

Segmented worms can inflict a lacerating bite with their tough chitinous jaws (e.g., the biting reef worm *Eunice aphroditois*). Envenomation, however, may take place through a puncture injury from bristles or setae along the body of the worm, hence the term bristle worm. The setae are paired structures associated with each segment of the worm's body and can inflict a painful sting when touched. The more common bristle worms are the sea mouse *Chloeia viridis*, the fire worm *Eurythroe complanta*, and the bristle worm *Hermodice carunculata*.

Symptoms from contact with bristle worm setae include local pain and minor swelling, and intense itching and numbness that often persist for weeks. Treatment consists of symptomatic relief of pain and immersing the extremity in hot water for 30 minutes, followed by rubbing dilute ammonia or isopropyl alcohol on the wound. After air drying, setae can be removed with adhesive tape. Local anesthetic ointments may be helpful, as well as steroid and antihistamine creams or lotions that may decrease the inflammatory response and intense pruritus. Delayed tissue necrosis and infection must be closely monitored. Antitetanus therapy and careful wound care follow-up should also be provided.

SPINE OR PUNCTURE WOUNDS OF VERTEBRATES

Dogfish Shark[1,4,8,9,14]

Sharks can inflict injury, as previously described, with their sharp teeth and sandpaperlike skin (dermal denticles). In addition, the dogfish shark *Squalus acanthias* and Port Jackson shark can inflict a dangerous spiny puncture wound resulting in a significant laceration as well as a toxic envenomation. The dogfish shark is a slender creature with a pointed snout and high spines anterior to each of its two dorsal fins. Dogfish sharks are relatively small creatures and as adults average 2 to 4 feet in length.

Spine-puncture wounds with envenomation may result in lacerations, hemorrhage, severe radiating pain, erythema, swelling, and serious systemic anaphylactoid reactions in addition to cardiopulmonary and neurologic failure.

Therapy for dogfish shark puncture wounds and envenomation include general principles of care previously outlined for local wounds, shock, and anaphylactoid reactions. Dogfish shark venom is heat-labile and soaking the affected area in hot water (45 to 50°C) can be very effective in inactivating this toxin. Appropriate use of analgesics is essential and tetanus toxoid immunization should be updated when necessary. Systemic antibiotics having efficacy against penicillinase-producing staphylococcus should probably be used for deep puncture wounds and significant lacerations.

Stingrays[1,4,6,8–10,14,21,39–42]

Skates and rays (phylum Chordata, class Chondrichthyes, order Rajiformes) compose the suborder Myliobatoidea and include the families Dasyatidae (stingrays), Potamotrygonidae (river rays), Gymnuridae (butterfly rays), Urolophidae (round stingrays), Myliobatidae (eagle rays), Rhinopteridae (cow-nosed rays), and Mobulidae (devil or manta rays).

Stingrays pose a threat to the bather, swimmer, diver, and fisherman alike. Stingrays vary in size from a few pounds (round stingray *Urolophus halleri*) to over 700 pounds (giant stingray of Australia *Dasyatis brevicaudata*). They inhabit the tropical and subtropical waters of the world, being found usually on sandy bottoms, near shallow reefs, lagoons, river mouths, and inlets. When swimming freely, the stingray generally poses no

threat; however, when partially submerged in the sand the stingray is well camouflaged and very difficult to spot. Only the very observant snorkeler or diver will notice its flat, partially sand-covered body and its vigilant protruding eyes.

The stinging apparatus (caudal appendage) of the stingray consists of a tail from which extends a stinger or spine. There are several types of caudal appendages (gymnurid type, mylibated type, dasyated type, urolophed type) varying according to the development of the spine and its location on the tail.

The gymnurid and mylibated types are poorly developed and usually present limited striking ability. The dasyated and urolophed types are well developed, having muscular tails and caudally placed spines permitting greater whiplike action and striking force.

The stinging spine has sharp recurved teeth along its length, thus forming an organ structurally similar to a fishhook with multiple barbs. The stinging spine is a cartilaginous structure containing grooves along its length harboring the glandular tissue and venom sacs that produce the stingray's toxic venom. The entire spine is covered with an integumentary layer, termed the integumentary sheath.

Injury from stingrays, therefore, consists of a lacerating puncture wound in which pieces of spine, glandular tissue, and integumentary sheath may be found. In most instances, wounds occur on the lower extremities when the organism is stepped upon by bathers wading in shallow water. Although rare, deaths have occurred secondary to envenomating abdominal wounds when the victims have fallen off rafts onto a stingray hiding in shallow water along sandy beaches.

Envenomation results from a heat-labile protein toxin. Localized reactions include severe, often excruciating, pain. Numbness may occur, eventually affecting the entire extremity. Systemic reactions include nausea, vomiting, diarrhea, diaphoresis, arrhythmias, cardiovascular collapse, and anaphylactoid reactions.

Pharmacologically, in laboratory animals, the venom seems to have cardiotoxic effects resulting in varying degrees of AV block, ST-T wave changes, cardiac standstill, interventricular conduction defects, ischemia, and premature ventricular contractions (PVCs). Toxicity to the CNS results in depression of medullary respiratory centers, behavioral changes, and convulsive seizures.

Therapy consists of careful wound care. At the scene, the wound should be irrigated with saltwater, except in cases of penetrating wounds of the head, chest, or abdomen. Every attempt should be made to remove any remnant of the integumentary sheath in the wound and most importantly, the extremity should be immersed for at least 90 minutes in hot water (45 to 50°C). The hot water inactivates heat-labile toxin, but should not be so hot as to scald the patient.

Emergency department management should include attention to the wound using local infiltration of xylocaine when necessary. In addition, systemic analgesia is usually required. The spine should be removed at this point. Extensive debridement and copious irrigation removing all foreign matter is often necessary. Drains should be placed prior to closure of extensive lacerations. Simple puncture wounds should not be sutured. In addition to the routine indications for surgery, patients who sustain penetrating abdominal or chest wounds should have exploratory surgery in order to remove intrathoracic or intra-abdominal pieces of integumentary sheath and to permit proper irrigation and debridement of devitalized tissue. Routine management of systemic reactions consisting of hypotension, respiratory depression, and anaphylaxis should be instituted.

Antibiotic therapy should be withheld initially; tetanus toxoid prophylaxis must be updated when appropriate. Prophylactic use of benadryl, 50 mg, intramuscularly (IM) in the adult, and methyl prednisolone sodium succinate, 40 mg IM, with oral doses of benadryl for 24 hours and decreasing oral doses of steroids for five days has been recommended for the prevention of anaphylactoid reactions. The most crucial therapeutic aspect in regard to stingray injuries is the inactivation of heat-labile toxin. This in concert with removal of any remaining integumentary sheath and attention to local wound care usually results in uncomplicated wound healing. Those patients not treated as indicated often have problems with subsequent infection, tissue necrosis, and abscess formation, and require extended medical care.

Ratfishes[1,4,6,14]

Ratfishes (class Chondrichthyes, order Chimaerae) are geographically distributed from the north temperate to south temperate zones. They have been found as deep as 1,400 fathoms and have been named sea cats. They can inflict a severe bite as well as produce injury and envenomation with their single long tapering dorsal spines. The venom is produced by glandular epithelium located along the spine and covered by an integumentary sheath. Very little is known about the venom of ratfishes.

Medically, symptoms include immediate pain which may lessen over several hours, but continue as a dull ache. Numbness followed by cyanosis and a dark discoloration may develop about the puncture site. Peripherally there is pallor, swelling, arthralgia, and lymphadenopathy. Treatment is similar to that for stingray injuries and the reader is referred to the previous section for details.

Catfishes[1,4,6,8,9,14,43]

Catfishes (class Osteichthyes, family Siluridae) comprise over 1,000 species. Most species vary in size and shape and are found in fresh water while the most venomous, the marine catfish *Plotosus lineatus* is a saltwater inhabitant. Its venom can cause death. The electric catfish *Malapterusus* sp. can repel attackers and kill prey by discharging electric currents through the water. The freshwater catfishes of North America include the brownhead *Ictalurus nebulosus*, the Caroline mudtom *Noturus furiosus*, the channel catfish *I. punctatus*, the blue catfish *I. fucatus*, and the white catfish *I. catus*.

The venom glands of catfishes are located along the spines of the dorsal and pectoral fins, which are covered by an integumentary sheath. The stingers are sharp, strong, and easily capable of puncturing skin and muscle. When the integumentary sheath is disrupted venom is released into the wound. The marine catfish's venom appears to have neurotoxic and hemotoxic properties causing muscle spasm, respiratory distress, and death when administered to laboratory animals.

Envenomation in human beings initially involves a severe, throbbing, burning pain which may radiate up the extremity, followed by pallor, swelling, and cyanosis around the puncture site; this is often accompanied by muscle spasms and lymphangitis. Paresthesias at the puncture site may occur and spread to the entire extremity. Systemic symptoms include generalized tremulousness, nausea, vomiting, hypotension, and shock leading to death. In most instances symptoms gradually resolve within a few hours.

Injury most frequently occurs when fishermen are handling catfish caught by rod and reel. Catfish have a very slimy body and are difficult to hold when attempting to remove them from fishhooks. Prevention of injury is critical and is usually possible if these fish are handled with gloves or towels. Fishermen who inadvertently hook a catfish would be advised to simply cut the line.

Treatment of a catfish sting consists of applying a venoconstrictive tourniquet to the affected extremity with suction applied to the wound (avoiding mouth to wound contact) followed by hot compresses or immersion of the extremity in hot water. These therapeutic modalities have not definitely been shown to result in removal or inactivation of venom, but empirically should be applied within the first ten minutes of injury. Local wound care and removal of stingers should be done under local anesthesia. Many species of catfish have recurved teeth on their spines which can cause severe lacerations. Proper irrigation and primary wound closure is indicated. If more serious disruption of tissue occurs, drains should be placed prior to wound closure. Systemic analgesia is usually necessary, tetanus toxoid immunization should be updated, and the patient should be placed on broad-spectrum antibiotics having effectiveness against penicillinase-producing staphylococci. Complications of catfish stings include tissue necrosis, gangrene, bacterial infections, foreign body reaction, and peripheral neuropathy.

Weevers[1,4,6,9,14,44]

Weevers are small fishes (phylum Chordata, class Osteichthyes, order Perciformes, suborder Percoidei, family Trachinidae) usually not obtaining lengths greater than 18 inches. The species of note are the greater weevers *Trachinus draco* and the lesser weevers *T. vipera*. They inhabit inshore waters of the eastern and northern Atlantic Ocean and the Mediterranean and Black Seas. They are located in soft, sandy, muddy areas living upon squid, worms, small fish, and crustaceans. Injuries to humans occur while wading or swimming in the areas they inhabit. Weevers are extremely toxic organisms, their venom apparatus being contained in their dorsal and opercular spines. The dorsal spines do not usually number more than seven and contain venom glands covered by an integumentary sheath. Weevers, although sedentary, are easily provoked and can strike very quickly, producing a puncture wound with envenomation.

Envenomation results in immediate local pain of a burning, stabbing, or crushing nature causing the patient to scream in agony, thrash about, and in many cases lose consciousness. The pain may spread to surrounding areas and is often associated with swelling, numbness, edema, and local vesiculation. Systemic symptoms include headache, delirium, nausea, vomiting, dizziness, sweating, cyanosis, arthralgias, lymphadenopathy, cardiac conduction disturbances, seizures, respiratory distress, shock, and death. Secondary infection and gangrene are not uncommon, and infection has been implicated as the ultimate cause of death in several patients. Full recovery often takes several months.

The venom is thought to contain serotonin as well as epinephrine, norepinephrine, histamine, a cholinesterase, and other proteins.

Since there is no known antidote for the weever's toxins, therapy is directed at symptomatic treatment as outlined for stingray injuries. Analgesia can be a major problem with weever envenomation. Intravenous morphine sulfate has not often been helpful in relieving pain. Intravenous injection of calcium gluconate and Demerol may be helpful as well as local infiltration of Xylocaine or procaine. In addition, in view of the frequent complication of infection, prophylactic antibiotic therapy should be initiated with broad-spectrum antibiotics having efficacy against penicillinase-producing staphylococci.

Scorpionfishes[1,4,6,9,14,21,45–49]

Scorpionfishes (family Scorpaenidae) comprise several hundred species categorized into three groups according to the anatomy of their venom apparatus: zebrafish type (*Pterois*), scorpionfish type (*Scorpaena*), and stonefish type (*Synanceja*).

Scorpionfishes are generally bottom dwellers inhabiting the rocks and crevices of the ocean floor (hence the term rockfish), but occasionally they can be found buried in the sand (stonefish type) or swimming freely about the coral reef (zebrafish type). They inhabit the temperate and tropical waters of the world, but some species are found in Arctic waters.

Scorpionfishes usually inflict injury during attempts to remove them from fishhooks or nets, after being stepped on by a swimmer's unprotected foot, or while being handled and touched in a home saltwater aquarium. The zebrafish *P. volitans* is so beautifully decorated by nature's camouflage that one almost feels compelled to reach out and fondle this venomous creature. *P. volitans*, also known as the lionfish, turkeyfish, tigerfish, featherfish, firefish, and scorpionfish, unfortunately, can be found on sale in tropical fish stores throughout the United States. Thousands of these fish are imported from the Philippines each year, ultimately residing in aquaria of tropical fish enthusiasts. Only one case of cardiovascular collapse secondary to *P. volitans* envenomation has been documented in the United States to date, and luckily no reported deaths.

The venom apparatus of scorpionfishes is located in dorsal, pectoral, pelvic, and anal fin spines. These spines have extremely sharp points, easily capable of puncturing tissue, glove material, and thin swinfins. Along the spines are venom grooves in which lie venom glands. An integumentary sheath covers the entire glandular and spiny structure. As previously mentioned, the structure of the venom apparatus—that is, fin spines, integumentary sheath, venom glands, and venom ducts— serves to classify rockfish into three distinct categories.

The venoms of rockfishes are heat-labile proteins varying in toxicity according to the species involved. In general, stonefish venom is more potent and more frequently associated with systemic symptoms than scorpionfish or zebrafish venom. However, the lionfish *Pterois volitans* and California scorpionfish *Scorpaena guttata* are capable of producing envenomation comparable to that of stonefish.

Rockfish stings usually cause local reactions of intense pain with radiation followed by swelling, erythema, edema, local cyanosis, and occasionally necrosis and sloughing of the tissues. Life-threatening reactions resulting from systemic absorption of toxin include nausea, vomiting, delirium, lymphangitis, lymphadenopathy, arthralgias, fever, hypotension, cardiovascular collapse, respiratory distress, and death.

Therapy consists of immediate proximal venoconstrictive tourniquet application, wound irrigation, and encouragement of bleeding from the puncture site in order to remove the toxin and limit systemic absorption. Inactivation of heat-labile toxin can often be accomplished by immersion of the affected extremity in hot water (45°C to 50°C) for 30 to 90 minutes. Local and systemic analgesia is usually required. Injection of local anesthetics and the addition of magnesium sulfate to the water bath have been variably beneficial in relieving pain. The use of systemic opiates is often required. Systemic reactions of hypotension and cardiovascular collapse have been successfully treated with IV fluids and epinephrine. The use of the MAST and adjunctive supportive therapy must be considered in severe reactions. Tetanus toxoid immunization and follow-up wound care may be required. Stonefish Antivenene is very effective in neutralizing all the observable toxic effects of stonefish envenomation, but is only available from the Commonwealth Serum Laboratories, Melbourne, Australia.

Prevention is the chief consideration in regard to all scorpionfish stings. When diving or snorkeling, one must resist the temptation of reaching into crevices of a coral reef, routinely wear thick gloves while diving, cut fishing lines if scorpionfish are hooked, and refrain from placing hands (even if gloved) in aquaria containing these creatures.

Toadfishes[1,4,8,9,14]

Of the toadfishes (family Batrachoididae) 15 species have been found to be toxic. Toadfishes, ugly and quite repulsive in appearance, inhabit the warm waters of the North American, European, African, southern Australian, and southern South American coastlines. They are also found in the cold waters of the North Sea and off the southern Canadian coast.

Toadfishes are bottom dwellers, preferring turbid water. They are usually found in rock crevices, under debris, hidden by seaweed, or buried in the sand. Their ability to change color gives them superb camouflage, and they are often very difficult to detect. The primary mode of injury is stepping upon these creatures in shallow sandy beach areas.

The highly developed venom apparatus of toadfishes is located on the dorsal and opercular spines. The sting apparatus consists of a hollow spine surrounded by a venom gland and covered almost completely by an integumentary sheath. Very little is known about the toxicology of toadfish venom.

Clinically, the symptoms associated with toadfish stings are stinging, burning, radiating pain accompanied by a typical inflammatory reaction of swelling, redness, and warmth. No known fatalities have been reported from a toadfish sting, and treatment consists of those modalities mentioned in regard to scorpionfish stings. Secondary infection from a toadfish sting may occur and follow-up care should be arranged.

Prevention consists of refraining from wading in sandy beach waters without thick-soled protective foot gear. In addition, a shuffling gait will disturb the sand and often cause a toadfish in the area to move to another location. If caught on hook and line, toadfishes should be released by cutting the line; handling these fishes can prove hazardous.

Surgeonfishes[1,4,6,9,14]

Surgeonfishes (family Ancanthuridae) are so named because of their sharp, lancelike spines located on either side of the tail at the base of the tail fin.

The spine lies within a groove, but may extend from the groove pointing cephalad when the fish is disturbed or becomes excited. The spine in relationship to the tail can be likened to a pocket knife when the blade is pulled from the closed position, if one imagines the body of the knife to simulate the tail of the fish, and the attachment of the proximal blade to the knife housing as the caudal part of the tail.

Surgeonfishes are abundant in the coral reefs of tropical waters but rarely pose a threat to swimmers, snorkelers, or divers. Most injuries occur when removing these fish from nets or hooks. In addition, only a few species appear to have venomous spines.

Lacerating, painful wounds can be inflicted by the tail lance. Envenomation may also occur either in association with the tail lance or spines on the caudal peduncle. Symptoms include an intense, radiating pain often lasting for several hours. The pain may continue with varying degrees of severity for up to one week. Associated symptoms include local swelling, and occasionally nausea. Treatment is the same as that for stings from scorpionfishes.

Marlin, Sailfish, Swordfish

Game fish can pose a significant danger to fishermen by direct injury or, indirectly, as a result of damage to their boats. Case reports of chest and neck swordfish impalement wounds have been documented. These puncture wounds are not envenomed; however, hemorrhage, tissue injury, and infection pose serious problems. Incidents of huge marlins ramming and puncturing boats below the waterline, although rare, have occurred.

Large game fish must be handled with extreme caution by experienced fishermen using proper equipment.

Attempts to handle sworded game fish should only be done after the fish is completely exhausted. Premature boating of these creatures is extremely dangerous and ill-advised.

Miscellaneous Fishes with Venomous Spines[4,6,9,14]

Several other families of fishes have or are reported to have venomous spines, but very little information is available in regard to the toxicological nature of the venom or the anatomy of their venom apparatus. The following is a list of these fishes in phylogenic order:

Common Name	*Family Name*
Deep sea scaly	Stomiatidae
Dragonfishes	
Squirrelfishes	Hollocentridae
Leatherbacks	Carangidae
(jacks, scard, pompano)	
Butterflyfishes	Chaetodontidae
Old wives	Enoplosidae
Majarras	Gerridae
Bugglerfishes	Histiopteridae
Snappers	Lutanidae
Fingerfishes	Monodactylidae
Perches	Percidae
Scats	Scatophagidae
Seabasses	Serranidae
Stargazers	Uranoscopidae
Rabbitfishes	Siganidae
Snake mackerels	Gemphylidae
Sculpins	Cottidae
Searobins	Triglidae
Flying gunardy	Dactylopteridae
Dragonets	Callionymidae
Goosefishes, anglerfishes	Lophiidae

INJURY FROM FANGS

Sea Snakes[1,4,6,8–10,14,50]

Sea snakes are air-breathing marine reptiles (family Hydrophiodae) comprising about 50 species, 14 of which have been reported to cause human envenomations. Sea snakes inhabit the tropical and subtropical waters of the Indo-Australian seas, and the Indian and Pacific Oceans. The more common dangerous species include:[48]

- Sea snake *Enhydrina schistosa*—Persian Gulf to Cochin China, north coast of Australia.

- Banded sea snake *Hydrophis Caerulescens*—Persian Gulf to Japan, Netherlands Indies.
- Hardwick's sea snake *Lapemis hardwicki*—southern Japan to the Merguri Archipelago, northern Australian coast.
- Yellow-bellied sea snake *Pelamis platurus*—eastern Africa, Indo-Australian area, Gulf of Panama.

Sea snakes are extremely venomous creatures capable of inflicting a lethal bite. They pose a significant threat to fishermen and bathers in areas such as Penang, Malaysia where the incidence is one bite per 270,000 bathing hours. Sea snake bites seem to be more prevalent in turbid water and at river mouths. The incidence may be affected by the time of year and the snake's breeding cycle, during which time they exhibit more aggressive behavior. Bites are most likely to occur when the victim is removing snakes from fishing lines or nets or wading or bathing.

The venom apparatus of sea snakes consists of venom glands, venom ducts, and fangs, the first two being located caudad and ventral to each eye, and the last consisting of one or two pairs located distally in the upper jaw. The venom apparatus of sea snakes is quite primitive in relationship to that of terrestrial snakes. Inflicting a usually painless bite, sea snakes are incapable of dislocating their jaws when striking. Envenomation may be incomplete or may not occur at all. Nevertheless, sea snakes must be considered lethal creatures and appropriate safeguards should be taken when in an aquatic environment inhabited by these serpents.

The venom of sea snakes is considered more toxic than terrestrial snake venom, such as that of rattlesnakes, copperheads, and kraits, but about equal in potency to cobra venom. Toxicologically, one drop of venom is sufficient to kill three adult humans. In animals, sea snake venom causes neurotoxicity acting upon neuromuscular junctions producing paralysis. In human beings, the venom causes myotoxic and hemotoxic effects in addition to neurotoxic symptoms. Sea snake venoms seem to contain a common antigen and, in general, the protein composition is less complex than venoms of other families of snakes. Notably fewer enzymes are contained in sea snake venoms than in venoms of terrestrial snakes.

Pharmacologically, sea snake venoms contain phospholipase A_2, phosphodiesterase, phosphomonoesterase, fibrinogen clotting, hyaluronidase, deoxyribonuclease, acetylcholinesterase, and leucine aminopeptidase, and have thrombinlike activity.

The clinical syndrome of envenomation usually occurs within 30 minutes to one hour after the bite. Symptoms of envenomation include generalized myalgias, stiffness, euphoria, anxiety, ascending paralysis, flaccidity, ptosis, trismus, dysphagia, nausea, vomiting, dryness of the mouth, thirst, diaphoresis, muscle spasms, fasciculations, cyanosis, mydriasis, hypotension, arrhythmias, cardiovascular collapse, respiratory arrest, and acute myoglobinuric renal failure. The overall fatality rate is 28 percent.

Treatment of sea snake bites initially includes proper diagnosis, which is based upon clearly establishing the opportunity for contact with sea snakes, the presence of a painless wound, the presence of fang marks, identification of the snake when possible, and the occurrence of symptoms of envenomation, including early complaints of muscle stiffness, ptosis, paralysis of the legs, and trismus.

Common goals of therapy, as with other types of envenomation injuries, include removal of venom at the site of injury, prevention of absorption of venom, neutralization of toxin, supportive therapy to treat toxic effects, and treatment of secondary complications.

In concert with these therapeutic goals, the recommendations for treatment of sea snake bites with envenomation are:

- Application of a venoconstrictive tourniquet using appropriate safeguards against producing extremity ischemia. Tourniquets may only be effective if applied within 30 minutes after the bite and should not be left on for more than four hours.
- Cleansing the wound thoroughly, removing fangs if present.
- Refraining from applying ice to the wound.
- Immobilizing the affected extremity and placing the victim at rest.
- Administering Sea Snake Antivenene (available from the Commonwealth Serum Laboratories, Melbourne, Australia) or any polyvalent snake antivenin containing krait (elapidae) fraction as directed, and only after appropriate skin or conjunctival allergy testing.
- Removing tourniquets upon administration of antivenin.
- Refraining from administering opiates for pain relief; worsening of respiratory status may occur.
- Institution of supportive therapy for hypotension, arrhythmias, respiratory arrest, and renal failure from hemoglobinuria or myoglobinuria.

INJURY FROM BEAKS

Octopuses[1,2,6,8–10, 14, 51–58]

Octopuses are strange-looking mollusks of the class Cephalopoda, which includes cuttlefishes and squids.

Cephalopods can inflict lacerations, avulsions, or crush injuries by biting and can cause envenomation with their salivary gland toxins, or poisoning, if their flesh is ingested. The following discussion centers upon octopuses but cuttlefishes and squids may produce similar types of injuries, envenomation, and poisoning.

Anatomically, octopuses have a body, within which are situated their eyes and two chitinous jaws that form a sharp beak. The beak is capable of inflicting a serious laceration. Radiating from the body are eight tentacles, having on their ventral surfaces numerous suction cups. The tentacles are used for clinging to and grasping underwater objects and prey. Occasionally, a diver's arm or body may be the object to which the octopus clings, leaving suction marks that are round and erythematous and exhibit petechial hemorrhages.

Octopuses vary in size, the largest reportedly (*Guinness Book of World Records*) weighing 6 to 7 tons and having tentacles reaching lengths of 200 feet. Most venomous octopuses are small, reaching sizes of only 8 to 12 inches. Usually, octopuses create a minor threat to divers, but the white *Octopus joubini* (Florida) and the blue-ringed octopus *Hapalochlaena maculosus* (Indo-Pacific region) are especially venomous. Three deaths have been reported in Australian waters as a result of bites from *Hapalochlaena* sp. One diver allowed a small octopus of unknown species (*H. lunulata?*) to crawl up his arm toward his neck, where he sustained a lethal bite. In spite of artificial ventilation he died within two hours of hospitalization.

The venom apparatus of octopuses consists of the anterior and posterior salivary glands, salivary ducts, buccal mass, and two jaws forming a beaklike structure. Envenomation is produced through a laceration caused by the bite. When feeding upon small crabs, however, the octopus apparently releases its toxin near the crab's gill cavity, which results in envenomation in the absence of a bite.

The venom of *H. maculosus*, maculotoxin, has been studied and found to be a neurotoxin chemically identical to tetrodotoxin. Maculotoxin selectively blocks nerve action potentials, producing paralysis and causing death from respiratory failure.

Envenomation in humans produces an initial local stinging sensation followed by swelling, redness, warmth, and pruritus at the wound site. Profuse local bleeding may occur and is thought secondary to interference with clotting mechanisms. Systemic reactions include tingling (lips, mouth, and tongue), vomiting, headache, chills, low-grade fever, abdominal pain, anorexia, blurred vision, loss of tactile sensation associated with a floating feeling, seizures, flaccid paralysis, respiratory difficulty, respiratory arrest, and death from respiratory failure.

Therapy of cephalopod bites consists of local irrigation and those modalities recommended for envenomation from stinging marine organisms. Healing is usually without incident and infection is rare, although delayed cellulitis infrequently occurs. Frequent observation for infection and granuloma formation is warranted and patients should be started on broad-spectrum antibiotics effective against antipencillinase-producing staphylococci. Tetanus toxoid immunization must be updated as well. Without a known antivenin, respiratory support may play a crucial role in survival after serious envenomation.

Divers should refrain from handling cephalopods so as to prevent injury from bites and envenomation even though the temptation may seem irresistible.

POISONING FROM INGESTING MARINE INVERTEBRATES

Bivalve Mollusks

Bivalve mollusks (clams, oysters, mussels, scallops) are plankton feeders that depend upon extracting food and oxygen from the aquatic environment. These invertebrates siphon and filter large volumes of water; studies of mussels have shown that they can filter up to 20 liters of water per day. However, the lack of selectivity in their filtering mechanism unfortunately enables them to concentrate in their visceral organs a significant quantity and wide variety of contaminants pathogenic for humans, including: bacteria, viruses, dinoflagellates, toxic metals, pesticides, hydrocarbons, chemicals, and radioactive material.

Bacterial[1,9,59–72]

Typhoid fever has in the past been linked to the ingestion of raw mollusks, particularly clams and oysters. In 1924 an epidemic of typhoid fever in which approximately 150 died was attributed to the ingestion of contaminated oysters. Comtemporary public health surveillance of shellfish harvesting and sanitation programs have essentially eliminated the threat of mollusk-borne typhoid fever in the United States.

In spite of current mollusk-associated public health measures, gastroenteritis has continued to plague the world's population, sometimes in epidemic proportions. Gastroenteritis caused by the ingestion of mollusks, fish, and crustaceans (especially shrimp) containing *Vibrio parahemolyticus* produces a clinical syndrome similar to *Salmonella* gastroenteritis. *V. parahemolyticus* is the etiologic agent in the most common type of summer-associated gastroenteritis in Japan; it has been a recognized inhabitant of Japan's coastal waters for some time. *V. parahemolyticus*, and poisoning epidemics as a consequence of its ingestion, have been identified worldwide. These areas include the coastal waters of the United States, the United Kingdom, and Australia and other areas of the Pacific Ocean.

Gastroenteritis produced by *V. parahemolyticus* usually follows a 12- to 24-hour incubation period, and clinical symptoms last from 24 to 48 hours, after which time complete resolution is the typical course of events. The symptom complex consists of explosive watery (sometimes bloody) diarrhea, nausea, vomiting, abdominal cramps, fever, headache, prostration, volume depletion, rectosigmoid ulceration, and fecal leukocytosis in severe cases. Although usually a self-limiting process, the disease may cause significant abdominal pain and volume depletion, requiring analgesics and IV administration of fluids and electrolytes. Hospitalization may be required for seriously ill patients. *V. parahemolyticus* is sensitive to chloramphenicol, gentamycin, and tetracycline, and in serious cases of gastroenteritis the patient should be started on oral tetracycline. Appropriate stool and blood specimens should be obtained for culture and sensitivity studies prior to the institution of antibiotic therapy. *V. parahemolyticus* is a halophilic (salt loving) bacterium requiring special bacteriological culture media containing at least 0.5% NaCl, such as TCBS (thiosulfate citrate bile salts sucrose) agar.

Vibrio cholera epidemics from ingestion of raw clams and mussels as well as other seafood products has been a problem in some European and Far Eastern countries, particularly Italy and Malaysia. People traveling to countries in which sanitation regulations for shellfish harvesting are ineffective or nonexistent must consider the consequences of eating raw mollusks.

Clostridium botulinum type E has been cultured from coastal waters off the United States and from the eastern oyster but no cases of botulism have been linked to ingestion of fresh mollusks.

Earampamoorthy and Koff[65] rightfully point out that bacterial contamination of mollusks is not limited to those concentrated from the aquatic environment but may also occur during packaging, transportation, storage, repacking, and display of the market product. Improper handling of shellfish may encourage the proliferation of bacteria and the production of toxic products.

Viruses[9,64,65,67,69,73–82]

Hepatitis is the disease process of major epidemiological importance causally linked to shellfish ingestion. The first recorded outbreak of shellfish-associated hepatitis A infection was reported in Sweden in 1955 in which 600 cases were documented following ingestion of sewage-contaminated oysters. No further cases were reported until 1961 when three major outbreaks of shellfish-associated hepatitis occurred in the United

States. Since 1961 sporadic occurrences have been reported in the United States and Germany. Clams are more dangerous than oysters in that they have a greater potential for concentrating hepatitis virus because they are capable of migrating to various aquatic environments, while oysters attach themselves to rocks, permitting more effective surveillence of their environment.

Hepatitis A infection has been associated with steamed clams; studies have shown that the internal temperature at "gaping" is insufficient to kill hepatitis A virus.

Hepatitis B surface antigen (HBsAg) has been isolated from a clam estuary contaminated by the raw sewage of a New England coastal hospital. However, there is no specific data presently link to HBsAg-contaminated shellfish with hepatitis B infection in humans.

A very interesting outbreak of oyster-associated hepatitis B occurred in the spring of 1980 in Baltimore, Maryland among a 13-member family group who gathered weekly for oyster eating parties. The oysters were placed in a cooler the nights prior to the parties and were refrigerated overnight until the parties began the following day. The Center for Disease Control's investigation (reported by Dr. Mark Cain April 19, 1982, at the Epidemic-Intelligence Service Conference Centers for Disease Control, Atlanta, Georgia) revealed that the individual who had cleaned the oysters and placed them in the cooler was a carrier of HBsAg and the index case. It was postulated that traces of his blood (secondary to scrapes and abrasions occurring while cleaning the oysters) had become mixed with the cooler water. Hepatitis B infection occurred in seven individuals and was associated with shucking the oysters that had been placed in the contaminated cooler water. Infection was believed to occur via scrapes and abrasions in the skin of those individuals shucking the oysters since several family members eating oysters but not shucking did not contract hepatitis B infection. Obviously, this outbreak of hepatitis B was related to circumstances involving oysters but not as a result of oyster-borne infection.

Non-A, non-B hepatitis may also play a role in infections associated with shellfish but information is lacking regarding this possibility.

Those patients who present with symptoms of clinical hepatitis must be questioned as to their history of shellfish ingestion within the four- to six-week period preceding the development of symptoms of the disease. The local public health authorities and the Center for Disease Control (Hepatitis Department, Phoenix, Arizona) should be informed of any patient thought to have shellfish-associated hepatitis.

In addition, patients diagnosed as having shellfish-borne gastroenteritis should receive immune serum globulin (0.6 mg/kg) initially and repeated in thirty days as prophylaxis against hepatitis A. Viral gastroenteritis has been reported as a result of ingestion of contaminated oysters from coastal beds in New South Wales, Australia, and is attributed to infection by the Norwalk virus.

In addition, poliovirus and echovirus have been isolated from shellfish in the Great South Bay, Long Island, New York, although no clinical human infections have been attributed to ingestion of infected mollusks. Other enteric viruses, including enteroviruses, adenoviruses, and reoviruses, are thought to be causally related to shellfish-borne gastroenteritis. Epidemiological data, however, to support this suspicion are lacking. Metcalf[77] points out:

> The virologic dilemma represented involved the formidable technical difficulties encountered in working with those enteric viruses causally associated with shellfish-transmitted enteric disease. . . . Shellfish virology research needs to take some new directions. A vigorous, imaginative program which places primary emphasis upon these enteric virus pathogens and conditions actually involved in shellfish transmitted disease is needed. . . . The end result of such a program would be better protection of public health in general, and a possibility that the number of shellfishing waters approved for the taking of shellfish could be increased.

Dinoflagellates[1,2,6,9,21,38,65,67,69,83–86]

Dinoflagellates (class Mastigophora, order Dinoflagellata) are predominantly free-living, unicellular protozoans forming part of the ocean plankton, synthesizing carbohydrates, proteins, and fats. These one-celled plant-animals when in high concentrations may produce yellow, brown, green, black, blue, red, or milky bioluminescence of the water. The most common color associated with "blooming" of dinoflagellates is red, hence the terms red tide, red current, and red water. The following list indicates the marine dinoflagellates incriminated in human intoxications as a result of shellfish ingestion:

Ptychodiscus brevis (formerly, *gymnodinium brevis*) (Gulf of Mexico and Florida)
Gy. sp. (South Africa)
Gonyaulax actenella (British Columbia)
G. catenella (Pacific coast of North America)
G. excavata
G. grindleyi (Capetown, South Africa)
G. tamarensis (eastern coast of North America)
Pyrodinium bahamense (Port Moresby, New Guinea)

P. phoneus (Belgium, North Sea)
Exuviaella mariae-lebouriae (Japan, British Columbia, California)

Those dinoflagellates suspected of causing human intoxication are:

Glenodinium foliaceum (Baltic Sea)
Amphidinium sp. (warm and cool temperate waters)
Cochlodinium catenatum (California, Japan)
Gy. galatheanum (Walvis Bay, southwest Africa)
Gy. mikomoti (Japan)
Gy. splendens (Washington, British Columbia)
Gy. veneficum (English Channel)
Noctiluca scinitillans (diffuse)
G. monilata (Florida)
G. polyhedra (southern California, Portugal, Australia)
Heterocapsa triquetra (Baltic Sea)
Peridinium trochoideum (Bay of Guanabara, Rio de Janeiro, Brazil)
Polykrikos schwartzi (Atlantic Ocean, north Baltic and Mediterranean Seas, California coast)
Euviaella baltica (Angola, western Africa)
Prorocentrum micans (California)
Prymnesium parvum (Mediterranean Sea)

Venerupin Shellfish Poisoning[1,2,6,9,22,69]

Venerupin shellfish (order Filibranchia) are found in Japanese, British Columbian, and Californian coastal waters. Venerupin shellfish poisoning has been limited to those mollusks inhabiting and harvested from the brackish waters of certain specific areas of Japan, namely, Lakes Hamana and Kanazawa. The venerupin shellfish producing human intoxication are *Venerupis semidecussata* or *Tapes semidecussata* (Japanese little neck) and *Crassostrea gigas* also known as *Ostrea gigas* (giant Pacific oyster, Japanese oyster). *Dosinia japonica* (Japanese dosinia) has been found to contain venerupin toxin, but no reports of human intoxication from this species of mollusk have been documented.

Venerupin toxin is heat labile and concentrated in the digestive organs and livers of venerupin shellfish. The toxin is believed to be derived from the dinoflagellate *Ex. mariae-lobouriae* (previously named *Provocentrum* sp.) upon which the shellfish have been feeding.

The syndrome produced by venerupin intoxication usually begins 24 to 48 hours after ingestion of the contaminated mollusks, but the incubation period may extend to one week. It results from a hemorrhagic diathesis combined with liver failure. Initial symptoms include anorexia, abdominal pain, nausea, vomiting, consti-

pation, and headache followed shortly thereafter by bleeding of the gums and nasal passages, petechial hemorrhages, ecchymoses, jaundice, ascites, delirium, coma, and death in 33 percent of the cases. Laboratory studies reveal anemia, leukocytosis, and abnormalities in blood clotting and liver function tests. Postmortem examinations reveal diffuse liver necrosis with hemorrhage and fatty degeneration as well as congestion and hemorrhage of heart, lung, and gastrointestinal tract.

Therapy consists of activated charcoal combined with purgatives (in a slurry) to prevent absorption and hasten elimination of toxin. Otherwise, supportive care to treat the hemorrhagic diathesis and liver failure is required.

The Japanese government has placed affected areas under quarantine during peak danger periods between January and April in order to prevent outbreaks of venerupin shellfish poisoning.

Paralytic Shellfish Poisoning[1,2,6,8,9,21,22,64,65,67,86–93]

Paralytic shellfish poisoning (PSP) is produced from ingestion of certain shellfish that have been feeding upon toxic dinoflagellates, specifically, *Gonyaulax* sp (*G. acatenella*, *G. catenella*, *G. grindleyi*, *G. tamarensis*), *P. bahamense*, and *P. phoneus*. Human PSP has a worldwide distribution including North America, Central America, Europe, Africa, Asia, Oceania, and the Pacific Islands.

During warm seasons—encouraged by high light, water temperatures of approximately 10°C, calm seas, water low in nitrogen and phosphorus—these dinoflagellates "bloom," producing bioluminescent tides, commonly called red tides. Dinoflagellate blooms have been associated with large mollusk, fish, and bird kills. At the Merrimack river estuary, Plum Island, off the Massachusetts coast (1972), 95 birds were found dead and autopsies revealed hemorrhage of their internal organs as well as mollusk shells in their stomachs. The poisoning (initially thought secondary to pesticide spraying of the area) was proved to be from mollusk-borne infestation with the dinoflagellate *G. tamarensis*.

The toxin from *G. catenella*, saxitoxin, was first isolated from the Alaskan butter clam *Saxidomus giganteus*, from which it received its name. The chemical structure of saxitoxin has been documented as shown in Figure 34–1.

Saxitoxin is a neurotoxin closely resembling tetrodotoxin but less potent. Saxitoxin appears to block sodium channels in nerve fibers, thereby inhibiting impulse conduction, which perhaps accounts for the deaths that result from respiratory paralysis. Saxitoxin is thought to be 50 times as potent as curare, and an ingestion of as little as 0.5 mg may be lethal. Intraperitoneal injection of bivalve extracts into mice serves as the basis for the bioassay of saxitoxin. A concentration of more than

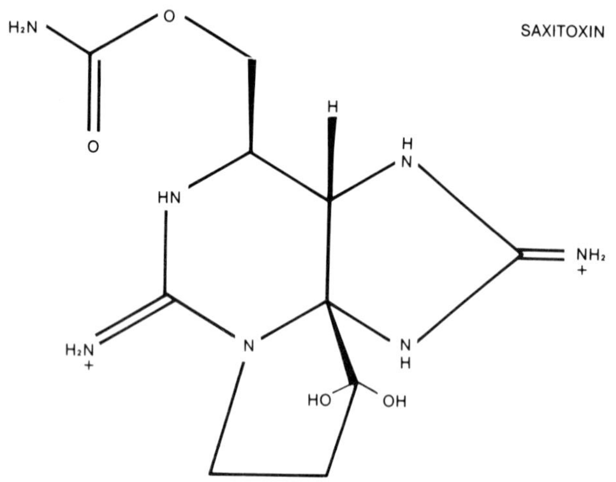

Figure 34–1 Saxitonin Chemical Structure.

80 μg/100 gm of tissue extract is thought dangerous for human consumption. Bioassay for saxitoxin facilitates epidemiological surveillance of shellfish. However, no direct assay is presently available.

The symptoms associated with PSP usually develop within 30 minutes of ingesting the poisonous mollusks. Initially perioral and acral paresthesias, diffuse erythema, nausea, vomiting, diarrhea, and abdominal pain occur, followed by ataxia, muscle weakness, sensations of floating, generalized motor incoordination, dysphonia, dysphagia, vertigo, nystagmus, headache, respiratory distress, and in approximately 8.5 percent of cases, death from respiratory failure.

Therapy consists initially of purgatives, cathartics (without magnesium, because elevated magnesium levels depress nerve conduction by changing cell membrane potentials, increasing resistance, and therefore, possibly aggravating symptoms of PSP), and saline enemas in order to promote elimination of unabsorbed toxin still present in the GI tract. If vomiting has not occurred, emetics should be administered and gastric lavage should be performed. Administration of IV solutions of normal saline or Ringer's lactate with added electrolytes (as indicated) may be necessary depending upon the patient's vital signs, urine output, and laboratory test results. Observation of the patient's respiratory status is critical.

In the presence of muscle weakness measuring FEV_1 (a portable spirometer can be used) and frequent arterial blood gas analysis to follow $PaCO_2$ levels may be extremely helpful in ascertaining when a patient may require mechanical ventilatory assistance. Paresthesias may indicate an alteration in the relationship of ionized and un-ionized calcium. Since saxitoxin is similar to tetrodotoxin, the latter thought to block sodium channels in nerve membranes, the administration of calcium

(as is suggested for neurotoxic shellfish poisoning and ciguatera fish poisoning) may increase the sodium channel blockade, thereby further decreasing neurotransmission of the action potential. Consequently, calcium administration is contraindicated in PSP.

Neurotoxic Shellfish Poisoning[1,6,9,38,64,84,88,93,94]

Neurotoxic shellfish poisoning is caused by the dinoflagellate *P. breve* producing red tides off both the Gulf and Atlantic coasts of Florida. Neurotoxic shellfish poisoning is far less severe than paralytic shellfish poisoning and in many ways resembles ciguatera fish poisoning. Symptoms occur within minutes to hours after ingestion of the toxic mollusks and include nausea, vomiting, paresthesias, reversal of hot and cold temperature sensation, diarrhea, ataxia, and rarely, paralysis.

One of the several toxins *P. breve* produces has been found to inhibit calcium uptake in endoplasmic reticulum of skeletal muscle. Theoretically this suggests treating severe cases with therapeutic doses of calcium; presently, this hypothesis remains experimental. Another toxin isolated stimulates post-ganglionic cholinergic nerve fibers and may be responsible for the diarrhea associated with neurotoxic shellfish poisoning. Therapy is directed toward eliminating any unabsorbed toxin using those modalities mentioned in reference to paralytic shellfish poisoning.

P. breve is an unarmored dinoflagellate capable of being disrupted in rough surf, thereby becoming aerosolized. This aerosolized mist when breathed by bathers or seashore inhabitants may produce a syndrome comprising copious rhinorrhea, conjunctival irritation, and nonproductive cough. This is usually a transient, rapidly reversible, self-limiting process requiring no therapeutic intervention.

Other Invertebrates[1,2,6,9,22,38,64,69]

Toxic ingestion may be caused by many other invertebrate organisms including univalve mollusks (whelks, ivory shells, turban shells, murex shells, abalone, sea hares), bivalve mollusks (callistin shellfish, Tridacna clam), cephalopods (octopuses, squids, cuttlefishes), and crustaceans (crabs, lobsters, shrimps). A complete description of these poisonings is beyond the scope of this chapter and for further information the reader is directed to the references cited.

POISONING FROM INGESTION OF MARINE VERTEBRATES

Poisonous fishes as defined by Bagnis et al. are " . . . fishes which, when ingested, cause a biotoxication in humans due to a toxic substance present in the fish.

Fishes that may become accidentally contaminated by bacterial food pathogens are not included."[23]

Ichthyotoxism is the term used to describe poisoning from ingestion of fish. The major classifications of ichthyotoxism include: ichthyosarcotoxism (poisoning from ingesting a toxin found within the flesh, viscera, or slime), ichthyootoxism (poisoning from ingesting a toxin limited to the gonads), ichthyocrinotoxism (poisoning from ingesting a toxin within or elaborated by glandular structures), and ichthyohematotoxism (poisoning from ingesting a toxin found in the blood).

Ichthyosarcotoxism[3,6,9,22,38,80,95]

Ichthyosarcotoxism is by far the most frequent and dangerous form of ichthyotoxism and poses the greatest public health hazard from ingestion of marine organisms. Halstead[3] classifies ichthyosarcotoxic fish poisoning into: (1) cyclostome poisoning (lampreys, hagfishes), (2) elasmobranch poisoning (sharks, skates, rays), (3) ciguatera poisoning (ciguatoxic fishes), (4) scombroid poisoning (scombroid and non-scombroid fishes), (5) puffer fish poisoning (tetraodontoid fishes), (6) gemphylid poisoning (gemphylidotoxic fishes), and (7) hallucinogenic fish poisoning.

Elasmobranch Poisoning[1,3,6,9,23]

Eating shark flesh has been known to cause a mild gastroenteritis (e.g., Greenland shark *Somniosus microcephalus*). Ingestion of shark liver may have lethal consequences, but toxic effects generally produce GI and neurologic symptoms. The composition and nature of the poison is unknown and therapy is purely symptomatic. Abstinence from shark products, unless a particular specimen is definitely known to be nontoxic is advisable.

Ciguatera Poisoning[1,3,5,6,9,11,21,38,64,67,85,88,95–117]

The term ciguatera was first used by the early Spanish settlers of Cuba. The word is derived from *cigua*, meaning snail, referring to the univalve mollusk *Turbo pica* (class Gastropoda), which is known to produce digestive and nervous disorders when ingested.

Ciguatera poisoning is the most commonly documented and reported poisoning from vertebrate fishes, and in fact is the most common form of food-borne disease related to seafood ingestion in the United States. During the ten-year period 1970 to 1980 the Center for Disease Control reported 94 outbreaks involving 418 cases of ciguatera poisoning. However, these figures probably do not reflect the true magnitude of the problem. Lawrence and coworkers[109] suggest a ratio of five cases per 10,000 population per year as a more accurate estimation of the true incidence of ciguatera poisoning.

It is very difficult to obtain data on ciguatera poisoning because minor symptoms may be attributed to a viral gastroenteritis or other enteric food poisoning, physicians and health professionals generally are unfamiliar with the syndrome, and many countries worldwide have no mandatory reporting laws. Furthermore, only over the last few years have papers on ciguatera poisoning been published in the general medical and emergency medical literature to alert physicians to this particular fish-borne illness.

Fishes associated with ciguatera poisoning inhabit the tropical waters of the world extending from 35°N to 34°S latitude. The greatest concentration of ciguatoxic fishes is in the Caribbean and Indo-Pacific. Ciguatoxic fishes are usually reef and bottom dwellers, and those weighing over 10 to 12 pounds are more likely to be toxic. In fact, Hessel and coworkers[117] reported that of the Pacific Ocean red snapper studied, 69 percent of those weighing over 2.8 kg (6.16 pounds) were found to be toxic, as compared with 18 percent of those under 2.8 kg. Furthermore, there seems to be a higher prevalence of toxicity in those fish whose habitats have been disturbed by natural or man-made destructive forces, such as storms, pier and wharf construction, beach excavations, and dredging.

The following orders of bony fishes (phylum Chordata, class Osteichthyes) have been reported as being ciguatoxic and include some 400 to 500 species:[3,9]

Clupeiformes:	herrings, anchovies
Myctophiformes:	lizardfishes, lanternfishes
Anguilliformes:	true eels, that is, conger eels, moray eels, snake eels
Beloniformes:	needlefishes, halfbeaks
Gasterosteiformes:	trumpetfishes, seahorses
Beryciformes:	squirrelfishes, soldierfishes
Perciformes:	perchlike fishes, that is, surgeonfishes, cardinal fishes, tangs, blennies, jack, pompano, permit, butterflyfishes, bannerfishes, angelfishes, dolphin, silverfishes, gobies, pacific sailfish, sergeant major fishes, grunts, parrotfishes, wahoo, tuna, bonito, king, mackerel, scorpionfishes, grouper, rabbitfishes, barracuda
Bothidae:	flatfishes, for example, flounder
Tetraodontiformes:	filefishes, triggerfishes, cowfishes, puffers, trunkfishes
Batrachoidiformes:	toadfishes
Lophiiformes:	goosefishes, frogfishes

Ciguatera fish poisoning is believed to result from toxins produced from a certain benthic alga dinoflagellate, *Gamberdiscus toxicus*, frequently found on the surface of brown and red seaweed. There is presently confirmed evidence that it produces both ciguatoxin and maitotoxin. The source of ciguatoxin in significant concentration to affect man is a consequence of a multiplicity of environmental factors interwoven with the food chain of marine organisms.

Many investigators have tried to elucidate the chemical nature, pharmacokinetics, and properties of ciguatoxin but the specific molecular structure has not yet been demonstrated. Present evidence indicates that ciguatoxin is an odorless, colorless, heat-stable, lipid-soluble, acid-stable lipid having a quaternary nitrogen atom, one or more hydroxyl groups, and a cyclopentanone moiety with the atomic formula $C_{35}H_{65}NO_8$. Ciguatoxin therefore is unaffected by cooking, freezing, or storage conditions and is not inactivated by gastric juices. These properties, coupled with its tasteless and colorless nature, make prevention of poisoning and detection of ciguatoxic fishes very difficult.

In the effort to detect ciguatoxic fishes, folkloric taboos prohibit eating a lone fish captured from a school, fish products that repel ants or that a pet turtle will not eat, thinly sliced meat not showing a rainbow effect when held up to sunlight, and fish products that tarnish a silver spoon when placed in a cooking pot. Upon close scrutiny, none of these suggestions has proved effective or valid.

Detection of ciguatoxin in tissue of suspected fishes by a radioimmune assay[107] has been possible since 1977. Presently, no methods are available for the detection of ciguatoxin in the blood or secretions of the poisoned victims. Ciguatera poisoning, however, is probably caused by a variety of toxins or other concomitant ichthyosarcotoxic processes, which accounts for the multiplicity of clinical signs, symptoms, and responses to therapy.

The clinical syndrome generally begins within six hours after ingestion but can occur as early as 15 minutes or be delayed as much as 30 hours. Approximately 75 percent of patients have symptoms within the first 12 hours after ingestion of the toxic fish. Initially, acral and perioral tingling, numbness, and prickly and burning sensations occur, followed by headache, vertigo, hypersalivation, metallic taste (rare), nausea, vomiting, watery diarrhea, and abdominal cramps. The GI symptoms may not occur but usually are present and may precede the onset of sensory disturbances.

Neurologic symptoms include the phenomenon of temperature dysesthesias (hot objects feel cold and cold objects feel hot), which usually appears two to five days after ingestion and is neither pathognomonic nor required for the diagnosis of ciguatera poisoning. However, it is an extremely valuable diagnostic clue. Hyperexcitability manifested as anxiety, nervousness, giddiness, apprehension, restlessness, shouting, hysteria, muscle stiffness or spasms, trismus, fasciculations, hyperreflexia, hallucinations, irrational behavior, generalized seizures, and opisthotonus may give way to fatigue, weakness, ataxia, muscular incoordination, aphonia, hyporeflexia, areflexia, inability to stand, cranial nerve palsies, ptosis, stupor, coma, flaccid paralysis, respiratory muscle paralysis, respiratory failure, and complete adynamism. Cardiovascular symptoms of bradycardia, hypotension, and conduction disturbances with heart block are particularly dangerous and indicative of severe poisoning. Sims points out, "Manifestations of extremely serious ciguatera fish poisoning include the following: severe bradycardia, severe hypotension, convulsions, severe generalized paresthesias, severe hypocalcemia, aphonia, bronchorrhea, unconsciousness, and progressive heart block."[1]

The mortality rate from acute poisoning has been reported from zero to as high as 80 percent, depending upon the series of cases reviewed. There have been two deaths in the United States from ciguatera poisoning, both in Hawaii in 1964.[1]

Chronic symptoms of ciguatera poisoning have been well known but generally poorly studied. A wide variety of problems involving cutaneous, GI, neurologic, cardiovascular, genitourinary, and psychic systems can be affected. Chronic symptoms can last for many years and become emotionally and physically debilitating.

Ciguatera poisoning may present as a diffuse multisymptom involvement or as a more limited process with one or more systems predominating. Bagnis in 1968[118] classified ciguatera poisoning according to the predominant symptoms: neurologic symptoms, digestive symptoms, itching, erythema, cardiovascular symptoms, neuromuscular symptoms, and sensory disturbances. This is a useful classification because it may help to predict the course of the patient's illness and degree of aggressiveness required in the therapeutic approach.

Therapy for ciguatera poisoning has included a wide range of modalities, including emetics, gastric lavage, and purgatives for elimination of toxin and prevention of absorption; chlorpromazine as an antiemetic; atropine and 2-PAM for GI, cardiac, and anticholinesteraselike symptoms produced by ciguatoxins; infusions of electrolyte solutions high in calcium, magnesium, potassium, chloride, and bromide, and the administration of EDTA for paresthesias and cardiac and neurologic symptoms; barbiturates, glucocorticoids, and cold showers for itching, paresthesias, and neurologic complaints; magnesium sulfate and sedatives such as phenobarbitol and Valium in order to control insomnia, hyperexcitability, and seizures; and vitamin supplements (particularly B and C complexes) to hasten recovery. All of these regimens have been recommended or condemned for various reasons.

The current therapeutic interventions are based upon the following concepts:

- Ciguatera poisoning is a consequence of multiple toxins and factors.
- Ciguatoxin is not an anticholinesterase.
- Ciguatoxin has been shown to affect sodium membrane permeability and resting membrane potentials by its action as a competitive inhibitor of calcium ions for receptor sites on the nerve membrane.

In consideration of these factors, the following recommendations are set forth for the treatment of ciguatera poisoning:

- Within six to eight hours after ingestion administer emetics (if vomiting has not occurred) or utilize gastric lavage to promote gastric emptying and elimination of any remaining fish products.
- Administer activated charcoal combined with a non-magnesium-containing cathartic in a slush to promote elimination of toxin.
- Administer atropine, 0.01 to 0.02 mg/kg IV every ten minutes if necessary (symptomatic heart rate less than 50 per minute).
- Administer dopamine infusion, 5 to 20 μg/kg per minute, for severe and prolonged hypotensive episodes or when cardiovascular symptoms predominate. Titrate to systolic blood pressure of 100 to 120 mm Hg.
- Administer IV calcium gluconate in doses of 15 mg/kg over 15 minutes, followed by a continuous infusion of 45 to 70 mg/kg of calcium gluconate daily for 5 days or until serum calcium is in mid-normal range. (This is used in severe poisoning to act as a substrate against competitive inhibition of calcium by ciguatoxin.)
- Administer diazepam for hyperexcitability and diazepam and phenytoin for convulsions; do not use barbiturates.
- Administer IV fluids utilizing normal saline and Ringer's lactate with additional electrolyte solutions, depending upon the patient's vital signs, urine output, amount of vomitus and diarrhea, and the results of laboratory studies.
- Administer large doses of multivitamins, and acetaminophen 5 to 10 mg/kg every six to eight hours if necessary for headaches.
- Provide mechanical ventilatory support and oxygen therapy for respiratory failure.
- Utilize transvenous cardiac pacing in the presence of refractory bradycardia or heart block.
- Provide diet containing no fish, shellfish, alcoholic beverage, or nuts.

While there have been no published studies on utilizing high dose calcium infusions for treatment of ciguatera poisoning, Sims has had encouraging results in several severely poisoned individuals with significant bradycardia, heart block or hypotension. In life-threatening situations, when all other modalities have been unsuccessful and the patient demonstrates deterioration in spite of routine therapy, high-dose calcium infusions should be considered.

Patients with chronic symptoms should be treated with oral administration of calcium gluconate, multivitamins, and acetaminophen and should refrain from ingesting fish, fish products, shellfish, alcohol, and nuts, all of which have been implicated in producing recurrent episodes of symptoms. Patients unfortunate enough to sustain a second episode of ciguatera poisoning frequently have more severe symptoms, and it has been postulated that this exaggerated response may be a consequence of immunologic sensitization.

Prevention of illness from ciguatera poisoning involves awareness of the syndrome, refraining from eating fishes in affected areas, ingesting only smaller reef fishes less than 5 pounds, and confirming that the 3 to 5 pound fish fillet, "snapper fingers," or fish sticks, purchased in the market or at a restaurant, are not small fillets or small pieces of a larger fish.

Scombrotoxism[1,3,6,9,22,38,64,67,87,119–125]

Scombroid fish poisoning is a consequence of the ingestion of poorly canned, refrigerated, or preserved scombroid fishes (suborder Scombroidei: tuna, albacore, mackerel, kingfish, wahoo, bonito, etc.) or nonscombroid fishes having red skeletal muscle or portions of red skeletal muscle, which have undergone the action of certain bacteria. Recently, mahi-mahi (*Coryphaena hippurus*), a nonscombroid fish, has been implicated in producing scombrotoxism.

This is the only form of ichthyosarcotoxism in which bacteria participate in the poisoning process. The organism usually incriminated in scombroid fish poisoning is *Proteus morgagni*, which is known to contain histadine decarboxylase activity. But *Alcaligenes metalcaligenes, Sarcina flara, Shigella dysenteriae, Clostridium perfringens*, certain *Escherichia coli*, and *Aerobacter aerogenes* have also been found capable of generating histamine. These bacteria, therefore, act upon the histadine in the flesh of the fish, converting it to histamine and a histamine-like substance called saurine, a heat-stable compound which has been found to include histamine dihydrochloride, histamine phosphate, and other substances.

A histamine-like reaction begins within minutes to a few hours after the ingestion of the toxic fish. Interestingly, the ingestion of large doses of histamine in humans does not usually result in poisoning unless the person is taking INH or other GI tract histaminase blockers. Healthy fish usually contain less than 0.1 mg of histamine per 100 gm of flesh. Increasing levels of histamine can be measured in fish that are left at room temperature for several hours.

Symptoms of scombroid fish poisoning include a toxic erythema or flushing (particularly involving the face, neck, upper trunk, and conjunctivae) often resembling a sunburn, burning sensation of the mouth and throat, nausea, abdominal cramps, diarrhea, headache, oral blistering, palpitations, dizziness, prostration, chills, thirst, pruritus, blurred vision, urticaria, swelling of the face, increased flatulence, tachycardia, and hyperactive bowel sounds.

The differential diagnosis includes alcohol ingestion associated with chloral hydrate, tyramine, monoamine oxidase inhibitors, Antabuse, and non-alcoholic-related flush syndromes of carcinoid, pheochromocytoma, the Zollinger-Ellison syndrome, and allergy. Other drugs capable of producing flushing are antimuscarinics, histamine releasers (e.g., opiates), nicotinic acid, and nitrites, all of which must be considered in the differential diagnosis of flush reactions.

Therapy for scombroid fish poisoning consists of subcutaneous injections of epinephrine, antihistamines IM or IV (diphenhydramine or hydroxyzine) and/or bronchodilators IV if epinephrine and antihistamines are insufficient in relieving bronchospasm. In order to hasten elimination and prevent absorption of histamine or saurine, emetics and cathartics should be used if vomiting and diarrhea have not occurred spontaneously. Corticosteroids may be required in rare cases.

Scombroid fish poisoning is very difficult to prevent, since surveillance is often lacking, toxins are heat stable, and the fish usually has no abnormal taste. Occasionally, the meat may taste peppery, which should alert the individual to the possibility of spoilage. Fishermen should make every effort to ensure proper refrigeration of their catch and fish allowed to remain in the sun for more than two hours should not be eaten. Furthermore, patients taking certain medications, particularly isoniazid, should refrain from eating scombroid fishes or fish with red skeletal muscle. It has been shown that isoniazid is a potent inhibitor of GI histaminase. Isoniazid in concert with only slightly elevated levels of histamine or saurine in scombroid fishes may have complementary effects, whereas each factor individually may be insufficient to produce poisoning.

Tetrodotoxism[1,3,6,9,22,38,57,64,67,88-90,116,126,127]

Pufferfish poisoning, or tetrodotoxication, is a very rare but serious and often fatal form of ichthyosarcotoxism. Pufferfish poisoning, also known as fugu poisoning, is generally found in the countries surrounding the South Indochina Sea and in Japan. Tetraodontiformes are also found in Californian, African, South American, and Australian waters. Tarichatoxin found in some California newts has been discovered to be identical to tetrodotoxin present in pufferfishes (suborder Gymnodontes). Other terms used to designate tetrodotoxin are: fugu poison, spheroidin, and tetraodontoxin. In Japan, where the fish is a delicacy, deaths from tetrodotoxism have been reported at 100 per year during the period 1886 to 1958. Public health measures have included the licensing of restaurants and handlers of tetrodon fishes sufficiently knowledgeable to clean and eviscerate the known toxic species without cutting the liver or roe where the toxin is very highly concentrated. In the United States, laws have specifically been established to prevent the sale of tetrodon fishes, markedly reducing the number of poisonings in this country.

Tetrodotoxin acts by reducing membrane permeability to sodium ions by blocking sodium influx and thereby interfering with production of action potentials in certain excitable cells.

Pufferfish poisoning produces symptoms within minutes of ingestion, characterized by paresthesias (initially of the mouth, tongue, lips, and face, progressing to involve the extremities and finally producing generalized numbness of the entire body), headache, general malaise, diaphoresis, nausea, vomiting, abdominal pain, dysphagia, and salivation; followed by neurologic symptoms of incoordination, weakness, muscle fasciculations, respiratory paralysis, generalized ascending paralysis, cyanosis, and dermatologic symptoms of blistering and severe scaling of the skin. Hypotension and cardiovascular collapse may occur and the mortality rate may be as high as 60 percent.

Therapy is directed toward maintaining airway, ventilation, adequate circulatory function, and monitoring and treating dysrhythmias. There is no known antidote for tetrodotoxin and treatment remains symptomatic and empirical.

OTHER DANGEROUS MARINE ORGANISMS[1-4,6,9,10,12,21,22,38,64,67,128-135]

Many other organisms are dangerous but cannot be described in detail in this chapter. They include: poisonous marine turtles; marine mammals such as sea lions, seals, polar bears, dolphins; marine animals that shock, such as electric rays and eels; parasitic catfish;

schistosomal organisms; algae; bacteria; and miscellaneous fishes and reptiles. The reader is referred to the references cited for information regarding these dangerous marine organisms.

REFERENCES

1. Sims JK: Harmful marine life, in Shilling CW (ed): *Physicians' Guide to Diving Medicine*. Washington, DC, Undersea Medical Society, in press.
2. Halstead BW: *Poisonous and Venomous Marine Animals: Invertebrates*. Washington, DC, US Government Printing Office, 1965, vol. 1.
3. Halstead BW: *Poisonous and Venomous Marine Animals: Vertebrates*. Washington, DC, US Government Printing Office, 1967, vol. 2.
4. Halstead BW: *Poisonous and Venomous Marine Animals: Vertebrates*. Washington, DC, US Government Printing Office, 1970, vol. 3.
5. Steinfeld AD, Steinfeld HJ: Ciguatera and the voyage of Captain Bligh, *JAMA* 228 (10):1270–1271, 1974.
6. Banner AH: Hazardous marine animals, in Tedeschi CG, Eckert WG, Tedeschi LG (eds): *Forensic Medicine: A Study in Trauma and Environmental Hazards*. Philadelphia, WB Saunders, 1977, pp 1378–1429.
7. Davies DH, Campbell GD: The Aetiology, Clinical Pathology and Treatment of Shark Attack. (Based on observations in Natal, South Africa.) *J Royal Med Service* 48:110–136, 1962.
8. Ellis MD (ed): *Dangerous Plants, Snakes, Arthropods and Marine Life: Toxicity and Treatment*. Hamilton, Ill, Drug Intelligence Publications, 1978.
9. Halstead BW, Courville DA: *Dangerous Marine Animals that Bite, Sting, Shock, Are Nonedible*, ed 2, Centreville, Md, Cornell Maritime Press, 1980.
10. Strauss MB, Orris WL: Injuries to divers by marine animals: A simplified approach to recognition and management. *Milit Med* 139:129–130, 1974.
11. Morton RA, Burklew MA: Incidence of ciguatera in barracuda from the west coast of Florida. *Toxicon* 8:317–318, 1970.
12. Tinker SW: *Fishes of Hawaii*. Honolulu, Hawaiian Services Inc, 1928.
13. Khlentzos CT: Seventeen cases of poisoning due to ingestion of an eel: *Gymnothorax flavimarginatus*. *Am J Trop Med* 30:785–793, 1950.
14. Sherman RT, Furste W: A guide to prophylaxis against tetanus in wound management. *Am Coll Surg*, 1972.
15. Taylor GD: The otolaryngologic aspects of skin and scuba diving. *Trans Amer Laryng Rhinol Otol Soc*, January 23–24, 1959, pp 409–459.
16. Sims JK, Irei M: Human Hawaiian sponge poisoning. *Hawaii Med J* 38(9):263–270, 1979.
17. Taylor L: Tetanus from a marine sponge. *J Otolaryngol* 72:762, 1958.
18. Yafee HS: Irritation from red sponge. *N Engl J Med* 282:51, 1970.
19. Burnett JW: An electron microscopic study of two nematocytes in the tentacle of *Cyanae capillata*. *Chesapeake Sci* 12(2):67–71, 1971.
20. Burnett JW, Calton CJ: Review article: The chemistry and toxicology of some venomous pelagic coelenterates. *Toxicon* 15:177–196, 1977.
21. Manowitz NR, Rosenthal RR: Cutaneous-systemic reactions to toxins and venoms of common marine organisms. *Cutis* 23:450–454, 1979.
22. Bagnis R, Berglund F, Elias PS, et al: Problems of toxicants in marine food products (marine biotoxins). *WHO* 42:69–88, 1970.
23. Weill R: Contribution a l'étude des cnidaireset de leurs nematocystes. *Trav Stat Zool Wimbereux*, 1934, vols 10–11.
24. Wittle LW, Middlebrook RE, Lane CE: Isolation and partial purification of a toxin from Millepora alcicornis. *Toxicon* 9:327–331, 1971.
25. Wittle LW, Scura ED, Middlebrook RE: Stinging coral (*Millepora tenera*) toxin: A comparison of crude extracts with isolated nematocyst extracts. *Toxicon* 12:481–486, 1974.
26. Arnold HL: Portuguese man-of-war (blue bottle) stings: Treatment with papain. *Straub Clin Proc* 37:30–33, 1971.
27. Burnett JW, Calton GJ: Sea nettle and man-of-war venoms: A chemical composition of their venoms and studies on the pathogenesis of the sting. *J Invest Derm* 62:372–377, 1974.
28. Freeman SE: Actions of *Chironex fleckeri* toxins on cardiac transmembrane potentials. *Toxicon* 12:395–404, 1974.
29. Freeman SE, Turner RJ: Cardiovascular effects of Cnidarian toxins: A comparison of toxins extracted from *Chiropsalmus quadrigatus* and *Chironex Fleckeri*. *Toxicon* 10:31–37, 1972.
30. Alsen C, Berress L, Tesseraux I: Toxicities of sea anemone (*Anemonia sulcata*): Polypeptides in mammals. *Toxicon* 16:561–566, 1978.
31. Hinegardner RT: The venom apparatus of the cone shell. *Hawaii Med J* 17(6):533–556, 1958.
32. Kohn AJ: Cone shell stings: Recent cases of human injury due to venomous marine snails of the genus *Conus*. *Hawaii Med J* 17(6):528–532, 1958.
33. Baden HP, Burnett JW: Injuries from sea urchins. *South Med J* 70(4):459–460, 1977.
34. Cracchiolo A III, Goldberg L: Local and systemic reactions to puncture injuries by the sea urchin spine and the date palm thorn. *Arthritis Rheum* 20(6):1206–1212, 1977.
35. O'Neal RL, Halstead BW, Howard LD: Injury to human tissues from sea urchin spines. *Calif Med* 101(3):199–202, 1964.
36. Rocha G, Frago S: Sea urchin granuloma of the skin. *Arch Dermatol* 85:146–148, 1962.
37. Unkles SE: Bacterial flora of the sea urchin *Echinus esulentus*. *Appl Environ Microbiol* 34:347–359, 1977.
38. Goldfrank L, Lewin N, Weisman R: The red snapper. *Hosp Physician* 17:36–54, 1981.
39. Bitseff EL, Garoni WJ, Hardison CD, et al: The management of stingray injuries of the extremities. *South Med J* April:417–418, 1970.
40. Cross TB: An unusual stingray injury: The skindiver at risk. *Med J Aust* 2:947–948, 1976.
41. Mullaney PJ: Treatment of stingray wounds. *Clin Toxicol* 3(4):613–615, 1970.
42. Russell FE, Panos TC, Kang LW, et al: Studies on the mechanism of death from stingray venom: A report of two fatal cases. *Am J Med Sci* 566–584, 1958.
43. Scoggin CH: Catfish stings. *JAMA* 231:176–177, 1975.
44. Russell FE, Emery JA: Venom of the weevers *Trachinus draco* and *Trachinus vipers*. *Ann NY Acad Sci* 90:805–819, 1960.
45. Cameron AM, Endean R: The venom apparatus of the Scorpion fish (*Notesthes robusta*). *Toxicon* 4:111–121, 1966.
46. Hunter AE: Lionfish sting—Nevada. *Morbid Mortal Week Rep* 83–84, 1979.
47. Schaffer RC Jr, Carlson RW, Russel FE: Some chemical properties of the venom of the scorpionfish *Scorpaena guttata*. *Toxicon* 9:69–78, 1971.

48. This lion doesn't roar. *JAMA* 242(1):17, 1979.

49. Weiner S: The production and assay of stonefish antivenene. *Med J Aust* 15:719, 1959.

50. Tu AT: Venoms of hydrophiidae, in Tu AT: *Venoms, Chemistry and Molecular Biology*. New York, John Wiley & Sons, 1977, pp 151–177.

51. Cage PW, Dulhunty AF: Effects of toxin from the blue ringed octopus (*Hapalochaena maculosa*), in Martin DF, Padilla GM (eds): *Marine Pharmacognosy*. New York, Academic Press, 1973, p 85.

52. Croft JA, Howden MF: Chemistry of maculotoxin: A potent neurotoxin isolated from *Hapalochlaena maculosa*. *Toxicon* 10(6):645, 1972.

53. Flecker H: Fatal bite from octopus. *Med J Aust* 2(9):329–331, 1955.

54. Mabbet H: Death of a skindiver. *Aust Skindiving Spearfishing Digest* 13:17, 1954.

55. Sheumack DD, Howden MEH, Quinn RJ, et al: Maculotoxin: A neurotoxin from the venom glands of the octopus *Hapalochaena maculosa* identified as tetrodotoxin. *Science* 199:188–189, 1978.

56. Sutherland SK, Brood AJ, Lane WR: Octopus neurotoxins: Low molecular weight nonimmunogenic toxins present in the saliva of the blue-ringed octopus. *Toxicon* 8(3):249, 1970.

57. Sheumack DD, Howden MEH, Spence I, et al: Tetrodotoxin in the blue-ringed octopus. *Med J Aust* 1:160–161, 1978.

58. Trethewie ER: Pharmacological effects of the venom of the common octopus, *Hapalochaena*. *Toxicon* 3(1):55, 1965.

59. Barlows A, Herman GJ, DeWitt WE: The isolation and identification of *Vibrio cholerae*: A review. *Health Lab Sci* 8:167–175, 1971.

60. Baross J, Liston J: Occurrence of *Vibrio parahemolyticus* and related hemolytic vibrios in marine environment of Washington state. *Appl Microbiol* 20:179–186, 1970.

61. Blake PA, Merson MH, Weaver RE, et al: Disease caused by a marine vibrio: Clinical characteristics and epidemiology. *N Engl J Med* 300(1):1–5, 1979.

62. Bolen JL, Zamiska SA, Greenough WB: Clinical features in enteritis due to *Vibrio parahemolyticus*. *Am J Med* 57:638–641, 1974.

63. Chatterjee BD, Neogy KN, Gorbach SL: Study of *Vibrio parahemolyticus* from cases of diarrhea in Calcutta. *Indian J Med* 58:234–238, 1970.

64. Dembert ML, Strosahl KF, Bumgardner RL: Disease from fish and shellfish ingestion. *Am Fam Physician* 24(2):103–108, 1981.

65. Earampamoorthy S, Koff RS: Health hazards of bivalve mollusk ingestion. *Ann Intern Med* 83(1):107–110, 1975.

66. Hollis DG, Weaver RE, Baker CN et al: Halophilic *Vibrio* species isolated from blood cultures. *J Clin Microbiol* 3:425–431, 1976.

67. Horwitz MA: Specific diagnosis of food-borne disease. *Gastroenterology* 73(2):375–381, 1977.

68. Lumsden LL, Hasseltine HE, Leake JP, et al: A typhoid-fever epidemic caused by oyster-borne infection: 1924–1925. *Public Health Rep* 50 (Suppl):1–102, 1925.

69. McMichael DF: Dangerous marine mollusco, in Evans JW: *Proceedings of the First International Convention on Life-Saving Techniques*. Bull Post Grad Comm Med Univ, Sydney, 1963, Scientific Section Suppl: Part III.

70. Sakazaki R: Halophilic *Vibrio* infections, in Riemann H (ed): *Food-Borne Infections and Intoxications*. New York, Academic Press, 1969, pp 115–129.

71. *Vibrio parahemolyticus* gastroenteritis—United States: 1969–1972. *Morbid Mortal Week Rep* 22:231–232, 1973.

72. Kaneko T, Colwell RR: Ecology of *Vibrio parahemolyticus* in Chesapeake Bay. *J Bacteriol* 113:24–32, 1973.

73. Follow-up on shellfish-associated hepatitis—southern United States. *Morbid Mortal Week Rep* 22:388, 1974.

74. Koff RS, Sear HS: Internal temperature of steamed clams. *N Engl J Med* 276:737–739, 1967.

75. Mahoney P, Fleischner G, Milliman I, et al: Australian antigen: Detection and transmission in shellfish. *Science* 183:80–81, 1974.

76. Mason JO, McClean WR: Infectious hepatitis traced to the consumption of raw oysters: An epidemiologic study. *Am J Hyg* 73:90–111, 1962.

77. Metcalf TG: Indication of viruses in shellfish growing waters. *Am J Public Health* 69(11):1093–1094, 1979.

78. Mosley JW, Galabos J: Viral hepatitis, in Schiff L (ed): *Disease of the Liver*, ed 4. Philadelphia, JB Lippincott, 1975, pp 527–528.

79. Murphy AM, Grohmann GS, Christopher PJ, et al: An Australia-wide outbreak of gastroenteritis from oysters caused by Norwalk virus. *Med J Aust* 329:332, 1979.

80. Shellfish-associated hepatitis: Massachusetts. *Morbid Mortal Week Rep* 21:20, 1972.

81. Vaughn JM, Landry EF, Viccale TJ, et al: Survey of human entero virus occurrence in fresh and marine surface waters of Long Island. *Appl Environ Microbiol* 38:290–296, 1979.

82. Collins C: Massachusetts Department of Health: The Red Tide—A public health emergency. *N Engl J Med* 288(21):1126–1127, 1973.

83. Kim YS, Padilla GM, Martin DF: Effect of *G. breve* toxin on calcium uptake and ATPase activity of sarcoplasmic reticulum vesicles. *Toxicon* 16:495–501, 1978.

84. McFarren EF, Tanabe H, Silva FJ, et al: The occurrence of a Ciguatera-like poison in oysters, clams and *Gymnodinium breve* cultures. *Toxicon* 3:111–123, 1965.

85. Popkiss ME, Horstman DA, Harpur D: Paralytic shellfish poisoning: A report of 17 cases in Cape Town. *S Afr Med J*:1017–1023, 1979.

86. Akiba: Study of poisoning by venerupis semidecussata and Ostera gigas and other poisonous substances (in Japanese, English summary). *Nisshen Igaku* 36(6):1–24, 1949.

87. Hughes JM, Merson MH: Current concepts: Fish and shellfish poisoning. *N Engl J Med* 295(20):1117–1120, 1976.

88. Kao CY: Tetrodotoxin, saxitoxin and their significance in the study of excitation phenomena. *Pharmacol Rev* 13(2):997–1049, 1966.

89. Narahashi T: Mechanism of action of tetrodotoxin and saxitoxin on excitable membranes. *Fed Proc* 31(3):1124–1132, 1972.

90. Prakash A, Medcof JC, Tennant AD: *Paralytic Shellfish Poisoning in Eastern Canada*. Ottawa, Fisheries Research Board of Health, 1971.

91. Schantz EJ, Schnoes HK: The structure of saxitoxin. *J Am Chem Soc* 97(5):1238–1239, 1975.

92. Wong JL, Oesterlin R, Rappoport H: The structure of saxitoxin. *J Am Chem Soc* 93:7344, 1971.

93. Grunfeld Y, Spiegelstein MY: Effects of *Gymnosinium breve* toxin on the smooth muscle of guinea pig ileum. *Br J Pharmacol* 51:67–72, 1974.

94. Trieff NM, Spikes JJ, Ray SM, et al: Isolation and purification of *Gymnodinium breve* toxin, in de Uries A, Kochva E (eds): *Toxins of Animal and Plant Origin*. New York, Gordon & Breach Science Publishers, 1972, pp 557–577.

95. Baratta RO, Tanner PA Jr: Ichthyosarcotoxism—Ciguatera intoxication. *J Fla Med Assoc* 57(57):39–42, 1970.

96. Bagnis R, Chanteau S, Chungue E, et al: Origins of ciguatera fish poisoning: A new dinoflagellate *Gambierdiscus toxicus*. Adachi and Fukuyo definitively identified as the causal agent. *Toxicon* 18:199–208, 1980.

97. Adochi R, Fukuyo Y: The tecal structure of a marine toxic dinoflagellate *Gambierdiscus toxicus* gen. et. sp. nov. collected on Ciguateral endemic areas. *Bull Soc Sci Fish* 45:67–71, 1979.

98. Bagnis R, Kuberslu T, Laugter S: Clinical observations on 3009 cases of Ciguatera (fish poisoning) in the South Pacific. *Am J Trop Med Hyg* 28:1067–1073, 1979.

99. Bagnis R: Concerning a fatal case of Ciguatera poisoning in the Tuamotu Islands (Symposium: Marine Biotoxicology). *Clin Toxicol* 3(4):579–583, 1970.

100. Banner AH, Shaw S, Alender C, et al: Fish intoxication: Notes on Ciguatera—Its mode of action and suggested therapy. *South Pac Comm Tech Pap* no. 141, 1964.

101. Banner AH; Ciguatera fish poisoning: A symposium—Ciguatera in the Pacific. *Hawaii Med J* 24(5):353–354, 1965.

102. Craig CP: It's always the big ones that get away. *JAMA* 244(3):272–273, 1980.

103. DeSylva DP, Deichmann WB: Toxins in the food chain. *Dev Toxicol Environ Sci* 4:433–440, 1978.

104. Gelb AM, Mildvan D: Ciguatera fish poisoning, *NY State J Med* 79:1080–1081, 1979.

105. Gudger EW: Poisonous fishes and fish poisonings, with special reference to Ciguatera in the West Indies. *Am J Trop Med* 10:43–45, 1930.

106. Heimbecker RO: Ciguatera poisoning: Snowbirds beware. *CMA J* 120:637–638, 1979.

107. Hokama Y, Banner AH, Boylan DB: A radioimmunoassay for the detection of Ciguatera. *Toxicon* 15:315–325, 1977.

108. Jones HR Jr: Acute ataxia associated with Ciguatera-type (Grouper) tropical fish poisoning.

109. Lawrence DN, Enriquez MB, Lumish RM, et al: Ciguatera fish poisoning in Miami. *JAMA* 244(3):254–258, 1980.

110. Li KM: Ciguatera fish poisoning: A cholinesterase inhibitor. *Science* 147:1580–1581, 1965.

111. Okihiro MM, Keenan JP, Ivy AC Jr.: Ciguatera fish poisoning with cholinesterase: Report of a case. *Hawaii Med J* 24(5):354–357, 1965.

112. Parc F, Ducousso R, Chanteau S, et al: Problems linked to the Ciguatera immunological detection. *Toxicon* 17 (Suppl. 1):137, 1979.

113. Rayner MD: Mode of action of Ciguatera. *Fed Proc* 31(3):1139–1145, 1972.

114. Russell FE: Short communication: Ciguatera poisoning—report of 35 cases. *Toxicon* 13:383–385, 1975.

115. Scheuer PJ, Takahashi W, Tsutsumi, et al: Ciguatera: Isolation and chemical nature. *Science* 155:3767:1267–1268, 1967.

116. Teravainen H: Myoneural ultrastructure and cholinesterases after tetrodotoxin treatment. *Acta Physiol Scand* 79:369–372, 1970.

117. Hessel DW, Halstead BW, Peckham NH: Marine biotoxins. I. Ciguatera poison: Some biological and chemical aspects. *Ann NY Acad Sci* 90:788, 1960.

118. Bagnis R: Clinical aspects of ciguatera (fish poisoning) in French Polynesia. *Hawaii Med J* 28:25–28, 1968.

119. Gilbert RJ, Jobbs G, Murray CK, et al: Scombrotoxic fish poisoning: Feature of the first 50 incidents to be reported in Britain (1976–1979). *Br Med J* 71–72, 1980.

120. Kim R: Flushing syndrome due to Mahimahi (Scombroid fish) poisoning. *Arch Dermatol* 115:963–965, 1979.

121. Merson MH, Beane WB, Gangarosa FJ, et al: Scombroid fish poisoning outbreak traced to commercially canned tuna fish. *JAMA* 228:1268–1269, 1974.

122. Taylor SL, Guthertz LS, Leatherwood M, et al: Histamine production by *Klebsiella pneumoniae* and an incident of Scombroid poisoning. *Appl Environ Microbiol* 274–278, 1979.

123. Uragoda CG, Kottagoda SR: Adverse reactions to isoniazid on ingestion of fish with a high histamine content. *Tubercle* 58:83–89, 1977.

124. Uragoda CG: Histamine poisoning in tuberculosis patients on ingestion of tropical fish. *J Trop Med Hyg* 81:243–245, 1978.

125. Zimmer L, Altman R, Thun M, et al: Scombroid poisoning—New Jersey. *Morbid Mortal Week Rep* 29:106–107, 1980.

126. Burklew MA, Morton RA: The toxicity of Florida gulf puffers, genus *Sphoeroides*. *Toxicon* 9:205–210, 1971.

127. Torda TA, Sinclair E, Ulyatt DB: Puffer fish (tetrodotoxin) poisoning: Clinical record and suggested management. *Med J Aust* 1:599–602, 1973.

128. Adams RM, Remington JS, Steinberg J. et al: Tropical fish aquariums: A source of *Mycobacterium marinum* infections resembling sporotrichosis. *JAMA* 211(3):457–461, 1970.

129. Cardellina JH II, Marner JF, Moore RJ: Seaweed dermatitis: Structure of lyngbyatoxin A. *Science* 204:193–195, 1979.

130. Flowers DJ: Human infection due to *Mycobacterium marinum* after a dolphin bite. *J Clin Path* 23:475–477, 1970.

131. Girard SM, Paik YK, Melton RJ, et al: *Clostridium perfringens* cultured from a Hawaiian sardine, *Sardinell marquesensis*. *Hawaii Med J* 38(11):317–329, 1979.

132. Johnson RM, Katarski ME, Weisrock WP: Correlation of taxonomic criteria for a collection of marine bacteria. *Appl Microbiol* 708–713, 1968.

133. Solomon AE, Stoughton RB: Dermatitis from purified sea algae toxin (Debromoaplysiatoxin). *Arch Dermatol* 114:1333–1335, 1979.

134. Williams CS, Riodan DC: *Mycobacterium marinum* (atypical acid-fast bacillus) infections of the hand. *J Bone Joint Surg* 55A(5):1042–1050, July 1973.

135. Yafee HS, Stargardter F: Erythema multiforme from Tedania Ignis. *Arch Dermatol* 87:107–108, 603, 1963.

Psychiatric Emergencies

"Substance Abuse" (Chapter 35) includes an in-depth discussion of the pharmacology of specific narcotics, stimulants, inhalants, hallucinogens, and sedatives; a review of overdose, intoxication, and abstinence syndromes; and the complications of chronic abuse. The reader interested in this topic may also wish to refer to "Poisoning and Drug Overdose" (Chapter 24).

In "Alcohol Abuse" (Chapter 36) alcoholism is presented as a "disease concept," and the author provides a succinct review of alcohol metabolism, tolerance, intoxication and overdose, addiction and withdrawal syndromes, and their treatment on an outpatient and inpatient basis. The interested reader may also wish to refer to "Seizures and Acute Confusion" (Chapter 47). "Depression, Anxiety, and Suicide" (Chapter 37) clearly outlines the recognition and management of patients with depression and anxieties, particularly the suicidal patient.

35. Substance Abuse

DANIEL SHINE, M.D.

Drug abusers are often difficult patients, medically and personally. The emergency department is frequently their principal source of medical care, and complaints may be acute or chronic. Patients present with any of several psychiatric, surgical, obstetric, and medical syndromes. These illnesses may result from acute intoxication, from abstinence, from the concomitant actions of several drugs, or from the contaminants, diluents, and vehicles found in drugs of abuse.

The physician evaluating an addict must take into account routes of drug administration, the effects of drugs on laboratory tests, the illnesses to which drug addicts are prone, and the possibility that a condition unrelated to drugs is being masked by the use of them. Moreover, symptoms and signs of many conditions may be artfully feigned by the patient seeking drugs.

In approaching diagnostic problems of such diversity and so complex an underlying disorder as drug abuse, the physician must seek a good working relationship with the patient. Such a relationship may be elusive. Drug abusers tend to be little educated (even about the drugs they use), "street wise" in their codes of behavior, and magical in their thinking. Patients may be manipulative in their efforts to obtain drugs or ambivalent about seeking medical care. In either case there may be a bewildering number of symptoms to evaluate.

Physicians, for their part, are often judgmental about their patients' life styles, annoyed by the chronicity of problems presented for immediate attention, and doubtful about the patients' willingness to comply with whatever treatment may be prescribed or referral arranged. Especially irksome to the physician, a professional inclined to take charge, is the suspicion of being manipulated.

The simplest and least satisfactory solution to these problems lies in the common practice of construing any interaction between patient and physician as a game of concealment and detection. As a result of this game either the patient emerges victorious with a prescription or the physician unmasks the addiction and summarily dismisses the addict.

In this sort of exchange both patient and physician find themselves performing familiar roles, and in a busy emergency department the resolution of such an encounter is clearly in sight and swiftly attained. In either outcome, however, the issue of treatment for the patient's addiction is avoided. Drug abusers, like alcoholics, are quick to defend their addicted life style even while they desire treatment. They are therefore unlikely to ask directly for help or to seek any more therapeutic alternatives than the traditional deception and detection. For many addicts even detection and brusque dismissal is preferable to a confrontation with possible change.

The detection game thus serves as a defense for both patients and physicians; however, it falls to the latter to refocus therapeutic issues. The physician should therefore:

- Avoid taking personally an addict's attempt to deceive;
- Avoid mistaking detection for treatment; and
- Attempt to address the underlying problem of addiction by making appropriate referral.

Despite the problems, care given to drug abusers can be thorough and the system of referral effective. Certainly, drug abuse is a chronic, relapsing condition that is difficult to treat. However, even when definitive cure is not effected by pharmacologic and psychosocial therapy, success is often achieved in stabilization of the patient's drug use, reversal of antisocial behavior, and intervention in potentially life-threatening crises. For these reasons it is essential not only that drug abuse be identified but also that abusers be referred for treatment.

The words addiction, abuse, and dependence are often used interchangeably, but they are not synonymous. Dependence (or addiction) is defined in terms of compulsive drug-seeking behavior, physiologic tolerance to increased doses of drug, and stereotyped signs and symptoms of withdrawal upon drug deprivation.[1] This definition is based on clinical observations drawn from several disciplines, and it reflects the lack of a unifying etiologic hypothesis. Work with opiate[2] and (more recently) benzodiazepine[3] receptors in the central nervous system (CNS) and elsewhere has not so far provided a biologic model of drug dependence. Nor has psychiatric investigation yielded an accepted psychosocial explanation of the development of addiction.[4] At this time, the definition of drug dependence is descriptive, and the therapies used to treat it are pragmatic.

Drug abuse, a less frequently defined term, implicitly compares the behavior of an "abuser" with the accepted conventions of psychoactive chemical use. The imprecision of the phrase permits its application to individuals who compulsively use large amounts of a drug that does not produce tolerance or stereotyped withdrawal. The distinction between "physical" and "psychological" dependence is another attempt to include under the general heading of addictive those compounds that do not produce a predictable syndrome of withdrawal.

The discussion that follows is concerned only with that minority of drug users whose style of life and whose health problems are largely determined by the use of drugs other than alcohol.

NARCOTICS

Narcotic addicts are more likely to use several opiates and nonopiates than was the case several years ago.[5] Although all opiates produce similar intoxication and withdrawal, the time courses, routes of administration, and associated complications differ. A knowledge of the different commonly used opiates is therefore of value.

Pharmacology

Heroin

Heroin (diacetyl morphine) varies greatly in purity and in the substances with which it is cut. One recent study found the modal concentration of heroin in street samples to be about 3 percent.[6] The mean concentration was higher due to the occasional appearance of good quality heroin. Even lower concentrations are also commonly reported.[7,8] The "cut" is now not exclusively quinine, and assays for quinine are therefore not always reliable in diagnosing heroin use. Talc, lactulose and other sugars, procaine, sodium bicarbonate, and even phencyclidine have been used to dilute heroin for street sale. Benzodiazepines and antihistamines have also been identified as diluents, creating problems of unwitting polydrug addiction. Heroin may be "stepped on" (diluted) many times by different dealers using different diluents.

Heroin comes in a brown form (usually Mexican), which is cheaper, less potent, and more likely to contain vegetable matter than white heroin. It may cause syndromes of thrombocytopenia and musculoskeletal pain. White heroin, usually from Asia, is the addict's preferred form. It may be powdered, crystalline, or clumped and is usually sold as fractions of a gram or "spoon." A heroin addict may use from one to ten or more "quarters" a day.

The heroin is mixed with water of variable purity, heated until dissolved, and sometimes strained through cotton (which may, at a time of need, be itself heated in water to release trapped heroin). The solution is then injected either intravenously (IV) or subcutaneously. Heroin, or fumes from heated heroin, may also be inhaled ("snorted"). It is, however, largely inactive when orally ingested because of incomplete absorption and first-pass hepatic metabolism.[9] Heroin is quickly transformed to morphine and monoacyl morphine in the liver. These metabolites account for heroin's effects and have half-lives of about two hours. They are not bound to plasma proteins.

Methadone

Methadone diverted from maintenance and detoxification programs is sold for about $1 per milligram on the street. It comes as a 40-mg scored disc ("biscuit") mixed with cellulose to form a sludge in water that is said to discourage parenteral use. The methadone is, however, easily filtered with a household apparatus. Methadone also comes as 5-mg and 10-mg Dolophine tablets ("Dolies" or "Dollies"), as a syrup (10 mg/ml), and as a solution (10 mg/ml).

Unlike most other opiates, methadone is well absorbed from the gastrointestinal (GI) tract and undergoes little first-pass metabolism. Parenterally, a single dose of methadone is slightly more potent than morphine on a weight basis.[10] Peak levels occur between two and four hours after ingestion. Methadone is long acting, with a half-life of about a day. The drug is highly protein bound and has a large volume of distribution. Methadone is both metabolized in the liver and excreted unchanged in the urine.[11] Plasma levels at steady state vary considerably from patient to patient and from day to day.[12] Acidification of the urine produces a statistically significant, but probably not clinically important, increase in clearance of parent drug.[13] Patients on methadone maintenance may be receiving more than 100 mg/day, however the current trend is toward lower doses (20 to 50 mg).[14]

LAAM

LAAM (L-α-acetyl methadol) is an experimental long-acting derivative of methadone. It is slightly less potent than methadone in single doses, but has a half-life of 1½ to 2 days and is therefore given three times a week. LAAM comes as a solution of 10 mg/ml. Absorption and metabolism are similar to methadone.[15]

Percodan

Percodan (oxycodone, aspirin, phenacetin, caffeine) and Percocet (oxycodone and acetaminophen) are common street narcotics. Although insoluble, Percodan may be crushed, shaken into a suspension, and injected IV ("cold shake"). Percodan is about 50 percent absorbed from the GI tract. The half-life of oxycodone is about two hours, and elimination occurs through the liver and kidneys. It is not uncommon for addicts to use 30 to 40 tablets a day and to present with signs of salicylism, acetaminophen-induced hepatic damage, GI hemorrhage, and local complications of "cold shaking" such as phlebitis, cellulitis, and skin abscesses.

Dihydrocodeinone

Dihydrocodeinone in cough syrups is commonly abused. Parenterally, dihydrocodeinone is equivalent to morphine in potency. Morphine, however, is far less well absorbed and subject to greater first-pass metabolism compared with dihydrocodeinone. The two preparations containing dihydrocodeinone without an antihistamine, anticholinergic, or catecholamine are Dicodid and Tussionex. Both a syrup (5 mg/ml) and tablets (5 mg) are available. The duration of action of these antitussives is similar to morphine's. Addicts may ingest 200 to 300 ml a day.[16]

Demerol

Demerol (meperidine) is not a common street narcotic but may be abused through forged prescriptions. The duration of action is somewhat shorter than morphine's. Demerol comes as injectable solutions of 2.5, 5.0, 7.5, and 10.0 percent and as 50-mg and 100-mg tablets. The accumulation of normeperidine, an active metabolite, may cause seizures in overdose and in patients with renal disease or cancer.[17] Pupillary dilation is sometimes seen after overdose. Although naloxone reverses all signs of opiate overdose due to meperidine, animal studies suggest that naloxone may not give complete protection against seizures.[18]

Darvon

Darvon (propoxyphene) is a common street drug, which is obtainable as the napsylate (Darvon-N) and the more soluble hydrochloride (Darvon). Propoxyphene is a weak opiate, irritating to the veins, and often taken orally by patients on methadone maintenance to "boost the methadone dose." Users may take 15 to 20 65-mg (napsylate) capsules a day. Propoxyphene is metabolized in the liver and has a variable half-life (three to eight hours). It does not completely suppress syndromes of abstinence from more potent opiates and itself produces only mild addiction, even after high-dose IV use.[19] In overdose, seizures and cardiac conduction defects may be added to the usual opiate signs and symptoms.[20]

Talwin

Talwin (pentazocine) is a partial opiate agonist which also produces abstinence signs in persons addicted to more powerful opiates. Pentazocine produces a mild addiction in those who use it regularly.[21] It is not a common street drug, but its presence among the list of medications to which a patient claims allergy may be a clue to opiate addiction.

Other Opiates

Other opiates which may be encountered are Dilaudid (hydromorphone) known as "DLS," a short-acting oral and parenteral opiate of greater potency than heroin; deodorized tincture of opium ("DTO"), a hydroalcoholic solution of 10 percent opium (1 percent morphine); Pantopon (opiate alkaloids); and Numorphan (oxymorphone), known as "blues."

Overdose and Intoxication

Opiate intoxication causes feelings of pleasant drowsiness and contentment. The user may describe a warm sensation in the abdomen and chest. Many chronic users claim that opiates produce in them only remission from abstinence symptoms, but signs of intoxication are often present.

For several seconds following IV injection, heroin and other powerful opiates produce intense euphoria ("rush" or "flash"), which may be accompanied by nausea and vomiting but is nevertheless pleasurable.[22]

On examination the patient may appear to be alternately dozing and waking ("nodding"). Vital signs are decreased, the pupils pinpoint, and speech becomes infrequent and slurred. Hypothermia may be severe in cold climates.

Overdose is usually accidental, a result of unexpectedly potent heroin or of waning tolerance. The use of pharmaceutical-grade opiates by heroin addicts tolerant to poor quality street heroin may produce overdose. Conversely, narcotic overdose is less common among methadone-treated addicts, presumably because of the consistent tolerance that daily methadone confers.

There appear to be two overdose syndromes. One results in death within minutes. The mechanism of death in this syndrome in unknown, but apparently it is toxic rather than allergic, and may in part be related to simultaneous alcohol ingestion. This sudden death syndrome occurs mainly among heroin users. The demonstration in chronic heroin addicts of ECG changes consisting of ST–T abnormalities and prolonged QT intervals suggests that arrhythmia may contribute to sudden death. Overdoses of this type are unlikely to be due to the "cut" or to respiratory depression alone.

The second type of overdose syndrome may occur after use of any opiate. Coma develops over minutes after parenteral use and over hours after oral ingestion. There is the classic picture of constricted pupils, shallow and infrequent breathing, hypotension, and occasionally pulmonary edema. Death results from hypoxia.[23]

The diagnosis of opiate overdose should be considered in any patient who is obtunded. Even trauma sufficient to account for unconsciousness may have been associated with opiate overdose. *All unconscious patients in whom the cause of coma is at all in doubt should receive Narcan (naloxone).*

Naloxone is a pure opiate antagonist that, unlike nalorphine, will not cause deepening of coma in cases that are not narcotic induced. The effect of naloxone on opiate-intoxicated patients is predictable, immediate (peak effect in about five minutes), and usually striking.[24] Naloxone is therefore both diagnostic and therapeutic. Although there have been reports of alcohol intoxication responding to naloxone, sedative hypnotic drugs do not respond.[25,26]

Before giving naloxone, pupil size, respiratory rate and depth, blood pressure, and pulse should be noted. Then 0.8 mg should be given by rapid IV injection. Patients in whom one of these parameters changes without a change in coma grade should be given an additional 0.4 mg naloxone every five minutes until ten doses have been given or coma is reversed. Although 0.8 mg will reverse most opiate intoxications, propoxyphene overdose in particular may require more.

Naloxone is also very effective intramuscularly (IM), although peak effect may not occur for 15 to 30 minutes.[27] If it proves difficult to find a peripheral vein, naloxone should be given IM in the same dose before attempting cut-down or central vein cannulation.

When mixed overdose, postictal confusion, sepsis, or cerebral anoxia (from hypoventilation, pulmonary edema, arrhythmia, or shock) are complicating factors, the response to naloxone may be partial. A complete response to naloxone, while not necessary to stabilize the patient, excludes the possibility that other conditions are contributing to coma.

Naloxone should not be considered as seizure prophylaxis in patients who have taken overdoses of propoxyphene or meperidine.[18] It is probably wise to admit such patients for observation.

Although response to naloxone is the best sign of opiate intoxication, evidence of chronic abuse may point to the diagnosis. Skin findings, sometimes hidden in tattoos, are usually present in parenteral narcotic users. Parallel punctate scars on either side of the vein ("tram lines") or a single row following the center of the vein ("tracks") are characteristic. Palpable sclerotic veins with overlying hyperpigmentation are sometimes found. Dried blood on the skin may indicate recent injection. Opiate-induced histamine release occasionally causes a localized urticaria.[28]

Signs of chronic venous insufficiency and obliteration of lymph channels are often present (puffy hands or feet). Healed ulcers and abscesses from subcutaneous administration ("skin popping," "skinning") or attempted IV injections ("misses") may also be seen. Digital amputations from arterial injections are not rare.

Gynecomastia may be present in males either as a result of marijuana or methadone-induced hypogonadism,[29,30] or from liver disease related to alcoholism or recurrent hepatitis. Injections into the breast tissue ("pseudogynecomastia") is a rare finding.[31]

Pulmonary pathology associated with chronic heroin use is not usually apparent clinically, although granulomas and bronchiectasis may be seen on chest roentgenogram, and signs of pulmonary hypertension may be present.[32] The spleen is sometimes enlarged and firm. Bowel sounds are characteristically diminished.

Acutely, narcotic overdose may be associated with pulmonary edema. Because cardiomegaly is not present and because infiltrates clear quickly with treatment, the pulmonary edema of opiate overdose has been compared with that of near-drowning. In near-drowning the acidosis is characteristically metabolic; opiate overdose manifests both respiratory and metabolic acidosis.[33] Increased intracranial pressure is often associated with heroin-induced pulmonary edema.[34]

Neurologic signs of opiate overdose apart from coma include middle cerebral artery syndromes with focal findings in a minority of patients. Some of these individuals have been found to have unexplained occlusions by arteriography.[34] Another, more common, sign of acute narcotic poisoning is pupillary miosis. This sign may be seen even in mild intoxications since tolerance to the pupillary effects of opiates is only slight. Miosis is therefore of no prognostic value. Moreover, sedative overdose may produce miosis, and mydriasis may be a feature of cerebral anoxia or meperidine poisoning.[35] Some addicts routinely self-administer long-acting mydriatics such as atropine; in such cases the pupils are unreactive.

Once considered, the diagnosis of uncomplicated opiate overdose is not difficult to make. Mixed overdoses and those that are complicated by neurologic damage require further work-up with urine screening, EEG, and CT scan.

When signs of chronic heroin use are present but the patient responds only partially to naloxone, consideration should be given to the following causes of coma related to drug abuse: seizure; tetanus; sepsis with or without emboli; neurologic sequelae of hepatitis; cerebral angiitis (associated with amphetamine and methylphenidate abuse); uremia from heroin-induced glomerulopathy, amyloidosis, or rhabdomyolysis with acute tubular necrosis (ATN); GI hemorrhage from Percodan ingestion; perforation of an abdominal viscus or pancreatitis masked by opiate analgesia; internal bleeding from heroin- or quinine-induced thrombocytopenia; and the effects of other drugs, including those with which heroin may have been cut. (See Chapter 45.)

The possibility should also be entertained that home remedies have been applied by fellow users. Intravenous salt solutions and forcibly administered oral liquids may contribute to obtundation. Application of ice to the genitals is a popular home remedy, and the finding of cold genitals may indicate that opiate overdose was considered the diagnosis by the patient's friends.

Occasionally heroin is used as a means of homicide. Battery acid scraped from the terminals, convulsants such as strychnine and nicotine, or even undiluted heroin are reliably fatal by the IV route.

The treatment of opiate overdose includes naloxone, supportive therapy, and only occasionally GI decontamination. Dialysis and hemoperfusion are not useful.

Removal of ingested opiates by emesis and charcoal with magnesium citrate is indicated within two to four hours of an oral ingestion, provided that the patient is alert or can be made so with the aid of naloxone. Naloxone antagonizes apomorphine-induced emesis, so syrup of ipecac should be used. Ipecac syrup is not arrhythmogenic and reliably produces emesis in over 90 percent of patients within 30 minutes of one or two 30-ml doses.[36]

Severe central nervous system depression or pulmonary edema may require endotracheal intubation. (See Chapters 56 and 59 for indications for intubation.) Overdose with propoxyphene or meperidine may call for intubation for lavage if the risk of seizures or arrhythmia is thought to outweigh the risks of intubation.

The half-life of naloxone is about 45 minutes, and its effects wear off after one to one and a half hours.[26,27] On the other hand, the CNS depressant effects of long-acting opiates such as LAAM may last for a week following large ingestions. Doses of naloxone may therefore have to be repeated, and IV infusions have been used with success. Once it has been shown that naloxone completely reverses coma, it is no longer necessary (and may from a management standpoint be undesirable) to keep the patient fully awake while the opiate is metabolized.

The abrupt withdrawal precipitated by naloxone may be accompanied by rage or even psychosis. These reactions are short-lived and do not require medication; however the patient should not be allowed to leave the hospital until it is clear that further naloxone is unnecessary. There are case reports of pulmonary edema and hypertensive reactions following abrupt reversal of opiate-induced coma.[37]

Treatment of narcotic-induced pulmonary edema should be with the usual means, but digoxin should not be used. Infiltrates and blood gases usually improve by the end of two days, although pulmonary function tests may be abnormal for weeks.[38] Shock usually responds to naloxone and IV fluids. Opiates may cause urinary retention and fecal impaction. These conditions should be looked for and treated.

A blood count, clotting studies, and measurement of blood gases, liver and renal function tests, an ECG, chest roentgenogram, electrolytes, and blood sugar should be included in the initial assessment of the serious opiate overdose. If Percodan or Percocet ingestion is suspected, early measurement of salicylate or acetaminophen in plasma is important. Plasma opiate levels are not useful in estimating prognosis because tolerance to opiates, not their concentration in the blood, determines the clinical state. Detection of opiates in urine may be helpful in some cases. Since hydrolysis of morphine from its glucuronide conjugate improves sensitivity of testing, the laboratory should be notified when heroin is being sought.

Findings that should encourage hospitalization of the patient with opiate toxicity include (1) a history or drug screen documenting overdose with a long-acting opiate, (2) a response to naloxone that is only partial, (3) a history or drug screen suggesting multiple drugs, and (4) the presence of serious problems related or unrelated to the overdose. It is unlawful to deny hospital admission to a drug addict because of his or her addiction.

Abstinence Syndromes

Daily administration of potent opiates for two to three weeks can produce tolerance and, upon deprivation, a marked abstinence syndrome.[39] Narcotic addicts deprived of drugs may present to emergency departments with complaints of withdrawal or, more likely, with specific somatic problems.

The appearance of drug craving precedes by 4 to 24 hours any objective signs of withdrawal. Only the stigmata of chronic IV opiate use may be present at this time. Subsequently, withdrawal signs occur in predictable and progressive stages over a time course determined by the duration of action of the opiate. Attempts to grade the severity of abstinence minimize the overlapping of stages, however the abstinence syndrome is usually progressive.

Grade 0 occurs within 2 to 6 hours after withdrawal of a short-acting narcotic and within 12 to 24 hours after long-acting narcotics are withdrawn. Craving and anxiety are the only symptoms and there are no specific signs.

Grade I occurs within 4 to 12 hours after withdrawal of a short-acting narcotic and after 24 to 48 hours without long-acting opiates. The patient feels irritable and may appear to be in a light, restless sleep ("yen sleep"). Yawning, lacrimation, rhinorrhea, and diaphoresis may be seen with elevations of pulse and blood pressure.

Grade II occurs 8 to 16 hours after withdrawal of short-acting and 48 to 72 hours after withdrawal of long-acting opiates. The patient is restless, nauseated, and suffers from insomnia and myalgias. Mydriasis, piloerection, tremors, and further elevation of vital signs are seen.

Grade III occurs 14 to 36 hours after withdrawal of short-acting narcotics. Aching bones and muscles, hot and cold flashes, further progression of symptoms appearing in Grade II, and abdominal pain are characteristic. The above signs progress and hyperpyrexia may occur. Symptoms are usually milder in withdrawal from long-acting opiates.

Grade IV is now rarely seen in this country because of the low potency of street drugs. Manifestations develop 16 to 36 hours after withdrawal of short-acting opiates. The patient complains of severe abdominal cramps and diarrhea, spontaneous ejaculation or orgasm, and vomiting. There may be marked weight loss, hyperglycemia, hemoconcentration, and leukocytosis with fever.[40]

It is important to realize that opiate abstinence syndromes, although uncomfortable, are almost always benign and self-limited. Withdrawal from short-acting opiates is complete within three or four days. Abstinence from longer-acting opiates is milder, but symptoms may continue for several weeks.

Consideration should be given to the possibility of withdrawal from more than one drug and to the probability that nonopiates or weak opiates (such as propoxyphene or codeine) have been used in an attempt to ameliorate abstinence symptoms. Alcohol is a popular home remedy for opiate withdrawal. Syndromes of abstinence from alcohol or sedatives share with opiate withdrawal signs of diaphoresis, anorexia, tremor, tachycardia, hypertension, and restlessness. Seizures and delirium, however, are unique to sedatives and alcohol. Combined withdrawal and intoxication may present a confusing picture requiring observation in the hospital.

When it is difficult but important to differentiate sedative or alcohol from opiate withdrawal, a trial dose of short-acting barbiturate (e.g., 200 mg oral pentobarbital) may be helpful. This maneuver will not reverse signs of opiate abstinence, but will markedly improve sedative or alcohol withdrawal. Similarly, small doses of a short-acting opiate (e.g., 10 mg subcutaneous morphine) will improve only the signs of opiate abstinence.

Addicts may submit to invasive procedures, even laparotomy, in order to obtain narcotics, so it is important that the abstinence syndrome be recognized. Other conditions in the differential diagnosis are viral respiratory and GI syndromes, tetanus, endocarditis, osteomyelitis, diabetic ketoacidosis, and abdominal conditions of surgical importance. Control of opiate abstinence syndromes should be with an oral medication, preferably methadone. Small, frequent doses (5 mg orally every hour until signs of abstinence resolve) allow close approximation to the patient's needs. If the parenteral route is unavoidable half to two-thirds the oral dose should be given IM.[10] Since an adequate dose of oral methadone can usually be delivered in a volume of less than 10 cc, parenteral methadone is rarely necessary, even in preoperative patients.

The decision to treat opiate abstinence syndromes is a difficult one, but if treatment is undertaken it should be with the aim of admitting the patient for detoxification or stabilization for transfer to definitive therapy. It is illegal for a practitioner or hospital to undertake maintenance therapy of drug addiction on an outpatient basis. Specialized facilities prepared to treat opiate addiction with methadone and/or psychotherapy offer the best hope for improvement. Referral thus becomes an important function of the emergency department treatment of opiate withdrawal. Aggressive intervention by social workers, counselors, or nurses skilled in interviewing techniques is more likely to result in adequate follow-up than is referral by the emergency physician. Close cooperation between social service and emergency department staffs is necessary for a functioning referral system.

Complications of Chronic Opiate Abuse

Lungs

Pulmonary complications of chronic opiate abuse include bronchiectasis and pneumonia, which may be related to recurrent episodes of pulmonary edema or to infection resulting from chronically depressed cough. Granulomatosis from talc or cotton particles may be a cause of pulmonary hypertension and cor pulmonale. Acute pulmonary angiitis may be associated with IV injection of oral preparations. There is some indication that chronic regional ventilation-perfusion mismatch as well as pulmonary function abnormalities may be partly due to the toxicity of heroin itself. Fever and multiple pulmonary infiltrates suggests tricuspid or (more rarely) pulmonic valve endocarditis.[41]

Liver

Hepatic disease, acute and chronic, is closely associated with heroin abuse. Transaminase elevations are demonstrable in up to 75 percent of addicts, however the nature of the pathology is a subject of controversy. Some investigators have found viral and chronic persistent or active hepatitis to be the predominant lesions, while others have observed alcoholic hepatitis on biopsy in the majority of patients.[42,43]

Methadone maintenance does not influence the prevalence or extent of hypertransaminasemia.[44] The prevalence of hepatitis surface B antigen positivity among asymptomatic heroin addicts appears to be between 10 and 40 percent.[42]

Kidneys

Renal disease may be secondary or primary. Secondary renal pathology includes that related to hepatitis, septicemia, endocarditis, and myoglobinuria. The existence of a primary heroin-induced glomerulopathy has been debated. Several reports of focal glomerular sclerosis, often progressing to end-stage renal disease, have been published. One large study suggested that glomerular sclerosis was 40 times more common among addicts than nonaddicted, age-matched controls. Blacks appeared to be at particular risk.[45] Other authors have found no predominant lesion in addicts with renal disease.[46]

Immunology

Immunologic abnormalities include a false-positive VDRL (20 to 30 percent of heroin addicts),[47] hypermacroglobulinemia, increases in titers of antibody to smooth muscle and to lymphocytes, and chronic eosinophilia.[48] Splenomegaly is common, as is increased susceptibility to infection, especially tuberculosis, pneumonia, cellulitis, endocarditis, and osteomyelitis. Recently several cases have been reported of unusual and severe opportunistic infections in drug abusers found to have markedly abnormal cellular immunity. *Pseudomonas* osteomyelitis is almost uniquely an addict's disease. The vertebrae are characteristically affected, and the illness may present blandly as back pain in an addict apparently simulating pathology to obtain narcotics.[49]

"Cotton fever" is an acute febrile illness lasting less than 24 hours that follows IV injection of cotton fibers. It is especially likely to occur in addicts who are boiling cotton filters to release trapped heroin.[50]

Eyes

Ophthalmologic complications include irreversible macular ischemia from talc emboli and quinine amblyopia. For some reason, the latter is rare in heroin addicts.[51]

Heart

Cardiac damage from heroin has recently been suggested.[52] Myofibrillar changes suggestive of toxic and anoxic damage may help explain sporadic reports of cardiomyopathies in heroin addicts.

The leading cardiac complication, however, is endocarditis. The tricuspid valve is most often involved. Murmurs may not be appreciated, and septic emboli may be the most prominent feature. By far the commonest organism is *Staphylococcus*, which is reliably cultured from venous blood even when the right side of the heart is involved. *Streptococcus viridans* is rare, and exotic organisms may be found. The dictum remains a good one that fever in a parenteral drug abuser is endocarditis until proved otherwise.[41]

Treatment of endocarditis does not require opiate withdrawal. Indeed, signs of opiate abstinence such as tachycardia and fever may be confused with those of continuing infection. Methadone does not interfere with the activity of antibiotics and vice versa. An exception is rifampin, which may accelerate methadone metabolism. Interaction between other opiates and antibiotics has not been reported.[53,54]

Blood

Hematologic abnormalities include thrombocytopenia and eosinophilia. Quinine-induced thrombocytopenia is well recognized (and not always associated with recoverable antibody), but recently a syndrome of thrombocytopenia apparently associated with brown heroin has been reported. The syndrome lasts a few days and responds to steroids.[55]

Nervous System

Neurological complications are diverse. A syndrome of delayed postanoxic encephalopathy has been reported following overdose.[34] Poisoning may also be accompanied by stroke without evidence of embolism. The etiology of such focal deficits is uncertain, but necrotizing cerebral angiitis (seen in stimulant abusers) is not the mechanism.

Acute transverse myelitis and a variety of peripheral nerve disorders (which may occur remote from injection sites) have been documented. Peripheral neuropathies have a predilection for the radial nerve and brachial plexus.[56]

Seizures are not a feature of opiate withdrawal or intoxication; however phenytoin may accelerate methadone metabolism and produce symptoms and signs of opiate abstinence syndrome.

Endocrine

Endocrine sequelae of narcotic abuse are recent findings. In males, methadone (and to a lesser extent heroin) lowers serum testosterone, sperm motility, and libido. Loss of libido is dose related. Gynecomastia is a possibly related finding. In females, secondary amenorrhea may be present in both heroin and methadone users, probably due to interference with hypothalamic releasing factors. Higher doses of methadone may cause a loss of libido in women.[57,58]

Edema, which is occasionally seen as a methadone side-effect, may in part be due to opiate augmentation of vasopressin release or function, but other factors are probably involved.

Thyroid function is normal, but total thyroxin levels may be elevated due to increases in thyroid binding globulin. A similar elevation has been noted in ceruloplasmin levels.[59]

Surgery

Surgical complications generally concern the extremities and abdomen. Acute embolic obstruction of a peripheral artery or intense vasospasm from intra-arterial injection may require prompt intervention. Mycotic aneurysms and arteriovenous fistulas are also seen. "Skin popping" can result in a necrotizing fasciitis requiring extensive debridement. The external appearance of these lesions may resemble that of simple cellulitis, but pain is usually disproportionate. Aggressive incisional biopsy and visual inspection of subcutaneous tissue should be employed if cellulitis is extensive or fever high.[60] Multilocular abscesses and ulcers are common. Recurrent cellulitis may cause contractures. Tetanus is an occasional complication of parenteral drug abuse which is included here because of the need for debridement as a primary mode of therapy.

An important condition with surgical implications is pseudobowel obstruction. This condition presents with distention, pain, obstructive bowel sounds, and dilated small bowel with air-fluid levels on roentgenograms. The obstruction is relieved by abstinence from narcotics, not surgery.[61]

Obstetrics and Gynecology

Obstetric and gynecologic manifestations of drug abuse include secondary amenorrhea, pelvic inflammatory disease, unwanted pregnancy, and syphilis. The first results from a direct toxic effect of opiates, and the others from the high rate of prostitution among addicts. Rectal and pharyngeal gonorrhea may be more common in both males and females.

It is unclear whether pregnant narcotic addicts who withdraw during the first trimester are at risk for spontaneous abortion. In the second and third trimesters, however, even slow withdrawal has been associated with fetal distress, elevated amniotic amines, and miscarriage.[62] Women who are maintained on low (20-mg) doses of methadone throughout their pregnancies appear to give birth to more mature infants of higher birthweight who do not usually undergo significant withdrawal.[63]

Women addicted to methadone have about twice the rate of obstetric complications as age-matched nonaddicted controls.[64] Meconium staining, anemia, premature rupture of membranes, abruptio placentae, placenta previa, and multiple births are among the more common complications.

Studies of chromosome breakages are conflicting and difficult to interpret [65,66] but there is no evidence that methadone or heroin predisposes to birth defects.

Mental Health

Psychiatric complications are common. Narcotic addicts coming into treatment today appear to be older, less educated, and more heavily involved with a number of drugs than addicts of several years ago. Arrests tend to predate drug involvement, and the extent and nature of associated psychopathology is a cause for concern.[5] Although opiate use was recently found to be unrelated to affective or cognitive disorders (unlike sedative and stimulant use),[67] other studies have found a high incidence of depression among opiate addicts.[68]

Psychological testing suggests no personality trait common among opiate abusers, and that psychopathology of all types occurs. Addicts withdrawing from opiates may be at increased risk of acute anxiety attacks, since plasma methadone levels appear to correlate roughly with anxiety.[69] Acute exacerbation of underlying psychopathology is often seen during withdrawal. Psychotic, manic, depressive, or neurotic manifestations may bring the patient to treatment.

In treating depressed opiate addicts it should be realized that monoamine oxidase inhibitors may potentiate the effects of some opiates by blocking nonspecific oxidases involved in narcotic metabolism.[70]

STIMULANTS

Cocaine, methyphenidate, and amphetamine derivatives are compounds that produce cortical arousal, anorexia, and sympathetic stimulation in a predictable, dose-related fashion. The user experiences a sense of energy, alertness, and euphoria that is variously described as feelings of omnipotence, excitation, or calm. Among these compounds cocaine has achieved popularity with the middle class in recent years, possibly because the drug is shorter acting and thought to induce less tolerance, milder withdrawal, and minimal toxicity. Each substance has its adherents, but users expressing a preference have difficulty in distinguishing their favorite from other drugs of the same type.

Much is known and hypothesized about the biochemical actions of stimulants on the nervous system. Both augmentation of central norepinephrine and an effect on dopamine receptors appear to be involved in the stimulating and psychotomimetic actions of these drugs.[71] A complete discussion is beyond the scope of this chapter.

Pharmacology

Amphetamine

Amphetamine ("speed," "uppers," "street whites") bears a close structural resemblance to norepinephrine. It is a white, water-soluble powder which may be injected IV, taken orally, or absorbed from mucosal surfaces. Peak plasma levels occur within two hours after oral ingestion, and the highest concentrations are found in the brain, lung, and kidney.[72]

Amphetamine is both metabolized in the liver and excreted unchanged by the kidney. It is not known whether the metabolites are centrally active, however formation of a false neurotransmitter may be partly responsible for the marked tolerance that develops to peripheral adrenergic effects. Plasma half-life varies from 8 to 30 hours depending upon the pH of the urine, and amphetamine may be found in alkaline urine up to a week following a large dose.[73]

Tolerance to the central and peripheral effects is considerable. Chronic users may use 10 to 20 times the usual starting dose. Withdrawal occurs within days of abstinence, and although physical signs are few there is a predictable period of lethargy, abnormal sleep patterns, and, often, craving for sedatives. During this period, which may persist for several months, patients frequently suffer from a depression that responds poorly to tricyclic antidepressants and may be complicated by suicide attempts.

Methamphetamine ("crystal") has more marked central effects than its parent compound. It is available illegally as a white powder and by prescription as 2.5-, 5.0-, 10.0-, 15.0-, and 20.0-mg capsules. Amphetamine is available in dosage forms from 5 to 30 mg. "Street whites" are illegally purchased tablets that often contain caffeine or ephedrine rather than amphetamine.

Cocaine

Cocaine ("coke," "blow," "snow") is a soluble white powder derived by hydroxylation and benzoylation from the coca leaf. Cocaine is a topical anesthetic and CNS stimulant. It may be inhaled, injected IV, or the fumes inhaled ("free based"). Intramuscular or subcutaneous injection is painful. Ingested cocaine is absorbed slowly but to the same extent as inhaled. Absorption is from the duodenum.[74] Massive ingestions by users swallowing bags of cocaine to avoid arrest have resulted in death.[75]

Effects are almost immediate by any route other than oral, and there appears to be concentration in the CNS after IV injection. Plasma half-life is about one hour, and effects usually last one or two hours. Cocaine is metabolized by esterases in the blood and liver. Excretion is not importantly dependent upon urine pH.[74]

Tolerance to the effects of cocaine may be considerable and is said to be lost only after a long period. Withdrawal is less marked than for amphetamines but similar in type. Cocaine is produced commercially in small quantities. Most street cocaine, however, is illegally imported from South America. Before sale, cocaine is usually diluted with other, noncentrally active, local anesthetics and with cornstarch or baking soda. Concomitant use of IV opiates and cocaine ("speed ball") is common. References to cocaine as a narcotic, however, are pharmacologically inaccurate and based on a legislative curiosity.[76]

Methylphenidate

Methylphenidate (Ritalin) is an amphetamine derivative used in the treatment of pediatric hyperkinesis, narcolepsy, and occasionally depression. Parenteral abuse is commonest among IV narcotic users. Oral abuse has also been reported. Methylphenidate is completely absorbed after ingestion, with peak levels in about two hours. The half-life of the parent compound is only one to two hours, but metabolites are apparently psychoactive and have half-lives of about seven hours. Subjective effects may last as long as 12 hours. The drug is deesterified in the liver, and the products are excreted by the kidneys. Methylphenidate is available as 5-, 10-, and 20-mg tablets.[77]

Overdose and Intoxication

Because of the development of tolerance, the size of an acute stimulant dose gives only a rough guide to the expected toxicity. Plasma levels are prognostically unreliable for the same reason. Stimulant intoxication presents as euphoria and talkativeness, hyperadrenergic signs, and occasionally as hallucinations.

On examination the patient is oriented. Typically there is mydriasis, increased blood pressure and pulse, tremor, and hyperreflexia. Mucous membranes are dry and there may be either pallor or flushing. Grinding of the teeth may be seen. The local anesthetic effect of cocaine on the pharynx may induce sniffing or repeated swallowing.

Symptoms of mild overdose include dizziness, headache, irritability, and tremulousness. After more serious overdoses symptoms may include chest pains and palpitations, nausea, and vomiting. Psychiatric symptoms may be prominent, with hallucinations in any sensory modality. Paranoid delusions, a hallmark of chronic stimulant abuse, may be present. Short- and long-term memory are intact and the response of these patients to the disturbing content of their hallucinations is more often one of concern than is the case in schizophrenia.[78] The precipitation of acute paranoid schizophrenia by stimulant abuse is a well-described event and must be differentiated from a toxic, and therefore transient, psychosis.[71]

Severe overdose is manifested by ventricular arrhythmias, convulsions, severe hypertension with the risk of intracranial hemorrhage, and hyperthermia. Extreme hyperpyrexia may cause a consumptive coagulopathy and acute tubular necrosis from myoglobinuria.[79,80]

The differential diagnosis of stimulant intoxication or overdose includes chronic paranoid schizophrenia, manic depression (manic phase), panic states, stimulant precipitated nontoxic schizophrenia, hyperthyroid crisis, pheochromocytoma, and other drug ingestions (principally hallucinogens). History and urine testing are the best methods of making the diagnosis. Signs of chronic abuse such as needle tracks (see the discussion of signs of parenteral abuse of narcotics, above), extreme weight loss, and stereotypic movements such as picking at the skin may be helpful clues. When the diagnosis of stimulant overdose is made, consideration should be given to the possibility that other substances, especially narcotics, may also be present.

The laboratory work-up of moderate to severe overdose should include baseline electrolytes, renal and liver function tests, clotting parameters, and urine analysis for cells, myoglobin (in the presence of high fever), and drugs. The laboratory should be notified that amphetamine is specifically being sought. An ECG and thyroid function tests may also be helpful.

Treatment of mild overdose consists of withdrawal of the stimulant (tapering is not necessary) and sedation if required. Butyrophenones, chlorpromazine, diazepam, and propranolol have all been advocated as the preferred sedative. The first two have been shown to increase the resistance of mice to fatal doses of amphetamine[81] and hold the theoretical advantage of acting on dopamine receptors, where psychotic effects are thought to originate. Hyperpyrexia and hypertension may also be responsive to these drugs. At effective doses, chlorpromazine (but not haloperidol) increases the half-life of amphetamine in rats.[82] There are, however, major species differences in amphetamine metabolism.[83] Both drugs lower seizure thresholds and, by their nonspecific antipsychotic action, may make the differentiation between drug induced and drug precipitated psychosis more difficult.

Diazepam has been advocated as providing sedation without lowering seizure thresholds or obscuring the distinction between functional and toxic psychosis.[71]

Propranolol has been reported to lower anxiety and arouse stuporous patients from overdoses of cocaine while reversing the cardiopressor response.[84] Propranolol does not increase the resistance of mice[81] or dogs[85] to fatal doses of amphetamine, and its use is open to the objection that unopposed α-adrenergic stimulation may, in the presence of propranolol, raise blood pressure dangerously.

A reasonable course might be to use diazepam (1 mg/minute IV until calm) for anxiety reactions, droperidol (2.5 mg/minute IV until control is effected),[86] or chlorpromazine (25 mg IM every hour until control is effected) for treatment of psychotic manifestations, and to reserve propranolol for the treatment of arrhythmias. The physician using propranolol should be prepared to treat a hypertensive reaction.

If the patient is seen within four hours of ingestion, an attempt at gastric lavage or (preferably) ipecac-induced emesis should be made. Charcoal and a saline cathartic should be used when emesis ceases.

In severe overdose, supportive and corrective treatment of temperature elevation, hypertension, hypotension, oliguria, and arrhythmia probably requires admission to an intensive care unit, continuous monitoring, and access to the central venous circulation. If urine output is adequate, acidification of the urine is advisable. Drug recovery may be increased by a factor of 10 to 20 in acid urine.[87] Urine flow is not so important in drug elimination, but a moderate diuresis (200 to 300 ml/hour) may help prevent ATN in the hyperpyrexic patient.

Ammonium chloride, 2.75 mEq/kg orally or IV (slowly) should be given every six hours as needed to maintain the urine pH below 6.0. Ascorbic acid, 1 to 2 gm IV over six hours, may be used in addition if needed. It is important to exclude phenobarbital and salicylate as contributory to the clinical state before urinary acidification is attempted, as clearance of these drugs may be markedly decreased in acid urine.

Hemodialysis effectively removes amphetamines in the anuric or clinically deteriorating patient.[87] Data on the efficacy of resin or charcoal hemoperfusion are lacking.

Hypertension not responding to sedation may be treated with an alpha antagonist (5 mg phentolamine IV), nitroprusside, or diazoxide. Hypotension in advanced overdose is probably best treated with a directly acting adrenergic drug such as dopamine rather than with agents which release endogenous catecholamines. Ventricular arrhythmias, seizures, and hyperpyrexia respond to the usual measures.

Complications of Chronic Stimulant Abuse

Medical complications of prolonged stimulant abuse include local and systemic sequelae of IV narcotic use already discussed, with a particular liability to abscess and phlebitis. Damage to and perforation of the nasal septum has been reported following chronic cocaine inhalation.[88,89]

A dose-related effect of chronic stimulant administration on brain microvasculature has been demonstrated in animals[90] and suspected in humans.[91] Necrotizing cerebral angiitis, cerebrovascular accident, and microaneurysms after chronic parenteral and oral stimulant abuse have been reported. Cornstarch emboli have been identified in the retinas of cocaine abusers. Cardiomyopathy may also be a consequence of stimulant abuse.

Amphetamines and methylphenidate appear to prolong the actions of tricyclic antidepressants, anticonvulsants, and anticoagulants, probably by interfering with their metabolism. Several reports have suggested that lithium-treated patients fail to experience the cocaine "high." Neither the mechanism of this effect nor the implication for treatment of cocaine abuse has been elaborated.[92]

Mental Health

Psychiatric complications of stimulant abuse include psychosis and sedative addiction. The psychosis of chronic stimulant abuse is likely to be delusional, paranoid, and accompanied by stereotypic behavior. Tactile hallucinations of bugs under the skin often accompany characteristic picking movements.[78] As previously mentioned, orientation, memory, and insight are usually well preserved and insight is better than in paranoid schizophrenia.

Visual hallucinations in chronic cocaine abusers may be similar to migrainous auras, with flashes of light or geometric shapes. They may also be organized and complex.

The depression that accompanies withdrawal of stimulants appears more likely to occur following abuse of amphetamine than of cocaine or methylphenidate. Symptoms may be severe, long lasting, and complicated by suicide attempts and sedative addiction. Response to antidepressants is often disappointing.

Obstetrics

Obstetric complications such as toxemia and premature rupture of membranes are not as common in stimulant abusers as in narcotic abusers. Case reports have linked maternal amphetamine abuse with cardiovascular and CNS malformations in the child. Neonatal withdrawal may be characterized by agitation or, more often, depression. Seizures may also occur in this variable syndrome which lasts several days. There is some evidence that narcotic abuse in the mother confers protection against hyperbilirubinemia in the infant; amphetamine abuse does not do so.[93]

Surgery

Surgical complications include local lesions related to parenteral stimulant use and poisoning after large ingestions of packaged stimulants. Packages should probably be recovered by laparotomy rather than by endoscopy, emesis, or waiting for them to pass.[75]

INHALANTS

The use of organic solvents as euphoric agents became widespread in the 1960s among teenagers; more recently alkyl nitrites have gained popularity. Both types of compounds are inexpensive and sold legally. Pharmacologic tolerance to these substances may or may not occur; however no specific withdrawal syndromes apart from craving have been described. Because of their lipid solubility and the route of administration, most of these drugs act quickly and briefly. Some, however, have active metabolites that are eliminated only after several days.

Solvents are usually sniffed directly from their containers, from a saturated rag, or from a plastic or paper bag. Nitrites are available in cotton-wrapped ampules designed to be crushed. The use of heat to raise vapor pressure and of large bowls to increase dispersion has been reported. Oral and parenteral use is rare but often rapidly fatal. Most inhaled solvents are mixtures of several substances.

The emergency presentation of inhalant abuse is likely to involve toxic effects related to chronic use or complications of acute intoxication rather than overdose or withdrawal. Some common inhalants are given below, however virtually any lipid soluble substance with a high vapor pressure has psychoactive properties.

Toluene is found in household, plastic, and model cements, in lacquer thinner, and in gasoline.

Hexane and other aliphatic hydrocarbons are present in gasoline and in some industrial solvents.

Fluorocarbons such as carbon tetrachloride, dihydrodifluoromethane, and trichlorofluemethane are constituents of aerosols, refrigerants, and cleaning fluids.

Acetone is present in fingernail polish, cements, and paint remover.

Naphtha is found in lighter fluids and in cleaning solutions.

Nitrites are not solvents or psychoactive compounds. Central effects depend upon their cardiovascular actions. Nitrites, principally amyl and isobutyl, are often sold under the guise of room deodorants to avoid drug laws. Ampules of 0.18 and 0.30 ml are also available.

Overdose and Intoxication

Intoxication with solvents resembles alcohol inebriation. Initially euphoria, dizziness, and auditory or visual hallucinations are typical. The patient may be observed to sneeze or cough, vomit, and avoid bright light. Flushing is common, but pupillary response is inconsistent. In the second stage tinnitus, confusion, diplopia, or blurred vision are prominent. The patient may appear pale and disoriented. In the third stage there is further mental clouding. Nystagmus, ataxia, slurred speech, and diminished reflexes appear. Inhalant intoxication is distinguished from alcohol intoxication by the characteristic odors, the rapidity with which stages evolve, and the presence of hallucinations.[94]

Acute delirium is best treated supportively with fresh air, and avoidance of excessive stimulation on one hand and of ambiguous stimuli (such as darkened rooms or whispering) on the other. The patient should not be left alone, but sedatives are rarely needed.

A prolonged toxic psychosis has been reported in association with cerebellar damage in chronic toluene abusers.[95] Chronic gasoline sniffing may present with delirium lasting several weeks and accompanied by choreiform movements.[96] Prolonged delirium has also been reported after chronic trichloroethylene exposure.[97]

Inhalant intoxication occasionally presents as suffocation or sudden death. Tightly fitting masks or bags may render the patient quickly unconscious with the device still in place. Trichloroethylene and fluorinated refrigerants were the substances most often implicated in over a hundred sudden deaths from inhalant abuse between 1960 and 1970.[98] The association of stress or strenuous activity with sudden death suggests that solvents may sensitize the heart to the arrhythmogenic action of catecholamines. Resuscitative efforts should therefore minimize the use of adrenergic drugs.

Nitrite intoxication causes vasodilation with a fall in blood pressure and pooling of blood in dependent parts. The drug is popular among homosexuals because of its action in relaxing the anal sphincter. Intoxication is rapid and consists of light-headedness, an intensification of sounds, and occasionally a throbbing headache. Nitrites also have a reputation as an aphrodisiac. Signs include flushing, fainting, and hypotension. Patients with cardiovascular disease that may become decompensated by drastic changes in venous return or systemic blood pressure are at risk from nitrite use.

A dose-related response to nitrites is the formation of methemoglobin. The mechanism by which a strong reducing agent effects this oxidation is obscure. Methemoglobin levels may be 20 percent after recreational inhalation, and much higher following oral ingestion. Infants and patients with anemia or heart disease are at particular risk for hypoxemia. The occasional patient with hemoglobinopathy or familial deficiency in hemoglobin reductase is also at risk.[99]

Cyanosis unresponsive to oxygen in a patient without pulmonary or cardiac disease suggests methemoglobinemia. Treatment, however, should be reserved for stuporous or comatose patients, since spontaneous reduction of methemoglobin occurs within one to three days. Methylene blue, 1 to 2 mg/kg given IV over five minutes as a 1 percent solution, is the treatment of choice. A second dose of 2 mg/kg may be given after an hour if needed, but the total dose should not exceed 7 mg/kg. The aim is to improve tissue oxygenation, not to abolish cyanosis, which may be present at low levels of methemoglobin.[100]

Complications of Chronic Inhalant Abuse

It is uncertain whether solvents have a predictable effect on cognition or on the EEG after chronic use. Certainly they have such an effect in some individuals.[101] Cerebellar and cerebral atrophy, vascular lesions of the basal ganglia, and prolonged psychosis have been reported.[102] Hexane apparently is unique in causing a peripheral and cranial neuropathy in some patients.[103]

Toluene, trichloroethylene, and carbon tetrachloride have been reported to produce hepatitis, pancreatitis, and renal tubular lesions after chronic use. The hepatitis, which may occur alone, is centrilobular and may progress to fibrosis. Renal involvement may also be solitary. It presents as acute tubular necrosis, renal tubular acidosis (distal) without osteomalacia or nephrocalcinosis, or as proteinuria. Alcohol use may sensitize the liver to solvent toxicity by facilitating entry to the hepatocyte or competing for metabolic enzymes.[104–107]

Lactic acidosis is a recognized complication of toluene inhalation.[108] Aplastic anemia and myeloid metaplasia have occurred after chronic sniffing of hydrocarbons, principally benzene. The risk may be greater in those with sickle cell disease.

Contaminants or additives may also cause complications. Lead toxicity is a recognized consequence of gasoline inhalation.[109] Metal fragments in fluorocarbons have caused pulmonary fibrosis.[110]

The effects of inhalant use on pregnancy are unknown.

HALLUCINOGENS

Hallucinogens form a chemically heterogeneous group of substances which predictably alter perceptions of sense, data, and time, produce illusions and hallucinations, and impair reality testing. They also share with other psychoactive compounds the ability to alter mood, thought, and behavior. Examples of hallucinogens are synthetic ergot alkaloids such as lysergic acid diethylamide (LSD), phenylalkylamines like mescaline, and indolealkylamines such as dimethyltryptamine (DMT) and psilocybin. Marijuana and phencyclidine, the two hallucinogens of greatest importance in the emergency department, in fact produce hallucinations only rarely.[111]

There has been a steady scientific interest in hallucinogens as models for and treatments of schizophrenia and as useful agents in the study of neurotransmission and hormonal organization in the brain. At the same time, there has been a rapid decline in the recreational popularity of these substances. The two exceptions to the generally waning interest in hallucinogens are phencyclidine and marijuana.

Marijuana appears to have found a permanent place in many segments of American society as a mild euphoriant of recreational use and occasional abuse. The ubiquitous presence of phencyclidine in street drugs sold under various more exotic names seems to be more a result of the drug's potency and ease of manufacture than any real public demand. Phencyclidine, marijuana, and, as a representative of other hallucinogens, LSD will be discussed.

Phencyclidine

Phencyclidine is the principal constituent of many substances sold illegally as LSD, THC (tetrahydrocannabinol, the major active compound in marijuana and hashish), psilocybin, mescaline, and peyote. It is also sold as "PCP" (PeaCe Pill), "Tic," "Tac," "animal (or hog or monkey) tranquilizer," "pig killer," "T," "peace," "CJ," "JK," "supergrass," or "rocket fuel." Originally used as a short-acting dissociative anesthetic, phencyclidine was dropped because of dysphoric effects on emergence from anesthesia. Ketamine (Ketalar) is a derivative used in veterinary practices.

In pure form, phencyclidine is a glistening white powder, soluble in water and alcohol. Street samples may be sold as an off-white powder, in tablets of various colors, as a liquid, or sprinkled on joints of marijuana or parsley. Phencyclidine may be smoked, inhaled, ingested, or occasionally injected IV.

Phencyclidine is an analgesic with sympathomimetic, anticholinergic, and CNS stimulant and depressant properties. It is rapidly absorbed by any route, is lipid soluble, and may undergo reexcretion into the stomach and bile. The volume of distribution is unknown, but the presence of high levels in CSF and RBCs and the persistence of effects after clearance from the blood suggest that the drug is not bound to plasma proteins and may be concentrated in the brain. Plasma levels above 100 μg/liter are associated with severe poisoning, and effects tend to be dose and level related. Half-life after low to moderate doses is about one hour, and the major hydroxy metabolite does not appear to be active.[112]

At variance with the excretion half-life, the duration of phencyclidine's effects may be prolonged. Coma after high doses may persist for 12 hours and psychosis for several days.[113] Moderate tolerance to chronic use occurs in animals, but species differences are considerable. There is no known withdrawal syndrome. In overdose the presence of a toxic by-product of synthesis may cause bloody diarrhea and vomiting.[112]

Overdose and Intoxication

Most authors consider doses above 10 mg as likely to produce serious intoxication. Doses of 100 to 200 mg have caused death.[113] Phencyclidine's psychiatric effects appear to be more closely dose related than is the case for other hallucinogens.

Symptoms of intoxication begin within minutes to several hours after acute dosing but psychiatric symptoms may have an insidious onset in chronic abuse. Low-dose intoxication produces euphoria, lability of mood, concreteness of thought, confusion, and distortions in body image. True hallucinations are unusual. With increasing doses marked anxiety, hyperacusis, hostility, depersonalization, and ultimately a cataleptic or stuporous state (characteristically with the eyes open) are seen.[114]

Physical signs are characteristic. Low doses usually produce hypertension and an increase in respiratory rate and depth. At higher doses hypotension may occur, but hyperpnea usually persists until coma is advanced or convulsions supervene.

Hyperreflexia and muscular rigidity are common even in coma. Pharyngeal reflexes may be increased, making endotracheal intubation difficult. Corneal reflexes, however, are usually depressed and ptosis may be seen. Purposeless movements, grimacing and sucking, ataxia, or catatonia may occur. Diminished pain perception is characteristic. Pupils may be constricted or in midposition, but light reflexes are decreased. Marked horizontal and vertical nystagmus occur on testing after low doses and in the primary position after higher doses. Hypersalivation and diaphoresis occur occasionally.

After serious overdoses, arrhythmias and shock result in part from the drug's direct myocardial action. Hyperpyrexia is sometimes present, and together with muscular rigidity it may contribute to the rhabdomyolysis with myoglobinuric renal failure which is sometimes seen.[115]

Low-dose manifestations may be distinguished from other hallucinogen intoxications by the absence of hallucinations or dilated pupils and by the presence of ataxia and nystagmus. Differentiation of moderate overdoses from sedative poisoning is facilitated by the presence of hypertension, hyperpyrexia, and hyperpnea. Some nonbarbiturate sedatives may, however, also cause hypertension. High-dose intoxication with phencyclidine may be difficult to distinguish from other causes of coma with convulsions. A history of any hallucinogen use in an agitated or mute patient should suggest phencyclidine intoxication.

Laboratory work-up should include urine drug screening and plasma levels. The drug may also be present in high concentration in vomitus or gastric aspirate. In advanced overdose, cardiac monitoring, renal function tests and urinalysis, and close observation of temperature are essential.

Treatment of mild overdose consists of sensory deprivation and diazepam, if needed. "Talking down"

probably has no place in phencyclidine intoxication. Optimal therapy consists of a darkened, quiet room with the patient on a pad on the floor and unobtrusive observation. Ear plugs have been used in noisy emergency departments. Phenothiazines may produce hypotension, intensify anticholinergic manifestations, and increase the risk of seizures. The decision to remove phencyclidine from the GI tract or to attempt enhancement of renal elimination depends upon balancing the risks of stimulation with the benefits of considerably improved elimination of the drug.

As a basic amine with a pKa between 8 and 9, phencyclidine reaches higher concentration in acid than alkaline urine. The extent of this ion trapping is unclear. Some authors claim a 200-fold increase in phencyclidine when the urine pH is below 5,[116] others a 20-fold increase,[117] and one study failed to find a correlation between urine acidity and concentration of drug.[118] It seems likely, however, that acidification can importantly increase excretion (see amphetamine, above, for methods of acidification). Claims that lowering blood pH promotes exit of phencyclidine from the brain await confirmation.[117] Attempts to lower blood pH are likely to require large volumes of fluid and, in a patient with respiratory alkalosis from hyperpnea, to complicate management of acid-base status. It is important to exclude phenobarbital and salicylate as contributory to the clinical state before urinary acidification is attempted, as clearance of these drugs may be markedly decreased.

Phencyclidine has a diuretic action at low concentrations but may cause oliguria at higher. A brisk (200 to 300 ml/hour) diuresis may help prevent tubular necrosis and increase elimination slightly. At higher urine volumes acidification may become difficult.

Because of a proposed gastric secretion of phencyclidine, continuous nasogastric suction has also been used, with clearances reportedly approaching that of urinary acidification.[117]

Treatment of severe overdose necessitates removal of the drug and may require therapy for seizures, hypertension, hyperpyrexia, arrhythmia, and rhabdomyolysis. Seizures and opisthotonus should be treated with diazepam. Hypertension appears to be caused by α-adrenergic properties of phencyclidine and may respond best to phentolamine (5.0 mg IV) or to diazoxide or nitroprusside. Hyperpyrexia should be vigorously treated with the usual means. Hypotension may be a result of direct myocardial toxicity. If a pressor is used, one that acts directly rather than by releasing endogenous catecholamines is probably preferable. Response to adrenergic agents may, however, be increased by phencyclidine. Respiratory distress requires intubation, which should be performed by an experienced practitioner prepared to encounter pharyngeal spasm and an increased gag reflex. Phencyclidine has been found to inhibit pseudocholinesterase and may therefore prolong the action of succinyl choline given in the course of surgery or to facilitate intubation.[114]

In the clinically deteriorating patient hemodialysis and hemoperfusion should be considered, although there is no great experience with them.

Severe psychiatric reactions to phencyclidine may require hospitalization for several days, however physiologic effects of the drug usually clear within 12 to 24 hours.

Complications of Chronic Phencyclidine Abuse

The insidious development of psychosis that may persist for several weeks is a rare complication of chronic phencyclidine abuse. Few of the chronic abusers who develop psychosis have a history of psychiatric disorders, but poor ego strength and inadequate adjustment to family, work, and school appear to be common. Unlike LSD-precipitated psychosis, the illness is accompanied by neurologic disturbances (chiefly nystagmus), severity is dose related, and resolution follows a predictable course. Phenothiazines and haloperidol appear to be effective.[119]

Marijuana

Marijuana ("pot," "dope," "grass," "smoke," "tea") describes the desiccated leaves and flowers of the plant *Cannabis sativa*. The compressed resin of the plant is hashish, which is more potent and, in this country, less common. Cannabis refers inclusively to marijuana and hashish.

The principal psychoactive constituent of cannabis is δ-9-tetrahydrocannabinol (THC), which is difficult to synthesize and therefore rarely obtainable illegally. Phencyclidine is frequently sold as THC. Marijuana is about 2 to 20 percent THC, and hashish 15 to 20 percent.[120]

Cannabis may be smoked in "joints" or ingested. After smoking, effects begin within a few minutes and last for an hour or two. When ingested, cannabis produces effects within one hour that may last for six. Ingested cannabis is absorbed about one-third as well as smoked, but effects appear to occur at lower plasma concentration.[121]

Inhaled THC is about 20 percent absorbed, extensively bound to plasma proteins, partly metabolized by the liver and lung to psychoactive metabolites, and excreted as inactive metabolites in the urine and bile. Cessation of the drug's effects are due to redistribution, mainly into fat, and not to metabolism. The half-life of THC is long (one to two and a half days), and metab-

olites can be detected in the urine for as long as a week.[122] Metabolic tolerance in the form of a slightly shorter half-life occurs in experienced users, but no typical withdrawal syndrome has been convincingly described. Cannabis has been extensively studied because of the enormous popularity of the drug. Derivatives of THC appear to hold great promise as antiemetics[123] and may have a place in the treatment of glaucoma.[124]

Unlike phencyclidine, cannabis produces CNS effects that depend a good deal on the user's expectation and experience. Effects are also much milder and more brief. Overdose is rare despite wide variations in the potency of cannabis. The emergency physician may encounter acute intoxication as an incidental finding or in the inexperienced user. Medical complications in the chronic user and (rarely) poisoning after parenteral use of cannabis may also present to the emergency department. In patients with cardiovascular disease, intoxication can produce decompensation by inhibiting sympathetic reflexes and raising the concentration of circulating catecholamines.[125]

Overdose and Intoxication

After one or two joints (50 to 1,500 mg of marijuana or 5 to 150 mg of THC), cannabis typically produces euphoria, suggestibility, relaxation, appetite stimulation, hilarity, and subtle changes in visual and auditory perceptions. Sedation and dysphoria are alternative reactions in some users. After larger doses confusion, paranoid ideation, and depersonalization may emerge, particularly in the inexperienced. Toxic psychosis has been reported.[126]

On examination, the mildly intoxicated patient may be talkative and gregarious or withdrawn and anxious, depending often on the perceived threat of the environment. There is usually mild tachycardia, dry and injected conjunctivae, and occasionally a mild tremor. The pupil size is not consistent. With more marked intoxication, postural changes in blood pressure, paranoid behavior, ataxia, confusion, and (rarely) hallucinations may be seen.

Intravenous injection of cannabis infusion represents an exception to the generally benign presentation of intoxication. Onset of symptoms is immediate, with throbbing headache, weakness, chills, abdominal pain, vomiting, myalgias, and weakness. These symptoms may persist for several days. On examination tachycardia, hypotension that may be extreme, and fever are found. Hyporeflexia and muscle weakness are characteristic, but the sensorium is usually clear. Hypoglycemia, thrombocytopenia, cardiac injury, hepatitis, pancreatitis, and transient renal failure may all complicate the course.[127]

Treatment of cannabis toxicity depends on symptoms. The mildly intoxicated, anxious patient needs only friendly, but not condescending, reassurance. Small oral doses of diazepam or a short-acting barbiturate may be used if necessary in the moderately intoxicated patient. Parenteral overdoses are likely to require intensive care. Attention to volume repletion, treatment of cardiac arrhythmias, maintenance of adequate blood sugar, and attention to renal function, hemostasis, and body temperature form the bases of therapy. The prognosis is good.

There are no data on hemodialysis or hemoperfusion in parenteral cannabis poisoning, but in the deteriorating patient charcoal or resin hemoperfusion may be more effective than dialysis in removing important quantities of a lipophilic drug like THC.

Complications of Chronic Cannabis Abuse

Although cannabis causes bronchodilation after a single inhaled dose, chronic use of five or more joints per day has been shown to increase airway resistance.[128,129] Gynecomastia and oligospermia are recognized complications of chronic high-dose cannabis use, probably as a result of both hypothalamic and testicular actions of the drug.[29] Early reports of cerebral atrophy in chronic users have been discounted, but there is some evidence of a contribution by marijuana to cases of pubertal arrest.[130]

The effects of cannabis on pregnancy and the fetus are unknown, and laboratory evidence of genetic damage has neither been confirmed nor correlated with birth defects in humans.[131]

Government attempts to destroy *Cannabis sativa* plants have included spraying with paraquat and other herbicides. Paraquat is concentrated in the lung, where it can produce pulmonary fibrosis with severe respiratory insufficiency. Patients in whom paraquat poisoning occurs should be treated promptly and vigorously.[132] Dysphoric reactions to cannabis, however, are unlikely to be due to contamination with herbicide.

Lysergic Acid Diethylamide

Lysergic acid diethylamide (LSD, "acid") is an amine alkaloid with predominantly central effects. It inhibits serotoninergic neurons in the midbrain, which in turn produces a stimulation of limbic and visual areas of the forebrain. A second, dopaminergic, action of LSD may modulate the intensity of these effects and possibly accounts for the extraordinary potency of the drug. It is active after oral doses of 0.5 to 1.0 µg/kg.[133]

LSD is well absorbed and reaches peak plasma levels about an hour after ingestion. It may also be injected parenterally. Clinical effects are maximal after two to five hours. The half-life is known to be about three hours, but investigations of the products and routes of elimination are conflicting. Clinical effects usually last about 12 hours. Street LSD is sold as tablets or capsules, on blotting paper, or in sugar. It is often diluted with phencyclidine, amphetamine, and strychnine.

Tolerance to the hallucinogenic properties of LSD occurs very rapidly, possibly with the first dose. Patients tolerant to LSD are also tolerant to mescaline and psilocybin. There is no known withdrawal syndrome, and tolerance is rapidly lost.[134]

Overdose and Intoxication

LSD produces perceptual, cognitive, affective, and somatic changes in a roughly dose-related fashion. Perceptual changes include intensification of colors and sounds, visual hallucinations, disturbances in the appreciation of time, and synesthesia (a substitution of sensory modalities or a blending of different modalities in response to stimuli). Cognitive effects include depersonalization, suggestibility, and problems with logical thought and reality testing. Affective disturbances consist of marked swings in mood from euphoria to panic. Somatic sensations may include dizziness, weakness, nausea, tremor, and blurred vision. Attempts have been made to distinguish psychedelic from psychotomimetic actions of LSD based on serotonin and dopamine activities and the differential development of tolerance to hallucinations and psychosis.

On examination the intoxicated patient shows signs of centrally mediated sympathetic activity, vasoconstriction, and poverty of expression or loose associations. There may be diffuse muscle weakness and mild hyperthermia. Creatinine clearance is slightly diminished. The EEG shows generalized arousal.

Emergency presentation of LSD abuse is likely to involve dysphoric reactions. Such reactions include "bad trips," toxic psychosis, LSD-precipitated psychosis, and "flashbacks." Distinguishing among these entities is often impossible on presentation, and the diagnosis is commonly retrospective. A bad trip is a panic state occurring during intoxication and characterized by frightening hallucinations, feelings of losing control, fear that the effects are permanent, and loss of insight in the presence of a clear sensorium. Bad trips occur in the novice or in the chronic user whose previous experiences may have been pleasant.

Unlike a bad trip, toxic LSD psychosis more typically presents with auditory hallucinations in the absence of panic. These reactions appear to be more common in chronic users, in those with preexisting personality disturbance, and among patients taking LSD in stressful surroundings. Psychotic reactions appear to be more common with LSD than mescaline. The psychosis subsides within 24 hours.[135]

It is unclear whether LSD-precipitated psychosis represents an idiosyncratic reaction or the unmasking of a previously subclinical schizophrenia. These reactions are uncommon but may be prolonged when they occur. They are indistinguishable at the outset from toxic psychoses.

"Flashbacks" are spontaneous recurrences, usually during times of stress, of previous LSD experiences. They are more commonly dysphoric than pleasurable and may last several hours. Recurrences for several months are not uncommon.

Treatment of bad trips consists of sensory deprivation and reassurance ("talking down") combined with orientation. If necessary, oral doses of diazepam or phenothiazines may be used. Psychotic reactions, both toxic and drug-precipitated, respond to phenothiazines. Flashbacks usually do not require treatment apart from reassurance.

Complications of Chronic LSD Abuse

Apart from an increased risk of psychotic reactions, chronic LSD abuse has few reported medical complications. LSD is chemically similar to ergot constituents and acts as a mild vasoconstrictor. In patients with peripheral vascular disease or cardiomyopathy, chronic use may lead to decompensation.

Possible genetic effects of LSD have been extensively investigated. Although *in vitro* concentrations of 100 μg/ml are clearly toxic to mammalian cells, the results of animal studies are as various as their methods.[136] Reports of malformations in the infants of LSD-abusing mothers have not been confirmed in systematic studies.[137] LSD appears to be less mutagenic than many substances widely regarded as safe.

SEDATIVES

Sedative-hypnotic drugs, although chemically heterogeneous, produce similar clinical effects, degrees of tolerance, and withdrawal syndromes. Most are anticonvulsants and antispasmodics and have similar effects on the EEG. Moreover, one sedative abolishes the withdrawal syndrome caused by abstinence from others (the phenomenon of cross tolerance). Because of these similarities, sedatives are conveniently discussed as a group. It should, however, be realized that important differences exist among these drugs in their toxic manifestations and liability to abuse.

Sedatives are more commonly obtained by prescription than from illegal factories, and more commonly taken orally than parenterally. The emergency presentation is therefore less likely to involve problems caused by diluents, contaminants, and local or systemic complications of parenteral injection.

Sedative abusers are frequently abusers of other drugs as well. They may also be using sedatives to offset withdrawal symptoms from other drugs, particularly stimulants. The "disinhibition euphoria" produced by sedatives may be sought by the addict to counteract a severe underlying depression.

Pharmacology

Barbiturates

Barbiturates are not such common drugs of abuse as they were a decade ago. They have to some extent been replaced by ethchlorvinyl (Placidyl), glutethimide (Doriden), methaqualone (Quaalude, Sopor), and benzodiazepines, chiefly diazepam (Valium).[138]

Barbiturates may be short-, intermediate-, or long-acting, but abuse is usually limited to intermediate-acting compounds. The most common of these are secobarbital (Seconal), pentobarbital (Nembutal), amobarbital (with secobarbital as Tuinal), and butalbital (Fiorinal and others).

These drugs are bitter white powders, soluble in hot water and alcohol, which are completely absorbed within four hours from the GI tract and distributed throughout the body water. Barbiturates of this type are little bound to plasma proteins. They are metabolized by the liver to inactive compounds that are excreted in the urine. Excretion is not importantly enhanced by alteration of urine pH, unlike the excretion of phenobarbital and other long-acting barbiturates. The half-life of intermediate-acting barbiturates is 12 to 40 hours, but duration of effect depends greatly on redistribution within the body. In new users sleep lasts six to eight hours after usual doses, but an effect on performance of complex tasks may be demonstrated for up to 24 hours. After four to six weeks of daily use there is little hypnotic effect.[139]

Tolerance develops both acutely and chronically. In acute overdose, patients may emerge from coma at plasma levels of drug that would otherwise render them unconscious. Tolerance to chronic dosing develops over weeks of daily use, but is less pronounced than for opiates. The induction of hepatic microsomal enzymes (which may also influence metabolism of many other drugs) is partly responsible for tolerance. Tolerance to a lethal dose, however, does not develop to the same extent as tolerance to an intoxicating dose (i.e., the "therapeutic window" narrows). Tablet or capsule strengths are usually 30 to 200 mg. Butalbital is produced as 50-mg doses in combination tablets.

Benzodiazepines

Benzodiazepines are an ever expanding group of antianxiety and hypnotic compounds that also act on synapses in the spinal cord to reduce muscle tone. These drugs are very commonly prescribed because of their safety in overdose and low liability to produce addiction. Like barbiturates, benzodiazepines may be short- or long-acting. Short-acting compounds include oxazepam (Serax) and lorazepam (Ativan). Long-acting benzodiazepines include diazepam (Valium), chlordiazepoxide (Librium), chlorazepate (Tranxene), and fluorazepam (Dalmane). All these compounds produce similar actions although some are said to be more effective as hypnotics. Idiosyncratic "rage reactions" have been reported to occur following use of all the major benzodiazepines except oxazepam.

Prolonged duration of action depends upon hepatic metabolism to an active product. Short-acting compounds are metabolized to inactive glucuronides which are excreted in the urine. They have half-lives of 8 to 12 hours. Long-acting compounds form desmethyl derivatives and have long half-lives which increase linearly with age and are importantly prolonged by liver disease.[140–141] They range from 30 to over 100 hours.

Benzodiazepines are completely absorbed, although with variable rapidity, by the oral route. Intramuscular absorption is erratic. These drugs are almost entirely bound to plasma proteins and attach to specific receptors in the CNS. Benzodiazepines do not induce hepatic enzymes. Tablet strengths vary from 2 mg (lorazepam) to 30 mg (chlordiazepoxide). Combination tablets with antidepressants are also available.

Methaqualone

Methaqualone (Quaalude, Sopor) has gained popularity because of its reputation for causing intoxication without drowsiness and for acting as an aphrodisiac. Like barbiturates, methaqualone is a sedative, a hypnotic, and an anticonvulsant. It is also an antitussive and may enhance opiate analgesia. Methaqualone is a lipophilic white powder, soluble in alcohol but not water, which is completely absorbed within two hours and distributed in a large volume. There is a considerable binding to tissues. The drug is metabolized by microsomal liver enzymes (which it stimulates) to compounds that are probably inactive and are excreted in urine and bile. Plasma half-life is about 19 hours, but because of redistribution in the body, sleep lasts five to six hours after usual doses. Tolerance is moderate. Methaqualone is available as 150-mg and 300-mg tablets.[142]

Glutethimide

Glutethimide (Doriden) is a sedative with some antiemetic properties. It is poorly water soluble and absorbed erratically by the oral route. Highly variable peak plasma levels are attained after one to six hours. Binding to plasma proteins is minimal, and the drug is distributed largely in fat. Metabolism is hepatic, with formation of inactive products and a 4-hydroxy metabolite that appears to contribute to the toxicity of glutethimide.[143] Half-life is about 12 hours, but may be longer in overdose. Redistribution, however, is largely responsible for termination of hypnosis after four to eight hours in new users at usual doses.

Moderate tolerance develops to the effects of glutethimide. Signs of toxicity and withdrawal may resemble each other (seizures and tremors), and signs of spontaneous withdrawal without a change in drug intake may occur in chronic users. This phenomenon may be due to fluctuating plasma levels associated with erratic absorption or to toxicity of the active metabolite.[144] Glutethimide markedly stimulates hepatic enzymes. Glutethimide is available as 250- and 500-mg tablets and 500-mg capsules.

Methyprylon

Methyprylon (Noludar) is chemically related to glutethimide but more water soluble and possibly better absorbed. The pharmacology of this sedative has not been well described, but it is liver metabolized, with a variable half-life of two to seven hours. Methyprylon stimulates microsomal enzymes. Methyprylon is available as 50- and 200-mg tablets and as 300-mg capsules.[145]

Ethchlorvinyl

Ethchlorvinyl (Placidyl) is an anticonvulsant and sedative-hypnotic that is rapidly absorbed (maximum plasma levels in about an hour). Clinical effects are brief after usual doses—probably because of rapid redistribution—and half-life is five to six hours due to rapid hepatic metabolism. In overdose, ethchlorvinyl may have a half-life of over 100 hours, however, and coma may be prolonged.[146] Induction of hepatic enzymes does not appear to occur.

The packaging of ethchlorvinyl as a liquid-filled gelatin capsule facilitates parenteral use. Intravenous doses of 1.5 gm have caused serious poisoning. Moderate tolerance occurs, and prolonged psychosis has been reported after abstinence. Ethchlorvinyl comes as 100-, 200-, 500-, and 750-mg capsules.

Meprobamate

Meprobamate (Miltown and others) is a commonly prescribed sedative that also occurs in combination with anticholinergics, antianginal compounds, and estrogens. The drug is well absorbed within four hours in usual doses but may form gastric concretions in overdose. Rate of absorption also depends on the formulation.[147] Meprobamate is liver metabolized to inactive products and induces microsomal enzymes. Half-life is about 11 hours after usual doses. Meprobamate comes as 200-mg and 400-mg tablets and capsules.

Chloral Hydrate

Chloral hydrate (Noctec and others) is often considered a mild soporific, but it can produce marked tolerance and a withdrawal syndrome resembling delirium tremens. In overdose, cardiac arrhythmias, renal failure, jaundice, GI bleeding, and respiratory depression occur.[148,149] Chloral hydrate is rapidly absorbed and converted to the active trichloroethanol. This compound is metabolized by the liver with a half-life of about eight hours. Trichloroethanol both stimulates hepatic microsomal enzymes and displaces many drugs from plasma proteins. Chloral hydrate is available as a liquid containing 50 to 160 mg/ml, in capsules containing 250 mg or 500 mg, and as rectal suppositories containing 300 to 900 mg.

Bromides

Bromides (Elixsed, Nervine, and others) are far less commonly abused now than a decade ago. Bromide salts are rapidly absorbed but only very slowly excreted by the kidneys (half-life, 400 hours). Excretion is markedly enhanced by diuretics and salt loading. Neither tolerance nor a withdrawal syndrome appears to occur. Intoxication often presents with irritability, emotional changes, and occasionally with hallucinations. An acneiform or bullous skin eruption occurs in 25 percent of users. The laboratory finding of increased serum chloride (caused by instrumental interference) should suggest bromism in an intoxicated patient.[150]

Overdose and Intoxication

Sedative intoxication resembles alcohol inebriation and presents as either euphoria or CNS depression. Glutethimide intoxication may also cause seizures.[143] As noted above, sedative overdose presenting as coma requires consideration of other metabolic and systemic processes that produce coma. Some sedatives produce characteristic signs in overdose. Alcohol intoxication is usually apparent from the characteristic odor, but sedatives and alcohol act synergistically and are often taken together. Apparently trivial sedative overdoses may be serious in the presence of alcohol, and, conversely, signs of grave sedative poisoning may improve as unsuspected alcohol is metabolized.

All sedatives produce CNS depression in overdose; however, nonbarbiturate sedatives characteristically cause less respiratory depression and more marked cardiovascular effects than barbiturates. Prolonged coma is associated with ethchlorvinyl[151] and glutethimide.[152] Signs of hypertonicity and extrapyramidal manifestations suggest methaqualone toxicity.[153] A fluctuating coma may be present after overdose with long-acting barbiturates, but is also characteristic of glutethimide poisoning and meprobamate overdose with a gastric drug mass.[154,155] Cardiac arrhythmias in the absence of circulatory compromise should suggest chloral hydrate (ectopy)[148] or ethchlorvinyl (bradycardia).[146] Signs of severe gastric irritation may be present after alcohol and chloral hydrate ingestion. Pulmonary edema is particularly a feature of ethchlorvinyl[156] and meprobamate[157] poisoning. Dermal bullae suggest barbiturates, acneiform facial eruptions occur with bromide intoxication, and dermographism has been reported after glutethimide.

Benzodiazepines do not usually produce profound coma except after massive doses or mixed ingestions.[158] The presence of deep coma or cardiovascular instability with a history of benzodiazepine ingestion should prompt a search for additional drugs.

The decision to attempt removal of ingested drug from the stomach depends on the history and clinical state of the patient. Virtually any alert patient relating a history of sedative overdose should be given ipecac followed by charcoal and a saline cathartic when emesis ceases. Gastric lavage in the unconscious patient is more problematic. With the exceptions of glutethimide and meprobamate, sedatives are absorbed within four to six hours, and biliary or gastric recycling is not a feature of their metabolism. When respiration is adequate and the gag reflex is intact, there is probably little to be gained by endotracheal intubation solely for the purpose of lavage. If lavage is performed, samples of stomach contents should be sent both for qualitative (diagnosis) and quantitative (presence of a drug mass) analysis.

There are reports based on a small number of observations that physostigmine reverses coma caused by diazepam and presumably other benzodiazepines.[159] The benign course of pure benzodiazepine overdose and reports of cardiac arrhythmia after physostigmine reversal of diazepam-induced coma militate against the use of physostigmine in this setting.

Treatment of a serious overdose includes attention to respiration, fluid balance, body temperature, liver and renal function, and cardiac rhythm. Periods of apnea should be anticipated in severe barbiturate and glutethimide overdose and may occur when the glutethimide-intoxicated patient is apparently improving. Permanent improvement must in general be differentiated from a fluctuating course.

Although a moderate diuresis (200 to 300 ml/hour) may help prevent ATN, no data support forced diuresis or pH manipulation in the treatment of toxicity from any of these drugs except bromide. Large volumes of fluid may also be dangerous in overdoses associated with the development of pulmonary edema.

Determination of serial drug plasma levels is prognostically useful, may reveal continuing absorption of the drug, and can help with the decision to use hemodialysis or hemoperfusion.

Most sedatives are more efficiently removed from plasma by charcoal or resin hemoperfusion than by hemodialysis.[160] Hemodialysis is preferred for bromide intoxication and when uremia, acid-base disturbance, or electrolyte problems complicate poisoning. In general, drugs with large volumes of distribution are not present in clinically important amounts in the plasma and are therefore only slowly removed by these methods.

With good supportive care and anticipation of likely complications, even serious poisonings usually do not require hemoperfusion or dialysis.[161] Clinically deteriorating patients in whom a drug mass has been ruled out may benefit from these techniques.

Abstinence Syndromes

Severe barbiturate withdrawal syndrome resembles delirium tremens but occurs over a longer period. Abstinence syndromes may occur after abrupt withdrawal of intermediate-acting barbiturates taken in daily doses exceeding 400 to 800 mg. Characteristically, the patient seems to improve for 12 to 16 hours as signs of intoxication resolve. Apprehension and weakness then gradually appear. Insomnia, abdominal pain, nausea, and vomiting occur by 24 hours, and weight loss may ultimately be marked. Tachycardia and hypertension are characteristic. Seizures occur in a large number of barbiturate addicts taking more than a gram daily. The seizures may be multiple and appear at any time during the first five days. Seizures are most common, however, between the first and second days. Clonic and athetoid movements are also seen and the EEG may be abnormal for two weeks.

Onset of delirium usually follows the appearance of seizures, occurring between the third and seventh days. Both auditory and (more commonly) visual hallucinations may be present, and patients usually become disoriented. Psychotic manifestations may abate within three or four days, but may also be prolonged for several weeks.[162]

Abstinence from nonbarbiturate sedatives causes identical signs and symptoms; their onset and duration is a function of the duration of action of the drug. Minimal daily drug use sufficient for the development of abstinence syndromes is not clearly established. Meprobamate causes marked withdrawal in the majority of patients using 3 to 6 gm for longer than six weeks and in some patients taking 2 to 2.5 gm daily for nine months. Glutethimide can do this after doses of 2.5 gm daily for three months. Ethchlorvinyl has produced seizures after chronic use of 2 gm per day. Methyprylon has caused seizures and deaths after chronic doses of 5 to 12 gm daily. Lower doses of these drugs produce milder syndromes of abstinence.[138]

There has been considerable controversy over the liability of benzodiazepines to produce tolerance and withdrawal syndromes. After high doses (100 to 600 mg/day of chlordiazepoxide or 120 mg/day of diazepam) for several weeks, withdrawal seizures and psychosis are common.[163] They do not occur until several days to a week after abstinence. There are a few case reports of sometimes bizarre withdrawal reactions (including coma) after prolonged use of benzodiazepines at apparently therapeutic doses.[164] In systematic, properly controlled studies it appears that a withdrawal syndrome consisting of anxiety, anorexia, faintness, and trembling can occur following abstinence from therapeutic doses of chlordiazepoxide (15 mg three times a day) given for periods longer than four to six months.[165] Short-acting benzodiazepines may be more likely to cause such syndromes.[166]

Like delirium tremens, sedative withdrawal is easier to prevent than to treat. In advanced withdrawal, the use of phenothiazines and butyrophenones such as Haldol can cause impairment of thermoregulation and seizures.[167] Phenytoin is not effective in the treatment of sedative withdrawal seizures.[168]

Barbiturates are probably the best choice for prophylaxis and treatment. In established withdrawal, intermediate-acting barbiturates should be given in small doses (200 mg) but at frequent intervals (every hour) until the patient is calm but not oversedated. When oral therapy is impossible the IM route may be used.[169]

The prevention of sedative abstinence syndromes depends upon an estimate of the patient's chronic daily drug use. History is often unreliable, and challenge with oral pentobarbital is a safe method of quantitating daily sedative requirement; 200 mg is given orally every hour until signs of intoxication occur (ataxia, nystagmus, dysarthria, somnolence). The total dose given may then be used as an estimate of the patient's daily barbiturate needs. Detoxification should proceed either by tapering the dose of pentobarbital (given on a thrice daily schedule) or, preferably, by transferring the patient to phenobarbital.[170]

Phenobarbital has a long half-life (48 to 96 hours in the adult) and a wide margin of safety.[171] It has been found to substitute reliably for pentobarbital. Phenobarbital at 30 mg for each 100 mg of pentobarbital required during challenge testing should be given daily in divided doses. After three or four days, tapering can begin at a rate of 10 percent per day.

Single-dose prophylaxis using phenobarbital at 0.03 mg/kg/minute IV in addicts with mild withdrawal represents an alternative method.[172] The infusion is continued until signs of mild intoxication appear. The advantages of such single-dose treatment, however, appear to be outweighed by the risk of withdrawal seizures in patients with unusually short phenobarbital half-lives. The technique of daily oral phenobarbital based on pentobarbital challenge appears to be the safest method.

Complications of Chronic Sedative Abuse

Chronic intoxication with barbiturates occurs at doses of 1 to 4 gm/day. Unlike opiate addicts, sedative abusers maintain an almost constant state of intoxication. The user becomes confused, unkempt, infantile in behavior, emotionally labile, and often depressed.[162] Suicide attempts are not uncommon. Hallucinosis is not a regular feature of chronic intoxication, and patients usually remain oriented to time and place. Prolonged abuse is associated with psychotic depression.

Medical complications of sedative addiction include trauma and burns due to chronic intoxication, local and systemic lesions, similar to those of narcotic addicts, due to parenteral injection, and interference with the actions of drugs that are metabolized by microsomal enzymes in the liver.

The effects of sedatives on the fetus are unknown, although malformations following maternal use of benzodiazepines and meprobamate have been reported.[173] Coagulopathy in the newborn following maternal use of barbiturates has also been noted. A neonatal withdrawal syndrome clearly occurs following prolonged (greater than three months) maternal use of diazepam in reported doses as low as 15 mg daily.[172] The syndrome resembles neonatal narcotic withdrawal but may last several weeks. Similar syndromes have been reported for other sedatives.

REFERENCES

1. Eddy N, Halbach H, Isbell H, et al: Drug dependence: Its significance and characteristics. *Psychopharmacol Bull* 3:1, 1966.
2. Collier H: Cellular site of opiate dependence. *Nature* 283:625, 1980.
3. Speth R, Bresolin N, Yamamura H: Acute diazepam administration produces rapid increases in brain benzodiazepine receptor density. *Eur J Pharmacol* 59:159, 1979.
4. Penk W, Fudge J, Robinowitz R: Personality characteristics of compulsive heroin, amphetamine, and barbiturate users. *J Consult Clin Psych* 47(3):583, 1979.
5. McClellan A, McGahan J, Druley K: Changes in drug abuse clients 1972–1978: Implications for revised treatment. *Am J Drug Alcohol Abuse* 6(2):151, 1979.
6. Brown J, Malone M: Status of drug quality in the street-drug market. *Clin Toxicol* 9(2):145, 1976.
7. Schnoll S, Vogel W: Analysis of "street drugs". *N Engl J Med* 284:791, 1971.
8. Primm B, Bath P: Pseudoheroinism. *Int J Addict* 8(2):231, 1973.
9. Way E, Young J, Kemp J: Metabolism of heroin and its pharmacologic implications. *Bull Narc* 17:25, 1965.
10. Beaver W, et al: A clinical comparison of the analgesic effects of methadone and morphine administered intramuscularly, and of orally and parenterally administered methadone. *Clin Pharmacol Ther* 8:415, 1967.
11. Verebely K, Volavka J, Mule S, et al: Methadone in man: Pharmacokinetic and excretion studies in acute and chronic dosing. *Clin Pharmacol Ther* 18(2):180, 1975.
12. Horns W, Rado M, Goldstein A: Plasma levels and symptom complaints in patients maintained on daily dosage of methadone HCl. *Clin Pharmacol Ther* 17(6):636, 1975.
13. Bellward G, et al: Methadone maintenance: Effect of urinary pH on renal clearance in chronic high and low doses. *Clin Pharmacol Ther* 22(1):92, 1977.
14. Service Research Notes. National Institute of Drug Abuse. December 1979.
15. Fraser H, Isbell H: Actions and addiction liabilities of alpha-acetyl methadols in man. *J Pharmacol Exp Ther* 105:458, 1952.
16. Jasinski D, Martin W: Assessment of the dependence-producing properties of dihydrocodeinone and codoxime. *Clin Pharmacol Ther* 8(2):266, 1966.
17. Szeto H, et al: Accumulation of normeperidine, an active metabolite of meperidine in patients with renal failure or cancer. *Ann Intern Med* 86:738, 1977.
18. Gilbert P, Martin W: The antagonism of the convulsant effects of heroin, d-propoxyphene, meperidine, normeperidine, and thebaine by naloxone in mice. *J Pharmacol Exp Ther* 192:538, 1975.
19. Tennant F: Complications of propoxyphene abuse. *Arch Intern Med* 132:191, 1973.
20. Gary N, Maher J, Demyttenaere M, et al: Acute propoxyphene hydrochloride intoxications. *Arch Intern Med* 121:453, 1968.
21. Jasinski D, Martin W, Hoeldtke R: Effects of short- and long-term administration of pentazocine in man. *Clin Pharmacol Ther* 11(3):385, 1970.
22. Burroughs W: *Junky*. New York, Penguin, 1977.
23. Greene M, Luke J, Dupont R: Acute opiate overdose: A preliminary report on mechanism of death. *Proceedings of the Fifth National Conference on Methadone Therapy*. National Association for the Prevention of Addiction to Narcotics. New York and Washington, 1973.
24. Jasinski J, Martin W, Haertzen C: The human pharmacology and abuse potential of N-allylnoroxymorphone (Naloxone). *J Pharmacol Exp Ther* 157:420, 1967.
25. Evans L, Roscoe P, Swainson C, et al: Treatment of drug overdosage with naloxone, a specific narcotic antagonist. *Lancet*: 452, 1973.
26. Sorensen S, Mattisson K: Naloxone as an antagonist in severe alcohol intoxication. *Lancet*: 688, 1978.
27. Berkowitz B: The relationship of pharmacokinetics to pharmacological activity: Morphine, methadone, and naloxone. *Clin Pharmacokinet* 1:219, 1976.
28. Ostor A: The medical complications of narcotic addiction. I. *Med J Aust* 1:410, 1977.
29. Olusi S: Hyperprolactinaemia in patients with suspected cannabis induced gynecomastia. *Lancet*: 255, 1980.
30. Cicero T, et al: Function of the male sex organs in heroin and methadone users. *N Engl J Med* 292(17):882, 1975.
31. Carlson R, Velez R, Roulin R: Pseudogynecomastia secondary to injection of heroin into breast tissue. *Arch Intern Med* 138:483, 1978.

32. Siegel H: Human pulmonary pathology associated with narcotic and other addictive drugs. *Hum Pathol* 3(1):55, 1972.

33. Raskin M: Pulmonary edema of acute overdose reaction and near drowning: some radiographic and physiologic comparisons. *South Med J* 69(8):1063, 1976.

34. Challenor Y, Brust J, Baden, M: Neurological complications of addiction to heroin. *Bull NY Acad Med* 49(1):4, 1973.

35. Mitchell A, Lovejoy F, Goldman P: Drug ingestions associated with miosis in comatose children. *J Pediatr* 89(2):303, 1976.

36. Boxer L, Anderson F, Rowe D: Comparison of ipecac-induced emesis with gastric lavage in the treatment of acute salicylate ingestion. *Pediatr Pharmacol Ther* 74(5):800, 1969.

37. Tanara G: Hypertensive reaction to naloxone. *JAMA* 288(1):25, 1974.

38. Frand U, Shim C, Williams H: Heroin induced pulmonary edema. *Ann Intern Med* 77:29, 1972.

39. Fraser H, Isbell H, Van Horn C: Effects of morphine and dia-minophenyl-thiazole (daptazole). *Anesthesiology* 18:531, 1957.

40. Goodman L, Gilman A (eds): *The Pharmacological Basis of Therapeutics,* ed 5. New York, Macmillan, 1975.

41. Reisberg B: Infective endocarditis in the narcotic addict. *Prog Cardiovasc Dis* 23(3):193, 1979.

42. Stimmel B, Vernace S, Heller E, et al: Hepatitis B antigen and antibody in former heroin addicts on methadone maintenance. Correlation with clinical and histological findings. *Proceedings of the Fifth National Conference on Methadone Treatment.* National Association for the Prevention of Addiction to Narcotics. New York and Washington, 1973, p 501.

43. Cherubin C, Rosenthal W, Stenger R, et al: Chronic liver disease in asymptomatic heroin addicts. *Ann Intern Med* 76:391, 1972.

44. Stimmel V, Vernace S, Tobias H: Hepatic function in methadone maintenance therapy. *Proceedings of the Fifth National Conference on Methadone Therapy.* New York and Washington, 1973, p 419.

45. Rao T, Nicastri A, Friedman E: Natural history of heroin associated nephropathy. *N Engl J Med* 290(1):19, 1974.

46. Tresor G, Cherubin C, Lonergan E: Renal lesions in narcotic addicts. *Am J Med* 57:687, 1974.

47. Boak R, Carpenter C, Miller J: Biologic false positive reactions for syphilis among narcotic addicts. *JAMA* 175:326, 1961.

48. Husby G, Pierce P, Williams R: Smooth muscle antibody in heroin addicts. *Ann Intern Med* 83:801, 1975.

49. Holzman R, Bishko F: Osteomyelitis in heroin addicts. *Ann Intern Med* 75:693, 1971.

50. Shragg T: "Cotton fever" in narcotic addicts. *J Am Coll Emerg Physicians* 7:279, 1978.

51. Friberg T, Gragoudos E, Regan C: Talc emboli and macular ischemia in intravenous drug abuse. *Arch Ophthalmol* 97:1089, 1979.

52. Rajs J, Falconer B: Cardiac lesions in intravenous drug addicts. *Forensic Sci Internat* 13:193, 1979.

53. Sheagren J, Barsoum I, Lin M: Methadone antimicrobial activity and interaction with antibiotics. *Antimicrob Agents Chemother* 12(6):748, 1977.

54. Kreek M, Garfield C, Gutjahr C, et al: Rifampin induced methadone withdrawal. *N Engl J Med* 294:1104, 1976.

55. Adams W, Rufo R, Talarico L, et al: Thrombocytopenia and intravenous heroin use. *Ann Intern Med* 89:207, 1978.

56. Loizou L, Boddie H: Polyradiculopathy associated with heroin abuse. *J Neurol Neurosurg Psychiatry* 41:855, 1978.

57. Cicero T, Bell R, Wiest W, et al: Function of the male sex organs in heroin and methadone users. *N Engl J Med* 292:882, 1975.

58. Crowley T, Simpson R: Methadone dose and human sexual behavior. *Int J Addict* 13(2):285, 1978.

59. Bastomsky C, Dent R, Tocis G: Elevated serum concentrations of thyroid binding globulin and ceruloplasmin in methadone-maintained patients. *Clin Biochem* 10(3):124, 1977.

60. Melluzzo P, Willsder M, Mason H, et al: Necrotizing fasciitis in narcotic addicts. *Am Surg* 42:252, 1976.

61. Geelhoed G: Surgical complications of drug abuse. *Rev Surg* 215, 1976.

62. Zuspan J: Maternal intrauterine amine alterations in the pregnant drug addict. *J Reprod Med* 20:329, 1978.

63. Ostrea E: A study of the factors that influence the severity of neonatal narcotic withdrawal. *Addict Dis* 2:187, 1975.

64. Ostrea E, Chavez C: Perinatal problems (excluding neonatal withdrawal) in maternal drug addiction: A study of 830 cases. *J Pediatr* 94:292, 1979.

65. Abrams C: Cytogenetic risks to the offspring of pregnant addicts. *Addict Dis* 2(1):63, 1975.

66. Amarose A: Chromosome aberrations in the mother and the newborn from drug addiction pregnancies. *J Reprod Med* 20:323, 1978.

67. McLellan A, Woody G, O'Brien C: Development of psychiatric illness in drug abusers. *N Engl J Med* 301:1310, 1979.

68. Khantuan E: Letter. *N Engl J Med* 302(15):809, 1980.

69. A comparison of level of anxiety, depression, and hostility with methadone plasma concentration in opioid-dependent patients receiving methadone on a maintenance dosage schedule. *Proceedings of the Fifth National Conference on Methadone Treatment.* National Association for the Prevention of Addiction to Narcotics. New York and Washington, 1973.

70. *American Pharmaceutical Association Steering Committee for the Evaluation of Drug Interactions,* ed 2. Washington, D.C., American Pharmaceutical Association, 1976, pp 142–144.

71. Wesson D, Smith D: A clinical approach to diagnosis and treatment of amphetamine abuse. *J Psychedelic Drugs* 10(4):343, 1978.

72. Sever P, Caldwell J, Dring G, et al: The metabolism of amphetamine in dependent subjects. *Eur J Clin Pharmacol* 6:177, 1973.

73. Davis J, et al: Effects of urinary pH on amphetamine metabolism. *Ann NY Acad Sci* 179:493, 1971.

74. Wilkinson P, Van Dyke C, Jatlow P, et al: Intranasal and oral cocaine kinetics. *Clin Pharmacol Ther* 27:386, 1980.

75. Suarez I, Abelardo A, Lester J: Cocaine-condom ingestion. *JAMA* 238(13):1218, 1977.

76. Harrison Act (narcotics), 26 U.S.C. §4701(1964) c.1, 38 Stat 785 (Dec. 17, 1914).

77. Bartlett M, Egger H: Disposition and metabolism of methylphenidate in dog and man. *Fed Proc* 31:537, 1972.

78. Ellinwood E: Amphetamine psychosis. *J Nerv Ment Dis* 144:273, 1967.

79. Espelin D, Done A: Amphetamine poisoning. *N Engl J Med* 278:1361, 1968.

80. Ginsberg M, Hertzman M, Schmidt-Norwara W: Amphetamine intoxication with coagulopathy, hyperthermia, and reversible renal failure. *Ann Intern Med* 73:81, 1970.

81. Davis W, Logston D, Hickenbottom J: Antagonism of acute amphetamine intoxication by haloperidol and propranolol. *Toxicol Appl Pharmacol* 29:397, 1974.

82. Lemberger, L, Witt E, Davis J, et al: The effect of haloperidol and chlorpromazine on amphetamine metabolism and amphetamine stereotype behavior in the rat. *J Pharmacol Exp Ther* 174(3):428, 1970.

83. Dring L, Smith R, Williams R: The fate of amphetamine in man and other mammals. *J Pharm Pharmacol* 18:402, 1966.

84. Rappolt R, Gay G, Inaba D: Propranolol in the treatment of cardiopressor effects of cocaine. *N Engl J Med* 295:448, 1976.

85. Catravas J, Waters I, Walz W, et al: Letter. *N Engl J Med* 297:1238, 1977.

86. Gary N, Saidi M: Methamphetamine intoxication, a speedy new treatment. *Am J Med* 64:537, 1978.

87. Gomolin I: Amphetamines. *Clin Toxicol Rev* 2(2):1, 1979.

88. Grinspoon L, Bakalar J: *Cocaine, A Drug and Its Social Evolution.* New York, Basic Books, 1976.

89. Rumbaugh C: *Cocaine and Other Stimulants.* New York, Plenum Press, 1975, p. 241.

90. Goodman S, Becker D: Intracranial hemorrhage associated with stimulant abuse. *JAMA* 212:480, 1970.

91. Rumbaugh C, Bergeron R, Fang H, et al: Cerebral angiographic changes in the drug abuse patient. *Radiology* 101:335, 1971.

92. Cronson A, Flemenbaum A: Antagonism of cocaine high by lithium. *Am J Psychiatry* 135:856, 1978.

93. Eriksson M, Larsson C., Winbladh B, et al: The influence of amphetamine addiction on pregnancy and the newborn infant. *Acta Paediatr Scand* 67:95, 1978.

94. Wyse, G: Deliberate inhalation of volatile hydrocarbons. A review. *Can Med Assoc J* 108:71, 1973.

95. Grabski, D: Toluene sniffing producing cerebellar degeneration. *Am J Psychiatry* 118:461, 1961.

96. Carroll H, Abel G: Chronic gasoline inhalation. *South Med J* 66:1429, 1973.

97. Ikeda M, et al: Excretion kinetics of urinary metabolites in a patient addicted to trichloroethylene. *Br J Ind Med* 28:203, 1971.

98. Bass M: Sudden sniffing death. *JAMA* 212(12):2075, 1970.

99. Blush not with nitrates, editorial. *Ann Intern Med* 92(5):700, 1980.

100. Smith R, Olson M: Drug induced methemoglobinemia. *Semin Hematol* 10:253, 1973.

101. Dodds J, Santostefano S: A comparison of the cognitive functioning of glue-sniffers and non-sniffers. *J Pediatr* 64(4):565, 1964.

102. *Psychiatry and Neurology* 148:110, 1964.

103. Gonzalez E, Downey J: Polyneuropathy in a glue sniffer. *Arch Phys Med Rehabil* 53:333, 1972.

104. Cornish H, Adefuin J: Ethanol potentiation of halogenated aliphatic solvent toxicity. *Am Ind Hyg Assoc J* 27:57, 1966.

105. Clearfield H: Hepatorenal toxicity from sniffing spot remover. *Am J Dig Dis* 15:851, 1970.

106. Dorden W, Chipman D: Gasoline sniffing complicated by acute carbon tetrachloride poisoning. *Arch Intern Med* 119:371, 1967.

107. Taher S, et al: Renal tubular acidosis associated with toluene sniffing. *N Engl J Med* 290:765, 1974.

108. Fishman C, Oster J: Toxic effects of toluene: A new cause of high anion gap metabolic acidosis. *JAMA* 241:1713, 1979.

109. Boeckx R, Postl B, Coodin F: Gasoline sniffing and tetraethyl lead poisoning in children. *Pediatrics* 60(2):140, 1972.

110. Smith H: Inhalation of volatile substances. *Pharm Chem Newslett* 5(2):1, 1976.

111. Davies B, Beech H: The effect of 1-arylcyclohexylamine (Sernyl) on twelve normal volunteers. *J Ment Sci* 106:912, 1960.

112. Morgan J, Solomon J: Phencyclidine: Clinical pharmacology and toxicity. *NY State J Med* 2035, 1978.

113. Burns R, et al: Phencyclidine—states of acute intoxication and fatalities. *West J Med* 123:345, 1975.

114. Showalter C, Thornton W: Clinical pharmacology of phencyclidine toxicity. *Am J Psychiatry* 134:11, 1977.

115. Cogen F, et al: Phencyclidine-associated acute rhabdomyolysis. *Ann Intern Med* 88:210, 1978.

116. Done A, et al: Pharmacokinetic observations on the treatment of phencyclidine poisoning, in Rumack B (ed): *Management of the Poisoned Patient.* Princeton, N.J., Science Press, 1977, p 79.

117. Aronow R, Done A: Phencyclidine overdose: An emerging concept of management. *J Am Coll Emerg Physicians* 7:2, 1978.

118. Bailey D: Phencyclidine abuse: Clinical findings and concentrations in biological fluids after non-fatal intoxications. *Am J Clin Pathol* 72(5):795, 1979.

119. Fauman B, et al: Psychiatric sequelae of phencyclidine abuse. *Clin Toxicol* 9(4):529, 1976.

120. Rizlin R, Gupta R, Lundberg G: Delta-9-tetrahydrocannabinol levels in street samples of marijuana and hashish: Correlation to user reactions. *Clin Toxicol* 15(1):45, 1979.

121. Ohisson A, et al: Plasma delta-9-tetrahydrocannabinol concentrations and clinical effects after oral and intravenous administration and smoking. *Clin Pharmacol Ther* 28(3):409, 1980.

122. Lemberger L, et al: Delta-9-tetrahydrocannabinol: Metabolism and disposition in long-term marijuana smokers. *Science* 173:72, 1971.

123. Sallan S, Zinberg N, Frei E: Antiemetic effect of delta-9 THC in patients receiving cancer chemotherapy. *N Engl J Med* 293(16):795, 1975.

124. Hepler R, et al: *The Pharmacology of Marijuana.* March Press, 1976, p 815.

125. Beaconsfield P, Ginsberg J, Raimsbury R: Marijuana smoking: Cardiovascular effects in man and possible mechanisms. *N Engl J Med* 287:209, 1972.

126. Weil A: Adverse reactions to marijuana—classification and suggested treatment. *N Engl J Med* 282:997, 1970.

127. Mims R, Lee J: Adverse effects of intravenous cannabis tea. *J Natl Med Assoc* 69(7):491, 1977.

128. Zwillich C, Doekel E, Hammil S, et al: The effects of smoked marijuana on metabolism and respiratory control. *Am Rev Resp Dis* 118:885, 1978.

129. Tashkin D, et al: Subacute effects of heavy marijuana smoking on pulmonary function in healthy men. *N Engl J Med* 294:125, 1976.

130. Copeland R, Underwood L, Van Wyk J: Marijuana smoking and pubertal arrest. *J Pediatr* 96(6):1097, 1980.

131. Abel E: Prenatal exposure to cannabis: A critical review of effects on growth, development, and behavior. *Behav Neural Biol* 29(2):137, 1980.

132. Paraquat poisoning, persevere, editorial. *Emerg Med* 185, 1976.

133. Jacobs B, Trulson M: Mechanisms of action of LSD. *Am Sci* 67:396, 1979.

134. Sullivan A, et al: The fate of LSD in the body: Forensic considerations. *J Forensic Sci Soc* 18:89, 1978.

135. Hollister L, *Handbook of Psychopharmacology.* New York, Plenum Press, 1978, p 389.

136. Cohen M, Shiloh Y: Genetic toxicology of LSD 25. *Mutat Res* 47:183, 1977.

137. McGlothlin W, Sparkes R, Arnold D: Effect of LSD on human pregnancy. *JAMA* 212:1483, 1970.

138. Essig C: Newer sedative drugs that can cause states of intoxication and dependence of the barbiturate type. *JAMA* 196:714, 1966.

139. Goodman L, Gilman A (eds): *The Pharmacological Basis of Therapeutics,* ed. 5. New York, Macmillan, 1975.

140. Choice of benzodiazepines. *Med Lett* 23:41, 1981.

141. Klotz U, et al: The effects of age and liver disease on the disposition and elimination of diazepam in adult man. *J Clin Invest* 55:347, 1974.

142. Nayak R, et al: Methaqualone pharmacokinetics after single and multiple dose administration in man. *J. Pharmacokinet Biopharm* 2:107, 1974.

143. Curry S. et al: Disposition of glutethemide in man. *Clin Pharmacol Ther* 12:849, 1971.

144. Hansen A, et al: Glutethemide poisoning. *N Engl J Med* 202:250, 1975.

145. Randell L, Ilieu V, Brandman O: Metabolism of methyprylon. *Arch Int Pharmacodynam* 106:388, 1956.

146. Teehan B, et al: Acute ethchlorvinyl intoxication. *Ann Intern Med* 72:875, 1970.

147. Heyman J, Krumholz W, Merlis S: The influence of different pharmaceutical preparations of meprobamate on the rate of absorption in humans. *Curr Ther Res* 4:416, 1962.

148. Gustafson A, Svensson S, Ugander L: Cardiac arrhythmias in chloral hydrate poisoning. *Acta Med Scand* 201:227, 1977.

149. Marshall E, Owens A: Absorption, excretion and metabolic fate of chloral hydrate and trichloroethanol. *Bull Johns Hopkins Hosp* 95:1, 1954.

150. Wenk R, et al: Serum chloride analysis, bromide detection, and diagnosis of bromism. *Am J Clin Pathol* 66:49, 1976.

151. Schultz J, Crowder D, Medart W: Excretion studies in ethchlorvinyl intoxication. *Arch Intern Med* 117:409, 1966.

152. Maher J, Schreiner G, Westervelt F: Acute glutethimide intoxication. *Am J Med* 33:70, 1962.

153. Aboud R, et al: Methaqualone poisoning with muscular hyperactivity necessitating the use of curare. *Chest* 65:204, 1974.

154. Decker W, Thompson H, Aneson L: Glutethimide rebound. *Lancet* 1:778, 1970.

155. Allen M, Greenblatt D, Noel B: Meprobamate overdosage: A growing problem. *Clin Toxicol* 11:501, 1977.

156. Glauser F, et al: Ethchlorvinyl-induced pulmonary edema. *Ann Intern Med* 84:46, 1976.

157. Schwarz H: Acute meprobamate poisoning with gastrotomy and removal of a drug containing mass. *N Engl J Med* 295:1177, 1976.

158. Greenblatt D, et al: Acute overdosage with benzodiazepines. *Clin Pharmacol Ther* 21:497, 1976.

159. Larson G, Hulbert B, Wingrad D: Physostigmine reversal of diazepam induced depression. *Anesth Analg* 56:348, 1977.

160. Winchester J, et al: Dialysis and hemoperfusion of poisoning and drugs—update. *Trans Am Soc Artif Intern Org* 23:762, 1977.

161. Rosenbaum J, et al: Resin hemoperfusion for acute drug intoxication. *Arch Intern Med* 136:263, 1976.

162. Isbell H, et al: Chronic barbiturate intoxication, an experimental study. *Arch Neurol Psychiatry* 64:1, 1950.

163. Hollister L, Motzenbecker P, Degan R: Withdrawal reactions from chlordiazepoxide. *Psychopharmacolgia* 2:63, 1961.

164. DeBard M: Diazepam withdrawal syndrome, a case with psychosis, seizures and coma. *Am J Psychiatry* 136:104, 1979.

165. Covi L, et al: Length of treatment with anxiolytic sedatives and response to their sudden withdrawal. *Acta Psychiatr Scand* 49:51, 1973.

166. Tyrer P, Rutherford D, Huggett T: Benzodiazepine withdrawal symptoms and propranolol. *Lancet* 520, 1981.

167. Greenblatt D, et al: Fatal hyperthermia following haloperidol therapy of sedative-hypnotic withdrawal. *J Clin Psychiatry* 39:673, 1978.

168. Okamoto M, Rosenberg H, Boisse N: Evaluation of anticonvulsants in barbiturate withdrawal. *J Pharmacol Exp Ther* 200:479, 197.

169. Wikler A: Diagnosis and treatment of drug dependence of the barbiturate type. *Am J Psychiatry* 125:758, 1968.

170. Smith D, Wesson D: Phenobarbital technique for treatment of barbiturate dependence. *Arch Gen Psychiatry* 24:56, 1971.

171. Waddell W, Butler T: The distribution and excretion of phenobarbital. *J Clin Invest* 36:1217, 1957.

172. Martin P, et al: Intravenous phenobarbital therapy in barbiturate and other hypnosedative withdrawal reactions: A kinetic approach. *Coin Pharmacol Ther* 26:256, 1979.

173. Rementeria J, Bhatt K: Withdtrawal symptoms in neonates from intrauterine exposure to diazepam. *J. Pediatr* 90:123, 1977.

36. Alcohol Abuse

WILLIAM D. CLARK, M.D.

Mr. A is a 38-year-old man who comes to the emergency department for a cough. The examining physician notes the odor of alcohol, a tremor, and a degree of hyperactivity. Mr. B, aged 43, comes to the emergency department for an ankle sprain sustained during a fall on the stairs to his cellar. The examining physician orders a blood alcohol level, which is 275 mg/dl. Miss C is a 27-year-old nurse in the respiratory intensive care unit at another hospital, who is brought in for an overdose of diazepam. Questioning reveals that this is a suicide attempt and that she has been confused and depressed over the past several months, regularly drinking heavily. Mr. D, a skid row man, visits the emergency department daily for unclear reasons. He is loud, inconsiderate, conniving, scruffy, and generally a nuisance. Professor E presents with a classical perforated peptic ulcer. While he is being prepared for surgery, he confides to the nurse that his wife's drinking has been the center of a family conflict. The couple has been engaged in an escalating cycle of sadomasochistic behavior which is interrupted only by his attacks of abdominal pain.

Alcoholism prevalence is high, affecting 5 to 10 percent of adults, depending on geography and the criteria used for definition of illness.[1] Mortality figures dramatize the human toll: the four leading causes of death among 25- to 44-year-old white men are accidents, homicide, suicide, and cirrhosis of the liver (among blacks hypertension is fourth and cirrhosis fifth). Each of these problems has been shown to be directly related to alcoholism.[2] In addition, alcohol-related illnesses account for a large number of visits to all emergency departments,[3] and 10 percent of all U.S. deaths may be related to alcohol.[4]

The word alcoholic evokes a certain personal image for each health professional based on past experiences and the media. The image is often negative, derived from training experiences in settings where the only alcoholic patients are those for whom treatment has been unsuccessful. Those who recover do not live on skid row, or mindlessly haunt emergency department waiting rooms late at night, or consume countless resources while suffering from pancreatitis, delirium tremens, and pneumonia. With the continuing barrage of problems related to alcohol seen in emergency departments, it is no surprise that personnel are discouraged and hostile when confronted with the next inebriate. In this day of holistic approaches to medical care everyone knows that care-givers' attitudes affect patients. How can one develop positive attitudes regarding alcoholism? Why are senior alcoholism clinicians so warm with patients, so helpful, and so hopeful?

Surely all care-givers begin with positive attitudes and want the best for patients with whom they have contact. Unfortunately, the negative training experiences as well as the absence of effective teaching about alcoholism in professional schools conspire to destroy these basic helpful inclinations. Without strong support and supervision, every care-giver eventually participates in the "no-win" games that are an essential element of the behavior of alcoholic patients. This chapter covers some basic conceptual material about the nature of the alcoholic process; the pharmacology of alcohol; the processes of tolerance and addiction; and complications. With this pathophysiologic background a rational framework for management of people with alcoholism is developed, discussing the specific situations faced by the patients described in the initial paragraph.

Making the diagnosis of alcoholism in difficult cases is not the point of this chapter but physicians must agree on the basics. Sharing an understanding of the common elements of the disease process will help physicians look beyond the obvious socioeconomic variables and give good treatment to all patients; the skid row alcoholic deserves no better or worse treatment than the alcoholic psychiatrist.

People with alcoholism arrive in emergency departments with a wide variety of problems. Emergency management of typical discrete complications of alcoholism such as pneumonia and other infections, trauma, bleeding, and so on, is discussed elsewhere in this book. However, in the cases cited above, appropriate management should include early attention to alcoholism itself. Specific problems addressed in this chapter include the following: metabolism and effects of alcohol, management of alcohol intoxication and overdose, the withdrawal syndromes, patients who are unexpectedly discovered to need attention for alcoholism, people who come for crisis counseling, and screening medical exams ("clearance").

THE DISEASE CONCEPT

The fundamental lesion in alcoholism is a repetitive but inconsistent and sometimes unpredictable loss of control of drinking which produces symptoms of serious dysfunction or disability, frequently including physical addiction. The afflicted person usually denies the presence of the illness for prolonged periods. Since Jellinek wrote *The Disease Concept of Alcoholism* in 1960,[5] a controversy has raged about the disease idea.[6-11] The conceptualization herein suggests that the physician approach persons with alcoholism as if they had a disease, and use familiar techniques to establish a diagnosis, initiate treatment, and encourage a fruitful physician-patient relationship.

What are the essential elements of this concept, and do they take account of such scientific data as are available on the nature of alcoholism? Does the concept encourage the maintenance and development of human dignity and mutual self-respect between patient and caregiver, and does it explain the repetitively self-destructive behaviors? The central idea in this concept is that persons with the alcoholism syndrome are unable to control their intake of alcohol. The lack of control is incomplete, inconsistent, and insidiously deceptive; sometimes the person can abstain and at other times drink in a controlled fashion. However (using a year as a time frame) the person sometimes drinks more than intended, or drinks when he or she had not intended to drink, and suffers as a result. The frequency and amount of uncontrolled drinking determine the severity and spectrum of symptoms. Some manifestations of alcoholism vary in response to socioeconomic factors; thus the lawyer, psychiatrist, active housewife, or retired clerk present distinct complaints. It is not clear whether differential susceptibility or differences in amount of alcohol account for individual variability in medical complaints, such as liver disease, pancreatitis, and delirium tremens.[12]

The essence of the alcoholism syndrome is similar to tobacco dependence, aspirin dependence, compulsive eating, or severe nail-biting, except that the pharmacologic properties of this sedative and addictive drug produce grave consequences as the amount of intake increases. Heavier drinking is higher risk drinking, although factors other than quantity of intake may be critical for the progression to alcoholism.

The disease concept suggests a discontinuity between alcoholic drinking and healthy drinking. No one sets out to develop alcoholism or to become "hooked" on alcohol (nor does the smoker set out to develop lung cancer). The nascent alcoholic person may begin drinking for the usual reasons. Whatever the factors that promote heavy drinking, as the amount and frequency of intake increases, some people gradually fail to always control their intake. A dependence develops, the person begins to drink for unclear reasons, and is now drinking alcoholically, with serious consequences.[13] The pharmacology of alcohol is one reason for the transition from "dog wagging tail" to "tail wagging dog" or from "person takes a drink" to "drink takes a person." Other factors are less clearly understood,[14] but the qualitative as well as quantitative difference between alcoholic drinking and healthy drinking is emphasized by the disease concept.

The disease concept serves as a reminder that the disorder has a "life of its own." The syndrome is integrated into the totality of a person's physical, emotional, and social being, while retaining some degree of independence. Diabetes may become visible or worsen during depression or infection, but is not caused by these factors; alcoholism is similarly independent and interdependent. The disease concept reminds care-givers, that addictive drinking will not disappear without a direct approach, any more than diabetes is cured by psychotherapy, better environmental conditions, exercise of will power, or not eating carbohydrates.

Three major hypotheses have been investigated in order to understand the etiology of alcoholism: the sociocultural, the biochemical-genetic, and the psychological. None has been effective at explaining *the* cause of alcoholism. A review summarizes the data as follows:

> . . . no explanation that involves a single class of etiological factors seems adequate to account for what is most likely an 'overdetermined' disorder with multiple causes and a complex developmental course.[15]

Like other illnesses such as hypertension, or even infectious diseases such as tuberculosis, a continuum of causal factors is usually present. Another way of stating this is to state two aspects of its unpredictability. First, if conditions are right, any person who drinks alcohol has the potential to move into alcoholic drinking, and second, which of 100 drinkers will develop alcoholism cannot specifically be predicted (just as it is impossible to predict which individual smokers will develop cancer). Recent long-term follow-up studies of healthy populations confirm these ideas.[16,17] Thus, available evidence suggests that the concept of alcoholism as a disease should be accepted. The disease model provides a framework for understanding the destructive dependence exhibited by millions of Americans who seek physical, emotional, and spiritual assistance from physicians. Current data suggest that the fundamental lesion (inconsistent inability to control alcohol intake) is determined or conditioned by an array of etiologic factors that may differ from person to person. The disease concept will not be proved or disproved; it is a way of looking at certain facts and ideas that is helpful, but not subject to a rational or logical proof per se. However, physicians' acceptance of the fact that alcoholism behaves as if it were an illness facilitates the adoption of helpful behaviors by physicians, patients, and society.

ALCOHOL METABOLISM

A background in the physiology and metabolism of alcohol is helpful, and definitions are important in developing a consistent approach. A standard drink is 1½ oz of liquor (about 40 percent alcohol), 12 oz of beer (about 5 percent), or 5 oz of table wine (about 12 percent). Each of these servings contains approximately the same amount of alcohol ($1½ \times 0.40 = 12 \times 0.05 = 5 \times 0.12$). Patients seldom report drinks in standardized terms; one's "drink" is another's quart of beer or pint of whiskey or double highball with beer chaser, greatly confounding history-taking. Blood alcohol peaks 30 to 40 minutes after a person with an empty stomach takes a drink of alcohol. The height of this peak depends slightly on individual factors, but drinking three to four drinks quickly on an empty stomach typically elevates the standard (70-kg) person's blood alcohol level (BAL) to about 100 mg/dl, legally set as the limit for drunkenness in many states.

Although responses to the first drink or two vary, once a BAL of 100 mg/dl is achieved individual differences are minimal and the manifestations are solely due to the pharmacologic effect of the drug on the central nervous system (CNS). At this level all persons show some signs of inebriation, namely, slurred speech, uncoordinated gait, poor judgment, and emotional lability. Hepatic alcohol dehydrogenases (ADH) metabolize alcohol, lowering the BAL about 15 to 25 mg/dl per hour—a rate not substantially affected by total dose or the starting BAL. Thus, recovery from mild intoxication (100 mg/dl) requires two to three hours (BAL of 50 mg/dl), and about five hours for complete elimination. Metabolic rate differs from person to person but no important racial or ethnic differences in the metabolic rate have been noted.[18] Although the oxidizing capacity of ADH does not change with regular exposure to alcohol, the liver's microsomal enzyme oxidizing system (MEOS) does become activated, producing metabolic rates at the high end (25 mg/dl per hour).[19] However, even people with severe longstanding alcoholism do not exceed this metabolic rate.

ALCOHOL TOLERANCE

Many physicians do not appreciate the dramatic clinical effects of tolerance; however, diagnostic assessment is incomplete if tolerance effects are ignored. The diminished effects of high alcohol levels noted in tolerant persons are produced by nerve tissue adaption. As stated, a BAL of 100 mg/dl produces signs of inebriation in any nontolerant person, whereas the tolerant person may behave in a normal fashion even at very high alcohol levels. For instance, one person who acted soberly and denied drinking had a BAL of 568 mg/dl, a datum which settled the immediate issue (whether the person had been drinking) and also established the diagnosis of alcoholism.

This very dramatic example emphasizes the fact that the person who is tolerant does indeed function quite well because of the ability of the nervous tissue to adapt to the presence of alcohol. The person who has a BAL of over 100 mg/dl but appears sober is tolerant, and usually has alcoholism. This is likely to be the case for Mr. B from the introduction. Typically, Mr. B and other tolerant patients do not show signs of intoxication at the usual blood levels, but the apparent sobriety in spite of the high BAL may mask a serious cognitive and emotional deficit. The cover-up may be so effective as to mislead experienced interviewers[3] if they fail to note the odor of alcohol. The person who says, "Oh, I just had a drink before I came in," is surprisingly often taken at face value, when the "drink" may have been a pint of whiskey or a bottle of sherry!

INTOXICATION AND OVERDOSE

Intoxication and overdose of alcohol is frequently encountered in emergency departments but seldom on other services. All degrees of intoxication may produce serious problems, from coma to disruptive behavior; moreover, a single patient may frustrate emergency department staff for many hours during expression of the various problems associated with different levels of inebriation. Life support may be necessary, or suturing impossible, or the patient's unruly behavior may disturb staff or patients. Nurse C from the introduction represents a fairly typical situation. In addition, too often the staff denies that these patients have alcoholism, not recognizing that perhaps 90 percent of adults who appear drunk in emergency departments do have alcoholism. If health care staff understand that healthy drinkers who "have had one too many" only rarely appear in emergency departments, they can more realistically adjust their attitudes, expectations, and treatment approach.

Although good statistics are not available on this point, it should be apparent that the alcoholic 10 percent of the population who are frequently drunk (for illustrative purposes assume a conservative average of once a week) should account for more intoxication-related problems than the 60 percent of the population who are healthy drinkers, infrequently drunk (assume once a year on average). Thus from a hypothetical population of 100, 30 abstainers yield no episodes of drunkenness, 60 healthy drinkers yield 60 episodes, and 10 alcoholics 520 episodes per year. Additionally the healthy drinkers seldom become as intoxicated and are more often drinking in controlled environments (where someone else can drive, for example).

A comatose person with a BAL of 400 mg/dl may require the supports needed with any sedative overdose, including intubation and ventilatory assistance. The patient would likely awaken gradually at a BAL of 200 to 250 mg/dl six to eight hours after the initial measurement. Rapid infusion of intravenous (IV) fructose will increase the degradation rate of ethanol. However, the increase is limited to 20 or 25 percent (or less if the rate is already maximal because of steady exposure) so that this treatment is not clinically useful.[20] Furthermore, large volumes of fluids must be given,

increasing the possibility of fluid or electrolyte disturbances.

Behavior of intoxicated individuals shows features well known to emergency department staff. People are usually disruptive, often obnoxious, sometimes combative and destructive, and always difficult to control. Often, they are brought to the emergency department against their wishes (by police or friends); or else they may have some specific needs such as getting off the streets, finding a meal or a warm friendly place; or they may simply be looking for whatever attention is available. What they seek, then, is not what the staff is equipped to deliver, resulting in escalating friction. Furthermore, staff behavior must be adjusted to the reality that negative attention is as valuable to the intoxicated attention-seeker as positive attention.

Staff sometimes believe that patients are totally out of control, but everyone has observed that patients respond very differently to the arrival of a police officer or an attractive young nurse. These changes in response emphasize that staff behavior may have dramatic influences on patients' behavior. Furthermore, patients must be held responsible for their actions even while "out of control." Appropriate limits can be set by knowledgeable staff even though the situation is tense, other matters press for attention, and time is frequently limited. Helpful generalizations concerning appropriate staff behaviors are difficult, but some useful procedures for setting limits can be described.

One typical frustrating situation involves the arrival in the emergency department of a "regular" whose disruptive routines are well known from frequent visits. Careful observation of the objectionable behaviors often discloses ones which are subject to modification through alterations in staff behavior. Physicians and nurses should find protected conference time for considered discussions; only careful planning can result in a coordinated approach and development of a satisfactory management plan. This process of identifying behaviors and developing management plans has been described in a recent publication from the Addiction Research Foundation.[21]

The violent or agitated patient often responds to skillful "talking down" in a calm environment. However, safety of everyone concerned, including staff, other patients, and the inebriate, must be the primary consideration. Adoption of a nonthreatening posture and attitude allowing the patient to ventilate rather than trying to induce sober or responsive behavior is a helpful start. Offering a cigarette, coffee, or a doughnut sometimes turns wrath and agitation miraculously into tranquillity, again demonstrating that emotional lability is a regular feature of drunkenness.

Keeping the patient seated is a helpful strategy and minimizes the potential for violence. However, physical or chemical restraints may be needed to protect personnel or the patient, and if physical restraints are used, chemical restraints are usually indicated, except in the case of severe head trauma. Intramuscular (IM) chlorpromazine in doses of 25 to 100 mg will control most situations. It is prudent to start with 25 mg, increasing subsequent doses as necessary. The hypotensive effects of this drug are as dramatic as the sedative effects, thus, patients should be kept supine. Intravenous diazepam in 5-mg doses is also effective. Neither drug should be given unless staff are prepared to provide respiratory assistance; this is an unstable situation where good judgment is necessary in weighing the potential dangers of violence against those of additional sedation.

Patients whose lacerations have been sutured or who have no other serious medical problems are often left to sober up in emergency departments. They should *always* be restrained on stretchers since they may wake up unexpectedly. Although commonly administered, caffeine may cause a more dangerous situation by producing a slightly more awake inebriate who is as uncoordinated and who has as poor judgment as previously.

After sobering up (if treatment for withdrawal is not indicated), the patient will be discharged from the emergency department. Before dismissal, all patients should have some counseling, with emphasis on a few principles. First, any patient in a blackout state which may persist well into his or her apparent "sobering up" phase will retain little of what is said; therefore any messages must be brief and must be simple. This is true also of the serious cognitive and emotional disarray (short of blackouts) present in many intoxicated people. Patients who are not regular visitors to emergency departments feel guilty and ashamed of their behavior. Universally such patients are fearful and anxious, and often seriously depressed. Because of these feelings and low self-esteem, they remember the tone of an interview much better than its content. Thus, the discussion must be couched in supportive terms. Frequently, a brief diagnostic interview makes it clear that the patient has alcoholism. The discussion must directly and supportively address this diagnosis, just as would be the case if cancer or diabetes had been discovered. Psychiatric support for Nurse C after her overdose should include these principles. Further guidelines for discussion are included in the section on crisis counseling below.

Development of working relationships with community alcoholism treatment facilities is useful. Working with "wet drop-in" centers, overnight shelters, and detoxification facilities of various kinds facilitates the effective and appropriate discharge of patients who otherwise might clog the emergency department for many hours, and even then leave with inappropriate treatment plans.

ADDICTION AND WITHDRAWAL

The presence of one of the various withdrawal syndromes associated with extended daily intake of alcohol defines physical addiction to alcohol. Prolonged daily heavy drinking inevitably produces addiction to alcohol and a subsequent withdrawal syndrome. The pioneering work of Isbell and colleagues demonstrated that this process can occur after a few weeks of steady, heavy drinking in people who had no prior history of alcohol addiction.[22] The clinical manifestations of the withdrawal syndrome suggest a hyperactive response of the oversedated CNS during its readjustment to sobriety. The biochemical details of the brain's response to the prolonged sedation and depression by alcohol are not entirely clear. Proposed mechanisms have included enzyme induction and receptor proliferation; more recently, membrane alterations; and most recently of all, endorphin stimulation within central nervous tissue.[23,24] Whatever mechanism is finally proved, it is the readjustment to the sober state that causes the most clinical difficulty.

It should be remembered that not all people with alcoholism are physically addicted to alcohol. Many alcoholic people whose drinking is not consistently controlled and who experience great suffering and dysfunction in their lives never develop the daily drinking pattern that produces addiction. Professor E's wife might be included in this group. A clear example of this situation is the person who drinks only from Friday through Sunday. Although severe adverse consequences (aggressiveness and abuse, or Monday absences) may be apparent, the brain has a chance to recover from Monday through Thursday and the molecular changes in nervous tissue that produce the withdrawal syndrome will not develop unless the person moves to a pattern of daily drinking. On the other hand, it is true that the physically addicted state is a serious health consequence; therefore, any person who experiences withdrawal symptoms must have alcoholism.

Newer data developed in clinical research units demonstrate the presence of a partial withdrawal syndrome and the ease of becoming readdicted.[25] Readdiction takes place after a few drinks or at most a day of steady drinking in the person whose nervous system has previously undergone the changes of alcohol addiction. The presence of a withdrawal syndrome in patients who have been sober for many weeks and then drink for a few days dramatizes the clinical importance of rapid readdiction. Furthermore, one of the more severe withdrawal syndromes can develop after as little as seven to ten days of alcoholic drinking. The brain apparently has a "memory circuit" for the addiction syndrome.[23]

Controlled studies in research unit conditions show that intoxication and withdrawal appear to be more "shades of gray" than black or white, clearly separable states, at least in addicted drinkers. More simply, unless the alcohol level is rising, the person is in withdrawal; furthermore, the presence of tolerance means that symptoms and signs of intoxication are unusual. The person has to drink very large quantities to become clinically intoxicated. This can be shown by administering alcohol in a programmed fashion to a person who has been addicted. After a few weeks of sobriety alcohol is given in controlled doses for 16 hours. If alcohol is then withheld withdrawal symptoms can be demonstrated. During the next 24-hour cycle (16 hours' drinking and 8 hours off) withdrawal symptoms worsen. By the third cycle, the person has withdrawal symptoms constantly between drinks, worsening steadily as drinking continues.[25]

Thus, symptoms do not just occur when people cease drinking, but severe symptoms are a regular occurrence during the time that a person is still drinking. At first, heavier drinking may overcome the symptoms, but such factors as gastritis, families, and lack of funds limit the amounts one can drink. Therefore, people actively drinking heavily may arrive in the emergency department with withdrawal symptoms, even severe syndromes. Clinicians must remember that neither recent heavy drinking, nor alcohol on the breath, nor a very elevated BAL rules out delirium tremens.

WITHDRAWAL SYNDROMES

The variety of clinical presentations of alcohol withdrawal is well known to most physicians.[26,27] The syndromes may be mild or severe, of early or late onset, and of low or high morbidity. The problems of mild to moderate severity have their onset within minutes to hours after the last drink. Symptoms include tremors, sweating, anxiety, nervousness, agitation, vague fears, stomach upset with nausea and pain, and extreme difficulty sleeping. Hallucinations occur frequently in mild to moderately severe withdrawal. Symptoms peak at 24 hours and then gradually decline over two to four days. Recognition of this syndrome is not difficult in the emergency department if the history of alcohol intake is apparent, as in Mr. A from the introduction. Without obvious clues to the diagnosis, mild to moderate withdrawal syndromes may be missed.

Treatment

Safe, efficacious pharmacotherapy is available,[28] and should be initiated in the emergency department. The pros and cons of many drugs suggested for this purpose are briefly considered.

Alcohol

Alcohol itself has been used by some physicians and, of course, by many patients who attempt self-treatment by "tapering off." Unfortunately, alcohol is a relatively short-acting drug and is also psychologically difficult for the patient to take or for nurses to administer. Furthermore, physicians rarely prescribe adequate amounts of alcohol, perhaps because of lack of understanding of the data already presented regarding the complex interrelationships among intoxication, addiction, tolerance, and withdrawal symptoms. Finally, continuing damage to the heart, brain, liver, bone marrow, and immune systems is promoted by alcohol. All of these considerations make it inappropriate to prescribe alcohol in any circumstance in the treatment of alcohol withdrawal syndromes. Effective drugs are available that are longer acting and thus provide smoother symptom relief; that are cross-tolerant in the CNS itself; and that are not toxic to alcohol-affected organs.

Chlordiazepoxide

The prototypical drug used for mild to moderate alcohol withdrawal is chlordiazepoxide.[29] Chlordiazepoxide has an effective half-life of more than 24 hours. Its onset of action is in about two hours and peak action does not occur until six to eight hours after the first dose. When administered in adequate dosage during the first 24 hours after the onset of withdrawal symptoms and tapered rapidly, its pharmacokinetics are ideal for the treatment of alcohol withdrawal. In the emergency department in otherwise uncomplicated patients the oral administration of 100 mg is an appropriate starting dose. Intramuscular chlordiazepoxide is contraindicated because of unreliable absorption from muscle sites. Complete treatment protocols are available.[26] For average severity 300 to 400 mg in the initial 24 hours is typical, with 150 to 200 in second 24 hours, and 75 to 100 in third 24 hours; the prolonged excretion results in a gradual decline in blood levels during days 4 to 7 or 8.

Phenobarbital

Phenobarbital is an effective drug for patients who are allergic to chlordiazepoxide or if a nasogastric tube or severe GI symptoms prevent the administration of chlordiazepoxide. It should be given in approximately milligram equivalent doses to chlordiazepoxide.

Oxazepam

Oxazepam has effects similar to chlordiazepoxide but is shorter acting and effectively eliminated in the presence of cirrhosis or acute hepatitis.[30] Thus, it has some theoretical advantages in the setting of known liver disease. Therefore, if a shorter-acting drug is desired in the presence of head trauma or other CNS problems, oxazepam is probably the drug of choice. The starting dose should be 30 to 60 mg.

Paraldehyde

Paraldehyde has been the drug of choice over many years. This drug, although probably the most dramatic and effective in relief of alcohol withdrawal symptoms, should nonetheless not be used. It is dangerous because of acidosis (from outdated lots) and rectal strictures.[31] It is very short-acting and thus produces extreme swings in symptom relief; the short period of action and high potency result in rapid addiction to it. There is disagreement as to whether its odor and taste are objectionable, but it is definitely inconvenient to administer.

Other Drugs

Many other minor tranquilizers or sedatives have been shown to be efficacious, but have little to recommend them in terms of effectiveness, convenience, safety or cost.[28]

Outpatient Treatment of Alcohol Withdrawal

The initiation of outpatient detoxification regimens in the emergency department may prove helpful and cost-effective.[32] Necessary prerequisites for ambulatory management are an environment where a responsible person can be alert for the development of complications (which occur infrequently but may not be recognized by the patient) and the ability to return for follow-up. If, in addition, circumstances suggest that mild withdrawal is likely, the use of an outpatient detoxification regimen is cheap and enlists patients and their family or friends in the early phases of treatment. Give 50 to 100 mg of chlordiazepoxide, and send the responsible person out with instructions to give 25 to 50 mg by mouth every four to six hours depending upon the severity of symptoms. Do not give more than 150 mg to take home. At follow-up the next day, medication can be given for one to two days and the patient can then enter a longer-term treatment program.

Alcoholic Hallucinosis

So-called alcoholic hallucinosis is a variant mild to moderately severe withdrawal syndrome. The patient typically has very few autonomic signs and may have mild to absent tremor and anxiety but be hallucinating vigorously. The onset of hallucinations occurs shortly after the cessation of drinking. Hallucinations are frightening, but *not* an indication of severe withdrawal by themselves. This syndrome responds well to the usual drug schedules, and does not need special treatment except for reassurance of patient, family, and friends.

Delirium Tremens

Severe alcohol withdrawal is a complication justifiably feared among patients and physicians. This terrifying disease carries a morbidity currently between 5 and 10 percent in the best circumstances. The onset is classically stated as 72 hours after the last drink of alcohol;[33] however, as previously described, delirium tremens may develop with no apparent change in drinking pattern.[25] Therefore, patients may appear in the emergency department who are drinking heavily and are also in active delirium tremens.

Onset may be abrupt and precipitous, or vague and insidious; the symptoms peak in one to eight hours. Delirium is the hallmark, while other symptoms mimic those listed for mild to moderately severe withdrawal. Hallucinations are usually but not invariably present and autonomic signs are typically worse with delirium tremens, sometimes including hyperventilation (with severe alkalosis), tachycardia, hyperthermia (105 to 106°F), and hypertension. The variability of presentations is confusing to the neophyte; agitation can be minor or extreme, autonomic abnormalities completely absent or dramatic, while derangements of thought content can be minor or as serious as in acute paranoid schizophrenia. This latter group may have a fixed delusional system with auditory or visual hallucinations, no autonomic signs and little of the violent anxiety and agitation usually associated with delirium tremens. The patients with the worst prognosis are those with striking autonomic findings; in particular, hyperventilation and alkalosis are associated with a poor outcome. This may be because of hypersensitivity of the medullary respiratory center to pharmacotherapeutic agents as well as to carbon dioxide.[34]

Severity and duration are difficult to predict; extremely heavy uninterrupted prolonged drinking (for example, 3 quarts of whiskey daily for four months) and past episodes of delirium correlate with more severe symptoms, but not invariably. "Impending" delirium tremens is a term of little clinical usefulness. Patients can be treated based on a diagnosis of mild to moderately severe withdrawal if delirium is not clearly present; the response over the next hour or two will determine whether treatment for mild to moderately severe withdrawal or for delirium tremens is more appropriate.

Treatment must be initiated promptly in the emergency department. The drug whose efficacy has been most convincingly proved by appropriately controlled study is diazepam.[35] Ten mg should be administered IV over several minutes and then 5 mg given every five minutes IV until the patient becomes calm. Doses higher than 150 mg may be necessary to induce a calm state. Maintenance doses of 5 mg IV as often as necessary are then given. The point of treatment is to calm patients enough that restraints are not necessary, except possibly a single restraint to preserve the IV line.

Patients should not be comatose, but drowsy and easily aroused. Treatment suppresses symptoms but has never been shown to have an effect on the duration of delirium tremens. An alternative regimen, which has not been studied in a controlled fashion, has proved useful at the Cambridge Hospital. Twenty-five mg of chlorpromazine is given IM as a test dose and then 25 to 100 mg is given IM every 45 to 60 minutes until the appropriate level of calmness is achieved. Even in the most severe cases 500 mg or less is a typical total induction dose. Hypotension due to peripheral vasodilatation is an expected side-effect; thus, this regimen should not be used in patients with acute myocardial infarction. Incidence of seizures has not been observed to increase with this protocol.

Although mild cases of delirium tremens with few autonomic signs and minimum agitation may respond to high doses of chlordiazepoxide or haloperidol, these should not be used as first-line drugs. Both drugs are of low potency for this illness, thus delaying efficacious treatment in some patients. Moreover, a patient who initially appears mildly ill may worsen quickly and eventually require a second drug such as diazepam or chlorpromazine.

Seizures

The patient who presents to the emergency department with alcohol withdrawal seizures raises many issues. The diagnosis of alcohol withdrawal may be unclear if the history is scanty, which is often the case when the patient's cognitive function is compromised during the postictal state. Furthermore, some patients have a seizure as the sole manifestation of withdrawal; absence of the typical shakes, sweating, anxiety, and so forth increases the diagnostic difficulty. Alcohol withdrawal seizures are *grand mal*, typically occurring 24 hours after the last drink.[33] However, early and late seizures (five to seven days is common and 14 days possible) do occur.

The presence of seizures does not predict severity of other withdrawal symptoms, but in patients who also have delirium tremens, seizures precede the onset of delirium tremens. Seizures may be single or multiple, but no controlled data are available regarding efficacy of anticonvulsive treatment after the first seizure. If more than one seizure occurs, the second may follow by as few as one or as many as eight hours. The data on usefulness of prophylactic treatment against seizures

in patients known to be undergoing alcohol withdrawal conflict; thus some physicians use phenytoin if a history of seizures during prior episodes of withdrawal is present, while others do not give medication.[36] Hospital admission is appropriate for patients who have not had prior seizures, so that appropriate diagnostic measures may be undertaken and patients and families counseled in an environment where the patient can be observed. In particular, the diagnosis of alcoholism can be pursued and an appropriate introduction to alcoholism treatment established. Considering the above statements, patients should never be discharged from the emergency department with anticonvulsants, with or without previous withdrawal seizure history. Also, patients should be held under observation for at least eight hours after any withdrawal seizure.

Differential Diagnosis of Withdrawal Symptoms

Occasionally, the differential diagnosis of the withdrawal syndromes may be challenging. Paradoxically, intoxication may be difficult to distinguish from withdrawal. As previously discussed, as a drinking episode is lengthened the time spent *not* in withdrawal is shortened, and drunkenness may be fleeting. Aggressive and anxious behaviors may be similar during drunkenness or withdrawal. A distinguishing feature is that emotional lability is more dramatic when inebriated than during withdrawal. Moreover, the agitation of drunkenness usually worsens with talking, whereas the agitation of withdrawal often responds and improves with "talking down." Further, if intoxicated people are left alone they may quiet down or go to sleep. Although people in withdrawal may calm down while alone, they do not drop off to sleep.

Wernicke-Korsakoff's syndrome may confuse some observers because the "global confusional state" appears similar to the delirium of delirium tremens.[37] Distinguishing features include dramatically less agitation for the degree of confusion during Wernicke's disease and the presence of ocular, cerebellar, and peripheral nerve findings. Delirious patients with hepatic failure are usually more somnolent than agitated, and asterixis is present; however, if spider angiomata, ascites, and jaundice are absent, this diagnosis may be missed.

Acute schizophrenic syndromes typically show fewer autonomic findings and more fixed hallucinations and delusions, but in the individual patient accurate differential diagnosis is sometimes impossible. The history of alcohol intake is essential, but final diagnosis may be delayed seven to ten days while the clinical course is observed.

Subdural hematoma, a frequent concomitant of alcoholism, often shows focal neurologic signs and usually has a more waxing and waning course than does delirium tremens. Because these signs are not prominent or overlooked, the subdural is too often missed.[38]

Meningitis, pneumonia, and cerebral vascular accidents can also cause difficulty in diagnosis if atypical syndromes are present, and this demonstrates the need to consider the spectrum of diseases, especially metabolic (uremia, hyponatremia) and toxic (bromides, steroids, amphetamines, psychedelics), that may cause delirium.[38] Withdrawal from other drugs may be concomitant with alcohol withdrawal, but since patients need specific appropriate treatment, they often give history correctly, so drug withdrawal is not mistaken for alcohol withdrawal. In people who abuse barbiturates or benzodiazepines with alcohol, the differentiation between withdrawal syndromes may be impossible in the emergency department. Blood levels of barbiturates and a test dose of barbiturate assist in determining appropriate therapy; however, initial treatment of minor tranquilizer withdrawal is not different from alcohol withdrawal treatment. (See Chapter 35.)

Emergency Department Diagnosis of Alcoholism

Many people who do not appear at first glance intoxicated or in withdrawal may have alcoholism. Typical clues for the examiner include the odor of alcohol, the nature of the situation (aggressive behavior, home accident, suicide attempt); or the presence of tremor or anxiety (such as Mr. A or B, or Miss C). These nonspecific signs should alert staff to consider a possible diagnosis of alcoholism.

The alcoholic patient is likely to be anxious, negative, and defensive, a difficult person to interview. While attempting to clarify the situation, the interviewer must be sensitive to the patient's concerns, individualize the approach, and remember that the patient is already in pain if alcoholism is present. In the absence of alcoholism, on the other hand, patients will not be offended by a brief and skillful exploration for other symptoms of alcoholism. A simple screening test is available which is adequate for initial interviews. The CAGE (a mnemonic) test is designed to ascertain whether the patient has experienced poor control or adverse consequences of drinking, and what feedback has been received regarding drinking:

CAGE Screening Test for Alcoholism[39]

Have you ever felt the need to	*C*ut down on drinking?
Have you ever felt	*A*nnoyed by criticism of drinking?
Have you ever had	*G*uilty feelings about drinking?
Have you ever taken a morning	*E*ye opener?

Note that the test does not focus on how much the patient drinks (or how often), but looks for negative consequences of drinking; if these effects are present, there is a high probability of alcoholism. Further confirmation can be obtained by using the National Council on Alcoholism's 26 questions (see Appendix A) as a structured interview for other adverse effects of drinking.

Many professionals express skepticism regarding the value of such efforts. However, every interview has therapeutic content, and health care staff generally strive to achieve maximum benefit from their encounters with patients. Consider for a moment the alternatives for interactions with patients in whom some clue to a diagnosis of alcoholism is present.

First, one might do nothing; however, this "conspiracy of silence" is frequently developed to a fine art by the patient's friends and family, and only rarely will further silence be helpful. Too often physicians and nurses join this conspiracy. Waiting for something to happen or the light to dawn on the patient is courting another accident, pancreatitis, overdose, or violent episode.

A second approach might be to chastise the patient for self-abusive behavior, to criticize the patient for disrupting others' lives, or to issue a reminder that more drinking will "rot out your liver." This approach is perceived as mean and nasty by the patient and amplifies feelings of guilt, shame, and low self-esteem. Patients often strike back with their own hostile, angry criticism, thus generating another futile imbroglio.

A third alternative is to pursue a rational and caring approach in spite of the apparent futility of a desperate and emotionally negative, tense situation. Whether the eventual yield is high or low, the last approach has a chance of being helpful and also has the virtue of feeling good to the provider, who has thus made a positive effort which calls upon our most human and humanitarian inclinations. Moreover, the outlook for these patients is not hopeless,[40] and care-givers should not feel helpless about their role. The visit to the emergency department may be only a tiny episode in the patient's life, but may have profound consequences if problems are confronted in a professional manner. Every crack in the wall of denial has the potential to bring it down and begin the recovery process, resulting in the achievement of abstinence from alcohol and the eventual recovery from its destructive effects.

EMERGENCY DEPARTMENT CRISIS COUNSELING

Some patients with alcoholism will be asking for help, either as the "chief complaint" or after a screening interview such as the CAGE test. Since patients may have little idea what alcoholism treatment is, they often ask for *help*, unable to be more specific. The usual options are limited to participating in a withdrawal program (if appropriate), beginning a program of outpatient counseling,[41] or going directly to Alcoholics Anonymous (AA). The skillful staff person will assist the patient in a brief exploration of the appropriateness of these options. Most important is the ability to listen carefully to the patient's thoughts and feelings regarding perception of the illness process, ability to ask for people to help, and commitment to doing something at the present time.

During this process, tone and style are probably more important than logic and rationale. The patients' behavior is more important than what they think at this stage and the counselor should not surrender to the tendency to present the most logical, rational, and incontrovertible argument possible. The interpretation must be individualized so as to assist the patient to effect positive behaviors after leaving the emergency department. Frankness, openness, and a forthright acknowledgment of the facts will make it safe for the patient.

Thus, the initiation of treatment is a straightforward but empathetically conducted discussion of the diagnosis, abstinence, and available avenues for treatment. This process is usually painful to the patient (and often to the care-giver) but not harmful. Remembering the distinction between pain and harm will help the care-giver maintain courage and empathy while assisting patients to accept the obvious facts and take appropriate action. This kind of confrontation can foster a transition into a more explicitly therapeutic relationship.

Most patients are reluctant to consider entering treatment, and especially to join AA.[42] All patients and most care-givers have misconceptions about the nature and operation of AA. It is free, available 24 hours, easy to find, and totally and exclusively committed to facilitating recovery of people with alcoholism. Its use should be encouraged far more frequently than is presently the case, and in spite of the patient's objections. This is where gentle, skillful, supportive counseling can be of most use. Frequently, the patient who finally gets to AA says essentially, "I spent so many years avoiding AA, trying every other avenue, and not willing to face the problem head on. If only my doctor had been more forceful or helpful in getting me to see the benefits of AA sooner. . . ."

When patients seem disinclined to discuss the available options, the talk should be kept brief (10 minutes or less). Long discussions about the patients' perceptions of why they drink too much, details regarding difficulties with job, family, and so on are never helpful, and certainly not while intoxicated. Even while apparently rational, patients may be in a blackout, and recall little or nothing a few hours later. Thus, a brief discussion of presently available alternatives will suffice, and keeping several AA principles in mind will help the counselor to be concise and straightforward; namely, "keep it simple," "don't drink today," "easy does it."

For patients whose illness is more advanced or for people who repeatedly come to the emergency department, an even more simplified approach may be necessary. In skid row situations like Mr. D's, the focus usually is on finding an appropriate (and swift) placement. Local facilities differ, but patients will usually go to a withdrawal unit or a shelter and sobering-up station.[21] Adjusting expectations to match the reality of the chronicity of the illness can be helpful when care-givers must repetitively manage the problems of chronic public inebriates. Acknowledging that a night off the streets or a warm meal with supplemental vitamins in the presence of someone who cares may be the best intervention facilitates making speedy arrangements in a positive frame of mind. Care-givers make similar short-term plans for patients with end-stage chronic lung disease or debilitating cancers when there is small likelihood of interrupting the course of the disease. In short, care-givers must "patch" and bandage in whatever human ways are possible under trying circumstances.

"CLEARING" FOR DETOXIFICATION

Frequently, units that offer lower levels of care than the acute hospital request that emergency personnel "clear" patients for discharge to that facility, often a detoxification unit. Patients who have acknowledged the presence of alcoholism wish to enter a therapeutic setting where withdrawal can proceed safely in skilled hands, and in a fashion integrated with a comprehensive program for alcoholism treatment. Many detoxification units have minimum medical coverage, and require that patients be declared fit for a stay in such an environment. Emergency department physicians should have a definite paradigm in mind to facilitate this examination.

When a patient is intoxicated or agitated, it behooves examiners to be brief and direct without being superficial. In addition to open-ended questions (the "what's the main problem now?" sort), certain specific questions can be used to establish a high probability that the patient does not have serious acute problems, and direct the emphasis of the physical examination. An adequate screening relies heavily on history and vital signs rather than a comprehensive physical examination, and a competent job can be expeditiously done with minimum facilities. (See Appendix B.) The most serious and prevalent problems to be considered include metabolic disorders, neurologic complications such as Wernicke's syndrome and subdural hematoma, serious bleeding, pneumonia, and decompensated liver disease.

The recent drinking history determines the likelihood of a serious withdrawal syndrome and the likelihood of other medical complications.[19,22,23,25] At highest risk is the person who has been drinking steadily for months, often previously not known to have alcoholism. The patient's prior experience with delirium tremens and seizures and the use of medications, particularly sedatives or tranquilizers, are relevant to withdrawal risk. Has the patient considered or attempted suicide? Does the patient know of serious liver disease, and has a liver biopsy ever been done? Are abdominal symptoms so severe as to suggest pancreatitis; has the patient recently vomited blood?

Serious gastrointestinal bleeding is uncommon, and when significant is usually the presenting complaint. For these statistical reasons, the lengthy practice of placing a nasogastric tube and obtaining a hematocrit and stool guaiac has been revised. The patient is asked about vomiting and retching since the reported episode of hematemesis. If the response is positive, and the vomitus was free of blood on one or more occasions, the likelihood of serious bleeding is minimal. If the patient has not vomited since the hematemesis, postural vital signs are taken and the abdomen is examined. If the abdominal exam does not show hyperactive bowel sounds, and postural vital signs are normal, no further work-up is done. Positive results call for the usual protocol, including passage of a nasogastric tube, hematocrit, observation for a period of time, and so on. Thus, since most people in alcohol withdrawal whose hematemesis is only apparent after direct questioning do not have serious bleeding, protocols that facilitate treatment while minimizing the time and discomfort should be used. (See Chapter 23.)

The intake of other sedative or intoxicating drugs is problematic. Alcohol withdrawal is more serious than withdrawal from other sedatives and tranquilizers, except for barbiturate addiction. Most patients who abuse other sedatives and tranquilizers can be safely managed in an alcohol "drying-out" facility; moreover, transfer to a hospital can be arranged if the later onset (typically 5 to 10 days) of tranquilizer withdrawal syndromes ensues. Abuse of benzodiazepines has increased, but diazepam dosage must exceed 40 mg daily for prolonged periods before serious withdrawal symptoms are produced. (See Chapter 35.)

The physical examination should be directed toward ascertaining that the patient is likely to be safe over the next several days. The vital signs should never be ne-

glected. Fever means that the patient must be examined in detail including a white blood cell count, chest roentgenogram, and other diagnostic tests as indicated. Tachycardia and hypertension are common but their presence need only be carefully noted; hypotension requires thorough examination. Examination of the sclerae for icterus and the eyes for nystagmus or paresis is mandatory. All patients should be checked for asterixis ("liver flap"), and gait should be checked for symmetry. Although many patients are staggering and detailed testing is not possible, the presence of an asymmetric gait is a warning that more thorough neurologic examination is necessary. Observation of a symmetric gait and unremarkable neurologic examination suggests that hidden trauma in the trunk and legs is unlikely.

Mental status is of course important, but difficult to describe since the range of behavior during intoxication and withdrawal syndromes is quite wide. The observer should be well enough trained to ascertain that the patient's mental status is consistent with drunkenness or withdrawal. The most common mistake is failing to take account of a severely depressed level of consciousness that might indicate hepatic decompensation, overdose, or other metabolic derangement.

The psychiatric states of schizophrenia and manic depressive illness are too frequently diagnosed. Many observers fail to acknowledge that a diagnosis of psychiatric illness can rarely be made until the acute effects of alcohol intoxication and withdrawal diminish. In patients with bona fide psychiatric decompensation, it may be difficult or impossible to distinguish which problem is producing the presenting symptoms, and the decision to place the patient in a psychiatric, medical, or alcoholism unit must be based on evaluation of the individual case and on local policies concerning these matters.

Two metabolic problems especially relevant to the management of patients with alcoholism are hypoglycemia and acidosis. Alcohol-induced hypoglycemia was described 15 years ago; patients with poor food intake and binge drinking sometimes arrived with profound hypoglycemia. Investigations have shown that the inhibition of hepatic gluconeogenetic pathways by alcohol during glycogen-depleted fasting states is partly responsible for the hypoglycemia.[43] If unrecognized, this serious condition may produce irreversible brain damage. This problem should be considered and treated with 50 percent glucose IV before definitive laboratory data are available in comatose patients and in patients whose degree of somnolence appears inconsistent with other signs of intoxication. Because acute Wernicke's syndrome may worsen with the administration of 50 percent glucose (glucose metabolism requires thiamine), thiamine must be given before IV glucose. Although few patients have both Wernicke's and hypoglycemia, thiamine can be life-saving, and is harmless in other conditions.

An equally important problem is the presence of metabolic acidosis. The pathophysiology of this syndrome is not entirely clear, but the clinical picture is one of more or less severe acidosis with variable amounts of ketosis.[44] Lactate levels are not high unless shock with hypoxia ensues, with production of lactic acid. The determination of arterial pH and electrolytes is essential for patients whose clinical condition is severe or where clinical findings are not completely consistent with intoxication or withdrawal. It must be emphasized that clinical indications of acidosis do not always include Kussmaul respirations and hypotension; most cases are discovered because the patient's general condition is such as to require the determination of electrolytes or blood gases. (See Chapter 18.)

Alcohol affects the metabolism of many drugs.[45] Some are eliminated more rapidly (barbiturates, meprobamate), others show delayed metabolism (warfarin). In other circumstances alcohol interferes with the action of a substance (folic acid), or may potentiate the toxic effects of a drug (carbon tetrachloride). The list is extensive, and the clinician must remember to check this list whenever the clinical situation warrants.

Paraprofessional personnel, nurses, or physicians' assistants can easily perform the screening examination. If the volume of patients with alcohol-related problems is sufficient, it may be cost effective for paraprofessionals to make initial decisions for patients with alcohol-related complaints. Often such personnel become better trained in alcoholism counseling and know community facilities more intimately. They can thus provide more appropriate management than the busy emergency department physician.

REFERENCES

1. Mendelson J, Mello N: *Diagnosis and Treatment of Alcoholism.* New York, McGraw-Hill, 1979, pp 2–7.
2. Waller J: Unintentional injury, in Kissin B, Begleiter H (eds): *The Biology of Alcoholism,* Vol 4. New York, Plenum, 1976, pp 307–350.
3. Holts, et al: Alcohol and the emergency service patient. *Br Med J* 281:638–664, 1980.
4. Fourth Special Report to the U.S. Congress on Alcohol and Health. U.S. Department of Health and Human Services, 1981.
5. Jellinek EM: *The Disease Concept of Alcoholism.* New Haven, Hillhouse, 1960.
6. Edwards G, Grant M (eds): *Alcoholism: New Knowledge and New Responses.* Baltimore, University Park Press, 1978.
7. Keller M: The disease concept of alcoholism, revisited. *J Stud Alcohol* 37:1694–1717, 1976.
8. Wikler A: On the nature of addiction and habituation. *Br J Addict* 57:73–79, 1961.
9. Szasz T: Bad habits are not diseases. *Lancet* 2:83–84, 1972.
10. Bateson G: The cybernetics of self: A theory of alcoholism. *Psychiatry* 34:1–18, 1971. (Also in Bateson G: *Steps to an Ecology of Mind,* New York, Ballantine, 1972).
11. Alcohol and alcoholism. *Report of a Special Committee of the Royal College of Psychiatrists.* London, Tavistock, 1979.
12. Turner T, Mezey E, Kimball AW: Measurement of alcohol-related effects in man: Chronic effects in relation to levels of alcohol consumption. *Johns Hopkins Med J* 141:235–248, 273–286, 1977.
13. Bacon S: The process of addiction to alcohol. *Quart J Stud Alcohol* 34:1–27, 1973.
14. Ludwig AM, Bendfeldt F, Wikler A, et al: 'Loss of control' in alcoholics. *Arch Gen Psychiat* 35:370–373, 1978.
15. Armor DJ, Polich JM, Stambul HB: *Alcoholism and Treatment.* New York, Wiley, 1978.
16. Vaillant G: Natural history of male psychological health: VIII. Antecedents of alcoholism and "orality." *Am J Psychiat* 137:181–186, 1980.
17. Vaillant G, Brighton J, McArthur C: Physicians' use of mood altering drugs: A 20-year follow-up report. *N Engl J Med* 282:365–370, 1970.
18. Reed TE: Racial comparisons of alcohol metabolism: background, problems, and results. *Alcoholism Clin Exp Res* 2:83–87, 1978.
19. Korsten M, Lieber C: Hepatic and gastrointestinal complications of alcoholism, in Mendelson J, Mello N (eds): *Diagnosis and Treatment of Alcoholism.* New York, McGraw-Hill, 1979, pp 20–21.
20. Woods H, Alberti K: Dangers of intravenous fructose. *Lancet* 2:1354–1357, 1972.
21. Cox A: Management of intoxicated and disruptive patients, in: *Emergency Department Training Manual.* Toronto, Addiction Research Foundation, 1979.
22. Isbell N, Fraser HF, Wikler A, et al: An experimental study of the etiology of "rum fits" and delirium tremens. *Quart J Stud Alcohol.* 16:1–33, 1955.
23. Mendelson J: Biological concomitants of alcoholism. *N Engl J Med* 283:24–32, 71–81, 1970.
24. Mendelson J, Mello N: Biologic concomitants of alcoholism. *N Engl J Med* 301:912, 921, 1979.
25. Gross M, Lewis E, Best S, et al: Quantitative changes associated with signs and symptoms of acute alcohol withdrawal: Incidence, severity, and circadian effects in experimental studies of alcoholics, in Gross M (ed): *Alcohol Intoxication and Withdrawal.* New York, Plenum, 1975, pp 615–631.
26. Sellers E, Kalant H: Alcohol intoxication and withdrawal. *N Engl J Med* 294:757–762, 1976.
27. Gross M, Lewis E, Hastey J: Acute alcohol withdrawal syndrome, in Kissin B, Begleiter H (eds): *The Biology of Alcoholism,* Vol 1. New York, Plenum, 1977, pp 191–263.
28. Greenblatt D, Greenblatt M: Which drug for alcohol withdrawal? *J Clin Pharmacol* 12:429–431, 1972.
29. Greenblatt D, Shader R: Benzodiazepines in clinical practice. New York, Raven Press, 1974.
30. Shull H, Wilkinson G, Johnson R, et al: Normal disposition of oxazepam in acute viral hepatitis and cirrhosis. *Ann Intern Med* 84:420–425, 1976.
31. Stanley J: Rectal disease in a patient with delirium tremens. *JAMA* 243:1749–1750, 1980.
32. Alsen M: Outpatient treatment of acute withdrawal states. *Br J Addict* 70(suppl 1):56–63, 1975.
33. Victor M, Adams R: The effect of alcohol on the nervous system. *Res Publ Assoc Nerv Ment Dis* 32:526–673, 1953.

34. Victor M, Wolfe S: Causation and treatment of the alcohol withdrawal syndrome, in Bourne P, Fox R (eds): *Alcoholism: Progress in Research and Treatment.* New York, Academic, 1973, 137–170.

35. Thompson W, Johnson A, Maddrey W: Diazepam and paraldehyde for treatment of severe delirium tremens: A controlled trial. *Ann Intern Med* 82:175–180, 1975.

36. Sampliner R, Iber F: Diphenylhydantoin control of alcohol withdrawal seizures. Results of a controlled study. *JAMA* 230:1430–1432, 1974.

37. Victor M, Adams R, Collins G: *The Wernicke-Korsakoff Syndrome: A Clinical and Pathological Study of 245 Patients, 82 with Post-Mortem Examinations.* Philadelphia, FA Davis, 1971.

38. Plum F, Posner J: *Diagnosis of Stupor and Coma,* ed 2. Philadelphia, Davis, 1972, pp 101–106.

39. Ewing J, Mayfield D: CAGE. *Am J Psychiat* 131:1121–1122, 1974.

40. Polich J, Armor D, Braiker H: *The Course of Alcoholism Four Years after Treatment.* Report #R–2433–NIAA of the RAND Corporation. Santa Monica, 1980.

41. Schuckit M: Treatment of alcoholism in office and outpatient settings, in Mendelson J, Mello N (eds): *Diagnosis and Treatment of Alcoholism.* New York, McGraw-Hill, 1979, pp 229–255.

42. Zinberg N, Fraser K: The role of the social setting in the prevention and treatment of alcoholism, in Mendelson J, Mello N (eds): *Diagnosis and Treatment of Alcoholism.* New York, McGraw-Hill, 1979, pp 374–382.

43. Arky R: Alcohol hypoglycemia, in Kissin B, Begleiter H (eds): *The Biology of Alcoholism,* Vol 1. New York, Plenum, 1971, pp 212–216.

44. Kreisberg R: Diabetic ketoacidosis: New concepts and trends in pathogenesis and treatment. *Ann Intern Med* 88:681–695, 1978.

45. Sexias F: Alcohol and its drug interactions. *Ann Intern Med* 83:86–92, 1975.

Appendix A

"26 Questions"

1. Do you occasionally drink heavily after a disappointment, a quarrel, or when the boss gives you a hard time?
2. When you have trouble or feel under pressure, do you always drink more heavily than usual?
3. Have you noticed that you are able to handle more liquor than you did when you were first drinking?
4. Did you ever wake up on the "morning after" and discover that you could not remember part of the evening before, even though your friends tell you that you did not "pass out"?
5. When drinking with other people, do you try to have a few extra drinks when others will not know it?
6. Are there certain occasions when you feel uncomfortable if alcohol is not available?
7. Have you recently noticed that when you begin drinking you are in more of a hurry to get the first drink than you used to be?
8. Do you sometimes feel a little guilty about your drinking?
9. Are you secretly irritated when your family or friends discuss your drinking?
10. Have you recently noticed an increase in the frequency of your memory "blackouts"?
11. Do you often find that you wish to continue drinking after your friends say that they have had enough?
12. Do you usually have a reason for the occasions when you drink heavily?
13. When you are sober, do you often regret things you have done or said while drinking?
14. Have you tried switching brands or following different plans for controlling your drinking?
15. Have you often failed to keep the promises you have made to yourself about controlling or cutting down on your drinking?
16. Have you ever tried to control your drinking by making a change in jobs or moving to a new location?
17. Do you try to avoid family or close friends while you are drinking?
18. Are you having an increasing number of financial and work problems?
19. Do more people seem to be treating you unfairly without good reason?
20. Do you eat very little or irregularly when you are drinking?
21. Do you sometimes have the "shakes" in the morning and find that it helps to have a little drink?
22. Have you recently noticed that you cannot drink as much as you once did?
23. Do you sometimes stay drunk for several days at a time?
24. Do you sometimes feel very depressed and wonder whether life is worth living?
25. Sometimes after periods of drinking, do you see or hear things that aren't even there?
26. Do you get terribly frightened after you have been drinking heavily?

Source: National Council on Alcoholism: The Modern Approach to Alcoholism.

Appendix B

Emergency Department or Walk-In Service Screening Examination

Patient name ________________________________

A) History
1. Uninterrupted drinking for how long?
2. Last drink when?
3. Last time sober (no alcohol) 1 month or more?
4. Previous detoxifications (yes, no)? Most recently (where, when)?

A) History (continued)	No	Yes		B) Physical Examination	No	Yes	
D.T.s in past?			*	Head trauma?			*
Fits? seizures?			*	Jaundice?			*
Liver trouble?			*	Pupils not reactive?			*
Hematemesis today?			*	Asterixis?			*
Taking pills/meds?			*	Consciousness unusual**?			*
Chronic illnesses?			*	Orientation not O.K.?			*
Other important				Hallucination?			*
symptoms/problems?			*	Agitation severe?			*
				Gait not symmetric?			*
				Other important findings?			*

C) Vital Signs
  Pulse   *if > 120
  Respirations   *if > 24
  BP   *if > 160/110
                or < 100/70
  Temp   *if > 99.9

D) Laboratory Exam
1. None done
2. CBC _________ Chemistry ____________ *
   X-Ray _______ EKG __________________

E) Conclusion/Summary

My screening examination at this time reveals the following:
_______ 1. Everything consistent with drunkenness/withdrawal in an otherwise healthy individual.
_______ 2. Evidence of other acute problems manageable at a free-standing unit.
_______ 3. Evidence of chronic problems which seem stable at this time.*

Date ____________________Time ______________   Signed ________________________________
                                              Checked ____________________________M.D.

* If you check "yes," use the back of this form for documenting details.
** Not consistent with drunkenness/withdrawal.
Source: The Cambridge and Somerville Program for Alcoholism Rehabilitation, Inc.

37. Depression, Anxiety, and Suicide

MERRILL-LYNN PAGE, R.N., M.N., C.S.

Patients with depression, mania, or anxiety generally seek emergency treatment for the somatic symptoms that accompany these disorders rather than for the disorders themselves. They are frightened of their unknown condition and view it as a physical condition that requires immediate attention. Through careful interview and examination, the clinician can differentiate the mental disorders from the possible physical illnesses by the clinical picture, the course of illness, and the family and personal history. Ultimate differentiation is made by the patient's response to appropriate treatment.

Treatment of affective illness, depression or mania, may be of a true emergency nature, such as evaluation of suicidal risk. Hospitalization may be required for the patient whose depression is debilitating or the patient whose judgment is severely impaired by manic illness. Seldom is anxiety a life-threatening condition, but it is a crisis to the person experiencing it, who fears loss of control or death. For those patients whose condition is not a true emergency, careful differential diagnosis, patient education about the illness and types of treatment, and plan for treatment is the care required in the emergency department.

DEPRESSIVE EPISODE

A 40-year-old woman is brought to the emergency department by her husband and sister who are con-cerned about the patient's withdrawal from usual activities and loss of weight. The patient looks tired, speaks softly and slowly, and says she has not liked herself for several weeks. She does not know why she feels so poorly.

Depressive disorders may be primary, occurring with no apparent cause, or secondary, occurring in response to other conditions, such as trauma, surgery, or debilitating physical illness. Whether primary or secondary, the symptom picture and treatment are similar.

The National Institute of Mental Health reports that 20 million adults, or 15 percent of the U.S. adult population, suffer a serious depressive disorder in any given year. Women outnumber men approximately 2:1 in cases of depression.[1] Fifty percent of the adults in the United States with a major depression have another episode at some time in their lives.[2] The onset of a major depression can occur at any age, but new case incidence seems to peak between the ages of 24 to 45; relapsing cases are probably responsible for high incidence after 40 years of age.[1]

Types of Depression

Depression may be a normal mood, a symptom accompanying another illness, or a specific condition. Feelings found in depression, i.e., sadness or despair, may accompany other medical or psychiatric illnesses, both neurotic and psychotic, but are not necessarily major elements in the condition. The illness of depression itself is seen in the emergency department as a situational reaction, as a chronic depression, or a moderate or severe depression. In assessing the type and severity of depression, the patient's description of symptoms with onset and course, precipitating events, family and personal social and psychiatric history lead the clinician toward the diagnosis.

Situational Reactions

In situational depressive reactions, the condition develops after a loss or disappointment in life. The patient often recognizes the cause of the distress. It is personal, but usually recognizable to others, such as the ending of a relationship, loss of status, loss of support system, or adjustment to an illness. Symptoms are a depressed mood, often with accompanying anxiety, and preoccupation with the loss. Biologic symptoms are not prominent, but an increase or decrease in sleep or appetite is occasionally reported. Family and personal history may indicate a similar reaction to loss in the past.

Treatment of a situational depressive reaction primarily involves short-term therapy. A supportive atmosphere in which the patient can ventilate and grieve the loss should be provided. When anxiety is significant, short-term use of an antianxiety agent can supplement therapy. With therapy, the patient should be able to return to previous functioning.

Chronic Depression

Another form of depression encountered in the emergency department is that of chronic depression. The patient has few, if any, of the biologic symptoms of depression, but reports being depressed for a great portion of life. This contrasts with the limited illness of other depressions. Chronic dissatisfaction with life, especially with the treatment received from others, dominates the picture. In behavior, the patient is often demanding and clinging, yet hostile and rejecting of offered help.

The treatment of chronic depression is a therapeutic relationship that offers a supportive and empathic environment. The goal is not cure, but helping the patient to cope with the dissatisfactions of life. Both clinician and patient should understand this to avoid disappointment and failure of treatment. Over time, the patient can be encouraged to broaden interests and to engage in new activities that add some pleasure and sense of control to life. Goals should be small and reasonable, visits should be regular and short. The important factors are the continuing relationship between the clinician and the patient, and the clinician's active involvement and acceptance of the patient's condition. The clinician does not try to change the patient, but rather to help make life more bearable for the patient.

Moderate and Severe Depressions

The symptoms are similar in moderate and severe depression, but the degree of incapacitation is different. Initial observations in both suggest the diagnosis of depression.

In the moderately depressed patient, the mood shows in the sadness and despair in the face. Psychomotor activity reveals either agitation or retardation. The patient is fidgety and appears uncomfortable, or is slowed in actions and responses. The patient may seek attention because of biologic or emotional symptoms or because of compromised daily functioning. In the interview, the patient complains of biologic symptoms, e.g., decreased appetite with weight loss; decreased sleep with early morning awakening; decreased energy, concentration, and interest. The patient finds nothing brings the pleasure it once did. When asked directly, the patient reports feeling helpless, hopeless, worthless, and, often, guilty. Thoughts of suicide may be elicited.

In addition to the clinical presentation, family and personal history support the diagnosis of depression. Careful exploration reveals previous similar episodes in the patient or a family member. Questions need to be directed to the possibility that parents, siblings, grandparents, or even peripheral blood relatives experienced depressions. A history of manic episodes also supports the affective illness diagnosis of depression.

When dysphoric mood and decreased interest are accompanied by four of the other symptoms, the syndrome has lasted for two weeks or more, and no other cause for the symptoms can be found, the diagnosis of a major depressive episode can be made.[2] The presentation of a patient with a severe depression is an elaboration of that of a patient with a moderate depression. It usually occurs in patients of middle age or older. The patient shows significant weight loss, fatigue, and lack of attention to self-care. Withdrawal from others may be extreme, with the patient talking little. Family members often must provide the history. Psychomotor agitation is significant with pacing, hand-wringing, and grimacing, or the retardation may be so great that the patient appears almost catatonic. Mood is one of total despair and pessimism.

When the illness is of psychotic proportions, hallucinations and delusions may be elicited. These hallucinations are based on feelings of guilt and worthlessness. The patient may say, "I have cancer; my body is rotting; I am being punished for my sins." The patient may have auditory hallucinations of a self-derogatory nature. The clinician must attempt to ascertain if the patient is having command hallucinations of self-injury or death. The patient should be asked if the "voices" are demanding the patient commit acts of self-mutilation or suicide.

A severe depression with psychotic features must be differentiated from a schizophrenic illness with depressive features. In depression, the psychotic manifestations are consistent with depressed mood, i.e., somatic, pessimistic, and guilt-oriented. Family and personal history should indicate previous depressive illness and generally good functioning between episodes. In contrast, the manifestations of schizophrenic illness are more persecutory, paranoid, and bizarre. Family and personal history indicate more psychotic illness, previous compromise of functioning, and a generally chronic course of illness.

Medical examination and history are needed to confirm the diagnosis of depression, determine the physical effects of the illness, and suggest a course of treatment. Many drugs, including reserpine, methyldopa, steroids, hypnotics, and perhaps oral contraceptives can cause depressive symptoms. Pernicious anemia, hypothyroidism, viral infections, multiple sclerosis, Wilson's disease, malignancy, systemic lupus erythematosus, and porphyria should be considered.[1] Depression may appear as dementia, or accompany it, in the elderly. Often treatment of the depression improves or clears mental functions.

Treatment of moderate and severe depressions in the emergency department involves evaluation of suicidal risk, patient education, and, usually, referral for continued treatment. A calm, understanding manner, adequate time, and provision for privacy begin the treatment process. The clinician draws a picture of a known, treatable illness for the patient, rather than the fearful unknown the patient has been experiencing. The patient should be interviewed alone at first; the family can be included later, with the patient's permission, to add their observations and receive an explanation of the illness and treatment recommended.

A major concern in any depressed person is suicidal potential. Clinicians may be reluctant to ask about suicide for fear of "putting ideas into the patient's head." Most often, however, the patient is relieved to have such frightening ideas verbalized by the clinician. Various approaches may be taken; for example, the clinician may ask if the patient has felt that life is not worth living or that the family would be better off if the patient were dead. Any positive response must be pursued as to plan, available means of carrying out the plan, and immediacy of intent.

Hospitalization is mandatory if the patient is actively suicidal. A recent attempt, particularly of a high-risk/low-rescue nature, or a stated intent with plan and available means requires hospitalization. It may also be needed to provide care for the severely depressed patient who is physically debilitated or health-endangered by malnutrition. If the illness has drained the patient and family of coping resources or if family attitudes contribute to the patient's feelings of worthlessness, hospitalization is recommended.

Any resistance to hospitalization should be explored; the need for rest, medication trial, and observation by staff should be explained. When the situation is life-threatening, the clinician may have to arrange for involuntary hospitalization of the patient, explaining the reasons for such a decision.

An explanation of the nature of the illness can relieve the guilt feelings of the patient and the family, who may feel they caused the illness. Although not everything is understood about the causes of depression, explanation may include a discussion of reactions to discernible stresses in the patient's life and/or a possible biologic vulnerability to depression, much as some people are vulnerable to diabetes or hypertension. The clinician should explain that, although the patient currently feels improvement is not possible, the patient can return to previous mood and functioning with time and treatment.

Therapy

Decision to begin medication therapy at the emergency department visit depends on the clinician's knowledge of antidepressants or the availability of a psychiatrist for consultation. If medication is to be given, the patient can be started on a beginning dose of an antidepressant with an explanation of its effects and side-effects and definite plans for follow-up. Referral may be made to a psychiatrist, or the emergency department clinician may provide follow-up through a primary care setting.

A continuing relationship is necessary to provide supportive therapy during the time required for medication to take effect, to monitor treatment effects and side-effects, and to observe the patient's progress through treatment. The emergency department clinician who assumes the ongoing care of the patient should have pharmacologic and psychiatric consultation available.

The primary medical treatments for depressive episodes are the tricyclic antidepressants, monoamine oxidase inhibitors, and electroconvulsive therapy. If the patient or a family member has responded to an antidepressant in the past, a similar response may be expected with the same drug.

Among the tricyclics frequently used are amitriptyline hydrochloride, imipramine hydrochloride, depoxin hydrochloride, and desipramine hydrochloride. Amitriptyline is the most sedating and most anticholinergic; desipramine, the least anticholinergic.[3] The usual medication regimen is an initial dose of 50 mg daily, with increases of 25 to 50 mg every two days until 100 to 150 mg daily is reached. This dosage is maintained for at least three weeks for an adequate trial of the medication.[3] With the elderly or infirm, smaller increments are required, and a final dosage of 100 mg daily may be adequate. Patients who do not respond to one tricyclic may respond to another, owing to the different biochemical effects of the drugs.

It is necessary to explain that sedation and calming are immediate but improvement in mood is delayed, or the patient may become discouraged and discontinue treatment. Total daily dosage at bedtime is convenient, but divided doses may be needed to decrease the anticholinergic and cardiotoxic side-effects, particularly in the elderly.

When psychotic symptoms are present in depression, antipsychotic medication is the first step in treatment. Among those antipsychotics commonly used are perphenazine, trifluoperazine hydrochloride, and haloperidol.[4] As the psychosis clears, an antidepressant may be added if depressive symptoms remain. Consideration must be given to the combined anticholinergic actions and the onset of extrapyramidal symptoms, as well as the possibility of acute dystonia. Explanation is essential.

Among the side-effects of the tricyclics are dry mouth, constipation, and blurred vision. The body usually adapts to these symptoms and develops some degree of tolerance. Other conditions that may occur include increase in intraocular pressure, glaucoma, urinary retention, paralytic ileus, cardiac dysfunction, and toxic delirium, especially in the elderly.[3] Thus, these patients must be carefully monitored for the development of these conditions.

Given the lethality of overdose with tricyclics, no more than one week of medication should be ordered at any time. This is especially true as the patient regains some energy, but mood has not improved, because the patient may then have the energy and means to act upon suicidal impulses.

Monoamine oxidase inhibitors are also effective in the treatment of depression, often in cases that are unresponsive to the tricyclics. They are not as widely used, perhaps because of the potential for serious interactions with foods and other drugs. Furthermore, the use of these drugs requires a clinician experienced in their use and a reliable patient.

In depressed persons whose illness is so severe that the time required for antidepressants to work is not available, who have not responded to medication, or who have conditions that prevent safe use of medications, electroconvulsive therapy is the usual treatment. Given a fear in the general public surrounding its use or past experience when treatment was less sophisticated, careful education of the patient and family is essential. Referral to a psychiatrist and an inpatient stay are usually required.

A final caution in the biologic treatment of depression must be emphasized. Such treatment may precipitate a manic episode in those with bipolar illness. The clinician should watch for this occurrence.

In addition to biologic treatment, the patient requires psychological support through recovery. The patient and the clinician should have regular, short meetings, weekly at first, with telephone contact as needed for problems. The clinician should avoid probing for psychological issues, but should express empathy about the patient's situation. The patient must receive constant encouragement that treatment can work, given enough time. Patient and family may need help to avoid feeling guilty or seeing the patient as weak of character. Expectations of the patient should be neither unrealistic, as "snap out of it," nor regressive, with pitying and catering to the patient. No major decisions should be made until the depression has resolved.

When the patient has recovered, consideration must be given to medication withdrawal or maintenance. Continuing the medication for six months after recovery is recommended; then the dosage can be gradually reduced. In instances of recurrent depressions, a low dose of prophylaxis may be advisable.[5]

Among the psychiatric illnesses, depression can be one of the most rewarding for the clinician to treat. When treatment is effective, both the patient and the clinician are gratified by the patient's return to normal functioning. The final step of treatment is to advise the patient of the possible recurring nature of the illness so that treatment can be sought at the earliest signs of depression.

MANIC EPISODE

A 27-year-old man, accompanied by his wife and father, arrives at the emergency department. He is talking fast, in a loud voice. He makes suggestive statements to the female nursing staff. He paces the waiting room area.

On the other end of the spectrum of affective illness is manic illness. In the adult population, 0.4 to 1.2 percent will experience a manic episode,[2] and about 75 percent of those will have more than one episode.[6] Although the number of persons experiencing a manic illness may seem small, it is not unusual to see such a patient in the emergency department, most often brought by others. The incidence of the illness is the same in both men and women, with the first episode usually occurring before the age of 30.[6]

Mania, like depression, is a disorder of mood. Patients feel extreme elation, well-being, and a great sense of their own abilities and value. Manic illness is seen in the emergency department as an acute manic episode, with or without psychosis, or as a hypomanic episode.

The person experiencing an acute manic episode is often heard before seen. By observation alone, the clinician can spot the primary symptoms of mania, i.e., expansive or irritable mood and hyperactivity. During the interview, the patient usually evidences an elated mood, although irritation may be shown toward those who insisted on the emergency department visit. Increased activity is apparent in movement, speech, and thought.

The patient may move quickly and frequently, giving a history of increased exercise, reckless driving, increased strength, and hypersexuality. The need for sleep is decreased, with the patient getting none to only a few hours each night, yet feeling energetic. Lack of attention to personal hygiene may be evident in a disheveled appearance, or the expansiveness of mood may be reflected in clothing and makeup that is colorful to bizarre.

Speech is rapid and constant, making the patient difficult to interrupt. Distractibility shows in abrupt shifts of subject that often seem to be precipitated by the current environment. Usually, the thought process can be followed, although at times this may be difficult. One word in a thought may be the connecting element to the next thought.

Thought content is usually grandiose, and judgment is impaired. The patient reports possessing uncommon abilities and strengths, and often feels invulnerable. The patient may engage in many activities with little appreciation of consequences, such as planning a business without appropriate funds, bringing strangers home, or going on spending sprees. This lack of judgment can endanger job, financial security, and personal relationships. Grandiosity can reach psychotic proportions, such as delusions of a special relationship with God or important public figures. If delusions are paranoid in content, they are based on the specialness of the patient; for example, the patient may claim to be sought by the Federal Bureau of Investigation (FBI) because of an ability to change the course of world politics. Auditory hallucinations, if present, also reflect the specialness of the patient.

When the mood change and three or four of the other symptoms are present for one week or more and there is no other discernible cause for the symptoms, the patient meets the criteria for manic illness.[2]

Hypomania is an attenuated form of mania that causes the same symptoms of mood, activity, and thought, but to a lesser degree and without psychosis. A careful personal and family history, as well as medical examination, are needed for the diagnosis. Differential diag-

noses include drug-induced states, as from amphetamines, steroids, L-dopa, cocaine, and bromides. Hyperthyroidism and multiple sclerosis may result in similar symptoms. Schizophrenic illness may be suggested if the patient's mood is one of irritation.[2]

Differentiating acute mania and schizophrenic illness can be difficult. In mania, the disorder is mainly one of mood, although it may include thought of psychotic proportions related to the patient's excessive sense of self-value or ability. Between episodes, the patient is usually symptom-free and resumes previous functional level. In schizophrenic illness, the disorder is mainly one of thought content, usually bizarre and persecutory, with mood change being more transient. Between acute episodes, some symptoms usually remain, causing a deterioration in functioning.

Episodes of mania or depression should be sought in family and personal history. Previously unrecognized hypomania may be found on careful questioning. Although a family member may have been diagnosed as schizophrenic in the past, careful examination of the symptom picture may show that the illness more closely resembled manic-depressive illness. The premorbid adjustment of such a family member was usually good, without demonstrating the progressive course of schizophrenic illness.

Treatment of the patient with a manic episode can prove difficult, as the patient seldom sees any need for treatment. When the illness has caused significant problems, however, the patient may accept treatment through family pressure. Hospitalization is recommended; it is required when the patient's condition is endangering to health or when the patient's judgment is so impaired that the patient's behavior carries physical, social, or financial risks.

If outpatient treatment is planned, family involvement is essential to assist in monitoring the patient's condition and compliance with medication. This is more feasible with hypomanic patients, especially those who recall the distress resulting from previous manic episodes.

Biologic treatment of manic illness may be with lithium carbonate and/or antipsychotics. Lithium requires adequate serum blood levels and takes about seven to ten days to become effective. Because the manic outpatient is seldom cooperative with the daily blood drawings needed in the early phase of treatment to determine when an adequate lithium level has been obtained, initial treatment is easier with an antipsychotic, such as haloperidol, to treat the hyperactivity and lack of sleep; thought content may remain the same, however.[6] Referral can be made for later lithium treatment, especially when a history of recurring episodes suggests that maintenance therapy is required. Lithium maintenance can decrease the frequency and/or severity of manic episodes. Attention should be given to the possible occurrence of depression as mania clears.

The psychological treatment of manic patients is mainly supportive and educational. The clinician must establish a trusting relationship and help patients accept treatment. Meetings are initially frequent and brief. As the mania resolves, patients need help to deal with the feelings that result from such loss of control and the effects of this behavior on themselves and others. Patients often feel guilt and shame, as well as lowered self-esteem.

Family members also need supportive and educational meetings in which they can ventilate angry and frightened feelings to an empathetic clinician. Education about the illness with emphasis on the fact that the illness is causing the behavior can help reintegrate the patient into the family. Both patient and family need education about the recurring nature of the illness and early signs that might indicate need for further treatment. Often a change in sleep pattern and activity level are first signs.

Although few patients with manic illness may be seen in the emergency department, proper diagnosis, education, and treatment can avoid a series of significantly disrupting episodes in such a patient's life.

ANXIETY STATES

A 32-year-old man is brought by a co-worker to the emergency department. He is sweating, trembling, breathing rapidly, and clutching his chest. He says he thinks he is having a heart attack. The symptoms came on suddenly at work.

Anxiety is a normal condition of human existence. It is a diffuse, unpleasant feeling of apprehension; a fear of the unknown usually related to unconscious process. It is a signal for "fight or flight" from an unknown assault, usually an assault on self-esteem. As a normal condition, it can be useful in preparing for performance, as anxiety prior to a test motivates a student to study well. It may also be pathologic, of such a degree that a person's ability to function is diminished or erased. With a sufficient degree of anxiety, ego functions are compromised so that the person cannot take in, process, or act upon available data in a rational manner.

Most people have some anxiety about their visits to the emergency department. Illness or debilitation is a threat to self-esteem and results in anxiety. Anxiety can precede some illnesses and may be associated with other illnesses; in addition, there are mental disorders in which pathologic anxiety is the core symptom.

The association of anxiety with many other illnesses makes the history and examination even more impor-

tant so that other treatable conditions will not be missed. In addition to a careful description of events that accompanied the onset and course of symptoms, and a medical history, including a review of systems, medication, and oral intake, and variation of symptoms with foods ingested may point to physiologic conditions that are causing the anxiety symptoms.[5] Family history may also indicate possible organic conditions, as well as anxiety conditions.

The mental disorders with anxiety as the core symptom that are most likely to be seen in the emergency department are panic or anxiety attacks and agoraphobia (fear of public places).

Panic Attacks

Panic disorders usually occur first in late adolescence or early adult life, although they may appear later. They are relatively common, but no statistics are currently available as to incidence.[2]

Panic attacks are characterized by the sudden, unpredictable onset of intense anxiety with accompanying sympathetic nervous system symptoms. These symptoms may include dizziness, sweating, hot and cold flashes, palpitations, chest pain, dyspnea, a choking sensation, or trembling. Paresthesias, a feeling of unreality, and fear of imminent death are also common.[2] The symptoms last for several minutes to hours and bring the patient to the emergency department with fear of having a heart attack, stroke, or some other life-threatening condition. Panic attacks may occur daily, monthly, or every few years. When the patient has experienced three such anxiety attacks within three weeks, with four or more of the accompanying symptoms, the diagnosis of panic disorder is suggested.[2]

The first step in the emergency department is to rule out that which the patient fears is occurring, most often a heart attack. Careful examination and a description of the onset and course of symptoms begin the assessment. Additional conditions to be considered include hypoglycemia, pheochromocytoma, hyperthyroidism, caffeinism, withdrawal from substance abuse, amphetamine use or abuse, and prepsychotic states.[2] Laboratory studies, personal history, and family history aid in diagnosis.

Panic attacks may occur with no apparent precipitant, or a precipitant may be found in the history. The event may have occurred in recent days or weeks, or the precipitant may be the anniversary of the original event, such as the anniversary of a parent's death. Features of precipitating events include separation or loss, fear of injury, fear of performance, or facing a test or a new experience.[5]

The prepsychotic patient can also appear in the emergency department with anxiety symptoms. Diagnosis is aided by a personal or family history that includes psychotic illness. The patient's thought content related to what is happening may also have a more unusual flavor, often paranoid. Affect is usually blunted, and patients show less range of emotion than do patients with panic disorders.

Treatment of panic attacks begins with the clinician's attitude of calmness, understanding of the patient's fear, and reassurance. In most situations, touching provides some reassurance. Having staff or family remain with the patient helps to keep the patient from feeling alone and helpless.

Quite often the patient begins to calm while telling the story of the panic attack. The clinician can explain anxiety, perhaps as an extreme of nervousness, and how it can cause the overwhelming symptoms the patient has been experiencing. If there is a precipitant, it can be explored with the patient as an illustration of the way emotions can lead to physical symptoms, with the symptoms escalating the anxiety. When hyperventilation is part of the anxiety attack, having the patient breathe into a paper bag will demonstrate how easily the symptoms are relieved. The patient can be advised to keep such a bag handy in the future.

If the patient does not begin to calm in the interview, the administration of an antianxiety agent, such as diazepam (10 mg by mouth), is recommended.[7] If the episode seems to be a prepsychotic state, an antipsychotic can be given in an attempt to avoid an acute psychosis.

Further treatment includes patient education about anxiety attacks, ways to cope with them, and often referral for psychiatric treatment. Such treatment may involve supportive therapy, behavior modification, or insight-oriented psychotherapy. Given the potential for the development of dependence on the antianxiety agents, their continued use is discouraged, unless they are used in the context of a therapy relationship. The successful use of tricyclics or monoamine oxidase inhibitors has been reported in anxiety states.[3]

Agoraphobia

Also an anxiety state, agoraphobia may occur with or without panic attacks. It is a phobia related to territory, involving a distance and space that the patient requires in order to feel comfortable. The patient has a fear of being alone or in public places from which escape may be difficult or help not readily available.[2]

The prevalence of agoraphobia is approximately 6.3/1,000 in the general population, with women having the greater incidence. The illness first appears when the patient is 18 to 35 years of age. Family history usually includes an increase in the incidence of emotional disorders, and the patient frequently experienced a school phobia.[8]

The patient seeks help for agoraphobia because of associated anxiety attacks or because of the condition's interference with a normal life. Family members are also involved, since they must accommodate the patient's illness. With a detailed history, the patient usually reveals that anxiety attacks have been experienced in various situations, causing the patient to develop an anticipatory fear of having an attack if certain boundaries are crossed. Usual activities have been decreased in order to remain free of anxiety. The effect may be minimal, such as always taking a certain route to work or shopping at certain stores during less crowded hours, or it may have progressed to the point that the patient is housebound and fearful when alone.

Differential diagnoses include schizophrenic illness, depression that has caused withdrawal, and obsessive-compulsive personality.[2] A careful history of the onset of symptoms, development of the phobia, and premorbid personality help make the diagnosis of agoraphobia. The phobia is usually preceded in history by anxiety attacks, and it precedes the onset of secondary depressive symptoms. Obsessive-compulsive traits are excessive in the premorbid personality. Schizophrenic symptoms are not present on examination or in history. The family may be able to provide additional information about the patient and onset of illness.

Treatment of agoraphobia in the emergency department consists mainly of patient education about the nature of the illness, in addition to treatment for the current anxiety attack. Most people have some awareness of phobias as fears of objects or situations, and this awareness can be used to begin an explanation of the illness. The clinician explains how the patient probably experienced spontaneous anxiety episodes associated with particular situations in the past. The patient then began to avoid those situations in fear of feeling anxiety again. It is easier for the patient to cope with an understandable illness than the unknown condition that has led to such unusual behavior.

Referral for continued treatment is made to psychiatric staff. Treatment may involve the use of the tricyclics or monoamine oxidase inhibitors in doses similar to those used for antidepressant treatment.[3] In addition, behavioral modification and desensitization techniques can be helpful. With some patients, insight-oriented psychotherapy to uncover the unconscious sources of anxiety may be recommended. As with other patients, a specific referral is usually more successful than simply telling the patient to contact a psychiatrist.

Education in the emergency department about anxiety as a normal part of life and the treatment available for that which is beyond the bounds of normal anxiety assist the patient in coping with the illness and seeking treatment. Untreated anxiety states can become severely limiting illnesses.

SUICIDE EVALUATION

Most people consider suicide at some stressful time in life. It may be thought of as an end to suffering, an escape from unbearable failure, a move to a better life, or a punishment for oneself or others. The person can see no end to an intolerable situation nor means of dealing with it. For most people, the thought is transient, an emergency action that is rejected; for 24,000 people per year in the United States, however, it is a thought taken to completion with death. This figure does not include those suicides that appear as vehicular accidents, homicides, or drownings.[9]

Men commit suicide at a rate three times greater than women, although women attempt it twice as often as men. The rate for men rises with age, while the rate for women peaks at 55 to 65 years of age. The frequency is lower among the married; unmarried people commit suicide twice as often as married people. The rate for widowed and divorced is five times that of the married. Suicide is the third leading cause of death for adolescents, and the second for college students.[9]

To dispel some popular myths about suicidal people: those who talk about it do commit suicide; asking about suicidal thoughts and plans does not make a person do it; people who make repeated attempts do kill themselves, with 60 percent of all suicides having made previous attempts.[9]

In the emergency department, the clinician sees patients who have attempted suicide or those who are thinking of suicide and seek help. Some suicide attempts are covert, such as accidents with vehicles, weapons, or ingestions, or failure to care for themselves by taking essential medications properly. Therefore, the clinician needs a keen index of suspicion about possible suicide attempts and skill in recognizing such patients. Any suicidal thought or attempt should be considered serious.

Suicide Risk

Among patients for whom suicide is a significant risk is the psychotic patient, especially a patient with command hallucinations to end his or her life or with delusions of being evil. Such a patient requires hospitalization for safety during treatment for the psychosis. Even when the psychotic patient does not have such symptoms, but has suicidal thoughts, hospitalization is recommended due to the risk factor of compromised judgment. Other patients at risk are those with severe biologic depression, a newly diagnosed major illness, chronic or debilitating illness, and those with a recent loss or life change, even one that seems positive, such as a promotion.

In patients who show signs of despair, depression, or sense of crisis, the possibility of suicide should be investigated. Hints may be provided by patients who make statements about wishing for relief, not knowing how much longer they can hang on, wishing for prolonged sleep, feeling at the end of their rope, feeling others would be better off without them, or thinking that they would be better off dead. If such hints are not forthcoming, the clinician should ask if such feelings have occurred and specifically if the patients have thought of suicide.

If a patient has suicidal thoughts, the clinician should ask about a plan, intent to act, and means of action, such as planning to take an overdose of medicine and having a supply available. A definite plan with stated intent and means to carry it out indicate a need for hospitalization. When the patient has suicidal thoughts, perhaps even with plan and means but without definite intent to commit suicide, the patient and clinician *may* be able to negotiate a treatment plan that does not require hospitalization. This usually requires a trusting relationship with the patient, availability of a support system of family or friends, and a commitment from the clinician to be available beyond the normal schedule.

The feelings and situation leading to the suicidal plan are explored, with agreement by both parties to work together to seek alternative ways of coping with them. The patient must make a commitment not to act on suicidal feelings; the support people agree to act as guardians, removing available means from the patient; and all agree that, at any hint of breaking the agreement, the patient will be returned to the emergency department for reevaluation. If these requirements cannot be met, hospitalization is necessary.

Meetings with the patient should be frequent, even daily, and telephone contact must be available. In addition to counseling, interventions may include prescribing medication for depression, anxiety, or pain; interceding with others in the patient's behalf; arranging psychiatric evaluation and treatment. Care must be taken in prescribing medication so that the supply is less than a lethal dose. In considering this contract approach, thought is given to the impulse control of the patient. Evidence of alcohol or drug use that would interfere with the patient's control or a history of impulsive behavior negate the patient's ability to keep a contract.

In order to avoid unrealistic expectations of rescue, the clinician, patient, and family should discuss the responsibilities of each and the limitations. The clinician cannot be expected to be all-knowing or all-present, but agrees to make reasonable efforts to be aware of the patient's condition and available for advice. The patient and family agree to report truthfully and quickly to the clinician.

These negotiations and commitments take extra energy from the clinician, and the clinician must be aware that the drain can lead to the wish to be rid of the patient. This self-awareness is necessary so that the wish is not communicated indirectly to the patient, who then may grant the clinician's wish dramatically. Consultation with psychiatric personnel or a trusted colleague can help with this stress. Within these limitations, the clinician's caring and concern can have an important effect upon the patient's progress.

Patients with suicidal thoughts but without a definite plan or stated intent need to explore, with the clinician, the situation causing the distress, to ventilate their feelings, and to discuss alternative means of coping. Continued counseling with the clinician or referral to psychiatric personnel should be offered. The patient, with agreement to not act on the thoughts, is advised to return to the emergency department if feeling in danger. Use of crisis centers or hotlines is recommended.

Suicide Attempt

When patients have already attempted suicide, after providing necessary medical treatment, the clinician evaluates the attempt, continued risk, and plan for treatment. Indexes to consider are the risk/rescue ratio of the attempt,[10] the patient's feelings about surviving, purpose of the attempt, and the support system available.

Risk is the likelihood of death by the method used; rescue, the likelihood of discovery before death or serious injury. A few pills taken in front of the family constitutes a low risk/high rescue ratio, whereas a bottle of pills taken when the family is on vacation has a high risk/low rescue ratio. High risk merits hospitalization. In some instances, patients who have made low risk/high rescue suicide attempts may be treated as outpatients if other factors are favorable. If there is any doubt, safety comes first. In low-risk attempts, for example, the patient may have thought the method was lethal.

Discussion of the attempt must include how the patient feels about rescue. If the patient is disappointed and still wishes to be dead, hospitalization is required. If the patient is relieved and feels the act was foolish or regretful, outpatient treatment may be negotiated. However, the clinician should ascertain what has changed in the patient's situation or feelings that would prevent another attempt. With this precaution, it is hoped that the clinician will not be deceived and allow a seriously suicidal person to try again. The same factors of an available support system and contract for safety apply to the negotiations.

Some suicide attempts and threats have a manipulative quality about them. Their purpose seems to be to obtain something or to change the behavior of others. For instance, a patient may say, "I'll kill myself if you don't give me drugs; sign my disability paper." The clinician must decide whether to grant an undesirable request, hospitalize the patient for the threat, try to negotiate another request/response, or refuse and hope the patient does not act on the threat. With genuine concern from the clinician and an explanation that granting the request would not be in the patient's best interest, an alternative plan may be found. These are not easy situations at best, but with experience and consultation, the clinician can become skilled in handling these confrontations. When the purpose is to change the behavior of others, such as a lover's plan to leave, the negotiated contract for treatment may be successful, since the patient wishes not so much to die as to achieve some change in others. However, if safety cannot be ensured, hospitalization is required.

In exploring the history and present situation of a suicidal patient, significant losses and dates, such as the anniversary of the death of significant others or the patient's and significant others' birthdays, must be noted. If a family member or friend committed suicide, the patient's feeling about it must be explored. Of special importance is the suicide of a same sex parent, because the patient may believe in a self-fulfilling prophecy or may feel guilt about outliving the parent. The presence of any of these factors suggests significant risk.

The covert suicide attempts that appear as accidents or failure to take appropriate care of oneself are more difficult to evaluate. Patients often deny the meaning of their actions and, indeed, may be unaware of the motives. Exploration of the accident and events, possible harm, and the patient's feelings about injury and death may give clues to covert suicidal wishes. Genuine concern from the clinician about the risk to the patient may facilitate the development of a relationship that will allow the patient to look at the destructive behavior. Follow-up with the clinician or psychiatric personnel should be offered.

Working, even briefly, with suicidal patients is stressful and frightening. Such patients touch the helpless and angry feelings of clinicians since their work goal is to promote life. Clinicians do best with empathy for the patients and themselves in these situations and a colleague who can share the burden. When the outcome is a living, relieved patient, the work is satisfying; when unable to help these patients, clinicians can only face their human limitations and learn for the next patient.

REFERENCES

1. Greist JH, Greist TH: *Antidepressant Treatment—The Essentials.* Baltimore, Williams & Wilkins Co, 1979.

2. *Diagnostic and Statistical Manual of Mental Disorders,* ed 3. Washington, DC, American Psychiatric Association, 1980.

3. Baldesarrini RJ: *Chemotherapy in Psychiatry.* Cambridge, MA, Harvard University Press, 1977.

4. Kline, N, Angst J: *Psychiatric Syndromes and Drug Treatment.* New York, Jason Aronson, Inc, 1979.

5. Lazare A (ed): *Outpatient Psychiatry: Diagnosis and Treatment.* Baltimore, Williams & Wilkins Co, 1979.

6. Shopsin B (ed): *Manic Illness.* New York, Raven Press, 1979.

7. Glick RA, et al: *Psychiatric Emergencies.* New York, Grune & Stratton, Inc, 1976.

8. Balis GU (ed): *Clinical Psychopathology.* Boston, Butterworth Publishers, Inc, 1978.

9. Freedman AM, et al (eds): *Modern Synopsis of Comprehensive Textbook of Psychiatry.* Baltimore, Williams & Wilkins Co, 1972.

10. Weismann AD, Worden JW: Risk-rescue rating in suicide assessment. *Arch Gen Psychiatry* 26:554, 1972.

Social and Behavioral Considerations

"Domestic Violence" (Chapter 38) deals with the impact of domestic violence as seen daily in the emergency department. Relevant material is also included in "Major Trauma" (Chapter 7), "Orthopedic Emergencies" (Chapter 8), "Minor Lacerations and Abrasions" (Chapter 10), "Burns" (Chapter 21), "Poisoning and Drug Overdose" (Chapter 24), "Child Abuse" (Chapter 26), "Sexual Abuse" (Chapter 27), "Rape and Sexual Assault" (Chapter 65), and "Head and Neck Emergencies" (Section XIII). The author dispels some myths of domestic violence, carefully summarizes the criminal and civil laws that relate to domestic violence, and identifies the theories that may help to explain this behavior. The management of patients of domestic violence and the various impediments to their care are presented. "Psychiatric Emergencies" (Section VII), and "Grief and Loss" (Chapter 41) might also be considered with this subject.

Social, economic, and cultural factors affect the practice of emergency care both subtly and overtly. Increasing numbers of patients with heterogeneous backgrounds may choose to utilize emergency departments. These two facts prompted the presentation of "Sociocultural Considerations" (Chapter 39). Folk medicine treatments that may initiate or aggravate medical conditions are discussed, and the various cultural factors and practices that influence a patient's response to pain, blood, body image, hospitals, and traditional medications are described.

The inclusion of "Emotional and Spiritual Support" (Chapter 40) and "Grief and Loss" (Chapter 41) is unique in a textbook of emergency medicine. In these chapters, the authors describe models of emotional and spiritual support for emergency care patients and their families.

38. Emergency Management of Domestic Violence

CARMEN GERMAINE WARNER, R.N., M.S.N., F.A.A.N.

Throughout the past decade emergency care professionals have witnessed a change in the identification and acceptance of victims of both social and domestic violence. Rape victims, for example, have benefited from improved standards of care, an increased level of understanding by professionals, and the efficiency of reporting and prosecuting. However, victims of domestic violence, including both men and women, are just now receiving better and more appropriate care as a result of enhanced public recognition and understanding. Considerable effort and attention must be generated to attain the level of excellence required to afford these patients the proper assessment and intervention required for both their physiologic and their psychological trauma.

Protocol design and implementation are being required to promote quality care. Concomitant with this mandate is the increased consciousness raising of personnel through the media and broad-based community education programs. As a result, there has been a greater understanding of the problem along with the acceptance that this need for improved quality care is evident in emergency departments throughout the country.

INCIDENCE OF DOMESTIC VIOLENCE

Professionals working with patients of domestic violence indicate that it is virtually impossible to assess accurately the incidence of domestic violence. Data collected to project an estimated degree of occurrence come primarily from crime reports, police files, and emergency department admittance reports. These results indicate that one-third to one-half of all family relationships experience some form of domestic violence, focusing on both male and female spouse abuse and assault.[1-3] Police records also note that domestic disputes and disturbances comprise the highest percentage of all police calls.[4]

The results of these numerous domestic encounters are observed in the emergency department daily. Some patients provide an accurate history of the real incident, the causative factors, and the resulting impact. Others mask, defend, and deny the implications and reality of the problem, presenting personnel with the difficulty of timely and appropriate assessment and intervention.

The examples shown below are presented to acquaint emergency care professionals with the reality of domestic violence. It is hoped that these statistics may serve as signals for inquiry of possible masked incidence of male and female domestic violence.

- Kansas City: 85 percent of domestic homicide cases involved persons who had previously required intervention by law enforcement personnel at least once.[5]
- Detroit: 63 percent of the homicides concerned conflicts related to perception of sex roles.[5]
- El Paso County Court: 72.3 percent of court complaints involved physical violence.[6]
- Baltimore: 65.5 percent of all murders involved people who were friends or relatives.[5]

- California: 33 percent of all female homicides in 1971 were committed by their husbands.[5]
- New York State: 14,000 wife abuse cases were taken to court in 1973.[5]
- Boston: 70 percent of all assault patients seen in the emergency department were attacked at home.[5]
- St. Paul: 100 cases of wife beating were reported each week (this includes just those women who choose to press charges).[5]
- Maryland: 50 percent of all marriages involved some degree of physical abuse.[7]
- Washington, D.C.: 35 percent incidence of domestic violence was noted in emergency departments.[8]

The dimensions of domestic violence strike a realistic note only when they touch our personal lives. Until that time, the existing myths remain just myths and must be consciously dealt with each time a patient enters the emergency department. Understanding these myths (Table 38–1) will aid personnel to better appreciate the dynamics of the problem.

TABLE 38–1   Domestic Violence Myths

Common Myths	Existing Facts
The incidence of female domestic violence is not a common occurrence.	In over 70 percent of domestic disturbance calls, the female is the complainant.[9]
Males are not beaten by their female partners.	There is an equal number of husbands battered by their wives as women abused by their husbands.[10]
Domestic violence is a lower-class phenomenon.	Domestic violence occurs in all classes; in fact, the higher the educational level, the greater the acceptance.[8]
These "occasional" family disputes result in minor slaps and shakings.	Seven percent of wives and 0.6 percent of husbands are victims of serious abuse.[10]
The man or woman must have done or said something to precipitate the assault.	Among 77 percent of women surveyed, the physical assault was not preceded by a verbal confrontation.[8]
Aggression is inherent in a person's nature.	Violent, aggressive behavior is a result of conditioning, reinforcement, and learned behavior.[11]
Abused individuals do not have to remain in the abusive situation.	Family commitment, financial needs, fear, and loneliness are factors that contribute to the need to remain in the relationship.[8]

LEGAL IMPLICATIONS

Professionals intervening in cases of domestic violence recognize that legal ramifications frequently arise and present problems similar to those in rape. Because more men and women are referring their domestic problems to a court of law, emergency care personnel are confronted with the need to recognize and participate in the legal process.

Each state addresses and enforces specific legal regulations that should be thoroughly examined and analyzed prior to becoming involved in the legal system. Recognizing the broad diversification of laws concerning domestic disputes, including those both minor and violent in nature, a summary of criminal and civil laws at the state level is provided in Appendix 38–A.

THEORIES OF DOMESTIC VIOLENCE

Several theories have been identified that attempt to explain the violent behavior of domestic violence.[12,13] These include conflict theory, cultural theory, psychopathology theory, general systems theory, resource theory, and status inconsistency.

Conflict Theory

Conflict theory emphasizes violence as a means of bringing about social change and, thereby, maintaining the viability of a social unit.[12] The conflict perspective views the struggles between individuals and groups as normal and necessary parts of individual growth and societal development. Because conflict and tension are usually considered to be detrimental to group cohesiveness, conflict theory is not a popular theory. Visible cases of abuse represent just the tip of the iceberg; underneath the surface is a vast amount of conflict and violence between family members. Rejection of the conflict theory serves to perpetuate an idealized myth of familial love and gentleness that, while useful in preserving the integrity of the family as an important institution, prevents recognition and analysis of the widespread occurrence of violence in the family setting.[12]

Cultural Theory

Cultural theory emphasizes approval of violence in the value system of society and the social norms that indicate under what circumstances violence is to be used. It has been emphasized that the present cultural approval of physical punishment is one of the factors that lays the groundwork for child abuse, with the solution to the problem being development of both informal and legal prohibitions of physical punishment and replacement of physical force in child rearing with nonviolent parenting.[14]

Psychopathology Theory

The psychopathology theory argues that violence between family members is the result of abnormal psychological characteristics of a particular family member. Despite the fact that researchers[15–17] have identified abusive nature with respect to psychopathology, there is strong opposition[12,18] to psychopathology theory and assertions that only a small portion of those using violence can be determined to be mentally ill.

General Systems Theory

The general systems theory views abuse as a systemic product rather than a product of individual behavior pathology. This theory specifies positive feedback processes, which produce an upward spiral of violence, and a negative feedback process, which dampens the spiral and helps maintain the level of violence within tolerable limits.

As noted by Straus,[19] violence tends to increase through such processes as:

- labeling persons as violent, thus encouraging them to play out the violent role through the expectations of other family members
- creating a secondary conflict over the use of violence to settle the original conflict
- reinforcing the use of violence if the violent person achieves desired results
- developing of role expectations and self-concepts such as tough or violent.

Any of these circumstances may perpetuate violence, which will then stabilize through the use of dampening processes or escalate until the family unit is destroyed by divorce, desertion, or murder.[19]

Resource Theory

Resource theory states that violence is a resource that tends to be used to achieve desired ends when other resources such as money, respect, shared goals, and love are lacking or insufficient.[20]

Status Inconsistency

In status inconsistency, which is closely related to resource theory, it is recorded that violence is most common in families in which the classically dominant member fails to possess the superior skills, talents, or resources on which one's preferred superior status is presumed to be legitimately based.

IMPACT OF SOCIOECONOMIC STATUS ON DOMESTIC VIOLENCE

Emergency care personnel addressing the needs of patients of domestic violence must keep in mind the cross-culture dynamics of this problem. Specific considerations to be applied by emergency care personnel throughout the assessment and intervention process are noted below:

- There is little difference between white and blue collar acceptance of domestic violence.[21]
- Income levels are not a predictable indicator of violent behavior, although a greater percentage of violence occurs in families having lower prestige jobs than their neighbors.[1]
- The prevalence of domestic violence is as common in upper and middle class as poor families. However, data are more readily available for poor families because they must utilize public services more frequently.[22] This influences the data, making it appear as if poor families possess a greater incidence of domestic violence when, actually, they do not.
- Wives from working class families appear to have stronger resources, have less fear, and have more control over their lives than middle-class women.[23] Middle- and upper-class women are concerned about society's reaction and maintain taboos against taking their husband to court, calling the police, or admitting they had been battered.

BARRIERS TO IDENTIFICATION AND TREATMENT

Despite the increased awareness of domestic violence, along with an expanded understanding of the related dynamics and influencing factors, there still are numerous inhibitors that affect the quality care provided in the emergency department. The presence of these inhibitors does, in fact, retard and impede the intervention process and must be realistically addressed.

Professionals should enjoy the privilege of maintaining their individual views and attitudes concerning society. Just as these views do not interfere with the quality care provided a trauma patient, a victim of domestic violence must also be treated as a complete person with physical injuries, psychological disruptions, and emotional fears and anxieties. Specific inhibitors that exist between emergency care personnel and these patients are discussed below.[24]

Family

Historically, the family's right to privacy has been rigorously protected in educational, legal, medical, and religious spheres. Emergency care professionals are reluctant to "invade" family boundaries, and family members hesitate to reveal problems as family centered, choosing instead to handle domestic disputes within the home. Consequently, professionals confronted with domestic violence may succumb to the dangerous belief that the sanctity of the family system dictates a position of noninvolvement. A healthier approach would be to recognize that the members of a dysfunctional family may not be able to help themselves without assistance from a skilled outsider.

Historical Precedent

There is a historical precedent for wives being treated as property or children. As such, wives become an acceptable target for corporal punishment. A consequence of this kind of thinking is that an abused woman is not viewed as having a problem other than her unwillingness to fulfill her obligation to please the man who "owns" her. Emergency care professionals who excuse violent occurrences because one of the spouses "asked for it" unwittingly sabotage treatment. The professional must help the patient distinguish between violent acts (always totally unacceptable) and contributing factors over which the patient has some control.

In some cases, violent outbursts are rationalized on the basis of cultural stereotypes, presuming that violence within a particular group of people is the norm. While some groups of people may tend to express themselves physically more often than others, the misinformed belief that violence is to be tolerated within certain groups falsely excuses professionals from intervening with the very people whose need may be most acute.

Definition of Violence

Individuals who are chronically exposed to extreme forms of violence, either in their job or personal milieu, tend to become impervious to lesser forms of violence. A slashed arm seems minor compared with a gunshot wound. Likewise, a kick in the abdomen may be perceived as trivial compared with the slashed arm. A person who has been repeatedly roughly shaken and pinched by a spouse may not be perceived as a victim of violence at all. This dulled state of perception is pathologic, particularly in terms of prevention, early identification, and treatment of domestic violence. A corollary of a dulled state of perception is the patient's tendency to use nonspecific descriptors and minimizing language to deny the seriousness of the situation to themselves and others. Although there are many psychosocial reasons for the patient's denial, what is most important is that imprecise language is used and that professionals must anticipate it, recognize it, interpret it, and validate it with the patient. A classic example is the woman who reports, "I yelled at my husband and then we had a fight." After persistent questioning, which required the victim to specify the details of her experience, it was learned that the victim yelled obscenities at her husband after he chased her from room to room threatening to kill her. The "fight" consisted of his kicking and punching her in the head, chest, and abdomen.

The Patient or Victim

Patients of domestic violence often impede helping agencies from mobilizing on their behalf. Along with requests for assistance, they simultaneously exhibit overwhelming dependency, passivity, and even open resistance to change, which can infuriate professionals who are independent, self-motivated, and efficient problem solvers. The thought of leaving a known but oppressive environment engenders a state of ambivalence within the victim, which may be interpreted as disinterest or laziness, rather than immobilizing psychic conflict. A female victim may fear leaving the relationship because she believes she is incapable of surviving outside of it; she dreads retribution by the assailant; the thought of single parenthood is intolerable; and, perceiving her partner's fragility, she fears his self-destruction if she leaves. Simultaneously, the patient fears remaining in the relationship because she can no longer cope with its chronic, unpredictable stress, she values her children's well-being, and she dreads continuing a potentially lethal relationship. Patients are often psychologically and physiologically debilitated by the time they seek professional help. They lack the energy to reflect objectively on the severity of their past history and cannot conceptualize an improved future. It is only through persistence and tenaciousness on the part of the emergency care professional that domestic violence patients can sufficiently restore their resources in order to choose healthy alternatives to their current situation.

Element of Blame

Most people believe that "you get what you deserve" and "you reap what you sow." Unfortunately, the world is not always a rational or logical place. It is rather unsettling to believe that events beyond our control could influence our lives in severely destructive ways. Adopting the "it could never happen to me" philosophy is a defense against the realization that everyone is susceptible to bad fortune and bad judgment. Believing that people get what they deserve and denying that the "innocent" may be victimized lead to the rationalization that patients must be blamed for their misfortunes.

The emergency care professional must assist the patient and others to distinguish between "blame-ability" and "response-ability." The fact that a woman chooses a series of abusive mates is not cause for blame. Each abusive encounter will reinforce the woman's own sense of worthlessness and the worthlessness of women in general. Masochistic behavior should not be reinforced by health care providers who subtly imply that it is the patient's fault for choosing such partners. Rather, professionals must communicate that these patients can get help in regaining control over their lives and assume responsibility for their actions.

Professional Impotence

A lack of education and training regarding current useful approaches for domestic violence patients, the general underdeveloped "state of the art," and a lack of community resources contribute to the professional's feelings of inadequacy in treating patients of domestic violence. Feelings of helplessness may be particularly aroused when treating a patient who has been in a violent situation for years and has already made several unsuccessful attempts to get help. While this patient might appear to have a poorer prognosis than the patient seeking help for the first time, many who eventually get out of abusive relationships are older, have been involved in abusive relationships longer, and have sought help before. Once professionals receive adequate education and training in this area, feelings of inadequacy in treating domestic violence patients should decrease.

Common Response

Domestic violence situations can be extremely affectively laden and may produce strong responses from the well-meaning but naive care giver. Overreaction by the helping person may result in frightening the patient into silence or, even worse, into defending the assailant. This prevents the patient from assessing personal feelings and needs. The patient's task is to recognize, express, and channel anger constructively. Therefore, treatment must remain focused on the patient, not on the outraged professional.

Excusing the Assailant

Domestic violence incidents too frequently evoke pity and compassion for the assailant. Observation of the assailant's solicitous concern and apologetic behavior toward the patient may result in professionals encouraging the couple to continue the relationship despite evidence of a long history of abuse. Recommending counseling while the couple continues living together is a risky option at best. Certainly, the assailant requires professional help, but this requirement in no way diminishes the patient's need to be extricated from the abusive situation.

MANAGEMENT OF PATIENTS OF DOMESTIC VIOLENCE

The physical and emotional trauma of both men and women is addressed by surgeons, obstetricians, internists, pediatricians, and psychiatrists, as well as emergency care personnel on a daily basis.

It has been noted that abused women seek medical attention more frequently than nonabused women, with the patient/physician interaction being the sole confidential contact possible for them.[25] This stresses the importance for emergency care personnel to assess and manage properly men and women who enter the emergency department as patients of domestic violence.

The necessity of this assessment/intervention process, occurring during the initial emergency visit, is concomitant with the belief that intervention as a result of a crisis is more likely to have impact, can prevent serious morbidity, and can aid in the resolution of the crisis if intervention occurs during the acute phase of emergency entrance.[26]

Assessment Process

Despite recognition that abused patients are seeking medical attention at an increasing rate, emergency care personnel must remember that not all patients will openly identify themselves as being abused. In fact, it is common for patients to disguise their apparent trauma and to correlate it with other nonrelated incidents. In order to assist emergency care personnel in the assessment process, several factors should be understood.

Identify the Profile of an Abused Woman

Emergency care personnel will discover portions of this profile to be helpful for many patients, but special consideration should be taken to assess each situation individually. Factors in the profile of an abused woman are noted below:[8]

- recurrent soft tissue injuries
- recurrent admissions to the emergency department
- identification as being accident prone
- injuries to specific parts of the "body map" (see Table 38–2)
- masking of true causes for injuries
- previously abused physically
- witnessed abuse of a parent when young
- sexually abused as a child
- record of being raped by a husband or boyfriend
- misuse of alcohol or drugs by patient or partner
- attempts at suicide
- feelings of depression
- frequent complaints of pain
- unstable marriage.

Identify the Profile of an Abused Man

The profile of an abused man may prove to be less defined than that of a woman and must be applied carefully as a base point for further assessment and problem identification. The incidence of male abuse is subject to considerable question, recognizing that the level of comfort in the reporting process is very low. Not until there exists an openness in seeking medical and psychological assistance will professionals witness an accurate data base. The profile of an abused man shown below should be carefully reviewed and used only as a basis for further questioning:

- manifests injuries primarily on legs, back, head, or shoulders
- presents with injuries reflecting use of a hard or sharp object, rather than general bruising or beating
- has serious injuries requiring emergency attention

TABLE 38–2   Body Indicators of Trauma

Domestic Violence Trauma	Nondomestic Violence Trauma
Head	Forearm
Face	Wrist
Chest	Hands
Breast	Lower legs
Abdomen	Ankle
Buttocks	Feet
Back	
Bodily injury during pregnancy	

- maintains strong, rigid expectations of each parent's specific role
- has body size or shape not relevant to the type or degree of injury
- indicates on questioning that verbal aggression led to physical aggression.

Outline Characteristics Affecting Abuse

Emergency care personnel throughout the intervention process, whether related to domestic violence or not, are responsible for instituting teaching and prevention techniques whenever possible. In an attempt to assess a family unit that might generate violent behavior, certain family characteristics should be noted.[13]

- the amount of time family members spend with each other. This time is known as "time at risk."
- the diversification and wide range of interests and activities involving family members. In essence, the greater the areas of interaction, the greater is the potential of opportunities for conflict.
- the appreciation of the fact that these numerous activities overlap, causing potential competition
- the intense level of emotional involvement in the family unit. Specific activities that are central to family interaction involve a great deal more frustration than other types of activities.
- the presumed right of family members to discuss and influence other members of the family. Comments and suggestions are much more fully interchanged among family members than nonfamily members.
- the varying outlooks on life that exist by the mere fact that men and women frequently experience different views on the same subject
- the fact that family roles are, to a certain degree, assigned on the basis of age and sex rather than on the basis of ability or interest
- the nature of family membership itself, that for children being completely involuntary and for spouses only semivoluntary. The commitment to family is basically very strong; even if there were no legal parameters, it would be difficult to end a marriage.
- the existence of privacy within a family. This is an important factor because, in essence, it insulates the entire unit from friends and relatives.

Awareness of some of these characteristics should aid emergency care personnel in understanding the existence of conflict concomitant with interpersonal support and love in each family seen in the emergency department. This understanding, laced with crisis intervention skills and awareness of community network systems, provides a critical part in the assessment/intervention process.

Clarify Specific Types of Injuries

It is essential that emergency care personnel accurately assess patients of domestic violence. In situations in which the patient freely admits his or her situation, minimal difficulty exists. However, when the patient masks the fact that domestic trauma has occurred, personnel should use other techniques of assessment (Table 38–2).

Special notation should be made of any injury occurring during pregnancy. A pending or completed miscarriage frequently occurs in battered women. The following incidence of reported miscarriage, abortions, and rape may be helpful to emergency care personnel throughout the assessment process:[25]

- Abused women experience a miscarriage at the rate of 1 in 4.
- Nonabused women experience a miscarriage at the rate of 1 in 15.
- Abused women of all socioeconomic backgrounds choose a legal abortion more frequently than nonabused women.
- Abused women are reported as "victims" of rape by boyfriends and husbands eight times as frequently as nonabused women.

Identify Psychological Aspects of Abuse

Very little is known about the complex psychological aspects of spouse abuse; yet it is essential for emergency care personnel to understand some of the factors that trigger it.

In a study involving 100 abused women, 71 were reported to be taking antidepressants or tranquilizers, presumably because they were depressed or distressed by a particular situation.[26] Of these 100 women, 21 were diagnosed as depressed, while 34 attempted to poison themselves. Other factors common to these women were:

- All had disastrous marriages.
- Fifty-eight percent had not experienced the traditional courtship and engagement routine.
- Eighty-five percent experienced premarital sexual interaction without the benefit of contraception.
- Sixty percent were pregnant prior to marriage.
- Twenty-five percent actually were abused prior to marriage.

Although these were characteristics of one particular study, other data that identify some of the common findings in abused women include:[27,28]

- has low self-esteem
- is dependent and fearful of loss of support
- manifests a passive personality
- has few friends
- maintains a terrible sense of insecurity
- is afraid to be alone
- is unable to resist abuse because this is foreign to their passive personalities
- believes all myths about battered relationships
- strongly believes in family unit
- accepts responsibility for the batterer's actions
- suffers from guilt, yet denies the terror and anger felt
- presents a passive face to the world but has the strength to manipulate enough to prevent further violence and to prevent being killed
- has severe stress reactions with psychophysical complaints
- uses sex as a way to establish intimacy
- believes that no one will be able to help resolve the predicament except themselves.

Patients seen in the emergency department do not exhibit a profile inclusive of all these characteristics; yet emergency care personnel can use these factors as indicators of potential abusive problems impacting on both men and women.

Apply Specific Questioning Techniques

Emergency care personnel who have gained an information base concerning patients of domestic violence may be better able to manage not only the patients who openly admit to being abused but also those who mask the real causative factors of the trauma. Personnel may be reluctant to inquire directly about the nature of the injury, assuming the patient does not wish to discuss it.

On the contrary, patients who have been abused are frightened, lonely, overwhelmed, embarrassed, and desperately need to share their dilemma with someone. This is evident even when they may deny its reality. Examples of direct questions that may be helpful when seeking information concerning possible abuse include the following:[24]

- Have you ever been in a relationship in which you have been hit, punched, kicked, or hurt in any way? Are you in such a relationship now?
- How does your mate act when he/she is drinking? Is he/she verbally or physically abusive?
- Have there been any times during your relationship when you have had physical fights?
- You have mentioned that your mate loses his/her temper with the children. How are things between the two of you?

- You seem to have some special concern about your mate. Can you tell me more about this? Are you fearful? Has he/she ever hurt you?
- Do your verbal fights also include physical contact?
- Many individuals tell me they argue with their boy/girl friends and later state they have been beaten. Could this be happening to you? Are you being beaten?
- Sometimes when mates are overprotective and as jealous as you describe, they react strongly and use physical force. Is this happening in your situation?
- I notice you have a number of bruises. Would you tell me how they happened?

SPECIAL CONSIDERATIONS OF THE OLDER ABUSED INDIVIDUAL

Instances involving abuse of the elderly, like other forms of abuse, are increasing in recognition, identification, and intervention. This form of abuse, similar to other abusive acts, involves not single attacks but recurring events. Older men are being battered and abused, but it is more common for older women to be abused. In these instances, the abusers are usually female. This pattern develops because there are more elderly women than men and most individuals caring for these women, despite the relationship, are younger women.

Certain factors contributing to the vulnerability of older people are that they are:

- less mobile than younger individuals
- dependent on the individual inflicting the abuse
- financially exploited by those caring for them
- being physically beaten as well as mentally abused
- being abused by individuals who themselves have serious problems
- afflicted with age-related diseases that may make their care more difficult
- unable to leave and uproot their present living situation
- afraid they will be sent to a nursing home
- fearful of being left alone
- not suited for the present design of shelters.

THE INTERVENTION PROCESS

To many patients their arrival at the emergency department is their first contact with any system. The initial support, understanding, and sensitivity provided by emergency care personnel will greatly influence whether these patients will obtain and maintain contact with the law enforcement, social service, and health care system.

Regardless of the length of the emergency department visit, it is essential for personnel to introduce materials covering appropriate referrals and information concerning filing a complaint. The greater the understanding of current problems confronting these patients, the easier it will be for personnel to design and implement appropriate methods of management. The following guidelines have been developed in an effort to assist emergency care personnel in assessing and designing appropriate referral and evaluation components of intervention.

Assessment

Assessment of pertinent data should be obtained from the patient, family, friends, law enforcement personnel, community violence advocates, and first responders.

Environmental Assessment

- condition upon arrival; whether patient is hesitant or open with personnel
- factors concerning admission (alone or accompanied by another)
- time span between incident and emergency department admission
- interaction between patient and accompanying family or friends
- level of comfort displayed by patient toward personnel
- existing lines of communication
- relationship of this incident with existing stressors in life
- comparison of this incident with previous abuse visits.

Physical Abuse Assessment

- repeated abuse on certain portions of the body, including the head and face
- noted recurrence of injuries and bruises on body parts frequently covered by clothing, such as buttocks, thighs, breasts, chest, and abdomen.

Emotional Assessment

- level and evidence of such emotions as fear, anger, guilt, depression, lack of confidence or self-esteem, shame, or despair
- manner of misdirecting their feelings in physical destruction rather than verbally.

Design

Designing the framework for establishing and coordinating priorities of care, along with preparation of personnel, equipment, and procedures, is a critical second step:

- Design and develop a special social and domestic violence team.
- Design and develop a management protocol for social and domestic violence patients.
- Conduct staff training and development, incorporating the knowledge and skills contained in the established protocol. Topics to be covered include commonalities of social and domestic violence; theoretical concept of violent behavior (myths, trends, and current studies); family systems theory; recommended assessment and management techniques; specific communication techniques; interviewing techniques; and networking with law enforcement, justice, legal, and community support systems.
- Require certification of personnel in the area of social and domestic violence.
- Implement protocol recommendations: special team on call and network of resources to activate immediately.
- Develop a monitoring system.
- Incorporate an evaluation and feedback component.
- Admit the patient immediately.
- Maintain total privacy for patient, family, and friends.
- Incorporate standards of quality care through approved protocols.
- Establish an environment of honesty, support, and trust.
- Stress the importance and worth of self.
- Gather information as privately as possible.
- Note the specific history and physical examination (Exhibit 38–1).
- Recognize the importance and legal requirements of photographs, patient teaching, and consent forms.

Intervention

Immediate stabilization and intervention of these patients must be fulfilled, recognizing the cause of the injuries as well as the cure. Special considerations for emergency care personnel include:

- Recognize the psychological state as being unique from other patients and attend to them immediately.

- Remain cognizant of nonverbal behavior. If personnel are hostile or biased, replace them with personnel who are open and comfortable dealing with these patients.
- Provide specific intervention for trauma-related problems.
- Notify the appropriate authorities if rape, a gunshot wound, or a stabbing occurred.
- Document specific verbal and nonverbal interaction, along with emergency personnel impressions and reactions.
- Record the patient's emotional state in addition to physical appearance.

An example of a physician's assessment and intervention report is noted in Figure 38–1.

Referral and Networking Procedures

Emergency care personnel must assess the need for the patient to be admitted, transferred, or referred. Regardless of specific transfer or referral, the hospital social service department must be contacted and a visit requested while the patient is still in the emergency department.

The potential for physical transfer to a psychiatric facility, a rehabilitation center, an emergency shelter, or a community center must be recognized, and the patient should be assisted in contacting crisis hotlines, shelters, and law enforcement personnel. Some or all of the following resources can be mobilized:

- medical institutions for birth control, abortions, and tubal ligations in the case of female victims, along with good medical and mental health care
- social service agencies for financial aid, child protective services, food stamps, clothing, day care, housing, and emergency shelter
- criminal justice agencies for protection against further violence
- legal aid for assistance with warrants, court procedures, separation, and divorce agreements
- vocational rehabilitation agencies for financial assistance and information about educational pursuits, job training, and employment counseling
- women's or men's groups for information, support, and shelter.

In addition, patient and family teaching sessions can be incorporated into the patient's follow-up care and preventive health maintenance ideas can be presented.

Evaluation

The level of excellence in care provided these patients must be monitored, being careful to note the patient's

Exhibit 38–1 Spouse Abuse Emergency Examination Protocol

I. History
  A. Present incident
    1. Day, time, and location of abuse
    2. Force applied
      a. Specific types of violence
      b. Verbal and nonverbal threats
      c. Use of restraints
      d. Use of alcohol or drugs (by assailant)
      e. Loss of consciousness
    3. Type of abuse
      a. Beatings (hand, object)
      b. Objects thrown at patient
      c. Patient being thrown against object
      d. Use of weapon
      e. Inflicted wound due to weapon
      f. Shaken, shoved, kicked, or hit
    4. Type of complaint
      a. Headaches
      b. Choking sensations
      c. Hyperventilation
      d. Gastrointestinal symptoms
      e. Allergic phenomena
      f. Asthma
      g. Chest pain
      h. Back pain
      i. Pelvic pain
    5. Present situation
      a. Location and safety of the children
      b. Notation of assailant's location
      c. Who accompanied the patient to emergency department
  B. Past incidents
    1. Repeat abuses and injuries
    2. Time, sequence of past abuse
    3. Pattern of injury
    4. Patient's response to each injury
    5. Whether patient returned home after each episode
    6. Attempted suicide
    7. Suspected child abuse by either parent
    8. Use of alcohol or drugs by patient
  C. Health history
    1. Current medications
    2. Allergies
    3. Current treatment or health care regimen
II. Physical Examination
  A. Assessment of airway, breathing, and circulation
  B. Inspection of outer garments for evidence of violence (e.g., torn clothing, blood, stains)
  C. Examination of skin for signs of bruises, lacerations, or contusions
  D. Examination of head, eyes, ears, nose, mouth, and throat for trauma
  E. Examination of extremities, ribs, and skull for evidence of fractures
  F. Examination of breasts, chest, back, abdomen, and pelvic regions for signs of trauma or internal injuries
  G. Examination of entire body for signs of hidden trauma
  H. Assessment of psychological stress
III. Laboratory
  A. Color photography
    1. Evidence of trauma or restraint while patient dressed
    2. Evidence of trauma or restraint while patient undressed
    3. Notation of who took the photographs, who is in the photographs, the day, date, and time
  B. Blood samples (as deemed appropriate)
    1. Complete blood cell count
    2. Blood chemistry profiles
    3. Drug and alcohol screen
  C. Urine samples (as deemed appropriate)
    1. Urinalysis
    2. Drug screen
IV. Radiography (as deemed appropriate)
  A. Skull radiographs
  B. Radiographs of extremities
  C. Chest radiographs
  D. Computerized axial tomographic scan

1. Date of Assault _______________________ .

2. Statement of Complaint (use patient's own words):

3. Description of Assault (use patient's own words):
   a. Specific detail and chronology of assault:
   b. Pain and symptoms mentioned:

4. Check physical findings:

	Contusions	Abrasions	Lacerations	Bleeding	Fracture	Other (Specify)
Head						
Ears						
Nose						
Cheeks						
Mouth						
Neck						
Shoulders						
Arms						
Hands						
Chest						
Back						
Abdomen						
Genitalia						
Buttocks						
Legs						
Feet						

5. Describe presence of trauma. Indicate location, appearance, and size. Indicate possible source such as teeth, cigarette burns, etc.:

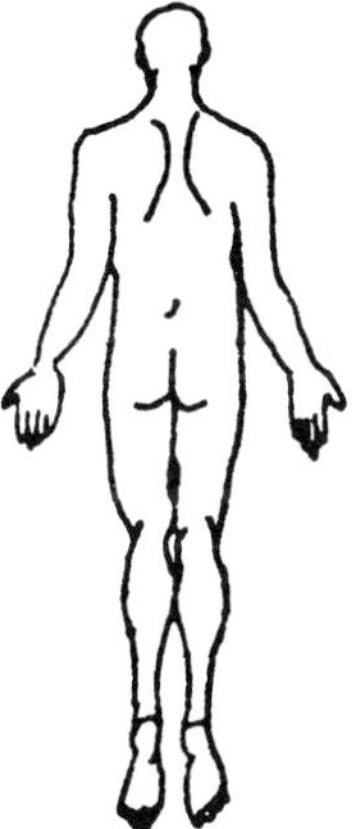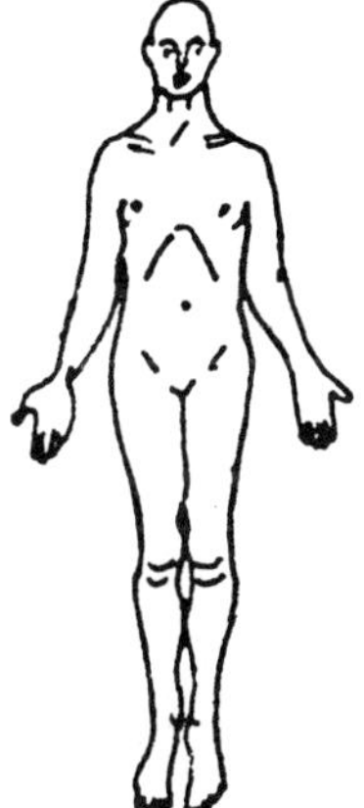

6. Internal injury:

7. Previous assaults (describe injuries and treatment):

8. Additional comments:

9. Assessment:

10. Consultations (service and consultant):

______________________________   ______________________________

______________________________   ______________________________

Figure 38–1   Domestic Violence Victim's Assessment and Treatment Report. (*Source:* Goldberg W, Carey A: Domestic Violence Victims in the Emergency Setting. *Topics in Emergency Medicine* 3: 71, 1982. Reprinted with permission of Aspen Systems Corporation, © 1982.)

Mental Health Consultant

I. *History of Current Abusive Relationship*	*Specific Comments*

I. *History of Current Abusive Relationship*
  A. Relationship to assailant (circle):
     Married   Friend
     Divorced   Ex-friend
           Separated
  B. Living arrangement (circle):
     Cohabit   Separate
  C. Length of relationship:
  D. Onset of abuse:
  E. Frequency of abuse:
     1) How often:
     2) Abuse pattern is (circle):
        Increasing   Staying the same
              Decreasing
  F. Types of abuse (circle):
     Verbal   Mobility Restriction
     Battering   Phone Restriction
     Sexual   Economic
           Other (specify)
  G. Instruments of abuse (circle):
     Gun   Fire
     Knife   Hot substance
     Blunt object   Cord
           Other (specify)
  H. Descriptive quality of assault (circle):
     Ritualistic   Slow rise in tension
     Impulsive   Other (specify)
  I. Coincidental Factors:

	Victim	Assailant
Alcohol		
Drugs		
Argument		
Omission		
Commission		
Other (specify)		

  J. Behavior after assault(s) (circle):
     Reconciliation   Terminate relationship
     Leave scene   Contact friend
     Contact relative Other (specify)
  K. Attempts to leave relationship (describe):
  L. Supportive resources (circle):
     Family   Employer
     Friends   Other (specify)
  M. The overall relationship is changing in the following way (circle):
     Much worse   Better
     Worse   Much better
           Same
II. *Education Level* (circle highest):
    1   2   3   4   5   6   7   8   9   10   11   12
    GED
    Post High School (specify) ___________________________________
    Graduate Education (specify) _________________________________
    Other Education (specify) ___________________________________
III. *Employment Summary*
    Current: ___________________________________
    Past: ___________________________________
IV. *Children*

Name	Sex	Date of Birth	Place of Residence	Well Being	Comments

Figure 38–1   continued

V. *Summary of Past Abusive Relationships*

   A. Adult: _______________________________________

   B. Child: _______________________________________

VI. *Mental Status* (circle)

above average intelligence   average intelligence   below average intelligence   mentally retarded   alert   disoriented   short-term memory intact   long-term memory intact   depressed   elated   fearful   angry   flat   passive   demanding   manipulative   labile   apathetic   agitated   bizarre   poverty of ideas   flight of ideas   loose associations   delusional   paranoid   suicidal   homicidal   drug abuse   alcohol abuse

Additional comments:

VII. *Alternative Place(s) of Residence*   _______ Yes   _______ No

   Name: Name:

   Address: Address:

   Telephone: Telephone:

VIII. *Contact Person(s)*

   Name: Name:

   Address: Address:

   Telephone: Telephone:

   Relationship: Relationship:

IX. *Victim's Goals*

   A. Short-term:

   B. Long-term:

X. *Assessment*

   A. Present danger:

   B. Problem solving ability:

   C. Needs:

   D. Readiness for intervention:

   E. General impressions:

XI. *Recommendations*

XII. *Victim's Plan* (if known)

XIII. *Final Disposition*

____
Signature

Figure 38–1   continued

---

reaction and interaction with implemented and proposed care. A follow-up intervention plan to determine quality and appropriateness of care and a procedure of quality assurance should be implemented while being careful to maintain a mechanism of patient evaluation and feedback.

Throughout this assessment, design, implementation, referral, and evaluation process, the underlying common thread is to develop a strong element of trust that will provide the foundation for cooperative, immediate, short-term and long-term intervention.

SUMMARY

Throughout the past decade emergency care professionals have witnessed an increase in the number of domestic violence patients who enter the emergency department. Concomitantly, personnel have experienced a consciousness raising that has alerted them not only to the sensitivities of this problem but also to the indicators leading to proper assessment and intervention techniques.

The professional growth occurring during these past years has not been without its barriers and resistance. Professionals, frequently experiencing similar personal situations, try to avoid caring for these patients because of the inner struggle it presents, while others unfamiliar with the reality of this problem find the problems of patients to be time consuming and annoying.

With the increase in recommended approaches for physical management comes the importance of understanding and implementing psychological and sociological considerations. Only through a consistent network of approaches addressing the total patient can there be any opportunity for rectifying the situation and preventing further violent episodes. Emergency care professionals must coordinate their role with that of their peers, the patient, family members, and the community to help minimize the devastating impact of domestic violence.

REFERENCES

1. Gelles R: *The Violent Home.* Beverly Hills, Calif, Sage Publishers, 1972.

2. Levinger G: Sources of marital dissatisfactions among applicants for divorce. *Am J Orthopsychiatry* 36:803–807, 1966.

3. Walker L: *The Battered Woman.* New York, Harper & Row, 1979.

4. Stephens DW: Domestic assault: The police response, in Roy M (ed): *Battered Women: A Psychosociological Study of Domestic Violence.* New York, Van Nostrand Reinhold, 1977.

5. *A Monograph on Services to Battered Women*, No. (OHDS) 79–05708. US Department of Health and Human Services, Office of Human Development Services, 1979, p 6.

6. Bunyard LK: *Battered Women: An Overview of the Problem in Colorado Springs.* Denver, Colorado Springs Police Department, 1977.

7. Langley R, Levy R: Wife abuse: Why will a woman stay and take it? *New Woman* 7:89–98 (July-August) 1977.

8. Appleton W: The battered woman syndrome. *Ann Emergency Med* 9:84–91 (February) 1980.

9. Martin D: *Battered Wives.* New York, Pocket Books, 1977, pp 11–12.

10. Steinmetz SK: The battered husband syndrome. *Victimology* 2:499–509, 1978.

11. Brazill J: Violence: Dynamics of learned behavior, in Warner CG (ed): *Conflict Intervention in Social and Domestic Violence.* Bowie, Md, Robert J. Brady Co, 1981.

12. Steinmetz SK, Straus MA: *Violence in the Family.* New York, Dodd, Mead & Co, 1974.

13. Straus MA: A sociological perspective on the prevention and treatment of wife beating. *Nursing Dimensions* 11:45–63 (Spring) 1979.

14. Gil DG: Violence against children. *Marriage Family* 33:637–648 (November) 1971.

15. Young L: Parents who hate, in Steinmetz SK, Straus MA (eds): *Violence in the Family.* New York, Dodd, Mead & Co, 1974.

16. Steele BF, Pallach CB: A psychiatric study of parents who abuse infants and small children, in Hefler RE, Kempe CH (eds): *The Battered Child.* Chicago, University of Chicago Press, 1968.

17. Kempe CH, et al: The battered child syndrome. *JAMA* 171:17–24, 1962.

18. Gelles RJ: Child abuses as psychopathology: A sociological critique and reformulation. *Am J Orthopsychiatry* 43:611–621, 1973.

19. Straus MA: A general systems theory approach to a theory of violence between family members. *Soc Sci Information* 12:105–123, 1973.

20. Goode WJ: Force and violence in the family. *J Marriage Family* 33:624–636, 1971.

21. Straus MA: Normative and behavioral aspects of violence between spouses. Research paper No. VA-2. Durham, NH, University of New Hampshire, 1977.

22. Grambs, M: Wife beating as an American law. *Behavior Today*, February 1977, pp 5–6.

23. Davidson T: *Conjugal Crime: Understanding and Changing the Wife Beating Pattern.* New York, Hawthorne Books, 1978.

24. Goldberg W, Carey A: Domestic violence victims in the emergency setting. *Topics in Emergency Medicine* 3:71–73 (January) 1982.

25. Flitcraft A: Battered women: An emergency room epidemiology with a description of a clinical syndrome and critique of therapeutics. Testimony before Subcommittee on Domestic and International Scientific Planning, Analyses and Cooperation. Washington, DC, February 18, 1978.

26. Gayford JJ: Wife beating: A preliminary survey of 100 cases. *Br Med J* 1:194–197, 1975.

27. Bell JN: Rescuing the battered wife. *Hum Behavior*, June 1977, pp 16–23.

28. Walker-Hooper A: Domestic violence: Assessing the problem, in Warner CG (ed): *Conflict Intervention in Social and Domestic Violence.* Bowie, Md, Robert J. Brady Co, 1981, pp 52–57.

APPENDIX 38–A

Summary of Criminal and Civil Laws That Relate to Domestic Violence

CRIMINAL SANCTIONS

Assault and Battery—Penal Code §§ 240, 242

An assault is an attempt to commit violent injury to another person, combined with the realistic ability to inflict the injury. A battery is the actual use of force or violence upon another person. Assault and battery is the most common criminal action arising from domestic violence situations.

Because assault and battery is a misdemeanor, a police officer cannot make an arrest unless the crime is committed in his or her presence, the victim has filed a complaint with the district attorney and a warrant has been issued, or the victim makes a citizen's arrest.

Assault with a Deadly Weapon or Force Likely to Produce Great Bodily Injury—Penal Code § 245

Assault with a deadly weapon is a felony. The officer need only have a reasonable belief that the crime has been committed, and that the person arrested committed it, in order to make an arrest. Although cases of battery do not usually involve weapons such as firearms or knives, a closed fist may be regarded as a deadly weapon or force under this statute. Actual injury is not required—only the *use* of a deadly weapon or force.

Assault with Intent to Commit Murder—Penal Code § 217

Assault with intent to murder is a felony. The prosecution must prove that the batterer *intended* to kill. This intent can be shown by threats, conversations, past behavior, the amount of force used, and any other similar evidence. Despite the fact that many victims of battery believe that their assailant intends to kill them, and the fact that one of eight homicides in the United States involves violence between spouses, arrests in this situation rarely occur under this statute. This is because the "intent to kill" is difficult to prove.

Mayhem—Penal Code § 203

Mayhem is the removal, disfiguring, or disabling of a part of another person's body, such as the fingers, hands, tongue, eyes, ears, lip, or nose. This crime is relevant to cases of domestic violence in which a person loses the use of part of the body during a beating.

Assault with Intent to Commit Mayhem—Penal Code § 220

This felony requires an intent to amputate, disfigure, or disable a part of the body. An attack and injury alone will not be enough to show the assailant's intent. However, any disfigurement, such as the loss of eyesight or fingers, or a permanent scar will infer the required intent.

Possession of a Deadly Weapon with Intent to Assault—Penal Code § 467

This statute is useful in the domestic violence situation in which there have been threats without actual harm. A deadly weapon may be a gun or a knife, as well as other objects, depending on the manner in which they are intended to be used, such as books, bats, and other heavy, blunt objects.

Because it is a misdemeanor, the victim must file a complaint. The statute can be used to prevent violent confrontation, if the assailant is arrested and taken into custody. It is more likely, however, that the assailant will be released on bail or released on personal recognizance. The original situation might be aggravated, and the likelihood of violence against the victim might be increased. If a victim intends to use this law, he or

559

she may wish first to contact a shelter to arrange for a safe place to stay.

Murder and Justifiable Homicide—Penal Code §§ 187, 198, 199

Murder is the killing of another person. In some situations, however, the killing of another person is justifiable because it is done in self-defense. Showing justifiable homicide is crucial to the defense of a victim of domestic violence who kills an assailant.

To prove justifiable homicide, a victim of domestic violence must show that there was:

- resistance to the assailant's attempt to kill or seriously injure
- fear of loss of life or severe injury
- danger that was immediate and impending
- no excessive force used in defense

The requirement of immediate and impending danger means that a person must be faced with attack before killing the batterer in self-defense can be justified. As a practical matter, a person's only opportunity for self-defense may be when the assailant is off guard. Recent court cases have suggested that killing in self-defense may be justifiable under certain circumstances, even if no imminent danger exists.

Some courts have found there was no defense of justifiable homicide when the person had an opportunity to escape an attacker and did not do so. In California, however, there is no "retreat" requirement; a person attacked in the home need not retreat, and may kill in self-defense anyone who breaks into the home with felonious intent.

A person may use only as much physical force as is necessary for self-defense. Simple assault and battery or threats by an attacker will not justify killing the attacker. The court will look at many factors, including the nature of the attack, to determine the necessity of killing in self-defense.

Woman Beating—Penal Code § 273.5

This statute makes it a felony for any person to use physical force on a person of the opposite sex with whom he or she is living. Since it is a felony, the officer can make an arrest even if the officer was not present at the time of the criminal act. Generally, injuries must be visible. Prosecution may be difficult if there are no marks of injury and no medical testimony about injury suffered by the victim.

District attorneys may be reluctant to charge an assailant in a domestic dispute with a felony. Factors considered are that the higher bail on felony arrests may strain a limited family budget and that longer jail sentences for felonies can worsen an unstable relationship and family economic problems.

Disturbing the Peace—Penal Code § 415

This statute makes threatening and fighting conduct, or the use of vulgar, profane, or indecent language in the presence of a child or a woman, a misdemeanor. Visible abuse is not required. The statute may be used as a preventive measure against some forms of violence.

Peace Bond—Penal Code § 706

When the court concludes that a person may "disturb the peace," the person complained of may be required to post a peace bond of up to $5,000, enforceable for 6 months and renewable. Failure to deposit the bond with the court may result in imprisonment. If the person disturbs the peace after the bond is posted, the penalties are loss of money and possible criminal action. The peace bond is rarely used in California because of questions about its constitutionality.

Burglary—Penal Code § 459

This statute makes the entering of any house or room with intent to commit a felony illegal. The crime must be committed by someone with no right to be in the room or building. Therefore, a man who enters his own home with the intent to commit a felony cannot be guilty of burglary. A woman who has separated from her spouse and lives in a separate dwelling, however, is protected by the statute if her husband attempts to break into her separate dwelling.

Unlawful Entry—Penal Code § 602.5

This crime is a lesser crime than burglary but also involves the unauthorized entry or presence in someone else's dwelling. If the person who enters a dwelling pays the rent on the premises, he or she cannot be guilty of unlawful entry. Since it is a misdemeanor, a woman who wishes a man off her premises must make a citizen's arrest or file a complaint.

Forcible Entry and Detainer—Penal Code § 418

Anyone using force or violence to gain entry to the premises of another is guilty of misdemeanor under this statute. Because the purpose of the statute is to keep the peace, a person might argue that another person's ownership of the property is irrelevant.

Malicious Mischief and Vandalism—Penal Code §§ 594, 603

Malicious mischief involves destruction of property belonging to another. Vandalism is a form of malicious mischief in which the criminal forcibly enters a dwelling belonging to another and damages or destroys any property in the dwelling.

In a domestic confrontation between spouses these sanctions rarely apply since any property damaged usually belongs to both husband and wife. For example, a man would be guilty of malicious mischief if the property destroyed belonged to the woman only.

Criminal Contempt—Penal Code § 166

It is a misdemeanor to disobey any orders issued by any court. This statute provides criminal sanctions against violating civil restraining orders. Restraining orders may be sought by victims of domestic violence to exclude an assailant from the premises in which the victim resides, to prohibit the assailant from disturbing the peace, or to determine the temporary custody of any children.

Law enforcement officers may be reluctant to arrest an assailant on the victim's premises in violation of a restraining order unless the victim produces clear proof of the violation and a certified copy of the restraining order.

Felony Child Stealing—Penal Code §§ 278, 278.5

It is a felony for any person who does *not* have legal custody rights over a child to take away, detain, or hide that child from the person who has lawful custody over the child. The child must be returned to the person with legal custody at the expense of the defendant. If there is no court order of custody, both parents have lawful custody over the child. In this case, for example, it is not unlawful for a woman to take her children with her if she must leave a violent home to protect her safety and that of her children.

Child Abuse

It is a crime for any person to physically abuse or sexually assault a child.

Imprisonment: Minimum and Maximum Penalties

The crimes discussed in this section are either misdemeanors or felonies. A misdemeanor is a less serious crime that is punishable by a fine or imprisonment in a county jail for a term of less than 1 year. A felony is a serious crime punishable by imprisonment in a state prison. Victims who decide to bring criminal charges against their attackers may discuss with the district attorney assigned to the case the probable sentence that the attacker will receive if convicted of a crime.

The Determinate Sentence Law of 1976 governs imposition of prison sentences for felony crimes. The majority of prison terms under the new law are determined by adding the "base term" and any "enhancements." Also, there are "limitations" set on the maximum term. Every crime covered by the new law carries a range of three possible terms: an upper, middle, and lower term. The judge must choose the middle term as the base term, unless there is a hearing in which aggravating or mitigating circumstances are shown; if this is the case, the upper sentence will be used as the base term, and if mitigating circumstances are shown, the lower sentence will be used. Once a base term is chosen for the particular crime charged, the sentence can be made longer if certain enhancements are found. The sentence will be lengthened if:

- the defendant was armed with a firearm or use of a deadly weapon (Penal Code § 12022)
- the defendant used a firearm (Penal Code § 12022.5)
- the defendant intentionally caused great bodily injury (Penal Code § 12022.7)
- the defendant caused great loss of property (Penal Code § 12022.6)
- there were prior prison terms actually served by the defendant (Penal Code § 667.5)
- consecutive sentences may be imposed (Penal Code §§ 669, 1170.1).

There are limitations on the total sentence, and these are covered by Penal Code §§ 1170.1(a), 1170.1(f), and 1170.1(d).

Probation

For the first offense, the defendant is usually released on probation. The victim may contact the district attorney about a supervised probation with mandatory therapy.

CIVIL REMEDIES

Assault and Battery

In California a victim of domestic violence can receive compensation for injuries from the spouse for civil assault and battery. This civil action in tort may be an inadequate remedy, in which the victim has had to leave his or her home, possessions, and children. The victim receives no assurance of safety and also may not be able to collect damages if the spouse has no money. If the victim is receiving alimony or child support from the spouse, a civil money judgment against the spouse may jeopardize the ability to make payments and result in bankruptcy. A victim who sues an attacker for civil damages will have to wait for the matter to come to trial, which may take several years.

Temporary Restraining Order—Code Civ. Proc. §§ 526, 627; Civil Code §§ 4359, 5105

Restraining orders are available under general civil laws and the California Family Law Act. The effects, for example, to prevent harassment, to prevent beating, and to keep a man out of a woman's home, are similar although the legal requirements differ. For more information, one must contact legal aid, a shelter, or a private attorney.

Civil Contempt—Code Civ. Proc. § 1209; Civil Code § 430(c)

If a temporary restraining order has been violated, civil contempt procedures may be used to enforce the order. Civil contempt may result in fine or imprisonment of the person who violated the restraining order. However, a victim should be aware that civil contempt procedures are slow and may have little effect on an attacker who has already violated the court's restraining order. The criminal contempt (Penal Code § 166.4) procedure may be used also.

Forcible Entry—Code Civ. Proc. § 1159

Forcible entry is the use of violence to gain entry onto any property. The law provides for compensation to the victim of forcible entry in the form of damages to the victim's property and for invasion of the victim's right to peaceful possession. This statute protects only property interests and does not protect the occupant from physical or mental injury, which limits the statute's usefulness in domestic violence situations.

Compensation for Victims of Violent Crimes

California provides compensation to victims of violent crimes for monetary losses, including necessary medical expenses, lost earnings, child care, and cost of job retraining. Compensation is limited to a maximum of $23,000. Attorneys' fees up to 10 percent of the award are also available. To receive this state compensation, the victim must have suffered physical injury or death as a result of a violent crime and must have been a California resident when the crime occurred. A victim of domestic violence may not receive compensation if he or she refuses to cooperate with the police in apprehending and prosecuting the batterer.

The amount of compensation the victim receives depends on financial need. The state decides whether the victim is able to meet basic expenses from any personal assets without serious financial hardship. Most state programs do not allow compensation to victims who are married to or living with their assailant because the assailant might indirectly receive the compensation and benefit from the crime. California, however, allows compensation to victims who live with the batterer.

Information and application forms about compensation to victims of violent crimes may be obtained from the State Board of Control in Sacramento, California, or from the police, sheriff's department, or other law enforcement agency involved in other states.

Dissolution Proceedings—Civ. Code §§ 3250 et seq.; §§ 4500 et seq.

In California a person may terminate a marriage (called "dissolution" of the marriage) without proving fault by either party. The two grounds for dissolution in California are irreconcilable differences and incurable insanity. If there is a record of violence in a marriage, a person wishing to dissolve the marriage would probably rely on irreconcilable differences as grounds.

The court granting a decree of dissolution does not have authority to award money damages to a spouse who was a victim of violence in the marriage. The domestic court may award an equal division of community property and spouse and child support, when appropriate. To obtain money damages for physical injuries suffered during the marriage, the victim would have to use either the civil tort action for assault and battery or seek state compensation for victims of violent crimes.

Child Custody

If there is no court order of custody in effect, the mother and father of the child have equal custody rights. A battered woman can take the child with her if she leaves home, but the father can legally take the child back or refuse to let the child be taken. This is true regardless of whether the woman and the father are married.

A custody order can be made in conjunction with a dissolution, legal separation, annulment, or paternity suit. Also, a parent can bring an action for custody independent of any other action. The court will determine the custody of the minor child according to the "best interests of the child." The child's wishes will be taken into account. Custody will be awarded in this order of preference: (1) either parent according to the best interest of the child; but if all things are equal, and the child is young, custody may be awarded to the mother; (2) the person with whom the child has been recently living; (3) another person deemed by the court to be able to provide proper care. A custody order can be enforced by calling the police or going back to court.

The court will award reasonable visitation rights to the parent who does not have custody, unless it is shown that such visitation would be detrimental to the best interests of the child. Third-party visitation with a neutral party, so that for instance the woman does not have to see the child's father, can be arranged. Shelters or attorneys can provide information about this.

Source: Handbook on Domestic Violence, Information Pamphlet No. 11. California Department of Justice, Office of Attorney General, April 1978.

39. Sociocultural Considerations

BEVERLY C. YIP, M.S.W.
ROBERTA PETERSON, M.S.S.W.

People throughout the world share the same anatomical and physiological systems, but race and culture provide humanity with a heterogeneity by differentiating humans into distinct groups. *Culture* is an all-encompassing term that refers to the behavioral contents of a society. It can be viewed as a system[1] or as a total configuration that shapes the norms, values, social structure, language, foods, and customs of a group as well as its medical beliefs and practices.[2,3] Because social and cultural factors influence the practice of medicine, it is of value for emergency care personnel to learn more about the cultures of the client populations served.

For emergency department personnel, knowledge of sociocultural perspectives is of particular importance because of the nature of emergency department situations. Patients and their families who are experiencing a crisis may be distraught and anxious. Communications may be adversely affected by emotional states even among those patients who are very familiar with medical systems and practices. It is not surprising, therefore, that patients and their families with language and cultural differences may view emergency departments and hospitals with fear and anxiety. Emergency department personnel need to be understanding and sensitive to ethnic differences. Awareness of the sociocultural factors that influence a patient's attitude and behavior toward treatment will result in better health care. The medical practitioner will be able to obtain greater cooperation on the part of the patient and the family and engender greater confidence in the care received. The intent of this chapter is to develop awareness among health care providers to the fact that patients of different ethnic backgrounds may have varying perceptions of health treatment and disease that should be considered for the delivery of optimum health care.

A review of the literature indicates that many countries and cultures share similar views about the etiology and treatment of disease. Many of the newer immigrants come from parts of the world where belief in magic in its various forms is prevalent and where indigenous medical systems persist along with modern medicine. Hispanic and Pacific-Asian cultures share many beliefs, especially those relative to the magicoreligious causes of disease and the hot-cold, or humoral, system of medicine.[4]

It is hoped that the material presented below will have value assisting medical personnel in working with and treating patients of different cultures who still adhere to indigenous medical practices whether they are newly arriving Southeast Asian refugees or acculturated Hispanics.[5] However, health care practitioners should not apply the knowledge provided in this chapter indiscriminately since no society is monolithic, nor can one generalize typical qualities to everyone. Readers should guard against stereotyping Hispanic and Pacific-Asian clients. The majority of these immigrants come from urbanized areas and are familiar with modern medical practices. Within each culture there will be individual variances, depending on such factors as generation, or ethnic background, or being an urban or rural dweller, or belonging to a particular social class.[6,7] There may be differences in degree of cultural solidarity even among members of the same family.

Medical personnel have a role in assisting patients of different cultural backgrounds to accept modern medical treatments more readily. This can be accomplished through the sensitive integration of cultural beliefs in health care delivery. In the words of Benjamin Paul, "Scientific measures must be put in harmony with local (indigenous) notions about spirits, taboos and herb doctors which customarily figure in healing and prevention of diseases."[1] Knowledge of cultural backgrounds and beliefs can be used as a means of developing rapport and cooperation between patients and health care professionals, thus improving the chances for successful treatment and better health care.

CONCEPTS OF DISEASE AND ETIOLOGY

Primitive medical systems believed that disease and illness could be caused by means other than natural phenomena, such as germs, viruses, hormonal imbalance, and physiologic malfunctions. Foremost among the cultures of Latin America and Asia is the belief that illnesses can be caused by the imbalances of elements such as hot and cold, wet and dry, and excess fluids or bad air. The hot-cold beliefs or humoral system of disease and treatment, because of its central position in the medical system, will be dealt with in more detail later in the chapter. In addition to the imbalance beliefs, illness could be caused by psychological or supernatural means. Sickness could be induced by anger, jealousy, or sadness. Illness could be caused by a malevolent glance from certain adults who have strong or electrical eyes, causing fright or "evil eye." Ancestors, gods, and/ or demons could cause illness and epidemics. Illness could be retribution for ancestral or past misdeeds. Through witchcraft, foods could be poisoned or foreign bodies entered into the body. Gods could possess the soul, or the soul could get lost. Violators of taboos and regulations could cause illness, as could emanations given off by a corpse.[4,8] A commonly held belief shared by Hispanics and Southeast Asians is that disease can be attributed to contagious infection of "bad body humor." This may be a substance that exudes with perspiration and causes autoinfection if one does not bathe enough because it reenters the pores and infects the blood, or it may infect others through close contact, sexual relations, or sitting on seats still warm from a previous occupant.[8,9]

ETHNOMEDICAL THERAPY

Indigenous medical treatments were responses that reflected the ideas expressed in the diagnostic statements about the illness. If the illness was attributed to an imbalance of elements that are considered "hot," treatment would consist of "cold" medicines. If the illness was attributed to malevolent sources of power, treatments would reflect a restoration of balance of power between the evil source and the victim.[10] Such treatment could neutralize or eliminate the malevolent sources of power by removing the poisonous object from the victim's body, for example, or through rituals or sacrifices imploring the demon to desist. Other treatments could augment or restore personal power to the victim through taking medicines and herbs or by rubbing and massaging with ointments and oils.

Some cures used a combination of treatments, such as that practiced in rural Mexico for fright, an illness that leaves children sad. This illness can be cured by *curanderos* who "lay the shadow" that affects the victim:[5]

> These curanderos keep a supply of powdered cedar, palm and blessed laurel which they throw on the forehead, breast, wrists, palms of the hand, nape of the neck, and into the nostrils of the sick child. While this is being done, the woman prays the Credo, and at the end holds the child's head and cries out that the shadow should withdraw and that the child no longer need be frightened.

The Chinese believe illness to be caused by the disturbances of the forces of Yin (female, cold, passive, moist, negative) and Yang (male, warm, active, dry, positive). Their healing methods include acupuncture, heat treatment of acupuncture points (called *moxa* treatment), massage, sucking or rubbing the surface of the skin, herbs, meditation, and breathing and other exercises.[7] Some of these traditional treatments have been mistaken by Western practitioners as abusive or masochistic, such as the practice of rubbing the skin with a coin or Chinese spoon until bruises appear. This treatment was believed to be effective in ridding the patient of "bad winds," which caused such symptoms as fever, chills, and headaches.[11] Other therapies resulted in skin burns, such as the moxa treatment in which combustible cones of powdered leaves were ignited on specific spots or the use of heated glass bottles to rid the body of "bad air."

Within the medical system, preventive medicine is also practiced. Prevalent throughout Latin America and Asia is the elaborate system of humoral or hot-cold beliefs that must be followed if health is to be maintained. For example, Guatemalan Mayans prevent chilling by advocating such measures as keeping oneself covered, avoiding cold water and foods that are classified as "cool," and avoiding getting caught in the rain.[12] Other preventive measures reflected the beliefs that spirits and evil powers could cause illness, such as changing the name of a child after someone in the family has suffered a fatal illness in order to hide the soul of the child by confusing the illness-causing spirits[13] or by protecting children from the evil eye by hanging unattractive objects on their clothing thus disguising their attractiveness from the evil eye.[14]

Indigenous practitioners have many names such as curanderos, abularyos, magicos, shamans, sorianos, diviners, herbalists, acupuncturists, midwives, and masseurs. Even astrologists, palmists, and monks qualified as dispensers of medical care and advice, which was appropriate since spiritual accreditation was frequently attributed to indigenous medical roles.[7,11,15] The curanderos of Latin America are primarily women, as are midwives. Some, like the Filipino abularyos and the Guamanian sorianos, are primarily men. Some practitioners are specialists dispensing only a specific type of treatment or treating certain parts of the anatomy. Qualifications for indigenous practitioners vary considerably from no formal training to long apprenticeships. This is especially true of Asian civilizations, which have a sophisticated literature going back to the beginning of the Christian era.[7,15]

CULTURAL BELIEFS AND PRACTICES

Humoral or Hot-Cold System

The humoral or hot-cold system of beliefs common to much of Latin America and South and Southeast Asia apparently had its roots in the Old World,[1,4,16] since mention of hot-cold proscriptions and prescriptions have been found in the writings of Greek scholars, notably Hippocrates. However, owing to the striking similarities between the Hippocratic doctrine and the older Yin-Yang philosophy of ancient China, there remains doubt as to the origin of this system of medicine.

The basic principle of the humoral or hot-cold system is that many things in nature are inherently hot, cold, or something intermediate quite apart from its physical temperature. Hot-cold labels can be placed on foods, liquids, medicines, body states, or illnesses as well as on inanimate objects. Health can only be maintained as long as the body's natural balance of hot and cold or wet and dry is not disrupted. For example, overconsumption of hot foods increases the body's normal heat content and causes illnesses thought to be hot in nature. Treatment would be to equalize the body temperature.[1,7,17] Hot-cold distinctions serve as a series of

avoidances and prescriptions that are not only used in maintaining health but also important in pregnancy, child rearing, food selection, and work habits. In addition, the entire medical patterning of disease and illness is involved: diagnosis, home medical care, convalescence, and prognosis.

There are variations of the hot-cold system as they are applied from culture to culture and even from household to household. Considerable disagreement exists on food classifications.[4,8,16] Logan classified the system used in Latin American cultures according to certain characteristics such as color, sex, origin, nutritive value, physiological effect, or medical use.[16] For example, darker-colored flesh such as beef is hot and lighter-toned flesh such as pork and fish are cold. Vegetables and fruit are cold, but unusually nutritious vegetables or fruits such as peanuts and avocados are hot. Foods that produce an allergic reaction such as hives are considered hot, as is the disease, but those that consistently produce diarrhea or other cold reactions are categorized as cold.

Hart found much similarity between the hot-cold classifications of the Philippines and Latin America, which he attributed to their common Spanish heritage.[4] Filipinos consider chocolate as hot and recommend it for chills.

Vietnamese and Chinese maintain strong beliefs in the Yin-Yang or hot-cold system.[7,18,19] There are proscriptions and prescriptions for foods and home remedies. Most vegetables and fruits are also considered cold, except for mangoes, which are considered hot. Although there may be similarities between Hispanics and Pacific Asians in their interpretations of the hot-cold principles, the variability both within one ethnic group and between ethnic groups is such that generalizations cannot be made.

Illnesses are defined as hot or cold according to such criteria as etiology, the treatment generally prescribed, symptomatic sensation, or the part of the body affected.[16] For example, evil eye causes hot illness; if the treatment for the particular illness is to avoid hot foods such as peppers and liquor, then that illness is a hot illness. If the body feels chilled, it is a cold illness and vice versa. If the illness affects a body organ that is considered hot, such as the liver, the illness is hot. Medicines that are used to treat illnesses must be contrastive in temperature. Aspirins are effective in treating symptoms associated with colds such as head colds and rheumatism and therefore are labeled hot medicines; Alka-Seltzer is labeled cold because it is used for treating fevers and stomachaches, which are considered hot illnesses. New medicines will be labeled the opposite of the temperature designation of the illness it was used for, or unknown illnesses will be classified opposite to the temperature designation of the medicine used in treatment.

It has been recommended that health care personnel, when treating patients who believe in the humoral or hot-cold system of medicine, accept and work within the existing system of cultural beliefs. If the cultural belief system is ignored, patients may reject prescribed medications.[1,16,20]

Response to Pain

Although the few studies on the influence of culture and the response to pain have not resulted in definitive answers, and the question as to whether or not there are basic differences between ethnocultural groups in their response to pain remains unanswered, there has been some evidence that attitudinal factors do influence the response to pain within cultural groups.[21,22]

According to a field study done in Thailand,[23] pain response is less demonstrative in the peoples of Islamic and Buddhist faiths. Islam links pain with sin, which may be overcome by prayer, pilgrimage, or other means; Buddhists believe that "pain is an inevitable product of cosmic retribution for past misconduct."

Chinese, Japanese, Koreans, and Filipinos tend to be less demonstrative in pain response because of the value placed on stoicism and maintenance of "face."[7] Normative behavior requires an individual to control expressions of pain and suffering. The inability to control self-expressions will result in loss of face and bring shame on the individual and family. This concept of "face" is referred to in several Asian languages as *haji* (Japanese), *mentzu* (Chinese), *chaemyn* (Korean), or *hiya* (Tagalog). In a clinical situation, medical personnel should bear in mind that the patient may be minimizing the degree of pain or masking the amount of suffering. It would be useful in such instances to be more inquisitive about the presence of pain than with more demonstrative patients.

Vietnamese, however, may be more demonstrative. There is no shame associated with crying or expressing pain. According to one source, Vietnamese may even exaggerate their pain because of the belief that when one goes to a physician or hospital, one must be very sick and have pain.

The Hispanic woman expresses pain freely as part of the birth process. While the American woman may practice natural childbirth techniques to overcome pain and be stoic in her approach to labor pains, the Hispanic woman, for example, can be heard loudly attesting to the pain she is experiencing.

Being more directive in ascertaining the presence of symptoms is required when interviewing patients who have great respect for physicians. Some attribute so much knowledge and authority to physicians that they feel it is not necessary to tell them anything about the symptoms since the physicians would know without being told.

Concept of Blood

Certain rural, less-educated people have a concept of blood that makes them fear such medical procedures as blood drawing for laboratory tests, transfusions, or surgery. They believe that blood is nonregenerative and that an individual has only a finite supply of blood that is available in the body. Once blood is lost either from a cut or blood drawing, it is believed that it is lost forever and that the individual is permanently weaker. This belief is shared by Guatemalan Indians, Cambodians, and Hmongs of Laos, as well as rural Vietnamese. In practice, they will consent to drawing blood for tests and do not mind if only a small quantity is taken. However, they do object if several vials are drawn, not only because they feel they are losing a very important part of their body, but also because they suspect that the hospital may be selling it. It is suggested that when blood is drawn, the patient should be asked to avert his or her eyes or the medical person should adequately explain that the lost volume is compensated for by the body.

Ethnic groups that place a high value on ancestors and bloodline are also fearful of blood transfusions. For example, Vietnamese and Hispanics do not like transfusions because they fear receiving "unknown" blood, which may be bad, thus introducing negative characteristics into the bloodline. In such instances, medical personnel need to ascertain and then allay the fears and take extra efforts in explaining to the patient the process and the benefits and effects of the procedure. Reassuring the patient that the blood is "good" or "clean" would be helpful.

Concept of Body and Image

Cultural concepts of the body and image are also factors influencing response to medical care. Although there is little available in the literature, a Thai field study noted that the varying perceptions of the body between Islamic and Buddhist subjects influenced how immunization programs were accepted.[23] Within Islamic concepts, the physical body contains both good and evil. Great stress is placed on purifying the body, and the body can be saved by removing the corruption from the body and the spirit. Islamic villagers believed in taking care of the body and in their concepts of corruption had ideas that were compatible with modern theories of disease. In contrast, Buddhist villagers considered the body as a source of contamination for the soul and a handicap to salvation. They believed that although the soul can be saved and purified by prayer and discipline, the body was beyond help.

Reincarnation is central to the Buddhist faith. Some Buddhists do not approve of autopsies because of the fear that in the event that an organ is lost or left out, it will prevent the deceased person from being reincarnated. Surgery to remove organs may cause similar fears, which will need to be addressed.

Rural, less-educated groups from Southeast Asia also have a fear of radiography. They believe that exposure to radiation will reduce their longevity. Fears are also due to unfamiliarity with radiograph machines. Once assured by a trusted community leader that the procedure is safe, they will usually be more cooperative.

When Western Physicians Are Consulted

Indigenous medical practice consists of self-help and use of traditional folk healing methods and practitioners. Younger, progressive members of a group may seek modern medical treatment first and resort to folk medicine as a last resort. Older more traditional members of a culture may approach their illness in the opposite manner, and only if folk remedies are ineffective are Western-trained physicians used.[7,11,23–25] For those who rely on folk medicine as their primary source of medical help, their visit to a Western practitioner may be only when they are in extremely serious condition, requiring a more extensive treatment plan, longer hospitalization, and more elaborate treatment than the patient who uses Western medicine as the primary treatment model.

Among the less urbanized areas of the Pacific Asian and Hispanic countries, illness is not recognized as a specific disease but in terms of symptoms. It is only as the symptoms get worse or prevent the individual from carrying on the daily routine that the patient and family discuss the problem and decide from which of the traditional folk healers they should seek help.[25] If the treatment of the first folk healer is ineffective, the family consults again and decides that the illness was misdiagnosed and consults another of the indigenous practitioners. They may exhaust all the available folk healers before they try the Western-trained physician. In the clinical setting, medical personnel should keep in mind that they will encounter more advanced conditions and chronic situations. Additionally, because patients may have used various medications, diagnosis may be complicated because of medicinal side-effects.[7]

Value of Modesty

Among Asians, especially women who were born and raised in Asia, the cultural value placed on modesty should be considered. It is generally a very stressful situation for Asian women to be examined by physicians who are non-Asian males.[7] The sense of shame or impropriety may hinder communication between physician and patient. Use of female medical personnel or female assistants in the examining process is helpful. In clinical settings that involve obstetrics and gynecology, preference is for female medical personnel. Vietnamese and Lao/Hmong women refuse to have breast or pelvic examinations by a male physician. Filipinos consider a "good doctor" one whose breast examination is so cursory that it seems to be "accidental," thus diminishing embarrassment.

An issue beyond that of modesty is that of virginity. To a woman of Guam, the Philippines, or a Hispanic culture, virginity is a significant aspect of her world and must be maintained until she is married. A pelvic examination jeopardizes the status of "virgin" and is, therefore, avoided by women of these cultures. An unmarried woman of any age from one of these cultures will consider a pelvic examination a threat to her reputation, marriageability, and standing in the community.

Modesty is not limited to women. Some Asian men are also very modest about disrobing. Dislike of modern medical practices extends to physical examinations and the need to disrobe for tests and diagnosis. It is believed that the practitioners of traditional medicine need only to take the pulse on both wrists in order to make a diagnosis.[19]

Fear of Hospitals

Hospitalization in Asian countries is reserved for patients with serious illnesses or injuries. Consequently, hospitals and hospitalization create greater anxieties among Asian patients than among American patients. In interviews with Vietnamese, Cambodian, and Lao/Hmong individuals, all spoke of fear of hospitals. Since hospitalization was used only for the very ill, many patients died in hospitals. Therefore, if hospitalization was needed, one must be very sick.

Hospitals are frightening places for other reasons besides indicating that one has a serious problem. For immigrant Hispanics and Pacific Asians, hospitals are huge, impersonal institutions. Sophisticated technology and its machines, even such mundane things as surgical masks, are frightening. Patients and their families may already be experiencing stress and anxiety over adjusting to a new country. With the added issue of a crisis or emergency situation, they may feel that their whole world is collapsing around them. Situational factors such as the lack of bilingual/bicultural staff or lack of insurance or resources to pay for services compound fear and anxiety. Immigrant families often lack support systems and have no extended family to assist them through the crisis.

Elder Samoans are especially wary of hospitals and consider a visit to a hospital as a last resort. The sentiment may be that an illness is God's will and should be left alone. Abdominal surgery is particularly repugnant to elder Samoans, and hospitalization for such treatment should be discussed with the family of a patient prior to talking it over with the patient to determine the best approach.

Emergency department personnel need to be sensitive to the enormity of the situation for Hispanics and Pacific Asians, especially if they have difficulty in understanding English. In order to allay the fear of hospitals, medical personnel need to carefully explain the reason for hospitalization, the process for admission, the projected length of stay, and any other information that would relieve some of the anxiety. One large teaching hospital continues to be viewed with fear and suspicion because the community blames the death of one of its members on the hospital. They believe that the hospital "practices" on patients because the patient who died was operated on several times within a short time. If the hospital or emergency department does not have a bilingual/bicultural staff, systems should be established that would make use of community people or leaders who are trusted to interpret and explain to the patient and the family the existing situation.

There is often great reluctance to leave a family member alone in the hospital. To people from Hispanic cultures, a stay in the hospital requires that the patient be accompanied by family members. Samoans also feel strongly about not leaving an ill relative alone, especially if there is a possibility that the patient may die. Samoan mothers attend their hospitalized children constantly and bring sleeping mats to spread on the floor beside the child's bed at night.[26] Relatives of the patient are likely to take turns to be assured that there is someone in attendance at all times.

In Asian hospitals, procedures regarding the family's participation in the care and feeding of the patient is less restrictive than in the United States. The fear of abandoning a member of the family is increased if the patient does not speak English. The association of hospitals with death can contribute to the fear of abandonment if the cultural norm is not to have any member of the family die alone. Hospital personnel should be sensitive to the family's unease and suggest ways the family can continue to maintain contact with the patient during hospitalization.

Medication

People in non-Western areas use Western medicines along with prescribed foods and herbal medicines.

Compliance with Western prescriptions may not be reliable since there may be a tendency to either overdose or underdose, depending on the individual. There is also a likelihood that foods being eaten concurrently with medications may be contrary to the medication's pH base. Some feel that if one pill is good, two is even better. Others believe that Western medicine is designed for a race of people characterized by larger physiques; therefore, their medicine is too strong for Southeast Asians who tend to be smaller. They will take less than the prescribed dosage or stop taking the medicine as soon as side-effects, such as dizziness, occur. In prescribing medicine, thorough instructions and explanations should be given.

A patient may take folk medicines simultaneously with prescribed medications, raising the possibility of complications. Often groups or families share medicine. If there is some medicine left over from when an individual had a chest pain, then a spouse or friends may use it for their pain, without benefit of medical advice.

Choice of Medical Treatment

Modern medicine generally has been established throughout Latin America and Asia. However, it has not displaced indigenous medical practices but rather has increased the medical options available to these populations. Traditional medical systems persist and exert a significant influence on the state of health and on medical decisions even among the most Westernized.[1,7,9,24] How then does one decide which medical system to use?

Observers have pointed out that people in developing areas where modern medical practice is another option for health care tend to distinguish which kinds of illness can be cured by a physician from those that will respond only to the therapy of indigenous healers.[5,15,24] Mestizo populations of coastal Peru and Chile divide diseases into five categories, two of which can be treated by physicians and three of which can be treated only by native healers.[24] Physicians are successful in treating obstructions of the gastrointestinal tract and illness due to exposure to heat or cold, but they are not successful in treating illnesses due to exposure to "bad air," severe emotional upset, or contamination by "unclean" persons because physicians do not know these illnesses and do not believe in them.

Curanderos and curanderas in the Hispanic cultures are employed to cure stomach pains and headaches with plants, herbs, and other substances naturally available to them. These substances are used in addition to prayer, which is also an integral part of the curandero's practice. The Guamanian soriano is much like the curandero in that he uses herbs and prayer. The soriano also uses massage, as do the healers in the Samoan culture. Filipino healers include abularyos (like curanderos and sorianos) and hilots (midwives). They use herbs, teas, and prayer to cure fever, shock, colic, menstrual maladies, skin eruptions, diarrhea, and burns.

Other criteria for deciding which medical system to use are the outcome of previous treatment for the same illness, the course of an illness, or other factors that may cause an individual to shift from one system to another.[15] Patients and their families usually try indigenous medical systems first and resort to a physician only after their native medicines fail.

Undoubtedly, indigenous medical systems are more popular because the treatments provide more gratification. People in non-Western areas have used modern therapy primarily for the effectiveness of its medicines for getting rid of symptoms but do not think much of its practices.[15] The efficacy of a physician's prescription for rest and relaxation cannot be compared to the rites and rituals of indigenous healers whom they believe will get rid of the basic cause of the disease. They perceive that modern medicines will alleviate the itch or the pain, but it is powerless in ridding the body of the evil spirit or "bad air." The abularyos, curanderos, and sorianos mentioned above go much further in treating the patient than does the Western practitioner. They treat the cause at the same time they cure the symptom.

Modern medicine thus suffers in comparison to native medical practices in regard to perceived effectiveness. Even when illnesses end in spontaneous recovery, the native healer is given the credit; or when both systems are tried and the physician cures the patient, the healer gets the credit. Misperceptions extend to modern medical practices as well as results, with the patient believing that the diagnostic measures are the treatment. After submitting to blood drawing and radiography, they do not feel better, thus reenforcing their beliefs that indigenous systems are better and increasing their skepticism toward modern medicine.

APPLICATION TO EMERGENCY CARE

Health care providers need to become familiar with the culture of the patient or group that they treat. They can become familiar with native concepts of illness and health and utilize them as a psychological means of gaining confidence, improving diagnosis, and ensuring improved health care. Knowing that a patient has a cultural bias against such practices as blood drawing or transfusion, the practitioner must be very sensitive as to how the patient will react to such procedures. The physicians must take special efforts to educate and reassure the patient and the family about the need, benefits, and consequences of the procedures. This explanation should also be couched in terms of the cultural context of the patient, that is, blood is drawn to find out if it is "good" or "bad," or if a blood transfusion is needed, "good" or "clean" blood is given. Failure to explain within the cultural framework may result in the patient or the family failing to cooperate or subsequently blaming any or all conditions to that procedure.

Similarly, understanding and appreciation of the hot-cold or humoral beliefs would result in greater cooperation in diagnosis and treatment. Physicians should be knowledgeable enough about the specific cultural interpretations of the system to understand when such beliefs would impede the administration of health care and to plan a course of treatment that would use the traditional system, such as classifying prescriptions according to the contrastive requisites of the system.

Observers of the social relationships between medical personnel and the groups that they serve state that the social distance between the practitioner and the patient affects the utilization of modern medicine.[15,24] Simmons states that mutual trust, respect, and cooperation vary inversely with the social distance between the practitioner and patient.[24] The difficulties in establishing rapport between physicians, who are predominantly from middle- and upper-class white segments, and ethnic minority immigrants, coupled with the attitudes of superiority toward native concepts of disease and treatment, underscores the effort conscientious practitioners must make to bridge the gap. This does not mean that practitioners should overcome social distance by being overly friendly, since in cultures where authority is stressed as in Latin America and Pacific Asian countries, maintenance of social distance may enhance rather than diminish confidence in the practitioner. Rather, because of the numerous elements that hinder communication so necessary for optimum health care, other means such as a culturally informed practice of medicine is suggested. Knowledge of such cultural traits as *enryo* (Japanese), *him huy* (Chinese), *kreng chai* (Thai), or *Pakikisama* (Tagalog), in which making demands of others or being a burden is avoided, can be important in the clinical setting. This trait, which is similar to the Western concept of reserve, may influence the patient not to create any inconvenience or trouble for the medical personnel and not to ask for clarification or to disagree. Many Hispanics and Pacific Asians are too polite to disagree and may agree or give consent even if they do not want to.

Physicians are viewed as knowledgeable and expert in treating illness and disease and placed in positions of authority. Because they are held in high esteem, they are expected to be able to diagnose the illness immediately and to treat it promptly. Some patients, especially female Asian patients, believe that the physician knows everything pertinent to the patient and the illness and that there is no need to describe symptoms or conditions of her body. Complete trust coupled with language barriers may make patients appear, to the untuned ear, as being apathetic to their own conditions.

Above all else, emergency department personnel should be cognizant of the attendant fear and anxiety that Hispanics or Pacific Asian patients and their families may be experiencing. They may not understand what is happening or what the medical staff is doing. They may not understand what people are saying or what they are signing. Empathy in all medical personnel is a significant necessity. Finally, medical personnel can help patients whose preference is for indigenous medical practice to obtain the best that modern medicine has to offer, if provided in a culturally sensitive manner, for they will select modern medical practices and discard old customs only if they can readily perceive the benefit for doing so.

In summary, when working with patients of Hispanic and Pacific Asian background, emergency department personnel should consider the following:

- Guard against stereotyping Hispanic and Pacific Asian clients. There are great variations within each culture and among individuals depending on such factors as the degree of acculturation, level of education, number of years in the United States, generation, social class, or former urban or rural background. Those that are least familiar with Western medical practice will require greater skill and patience on the part of medical personnel.

- Be cognizant of the fear and anxiety generated by crisis situations and emergency/hospital facilities. For new immigrants and refugees, the crisis situation comes on top of problems and stresses of adjusting to a new country. The lack of bilingual/bicultural staff or the lack of resources to pay for the services compounds fear and anxiety.

- Ascertain whether the patient or the family speaks English sufficiently to comprehend or understand questions, explanations, or instructions. Frequently, in cases in which English is a second language, the individual may speak enough English for basic needs but not comprehend complex English sentences nor technical terms. If the patient or family speaks only limited English, ascertain which language or dialect is used and enlist the help of a bilingual/bicultural translator. Emergency departments should have available a list of bilingual/bicultural staff or community resources that can be called to provide interpretation or translation in the languages represented. These bilingual/bicultural resources should be available 24 hours a day, 7 days a week. Additionally, staff must be provided training so that they can provide cross-cultural communication between the medical system and the patient.

- Assign female medical personnel to perform physical examinations of women patients, if possible. This is preferred especially for pelvic and breast examinations. Examinations by men and non-Asians are stressful situations for women who were born and raised in Asia.

- When communicating with the patient or family, speak in simple terms and speak slowly. Explain what is happening in lay terms, what tests or procedures need to be done, and what to expect. Permit family members to remain with the patient, if at all possible.

- Be explicit in ascertaining the presence or absence of symptoms. Some Asian groups tend to be less demonstrative in pain response because of the value placed on stoicism and on the maintenance of "face." Because physicians are attributed with so much knowledge and authority, patients may not reveal the presence of symptoms, believing that the physician knows without having to be told.

- Ascertain whether the patient has received treatment from other sources or has engaged in self-treatment. Shifting between native and Western medical practices and consulting more than one physician are acceptable practices among Hispanics and Pacific Asians.

- When giving explanations or instructions, physicians should take into consideration the patients' cultural belief system. Some patients believe that blood is nonregenerative, so extra care should be taken to explain the procedure so that fears will be allayed. When prescribing medication, explain the medication within the contrastive hot-cold system if that is part of the patient's belief system. For example, if the patient has a fever, which is considered a hot illness: medicine to treat it would be considered cold.

Social work consultation should be considered by emergency departments who are interested in improving services to Hispanics and Pacific Asians. Social work consultation would be beneficial in terms of diagnosis and treatment. Such consultation could be focused on the specific cultures endemic to the locale and provide in-depth and practical information. Social workers knowledgeable and experienced in working with Hispanics and Pacific Asian populations could provide valuable in-service training to the department personnel. In addition, social workers knowledgeable about the community could provide useful linkages to community-based resources for aftercare and follow-up on discharge of the patient.

Individual social work consultation should also be considered for patients who present multiple problems. These could include a complex or complicated medical problem beyond the ability of a lay interpreter to assist with. In addition to the complexity of the medical problem, the absence of a support system or the presence of multi-faceted environmental problems may require the help of a consultant. Care, however, must be taken to ensure that the social worker is knowledgeable and experienced in working with the particular ethnic group of the patient.

REFERENCES

1. Paul BD (ed): *Health, Culture & Community: Case Studies of Public Reactions to Health Programs.* New York, Bantam Books, 1955.
2. Benedict R: *Patterns of Culture.* Boston, Houghton-Mifflin, 1934.
3. Ackerknecht EH: Primitive medicine and culture pattern. *Bull History Med* 12:545–574, 1942.
4. Hart DV: *Bisayon Filipino & Malayan Humoral Pathologies: Folk Medicine and Ethnohistory in Southeast Asia.* SE Asian Program, data papers #76. Ithaca, NY, Department of Asian Studies, Cornell University, 1969.
5. Lewis O: Medicine and politics in a Mexican village, in Paul BD (ed): *Health, Culture and Community.* New York, Russell Sage Foundation, 1955.
6. Suchman EA: Sociomedical variations among ethnic groups. *Am J Sociol* 76:319–331 (November) 1964.
7. True RH: *Health Care Issues for Asian Americans.* San Francisco, Division of Alcohol, Drug Abuse, and Mental Health Administration, Department of Health, Education and Welfare, region IX, July 1979.
8. Foster GM: Relationships between Spanish and Spanish American folk medicine. *J Am Folklore* 6:201–219, 1953.
9. Erasmus CJ: Changing folk beliefs and the relativity of empirical knowledge. *Southwestern J Anthropology* 8:411–428, 1952.
10. Glick LB: Medicine as an ethnographic category: The Gimi of the New Guinea Highlands. *Ethnology* 6:31–56, 1976.
11. Silverman ML: *Vietnamese in Denver: Cultural Conflicts in Health Care.* New Haven, Conn, Yale University, Department of Epidemiology and Public Health, October 1979.
12. Adams RN: *An Analysis of Medical Beliefs and Practices in a Guatemalan Indian Town.* Guatemala Pan American Sanitary Union, 1953.
13. Hughes C: Public health in non literate societies, in Gladston I (ed): *Man's Image in Medicine and Anthropology.* New York, International Universities Press, 1963.
14. Ozturk OM: Folk treatment of mental illness in Turkey, in Kiev A (ed): *Magic, Faith and Healing.* New York, The Free Press, 1964.
15. Lieban RW: Medical anthropology, in *Handbook of Social and Cultural Anthropology.* Chicago, Rand, McNally & Co, 1974.
16. Logan MH: Humoral medicine in Guatemala and peasant acceptance of modern medicine. *Human Organizations* 32:385–395, 1973.
17. Wellin E: Theoretical orientations in medical anthropology: Continuity and change over the past half century, in Landy D (ed): *Culture, Disease and Healing.* New York, Macmillan, 1977.
18. Hessler RM, Nolan MF, Ogbru B, New PK: Intraethnic diversity: Health care of the Chinese Americans. *Human Organization* 34(3):253–262, 1975.
19. Le TR: *Modern and Traditional Medical Practices of Vietnam.* San Francisco, International Institute, 1978.
20. Harwood A: The hot-cold theory of disease: Implications for treatment of Puerto Rican patients. *JAMA* 216:1153–1158, 1971.
21. Zborowski M: Cultural components in responses to pain, in Jaco EG (ed): in *Patients, Physicians and Illness.* Glencoe, Ill, Free Press, 1958, pp 256–268.
22. Wolfe BB, Langley S: Cultural factors and the response to pain, in Landy D (ed): *Culture, Disease and Healing.* New York, Macmillan, 1977.
23. Hanks LM, Jr, Hanks JR: Diphtheria immunization in a Thai community, in Paul BD (ed): *Health, Culture and Community.* New York, Russell Sage Foundation, 1955, pp 155–185.
24. Simmons OG: Popular and modern medicine in mestizo communities of coastal Peru and Chile. *J Am Folklore* 68:57–71, 1955.
25. Nurge E: Etiology of illness in Guinhangdan. *Am Anthropologist* 60:1158–1172, 1958.
26. Gerber ER: *The Cultural Patterning of Emotions in Samoa.* San Diego, University of California, 1975.

40. Emotional and Spiritual Support

RUTH I. STOLL, B.S.N.Ed., M.S.N.

Many members of the emergency department staff have the skills and techniques to provide emotional support to patients and their families, but their ability to apply these skills and techniques may be constrained by time, organization, or role. Often nurses in the shock-trauma units of large metropolitan hospitals feel they are just too busy to provide this emotional support. "We have all we can do to work with the patients. We call the chaplain or liaison nurse to come and help with the families now, and patients later." Such comments indicate that these nurses are aware of the need for another dimension of care but that they do not see such care as a part of their domain. It has been delegated to another.

Emotional and spiritual support should be, and can be, an integral part of the care available to any patient or family needing emergency care. "Nursing is an interpersonal process because it is always concerned with people either directly or indirectly"[1p3] The staff's beliefs about people who are patients directly influence this interpersonal process. The way in which the health care givers view themselves is also important, since they share with patients the common bond of being human. Such a view necessitates some understanding of people as humans and as patients.

HOLISTIC MODEL

The Person as a Whole Being

The person who is the patient has been described by almost every discipline. Each has a unique point of view, and most focus on one dimension or another. Health care givers need a holistic view. The patient is a whole person who cannot be separated into segments for diagnosis and care. People are more than the sum of their parts. Recent emphasis in psychosomatic medicine reveals that our beings—body, soul, and spirit—are integrally related, one part affecting and being affected by the other parts. To be in pain means, "I feel pain in my body, mind, emotions and spirit . . . or as one person said . . . '*I am* in distress; my eyes are red from weeping; my health is broken from sorrow; I am pining away with grief . . . my sins have sapped my strength' " (Psalms 31:9–10).

Health care givers are very aware of the person's body, but they must be equally aware of the fact that the body houses another dimension, the spirit, "which is the real person, the part of us nobody can see, the part that doesn't die . . . it's the inside you!"[2] The spirit is the part of a person that allows God-consciousness and the possibility of relatedness to God, however "God" is defined. The model shown in Figure 40–1 is an illustration of this concept.

At least five characteristics emerge from the holistic view of a person and directly influence the health care giver's relationship to a patient:

1. A person is a conscious, rational being who has the right to choose and is morally responsible for personal decisions and behavior.
2. A person has the potential for growth and change, especially at times of crisis.

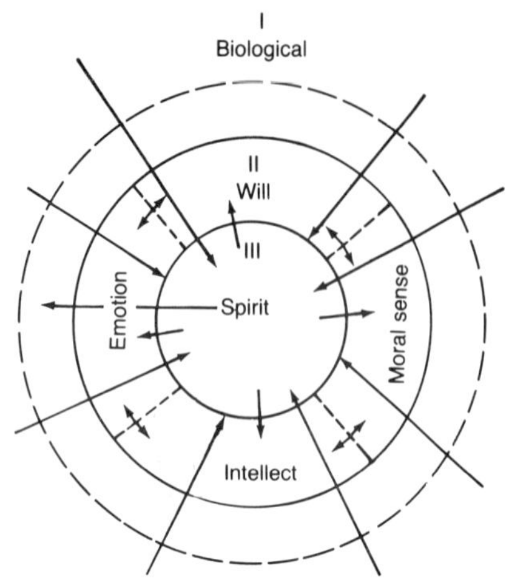

I. Biological: Five senses, world-conscious.
II. Psychosocial: Soul, self-conscious; self-identity.
III. Spirit: God-conscious, relatedness to deity. Incoming arrows are examples of life experiences penetrating the spirit:
Via intellect: unanswered philosophical and religious questions.
Via emotion: relationships of love and hate.
Via will: decisions regarding job, marriage, divorce, births, deaths, deity.
Via moral sense: support of personal convictions or inability to support personal convictions.
Outgoing arrows are examples of spirit responses:
Via intellect: statements of affirmation or doubt about God.
Via emotion: joy, peace, fear, loneliness, anxiety.
Via will: decisiveness or instability.
Via moral sense: integrity or guilt.
Via biological: energetic activity or perhaps illness related to stress (i.e., peptic ulcer, ulcerative colitis, overindulgences in food and drugs).

Figure 40–1   Conceptual Model of Nature of Man. (*Source:* Reprinted with permission from Beland IL, Passos J: *Clinical Nursing: Patho-physiological and Psychosocial Approaches,* ed 3. New York, Macmillan, 1975, p. 1087, Copyright ©1975 by Macmillan Publishing Co., Inc.)

3. Each person is a unique individual seeking self-esteem and autonomy, and simultaneously needing to live with others and with God (a higher being).
4. Each person has a life style of patterns, ways of "coping," that are more or less effective in stressful situations or crises.
5. Each person has values, beliefs, and goals that affect and give meaning to behavior and experiences.

The Person as a Patient

The person who comes to the emergency department brings along a perspective of need. Needs and problems are a part of everyone's life. Maslow suggested a hierarchy of needs composed of safety-oriented needs and growth-oriented needs that motivate each person's behavior.[3] Safety-oriented needs are those that are essential to the preservation and development of life and health; growth-oriented needs are those that lead to self-actualization. The emotional and spiritual well-being of a person is affected by the fulfillment of all these needs. Four general situations that arise in the emergency department reflect unmet human needs.

First, an immediate threat to life and health because of accident, trauma, or illness may also threaten a person's sense of control. The person feels unable to cope with the present circumstances. This situation might result from the accumulated stress of unemployment or responsibility for the care of a chronically ill family member whose care just got to be "too much."

Second, the need might reflect a lack of available and/or accessible resources. Frequent use of the emergency department is often due to inability to locate a private physician or to inadequate funds. It may be that patients are not familiar with available resources because they are traveling through a town or have only recently moved into a new community. At other times, patients have no choice but to go where taken by ambulance or emergency squad. Scarcity of resources with concomitant dependency on others can be a frightening experience.

Personal limitations or neglect might be a third area of need. When a person is asked, "Why didn't you come to the emergency department sooner?" an explanation of "I didn't think it was serious" or "I thought it would go away" may be given. This suggests procrastination, denial of any need, or a lack of knowledge or motivation on the part of the responsible person. Fear of the consequences of personal limitations or neglect can create guilt, which may easily be reinforced by thoughtless care givers.

Finally, the emergency department may be used because of societal requirements. Behavior due to alcohol abuse, drug misuse, or even the aging process may appear bizarre and unacceptable to the community. Or, a person may be the victim of another's deviant behavior (e.g., sexual assault). In such situations, society responds by assuming responsibility for the person unable for some reason to assume responsibility for personal behavior or the effects of asocial behavior.

Such situations of need not only produce stress but also are potential crises. Lazarus suggests that stress can refer to "any demands which tax the system, whatever it is, a physiological system, a social system, (a spiritual system), or a psychological system."[4] Barut writes that

> the distinguishing feature of psychological stress is that the individual's reaction is dependent upon how the individual consciously or unconsciously *interprets* the significance of a harmful or challenging event. Lazarus suggested that the major intervening variable in the study of psychological stress is the concept of threat.[5]

Inherent in the nature of a threat is the suggestion of approaching danger or challenge. It triggers a person's alarm system, thereby arousing fear.

Francis and Munjas suggest that "anxiety occurs as a result of threat to the self-system and alters one's behavior. It can be a disrupting force to a person's homeostasis or dynamic equilibrium."[6[p36]] Simultaneously, depending on the amount and the individual's response, anxiety can be the positive energy force that thrusts a person into change and growth. Mild anxiety seems to alert a person's senses and to increase that person's awareness of options and solutions to enhance problem solving. With even moderate anxiety, however, perception is narrowed and attention is decreased.

Fink defines a crisis as "the experiencing of an acute situation where one's repertoire of coping responses are inadequate in effecting a resolution of the stress."[7] Crisis can be viewed as a turning point, turning people toward or away from growth and wholeness, depending on whether they are able to reorganize their self-system and bring order back into their life. The existence of a crisis is determined by the meaning people give the event and what resources they have to cope with it. Whether a crisis exists for a person can be assessed by determining the answers to the following questions:

- What is the nature of the precipitating threat?
- What is the meaning of this experience to the person? To the family?
- How does the person feel about himself or herself? His or her ability to cope?
- How is the person coping with the experience?
- What does the person feel he or she is receiving from others?
- What does the person feel he or she needs?
- Is the person able to use the available resources?

COMMON EMOTIONAL DISTRESS EXPERIENCED IN CRISIS

Although each person reacts differently to the stress of an emergency, some common feelings can be iden-

tified. Stress can cause one to fear—fear of unknowns concerning the outcome of trauma, the upheaval of the normal routines of life, and the overwhelming newness of the emergency department itself. Fear of death and the termination of life is consciously or unconsciously present.

Feelings of helplessness and inadequacy arise when people are uncertain that competent help is available to meet the stress. This is especially true for people who normally function independently or have no significant others to assist them. When they themselves lose control, they feel they must find someone or something who is or can be in control of the situation. Control gives order to life, providing stability and security. Without it, people feel lost.

Stress causes feelings of isolation and loneliness, as if no one else has ever been in a similar situation. Stress can also disarrange a person's thought patterns, making it difficult for the person to separate fears and fantasies from reality. Personal objectivity is so distorted that what is real seems less real than what is feared or imagined. Many of these feelings contribute directly to a sense of hopelessness.

SPIRITUAL DISTRESS EXPERIENCED IN CRISIS

Spiritual needs may or may not be identified with a person's religion. They do include "any factor(s) necessary to establish and/or maintain one's relationship to God, as defined by that person."[8] Sherrill believes that "the circumstances which confront a man and require of him a decision to grow, or to stay as he is, or to regress are . . . (very often) . . . the garments which God wears when confronting men."[9] In theological terms, this suggests that people may perceive spiritual issues in their crisis experience. The very common question "Why is this happening, and why now?" is a significant spiritual question. It raises the issue of meaning and purpose. Duncan writes that "the meaning and purpose of life is the ultimate concern of a religion of faith."[10] Travelbee suggests that no illness or crisis has meaning in itself.[1[p12]] The person experiencing it gives it meaning. Even people who have faith in a personal God, a God whom they believe is in control of their life, may question the way in which their human experience fits into the context of a whole purpose. They seek constructive ways of fulfilling the purpose of their lives. Frankl believes meaning and purpose are spiritual values that provide a reason for living when work, health, or other values cannot be fulfilled.[11]

People have different personal beliefs about, and experience with, God as they define God. Jourard suggested that "whatever a person takes to be the highest value in life can be regarded as his God . . . the focus and purpose of his time and life."[12] A person may not give much time or thought to God until an emergency or crisis occurs. Even then, for some people, God remains a nonentity and does not have a role in the crisis. They feel able to cope with everything alone. Their trust in themselves and their significant human relationships certainly must be respected. However, for many others, God is a very real Being and is involved in human experience.

Spiritual trust is the confident expectation that God will meet human needs. An individual's needs depend on the individual's beliefs about God and the depth of the individual's personal involvement with God. Spiritual trust implies that there is a measure of consistency in how God relates and responds to a person. Feeling that God cares what is happening, the person perceives a sense of order and predictability about the events in and directions of his or her life. Crisis can distort or limit a person's sense of reality or awareness of God, however. The patient who is suffering, is in pain, or has experiences identified as "out of context for me" may begin to feel that God is lost or inconsistent in the relationship. As a result, the patient's sense of trust and confidence in God's "thereness" and relationship is lost. The patient may or may not be consciously aware of this feeling.

An emergency situation, then, can be a spiritual crisis. Holcomb defines a spiritual crisis as an experience "in which one feels or perceives that significant meaning or values are threatened or are being lost."[13] The grief associated with any loss, whether of relationships, aspirations, occupation, or body image, can disrupt spiritual trust. Campbell lists some other possible causes of disrupted spiritual trust:[14]

- projected blame
- refusal to accept illness (or trauma, prognosis)
- diminished positive self-image
- inability to find satisfactory reasons for crisis or disaster . . . (unresolved guilt . . . separation from one's spiritual supports)

The emotional distress discussed earlier can affect in great measure a person's relationship with God and personal spiritual well-being as reflected in physical, emotional, moral, and intellectual behavior. As the health care giver assesses the possibility of spiritual distress, these behaviors must be kept in mind. Such an assessment can be facilitated by these suggested questions:[15]

- How significant is God or religion to the patient?
- What is the patient's source of strength or hope?
- What helps most when supportive help is needed?

- What religious practices are important to the patient? How meaningful is prayer to the patient? Would it help now?
- What does the patient think is going to happen now?
- Has this experience affected the patient's feelings about God and faith?
- Would a spiritual counselor be meaningful to the patient now?

SUPPORT

Patients need comfort and support. In the sense of support, to comfort means to keep from fainting, yielding, or losing courage. It means to strengthen and give hope, to encourage as well as to lessen pain. To be comforted is to feel relief or encouragement, to have one's spirits lifted, to be supplied with what is needed to accomplish an end.

Patients must define their own needs for comfort and support. It is not the responsibility of the care giver to decide what a particular patient requires. Instead, the care giver helps the patient and family to identify their needs. The term *helper,* as used in the rest of this chapter, is defined as any person, physician, nurse, chaplain, or social worker who is available, is willing, and has the skills to provide emotional and spiritual support as described.

Many people can and do provide support, some more significantly than others. These are people who have intuition and sensitivity. People who have lived through a crisis experience and received comfort themselves can convey a unique empathy to someone in a similar situation. Participants of self-help groups, such as Make Today Count and Alcoholics Anonymous, are examples. "When others are troubled, needing our sympathy and encouragement, we can pass on to them this same help and comfort . . . given us" (II Corinthians 1:4). Some people may use the helper's role to work out their own unresolved problems. This can be detrimental to the patient, however, and such helpers should not be encouraged. Helpers should work to develop personal characteristics that, integrated with knowledge and skill, provide sensitive and significant comfort.

As noted by Brammer, an increasing body of knowledge reveals that "the person of the helper is as significant for positive growth in . . . patients . . . as are the methods the helper uses."[16[p18]] It is the unique combination of knowledge and skills in a person that provides appropriate comfort for the resolution of crisis and facilitates patients' growth. The ultimate goal of the helper is to enable the patient to grow.

Four elements enable the helper to provide emotional and spiritual support: (1) therapeutic use of self, (2) process, (3) skills, and (4) resources.

Therapeutic Use of Self

The most significant instrument helpers have to assist a patient is themselves. In order to use themselves therapeutically, they must be aware of, and increasingly comfortable with, their own identity. Although Travelbee refers to nurses, her ideas can apply to anyone desiring to be a helping person.[1(p19)]

> To use one's self therapeutically means to use one's personality consciously . . . it implies that, the nurse possess a profound understanding of the human condition . . . to realize that one's spiritual values, or . . . philosophical beliefs about human beings, illness and suffering will determine the extent to which she is able to help others find meaning (or no meaning) in these situations.

Self-awareness implies a sensitivity to one's own behavior and the potential impact of that behavior on others. The helper may unconsciously communicate a defensive attitude toward patients or an impatience with their repeated requests for instructions and information. Defensiveness might be the helper's way of providing protection against sensory overload or painful involvement with patients. However, it is interpreted by patients as rejection, which undermines patients' self-esteem and causes them to withdraw. Helpers must be aware of their own needs and coping behavior; when those behaviors interfere with their helping abilities, they must be willing to seek assistance in developing alternate coping strategies. Recognizing that one's own behavior can be a "hot line" of unspoken messages to patients and families is a vital part of being a supportive person.

Because helpers cannot give what they do not possess, helpers must be aware of their own inadequacies. Sensitive evaluation of their interactions with patients can enable them to define areas in which disciplined effort and study will develop the knowledge and skill that are lacking. Helping includes the development of "discipline as well as self-insight, reasoning as well as empathy, logic as well as compassion."[1(p19)] Art and science are melded together in an educated heart.

Before they can establish a helping relationship with another, helpers must acknowledge their own vulnerability and humanity. They must recognize human finiteness, personal strengths and limitations, personal capacities and resources, and a susceptibility to pain and crisis similar to that of the patients. Vulnerability implies that helpers must allow themselves to feel along with patients, yet not be overcome by patients' feelings and situation. With this type of empathy, helpers can maintain an objective sensitivity and use problem-solving skills to help patients work through their own experience. Fish and Shelly believe that "vulnerability means to offer ourselves as a resource . . . lending people our strength until they can regain their own strength . . . willing to open oneself up to rejection, and criticism . . . as well as to the joy and praise of other people."[17(p91)] By showing this vulnerability, the helper says to the patient, "I am like you in some ways, but what I have I want to share with you, and I want you to share what you have with me. We'll carry this burden together!"

Brammer concludes that helping is emotionally, and I would add spiritually, draining, even when not of an intense nature. It demands the full mobilization of the helper's total faculties. Therefore, "some provisions must be made for the helper to recharge his own battery."[16(p23)] Taking time for reflection and meditation is essential for personal restoration as well as development of self-awareness. Even a five-minute coffee break allows for emotional and spiritual regrouping. One chaplain assigned to an emergency department believes that emotional and spiritual support must frequently be provided to the staff as well as to the patients and families.

Process

A basic process in helping is paying attention, or attending, which may be the best indication to a patient or family that the helper really cares. Attentive behavior means an openness to the patient who comes to the emergency department. It means making a concerted effort to eradicate preconceived notions and classifications, be they cultural, social, religious, or medical. It is so much easier to "pigeonhole" people by diagnosis or priorities, even by triage, than it is to be as open as possible to the person's problem. The Good Samaritan in the well-known story *saw* with a sharp mind, an empathic spirit, and practical assessment skills an ill man. Although he belonged to a group despised by the Samaritan's peers, the man needed what the Samaritan had to offer—therefore, the Samaritan took action.

Meserve notes that "attend and attention come from the same root, the Latin *attendere,* which means 'to stretch out toward.' "[18] The helper moves toward the person. Elder reports a study of patient communication.[19] She describes how a patient asked her physician and all the different nurses who came to her room the same question. All quickly gave her an answer and left the room. Finally, Elder approached the patient and inquired about the meaning of the repetitive behavior—something still must be wrong. Because Elder stayed, the patient expressed clearly her real concerns and fears. Elder paid attention, validated her perceptions and questions, and was able to assist. Elder concludes that "patients do not communicate their needs clearly or adequately to nursing personnel . . . patients tended to move from expressing needs . . . involving concrete help to the expression of those which are frequently categorized as emotional."[19]

It is possible to be physically close to a patient but to remain out of reach emotionally and spiritually. Attending requires concentration on the patient and the patient's problems *now*. Rogers calls this congruence.[20] Helpers seek to reflect to patients what they are and what they are feeling. Helpers should feel no conflict regarding their responsibility to patients or how the conversation should proceed. Genuine congruent behavior requires helpers to filter their emotions and to bring them into some measure of objective control.

There are circumstances in which it is not possible to spend extended time with a patient or family. At such times, congruity requires the helper to acknowledge honestly to the patient the rush and situational constraints and to state clearly what help is possible. The helper may be able to return at a later time or to provide another resource. Helper and patient must know the boundaries of the help available; this knowledge provides security.

Helpers must be ethically honest and responsible during the attending process. They must define their relationship to the patient and family as clearly and concretely as possible. Patients may begin to "unload" more of their emotional and spiritual hurts than any helper can handle, given the constraints of the immediate problem. These "unloadings" could leave patients emotionally and spiritually naked and embarrassed. A responsible helper is sensitive to this and helps patients share within the appropriate boundaries.

The helper does not assume the decision-making responsibility of patients. Patients' self-esteem is undermined when it is presumed that, because of the crisis, they cannot do anything for themselves or, conversely, that they have more than enough resources to cope with the situation. If the helper cooperates with patients in identifying what they can and cannot do, what resources they do or do not have, the helper demonstrates respect for the patients. The message conveyed is, "You are not totally out of control. You are able to cope."

Truthfulness means consistency with reality. Truth is a major antidote to anxiety. It is possible to cope with truth. It is unreality or the unknown for which a patient has no defense.[6[p67]] Keeping patients informed of their condition or outcomes does not necessarily mean giving them all the details, however.

One chaplain said that, in her experience, the family wanted to hear, "Yes, it is bad, but we are doing every-

thing we can." Such a message from the nurse or physician, together with the presence of the chaplain, is both realistic and comforting. The chaplain can help the family to reflect verbally or nonverbally on the meaning of that message.

Problem solving is a logical process evident throughout helper-patient interactions. It is important to gain, interpret, and organize information in a manner that enables helper and patient to form conclusions, set priorities, and take actions. Evaluation is inherent throughout. The problem-solving process can become a cold, diagnostic process. If the patient and the patient's concerns remain central, however, the helper can use the process both to guide and to follow the patient.

Skills

Three skills are basic and essential in providing emotional and spiritual support: (1) listening, (2) joint exploration, and (3) providing hope. They are not formulas for success. Rather, these skills are helpful only when they are adapted to individual helper styles. They must be the servants of the person using them. They must be chosen to accomplish a purpose—means to an end, not ends in themselves.

Listening

One of the key skills, listening, allows patients to verbalize their feelings and reactions. It helps patients understand and be understood. Listening is an active process whereby the helper tries to see things from a patient's point of view. Listening requires the use of more than one human sense. It means making eye contact and observing the patient's body movements, body position, and facial expressions. It means hearing basic or underlying messages; relevant omissions, patterns, or themes; and the confusion that may distort facts. Touch enables the helper to "listen" to physiological reactions as well. Trembling, body rigidity, or cold, clammy hands may be felt by a gentle touch.

Three levels of communication can occur in the helper-patient interaction. The first level is communication of facts, the second level is communication of opinions, and the third level is communication of feelings. The level at which feelings are communicated is closest to the disclosure of the real person. While listening to the patient, the helper may detect what is occurring in the relationship.

Listening includes paraphrasing and clarifying what the patient or family has expressed. This does not mean parroting what they have said in a mindless manner but seeking to understand what they mean. Helpers must validate what they see, hear, and feel from the patient to be certain that what the patient desires to convey is really understood.

Barriers can obstruct sensitive listening. Selective hearing occurs: only what the helper wants to hear is heard. This is especially true when strong emotions, such as anger and despair, or spiritual needs are expressed by the patient. The helper may believe that spiritual needs are of professional concern only to the chaplain, and this belief creates a barrier. The word barriers *God*, *prayer*, or *rosary* may cause a defensive response within the helper. The constraints of time and professional duties have already been mentioned. Because of their own bias and values, helpers have often tuned out people with socially unacceptable problems, such as alcoholism. Fish and Shelly suggest that "to listen with sensitivity does not require that we condone behavior which violates our moral values, but it does enable us to empathize with people."[17[p88]]

Joint Exploration

The helper using the skill of joint exploration does not violate a patient's integrity by forcing the exposure of feelings and thoughts prematurely. Respecting a patient's reticence, the helper seeks to build a bridge of trust and tactfully invites the patient to share at whatever level is comfortable for that patient. Initially, remarks such as "It must really hurt" or "You really look so concerned. Let's talk about it" may facilitate patient exploration. Another approach might be inquiring "What helps you cope?" For some patients, sitting quietly with them, touching them on the forearm, or offering to say a prayer with or for them may remind them that a human presence and/or God is with them. Even in the initial history-taking process the helper can communicate personal concern.

If the patient appears to be receptive, the helper can provide an opportunity to externalize and sort out the feelings and thoughts hidden and disorganized within the patient. Both emotions and thoughts must be released. It is difficult to say which of these comes first, since each person responds differently. Crying should certainly be accepted, perhaps even encouraged. Anger must be accepted as well. Open-ended questions and reassuring gestures or phrases encourage the patient and/or family to continue recounting events and perceptions. During this process, patients begin to recognize their situation. They may be able to shed their denial of reality or acknowledge the pain of loss. It may mean trying to identify and connect fact with fact, search out the meaning these facts have for them personally, and interpret the implications for both present and future living. Ultimately, the patient or family may be able to say "Here I stand. What now?"

Exploration is work—emotional, cognitive, and spiritual work that only the patient and/or family can do. The helper cannot do it for them. However, the helper can be a sounding board, thereby helping them to confront reality. It cannot be stated dogmatically which helpers should be designated to assist the patient or family in this exploratory work. Also, it may not be the same helper for each patient. It does seem important that the helper who has the initial contact with the patient or family begin the exploratory work. Then, if necessary, that helper can refer the patient to another for continuity of care.

In exploration, there is a danger that the helper will prematurely cap the patient's sharing of emotional or spiritual distress. Reassurance given too abruptly may cut off the release of inner tensions before the patient has finished the process. The patient may express guilt or a feeling of being judged on past life and punished. "Why is God allowing this?" Statements of this nature often make the helper uncomfortable. Prayer or reassurances may be offered by the helper more to cover this personal discomfort than to assist the patient. A more supportive gesture might be to ask for further description or clarification of feelings, giving the patient an opportunity for release or confession. Then words of hope, a prayer of forgiveness, or a chaplain referral might be appropriate.

Providing Hope

Previously, the questions "What is this patient's source of hope and strength?" and "Who or what resources are available to the patient?" were suggested. Lynch has written that hope is "a sense of the possible, that what we really need is possible, though difficult . . . what I hope for, I do not yet have or see; it may be difficult; but I can have it . . . it is possible."[21] Hope is neither wishful thinking nor a strong desire for something. Hope is the ability to see a way through, to have a sense of confidence that there is an anchor or that there are some alternative options and possibilities. When a patient has experienced an emergency situation and become emotionally, cognitively, and spiritually disoriented owing to the stress, hope may be lost. It is impossible to see anything beyond the present moment, and that may be overwhelming. Depression and despair are likely to occur. Based in reality, hope means the mobilization of available resources, the patient, and significant others so that realistic action can be taken by the patient for reorganization of life patterns.

Hope is fostered in the context of mutuality. Patients draw hope from the helper who believes in their abilities and who encourages them to use the energy remaining within them. Hope springs from the assurance that the helper will deliver the help promised and periodically provide feedback to patients and family of what is being given.

Setting short-term achievable goals with patients increases hope. This may mean planning for the next one or two hours: Who needs to be called? Were children left alone? Can I have relief now or when? Allowing patients to participate in the decision-making process and action enhances feelings of hope.

Resources

Emergency care is limited by its very nature. It is not intended to be indefinite or long term. Emotional and spiritual support often is needed for weeks or months following the emergency, however. Patients and families must be put in touch with present and ongoing resources. Three resources should be mentioned: (1) prayer and other religious rituals meaningful to patients and/or families, (2) significant others, and (3) community-liaison networks.

First, prayer is a part of all religions. It brings perspective, strength, and remembrance of God to the fearful person. Many families with a variety of religious beliefs desire to pray or have the chaplain pray with them in the crisis. Since prayer is considered a private expression of one's intimate relationship with God, providing privacy for the chaplain and/or the family will be most appreciated. If a long wait in the emergency department is expected, use of the hospital chapel might be considered. The use of familiar religious symbols, such as a cross or rosary, or the reading of a familiar psalm may have a calming effect on the waiting patient and/or family. Different religious beliefs have specific prayers and rituals. For example, the sacraments are first in importance to Catholic patients.[22] It is important to be familiar with the major spiritual beliefs of people because these beliefs provide continuity from the past to the present and into the future.

People significant to patients can be a second source of assistance. The family comes to mind immediately, but the immediate family members are often in need of support themselves. The helper should identify those members of the family who seem to communicate strength and hope to the others. They should be mobilized and encouraged to utilize their strengths. Providing the opportunity and a *place* for the family to work through as a group much of what has been suggested for the patient is also extremely helpful. The family should be asked if they have a minister, priest, or rabbi who is a pastoral counselor to them. Should he or she be called? Is there someone else who functions as a family friend or counselor? It may be as significant for such a person to be present as the family members themselves. The helper should not forget that a significant other may be a neighbor or even a pet for some elderly person. The helper in the emergency department can initiate a network of helping relationships for support.

The last group of resource persons may be hospital or community based and might include chaplains, social workers, and liaison psychiatric nurses. Their specific role is dependent on the setting and the particular model of supportive care they choose to follow. In one study, members of the clergy were identified by patients as the most significant people for spiritual support. It was the recommendation of another study that "a question inquiring whether a patient desires to see a clergyman be part of an admission procedure."[17[p165]]

It is important that clear, collaborative relationships be established with hospital- or community-based resource helpers so that care can be uninterrupted. The support in the emergency department must be complementary to, rather than competitive with or independent of, other resource helpers. Open communication must be encouraged. If any of these resource helpers are not available in the emergency department, some type of on-call assistance should be established.

Emotional and spiritual support usually is given by the chaplain and/or the social worker. Nurses and/or physicians who feel comfortable in these areas and know the meaning of such support should choose to provide it, following sensitive assessment of the patient's and family's needs. Any professional care giver can be educated to a more sensitive and accurate assessment of these dimensions in patient care.

REFERENCES

1. Travelbee J: *Interpersonal Aspects of Nursing*, ed 2. Philadelphia, FA Davis Co, 1971.
2. Bayley J: *The View From a Hearse*. Elgin, Ill, David C, Cook, 1969, p 47.
3. Goble F: *The Third Force*. New York, Pocket Books, 1971.
4. Lazarus RI: The concepts of stress and disease, in Levi L (ed): *Society, Stress and Disease*. London, Oxford University Press, 1971, p 54.
5. Barut CJ: *A Descriptive Study of Potential Sources of Stress as Reported by Nurses Working in Critical-Care Units and on General Medical-Surgical Floors*, doctoral dissertation. University of Toledo, 1978, p 17.
6. Francis GM, Munjas B: *Promoting Psychological Comfort*, ed 3. Dubuque, Iowa, William C. Brown, 1979.
7. Fink SL: Crisis and motivation: A theoretical model. *Arch Phys Med Rehab*, November 1967, p 592.
8. Beland IL, Passos JY: *Clinical Nursing: Pathophysiological and Psychosocial Approaches*, ed 3. New York, Macmillan, 1975, p 1088.
9. Sherrill LJ: *The Struggle of the Soul*. New York, Macmillan, 1963, p 39.
10. Duncan F: Pastoral care of disabled persons, in Oates W, Lester A (eds): *Pastoral Care in Clinical Human Situations*. Valley Forge, Pa, Judson Press, 1969, p 154.

11. Frankl VE: *The Doctor and the Soul*. New York, Alfred Knopf, 1955, pp 154–157.

12. Jourard S: *Healthy Personality*. New York, Macmillan, 1974, pp 306–307.

13. Holcomb WL: Spiritual crisis among the aging, in Spencer MG, Dorr CJ (eds): *Understanding Aging: A Multidisciplinary Approach*. New York, Appleton-Century-Crofts, 1975, p 235.

14. Campbell C: *Nursing Diagnosis and Intervention in Nursing Practice*. New York, John Wiley & Sons, 1978, p 1236.

15. Stoll R: Guidelines for spiritual assessment. *Am J Nursing* 79:1574–1576, 1979.

16. Brammer LM: *The Helping Relationship: Process and Skill*. Englewood Cliffs, NJ, Prentice-Hall, 1973.

17. Fish S, Shelly J: *Spiritual Care: The Nurse's Role*. Downers Grove, Ill, Inter Varsity Press, 1978.

18. Meserve HC: Attention. *J Religion Health* 18:4. (January) 1979.

19. Elder RG: What is the patient saying. *Nursing Forum* 2(1):29, 1963.

20. Rogers C: *On Becoming a Person*. Boston, Houghton-Mifflin, 1961.

21. Lynch WF: *Images of Hope*. Baltimore, Helicon Press, 1965, p 24.

22. Weiler: Patients' evaluation of pastoral care. *Hosp Prog* 56:34–38 (April) 1975.

41. Grief and Loss

CLARICE A. SCHULTZ, R.N., B.S.N.

Grief is a state that follows the loss of a loved one in which the bereaved feels shock and numbness, followed by searching, yearning, depersonalization, and disorientation. It is a time when there is a loss of confidence and a loss of a sense of future.

Immediate mental health care intervention during a crisis can do much to initiate a constructive grief process. To facilitate this, an individual who is trained to deal with grief must become acquainted with the normal dynamics of postcrisis grief. These workers may be nurses, physicians, chaplains, clergy, social workers, psychologists, teachers or trained lay volunteers. In an emergency department setting one sees the family in crisis but usually is not able to see the progress or resolution of their grief 6 months or 1 or 2 years later. It is essential that emergency care be adapted to meet the needs of grievers in the months to come.

One of the most effective things the health care professional can do in this setting is provide correct information and as many details as possible during a crisis and later during postcrisis visits. Reality is difficult for the griever, but not knowing what is happening is often worse than the actual event.

Occasionally, a griever will take a 2-week vacation after the death of a loved one with the intention of crying it out and being done with it. However, grief cannot be hurried; it is an ongoing process. The grieving period usually includes all the seasons, holidays, and anniversaries once shared intimately with the dead loved one. Usually, the grief resolution process takes at least a year. When grief resolution is arrested it often causes emotional and physical stress. A helping person can give two important keys to successful resolution of the grief: permission and forgiveness. Grievers need permission to cry, to be angry, and to talk about the loss. They must learn to forgive the dead person for causing pain, to forgive family and friends for difficulties arising during stress, and most of all to forgive themselves for real or imagined guilt concerning their relationship with the deceased.

NEED FOR ESTABLISHING A PROTOCOL

Grief is a natural phenomenon. However, if grief is to be overcome successfully, early intervention and guidance is sometimes needed. The griever finds it difficult to ask the right questions or define what is needed in order to complete the grief process. Therefore, these needs must be anticipated by the health care professional.

An obvious source of a grief reaction is the death of a loved one. However, any loss may initiate the grieving process. For example, divorce and moving from an established home to a new one are serious losses. Such losses are often denied by the client because they result from choice. In fact, the choice may have been a good one.

For some persons, losing a mate through divorce is as complete a loss as if death had occurred. Divorce is frequently accompanied by the loss of the family home, a move to another geographic area, and a change of economic and social status. This necessitates dealing with each loss individually. Two losses incurred at one time are not the same as one big loss. When a mate dies and the survivor must relocate there is grief not only for the dead mate but also for the loss of the home they shared. This is why a griever should be advised not to make significant changes in life style for at least a year after a death.

Many griefs are greater than the precipitating event. If a child is killed, it is a great grief. If the child was murdered, the grief becomes more complicated. Also, if the child was murdered while disobeying the parents, the situation worsens. Add to this the fact that the murderer may be brought to trial and released because of a legal technicality. It is unfortunate that there are so few professionals available to help grievers involved in such situations.

Consider how difficult it must be to make the kinds of significant decisions that grievers are called on to make in our society, especially at a time when there is a loss of confidence as well as a loss of a sense of future. Many people are emotionally crippled, sometimes for life, because of poor decisions that they made by themselves or with the assistance of well-meaning but mistaken or inept individuals acting in their behalf.

Because grief renders an individual socially and emotionally disoriented, there is a diminished ability to cope with stress. Therefore, it is necessary that some mechanism for coping with the dynamics of death is established. Every society throughout history and throughout the world has done this. In the United States, unfortunately, we are in a period of cultural development in which there is no readily understood pattern for dealing with death.

Our grandparents coped with dying and grief in a manner that is probably inappropriate for us. This is because the manner of dying and grieving is significantly different in a mobile and technological society than it was two generations ago.

DEVELOPMENT OF A PROTOCOL FOR RELIEVING GRIEF

Developing a methodology for identifying, evaluating, and resolving grief would require not only research of current scientific publications but also an in-depth and intimate interaction with individuals and families who had experienced the loss of people who were close to them.

Significant insight into the normal dynamics of grief resolution has been developed by the Society of Compassionate Friends, a self-help organization with chap-

ters throughout the United States. The purpose of this society is to aid parents in the resolution of grief experienced after the death of a child and to foster the physical and emotional health of the bereaved parents and siblings.

The insight gained from meeting with members of this group is particularly beneficial because individuals are able to identify needs and feelings experienced after learning of the death of their child from medical personnel in the emergency department. Finally, they are able to assess their grief 6 months, 1 year, 18 months, and 3 years after the loss.

ROLE OF THE GRIEF WORKER

When death of a patient appears imminent, the emergency department staff must change its perspective. The family becomes the patient. While there is little more that can be done for the patient, the family's needs are just beginning. Many families said it felt like an invisible wall came down and separated them from the medical staff as soon as death of the patient occurred. They sensed a need to be rushed away, as though the taboo of death remained until they and the body had been removed. This is particularly true for family members who frequently accompanied the patient to the emergency department before the death occurred and always felt welcome. They had perceived it as a safe place and now when they most needed the caring support of the staff they were confronted with such questions as, "Where do you want the body sent?"

If a patient is dead on arrival or dies in the emergency department, the family must be contacted. Families express tremendous anger and bitterness at being deceived. Yet, they clearly remember words of caring and kindness expressed over the telephone. The majority of families interviewed said they knew there was no hope regardless of what they were told over the telephone. Yet, each maintained an unreal sense of hope until they were told in the emergency department that their loved one was dead. Even then the hope stayed until they saw the body.

Grief workers should be waiting at the door to greet the family. They should introduce themselves and explain their role. In addition to trained health care professionals, grievers who have successfully resolved their own grief at least a year after a crisis often make competent grief workers.

The family and friends should be escorted to a private, comfortable room that has water, coffee, tea, and snacks available. This room preferably should be in the emergency department. Designating a private room for families in crisis is important. Many families have stated they were embarrassed to have their grief on public display.

If lifesaving measures are in progress, grief workers should act as a communication link between the treatment room and the family. These grief workers should provide as many details as possible (e.g., number of medical staff involved, what the injuries appear to be, which medications are being given, and what equipment is being used). This prepares the family for what is to come.

In the months following the death the grievers will seek out every possible detail. They will spend hours going over the experience and the information they received. They will talk with other physicians, nurses, firefighters, and police. They will check the story over and over. By all means be truthful. The grief worker can best assuage the family's pain by conveying information in a caring manner.

Informing the Family

A physician should make every effort to be present and tell the family of a death. Even though physicians may be uncomfortable with this responsibility, they should offer assistance and tell the family to contact them if there is a need. The family seldom calls the physician, but they do remember if help was offered. It is important that the physician make an appearance soon after the death. It is unfair to the family as well as to the rest of the staff to wait for an extended period.

News of the death should be given directly and honestly. There is only one word for dead and that is *dead*. Frequently, professionals think they have conveyed the news of the death to a family only to have another professional say, "What we really meant was . . ." Words such as expired, passed away, we lost him, or he didn't make it are not acceptable. There is no easy or painless way to convey the news of death. All that is necessary, for example, is a simple, "I am sorry, your son is dead."

State concern for the family's well-being and willingness to be of further help. They will never forget this honest and concerned approach even if at the moment all they can express is anger.

Reaction to the News of Death

Reactions to the news of death are many and varied. All are proper, and probably none is a measure of the love an individual had for the dead person.

Some grievers act numb and show no reaction. It is difficult to know if they heard the message or if it had any meaning. When asked if they understand what has been said, they often answer "Yes." They give the impression they do not care about the person who died.

Gently reinforce reality with, "I'm so sorry, it's hard to lose your husband . . ." They are less likely to deal with this message if they are not given adequate time or if they leave without viewing the body.

Other grievers react mechanically. If asked for their driver's license they will reach into the pocket where it is always kept. If it is not there they will have no idea where to look. These grievers need regressive care. Suggest they look in another pocket. Ask if they had the billfold when they left home. Bear in mind they are disoriented and cannot function logically at present. Someone should bring them a drink even if they are not thirsty. The hot or cold liquid acts as a stimulant and helps them get in touch with the present. If a telephone call is necessary, they may need assistance with the numbers as they dial. If dialing the telephone is more than they can handle, this may have to be done for them. Give them time to struggle with the message but be there to give reassurance. Perhaps someone will have to take the phone and summarize the message and answer questions. However, let them do whatever they can do for themselves.

Some grievers react with a loud cry. They may want to throw themselves on the body and breathe life into it. They may scold the body or beg the dead one to wake up and tell them it is not true. Give them all the time they need to deal with the message they have just received. If you are in a hospital hallway, do not try to silence the griever or be concerned about the likes or dislikes of other people. Rather, let the others know you are with the griever and will help see this through. Show by a calm and accepting attitude that this is the normal procedure in interacting with a grieving individual and let your own tears flow if they come naturally.

Other grievers engage in activity. These individuals are looked on as being mature. However, they are no more accepting the death than are the ones who are numb or sobbing. They are delaying the acceptance by occupying time with appropriate activity. They may call relatives or they may make funeral arrangements. Eventually they will need to talk about the death and then they will do their crying. It is not surprising to hear someone is "going to pieces" 6 months after a death when they seemed so accepting when it occurred. This indicates they are just beginning the process of overcoming their grief.

Grievers often seek health care because they experience vague physical symptoms or because they think they are losing their minds. They need to be reassured that this is a normal response to loss. Health care personnel can be most effective by interacting with the griever's emotional time clock rather than with the chronological time clock. If the griever appears to be standing beside an open casket, the professional should respond as though the event occurred recently rather than perhaps 6 months previously.

Feelings

Anger is part of every grief reaction, and sooner or later it will surface. The griever directs anger at the dead person for inflicting such pain. In the beginning such feelings are unacceptable to the griever, and these feelings develop into free floating anger. It is often directed against expendable persons at the death scene. Typical targets include police, ambulance personnel, emergency department personnel, morticians, and ministers. Each is necessary initially but is expendable after the crisis is over. Such anger helps to disperse the intense feelings without jeopardizing the primary support group. An understanding of this phenomenon will enable a grief worker to accept such anger.

Protect an angry person from doing any physical harm. A common reaction is to punch the fist through glass. Protect others from this anger, and help to mend strained feelings among the support group. Reflective feelings are helpful. The grief worker may say, "That's a good reason to be angry." When anger is directed at a dead person, grievers are usually hushed and quickly removed from the area. Intervene and let them express this feeling.

Later, anger turns to severe criticism of the professionals or others who were somehow involved in the death. In time it must be directed at the source, which justifiably might be emergency care personnel or the dead person for causing such pain. This is reflected in remarks such as, "My husband died and didn't leave me a penny's worth of insurance."

Guilt is part of grief and the griever must ask himself all those torturous questions, "If only" or, "Why didn't I?" There is a yearning to repeat events leading to the death. Guilt is especially severe if death was by suicide. Relief will come from believing loved ones have the right to live their own lives, to make their own choices, and, if necessary, to choose their own style of death, even though this style of death is not acceptable to the griever.

In order for healing to occur, grievers must forgive the dead person. The professional quickly tends to assure the griever that the dead person would have understood. This we cannot know. Grievers must forgive themselves before they can accept another's forgiveness.

The process of forgiveness starts with confession. Only after they believe they have confessed enough and have been heard can they accept forgiveness. Therefore, the best one can do for grievers is to reflect their feelings and let them know they were heard. A major problem with accepting forgiveness is that one must then go on with life—a very distasteful thought for one in deep grief. It may take months before an individual is ready to work it through.

Physical Symptoms

Grievers bring to the emergency department complaints that are difficult to evaluate by clinical tests. It is wise to take a "grief" history whenever the symptoms seem inappropriate. Ask the client if any major losses have occurred during the past year. For example, did the client move, lose a primary person, break an engagement, or lose a job? Ask if they know anyone who had similar symptoms. Often they will answer, "Yes, just like Dad when he had his heart attack." This is a clue that the symptoms may be a grief reaction or may have been triggered by grief.

The impact of grief on the elderly is often misunderstood. It is often said that the elderly can take grief in stride. Do not let their calm exterior be misleading, since it may not be a measure of the depth of their grief. Be gentle and if possible call someone to be with them. Even with your best efforts they will often give up on life.

Physical expressions of grief are seen in the general population. At a time of crisis it is usually experienced as pain in the pit of the stomach. If death of a loved one resulted from a blow on the head, the griever may experience pains in the head. Encourage these individuals to accept this as normal grief and to talk about their concerns and about the pain they think their loved one felt when dying.

Unresolved grief may cause sleep disturbances, eating problems, free floating anxiety, bitterness, and displaced anger directed toward innocent family members or coworkers.

Attention Span

Some people deal with increments of their grief and only for short time spans. This means of dealing with death is most prevalent in children. For a short time they will express intense grief and just as quickly they will return to play. Adults show a lack of understanding of child growth and development when they say, "It's so nice to be children; see how quickly they forget." Do not be misled. A child never forgets a primary grief. It is essential that children be included in all grief processes. If adults show confidence that the child has the inner resources to see it through, the child learns there is nothing wrong with having feelings of great sadness. Instead, it is worthwhile to invest in relationships again, to love deeply, and to risk the inevitable pain of another loss.

A child who is quickly given to a baby sitter and isolated from the grieving family perceives there is something wrong with having deep feelings. If children are denied the opportunity to grieve, they will imagine occurrences that are far worse than any reality they might experience.

Prepare the Family to View the Body

Before families view the body of their loved one, suggest they call their minister, priest, or rabbi if this has not already been done. Families are reluctant to call their minister, thinking it will be too much of a bother. They tend to see a minister as a participant in the funeral but not as a grief worker. And yet, the minister may be the only professional who will relate to them into the postgrief period. The minister's effectiveness will be enhanced if there is personal involvement. Ministers are part of the family's support group and will relate to the family members in the future. There is value in the minister's mere presence.

The grief worker should show an expectation that the family will want to view the body. If they say "No," it is best not to hear the first or second "No." It is clear that seeing the body is an important factor because it results in perceptual confirmation and ensures healthy grief work.

Most people who do not view the body at the time of death or in the emergency department are sorry later. Until they see and touch the lifeless body the news is too unbelievable to accept. Once the body is seen and touched, death is hard to deny and then the family can muster the courage to do what must be done. They can bury their loved one and eventually let go. If the death is not accepted, then letting go is impossible and the family will be condemned to a lifelong search. Many hours must be invested in fantasizing about whether the person is really dead. Whatever the griever sees at the scene of death or in the emergency department is real. It is a picture that may be horrible but is still reality.

One father who is a member of the Society of Compassionate Friends said, "They called from the hospital and said my son was dead. They were crazy. I knew he wasn't dead because I had just seen him. I went to the emergency department and there were people running around and they all told me my son was dead. Then they took me to see him. I held my boy and knew he was dead. Then I could do what had to be done. I could have him put in the ground." That says it all. There was accepting peace in that man's deep sorrow.

Another member, a young woman, was called by the hospital and was told her husband had been electrocuted on the job and she should come in as soon as possible. She lived nearby and was at the emergency department within 10 minutes after the call. A nurse met her and said, "I am sorry, your husband was dead on arrival. Would you like to see his body?" The woman answered "No." She said her insides just screamed out to the nurse yet she could make no audible sound. The young woman said she could not believe the nurse just walked away. When asked what she wanted from the nurse she said, "I wanted to tell the nurse I was afraid to go in alone. I was afraid I would faint or vomit. I didn't know what it looked like to be burned. I thought maybe he was all charred. Later, I found there were only two little marks on him. I felt so cheated. I wanted to hold and caress him. I wanted to weep on him and run my fingers through his hair. I couldn't believe the nurse just walked away. Didn't the nurse understand I meant I don't want to see him dead? I want to see him alive."

If, after a suitable time, the grievers are unwilling to view the body, honor their decision. However, be certain one refusal does not speak for the entire family. The brothers, sisters, or children of the deceased may need to spend time with the body, and they should be encouraged to do so. Later grief work is facilitated if even one member of the family or perhaps a minister sees the body. That one person can share what they saw and reassure the other grievers it was indeed their loved one who was dead.

Some families who chose not to view the body did so because they were afraid of what they might see. Countless others were angry because they were advised not to see the body because the injuries were "too severe." Later, during the searching phase they questioned firefighters, police, and the mortician as well as every available bystander and found they were denied seeing the body because an arm was missing or there was a large gash on the face. In reality, these injuries were minor compared to what they imagined. They were angry because they were denied the right to see the body of the loved one and were given misinformation about the extent of the injuries.

Emergency care personnel should be aware of the normal dynamics of grief and realize that in time these extensive injuries will give comfort to the grievers because it gives a reason for the death. Death is often more difficult to accept when there are no external injuries.

Prepare the Body for Viewing

There is a need to see the body at peace, and most cultures have methods to accomplish this task. Regardless of the magnitude of an illness or accident, seeing a body at peace brings solace to the grievers. There is a need to honor the body with the respect the dead person gave to it in life.

One of the most intense sorrows expressed by a majority of families was that they were not asked to donate organs of their dead loved one. It appears to be a comfort to many people to know a part of someone they loved is improving the quality of life for another. Often they had discussed this with the dead person and had planned to donate the organ, but in the disorientation of the crisis, they forgot. Also, it may be that the reluctance of medical personnel to approach the family of a dead person results in a shortage of viable organ donations. The medical staff needs to understand that in time the family will gain great comfort knowing that a part of a loved one lives on.

Immediately after the death, slightly raise the head of the cart or bed to prevent pooling of blood in the face and head. Tubes and equipment may be removed but need not be put away. Some of those interviewed said the presence of equipment was comforting because they knew extraordinary efforts were used in an attempt to save the life.

The family can understand the body has been through a lot. Usually at least a portion of the body can be uncovered. For example, the hands of a loved one are readily recognized by the family. Bandage or cover any mutilated parts and place the least injured side toward the door. Check to see that the hands are in a restful position, the head is on a pillow, and the sheets are neatly arranged.

Viewing the Body

Ideally, the body should be taken to a viewing room. Every hospital should honor the dead by having a private viewing room that is comfortably furnished and peacefully decorated.

Take the family in to view the body. Encourage them to touch the body, to talk to the body, and to tell the body how they feel. Suggest that before they leave they say "Good-bye." Families said they wanted to say these things as well as to scold or love the dead one but were embarrassed. It is very important for the medical staff to verbalize these permissions. Show your acceptance of the body by touching it. Gently caress the cheeks and the arms. Run your fingers through the hair. These nonverbal permissions will do more to comfort them than any words.

It is interesting to note that many people donate a body to science to escape the need for dealing with the body. The final disposition brings a sense of completion to the family. When the body is donated, this completeness, this finishing, this sense of placement in a final resting place is missing. When this occurs, there is a tendency to wait for the dead one to return. Therefore, the grief work is retarded.

There are ways to help the family in such instances. For example, the body can be displayed in a natural position in the hospital bed, even hours later when the family arrives from out of town. They can even hold a simple religious or memorial service at the bedside. Such activities will greatly facilitate grief work.

A severely mutilated body can complicate the grieving process because in some cases the body cannot be shown. However, there are things that can be done. One of the principal things the family needs is time. Spend as much time with identifying material as you would with the body if it could be shown. For example, a lock of hair could be given to the family. Identifying dental films could be shown to the family for comparison. Show exactly why they are the same. Spend time looking at identifying jewelry. Explain where it was on the body, what the trauma did to the jewelry, and any information that you can share with the family. That is all they have.

Families who do not see the body find it difficult to believe it was their loved one who was dragged from the lake or who was in the airplane when it crashed. Somehow, it is all a mistake and a part of them waits forever for the return of their loved one. Their fantasies are fed and encouraged by news articles about people who were given up for dead and then returned years later.

Many people said they wished they could have spent some time alone with their loved one. If possible, give the family some private time with the body. Tell them where you will be and that you want to see them before they leave.

Anger is very near the surface in acute grief, and it is common to have someone shout that what you are doing or what has been done is wrong. Try to understand this anger.

Follow-up

When the family is ready to leave, express your concern and sympathy. Tell them you care and would like to hear from them again. A verbal invitation is not sufficient because they will not believe you are serious. Instead, give them a card with your name and a date about 3 weeks away on which you would like to see them. Request them to come back for a visit so you can see how they are doing. Assure them that when they return you will attempt to answer any questions that they might have.

In 3 weeks they will have many questions that did not occur to them at the time of the crisis, questions that if unanswered will haunt them and greatly impede the grieving process. The questions should be answered simply and honestly. Typical questions are: "Was he in a lot of pain?" "Would it have helped if there was a specialist at the hospital?" "Did he ask for me?" If you do not know the answer to their questions, give whatever information you have concerning the matter. Let them know these questions are a sign of the normal grief process and that searching for the facts is normal. They are compelled to continue the search. This stems from a basic desire to find the dead person. The facts surrounding the death help the griever come to terms with the reality of death and the fact that the loved one will never return.

Use of Drugs

The members of the Society of Compassionate Friends who were interviewed state that they do not advocate the use of drugs for the purpose of allaying grief. One mother said she was given a prescription for amitriptyline (Elavil) and diazepam (Valium). These drugs were prescribed when her child was killed and the prescription was continually refilled. Now, 3 years later she cannot remember the wake, the funeral, nor the memorial service. She has not completed the grief process, has no memories of her loved one to help her, and she has become addicted to the prescription drugs.

Countless numbers of grievers are given drugs to overcome a fear of losing their minds, to minimize illusions of seeing the dead person, and to alleviate physical pains. Instead of being given drugs to mask feelings, grievers should be encouraged to experience these feelings. Grievers should be taught that illusions, jealousy, anger, the wish to kill, and thoughts of suicide are part of normal grief. They should be taught methods of dealing with these feelings rather than drugged to make their already confused world even more foggy. Health care professionals accept the fact that while the use of medication for the treatment of anxiety sometimes may be indicated, alternate methods of treatment of grief are preferred.

NEEDS OF THE GRIEF WORKER

After investing a great deal of time and a great deal of themselves, grief workers will feel drained. There may be a need to spend time walking in the fresh air or perhaps to find a friend and share feelings. It is important that time be set aside to unwind and revitalize. It is unwise to go from one intense grief crisis to another without a time interval. If a helping person is both a full-time professional as well as a part-time grief worker, the professional duties should be structured in such a way that provision will be made for this essential change of pace.

SUMMARY

We live in a society that in some ways denies death and grief. Other societies have developed rituals that carry the disoriented griever through the necessary steps of disposing of the body and resolving grief. Our society is a mixture of cultures, therefore, no one method is acceptable to the general population. Our highly mobile society separates grievers from their support groups, and our technology makes the dying and grieving processes different today than they were for our forefathers. As a result, grievers remain in a state of disorientation longer and have to struggle through their grief without the benefit of rituals.

Since grief is often thought to last only 2 weeks to 2 months, the grieving family is thoroughly confused by the natural dynamics of grief that occur months and years later. Normal grief reactions are interpreted as abnormal depressions and a losing of touch with reality. Physical symptoms are not recognized as having their origins in grief, and a great deal of emotional suffering could be eliminated if we as a society understood the normal dynamics of grief. These dynamics of grief are the same as the dynamics of any significant loss we experience throughout our lives.

To assist other humans through the stages of grief, to help them avoid crippling emotional problems, and to aid in their healing so they may be willing to reinvest in life and love is truly a beautiful thing to do.

BIBLIOGRAPHY

Davidson GW: *Understanding Death of the Wished-For Child*. Springfield, Ill, OGR Service Corporation, 1979.

Grollman EA: *Talking About Death—A Dialogue Between Parent and Child*. Boston, Beacon Press, 1970.

Hewett JH: *After Suicide*. Philadelphia, Westminster Press, 1980.

Kavanaugh RE: *Facing Death*. Baltimore, Penguin Books, 1972.

Kliman AS: *Crisis—Psychological First Aid for Recovery and Growth*. New York, Holt, Rinehart & Winston, 1978.

Kubler-Ross E: *Questions and Answers on Death and Dying*. New York, Collier Books, 1974.

LeShan E: *Learning to Say Good-By: When a Parent Dies*. New York, Avon Books, 1978.

Schiff HS: *The Bereaved Parent*. New York, Crown, 1977.

Alterations of Central Nervous System Functions

Despite the great strides made during the last decade in providing emergency care to the ill and injured, death from central nervous system processes remains a common cause of death. The prehospital care of the patient with central nervous system injuries, particularly head and neck injuries, is emphasized, since the initial care of these patients is critical in determining subsequent morbidity and mortality. In "Head Injuries" (Chapter 42), precise protocols for the prehospital management of the head-injured patient and a general review of the priorities in establishing the airway, breathing, and ensuring circulation are presented. A scale utilized to measure the important parameters of change in the level of consciousness is presented. The use of diagnostic tests, management, and treatment of head injuries in the emergency department are explored.

"Cervical Spine Injuries" (Chapter 43) is devoted to injuries of the cervical spine, because the early recognition, appropriate management, and treatment of such injuries are essential to prevent serious spinal injury and subsequent prolonged disability. The reader concerned with the patient with hypothermia secondary to spinal cord injury is referred to "Hypothermia" (Chapter 30). The reader interested in traumatic injuries of the head and neck is referred to "Head and Neck Emergencies" (Section XIII), "Shock" (Chapter 6), and "Major Trauma" (Chapter 7).

In "Headache" (Chapter 44), the incidence, etiology, and differential diagnosis of headaches are discussed. A carefully constructed decision tree is provided to assist the reader in approaching the patient. Traumatic and nontraumatic causes are reviewed.

In "Coma" (Chapter 45), the author reviews the etiologic classification of coma, including the traumatic and nontraumatic causes; addresses the basic neuroanatomy and physiology; and then provides an organized approach to the patient with coma. Special diagnostic procedures are explored, and the therapeutic options available in the prehospital emergency setting and in the emergency department are discussed. The same approach is used in "Cerebrovascular Accidents" (Chapter 46). Finally, in "Seizures and Acute Confusion" (Chapter 47), the central nervous system process and systemic processes that may present as seizures or acute confusional states are reviewed. Prehospital and emergency department treatment of adults and children is reviewed.

The reader interested in the patient with confusion or coma is also referred to "Alcohol Abuse" (Chapter 36), "Substance Abuse" (Chapter 35), "Metabolic and Endocrine Emergencies" (Section III), "Poisoning and Drug Overdose" (Chapter 24), and "Psychiatric Emergencies" (Section VII). Physicians treating patients with alterations of central nervous system function, shock, and trauma may also wish to consult "Shock" (Chapter 6), "Major Trauma" (Chapter 7), "Orthopedic Emergencies" (Chapter 8), "Transfusion Therapy" (Chapter 9), and "Minor Lacerations and Abrasions" (Chapter 10). "Head and Neck Emergencies" (Section XIII) may also be of interest.

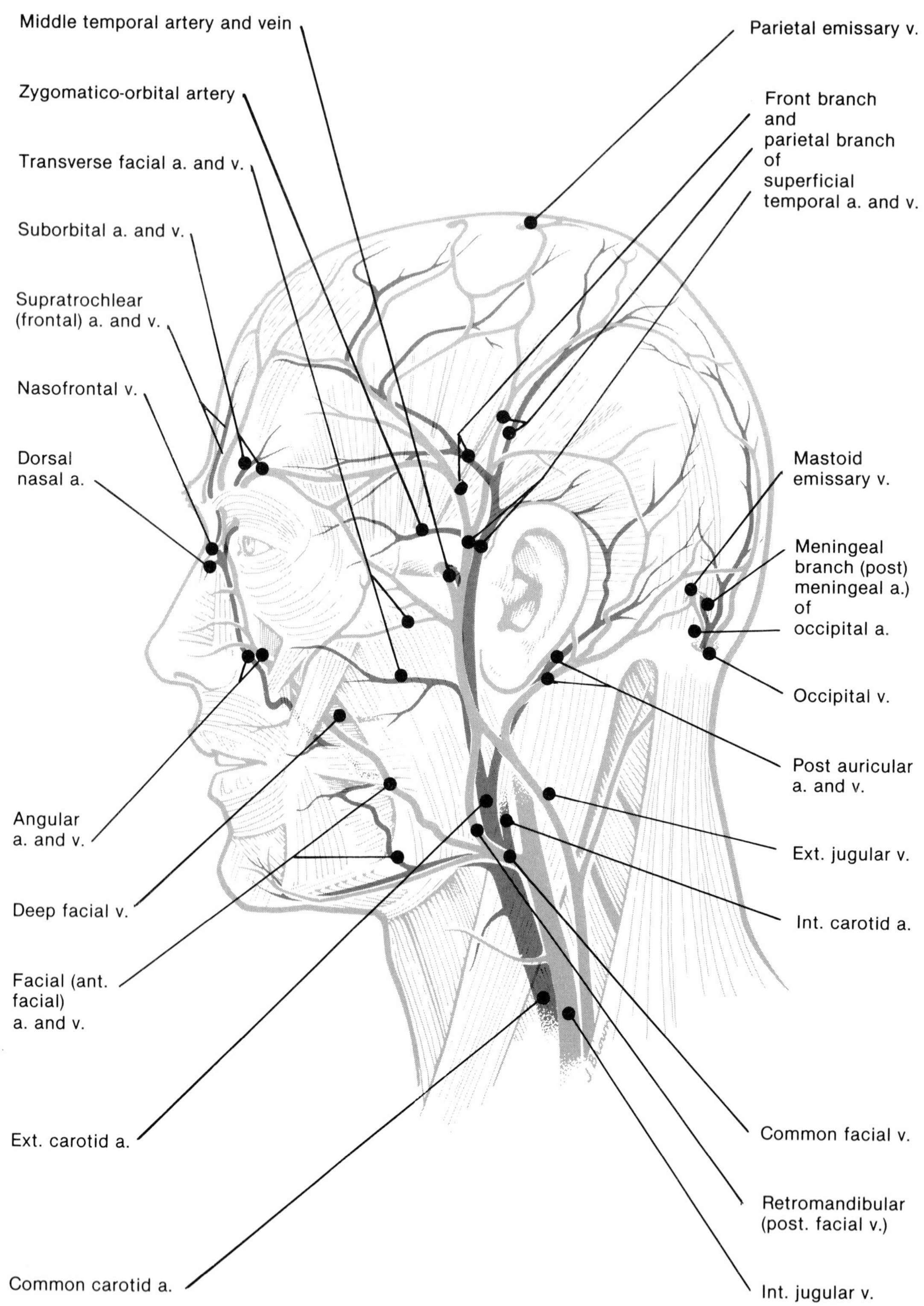

Normal Extracranial Vascular Structures of the Scalp

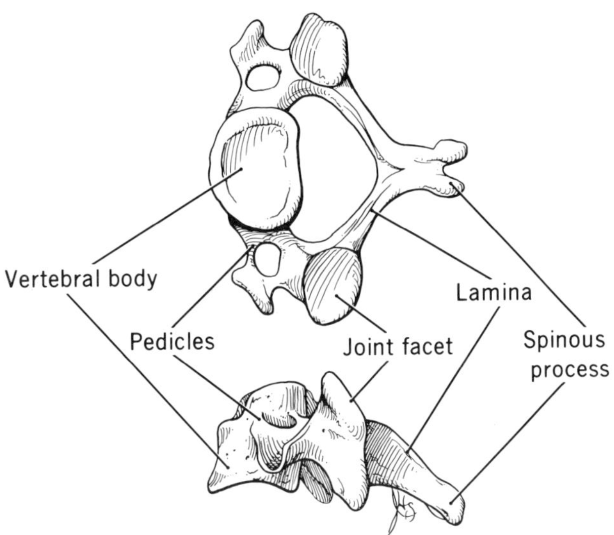

Anatomy of the Cervical Spine

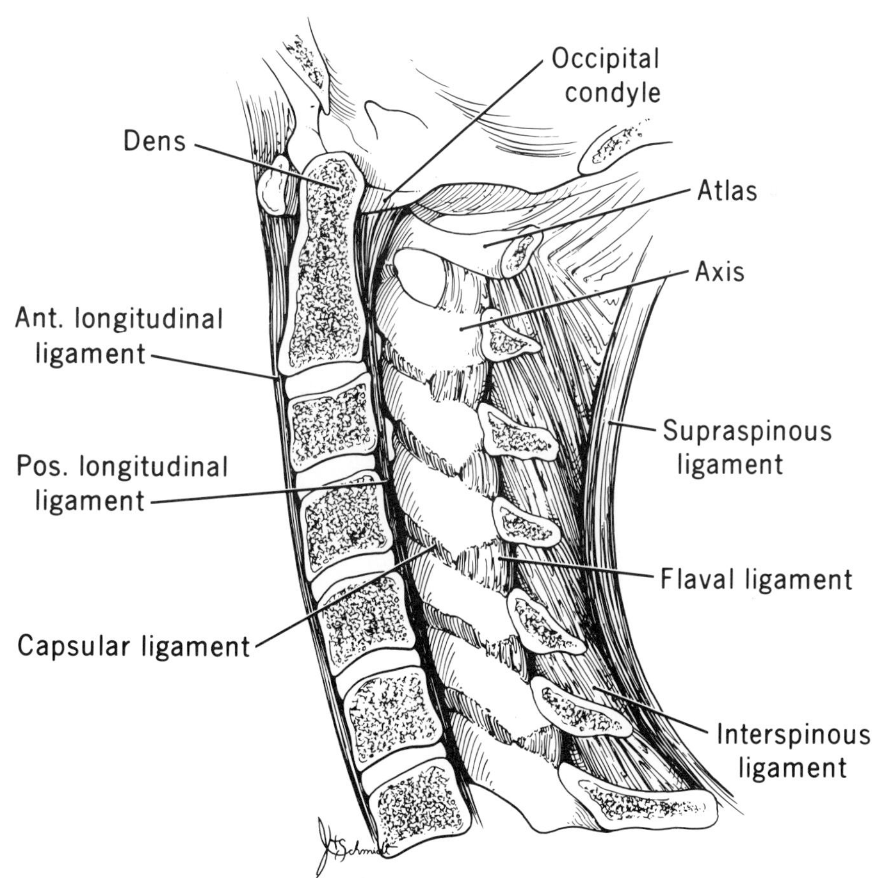

Ligamentous Anatomy of the Cervical Spine

42. Head Injuries

REBECCA W. RIMEL, R.N., B.S.N., N.P.
GEORGE W. TYSON, M.D.
JOHN A. JANE, M.D., Ph.D.,

In recent years, there has been a steady increase in the number of persons sustaining injury to the central nervous system (CNS). More patients die each year in automobile accidents than were lost in the whole Vietnam conflict, and CNS trauma is the single most common cause of death in these accidents. The head is injured in more than two-thirds of all automobile accidents, and brain injury is the cause of death in about 70 percent of fatalities. The severity of CNS injuries, as well as the high rate of morbidity and mortality, has fostered much research in the area of medical and surgical management. Together, neurosurgeons and neurosurgical nurses have been looking for better ways to handle problems such as increased intracranial pressure and respiratory difficulties, and to rehabilitate patients with head and spinal cord injuries. Little attention has been paid, however, to the prehospital and emergency department management of these patients. Because mortality as a direct result of CNS trauma usually occurs within the first two or three days after injury, the initial care of these patients is critical. Therefore, with early prehospital intervention and improved emergency management, the morbidity and mortality of CNS trauma patients presumably can be greatly reduced.

The optimal management of patients with major craniocerebral injuries involves an aggressive multidisciplinary approach to diagnosis and treatment. Not only must continuous neurosurgical supervision be provided, but specialized support personnel such as neuroanesthesiologists and nurses with special neurosurgical training must be available. The intensive care unit (ICU) must have equipment for continuous monitoring of such vital parameters as intracranial pressure and arterial blood gases. For long-term care, inpatient rehabilitative services must include neuropsychiatric evaluation and counseling, and physical and occupational therapy.

PREHOSPITAL ACUTE CARE OF THE HEAD-INJURED PATIENT

The goal for each CNS trauma patient is stabilization of all vital systems, prevention of further injury, and reduction of brain and/or spinal cord edema. The following protocol for prehospital management, developed at the University of Virginia, is directed to the prehospital emergency care personnel:

1. Check for responsiveness. If the patient is unresponsive, determine if the patient is breathing. If the patient is responsive, check for bleeding.
2. Treat breathing difficulty.
3. Establish circulation. If the patient has no carotid or femoral pulse, begin cardiopulmonary resuscitation (CPR). Shock is seldom a complication of head injury. In the event of hypotension, search for and treat other causes. Begin intravenous administration of 5 percent dextrose in Ringer's lactate, using a #8 percutaneous plastic catheter.
4. Look for and control obvious bleeding.

5. Obtain a history, and determine the mechanism of injury. If the patient is conscious, ask the location of any pain, particularly in the back or neck. Ask if the patient has any numbness. Ask if the patient has any medical problems. Has the patient ingested any alcohol? Drugs? Does the patient take any medications? If the patient is unable to give this history, ask a witness and/or relative the same questions.
6. Conduct a neurologic examination.
7. Record vital signs.
8. Immobilize the patient before transport.
9. Search for other injuries.
10. Treat open head injuries.
11. Transport the patient to an appropriate medical facility.
12. Prevent aspiration pneumonia.
13. Contact the hospital base station.

Many accident victims suffer damage to the skull and underlying brain tissue. The most important symptom in a patient with a head injury is a change in the level of consciousness. All patients with a head injury must be treated as if they actually had an unstable spine and a spinal cord injury.

A patient with damaged brain function may lose the gag and cough reflexes, and the tongue may fall back against the throat, obstructing the airway. If this occurs, the airway can be opened by means of the modified jaw thrust maneuver. If the patient is still not breathing, four quick breaths should be given. If the chest does not rise, the chin lift maneuver, in conjunction with as much extension of the neck as necessary, should be used to open the airway. After the airway is established, breathing can be assisted by mouth-to-mouth ventilation. The unconscious patient can also be artificially ventilated by means of a bag mask resuscitator at a rate of 24 breaths/minute. Prior to ventilation, however, an oropharyngeal airway must be inserted to prevent the relaxed tongue from obstructing the airway; when the patient regains consciousness, the oral airway must be removed immediately. Careful attention must be given to the accumulation of fluid in the throat of the unconscious patient. Blood from the mouth and nose can flow back into the throat, subsequently entering the lungs. Periodic suctioning of the throat is essential to remove this blood and thereby prevent aspiration pneumonia. In the conscious patient who is breathing, humidified oxygen can be administered via a reservoir mask. (See Chapter 56.)

The Glasgow Coma Scale can be used as an objective measure of the extent and progression of neurologic injury. The victim's response to three specific requests of the rescuer is assigned a number. The highest score is 15, and the lowest score is 3. The higher the score, the more responsive the victim is to the rescuer's commands. (A complete discussion of the Glasgow Coma Scale is included in the discussion of emergency department management of the head-injured patient.)

Blood pressure, pulse, and respirations should be monitored; bradycardia (<70 beats/minute) and hypertension are signs of increased intracranial pressure. The character of the respirations also has considerable diagnostic importance. The appearance of any respiratory abnormality may indicate brain injury.

Open head injuries include lacerations of the scalp and fragmentation of the skull from a fracture; in addition, lacerations of the membranes that cover the brain may extend into the brain. A few of these conditions and their treatments are

- scalp bleeding. If blood quickly soaks through the sterile pressure dressing, then apply minimal direct hand pressure.

- bleeding or drainage of cerebrospinal fluid from the ear or nose. Do not attempt to stop bleeding. The ear should never be packed, but a loose dressing may be applied gently to cover the external portion of the ear. Brush hair and dirt away from the ear. If drainage of cerebrospinal fluid is indicated by waterlike fluid in the ears or nose, no attempt should be made to block the flow.

- open (compound) skull fracture. Cover the wound with a sterile dressing without cleaning it.

- foreign body. Immobilize the foreign body with tape and a dressing without removing it.

The patient's vital signs should be monitored every 15 minutes. Signs of airway obstruction are particularly important, since obstruction of the airway will result in accumulation of carbon dioxide (CO_2) in the blood. Elevation of the CO_2 level in the blood is extremely dangerous; it increases the intracranial pressure, which exacerbates the head injury. Intracranial pressure can be reduced by an injection of methylprednisolone (Solu-Medrol). The following regimen is recommended:

15 years and older: 2 gm IV
5–15 years: 1 gm IV
5 years: 0.5 gm IV

Frequently, the patient with traumatic injuries becomes nauseated and vomits. When a patient aspirates the vomitus into the lungs, aspiration pneumonia may ensue. A portable suction apparatus should be at the patient's side at all times, and the emergency care personnel should be prepared to suction all vomitus from the patient's mouth. In the unconscious patient, an esophageal airway can frequently protect the patient from aspiration of gastric juices.

Pertinent information to be communicated to the hospital base station includes patient's age and sex, mechanism of injury, vital signs, brief history, results of neurologic examination, Glasgow Coma Scale score, findings after pupillary examination, other injuries, and treatment that has been rendered.

INITIAL CARE OF THE HEAD-INJURED PATIENT IN THE EMERGENCY DEPARTMENT

The emergency department physician often has a more significant impact on the outcome of major head injuries than does the neurosurgeon. Less than an hour's attention to the principles of basic life and brain support in the emergency department may reduce the cost of subsequent treatment by hundreds of days, thousands of personnel hours, and tens of thousands of dollars. More importantly, appropriate critical care at the right time can conserve human faculties that would otherwise be lost forever to the victim, the victim's family, and the community. The time to initiate this care is as soon as possible after the injury to the CNS. The emergency department physician is therefore critical to the outcome of any head-injured patient.

Basic Life and Brain Support

Although the neurosurgeon's primary concern may be treatable intracranial hematomas, there are other causes of significant injury to the already injured brain, such as hypotension, hypoxemia, and anemia. These insults must be corrected during the initial phase of head injury treatment in order to prevent further injury that would increase the ultimate functional disability. Attention to the head injury itself should be delayed until all organ systems—including the CNS—are well perfused with adequately oxygenated blood. Resuscitation and subsequent stabilization of vital functions accordingly take precedence over any specific treatment of the head injury itself. Care must always be exercised, however, to minimize the possibility of inadvertent spinal cord injury during the resuscitation period. All patients with head injuries must be considered to have a concomitant cervical spine injury until proved otherwise, but the demands of resuscitation need not compete with the need for cervical stability.

Establish and Maintain a Clear Airway

Initially, the mouth and oropharynx should be digitally cleared of foreign bodies, including dentures. As soon as possible, the trachea should be suctioned in order to remove material that has already been aspirated. An oral airway should be inserted in order to prevent the flaccid tongue of a supine, unconscious patient from falling backward and occluding the oropharynx.

Although the supine position is probably the safest position for a patient in whom a cervical injury has not yet been excluded, it is a poor position for airway maintenance in an unconscious patient. Airway obstruction by bronchial secretions, which may become profuse within hours of head injury, and aspiration of oral secretions or vomitus are hazards of the supine position. Only constant vigilance and repeated oropharyngeal and tracheal suctioning can prevent airway obstruction without inserting a mechanical airway. An adequate airway is better guaranteed by passage of a cuffed endotracheal tube. Unless a cervical spine injury has already been excluded, the neck should be extended only minimally, if at all. A "blind" nasotracheal intubation is the safest technique. In the obtunded patient with intact pharyngeal reflexes, intubation—particularly when difficult—may cause a deleterious increase in intracranial pressure. This effect can be diminished by first hyperventilating the patient for several minutes through a "bag and mask" apparatus. (See Chapter 56.)

Vomiting is common following head injury, especially when ethanol intoxication is superimposed. With brain concussion, it characteristically occurs as the patient begins to regain consciousness. The stomach of all unconscious patients should be emptied with a #18 sump tube. If a fracture of the anterior fossa is suspected, the sump tube should be passed through the mouth (by means of a laryngoscope) in order to avoid the risk of passing the nasogastric tube into the brain through the fracture site.

If intubation is necessary for airway protection, the procedure should be performed before the stomach is emptied. Passage of a nasogastric tube may induce vomiting in an unconscious patient, but regurgitation and aspiration during intubation may be prevented by depressing the cricoid cartilage, which partially occludes the esophagus. After intubation, the gastric contents should still be drained since aspiration occasionally occurs around an "inflated" cuff.

The unconscious patient who cannot be adequately supervised or successfully intubated should be cared for in the lateral decubitus or even the semiprone position as these positions decrease the possibility of aspiration. Proper application of a bulky soft cervical collar discourages inadvertent flexion or extension of the cervical spine. The limbs of an obtunded but restless patient should never be restrained while the patient is in the supine position. Physical restraint alone is an improper treatment of agitation in the head-injured patient whose consciousness is impaired. Investigation of the underlying cause of agitation is mandatory.

Ensure Adequate Respiration

Delay in diagnosis or inadequate treatment of hypoxemia are probably the most common major errors in the initial management of head injuries. Clinical signs of hypoxemia are often ambiguous or lacking in this group of patients. Significant hypoxemia without cyanosis is common. In addition, a hyperventilatory respiratory pattern cannot be assumed to provide adequate gas exchange and may, in fact, be due to hypoxemia or metabolic acidosis. Hypoxemia must be excluded before hyperventilation can be attributed to the brain injury itself. The injured brain is very sensitive to even mild or transient hypoxemia or hypercapnia. Therefore, the severity of cerebral injury is often increased by aberrations in the levels of arterial blood gases that may not necessarily be deleterious to other organs.

The levels of arterial blood gases should be determined in all unconscious patients, even those who display grossly normal, spontaneous ventilation. High-flow (10–12 liters/minute) humidified oxygen should be given by mask until the results of blood gas analysis are known. A grossly inadequate ventilatory pattern, asymmetric movement of the thoracic cage, or pulmonary edema (which may be neurogenic) all demand immediate intubation and positive pressure ventilation by Ambu bag or, preferably, by mechanical ventilation. The unconscious patient should also be intubated and artificially ventilated if the arterial pCO_2 is greater than 35 mm Hg or if the pO_2 cannot be maintained above 80 mm Hg by high-flow oxygen supplied by mask. (See Chapter 59.)

Subsequent neurologic deterioration should prompt redetermination of the arterial blood gas content, since respiratory insufficiency is a common cause of neurologic deterioration in the emergency department. Altered levels of blood gases alert the emergency department physician to a cause of deterioration that can be immediately and effectively treated. Aspiration commonly occurs in head-injured patients prior to arrival in the emergency department, and delayed respiratory insufficiency may occur after a normal chest roentgenogram and blood gas analyses have been obtained. As a rule, the burden of proof that the respiratory status of a head-injured patient is satisfactory is on the physician.

Establish Adequate Circulation

Arterial hypotension in head-injured patients should usually be treated by rapid infusion of 5 percent dextrose in Ringer's lactate through a large bore (#18 gauge

or larger) intravenous catheter. However, overhydration should be avoided, since this may exacerbate any predisposition to post-traumatic cerebral edema or to adult respiratory distress syndrome ("shock lung"). In addition, not all causes of shock in head-injured patients respond to volume expansion. For example, trauma-induced atrial fibrillation with congestive heart failure requires a very different treatment, as does pericardial tamponade. In such cases, physical findings usually suggest the correct diagnosis.

It is exceptional for brain injury alone to cause sustained hypotension; even in these cases, respiration usually fails first. Spinal cord injury may cause shock secondary to loss of sympathetic innervation of vascular smooth muscle. More commonly, however, the hypotensive head-injured patient harbors an occult intrathoracic, intra-abdominal, pelvic, or long bone injury. Intracranial hematomas in adults do not reach a volume sufficient to cause hypovolemic shock, but intracranial or even subgaleal loss of blood from the circulatory system may cause profound hypotension in infants. Scalp lacerations are potential sources of significant blood loss in any age group. The physician should not be misled by the fact that, because of systemic hypotension and local clot formation, active scalp bleeding may have ceased by the time the patient arrives in the emergency department. Questioning prehospital emergency care personnel and inspecting the stretcher used to transport the patient may disclose evidence of extensive external hemorrhage. Active hemorrhage from the scalp can sometimes be temporarily controlled by direct compression; rapid through-and-through single layer closure of scalp lacerations—without debridement—provides immediate control of severe bleeding. Debridement and definitive suturing of lacerations should be deferred until other emergency therapeutic and diagnostic measures are completed.

As in hypoxemia, the profound effects of arterial hypotension on the injured brain are easier to prevent than to treat. Monitoring urine output to determine peripheral perfusion is thus an essential part of the emergency management of multiply traumatized, head-injured patients. After a Foley catheter has been inserted, urine output should be recorded at least hourly. Even when extracranial trauma can be excluded, early institution of continuous urinary drainage is mandatory since bladder distention is a physiological stress that can indirectly increase intracranial pressure.

Exclude Major Extracranial Injuries

Having treated airway obstruction, respiratory insufficiency, and arterial hypotension, the physician should search for extracranial injuries that may compromise the effectiveness of initial treatment. Thirty percent of all patients with major head trauma also have significant extracranial injuries. Twenty-five percent of these injuries are themselves life-threatening.

Facial Injuries. Although blood loss from facial injuries is seldom severe enough to cause hypovolemic shock, soft tissue swelling and continued hemorrhage from the nasopharynx may compromise the patient's airway. Intubation of a tenuous airway is usually feasible and should be performed electively when the patient's airway is still patent. This is always preferable to emergency tracheostomy.

Thoracic Injuries. As noted earlier, physical signs of hypoxemia are more elusive than those of hypotension. The emergency department physician must therefore maintain a high index of suspicion for thoracic injury in all unconscious trauma patients. A supine roentgenogram of the chest is probably the second most important radiographic study in patients with head injuries. If intubation and positive pressure ventilation are utilized to treat the patient with rib fractures, the emergency department physician should be alert to the possible development of a tension pneumothorax.

Abdominal Injuries. Tenderness to palpation cannot be observed in a truly comatose patient. Abdominal rigidity should not be attributed to head injury unless the limbs are similarly rigid. Finally, ileus should not be ascribed to head trauma until primary abdominal and spinal injuries have been excluded.

Cervical Spine Injuries. In a conscious patient, local tenderness to palpation of the spinous processes is the most useful sign of an acute cervical injury. Although this finding may occur with only soft tissue injury, it virtually always occurs in the presence of fracture or dislocation. An abnormal head tilt should also raise suspicion of a cervical injury, as should limitation of voluntary movement. The neck of a head-injured patient should never be passively flexed or extended by the physician, particularly if the patient is not fully conscious.

In comatose patients with cervical subluxations, palpation may reveal an abnormal distance between two adjacent spinous processes or a lack of resistance to digital pressure over the space between them. In addition, areflexia, an atonic anal sphincter, and diaphragmatic breathing suggest cervical spinal cord injury. Injuries of the upper cervical spine are often associated with signs of facial, particularly mandibular, trauma. When unconscious patients are moved, there should always be one person responsible solely for support of the head and neck. (See Chapter 43.)

THE NEUROLOGIC HISTORY AND EXAMINATION

Determination of the exact nature and location of the primary brain injury is not the responsibility of the emergency department physician. Instead, the emergency department physician must anticipate, diagnose, and treat major extracranial causes of secondary cerebral insult, such as hypoxia and hypotension, and must rapidly assess the severity of the head trauma in order to dictate the direction of the post-traumatic clinical care. Most importantly, this physician should record parameters of neurologic function that might subsequently be the basis for neurosurgical decisions.

History

Historical data obtained from even the most lucid head-injured patient is often of limited value. The patient's own judgment of the occurrence or duration of unconsciousness may not agree with the reports of witnesses. Thus, the patient's denial of unconsciousness at the time of the trauma is, by itself, insufficient grounds for dismissing the possibility of concussion.

When unconscious patients have obvious cranial and/or extracranial injuries, attempts to obtain a history from witnesses are often perfunctory. The most valuable (and accessible) witnesses are members of the rescue squad. They should be questioned concerning the

- mechanism of injury. For example, the use of automobile lap belts without shoulder restraints may be associated with an otherwise unsuspected fracture of the lumbar spine or ruptured abdominal viscus. A shattered steering wheel may indicate a deceleration injury of the thoracic aorta.

- post-traumatic clinical course. Rescue squads are now being trained to perform relatively sophisticated serial neurologic examinations, and the patient may be mismanaged if the record of their observations is not obtained. For example, a patient whose best performance upon arrival in the emergency department is to open the eyes, flex the arms, and vocalize in response to noxious stimuli may require only close observation if the patient was totally unresponsive to all stimuli shortly after the accident. Immediate referral to a head injury center would be required, however, if this same patient had been alert and conversant when first evaluated by the rescue squad.

External Signs of Cranial Trauma

Scalp Wounds

Lacerations, ecchymoses, and hematomas of the scalp all draw attention to the fact that the patient has sustained a head injury and indicate the foci of trauma. (See Fig. 42–1.) Not all neurologic deficits associated

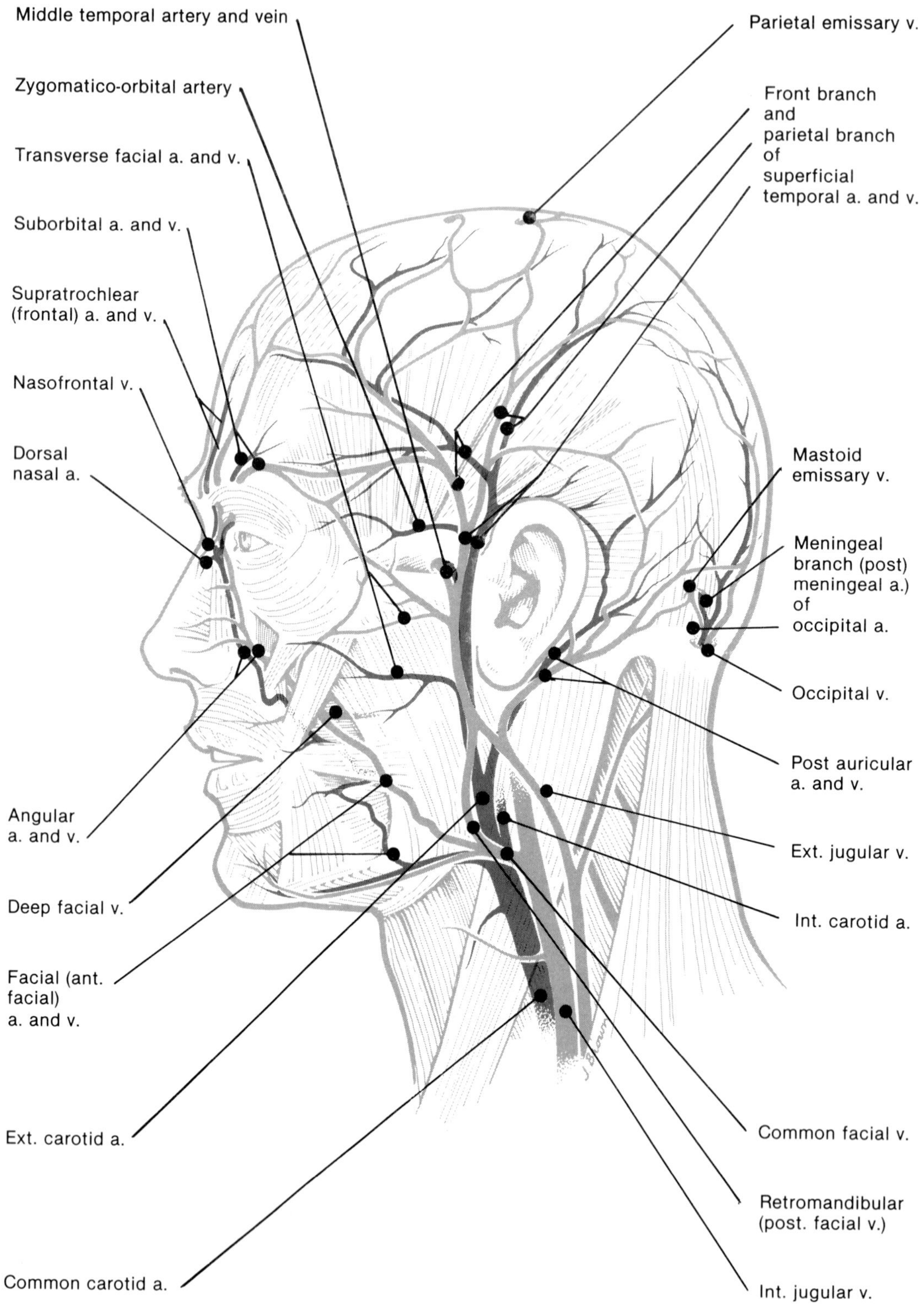

Figure 42–1   Normal Extracranial Vascular Structures of the Scalp.

with external (or radiographic) signs of recent head trauma are due to traumatic brain injury, however. Such deficits can also occur, for example, when (1) epileptics strike their heads during the course of a seizure and develop postictal hemiplegia, and (2) patients fall at the onset of a cerebral vascular accident (CVA). Although initially treating the patient for a head injury alone would probably do no harm, vital therapeutic measures are omitted if inadequate attention is paid to atypical aspects of an accident. For example, myocardial infarction or insulin-induced hypoglycemia may cause an unintoxicated patient to lose consciousness and drive a car off the road even when driving conditions are good.

Scalp wounds may also provide a portal of entrance of bacteria and subsequent intracranial infection. Skull roentgenograms should be scrutinized for fracture lines in areas that underlie scalp lacerations. Compound fractures are more prone to intracranial infection and require debridement of the margins of the laceration, including the pericranium. Small scalp lacerations associated with underlying vault fracture may be safely debrided in the emergency department. Because it is more difficult to maintain hemostasis during debridement of larger scalp wounds, these are better treated in the operating room. Temporary scalp closure without debridement should be performed in the emergency department if any delay is anticipated before surgery can be performed. Early closure diminishes the chance of local or intracranial infection and prevents further blood loss. Scalp lacerations that are not associated with underlying skull fractures can be closed after only minimal debridement. Hair should be shaved from the margins of the wound, except where the eyebrows are involved.

Copious irrigation is the most effective means of removing foreign material and minimizing the risk of infection. A single-layer closure leaves no foreign material within the scalp once the sutures are removed. Removal of foreign bodies that project from the skull should be performed only as part of a definitive operative procedure if penetration of the cranial vault is suspected. (See Chapter 10.)

Basal Skull Fractures

Unlike fractures of the cranial vault, basal fractures are more often diagnosed by physical rather than radiographic examination. (See Fig. 42–2.) These fractures are inevitably compound (involving the paranasal sinuses or middle or external ear) and are thus a potential source of intracranial infection. A basilar skull fracture may also be associated with a tear of the middle meningeal artery and the subsequent development of an epidural hematoma. (See Fig. 42–3.)

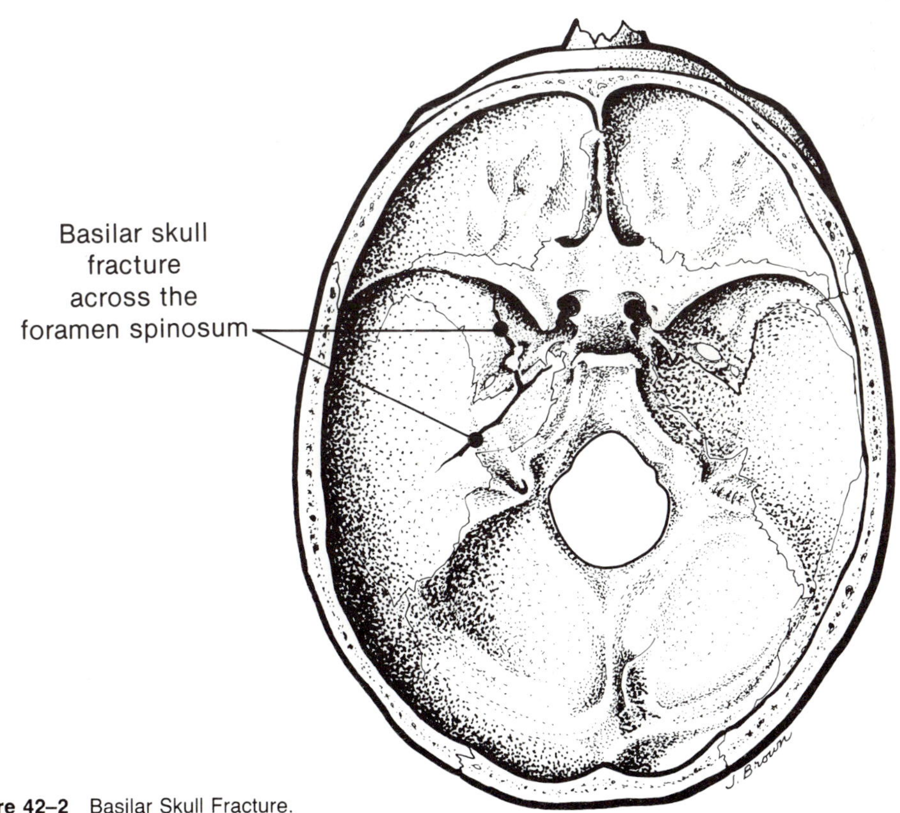

Figure 42–2 Basilar Skull Fracture.

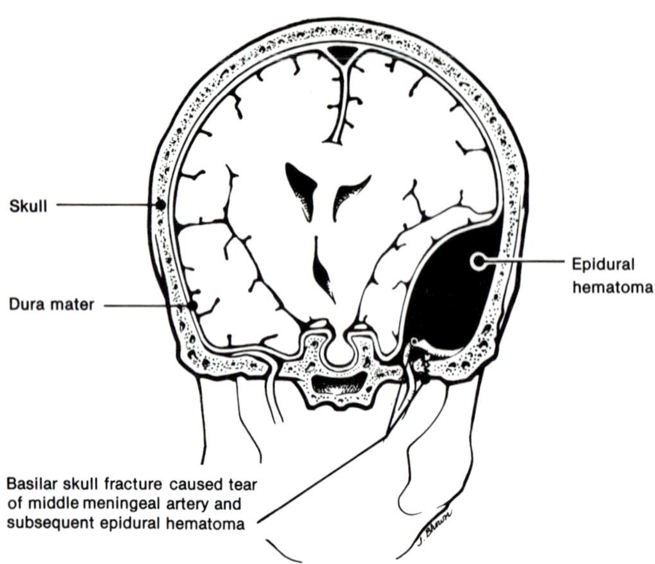

Figure 42–3   Epidural Hematoma.

Signs of fracture of the anterior cranial fossa include cerebrospinal fluid rhinorrhea, often combined with epistaxis; subconjunctival hemorrhage; and periorbital ecchymosis (raccoon eye). The latter two signs are also seen with direct orbital trauma. In general, basal fractures should be suspected when subconjunctival hemorrhage extends toward the back of the globe or when a periorbital ecchymosis has a sharply defined margin. Hyphema, unilateral limitation of upward gaze (seen with fractures of the orbital floor), and traumatic iridoplegia suggest direct orbital injury. Unilateral or bilateral anosmia may occur with anterior fossa fracture, but results of testing for this are usually unreliable in the acutely traumatized patient.

Fractures of the petrous bone produce hematotympanum or, less commonly, cerebrospinal fluid otorrhea. In the absence of an obvious laceration, bleeding from the external auditory canal usually signifies a petrous fracture. In such cases otoscopy may increase the risk of intracranial infection. For the same reason, irrigation of the external canal to remove blood and packing the nose or ear to prevent further egress of either cerebrospinal fluid or blood are contraindicated.

Sensorineural hearing loss may occur with petrous fracture and may be associated with signs of vestibular dysfunction (e.g., vertigo, nausea, or nystagmus) or even a peripheral facial palsy. More often, however, hearing loss after head trauma is of the conductive type and is attributable to blood in the middle or external ear, rupture of the tympanic membrane, or disruption of the ossicular chain. Since these are potentially correctable lesions, all conscious patients with head injury should be carefully examined for hearing loss and suspicious cases referred to an otolaryngologist.

A minor but important point should be made about Battle's sign, an ecchymosis over the mastoid process that is associated with petrous bone fracture. Since this sign does not develop for 24 to 36 hours, it is seldom seen in the emergency department. A patient who has this physical finding immediately after an accident has certainly sustained trauma to the mastoid area but has not necessarily sustained a petrous fracture.

Memory Function

The patient in the emergency department who is otherwise intact neurologically, but exhibits amnesia for the trauma even though there is no history of loss of consciousness, is a candidate for the diagnosis of "concussion." Furthermore, the duration rather than the severity of a memory deficit determines the prognosis. Many patients who appear "awake, alert, and fully oriented" on casual examination demonstrate ongoing impairment of recent memory function on subsequent specific testing. When this post-traumatic amnesia persists for more than 24 hours, the concussion is regarded as severe.

Level of Consciousness

A change in the level of consciousness is the earliest sign of neurologic deterioration following head injury. Unfortunately, meaningful evaluation of consciousness has been hampered by use of nonstandardized and purely descriptive terminology. In order to designate the severity of head injury quantitatively and predict outcome, Teasdale and Jennett developed the Glasgow Coma Scale, which relates consciousness to the parameters of responses, verbal responses, and eye opening. In each of these test categories, the examiner determines the best response the patient can make to a set of standardized stimuli. An increasing number of points are assigned to responses indicative of increasing degrees of arousal. The components of the best three test categories are as follows:

1. best motor response. The examiner determines the best motor response the patient can make with either arm:
   a. *obeys commands (6 points):* The patient, once aroused, raises an arm on request or holds up a specified number of fingers. Grasping the examiner's fingers on request is an unreliable test because of "tonic grasp" reflexes. However, ordering the patient to release the grip is a valid test.
   b. *localizes noxious stimuli (5 points):* The patient fails to obey commands, but moves either arm

toward a noxious cutaneous stimulus and eventually "finds" it with the hand. The stimulus should be maximal in intensity and should vary in site of application (e.g., pinch trapezius muscle; apply knuckle to sternum) in order to exclude stereotyped flexor movements.

c. *flexion withdrawal (4 points):* In response to a noxious stimulus, the patient briskly flexes either arm but does not manually localize the irritant.

d. *abnormal flexion (3 points):* In response to a noxious stimulus, the patient slowly adducts the shoulder, flexes and pronates the arm, flexes the wrist, and makes a fist. This stereotyped posture is tantamount to "decorticate rigidity."

e. *abnormal extension (2 points):* The patient adducts and internally rotates at the shoulder, extends the forearm, flexes the wrist, and makes a fist ("decerebrate rigidity").

f. *no motor response (1 point):* To be accurate, the examiner must have excluded spinal cord injury and be sure that the stimulus is sufficiently noxious.

2. best verbal response. The best verbal response that a patient can make after being maximally aroused (by noxious stimuli, if necessary) is determined. If the patient cannot respond because of intubation, oral injuries, or dysphasia, this test category is omitted and the letter *V* or *T* is placed after the total score from the other two test categories.

a. *oriented (5 points):* The patient carries on a conversation and can correctly give name, place, the year, and the month.

b. *confused (4 points):* The patient is conversant but is not fully oriented or shows other signs of confusion.

c. *verbalizes (3 points):* The patient cannot be engaged in sustained conversation, but utters intelligible words in an exclamatory (curses) or disorganized manner.

d. *vocalizes (2 points):* The patient makes sounds (moaning or groaning), but they are not recognizable as words.

e. *no vocalization (1 point):* The patient utters no sound even in response to noxious stimuli.

3. eye opening. The minimum stimulus sufficient to cause opening of one or both eyes is determined. If the patient is physically prevented from opening either eye (bandage or lid swelling), the letter *E* is recorded after the Glasgow Coma Scale score.

a. *eyes open spontaneously (4 points).*

b. *eyes open to speech (3 points):* The command to open the eyes is an acceptable stimulus, as is calling the patient's name.

c. *eyes open to noxious stimuli (2 points):* The stimulus applied may be the same as that used to determine the best motor response.

d. *no eye opening (1 point).*

The scores from each of the three test categories are added to determine the total Glasgow Coma Scale score. Provided all three categories can be evaluated, possible scores range from 3 to 15. Coma is defined by Teasdale and Jennett as (a) no response to command, (b) no comprehensible verbal response, and (c) no eye opening. According to these criteria, all scores of 7 or less, but no scores of 9 or more, constitute coma.

Focal and Lateralizing Neurologic Signs

Focal neurologic signs are indicative of dysfunction in specific regions of the brain, and these can provide the physician with information about the nature and evolution of local pathologic processes. (See Chapter 45.)

Pupils

Although much attention is given to pupillary asymmetry following trauma because of the significance of the unilateral "fixed and dilated" pupil, abnormalities of pupillary size, reactivity, and symmetry do not always signify the presence of an intracranial space-occupying lesion. Almost 20 percent of the population has a "subjective" (nonmeasurable) pupillary asymmetry, and almost 5 percent have a measurable (greater than 1 mm) difference in pupil size.

There are several reasons that a pupil may be abnormally small or large. Direct orbital trauma should be suspected in patients with other signs of orbital injury, particularly when pupillary asymmetry is associated with little or no impairment of consciousness. Spontaneous, symmetric variation in pupillary size and reactivity is common, even in patients who have not sustained a head injury. Opiates cause abnormally small pupils; glutethimide (Doriden) and amphetamines produce abnormally large pupils. Since ingestion of these drugs may predispose to falls or motor vehicle accidents, they may occasionally confuse the neurologic findings after head injury. The pupils may become dilated during an epileptic seizure and, during the postictal period, there may be transient anisocoria.

The larger pupil is not necessarily the abnormal one. A small, reactive pupil associated with a mild lid ptosis and a contralateral hemiparesis may signify cerebral infarction secondary to carotid thrombosis. The small pupil in this instance is due to sympathetic dysfunction (Horner's pupil).

Equal, midposition, nonreactive pupils may be due to a light stimulus of insufficient intensity or to ethanol or barbiturate intoxication.

The more depressed the level of consciousness, the more likely a unilateral "fixed and dilated" pupil represents herniation of brain structures secondary to increased intracranial pressure.

Eye Movements

Tonic Conjugate Deviation. Occasionally after head trauma, the eyes tonically deviate to one side. During a seizure, the eyes usually deviate to the side opposite the focus; during the immediate postictal period, they usually deviate to the side of the focus. Sustained tonic deviation that can be overcome by cold water irrigation of the contralateral ear is usually associated with a destructive or compressive lesion of the hemisphere toward which the eyes deviate. The level of consciousness in patients with such injuries is almost invariably severely depressed, and hemiplegia is usually present.

Brain stem injuries may also cause tonic eye deviation; but, in these cases, cold water irrigation of the contralateral ear produces little or no effect.

Reflex Eye Movements. Determination of reflex eye movements is the most useful bedside test of the functional integrity of the brain stem in unconscious patients. Quite often, the emergency department physician can reasonably decide that a head-injured patient should be transferred to a regional center without testing this parameter of neurologic function; however, a baseline determination of reflex eye movements provides the neurosurgeon with data that not only influence the therapeutic plan but also permit an evaluation of its efficacy. Transfer of the patient is seldom, if ever, delayed by taking the time to test oculocephalic and oculovestibular reflexes.

Testing for oculocephalic reflexes, known as doll's eyes phenomenon and proprioceptive head-turning, in the unconscious patient is based on the fact that sudden rotation of the head to one side normally causes brisk conjugate eye deviation to the opposite side, followed by slow restoration of the eyes to midposition. (See Fig. 42–4.) This reflex is usually suppressed in conscious patients. The test should be performed by rotating the head first to one side and then the other. The responses should be graded as normal (conjugate deviation), abnormal (dysconjugate or asymmetric eye movement), or absent (no movement of either eye). Brain stem and peripheral nerve injuries—but not hemispheric lesions—cause disorders of these reflexes. Like pupillary reflexes, ocular reflexes disappear late in the course of metabolic encephalopathy; therefore, encephalopathy should be considered in all comatose patients who display major respiratory and motor abnormalities, even those who retain their ocular and pupillary reflexes. (See Chapter 45.)

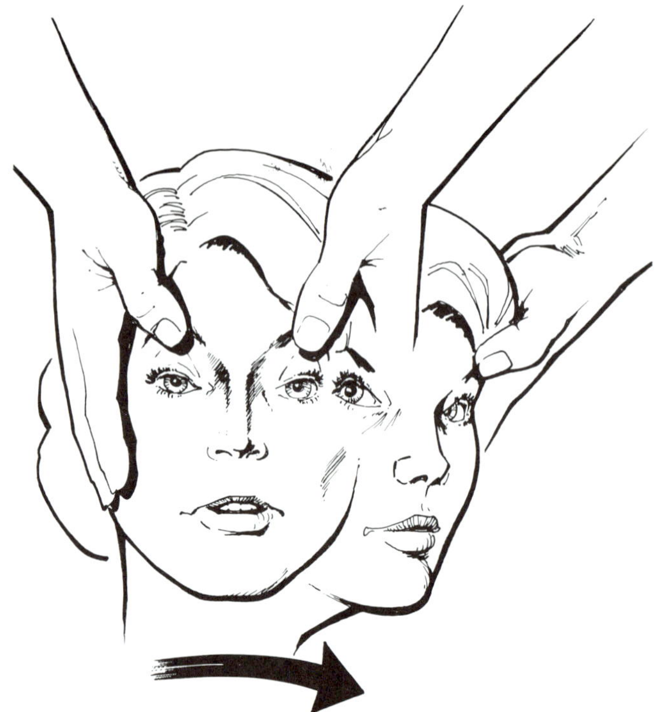

Figure 42–4   Oculocephalic Reflex.

Because cervical spine injury must be excluded before the head is rotated, and because proprioceptive head-turning is weaker than caloric stimuli in evoking ocular reflexes, oculovestibular testing is preferred.

The oculovestibular reflexes (cold caloric) test is dependent on brain stem pathways similar to those involved in proprioceptive head-turning, but it takes advantage of the fact that the lateral semicircular canal, which is adjacent to the innermost portion of the external auditory canal, controls horizontal gaze. The head of the bed or stretcher is elevated 30° to bring the lateral semicircular canal into a vertical position and after making sure there is no tympanic laceration 20 cc of ice water is irrigated against the tympanic membrane through an otoscope speculum. In an unconscious patient, a normal response is a tonic conjugate deviation of the eyes toward the side that is irrigated. (See Fig. 42–5.) This occurs after a latency of up to 30 seconds. Nystagmus, with the fast component away from the irrigated ear, occurs in less obtunded patients. The test should not be performed on the side of a suspected fracture of the petrous bone or laceration of the tympanic membrane. Several minutes should be allowed to elapse before the opposite ear is tested. Responses are graded as they are in the oculocephalic test. The examiner must be certain that the jet of water reaches as far as the tympanic membrane before declaring the reflex absent.

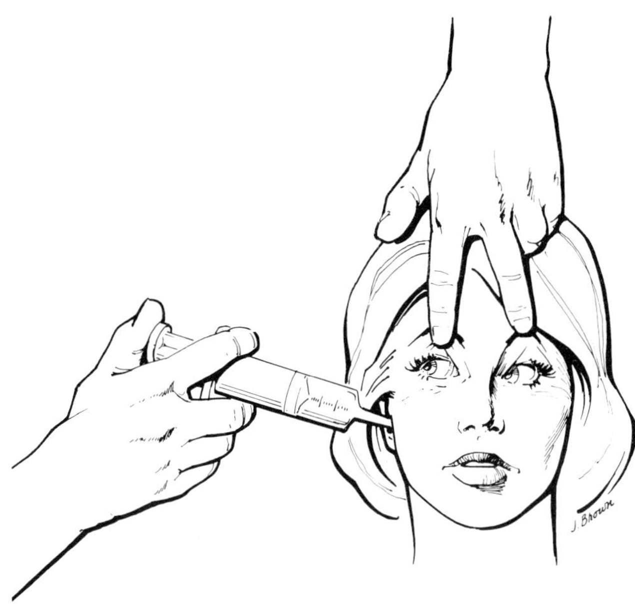

Figure 42–5 Oculovestibular Reflex.

Motor Activity

Mild paresis may be demonstrated—if the patient is able to cooperate—by having the patient close the eyes while holding both arms outstretched in front of the body. Gradual downward drift of one arm is a reliable sign of paresis, provided that maintenance of the posture causes the patient no musculoskeletal pain. Adventitious movements of the extended arms are common in children, and thus walking and even running are better tests of hemiparesis in younger patients. Hopping, first on one foot and then the other, can be used in adults to exclude lower extremity paresis, as well as cerebellar or proprioceptive incoordination, but many normal children cannot hop on each foot. Reflex asymmetry without demonstrable weakness is seldom due to head injury in fully conscious patients.

In obtunded patients, hemiparesis may be indicated by a paucity of spontaneous movement of the limbs on one side of the body or by a similarly asymmetric response to noxious stimuli. If a patient moves one arm preferentially when a noxious stimulus is applied to the trunk, the existence or the degree of hemiparesis may be further evaluated by reapplying the stimulus with the more "active" extremity restrained. Unilateral hyperreflexia, particularly when accompanied by pathologic reflexes (for example, Babinski's sign), is usually indicative of hemiparesis in unconscious patients. Passive external rotation of one leg at the hip, causing the toes to point more laterally on one side than on the other, has a similar connotation. The same phenomenon is often observed in hemiplegia due to spinal cord injury, however.

Vital Signs

In the acutely traumatized patient, vital signs must be recorded at frequent intervals (at least every 15 minutes) since changes in vital signs are of the greatest diagnostic value. The patterns of vital sign changes in patients with increasing intracranial pressure are often nonspecific. Therefore, neurologic deterioration associated with a major change in vital signs should not be attributed to an expanding intracranial mass lesion until primary cardiopulmonary and metabolic abnormalities have been excluded or corrected. The classic Kocher-Cushing changes of bradypnea followed by bradycardia and widening pulse pressure (owing primarily to systolic hypertension) are seldom seen in head-injured patients, and thus diagnosis of increasing intracranial pressure should not await the appearance of this triad. As noted earlier, when neurologic deterioration is due to a primary intracranial lesion, deterioration in the level of consciousness usually precedes major changes in vital signs.

Immediately after head injury, vital signs may be reduced to a minimum. The pulse may be slow, irregular, and faint (owing to profound hypotension); respiration may be shallow, irregular, and infrequent. Body temperature may fall. During this state, neurologic function is often profoundly depressed. The patient may demonstrate flaccid quadriplegia, areflexia, dilated and unreactive pupils; ocular reflexes may be absent. If the patient has sustained a concussion, these signs usually resolve by the time the patient arrives in the emergency department. Transient lateralizing signs may be observed as recovery proceeds. For example, the plantar responses may briefly be bilaterally extensor before one and then the other becomes flexor.

Even after mild concussion, the patient may have a tachycardia during the period of hospital observation. However, sudden precipitous rises in pulse rate demand further explanation. Tachycardia associated with hypotension should raise suspicion of occult internal hemorrhage. When hypotension is due to an acute spinal cord injury, bradycardia rather than tachycardia may be observed. However, progressive bradycardia and obtundation demands exclusion of increased intracranial pressure.

Abnormal respiratory patterns are only occasionally of value in localizing an acute head injury and predicting its outcome. For example, Cheyne-Stokes respiration and most other forms of periodic breathing are not necessarily indicative of an unfavorable outcome. North and Jennett found that only persistent spontaneous tachypnea (rate greater than 24/minute) combined with arterial hypocapnia (pCO_2 less than 30 mm Hg) is consistently associated with a poor prognosis. Furthermore, only grossly erratic patterns of breathing are of localizing value (pontomedullary dysfunction). It must be emphasized that cerebral injury is not the cause of all abnormal respiratory patterns after head trauma; upper airway obstruction has been observed to cause a periodic breathing pattern.

Body temperature often falls immediately after head injury, but it may subsequently rise to around 38°C and remain at this level for 24 to 36 hours. A more protracted hyperpyrexia may be due to traumatic subarachnoid hemorrhage, in which case nuchal rigidity often becomes demonstrable. Intracranial or extracranial infection must be excluded when the temperature remains above 39°C or when hyperpyrexia is associated with neurologic deterioration. Abrupt marked hypothermia or rapid early rise in temperature may indicate a poor prognosis.

Restlessness

Restlessness or agitation is often seen during the early recovery phase of concussion, but increasing headache due to an enlarging extradural hematoma may produce a similar picture. In the former case, restlessness is associated with a progressive increase in the Glasgow Coma Scale score; in the latter case, however, the score relentlessly decreases. More commonly, agitation in the unconscious patient results from hypoxemia, hypotension, painful musculoskeletal injuries, or simply a distended urinary bladder.

Other Diagnostic Tests

Metabolic Studies

Not all neurologic impairment following head trauma is structural in origin. Ethanol intoxication in a head-injured patient may profoundly depress the level of consciousness, respiration, and eventually ocular and pupillary reflexes. However, alcoholic intoxication does not generally cause focal or lateralizing neurologic signs unless associated with a seizure. A serum concentration of ethanol of less than 0.3 percent is not likely to cause coma, and a level less than 0.2 percent is not likely to cause significant confusion.

All known diabetics who sustain a head injury and arrive in the emergency department unconscious should be given 50 cc 50 percent glucose immediately after blood is drawn for metabolic studies. If the patient is hyperglycemic, this dose of glucose will seldom, if ever, cause further harm; if the patient is hypoglycemic, this dose may be both life-saving and diagnostic.

Funduscopic Examination

Even in the presence of a rapidly expanding intracranial hematoma, papilledema is seldom observed. Therefore, the absence of this sign in the hours immediately after head injury is no assurance that significant intracranial hypertension does not exist. Sudden compression of the thorax or of the neck, as occurs with impaction of the chest on a steering wheel or with strangulation, produces a sudden increase in intracranial venous pressure that may be associated with retinal venous hemorrhages similar to those seen with papilledema. Because similar hemorrhages occur in the brain, retinal venous hemorrhages may suggest intracranial hypertension even though there is no direct causal relationship. Subhyaloid hemorrhages are associated with subarachnoid hemorrhage, either spontaneous or traumatic. These hemorrhages are round and sharply circumscribed and thus are not readily confused with other types of hemorrhages of the posterior pole of the eye.

Lumbar Puncture

Not only does lumbar puncture have no value in the diagnosis or treatment of head trauma, it may be harmful, since cerebral herniation and death may follow increased intracranial pressure. Blood is commonly present in the cerebrospinal fluid of patients who have sustained head trauma, including many patients with no clinical signs of neurologic dysfunction. Conversely, some patients with extracerebral hematomas have few or no red blood cells in their cerebrospinal fluid. Only if meningitis is a serious possibility should a patient who has sustained recent head trauma undergo lumbar puncture.

Radiographic Studies

Obtaining roentgenograms of head-injured patients is often a hazardous undertaking. Too often, a thorough physical examination is deferred in favor of "total body" roentgenogram studies. Furthermore, the patient is usually monitored only sporadically during the period of time in which the roentgenograms are being taken, and valuable time is wasted obtaining roentgenograms that are of minor importance in the emergency management of the patient. For example, multiple views of a fractured extremity are extraneous if emergency treatment is to consist only of splinting. If the results of a particular roentgenogram will not change the emergency department management of a clinically unstable patient, then the roentgenogram should be deferred.

Cervical Spine. A cross table lateral roentgenogram of the cervical spine should be the first obtained in an unconscious patient with a head injury. Ideally, this should be obtained while the patient remains on the emergency department stretcher. If all seven cervical vertebrae are visualized and alignment appears normal, the patient can then be moved onto a table for subsequent studies. The fact that alignment is normal with the neck in neutral position does not guarantee that the spine is stable, i.e., that subluxation will not occur if the neck is flexed or extended, just as the fact that no fractures appear on a single lateral view of the cervical spine does not exclude certain fractures of the upper cervical vertebrae. Therefore, caution is still warranted in moving the patient.

Chest. It is the chest roentgenogram rather than the skull roentgenogram that usually reveals potential sources of secondary insult to the injured brain. Even if the chest roentgenogram is normal, however, there is a possibility of hypoxemia. Since no roentgenogram should be obtained before acute resuscitative procedures are completed, the chest roentgenogram can also be examined for proper positioning of the central venous pressure catheter and the endotracheal tube. The thoracic spine is shown with variable degrees of clarity on a chest roentgenogram, and gross lateral displacements can usually be discerned. These findings are almost invariably associated with paraplegia.

Skull. A lateral and anteroposterior view of the skull should always be obtained. There is no fracture pattern or location that is pathognomonic of extracerebral hematoma. Nevertheless, a fracture line across the temporal region or along the more distal portion of the groove for the middle meningeal vessels should increase the physician's watchfulness for development of an extradural hematoma. Arterial extradural hematomas seldom occur in the absence of overlying fracture and almost never occur contralateral to one, unless there are bilateral fractures. Most fractures across the middle meningeal groove produce no clinically significant epidural lesion. Fractures across the vertex or those extending into the occiput may be associated with venous extradural hematomas due to laceration of dural venous sinuses. These occur more frequently in children than in adults, as do extradural hematomas resulting from diploetic hemorrhage. The latter may occur with extensive skull fractures in infants, particularly when there is an unusual degree of separation between the edges of the fracture.

Intracranial air or air fluid levels in the paranasal sinuses usually indicate fracture of the base of the skull. These radiographic findings have the same clinical significance as the external stigmata of basal skull fracture discussed earlier. A focal double density over the convexity of the skull may indicate a depressed skull fracture, and a tangential roentgenogram of the lesion may confirm the diagnosis. The presence of a depressed fracture may sometimes be ascertained by palpating the skull through a scalp laceration with a sterile-gloved hand. In such cases, the tangential roentgenogram may reveal more severe depression than was indicated by palpation. Quite often, the inner table is depressed more than the outer table. Note should be made of any intracranial bone fragments or foreign bodies seen on the roentgenogram.

Both the lateral and the anteroposterior projection should always be specifically examined for pineal calcification, which occurs in approximately 40 percent of patients over age 20. Any calcification that is not seen in both views should not be considered the pineal body. A shift of greater than 3 mm to either side of the midline in the anteroposterior projection is considered significant, but does not always indicate an extracerebral hematoma. Nevertheless, in the symptomatic patient, such a shift demands immediate further investigation, provided that the patient's vital signs are stable enough to permit further diagnostic tests outside the emergency department. For the nonradiologist, the amount of pineal displacement is most easily determined by drawing a line from one outer table to the other at the level of the pineal gland. The distance between the midpoint of this line and the center of the pineal calcification is the measurement of pineal shift.

SPECIFIC TREATMENT OF HEAD INJURIES

Steroids

In patients with Glasgow Coma Scale scores of 12 or less, 2 gm methylprednisolone (1 gm for ages 5 to 15 and 0.5 gm for children under 5 years) can be given IV and the dose repeated in six hours if there has been no clinical improvement. Since the longer the initiation of treatment is delayed, the less effect there is on cerebral edema, steroid treatment should be begun as soon as possible after the arrival of the patient in the emergency department.

Hyperventilation

Induction of moderate hypocapnia (arterial pCO_2 of 25 to 30 mm Hg) by controlled hyperventilation reduces intracranial pressure by decreasing cerebral blood flow and thus cerebral blood volume. In addition to these specific actions, controlled ventilation via endotracheal tube ensures good pulmonary alveolar oxygenation. Hyperventilation should be routinely employed in the acute management of any patient who arrives in the emergency department with a Glasgow Coma Scale score of 8 or less or displays progressive deterioration in the level of consciousness.

Neurogenic pulmonary edema occasionally occurs after a severe head injury. The most important therapeutic maneuver is to intubate the patient and initiate continuous positive pressure ventilation. (See Chapter 48.)

Elevation of the Head of the Bed

If the patient's cardiovascular status permits, intracranial venous pressure may be diminished by elevating the head of the bed to 60°. In addition, care should be taken to avoid compression of the jugular veins, which often occurs when the head passively falls to one side or when the tapes that hold a tracheotomy tube in place are tied too tightly.

Control of Temperature

Hyperpyrexia increases intracranial pressure and thus should be aggressively treated in those patients who require hyperventilation. Acetaminophen suppositories should be used initially, and even a cooling blanket should be utilized, if necessary. The goal of therapy is to reduce the patient's body temperature to 36°C or 37°C.

Mannitol

Use of a therapeutic trial of mannitol in the emergency department should be discouraged. Under these circumstances, it is impossible to determine whether a subsequent clinical improvement reflects the natural history of the injury or is instead due to a temporary decrease in intracranial pressure that masks an intracranial mass lesion. The use of mannitol thus commits the physician to performing a definitive diagnostic test, usually an angiogram or a computerized axial tomography (CT) scan. This drug should be used in the emergency department only as a temporary, life-saving measure and then only after other therapeutic modalities have failed to halt progressive neurologic deterioration. The dose under these circumstances is 1 to 2 gm/kg body weight. Thus, for a 70-kg man, an entire 500-cc bottle of 20 percent mannitol should be used. It should be infused as rapidly as possible.

Mannitol should not be used in the presence of hypovolemic shock, congestive heart failure, or preexistent dehydration. It is also contraindicated in the presence of neurogenic pulmonary edema, despite the fact that this syndrome is usually due to increased intracranial pressure. Acute expansion of the intravascular volume only exacerbates the edema.

Maximum reduction of brain water occurs at a serum osmolality of approximately 310 mOsm/liter, and dehydration much beyond this point is both unproductive and dangerous.

Insertion of a Foley catheter is mandatory if mannitol is given. However, infusion of mannitol should not be delayed if the catheter is not immediately available.

Anticonvulsants

If a patient regains consciousness after a single post-traumatic seizure and is then neurologically stable, anticonvulsant drugs are not indicated. Immediate initiation of anticonvulsant therapy is indicated, however, for patients

1. who have a penetrating head injury, regardless of whether they have already had a seizure
2. who have had a single post-traumatic seizure but show no postictal signs of neurologic recovery
3. in whom a seizure is associated with neurologic deterioration
4. who have multiple seizures
5. who have depressed skull fractures located near the motor cortex (approximately midway between the front and back of the head)
6. whose level of consciousness is severely depressed (Glasgow Coma Scale score of less than 8)

Diphenylhydantoin (Dilantin) may be used in the acute treatment of seizures associated with head trauma. With an intravenous loading dose of 10 mg/kg body weight, a therapeutic blood level is reached almost immediately and lasts approximately 24 hours. The drug must be given in normal saline that contains no other medications. The rate of infusion should not exceed 50 mg/minute, and the electrocardiogram (ECG) and blood pressure should be monitored. If bradycardia, hypotension, or prolongation of QRS or PR intervals occurs, the infusion should be interrupted until vital signs and ECG are again normal. When resumed, infusion should be at a slower rate. Clinically significant respiratory depression or sedation occurs infrequently.

Diazepam (Valium) is useful in the treatment of status epilepticus. The intravenous dose in small children is 0.1 mg/kg body weight. Adults may require up to twice the calculated dose (.15 to .20 mg/kg body weight infused no faster than 5 mg/minute). The dose may be repeated once or twice at ten-minute intervals, but only the minimum amount necessary to stop the seizures should be given. High cumulative doses cause hypotension and respiratory depression. Intubation may become necessary in the course of treating status epilepticus. After the seizures have been controlled with this medication, the patient should be given a loading dose of diphenylhydantoin as outlined previously. (See Chapter 47.)

Antibiotics

Meningitis following basal skull fracture is usually due to pneumococci, and thus many prophylactic regimens consist of low-dose penicillin and/or sulfa for seven to ten days. For example, sulfisoxazole (Gantrisin), 2 gm/day, is given only with frank cerebrospinal fluid rhinorrhea or otorrhea. With open or penetrating injuries of the cranial vault, an initial 2-gm intravenous dose of nafcillin is recommended.

Criteria for tetanus prophylaxis with wounds of the scalp are the same as those for other soft tissue injuries.

Analgesics

Narcotic analgesics and sedatives obscure the post-traumatic clinical course by altering pupillary size and reactivity and by depressing the level of consciousness. These drugs may also suppress spontaneous ventilation, which causes CO_2 retention and an increase in cerebral blood volume, which in turn may increase intracranial pressure. For these reasons, only aspirin or acetaminophen are recommended in cases of post-traumatic headache.

THE DISPOSITION OF THE HEAD-INJURED PATIENT

The emergency department physician can (1) send a head-injured patient home, (2) admit the patient to the hospital at which he or she is being treated, or (3) transfer the patient to a regional head injury center. There are no rigid triage criteria simply because therapy must be individualized. In addition, the therapeutic and diagnostic resources of different medical communities vary. Therefore, the following head injury triage classification should be used as a flexible guideline.

Discharge from Emergency Department

Patients with a scalp injury but no signs or symptoms of craniocerebral injury can be discharged. Obvious exceptions include those patients who suffer major blood loss from scalp lacerations and those whose scalp wounds cannot be satisfactorily closed in the emergency department.

Asymptomatic patients whose concussions have resolved by the time they arrive at the emergency department can also be discharged. Such patients are fully ambulatory and conversant, and the results of a neurologic examination are completely normal. They complain of little more than mild headache. Memory for events immediately preceding the accident should be returning, although memory of some events immediately succeeding the accident may be permanently lost. Most important is the fact that storage and retrieval of new memories is intact at the time of examination. Ideally, such patients might be admitted for overnight observation, but they can be discharged from the emergency department provided that they can be brought back to the hospital if increasing headache, vomiting, or obtundation supervene.

Admit to the Local Hospital for Observation

Patients with an unresolved concussion should be admitted for observation until they are fully oriented and can consistently demonstrate normal immediate recall and recent memory. They need not remain in the hospital until the headache resolves, provided that it is diminishing. Most patients in this category can be discharged within 24 hours.

Preschool age children, even if the results of a neurologic examination are normal, should be kept in the hospital for observation because this age group often reacts atypically to head trauma. Intermittent somnolence, agitation when aroused, and vomiting are seen after both trivial and major injuries. A child with an extracerebral hematoma may periodically appear quite alert. The degree of severity of the head injury is usually apparent after a day of observation.

Stuporous patients, i.e., those with a Glasgow Coma Scale score of 11 or greater, who have no focal or lateralizing signs and are improving neurologically should be admitted. A significant number of patients in this category have a concussion with superimposed ethanol intoxication. They merit close inpatient observation, but require nothing more than supportive treatment as long as they continue to improve.

Patients with basal or convexity skull fracture, even those with no neurologic deficit, should be admitted for observation simply because skull fracture indicates a relatively great force was applied to the head. These patients are usually observed for 24 to 48 hours.

Transfer to Regional Head Injury Center

The following types of patients should be transferred to a regional head injury center:

1. severely obtunded patients (Glasgow Coma Scale score less than 11).
2. patients with deterioration in level of consciousness.
3. patients with focal or lateralizing neurologic signs.
4. patients with a penetrating cranial injury or a depressed skull fracture.
5. preschool age children with any skull fracture.
6. patients with cerebrospinal fluid rhinorrhea or otorrhea.
7. patients with post-traumatic seizures who are not known to be epileptic.
8. head-injured patients with painful extracranial lesions that require narcotic analgesics. In multiple trauma patients, narcotic analgesics are usually indicated to relieve the pain of major skeletal injuries (e.g., fractured femur) or to enhance the effectiveness of artificial ventilation by depressing the patient's own respiratory drive.

TRANSPORTATION OF HEAD-INJURED PATIENT TO THE REGIONAL HEAD INJURY CENTER

Transporting the head-injured patient to another hospital often poses difficult problems. The patient is most in need of continuous medical attention during transfer, but is often least able to obtain it at this time. During this period, unrecognized airway obstruction, improper ventilation, and inadequate fluid volume replacement cause further brain damage more often than extracerebral hematoma does. The standards for adequate resuscitation and stabilization are never more important than when an emergency department physician even temporarily removes an acutely injured patient from expert medical supervision. The following guidelines should be adhered to if permanent neurologic damage from the transport procedure is to be avoided.

Except under the most exceptional circumstances, no patient can be transported who does not have

1. a patent airway
2. satisfactory spontaneous or artificial ventilation
3. adequate blood pressure

As has been emphasized repeatedly, resuscitation and stabilization are always more important than specific treatment of any head injury.

The patient who is leaving the emergency department must be prepared for the transfer:

1. The neck should be immobilized in a neutral position if a cervical spinal injury has not been excluded.
2. Continuous patency of the airway must be guaranteed. In an unconscious patient, this almost always necessitates intubation. If the emergency department physician is unsuccessful in this procedure, it is usually a judicious expenditure of time to call in an anesthesiologist. Suctioning equipment must be available during transport.
3. A route for bag ventilation must be available. Again, this usually involves passage of a cuffed endotracheal tube.
4. A route for fluid resuscitation must be established. An intravenous catheter (#18 gauge or larger) must be inserted prior to transport. The emergency care personnel should be instructed to infuse 5 percent dextrose in Ringer's lactate at either a "wide open" or "keep vein open" rate, depending upon whether the systolic blood pressure falls below 100 mm Hg.
5. A Foley catheter should be inserted in all unconscious patients.

6. The neurosurgeon at the regional head injury center should be called before the patient is placed in the ambulance. No patient is so critically ill that transport cannot be "delayed" for the time necessary to obtain the advice of the neurosurgeon. On the contrary, the more severe the injury, the more important such advice may be. Mannitol should sometimes be given during transport, but this decision should be made only after consultation with the neurosurgeon.
7. Complete medical data should be transferred with the patient. A transfer record, a copy of the emergency department record, and all roentgenograms should be sent with each head-injured patient.

CONCLUSION

Sophisticated care of the head-injured patient in the emergency department does not demand sophisticated knowledge of neurosurgery. Instead, it depends upon

1. meticulous attention to the fundamental principles of resuscitation.
2. prevention of secondary cardiopulmonary abnormalities that can further injure the traumatized brain.
3. performance of serial neurologic examinations. In the case of acute head injury, a simple neurologic examination performed repeatedly usually provides the physician with more useful information than a more elaborate examination performed only once.
4. consultation with the neurosurgeon. If there is any possibility that neurosurgical consultation might enhance the emergency department management of the patient, the emergency department physician should not hesitate to contact the appropriate neurosurgical staff member.

There is no question that protocols for any phase of emergency management of CNS trauma are of no value unless there is a high degree of compliance. This can only be achieved through training paramedics, emergency medical technicians, nurses, and physicians in the optimal care that can be afforded these patients. If the morbidity and mortality of the CNS trauma patient are to be decreased, those involved in emergency medicine must take an active role in training programs, seminars, and clinical practice for physicians, emergency department nurses, paramedics, and emergency medical technicians.

BIBLIOGRAPHY

Carlsson CA, Von Essen C, Lofgren JC: The factors affecting clinical course of patients with severe head injuries. *J Neurosurg* 29:242–251, 1968.

Decker TB, Blaylock RLD, Perot PL: Emergency care of patients with cerebral injuries. *Postgrad Med* 55:102–110, 1974.

Galbraith S, Murray WR, Patel AR, et al: The relationship between alcohol and head injury and its effect on the conscious level. *Br J Surg* 63:128–130, 1976.

It's an Emergency. *Newsweek,* November 21, 1977, pp 105–108.

Jennett B, Teasdale G, Galbraith SL, et al: Severe head injuries in three countries. *J Neurol Neurosurg Psychiatry* 40:291–298, 1977.

Kraus JF: Epidemiologic features of head and spinal cord injury. *Adv Neurol* 19:261–280, 1978.

McDowall DG, Norman JB: Symposium on neurosurgical anesthesia. *Br J Anaesth* 48:719–804, 1976.

North JB, Jennett S: Abnormal breathing patterns associated with acute brain damage. *Arch Neurol* 31:338–344, 1974.

Perot PL: Trauma at first site: Craniocerebral injuries. *Postgrad Med* 55, 1974.

Plum F, Posner JB: *The Diagnosis of Stupor and Coma,* ed 2. Philadelphia, FA Davis, 1972.

Teasdale G, Jennett B: Assessment of coma and impaired consciousness: A practical scale. *Lancet* 2:81–84, 1974.

43. Cervical Spine Injuries

DAVID J. DULA, M.D.

Traumatic injuries to the cervical spine must be recognized as soon as possible and managed properly if the catastrophic complications of such injuries are to be avoided. Conservative estimates place the number of serious spinal cord injuries at approximately 5,000/year, with an additional number of spinal injuries that do not involve the cord.[1] Statistics show that less than 50 percent of the patients with significant injury to the bony cervical spine have injuries to the cord. Of cord injuries, less than 50 percent are complete injuries (total loss of cord function distal to the lesion); the majority are partial (some remaining cord function distal to the lesion) and these patients have an excellent prognosis for recovery.[2]

It is estimated that up to 10 percent of patients with an underlying cervical spine injury develop paralysis as the result of unprotected manipulation of the head and neck during their initial medical care.[3] Because of the devastating nature of spinal cord injuries and the prolonged disability that results, it is vital to develop a system of care for such patients that will prevent any additional cord injury and provide the best chance for recovery. To achieve this goal, emergency care personnel must be trained to recognize and treat injuries of the cervical spine. Of special importance is the detection of partial cord injuries, because these injuries are the most difficult to detect and have the greatest potential for recovery. The development and utilization of regional spinal cord centers, along with good prehospital and emergency department care, provide patients with cord injuries optimal care.

ANATOMY

The cervical spine is composed of seven vertebrae; the first, the atlas, articulates with the occipital condyles superiorly and the odontoid process and superior facets of the second vertebra body inferiorly. It is a ringlike structure and is different from the other six cervical vertebrae in that it has no vertebral body. The remaining six cervical vertebrae have a vertebral body, pedicles, laminae, and a spinous process (Fig. 43–1). The second cervical vertebra, the axis, has a bony strut (the odontoid) attached to its vertebral body that permits both stable articulation with the atlas and rotational mobility. The remaining cervical vertebrae articulate with each other by way of the facet joints.

The ligamentous structures of the cervical spine are vitally important to its stability. The major ligaments include the supraspinous ligament and the interspinous ligament, the articular capsule of the facet joints, the ligamentum flavum, the posterior longitudinal ligament, the anterior longitudinal ligament, and the transverse ligament (Fig. 43–2). The anterior longitudinal ligament is a strong, narrow band of dense fibers connected to tissue that is attached to the anterior margins

I would like to give special thanks to Donna Rentzel for her help and encouragement in preparing this manuscript and to James Schmidt for his help in providing the illustrations used in this chapter.

of the vertebral body and the intervertebral disks; it maintains stability when the cervical spine is extended. The posterior longitudinal ligament courses along the posterior aspect of the vertebral bodies and disks and forms the anterior boundary of the spinal canal. The capsular ligament is a thin, loose structure that attaches to the margins of the articular processes of the facet joints. The ligamentum flavum is a thick, dense ligament that connects with the lamina of each vertebral body and forms the posterior ligamentous margin of the spinal canal. The supraspinous ligament and the interspinous ligament connect the spinous processes of the vertebral bodies and impart stability to the cervical spine during flexion maneuvers. The transverse ligament maintains the odontoid in its fixed position within the atlas.

The combination of these vertebrae and ligaments allows the cervical spine to maintain its stability despite its high degree of mobility.

PATHOPHYSIOLOGY

Traumatic injuries to the bony cervical spine and cervical cord are often interrelated (Table 43–1). However, to understand the different injuries that can occur to the cervical spine and cord, it is easier to consider them separate entities.

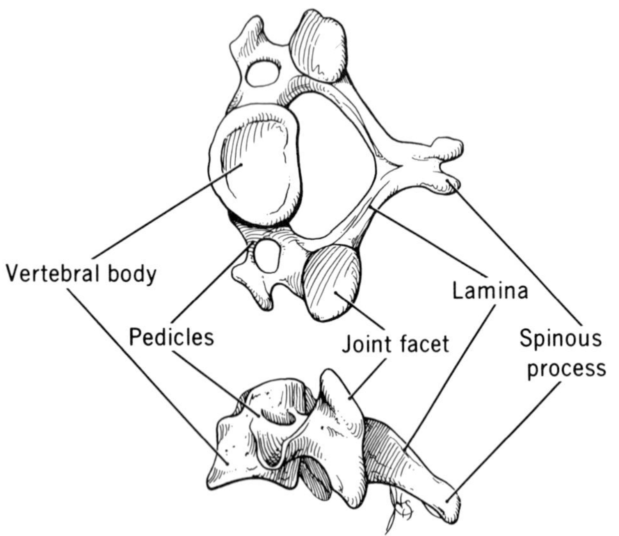

Figure 43–1   Anatomy of the Cervical Vertebrae.

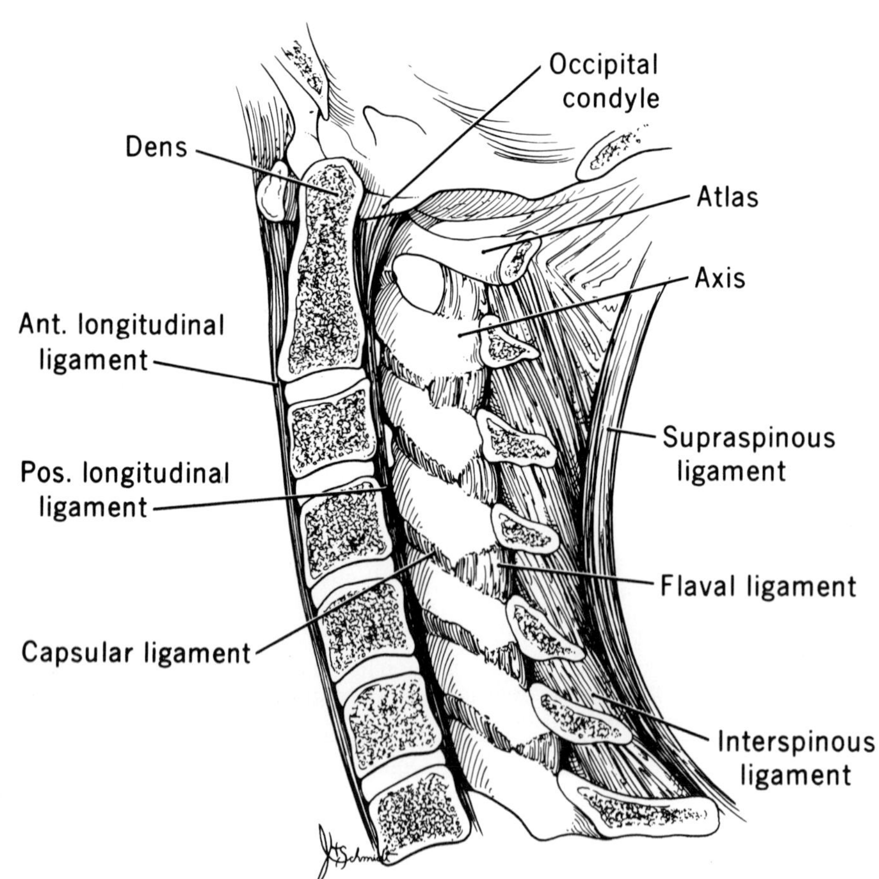

Figure 43–2   Ligamentous Anatomy of the Cervical Spine.

Cervical Spine Injuries

Trauma to the cervical spine from either direct or inertial forces most commonly results from motor vehicle accidents, but such an injury can also occur in falls, sports, and incidents involving projectiles (Table 43–2). Inertial forces play a prominent role in an automobile accident, for example, when the driver is wearing a shoulder harness and a seatbelt. The thorax is secured to the seat of the car, whereas the head and neck remain mobile and are subjected to inertial forces that may result in a flexion or extension injury to the cervical spine.[4] Whether the cervical spine is traumatized from a direct blow or from an inertial event, the injury results from a combination of several forces—flexion, rotation, compression, and extension.

- A. Flexion Injuries
    1. Anterior subluxation
    2. Bilateral interfacetal dislocation
    3. Clay shoveler's fracture
    4. Flexion tear drop fracture
- B. Rotation Injuries
    1. Unilateral interfacetal dislocation
- C. Vertical Compression Injuries
    1. Bursting fracture
        a. Jefferson fracture of atlas
        b. Burst fracture, lower cervical vertebrae
- D. Extension Injuries
    1. Extension tear-drop fracture
    2. Hangman's fracture (deceleration, hyperextension)

TABLE 43–1   Relation of Cervical Spine Injuries to Cervical Cord Injuries

Type of Spine Injury	No.	(%)	Total Cord	Partial Cord
Stable Fracture	20	(22)	0	3
Unstable fracture	63	(69)	19	13
No Fracture	8	(9)	0	8
Total	91	(100)	19 (21%)	24 (26%)

TABLE 43–2   Trauma to Cervical Spine

	No.	(%)
Auto	65	62.5
Falls	24	23.0
Motorcycle	5	4.8
Dive	5	4.8
Sport	2	1.0
Missile	1	1.0
Other	2	1.9

These forces may cause injury to either the ligaments or the osseous structures of the cervical spine.

Flexion injuries to the cervical spine may disrupt the posterior longitudinal ligament, resulting in various degrees of anterior subluxation and cervical instability. A severe flexion force may produce additional subluxation and dislocation of the facet joints (Fig. 43–3). When the posterior longitudinal ligament tears, separation or fanning of the spinous processes results, an important finding that can be seen on the lateral cervical spine roentgenogram. A simple wedge fracture or teardrop fracture of the vertebral body results from compressive forces exerted on the anterior portion of the vertebral body during extreme flexion (Fig. 43–4). A clay shoveler's fracture (Fig. 43–5) is defined as an avulsion type of fracture of the proximal portion of the spinous process, usually occurring at C6, C7, or T1 as a result of an abrupt flexion of the head against the tensed posterior ligaments.

A flexion-rotation mechanism of injury may result in a unilateral facet dislocation. This injury occurs when the flexion force is great enough to cause one facet to move across its adjacent inferior facet and come to rest in a dislocated position (Fig. 43–6). The posterior ligament complex and capsule of the involved joint is disrupted, and the posterior longitudinal ligament is partially disrupted. In this position, the vertebral bodies are locked, however, and the fracture is therefore considered to be stable.

A compressive force to the cervical spine results in several classical injuries, such as a Jefferson fracture of the atlas (Fig. 43–7). This injury is the result of a force transmitted through the occiput to the lateral masses of the atlas. The force drives the articular masses laterally, producing bilateral fractures of both the anterior and posterior arches of C1, and disrupting the transverse atlantal ligament. A bursting fracture of the lower cervical bodies may result from vertical compression forces transmitted to the cervical spine (Fig. 43–8). This is the result of the nucleus pulposus being imploded into the vertebral body, resulting in the characteristic comminuted fracture of the cervical vertebral body. The posterior fragments of the vertebral body are usually displaced posteriorly.

Extension injuries of the cervical spine frequently cause injuries to the cord without evidence of injury to the cervical vertebrae. Buckling of the ligamentum flavum posteriorly and compression of the cord against the spurs of the vertebral body anteriorly cause a temporary compression of the cord (Fig. 43–9). Additionally, hyperextension of the neck can cause fracture dislocations of the cervical spine, posterior atlantal arch fractures, or extension teardrop fractures of the cervical spine. The teardrop deformity results from an avulsion of bone by the stressed anterior longitudinal ligament

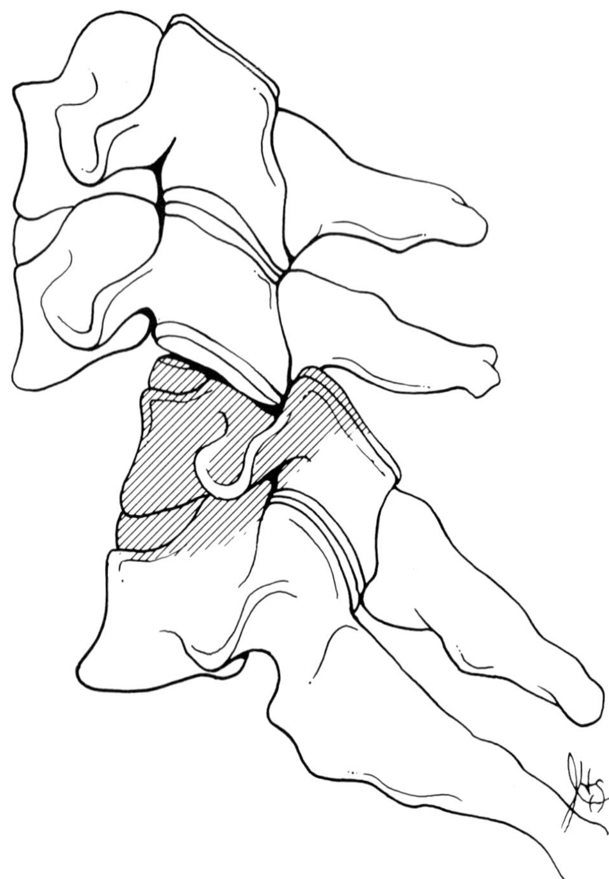

Figure 43–3 Interlocking Articular Facets.

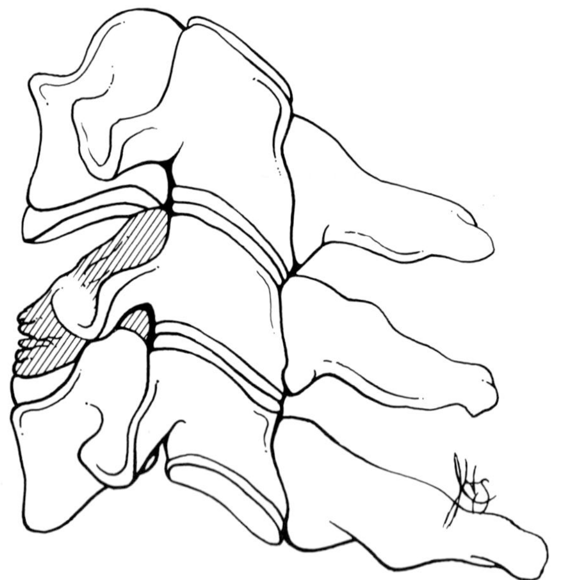

Figure 43–4 Wedge Fracture of a Cervical Vertebra.

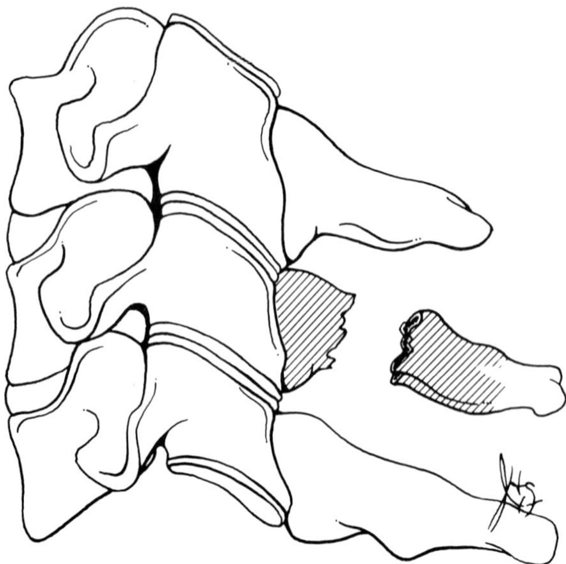

Figure 43–5 Clay Shoveler's Fracture.

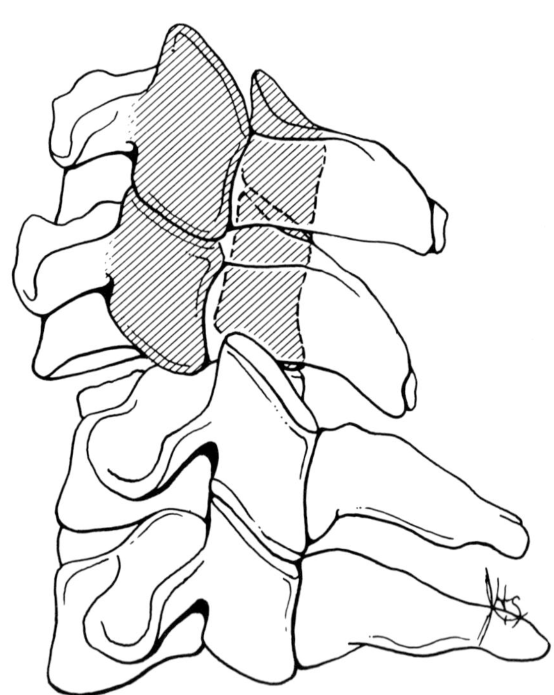

Figure 43–6 Unilateral Locked Facet.

during extension (Fig. 43–10). Another type of hyperextension injury is the hangman's fracture, which derives its name from the fact that its pathologic skeletal characteristics are similar to those caused by judicial hanging.[5] This fracture is a bilateral fracture of the pedicles of the axis associated with a subluxation of C2 on C3 (Fig. 43–11).

Shearing forces acting on the first and second vertebrae may cause fracture of the odontoid and/or disruption of the transverse ligament—the fibrous band that retains the odontoid in its proper anatomical position within the ring of the atlas (Fig. 43–12). These injuries are highly unstable and require immediate care to prevent injury to the cord.

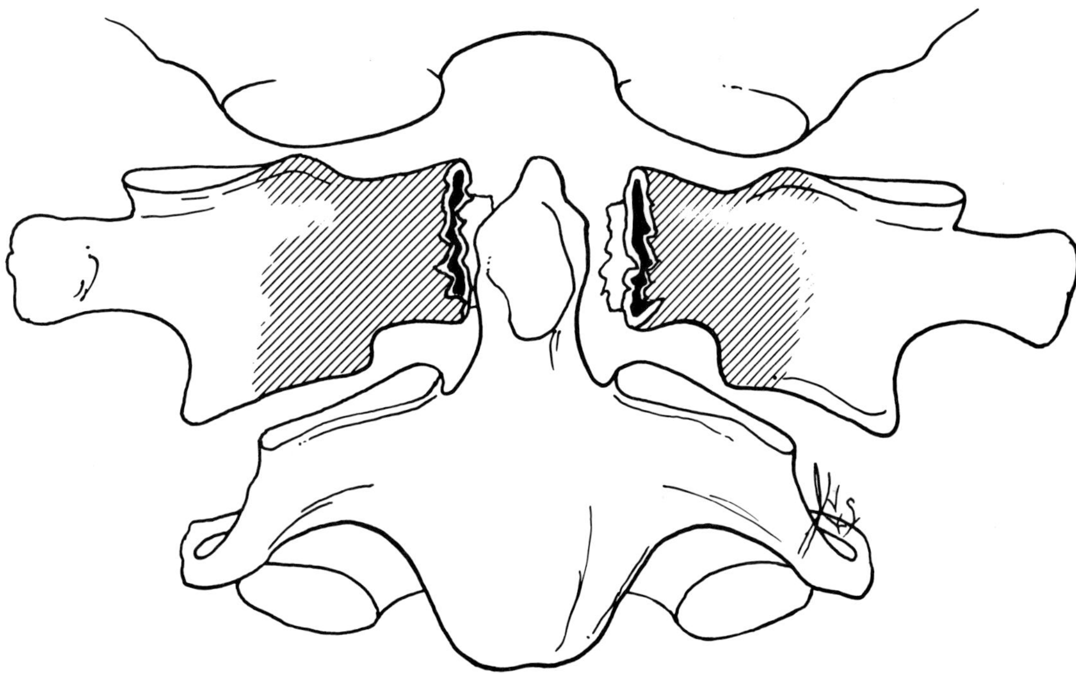

Figure 43–7   Jefferson Fracture with Bursting of the Ringlike Structure of the Atlas.

Other types of fractures, dislocations, and subluxations can best be understood in relation to the anatomical structures involved. It is difficult to determine with certainty whether any cervical fracture is stable or unstable, and a realistic approach may be to divide types of fractures into those that have a high probability of being stable and those that have a high probability of being unstable. Some cervical spine injuries may be unstable only in certain positions, such as flexion instability in posterior longitudinal ligament tears, while others may represent gross instability in any position, such as hangman's fracture or fractures of the odontoid.

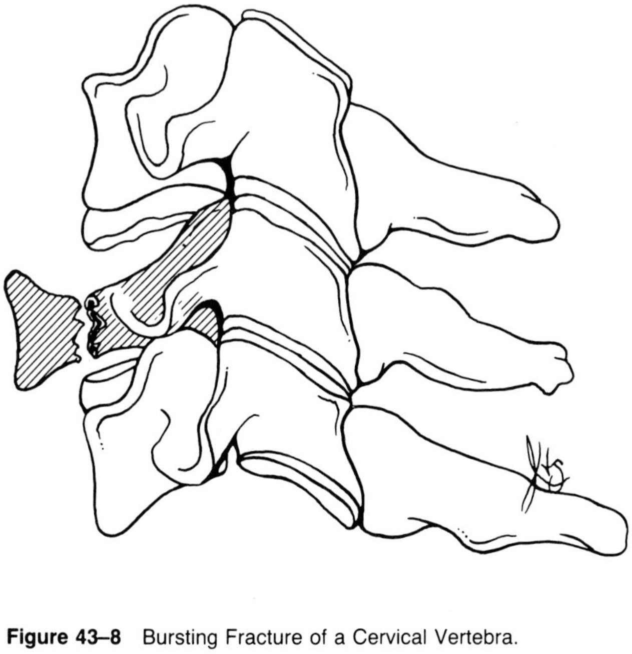

A. Stable
   1. Anterior subluxation
   2. Unilateral interfacetal dislocation
   3. Simple wedge fracture
   4. Burst fracture, lower cervical vertebrae
   5. Clay shoveler's fracture
B. Unstable
   1. Bilateral interfacetal dislocation
   2. Flexion tear-drop fracture
   3. Extension tear-drop fracture (stable in flexion, unstable in extension)
   4. Hangman's fracture
   5. Jefferson fracture of atlas
   6. Hyperextension fracture-dislocation

Even stable cervical spine injuries require care, since exaggerated motion of the neck may exacerbate a partial cord injury. A review of the anatomy of the cervical cord and its position within the bony network of the cervical spine makes it clear how the cord can be injured (Fig. 43–13). Disruption of the bony framework, herniation of disk material, or compromise of the vascular supply to the cord may all result in an insult to the cervical cord. Hyperextension may temporarily compress the cord. Inertial forces acting on the cervical cord

Figure 43–8   Bursting Fracture of a Cervical Vertebra.

may result in areas of contusion to the cord, while a severe injury may result in anatomical transection of the cord.

Cervical Cord Injuries

The variety of clinical conditions that result from trauma to the cervical cord can be classified as partial or complete cord injuries, depending on the degree of damage to the cord. A *complete* cord injury is defined as the absence of any sensory, motor, or autonomic neurologic function below the level of the lesion.[6] A *partial* cord injury is defined as a partial loss of cord function below the level of the lesion, i.e., some sensory, motor, or autonomic nervous system function remains. In a study of 91 cases of injury to the cervical spine, the cord was injured in 47 percent of the cases; 21 percent were complete cord injuries, whereas 26 percent were partial.[2]

Partial cord injuries can be further subgrouped into three major clinical presentations: (1) central cord injury, (2) anterior cord injury, and (3) the Brown-Séquard syndrome. Central cord injury results in motor weakness of the arms greater than that in the legs, loss of urinary bladder function, and varying degrees of sensory loss secondary to the injury.[7] The anterior cord injury is characterized by an immediate paralysis with hypoesthesia and hypalgesia up to the level of the lesion, although touch, motion, position, and vibratory sensation are spared.[8] The Brown-Séquard syndrome results from a cord injury that impairs motor function on one side of the body and pain and temperature perception on the contralateral side of the body below the level of the lesion.[9] An anatomical analysis of the cervical cord (Fig. 43–14) shows that total disruption or necrosis of the cervical cord and thus of all pathways through the cord results in complete loss of sensation, motor function, and autonomic nervous system function below the level of this lesion. The most evident autonomic effects are the absence of sweating, difficulties with vasomotor control, and priapism.

The acute central cord syndrome is caused most often by hyperextension of the cervical spine; injury to the cord results from posterior compression by bulging of the ligamentum flavum and anterior compression by the vertebral bodies (see Figure 43–10). The unique pattern of muscle weakness, combined with a history of hyperextension to the cervical spine, should make the

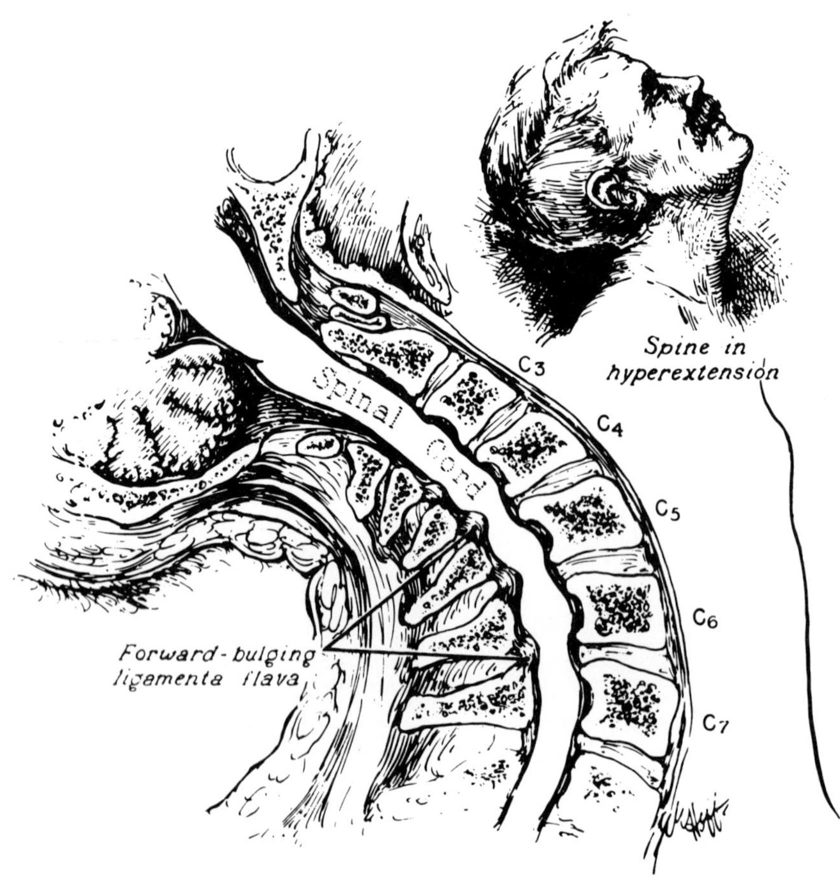

Figure 43–9   Mechanism of Cord Compression in Hyperextension Injuries of the Cervical Spine.

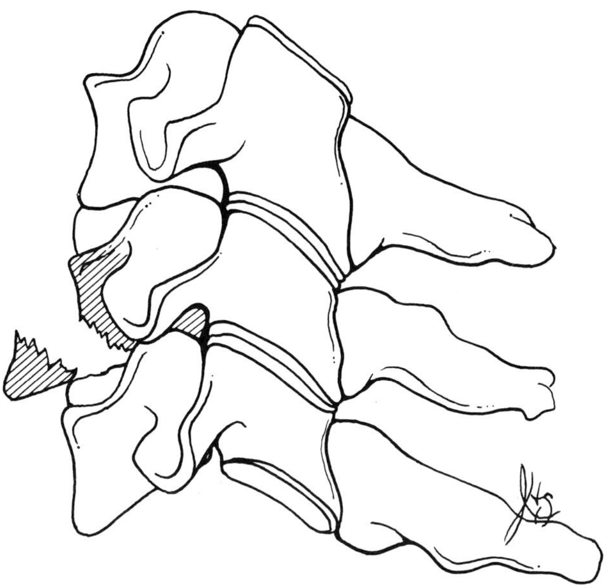

Figure 43–10 Teardrop Fracture of the Cervical Vertebrae.

emergency department physician highly suspicious of this entity. This lesion is associated with varying degrees of edema and/or contusion, hemorrhage, or necrosis of the central portion of the cord. Since fibers in the lateral cortical spinal tract are laminated with the upper extremity fibers, which are located medially, and the lower extremity fibers are located more peripherally, the fibers supplying motor function to the arms are more susceptible to this type of injury (Fig. 43–15). The recovery from this injury usually follows the same laminar pattern in that leg strength is recovered before arm strength; finger and fine hand movements are usually the last to be recovered. Depending on the amount of central cord destruction, the degree of recovery may vary. The neurologic deficit may have occurred at the time of the injury and may have already cleared by the time emergency care personnel arrive. This is especially common with football players, who may have only temporary paresthesias or dysesthesias of the hands after suffering an injury to the neck.[10]

The differential diagnosis of the central cord injury should include cruciate paralysis of Bell and a bilateral brachial plexus injury. Cruciate paralysis results from an injury to the atlanto-occipital area with subsequent injury to the cord in the area of the pyramidal decussation.[9] A lesion in this area presents a clinical picture similar to that of the central cord syndrome. For this reason, roentgenograms of the odontoid are important in the evaluation of physical findings consistent with a central cord injury. Bilateral brachial plexus injury may also simulate a central cord injury, although the neurologic deficit in this entity is confined to the nerve roots and is usually associated with absence of deep tendon reflexes.

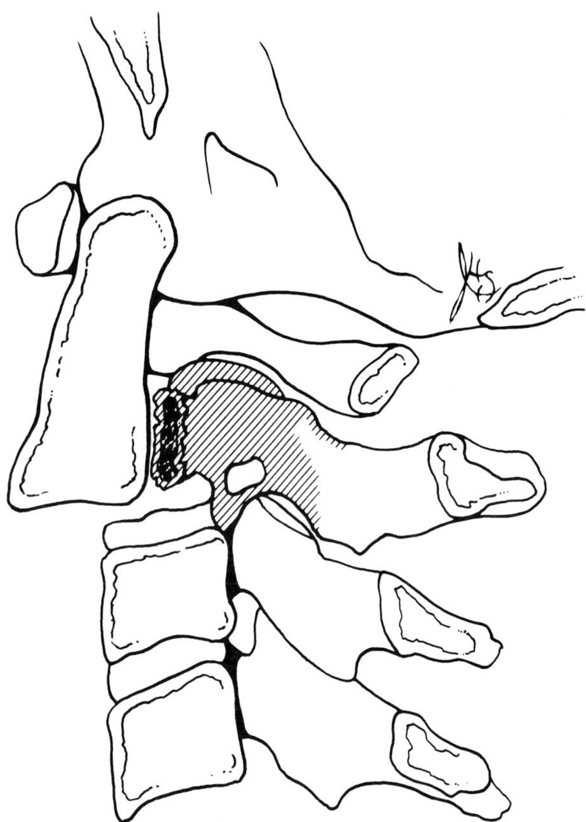

Figure 43–11 Hangman's Fracture with Anterior Subluxation of C2 on C3 and Bilateral Pedicle Fractures of C2.

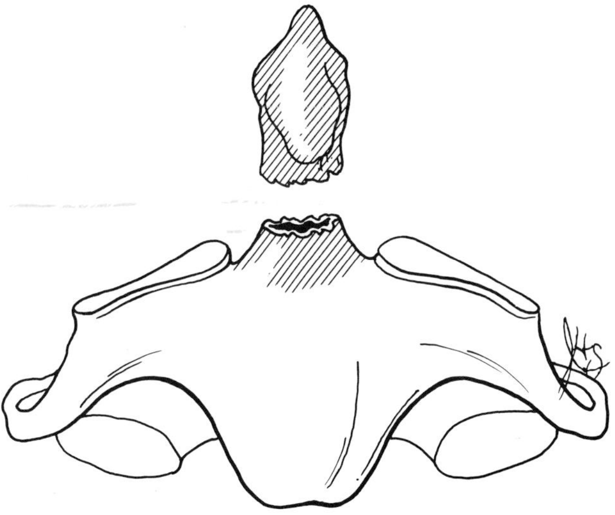

Figure 43–12 Fracture of the Odontoid.

The syndrome of acute anterior spinal cord injury usually results from compressive forces to the anterior portion of the cord by either a bony fragment or a herniated disk. The clinical findings of this lesion can be understood by noting the area of the cord that is injured (Fig. 43–16). The uninjured area is that of the

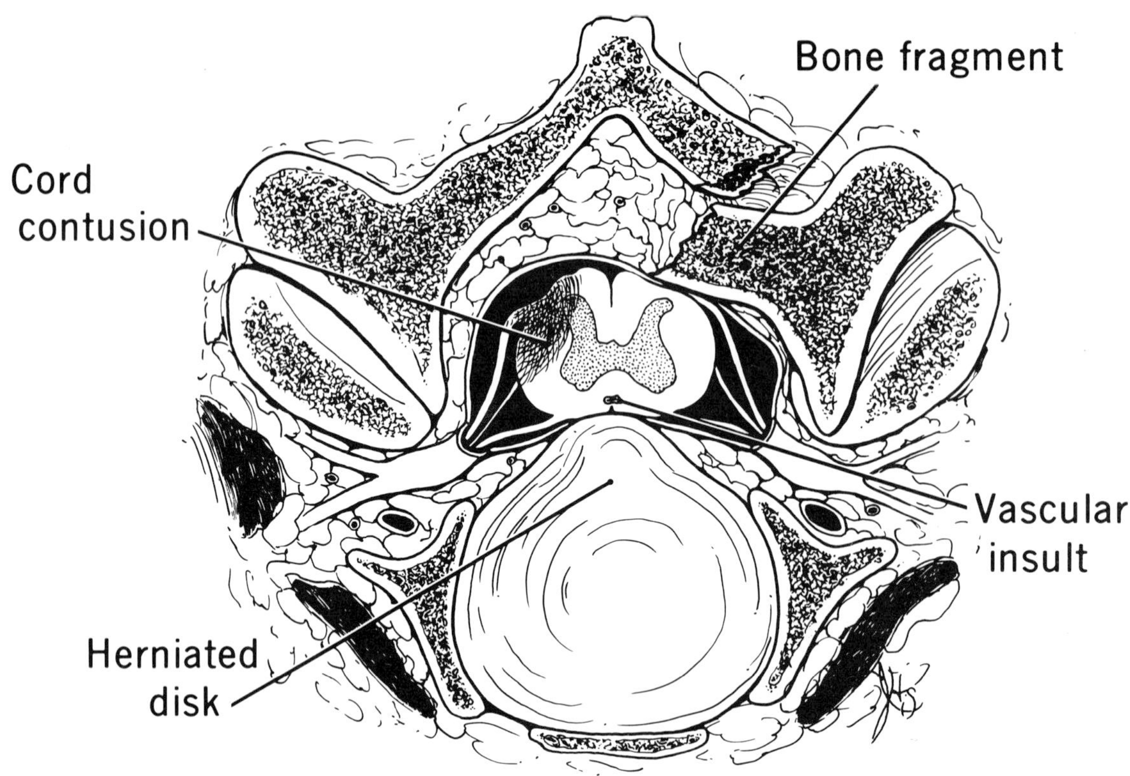

Figure 43–13 Mechanisms of Cord Injury Associated with Trauma.

posterior columns, which are the tracts that convey touch, motion, position, and vibratory sense. This lesion may occur in the absence of any fracture or dislocation; for example, it may be caused by a herniated disk.

The Brown-Séquard syndrome can also be understood by observing the area of cord that is injured and the tracts that have been disrupted (Fig. 43–17). Since sensory tracts cross at the cord level and motor tracts cross at the pyramidal decussation, a lesion of this type results in a loss of sensation and temperature sense on one side of the body (contralateral to the cord lesion) and a resultant weakness on the opposite side of the body (ipsilateral to the lesion).[11] This lesion may result from a lateral compressive force to the cervical cord as a result of disk or bony disruption of the cervical spine.

DIFFERENTIAL DIAGNOSIS

Other entities that may be considered in the differential diagnosis of cervical cord injuries are hysterical paralysis and brachial plexus injuries. Hysterical paralysis may be difficult to distinguish from an acute cervical cord injury, especially when the complex clinical manifestations of the partial cord syndromes are considered. In hysterical paralysis, the motor and sensory deficits usually do not follow any known anatomical patterns, but caution must be used to exclude any possibility of a partial cord syndrome. In true cord injuries, reflexes are usually lost; however, they are retained in hysterical paralysis.[12] If the patient has a weakness of one leg, the Hoover test may be applied; the physician places a hand below each of the patient's heels, and the patient is asked to raise the paralyzed leg. If the nonparalyzed leg is not pushed down against the hand during such an effort, the patient is not trying to lift the so-called paralyzed leg. Thus, the suspicions of hysteria are strengthened.[12]

Traumatic injuries to the brachial plexus may mimic a cord injury. The injury may be partial or complete, and the patient may have a sensory and motor deficit that corresponds to the injured nerve roots. Rarely, bilateral brachial plexus injury may be difficult to distinguish from a central cord injury. With brachial plexus injuries, however, the deficit should be confined to the extremity of the injured brachial plexus, and there should be no true cord deficit demonstrated on neurologic examination.[13,14]

Nontraumatic conditions may also cause spinal cord injury and should be considered in patients with acute spinal cord injuries. For example, ischemia of the spinal cord may occur because atherosclerotic disease, thrombosis, or dissection of the thoracic aorta has occluded the spinal cord circulation.[11] An oncologic emergency

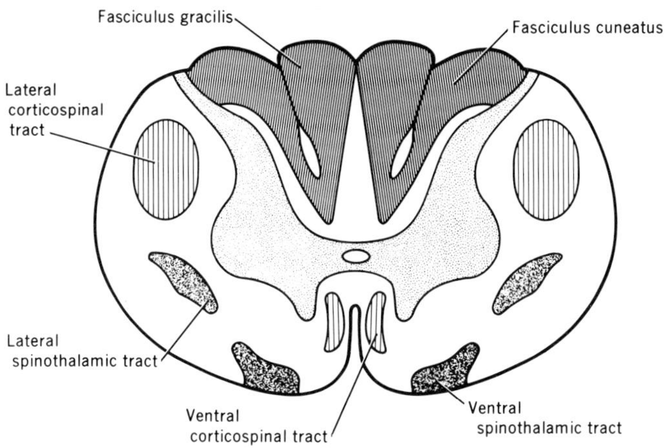

Figure 43–14   Anatomy of the Cervical Cord.

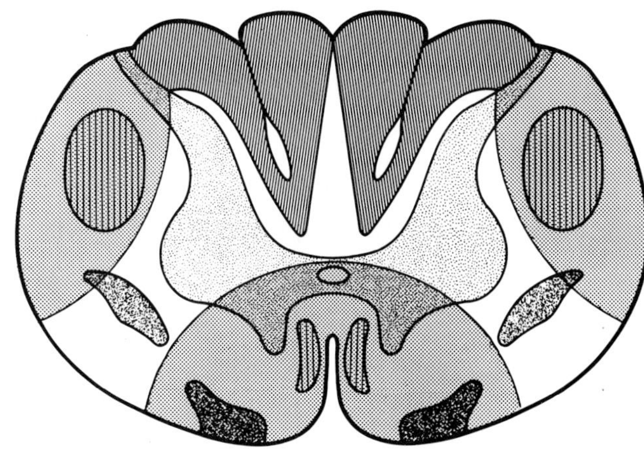

Figure 43–16   Anterior Cord Syndrome.

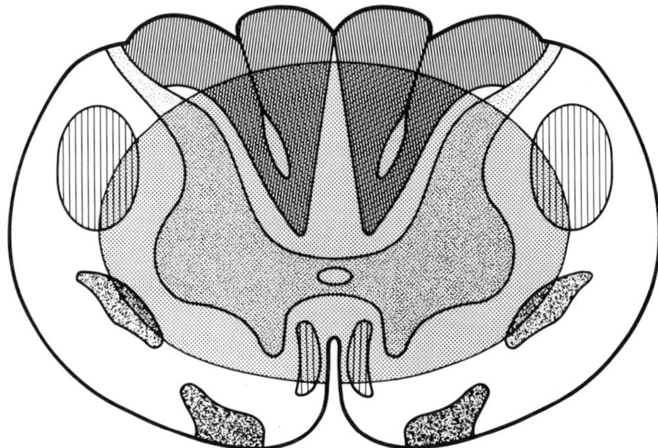

Figure 43–15   Central Cord Syndrome.

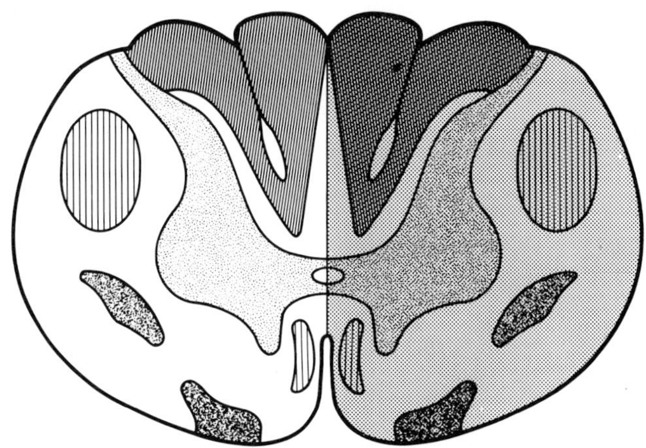

Figure 43–17   Brown-Séquard Syndrome.

may arise when a tumor encroaches on the spinal cord and causes neurologic dysfunction. This condition may manifest itself suddenly, and its consequences may be devastating if it is not diagnosed and treated rapidly.[15] Hematomas may occur around the spinal cord, especially in patients receiving anticoagulants, and cause spinal cord compression.[16] Osteoarthritis and ankylosing spondylitis of the cervical spine may cause bony encroachment on the spinal cord and make it more susceptible to injury, even from trivial trauma.[12,17]

CLINICAL MANIFESTATIONS

The condition of patients with traumatic injuries to the cervical spine should be evaluated by an appropriate history and physical examination. The physician should suspect cervical spine injury in any patient who suffers significant trauma, especially one who has suffered injury to the head or neck or who has lost consciousness. The absence of a head injury does not exclude a cervical spine injury, however; those wearing shoulder har-

nesses may be protected from injury to the head, although the inertial forces may cause flexion or extension injuries to the cervical spine.[4] Complaints of neck pain, stiffness, paresthesias, or radicular pain of the extremities may indicate cervical spine injury. The ability of patients to walk after their accident does not exclude the possibility of significant cervical spine or cervical cord injury, as 17 percent of patients with serious injury to the cervical spine have been reported walking at the scene of their accident.[2]

Palpation of the spinous processes of the cervical spine may reveal significant tenderness or deformity that may make the emergency department physician suspect cervical spine injury. In addition to examining patients for possible bony injuries to the cervical spine, the clinician must check for any evidence of cord injury. Cursory examinations are to be condemned, as they may reveal only a total cord injury and miss the partial cord injury. Physical examination must include examination of the motor and sensory functions of the cord. Strength of the arms and legs must be assessed and any differences

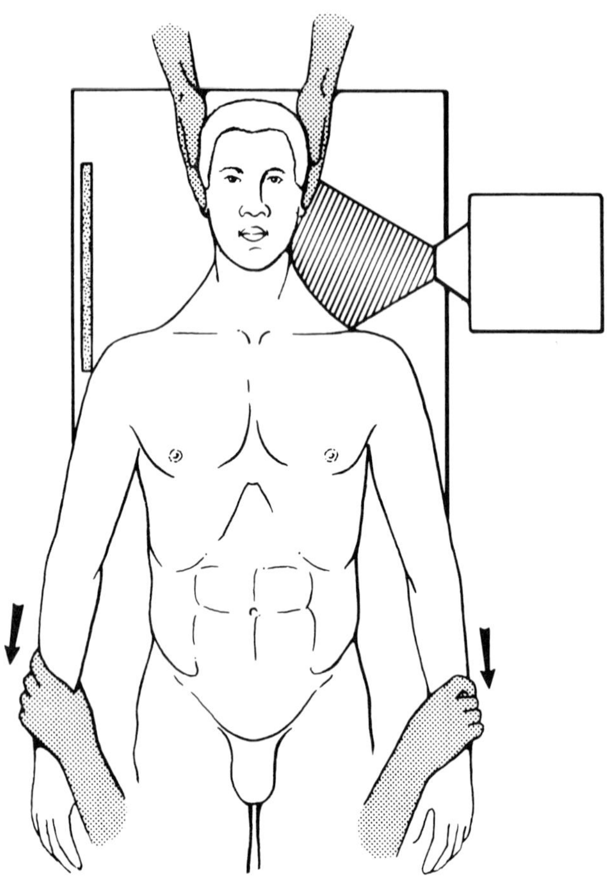

Figure 43–18 Method of Obtaining Lateral Roentgenogram of the Cervical Spine with Downward Traction on the Patient's Arms to Expose All Seven Cervical Vertebrae.

in strength noted. A quick sensory examination can be performed to determine any level of sensory deficit. Once the examination has been completed, the findings should indicate whether there has been any cord injury.

RADIOLOGY

Early roentgenogram evaluation of the cervical spine is an important step in the management of the traumatized patient suspected of having a neck injury. It should be done in a way that permits adequate evaluation of all seven cervical vertebrae without adding further insult to a potentially unstable cervical spine. This goal can be met by performing a portable cross table lateral roentgenogram of the cervical spine with downward traction on the patient's arms (Fig. 43–18).[18] A cross table lateral view, anterior posterior view and view of the odontoid constitute a minimum roentgenologic evaluation of the cervical spine, as 17 to 25 percent of injuries to the cervical spine may be missed by limiting studies to the cross table lateral view alone.[19] In patients with a suspected neck injury, a full cervical spine series

should be taken—including careful flexion and extension views if the spine is stable—as only with these latter roentgenograms can ligamentous injuries be fully evaluated.[18] Tomography and scan of the cervical spine by computerized axial tomography (CT) are useful adjuncts in the radiologic evaluation of the cervical spine when findings are equivocal.

In general, roentgenogram evaluation may underestimate the degree of injury as ligamentous injury may be difficult to detect and cord injury may be present despite a negative roentgenogram (see Table 43–1).

SPECIAL PROBLEMS

Immediate problems associated with cervical cord injuries include disorders of temperature regulation and blood pressure control. In the normal, intact nervous system, alterations in body temperature can be corrected by impulses traveling through the autonomic nervous system under the control of the thermal regulatory center in the hypothalamus. These impulses are conducted mainly by the sympathetic nervous system, which is involved in vasomotor control of blood vessels in the skin, muscular shivering, and sweating. Disturbances of thermal regulation seem to be most prominent with lesions at the T8 level and above. A patient with a nervous system intact to the T8 level retains sufficient thermal regulatory response to maintain an adequate body temperature, despite fluctuations in the ambient temperature.[20] The disturbances of thermal regulatory mechanisms in patients with spinal cord injuries make them prone to both hypothermia and hyperthermia, but the former is more common. Patients with spinal cord lesions below the cervical level are at much less risk for thermal regulatory disorders not only because they have more active voluntary muscle, but also because they retain some normal sympathetic activity related to sweating and vasomotor control.

Hypothermia is considered to be a core body temperature at or below 35°C.[21] Severe hypothermia is particularly likely to occur soon after injury to the spinal cord as a result of the cutaneous vasodilatation and subsequent heat loss that takes place during this stage of the injury. (See Chapter 30.)

Hyperthermia may occur after spinal cord transection and is likely to develop in hot climates or in the presence of infection. Hyperthermia occurs because of the body's inability to lose body heat through the vasodilatation and sweating that is normally mediated by the sympathetic nervous system. Although sweating and heat loss may occur in the skin that is still normally innervated, thus allowing some degree of temperature control, this limited degree of thermoregulation may not be sufficient to maintain a normal body temperature.[20] (See Chapter 29.) Clinical management involves recognizing that substantial alterations in body temperature may occur in patients with spinal injuries. A temperature probe that records wide fluctuations in core body temperature is extremely useful.

Hypothermia is best treated by passive rewarming measures when it is mild and the patient is stable; active rewarming measures, such as the use of a heated aerosol oxygen mask, may be needed if the hypothermia is severe, however.[20] Treatment for mild hyperthermia requires keeping the patient in a cool place, while severe cases, e.g., those with core body temperatures above 40.5°C, may require immediate treatment similar to that used in managing heat stroke. When the patient's body temperature is stabilized, the patient should be warned that precautions to prevent the recurrence of hypothermia or hyperthermia must be taken.

Cervical cord injuries may also disrupt the normal blood pressure regulation owing to the loss of sympathetic innervation distal to the cord lesion.[22] As a result, severe orthostatic hypotension may occur in "spinal man" and result in syncope in the head-up posture. This phenomenon usually diminishes with time as the body adapts to the hypotensive change caused by the head-up position. Any symptomatology or severe orthostatic hypotensive change that occurs can be quickly resolved by putting the patient in the supine position.

Although patients with cervical cord injuries have a lower resting blood pressure, they manifest paroxysmal increases in blood pressure during certain physiologic stimuli, such as defecation, urinary bladder distention, muscle spasms, distention of the rectum, or cutaneous stimuli. This rise in blood pressure, which may be associated with sweating, flushing of the face, and headache, was described as a distinct syndrome by Head and Riddoch in 1917.[16] Known as autonomic hyper-reflexia or autonomic dysreflexia, it seems to be the result of an exaggerated reflex of the sympathetic nervous system in victims of spinal cord injury. Autonomic dysreflexia can have damaging effects on the body and requires urgent treatment. The most important therapeutic measure is to alleviate the precipitating causes. This would entail emptying the urinary bladder correctly, preventing fecal impactions, and treating severe muscle spasms with diazepam (Valium).[21] If the precipitating cause cannot be identified and removed, then the head-up position may be used to help lower the blood pressure. In severe cases, an infusion of trimethaphan camphorsulfonate (Arfonad) may be carefully used to control blood pressure.

TREATMENT

It is vital that all emergency care personnel maintain a high index of suspicion regarding cervical spine injuries. Initial management begins in the field, where stabilization of the cervical spine is most important in the prehospital care of these patients. This may be accomplished by use of long or short spine boards, a cervical collar, and/or sandbags; if none of these are available, a rolled Turkish towel can be wrapped around the patient's neck and taped in place to serve as a substitute for a formal cervical collar. Patients with injury to the cervical cord may require respiratory support in the field. Furthermore, these patients may develop an ileus that will predispose them to vomiting and subsequent aspiration. For these reasons, cervical spine immobilization should be accomplished in a way that permits personnel to deal rapidly with life-threatening problems, such as airway compromise or respiratory failure.

The patient should be kept flat to avoid problems associated with neurogenic shock, which frequently results from the loss of vasomotor control that occurs when a cervical cord injury has disrupted the autonomic nervous system. These patients are extremely sensitive to change in position and may become frankly hypotensive if placed in a head-up or seated position. In addition, the body temperature should be monitored in order to detect hyperthermia or hypothermia. Reasonable care should be taken to avoid having the patient lie on hard objects in order to avoid the development of pressure sores.

When the patient arrives in the emergency department, stabilization of the cervical spine should be continued while care for the airway, respiratory system, and cardiovascular system is provided and a history of spinal cord deficit and any changes during transport is obtained. A physical examination should be done in the emergency department to detect partial cord injury, for this is the most common type of cord injury. Injury to the cervical spine often occurs without neurologic deficit, and stabilization of the cervical spine should be continued even though the patient shows no sign of cervical spine injury. Furthermore, although the cervical spine roentgenograms may be normal, the possibility of cord injury still exists. It has been reported that 10 of 91 patients in a retrospective study had cord injury without any evidence of bony damage to the cervical spine.[2] Unnecessary manipulation of the head and neck should be avoided until the condition of the cord is fully evaluated. Airway support can be done either by nasotracheal intubation or oraltracheal intubation, using a laryngoscope and manual traction on the head to maintain the axis of the cervical spine. If these measures are unsuccessful, a cricothyreotomy or intubation of the trachea over a fiberoptic laryngoscope can be considered.

Once instability of the cervical spine is diagnosed, a more permanent means of stabilization is required. An easy, effective procedure that can be performed in the emergency department is the application of Gardner-Wells tongs with about 10 to 15 pounds of traction.[23,24] Hypotension resulting from neurogenic shock can usually be resolved by putting the patient in a flat or slight degree of Trendelenburg position. Respiratory insufficiency is common and may require timely ventilatory support as dictated by the patient's clinical status, arterial blood gas levels, and spirometry. Gastrointestinal ileus requires the use of a nasogastric tube to empty gastric contents and reduce the risk of aspiration. Urinary retention requires the use of a Foley catheter, and measures should be instituted early to prevent development of decubital ulcers. There is no real evidence to suggest that steroids are of value in the treatment of cord trauma, but their use is generally advocated.[23,25] Such therapy should be initiated in the emergency department with a bolus of 10 mg dexamethasone (Decadron IV) for an adult patient or at a dosage of 0.2 mg/kg in the pediatric age group.[23,25,26] Definitive care of such patients should be provided by neurosurgical and/or orthopedic subspecialties. Referral of such patients to a regional spinal cord center for management of their acute problems and rehabilitation is ideal.

REFERENCES

1. Talbot HS: Spinal cord injury. *Arch Surg* 102:539–540, 1971.
2. Dula DJ: Trauma to the cervical spine. *JACEP* 8:504–506, 1979.
3. Rogers WA: Fractures and dislocations of the cervical spine: An end result study. *J Bone Joint Surg* 39A:341, 1957.
4. Huelke DF: Cervical fractures and fracture dislocations sustained without head impact. *J Trauma* 18:533–538, 1978.
5. Wood JF: The ideal lesion produced by judicial hanging. *Lancet* 1:53, 1913.
6. Stauffer ES: Diagnosis and prognosis of acute cervical spinal cord injury. *Clin Orthop* 112:9–15, October 1975.
7. Schneider RD, Charie G, Pantek H: The syndrome of acute central cervical spinal cord injury. *J Neurosurg* 11:546–577, 1954.
8. Schneider RD: The syndrome of acute anterior spinal cord injury. *J Neurosurg* 12:95–122, 1955.
9. Schneider RD, Crosby EC: Traumatic spinal cord syndromes and their management. *J Clin Neurosurg* 20:424–492, 1972.
10. Maroon JC: Burning hands in football spinal cord injuries. *JAMA* 238:2049–2051, 1977.
11. Vick NA: *Grinker's Neurology*. Springfield, Ill, Charles C Thomas, 1976.
12. Youmans JR (ed): *Neurological Surgery*, ed 3. Philadelphia, WB Saunders, 1973; pp 1049–1066.
13. Taylor E: Traumatic intradural avulsion of nerve roots of the brachial plexus. *Brain* 85:579–602, 1962.
14. Dula DJ: Traumatic avulsion injury of the brachial plexus. *Ann Emergency Medicine* 10:45–48, 1981.
15. Nissenblatt MJ: Oncologic emergencies. *American Family Physician* 20:104–114, August 1979.
16. Head H, Riddoch G: The autonomic bladder, excessive sweating and some other reflex conditions in gross injuries of the spinal cord. *Brain* 40:188–263, 1917.
17. McCarty DJ: *Arthritis in Allied Conditions*, ed 9. Philadelphia, Lea & Febiger, 1979, p 626.
18. Kimball M, Sachagello CR: Avoiding a pitfall in resuscitation: The painless cervical fracture. *South Med J* 70:477–478, 1977.
19. Shaffer MA, Doris PE: Limitation of the cross table lateral view in detecting cervical spine injuries. *Ann Emergency Medicine* 10:508–513, 1981.
20. Johnson RH: Temperature Regulation and Spinal Cord Injuries in Vinken PJ, Bruyn GW: *Handbook of Clinical Neurology 26.* Amsterdam, North Holland, 1976, pp 355–373.
21. Reulen JB: Hypothermia: Pathophysiology, clinical setting and management. *Ann Intern Med* 89:519–527, 1978.
22. Frankel H, Mathias C: Cardiovascular Systems in Tetraplegia and Paraplegia in Vinken PJ, Bruyn GW: *Handbook of Clinical Neurology 26.* Amsterdam, North Holland, 1976, pp 313–334.
23. Schwartz GR: *Principles and Practice of Emergency Medicine.* Philadelphia, WB Saunders, 1978, pp 436, 437, 623–625.
24. Gardner WJ: The principles of spring-loaded points for cervical traction. *J Neurosurg* 39:543, 1973.
25. Wilkins EW: *MGH Textbook of Emergency Medicine.* Baltimore, Williams & Wilkins, 1978, pp 501–516.
26. Kempe CH: *Current Pediatric Diagnosis and Treatment*, ed 5. Philadelphia, Lange, 1978, p 553.

SUGGESTED READINGS

Gerlock AJ, Kirchner SG, Heller RM, Kaye JJ: *Advanced Exercises in Diagnostic Radiology—The Cervical Spine in Trauma.* Philadelphia, WB Saunders, 1978.

Harris JH Jr: *The Radiology of Acute Cervical Spine Trauma.* Baltimore, Williams & Wilkins, 1978.

Rockwood CA Jr, Green DP: *Fractures, 2.* Philadelphia, JB Lippincott, 1975.

Vinken PJ, Bruyn GW: *Handbook of Clinical Neurology—Injuries of the Spine and Spinal Cord, Part I.* Amsterdam, North Holland, 1976.

Vinken PJ, Bruyn GW: *Handbook of Clinical Neurology—Injuries of the Spine and Spinal Cord, Part II.* Amsterdam, North Holland, 1976.

Youmans JR: *Neurological Surgery 2.* Philadelphia, WB Saunders, 1973.

44. Headache

E. JOHN GALLAGHER, M.D.

Headache exceeds low back pain and rivals the common cold as one of the ubiquitous afflictions of the human race. It is one of the most common reasons for visits to the emergency department. Although there are numerous ways to classify the causes of pain in the head, a simple classification is probably the most useful to the emergency department physician.

An adaptation of one classification of Diamond and Dalessio divides all headaches into five categories[1]:

1. muscle contraction headache
2. vascular headache
3. traction headache
4. inflammatory headache
5. headache secondary to disease of individual extracranial structures

These categories are characterized by differences in mechanisms of pain production. Before the pathophysiology of head pain can be discussed, however, it is necessary to understand what cranial structures are pain-sensitive.

Pain-sensitive structures can be either extracranial or intracranial. Extracranial structures include the periosteum of the skull and all structures superficial to it: (1) the musculature, i.e., the frontalis, temporalis, occipitalis, and paraspinal cervicals; (2) the blood vessels of the scalp; (3) the skin; and (4) the cranial appendages, i.e., ears, eyes, teeth, nose, and bony sinuses. Intracranial structures that are pain-sensitive include (1) blood vessels, i.e., dural arteries, intracerebral arteries, and venous sinuses; and (2) perivascular dura. It is notable that the parenchyma of the brain and most of its meningeal covering are *not* pain-sensitive.

BASIC PATHOPHYSIOLOGY AND CLASSIFICATION OF HEADACHE

Anatomical structures that are pain-sensitive produce pain by one of four different mechanisms:

1. In the muscle contraction or "tension" headache, the pain is thought to be caused by the sustained contraction of pericranial musculature, specifically the frontalis, temporalis, occipitalis, and posterior paracervical muscles. Patients often describe this type of headache as "squeezing, bandlike, or tight."
2. The vascular variety of headache is caused by vasodilation of extracranial and intracranial arteries. The consequence of this vasodilation is a "pounding, pulsing, or throbbing" quality of pain. Because the vasodilation of arteries that occurs at other times, such as during exercise, is not generally painful, it appears that concomitant increased permeability, edema, and localized perivascular inflammation are necessary in order to account for the pain of these headaches. Some of these headaches, such as a migraine (which might be conceptualized as a kind of "transient vasculitis") appear to be mediated by vasoactive sub-

stances such as serotonin, histamine, the kinins, and others.

3. Traction headaches include head pains caused by traction on intracranial vascular structures. The quality of pain may vary from the dull ache caused by a mass lesion (such as a subdural hematoma or a tumor) to the sudden, excruciating pain of a subarachnoid hemorrhage.

4. Inflammatory headaches are caused by inflammation within and around pain-sensitive vascular structures. This category includes headaches associated with meningitis and arteritis.

5. In disease of isolated extracranial structures, headaches are produced by a combination of traction, inflammation, and muscle contraction. Because these headaches do not fall within any category, yet represent a significant portion of the headaches seen in the emergency department, they warrant a separate classification. They include headaches secondary to pathology in the eye, sinuses, cervical spine, ear, temporomandibular joint, teeth, and certain cranial nerves.

THE HEADACHE HISTORY

In the assessment of headache, even more than in other conditions seen in clinical medicine, the history is crucial. This is true not only because pain by its very nature is subjective, but also because the vast majority of headaches are not associated with physical findings. With the other pains commonly experienced by patients in the emergency department, such as abdominal pain and chest pain, the physician can be reassured by the finding of a soft abdomen or aided by the abnormal electrocardiogram (ECG). When physical findings are associated with headache, a diagnosis and/or decisions regarding further studies can also be readily made. This, however, is the exception rather than the rule with headache; therefore, great emphasis is placed upon obtaining a careful headache history.

1. chronicity. The first and most important question is whether this is the first time the patient has had such a headache or whether such headaches are familiar and episodic. Any headache not previously experienced by the patient deserves immediate attention. If the headaches are chronic, then the physician must investigate the pain pattern, as detailed under Question 9.

2. onset. Whether the pain was sudden or gradual in onset is important. An unfamiliar headache of abrupt onset (especially during exertion) is considered to be caused by a subarachnoid hemorrhage until proved otherwise.

3. duration. Although obviously linked to chronicity and abruptness of onset, the question of duration has a slightly different emphasis. The physician must determine how long the patient has had this headache and, if previously experienced, how long it usually lasts.

4. severity. Most persons, in order to justify their presence in an emergency department, exaggerate the severity of their headache. The inquiry, Is this the worst headache of your life? must therefore be put very gently to the patients. If asked in a challenging way, the question becomes rhetorical and many unnecessary lumbar punctures result, often with patients returning on yet another day complaining of post-lumbar puncture headaches. In general, the most severe headaches are caused by vascular conditions (cluster/migraine), subarachnoid hemorrhage, and trigeminal neuralgia. Severity of pain, however, is poorly correlated with severity of underlying disease.

5. location. Hemicranial or localized pain is generally of greater concern than pain that is circumferential or involves the entire head. Pain of the latter variety is usually secondary to a muscle contraction headache or toxic vascular headache, although increased intracranial pressure, meningitis, and subarachnoid hemorrhage can produce a similar generalized headache.

6. associated symptoms. Migraine commonly has associated nausea and vomiting, while cluster headache may be associated with a partial Horner's syndrome. Subarachnoid hemorrhage and meningitis are frequently, though not invariably, seen in conjunction with nuchal rigidity. Focal findings associated with a headache, unless part of a migrainous prodrome, are of great concern.

7. quality of pain. Vascular headaches are usually throbbing, while muscle contraction headaches are often described as "tight" or "squeezing." Traction headaches vary greatly and include such disparate kinds of head pain as the dull ache of a mass lesion and the severe pain of subarachnoid hemorrhage. Inflammatory headaches include the generalized pain of meningitis and the localized pain of temporal arteritis.

8. prodrome. Only the classic migrainous headaches have true prodromata. These are usually visual, but may vary from peculiar sensations to a hemiparesis.

9. pattern. If the headache is one previously experienced by the patient, it is useful to know the
   a. frequency with which the headache occurs—daily, with menses, seasonally, sporadically, or constantly.
   b. duration. Trigeminal neuralgia is momentary;

cluster headaches do not last more than four hours. Untreated migraine commonly lasts at least six hours. Muscle contraction headaches are frequently constant.

   c. precipitating features. Fever commonly causes toxic vascular headache, as can hypoxia, nitroglycerin, indomethacin, and oral contraceptives. Migraine may be precipitated by tyramine-containing foods. Subarachnoid hemorrhages are often precipitated by exertion.

   d. usual time of onset. Migraines are usually daytime headaches, while cluster headaches are nocturnal. Cluster headaches tend to occur repeatedly at the same time of day or night, often awakening patients from sleep. Brain tumor headaches are frequently worse upon awakening.

   e. age at onset. Migraines commonly begin in adolescence, while cluster is a headache of middle age. Temporal arteritis is a headache of the elderly.

   f. family history. A tendency to experience migraines is often inherited.

   g. types. In patients with recurrent headache, it is important to ask how many different kinds of headaches a person has, since there are probably headache-prone personalities, e.g., patients with migraine frequently suffer from muscle contraction headache as well.

PHYSICAL EXAMINATION

Since most headaches are not associated with physical findings, the history is far more important than the physical examination. Nevertheless, in every patient, a goal-directed neurologic examination must be performed. As with all other examinations performed in the emergency department, the history dictates the focus and extent of the physical.

The following areas must be included: (1) vital signs, especially blood pressure and temperature; (2) presence or absence of nuchal rigidity; (3) mental status, especially alterations of consciousness; (4) tenderness of the scalp, paracervical muscles, sinuses, and temporal arteries; (5) presence or absence of focal findings, especially as reflected in the cranial nerves; (6) functional testing of drift, gait, and station; (7) funduscopic examination; (8) visual acuity; and (9) any sign of trauma, such as palpable hematomas, lacerations, scalp edema, "racoon sign," "Battle's sign," rhinorrhea, or otorrhea.

MUSCLE CONTRACTION HEADACHE

The most common variety of head pain for which patients seek the care of a physician is a muscle contraction headache. When patients state that they have the headache "all the time" and have had it "for years," the probability that these patients have a muscle contraction headache is quite high. Since the majority of these headaches are relieved with aspirin, those who seek care usually represent a subpopulation whose headache has not responded to nonprescription analgesics.

Muscle contraction headaches appear gradually and are rarely of such severity that patients go to the emergency department within hours of onset. The pain is usually in a bandlike or caplike distribution, with a prominent occipital, suboccipital, and paracervical component. Typically, the pain is described as "tight," "pressing," or "heavy" and is often associated with pain upon combing the hair. The main area of discomfort may be bifrontal, bitemporal, biparietal, or occipital, but it is usually bicranial rather than hemicranial. A common physical finding is scalp tenderness and pain upon palpation of the paracervical muscles. Although these patients may appear to have nuchal rigidity, their pain occurs not only with flexion of the neck, but also with cervical rotation; this distinguishes it from that of meningeal irritation. Scalp and muscle tenderness is the only physical finding associated with muscle contraction headache.

A surprising number of patients link the beginning of their headache to a specific incident, frequently an episode of head trauma. The vast majority of patients who experience a post-traumatic headache that persists more than six months following trauma have no discernible intracranial pathology and probably have a muscle contraction headache.

Associated symptoms are frequently, though by no means uniformly, those of agitated depression with alterations of mood and a disturbance of the patient's sleep cycle. Viewing muscle contraction headaches as "depressive equivalents" is a helpful clinical approach so long as the physician does not expect to discover an underlying depression in every instance. Often these headaches are merely somatic manifestations of transient life stresses (ergo, their colloquial designation as "tension headaches"), and the patient may be looking only for an opportunity to ventilate and, perhaps, for some reassurance.

It has long been assumed that the pain of muscle contraction headache is secondary to sustained contraction, and perhaps ischemia, of pericranial musculature. Although this is a useful pathophysiological model, it is difficult to demonstrate this consistently electromyographically. Gaps in current knowledge, once filled, may explain the not infrequent appearance of vascular complaints in a headache that is, in all other respects, a "typical" muscle contraction headache.

Treatment of a muscle contraction headache should always begin with explanation and end with reassurance. Many of these patients are fearful that they have a brain tumor, and a few words about the relationship between tension and its literal manifestation as a headache is often sufficient. Mild analgesia is also appropriate but should be limited to nonsteroidal anti-inflammatory agents. Mild tranquilizers, although occasionally appropriate, should generally not be prescribed by the emergency department physician, who sees the patient at only one point in the course of an illness. Opiates should never be used for muscle contraction headaches. If the patient appears significantly depressed, no tricyclics should be given, but a psychiatric referral may be appropriate.

A variety of nonpharmacologic interventions are intuitively appealing and have met with some success in various treatment centers. These include acupuncture and the use of biofeedback and stimulus pairing that involves electromyograms of the pericranial musculature, as well as more meditative means of eliciting the relaxation response. Although it is difficult to study such methods because of a significant placebo effect, nonpharmacologic intervention may hold great promise, especially in light of recent developments in our knowledge about endorphins.

VASCULAR HEADACHES

Characterized by painful vasodilation of intracranial and extracranial arteries, vascular headaches can be divided into those that are bicranial and those that are hemicranial, depending upon whether the pain is on both sides of the head or localized to one side.

Bicranial Vascular Headache

The bicranial headache, which reflects a systemic abnormality affecting both carotid arteries and their tributaries, may be further divided into two categories: (1) toxic vascular headaches in which an endogenous or exogenous toxin produces painful vasodilation and (2) hypertensive headaches in which there is either a sustained marked elevation of diastolic blood pressure or a rapid rise in blood pressure as seen with pheochromocytoma.

Toxic Vascular Headache

Fever, probably the most common cause of the toxic vascular headache, is related to the vasodilation of the

febrile state. Thus many, if not most, patients with a fever higher than 102°F (38.9°C) will have a pulsatile bicranial headache as part of their illness.

Abnormalities of blood gases, namely hypoxia and hypercapnia, cause headache by producing vasodilation of cerebral vessels. Carbon monoxide, by producing cellular hypoxia, causes a headache in most patients when the level of carboxyhemoglobin is in excess of 20%. Headache is, in fact, one of the most reliable indicators of early carbon monoxide toxicity. The headache of altitude sickness, rarely seen at elevations below 8,000 feet, is also thought to be related to hypoxia, although the headache is not relieved by O_2 but rather, like altitude pulmonary edema, responds to descent.

Some of the common medications that often produce headache include oral contraceptives, indomethacin, and nitroglycerin. The mechanism is thought to be related to vasodilation, although the evidence is clearest in the case of nitroglycerin and its derivative. Insulin-requiring diabetics may develop throbbing afternoon headache as the earliest symptom of hypoglycemia. Whether the so-called hunger headache is secondary to hypoglycemia, however, is speculative.

Among the common foods and beverages that cause headache secondary to vasodilation are (1) ethanol, which produces the common "hangover" headache relieved by vasoconstrictors such as caffeine; (2) monosodium glutamate, which causes the head pain and flushing characteristic of the "Chinese restaurant syndrome;" and (3) sodium nitrite, which is a cured meat preservative responsible for the so-called "hot dog headache." Abrupt caffeine withdrawal in persons who drink large quantities of coffee, tea, or colas may, by inducing reflex vasodilation, cause a throbbing vascular headache.

Postictal distention of the vasculature occurs in many patients following a generalized seizure, and patients who suffer from this syndrome recognize headache as a usual component of their postictal state. The headache rarely persists more than a few hours and is of no pathologic significance. A patient who has an unfamiliar headache following a seizure, however, requires careful observation and may warrant computerized axial tomography (CT scan).

Other decidedly uncommon toxic vascular headaches include "exertional headache" and "orgasmic headache." These are of note because of the difficult diagnostic problems that they present to the emergency department physician. Both are benign syndromes, but they must be distinguished, respectively, from a brain tumor and a subarachnoid hemorrhage.

The treatment of the toxic vascular headache is that of the underlying disease. For example, a febrile headache requires antipyretics, and the headache caused by carbon monoxide toxicity responds to breathing 100 percent O_2.

Hypertensive Headache

Hypertension is a much overdiagnosed cause of headache, especially among patients with mild to moderate elevation of blood pressure. The throbbing occipital headache that may be associated with *severe* hypertension is commonly confused with the squeezing headache of muscle contraction occurring in the same anatomical location. Muscle contraction headaches and high blood pressure are both common, and the coincident occurrence of both entities in the same individual cannot be assumed to show cause and effect.

There is evidence in support of coincidence rather than causality. If patients with high blood pressure are compared with nonhypertensive matched controls, the occurrence of headache in both groups is *not* significantly different until diastolic blood pressure exceeds 130 mm Hg. Above this level, however, hypertensive patients do suffer from headache more commonly than nonhypertensive controls.

Circumstances under which hypertension actually produces headache are few in number, but are serious and generally in need of immediate attention. In addition to sustained diastolic elevations in excess of 130 mm Hg, the other entities in which hypertension causes headache have in common rapid elevations of blood pressure:

- pheochromocytoma. Paroxysmal outpouring of catecholamines in the blood produces pounding headache in most patients with these tumors.

- hypertensive encephalopathy. This headache appears to be secondary to both vasodilation and cerebral edema, and thus has a combination vascular and traction etiology.

- toxemia of pregnancy. Rapid blood pressure elevations may produce headache in women who are pre-eclamptic. Because the prepregnant blood pressure in young women is often low (90/70), a moderately high blood pressure (140/100) may represent a substantial increase in mean arterial pressure. The pain here, as in hypertensive encephalopathy, is probably related to a combination of brain swelling and vasodilation.

In all of the hypertensive headaches, blood pressure control should alleviate the headache. (See Chapter 52.)

Hemicranial Vascular Headaches

The hemicranial vascular headaches include the migraine and cluster syndromes. The pain in both is thought to be related to vasodilation which, for unknown reasons, selectively involves the cranial vessels on one side of the head. In the case of migraine, *both* intracerebral and extracerebral vessels are dilated. In cluster, the vasodilation appears to be more discrete, selectively involving the external or internal carotid artery, or just the orbital and periorbital vasculature of one eye.

Migraine

The term *migraine* is derived from the Greek word *hemicrania* and may be defined as an episodic, usually hemicranial, headache of throbbing quality, sometimes preceded by an aura. There are two kinds of migrainous headaches, depending upon the presence of a prodrome. Classic migraine, which constitutes about one-third of all migraines, is preceded by an aura. Common migraine, which constitutes the remaining two-thirds, develops with little or no warning.

In classic migraine, the prodromata are almost always visual, varying from "scintillating scotomata" (flashing lights with blind spots) to "fortification spectra" (jagged, wavy lines). The patient may also have illusory visual distortions, and less commonly, hallucinations. Very rarely in classic migraine, the patient may have an episode of ophthalmoplegia or hemiplegia as part of an aura. In ophthalmoplegic migraine, the absence of pupillary dilation excludes an aneurysm; in hemiplegic migraine, the patient usually has a family history of this syndrome that can be relied upon to distinguish the event from a stroke.

The generally accepted pathophysiology of migraine suggests that the syndrome occurs in two stages: (1) an initial vasoconstrictive stage produces a well-defined aura in some patients and, at the very least, a "peculiar feeling" in most patients; and (2) the painless vasoconstrictive phase is followed by painful vasodilation as the prodrome gives way to a hemicranial headache.

The aura is probably secondary to hypoperfusion of the optic radiations of one hemisphere. Because these fibers represent the temporal half of the ipsilateral retina and the nasal half of the contralateral retina, the aura will generally appear in the visual field contralateral to the vasoconstricted carotid artery. The subsequent dilation of this vessel produces a hemicranial headache on the ipsilateral side of the head. Thus, a patient with classic migraine may see scintillating scotomata to the left and then experience a throbbing headache occurring on the right side of the head.

Migraines last at least four hours, if untreated, and may last an entire day or more. They rarely occur daily. They develop slightly more often in women, are commonly exacerbated by menses, and diminish with the menopause and the third trimester of pregnancy. They are usually associated with nausea and vomiting. Often, there is a family history of migraine.

There are four major modalities available for the treatment of migraines: (1) abortive, (2) prophylactic, (3) analgesic, and (4) sedative. Ergotamine tartrate, a vasoconstrictor, is the mainstay of management in migraine. It is most effective if taken in the prodromal or vasoconstrictive phase of the headache because it prevents the reflex vasodilation that follows vasoconstriction; thus, the headache may be aborted. Because of its intense vasoconstrictive properties, however, the drug is contraindicated in patients with coronary artery disease, peripheral vascular disease, hypertension, and pregnancy. Patients with migraine frequently vomit, and the most common reason for therapeutic failure with Cafergot (caffeine 100 mg, ergotamine tartrate 1 mg) is failure of the drug to be absorbed. Consequently, the rectal suppository, sublingual preparation, or inhaled ergotamine is often preferable. Parenteral preparations are also available, but use of these may be hazardous because of the potential for intense vasoconstriction. Cafergot by mouth is taken at 30-minute intervals, but the total dose is not to exceed 6 mg. The suppositories are taken one hour apart, not to exceed two doses. Cafergot may also be used prophylactically, taken twice a day, not to exceed 10 mg/week. Propranolol, which is safer in patients with coronary artery disease and high blood pressure, may also be used prophylactically in doses of 20 to 120 mg every six hours, but it has no demonstrable effect when used abortively.

Many patients with migraine go to the emergency department only when their therapeutic regimen has failed. These patients are usually in severe pain and must be treated either with opiate analgesics or sedatives. Because of the significant problem of opiate addiction in chronic recurrent headache disorders, chlorpromazine orally in doses sufficient to induce sleep (50 to 300 mg) may be a preferred alternative to meperidine hydrochloride or morphine.

Cluster Headache

Named because of their tendency to "cluster" about short spans of time, cluster headaches occur in bouts that are interspersed with pain-free intervals. They may occur nightly for a few weeks and then disappear for months. They are hemicranial headaches, usually involving the eye, with supraorbital or infraorbital radiation. They last usually an hour; rarely, longer than four hours. They typically occur in middle-aged men who smoke heavily, usually awakening them from sleep. Unlike the pain of many other headaches, the pain has a "colicky" quality that causes patients to move about (in contrast to patients with subarachnoid hemorrhage who have equally severe pain but generally remain as still as patients with peritonitis). Although the pain is vascular in origin, it is often described as "boring."

As a reflection of the marked alteration in autonomic discharge, about one patient in five with a cluster headache develops a partial ipsilateral Horner's syndrome (ptosis, miosis) associated with lacrimation, conjunctival injection, and rhinorrhea. The intraocular vasodilation associated with cluster headache may elevate the intraocular pressure, though generally not so high as in narrow angle glaucoma. Other means of distinguishing between narrow angle closure and cluster headache in a patient with a painful red eye is the absence of a steamy cornea and the retention of pupillary reactivity in cluster. Visual acuity should be normal in cluster but diminished in narrow angle closure glaucoma.

With cluster headache, in contrast to migraine, there is no warning prodrome, no nausea and vomiting, and no significant family history.

Cluster headaches are more difficult to treat than migraines because of their sporadic nature and the absence of a warning prodrome. The severity of the pain and the marked anxiety that accompanies these headaches creates a sense of urgency that generally is not present in migraine. A patient with a migraine attack is often pain-free following a headache, at least for a few days, whereas a patient with cluster, once the attacks begin, may have several more over a period of 24 hours. The following drugs have been used with some, though limited, success in the management of cluster headache:

1. ergotamine, 1 mg at bedtime as needed.
2. propranolol, 80 to 480 mg daily.
3. lithium carbonate, 900 to 1,800 mg daily with careful monitoring of blood levels.
4. prednisone, 30 to 60 mg daily to be tapered over weeks.
5. methylsergide maleate, 4 to 12 mg daily. Because of reported complications of retroperitoneal and mediastinal fibrosis, this drug should not be used for more than three months at a time.
6. chlorpromazine, 100 to 1,000 mg daily.
7. tricyclic antidepressants (amitriptyline hydrochloride), 25 to 200 mg at bedtime.
8. cyproheptadine hydrochloride, 4 to 8 mg four times a day.

When patients suffering from a cluster headache appear in the emergency department, they require either an opiate analgesic or a sedative such as chlorpromazine, 50 to 300 mg. When they are pain-free in a few hours, they can begin one of the prophylactic regimens.

TRACTION HEADACHE

Displacement and traction upon pain-sensitive structures, usually the vasculature, can cause headache that may vary in severity from mild and intermittent to excruciating and constant. There are five broad categories of traction headaches: (1) subarachnoid hemorrhage; (2) mass lesions, such as traumatic hematomas, some cerebral vascular accidents (CVAs), and tumors; (3) vascular anomalies; (4) post-lumbar puncture and post-concussive headache; and (5) pseudotumor.

Subarachnoid Hemorrhage

Headache caused by subarachnoid hemorrhage is characterized principally by two features: its severity and its abrupt onset. Typically, the cause is a congenital berry aneurysm that ruptures spontaneously, often during exertion. Because the aneurysm is situated within the subarachnoid space, focal findings are not usually seen. Nausea and vomiting frequently accompany subarachnoid hemorrhage, and there may also be a low-grade fever. When the temperature is initially greater than 101°F (38.3°C) rectally, however, the physician should seek another cause for the headache.

Just as blood in the peritoneum produces peritonitis relatively slowly, blood in the cerebrospinal fluid may not immediately cause nuchal rigidity. The pain of subarachnoid hemorrhage is initially due to sudden displacement of vessels; in time, a chemical meningitis that produces pain by an inflammatory mechanism results from the hemorrhage.

Although high resolution CT scanners will detect the vast majority of subarachnoid hemorrhages, the "gold standard"—especially in institutions that lack CT scanners—remains the lumbar puncture.

Mass Lesions

Hematomas (Traumatic)

A hematoma anywhere in the brain may, if it places traction on pain-sensitive structures, cause pain. These mass lesions may be located in the epidural and subdural spaces or within the brain parenchyma itself. In each of these syndromes, headache is a feature, though not necessarily the most prominent symptom.

When awake, patients with an epidural hematoma (Fig. 44–1) almost invariably have headache and usually have roentgenographic evidence of a fracture line through the middle meningeal groove. As they expand, these hematomas may produce an uncal herniation syndrome (see Chapter 45, Coma).

Patients with acute subdural hematomas (Fig. 44–2) are usually too obtunded to complain of headache, but those with subacute and chronic subdural hematomas commonly have headache. Because they are extra-axial lesions, the hallmark of subdural hematomas is a depression of consciousness out of proportion to focal

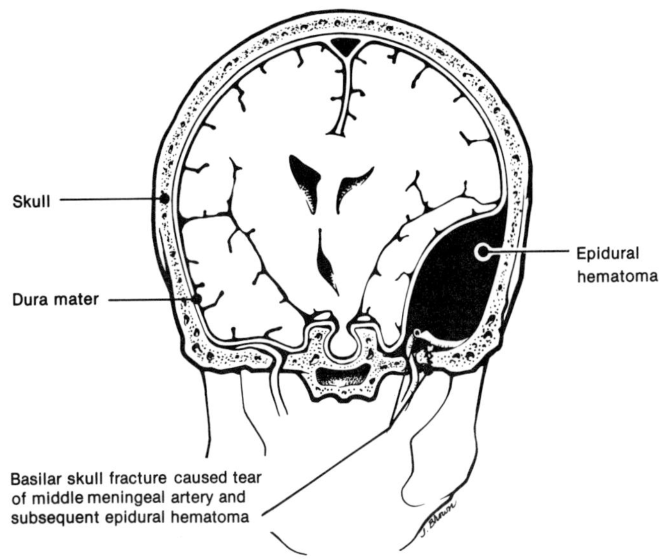

Figure 44–1   Epidural Hematoma.

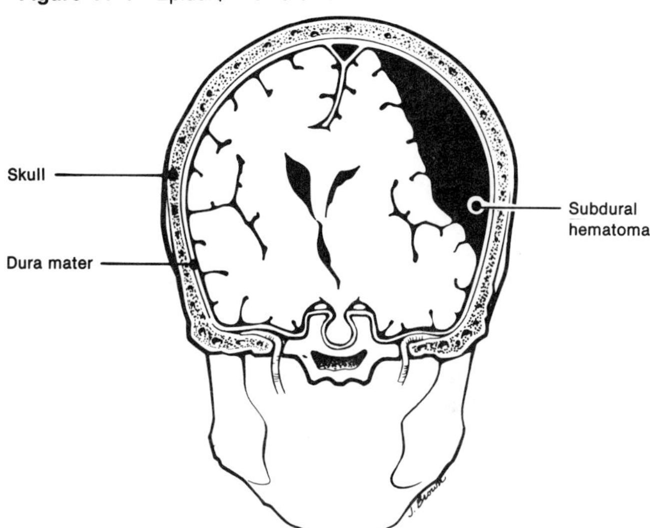

Figure 44–2   Subdural Hematoma.

findings. Because the patient often cannot recall the traumatic episode, which in the alcoholic or the elderly may have been trivial, these patients must be approached with a high index of suspicion. This is one reason for recommending a head CT scan in all patients with headache who have a focal finding or an abnormal mental status.

The treatment of most hematomas is surgical evacuation.

Cerebral Vascular Accidents

With the advent of the CT scan, much of the classic teaching with regard to the relationship between CVAs and headache has had to be revised:

- Approximately one-third of patients with nontraumatic intracerebral hematomas have headache at the time of onset. The headache may be overshadowed by the focal findings.

- Less than 15 percent of patients with large artery thromboses complain of headache. Again, focal findings are the prominent feature.

- Lacunar CVAs and embolic CVAs uncommonly produce headache.

- Expanding lesions in the posterior fossa (subtentorial lesions) usually cause occipital headache. Because an expanding posterior fossa lesion can rapidly lead to death, any patient with an occipital headache of sudden onset and cerebellar or brain stem findings should be CT-scanned immediately to determine if surgical decompression is indicated.

Brain Tumors

Expanding lesions *above* the tentorium produce pain that refers anteriorly to the frontal region or vertex; subtentorial lesions, i.e., those in the posterior fossa, cause pain that refers posteriorly to the occipital region.

The vast majority of headaches that the emergency department physician see are *not* caused by mass lesions. However, because half of the patients with brain tumor complain of headache, a space-occupying lesion must always be considered in the differential diagnosis of head pain, although such an etiology usually appears at the bottom of the list of possible causes. Certain key features of a headache increase the physician's index of suspicion and may mandate further work-up. Some of these are (1) pain that awakens the patient from sleep earlier than usual, (2) pain that is worse with Valsalva's maneuver (cough, bending), and (3) new or unfamiliar headache associated with nausea and vomiting. Clearly, however, there is a substantial overlap of the headache of a brain tumor with other headaches. For example, (1) muscle contraction headache may be associated with early morning awakening as part of a depressive sleep cycle, and patients may feel that the headache wakes them; (2) vascular and muscle contraction headache may worsen with Valsalva's maneuver; and (3) most migraines are associated with nausea and vomiting.

To make matters more difficult, most brain tumor headaches are only moderately painful, usually intermittent, and often relieved with aspirin. The presence of focal findings, an abnormal mental status, or funduscopic changes obviously alerts the physician to the need for further work-up. If, however, the results of an examination are normal, the diagnosis of a brain tumor is often legitimately missed at first. The nonspecific quality of brain tumor headache is one of the reasons that the emergency department physician must arrange follow-up for all patients in whom the cause of headache cannot be determined with a reasonable degree of diagnostic confidence.

Vascular Anomalies (Unruptured)

Congenital arterial aneurysms (berry aneurysms) and arteriovenous malformations are vascular anomalies traditionally associated with headache. However, arterial aneurysms generally do not cause headache until they rupture, at which time they produce the sudden, excruciating headache characteristic of a subarachnoid hemorrhage.

Arteriovenous malformations may produce headache of either the vascular or traction variety, but this is unusual if there is no leakage of blood. In particular, the association between unruptured arteriovenous malformations and migraines appears spurious and coincidental. Although migraine headaches usually alternate from one side of the head to the other, a constantly unilateral episodic vascular headache is far more likely to be a migraine than an unruptured or leaking arteriovenous malformation. The persistence of a migrainous aura well into or beyond the headache does, however, suggest an arteriovenous malformation, especially if accompanied by a history of seizures or the presence of a cranial bruit.

Post-Lumbar Puncture and Postconcussive Headaches

Because of their striking postural characteristics, these two types of headache are grouped together. When the patient is upright, these headaches can be quite severe, but they are ameliorated and often eliminated when the patient assumes the recumbent position.

The post-lumbar puncture headache appears hours after the procedure, is bicranial, and may be pulsatile. It may be secondary to a cerebrospinal fluid leak that produces relative intracranial hypotension and downward traction on pain-sensitive structures that worsens when the patient is upright. This may be associated with a false localizing abducent (VI) cranial nerve palsy, also thought to be secondary to traction placed on the nerve by downward displacement.

A postconcussive headache may follow head trauma after an interval of hours to a few days. It is frequently accompanied by vertigo, nausea, and vomiting, much of which is relieved by lying down. These headaches are associated with a normal CT scan at two weeks post-trauma, a normal neurologic examination, and an excellent prognosis. Usually, there is a history of a loss of consciousness, but occasionally the antecedent trauma is surprisingly trivial. Since these headaches rarely last more than a few weeks, patients with post-traumatic headache that continues for months usually are found to have a muscle contraction headache, especially if the symptoms are associated with a normal CT scan.

Pseudotumor Cerebri

The headache associated with pseudotumor is a diffuse, dull discomfort, much like a muscle contraction headache. The distinguishing clinical feature is the evidence of increased intracranial pressure revealed by funduscopic examination. The slitlike ventricles and the absence of a mass effect on CT scan in a patient with papilledema and headache strongly suggest benign intracranial hypertension. The elevated cerebrospinal fluid pressure, often above 500 mm H_2O, with otherwise normal fluid is confirmatory. Because of pressure on the optic nerves, the syndrome is not entirely benign and requires treatment with repeated lumbar punctures, acetazolamide to decrease cerebrospinal fluid production, or steroids. Visual fields should be carefully followed.

INFLAMMATORY HEADACHES

Those headaches caused by inflammation within or around pain-sensitive structures, usually vessels, are classified as inflammatory headaches.

Meningitis

Since most of the meningeal covering of the brain is not pain sensitive, the pain of meningitis probably originates from perivascular areas of the meninges at points where the cerebral and dural arteries are in contact with the inflamed tissue. This may be the reason that these headaches often seem to be vascular or pulsatile in character.

The headache of meningitis usually involves the entire head and is associated with significant fever and nuchal rigidity. Retro-orbital pain that is exacerbated by ocular movement is highly suggestive of meningitis. Although patients with bacterial meningitis appear to be more seriously ill than patients with viral meningitis, the two entities can only be reliably distinguished by a Gram stain of the centifuged cerebrospinal fluid. If the white blood cell count in the cerebrospinal fluid is more than 500, if polymorphonuclear leukocytes predominate, and if the level of cerebrospinal fluid glucose is low, the most likely diagnosis is bacterial meningitis. Because toxic vascular headaches and meningitis are both associated with fever, it must be determined whether a febrile patient's headache is the consequence of the febrile state or of meningitis. A reasonable rule of thumb is that any febrile patient who has a headache and lacks a clear source for a significant ($> 101°F$ (rectal)) fever should have a lumbar puncture.

The treatment of bacterial meningitis usually involves a choice of penicillin, ampicillin, or chloramphenicol, depending on the centrifuged cerebrospinal fluid Gram stain, patient age, allergic history, and geographical location. Viral meningitis does not necessitate treatment unless antibiotics have been taken, in which case it must be managed as a partially treated bacterial meningitis. Patients with clear-cut viral or aseptic meningitis, especially during an epidemic, may not require hospitalization. (See Chapter 20.)

Arteritis

The headache of arteritis is due not to vasodilation but to inflammation within the walls of medium- to large-sized arteries. Because of this, the head pain of arteritis is generally caused by either cranial (temporal) arteritis or polyarteritis nodosa. The cerebral vasculitis of systemic lupus erythematosus involves the arterioles and smaller vessels that are not pain-sensitive, therefore, central nervous system involvement in this condition does not generally cause headache.

Cranial arteritis usually occurs as unilateral headache associated with temporal artery tenderness and an increased erythrocyte sedimentation rate in the elderly. If either the patient's age or the erythrocyte sedimentation rate is below 50, the diagnosis is unlikely. Because of the involvement of the ophthalmic artery in cranial arteritis, there may be visual symptoms that can result in blindness if untreated. These patients should be hospitalized for a temporal artery biopsy, which may be falsely negative, and for treatment with corticosteroids, which are highly efficacious.

Polyarteritis is a much less common variety of necrotizing vasculitis. Headache is rarely the first symptom of this systemic illness, which carries a poor prognosis.

HEADACHE SECONDARY TO DISEASE OF INDIVIDUAL EXTRACRANIAL STRUCTURES

Headache from *intra*cranial disease is often referred pain. In contrast, headache from *extra*cranial structures, such as the eye or bony sinuses, usually localizes the pathology for the examiner.

Cranial Neuralgias

The cranial neuralgias are of two distinct varieties: those that involve the fifth cranial nerve (trigeminal neuralgia) and those that involve the ninth cranial nerve (glossopharyngeal neuralgia). The pain is hemicranial or hemifacial in the corresponding distribution of one of the branches of the involved cranial nerve and is characterized by an excruciating, lancinating pain, usually lasting moments. In trigeminal neuralgia, the attack occurs in either the ophthalmic, maxillary, or mandibular branch and may be triggered by a touch on the face, chewing, or even by a draft of cold air. The pain of glossopharyngeal neuralgia occurs in the tonsil, throat, or ear and is triggered by yawning or swallowing. Patients with cranial neuralgias will go to great lengths to avoid stimulating their trigger zone.

Medical therapy is directed at diminishing afferent stimuli from the trigger zone, which, according to one theory, produces pain by summating impulses in an aberrant fashion. In therapeutic doses, carbamazepine (Tegretol) or phenytoin (Dilantin) usually reduces attacks of neuralgia by raising the threshold for stimulation, much as they do for seizures. If this fails, however, there are a number of very good neurosurgical procedures available.

Ocular Etiology of Headache

Conjunctivitis, keratitis, and other superficial ocular inflammatory processes do not usually enter into the differential diagnosis of headache. Ocular causes of headache that provide the emergency department physician with more of a challenge include (1) acute glaucoma, (2) deep ocular inflammation, and (3) eyestrain. (See Chapter 66.)

Acute Glaucoma

Narrow angle glaucoma is defined as intraocular hypertension associated with a closed angle. It is characterized by pain in and around the orbit; diminished visual acuity; a fixed, midposition pupil; perilimbal injection; a steamy, edematous cornea; a shallow anterior chamber; and, often, nausea and vomiting. Treatment involves topical miotics, osmotic diuretics, and immediate ophthalmologic consultation.

Ocular Inflammation

While superficial ocular inflammation, such as conjunctivitis or keratitis, is usually self-evident, deeper inflammatory processes may easily be overlooked. For this reason, all patients being examined in the emergency department for headache must have their visual acuity and pupillary reactivity checked. The two major deep ocular inflammations are uveitis (usually manifest as iritis) and optic neuritis. Both are characterized by pupillary abnormalities and by diminished visual acuity.

Iritis, which is usually idiopathic or traumatic, is associated with ocular pain, photophobia, a poorly reactive pupil, perilimbal injection, and decreased visual acuity. Photophobia is usually direct and consensual. Consensual photophobia is a very specific, though relatively insensitive, test for iritis. Cells and flare may be seen in the anterior chamber on slit-lamp examination. Treatment usually involves mydriatics to diminish pain and prevent synechiae.

Optic neuritis is characterized by a "Marcus Gunn" pupil, i.e., the pupil of the involved eye paradoxically dilates when a swinging light source moves from the normal eye to the involved eye. This merely reflects the fact that the consensual pupilloconstrictor response (originating from the normal eye) is stronger than the direct pupilloconstrictor response in the involved eye; the normal eye "sees" more light than the involved eye since the latter has been relatively deafferented by the inflammation. As a concomitant of this, visual acuity is usually reduced. If the inflammation in optic neuritis involves the surface of the disc, there will be evidence of papillitis, which is distinguished from papilledema by the fact that visual acuity is normal in papilledema. If, on the other hand, the inflammation is behind the disc, as in retrobulbar neuritis, the fundi will appear normal in spite of the diminished visual acuity and Marcus Gunn pupil. For this reason, it is said that in retrobulbar neuritis "the patient sees nothing, and the doctor sees nothing." Most cases of optic neuritis are, like cases of iritis, idiopathic. Contrary to what is often taught, most patients with optic neuritis do *not* subsequently develop multiple sclerosis.

Eyestrain

Eyestrain is a much overdiagnosed cause of headache, but it may be a cause of headache in the case of (a) certain refractive errors or (b) a muscle imbalance. The refractive errors in which accommodation may offer partial compensation, namely hyperopia and astigmatism, are the only ones associated with headache because accommodation, i.e., increasing the curvature of the lens, involves a sustained contraction of the ciliary muscle that may produce a muscle contraction headache. For these same reasons, compensation for myopia alone does *not* appear to cause headache. Sustained contraction of the extraocular muscles in an attempt to maintain parallel visual axes and compensate for a convergence insufficiency is the other common circumstance in which eyestrain may produce headache, again of the muscle contraction variety.

In order to demonstrate a causal relationship between eyestrain and headache, however, the head pain must disappear with corrective lenses.

Ear Pain

Pain arising from the ear is usually a relatively straightforward problem in the adult. Otitis externa or acute otitis media are visible with the otoscope. Serous otitis media, which occurs primarily in children, can be a more difficult diagnosis and may require further investigation or a therapeutic trial with decongestants and antibiotics. (See Chapter 67.)

Referred pain to the ear may occur with dental problems, temporomandibular joint disease, and early in a Bell's palsy, often associated with hyperacusis.

Sinusitis

Characterized by fever, local pain, and percussion tenderness, acute sinusitis does not usually cause diagnostic problems. It is aggravated by Valsalva's maneuvers and is often most bothersome when the patient arises in the morning. The common forms of acute sinusitis are (1) maxillary sinusitis, in which a roentgenogram (upright Water's view) of the antrum is usually diagnostic; and (2) frontal sinusitis in which roentgenograms may be negative. The treatment is decongestants (sympathomimetics and antihistamines) and antibiotics, a common combination being ampicillin and Actifed. The patient should be referred to an otolaryngologist for follow-up and for drainage if medical management fails. Some otolaryngologists feel that all patients with frontal sinusitis should be hospitalized.

Chronic sinusitis is also an overdiagnosed cause of headache.

The vast majority of patients who complain of chronic "sinus headache," when questioned further, describe the sensation as a diffuse "fullness" in the forehead, between the eyes, and in the infraorbital region. This is often secondary to perennial or seasonal rhinitis causing intermittent obstruction of sinus drainage. The focus of treatment should be decongestants.

Temporomandibular Joint Pain

A relatively common and benign condition, temporomandibular joint pain is usually secondary to periarticular spasm of masticating muscles, although it is also seen in rheumatoid arthritis. It may be caused by chewing, recent dental work, dentures, an asymmetric bite, or nocturnal grinding of teeth (bruxism). It is usually self-limited and appears to respond to occlusive exercises. Patients should generally be referred to a dentist.

This entity is distinct from dislocation of the temporomandibular joint in which patients are unable to close their mouths.

Headache Secondary to Cervical Spine Disease

Distinguishing a primary muscle contraction headache from one secondary to disease of the cervical spine may be impossible. Because of the prevalence of cervical spondylosis in the asymptomatic adult population, finding an abnormality on a roentgenogram of a patient with occipital or paracervical pain does not necessarily implicate cervical spine disease as the cause. There are, in fact, only a few circumstances in which pain in the back of the neck can be clearly linked to pathology in the cervical spine.

Whiplash injury may be defined as hyperextension followed by hyperflexion, which tears muscle fibers and sometimes produces brain stem symptoms but no findings. It is usually seen in the occupants of vehicles that have been struck from the rear. Pain is generally worse on the day following the accident than at the time of impact. Persistence of the paracervical pain and tenderness beyond a few months suggests that the syndrome may be blending with a primary muscle contraction headache.

Patients with ankylosing spondylitis and rheumatoid arthritis may develop atlantoaxial subluxation. Because of this, any patient with either of these illnesses who develops neck pain must be evaluated appropriately with great care.

Patients with cervical radiculopathy who have occipital pain probably have both as a consequence of cervical spine disease.

DIAGNOSTIC PROCEDURES IN THE EMERGENCY DEPARTMENT

In patients who appear, on the basis of a thorough history and goal-directed physical examination, to have a headache of the muscle contraction or vascular variety, no further diagnostic studies are indicated.

In patients in whom a traction type headache is suspected, a CT scan is the next appropriate diagnostic procedure. The CT scan may not visualize some vascular anomalies, but it is still an indicated procedure prior to angiography. In the postconcussive headache, as with trauma in general, a negative CT scan is associated with an excellent prognosis. In a patient with a clear history of a post-lumbar puncture headache, a CT scan is probably unnecessary.

In patients who appear to have inflammatory headache, a lumbar puncture is indicated immediately in a case of suspected meningitis and an erythrocyte sedimentation rate should be obtained in a case of suspected arteritis. The patients with disease of isolated extracranial structures require further diagnostic work-up pertinent to the organ system involved, as detailed earlier.

The role of skull roentgenograms in the work-up of headache in the emergency department is a controversial subject. The only circumstances in which they are clearly indicated is when disease of the calvarium, e.g., fractures, and primary bone disease are suspected. Thus, in many headache work-ups, the next appropriate diagnostic procedure is the CT scan. However, in the majority of patients, nothing beyond a meticulous history and goal-directed physical examination is immediately indicated in the emergency department.

REFERENCE

1. Diamond S, Dalessio DJ: *The Practicing Physicians's Approach to Headache*, ed 2. Baltimore, Williams & Wilkins, 1978.

BIBLIOGRAPHY

Caviness VS Jr, O'Brien P: Headache: Current concepts. *N Engl J Med* 302:446–450, Feb 21, 1980.
Friedman AP (ed): Symposium on headache and related pain syndrome. *Med Clin North Am* 62:3, 1978.

45. Coma

E. JOHN GALLAGHER, M.D.

Consciousness implies a certain cognizance of one's self and surroundings. Loss of consciousness includes physiologic states such as sleep and pathologic ones such as coma. That state of pathologic unconsciousness known as coma can be defined simply as unarousable unresponsiveness, while stupor can be defined as arousability only in response to a noxious stimulus. In order to avoid fine semantic distinctions that are not clinically useful, the term *coma* as used in this chapter encompasses the definition of stupor as well.

Etiology of Coma

In evaluating the comatose patient in the out-of hospital setting or the emergency department, the clinician should constantly keep in mind the etiologic decision tree shown in Figure 45–1. This diagram divides comatose patients into those with and those without evidence of significant head trauma. While this distinction cannot always be made with ease, it must be considered at the outset in order to protect the cervical spine in the event of a fracture. Once trauma has been tentatively ruled out, the nontraumatic causes of coma can then be divided into two categories:

1. organic, which produces more than 95 percent of all coma
2. functional, or psychogenic

The organic causes of coma can then be subdivided into those due to

1. the presence of a toxin or metabolite (toxic-metabolic)
2. structural disease

Toxic-metabolic processes that cause coma can be further subdivided into exogenous (overdoses) or endogenous metabolic abnormalities. Structural lesions can be divided into those located above and those located below the tentorium, namely, (1) supratentorial structural lesions, which include the herniation syndromes of either the uncal or central variety; and (2) subtentorial structural lesions, which are either compressive within the posterior fossa or destructive of brain stem tissue.

The distinction among these different groups and subgroups is not merely academic, but rather dictates very different modalities of management in the field and in the emergency department. The object of the initial evaluation, then, is to determine by means of a systematic examination the limb of this decision tree upon which the comatose patient lies. It is unnecessary for emergency care personnel to proceed beyond the boundaries of Figure 45–1 in order to formulate rational treatment plans and appropriate disposition. In fact, they can do this with relative ease if they keep in mind a modicum of basic anatomy and physiology.

BASIC ANATOMY AND PHYSIOLOGY

As noted in Figure 45–2, the brain is divided by the tentorium cerebelli into two compartments: supraten-

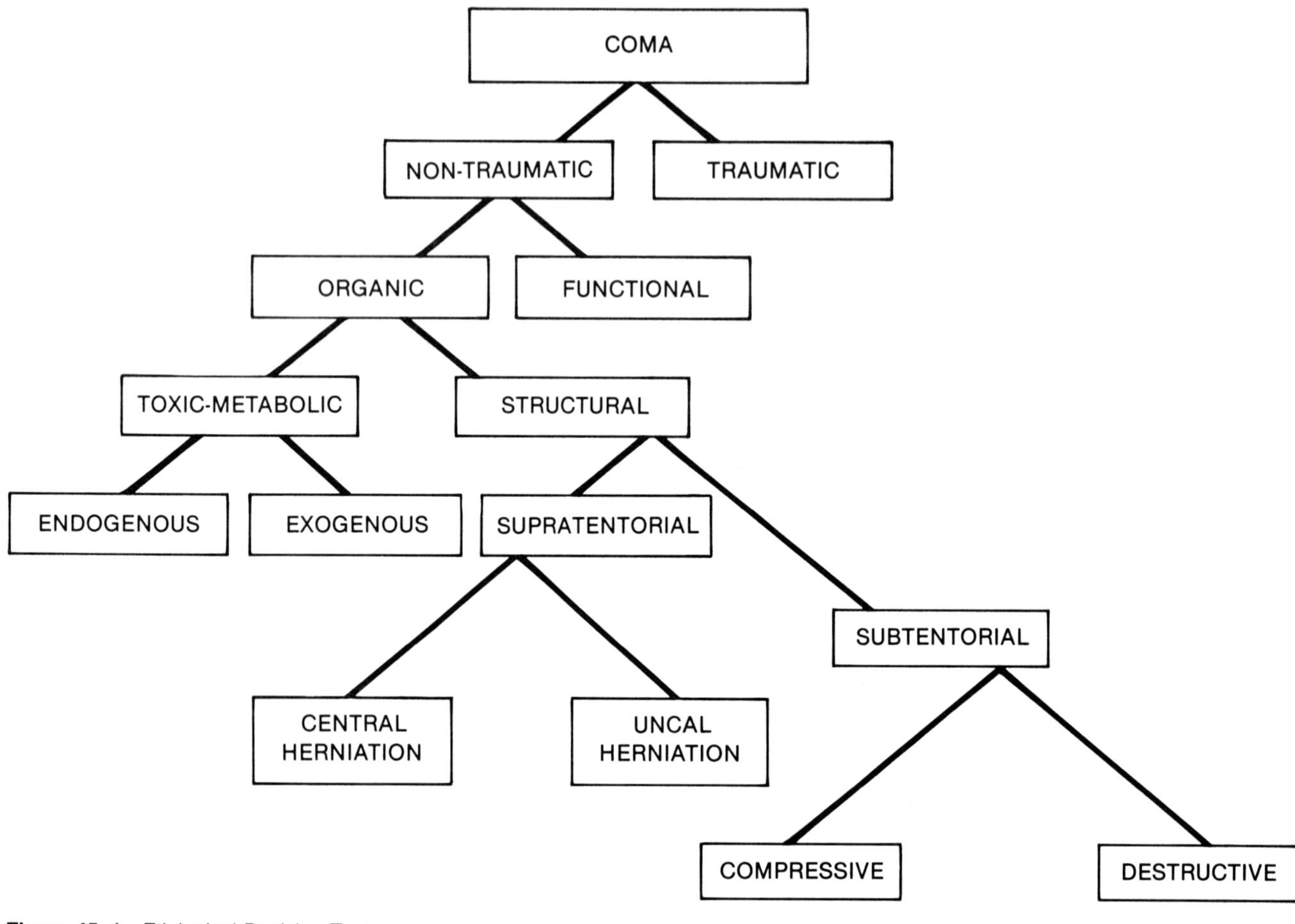

Figure 45–1   Etiological Decision Tree.

torial and subtentorial. A meningeal reflection of the dura, the tentorium forms both the roof of the cerebellum and the floor of the posterior portion of the cerebrum. It separates the cerebral hemispheres and diencephalon in the supratentorial compartment from the midbrain, pons, cerebellum, and medulla in the subtentorial compartment.

Anteriorly, the tentorium bounds an oval opening, the incisura, through which the brain stem passes from the supratentorial into the subtentorial compartment. Sitting on the edge of the incisura is the uncus, a portion of the temporal lobe, which plays an important role in uncal herniation.

Empirically, it appears that two anatomical structures are necessary for consciousness: (1) at least one hemisphere and (2) an intact ascending reticular activating system (ARAS), which is an ill-defined core brain stem structure coursing from the diencephalon to the mid-pons. Note that *both* are necessary for consciousness. From this it follows that there are essentially two ways to render a patient unconscious or comatose:

1. Involve both hemispheres by widely depressing brain functions.
2. Encroach upon the arousal mechanism (ARAS) in the brain stem.

Thus, there are essentially *two* kinds of coma. In the coma caused by toxic-metabolic conditions, both hemispheres are diffusely depressed by the presence of circulating toxins or metabolites that have crossed the blood-brain barrier. The coma produced by a structural condition develops when the brain stem ARAS is encroached upon by an anatomically definable lesion. If the pathologic process involves the brain stem *directly*, as in a brain stem cerebral vascular accident (CVA), it is classified as subtentorial. If, however, the structural lesion involves the brain stem indirectly, as an intracerebral hematoma above the tentorium, this is classified as supratentorial.

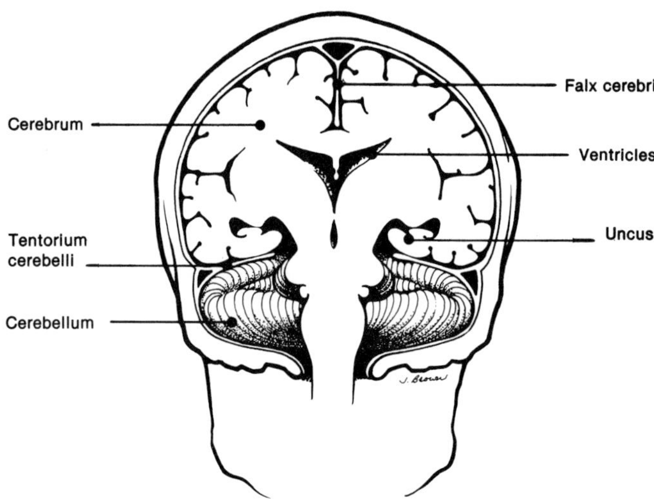

Figure 45–2 Cerebelli Compartments: Supratentorial and Subtentorial. (*Source*: Reprinted with permission from Plum F, Posner JB: *Diagnosis of Stupor and Coma*, ed 2. Philadelphia, FA Davis, 1972, 70.)

SYSTEMATIC APPROACH TO THE PATIENT WITH COMA

Initial assessment of the comatose patient follows the American Heart Association (AHA) guidelines for any patient who is potentially in full cardiopulmonary arrest. (See Chapter 55.) Procedures include stimulating the patient to verify unresponsiveness; opening the airway; assessing and, if necessary, assisting ventilation; and assessing and, if necessary, assisting circulation. Further management is described in the section on treatment later in this chapter.

As soon as the patient's vital signs have been stabilized and the tentative diagnosis of coma confirmed by application of a noxious stimulus, blood is drawn for an SMA-6 (glucose electrolytes, and BUN); toxicologic studies; and determinations of osmolality, calcium level, and a prothrombin time. In addition, 25–50 gm glucose and 0.8–2 mg naxolone hydrochloride (Narcan) are administered intravenously (IV). The $D_{50}W$ is given on the assumption that all comatose patients are hypoglycemic until proved otherwise. Patients who are comatose because of hyperosmolality secondary to hyperglycemia are not significantly harmed by an additional glucose load; however, in those who are hypoglycemic, the $D_{50}W$ is diagnostic as well as immediately therapeutic. If glucose cannot be given IV in the field, glucagon given intramuscularly (IM) or subcutaneously (sc) in a dose of 1 mg may be administered as a second-line choice. Narcan is an extremely safe opiate antagonist that, because it has virtually no agonistic properties, can be given with relative impunity. Although 0.8 mg will reverse most opiate overdoses, up to 2 mg may be

necessary. On the theory that an acute Wernicke's encephalopathy may be either the cause of the coma or may be precipitated by the large glucose load, 100 mg thiamine IV may also be given. Occasionally, the mannitollike effect of the hypertonic $D_{50}W$ will cause a transient improvement in the level of consciousness in patients who are undergoing herniation from a mass lesion. The response of a hypoglycemic patient to $D_{50}W$ is generally more dramatic and permanent.

Following this "blind" therapy, an arterial blood gas and pH should be measured in all patients. A Foley catheter should be inserted because many of these patients, especially those who are comatose as a result of an overdose, may experience acute urinary retention. Because arrhythmias of all types are common in comatose patients, cardiac monitoring begun in the field should be continued in the emergency department.

History

As in all clinical circumstances, the evaluation should begin with a history. While it is self-evident that patients in coma can offer no history, a great deal of useful information can be obtained from the emergency medical technicians, paramedics, police, friends, or family. Inquiries concerning medical history, medications being taken, prior health status, antecedent headache, or recent trauma can be very helpful. Whether the onset of coma was witnessed or unwitnessed is also extremely useful information. A quick search of a patient's pockets, purse, or wallet is an essential part of the initial assessment. Finally, it is essential to check for Medalert tags.

Physical Examination

Having stabilized the vital signs, ordered laboratory studies, given $D_{50}W$ and Narcan, and made an effort to get a history, the physician is ready to begin the actual physical assessment.

COMA SECONDARY TO HEAD TRAUMA

The first question that must be asked is, Is there evidence of trauma? To answer this, the physician must inspect and palpate the skull carefully for lacerations, hematomas, and scalp edema. It is especially important to look for evidence of basal skull fractures, since these, unlike fractures of the cranial vault, are frequently difficult to see on a skull roentgenogram. Signs of basilar fractures correlate with two major anatomical areas:

1. anterior fossa
   a. subconjunctival hemorrhage extending toward back of globe
   b. sharply demarcated medial periorbital ecchymoses ("raccoon sign")

    c. cerebrospinal fluid rhinorrhea (with or without epistaxis)
2. petrous fractures
    a. mastoid ecchymoses (Battle's sign)
    b. hemotympanum
    c. cerebrospinal fluid otorrhea (with or without bleeding from external ear)

Unfortunately, virtually all of these signs have more than one cause: subconjunctival hemorrhages and periorbital ecchymoses are associated with direct ocular trauma; direct trauma to the nose and ear can readily produce bleeding; and Battle's sign, which requires about a day to develop, may be the consequence of direct mastoid trauma.

If it appears that the etiology of coma may be traumatic, the physician must immediately stabilize the patient's cervical spine and score the patient according to the Glasgow Coma Scale:

Best Verbal Response	
None	1
Incomprehensible sound	2
Inappropriate words	3
Confused	4
Oriented	5
Eye Opening	
None	1
To pain	2
To speech	3
Spontaneously	4
Best Motor Response	
None	1
Abnormal extensor	2
Abnormal flexion	3
Withdraws	4
Localizes	5
Obeys	6
Total Coma Scale:	15

Designating this as a "coma" rather than a "head trauma" scale is an unfortunate turn of phrase, since (1) the scale is *not* necessarily applicable to nontraumatic coma (especially toxic-metabolic) and (2) a patient scoring 15 on the Glasgow Coma Scale would be awake and oriented, not comatose. Nevertheless, this scale has a high degree of interobserver and cross-cultural reliability and has contributed significantly to the management of the head-injured patient. It is essential that all emergency department physicians, nurses, paramedics, and emergency medical technicians become conversant with the Glasgow Coma Scale.

After being assigned a score from the Glasgow Coma Scale, the patient should have a lateral cervical spine roentgenogram, preferably taken with portable equipment that makes it unnecessary to move the patient. The association of traumatic coma with cervical spine injury obligates the physician to exclude this entity first; since the signs of spinal cord injury are often masked by coma, the most reliable means of assessing integrity of the cord after blunt trauma is by viewing its bony casing. The neck must be stabilized with a cervical collar to prevent flexion, and the head taped and flanked by sandbags to prevent rotation and lateral movement. Once the entire cervical spine is seen to be normal, including C7, a series of skull roentgenograms may be obtained.

As will be seen subsequently, the decision tree in Figure 45–1 is constructed in such a way that, in patients who have suffered occult trauma, e.g., a chronic subdural hematoma, findings will be compatible with structural disease. This will lead the physician, albeit by a more circuitous route, to the correct diagnosis.

NONTRAUMATIC COMA

Plum and Posner[1] in their classic monograph have identified five parameters to aid the physician in arriving at a working diagnosis for a comatose patient.

1. level of consciousness
2. pupils
3. extraocular movements
4. motor response
5. respiratory pattern

Of these five, the eye findings are the most helpful. For this reason, *it is suggested that the clinician begin with and focus largely upon the eyes of the comatose patient.*

Pupils

The pupils are observed in a darkened room for

1. reactivity to light
2. equality
3. absolute size in millimeters
4. roundness or irregularity

The remarkable, though unexplained, resistance of the pupillary light reflex to a large number of toxic-metabolic insults generates an axiom:

Rule I: The response of the pupils to light is preserved in toxic-metabolic coma.

This preservation of pupillary reactivity is so uniform that the few known exceptions to this rule are worth noting:

1. anoxia: pupils fixed and dilated
2. anticholinergic agents: pupils fixed and dilated
3. cholinergic agents: pupils fixed and pinpoint—unusual
4. opiates: pupils fixed and pinpoint
5. hypothermia: pupils fixed and midposition
6. barbiturate: pupils fixed and midposition—unusual
7. glutethimide (Doriden): pupils fixed and mid to large position

The fixed pupillary dilation of anoxia is well known, though poorly understood. The atropinic agents (commonly, tricyclic antidepressants) fix and dilate pupils because the loss of tonic input from the pupilloconstrictor portion of the third cranial nerve allows unopposed sympathetic overdrive. The use of atropine to treat bradycardia, either in the field or in the emergency department may by this same mechanism cause pupils to be transiently fixed and dilated. The opposite circumstance occurs in the case of cholinergic overdrive, as seen in organophosphate poisoning. Acetylcholine excess may result in such intense pupilloconstriction that the response to light appears to be lost because the pupil cannot become more miotic. Opiate pupils are generally reactive but are so tiny that further constriction in response to light is difficult to observe. Extreme hypothermia (core temperature < 85°C) may lead to fixed pupils. Patients who are apneic and hypotensive as a result of severe barbiturate overdoses may have fixed pupils, although most retain some type of pupillary reflex activity. Glutethimide (Doriden®) will fix the pupils in mid to large position.

Finally, it is important to remember that pilocarpine eye drops, commonly used for management of wide-angle glaucoma, cause pinpoint pupils. Conversely, mydriatics, although used less commonly, can produce pupils that are fixed and dilated.

It is noteworthy that these few exceptions can often be recognized in the emergency department or in the field. For example, anoxia is suggested by an antecedent history of hypoxia, usually a cardiopulmonary arrest. If there is a reason to believe that an anticholinergic syndrome is the cause of the coma (warm, dry, tachycardic patient with dilated nonreactive pupils), 2 mg physostigmine *slowly* IV *may* be warranted as a diagnostic/therapeutic intervention. This, however, is a potent drug and should *not* be given routinely. With a possible cholinergic syndrome (diaphoresis with evidence of poor bowel and bladder control, nausea, vomiting and diarrhea in association with hypoventilation and small pupils), atropine is warranted. However, many patients with this syndrome do not have pinpoint pupils. Opiate overdoses should not be a diagnostic problem if Narcan is given initially according to the protocol. Hypothermia should be self-evident if vital signs are done routinely. Barbiturate and glutethimide levels can be obtained from the toxicology laboratory if either of these drugs appears to be the cause of coma.

Extraocular Movements

Examination of the extraocular movements is done initially by testing oculocephalic reflexes, employing the "doll's eye" maneuver. Because this involves head-turning, it is contraindicated after trauma until injury to the cervical spine has been ruled out. Doll's eyes, or oculocephalic reflexes, are said to be "positive" or "present" if, when the head is turned in one direction, the patient's eyes move conjugatively in the opposite direction (Fig. 45–3). Thus, doll's eyes are present bilaterally if both eyes move to the extreme left when the head is turned to the right, and to the extreme right when the head is turned to the left.

When this maneuver is performed on a comatose patient, one of three things can happen: (1) presence of oculocephalic reflexes as described, (2) asymmetry of response (only one eye moves or both eyes move in only one direction), or (3) absence of response (eyes remain immobile). Present oculocephalic reflexes suggest that, as a gross first approximation, the brain stem

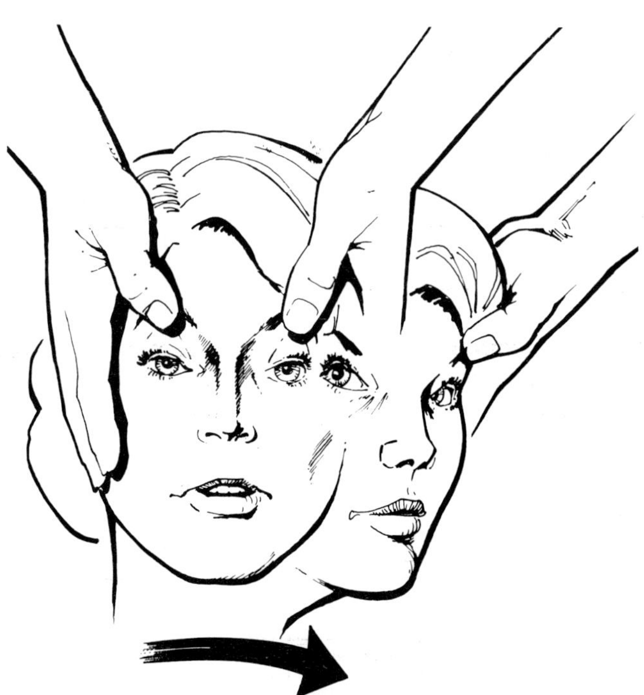

Figure 45–3 Oculocephalic Reflexes.

is intact. Asymmetry of response is a focal finding, suggestive of a structural lesion. If however, the eyes remain immobile, there are two possible explanations for this:

1. Brain stem dysfunction, or
2. Psychogenic unresponsiveness. (Awake patients do not possess the oculocephalic reflex.)

If there is an asymmetric response or no response to oculocephalic testing, it is necessary to proceed to oculovestibular testing, or "cold caloric" testing. This clinical test is the more reliable of the two tests of extraocular movement, probably because irrigation of the ear with ice water is a more potent stimulus than headturning. If the oculocephalic reflexes are clearly present, however, there is no need to proceed to oculovestibular testing, as the doll's eyes maneuver may produce false-negative results but not false-positive results.

The cold caloric test is done after the ear has been examined to verify the integrity of the tympanic membrane and to ensure that no cerumen is occluding the canal. The patient is then placed with the head elevated 30° from the horizontal and the canal irrigated with up to 200 cc ice water. It is necessary to wait ten minutes for the labyrinth on the irrigated side to return to its ambient temperature before the opposite ear can be irrigated; otherwise, false-negative results may be obtained.

There are four possible outcomes to the cold caloric test:

1. Eyes deviate conjugatively *toward* the irrigated ear, i.e., oculovestibular reflexes are present or positive (Fig. 45–4).
2. Eyes deviate asymmetrically; only one eye moves, or both eyes move toward one ear when it is irrigated but remain stationary when the opposite ear is irrigated.
3. Eyes remain stationary, i.e., oculovestibular reflexes are absent or negative.
4. Nystagmus, a fast phase toward the nonirrigated ear, is evoked.

Because the pathways involved in the oculovestibular reflex traverse much of the brain stem, integrity of this reflex suggests that a substantial portion of the brain stem is intact. The following is a more precise statement of this principle:

Rule II: In coma, loss of oculovestibular reflexes suggests brain stem dysfunction.

An asymmetric response implies focality and probable structural disease. Horizontal nystagmus with the fast

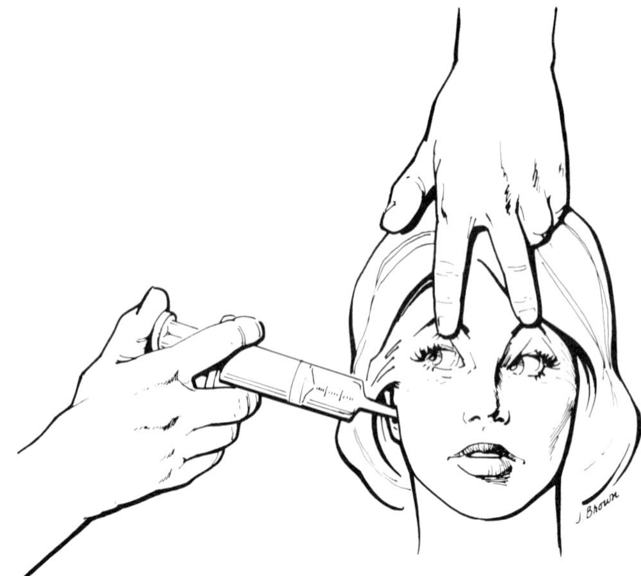

Figure 45–4   Oculovestibular Reflexes.

phase in the direction of the nonirrigated ear requires cortical participation; therefore, this finding in coma is considered to be diagnostic of *psychogenic unresponsiveness*. It serves as the operational definition of functional coma, as delineated in Figure 45–1. The differential diagnosis of this rare but extremely interesting entity includes catatonic stupor, major (vegetative) depressive disorder, somatoform illness (conversion disorder), and, uncommonly, malingering. Further distinctions among these possibilities can be accomplished by the use of sodium amytal.

If the eyes are deviated at rest, it is extremely likely that a structural lesion is the cause of coma. In general, there are only three causes for conjugate gaze deviation, i.e., deviation of the eyes from the midline such that *both* eyes appear to be "looking" in the same direction:

1. a silent or "dead" lesion in one hemisphere (CVA, mass) in which case the eyes look *toward* the lesion
2. a seizure or irritative focus in which case the eyes deviate *away* from the lesion
3. a lesion in the pons ("gaze center") in which case the eyes deviate *away* from the lesion

In the first two instances, the gaze palsy can be "broken" with cold caloric testing because the brain stem is intact. In lesions of the pons, however, the eyes usually do not move in response to cold calorics, in keeping with Rule II.

Significant dysconjugate gaze at rest implies not only structural disease but structural brain stem disease.

Motor Responses

The physician should attempt to elicit, by application of a noxious stimulus, a motor response. The painful stimulus should not be unduly noxious, however. Mentioned only to be condemned is the use of surgical clamps, the sternal "washboard," the nipple "pinch," or the testicular "twist." Patients are often understandably upset when, on the day following admission, they awaken to find presternal and periareolar ecchymoses as a consequence of a "vigorous" examination in the field or emergency department. Supraorbital ridge pressure is acceptable, as is pinching the Achilles tendon or twisting the loose skin on the inner aspect of the upper arm.

When a noxious stimulus is applied, there are three possible motor responses:

1. appropriate, varying from localization to withdrawal
2. stereotypic, i.e., either (a) *decortication* (flexion at fingers, wrist, and elbow with internal rotation at shoulder) or (b) *decerebration* (decortication with *extension* at elbow)
3. absent or flaccid

Because the corticospinal tracts are at a greater distance from the ARAS than the pathways that control pupillary reactivity and extraocular movements, motor responses in coma are not as reliable in determining levels of brain stem function as are the eye findings. Nevertheless, they are very helpful in determining asymmetry, which is useful in the following way:

> *Rule III:* Asymmetry of motor findings (focal or lateralizing signs) suggests that the etiology of coma is structural.

STRUCTURAL VS. TOXIC-METABOLIC ETIOLOGY OF COMA

After data on pupils, extraocular movements, and motor responses have been systematically gathered, the physician must assemble these findings in order to arrive at a working diagnosis. The work-up thus far has progressed to the third tier of the etiologic decision tree shown in Figure 45–1. Coma associated with significant head trauma has been distinguished from nontraumatic coma and dealt with separately. Coma with an organic etiology has been separated from the rare entity of "functional" coma, by virtue of the finding of horizontal nystagmus in response to cold water in the latter.

The major diagnostic question to be answered now is, Is the etiology of coma structural or toxic-metabolic?

Table 45–1 summarizes the general differences between coma with a structural etiology and coma with a toxic-metabolic etiology and places these distinctions in the context of the three parameters thus far examined. It is apparent that, as a corollary to Rule III, asymmetry of pupillary reactivity and of extraocular movements is also highly suggestive of structural disease. This is due to the focal nature of the pathologic process, in contrast to the diffuse nature of toxic-metabolic disease. Care must be used, however, in applying Rule III. Although asymmetric findings strongly suggest a structural process, symmetric findings do not exclude a structural lesion. In fact, early in the evolution of a structural process, depending on the location of the lesion, the examination may reveal few localizing findings. If the examination reveals no asymmetry of pupils, extraocular movements, or motor responses, the clinician cannot assume that the coma is, by exclusion, toxic-metabolic in origin; although it is suggestive. In order to make the diagnosis of a toxic-metabolic process with certainty, it is necessary to demonstrate findings that are not only symmetric, but also dissociated. This concept will be discussed later in this chapter.

Structural Lesions

Having determined that a structural lesion is the probable etiologic agent, the physician must then determine whether the process is encroaching upon the brain stem indirectly, i.e., from the supratentorial compartment via one of the herniation syndromes, or directly, i.e., from the subtentorial compartment. In either circumstance the following rule applies:

> *Rule IV:* In order for structural disease to cause coma, it must encroach, directly or indirectly, upon the brain stem.

TABLE 45–1   Structural vs. Toxic-Metabolic Etiology of Coma

	Structural	Toxic-Metabolic
Pupils	Asymmetric or nonreactive	Pupils Equal, Round, React to Light (PERRL) (with exceptions noted in discussion of Rule I)
Extra-ocular Movements	Asymmetric or absent	Symmetric or absent
Motor	Asymmetric or absent	Symmetric or absent

Supratentorial Structural Lesions

From Rule IV it can be seen that supratentorial structural lesions can cause coma only by producing an increase in intracranial pressure that, because the skull is a closed nonexpansile space, is transmitted to the brain stem through the incisura of the tentorium. This is the process of herniation, which, as noted in Figure 45–1, takes one of two forms: (1) central herniation, a relatively orderly rostrocaudal (top to bottom) process that occurs in four stages or levels (Table 45–2), and (2) uncal herniation, a process that occurs in two stages (Table 45–3).

Although other forms of herniation exist, such as cingulate and tonsillar herniation, unless otherwise specified the term *herniation* will be used here to describe the dynamic process whereby supratentorial structural lesions cause coma by encroaching upon the brain stem.

The diencephalic stage of central herniation and the early stage of uncal herniation are the treatable stages. Once significant midbrain damage has occurred, return of function (in adults) is improbable.

In contrast to toxic-metabolic syndromes, both herniation syndromes produce loss of pupillary reactivity to light, in one or both eyes, early in the evolution of the pathologic process. In the uncal herniation syndrome, the eye findings are usually ipsilateral to the lesion; in the early stages, the motor findings are usually contralateral. Later, as impairment of the third cranial nerve (CN III) progresses from a partial to a complete paralysis, i.e., from pupillary dilation to loss of oculovestibular reflexes, a Kernohan's notch develops as the cerebral peduncle is pressed against the opposite tentorial edge. This produces ipsilateral motor findings but this is usually late in the herniation process.

In the central herniation syndrome, depression of mental status is the earliest finding. In the uncal syndrome, the diencephalic stage may be omitted, and the earliest reliable finding is then the relative dilation of the pupil due to CN III compression by the uncus ipsilateral to the lesion.

Because respiratory patterns overlap from one level to another, as they do with toxic-metabolic coma, they are not as helpful diagnostically as pupillary responses, extraocular movements, and motor responses. Nevertheless, the following terms are in common usage:

- Cheyne-Stokes respiration: a cycle of apnea followed by a smooth crescendo of increasing respiratory rate and tidal volume, peaking with a hyperpneic phase, followed by a smooth decrescendo

TABLE 45–2   Central Herniation

Level	Level of Consciousness (LOC)	Pupils	Extraocular Movements (EOM)	Motor Responses	Respiration
Diencephalon	±	+	+	Appropriate or decorticate	± Cheyne-Stokes
Midbrain	–	–	±	Decorticate or decerebrate	± Central neurogenic hyperventilation
Pons	–	–	–	Decerebrate or flaccid	Apneusis
Medulla	–	–	–	Flaccid	Cluster ataxic apnea

TABLE 45–3   Uncal Herniation

Level	Level of Consciousness (LOC)	Pupils	Extraocular Movements (EOM)	Motor Responses	Respiration
Early	Lethargic or awake	Sluggish and unequal	Normal or dysconjugate	Appropriate or asymmetric	Normal
Late	Coma	Unequal or fixed	Dysconjugate or absent	Decerebrate or decorticate	Cheyne-Stokes respiration (CSR) or central neurogenic hyperventilation (CNH)

of respiration, returning to apnea. It is seen with toxic-metabolic coma and structural lesions located anywhere from the cerebral hemispheres to the upper pons.

- central neurogenic hyperventilation: sustained hyperventilation in patients with low midbrain and upper pontine damage. It cannot be distinguished from the Kussmaul breathing of metabolic acidosis without measurement of arterial blood gas and pH.

- apneusis: (involuntary) breath-holding at end-inspiration. It suggests pontine damage.

- ataxic breathing: irregular, disorganized respirations that reflect medullary damage.

Cushings reflex, i.e., hypertension and bradycardia as a result of increased intracranial pressure, is a relatively late finding in adults undergoing herniation and therefore not of much help diagnostically.

There is no substitute for observing the comatose patient over time. Frequent reexamination will often clarify a questionably nonreactive pupil or asymmetric motor response. Perhaps most important, the physician must recognize that Tables 45–2 and 45–3 are idealized schematics. A myriad of brain stem findings may occur at *multiple* neuraxial levels once herniation is under way. Nevertheless, the generalizations mentioned earlier are applicable to the vast majority of cases.

Supratentorial causes of coma include

1. CVAs
   a. hemorrhage
   b. infarct
2. trauma (hematoma)
   a. subdural (chronic) (See Fig. 45–5.)
   b. epidural (See Fig. 45–6.)
3. tumors

CVAs that cause coma are generally, but by no means exclusively, hemorrhagic. The prognosis for such patients is poor. In coma caused by trauma, however, the possibility of finding a surgically treatable extra-axial hematoma, such as a chronic subdural or acute epidural hematoma, affords a brighter prognosis—brain tissue is frequently normal beneath the clot. Supratentorial tumors cause coma less commonly than do either CVAs or trauma, accounting for 15 percent of all supratentorial mass lesions that cause coma.

Distinguishing among these various supratentorial lesions, however, is beyond the purview of the emergency department physician. In order to formulate appropriate short-term management, this physician need only decide that a herniation syndrome is causing the coma.

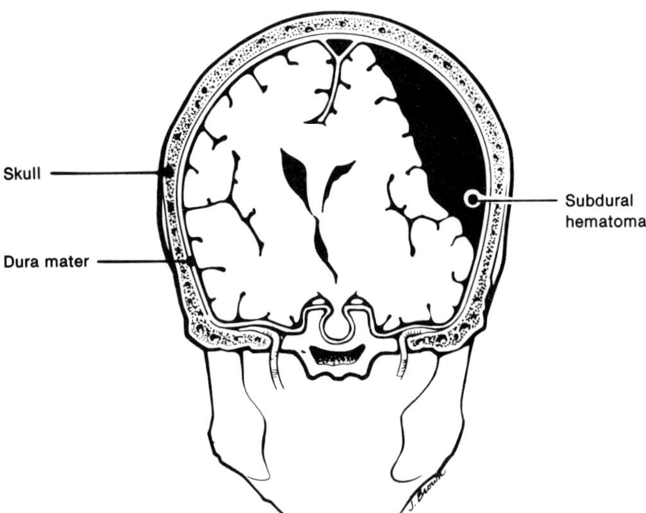

Figure 45–5 Subdural Hematoma.

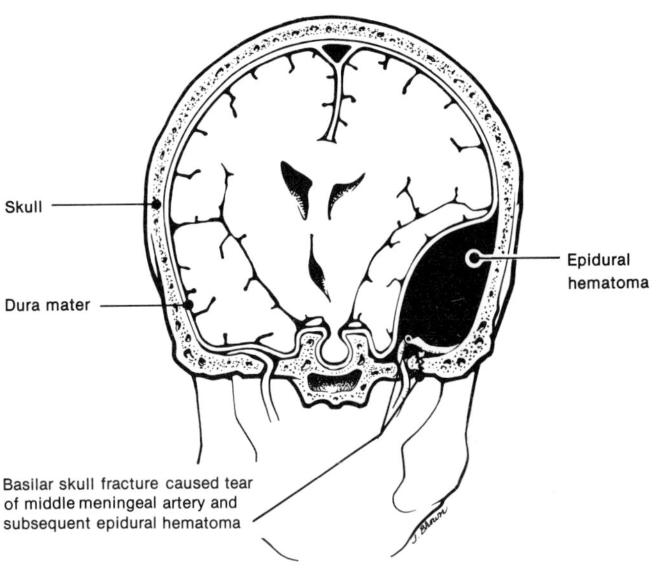

Figure 45–6 Epidural Hematoma.

Subtentorial Structural Lesions

The three salient characteristics of coma due to subtentorial structural lesions are

1. an absence of the dissociation of findings characteristic of toxic-metabolic coma (see Toxic-Metabolic Causes of Coma).
2. an asymmetry of pupils, motor responses, and especially extraocular movements. (Subtentorial lesions that cause coma rarely leave the oculovestibular reflexes intact.)
3. an absence of the orderly sequence of rostrocaudal deterioration so characteristic of the uncal or central herniation syndromes that mark coma-causing supratentorial lesions.

In the subtentorial space, or posterior fossa, there are lesions, as noted in Figure 45–1, that compress or destroy the brain stem.

Destructive Subtentorial Lesions. Unfortunately, the majority of subtentorial lesions that produce coma are destructive, usually brain stem infarcts that produce pupillary findings and abnormalities of extraocular movements not commonly seen in rostrocaudal deterioration. The best example of a physical finding that is virtually diagnostic of a destructive brain stem lesion is internuclear ophthalmoplegia, i.e., failure of the eye ipsilateral to the lesion to *adduct* when the other eye *abducts* appropriately in response to the cold caloric test. In addition, there are other cranial nerve findings that localize the pathologic process to the brain stem. Next in order of probability, but less common, is the pontine hemorrhage, which also presents a fairly characteristic clinical picture of pinpoint pupils, abrupt onset of coma, and loss of oculovestibular reflexes and responses.

Compressive Subtentorial Lesions. Lesions in the posterior fossa may compress the brain stem at (1) a midbrain level, upward through the tentorium; (2) a pontine level directly; or (3) a medullary level, causing a herniation of the cerebellar tonsils downward through the foramen magnum.

Among the most treatable of the compressive lesions is the cerebellar hemorrhage, which produces a syndrome of headaches, vomiting, truncal ataxia, and nystagmus. The posterior fossa must be explored before coma supervenes if the patient is to be salvaged, however.

When the physician in the emergency department sees a patient with brain stem findings (often pupillary or oculovestibular), it may be difficult to determine whether they are caused by an evolving supratentorial herniation syndrome or a subtentorial process. (See Fig. 45–7.) If in doubt, the emergency department physician should treat the patient as if herniation is taking place, at least until a decision can be made concerning further diagnostic or therapeutic intervention.

Toxic-Metabolic Causes of Coma

In Table 45–1, coma caused by structural disease was contrasted with that caused by toxic-metabolic disease and the differences catalogued in terms of pupillary reactivity, extraocular movements, and motor responses. A more general statement can now be made:

Rule V: If the hallmark of coma caused by structural disease is an asymmetry of findings, then the hallmark of coma caused by toxic-metabolic disease is a dissociation of findings.

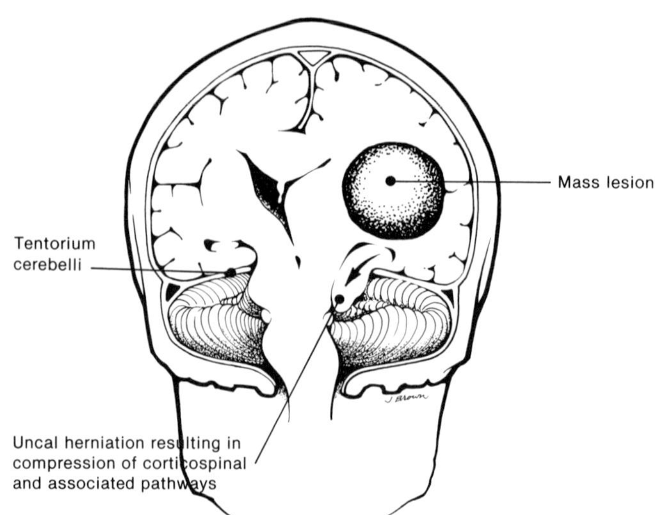

Figure 45–7 Supratentorial Mass Lesion Demonstrating an Effect on Subtentorial Structures.

The notion of asymmetric findings is not difficult to grasp, but the concept of dissociated findings is somewhat more elusive. The term *dissociation* refers to the tendency of toxic-metabolic processes to produce partial dysfunction at a number of levels of the neuraxis in a way that makes anatomical "non-sense"; that is, the process does not conform to an orderly rostrocaudal deterioration in which the brain stem is rendered dysfunctional level by level (as in a herniation syndrome), nor does it suggest a subtentorial lesion.

Most of the dissociated findings of toxic-metabolic coma involve both an intact pupillary light reflex and one of the following:

1. loss of oculovestibular reflexes
2. abnormal or absent motor responses that are usually symmetric
3. loss of respirations

Any one of these combinations is highly suggestive of coma with a toxic-metabolic etiology. At this point, in fact, the physician should check the results of laboratory studies ordered at the beginning of the work-up. Often there is a clue that suggests whether the toxin or metabolite is of endogenous or exogenous origin, since many common toxic-metabolic encephalopathies of both endogenous and exogenous cause are associated with characteristic laboratory abnormalities:

- Endogenous
  - A. Electrolyte disorders
    1. Hyponatremia
    2. Hyperosmolality
    3. Azotemia
    4. Hypoglycemia
    5. Hypercalcemia

6. Hyperkalemia*
B. Arterial blood gas abnormalities
  1. Increased pCO_2
  2. Decreased pO_2
  3. Metabolic acidosis*
    a. Postictal
    b. Hypoperfusion
    c. Renal failure
    d. Diabetic ketoacidosis
C. Elevated prothrombin time (hepatic encephalopathy)
D. Bloody cerebrospinal fluid
E. Endocrine
  1. Hypopituitarism
  2. Addison's disease
  3. Primary hypocortisolism
  4. Hypothyroidism
- Exogenous
  A. Toxins
    1. Antidote-responsive (immediate)
      a. Opiates (Narcan)
      b. Anticholinergics (physostigmine)
      c. Cholinergics (atropine)
    2. Acidosis-producing
      a. Aspirin (may also be alkalemic)
      b. Carbon monoxide
      c. Methanol
      d. Ethylene glycol
      e. Cyanide
      f. Iron
      g. Ethanol
      h. Paraldehyde
      i. Isoniazid
      j. Carbon Tetrachloride
    3. Serum level determination required
      a. Aspirin
      b. Barbiturates
      c. Ethanol
      d. Carboxyhemoglobin
      e. Lithium
      f. Iron
      g. Phenytoin
  B. Meningitis/encephalitis
  C. Thermoregulatory disorders
    1. Decreased temperature (less than 90°F)
    2. Increased temperature (more than 105°F)

It is essential to remember the following principle:

Rule VI: Laboratory values that are significantly abnormal strongly suggest a toxic-metabolic etiology of coma.

---

*Does not in and of itself cause coma.

Notable exceptions to this rule include (1) respiratory alkalosis, which is often seen in patients with structural lesions, e.g., central neurogenic hyperventilation, and (2) elevated blood ethanol levels, since these are frequently found in patients with head trauma.

Endogenous Causes of Toxic-Metabolic Coma

As noted, the endogenous causes of toxic-metabolic coma are frequently reflected in electrolyte disorders, arterial blood gas abnormalities, an elevated prothrombin time, bloody cerebrospinal fluid, or signs of endocrine failure.

Electrolyte Disorders. The following are the most common electrolyte disorders and the approximate levels that indicate the presence of a significant disorder:

1. hyponatremia (< 115 mEq/liter)
2. hyperosmolality (> 350 mOsm/liter)
3. azotemia (blood urea nitrogen determination > 100)
4. hypoglycemia (blood sugar < 35 mg/dl)
5. hypercalcemia (Ca^{++} > 12 mg/dl)

Hyponatremia is usually due to inappropriate "free water" reabsorption in the distal nephron. This is a consequence of excessive antidiuretic hormone (ADH) secretion, end-organ hypersensitivity to ADH, lack of cortisol (as in hypopituitarism or Addison's disease), or excessive water intake.

Hyperosmolality usually occurs as a result of dehydration. It is reflected as hypernatremia unless there is concomitant hyperglycemia or hyperlipemia, in which case there is a "pseudohyponatremia."

Azotemia reflects either renal failure or marked dehydration. The degree of hypernatremia, acidosis, urine/plasma creatinine ratio, and urinary sodium can be helpful in distinguishing prerenal azotemia from renal shutdown.

Hypoglycemia is a diagnosis that should be made on the basis of the patient's response to $D_{50}W$ and confirmed by determination of the serum glucose. Dextrostix should not be relied upon.

Hypercalcemia, frequently secondary to metastatic bone disease, is an increasingly common cause of an altered mental status. Hypocalcemia rarely, if ever, causes coma, however. (See Chapter 14.)

Arterial Blood Gas Abnormalities. Alterations of pH probably do not produce coma. Nevertheless, the causes of pH abnormalities, especially acidosis, are often responsible for profound changes in mental status. Thus, measurement of arterial blood gases and pH serves as a valuable marker.

Respiratory acidosis (elevated pCO_2, decreased pH) appears to cause coma by a combination of CO_2 narcosis and hypoxemia. Hypoxemia ($PO_2 < 50$) produces cerebral anoxia, which is usually accompanied by a metabolic acidosis. Significant metabolic acidosis (decreased pCO_2 and decreased pH) is usually of the anion gap variety (lower than serum $HCO_3 < 15$, $\Delta > 15$) and is frequently a clue to

- an antecedent seizure producing postictal coma and a rapidly resolving lactic acidosis
- antecedent hypoxia or hypoperfusion, which also produces a lactic acidosis
- renal failure
- diabetic ketoacidosis (although these patients are generally not comatose unless they are also hyperosmolar)
- a toxin ingestion

Prothrombin Time Elevation. Although also seen with aspirin overdose and with sodium warfarin (Coumadin), an elevated prothrombin time may be the only clue to hepatic coma, since the asterixis and multifocal myoclonus characteristic of toxic-metabolic encephalopathies in their earlier stages are lost when coma supervenes. An elevated prothrombin time should prompt the physician to look more carefully for other signs of liver failure, such as scleral icterus, spider angiomas, ascites, hepatomegaly, and splenomegaly, none of which are invariably present in hepatic coma. Quite commonly, there is an accompanying respiratory alkalosis, but this is also very nonspecific.

Subarachnoid Hemorrhage. The sine qua non of a subarachnoid hemorrhage is bloody cerebrospinal fluid, distinguished from a traumatic lumbar puncture by (1) the persistence of xanthochromia in the supernatant following spinning of the spinal fluid and (2) the failure of the fluid to clear between the first and third tube. Patients with evidence of increased intracranial pressure due to a mass lesion should be scanned by computerized axial tomography (CT) before a lumbar puncture is done because of the potential danger of herniation. The only exception to this rule arises when there is a suspicion of meningitis.

Endocrine Disorders. Panhypopituitarism and hypocortisolism can be tentatively distinguished from Addison's disease in the emergency department by means of electrolyte determinations. Because of the loss of both glucocorticoid and mineralocorticoid in Addison's disease, hyponatremia is accompanied by hyperkalemia. This is in contrast to adrenal failure secondary to hypopituitarism (or withdrawal of long-term steroid therapy) in which the absence of cortisol allows excessive ADH-independent back diffusion of free water, producing hyponatremia. Because aldosterone is unaffected, there is no accompanying hyperkalemia. Evidence of hypothyroidism in addition to evidence of glucocorticoid deficiency or loss of secondary sexual characteristics strongly suggests hypopituitarism.

Hypothyroidism (primary or secondary) is suggested in the emergency department by an increase in arterial pCO_2 and a decrease in temperature (both of which may be slight), accompanied by bradycardia and so-called "hung up" reflexes. The necklace scar of a thyroidectomy should be sought.

Exogenous Causes of Toxic-Metabolic Coma

The vast majority of exogenous, nontraumatic causes of toxic-metabolic coma are overdoses, followed by infections and disorders of thermoregulation.

Toxins. The coma-causing toxins are grouped according to whether or not they are (1) immediately antidote-responsive (in which case, diagnosis and therapy coincide), (2) acidosis-producing, or (3) detectable only by serum level.

Although there are a number of other antidote-responsive toxins in addition to the opiates, anticholinergics, and cholinergics, they are not listed here either because their response to the antidote is not rapid enough to be immediately diagnostic (sodium nitrite/thiosulfate in cyanide) or because coma is not a common presentation of that particular overdose (acetaminophen and *N*-acetyl cysteine).

Common toxins that may produce coma and metabolic acidosis include salicylates (which may also produce a respiratory alkalosis) and carbon monoxide. Less commonly, methemoglobinemia and cyanide poisoning produce cellular hypoxia and acidosis. Methanol and ethylene glycol produce organic acids when oxidized to their toxic intermediates and characteristically generate large anion gaps and high osmolality associated with negative serum ethanol levels.

Patients with a metabolic acidosis often demonstrate a Kussmaul respiratory pattern unless they have superimposed ventilatory failure. Many drug overdoses involve drugs that also depress respiration, and it is important to be on the alert for this hypoventilation; it can be especially devastating in a patient who is already acidotic on a metabolic basis. A useful rule of thumb is that the last two numbers in the pH should equal the pCO_2 in a pure metabolic acidosis with appropriate respiratory compensation. For example, a patient with pH of 7.15 on a metabolic basis should have a pCO_2 of about 15 mm Hg. A higher pCO_2 may be the first clue that the patient is tiring, and the physician should prepare for intubation. To wait until the pCO_2 exceeds a "normal" of 40 mm Hg may have disastrous consequences in the context of a metabolic acidosis. (See Chapter 59.)

Finally, the blood levels of a number of coma-producing toxins can be measured. The most common are the barbiturates and ETOH. The latter is often mixed with other drugs and, unless the level is very high, should not be assumed to be the sole cause of coma. Because some people develop a marked tolerance to barbiturates and ETOH, levels of both these drugs may be difficult to interpret. Glutethimide has been mentioned previously because of its notorious ability to fix the pupils; the blood level of this drug can also be determined. The use of glutethimide appears to be decreasing, and it is being replaced by other sedative-hypnotic drugs, such as methaqualone (Quaalude) and ethchlorvynol (Placidyl). Elevated aspirin and carboxyhemoglobin levels might be anticipated on the basis of arterial blood gas and pH abnormalities but must be confirmed by the toxicology laboratory. Lithium overdoses are becoming more common as this drug is increasingly utilized in the treatment of affective disorders. Iron overdoses, on the other hand, are on the decline and seem to be confined to the pediatric age group.

If taken in sufficient quantity, many other drugs, especially sedative-hypnotics, readily produce coma on a toxic-metabolic basis. Although these cannot be identified by assay, knowledge of a specific toxin is rarely crucial to management. In fact, once certain agents have been excluded, the treatment of most sedative-hypnotic overdoses is identical.

Infections. The infectious causes of coma include meningitis, which is usually bacterial, and encephalitis, which is usually viral.

In addition to a fever, bacterial meningitis that has not been treated is invariably accompanied by a positive Gram stain of cerebrospinal fluid. Because the bacteria may precede the presence of white cells, all cerebrospinal fluid must be centrifuged for five minutes and Gram-stained before it can be declared negative. More than three to five white blood cells is worrisome, especially if they are polymorphonuclear; in bacterial meningitis, the count is usually in the hundreds to thousands, accompanied by a low glucose level (less than 50 percent serum glucose) and elevated protein.

Viral encephalitis produces white blood cells, usually lymphocytes with a negative Gram stain, elevated protein, normal sugar, and, often, red blood cells. (See Chapter 20.)

Thermoregulatory Disorders. Temperatures below 85°F and above 105°F can produce coma. Both hypothermia and heat strokes are diseases of the elderly, the alcoholic, the addict, and the patient on phenothiazines or tricyclics. In comatose patients with temperatures between 85°F and 105°F, a nonthermal cause for coma should be sought. (See Chapters 29 and 30.)

SPECIAL DIAGNOSTIC PROCEDURES IN COMA

Skull Roentgenograms

With the advent of the CT scanner, which depicts tomographic cuts of the *brain*, the need to rely on inferential data obtained from roentgenograms of the *skull* naturally diminishes. As the technology improves, offering more efficient, rapid scans at a lower cost and with less irradiation, it is conceivable that skull roentgenograms may disappear altogether from some emergency departments. At the present time, there is much debate surrounding the indications for skull roentgenograms, and it is difficult to draw any meaningful conclusions. In general: (a) if a CT scan is indicated, skull roentgenograms are probably superfluous; and (b) if the patient does not require a CT scan, skull roentgenograms rarely provide information that alters treatment.

The need for a good lateral roentgenogram of the cervical spine in cases of suspected trauma has been mentioned previously. This is more important in the comatose patient than skull roentgenograms.

Lumbar Puncture

Evidence of increased intracranial pressure is a *relative* contraindication to a lumbar puncture in a comatose patient because of the possibility of inducing herniation. For the same reason, a spinal tap is contraindicated in coma that is believed to be secondary to trauma. In these types of patients, a CT scan is indicated prior to a lumbar puncture. On the other hand, in a patient in whom the diagnosis of meningitis is being seriously considered, there is no contraindication to a lumbar puncture.

The laboratory analysis of cerebrospinal fluid includes obtaining a spun Gram stain and determining an opening pressure, a white blood cell count with differential, a red blood cell count, as well as the protein and glucose levels. If there is an elevated white blood cell count without apparent explanation, the cerebrospinal fluid should be sent for tuberculosis and fungal cultures.

CT Scan

Computerized tomography of the head is a technique in which the brain is radiographically sectioned into multiple slices, generating attenuation profiles that are computer analyzed and then restructured anatomically. A CT scan may be done without or, preferably, with contrast enhancement. Small differences in coefficients of absorption in contiguous structures, which are indistinguishable from one another by means of conventional radiography, become apparent on the CT scan. For example, fresh bleeding into the ventricular system cannot be discerned on plain skull roentgenograms because it blends into the tissue "fluid density" of the brain, but it is grossly apparent on the CT scan. For this reason, it has largely replaced the more invasive procedures, such as angiography and pneumoencephalography, and has become the primary diagnostic radiographic procedure in coma.

The CT scan figures heavily in the management of coma suspected to be due to structural disease, including trauma, and is now indispensable in determining whether neurosurgical intervention would be appropriate. Essentially, the comatose patients who should be considered candidates for CT scan from the emergency department are those

1. with supratentorial mass lesions in which herniation seems likely
2. with subtentorial mass lesions that may be of the compressive variety (e.g., cerebellar hematomas)
3. any head trauma with altered mental status or focal findings
4. in whom the diagnosis is seriously in question

It is perhaps in coma of traumatic etiology that the CT scan plays the greatest role in the emergency department. In this setting, extra-axial hematomas, such as acute epidural and subdural hematomas, are well visualized and can be reliably distinguished from intracerebral hematomas, contusions, and edema (much of which is missed on angiography). The subacute and chronic subdural hematomas may present a problem, as they evolve through an isodense phase in which a mass effect may be the only clue to their presence. Conversely, a normal CT scan in head trauma suggests an excellent prognosis, if brain stem contusion can be excluded clinically.

Other Diagnostic Procedures

Funduscopic Examination

Although a funduscopic examination is helpful in the assessment of coma, it is often misleading. When rapid increases in intracranial pressure occur, the loss of spontaneous venous pulsation and the subsequent appearance of papilledema may not take place for some time. Because of this, the funduscopic examination, especially in the emergency department, can be quite specific for increased intracranial pressure, though it lacks sensitivity. Since it appears that it is not the increased pressure per se that produces herniation, but rather the *shifts* in structures caused by the expanding lesions,

pupillary reactivity is a better marker of the progress of rostrocaudal deterioration than the funduscopic examination. The funduscopic examination may lead directly to a diagnosis, however, when a subarachnoid hemorrhage produces characteristic subhyaloid (preretinal) hemorrhages. Because the blood is superficial and lies just beneath the internal limiting membrane, it obscures the retinal blood vessels.

Electrocardiogram

The electrocardiogram (ECG) in coma may provide an early clue to hypercalcemia (shortened QT interval) or hyperkalemia (peaked T waves). Subarachnoid hemorrhage may produce giant, symmetric T-wave inversion across the precordium. Tachycardia should cause the physician to suspect an anticholinergic overdose, especially if sinus and faster than 220 minus the patient's age.

Electroencephalogram

The usefulness of the electroencephalogram (EEG) is primarily in toxic-metabolic disorders, and it may be the only means of diagnosing electrical status epilepticus. Although a normal EEG essentially excludes a toxic-metabolic etiology of coma, it is not part of most routine coma work-ups and may not be immediately available in the emergency department.

TREATMENT

Out-of-Hospital Phase

The care of comatose patients begins in the street with the paramedic. In order to protect the cervical spine, the jaw thrust or chin lift are the best airway maneuvers, followed by a log roll of the patient to one side in order to clear the oropharynx of secretions or vomitus. If, following this, the patient is breathing adequately, an oral or nasal airway should be inserted to keep the tongue forward. If the patient is not breathing adequately but is moving air, endotracheal intubation is the procedure of choice both in the field and in the emergency department. Skilled physicians or paramedics can intubate the patient without moving the cervical spine. Bag and valve mask and the esophageal obturator (or its gastric modification) are alternative but less secure means of ventilation. (See Chapter 56.)

Unless the loss of consciousness is known to be nontraumatic, a cervical collar should be placed and the patient transported on a spine board. Pupils should be checked for reactivity to light and equality. An intravenous line should be inserted and, after a blood sample for glucose has been drawn, $D_{50}W$ and Narcan should be administered. If there is evidence of significant trauma, the patient must be assessed on the Glasgow Coma Scale.

A suggested paramedic head trauma protocol might read as follows:

1. If the Glasgow Coma Scale score is less than 8, the patient should be intubated (nasotracheal) and hyperventilated.
2. If the Glasgow Coma Scale score is less than 12, dexamethasone (Decadron) (10 to 100 mg) should be given IV.
3. If the pupils are unequal or nonreactive, the base station should be contacted concerning the use of mannitol.
4. The patient should then be transported directly to the closest appropriate facility where definitive therapy is available.

Treatment in the Emergency Department

When the patient arrives at the emergency department, the systematic assessment of the patient's condition according to the decision tree depicted in Figure 45–1 is begun. In order to determine appropriate treatment at the emergency department level, it is necessary to go only as far as the bottom tier of this decision tree.

Traumatic Etiology

If the etiology of the coma is believed to be traumatic, a cervical spine injury must be radiographically ruled out. The patient's Glasgow Coma Scale score is then assessed and a treatment decision made on the same criteria as that used in the field:

> Score on Glasgow Coma Scale < 12—10 to 100 mg Decadron
> Score on Glasgow Coma Scale < 8—Intubation with hyperventilation (pCO_2 of 25)

Whether high-dose steroids are of greater benefit than low-dose steroids is controversial. Hyperventilation, however, very effectively diminishes cerebral blood flow and decreases intracranial pressure.

Mannitol should be reserved solely for circumstances in which the brain stem is threatened with irreversible damage (usually from herniation). This occurs at some point between the development of a sluggish pupillary reflex and the loss of oculovestibular reflexes. Use of mannitol is indicated to gain additional time in the hope that the patient may have a surgically correctable lesion.

As noted earlier, any head trauma patient with altered mental status *or* focal findings should be CT-scanned. If the patient becomes agitated, it is worth the risks and problems of sedation in order to avoid image degradation on the scan. Sedation with an opiate is preferable, since it can be reversed safely and rapidly with Narcan.

Toxic-Metabolic Etiology

The emphasis for treatment of coma with a toxic-metabolic etiology is upon support of vital signs with specific intervention in selected circumstances. Certain disorders require immediate intervention.

Hyponatremia. Normal saline is usually satisfactory unless the patient is *in extremis* in which case 3 percent saline can be given *very slowly*, and 200 mg Solu-Cortef (or equivalent) intravenous push may also be given on the theory that the hyponatremia might reflect hypocortisolism secondary to hypopituitarism, Addison's disease, or long-term steroid therapy with abrupt withdrawal. (See Chapter 12.)

Hyperosmolar Syndromes. Dilute solutions ($< \frac{1}{2}$ normal saline) are used to treat hyperosmolar syndromes unless the patient is hypotensive in which case normal saline is used. Whether or not 5 percent dextrose is used depends upon whether or not hyperglycemia is contributing to the hyperosmolarity.

Azotemia. If azotemia is the result of renal failure, the emergency department physician need act immediately only if this is associated with life-threatening hyperkalemia, acidosis, or pulmonary edema.

Hypercalcemia. Beginning treatment of hypercalcemia in the emergency department involves volume expansion with saline followed by loop-blocking diuretics, such as furosemide (Lasix). Digitalis is, of course, contraindicated.

Hypokalemia. Under no circumstances can hypokalemia be treated rapidly.

Hypercapnia or Hypoxia. If acute hypercapnia occurs, the patient may require intubation; however, this is to be avoided in patients with chronic lung disease, if at all possible. (See Chapter 60.)

Metabolic Acidosis. Unless the pH is less than 7.10, depending on etiology, the patient need not be given sodium bicarbonate. Postictal lactic acidosis need not be treated unless the patient is in status epilepticus. Treatment of the lactic acidosis of shock requires therapy for the blood pressure and the underlying cause. In renal failure, the acidosis should not be treated unless it is life-threatening or associated with severe hyperkalemia. In diabetic ketoacidosis, it is preferable to avoid bicarbonate and start with small amounts (10 units regular) of intravenous, intramuscular, or subcutaneous insulin.

Hepatic Encephalopathy. Neomycin or lactulose enemas are frequently employed, but they need not be started in the emergency department. (See Chapter 23.)

Endocrine Disorders. As mentioned earlier, hypopituitarism, Addison's disease, and primary hypocortisolism may have hyponatremia and hypotension in common. Because a bolus of steroid does little harm and may be life-saving, after a blood sample has been drawn for a determination of plasma cortisol, any patient in coma with significant hyponatremia or hypotension should be given 200 mg Solu-Cortef or its equivalent.

The treatment of myxedema coma is highly controversial and beyond the scope of this chapter. The hypercapnia and hypothermia that frequently accompany this disorder must be treated very gingerly, as these patients are extremely brittle.

Reactions to Toxic Substances. Patients with toxic ingestions should be gastric lavaged with 15 liters in 200 cc increments using a forty French orogastric tube, followed by activated charcoal and magnesium sulfate. Classical teaching dictates that the airway be protected with an endotracheal tube to facilitate lavage. The use of antidotes is discussed more extensively elsewhere in this text; in brief, Narcan may be used with impunity, and physostigmine and atropine should be used conservatively.

In salicylate toxicity (> 50 mg/dl at six hours postingestion), bicarbonate should be started in the emergency department to enhance urinary excretion. In patients with carboxyhemoglobin levels greater than 20 percent, or in symptomatic patients, 100 percent O_2 is indicated. In cyanide toxicity, the Lilly Kit (containing amyl nitrite, sodium nitrite, and sodium thiosulfate) is recommended. In methanol and ethylene glycol toxicity, ethanol should be started immediately and dialysis considered. In lithium toxicity, a saline diuresis should be begun and dialysis considered. In iron toxicity, a decision about deferoxamine should be made in consultation with a pediatrician.

Bacterial Meningitis. One of the few indications for starting antibiotics in the emergency department is bacterial meningitis. After cultures of cerebrospinal fluid, blood, and nasopharynx have been taken, the physician has a choice of penicillin, ampicillin, or chloramphenicol, depending on Gram stain, patient age, geographical area, and allergic history.

Thermoregulatory Disorders. The physician should externally cool heat stroke as rapidly as possible to 102°F, but no lower if overshoot is to be avoided. The treatment of hypothermia involves passive external rewarming unless it becomes necessary to institute active core rewarming. (See Chapter 30.)

Structural (Nontraumatic) Etiology

If it has been determined that the lesion is structural rather than toxic-metabolic, it must then be determined whether the lesion is supratentorial or whether it is subtentorial. In this circumstance, any patient who appears comatose because of a supratentorial lesion should be treated as if the coma resulted from a herniation syndrome. Therefore, the use of steroids can be justified in any patient who is comatose because of a structural condition. Intracranial pressure should be further reduced as soon as there is evidence of additional encroachment upon the brain stem. The earliest indicator of this is likely to be a sluggish pupillary reaction to light, with or without asymmetry. At this point, the patient should be intubated, hyperventilated to a pCO_2 of 25, and considered a candidate for (warm) mannitol. In general, however, mannitol is used only if the brain stem may be undergoing irreversible damage and, if possible, in consultation with a neurologist or neurosurgeon. The patient should be CT-scanned immediately, unless the patient is deteriorating so rapidly that it is necessary to make parieto-occipital burr holes while the patient is in the emergency department. In experienced hands, the latter is a safe procedure; and, if the holes are well placed, the procedure may be diagnostic as well as therapeutic for certain extra-axial hematomas. This is now done only under the most extreme circumstances, however. Although most comatose patients with structural disease should have a CT scan, those with suspected supratentorial lesions and compressive posterior fossa lesions should receive preference over those with suspected destructive brain stem lesions since the latter are less visible on CT scan and less amenable to treatment.

Conclusion

Employing the principles mentioned, it should be possible to distinguish the toxic-metabolic from the structural etiology of coma. The physician can then focus further diagnostic work-up on either the laboratory or the CT scanner. From the laboratory studies, including those from the lumbar puncture, it is usually possible to determine whether the toxic-metabolic process is endogenous or exogenous and to order appropriate treatment in the emergency department if this is indicated. In structural disease, the CT scan can usually verify a diagnostic impression and indicate whether surgical intervention is warranted.

If, in toxic-metabolic coma, the patient begins to deteriorate, conservative management with support of vital signs is indicated. Electrolytes and acid-base status are monitored and dialysis considered, although this is rarely necessary. If a patient with a structural lesion begins to deteriorate, the physician should proceed more aggressively. Intubation with hyperventilation, high-dose steroids, mannitol, and neurosurgical consultation are in order on the assumption that the patient may be herniating and have a surgically correctable lesion.

REFERENCE

1. Plum F, Posner B: *The Diagnosis of Stupor and Coma*, ed 3. Philadelphia, FA Davis Company, 1980.

SUGGESTED READING

Redelman K (ed): Neurological injuries. *Critical Care Quarterly* 2: 1979.

46. Cerebrovascular Accidents

E. JOHN GALLAGHER, M.D.

A cerebrovascular accident (CVA) occurs as a result of either the occlusion or rupture of a blood vessel in the brain (Fig. 46–1). It is characterized by the relatively abrupt appearance of a neurologic deficit. While tumors and traumatic hematomas are commonly included in the differential diagnosis of CVAs they are not primary vascular events and thus will not be discussed in detail in this chapter.

Since CVAs are the most common serious neurologic problems encountered in the emergency department, it is essential that emergency department physicians have a coherent and logical approach to the evaluation of this condition. Such an approach is facilitated by classifying any suspected CVA into one of five etiologic categories. The practical value of such a classification scheme lies in the fact that each category dictates a different work-up, requires a different plan of initial management, and has a different prognosis. The five categories of CVAs include

1. large artery thrombosis
2. embolism
3. lacunae
4. intracerebral hematoma
5. subarachnoid hemorrhage

Although these syndromes have in common the abrupt onset of a deficit that marks the event as vascular, they can be distinguished from one another on the basis of history, neurologic examination, radiographic findings, and laboratory studies.

LARGE ARTERY THROMBOSIS

Pathophysiology

Atheromas, which form at areas of turbulent blood flow, may be associated with superimposed thrombi that narrow the arterial lumen further. As the thrombus increases in size and the stenosis progresses, at least half of the patients will have a transient ischemic attack (TIA) before they develop a CVA. When the thrombus totally occludes the lumen, a distal infarction results. The signs and symptoms of both the prodromal TIA and the CVA correlate with the anatomical area of the brain perfused by the compromised vessel. The large arteries most often affected are the internal carotid; vertebrobasilar; and anterior, middle, and posterior cerebral.

History

Because vascular events have a characteristic course of evolving symptomatology, a precise history of the sequence of events is essential to diagnosis. A large vessel thrombosis is characterized by

1. antecedent TIAs in the *same* vascular territory
2. a *stuttering* development of neurologic deficit over hours to days, rarely more than a week

Commonly, there is evidence of vascular pathology elsewhere, such as coronary artery or peripheral vascular disease, often associated with high blood pressure.

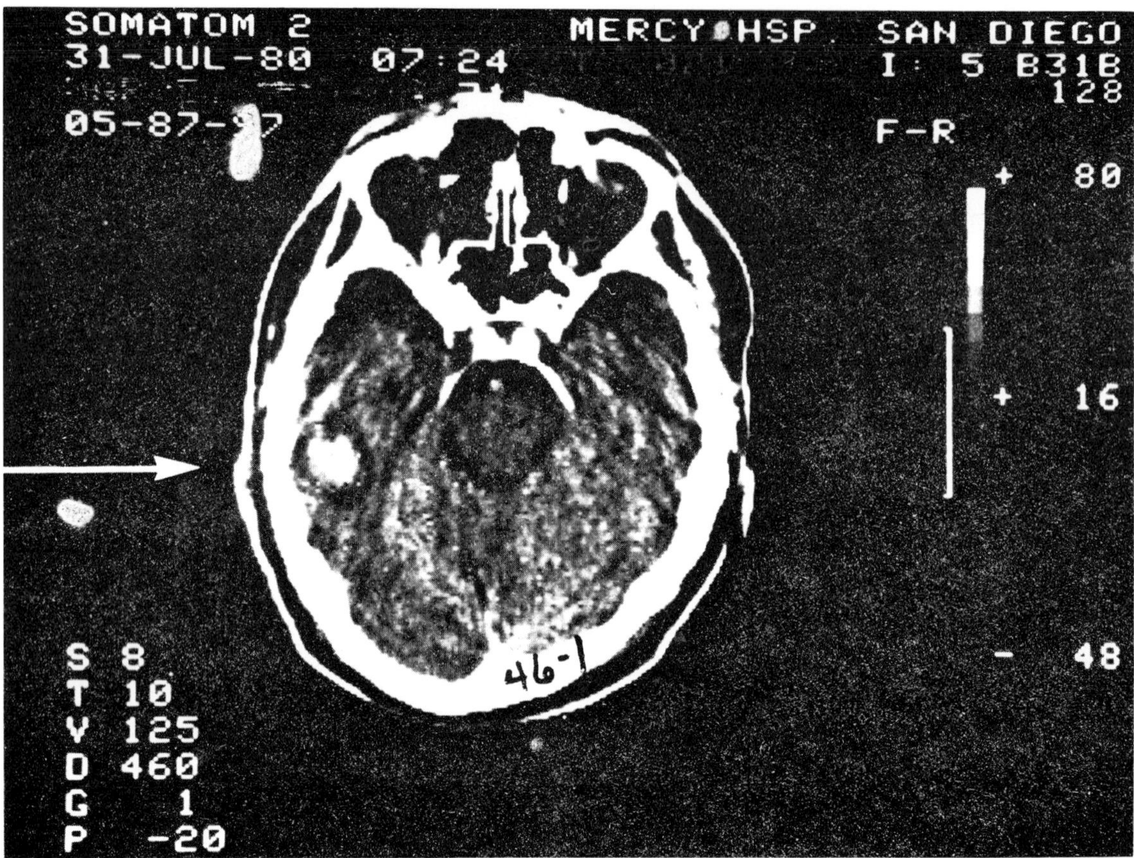

Figure 46–1   CT of the Head Showing Hemorrhage in the Posterior Left Temporal Lobe.

Neurologic Findings

The specific CVA syndromes produced by thrombosis of a large artery depend upon the anatomical area of the brain that is rendered ischemic by occlusion of that particular vessel. Although the possibilities are numerous and highly variable, a few common syndromes can be identified. In disease of the anterior circulation, i.e., the carotids, the findings are usually localized to a single hemisphere, producing lateralizing signs and symptoms. In disease of the vertebrobasilar artery, bilateral, often "crossed," brain stem findings are commonly seen.

Anterior Circulation

Middle Cerebral Artery Syndrome. Findings that can be localized to the vascular territory of the middle cerebral artery are usually the result of occlusion of the internal carotid artery. This affects most of the *lateral* portion of each hemisphere and produces a clinical picture characterized by

1. contralateral hemiparesis, with face and arm worse than the leg, owing to involvement of the lateral part of the motor strip
2. contralateral hemianesthesia, owing to involvement of the lateral part of the sensory strip
3. conjugate eye deviation such that the eyes look *toward* the involved hemisphere, owing to involvement of the frontal eye fields
4. homonymous hemianopsia, owing to involvement of the optic fibers posterior to the chiasm
5. aphasia if the dominant (usually left) hemisphere is involved, owing to involvement of the speech centers
6. denial or seeming unawareness of paralyzed side of body if the nondominant (usually right) hemisphere is involved

Posterior Circulation

Posterior Cerebral Artery Syndrome. The inferior portions of the temporal and occipital lobes, including the visual cortex, are supplied by the posterior cerebral artery. This vessel also gives branches to the thalamus. Any or all of the following findings are characteristic of proximal thrombosis:

1. Homonymous hemianopsia, owing to involvement of the visual cortex, is the most constant finding.
2. Contralateral hemisensory defect, owing to thalamic involvement, may also occur.
3. There is little or no hemiparesis.
4. Dominant hemisphere posterior cortical findings include
   a. amnesic aphasia (patients are able to describe and use an object though unable to name it)
   b. loss of recent memory
   c. alexia without agraphia, which may be so severe that patients cannot read what they have written.

Vertebrobasilar Artery Syndromes. Because the vertebrobasilar system supplies most of the brain stem and cerebellum, either directly or by way of bifurcation into the posterior cerebral artery, occlusion may produce an enormous variety of clinical findings, depending on whether the main trunk or one of its many branches is occluded.

Because there are two vertebral arteries, occlusion of one may produce no discernible abnormality unless the other has been previously compromised. Unfortunately, this is not uncommon. The vertebrals are the main vascular supply to the medulla so that thrombosis, when it occurs, produces lower brain stem syndromes, of which the most common is the lateral medullary syndrome. Although this is often called the posterior inferior cerebellar artery (PICA) syndrome, in most cases the occlusion is in the vertebral artery. The findings include

- loss of ipsilateral facial pain and temperature sense, owing to involvement of the descending tract of the trigeminal nerve, coupled with loss of contralateral pain and temperature sense over the remainder of the body, owing to involvement of the spinothalamic tract

- ipsilateral Horner's syndrome, owing to involvement of sympathetic fibers

- ipsilateral ataxia, owing to involvement of cerebellar fibers

- vertigo, nausea, vomiting, nystagmus, owing to vestibular involvement

- hoarseness, dysphagia, ipsilateral paralysis of palate, and diminished gag reflex, owing to involvement of the ninth and tenth cranial nerves

Just as vertebral thrombosis results in medullary abnormalities, basilar occlusion produces pontine and cerebellar findings that can be deduced from a knowledge of neurovascular anatomy. The complete basilar syndrome consists of coma with quadriplegia and variable cranial nerve abnormalities. The coma is secondary to involvement of the ascending reticular activating system, and the quadriplegia is a consequence of bilateral involvement of the pyramidal tracts. Incomplete basilar occlusion, as seen in the basilar branch syndromes, is a variety of CVA that is being recognized with increasing frequency. Such syndromes may be classified more correctly as lacunar CVAs, but they can also be considered large vessel thrombosis because they may be harbingers of complete basilar occlusion.

The basilar artery has three kinds of branches, numbering 15 to 20 on either side. Their occlusion produces three major varieties of findings:

1. Occlusion of the paramedian arteries produces lesions in the medial pons, characterized by
   a. contralateral hemiplegia, owing to pyramidal tract involvement.
   b. abnormalities of extraocular movements, either a conjugate gaze palsy in which the eyes look *away* from the lesion, owing to involvement of the pontine gaze center, or internuclear ophthalmoplegia, owing to involvement of the medial longitudinal fasciculus. An internuclear ophthalmoplegia is defined as an inability to *ad*duct the ipsilateral eye completely, accompanied by nystagmus in the *ab*ducting eye, when the patient looks to the side contralateral to the lesion.
2. Occlusion of the short circumferential arteries produces lesions in the lateral pons, which results in prominent contralateral sensory loss, owing to involvement of the lateral spinothalamic tracts.
3. Occlusion of the long circumferential arteries that embrace the pons on the way to the cerebellum produces lesions characterized by ipsilateral cerebellar findings. These may be associated with either medial or lateral pontine findings.

Anterior vs. Posterior Findings

Some general principles may aid the emergency department physician in distinguishing anterior circulatory (carotid territory) CVAs from those that are posterior circulatory (vertebrobasilar territory or brain stem):

- Bilateral findings argue strongly for a brain stem CVA, although unilateral findings in no way exclude a brain stem vascular event.

- Crossed findings, either sensory or motor, strongly suggest brain stem pathology. An ipsilateral facial hemisensory or motor deficit may be coupled with a contralateral hemisensory deficit or hemiparesis involving the rest of the body, for example.
- Eye movements can be helpful in a number of ways:
  - If a conjugate gaze palsy exists, the eyes look *toward* a destructive supratentorial lesion and *away* from a brain stem (pontine) lesion. Thus, in a right middle cerebral artery thrombosis, the eyes would be conjugately deviated to the right in association with a left hemiparesis; in a right (medial) pontine lesion, the eyes would be conjugately deviated left in association with a left hemiparesis.
  - If the eyes are dysconjugate or if there is an internuclear ophthalmoplegia, the lesion is in the brain stem.
- A hemiparesis accompanied by a hemisensory deficit on the same side of the body is more likely to be anterior than posterior.
- A dissociation of sensory findings may be helpful, i.e., when position and two-point discrimination are affected more than pain and temperature perception, a cortical lesion is likely (and vice versa).
- Cerebellar signs suggest a posterior lesion.
- The common motor aphasias suggest an anterior lesion.
- Pupillary inequality, because of the involvement of the third cranial nerve in the midbrain, or Horner's syndrome, because of the involvement of sympathetic fibers lower down, both suggest a brain stem lesion.
- True vertigo, if central rather than peripheral, is a brain stem symptom.

Laboratory Findings. A lumbar puncture is not necessary, but if performed will be normal in cases of large artery thrombosis.

Radiographic Findings. A computerized axial tomography (CT) scan may reveal a nonhemorrhagic infarction that is not within the territory of a single small artery and is compatible with a large artery thrombosis. Brain stem events often cannot be detected however, and the CT scan may appear normal.

Occlusion of a large vessel, such as the internal carotid artery or the anterior, middle, or posterior cerebral arteries, can be identified by angiography. The majority of middle cerebral artery thromboses, which are the most common, are actually due to stenosis at the level of the carotid artery.

Treatment and Prognosis

Because thrombotic CVAs evolve slowly and often unpredictably, there is no basis for prognostication early in their course. Early mortality is often due to herniation secondary to brain edema. Coma is a poor prognostic sign, since it suggests that core brain stem structures are either involved directly (as with a basilar occlusion) or compressed by an expanding mass (as with a large middle cerebral artery infarct).

The treatment for any "sleepy stroke," with or without CT scan documentation, must at the very least include treatment for brain edema. Whether to proceed with intubation, hyperventilation, and IV mannitol depends upon whether irreversible brain stem damage seems inevitable. Antihypertensive medications have no place in the early management of CVA unless the neurologic deficit is believed to be secondary to hypertensive encephalopathy, which is uncommon. Blood pressure control as a long-term means of preventing CVA is no longer a matter of debate—it is probably advantageous to control even *mild* hypertension. Anticoagulation therapy, however, is a highly controversial subject. There is general agreement on only a few items: (1) completed CVAs do not benefit from anticoagulation therapy, and (2) sodium warfarin (Coumadin) probably diminishes the likelihood of large vessel thrombosis following a warning TIA. (3) Antiplatelet therapy with aspirin may also decrease the incidence of thrombotic CVA in men. (4) There is no evidence that cerebral vasodilators are of therapeutic value.

In the majority of large vessel thromboses, surgery is not indicated. In selected cases of carotid occlusion, however, endarterectomy is beneficial if undertaken at the stage of TIAs or early in the course of an evolving thrombus.

Seizures following thrombotic CVAs are rare, but when they do occur should be treated with phenytoin (Dilantin). Physical therapy and rehabilitation are important considerations following stabilization of the neurologic deficit, but are outside the purview of the emergency department physician.

EMBOLISM

Pathophysiology

The vast majority of emboli to the brain originate either from the heart or large arteries. Although they may consist of bits of tumor, fat, or septic vegetations, cerebral emboli are almost invariably blood clots that have broken free from a larger thrombus downstream.

Most emboli derive from the left atrium, usually in association with paroxysmal or chronic atrial fibrillation, on either a rheumatic or idiopathic basis. Patients with valvular heart disease, certain prosthetic valves, recent myocardial infarction, or endocarditis are also at risk for cerebral emboli. Finally, it has recently been demonstrated that mitral valve prolapse is associated with an increased incidence of CVA in young patients.

Among the noncardiac sources of emboli are thrombi that originate in the aortic arch or great vessels in the neck. These thrombi, like those that form during the healing phases of a myocardial infarction, are presumed to be loosely adherent to an ulcerated endothelium. For this reason, carotid massage may be inadvisable in patients over 50 years of age (especially in view of the fact that "gentle" carotid massage is a contradiction in terms).

In the brain, emboli are evenly distributed between the two cerebral hemispheres, but show a striking predilection to enter the middle cerebral artery on either side. Because the clots are usually relatively small, they tend to migrate peripherally and produce discrete focal, often cortical, findings. There may be warning TIAs, but they are distinct from those that precede large vessel thrombosis in that emboli from the same source are statistically unlikely to lodge in precisely the same distal location. Thus, the TIAs that warn of an impending *embolic* CVA are often in *different* anatomical areas, while TIAs that precede *thrombotic* stroke are usually in the *same* anatomical area.

In the evolution of a thrombotic occlusion, there is time for collateral circulation to develop; ischemia waxes and wanes, producing a stuttering progression. In embolic stroke, however, occlusion is usually sudden, producing a deficit that is both abrupt and *maximal at onset*. The area of infarction is bland in the majority of cases, but it may be hemorrhagic about one-third of the time. Subsequently, the embolus may dissolve or disperse; depending on the duration of ischemia, the neurologic deficit may persist or resolve.

History

The most striking feature of a cerebral embolus is the sudden onset of maximal deficit, usually without warning. Only about 10 percent of patients who suffer embolic CVAs have antecedent TIAs, as has been mentioned. Atrial fibrillation; valvular heart disease, including mitral valve prolapse in young people; and recent myocardial infarction are common historical risk factors that have been discussed earlier. Occasionally, the history includes an arterial embolus to an extremity or some other peripheral location.

Neurologic Findings

The onset of the deficit is sudden, and 80 percent of the time it is maximal within moments. This is in contrast to the stuttering development of a thrombotic CVA (large vessel or lacunar) or the smooth evolution of a cerebral hematoma. Although emboli may occlude vessels in either the anterior or the posterior circulation, the middle cerebral artery and its distal branches are affected in 75 percent of the cases. In decreasing order of frequency, the posterior cerebral, basilar, and anterior cerebral territory are involved.

The middle cerebral artery syndromes produced by an embolus are, as would be expected, more focal than those produced by a large artery thrombus. Like those of a lacunar CVA, the findings are discrete. Unlike the lacunar CVAs, however, which represent occlusion of deep penetrating arteries, embolic CVAs result from occlusion of superficial cortical arteries. The clinical consequences of such an occlusion in the middle cerebral artery territory may include

- in the dominant hemisphere, a Broca's aphasia (nonfluent, associated with hemiparesis) or a Wernicke's aphasia (fluent, but unable to comprehend or to repeat, associated with minimal or no hemiparesis)
- in the nondominant hemisphere, denial of the paralyzed side
- in either hemisphere, a hemiparesis or monoplegia

In the posterior circulation, an embolus that lodges in the basilar artery may produce coma and a flaccid paralysis. This is one of the rare circumstances in which embolic CVAs may precipitate coma. If, as is more usual, the embolus passes into the posterior cerebral artery and causes an infarct in an area of the occipital cortex, a homonymous hemianopia is produced and, if it occurs in the dominant hemisphere, alexia without agraphia is observed. A recent memory deficit may also accompany occipital cortical lesions.

Laboratory Findings

Cerebrospinal fluid obtained by a lumbar puncture is either normal or, in those with a hemorrhagic infarction, xanthochromic or, rarely, grossly bloody. If the embolus is septic, there is, in addition, a cerebrospinal fluid pleocytosis, with an elevated protein level, normal glucose content, and negative bacterial cultures.

Radiographic Findings

Because a significant percentage of hemorrhagic (embolic) infarcts do not communicate with the cerebrospinal fluid, the CT scan is a more sensitive indicator of the presence of blood than the lumbar puncture. The infarction, whether hemorrhagic or bland, appears as a superficial lesion of, respectively, high or low density. (See Figure 46–1.)

Angiography may be indicated in patients without a plausible cardiac source, in whom surgical management might be beneficial. A peripheral occlusion in the vascular supply to the clinically involved area suggests an embolism, especially if a potential source is identified in a more proximal vessel.

Treatment and Prognosis

With the exception of the rare basilar occlusion, most patients survive embolic CVAs, which may clear rapidly. The majority, however, will suffer subsequent CVAs unless anticoagulant prophylaxis is begun (especially those patients with atrial fibrillation). The immediate therapeutic question concerns *when* anticoagulation therapy should be initiated. Fortunately, it is no longer necessary to rely on the lumbar puncture, which reflects a hemorrhagic infarct only if blood has leaked into the cerebrospinal fluid. If the CT scan shows no evidence of blood, then IV heparin may be started immediately, to be followed by oral Coumadin. The purpose of this treatment is not to alter the course of the present CVA, but rather to prevent the next one. In patients with endocarditis, however, anticoagulation therapy should be withheld.

Certain patients with carotid lesions and no cardiac source may be candidates for endarterectomy. Embolectomy does not appear to be of value.

About one patient in five with an embolic cortical infarct develops a seizure disorder at some later date.

LACUNAR CVAs

Pathophysiology

In contrast to large artery thrombosis, thrombotic occlusion of *small* penetrating arteries of the cerebrum and brain stem may produce distinct areas of infarction that, upon healing, leave behind discrete cavities or lacunae deep in the brain.

History

The temporal profile of lacunar CVAs is, as might be expected, very similar to that of large artery thrombosis. The deficit has a relatively sudden or stuttering development over hours to days. These CVAs, however, are preceded by TIAs in only about 25 percent of the cases. Headache and vomiting are rarely seen. The patients are usually hypertensive prior to and at the time of the CVA.

Neurologic Findings

At least four lacunar CVAs have been recognized, but the first is by far the most common:

1. Pure motor CVA may be secondary to an occlusion in (a) the internal capsule or (b) the pons. Hemiparesis variably affects the face, arm, and hand, but there are no sensory abnormalities, no gaze palsies or visual field cuts, no alterations of sensorium, and no deficits, such as aphasia or apractagnosia.
2. Pure sensory CVA is the sensory analogue of a pure motor hemiparesis. A discrete lesion in the thalamus produces a lone hemisensory deficit.
3. The dysarthria-clumsy hand syndrome is produced by a pontine lesion. As the name suggests, it is characterized by unilateral facial weakness, a clumsy hand on the same side, and slurred speech.
4. Crural paresis and ataxia may involve only one leg. Like the pure motor CVA, this results from a lesion in either (a) the internal capsule or (b) the pons.

Laboratory Findings

A lumbar puncture is not necessary; if one is performed, the results are normal. A lumbar puncture in a patient with an uncomplicated CVA is rarely necessary in the emergency department.

Radiographic Findings

If the lacuna is less than 1 cm in diameter, or in the brain stem, the CT scan is normal. If greater than 1 cm, the lesion can be seen deep in the hemispheres as an area of low density, compatible with a bland infarction.

Angiography is not necessary; it usually discloses no abnormality in the anatomical region that is implicated clinically.

Treatment and Prognosis

Control of blood pressure is the only treatment necessary, and this should be done gradually. No further medical or surgical intervention is warranted. These patients generally do very well, since only a small amount of tissue has been destroyed.

INTRACEREBRAL HEMATOMA

Pathophysiology

Penetrating arteries, the walls of which are weakened by long-standing, severe hypertension, may rupture *within* brain parenchyma. Such a rupture produces a circumscribed, expanding hematoma that generally displaces contiguous structures in an orderly fashion. Consequently, there is a smooth and gradual deterioration typically seen clinically. Hemorrhages are most commonly seen in the putamen, thalamus, cerebellum, and pons. The location and size of the lesions dictate signs and symptoms.

History

The onset, as is characteristic of all CVAs, is relatively abrupt. In some cases, the deficit is maximal at the outset; in most, however, there is *steady* deterioration over hours. The vast majority of patients have a background of moderate to severe high blood pressure. Warning TIAs are decidedly unusual. About one-half the patients vomit, especially those with cerebellar hematomas. About one-third have headaches. Presumably because of the involvement of the ascending reticular activity system in the brain stem, about one-quarter of the patients arrive at the emergency department in coma. This is in striking contrast to patients with thromboembolic (nonhemorrhagic) CVAs who rarely arrive in coma.

Neurologic Findings

Four anatomical areas of the brain appear to be predisposed to hemorrhagic CVAs:

1. Putaminal hemorrhage is by far the most common, accounting for about one-half of the "deep bleeds." Findings include a contralateral hemiparesis with conjugate deviation of the eyes *toward* the lesion in about one-half of the patients. As the lesion expands and extends in one direction, cortical findings may develop and the paresis may become a complete paralysis. The patient may become sleepy, eventually becoming comatose. At this juncture, many patients demonstrate pupillary inequality.
2. Thalamic hemorrhage is characterized by a marked hemisensory deficit, out of proportion to motor findings; in fact, there may be no motor findings at all. Thalamic bleeds produce an array of disturbances of ocular motility, most notably a tendency for the eyes to look down at the nose. The pupils are typically small and poorly reactive.

3. Pontine hemorrhage presents a very characteristic picture of coma with pinpoint, microreactive pupils. Unlike disorders of ocular motility produced by cortical and subcortical lesions, gaze palsies produced by pontine lesions cannot be broken by the doll's eyes maneuver or by cold calorics testing. (See Figures 45–3 and 45–4 in Chapter 45.) These patients are often decerebrate when first seen and usually die shortly after losing consciousness.
4. Cerebellar hemorrhage typically produces headache and, almost invariably, vomiting. The patient may be unable to stand or often, even to sit upright. At this stage, a cerebellar hemorrhage may be easily mistaken for acute labyrinthitis, although vertigo is usually more prominent in the latter condition. Appendicular cerebellar signs may be conspicuously absent, in contrast to the striking truncal ataxia. There may be a gaze palsy, with the eyes deviating *away* from the hematoma, although often there is only a "reluctance" to look into the ipsilateral visual field. Many patients do not have nystagmus.

An example of an intracerebral hemorrhage, displacing the falx cerebri and ventricles, is shown in Figure 46–2.

Laboratory Findings

A lumbar puncture, if one is performed, reveals bloody fluid in about three of four patients. Although blood is

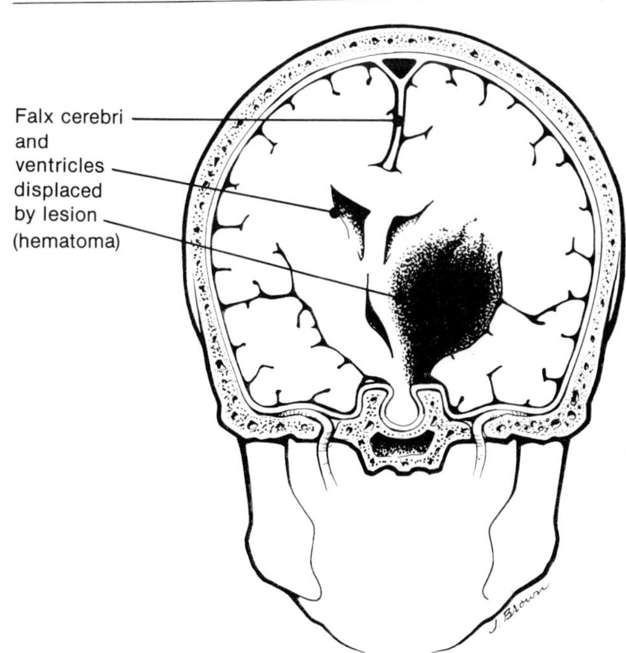

Figure 46–2 Intracerebral Hemorrhage.

grossly evident, the fluid is not generally as bloody as that observed in a subarachnoid hemorrhage.

A lumbar puncture that shows no blood, however, does not rule out an intracerebral hematoma; it indicates only that the hematoma has not extended into the ventricular system. For this reason, and because of the possibility of inducing herniation and death, patients suspected of having an intracerebral bleed should *not* have a lumbar puncture in the emergency department unless (1) a central nervous system (CNS) infection is a serious possibility or (2) a CT scan cannot be obtained and the results of a lumbar puncture will influence immediate management.

Radiographic Findings

A mass of increased density without contrast enhancement on a CT scan is diagnostic of a fresh bleed. Because of their size and location, pontine hemorrhages may be missed on CT scans, but cerebral and cerebellar hematomas are diagnosed with an accuracy that surpasses that of angiography.

Angiography is usually not necessary, but if performed shows a mass effect without evidence of arterial occlusion.

Treatment and Prognosis

Surgical evacuation of a cerebellar hematoma is the treatment of choice *if* the diagnosis is made prior to onset of coma. Once the patient loses consciousness, however, the probability of survival is markedly diminished. In the case of intracerebral hematomas, surgical intervention does not appear to alter outcome.

When a suspected cerebellar or cerebral hematoma appears to be associated with herniation, the patient should be treated as any other patient whose brain stem may be undergoing irreversible damage secondary to extrinsic compression would be treated:

1. endotracheal intubation and hyperventilation to a pCO_2 of 25 mm Hg
2. mannitol, 20 to 100 gm given intravenously (IV)
3. dexamethasone (Decadron), 10 to 100 mg IV

This should be done in the emergency department, prior to CT scan if necessary, and preferably in consultation with a neurosurgeon or neurologist. Such a patient is usually comatose with an asymmetry of findings, most notably pupillary abnormalities.

The argument for such a treatment plan is as follows: Patients who bleed into brain parenchyma have a 75 percent mortality within the first month. Those admitted in coma have an even higher mortality. It can be argued that, because tissue is not infarcted but rather compressed by an expanding hematoma, patients have a reasonable chance, not only of recovery, but of good return of function if herniation can be prevented. The risk of exacerbating the effects of a bleed by shrinking the space occupied by normal brain, however, is the theoretical argument against instituting such treatment. Thus, patients with small hematomas who are awake and do not appear to be deteriorating should be managed conservatively.

Blood pressure control is of value primarily as a preventive measure. Once the CVA is under way, it is unwise to attempt to lower blood pressure precipitously. Certainly, nothing should be done to lower blood pressure in the emergency department, unless it is suspected that the patient is suffering from pre-eclampsia or hypertensive crisis. Because it is not uncommon to observe patients with deep bleeds who have diastolic pressures to 140 mm Hg, these blood pressure levels should, in general, be left untreated until the neurologic findings have stabilized.

There is no treatment for pontine hemorrhage, medical or surgical, and most patients succumb. The prognosis of thalamic bleeds is slightly better than the others, possibly because these hematomas are generally smaller.

SUBARACHNOID HEMORRHAGE

Pathophysiology

Subarachnoid hemorrhage is caused primarily by rupture of berry aneurysms or arteriovenous malformations. Berry aneurysms are not congenital, but result from a developmental defect in the arterial wall that weakens with time and usually bursts in middle age. They occur at branch points in the circle of Willis, almost always anteriorly. When rupture occurs, a jet of blood under arterial pressure is released into the subarachnoid space, producing a sudden headache. Arteriovenous malformations are thin-walled shunts between arteries and veins. They usually occur within cerebral tissue; therefore, when they bleed, they do so not only into the subarachnoid space, but also into brain parenchyma.

History

Asymptomatic prior to rupture, berry aneurysms rupture without warning, often during exertion, producing a sudden, excruciating headache. This is usually accompanied by collapse, with or without a loss of consciousness. Vomiting is common.

Arteriovenous malformations prior to rupture may cause seizures and, less often, headache. When hemorrhage occurs, however, the clinical picture is very similar to that produced by a ruptured aneurysm.

Hypertension is unusual in the history of patients with either aneurysm or arteriovenous malformation.

Neurologic Findings

Berry aneurysms, because they are within the circle of Willis, bleed into the subarachnoid space when they rupture and generally do not produce focal neurologic findings. Any neurologic deficits that occur are thought to be secondary to a spasm or clot and may be transient.

Because of their location, arteriovenous malformations may bleed into cerebral tissue as well as into the subarachnoid space when they rupture, frequently producing focal or lateralizing signs. While consciousness is often lost, it is usually regained within minutes to hours. Because the chemical meningitis produced by blood evolves over hours, if the patient is seen a short time after the onset of bleeding, nuchal rigidity may be absent.

Subhyaloid hemorrhages may be seen on funduscopic examination. Because the blood is preretinal, these hemorrhages characteristically obscure the vessels.

A previously well person who suffers the sudden onset of "the worst headache I've ever had in my life," associated with collapse, has a subarachnoid hemorrhage until proved otherwise.

Laboratory Findings

A grossly bloody cerebrospinal fluid confirms the diagnosis.

Radiographic Findings

Blood in the subarachnoid space or a *normal* CT scan is compatible with a subarachnoid hemorrhage. Because the CT scan may not detect some subarachnoid bleeds, the lumbar puncture must still be relied upon in these cases to confirm the diagnosis.

Angiography is the only means of consistently demonstrating aneurysms. An arteriovenous malformation may be delineated clearly by angiography—if it has not been obscured by the bleeding. Patients with a normal angiogram following a bleed have a better prognosis than those in whom a lesion is seen.

Treatment and Prognosis

The initial management of patients in the emergency department with a subarachnoid hemorrhage is conservative, and the blood pressure should not be reduced.

Surgery, if undertaken, should be delayed until at least one week posthemorrhage. At that time, aneurysms may be clipped, ligated, or wrapped. Arteriovenous malformations may be ligated, resected, embolized, or irradiated. Because these malformations may be symptomatic prior to bleeding, they can sometimes be resected before hemorrhage occurs. Aneurysms are usually clinically silent prior to rupture, however, so that preventive resection is generally not an option with these lesions.

Both berry aneurysms and arteriovenous malformations tend to rebleed, although the latter are less likely to do so. The six-month survival following subarachnoid hemorrhage secondary to an aneurysm is 50 percent; with arteriovenous malformations, it is approximately 85 percent, although a small percentage of these continue to rebleed annually.

Patients in coma with a subarachnoid hemorrhage secondary to an aneurysm or an arteriovenous malformation have an especially poor prognosis, as is true of most patients who are comatose as a result of CVAs.

TRANSIENT ISCHEMIC ATTACKS

A TIA is a neurovascular event that results in a neurologic deficit that lasts less than 12 hours. Like crescendo angina, TIAs provide the emergency department physician with an opportunity to prevent reversible and transient ischemia from becoming irreversible and permanent infarction.

There are at least two kinds of TIAs: thrombotic and embolic. In the former, the signs and symptoms repeatedly affect the same vascular territory, denoting an ongoing occlusion of a particular artery by an accumulating thrombus. In the embolic TIA, the clots derive from a more proximal source, such as the left atrium or carotid bifurcation, so that a different vascular territory is likely to be involved on successive occasions.

Large artery thrombosis is preceded by a TIA at least 50 percent of the time. Lacunar CVAs, which are essentially small artery thromboses, are preceded by TIAs about 25 percent of the cases. Embolic CVAs are preceded by TIAs about 10 percent of the time. In each of these circumstances, identification of a TIA allows the emergency department physician to identify a population at risk. Although TIAs, by definition, last less than 12 hours, most last only a few minutes (5 to 30 minutes). Therefore, the results of a neurologic examination will be normal for a substantial proportion of patients with a TIA by the time they reach the emergency department. Thus, the diagnosis may often be missed unless the physician is prompted, by a high index of suspicion, to take a *meticulous* history.

On the basis of a history alone, it is frequently possible to localize the TIA to either the anterior (carotid) or posterior (vertebrobasilar) circulation. Clearly, accompanying physical findings make the task much easier, although they are not required for the diagnosis. An anterior circulatory TIA in the middle cerebral artery territory, for example, produces contralateral weakness and numbness, with or without aphasia or nondominant cortical findings; often, only a hand or one side of the face is affected. When the carotid circulation is involved, however, the findings, whatever they may be, are unilateral since only one hemisphere is involved at a time. Anterior TIAs may cause a transient monocular blindness or *amaurosis fugax*, i.e., the sudden onset of painless loss of vision followed by return of sight, often described as the "lifting of a torn curtain." The episode usually lasts less than one-half hour and is symptomatic of disease in the ipsilateral carotid.

Brain stem TIAs are extremely varied and especially difficult to identify, because the complaints are often vague and can be produced by other more benign entities. Dizziness or vertigo is a common symptom and may be associated with diplopia or dysphagia. Crossed motor or sensory findings (left facial and right arm numbness) are specific for an episode of brain stem ischemia. In contrast to carotid TIAs, vertebrobasilar TIAs often produce bilateral findings.

While TIAs are often included in the differential diagnosis of fainting or loss of consciousness, true syncope rarely has a primarily neurologic etiology.

The treatment of TIAs may be divided into three approaches:

1. *surgery.* In selected cases involving the anterior circulation, endarterectomy and extracranial-intracranial anastomosis may be of benefit. In the posterior circulation, surgery has not been demonstrated to be of value.
2. *anticoagulation.* Initial therapy with IV heparin, changed in a few days to oral Coumadin, although still controversial, appears to be of benefit. Before starting anticoagulation therapy, a CT scan should be obtained to make sure there is no bleeding, tumor, or subdural hematoma. In the case of emboli, anticoagulation therapy is recommended as prophylactic treatment for all patients with chronic or paroxysmal atrial fibrillation.
3. *antiplatelet therapy.* Aspirin appears to decrease the incidence of repeated CVA (and death) in men only.

DIFFERENTIAL DIAGNOSIS OF CVA IN THE EMERGENCY DEPARTMENT

The unmistakable signature of a CVA is its abrupt onset. In distinguishing cerebrovascular disease from other intracranial pathology, the emergency department physician must rely heavily upon the history in general and the type of onset in particular. The following are some of the entities with which a CVA may be confused:

- *brain tumor.* The symptoms of a brain tumor rarely have an abrupt onset, unless the presentation is that of a seizure (which is a rare presentation of a CVA). Usually, there is a slow deterioration of mental function or slow onset of headache rather than an abrupt onset of focal findings and/or headache. The CT scan is extremely helpful in verifying the physician's clinical impression.

- *traumatic hematoma.* In most cases of acute trauma, the cause of the neurologic problem is self-evident. Occasionally, however, a patient suffers a CVA and collapses, sustaining secondary head trauma. Alternatively, a history of trauma in the past may have been forgotten. In general, head trauma produces confusion and/or depression of consciousness out of proportion to focal or lateralizing findings, while CVAs produce the opposite, i.e., striking focality in a setting or relative mental clarity. This is especially true of extra-axial hematomas, such as epidural and chronic subdural hematomas, since there is often normal brain parenchyma that is being compressed underneath the hematoma. Thus, a mild hemiparesis may be accompanied by extreme drowsiness secondary to impending herniation. Nevertheless, there are many exceptions to this generalization; in comatose patients the distinction may be impossible without a CT scan.

- *CNS infection (meningitis, encephalitis, brain abscess).* If a fever is associated with an apparent CVA, the physician should suspect a CNS infection. If there is no evidence of increased intracranial pressure, a lumbar puncture should be done in the emergency department. If there is reason to believe that herniation may occur if fluid is withdrawn, then a CT scan must be obtained immediately. If this is not possible, it seems wiser to risk herniation than to miss a treatable illness, such as bacterial meningitis. (See Chapter 20.)

- *coma of other etiology.* The patient with a CVA who arrives at the emergency department in coma falls into the category of structural (nontraumatic) coma and should be treated accordingly (see Chapter 45). The prognosis for these patients is poor.

- *postictal hemiparesis (Todd's paralysis)*. Seizure as a presentation of CVA is rare. The history is critical and may reveal that the seizure is secondary to an old (embolic) CVA. In some patients, only observation over time will reveal the diagnosis.

- *old CVA with superimposed toxic-metabolic process*. Occasionally, a toxic-metabolic process unmasks an old neurologic deficit and the patient appears to be in coma as a result of a CVA. The presence of dissociated findings so characteristic of toxic-metabolic coma (such as preserved pupillary light reflexes but no reaction to cold caloric testing) should alert the emergency department physician to this possibility. These patients should, however, have a CT scan for confirmation of diagnosis.

- *migrainous aura*. Again, a past history of vascular headache is the distinguishing feature. Most patients recognize these prodromes quite readily. Even the rare patient with hemiplegic migraine usually has a family history of this. Also, the mean age for patients with migraines is quite different from the mean age for patients with CVA.

- *labyrinthitis/Meniere's disease*. This question frequently arises in the emergency department in regard to whether dizziness (vertiginous type) is central or peripheral in origin. The most important lesion to rule out is a cerebellar hematoma, since this must be surgically evacuated before irreversible brain stem damage occurs. Headache is a highly constant feature of this lesion, and any patient with true vertigo associated with a significant suboccipital headache should have a CT scan immediately. Other *central* causes of vertigo are associated with brain stem signs and symptoms such as dysphagia, diplopia, and specific cranial nerve abnormalities. The nystagmus often appears out of proportion to the vertigo. Vertical nystagmus in patients not on sedatives or minor tranquilizers suggests brain stem disease. *Peripheral* lesions may be associated with deafness and tinnitus, which are less common in central lesions. Finally, the severity of the vertigo may appear to be out of proportion to the nystagmus, which is often slight, may be rotatory, and fatigues on repeated stimulation.

BIBLIOGRAPHY

Mohr JP, Fisher CM, Adams RD: Cerebrovascular diseases, in *Harrison's Principles of Internal Medicine*, ed 9. New York, McGraw-Hill, chap. 365.

Mohr JP, et al: The Harvard cooperative stroke registry: A prospective registry. *Neurology* 28:754–762.

Weisberg LA: Computed tomography in the diagnosis of intracranial disease. *Ann Intern Med* 91:87–105, July 1979.

47. Seizures and Acute Confusion

GREGG T. HUSK, M.D.

APPROACH TO THE PATIENT WITH SEIZURES

Seizures commonly result in an emergency department visit. Approximately 1 million Americans suffer from epilepsy, and a seizure is the presenting symptom in 2 to 4 percent of emergency visits. In one patient, a grand mal seizure may represent life-threatening trauma; yet, in another, it may simply be an isolated fit that briefly interrupts a normal life span. The emergency department physician must quickly identify the critically ill patient; attempt to define etiology and reversible precipitants; make therapeutic decisions, often based on little history; and decide on inpatient or outpatient therapy.

The initial contact with the patient and witnesses offers a unique opportunity to obtain a history. What is called a seizure may be a simple faint or syncope from a profound bradycardia. (See Chapter 50.) Hence, exactly what was observed is of key importance. Past medical history, medications (and whether or not they have been used as prescribed), and trauma, either before or during the seizure, should be elicited. Seizures are dramatic events that have a variety of presentations, each of which demands a particular approach.

DEFINITIONS

A *seizure* is a temporary alteration in behavior due to abnormal electrical activity in the brain. *Epilepsy*, which refers to recurrent seizures, can be classified as *idiopathic* when no cause has been identified or as *symptomatic* when there is a known underlying condition. In adults, the most common type is *grand mal*, in which a patient suddenly loses organized muscle tone and becomes unresponsive; the patient may also undergo a sequence of extensor tone and apnea lasting seconds, followed by bilateral clonic motions lasting a few minutes. This sequence is followed by a period of depressed consciousness with stertorous breathing that resolves over minutes. Repetitive grand mal seizures without interictal recovery of consciousness is termed *grand mal status.* See Table 47–1 for a summary of causes of grand mal seizures.

MECHANISMS OF MORBIDITY

Patients with grand mal seizures can be injured in a number of ways. The cause of the seizure, e.g., an intracerebral hemorrhage due to trauma, may carry short-term morbidity. The seizure itself, however, by depriving the patient of normal protective movements, may result in burns, drowning, or a variety of traumatic injuries. Vomiting with aspiration can lead to pneumonia. With frequent seizures, intellectual deterioration can occur.

With grand mal status, there are additional risks. Disorganized neuronal activity with resultant increased cerebral oxygen consumption is coupled with poorly coordinated respiratory motions and upper airway ob-

TABLE 47–1   Etiologies of Grand Mal Seizures

Idiopathic grand mal epilepsy is called *primary epilepsy;* epilepsy caused by central nervous system or systemic processes is called *secondary epilepsy.* Central nervous system processes that can lead to epilepsy are

- birth injuries
- trauma
- craniotomy
- infection (meningitis, encephalitis, tuberculosis)
- tumor
- cerebrovascular accident (CVA)
- subarachnoid hemorrhage

Systemic processes that can cause epilepsy are

- medication noncompliance in an epileptic
- hypoglycemia
- uremia
- hyponatremia
- hypocalcemia
- hypoxia
- drug ingestions
- drug withdrawal
- malignant hypertension
- toxemia
- fever

---

struction from secretions or the tongue. Hypoxia may result in brain damage with cerebral edema. Increased motor activity can cause hyperthermia, which can lead to further complications. Electrolyte disturbances and profound acid-base abnormalities are common. Hypotension and arrhythmias can be produced by hyperemia, acidosis, and hypovolemia. Pathologists often find evidence of anoxic encephalopathy, in addition to a predisposing structural lesion. Morbidity and mortality have been described within the first 30 minutes of status, although most patients succumb after many hours of uncontrolled seizures.[1]

GRAND MAL STATUS

Clinicians recognize grand mal status separate and apart from isolated seizures because of the 3 to 30 percent short-term mortality and substantial long-term morbidity that these patients sustain. Most often, grand mal status is associated with a definable etiology or reversible precipitant. Hence, symptomatic epilepsy is more likely to result in status than is idiopathic epilepsy. In recent years, medication noncompliance has been recognized as the most common precipitant of status. Because clonic motions depend on the integrity of cortical neurons and subcortical pathways, many patients with large, destructive lesions may appear to have focal

or predominantly unilateral seizures and coma—the emergency department physician must recognize this as true grand mal status and treat it accordingly. (See Chapter 45.)

Diagnostic questions are generally interspersed with therapeutic interventions. At the outset, the primary examiner should dispatch someone to obtain a history from witnesses, relatives, and friends. The patency of the patient's airway should be ensured and vital signs measured. Oxygen (100 percent) should be administered by rebreather mask. Although the timing of endotracheal intubation is often debated, it becomes pressing with the passage of time and the administration of drugs that are respiratory depressants. Many clinicians intubate early, the interictal period being used of necessity. An intravenous line is placed, and blood is drawn to determine the levels of glucose, sodium, urea, anticonvulsants, and calcium. Fifty milliliters of a 50 percent glucose solution ($D_{50}W$) are given, and 100 mg of thiamine are administered IM if the patient appears malnourished or is an alcoholic. Arterial blood gases are measured to ensure adequate oxygenation and assess acid-base status. (See Chapter 56.)

The clinician must then shift attention to the ongoing seizure activity. The ideal drug is one that controls seizures quickly, has no depressant properties that will cloud the return to a premorbid mental state, and has no major short-term side-effects. Most clinicians use diphenylhydantoin alone, or diazepam followed by diphenylhydantoin as an initial regimen. If barbiturate withdrawal is suspected, phenobarbital is a first choice; otherwise, its sedative effects have led many clinicians to consider it a second-line drug. Diazepam given in 2.5-mg increments per minute up to 15 mg aborts seizures in the majority of patients. As it can cause respiratory depression and hypotension, however, vital signs must be monitored during its administration. Patients who initially respond to diazepam may have a resumption of seizures within 30 to 60 minutes. To avoid this, diphenylhydantoin may be added: a loading dose is given intravenously (IV) at 25 to 50 mg/minute up to a total dose of one gm. Bradycardia, hypotension, and, occasionally, respiratory depression can complicate the rapid infusion. Electrocardiographic monitoring and frequent checking of the patient's vital signs minimize risks. Diphenylhydantoin can form crystalline precipitates and should be given through a freely flowing intravenous line. Because intramuscular absorption is erratic, medication should not be administered intramuscularly (IM). Dosage modifications should be made if the patient is known to be currently *taking* the drug or if seizures can be controlled at a lower dose. Barbiturates may be added if diphenylhydantoin is ineffective, although many patients who fail to respond to diphenylhydantoin continue to have seizures as barbiturates are administered. Paraldehyde or general anesthesia remain as subsequent therapeutic options (Table 47–2).

When grand mal status is controlled, etiology can be investigated. The laboratory results may provide a clue, and specific therapy may succeed when anticonvulsants have failed, as in hyponatremia. A general physical examination is performed, with special attention to fever, marked hypertension, trauma, evidence of drug abuse, and tumor. A funduscopic examination may show signs of increased intracranial pressure. The neurologic examination may suggest an underlying structural lesion, such as tumor or CVA, or multiple areas of dysfunction, as in drug ingestion or encephalitis. If meningitis is suspected because of fever, meningism, or a petechial eruption, a lumbar puncture should immediately be performed. In some settings, the lumbar puncture can be deferred until a computerized axial tomography (CT) scan is obtained in order to minimize risk of transtentorial herniation.

The pace of drug administration and work-up must respect the pace of morbid events. As mentioned earlier, status that continues for hours has a high mortality and morbidity. This has encouraged some to suggest that diphenylhydantoin should be the first-line drug. Yet, morbidity and, occasionally, mortality are seen when status is successfully aborted within the first hour. In addition, the practical problems of placing a stable intravenous catheter and administering the drug at a tightly controlled infusion rate support a role for diazepam. This is particularly true for prehospital therapy, in which a 20-minute loading regimen for diphenylhydantoin seems undesirable.

A few distinctions can be drawn between the prehospital and emergency department phases of treatment of status. Because of the occasional early mortality associated with status, there is often a role for field treatment. The airway management skills of paramedics are generally excellent so that the potential side-effects of field treatment can be effectively managed. The general guidelines listed earlier are also applicable in the field. Certainly airway management, oxygen administration, assessment of vital signs, placement of an intravenous line, obtaining blood for glucose determination, and subsequent administration of $D_{50}W$ are mandatory. Diazepam should be considered when transport times are long or the status has persisted beyond one-half hour.

ISOLATED GRAND MAL SEIZURES

In contrast to the patient in status, a patient who has had a single grand mal seizure but who is returning to a normal level of consciousness requires different evaluation and management.

If there is significant confusion or depression of consciousness, the vital signs should be checked, and $D_{50}W$ should be given after blood has been drawn. The levels of glucose, urea nitrogen, calcium, sodium, and anticonvulsants should be determined. A history should be elicited from the patient. Retrograde amnesia may cloud memories of focal onset to a seizure, and witnesses may provide important additional information. If possible, however, the history should cover the events immediately preceding the seizure, focal movements or sensory experience, the duration of movement and postictal state (duration of coma and confusion), and incontinence.

TABLE 47–2   Intravenous Drugs Useful in Status Epilepticus

Drug	Dosage		Precautions	Miscellaneous
	Adult	*Pediatric*		
Diphenylhydantoin	50 mg/min up to one gm	15–20 mg/kg given evenly over 20 min	Hypotension; bradycardia; rarely, respiratory depression; need to monitor heart and vital signs	Given IV through rapidly flowing line, with normal saline, avoiding extravasation
Diazepam	5–15 mg at a rate of 2.5 mg/min	0.3 mg/kg at a rate of 0.5–2 mg/min	Respiratory depression; occasional hypotension; need to monitor vital signs	Side-effects much more common if phenobarbital is also given
Phenobarbital	130 mg every 10–15 min up to 1 gm	10–20 mg/kg over 20 min	Respiratory depression; hypotension; need to monitor vital signs	Drug of choice if barbiturate withdrawal is suspected
Paraldehyde	1–4 cc IV or 5–10 cc IM	0.5–4 cc IV	Occasional hypotension	Can be used only with glass syringes and metal needles

This helps to establish whether a seizure did occur and whether a focal onset was noted. Etiologic inquiries should include preexistent medical conditions, specifically diabetes and renal disease; medication history; barbiturate, alcohol, or other drug ingestions; head trauma; operations; CVA; tumor; and headaches. If the patient is known to have epilepsy, questions on medication compliance and prior evaluation should be included. Did the patient sustain injuries during the seizure? Thus, questions should concern etiology, precipitants, and complications.

The physical examination addresses the same areas. Is there evidence of dysfunction that establishes an etiologic diagnosis or the presence of complications? If the patient is known to be epileptic, the examination should include measurement of vital signs; a survey for trauma; an assessment of the patient's level of consciousness, memory, and orientation; and an examination of the cranial nerves. Muscle strength and cerebellar function can be screened by means of an upper extremity drift test, an assessment of tandem gait, finger-to-nose test, and a Romberg maneuver. Discovery of any abnormalities mandates more detailed testing. A patient with a first seizure requires a full neurologic examination. The decision to hospitalize adult patients with a first seizure is justified because 10 percent of patients who have their first seizures after age 20 have an underlying brain tumor. This remains a possible etiology even with a normal neurologic examination. Recent studies[2] suggest that a much smaller fraction, perhaps 1 or 2 percent, have a tumor as the underlying cause of a first seizure in adulthood—if the examination and history are nonfocal. Most experts hospitalize adults with first grand mal seizures. This allows for the initiation of drug therapy as well as the performance of diagnostic studies, such as a CT scan, electroencephalogram (EEG), and, if no mass lesion is found, a lumbar puncture. A focal onset mandates an inpatient work-up.

If a patient with known epilepsy is brought to the emergency department for a rare breakthrough seizure, the drug regimen should not be changed. Measuring the levels of anticonvulsants and providing this information to the patient's primary physician is the usual disposition for these patients.

Patients with frequent single seizures or patients who are noncompliant may require a dosage adjustment; at times, a new medication may be necessary. If possible, this should be done after consultation with the patient's primary physician. Regarding patients with repetitive grand mal seizures (with interictal recovery of consciousness), the emergency department clinician must remember that it requires many hours for both phenobarbital and diphenylhydantoin to achieve therapeutic blood levels with an oral loading regimen. These patients often require hospitalization.

Seizures Associated with Drug Withdrawal

Grand mal seizures commonly occur as part of the early alcohol withdrawal syndrome. Ninety percent of patients who have seizures for this reason do so from 6 to 48 hours after a decrease in alcohol consumption. Most often, these patients experience one to four seizures with interictal recovery of consciousness. They generally show tremulousness and agitation. Their sensorium is usually clear once the postictal state resolves. The great difficulty with these patients is that they have an increased risk of developing a structural reason for their seizures, owing to their propensity for trauma. Furthermore, administration of anticonvulsants to a patient of questionable reliability adds risk to therapy. For these reasons, it is very difficult to make judgments about admission and work-up of these patients. Any focality revealed by examination or history mandates a careful search for a mass lesion with a CT scan and an EEG. Many physicians admit patients who appear to be having an alcohol withdrawal seizure. Therapy also is unclear. Alcohol and the benzodiazepines exhibit cross tolerance, and appropriate therapy of alcohol withdrawal with diazepam or chlordiazepoxide decreases the risk of seizures. For patients who want to stop drinking, inpatient detoxification can be an alternative to medical hospitalization. (See Chapter 36.)

Barbiturate withdrawal results in grand mal status more frequently than does alcohol withdrawal. These patients should be hospitalized on a medical service. A similar syndrome has been described with many other sedative-hypnotic drugs.

Focal Epilepsy

Some patients have sensory symptoms, focal motor seizures, or a disturbance of consciousness associated with bizarre behavior. The latter, psychomotor epilepsy, is often followed by postictal confusion. These disturbances generally last from seconds to a few minutes. Many of these patients also have grand mal seizures, but focal seizures carry less short-term risk than do grand mal seizures. Etiologic concerns are similar to those associated with grand mal seizures, but the probability of finding a structural abnormality is higher with focal seizures. In adults, metabolic factors rarely produce focal seizures. The evaluation of a patient with a new focal seizure requires hospitalization because a focal seizure suggests focal brain disease.

Febrile Seizures

Up to 5 percent of children between the ages of 6 months and 6 years have a seizure associated with a febrile illness. These are typically generalized, and the history and examination do not disclose previous or current neurologic dysfunction. The diagnosis is made only if the spinal fluid is normal. Anticonvulsant therapy is controversial, and this decision appropriately belongs to the patient's primary physician. Emergency department therapy consists of cooling the child with antipyretics and sponging, and ruling out the presence of a bacterial infection.

APPROACH TO THE CONFUSED PATIENT

Patients are frequently brought to the emergency department for evaluation of bizarre behavior or manifest confusion. The physician then faces a patient who may be difficult to examine, and the available history may be very limited. Owing to these limitations, management decisions are often based on the presenting syndrome rather than a specific, established diagnosis. An approach that respects the morbid nature of many of the possible causes is required. The most common serious error in this instance is to decide, based on limited data, that the patient's condition is due to a psychiatric state and to transfer the patient to a psychiatric facility that may lack medical and neurologic facilities. Unless the history and examination speak strongly for a psychiatric diagnosis, initial hospitalization in a medical facility is indicated.

A wide variety of conditions can disturb the patient's capacity to perceive and integrate perceptions appropriately. Previous brain disease, especially diffuse disease, can increase the likelihood that as minor an insult as patching a patient's better eye will result in confusion. Young patients are most often confused because of a drug ingestion or a psychiatric process. With these patients, rarely is a diagnostic and therapeutic plan completed in the emergency department.

DEFINITIONS ASSOCIATED WITH CONFUSION

A patient who shows evidence of disordered thought processes is said to be *confused*. *Delirium* refers to grossly distorted perceptions in a patient with autonomic, motor, and emotional overactivity. This state is acute in onset and self-limited. *Dementia* refers to a slowly evolving loss of all categories of cognitive functioning, generally without clouding of consciousness. Usually, these features permit a clear distinction between dementia and acute confusion.

ETIOLOGY

Infection

Systemic and central nervous system infections can result in confusion. Most often, this takes the form of a delirium, although patients may show a depressed sensorium. Bacterial sepsis, meningitis, pneumonia, and viral encephalitis are the common causes. The patient's temperature, general appearance, and white blood count are the most important clues to this category of diagnoses. A lumbar puncture should be performed in the emergency department if meningitis is suspected so that therapy can be initiated as early as possible.

Metabolic Disturbances

As a rule, metabolic disturbances produce confusion with a depressed sensorium and no lateralizing findings. Hypoxia can at times produce a delirium, however. Hypoglycemia merits special concern, as it is a common cause of confusion and routine therapy of the confused patient with $D_{50}W$ is safe and effective. Plum and Posner[3] found a number of patients with hypoglycemia and lateralizing neurologic findings. Marked hyperglycemia with hyperosmolarity, and diabetic ketoacidosis are commonly associated with confusion.

Acute changes in serum sodium are likely to cause confusion. This usually occurs with substantial abnormalities (sodium less than 128 mEq/liter or greater than 155 mEq/liter). Hypercalcemia can produce polyuria, constipation, dehydration, and a confused state. Renal failure and liver disease are often associated with confusion. Asterixis can be seen with almost any of the metabolic encephalopathies. (See Chapter 14.)

Drug Ingestions

Many young people in a confusional state are manifesting a drug effect. The history may be useful, but specific accurate details of the quantity and identity of the ingested drug are difficult to obtain. Some ingestions may be suggested by a specific clinical syndrome. The anticholinergic syndrome, for example, consists of tachycardia; dry skin; fever; large, unreactive pupils; and visual hallucinations. Sympathomimetics can produce delirium with tachycardia; large, reactive pupils; and moist skin. Alcohol and the sedative-hypnotics generally produce a depressed sensorium, ataxia, nystagmus, and "drunken" speech. A diagnosis of a drug ingestion makes it possible to institute general supportive therapy; at times, specific measures are indicated.

Drug Withdrawal

In patients with narcotic withdrawal, the sensorium is clear. In early alcohol withdrawal, the patient is usually coherent, although intermittent visual or auditory hallucinations may interrupt the patient's lucid state. The patient may be tremulous and diaphoretic. This condition usually occurs hours to a few days after a decrease in alcohol consumption. Late alcohol withdrawal, or delirium tremens, usually develops three to five days after decreased consumption. The patient shows physical, autonomic, and emotional overactivity, hallucinates, and often verbalizes fearful perceptions. Withdrawal from barbiturates and other sedative hypnotics can produce a similar state.

Trauma

Patients who have sustained a concussion may show a delirious behavior during recovery. Patients with extra-axial collections of blood within either the subdural or the epidural spaces tend to show changes in consciousness out of proportion to focal findings. A confusional state, usually with a depressed sensorium, is common. The pupillary findings and progressive deterioration of responsiveness indicate the critical state of the patient's brain dysfunction. With chronic subdural hematomas, there may be no history of trauma, and the findings evolve more insidiously. (See Chapter 45.)

Postictal Confusion

Confusional states are common after grand mal or psychomotor seizures. The diagnosis is usually established by the history, coupled with the rapid return to a normal sensorium. If the sensorium remains disturbed or deteriorates, alternative diagnoses, e.g., a head injury or medication intoxication, should be considered.

Wernicke-Korsakoff Syndrome

Chronic alcoholics and other malnourished patients may develop acute confusion because of a thiamine deficiency. Extraocular palsies, nystagmus, truncal or appendicular ataxia are commonly associated. With appropriate therapy, these patients can show improvement in eye findings, cerebellar function, and sensorium. They are often left with residual memory impairments.

Focal Brain Disease

Occasionally, CVAs, brain tumors, or brain abscesses produce apparent confusion. A detailed examination generally demonstrates the focal nature of the process.

Psychiatric Processes

Schizophrenia can produce bizarre behavior and apparent confusion in young patients. The mental status examination usually demonstrates intact cognition. In older adults with no prior psychiatric history, schizophrenia is very unlikely. Depression may occur with many features that suggest a dementia. Detailed mental status and psychological testing may be required to differentiate these conditions.

Assessment

The first step with an obviously confused patient is to measure the vital signs. Any abnormality will dictate the pace and direction of further evaluation, for the vital signs provide the most significant clues to sepsis, meningitis, and malignant hypertension. An attempt should be made to explain all procedures to the patient. Blood should be drawn to determine the levels of glucose, urea, sodium, and calcium; a complete blood count should be obtained. If the sensorium is depressed, $D_{50}W$ should be given and thiamine considered. Arterial blood gases are measured. Relatives, police, or ambulance crew can often provide needed history. Has the patient had previous health problems? Is there a history of diabetes, liver, lung, or kidney disease? Has the patient had seizures, a psychiatric history, or a history of drug or alcohol use? Does the patient take any medicines regularly? How was the confusion first noted, and were there any signs of illness during the previous days? Was there any trauma?

The general examination should be completed, with particular emphasis on any evidence of trauma, drug abuse, meningism, lung disease, cardiovascular disease, or stigmata of chronic liver disease. The neurologic examination begins with an evaluation of mental status, which is a sequential evaluation of cognitive functioning. It consists initially of ascertaining the patient's level of consciousness. Evaluation is made of the patient's orientation. Attention span is checked by having the patient repeat sequences of numbers of increasing length. Language function is evaluated by examining the patient's capacity to name, repeat, and comprehend. Memory is checked by means of questions about events of public record, and the patient is asked to remember three unrelated words for five minutes. Constructional capacity can be assessed by having the patient write, or draw and copy familiar objects. Arithmetic problems and questions on proverb interpretation can be used to assess higher cortical functioning and abstract thinking. Behavioral observations should be recorded. This evaluation cannot be neglected, as it is the key to distinguishing psychiatric from organic illness. Psychiatric diseases tend to produce dysfunction in particular areas, while organic diseases tend to produce global dysfunction. The remainder of the neurologic examination may show evidence of increased intracranial pressure or focal cortical dysfunction. Finally, the physician checks for asterixis.

If the patient will not cooperate for an examination, the physician must consider the etiology to be organic. Some clinicians use an amobarbital interview if they strongly suspect that a confused patient is having a hysterical conversion reaction, but the emergency department use of this technique remains controversial. The patient whose initial examination suggests organic disease should have a lumbar puncture and a CT scan. The order of these tests depends on the likelihood of meningitis. These tests can be omitted if the history and examination suggest a specific diagnosis, and the patient is improving with appropriate therapy. Additional laboratory tests, appropriate to the antecedent work-up, may be useful.

With confused patients, the emergency department clinician's role is often limited. With young, previously healthy patients, a specific diagnosis and treatment plan often can be completed and the patient discharged. In other settings the focus shifts; the physician should provide immediate general supportive therapy, initiate diagnostic studies, and decide which inpatient specialists should be consulted to complete the diagnostic and therapeutic program.

REFERENCES

1. Rowan AJ, Scott DF: Major status epilepticus. *Acta Neurol Scand.* 46:573–584, 1970.
2. Livingston S: Etiologic factors in adult convulsions. *NEJM* 254:1211–1216, 1956.
3. Plum F, Posner J: *The Diagnosis of Stupor and Coma.* Philadelphia, FA Davis, 1970, p 177.

SUGGESTED READINGS

Hunter R: Status epilepticus, history incidence and problems. *Epilepsia* 1:162–188, 1959.
Penry J: The use of antiepileptic drugs. *Ann Intern Med* 90:207–218, 1979.
Solomon G, Plum F: *Clinical Management of Seizures, A Guide for the Physician.* Philadelphia, WB Saunders, 1976.
Strub R, Black F: *The Mental Status Examination in Neurology.* Philadelphia, FA Davis, 1977.

Alterations of Circulatory System Functions

One of the most common reasons that patients seek medical care at an emergency department is the symptom of dyspnea and/or chest pain. Certainly one of the most difficult differential diagnoses for emergency care personnel is to distinguish dyspnea that is primarily of cardiac origin (left ventricular heart failure) as noted in "Dyspnea and Pulmonary Edema" (Chapter 48) and that which is due to alterations of the respiratory system. "Obstructive Lung Diseases" (Chapter 57), "Pulmonary Embolism" (Chapter 58), "Respiratory Failure" (Chapter 59), and "Miscellaneous Respiratory Emergencies" (Chapter 60) may be helpful in approaching a patient with these complaints.

In patients with chest pain and a history of trauma, the reader is invited to review "Shock" (Chapter 6), "Major Trauma" (Chapter 7), and "Chest Trauma" (Chapter 61). In patients with chest pain without a history of trauma, the differential diagnosis is even more difficult. Myocardial infarction, as discussed in "Acute Myocardial Infarction" (Chapter 49), and its sequelae, "Disturbances in Cardiac Rhythm" (Chapter 50), are areas in which lay personnel, prehospital care personnel, and emergency department physicians and nurses have by their intervention made an important contribution in decreasing subsequent morbidity and mortality. Since the metabolic milieu of the heart is important in disturbances in cardiac rhythm, the reader is also referred to "Electrolyte Abnormalities" (Chapter 14), "Acid-Base Disturbances" (Chapter 18), and "Congestive Heart Failure" (Chapter 51). "Hypertensive Emergencies" (Chapter 52) provides a review of the etiology and treatment of common hypertensive processes encountered in the emergency department.

Emergency care personnel interested in "Vascular Injuries" (Chapter 53) and "Heart and Great Vessel Emergencies" (Chapter 54) may also wish to refer to "Shock" (Chapter 6), "Major Trauma" (Chapter 7), and "Chest Trauma" (Chapter 61). Finally, "Cardiopulmonary Resuscitation" (Chapter 55) provides an outline based primarily on the recommendations of the American Heart Association for the resuscitation of patients with cardiopulmonary arrest.

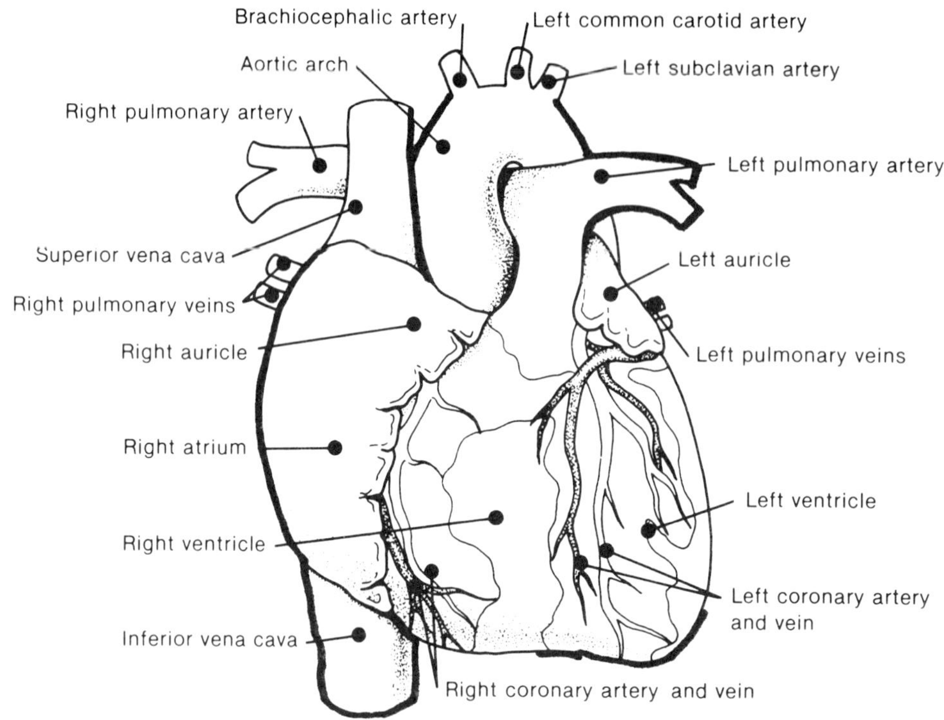

External Structures of the Heart

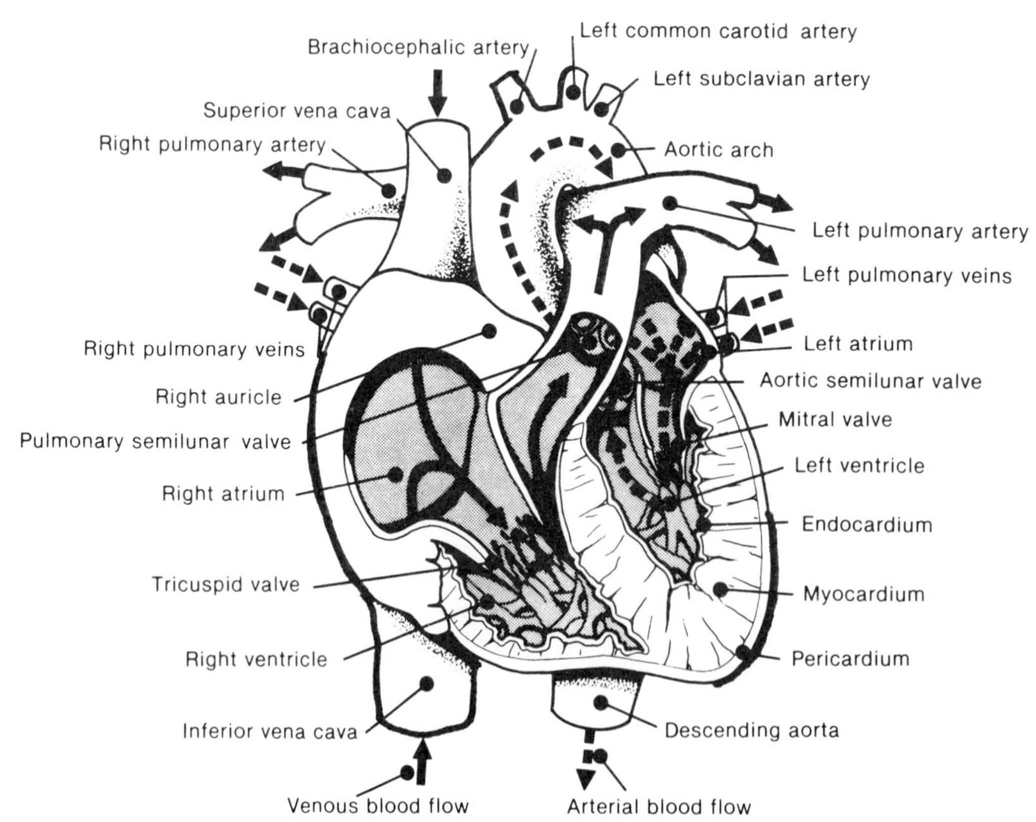

Internal Structures of the Heart

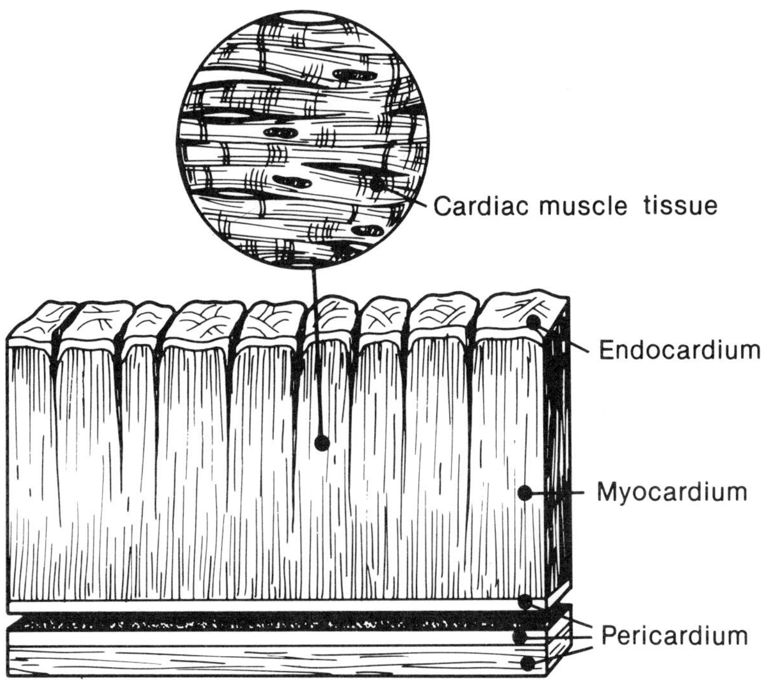

Heart Pericardium, Myocardium, and Endocardium

48. Dyspnea and Pulmonary Edema

GEORGE L. STERNBACH, M.D.

DYSPNEA

Shortness of breath or difficulty in breathing is a symptom of a variety of illnesses and conditions. The cause of dyspnea may be primarily respiratory, cardiac, neuromuscular, metabolic (e.g., acidosis), hematologic (anemia), or psychogenic (primary hyperventilation). The stage at which dyspnea is experienced varies from individual to individual. In a person with normal breathing capacity, a large increase in ventilation may be required to produce dyspnea. On the other hand, a relatively small ventilatory increase from the normal state may induce shortness of breath in an individual with a low breathing capacity.

Patients can experience dyspnea even when 70 percent of their maximum breathing capacity is not in use.[1] Dyspnea results from increased respiratory work and respiratory muscle dysfunction. The elastic resistance of the lung to stretch, airway resistance to gas flow, and tissue friction must be overcome in the work of breathing. At normal respiratory rates, elastic resistance is the most significant of these factors; at rates higher than 15 breaths/minute, however, resistance to flow in the airways assumes greater importance.

When muscular work is increased, the amount of oxygen required is increased. The oxygen costs of breathing itself increase disproportionately with increased ventilation. The resting state oxygen requirement may be trebled in patients who are tachypneic as a result of pulmonary vascular congestion.

Of the systemic stimuli to the respiratory control center, the most profound is arterial CO_2 tension. An increase in pCO_2 of 1.5 mm Hg from the normal level of 40 may cause a doubling of ventilation. Other factors that significantly influence ventilation are pH and arterial oxygen tension. Dyspnea in patients with chronic respiratory disease is well correlated with breathing reserve, which is the amount of ventilatory capacity available in excess of actual ventilation. The patient with pulmonary edema experiences dyspnea for a variety of reasons, even when breathing reserve is well maintained.

CARDIOGENIC PULMONARY EDEMA

Failure of the left ventricle to eject a normal amount of blood, which causes fluid to accumulate in the pulmonary interstitium, alveoli, bronchioles, and bronchi, may produce cardiogenic pulmonary edema. Paroxysmal nocturnal dyspnea is probably a milder, self-limited form of pulmonary edema. When bronchospasm is a prominent component, an episode may be referred to as "cardiac asthma," but this condition is not a distinct entity on the basis of its pathophysiology or etiology. (See Chapter 51.)

Etiology

The most common cause of acute pulmonary edema is coronary artery disease.[2] Acute myocardial infarction frequently causes pulmonary edema, especially if myocardial damage is extensive. Pulmonary edema may be an early or late complication of myocardial infarction and is often the presenting form, particularly among elderly patients. It is also a frequent presenting form of acute myocardial infarction in hypertensive patients, even though uncontrolled hypertension is not now as common a cause of acute pulmonary edema as it was in the past. (See Chapter 49.)

Pulmonary edema accompanies the terminal stages of chronic renal failure. It occurs in patients on hemodialysis, even those whose disease is relatively stable. (See Chapter 63.)

Stenosis of either the mitral or aortic valves may cause pulmonary edema, but mitral or aortic insufficiency is a more common cause. Acute severe aortic insufficiency is most often the result of bacterial endocarditis, dissecting aortic aneurysm, spontaneous rupture of an abnormal aortic leaflet, and blunt chest trauma. Of these, bacterial endocarditis is by far the most frequent cause.[3] Acute mitral insufficiency is usually the consequence of rupture of the chordae tendineae or papillary muscles. Chordae tendineae rupture may be due to rheumatic valvular disease, bacterial endocarditis, or blunt thoracic trauma. Rupture of a papillary muscle is most frequently a complication of acute myocardial infarction.[3]

Pathology

At autopsy, the lungs are noted to be heavy and pale or hemorrhagic. The normal tissue elasticity is lacking, and the lungs pit when pressure is applied. Frothy fluid emanates from the cut edges of the lungs, as well as from the bronchi.

Pathophysiology

An increase in hydrostatic pressure, caused by left ventricular failure or fluid overload, is the first step in the pathogenesis of pulmonary edema. Fluid begins to leave the vascular space when the capillary hydrostatic pressure exceeds the colloid osmotic pressure. Initially, the fluid collects in the perivascular interstitial connective tissue. Edema becomes significant when the rate of transudation exceeds the ability of the pulmonary lymphatics to remove fluid from the lung. As fluid continues to accumulate, it fills the alveolar spaces; it becomes more difficult to inflate the lungs, owing to diminished lung volume and reduced elasticity. Because of the nonuniform distribution of edema within the lungs, areas that are poorly ventilated are perfused, resulting in arteriovenous shunting. Peribronchial and bronchiolar edema results in narrowing and eventual collapse of

small airways. This leads to increased resistance to air flow both in inspiration and expiration.

Systemic arterial pressure is usually elevated. Cardiac output may be normal, decreased, or increased. Left ventricular end-diastolic pressure is markedly increased, resulting in an elevated pulmonary capillary wedge pressure that changes pulmonary regional blood flow. The apical portions of the lung, normally underperfused, receive greater than their normal flow of blood.

Arterial CO_2 tension depends on the balance between alveolar ventilation in the affected and unaffected regions of the lungs. In many patients, the pCO_2 is normal or low, reflecting increased total ventilation.[4] With extensive pulmonary edema or significant underlying pulmonary disease, alveolar hypoventilation occurs, resulting in CO_2 retention. Hypoxemia of a moderate or severe degree is almost invariably present.

Narrowing, obstruction, or closure of small airways results from increased interstitial pressure. Edema of the bronchial mucosa and reflex bronchospasm add to changes in air flow dynamics. In severe pulmonary edema, fluid-filled conducting airways also reduce air flow.

Diagnosis

Patients are usually anxious or restless during the early phase of pulmonary edema. They may be struck by a profound sensation of suffocation, which forces them to sit upright in order to breathe. In a severe attack, patients may be drowsy, uncooperative, or stuporous. The skin is cool and clammy, and cyanosis may be evident. The blood pressure is characteristically slightly elevated; the pulse, rapid and thready. Pulsus alternans may be present. The respiration rate is 30 to 40 breaths/minute.

The jugular veins are distended, and hepatojugular reflux is usually present. The chest examination may reveal only a few crepitations during the early phase of the illness. Typically, however, bubbling rales and wheezes are heard diffusely over the lung fields. Cardiac auscultation is difficult, owing to the volume of the respiratory sounds. A third heart sound may be audible.

In pulmonary edema caused by acute aortic insufficiency, the classic peripheral signs of chronic aortic insufficiency—such as Corrigan's pulse—are absent. This is because the signs of chronic insufficiency are the result of wide pulse pressure, which is not present in the acute condition. The aortic insufficiency murmur is short, typically ending in mid-diastole. A soft systolic aortic flow murmur may be heard. The patient is acutely, severely ill, and tachycardia is a consistent finding.

The patient with acute mitral insufficiency secondary to ruptured chordae tendineae displays the characteristic murmur of mitral insufficiency. It is commonly crescendo-decrescendo, however, rather than holosystolic. The murmur is heard at the apex and radiates to the left axilla or posterior left hemithorax. The precordium is hyperdynamic. A third heart sound is invariably present.[5] Echocardiography may be a useful diagnostic procedure.

Rupture of a papillary muscle may produce a similar clinical picture, although the murmur may be soft or even absent. The diagnosis is suggested by the abrupt appearance of heart failure in a patient during the first week following acute myocardial infarction.

The chest roentgenogram is a valuable tool in the diagnosis of pulmonary edema. The earliest radiographic change consists of a dilatation of the upper lobe vessels.[6] This is a reliable finding on an upright roentgenogram only, however, as redistribution of blood to the upper lobe vessels is seen on the supine chest roentgenogram of the well patient.[7] The next most important early finding is an increase in interstitial markings. Kerley A and B lines represent interlobular septa distended with edema fluid.[7] Kerley B lines are 1 to 2 cm long and appear perpendicular to the costal, diaphragmatic, or mediastinal pleura; Kerley A lines are longer and more centrally located.

Edema of the connective tissue surrounding the bronchi and blood vessels causes blurring of normally sharp vascular margins and later peribronchial and perivascular cuffing. As edema progresses to alveolar flooding, the roentgenogram shows dense opacification of the central portions of the lung fields with symmetric infiltrates that spare the periphery. Patchy, asymmetric, or unilateral patterns are commonly seen. Cardiomegaly is frequently present.

Radiographic changes have been found to be closely correlated to pulmonary capillary wedge pressure in many cases of acute pulmonary edema: at a pressure of less than 12 mm Hg, the roentgenogram is normal; when the pressure reaches 12 to 18 mm Hg, upper lobe vascular redistribution occurs; at 18 to 22 mm Hg, evidence of interstitial edema appears; and at pressures greater than 25 to 30 mm Hg, the full radiographic pattern of pulmonary edema is manifest.[8]

Differential Diagnosis

Entities that should be considered in the differential diagnosis include acute respiratory failure due to chronic obstructive pulmonary disease; acute infectious, toxic, or aspiration pneumonitis; pulmonary embolus; and pneumothorax. History, physical examination, and chest roentgenogram generally provide sufficient information for the physician to make distinctions. The most difficult differentiation is that between pulmonary edema and acute respiratory failure in a patient with chronic obstructive airway disease; not only may physical findings be similar—e.g., dyspnea, tachycardia, cyanosis, rales, and wheezes—but the presence of preexisting disease may so alter pulmonary architecture that the radiographic appearance of pulmonary edema is atypical. Areas of lung that have lost their vascularity, for example, do not display the classic radiographic findings of pulmonary edema.

Noncardiogenic pulmonary edema and the adult respiratory distress syndrome should also be considered in the differential diagnosis. Although these entities do not produce cardiomegaly or the typical radiographic findings of cardiogenic pulmonary edema, differentiation may be difficult on clinical grounds.

Treatment

Prehospital treatment of cardiogenic pulmonary edema has as its therapeutic goals the improvement of oxygenation and the reduction of cardiac workload. To these ends, it involves the proper positioning of the patient, cardiac monitoring, administration of oxygen, application of rotating tourniquets, and the use of diuretics and morphine. The patient should be placed in a sitting position with the legs dependent, because this position increases lung volume and vital capacity, decreases venous return to the heart, and diminishes the work of respiration. In fact, patients themselves will assume this position, if they are able to do so.

The patient should be monitored for the appearance of cardiac dysrhythmias. Oxygen should be administered by nasal cannula or mask at a rate of 4 to 6 liters/minute in order to augment oxygen delivery to ischemic tissues. (A lower flow rate should be considered in the patient with concomitant or suspected chronic obstructive pulmonary disease.) Because a large portion of hypoxemia in pulmonary edema is due to arteriovenous shunting, however, hypoxemia will not be corrected by the inhalation of supplemental oxygen alone.

Rotating tourniquets may be applied to the extremities in an effort to reduce venous return and thereby diminish central blood volume. The tourniquets are to be applied at greater than venous but less than arterial pressure. The tourniquet on one extremity should be released every 20 minutes. Application of tourniquets may be detrimental to the hypotensive patient, however.

The beneficial effects of morphine in pulmonary edema are incompletely understood. It is known that, by dilating the capacitance vessels of the peripheral venous bed, morphine reduces venous return to the central circulation. This diminishes the preload—ventricular diastolic filling pressure—of the heart. In addition, morphine has a sedative effect, decreases musculoskeletal and respiratory activity, and has mild arterial vasodilating effects. Five to 10 mg should be administered intravenously (IV) and subsequent dosage adjusted as needed. Consequent hypotension or respiratory depression may be reversed by the administration of naloxone hydrochloride.

Diuretic agents reduce the fluid volume of the body by renal excretion. Furosemide (Lasix), the agent of choice, effects a diuresis that begins about 20 minutes after intravenous administration. A more immediate effect of this drug is a reduction of pulmonary arterial and capillary wedge pressures, probably as a result of systemic venous dilatation.[9] As such, furosemide may be used even in patients with chronic renal failure, in whom a profound diuresis is not expected. The initial dose is 20 to 40 mg given IV.

Emergency department treatment should continue as described to improve oxygenation and reduce cardiac workload. If bronchospasm is a prominent feature, aminophylline may be administered. An intravenous loading dose of 5.6 mg/kg should be given, followed by an infusion of 0.35 mg/kg/hour. (A further discussion of this drug is found in Chapter 57.)

Oxygen should be administered, and this may be passed through 50 percent ethyl alcohol if substantial frothy sputum is present. The alcohol vapor has an antifoaming action that may improve gas exchange through the airways. In some cases, suction may be an equally efficient method of sputum elimination.

Intermittent positive pressure breathing (IPPB) is effective in the treatment of pulmonary edema, probably because it impedes venous return to the heart by increasing intrathoracic pressure. Additionally, IPPB may help to regulate respirations, provide more uniform ventilation, and decrease arteriovenous shunting. The presence of severe respiratory acidosis is an indication for IPPB or continuous positive pressure breathing.[4] Endotracheal intubation should be considered if the pO_2 cannot be maintained above 50 mm Hg with the methods that have been mentioned or if there is persistent severe CO_2 retention. (See Chapter 59.)

Nitroglycerin may be used for both its peripheral venous and arterial dilating actions. Although it is primarily a venodilator, its modest arterial dilating effect may substantially improve cardiac output in the presence of severe heart failure.[10] The dosage is 0.3 to 0.6 mg sublingually or 1 to 4 inches of ointment applied topically. Nitroglycerin may be detrimental to patients with hypotension, because it can reduce coronary perfusion pressure, potentially enhancing myocardial ischemia.[11]

Potent vasodilators may be used to reduce resistance to ventricular ejection—afterload—in instances of intractable pulmonary edema. This results in an increased ejection fraction and improved cardiac output. The drug of choice is sodium nitroprusside, a short-acting drug that dilates both arterial and venous vessels. Required

dosage varies, but intravenous infusion should be begun at 20 µg/minute and adjusted as needed.[12] Profound hypotension is the result of overmedication. Therefore, blood pressure should be monitored closely, preferably by means of an indwelling arterial catheter.

Phlebotomy may be a useful treatment for difficult cases, especially in patients with chronic renal failure. Preferably via a blood bank phlebotomy apparatus, 300 to 500 ml blood should be removed rapidly. If the patient is anemic, the cellular components may be banked and reinfused at a later time. Care must be taken, as phlebotomy may produce hypotension.

Once the primary goals of therapy have been achieved, efforts should be continued to improve cardiac contractility, to monitor and maintain the stability of the patient's condition, and to ascertain an etiology for the episode of acute heart failure. Digoxin is the drug of choice for increasing myocardial contractility. Unfortunately, it does not raise cardiac output rapidly enough to be of use as a primary drug for pulmonary edema. Once treatment has been started, however, the patient not previously taking this drug should be digitalized. An intravenous bolus of 0.5 to 1 mg should be administered, with an additional dose of 0.25 mg given every six hours to a total of 3 to 4 mg. Maintenance digoxin should then be started. However, the use of digoxin may be detrimental in the immediate postmyocardial infarction period, and its administration should be delayed in the patient with acute myocardial infarction.

The patient should be admitted to a coronary or intensive care unit for monitoring and further treatment. Certain patients benefit from early surgery. The patient with aortic insufficiency and intractable heart failure requires early valve replacement, even if infection is present.[13] In acute mitral insufficiency, surgery is often not urgent, and the patient's heart failure may be treated by conventional means and afterload reduction. Antibiotics should be instituted in endocarditis. Cardiac catheterization may indicate whether surgical intervention is needed.[3]

NONCARDIOGENIC PULMONARY EDEMA

Noncardiogenic pulmonary edema is characterized by increased pulmonary alveolar and interstitial fluid accumulation without left ventricular failure.

Etiology

Noncardiogenic pulmonary edema can result from a wide variety of systemic and pulmonary insults:

- airway obstruction
- central nervous system lesions
- diabetic ketoacidosis
- drugs
- fat embolus
- gastric content aspiration
- high altitude
- hypoglycemia
- infection/sepsis
- near-drowning
- organophosphate insecticides
- pancreatitis
- paraquat ingestion
- lung reexpansion
- trauma
- pulmonary embolus
- smoke inhalation
- transfusion reaction
- toxic inhalation
- uremia

High-altitude pulmonary edema is an entity that occurs only at altitudes greater than 8,000 feet above sea level. It generally affects young, healthy, high-altitude inhabitants who return from low-altitude exposure and unacclimated individuals who ascend rapidly and engage in strenuous physical exertion.[14] There is a latent period of 12 to 72 hours after ascent before pulmonary edema appears.[15] (See Chapter 31.)

Opiate-induced pulmonary edema has been recognized for nearly a century. Pulmonary edema appears to be universally present in patients who die of narcotic overdose; it may be induced by the intravenous injection, inhalation, or oral ingestion of narcotics.

Neurogenic pulmonary edema is associated with central nervous system pathology, including head and cervical spinal cord injury, subarachnoid hemorrhage, cerebrovascular accident, encephalitis, meningitis, brain tumor, Guillain-Barré syndrome, and grand mal seizures.[16–21] The rapidity with which neurogenic pulmonary edema develops is variable. It can occur within minutes of central nervous system insult, as demonstrated by its presence in head-injured battle casualties who succumbed instantaneously.[22]

Numerous nonnarcotic medications cause pulmonary edema in either overdose or therapeutic use:[23–27]

- barbiturates
- chlordiazepoxide hydrochloride (Librium)
- ethchlorvynol (Placidyl)
- methaqualone-diphenhydramine (Mandrax)
- opiate analgesics
- pentazocine (Talwin)
- propoxyphene hydrochloride (Darvon)
- salicylates
- thiazide diuretics

Salicylate-induced pulmonary edema may accompany aspirin overdose. Pulmonary edema may occur not only with salicylism,[28] but conversely, it may occur with therapeutic salicylate levels.[29]

Pulmonary edema is thought to be common in poisoning with organophosphate insecticides. These substances are rapidly absorbed through the skin, mucous membranes, gastrointestinal tract, and tracheobronchial tree. Pulmonary edema has been attributed to the muscarinic effects of the pesticides on vascular smooth muscle. When intoxication has been successfully treated, pulmonary edema has been resolved within hours.[30] (See Chapter 24.)

Pulmonary edema is observed in approximately three-quarters of near-drowning victims.[31] It appears with equal frequency in fresh and salt water near-drownings. Edema may be present at the time the victim is initially treated or it may be delayed in onset for as long as 48 hours. Near-drowning does not generally involve massive aspiration of liquid; pulmonary edema is usually the result of anoxic damage to alveolar capillary epithelium, owing to upper airway closure. (See Chapter 32.)

Inhalation of various noxious gases causes pulmonary edema by direct toxic effect. These gases include carbon monoxide, nitrogen dioxide, ozone, beryllium salts, cadmium oxide, phosgene, sulfur dioxide, ammonia, mercury vapor, and the halogens. Toxins are released by the combustion of modern synthetic materials as well as wood.

Pulmonary edema unrelated to circulatory overload may develop following blood or blood component transfusion. Symptoms begin abruptly or insidiously several hours after the institution of transfusion. Whole blood, packed red blood cells, fresh-frozen plasma, and platelet concentrates have all been associated with this reaction. Most of the cases reported have been associated with leukoagglutinins in donor or recipient serum.[32] (See Chapter 9.)

A variety of septic processes may be associated with pulmonary edema, including viral pneumonia, *Pneumocystis carinii* pneumonia, gonococcal septicemia, miliary tuberculosis, and malaria. Pulmonary edema is frequently an ominous complication of malaria, since, in this instance, it is generally unresponsive to therapy and rapidly fatal.

Noncardiogenic pulmonary edema has been known to follow upper airway obstruction, particularly that due to epiglottitis. The cause may be related to an increase in negative interstitial pressure, although hypoxia, bacteremia, or endotoxemia may also play a role. (See Chapter 57.)

Reexpansion of a lung following evacuation of pleural fluid or air has long been known to be associated in some cases with the development of pulmonary edema. This generally occurs on the same side as the pleural pathology, although contralateral pulmonary edema following reexpansion of pneumothorax has been reported.[33]

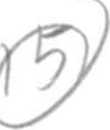

Pathology

The major pathologic finding in noncardiogenic pulmonary edema is excess fluid in the alveolar and interstitial spaces. Some forms, such as those due to airway obstruction, reexpansion, transfusion, and neurogenic insult, are benign and self-limiting.[34, 35] If appropriately treated, they seldom come to pathologic examination. Others, such as opiate-induced pulmonary edema, may be severe enough to lead to the patient's demise. Osler, who reported the initial case of opiate-induced pulmonary edema in 1880, described lungs containing "an extraordinary amount of bloody serum."[36] More recent pathology reports of deaths from narcotic overdose describe "intense congestion and edema, with frothy edema fluid oozing from the cut surfaces and cut ends of the bronchi." In hyperacute cases, there is "tremendous pulmonary congestion and edema which cause the lungs to become very heavy and large to such an extent that their anterior margins meet in the midline and completely overlap the pericardial sac."[37]

Pathophysiology

The common feature of noncardiogenic pulmonary edema appears to be damage to the alveolar-capillary membrane, which results in increased permeability and exudation of fluid into the interstitial and alveolar spaces. The edema fluid is rich in plasma protein, frequently equaling the protein concentration of serum.

In some instances, the alveolar-capillary membrane is damaged by direct action of toxic agents. In others, the exact mechanism of injury is less well understood. The role of hypoxia is frequently cited, and it is undoubtedly a factor in the pathogenesis of some entities, particularly pulmonary edema associated with near-drowning, smoke inhalation, high altitudes, and opiates. Nevertheless, it is clear that hypoxia alone does not disrupt alveolar membrane integrity; additional factors must be present in order to produce pulmonary edema.[38,39] The pulmonary release of vasoactive substances, such as histamine, serotonin or bradykinins, may also play a role in the development of noncardiogenic pulmonary edema.

In many instances, the initial site of fluid accumulation is the interstitial space. This decreases lung compliance and causes dyspnea, but auscultation of the lungs at this time fails to elicit any abnormal findings. As edema progresses, the patient's respiratory distress increases and signs of hypoxia become more apparent. Compliance and lung volume decrease further. Small airways, especially at the lung bases where pleural pressure is highest, are closed, and fine rales can be heard over the lower lobes because of the abrupt opening of these small airways during inspiration.

Hypoxia, undoubtedly the initiating factor of high-altitude pulmonary edema, acutely constricts pulmonary arteries by a direct effect on smooth muscle. This occurs in normal individuals as well as—to a much greater degree—those susceptible to high-altitude pulmonary edema. Hemodynamic studies in patients in the acute stage of high-altitude pulmonary edema reveal pronounced elevation of pulmonary artery pressure, normal pulmonary wedge pressure, and a normal or low cardiac output.[40] It has been postulated that this pulmonary arteriolar vasoconstriction is not uniform in all portions of the lung and that this asymmetry causes hyperperfusion of some portions of the pulmonary arterial vasculature, resulting in transcapillary exudation of fluid.[41]

The etiology of opiate-induced pulmonary edema is far from clear, though a direct cardiogenic cause has been excluded by the presence of normal pulmonary capillary wedge pressure. Hypoxia, hypersensitivity reaction, a toxic effect of narcotics, release of vasoactive substances, and neurogenic factors have all been proposed as mechanisms, but major objections have been posed to each of these hypotheses. Research is hampered by the lack of an experimental animal model.

Evidence suggests that the development of neurogenic pulmonary edema is mediated via the alpha-adrenergic sympathetic system in response to a massive hypothalamic discharge. The hemodynamic changes associated with the initial stages resemble those that follow high-dose infusion of epinephrine and can be prevented by pretreatment with alpha-adrenergic blocking agents. Increases in systemic and pulmonary arterial and venous pressures are profound and are followed by a significant shift of blood from the systemic to the pulmonary circulation. This results in pulmonary capillary hypertension, which in turn leads to pulmonary edema. Injury to pulmonary capillaries perpetuates the egress of water and solutes, even after pulmonary capillary pressure has been reduced.[42]

The pathophysiology of smoke inhalation injury has been well documented. It consists of progressive hypoxemia, reduced compliance, and leakage of fluid across the pulmonary capillary membrane. Intrapulmonary shunting develops. Even after edema has subsided, progressive fibrosis of the airways may lead to death or permanent disability.[17] (See Chapter 48.)

The direct action of infecting organisms, endotoxins, or other biologically active substances may also increase capillary permeability and thus result in pulmonary edema. The magnitude of the pulmonary capillary leak may be quite substantial. Dextran (molecular weight 500,000) has been identified in pulmonary edema fluid of patients with endotoxemia.[43]

Diagnosis

The clinical picture is one of respiratory distress with a variety of other findings. Cardiomegaly and jugular venous distention are not present as a rule. The patient may experience inspiratory chest pain or substernal discomfort, tachypnea, and a dry or productive cough. Cyanosis, tachycardia, hyperpnea, and hypotension may be present. Wheezing, rhonchi, or crepitant rales may be audible diffusely over both lungs, or such findings may be localized to portions of the thorax. Determination of arterial blood gas levels usually reveals hypoxemia and respiratory alkalosis.

The typical patient with opiate-induced pulmonary edema is seen within 2 hours of heroin injection or 6 to 12 hours following methadone ingestion. Coma, miosis, and cyanosis may be present. Respirations are typically depressed—sometimes profoundly so—though occasionally the patient is tachypneic. On occasion, a patient has no symptoms or clinical signs of pulmonary edema, and the diagnosis is made radiographically.

A roentgenogram of a patient with noncardiogenic pulmonary edema typically shows bilateral pulmonary vascular congestion and infiltrates, along with a cardiac silhouette of normal size. Many variants may be seen, however, including asymmetric and unilateral patterns. Although a normal cardiac silhouette is characteristic, the picture may be confused by preexisting cardiomegaly.

Severity of pulmonary edema seen on the chest roentgenogram roughly parallels the clinical severity of the condition. Patchy, irregular, unilateral or bilateral infiltrates are seen in mild cases, most prominently in the mid-lung areas. In more severe cases, the infiltrates may entirely fill both lung fields.

In near-drowning and toxic inhalation, the chest roentgenogram may be normal at the time of the patient's initial examination, but this is not a reliable indication of subsequent developments. Patients who have suffered near-drowning should be admitted to the hospital after initial resuscitation so that they can be monitored for the possible development of pulmonary edema.

Differential Diagnosis

With noncardiogenic pulmonary edema, the differential diagnosis is that of any patient in acute respiratory distress. It includes those entities listed in the differential diagnosis of cardiogenic pulmonary edema.

Treatment

Given the variety of conditions that cause noncardiogenic pulmonary edema, individualization of therapy is essential. When there is a clearly defined underlying condition, primary attention must be directed toward treatment of that condition. For example, airway obstruction should be overcome, intracranial lesions evacuated, sepsis treated, narcotic antagonists administered, or metabolic abnormalities corrected, as indicated. In the face of hypovolemia, resuscitation with crystalloid solutions is probably preferable to the use of colloids, as colloid infusion may increase water content of the lung.

Traditional therapeutic modalities useful in cardiogenic pulmonary edema—diuretics, morphine, and rotating tourniquets—have no place in the treatment of noncardiogenic pulmonary edema. Diuretics particularly may exacerbate the course of this condition, causing hypovolemia and hypotension.[44]

The mainstays of noncardiogenic pulmonary edema treatment are oxygen administration and—when necessary—mechanical ventilation. Oxygen reduces pulmonary artery pressure, a prime factor in increased pulmonary vascular permeability. Mechanical ventilation enhances oxygenation and reduces atelectasis. Positive end-expiratory pressure (PEEP) may be used to increase functional residual capacity, increase pulmonary compliance, and reduce pulmonary arteriovenous shunting. This therapeutic modality should be added to mechanical ventilation specifically to achieve these goals, rather than to reduce pulmonary edema directly, because it effects no primary reduction in pulmonary water content even when it significantly improves pulmonary function.

The prognosis for the patient with noncardiogenic pulmonary edema varies greatly, depending on the underlying cause. In some instances, the course is predictably benign; in others, fatalities are common. Mild forms of high-altitude pulmonary edema, for example, have been successfully treated with bed rest alone.[45] With appropriate management, patients with noncardiogenic pulmonary edema may eventually recover normal pulmonary function, even after an episode of severe respiratory impairment.

REFERENCES

1. Baldwin ED, Cournand A, Richards DW, Jr: Pulmonary insufficiency. *Medicine* 27:243–278, 1948.
2. Jackson F: Pulmonary oedema. *Practitioner* 219:656–663, 1977.
3. Simpson PC Jr, Bristow JD: Recognition and management of emergencies in valvular heart disease. *Med Clin North Am.* 63:155–172, 1979.
4. Robin ED, Cross CE, Zelis R: Pulmonary edema. *N Engl J Med* 288:292–304, 1973.
5. Luther RR, Meyers SN: Acute mitral insufficiency secondary to ruptured chordae tendineae. *Arch Intern Med* 134:568–578, 1974.
6. Cunningham JH, Richardson RH, Smith JD: Interstitial pulmonary edema. *Heart Lung* 6:617–623, 1977.

7. Grainger RG: The radiological diagnosis of interstitial pulmonary oedema. *Br J Radiol* 50:161–163, 1977.

8. McHugh TJ, Forrester JS, Adler L, et al: Pulmonary vascular congestion in acute myocardial infarction: A hemodynamic and radiologic correlation. *Ann Intern Med* 76:29–33, 1972.

9. Biddle TL, Yu PN: Effect of furosemide on hemodynamics and lung water in acute pulmonary edema secondary to myocardial infarction. *Am J Cardiol* 43:86–90, 1979.

10. Cohn JN, Franciosa JA: Vasodilator therapy of cardiac failure: I. *N Engl J Med* 297:27–31, 1977.

11. Bussmann WD, Schupp D: Effect of sublingual nitroglycerin in emergency treatment of severe pulmonary edema. *Am J Cardiol* 41:931–936, 1978.

12. Cohn JN, Franciosa JA: Vasodilator therapy of cardiac failure: II. *N Engl J Med* 297:254–258, 1977.

13. Morganroth J, Perloff JK, Zelois SM, Dunkman WB: Acute severe aortic regurgitation. *Ann Intern Med* 87:-223–232, 1977.

14. Scoggin CH, Hyers TM, Reeves JT, et al: High-altitude pulmonary edema in the children and young adults of Leadville, Colorado. *N Engl J Med* 297:1269–1272, 1977.

15. Hultgren HN, Spickard WB, Hellriegel K, et al: High-altitude pulmonary edema. *Medicine* 40:289–313, 1961.

16. Shanies HM: Noncardiogenic pulmonary edema. *Med Clin North Am* 61:1319–1337, 1977.

17. Overland ES, Severinghaus JW: Noncardiac pulmonary edema. *Adv Intern Med* 23:307–326, 1978.

18. Cohen HB, Gambill AF, Eggers GWN, Jr: Acute pulmonary edema following head injury: Two case reports. *Anesth Analg* 56:136–139, 1977.

19. Ciongoli AK, Poser CM: Pulmonary edema secondary to subarachnoid hemorrhage. *Neurology* 22:867–870, 1972.

20. Bloom S: Pulmonary edema following a grand mal seizure. *Am Rev Respir Dis* 97:292–294, 1968.

21. Poe RH, Reisman JL, Rodenhouse TG: Pulmonary edema in cervical spinal cord injury. *J Trauma* 18:71–73, 1978.

22. Simmons RL, Heisterkamp CA III, Collins JA, et al: Acute pulmonary edema in battle casualties. *J Trauma* 9:760–775, 1969.

23. Schoenfeld MR: Acute pulmonary edema caused by barbiturate poisoning. *Angiology* 15:445–453, 1964.

24. Bogartz LJ, Miller WC: Pulmonary edema associated with propoxyphene intoxication. *JAMA* 215:259–262, 1971.

25. Glauser FL, Smith WR, Caldwell A, et al: Ethchlorvynol (Placidyl)-induced pulmonary edema. *Ann Intern Med* 84:46–48, 1976.

26. Oh TE, Gordon TP, Burden PW: Unilateral pulmonary oedema and 'Mandrax' poisoning. *Anaesthesia* 33:719–721, 1978.

27. Richman S, Harris RD: Acute pulmonary edema associated with Librium abuse. *Radiology* 103:57–58, 1972.

28. Davis PR, Burch RE: Pulmonary edema and salicylate intoxication. *Ann Intern Med* 80:553–554, 1974.

29. Bowers RE, Brigham KL, Owen PJ: Salicylate pulmonary edema: The mechanism in sheep and review of the clinical literature. *Am Rev Respir Dis* 115:261–268, 1977.

30. Bledsoe FH, Seymour EQ: Acute pulmonary edema associated with Parathion poisoning. *Radiology* 103:53–56, 1972.

31. Knudson RD: Drowning and near-drowning. *Rocky Mt Med J* 69:67–68, 1972.

32. Carilli AD, Ramanamurty MV, Chang Y-S, et al: Noncardiogenic pulmonary edema following blood transfusion. *Chest* 74:310–312, 1978.

33. Trapness DH, Thurston JGB: Unilateral pulmonary oedema after pleural aspiration. *Lancet* 1:1367–1369, 1970.

34. Waqaruddin M, Bernstein A: Re-expansion pulmonary oedema. *Thorax* 30:54–60, 1975.

35. Soliman MG, Richer P: Epiglottitis and pulmonary oedema in children. *Can Anaesth Soc J* 25:270–275, 1978.

36. Osler W: Oedema of left lung—morphia poisoning. *Montreal Gen Hosp Rep* 1:291–292, 1880.

37. Halpern M, Rho YM: Deaths from narcotism in New York City. *NY State J Med* 63:2391–2408, 1966.

38. Staub NC: Pulmonary edema. *Physiol Rev* 54:678–811, 1974.

39. Whayne TF, Severinghaus JW: Experimental hypoxic pulmonary edema in the rat. *J Appl Physiol* 25:729–732, 1968.

40. Hultgren HN: High altitude medical problems. *West J Med* 131:8–23, 1979.

41. Kleiner JP, Nelson WP: High altitude pulmonary edema. *JAMA* 234:491–495, 1975.

42. Theodore J, Robin ED: Pathogenesis of neurogenic pulmonary oedema. *Lancet* 2:749–751, 1975.

43. Robin ED, Carey LC, Grenvik A, et al: Capillary leak syndrome with pulmonary edema. *Arch Intern Med* 130:66–71, 1972.

44. Hultgren HN: Furosemide for high altitude pulmonary edema. *JAMA* 234:589–590, 1975.

45. Marticorena E, Hultgren HN: Evaluation of therapeutic methods in high altitude pulmonary edema. *Am J Cardiol* 43:307–312, 1979.

49. Acute Myocardial Infarction

LESTER B. JACOBSON, M.D., F.A.C.C., F.A.C.P.

Coronary artery disease continues to plague a large segment of the American population. Some of these patients are asymptomatic, but others suffer from angina pectoris, congestive heart failure, and arrhythmias. Both asymptomatic and symptomatic patients are at risk for acute myocardial infarction and sudden death, events that occur with frightening unpredictability. While the statistical likelihood that patients with coronary artery disease will suffer acute myocardial infarction within a specified time period can be predicted from the responses of their ST segments and blood pressure to treadmill exercise testing, the occurrence and time of occurrence of the event in an *individual* patient cannot be prognosticated.

Acute myocardial infarction is a dramatic event. Neither the clinical course nor the short- and long-term prognoses can be predicted in an individual at the time of its onset. Patients with acute myocardial infarction are generally impressed with their symptoms, and those around the patients are generally impressed by their critically ill appearance. The gravity of the situation is underscored by the seriousness of purpose exhibited by the physician and other health care personnel in attendance. Their attentiveness reflects their appreciation of the fact that patients with acute myocardial infarction can suddenly and unpredictably develop catastrophic, potentially fatal arrhythmias that require immediate treatment.

PATHOGENESIS OF ACUTE MYOCARDIAL INFARCTION

Myocardial ischemia occurs when the myocardial oxygen demand, i.e., the amount of oxygen needed per minute per gram of cardiac tissue to maintain the functional and structural integrity of the heart, exceeds the oxygen supply to the myocardium for a period of time. Myocardial infarction occurs when this demand exceeds supply for so long a time—generally several minutes—that necrosis of cardiac tissue occurs.

Three major determinants account for about 80 percent of the myocardial oxygen demand: (1) the heart rate, (2) the contractile state of ventricular muscle, and (3) the left ventricular wall tension. Wall tension is directly proportional to the product of the pressure developed within the left ventricular myocardium and the radius of the left ventricle as it generates pressure; it is inversely proportional to the left ventricular wall thickness.

Myocardial oxygen supply also has three major determinants: (1) the coronary blood flow, (2) the oxygen-carrying capacity of the blood, and (3) the shape of the hemoglobin-oxygen dissociation curve. The coronary blood flow depends on the size of the coronary arteries, which may be altered by anatomical stenoses and vasomotor influences; the coronary vascular resistance; and the aortic and left ventricular pressures during diastole. The oxygen-carrying capacity of the blood depends predominantly on the hemoglobin concentration. The shape of the hemoglobin-oxygen dissociation curve depends on metabolic factors.

While almost all patients (more than 95 percent) who suffer an acute myocardial infarction have significant anatomical stenoses in the coronary artery distribution to the infarcted myocardium, a few such patients have normal coronary arteries. In view of this latter finding, it has been suggested that prolonged, severe vasoconstriction of the vessel, or thromboembolism, or in situ thrombosis with subsequent lysis of the thrombus is the mechanism of infarction in some individuals. Constriction of a coronary artery to such a degree that little or no blood flows through it, i.e., spasm, has been documented to occur in normal as well as in pathologically (atherosclerotically) narrowed vessels.[1,2] Spasm may occur spontaneously, as a result of mechanical stimulation (e.g., catheter), or in response to specific pharmocologic agents, of which ergonovine maleate is the most commonly used.

It is difficult to know exactly why acute myocardial infarction occurs when it does in patients with coronary artery disease, for the overwhelming majority of patients have the infarction at times of inactivity, when there is no clear increase in the myocardial oxygen demand. Thus, it has been hypothesized that the event is initiated by a decrease in myocardial oxygen supply, presumably because of a decrease in coronary blood flow. It is not possible in an individual patient to identify the exact event(s) responsible for diminished flow, but the most plausible mechanism is a decrease in the size of the supplying artery lumen because of intraluminal thrombus formation,[3] dissection into the base of an atherosclerotic plaque, or an increase in vasomotor tone that causes vasoconstriction. This last possibility is supported by coronary angiograms performed in the first few hours after an acute myocardial infarction. These angiograms showed that intravenous nitroglycerin administration may reestablish flow through a previously totally occluded segment of an artery that supplies the infarcting myocardium.[4]

It has been discovered during the past decade that myocardial infarction evolves over a period of several hours and that the size of the infarction is not determined at the time of the onset of the event.[5] Rather, extensive laboratory studies in experimental animals have shown that the size of an evolving myocardial infarction may be altered by maneuvers and medications that alter the balance between myocardial oxygen demand and supply. Interventions that decrease demand or increase supply have been demonstrated to lessen the size of an evolving infarct, while those that increase demand or decrease supply increase the size of the necrotic area (Fig. 49–1). Clinical studies aimed at determining the applicability of these principles to infarction in humans are now under way.[6]

CONSEQUENCES OF MYOCARDIAL ISCHEMIA

The metabolic abnormalities that occur with myocardial ischemia result in dramatic alterations in the electrical and mechanical properties of the heart. Changes in conduction velocities and refractory periods of cardiac electrical tissue predispose to the development of ventricular arrhythmias, and may result in intraventricular and atrioventricular (AV) conduction abnormalities. Changes in mechanical properties of the heart, such as an increase in the stiffness of the myocardium in diastole or a tendency for cardiac muscle to expand rather than contract during mechanical systole, contribute to the increase in left ventricular diastolic pressure and the decrease in left ventricular stroke volume that accompany myocardial ischemia.

SYMPTOMS OF ACUTE MYOCARDIAL ISCHEMIA AND INFARCTION

Patients with acute myocardial ischemia and infarction may or may not have symptoms to suggest what is occurring. The classic symptom is a discomfort that, in most patients, is located in the precordial area, but may be located in the epigastrium, the neck, the mandible, the shoulders, the arms, or the back. The discomfort is usually described as a pressure, tightness, or weightlike feeling; however, it may be described as a true pain with an aching or sharp, stabbing quality. Occasional patients complain of gastrointestinal symptoms that they commonly term "indigestion."

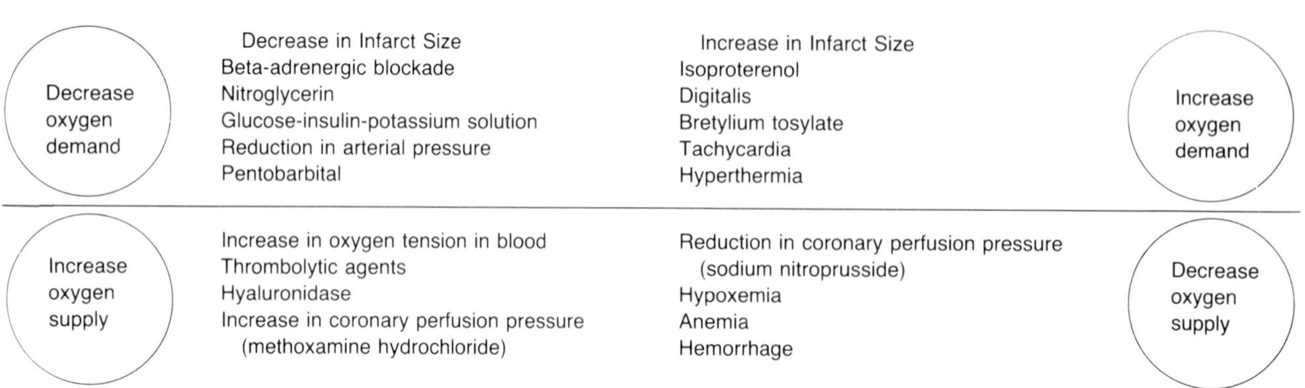

Figure 49–1 Interventions That Alter the Size of an Experimental Myocardial Infarction.[6]

Some patients with acute myocardial infarction simply collapse and die suddenly before any symptoms occur. Others complain of a feeling of weakness that may be mild to profound. Lightheadedness, with or without an awareness of cardiac activity, diaphoresis, nausea, vomiting, and a sense of impending doom are also commonly mentioned symptoms. In unusual patients, the abrupt onset of congestive heart failure symptoms may be the only manifestation of acute myocardial infarction.

PHYSICAL EXAMINATION FINDINGS

Patients with acute myocardial infarction usually appear seriously ill and uncomfortable. If their cardiac output is low, they may have an ashen, dusky coloration, and their skin may be cool and clammy. These signs, which are attributable to the large amounts of catecholamines secreted in response to the hemodynamic and psychological stresses of the event, may be masked to variable degrees in patients taking adrenergic blocking or depleting medications, such as propranolol and reserpine. Patients with acute myocardial infarction may be tachypneic. If so, they generally breathe small tidal volumes rapidly in response to pulmonary congestion and/or emotional stress.

The pulse may be rapid, normal, or slow, depending on the hemodynamic stress of the event, the responses of the autonomic nervous system, and the ability of the cardiac conduction system to respond to the hemodynamic and metabolic stimuli. The arterial pulses may be bounding, normal, or thready, depending on the stroke volume. The blood pressure may be high, normal, or low, depending on the cardiac output and the systemic vascular resistance. The jugular venous pressure may be high, normal, or low, depending on the circulating blood volume, the venous tone, and the cardiac performance.

The heart, on palpation, may be normal size or large. Its movement may seem to be normal or abnormal, depending on its condition prior to the acute infarction and on the anatomical and functional magnitude, as well as the location, of the evolving infarction. A fourth heart sound is commonly heard; in the presence of congestive heart failure, a third heart sound may also be audible. When the heart rate is rapid, the third and fourth heart sounds may fuse into a single sound and result in a triple cadence termed a *summation gallop*. Mitral insufficiency, typically across the posterior mitral valve leaflet, may occur as a result of ischemia or infarction that involves, generally, the inferior wall of the left ventricle. The resultant murmur may be pansystolic, midsystolic, or late systolic, depending on the systolic timing and the severity of the left ventricular wall motion abnormality. The mitral insufficiency murmur may be heard best at the base of the heart, at the left lower sternal edge, or at the apex; in contrast, the murmur of rheumatic mitral insufficiency, which is due almost exclusively to regurgitation across the *anterior* mitral valve leaflet, is almost always heard best at the apex. Ventricular septal rupture, a rare event in the early hours of acute myocardial infarction, may be recognized by a harsh, loud pansystolic murmur that is heard best at the left lower sternal edge and is accompanied by a prominent thrill in the area where the murmur is heard with maximum intensity.

A pericardial rub attributable to acute myocardial infarction only rarely occurs in the first hours of an infarction, although it commonly occurs during the second through fourth days of the event. As rubs are generally heard only in patients whose infarction involves the epicardium, they are most commonly heard in patients whose electrocardiograms (ECGs) suggest transmural myocardial infarction, i.e., show pathologic Q waves in addition to abnormalities of the ST segments and T waves. However, pericardial rubs are occasionally heard in patients whose ECGs do not show evidence of transmural myocardial infarction, presumably because transmural and epicardial infarctions are not always accompanied by pathologic Q waves.

ECG Evidence of Acute Myocardial Infarction

Specific ECG findings that suggest the presence of acute myocardial ischemia or infarction include peaked T waves, elevations and depression of the ST segments, pathologic Q waves, T-wave inversions, and atrioventricular and/or intraventricular conduction abnormalities. One of the earliest ECG abnormalities in acute myocardial infarction is a change in the contour and amplitude of the T wave, which may become tall and sharply peaked. This hyperacute pattern usually lasts for only a few minutes and is not generally seen because patients rarely have ECGs taken in the early minutes of an acute myocardial infarction (Fig. 49–2). ST segment elevations which are convex upward define the epicardial injury pattern, which is a reliable sign of extensive ischemic myocardial injury (Fig. 49–3). Leads vectorially opposite to those exhibiting ST elevations often show ST depressions, which are termed reciprocal changes or abnormalities. In some patients, the ST segment depressions are more marked than the ST segment elevations (Fig. 49–4); and changes in the contours of T waves may or may not accompany ST segment changes. In other patients, especially those with previous myocardial infarctions or with left ventricular hypertrophy, changes in previously abnormal ST segments may be the only ECG evidence of acute ischemia or infarction (Fig. 49–5).

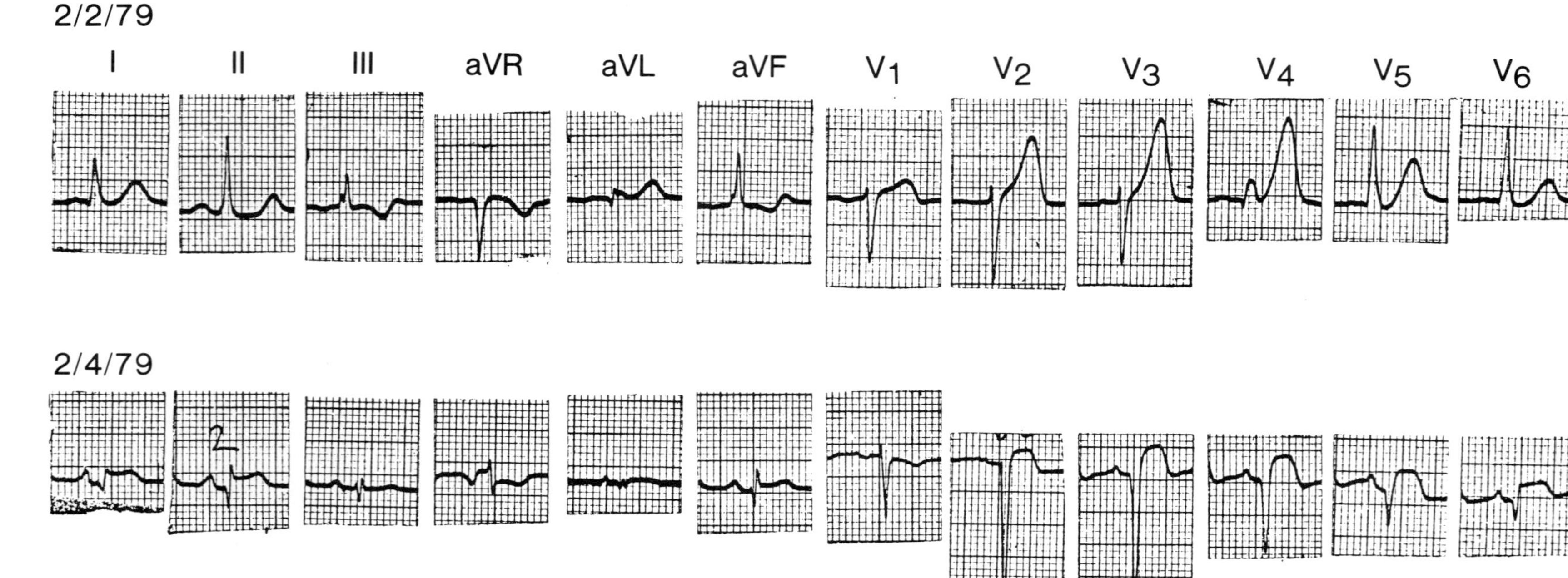

Figure 49–2   ECGs Showing Evolution of an Acute Myocardial Infarction from the Hyperacute T-Wave Pattern (top) to the Pathologic Q-Wave and ST Segment and T-Wave Abnormality Pattern (bottom). *Note:* The 12-lead ECG at top was recorded from a patient about 20 minutes after the onset of symptoms suggesting acute myocardial infarction. Leads V_2 through V_5 most clearly display the prominent hyperacute T-wave contours. The T waves in leads I, aVL, and V_6 are also abnormally tall, but less so. The 12-lead ECG (bottom), which was recorded two days later in the same patient, shows pathologic Q waves and ST segment and T-wave abnormalities indicating transmural infarction of myocardium seen by the leads in which the hyperacute T-wave abnormalities had been present. (ECG shown at 96% of original.)

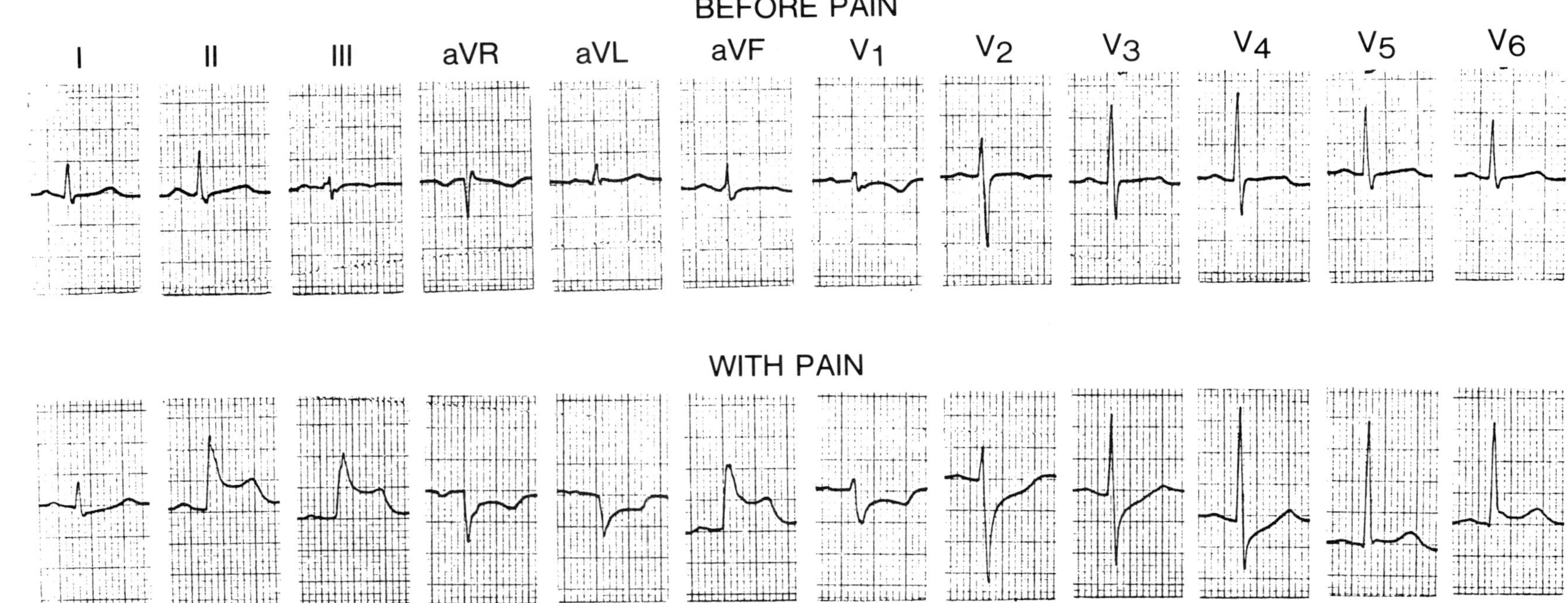

Figure 49–3   ECGs of Patient with Reversible Myocardial Ischemia Due to Coronary Artery Spasm. *Note:* These 12-lead ECGs were recorded from a 54-year-old man with normal coronary angiogram before and after (*top*) and during (*bottom*) an episode of reversible myocardial ischemia due to coronary artery spasm. During the pain, the ST segments in leads II, III, aVF, and V_6 are markedly elevated, displaying the epicardial injury pattern. Leads I, aVR, aVL, and V_1 through V_4 show reciprocal ST segment depression. Only minor T-wave abnormalities are present in the top tracing. (ECG shown at 93% of original.)

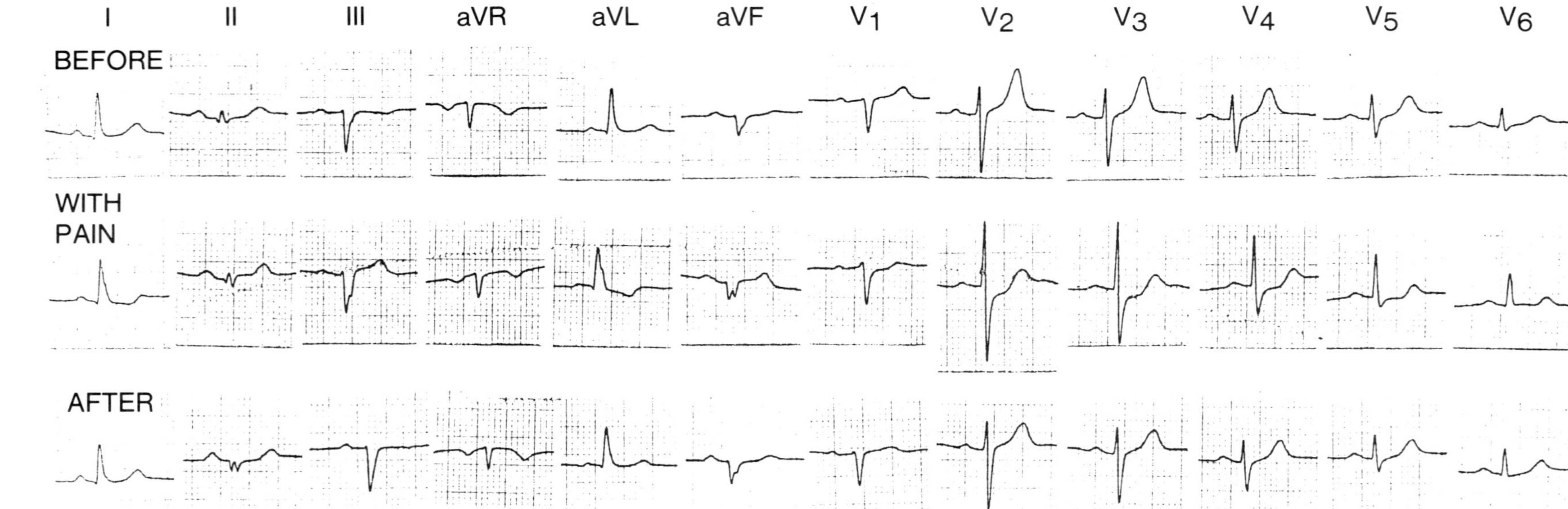

Figure 49–4   ECGs Showing Transient Depressions of ST Segments and Diminutions in the T-Wave Amplitudes during Myocardial Ischemia. *Note:* These 12-lead ECGs were recorded from a 58-year-old man with severe three vessel coronary artery disease before (*top*), during (*middle*), and after (*bottom*) an episode of nocturnal chest discomfort. During pain, transient depression of the ST segment and diminution in the T-wave amplitude occur in leads I, aVL, and V_2 through V_4. Both ST segment and T-wave contours return to baseline following relief of the chest discomfort. (ECG shown at 84% of original.)

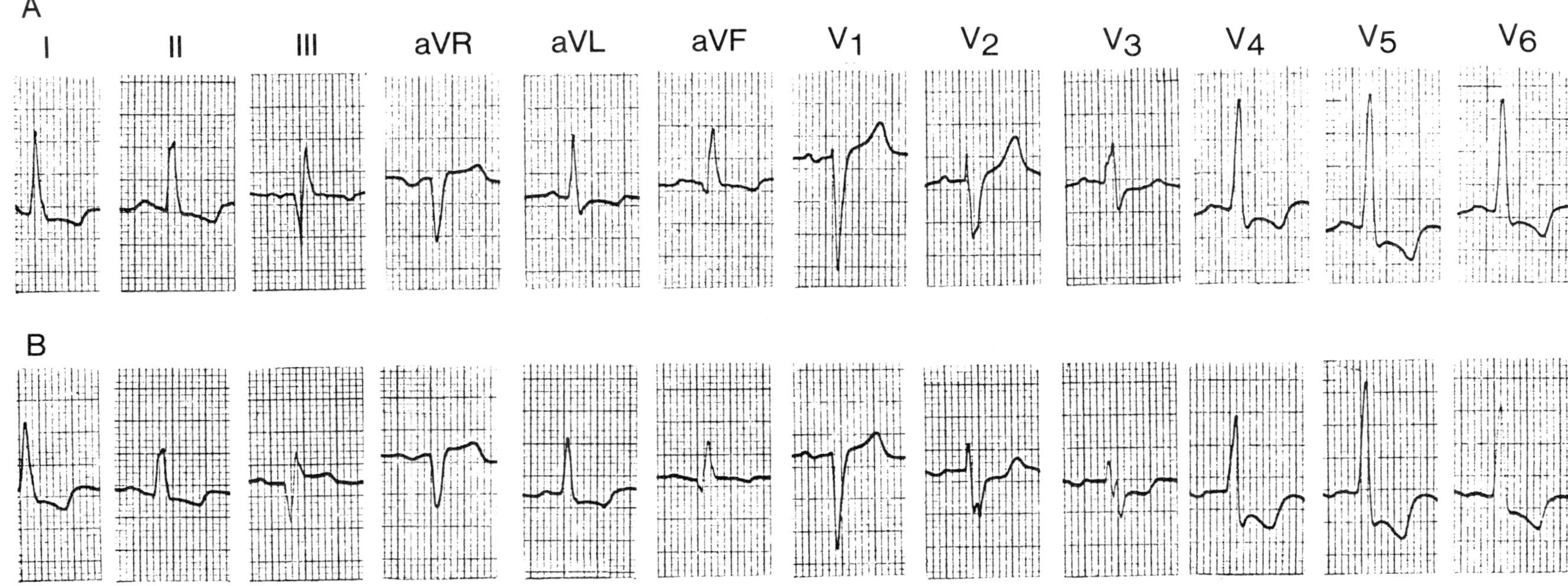

Figure 49–5   ECGs Showing Changes in ST Segment Contours as the Only Manifestations of Acute Myocardial Infarction. *Note:* These 12-lead ECGs were recorded from a man with hypertension and previous myocardial infarctions at a time when he was feeling quite well (*A*) and two weeks later, several hours after the onset of symptoms suggesting acute myocardial infarction (*B*). The ST segments in the later ECG are much more depressed in leads I, aVL, and V_2 through V_5. The patient died two days later in profound heart failure. At autopsy, extensive evolving myocardial infarction was found. (ECG shown at 95% of original.)

In some patients, changes in the direction of T waves may be the only signs of myocardial ischemia and infarction. If the T waves were initially normal, the ECG may show only T-wave inversion; however, if the T waves were initially abnormal, then the ECG may look more "normal" despite the occurrence of a new ischemic event (Fig. 49–6).

Pathologic Q waves, which reflect the absence of cardiac electrical activity from those portions of the heart "seen" by the leads in which they occur, may appear within 8 to 24 hours of the onset of symptoms of acute myocardial infarction (Fig. 49–2, *bottom*). However, as pathologic Q waves rarely appear earlier than 8 hours after the onset of symptoms, such Q waves in an ECG recorded shortly after the onset of symptoms suggest that a myocardial infarction has occurred earlier, but does not help assess whether or not a new infarction is occurring. ECGs showing pathologic Q waves are said to indicate transmural infarction, because the presence of Q waves correlates anatomically with infarction that extends from the endocardium through the epicardium, i.e., is transmural.

Certain ECG patterns make it difficult, if not impossible, to confirm an acute myocardial infarction electrocardiographically. In patients whose ventricular rhythm is completely paced by an artificial cardiac pacing system, the QRST complexes may show little, if any, change when infarction occurs. This may also be the case when a myocardial infarction has occurred previously (Fig. 49–5). Difficulty also arises when no previous tracings are available for comparison in a patient with Wolff-Parkinson-White syndrome, in whom atrioventricular conduction occurs exclusively via the accessory atrioventricular conduction pathway, for in such patients the ECG may show dramatic QRST abnormalities even in the absence of an ischemic event (Fig. 49–7). In patients whose ECGs show left bundle branch block prior to the onset of acute myocardial infarction, changes of variable degrees usually occur in the ST segment and T-wave contours during the acute event. However, the ST segments and T waves usually return to their preinfarction contours as the infarction evolves, and new Q waves do not usually appear. Thus, in a patient with left bundle branch block, an ECG taken before an infarction may be identical to one taken after the infarction. In contrast, patterns indicating right bundle branch block or left anterior fascicular block occurring prior to, or developing in the course of, acute myocardial infarction do not interfere with the evolution of the typical ECG abnormalities associated with the event (Fig. 49–8).

Complicating the ECG interpretation of myocardial infarction are the occurrences of ECG patterns that simulate ischemic events although the patients' coronary arteries and myocardium are structurally normal. As mentioned earlier, one such pattern occurs in patients with accessory atrioventricular conduction pathways. When AV conduction occurs via the accessory pathway, a negatively directed delta wave may simulate a pathologic Q wave and prompt the incorrect diagnosis of myocardial infarction (Fig. 49–9). Another complicating pattern is seen in patients with intermittent left bundle branch block; when intraventricular conduction is normal, the T waves in the anterior precordial leads may at times have deeply inverted, symmetrical contours like those seen in anterior wall ischemic events (Fig. 49–10). A third pattern occurs in patients whose ventricles have been paced for periods of hours to years. In such patients, the nonpaced QRS complexes that are stimulated by supraventricular impulses may show ST segment and T-wave contour abnormalities suggesting an ischemic event (Fig. 49–11). The mechanism of the development of such postpacing T-wave changes remains unclear.

In some patients, the development of bundle branch or fascicle blocks, or of first-, second-, or third-degree AV block may be a clue to the occurrence of acute myocardial infarction.

While virtually any arrhythmia may occur in the presence of acute myocardial infarction, the only arrhythmia that is essentially diagnostic of this event is the so-called accelerated ventricular rhythm. (See Chapter 50, Fig. 50–24.)

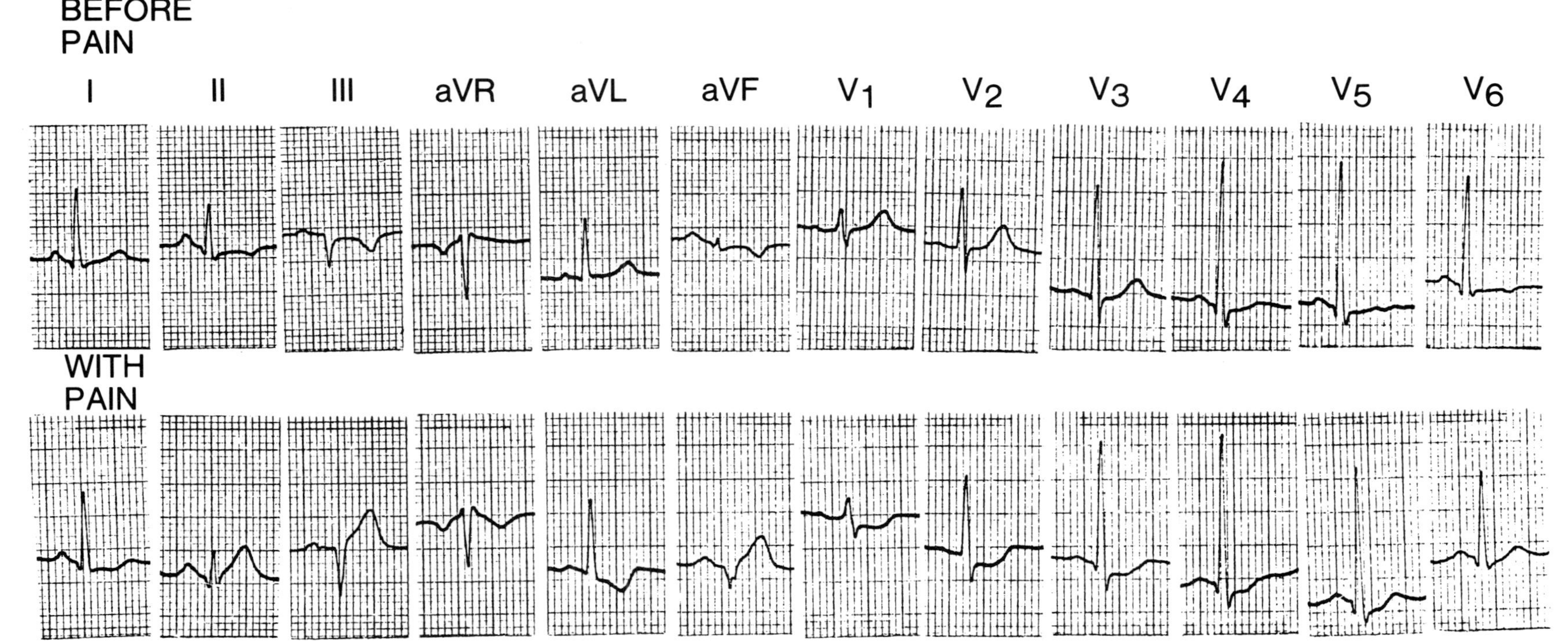

Figure 49–6 ECGs Showing Changes in Q Waves, ST Segments, and T Waves during Pain of Myocardial Ischemia. *Note:* These 12-lead ECGs were recorded before (*top*) and during (*bottom*) chest discomfort in a 48-year-old man with acute inferior and true posterior wall myocardial infarction three days earlier. The top strip, showing Q waves and ST segment and T-wave abnormalities in leads II, III, and aVF, as well as R > S with an upright T wave in lead V_1, is compatible with inferior wall and true posterior wall myocardial infarctions of uncertain age. During pain of myocardial ischemia, ST segment and T wave changes occur in all leads, and the T-wave direction becomes "normal" in the inferiorly directed leads and in lead V_1.

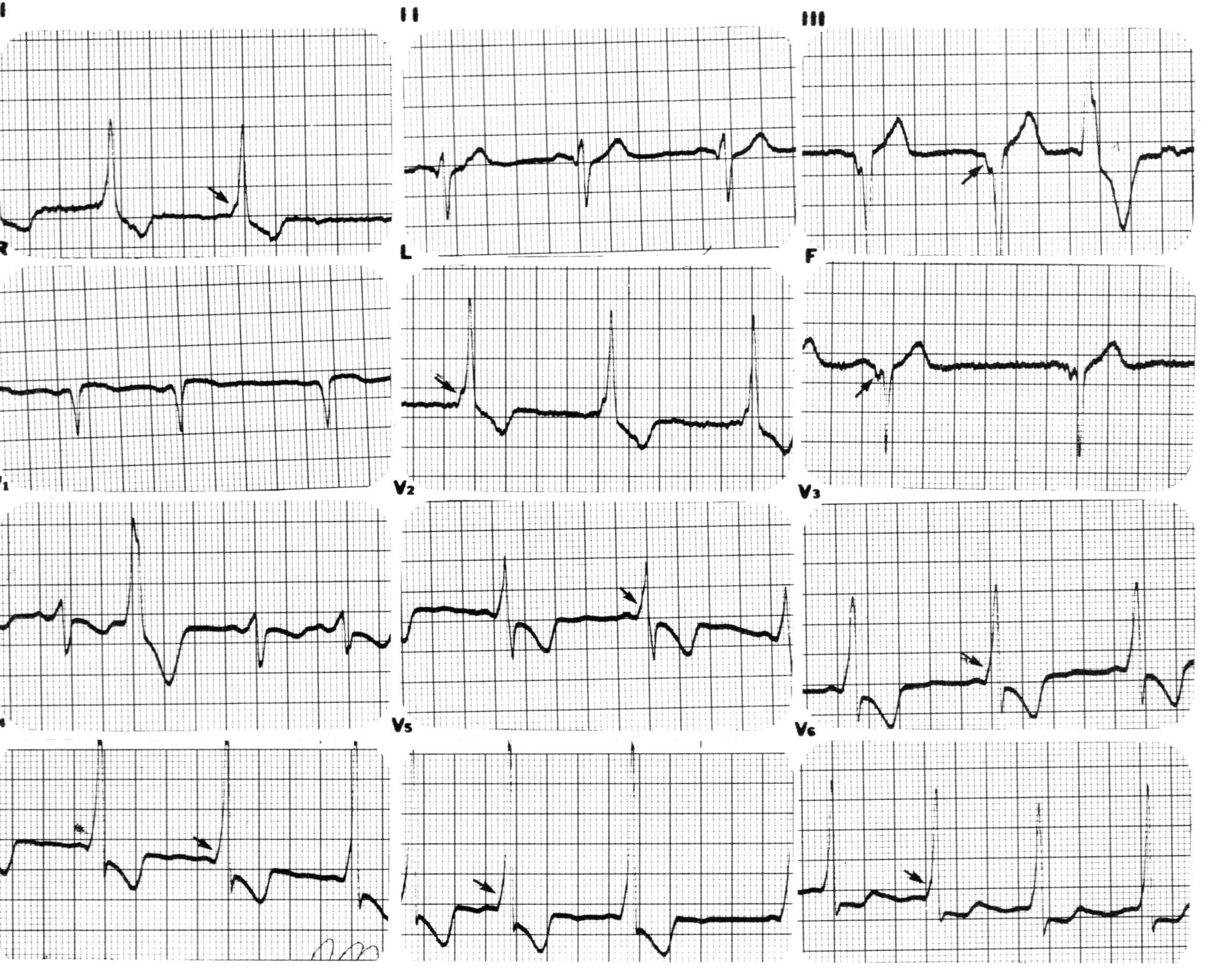

Figure 49–7   ECGs Showing QRST Abnormalities in a Patient with Wolff-Parkinson-White Syndrome during Accessory Pathway Conduction. *Note:* This 12-lead ECG was recorded from a 67-year-old woman with angina pectoris and Wolff-Parkinson-White syndrome during accessory pathway conduction. The PR interval is at the lower limit of normal (0.12 second), the QRS duration is abnormally long (0.13 second), and delta waves (*arrows*) are present. The dramatic ST segment and T-wave abnormalities might simply reflect an abnormal sequence of ventricular repolarization resulting from the abnormal sequence of ventricular activation via the accessory pathway, but they could conceivably reflect myocardial ischemia.

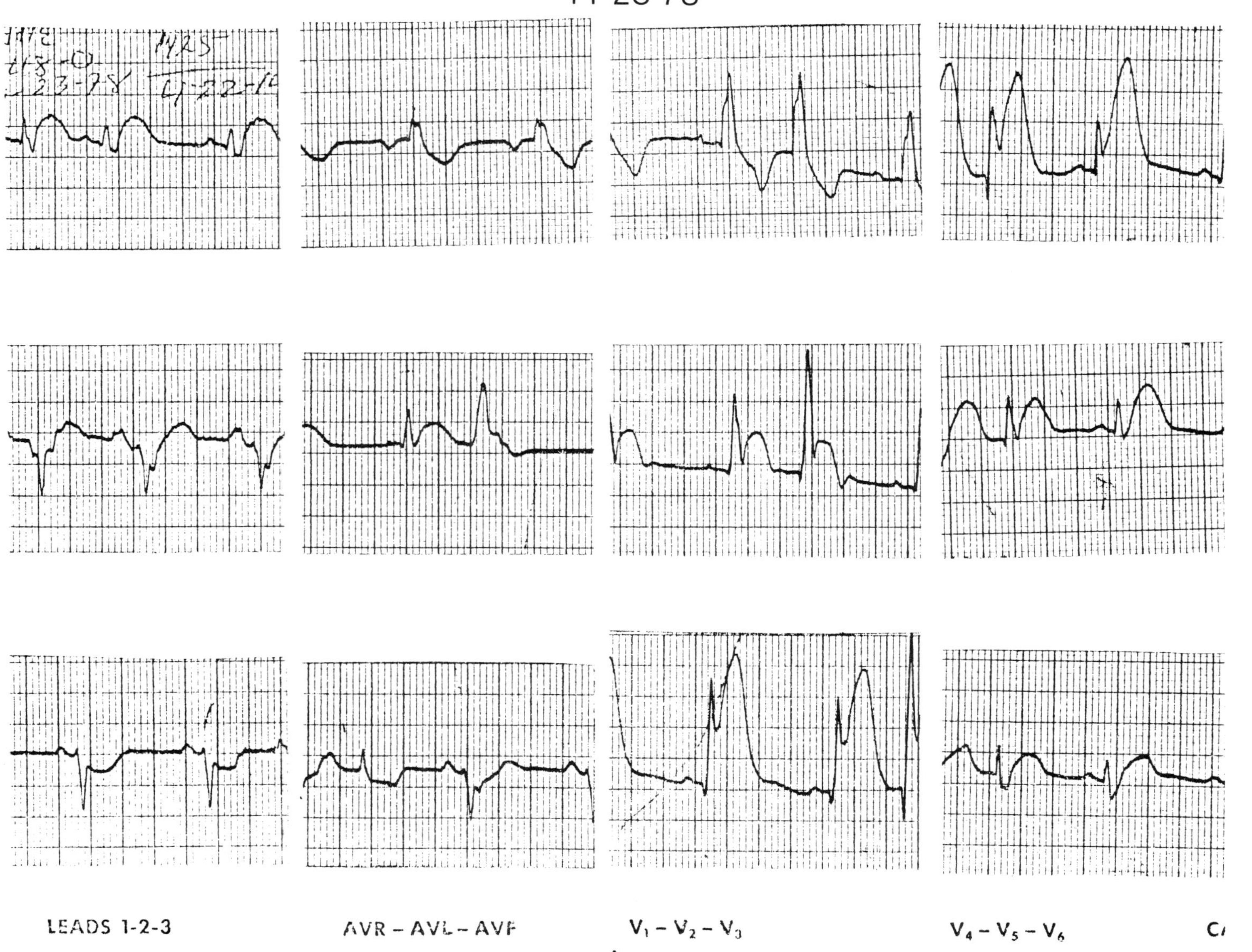

Figure 49–8   ECGs Showing Evolutionary Changes of Acute Myocardial Infarction in Patient with Preexisting Right Bundle Branch Block and Left Anterior Fascicular Block. *Note:* These 12-lead ECGs were recorded from a patient with preexisting right bundle branch block and left axis deviation attributable to left anterior fascicle block (A) three hours after the onset of symptoms suggesting acute myocardial infarction and (B) 15 days later. Despite the intraventricular conduction abnormalities, extensive ST segment elevations reflecting ischemic injury are seen in A, and pathologic Q waves with ST elevations and T-wave inversions indicative of transmural anterior wall myocardial infarction are clearly seen in B.

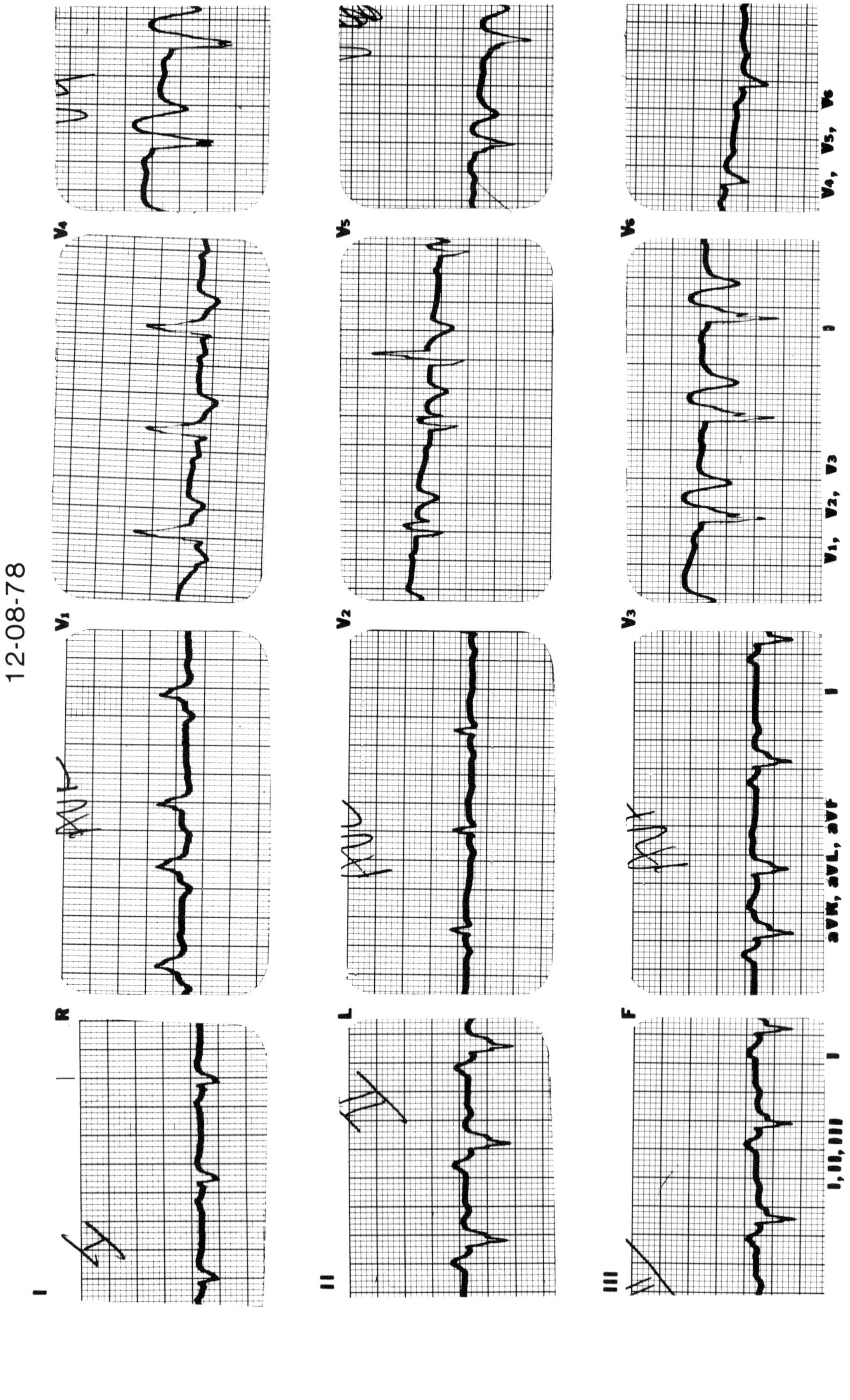

Figure 49–8 continued

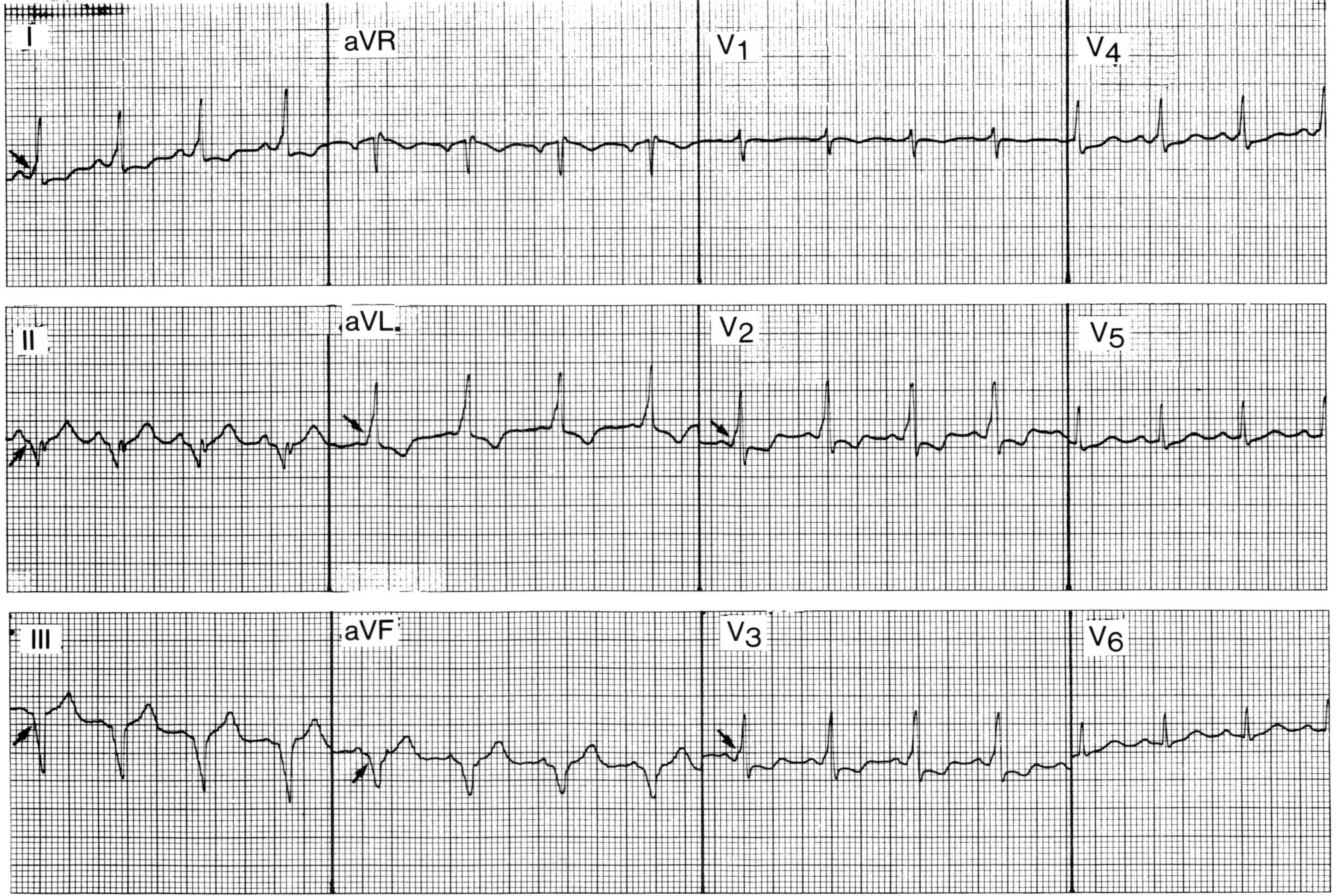

Figure 49—9 ECG Showing Pseudoinfarction Pattern in a Patient with Wolff-Parkinson-White Syndrome. *Note:* This 12-lead ECG was recorded from an asymptomatic 30-year-old man with an accessory atrioventricular conduction pathway that causes ventricular preexcitation. The PR interval is abnormally short (0.11 second), the QRS duration is abnormally long (0.12 second), and delta waves (*arrows*) are present. The negatively directed delta waves in leads II, III, and aVF simulate pathologic Q waves and suggest myocardial infarction. As this patient has no evidence of coronary artery disease or myocardial infarction, the pattern is referred to as a pseudoinfarction pattern.

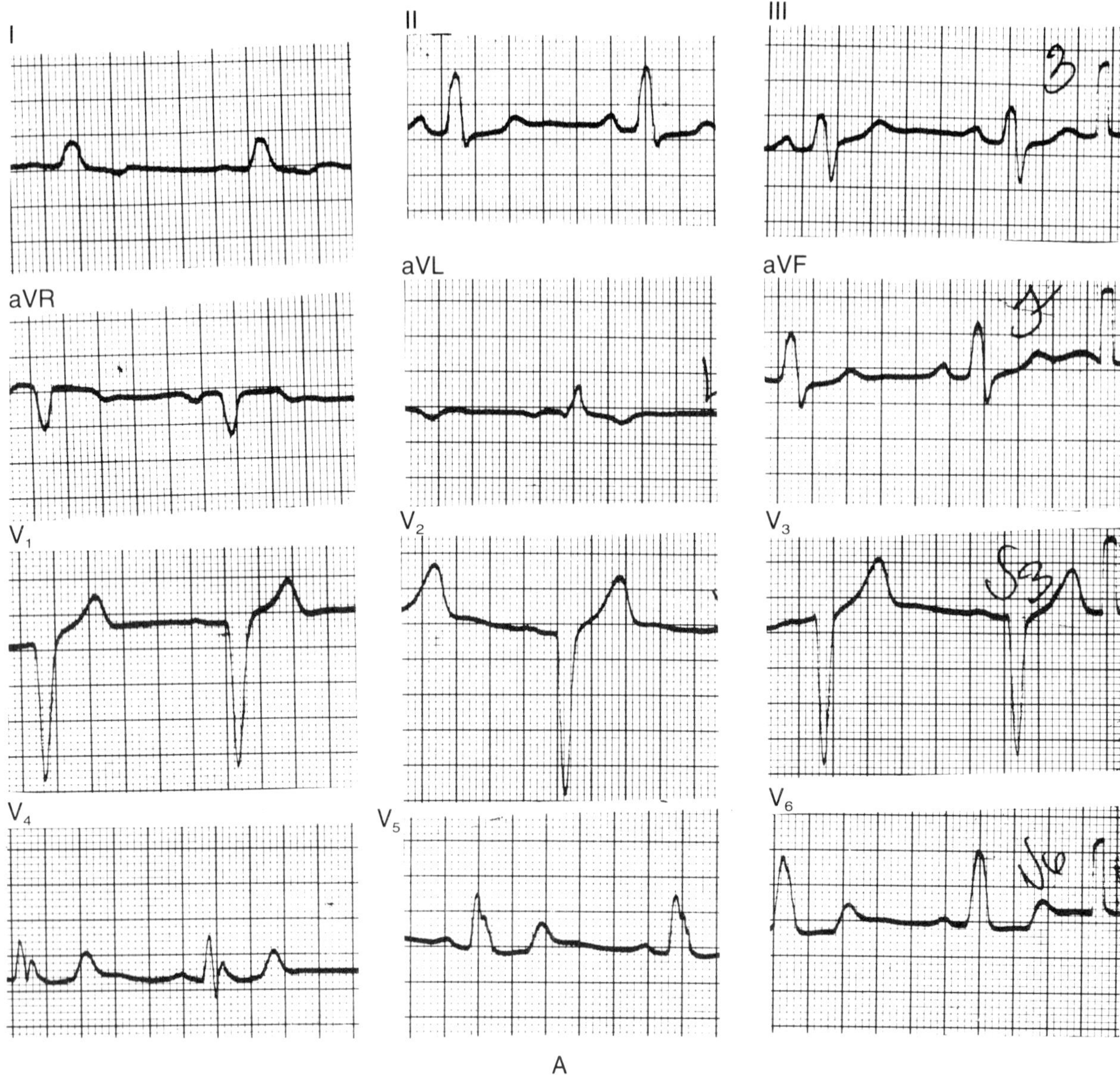

A

Figure 49–10 ECGs in a Patient with Intermittent Left Bundle Branch Block. *Note:* These ECGs were recorded from a 70-year-old woman with intermittent left bundle branch block and no evidence of coronary artery disease. *A* This 12-lead ECG was recorded during left bundle branch block. *B* Twelve-lead ECG during normal intraventricular conduction shows nonspecific T-wave contour abnormalities, most suggesting an ischemic process, in leads V_2 and V_3. *C.* Lead V_2 shows the transition from normal to left bundle branch block type of intraventricular conduction pattern.

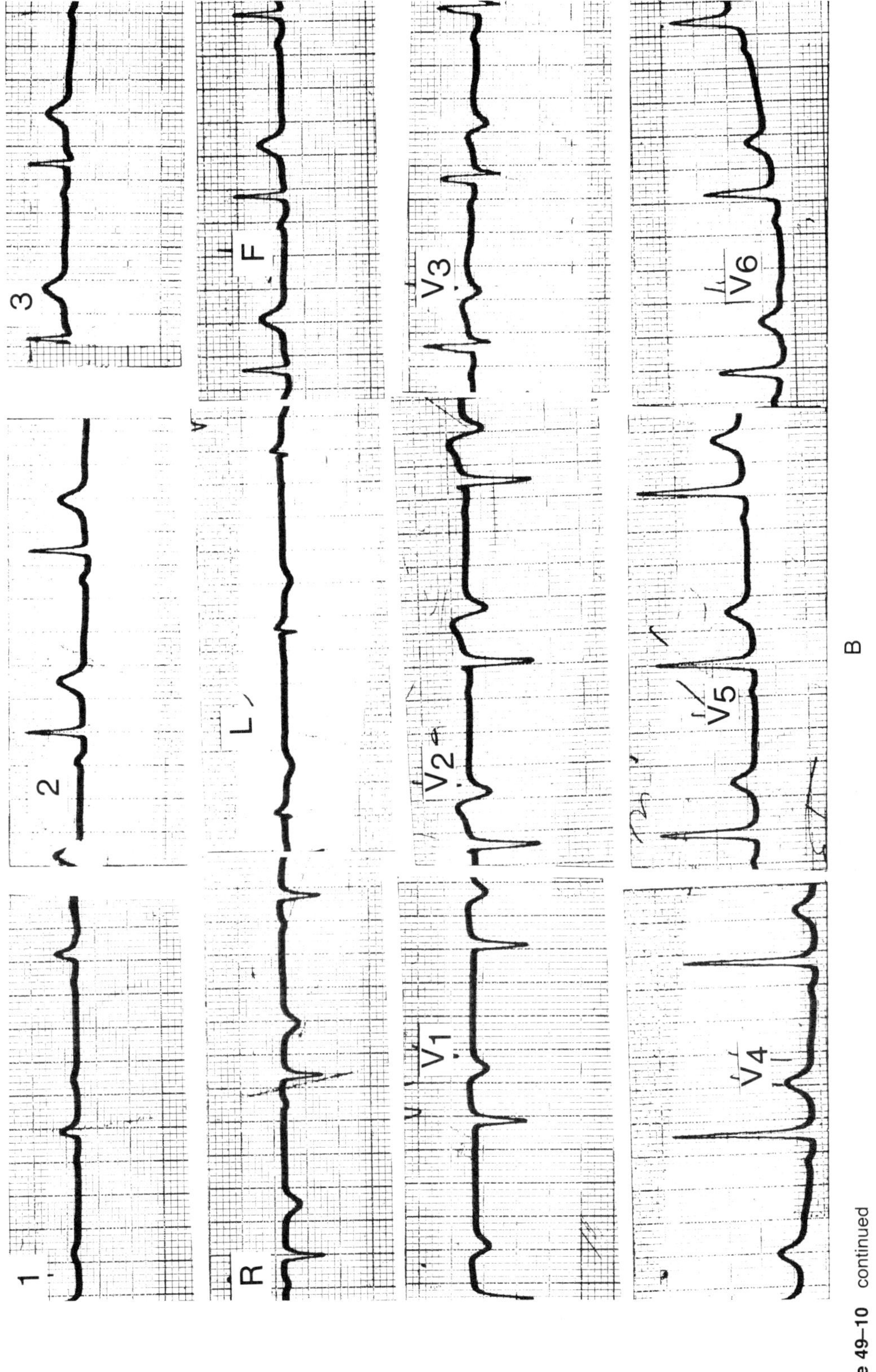

Figure 49–10 continued

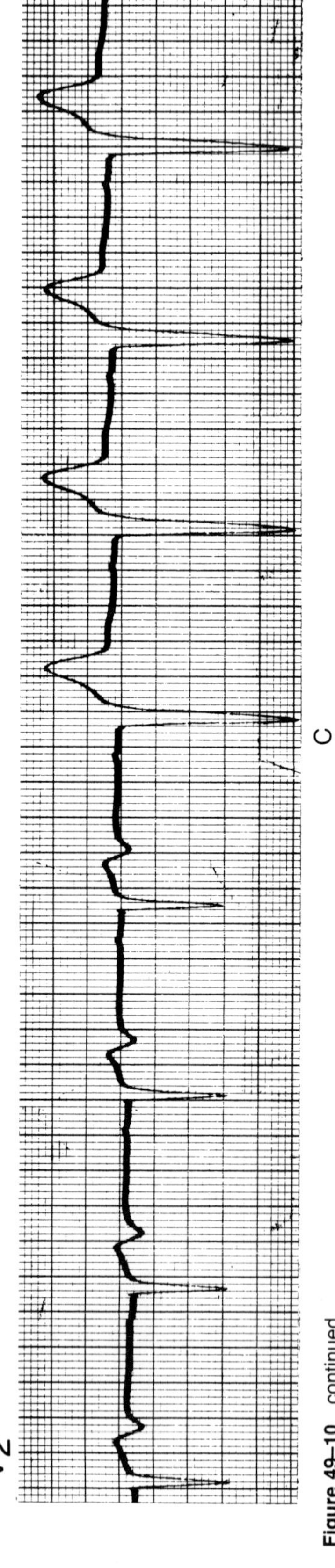

Figure 49–10 continued

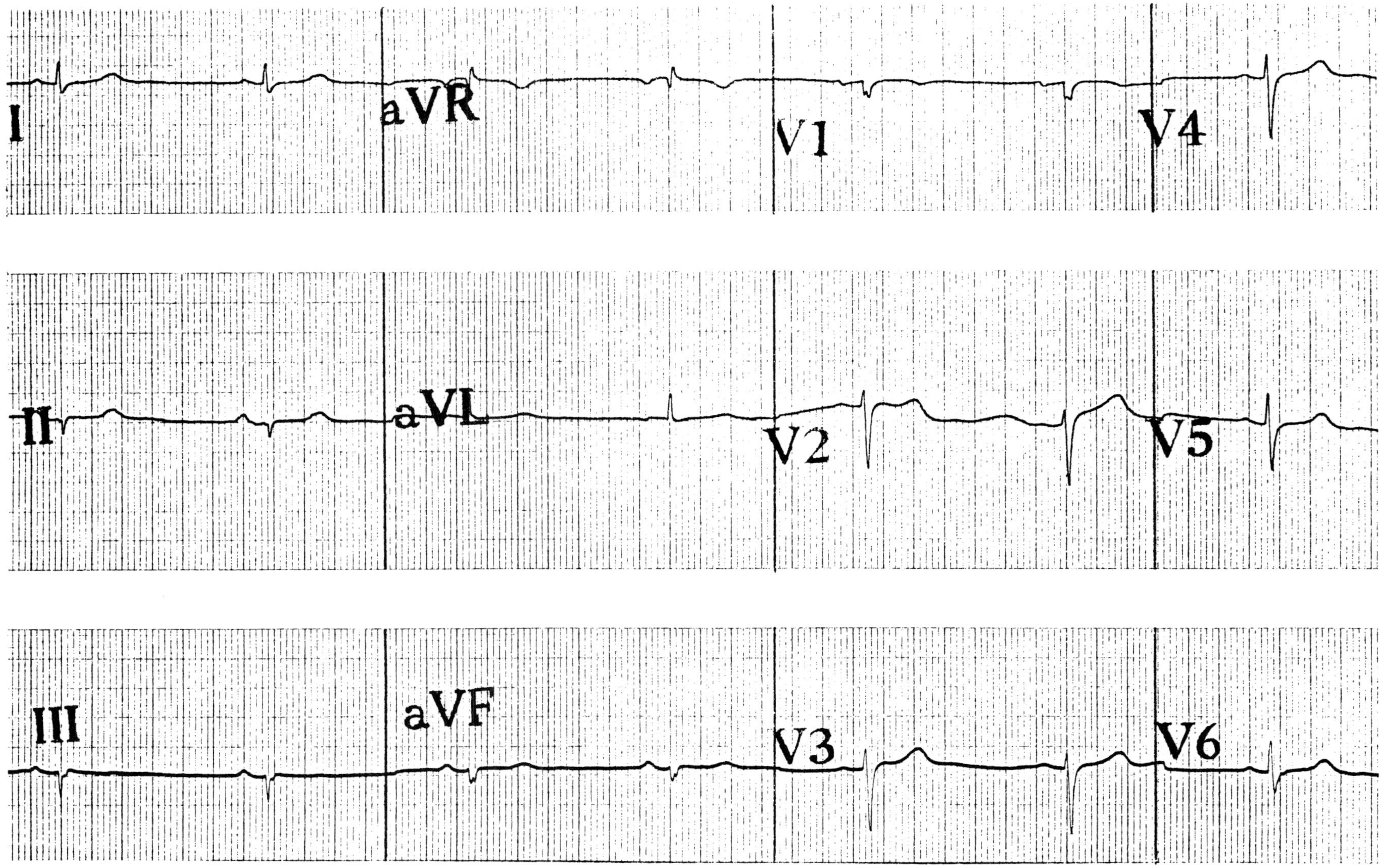

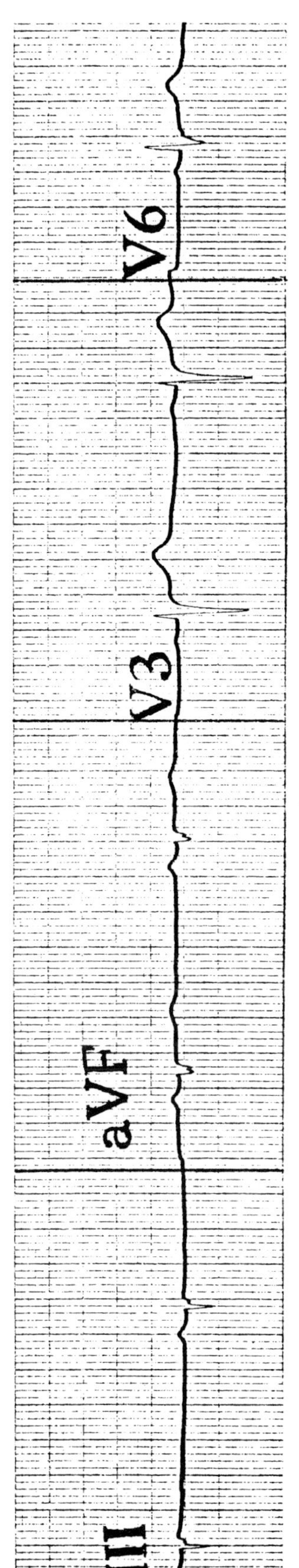

Figure 49–11 ECGs Illustrating the Phenomenon of Postpacing T-Wave Changes. *Note:* These 12-lead ECGs were recorded from a 72-year-old woman before (*A*) and one week after (*B*) implantation of a permanent demand right ventricular endocardial pacing system. The nonspecific inversion of the T waves in leads II, III, aVF, and V₃ through V₆ suggests an interval ischemic process, although none had occurred. Such T-wave abnormalities occurring following a period of ventricular pacing are termed postpacing T-wave changes.

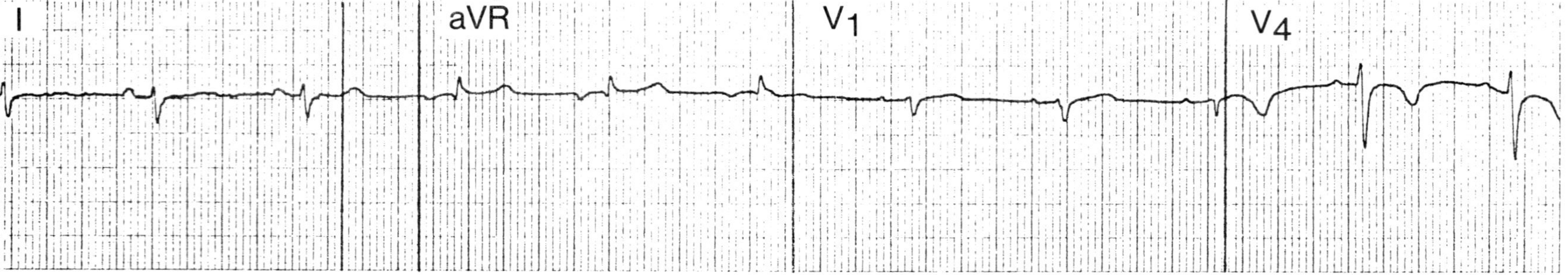
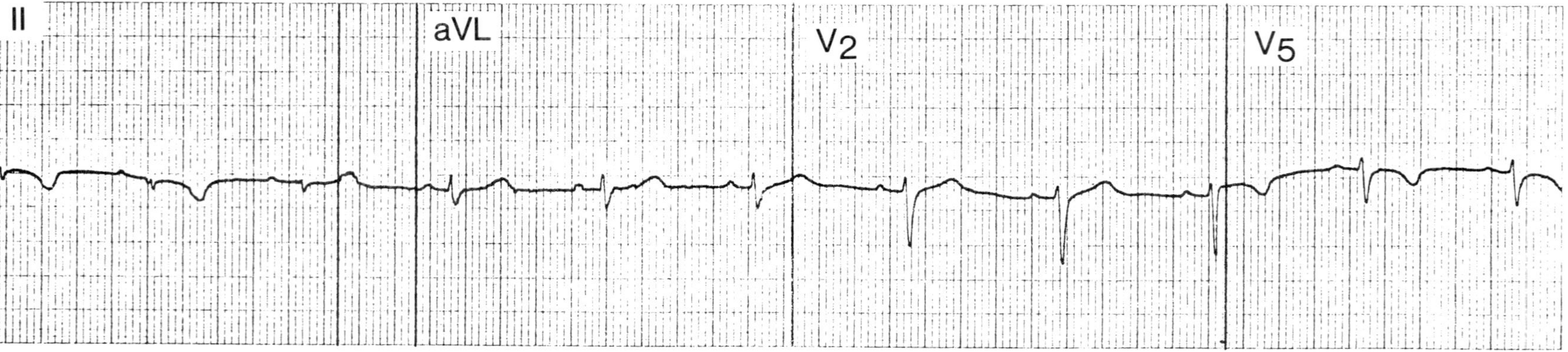
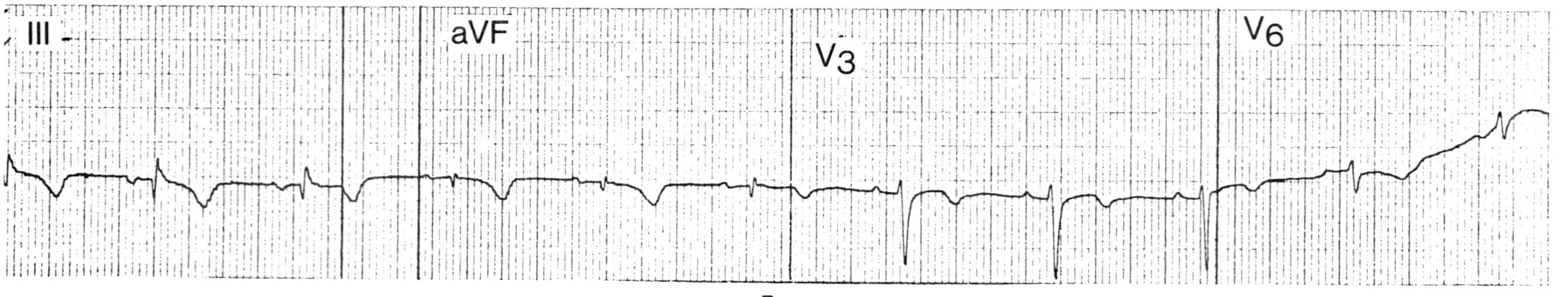

Figure 49–11   continued

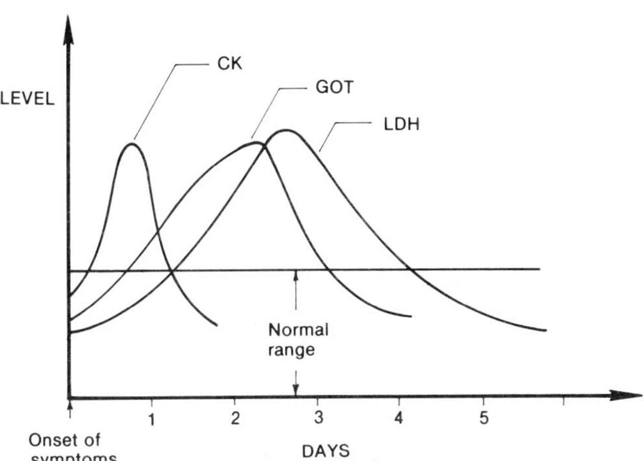

Figure 49–12 Time Courses of Serum Enzyme Levels in a Patient with Acute Myocardial Infarction.

Serum Enzyme Levels

Determination of the serum levels of enzymes that originate in the myocardium may help establish the presence of recent myocardial necrosis. The enzymes commonly measured are the creatine kinase (CK), glutamic-oxalacetic transaminase (GOT), and lactic dehydrogenase (LDH). As shown in Figure 49–12, however, the time courses of the levels of these enzymes is such that all may be within normal limits within the first several hours of acute myocardial infarction. Furthermore, CK also exists in skeletal muscle, brain, and kidney; GOT, in skeletal muscle, brain, kidney, and liver; and LDH, in red blood cells, skeletal muscle, kidney, and liver. Therefore, elevations in the serum levels of one or more of these enzymes may reflect skeletal muscle, cerebral, renal, hepatic, or erythrocyte injury rather than myocardial necrosis. A firm diagnosis of evolving myocardial infarction may require determination of the serum levels of the myocardium-specific isoenzymes (CK, MB, and LDH_1), measurements that are expensive and usually take several hours to perform. For these reasons, the decision on admitting a patient to the hospital with a suspected acute myocardial infarction should not depend on the results of serum enzyme determinations alone.

EMERGENCY DEPARTMENT MANAGEMENT OF THE PATIENT WITH ACUTE MYOCARDIAL INFARCTION

Cardinal in the management of the patient with acute myocardial infarction is early consideration of the diagnosis, for the overwhelming majority of deaths from infarction occur within the first three to four hours of the onset of symptoms. Once the diagnosis has been established or is considered likely, attention must be directed toward (1) prevention, detection, and treatment of arrhythmias; (2) relief of symptoms; (3) maintenance of adequate circulation.

Clearly, a confident and reassuring manner on the part of the physician and other health care personnel who are attending the patient will be of inestimable value in the management of the patient's anxiety and discomfort. The physician should discuss the suspected diagnosis with the patient in simple terms, stating that, since the patient is in the hospital and under close observation, the outlook for survival and meaningful recovery is excellent. It should be explained that medications will be given to relieve the symptoms until they disappear spontaneously within the ensuing 12 to 24 hours and that plans are being made for admission to the coronary care unit as soon as practical. The usual treatments and environment to which the patient will be subjected in the coronary care unit should also be discussed.

ARRHYTHMIAS

Because arrhythmia is the most common cause of death from acute myocardial infarction, the cardiac rhythm must be continuously monitored. An intravenous infusion should be started immediately in case rapid antiarrhythmic medication administration is subsequently required. An electrical defibrillator should be positioned in close proximity to the patient. (See Chapter 55.)

Although initial experiences with cardiac rhythm monitoring of patients with acute myocardial infarction suggested that the occurrence of ventricular tachycardia and ventricular fibrillation could be anticipated from the occurrence of premature ventricular complexes, more recent studies suggest that they more commonly occur without any "warning" arrhythmia. This has prompted the practice of administering prophylactic lidocaine to all patients with documented or strongly suspected acute myocardial infarction.[7] Specifically, lidocaine is administered intravenously (IV) in an initial bolus dose of 1 to 1.5 mg/kg over approximately one to three minutes; then an IV infusion of about 30 μg/kg/minute is started. For the average 70-kg person, this translates into an initial dose of 70 to 100 mg and a continuous infusion of about 2 mg/minute. Lidocaine in these doses may prevent the occurrence of ventricular tachycardia and fibrillation without much risk of serious side-effects.

If premature ventricular complexes appear despite these doses of lidocaine, the administration of the medication changes from prophylactic to therapeutic; therefore, a repeat bolus of 1 to 1.5 mg/kg (70 to 100 mg) over one to three minutes and an increase in the rate of infusion to about 55 µg/kg/minute (4 mg/minute) is advised. However, these quantities of lidocaine may induce serious side-effects, such as tinnitus, acute loss of hearing, diplopia, blurred vision, paresthesias, light-headedness, disorientation, twitching, convulsions, respiratory depression, and hypotension.

If premature ventricular complexes or brief (i.e., several second) runs of ventricular tachycardia occur even after the patient has received the above-mentioned doses of lidocaine, then procainamide is administered in a loading dose of about 5 to 15 mg/kg (350 to 1,000 mg for the 70-kg person) at a rate of about 25 to 50 mg/minute. After the loading dose has been given, the procainamide may be administered by continuous IV infusion at a rate of about 30 to 40 µg/kg/minute (2 to 3 mg/minute for the 70-kg person). Usually, the only serious side-effect encountered with the IV administration of procainamide is hypotension. The hypotension is due to vasodilatation, which is generally successfully reversed by slowing the rate at which the medication is being given or by stopping it altogether. In rare instances, however, restoration of adequate blood pressure may require the administration of IV fluids or vasoconstrictor medications, such as dopamine and norepinephrine.

If ventricular tachycardia occurs prior to the administration of antiarrhythmic medication, the lidocaine or procainamide should be administered in the previously discussed dosages so long as the patient's hemodynamic state is adequate. During this time, a sharp blow may be given to the precordium, for this maneuver occasionally terminates ventricular tachycardia. If ventricular tachycardia persists despite the IV administration of lidocaine and procainamide, and despite the precordial blow, then direct current cardioversion is in order. The patient should be given the minimum amount of IV diazepam (Valium) or thiopental (Pentothal) needed to achieve amnesia. If the patient is hemodynamically stable, a 10 to 50 watt-second electrical discharge synchronized to the QRS complex may be applied across the chest, as it will usually restore sinus rhythm. However, if ventricular tachycardia is causing severe hemodynamic deterioration, a 400 watt-second *nonsynchronized* discharge should be applied across the chest. If this shock precipitates ventricular fibrillation, the ventricular fibrillation can usually be terminated by immediately repeating the 400 watt-second nonsynchronized discharge.

If ventricular fibrillation that occurs spontaneously or in response to an attempted electrical termination of ventricular tachycardia cannot be terminated with repeated 400 watt-second nonsynchronized electrical discharges, then chemical defibrillation may be attempted by giving bretylium tosylate (Bretylol), 5 to 10 mg/kg (about 350 to 700 mg for the 70-kg person), IV as rapidly as possible while the patient is treated for cardiac arrest with closed chest cardiac massage, respiratory support, correction of metabolic abnormalities, and repeated precordial shocks. If ventricular fibrillation still cannot be terminated, or if it recurs after initial termination, another dose, 5 mg/kg (about 350 mg), may be given IV as rapidly as possible. Doses of up to 10 mg/kg (about 700 mg) may be given rapidly every 15 to 30 minutes, up to a total dose of 30 mg/kg (about 2,100 mg) before the patient is considered untreatable.

Bretylium tosylate may also be useful in preventing recurrences of ventricular tachycardia and ventricular fibrillation when lidocaine and procainamide fail to do so. In this situation, it is recommended that a loading dose of 5 to 10 mg/kg (350 to 700 mg) be given IV over a period of more than eight minutes; the slow rate of administration is aimed at minimizing the nausea and vomiting that may occur with more rapid injection. Maintenance dosage may be given by continuous IV infusion at rates of 1 to 2 mg/minute or by six hourly boluses of 5 to 10 mg/kg (350 to 700 mg) over a period of more than eight minutes.

Bretylium tosylate administration may initially result in transient increases in blood pressure and ventricular ectopy, usually lasting for periods of several minutes. The drug's most serious undesirable effect is significant hypotension, which may occur with dosages inadequate for suppression of ventricular arrhythmias; since this effect is due to vasodilatation, it is often exacerbated by the upright position. For these reasons, it seems prudent to restrict use of this medication to the treatment of hospitalized patients, except in the prehospital treatment of intractable and recurrent ventricular fibrillation.

Slowing of the sinus rate often occurs within minutes to hours after the onset of acute myocardial infarction involving, usually, the inferior wall of the heart. The mechanism is presumably enhanced parasympathetic input into the sinus node, for appropriate acceleration of sinus rate usually follows atropine administration. Therefore, if slow sinus rates are contributing to inappropriately low cardiac output or blood pressure, or to the predisposition to ventricular arrhythmias, atropine may be administered rapidly IV in doses of 0.5 to 2 mg. The few reported instances in which ventricular fibrillation occurred soon after the IV administration of atropine to patients with acute myocardial infarction should not preclude the use of this medication when slow heart rates are responsible for significant problems.[8] If cardiac standstill (an event that carries about an 85 percent mortality) occurs, the treatment of cardiac arrest should be commenced.

Disadvantageously slow ventricular rates may also

occur in the early hours of acute myocardial infarction because of second- and third-degree atrioventricular block. The appearance of second-degree atrioventricular block heralds the onset of complete atrioventricular block, which may occur within minutes to hours. In inferior wall infarction, the site of atrioventricular block is usually the atrioventricular node, and the second-degree atrioventricular block is of the Mobitz Type I (Wenckebach) variety; during complete atrioventricular block, the emerging escape pacemaker originates within the atrioventricular junction (His bundle) and has an automatic rate of about 35 to 45/minute (Figs. 49–13 and 49–14). If the ventricular rate occurring during the second- or third-degree AV block in inferior wall myocardial infarction is judged to be inadequately slow, atropine, 0.5 to 2 mg IV "push," or isoproterenol, 0.5 to 4 µg/minute by continuous IV infusion may be administered. Either medication may effect either an improvement in atrioventricular conduction or a mild to modest acceleration of the junctional rhythm. However, serious consideration should be given to establishing temporary demand ventricular pacing, which is the safest and most effective therapeutic modality for ensuring adequate ventricular rates in this setting in which the conduction disturbance is almost always transient and the left ventricular performance is not usually severely depressed.

In anterior wall myocardial infarction the sites of second- and third-degree atrioventricular block are usually the proximal portions of the bundle branches that lie within the infarcting myocardium. The second-degree atrioventricular block is Mobitz Type II; during complete atrioventricular block, the emerging escape pacemaker originates in the distal portion of a bundle branch or fascicle, or in Purkinje fibers, and usually has a dangerously slow rate of about 20 to 40/minute (Fig. 49–15). While isoproterenol administered in doses of 0.5 to 4 µg/minute by continuous IV infusion may rarely improve atrioventricular conduction or increase the rate of the escape pacemaker to an adequate level, this medication should be used only as a temporizing measure— a temporary ventricular pacing system should be established with dispatch. The majority of patients with anterior wall myocardial infarction complicated by complete atrioventricular block have cardiogenic shock related to extensive myocardial necrosis; thus, the mortality rate in these patients is high even when bradycardia is prevented by pacing.

MANAGEMENT OF SYMPTOMS

Most patients with acute myocardial infarction suffer chest discomfort that may be only bothersome, but more commonly is quite severe. Relief of the discomfort and alleviation of the anxiety that usually accompanies acute myocardial infarction are important not only for humanitarian reasons, but also for medical reasons. A reduction in pain and anxiety results in a decrease in the secretion of catecholamines, which predispose to arrhythmias and increase myocardial oxygen demand by increasing heart rate, contractile state, and wall tension (via their peripheral vasoconstrictive effects).

Morphine sulfate continues to be the most widely used analgesic for patients with acute myocardial infarction and is generally administered IV in doses of 2 to 3 mg every four to five minutes until pain relief is adequate, or until blood pressure falls to undesirably low levels. Usually, 8 to 25 mg are required as an effective initial dose. Meperidine hydrochloride (Demerol) is also widely used in this setting and is generally administered IV in doses of 15 to 20 mg every four to five minutes to the same end points. Both morphine sulfate and Demerol must be used with great caution in patients who have hypotension and/or bradycardia, for these medications may exacerbate the abnormalities. Furthermore, presumably because of their effects on vagal nuclei, both medications may result in bradycardia, hypotension, nausea, and vomiting. These drug-induced problems can generally be reversed within seconds to minutes by the IV administration of atropine in doses of 0.5 to 2 mg. Atropine appears to be more effective than the phenothiazine antiemetic medications in abolishing nausea related to the administration of morphine and Demerol; clinical experience suggests that this medication does not measurably increase the predisposition to ventricular tachycardia and fibrillation.

Diazepam (Valium) may be useful in the management of the patient who manifests an unacceptably high level of anxiety despite adequate relief of chest discomfort. In the acute situation, this medication may be administered IV in doses of 1 to 5 mg at a rate no more than 1 mg every two to three minutes. More rapid IV administration may result in hypotension, respiratory arrest, obtundation, and undesirably long periods of oversedation. In the less acute situation, Valium may be given orally in doses of 2 to 10 mg, depending on the level of anxiety, the age of the patient, the presence of associated diseases that might alter metabolism of the medication, and the hemodynamic state.

Currently, the sublingual and IV administration of nitroglycerin is gaining wider usage in patients with acute myocardial infarction. The theory is that nitroglycerin may favorably alter the balance between myocardial oxygen supply and demand, and thereby diminish the area of myocardial ischemia and the chest discomfort related to the ischemia. While the beneficial effect of nitroglycerin in the relief of chest discomfort due to reversible myocardial ischemia is clearly documented,

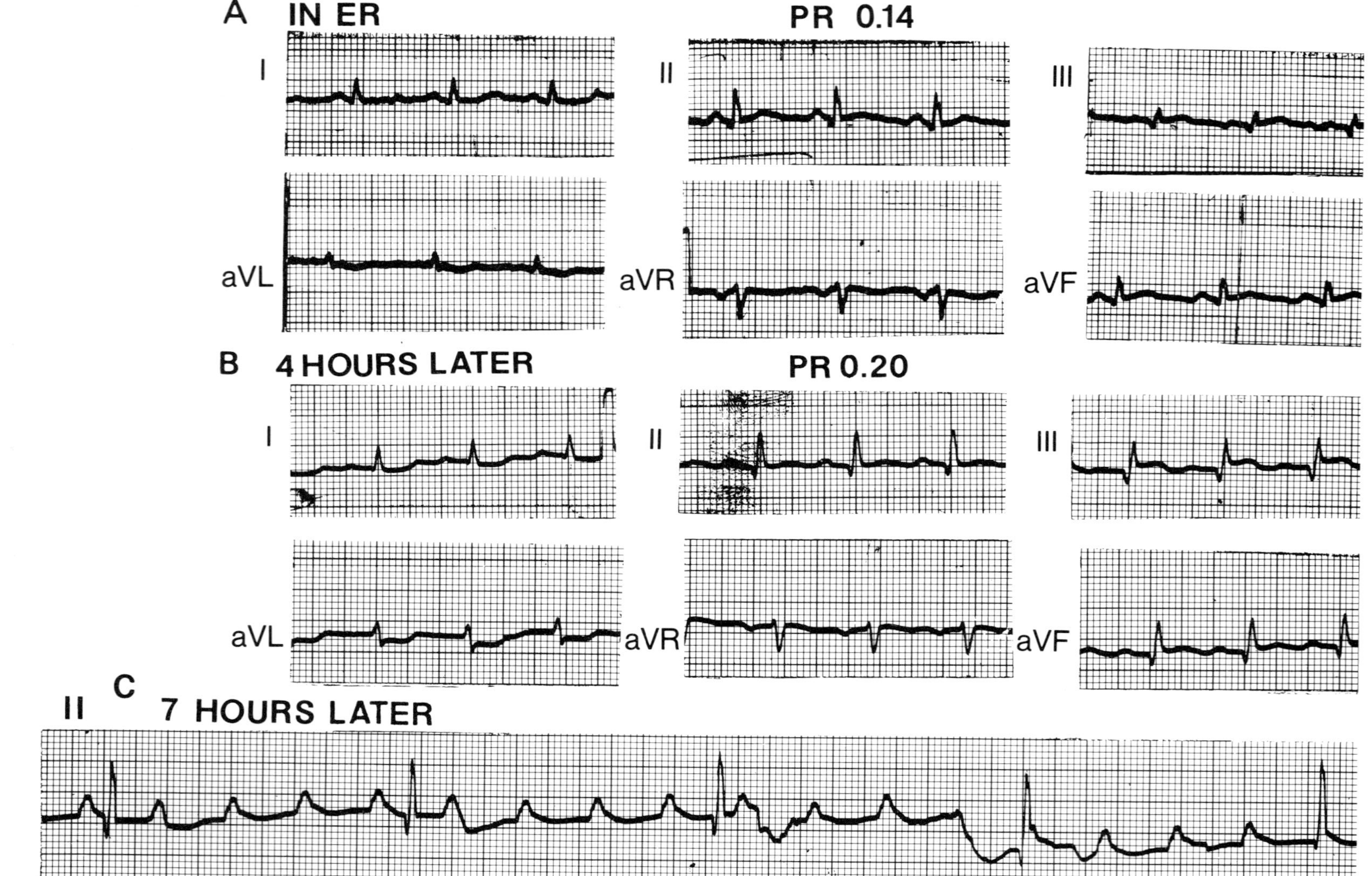

Figure 49–13   ECGs from a Patient with Acute Inferior Wall Myocardial Infarction. *Note:* These ECGs were recorded from a 44-year-old man with an acute inferior wall myocardial infarction. *A* When the patient was first seen in the emergency department, there were mild ST segment elevations in leads II and III, and mild ST segment depressions in leads V_2 and V_3, compatible with an acute ischemic process. *B* The same leads, recorded four hours later, show more dramatic ST segment abnormalities and document an increase in the PR interval from 0.14 to 0.20 seconds. *C* Seven hours later, there is complete atrioventricular block with a junctional rhythm occurring at a rate of about 31 beats/minute. The sinus rate is now very rapid, about 130 beats/minute, because atropine and isoproterenol have been administered in an unsuccessful attempt to improve AV conduction and to increase the rate of the junctional rhythm.

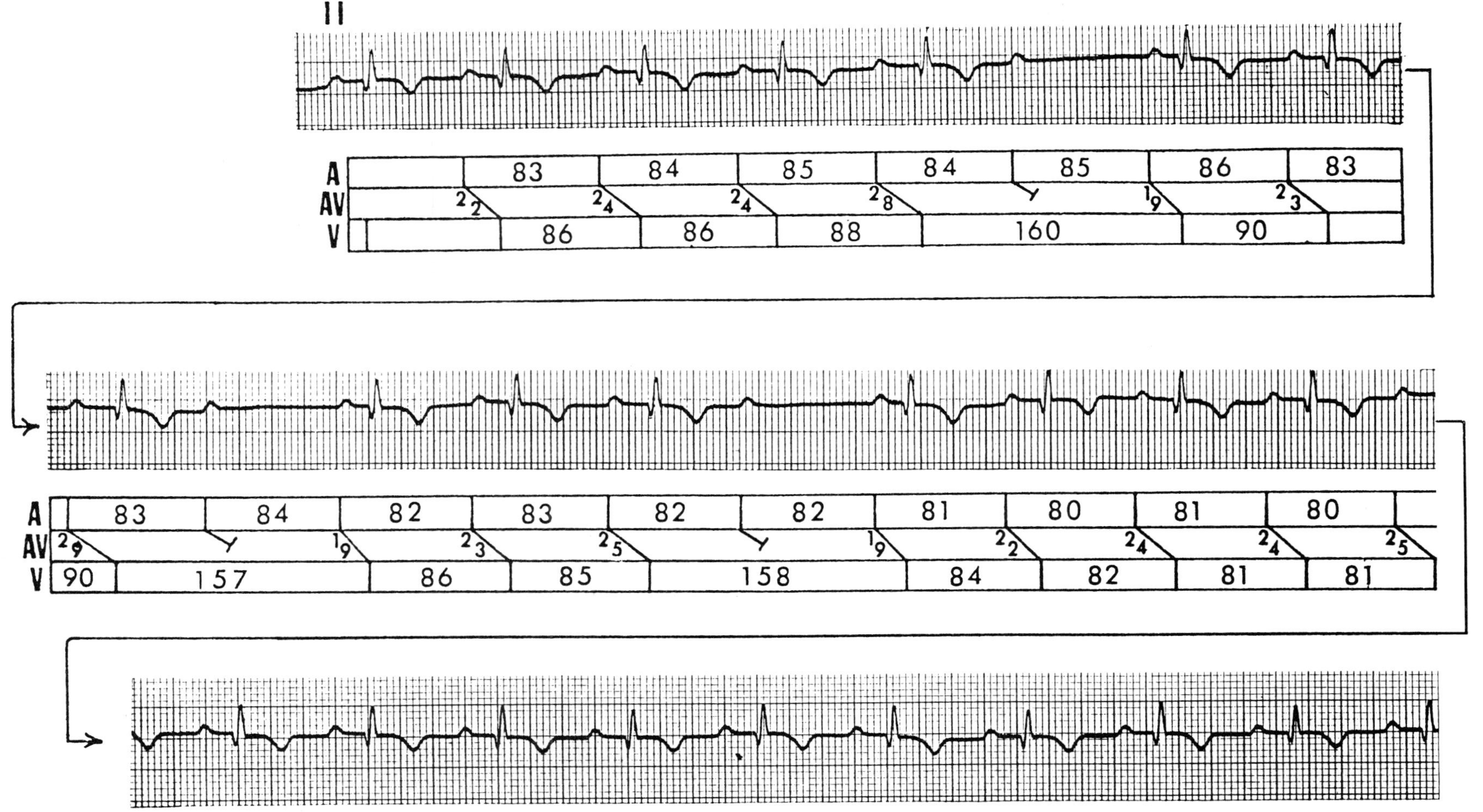

Figure 49–14 AV Wenckebach Periods Occurring in a Man with an Inferior Wall Myocardial Infarction. *Note:* These three continuous strips were recorded nine days later from the same patient whose ECGs are displayed in Figure 49–13. Atrioventricular conduction has returned, but there are periods of Mobitz Type I (Wenckebach) second-degree atrioventricular block. (*Source:* Reprinted with permission from Jacobson LB, Goldschlager N: *Arrhythmias: Case Studies.* Garden City, NY, Medical Examination Publishing Co, 1978.)

A ON ARRIVAL IN ER

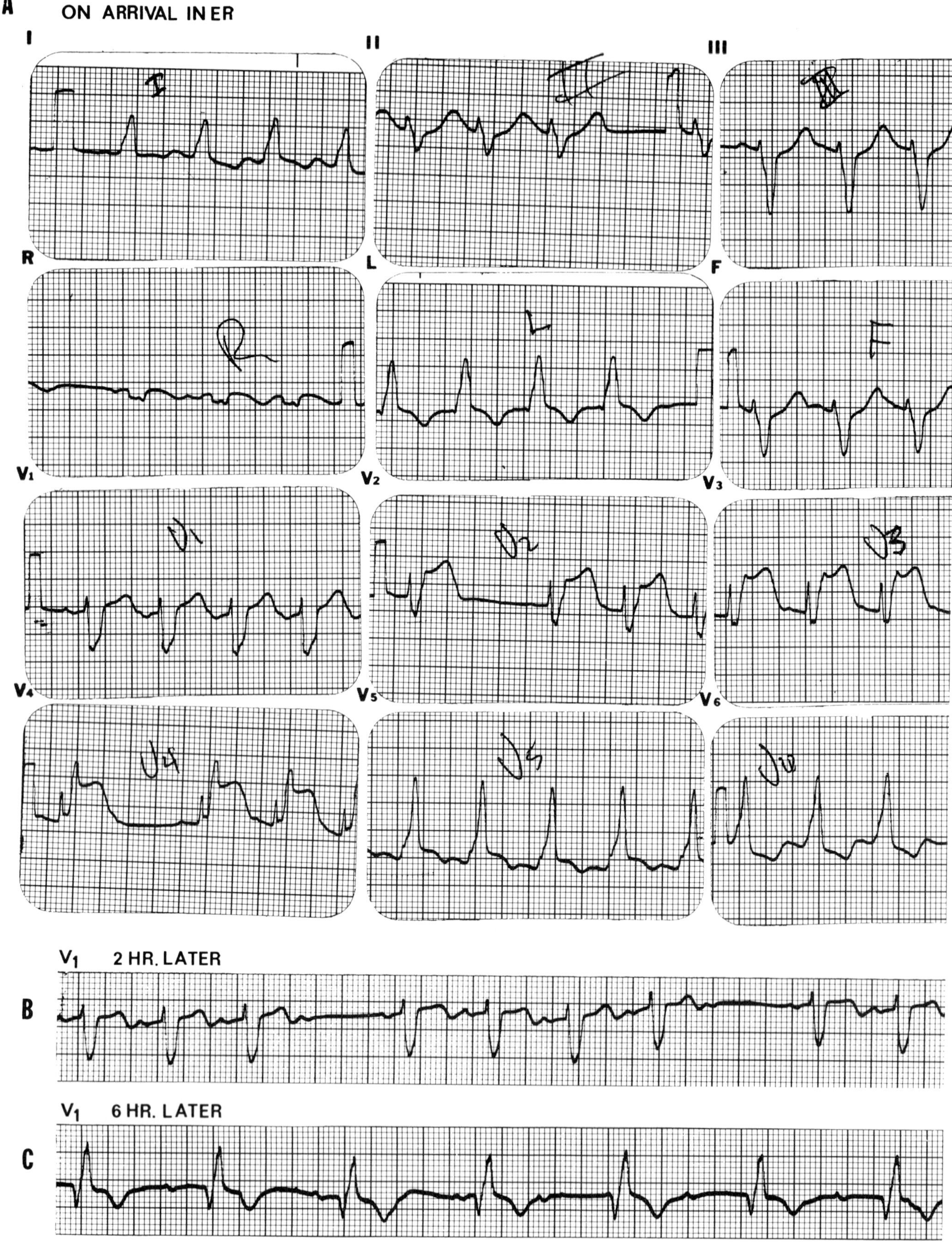

Figure 49–15

its effectiveness in relieving chest discomfort in patients with acute myocardial infarction is still unclear.

MANAGEMENT OF HEMODYNAMIC ABNORMALITIES

The prime function of the cardiovascular system is to provide adequate blood flow at appropriate perfusion pressure to the tissues of the body. The cardiac output (i.e., the volume of blood ejected into the circulation by the heart in a minute's time) is the product of the stroke volume (i.e., the volume of blood ejected by the left ventricle with each systole) and the heart rate. The systemic arterial blood pressure is the product of the cardiac output and the total systemic arterial resistance (TSR). The complex mechanisms that regulate heart rate, stroke volume, and TSR may be dramatically altered by endogenous physiologic events such as occur with acute myocardial infarction and by therapeutic interventions.

In sinus rhythm, heart rate depends on the intrinsic function of the sinus node and on the responses of the sinus node to neurohumoral autonomic nervous system traffic. Sympathetic stimuli increase and parasympathetic stimuli decrease the automatic firing rate of the sinus node, while beta-adrenergic blocking agents slow and parasympatholytic agents accelerate it. Thus, heart rate can be altered by modifying the autonomic milieu.

TSR is determined by the sum total of the cross-sectional areas of arterioles perfusing all body tissues. The size of an arteriole perfusing a particular tissue is regulated by the relative influences of vasoconstrictor and vasodilator stimuli acting in response to events that may originate within or distant from the particular tissue. As the stimuli mediating local vascular events may be neurohumoral transmitters (e.g., adrenalin, noradrenalin, acetylcholine) released by the autonomic nervous system or vasoactive materials (e.g., adenosine, histamine, hydrogen ion, potassium, angiotensin) produced by metabolic events, therapeutic alteration of TSR generally involves the administration of medications that antagonize the effects of endogenous vasoactive materials.

The left ventricular stroke volume has three determinants: (1) the preload, (2) the contractile state, and (3) the afterload. The preload is the size, or volume, of the left ventricle at end diastole, when the myocardium begins to develop its systolic tension. The end diastolic volume is highly dependent on the circulating blood volume, the systemic venous tone, and the TSR, being higher when blood volume is elevated and venous tone and TSR are high, and lower when blood volume is decreased and venous tone and TSR are low. The contractile state of the left ventricular myocardium will be defined below. The afterload is the tension that the left ventricular myocardium must generate in order to open the aortic valve and eject blood into the aorta. Left ventricular wall tension is inversely proportional to the thickness of the left ventricular myocardium, and it is directly proportional to the product of the pressure generated by the left ventricle and its radius during preejection and ejection periods. Because left ventricular wall tension is related to the size of the left ventricle, it follows that afterload is dependent on preload. Furthermore, as the pressure that the left ventricle must generate is directly related to the diastolic pressure in the aorta at the onset of ejection, it follows that afterload is highly dependent on TSR.

The relationship of stroke volume to preload, contractile state, and afterload are shown in the ventricular function curves of Figures 49–16 through 49–18. In Figure 49–16, the contractile state of the left ventricle is defined in terms of stroke volume and end diastolic volume. At any end diastolic volume, the greater the stroke volume, the better the contractile state of the left ventricle. Figure 49–16 also illustrates the Frank-Starling phenomenon, i.e., that stroke volume increases with increments in end diastolic volume in both normal and depressed contractile states. However, for a given increment in end diastolic volume, the increment in stroke volume is greater with better contractile function.

Acute myocardial ischemia and infarction, by reducing the amount of functioning left ventricular myocardium, depresses left ventricular performance; the left ventricle then operates on a ventricular function curve that lies below that on which it was operating prior to the ischemic event. The degree of depression of left ventricular performance is generally proportional to the amount of infarcted tissue, although the location of the

---

Figure 49–15   ECGs from a Patient with Acute Anterior Wall Myocardial Infarction. *Note:* These ECGs were recorded from a 72-year-old woman with acute anterior wall myocardial infarction. *A.* This 12-lead ECG, which was recorded shortly after the patient's arrival in the emergency department, shows an extensive anterior wall injury pattern, suggesting the acute infarction. In addition, there is left bundle branch block with left axis deviation and pauses in QRS rhythm due to Mobitz Type II second-degree atrioventricular block. *B.* Two hours later, the sinus rate is slightly slower, allowing the Mobitz Type II block to be seen more clearly. *C.* Six hours later, there is complete atrioventricular block with a ventricular escape rhythm occurring at a rate of about 58 beats/minute. The somewhat rapid rate of this escape rhythm (which, showing a right bundle branch block pattern, probably originates near the left bundle branch) is probably contributed to by the high doses of isoproterenol and dopamine that the patient was receiving to support her circulation.

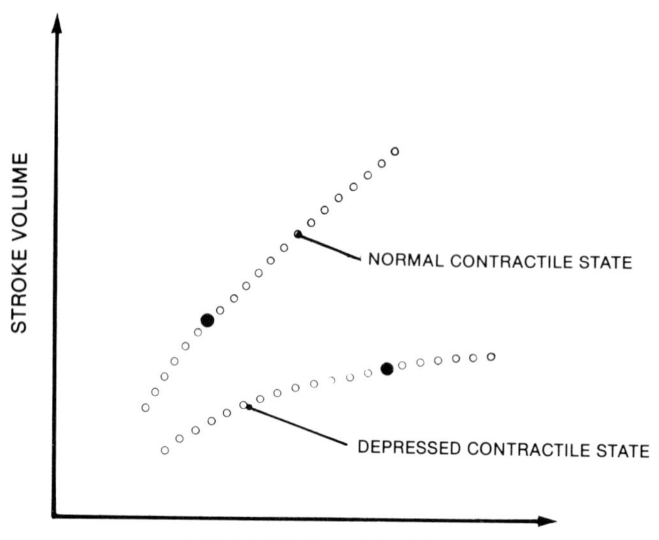

Figure 49–16 Ventricular Function Curves. *Note:* Ventricular function curves, constructed by plotting left ventricular stroke volume as a function of left ventricular end diastolic volume, illustrate the Frank-Starling mechanism of cardiac performance and define the contractile state of the left ventricle. The ventricular function curve of the left ventricle with depressed contractile state is flatter than and lies below that of the left ventricle with normal contractile state. The large, closed circles on each curve represent the stroke volume and end diastolic volume at which left ventricles with normal and depressed contractile states usually function in the basal resting state. The left ventricle with depressed contractile state usually operates at a higher end diastolic volume yet ejects a smaller stroke volume than the left ventricle with normal contractile state.

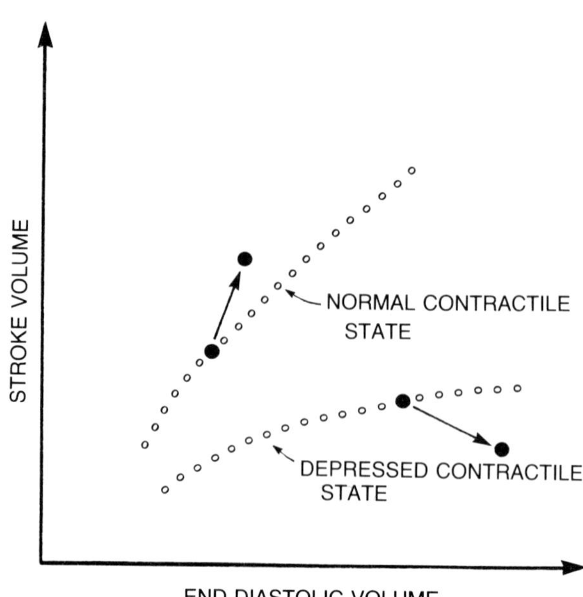

Figure 49–17 Ventricular Function Curves Showing the Effects of Increasing Afterload on the Relationship of Stroke Volume to End Diastolic Volume. *Note:* Ventricular function curves showing the effects of increasing afterload (by increasing arteriolar resistance) on end diastolic volume (EDV) and stroke volume (SV). Regardless of the contractile state of the left ventricle, increasing the afterload results in a larger end diastolic volume. However, whereas the increment in end diastolic volume effects an increase in stroke volume if the left ventricle has normal contractile function, it effects a decrease in stroke volume if the left ventricle has depressed contractile function.

infarction also appears to be important, with involvement of the interventricular septum and anterior wall appearing to have a greater depressant effect on performance than infarction of the inferior wall of comparable magnitude.

The closed circles in the normal and depressed ventricular function curves of Figure 49–16 represent the stroke volume and end diastolic volume usually present in the basal resting state of patients with normal and with chronically depressed left ventricular contractile function. The left ventricle with depressed contractile state generally performs at an end diastolic volume that is much larger than normal, yet ejects a stroke volume that is somewhat less than normal. Presumably, the left ventricle operates at the larger end diastolic volume in an attempt to normalize stroke volume. However, functioning at high end diastolic volume has deleterious consequences. Figure 49–19 displays the exponential relationship of diastolic left ventricular pressure to the diastolic volume of the chamber. When the left ventricular diastolic volume is normal, left ventricular diastolic pressure is low. As diastolic volume increases above normal, the diastolic pressure rises; the greater the initial volume, the greater will be the increment in pressure for a given increment in volume. At high diastolic volume, even small increments in volume result in dramatic rises in diastolic pressure to extremely high levels. As pressure in the pulmonary veins must exceed the diastolic left ventricular pressure if blood is to flow in the proper direction, the pulmonary venous pressure may rise to levels at which pulmonary congestion and pulmonary edema occur.

The exponential shape of the diastolic pressure-volume curve has important therapeutic implications, for at very high filling pressures even small decrements in diastolic volume, which may be achieved by venodilatation, diuresis, phlebotomy, or reductions in TSR, dramatically decrease left ventricular diastolic and pulmonary venous pressures. Acute myocardial infarction generally causes a shift of the left ventricular diastolic pressure-volume curve upward and to the left. The magnitude of the displacement is roughly proportional to the magnitude of infarcted tissue. Thus, at any given diastolic volume, diastolic pressure is higher with an

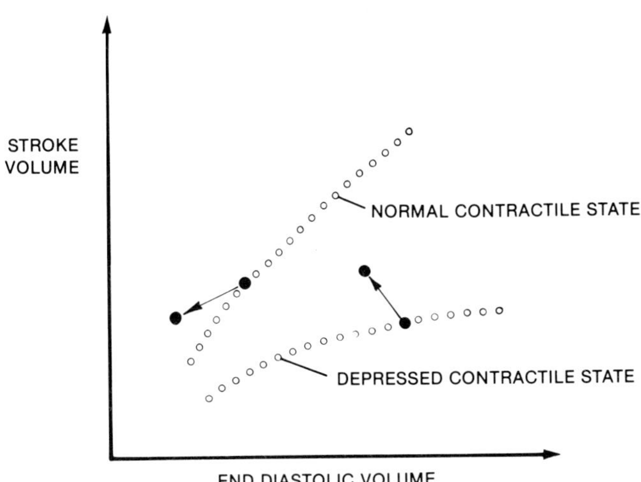

Figure 49–18   Ventricular Function Curves Showing the Effects of Decreasing Afterload on the Relationship of Stroke Volume to End Diastolic Volume. *Note:* Ventricular function curves showing the effects of decreasing afterload (by decreasing arteriolar resistance) on EDV and SV. Regardless of the contractile state of the left ventricle, decreasing afterload results in a smaller end diastolic volume. However, whereas the decrement in end diastolic volume effects a slight decrease in stroke volume when left ventricular contractile state is normal, it effects an increase in stroke volume when left ventricular contractile state is depressed.

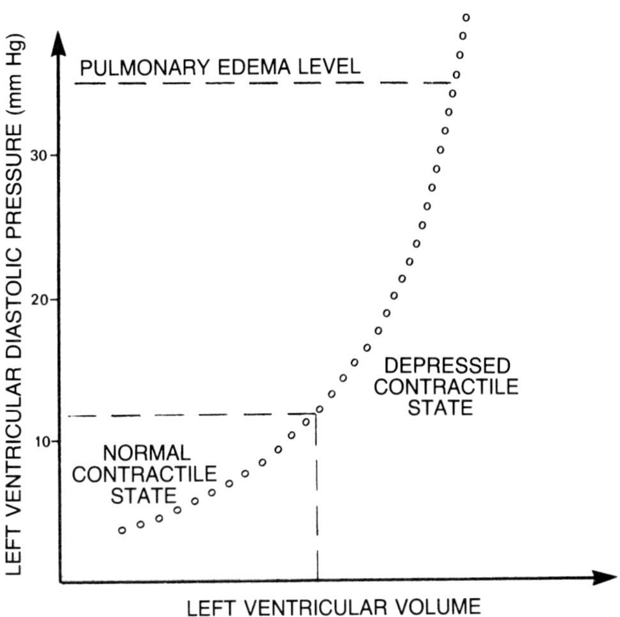

Figure 49–19   Exponential Relationship of Pressure to Volume in the Left Ventricle during Diastole. *Note:* The left ventricle with normal contractile state operates at lower diastolic volume and, therefore, at lower diastolic pressure than does the left ventricle with depressed contractile state. For a given increment in volume, the increment in pressure is greater if the initial volume is higher.

ischemic event than it was prior to the event. The larger the infarcted area, the greater the increment in pressure.

The ventricular function curves in Figure 49–18 display the relationships of stroke volume and end diastolic volume to increases in afterload achieved by raising TSR. Such increases in afterload effect increases in end diastolic volume regardless of the contractile state of the left ventricle. However, the rise in end diastolic volume is accompanied by an increase in stroke volume when contractile state is normal, but by a decrease in stroke volume when contractile state is depressed. Reducing afterload by lowering the TSR has the opposite effects, as shown in Figure 49–19. While it results in a reduction in end diastolic volume regardless of the contractile state, the reduction in end diastolic volume is accompanied by a fall in stroke volume when the contractile state is normal, and by a rise in stroke volume when the contractile state is depressed. Reducing TSR is the most effective intervention for lowering the diastolic pressure in and increasing the stroke volume from a left ventricle with depressed contractile state that is operating at high end diastolic volume.

Essential in the management of the patient with acute myocardial infarction is the achievement and maintenance of a hemodynamic state in which tissue perfusion is adequate and pulmonary venous pressure is not unduly elevated. The adequacy of tissue perfusion is generally assessed by measurement of the arterial blood pressure, palpation of the central (femoral and carotid) and peripheral (brachial, radial, tibial) pulses to determine their volume and contour, by examination of the skin on the trunk and on the extremities to assess its temperature and to observe its color, by verbal interaction with the patient to evaluate cerebral function (which reflects cerebral blood flow), and by measurement of urine output (which reflects renal perfusion). If the blood pressure is normal; the pulses of normal contour and volume; the skin pink, warm, and dry; the patient responding clearly and making urine, tissue perfusion may be judged to be adequate. On the other hand, if the blood pressure is low; the pulse thready; the skin pale, cool, and moist; the patient lethargic; and the urine output low, tissue perfusion is clearly inadequate.

Clinical assessment of the level of the pulmonary venous pressure is at best crude, as the physician is only able to observe the respiratory pattern and to examine the chest. Generally, if the respiratory pattern and the results of the chest examination are normal, the pulmonary venous pressure is probably not extremely high; if signs and symptoms of pulmonary edema are present, the pulmonary venous pressure is usually extremely elevated (greater than 30 mm Hg). However, the respiratory pattern and the results of the chest examination may be normal when the pulmonary venous pressure is significantly elevated (25 to 30 mm Hg) or even extremely low (less than 6 mm Hg). Also, when cardiac output is very low, and especially if acidemia is present, a patient may be tachypneic and dyspneic even when the pulmonary venous pressure is very low. Furthermore, the chest roentgenogram is of relatively little value in assessing the pulmonary venous pressure, partly because radiologic abnormalities often do not appear until several hours after a rise in and do not disappear until several days after a fall in the pulmonary venous pressure. For these reasons, and because the pulmonary venous pressure may be dramatically and abruptly altered by spontaneous or therapy-induced changes in left ventricular performance, TSR, venous tone, and circulating blood volume, accurate measurements of pulmonary venous pressure require direct measurement of the pulmonary artery wedge pressure. For this purpose, a balloon tipped end hole catheter (e.g., the Swan-Ganz catheter) is most commonly used. (See Chapter 71.)

Because the changes in hemodynamic state that accompany acute myocardial infarction depend on a multitude of interrelated factors, such as the circulating blood volume, the size of the infarction, the left ventricular performance prior to the event, and the autonomic nervous system responses to the event (i.e., in terms of altering heart rate, systemic venous tone, and TSR), frequent thorough reevaluations of the patient are essential.

MANAGEMENT OF HYPOTENSION AND INADEQUATE CARDIAC OUTPUT

Hypotension often occurs in the early hours of acute myocardial infarction, and its management depends on its mechanism. When hypotension reflects vasodilatation and bradycardia due to inappropriately high parasympathetic nervous system activity, atropine in doses of 1 to 2 mg IV usually resolves the problem. Leg raising and the IV administration of intravascular volume expanding fluids, such as normal saline, are helpful when vasodilatation and/or volume depletion is the mechanism. When hypotension occurs in the presence of normal heart rate and normal to elevated circulating blood volume and venous tone, the hypotension presumably reflects depressed left ventricular performance. In this case, the cautious administration of dopamine, a catecholamine with very strong alpha (i.e., peripheral vasoconstricting), very strong beta$_1$ (i.e., cardiac stimulating), and moderately strong beta$_2$ (i.e., peripheral vasodilating) properties may be used to raise the arterial

blood pressure to an acceptable level. Dopamine (Intropin) is administered by continuous IV infusion, beginning with 2 to 5 µg/kg/minute (150 to 350 µg/minute) and increasing the dose every one to two minutes until either an acceptable arterial pressure is achieved or a dose of about 50 µg/kg/minute (3,500 µg/minute) is reached. Higher doses do not generally improve the hemodynamic state and may predispose the patient to ventricular arrhythmias. When hypotension persists despite an adequate heart rate, normal to high circulating blood volume, adequate venous tone, and the administration of dopamine, norepinephrine may be given.

Norepinephrine (Levophed), a catecholamine with very strong alpha and beta$_1$ properties but no beta$_2$ activity, is administered by continuous IV infusion, starting with a dose of 1 to 2 µg/minute. The dose is increased by about 0.5 µg/minute every three to four minutes until either an adequate arterial blood pressure is achieved or a dose of 10 µg/minute is reached. Doses of norepinephrine in excess of 10 µg/minute are not likely to improve the hemodynamic state and may produce such severe vasoconstriction that the cardiac output falls and perfusion of vital organs is dramatically reduced. Normovolemic patients who remain hypotensive despite high doses of dopamine and norepinephrine have a very poor prognosis, because left ventricular performance is severely depressed. As both norepinephrine and dopamine may cause tissue necrosis if they extravasate, these medications are delivered into the central, rather than the peripheral, venous circulation.

Dobutamine (Dobutrex) is a synthetic catecholamine with very weak alpha, very strong beta$_1$, and moderately strong beta$_2$ properties. It has been shown to increase cardiac output and arterial blood pressure significantly when administered to patients who have low cardiac output and high intracardiac filling pressures in the settings of cardiac surgery and chronic left ventricular dysfunction of various etiologies.[9,10] While it has been documented to have similar beneficial effects in patients with acute myocardial infarction who are not hypotensive and whose cardiac outputs are not very low, documentation of its effects in acute myocardial infarction complicated by hypotension and severely depressed cardiac output is presently inadequate.[11]

A somewhat unusual cause of hypotension and inadequate cardiac output in the presence of high systemic venous pressure is infarction involving predominantly right ventricular myocardium. In this instance, the pulmonary venous pressure may be very low, presumably because the right ventricle cannot adequately eject blood through the pulmonary circulation into the left ventricle. Management involves IV fluid administration in volumes that ensure enough blood is delivered to the left ventricle to increase the left ventricular stroke volume. The diagnosis of right ventricular infarction as the cause of hypotension can be made *only* by direct measurements of intracardiac filling pressures.

MANAGEMENT OF CONGESTIVE HEART FAILURE

Acute myocardial ischemia and infarction may so profoundly depress left ventricular performance that left ventricular end diastolic pressure rises dramatically and results in pulmonary congestion or even pulmonary edema. The severe depression of left ventricular performance may be due to a very large area of ischemia in a previously normal heart, or to a small area of ischemia in a heart that previously had been functioning poorly. Patients with severe pulmonary venous hypertension are generally tachypneic and dyspneic because the interstitial and intra-alveolar edema results in abnormal lung compliance. If pulmonary edema is severe, blood gas exchange may be markedly impaired, resulting in severe hypoxemia and even hypercapnia. Patients with congestive heart failure may have high, normal, or low cardiac output, depending on the circulating blood volume, the systemic vascular resistance, and the degree to which left ventricular function is depressed. Those with dramatically low cardiac output and high intracardiac filling pressure qualify as having cardiogenic shock. (See Chapter 51.)

Treatment of the patient with pulmonary congestion involves ensuring adequate blood gases by the administration of

1. supplemental inspired oxygen
2. diuretics (such as Lasix, 20- to 80-mg IV push) in order to decrease the circulating blood volume, lower intracardiac filling pressures, and draw the intra-alveolar and pulmonary interstitial fluid back into the circulation
3. venodilators (such as sublingually administered nitroglycerin or isosorbide dinitrate, or intravenously administered Lasix) in order to diminish venous return to the heart and thereby diminish intracardiac filling pressures
4. arteriolar dilating agents such as sodium nitroprusside or trimethaphan camphorsulfonate (Arfonad) to reduce the impedance to left ventricular ejection, especially in the presence of hypertension or mitral regurgitation

Rotating tourniquets may be applied to the extremities to diminish venous return. The exact medications and maneuvers used should be selected on the basis of the severity of the pulmonary congestion, the degree of depression of cardiac output, and the arterial pressure. In the most ominous situation of extensive pulmonary

edema with respiratory depression, assisted or controlled ventilation with endotracheal intubation is appropriate.

Sodium nitroprusside (Nipride) is a rapidly acting, potent vasodilator that alters both venous and arteriolar tone. Its venodilating effect allows rapid lowering of intracardiac filling pressures; its arteriolar dilating effect rapidly lowers the impedance to left ventricular ejection, making it extremely useful in increasing forward stroke volume and reducing regurgitant volume when there is mitral insufficiency. It is also extremely useful in the treatment of pulmonary edema in the hypertensive patient. This medication is most widely used, however, in the management of acutely ill patients with high intracardiac filling pressures, low cardiac output, and poor left ventricular performance attributable to acute myocardial infarction or to a period of cardiopulmonary bypass during cardiac surgery.

Sodium nitroprusside is administered by continuous IV infusion, starting with a dose of 0.5 μg/kg/minute (35 μg/minute) and increasing the dose by about 0.5 μg/kg/minute every 5 to 10 minutes until the desired hemodynamic state is achieved or until the arterial pressure becomes undesirably low. In order to allow recognition of the achievement of an optimum hemodynamic state, and to avoid reaching an even more deleterious state than that present prior to administering this medication, it is essential to continuously monitor the arterial pressure and the left ventricular filling pressure (i.e., mean pulmonary artery wedge or pulmonary artery diastolic pressure). The maximum recommended dose of sodium nitroprusside is 10 μg/kg/minute (700 μg/minute), for doses in excess of this may result in tinnitus, blurred vision, and delirium related to thiocyanate toxicity. Higher doses than this may cause cyanide poisoning.

MANAGEMENT OF HYPERTENSION

A small percentage of patients with acute myocardial infarction have abnormally elevated blood pressures, which predisposes them to cardiac rupture and may increase the size of the evolving infarct by increasing myocardial oxygen demand. In many patients, the hypertension occurs in response to pain and anxiety, and the blood pressure falls to normal levels as analgesic medications relieve the pain and anxiety. When rapid lowering of the blood pressure is felt to be advisable, the cautious IV administration of sodium nitroprusside or Arfonad may lower blood pressure to a desirable level within minutes. Continuous monitoring of arterial pressure with an intra-arterial catheter is advised when such potent antihypertensive agents are used, however. In general, the hypertension that occurs in acute myocardial infarction lasts for only a few hours; thus, the oral or intramuscular administration of antihypertensive medications is inadvisable. Absorption may make them unavailable when needed, or their effects may become apparent at a time when they are not needed and are even perhaps detrimental.

THERAPIES OF DEBATABLE VALUE IN ACUTE MYOCARDIAL INFARCTION

Supplemental Inspired Oxygen

The administration of supplemental inspired oxygen to the patient with acute myocardial infarction has been a tradition and is likely to continue, even though its clinical benefit is unproved. However, it appears to be justified by the fact that hypoxemia is common in these patients. The hypoxemia generally reflects ventilation-perfusion ratio abnormalities within the lung. These abnormalities may be the result of (1) pulmonary interstitial and intra-alveolar edema; (2) the rapid small tidal volume respiratory pattern that occurs as a response to the discomfort or anxiety of the situation, or to pulmonary congestion or edema; and (3) the low pulmonary blood flow that may occur in the presence of low cardiac output or hypotension.

The aim of supplemental inspired oxygen administration is to ensure "adequate oxygenation," which generally means a systemic arterial oxygen saturation of greater than 95 percent (pO_2 greater than 70 mm Hg). Experimental studies of the effects of arterial oxygen tension on the size of an experimentally induced acute myocardial infarction suggest that the size of the infarct can be diminished when arterial oxygen tension is greater than normal. This beneficial effect has yet to be documented in the clinical setting, however. Of course, the administration of supplemental inspired oxygen to the patient with chronic obstructive pulmonary disease may result in CO_2 narcosis, so its use in such patients with acute myocardial infarction must be closely monitored.

Nitroglycerin

The effects of nitroglycerin in patients with acute myocardial infarction are currently being defined. When administered sublingually, this medication may act in one or two ways: (1) it may dilate systemic veins, causing venous pooling and decreased venous return to the heart; (2) it may dilate coronary arteries and thereby, perhaps, relieve obstruction in a vessel that has been totally occluded by a functional constriction in an area of severe anatomical stenosis. The systemic venodilating effect tends to decrease myocardial oxygen demand

by decreasing preload and wall tension; the coronary arterial dilating effect tends to increase coronary blood flow. Both effects should be beneficial to the patient with acute myocardial infarction. The potential risks of nitroglycerin administration are hypotension and vasovagal episodes, both of which may unpredictably accompany its use. It is still unclear whether nitroglycerin contributes to relief of chest discomfort associated with acute myocardial infarction, although it does help to relieve chest discomfort due to reversible myocardial ischemia, i.e., angina pectoris.

TRANSFER TO THE CORONARY CARE UNIT

Patients with suspected or documented acute myocardial infarction should be transferred to the coronary care unit (CCU) as soon as the CCU staff is prepared to assume responsibility for their care, but only when they are stable enough for the transfer. Patients who are having recurrent ventricular tachycardia or fibrillation that requires repeated electrical conversions should not be transferred, for the CCU offers no advantage over the emergency department in the management of a patient who is requiring almost continuous resuscitation.

Cardiac arrest occurs all too often in transit from the emergency department to the CCU, and the disadvantages of resuscitating a patient in a hallway or elevator are minimized if a transfer routine has been well rehearsed. Specifically, there must be at least two persons trained in cardiopulmonary resuscitation with the patient. The cardiac rhythm must be clearly displayed on an oscilloscope that is constantly in view of the accompanying personnel. Some monitoring devices generate an audible pulse of sound whenever a QRS complex is sensed, allowing auditory as well as visual monitoring of cardiac rhythm. The patient must be able to exercise reasonable self-control and to cooperate, or else be adequately sedated; the patient must not be thrashing about because of the risk of interfering with the ECG monitoring and with treatment. A portable defibrillator with electrode jelly must be placed on the bed or gurney so that it is immediately accessible if needed. An IV infusion must be functioning, and medications, such as lidocaine, atropine, and sodium bicarbonate must be readily available in clearly marked syringes. A portable oxygen tank, as well as equipment for endotracheal and nasotracheal intubation and for suction, must accompany the patient. The CCU staff should be informed of the time the patient departs from the emergency department in order to make themselves immediately available when the patient arrives.

REFERENCES

1. Maseri A, Severi S, DeNes M, et al: "Variant" angina: one aspect of a continuous spectrum of vasospastic myocardial ischemia. Pathogenetic mechanisms, estimated incidence and clinical and coronary arteriographic findings in 138 patients. *Am J Cardiol* 42:1019–1035, 1978.

2. Gunther S, Muller JE, Mudge GH Jr, et al: Therapy of coronary vasoconstriction in patients with coronary artery disease. *Am J Cardiol* 47:157–162, 1981.

3. Rentrop P, Blanke H, Karsch KR, et al: Selective intracoronary thrombolysis in acute myocardial infarction and unstable angina pectoris. *Circulation* 63:307–317, 1981.

4. Oliva PB, Breckinridge JC: Arteriographic evidence of coronary spasm in acute myocardial infarction. *Circulation* 56:366–374, 1977.

5. Braunwald E, Sobel BE: Coronary blood flow and myocardial ischemia, in Braunwald E (ed): *Heart Disease*. Philadelphia, WB Saunders Co, 1980, pp 1299–1301.

6. Rude RE, Muller JE, Braunwald E: Efforts to limit the size of myocardial infarcts. *Ann Intern Med* 95:736–761, 1981.

7. Harrison DC: Should lidocaine be administered routinely to all patients after acute myocardial infarction? *Circulation* 58:581–584, 1978.

8. Massumi RA, Mason DT, Amsterdam EA, et al: Ventricular fibrillation and tachycardia after intravenous atropine for treatment of bradycardia. *N Engl J Med* 287:336, 1972.

9. Leier CV, Webel J, Bush CA: The cardiovascular effects of the continuous infusion of dobutamine in patients with severe cardiac failure. *Circulation* 56:468–472, 1977.

10. Bendersky R, Chatterjee K, Parmley WW, et al: Dobutamine in chronic ischemic heart failure: alterations in left ventricular function and coronary hemodynamics. *Am J Cardiol* 48:555–558, 1981.

11. Gillespie TA, Ambos HD, Sobel BE, et al: Effects of dobutamine in patients with acute myocardial infarction. *Am J Cardiol* 39:588–594, 1977.

50. Disturbances in Cardiac Rhythm

LESTER B. JACOBSON, M.D., F.A.C.C., F.A.C.P.

Disturbances in cardiac rhythm are among the most common problems seen by emergency department physicians today. Arrhythmias may occur in infants as well as in the elderly, and in otherwise healthy persons as well as in the chronically or seriously ill. The arrhythmia may be of no clinical significance, or it may be of catastrophic proportions. Faced with a patient who may be having arrhythmias, the emergency department physician must (1) determine whether the patient has an arrhythmia at that moment and, if not, assess the likelihood that the patient has had an arrhythmia in the recent past or is likely to have one in the near future; (2) establish an accurate electrocardiographic diagnosis of the arrhythmia; (3) predict the clinical course of the arrhythmia in the individual patient; and (4) plan a course of management based on these considerations and on the patient's clinical condition and underlying cardiovascular status.

SYMPTOMS ATTRIBUTABLE TO ARRHYTHMIAS

Many symptoms are attributable to arrhythmias. Some patients simply have an awareness of cardiac action, commonly termed *palpitation*. The sensation may be a single pumping feeling in the chest that is due to premature beating, a fluttering in the chest that reflects premature beats occurring in rapid succession, cardiac irregularity that is due to the irregularity of the underlying rhythm as in atrial fibrillation, or a pounding in the chest that may occur with slow as well as rapid heart rates. It is clear that the regularity or irregularity, and the rapidity or slowness of the rhythm, as sensed by the patient may have little relationship to the exact cardiac cadence that is occurring.

Some patients with arrhythmias may be totally unaware of cardiac action, but rather complain of transient presyncope (lightheadedness, dimming of vision, nausea, loss of balance) or frank syncope. Others complain of paroxysmal or persistent and progressive shortness of breath, with or without signs and symptoms of obvious congestive heart failure. Still others experience chest discomfort suggesting myocardial ischemia. Some patients with arrhythmias, be they rapid or slow, paroxysmal or sustained, have no symptoms; rather, their arrhythmia may have been detected on a routine examination or a routine electrocardiographic tracing.

THE HEMODYNAMIC CONSEQUENCES OF CARDIAC ARRHYTHMIAS

While an awareness of cardiac action may be the major reason that a patient with an arrhythmia seeks medical assistance, it is the hemodynamic consequence of the arrhythmia that determines the morbidity and mortality associated with it. The prime function of the cardiovascular system is to provide adequate blood flow at appropriate perfusion pressure to the tissues of the body. The cardiac output, i.e., the volume of blood ejected into the circulation by the heart in a minute's time, is the product of the volume of blood ejected with each systole [stroke volume (SV)] and the heart rate

(HR). Thus, maintenance of adequate cardiac output requires an adequate stroke volume times heart rate product. Arterial blood pressure is the product of the cardiac output and the total systemic resistance (TSR). Thus, maintenance of adequate arterial pressure requires maintenance of an adequate SV × HR × TSR product.

As the ability of the heart to increase stroke volume is limited, a dramatic fall in heart rate (generally from normal to less than 30 to 40 beats/minute) may result in a sudden fall in cardiac output and, therefore, in blood pressure. Also, with the sudden onset of tachycardia (either supraventricular or ventricular) the stroke volume may fall so dramatically that cardiac output and, thus, blood pressure may fall to catastrophically low levels before reflex adjustments in capacitance (venous) and resistance (arteriolar) vessels can be made. The compensatory mechanisms include an increase in venous tone, which will increase intracardiac volume and thus stroke volume, and an increase in arteriolar resistance, which will increase the blood pressure.

In any individual patient, the hemodynamic consequences of and the symptoms related to a cardiac rhythm disturbance depend on many factors. These include the rate of the arrhythmia, the atrial and ventricular relationships during the arrhythmia, the functional state of the heart, the presence of coronary artery and cerebral vascular disease, the amount of extracellular fluid, the patient's posture and level of consciousness at the time the arrhythmia occurs, and the ability of the autonomic nervous system to make rapid adjustments to the alteration in cardiac rhythm, a response that may be vitally affected by vasoactive medications, such as vasodilator and antihypertensive agents. Symptoms attributable to the hemodynamic consequences of cardiac arrhythmias may be separated into three categories: (1) presyncope, syncope, and seizure, which reflect a sudden catastrophic fall in cerebral blood flow; (2) chest discomfort, which reflects myocardial ischemia; (3) dyspnea, which reflects pulmonary congestion due to high pulmonary venous pressure.

THE CARDIAC CONDUCTION SYSTEM

The cardiac conduction system may be viewed as having two portions. The upper, or supraventricular, part consists of the sinus node and the atrioventricular (AV) junction, which is comprised of the AV node and the bundle of His. The lower, or intraventricular, part consists of the bundle branches and their fascicles, which terminate in the Purkinje fibers that activate the ventricular myocardium.

Under normal circumstances, the sinus node, which lies at the junction of the superior vena cava with the right atrium, has the most rapid automatic firing rate of all cardiac electrical tissues. Thus, the cardiac depolarization process is normally initiated by electrical impulses arising in the sinus node. Impulses exiting the sinus node enter the right atrium, where they initiate an orderly sequence of depolarization of both right and left atrial tissue, right atrial activation beginning about 0.01 seconds before left atrial activation. The contour and duration of normal P waves reflect the normal atrial activation sequence. Abnormal anatomical sequences of atrial depolarization may result in P waves with contours and durations that differ from the norm.

Impulses traversing atrial tissue reach and enter the superior portion of the AV node, which lies near the tricuspid valve in the lower portion of the interatrial septum and the upper portion of the interventricular septum. It is still unclear whether atrial impulses travel from the sinus node to the AV node solely in atrial muscle or whether they also travel in specialized conduction pathways termed *internodal tracts*. The impulses travel in orderly fashion from the upper to the lower portion of the AV node. At the inferior portion of the AV node, the impulses enter the bundle of His, through which they travel to enter fibers of the right and left bundle branches. Fibers of the right bundle branch, which functionally consists of one fascicle, terminate in right ventricular myocardium. Fibers of the left bundle branch, which functionally consists of anterior, posterior, and sometimes septal fascicles, terminate in left ventricular and interventricular septal myocardium. Under normal circumstances, ventricular tissue is depolarized by impulses arriving via both right and left bundle branches. Ventricular activation by the left bundle branch fibers begins about 0.03 to 0.04 seconds before that by the right bundle branch fibers.

Ventricular tissue is initially depolarized simultaneously in three distinct areas: (1) the central portion of the left side of the interventricular septum, (2) the paraseptal anterior free left ventricular wall, and (3) the paraseptal posterior left ventricular wall. The depolarization process then spreads to involve the right side of the interventricular septum, the free right ventricular and free left ventricular walls, and finally the high lateral and posterior portions of the left ventricle. The contour and duration of normal QRS complexes reflect the normal anatomical sequence of ventricular activation. Abnormal sequences of ventricular depolarization may produce QRS complexes with contours and durations that differ from the norm.

Some patients have, in addition to the normal AV node-His-Purkinje system, another (accessory) pathway connecting atrial to ventricular tissue. Some accessory AV conduction pathways are capable of transmitting impulses from atrium to ventricle as well as from ventricle to atrium, while others can conduct impulses in only one direction. The tissue that comprises the accessory AV conduction pathways usually has properties similar to those of His-Purkinje system tissue and very different from those of the normal AV nodal tissue. Consequently, accessory AV conduction pathways may be able to conduct impulses more rapidly or in more rapid succession than the normal AV conduction system. (For further discussion of accessory AV conduction pathways, see The Wolff-Parkinson-White Syndrome.)

DIAGNOSIS OF THE ARRHYTHMIA

Accurate diagnosis of an arrhythmia is facilitated by first defining the ventricular (QRS) rhythm, then defining the atrial rhythm, and, finally, determining the relationships between the ventricular and atrial rhythms. From a practical point of view, it is helpful to determine whether an arrhythmia consists of ectopic beats, a bradycardia, or a tachycardia; and then whether the arrhythmia arises in supraventricular (sinus node, atrium, AV node, His bundle) or ventricular (bundle branch, ventricle) tissue. However, the emergency department physician facing a patient who appears to be seriously ill because of an arrhythmia that is not clearly definable may have to make an educated guess concerning the type of arrhythmia. In this endeavor, the clinical setting of the patient is of utmost importance, because specific arrhythmias occur with greater frequency in specific clinical settings. Table 50–1 indicates the arrhythmias that are more likely and that are less likely to occur in specific clinical settings.

ECTOPIC BEATS

P waves or QRS complexes that are stimulated by impulses arising outside the sinus node are termed *ectopic* complexes or beats. The contours of these ectopic P waves or QRS complexes initiated by ectopic impulses generally differ from the norm because the ectopic impulse results in an abnormal anatomical sequence of atrial or ventricular activation. The duration of an ectopic P wave is generally similar to that of a sinus-stimulated P wave, presumably because both sinus impulses and ectopic atrial impulses initially activate one small area from which depolarization must spread throughout atrial tissue. The duration of an ectopic QRS complex, however, is generally longer than normal, because it takes longer for all ventricular tissue to be activated when depolarization is initiated at a single site than it does when several different areas are activated almost simultaneously, as normally occurs with initial ventricular depolarization via a bundle branch.

TABLE 50–1 Arrhythmias Encountered in Specific Clinical Settings

Clinical Setting	More Likely	Less Likely
Acute myocardial infarction	PVCs, VT, VF, AV block	Atrial FIB, flutter, APCs, PSVT
Sick sinus syndrome	Sinus arrest, pauses, atrial FIB, flutter, APCs, PSVT	PVCs, VT, VF, AV block
Wolff-Parkinson-White syndrome	PSVT, atrial FIB, flutter	VT, VF, AV block

Key: APCs, atrial premature complexes; AV, atrioventricular; FIB, fibrillation; PSVT, paroxysmal supraventricular tachycardia; PVCs, premature ventricular complexes; VF, ventricular fibrillation; VT, ventricular tachycardia.

Atrial (Supraventricular) Premature Complexes or Beats

Ectopic atrial beats may occur one at a time as isolated events, in pairs, or in brief runs. They may initiate supraventricular tachyarrhythmias, or a brief or prolonged period of cardiac standstill. It is crucial to determine whether the ectopic atrial beat is premature and therefore indicates abnormal atrial irritability, or whether it occurs after a pause in atrial rhythm and thus is an escape mechanism that prevents prolonged pauses in rhythm.

An atrial premature complex (APC) can be recognized in the surface electrocardiogram (ECG) by the appearance of a P wave before the next sinus P wave is expected to occur (Fig. 50–1). While prematurity is quite easy to define when the sinus rhythm is reasonably regular, the presence of dramatic sinus arrhythmia makes the diagnosis of prematurity more difficult. The contours and axes of premature P waves are usually different from those of sinus P waves unless the premature atrial impulse arises in or near the sinus node, in which case it resembles the sinus P wave. The identification of a premature P wave may be difficult if the P wave falls in the ST segment or TU wave of the preceding QRSTU complex and is obscured by it, or if the sequence of atrial depolarization causes the P wave to be diminutive or isoelectric in the surface ECG lead being examined. Thus, it may be necessary to record more than one surface ECG lead in order to see premature P waves accurately (Fig. 50–1).

While isolated APCs may be bothersome to the patient because they cause an unpleasant awareness of cardiac action, they are rarely of great hemodynamic consequence per se. Rather, their significance relates to the ability of the APCs to initiate sustained atrial

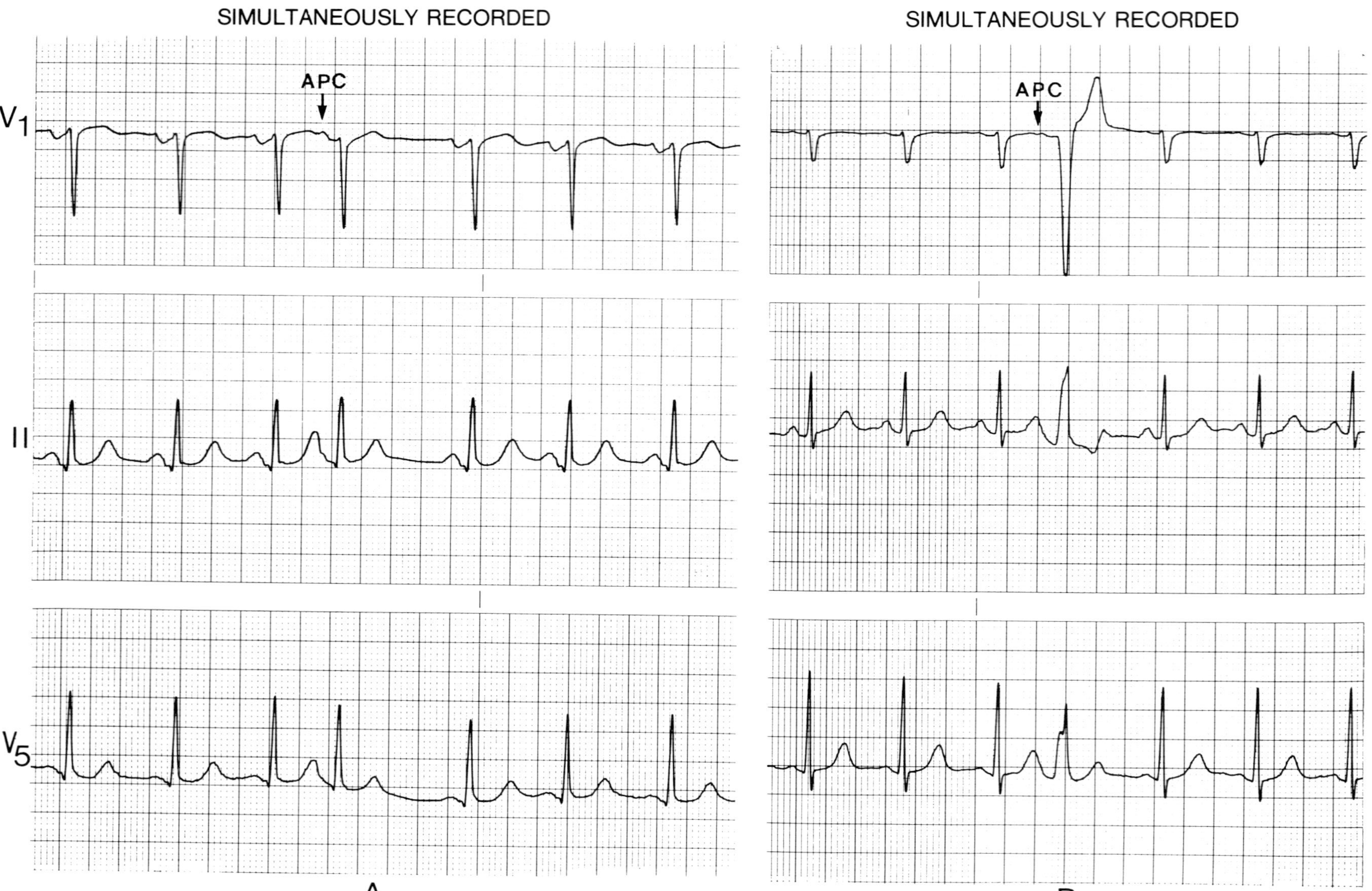

Figure 50–1 ECGs Showing Atrial Premature Complexes. *Note:* The ECG in *A* shows an atrial premature complex (APC) stimulating a QRS complex that has a contour essentially identical to that of the sinus-stimulated QRS complexes. In *B*, an APC stimulates a QRS complex with a left bundle branch block pattern, whereas sinus-stimulated QRS complexes have normal contours. In *A*, the APC is clearly seen in leads V₁ and II, but not in lead V₅; in *B*, the APC is clearly seen only in lead V₁.

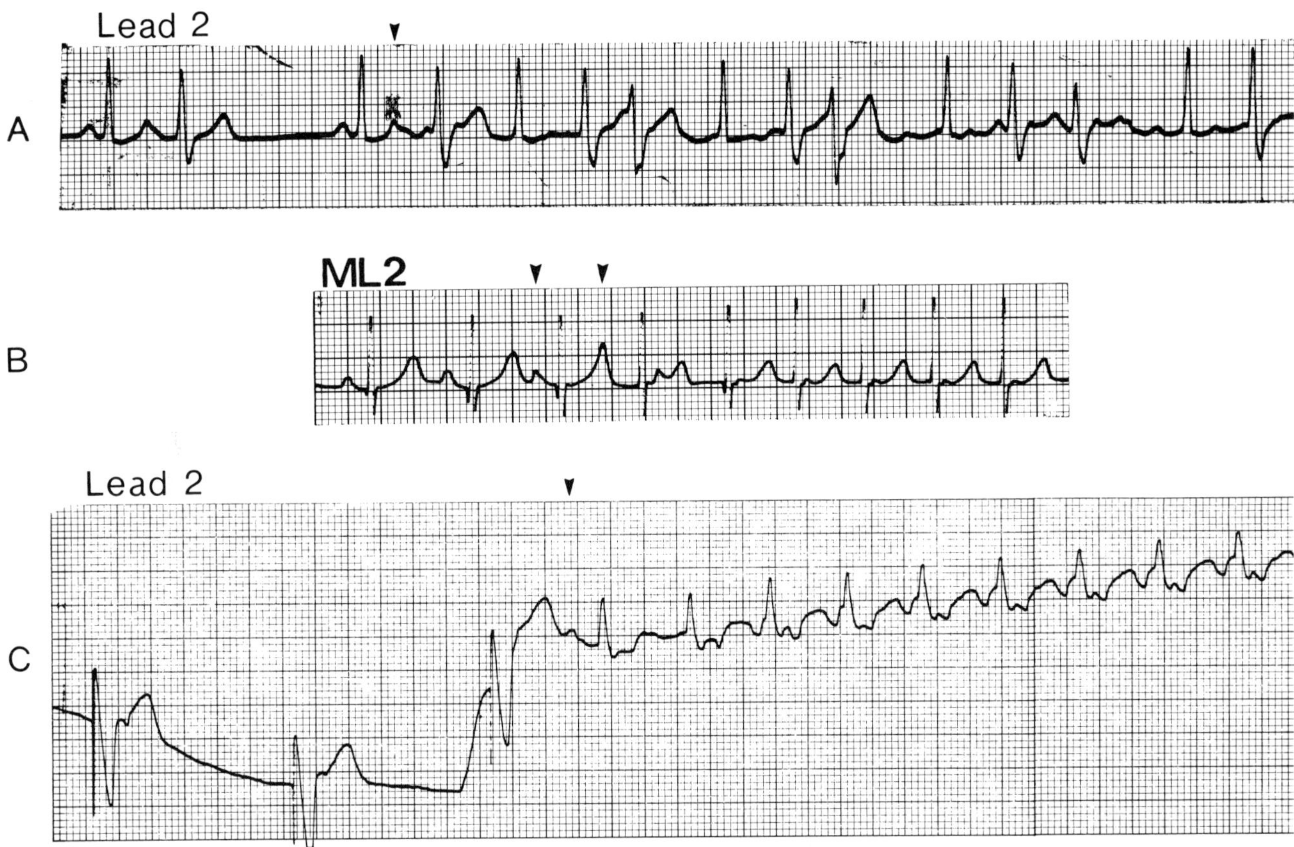

Figure 50–2 ECGs Showing the Onsets of Three Atrial Tachyarrhythmias. *Note: A* An atrial premature beat (*arrow*) initiates atrial fibrillation. *B* Sustained AV nodal reentrant paroxysmal supraventricular tachycardia is established following two atrial premature beats (*arrows*). *C* An atrial premature complex (*arrow*) initiates atrial flutter, during which there is 2:1 AV conduction. (ECG at 90% of original.)

tachyarrhythmias, such as fibrillation, paroxysmal supraventricular tachycardia (PSVT), and flutter (Fig. 50–2) and to the ability of the patient's cardiovascular system to tolerate the tachyarrhythmias. The emergency department physician must (1) assess possible factors predisposing the patient to a supraventricular tachyarrhythmia, (2) determine the underlying cardiovascular status of the patient to help predict whether an atrial tachyarrhythmia will result in significant problems, and (3) then decide what specific management is appropriate for that individual patient.

The physician confronted by the patient with even isolated APCs, however, should attempt to evaluate the factors predisposing to their ectopy. In some patients, the APCs may simply be a reflection of anxiety or emotional stress. In others, they may be a reflection of (1) large left atrial volume or high left atrial pressure, as seen in atrial septal defect, mitral stenosis, mitral insufficiency, or congestive heart failure; or (2) large right atrial volume or high right atrial pressure, as seen in atrial septal defect and chronic obstructive pulmonary disease. Furthermore, because of their stimulant ef-

fects, alcoholic beverages, caffeine, cigarette smoking, and medications such as thyroid hormone, bronchodilators, and sympathomimetic amines may be contributory factors. Finally, APCs may reflect pericardial irritation or inflammation, as may occur in acute myocardial infarction or renal failure, and primary pericarditis of other various etiologies. Patients who tolerate atrial tachyarrhythmias poorly include

- those with mitral stenosis in whom the rapid ventricular rate may result in dramatic elevation of left atrial pressure and the precipitation of pulmonary edema, and in whom the ineffective atrial mechanical activity may predispose to thromboembolism
- those with severe congestive heart failure or severe left ventricular hypertrophy (such as is seen with valvular aortic stenosis and hypertrophic cardiomyopathy) who need the properly timed atrial contribution to ventricular filling
- those with the bradycardia-tachycardia variant of the sick sinus syndrome in whom termination of

tachycardia is followed by prolonged cardiac stand-still

- those with rapidly conducting accessory AV conduction pathways.

Management of the patient with APCs must be based on the total clinical picture. If anxiety or sleep deprivation is playing a major role in an otherwise healthy patient, a supportive discussion and possibly a minor tranquilizer or soporific medication might be appropriately prescribed. Discontinuation of stimulants should be advised and dosages of potentially inciting medications reduced. Therapeutic maneuvers aimed at controlling congestive heart failure should be optimized. In some patients with mitral stenosis, aortic stenosis, or idiopathic hypertrophic subaortic stenosis, the onset of APCs raises the possibility that the cardiac lesion is serious enough to warrant consideration of cardiac surgery. Thus, thorough cardiologic evaluation is advisable at this time.

Several antiarrhythmic medications are available for treating the patient with APCs. As the treatment of APCs is rarely an emergency, the oral route of administration is preferred. Quinidine preparations, procainamide (Pronestyl, Procan), propranolol (Inderal), and disopyramide (Norpace) are all reported to be effective in suppressing atrial premature beats. As the relative efficacy of these different agents in suppressing APCs is unclear, selection of a specific drug generally depends on the potential side-effects of the drug in an individual patient, the necessary dosage schedule, and the cost. For example, a beta-blocking medication, such as propranolol, would be ill-advised for the patient with bronchospastic lung disease, poor left ventricular function, or insulin-dependent brittle diabetes mellitus; but it is often extremely effective and well tolerated by young, otherwise healthy patients with APCs. Disopyramide, which may have a significant depressant effect on cardiac performance, would be ill-advised for the patient with poor left ventricular function; furthermore, its anticholinergic properties often cause urinary retention in older males and constipation in older patients of both sexes. Quinidine preparations may cause significant diarrhea. Procainamide preparations must be administered at four- to six-hour intervals to achieve effective serum levels consistently. On long-term administration it results in positive antinuclear antibody and lupus erythematosus cell tests in a high percentage of patients, and a bothersome, often prolonged, lupuslike polyarthritis in a few.

Supraventricular beats may originate in the AV junction as well as in the atrium. An AV junctional premature beat (JPC) may be recognized by the premature occurrence of a normal-appearing QRS complex with an abnormal-appearing P wave either preceding it at an unusually short interval (less than 0.11 seconds) or occurring within it or shortly after it. The abnormal contour and axis of the P wave reflect the abnormal sequence of atrial depolarization that is due to the initiation of atrial activity near the upper portion of the AV node, well away from the sinus node. Junctional premature complexes appear to occur much less frequently than APCs, but their clinical significance and management do not appear to be different from those of APCs.

Ventricular Ectopic Beats

Impulses arising in the bundle branches or in ventricular tissue stimulate QRS complexes that are called ventricular ectopic beats (VEBs). VEBs may be recognized by their abnormal, often bizarre contours and by their prolonged duration (Fig. 50–3). When VEBs follow normal QRS complexes at intervals shorter than expected on the basis of the preceding rhythm, they are called premature ventricular complexes or beats (PVCs). When they follow pauses in QRS rhythm of more than about 1.2 seconds, they are called ventricular escape complexes or beats.

PVCs may arise in both healthy and diseased hearts. They are more likely to occur in association with ischemia, hypokalemia, digitalis excess, hypoxemia, congestive heart failure, and the administration of catecholamines, sympathomimetic amines, phenothiazines, and tricyclic antidepressants. PVCs may occur singly, in pairs, or in brief runs, and they may initiate paroxysmal or sustained ventricular tachycardia or ventricular fibrillation (Fig. 50–3 and 50–4).

While isolated PVCs may cause an unpleasant awareness of cardiac action, they generally do not contribute to hemodynamic deterioration unless they occur very frequently. Such might be the case in a bigeminal rhythm in which a PVC follows each sinus beat at an interval so brief that the PVC is mechanically ineffective, i.e., does not produce adequate stroke volume (Fig. 50–3, D). PVCs generally assume clinical importance when they initiate repetitive ventricular beating, sustained ventricular tachycardia, and ventricular fibrillation, hemodynamically disadvantageous and often disastrous rhythms that occur only rarely in the absence of heart disease—although the heart disease may not be clinically apparent prior to the occurrence of the catastrophic arrhythmia. So, faced with a patient having PVCs, the emergency department physician must attempt to determine whether the patient has cardiac disease. In this pursuit, it is essential to obtain a detailed medical history and family history, to perform a thorough physical examination, and to review a 12-lead ECG. In selected patients, chest roentgenogram, echocardiogram, and treadmill exercise test may be necessary.

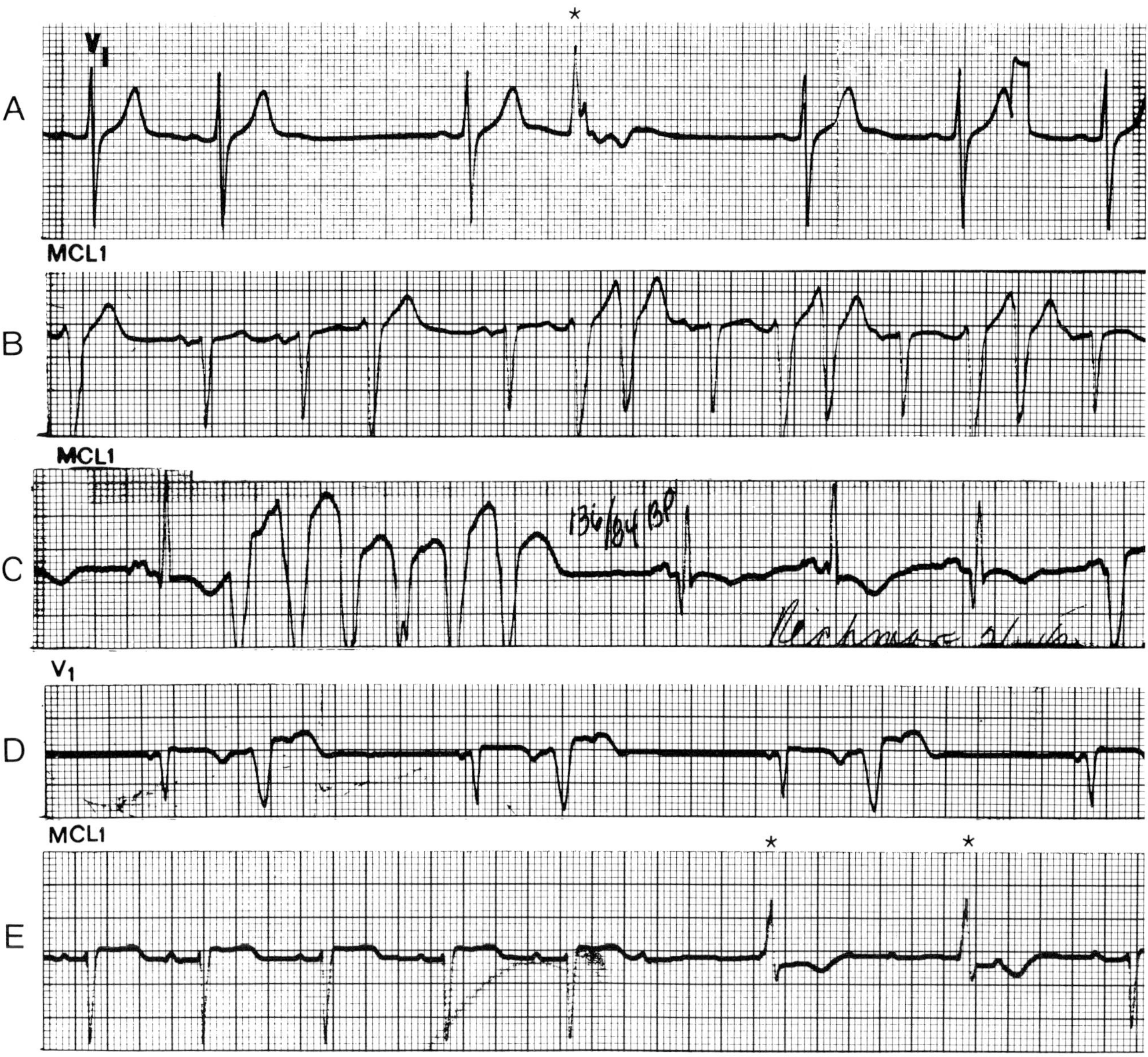

Figure 50–3   ECGs Showing Ventricular Ectopic Beats. *Note: A* The fourth QRS complex (*asterisk*) is a premature ventricular complex (PVC). *B* PVCs are occurring both singly and in pairs. *C* A brief (1.8 second) run of ventricular premature beats at a rate of about 170/minute. *D* Bigeminal rhythm in which a PVC follows each sinus-stimulated (or AV junction-stimulated) QRS complex. *E.* Ventricular escape beats (*asterisks*) terminate pauses in QRS rhythm occasioned by a brief period of AV block.

Antiarrhythmic medication need not be prescribed for patients with asymptomatic PVCs if there is no evidence of cardiac disease; it may be offered to normal patients with symptomatic PVCs after discussing with them the potential benefits and risks of specific antiarrhythmic medications. However, PVCs in a patient with a history or symptoms of coronary artery disease should be looked upon as a potentially serious problem and should be treated with specific antiarrhythmic medication unless hypokalemia, hypoxemia, congestive heart failure, or medications (e.g., digitalis, phenothiazines, tricyclic antidepressants) are clearly playing a role. If such contributory factors are present, they should be addressed before specific antiarrhythmic medication is administered. It is advisable to prescribe antiarrhythmic medication for PVCs in a patient with obvious ventricular aneurysm, which is almost always a reflection of coronary artery disease with previous myocardial infarction. Patients with unstable angina pectoris and PVCs should probably be admitted to the hospital for observation of their cardiac rhythm while antianginal therapy is administered.

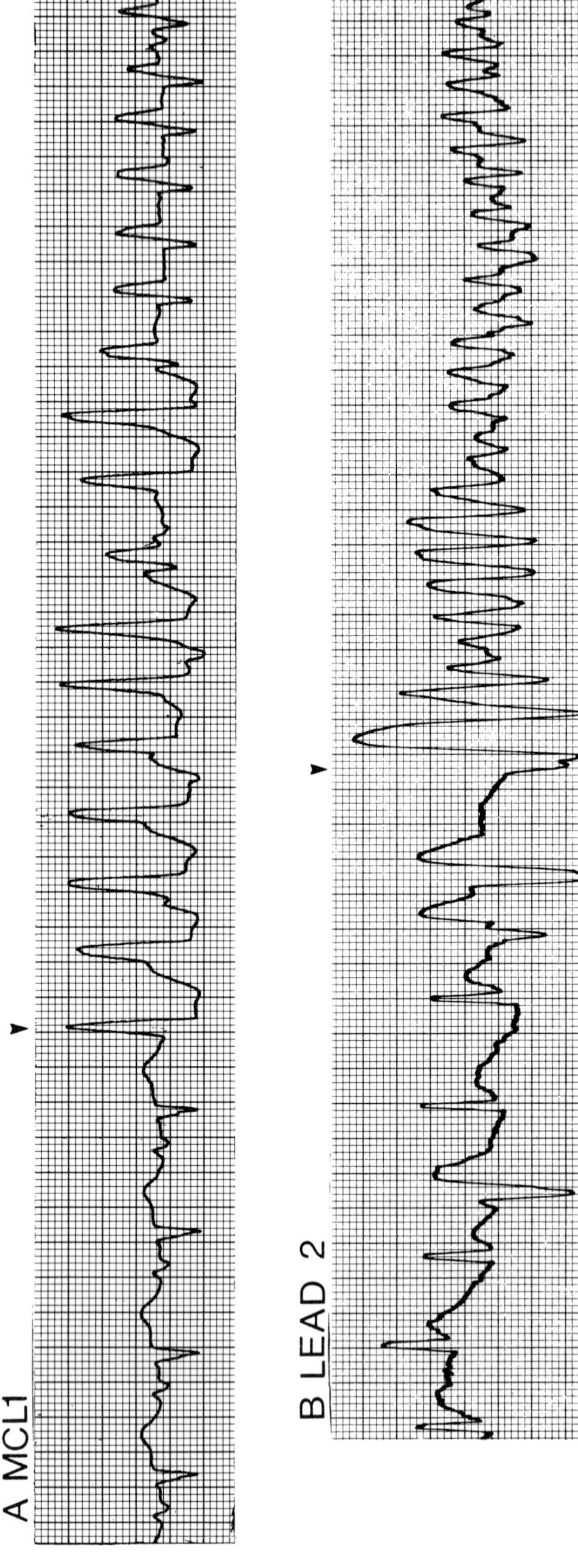

Figure 50–4 ECGs Showing the Onsets of Ventricular Tachycardia and Ventricular Fibrillation. *Note:* *A* A premature ventricular complex (*arrow*) initiates sustained ventricular tachycardia during which there is AV dissociation. *B* A premature ventricular complex (*arrow*) initiates ventricular fibrillation.

PVCs are very common in patients with the mitral valve prolapse, or click-murmur, syndrome. In these patients, the mitral valve and/or its supporting structures typically have abnormalities that may be detected clinically by the presence of systolic click(s) and systolic murmurs; the clicks and murmurs may vary in intensity and timing with changes in body position, as well as in response to respiration and to vasoactive medications, such as amyl nitrite. Sudden death has been reported to occur in a small number of patients with the mitral valve prolapse syndrome, suggesting that a fatal ventricular arrhythmia was initiated by the PVCs. However, the reported high frequency with which mitral valve prolapse has been detected echocardiographically and the small number of patients with this syndrome who suffer sudden death make it as yet unclear whether it is advisable to treat asymptomatic (or even symptomatic) isolated PVCs in these patients. As the few patients with mitral valve prolapse reported to have died suddenly had either dramatic anatomical abnormalities of the mitral valve apparatus, long QTU intervals, or nonspecific ST segment and T-wave abnormalities in the inferior and lateral precordial leads of a resting ECG, it would seem reasonable to prescribe specific antiarrhythmic medication to patients with mitral valve prolapse syndrome and isolated PVCs if they have physical examination or echocardiographic evidence of dramatic anatomic abnormalities of the mitral apparatus, or these ECG abnormalities.[1]

PVCs may initiate serious ventricular arrhythmias in patients whose ECGs show long QTU intervals. A few patients with long QTU intervals may have a congenital predisposition to this abnormality; some may have congenital hearing loss and a history of recurrent episodes of presyncope or syncope. However, the majority of patients with long QTU intervals either have coronary artery disease, hypokalemia, or mitral valve prolapse syndrome; or they are taking phenothiazines, tricyclic antidepressants, quinidine, procainamide, or disopyramide.

As a general principle, treatment of a patient with PVCs is initially directed to correcting metabolic, hemodynamic, and drug-related abnormalities, unless the PVCs are presently initiating hemodynamically deleterious arrhythmias, in which case specific antiarrhythmic medication might be administered immediately. Antiarrhythmic medications may be administered orally or intravenously, depending on the urgency of the clinical situation and the specific drug selected. The choice of a specific medication depends on the predicted effectiveness and potential side-effects of the drug, the route of administration available, the dosage schedule, and the clinical condition of the patient. Beta-blocking medications, such as propranolol, metoprolol* (Lopressor), atenolol (Tenormon,) and nadolol (Corgard),

would be ill-advised for the patient with poor left ventricular function, congestive heart failure, sick sinus syndrome, AV nodal conduction abnormalities, and bronchospastic lung disease; but they might be useful in the otherwise healthy patient, the anxious patient, the thyrotoxic patient or the patient with mitral valve prolapse syndrome. Administration of quinidine and procainamide might be dangerous in the patient with long QTU intervals, for these medications may lengthen the interval even further and thereby worsen ventricular arrhythmias. Furthermore, because recent studies suggest that the administration of a quinidine preparation to a patient on digoxin may result in a dramatic rise in the serum digoxin level and an increase in ventricular arrhythmias, particular care must be taken to administer quinidine less frequently and in lower dosage than normal to a patient with digitalis-related ventricular arrhythmias.[2] Disopyramide, also, is best avoided in long QTU syndromes, as it has been reported to lengthen the QTU interval, and to result in more serious ventricular arrhythmias in this situation. It is also prudent not to use disopyramide in the presence of severe congestive heart failure and poor left ventricular performance, as it has been reported to cause even more profound depression of left ventricular performance in such patients. Lidocaine is generally the drug of first choice when rapid suppression of PVCs is in order, as in the patient with acute myocardial infarction (see Chapter 49); it usually has few side-effects if administered in the recommended dosages. Diphenylhydantoin (Dilantin) is reported to be effective in suppressing PVCs in patients with long QTU intervals, and in patients whose PVCs are digitalis-induced or digitalis-related.

PARASYSTOLE

While the occurrence of most premature ectopic beats is somehow dependent on the basic underlying rhythm, the occurrence of some premature beats is totally independent of the basic underlying rhythm. The concurrent occurrence of two independent rhythms within the same part of the heart is termed *parasystole*, and the complexes stimulated by the ectopic impulses comprise the *parasystolic rhythm*. Parasystolic rhythms most commonly originate in ventricular tissue, although they occasionally arise in the atrium or AV junction. A parasystolic focus generates impulses at constant intervals, regardless of the underlying rhythm; whenever an impulse finds surrounding tissue in a nonrefractory state, it initiates depolarization of the tissue. The parasystolic focus cannot be entered or depolarized by impulses

---

*Metoprolol and atenolol may be used with caution in patients with bronchospastic lung disease.

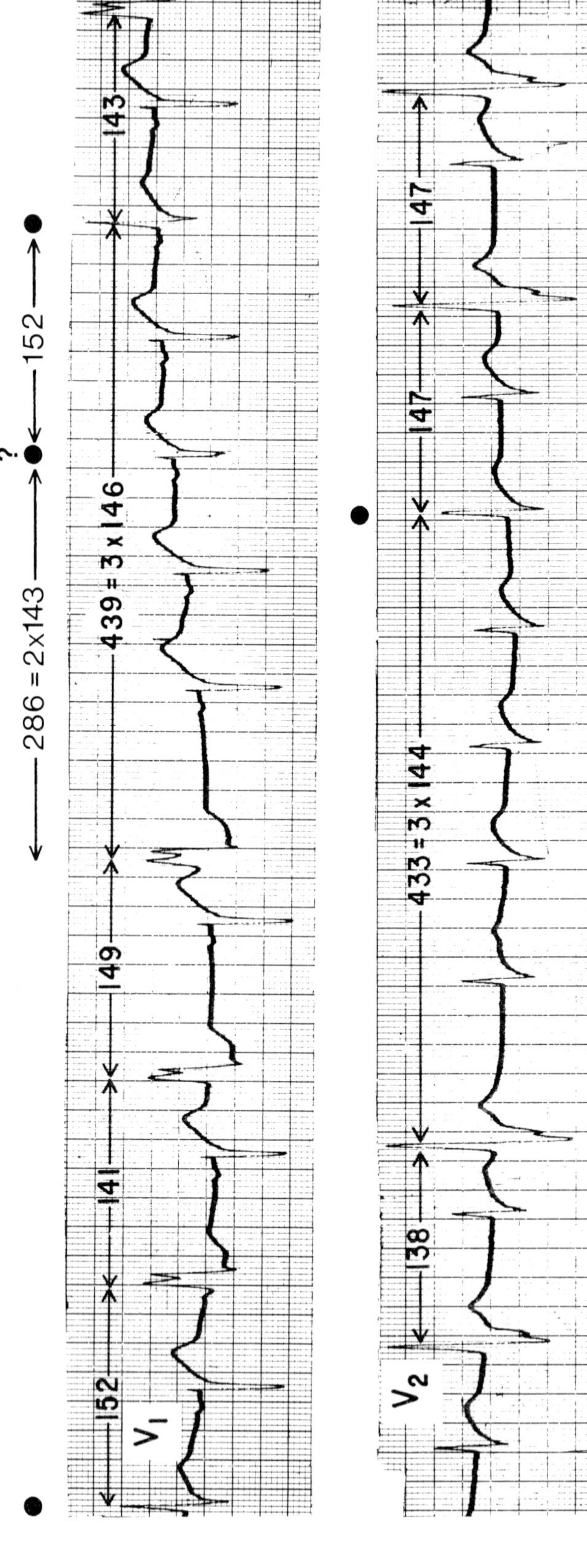

Figure 50–5   ECGs Showing Ventricular Parasystole. *Note:* The wide, bizarre QRS complexes occurring at variable coupling intervals and at intervals that are multiples of a common interval establish the diagnosis of ventricular parasystole. Fusion complexes (●) occur frequently. Times noted are the intervals in hundredths of a second between consecutive parasystolic complexes. (ECG at 81% of original.)

arising outside it, a property termed *protection*, which allows the focus to remain independent of the underlying rhythm.

Parasystolic beats may be recognized by their occurrence at regular intervals and by their temporal independence from the underlying rhythm, which results in (1) variable coupling intervals of the parasystolic complexes to the complexes of the underlying rhythm; (2) consecutive parasystolic complexes occurring at intervals that are multiples of a common interval; and (3) the frequent appearance of fusion complexes in which both a parasystolic impulse and an impulse of the underlying rhythm contribute to ventricular activation (Fig. 50–5). Obviously, long rhythm strips are necessary to establish the diagnosis of a parasystolic rhythm. Accurate diagnosis of parasystole is important, for ventricular parasystolic beats have *never* been reported to precipitate ventricular fibrillation, and only once have they been reported to initiate ventricular tachycardia. Thus, they are generally of little hemodynamic significance and ought to be treated only if they are causing symptoms. When treatment, i.e., suppression, of a parasystolic rhythm is felt to be appropriate, the usual antiarrhythmic medications may be prescribed.

ABERRATION VS. ECTOPY

The typical contour, axis, and duration of QRS complexes reflect the normal anatomical ventricular activation sequence via both left and right bundle branches. Abnormal sequences of ventricular activation may result in QRS complexes that have abnormal contours and durations. The adjective *aberrant* means deviating or straying from normal; in its strictest sense, then, the phrase *aberrant intraventricular conduction* refers to impulses that activate the ventricular myocardium in an abnormal temporal sequence, resulting in an abnormal anatomical sequence of ventricular depolarization. This abnormal course of events may be manifested on surface ECG tracings by the appearance of a QRS complex that differs from normal in contour, duration, or mean frontal plane axis. In this sense, aberrant intraventricular conduction could be initiated by impulses arising in supraventricular *or* in ventricular tissue. In clinical practice, however, the term *aberrant intraventricular conduction* is generally reserved for the phenomenon in which a supraventricular (sinus, atrial, or junctional) impulse activates the ventricles in an abnormal sequence, resulting in a QRS complex with a contour different from those generally stimulated by supraventricular impulses *in that same patient*—regardless of whether or not the patient's usual QRS complexes are of normal or abnormal contour or duration. It is *not* used to describe abnormal QRS complexes that result

from ectopic impulse formation within the ventricles themselves, even though such ectopic impulses result in an abnormal sequence of ventricular activation.

Application of the adjective *aberrant* to an unusual appearing QRS complex indicates that the complex is stimulated by an impulse arising in supraventricular rather than ventricular tissue. In fact, the concept of aberrant intraventricular conduction assumes clinical relevance because it is critically important prognostically and therapeutically to know whether an abnormal QRS complex results from aberrant intraventricular conduction of a supraventricular impulse or from ectopic ventricular impulse formation.

Aberrant intraventricular conduction of a supraventricular impulse occurs when a supraventricular impulse reaches the intraventricular conduction system (the bundle branches and their fascicles) at a time when one or more portions of the system cannot conduct the impulse either as rapidly as usual or at all, because it is still refractory (i.e., still recovering its excitability from having been recently depolarized). Thus, ventricular activation occurs via those portions of the intraventricular conduction system that are nonrefactory when the supraventricular impulse reaches them. The contours of aberrantly conducted supraventricular impulses generally show rather characteristic right bundle branch block, left bundle branch block, or left anterior fascicle block patterns, probably because the proximal portions of the bundle branches (or fascicles) have the longest refractory periods of the intraventricular conduction system tissue. In contrast, PVCs generally do *not* have a pure bundle branch block or fascicle block contour, but are more bizarre because ectopic ventricular impulse formation usually results in an anatomical sequence of ventricular depolarization different from that occurring in bundle branch or fascicle blocks (Fig. 50–6, D and E). Furthermore, PVCs are usually wider than QRS complexes with pure bundle branch or fascicle block patterns, probably because depolarization of the entire mass of ventricular myocardium from one small area of peripheral Purkinje fiber takes more time than does depolarization from a bundle branch or fascicle which depolarizes several areas of ventricular myocardium almost simultaneously. In the unusual event that an ectopic ventricular impulse arises in the proximal portion of a bundle branch or fascicle, the contour of the resultant PVC may have a pure bundle branch or fascicle block pattern (Fig. 50–6, F). In this instance, the contour of the abnormal QRS complex does not accurately reflect the mechanism of its occurrence.

In the presence of sinus rhythm, evaluation of the P wave preceding an abnormal premature QRS complex may be helpful in the differential diagnosis of aberration versus ectopy. When a premature abnormal QRS complex is preceded by a *premature* P wave, the QRS com-

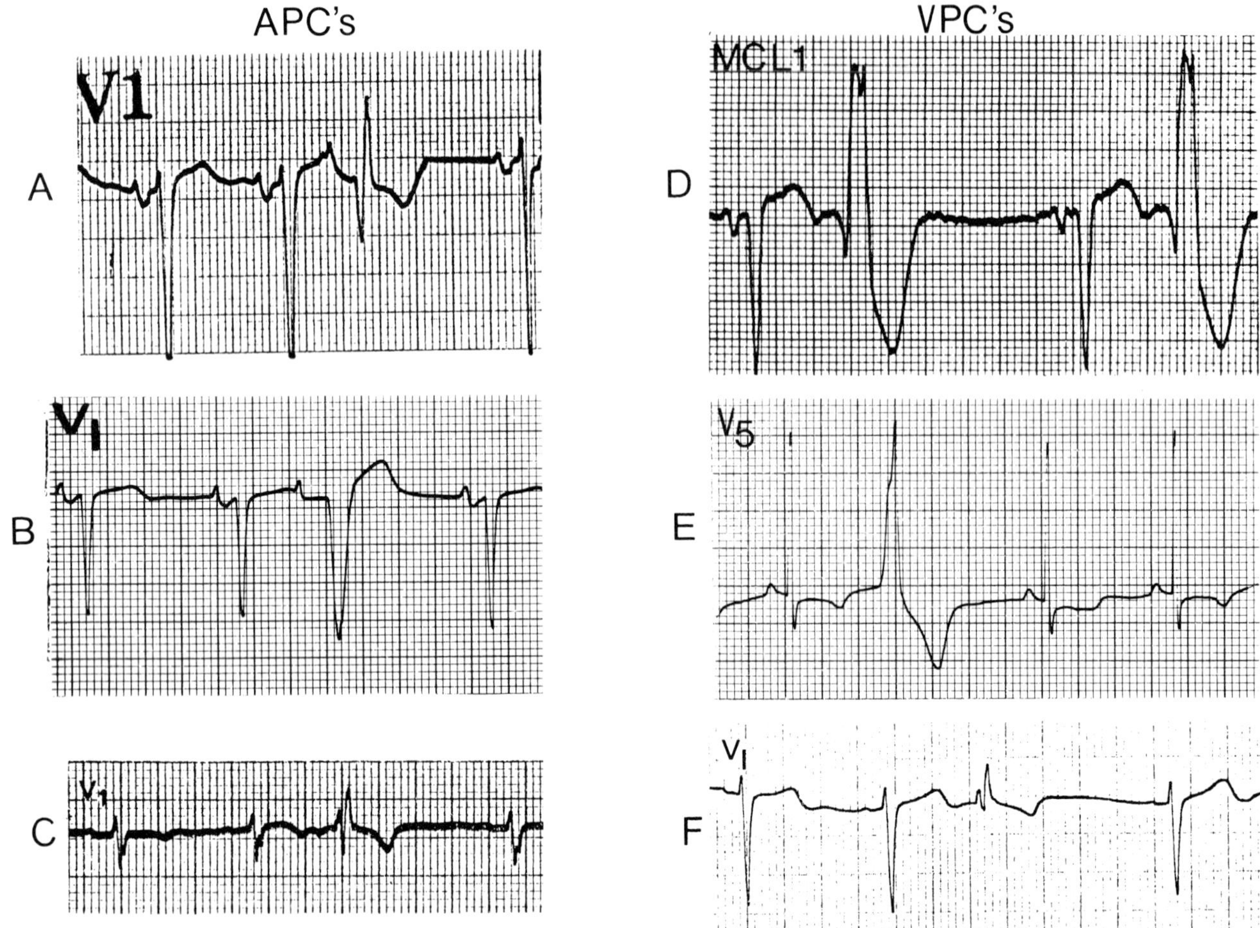

Figure 50–6   ECGs Showing Atrial and Ventricular Premature Complexes. Note: Tracings show atrial premature complexes (APCs) conducted with right bundle branch block (*A*), left bundle branch block (*B*), and mild right bundle branch conduction delay patterns (*C*). The ventricular premature complexes (VPCs) in (*D* and *E*) probably originated in distal Purkinje fibers. The VPC in *F* probably originated within the left bundle branch, as it has a "pure" right bundle branch conduction delay pattern and is only mildly widened.

plex is most likely to be supraventricular in origin, either stimulated by the preceding P wave or by an AV junctional impulse that has initiated depolarization of the atrium before the ventricles. It is always possible, of course, to explain a premature P wave preceding a premature abnormal QRS complex as the result of the fortuitous occurrence of sequential atrial and ventricular ectopic impulses, but this seems to occur only very rarely. Impulses arising in the intraventricular conduction system activate ventricular tissue well in advance of atrial tissue, since the atrium can be reached only after the impulse retrogradely traverses the AV node, which conducts impulses much more slowly than does the intraventricular conduction system. Preceding P wave criteria obviously are useless in the presence of atrial fibrillation in which atrial activity is so rapid and disorganized that the relationships of atrial to ventricular activity cannot be defined.

In the presence of atrial fibrillation, the differential diagnosis of aberration versus ectopy is facilitated by an evaluation of the relationship of the coupling interval of the abnormal QRS complex (i.e., the interval between the abnormal QRS complex and the immediately preceding typical one) and the preceding cycle length (i.e., the interval between the two QRS complexes immediately preceding the abnormal QRS complex in question). As the refractory periods of different portions of the intraventricular conduction system are set on a beat-to-beat basis and shorten with increasing heart rate (i.e., following shorter R-R intervals), an abnormal QRS complex occurring at a coupling interval longer than the preceding cycle length is more likely to be due to ectopic ventricular impulse formation than to aberrant intraventricular conduction of an atrial fibrillatory impulse. In contrast, a wide QRS complex occurring at a short coupling interval relative to the preceding cycle length is more likely to be due to aberrant intraventricular conduction. If the preceding cycle length is *very* long, however, the propensity for ventricular ectopy is enhanced, a phenomenon termed the *rule of bigeminy*. Ventricular ectopy is also likely to be the mechanism of essentially identical abnormal QRS complexes occurring at *constant* coupling intervals, despite variable preceding cycle lengths during atrial fibrillation. The term *Ashman phenomenon* refers to a brief run, during rapid atrial rhythms, of aberrantly conducted supraventricular impulses that simulate ventricular tachycardia. The first abnormal QRS complex in such a run usually occurs at a short coupling interval relative to the preceding cycle length. Figure 50–7 displays several rhythm strips that illustrate these points.

BRADYARRHYTHMIAS*

While it is well recognized that heart rates in the range of 40 to 50 beats/minute may occur in normal, healthy adults and that heart rates as low as 30 beats/minute may be seen in very well trained athletes, a sudden fall in heart rate to these levels or pauses in ventricular rhythm lasting more than a few seconds may have serious, even disastrous, clinical consequences. The presyncopal symptoms, syncope, seizure, and sudden death that may occur at times of bradycardia reflect inadequate cerebral perfusion resulting from low cardiac output and low systemic arterial blood pressure.

An acute fall in ventricular rate may occur because of failure of either impulse formation or impulse conduction (Table 50–2). When the sinus node does not activate the atrium, either because the sinus impulse is not generated appropriately (i.e., sinus arrest) or because the generated impulse cannot be conducted into the atrium (i.e., sinoatrial exit block), subsidiary automatic tissue in the AV junctional area would be expected to terminate the pause within one to two seconds by generating a stable rhythm that would gradually increase its rate to about 45 to 55 beats/minute. Following resumption of an atrial rhythm whose rate exceeds the junctional rate, the lower AV junctional pacemaker would be overdriven and would then become dormant. This expected course of events is shown in Figure 50–8. If, however, the AV junctional tissue fails to generate an impulse, automatic tissue in the fascicles or Purkinje fibers of the intraventricular conduction system would be expected to begin to initiate ventricular activation within a few seconds and to maintain a stable rhythm

at a rate of about 30 to 40 beats/minute. Thus, clinically important bradycardias would not be expected to follow the sudden cessation of sinus or atrial activity, because of the availability of subsidiary pacemakers. This is not always the case, however, and prolonged cardiac standstill may ensue (Fig. 50–9).

Since patients in whom the expected escape rhythm does occur are not likely to be symptomatic and, therefore, not likely to come under clinical observation, it is unclear how often the expected AV junctional escape mechanism prevents clinically symptomatic bradycardia related to sinus or atrial arrest, or sinoatrial exit block. Prolonged junctional arrest in patients with sinus arrest or sinoatrial exit block may be related to concomitant disease in the approaches to and body of the AV node and His bundle, and/or to increased parasympathetic traffic or decreased sympathetic traffic into this subsidiary automatic tissue.

Sudden Sinus or Atrial Standstill

A diagnosis of sinus or atrial standstill is established by the sudden disappearance from the electrocardiogram of atrial activity, i.e., P waves, flutter waves, or fibrillatory waves. Sinoatrial exit block should be suspected when the length of a pause in sinus rhythm is a multiple of the spontaneous sinus cycle length at that time (Fig. 50–10). When the pause is not a multiple of the spontaneous sinus cycle length, the pause is referred to as a sinus pause or, when overly prolonged, a period of sinus or atrial standstill, or arrest (Fig. 50–9).

While these bradyarrhythmias may be associated with acute myocardial infarction or electrical termination of atrial and ventricular tachyarrhythmias, they are most commonly seen in patients with the so-called sick sinus syndrome, in which APCs, atrial tachyarrhythmias, slow sinus rhythm, sinoatrial exit block, and sinus arrest may occur at different times. In many patients with sick sinus syndrome, the occurrence of atrial standstill is totally unpredictable (Fig. 50–9), while in other patients it may predictably follow the spontaneous cessation of an atrial tachyarrhythmia (Fig. 50–11). Regardless of the events preceding atrial standstill in the sick sinus syndrome, the period of asystole rarely lasts more than five to ten seconds and is usually terminated by atrial or junctional complexes. Sudden death is not common in patients with sick sinus syndrome because the bradycardia that occurs is usually neither profound nor persistent.

The management of the patient with transient sinus or atrial standstill involves stimulating the sinus node or AV junctional automatic tissues so that they will generate impulses. This can usually be achieved with one or more blows to the lower sternal area or by alteration of the autonomic nervous system traffic into

---

*Portions of this section have, with permission of the publisher, been modified and reprinted from Jacobson LB, Lester RM, Scheinman MM: Management of acute bundle branch block and bradyarrhythmias. *Med Clin North Am* 63:93, 1979.

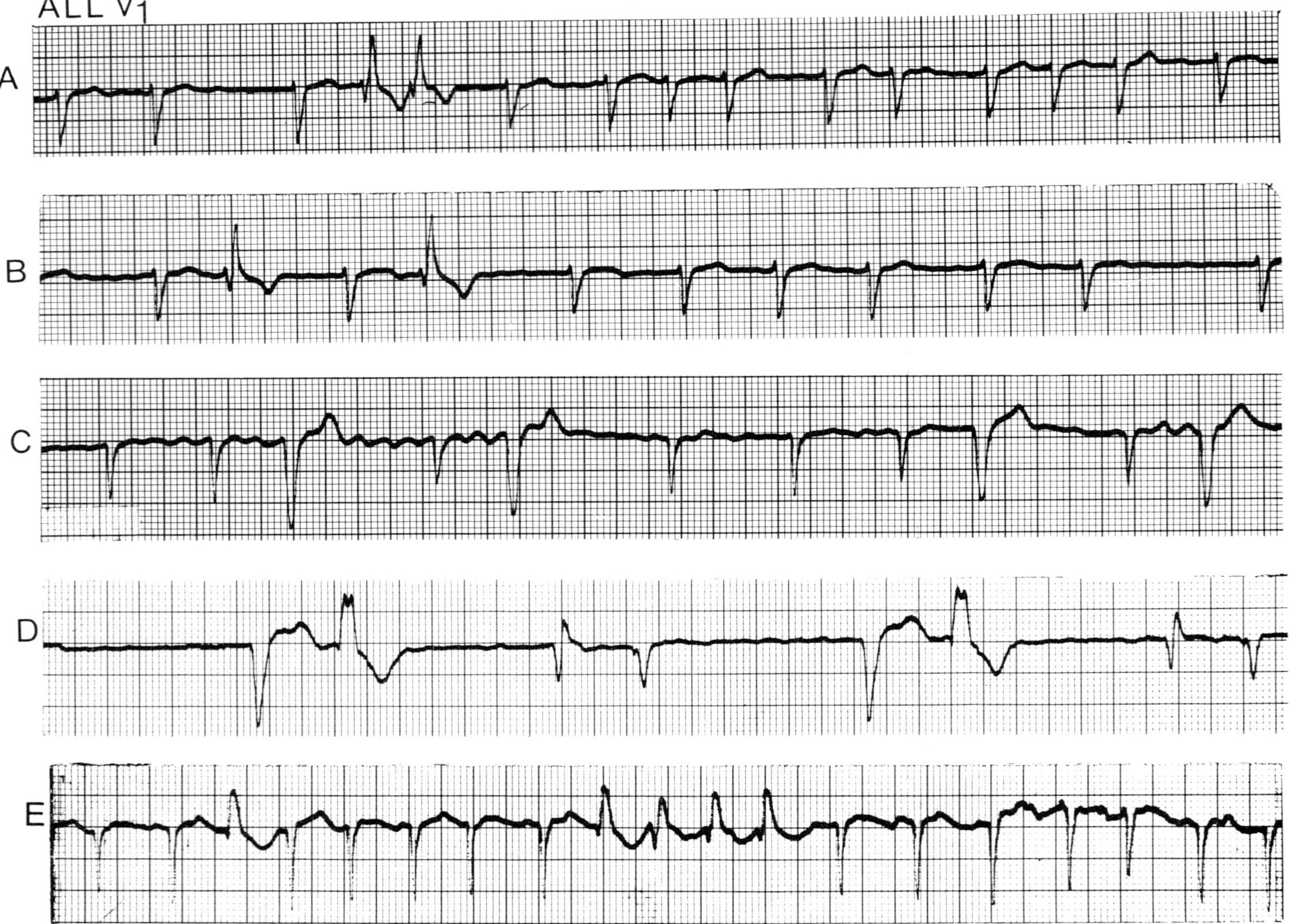

Figure 50–7   *Note:* In *A* and *B*, the rsR′ complexes occur at short coupling intervals relative to the preceding cycle lengths and have a "pure" right bundle branch block type pattern, suggesting they are aberrantly conducted fibrillatory impulses. In *C*, the wide QRS complexes are most likely ventricular ectopic beats because although they occur at short coupling intervals relative to the preceding cycle lengths, the coupling intervals are identical. In *D*, there is a bigeminal rhythm in which the QRS complexes that terminate very long pauses are followed by different and even more bizarre QRS complexes that occur at short cycle lengths. The QRS complexes occurring at short cycle length are probably ventricular ectopic beats because their contours are very abnormal and because they occur at very short coupling intervals after QRS complexes that terminate long pauses. The events in *D* illustrate the rule of bigeminy. In the middle of strip *E*, an abnormal QRS complex occurring at a short coupling interval relative to the preceding cycle length is followed by a run of three similarly abnormal QRS complexes. This brief run of aberrantly conducted supraventricular impulses that simulate ventricular tachycardia illustrates the Ashman phenomenon.

TABLE 50–2   Mechanisms of Bradycardias

Abnormal Impulse Formation	Abnormal Impulse Conduction
Sinus Arrest	Sinoatrial exit block
Spontaneous	AV nodal block
Following termination of tachycardias	His-Purkinje system
Artificial cardiac pacemaker malfunction	block

Source: Modified and reprinted with permission from Jacobson LB, Lester RM, Scheinman MM: Management of acute bundle branch block and bradyarrhythmias. *Med Clin North Am* 63:93,1979.

these pacemaker tissues. Parasympathetic stimuli and beta-adrenergic blocking agents slow the automatic rate of the sinus node and decrease the ability of sinus impulses to traverse the sinoatrial junction into atrial tissue; while parasympatholytic agents and beta-adrenergic stimulating agents enhance sinus node automaticity and the ability of a sinus impulse to traverse the sinoatrial junction. Thus, it might be expected that intravenously (IV) administered atropine or isoproterenol would be effective in managing sinus arrest or atrial standstill in patients with recurrent bouts of bradycardia; however, the time required to administer these medications usually exceeds the period of cardiac standstill, spontaneously, making the use of such medications unsatisfactory in an emergency. Atropine is generally administered in a dose of 1 to 2 mg IV as rapidly as possible, while isoproterenol is administered in a dose of 1 to 3 μg/minute by continuous IV infusion of a solution containing 1 mg isoproterenol in 250 ml of 5 percent dextrose in water. Because some patients with sick sinus syndrome have blunted responses to autonomic interventions, these medications are often inef-

fective even in clinically significant bradycardias. In such instances, the institution of temporary atrial or ventricular pacing is required immediately to ensure an adequate heart rate. Permanent atrial or ventricular pacing is the only reliable and effective treatment for the patient with recurrent clinically significant supraventricular bradyarrhythmias.

Atrioventricular (AV) Block

Abnormalities in conduction of impulses from atrium to ventricle are termed AV blocks. AV blocks are categorized as first degree (1°), second degree (2°), or third degree (3°); the higher the degree of block, the greater the impairment in AV conduction. A 1° AV block is said to be present when all sinus impulses are conducted to the ventricles, but AV conduction takes longer than normal. Thus, the presence of 1° AV $\pm$ block is recognized when all P waves are followed by QRS complexes that they stimulate, but the PR interval exceeds 0.20 seconds.

In 2° AV block, some, but not all, sinus impulses are conducted into the ventricles. A 2° AV block is recognized by the intermittent failure of a QRS complex to follow a sinus P wave. Second-degree AV blocks are divided into Mobitz Types I and II. A Mobitz Type I 2° AV block, also known as a Wenckebach Type 2° AV block, is characterized by progressive PR interval prolongation in the conducted beats preceding the P wave that fails to stimulate a QRS complex (Fig. 50–12, A). Mobitz Type II 2° AV block is characterized by constancy of the PR intervals in the beats preceding and following the nonconducted sinus P wave (Fig. 50–12, B). Mobitz Type I block is almost always due to depressed conduction in the AV node, while Mobitz Type II block is almost always due to depressed conduction in the bundle branches or in the His bundle. The term *high-*

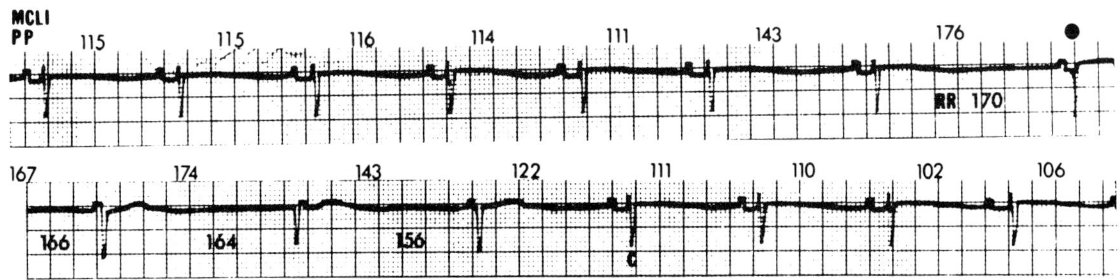

Figure 50–8 Continuous ECG Strips Showing the Expected Response to Sinus Slowing. *Note:* In the top strip, the sinus rate suddenly slows (PP intervals lengthen), and a junctional escape beat (●) terminates the resultant pause. The first three QRS complexes in the bottom strip are dissociated from the P waves and are junctional escape beats. These escape beats occur at progressively shorter intervals, demonstrating the warm-up phenomenon of a subsidiary pacemaker. As sinus rate accelerates (PP intervals shorten), sinus impulses again capture the ventricles. C denotes the first capture beat that reintroduces AV association. Numbers denote time in hundredths of a second. (*Source:* Reprinted with permission from Jacobson LB, Lester RM, Scheinman MM: Management of acute bundle branch block and bradyarrhythmias. *Med Clin North Am* 63:93, 1979.)

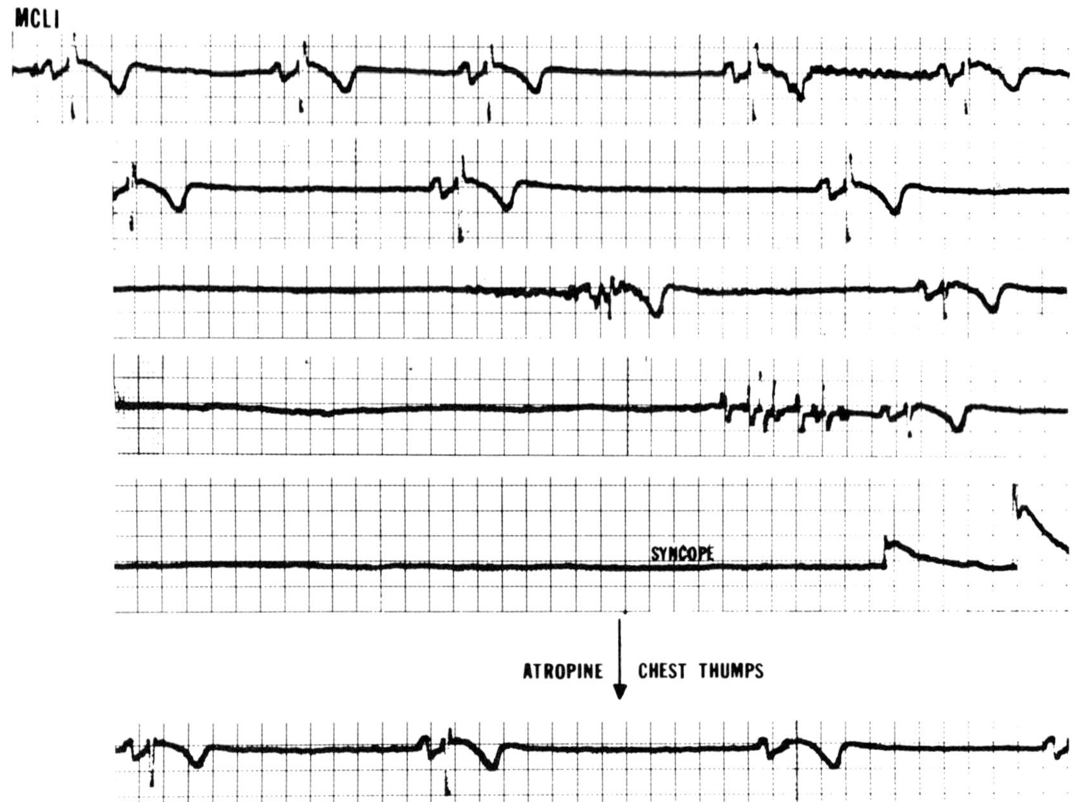

Figure 50–9 ECGs Showing Sinus Slowing Followed by Cardiac Standstill, but No Escape Rhythm. *Note:* The top five continuous ECG strips show profound sinus slowing and sinus arrest or atrial standstill, followed by complete cardiac standstill. No escape beats appear despite a pause of at least ten seconds. Following blows to the precordium and the intravenous administration of atropine, very slow sinus rhythm (at a rate of about 20 beats/minute) resumes, as shown in the bottom strip. (*Source:* Reprinted with permission from Jacobson LB, Lester RM, Scheinman MM: Management of acute bundle branch block and bradyarrhythmias. *Med Clin North AM* 63:93, 1979.)

grade 2° AV block refers to the failure of two or more consecutive sinus P waves to be conducted to the ventricles; this may occur when the block is Mobitz Type I or II. First- and second-degree AV blocks are defined only when the atrial rhythm is sinus.

Third-degree or complete AV block is said to be present when atrial impulses are never able to be conducted to the ventricles. In this event, the ventricular rhythm must be stimulated by impulses arising in automatic tissue below the level of block, which may be in the AV node, the His bundle, or the proximal portions of the bundle branches. Such escape rhythms are usually regular and have rates of 30 to 50 beats/minute. QRS rhythms arising in the AV junction (His bundle) generally have more normal contours and more rapid rates than those arising in the bundle branches or in Purkinje fibers. Third-degree AV block is recognized by the occurrence of a QRS rhythm that is temporally independent of the atrial rhythm, even though atrial impulses occur at times when they would normally be able to traverse the AV conduction system. The total independence of atrial and ventricular rhythms allows the diagnosis of third-degree AV block to be made regardless of whether the atrial rhythm is sinus, fibrillation, flutter, or ectopic tachycardia (Fig. 50–13).

When there is a sudden failure of impulse conduction from atrium to ventricle, i.e., when there is AV block, there will be a pause in ventricular rhythm until either AV conduction resumes (Fig. 50–14, A) or an escape rhythm emerges (Fig. 50–14, B). It is at the time of onset of AV block and of cessation of firing of an escape pacemaker that patients with paroxysmal or chronic AV block may experience presyncope, syncope, seizure, or sudden death. The severity of the symptoms is roughly related to the duration of ventricular standstill, the rate and stability of the emerging escape rhythm, the posture and activities of the patient at the time, and the presence of cardiovascular disease.

When AV block occurs within the AV node, the emerging escape pacemaker usually arises in the His bundle. Such junctional pacemakers usually emerge within a few seconds and initiate a stable rhythm at a

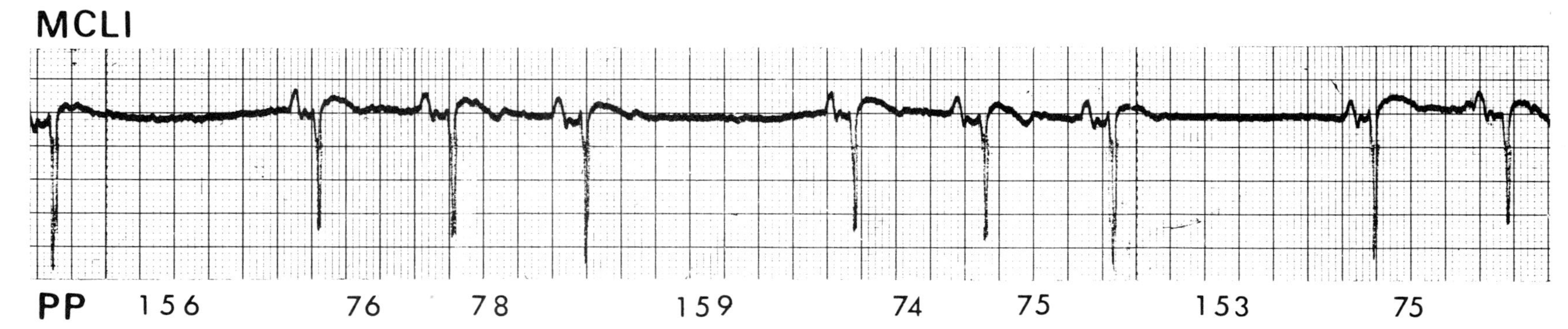

Figure 50–10   ECG Showing 4:3 Sinoatrial Exit Block. *Note:* The group beating is attributable to 4:3 sinoatrial exit block, for the PP intervals during the pauses are almost exactly twice the shorter PP intervals. Times are in hundredths of a second. (*Source:* Reprinted with permission from Jacobson LB, Goldschlager N: *Arrhythmias: Case Studies.* Garden City, NY, Medical Examination Publishing, © 1978.)

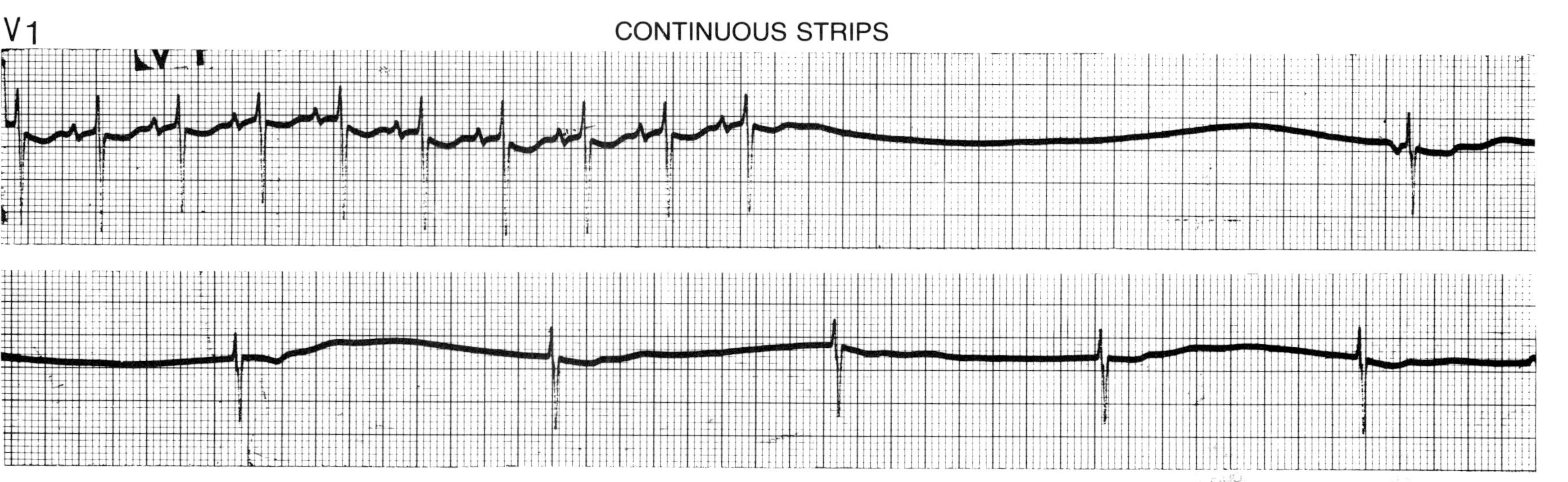

Figure 50–11   ECG Showing Transient Cardiac Standstill after Termination of a Supraventricular Tachyarrhythmia. *Note:* Following spontaneous termination of a supraventricular tachyarrhythmia, there is a 3.9-second period of cardiac standstill that is terminated by a junctional or atrial escape beat. About 3.6 seconds later, there emerges a junctional escape rhythm that gradually increases its rate until, in the next to the last beat in the bottom strip, it is suppressed by emergence of a more rapid atrial rhythm. These strips were recorded from a patient with the bradycardia-tachycardia variant of the sick sinus syndrome.

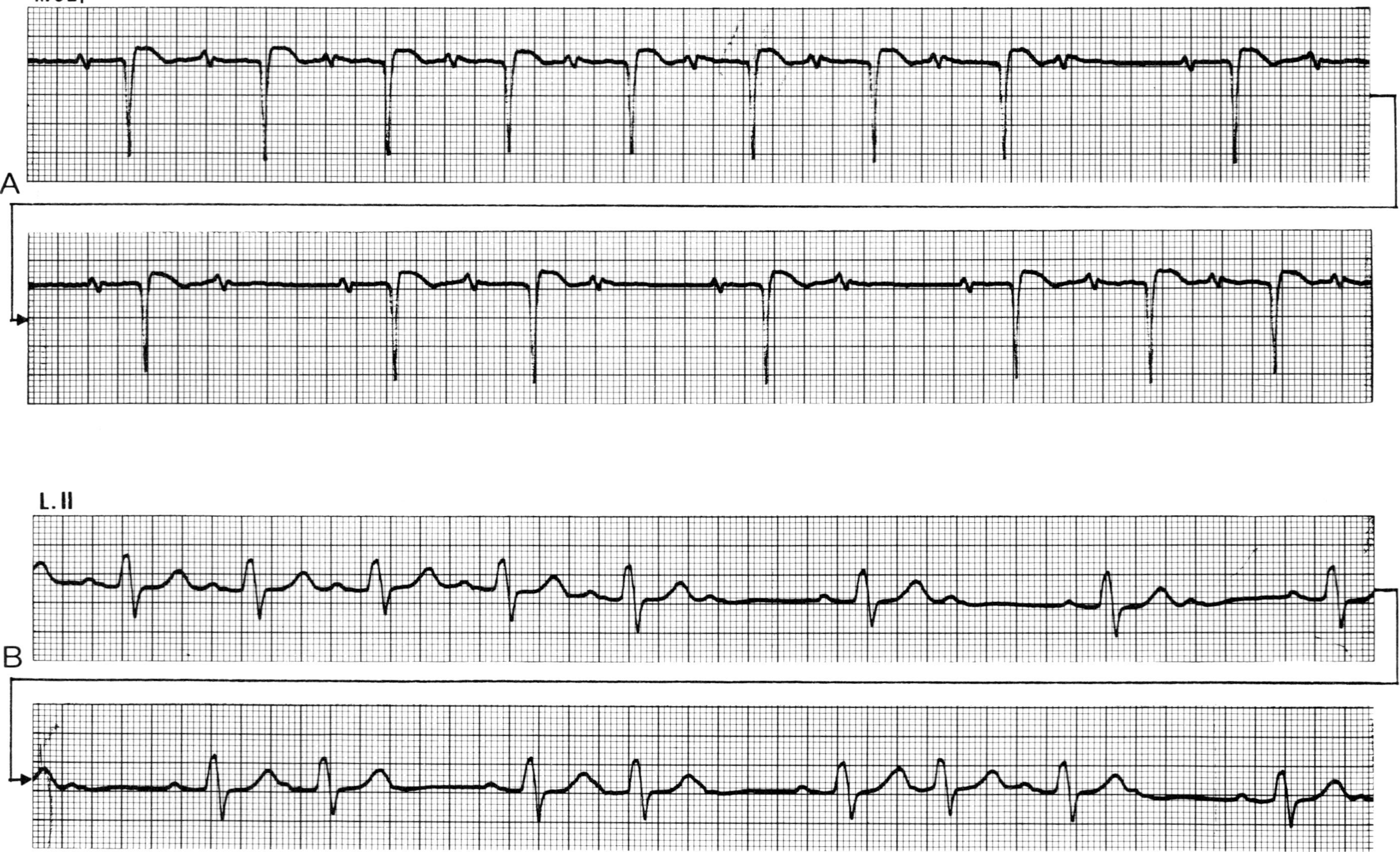

Figure 50–12   ECGs Showing Mobitz Types I and II Second Degree AV Blocks. *Note: A.* These two continuous lead MCLI rhythm strips were recorded from a 74-year-old woman with digitalis intoxication. Sinus P waves, which occur with regularity at a rate of about 72/minute, intermittently fail to stimulate QRS complexes. The progressive PR interval prolongation in the conducted beats that precede the nonconducted P waves establishes the diagnosis of Mobitz Type I or Wenckebach Type second-degree AV block. *B.* These two continuous lead II rhythm strips were recorded from an 82-year-old woman with paroxysmal presyncopal symptoms and dyspnea. Sinus P waves occur with reasonable regularity, but they intermittently fail to stimulate QRS complexes. The constancy of the PR intervals in the conducted beats that precede and follow the blocked P waves establishes the diagnosis of Mobitz Type II second-degree AV block. During the period of block, there is some mild irregularity in the P-wave rhythm, perhaps owing to autonomic nervous system mediated beat-to-beat changes in sinus rate or to atrial premature complexes.

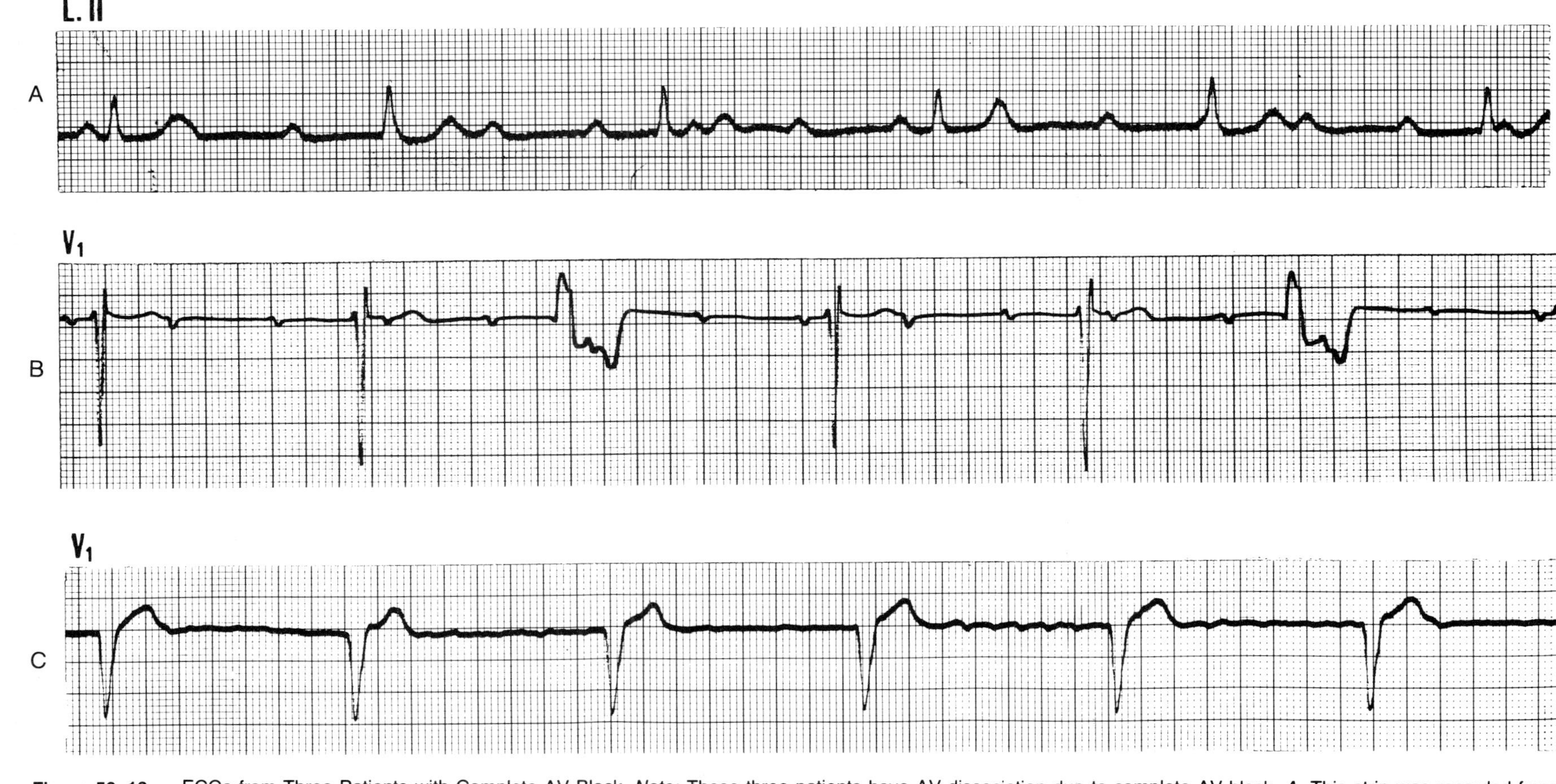

Figure 50–13   ECGs from Three Patients with Complete AV Block. *Note:* These three patients have AV dissociation due to complete AV block. *A.* This strip was recorded from a 15-year-old boy with acute rheumatic fever. The atrial rhythm is sinus. The QRS complexes, which occur with regularity at a rate of about 32/minute, have normal contours, except when P waves are superimposed upon them. The normal QRS contours suggest that this escape rhythm arises in the AV junction (His bundle). *B.* This strip was recorded from an 82-year-old woman with recent onset of weakness, fatigue, paroxysmal lightheadedness, and congestive heart failure. The atrial rhythm is sinus. There is group beating of the QRS complexes; two escape complexes which have a right bundle branch block type contour, indicating that they probably originate near the left bundle branch, are followed by a ventricular ectopic beat. The average ventricular rate is about 40 beats/minute. *C.* This strip was recorded from a 66-year-old man with chronic atrial fibrillation and complete AV block contributed to by digoxin. The QRS complexes, which occur with regularity at a rate of about 39/minute, show a left bundle branch block pattern, suggesting that they originate in or near the right bundle branch.

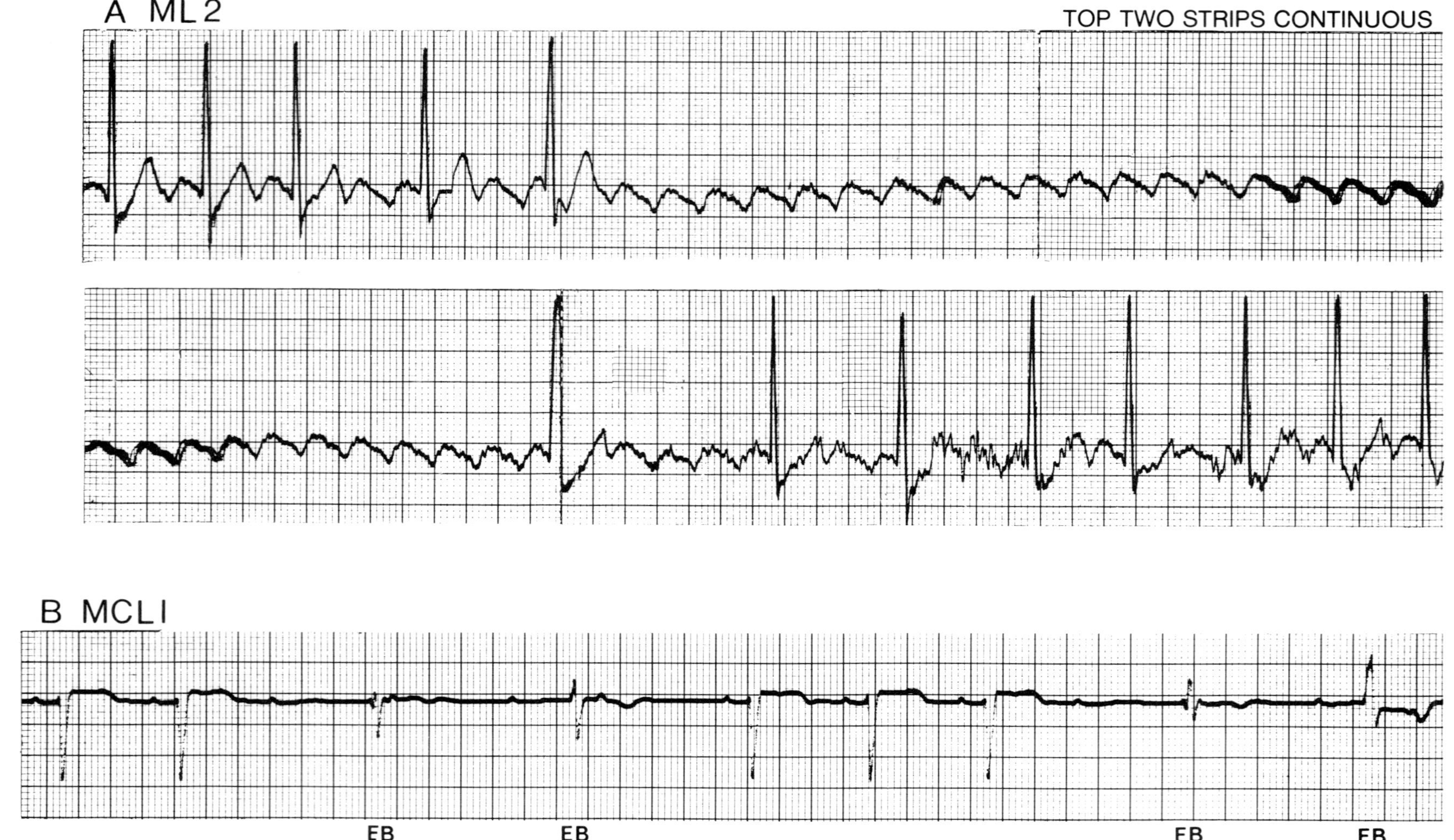

Figure 50–14   ECGs Showing Transient AV Block. *Note: A* During atrial flutter, a nine-second period of ventricular standstill due to AV block is terminated when AV conduction resumes. *B* Pauses in QRS rhythm occasioned by periods of Mobitz Type II second-degree AV block are terminated by fascicular or ventricular escape beats (*EB*).

rate of about 40 to 50 beats/minute. When AV block occurs within or below the His bundle, however, the emerging pacemaker must arise in the fascicles or Purkinje fibers of the intraventricular conduction system. Such *infra-Hisian* pacemakers usually take several seconds to emerge, initiate a rhythm at a rate of about 20 to 40 beats/minute, and may unpredictably cease to fire for many seconds for no apparent reason.

While transvenous ventricular pacing is the safest, most effective, and most reliable therapy for bradycardia related to AV block, attempts to establish temporary pacing in an emergency department that has no fluoroscopy capability is impractical and risky. Thus, the emergency department management of the patient with paroxysmal or persistent AV block generally involves attempts to ensure an adequate ventricular rate by administering medications that enhance AV conduction or increase the rate and stability of the escape pacemaker.

When the site of AV block is in the AV node, AV conduction can usually be improved by atropine and isoproterenol; both medications, but especially the latter, may also increase the rate of a junctional pacemaker. Thus, in Wenckebach (Type I) second-degree AV block and complete AV block that occurs in acute inferior wall myocardial infarction or with digitalis excess, atropine and isoproterenol may result in more rapid ventricular rates (Fig. 50–15, A). When the site of the AV block is within or below the His bundle, as in Mobitz Type II second-degree AV block or complete AV block that occurs in acute anterior wall myocardial infarction, isoproterenol, but not atropine, might increase the ventricular rate (Fig. 50–15, B).

Although atropine and isoproterenol *may* be useful in increasing ventricular rate in AV block, their administration should be viewed as a temporizing measure to be used while plans are being made for the institution of ventricular pacing. In the most urgent situation of ventricular standstill, "blind" attempts to achieve ventricular pacing may be made with a standard or a balloon tip "flow-directed" electrode catheter inserted into a vein, or with a wire electrode inserted percutaneously through the chest wall or epigastrium into the right or left ventricular chambers.

TACHYARRHYTHMIAS

Tachycardia is said to be present when the rate of a rhythm exceeds a particular, but arbitrarily chosen, limit. Tachycardias may be clinically significant because of the adverse hemodynamic effects of the rapid heart rate and, often, the accompanying changes in atrial and ventricular contraction sequences; or because of their ability to degenerate into even more rapid and, therefore, more hemodynamically disadvantageous arrhythmias.

The management of the patient with a tachyarrhythmia depends on the immediate hemodynamic effects of the arrhythmia, the projected clinical course of the arrhythmia with and without specific therapeutic interventions, the underlying cardiovascular status of the patient, and the nature of the arrhythmia itself. It is, therefore, critical in evaluating a patient with a tachyarrhythmia to answer the following questions:

1. Is the tachyarrhythmia causing a serious problem at the moment, or is its continuation likely to?
2. What, exactly, is the tachyarrhythmia?
3. What is the patient's underlying cardiovascular status, i.e., does the patient have evidence of heart disease?
4. What is the most prudent way to terminate the arrhythmia or to attenuate its adverse effects?

Supraventricular Tachyarrhythmias

Supraventricular tachyarrhythmias are unusually rapid rhythms that arise in sinus nodal, atrial, or AV junctional tissue. The arrhythmia may result from either enhanced automaticity or reentry within supraventricular tissue. In supraventricular tachyarrhythmias, the ventricular rhythm is stimulated by supraventricular impulses. The tachyarrhythmias may have adverse hemodynamic effects because the resultant ventricular rate is quite rapid, because atrial contraction becomes ineffective, and/or because the normal atrial and ventricular contraction sequence has been lost. Essential to the management of patients with supraventricular tachyarrhythmias is an assessment of the relative significance of these factors, for therapeutic maneuvers aimed simply at slowing the ventricular rate may be quite different from those aimed at terminating the tachyarrhythmia in order to restore the normal atrial and ventricular contraction sequence.

The specific supraventricular tachyarrhythmias are

- sinus tachycardia
- ectopic atrial tachycardia (EAT)
- multifocal atrial tachycardia (MAT)
- atrial fibrillation
- atrial flutter
- paroxysmal supraventricular tachycardia (PSVT)
- nonparoxysmal junctional tachycardia (NPJT)

The mechanistic similarities and differences of these tachyarrhythmias have important diagnostic and therapeutic implications (Fig. 50–16). For example, in most supraventricular tachyarrhythmias, a rapid independent atrial rhythm stimulates the ventricular rhythm. In paroxysmal supraventricular tachycardia (PSVT) due to

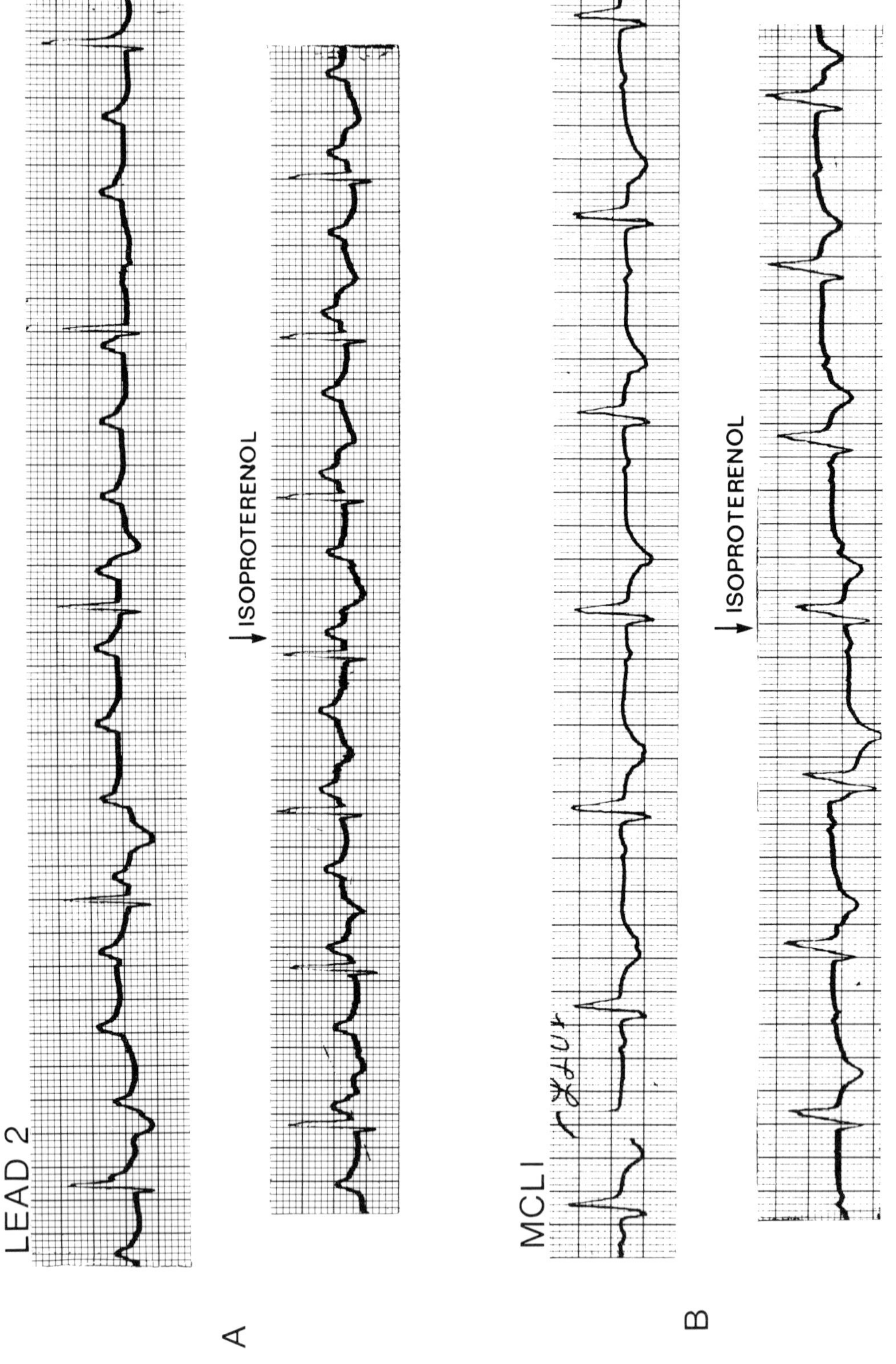

Figure 50–15 ECGs Showing Effect of Isoproterenol in AV Complete Block. *Note:* In strips *A*, which were recorded from a patient with an acute inferior wall myocardial infarction, there is complete AV block. The atrial rhythm is sinus tachycardia; the QRS rhythm is junctional in origin and occurs at a rate of about 35 beats/minute. During the intravenous administration of isoproterenol, AV conduction occurs with a 2:1 ratio. In strips *B*, recorded from a patient with an acute anterior wall myocardial infarction, there is complete AV block with an atrial rate of about 100 beats/minute, and an idioventricular or fascicular rhythm at a rate of about 50 beats/minute. The intravenous administration of isoproterenol increases the rate of the idioventricular or fascicular rhythm, but does not improve AV conduction.

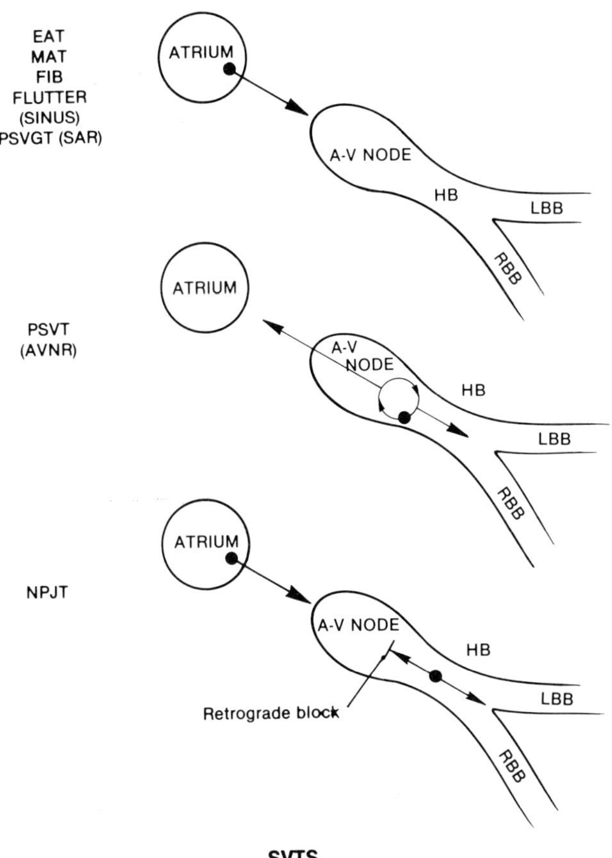

Figure 50–16 Mechanisms of Supraventricular Tachyarrhythmias. *Key: AVNR,* AV nodal reentry; *EAT,* ectopic atrial tachycardia; *FIB,* fibrillation; *HB,* His bundle; *LBB,* left bundle branch; *MAT,* multifocal atrial tachycardia; *NPJT,* nonparoxysmal junctional tachycardia; *PSVT,* paroxysmal supraventricular tachycardia; *RBB,* right bundle branch; *SAR,* sinoatrial reentry.

the mechanism of AV nodal reentry (AVNR), however, both atrial and ventricular rhythms are dependent on AV nodal reentrant impulses. In nonparoxysmal junctional tachycardia, the atrial rhythm is independent of the more rapid AV junctional pacemaker that stimulates the ventricular rhythm; but, because of retrograde AV nodal conduction block, the junctional impulse cannot stimulate the atrium.

Sinus Tachycardia

The sinus node is strongly influenced by the autonomic nervous system, circulating catecholamines, the temperature of the circulating blood, and thyroid hormone. The automatic firing rate of the sinus node is increased by stimulation of the sympathetic portion of the autonomic nervous system, as well as by circulating catecholamines, elevation of body temperature, and thyroid hormone. Its automatic firing rate is decreased by stimulation of the parasympathetic nervous system,

beta-adrenergic blocking agents, decrement in body temperature, and deficiency of thyroid hormone.

Sinus rhythm at rates in excess of 100 beats/minute is said to be abnormal; this tachyarrhythmia is termed *sinus tachycardia.* Since the normal sinus mechanism is operating, sinus tachycardia is an arrhythmia only by virtue of its rate. Thus, sinus tachycardia should not be looked upon as an arrhythmia per se, but rather as a response to certain events. It is the responsibility of the physician to search for the specific event causing the tachycardia.

Sinus tachycardia is commonly seen in patients with infection, heart failure, acute anxiety reactions, asthmatic attacks, and intravascular volume depletion that is, most often, due to hemorrhage or gastrointestinal fluid loss. In some patients, medications such as thyroid hormone, bronchodilators, or vasodilators (e.g., hydralazine hydrochloride) contribute to the rapid rate. Rarely, sinus tachycardia at rates as high as about 140 beats/minute may occur chronically for no identifiable reason. Only in the rarest instances, for example, thyrotoxicosis, are specific medications (generally beta-blocking agents) administered in an attempt to slow the heart rate.

Ectopic Atrial Tachycardia

Ectopic atrial tachycardia (EAT) is a rare arrhythmia in which an ectopic atrial pacemaker discharges at a reasonably constant and rapid rate. While in most clinically encountered ectopic atrial tachycardias, the atrial rate is in the range of 160 to 190 beats/minute, cases have been observed in which the atrial rate is only slightly more than 100 beats/minute, or as rapid as about 240 beats/minute. Most ectopic atrial tachycardias are seen in patients with severe heart disease during a period of profound congestive heart failure; in some patients, it may be a manifestation of excessive digitalis.

The ventricular (QRS) rate and rhythm in ectopic atrial tachycardia depend on conduction of the atrial impulses through the AV conduction system, the slowest conducting portion of which is almost always the AV node. At times, there may be consistent 1:1 or 2:1 AV conduction; at other times, AV Wenckebach periods (e.g., 3:2, 4:3, 5:4) may occur (Fig. 50–17, A). The AV conduction ratio generally depends on the atrial rate, conduction being "better" at lower atrial rates, and on the conduction properties of the AV node, which can be altered by medications and by autonomic nervous system traffic.

The P waves in ectopic atrial tachycardia are generally of abnormal contour and duration, being sharply pointed and narrow (Fig. 50–17, B). When the atrial rate is rapid and 1:1 AV conduction is present, P waves may not be seen easily. However, when AV conduction

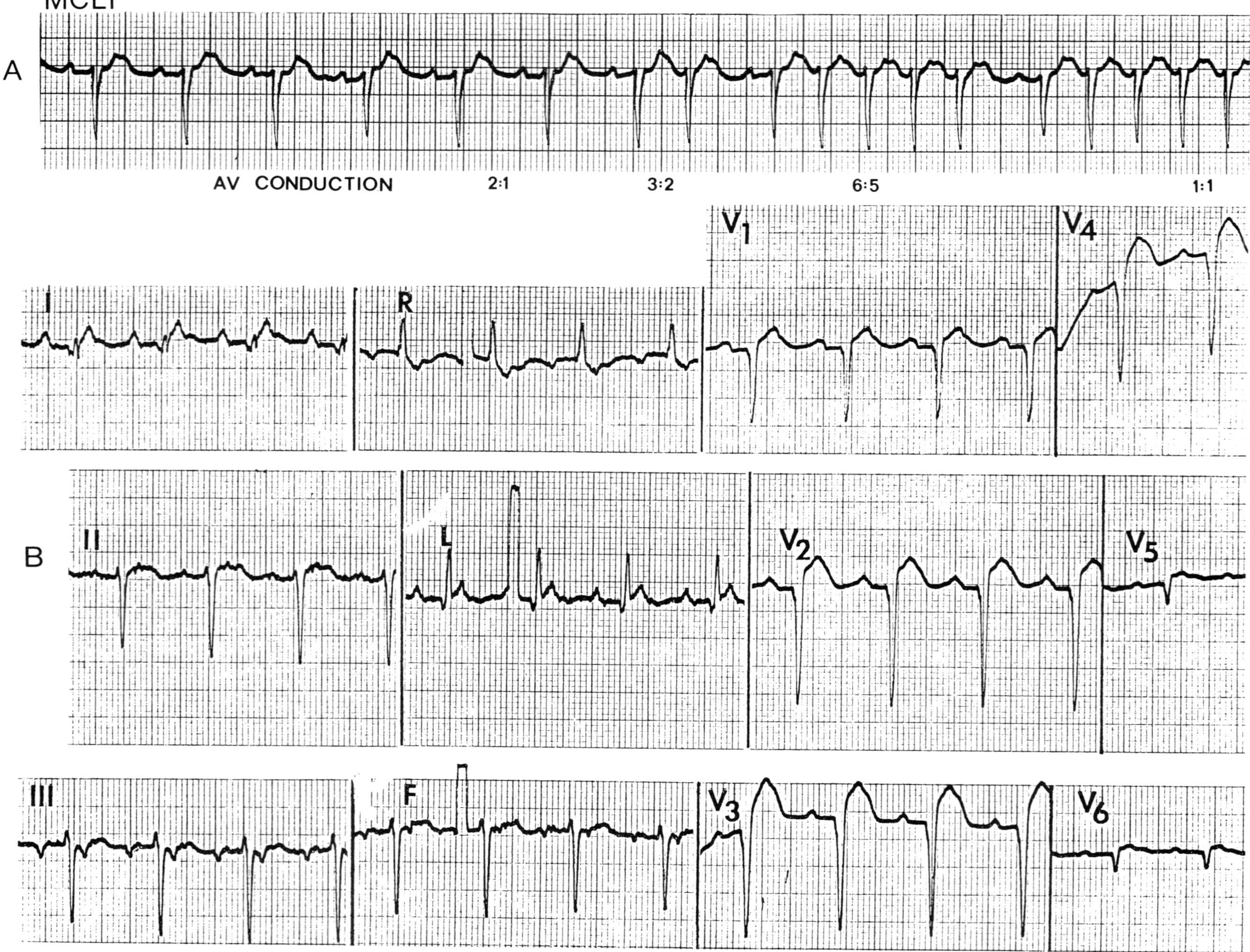
MCLI
A
AV CONDUCTION
2:1
3:2
6:5
1:1
I
R
V1
V4
B
II
L
V2
V5
III
F
V3
V6

is less than 1:1, as may occur spontaneously or in response to carotid sinus massage or medication, e.g., edrophonium chloride (Tensilon) or digitalis, P waves may be clearly seen.

The adverse hemodynamic effects of ectopic atrial tachycardia relate predominantly to the rapidity of the ventricular rate, for the *atrial kick* is maintained by the organized atrial rhythm. When AV conduction is 1:1, the patient may be profoundly ill, and treatment aimed at slowing the ventricular rate by slowing AV nodal conduction is in order. If digoxin is *not* the cause of the arrhythmia, then digoxin may be given, preferably intravenously, in doses of 0.125 to 0.375 mg. Even if the arrhythmia *is* digoxin-related, more digoxin may be given to slow the ventricular rate when AV conduction is 1:1. However, it should be administered only in very small doses of about 0.0675 to 0.125 mg. It should be used simply to achieve slower ventricular rate while the heart failure, which predisposes to the ectopic atrial tachycardia, is brought under control. Beta-blocking agents and verapamil, a calcium blocking agent, should rarely, if ever, be used in these patients, as they may worsen the already usually profound heart failure state.

If AV conduction of the ectopic atrial tachycardia is 2:1, the ventricular rate is usually about 100 beats/minute and the rhythm is not a problem per se. Such patients probably should be admitted to the hospital for treatment of heart failure, however, and for monitoring of the cardiac rhythm, especially if digoxin is causing or contributing to the arrhythmia. Digoxin should *not* be given to patients with ectopic atrial tachycardia when the AV conduction ratio is 2:1 or greater, for such an intervention may result in higher grades of AV block and in ventricular arrhythmias that are often fatal.

If due to digoxin excess, ectopic atrial tachycardia may be terminated by the cautious IV or oral administration of potassium chloride (KCl), even if the serum potassium level is normal. KCl usually produces a gradual slowing of the atrial rate by about 10 to 20 beats/minute, an event that has the undesirable effect of increasing the tendency for AV conduction to become 1:1. However, while the resultant increase in ventricular rate may worsen the patient's hemodynamic state, the deterioration is usually transient, for the ectopic atrial tachycardia generally terminates shortly (minutes to an hour or so) after such slowing of the atrial rate. Direct current cardioversion of ectopic atrial tachycardia, especially if digitalis-related, is ill-advised because of the severe, and occasionally disastrous ventricular arrhythmias that may follow.

Multifocal (Chaotic) Atrial Tachycardia

Multifocal atrial tachycardia is characterized by the occurrence, during sinus rhythm, of APCs of several

Figure 50–17 ECGs Showing Ectopic Atrial Tachycardia. *Note: A* Rhythm strip recorded during ectopic atrial tachycardia shows the effects of variable AV conduction on the QRS rhythm. *B* Twelve-lead ECG recorded from the same patient whose rhythm strip is seen in *A* shows consistent 2:1 AV conduction and abnormal P-wave contours. This tracing also shows extensive anterior wall myocardial infarction and left axis deviation attributable to left anterior fascicle block.

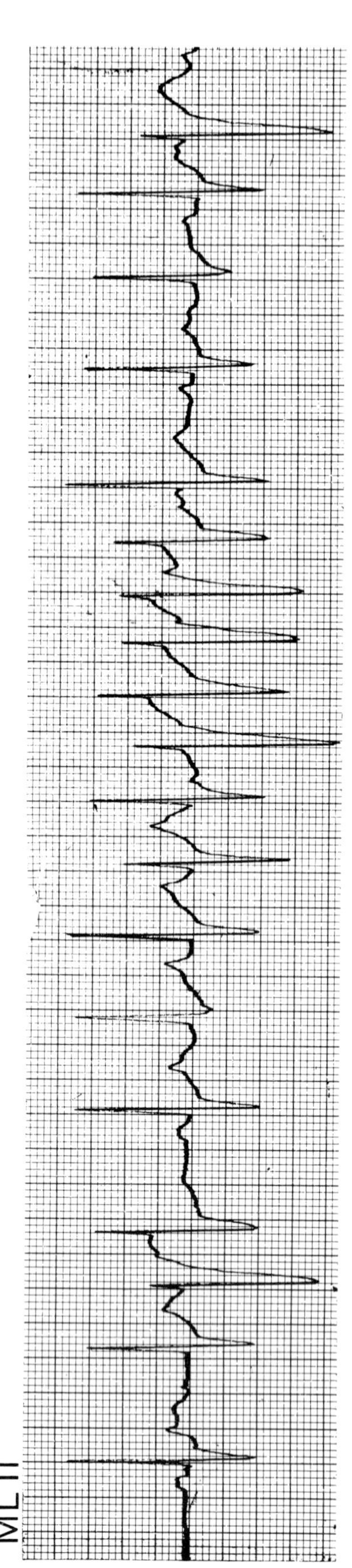

Figure 50–18 ECG Showing Multifocal Atrial Tachycardia. *Note:* The occurrence of P waves of several different contours at variable and brief intervals establishes the diagnosis of multifocal atrial tachycardia. The variability in the contours of the QRS complexes reflects different degrees of aberrant intraventricular conduction.

contours at rapid rates, at variable coupling intervals, and in salvos (Fig. 50–18). The APCs may be conducted normally or aberrantly, or they may be blocked within the AV conduction system.

Multifocal atrial tachycardia is seen almost exclusively in patients with respiratory failure related to acute and chronic pulmonary disease, although it occasionally occurs in patients with end-stage heart disease. Hypoxemia, acidemia, hypercapnia, and the high state of sympathetic stimulation attributable to abnormal respiratory function are predisposing factors. The rhythm presumably reflects high right atrial pressures and volumes that occur in those patients with severe right ventricular hypertension. The rhythm per se is rarely, if ever, of hemodynamic consequence. Rather, it is a marker of the precarious respiratory status of the patient, and it mandates immediate attention to the respiratory problem. Therapy is directed at improving the arterial blood gas levels and correcting metabolic abnormalities, which may require the use of bronchodilators, supplemental inspired oxygen, antibiotics, chest percussion and postural drainage, and even assisted or controlled ventilation with a respirator. As the arterial blood gas and metabolic abnormalities improve, multifocal atrial tachycardia typically abates and disappears, occasionally leaving isolated APCs. Specific antiarrhythmic medications should not be administered to these patients, because their blood gas and metabolic abnormalities predispose them to the toxic effects of these medications. (See Chapter 57.)

Atrial Fibrillation

Atrial fibrillation is characterized by a fine or coarse irregular baseline, which reflects disorganized atrial activity, and, in the presence of adequate AV conduction, an irregular ventricular (QRS) rhythm attributable to more or less random temporal conduction of the fibrillatory impulses through the AV conduction system (see Figure 50–16). The rate of the ventricular rhythm in atrial fibrillation is determined by the conduction properties of the AV node, which may be altered by medications and by changes in autonomic nervous system traffic. In the presence of normal AV nodal function, the ventricular rate during atrial fibrillation is in the range of 160 to 180 beats/minute; when AV nodal function is depressed, the ventricular rate is slower. In patients with accessory AV conduction pathways that conduct rapidly and have short refractory periods, the ventricular response during atrial fibrillation may be much faster, occasionally, as rapid as 300 beats/minute (see discussion of Wolff-Parkinson-White syndrome).

Although atrial fibrillation may occur episodically in otherwise healthy patients, it is generally seen in patients with structural cardiac disease and/or progressive degenerative disease of the supraventricular portion of the cardiac conduction system. The rapid ventricular rate associated with atrial fibrillation generally results in symptoms and in hemodynamic deterioration, and the loss of the atrial contribution to ventricular filling may dramatically depress ventricular performance in patients with significant left ventricular dysfunction. In still other patients, especially those with large left atria, mitral stenosis, idiopathic hypertrophic subaortic stenosis, and congestive heart failure, atrial fibrillation predisposes to the formation of left atrial thrombi and, therefore, to arterial embolism.

Management of the patient with atrial fibrillation begins with an assessment of the relative deleterious effects of the rapid ventricular rate and the loss of atrial contraction on the hemodynamic state, the reversibility of the circumstances that predisposed to or precipitated the onset of the arrhythmia, and the likelihood that sinus rhythm can be restored and maintained. The aim of treatment is to convert the rhythm to sinus, but if this is not advisable or not likely to be achievable, to slow the *resting* ventricular rate to about 70 to 80 beats/minute and to prevent excessively rapid ventricular rates from occurring with effort.

If the patient with atrial fibrillation and rapid ventricular rate is critically ill, because of either the rapid rate itself or the loss of atrial contraction, direct current cardioversion to sinus rhythm may be attempted and can usually be achieved with a 100 to 400 (but occasionally only a 50) watt-second electrical discharge, which should be synchronized to the spontaneous QRS complexes. In the less seriously ill patient, the oral or IV administration of digoxin or beta-blocking medication generally slows the ventricular rate over a period of minutes to hours; verapamil given IV will slow the ventricular rate in minutes. However, the heightened sympathetic nervous system stimulation that is often present in patients with congestive heart failure, acute or recent myocardial infarction, pericarditis, pulmonary embolus, or pulmonary parenchymal processes may oppose the rate-slowing effect of the medications. Atrial fibrillation of recent onset may abruptly terminate spontaneously, or as the ventricular response slows in response to medications. If atrial fibrillation persists despite achievement of a reasonably slow ventricular rate, plans should be made to perform direct current cardioversion. Quinidine or procainamide should be administered in the usual therapeutic doses for 24 to 48 hours prior to the electrical conversion attempt, for these medications may themselves convert the rhythm to sinus (or to atrial flutter). Furthermore, they seem to aid in maintaining sinus rhythm once it is restored. It is inadvisable to attempt direct current cardioversion in the presence of electrolyte, metabolic, or blood gas abnormalities, or digitalis excess, because more serious arrhythmias may emerge within seconds to minutes after the electrical discharge. It is often difficult to restore and impossible to maintain sinus rhythm if right or left atrial enlargement is extreme, or if the fibrillation has persisted for more than a few months. As conversion to sinus rhythm in patients with severe mitral valve disease, idiopathic hypertrophic subaortic stenosis, and low cardiac output from any cause courts the disaster of systemic embolism from a left atrial thrombus, many cardiologists feel that such patients should be anticoagulated for at least a few weeks prior to any conversion attempt.

It may be necessary to manage atrial fibrillation differently in patients with accessory AV conduction pathways, for the accessory pathway is composed of tissue with properties different from those of AV nodal tissue and much more like those of His-Purkinje system tissue. If AV conduction is occurring predominantly by the accessory pathway, digitalis, beta-blocking medications, and verapamil are usually *not* effective in slowing ventricular rate, but procainamide, quinidine, or disopyramide might be. (This topic is discussed in more detail in the section on the Wolff-Parkinson-White syndrome.)

Atrial Flutter

Atrial flutter is recognized by the regular occurrence of saw-toothed waves, seen best in leads II, III, and aVF of the surface ECG (Fig. 50–14, A, and 50–19). The usual rate of these flutter waves is about 300/minute, but it may be as slow as 220/minute or as rapid as 340/minute. The ventricular rate and rhythm in atrial flutter depend on conduction of the flutter impulses through the AV node. In most clinical circumstances and at most flutter rates, the normal AV node conducts every other flutter impulse into the ventricles, resulting in the regular appearance of QRS complexes of the usual contour at a rate exactly one-half the flutter rate. Diseased AV nodes conduct the flutter impulses less well, and the resultant ventricular rate is slower. One-to-one AV conduction of flutter impulses may be seen in infants, in patients with accessory AV conduction pathways that have short refractory periods (see Wolff-Parkinson-White Syndrome), and in patients with relatively slow flutter rates of about 220 to 240 per minute. AV nodal conduction of the flutter impulses may be enhanced by beta-adrenergic stimulating drugs, bronchodilators, and vagolytic medications or maneuvers; it may be inhibited by digitalis glycosides, parasympathetic stimulation, vagotonic medications and maneuvers, and beta-adrenergic blocking agents, and verapamil.

Atrial flutter generally occurs in patients with structural cardiac disease, and it may be the only manifes-

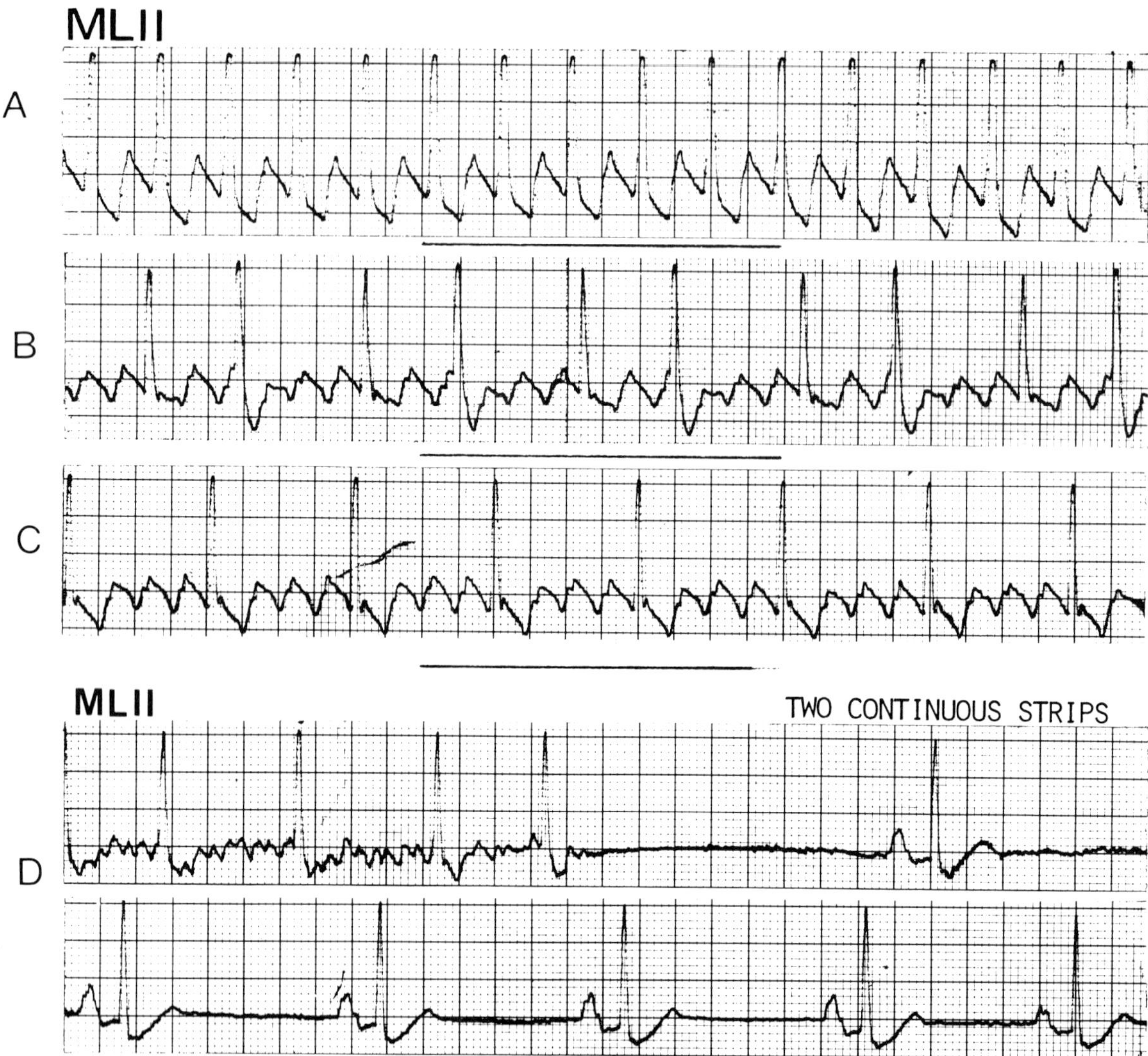

Figure 50–19   ECGs Showing Effects of Digoxin and Propranolol in Atrial Flutter. *Note: A, B,* and *C* were recorded serially, following the oral administration of digoxin and propranolol to a patient with atrial flutter. These medications effect a change in AV conduction from 2:1 in *A* to 4:1 in *C*. About two hours after the strip in *C* was recorded, the strips in *D* were recorded; they show the spontaneous termination of atrial flutter to cardiac standstill and the resumption of sinus rhythm that gradually increases in rate.

tation of disease of the sinus node and atrial tissues, in which case it would be considered a manifestation of the sick sinus syndrome. Atrial flutter generally causes hemodynamic deterioration by virtue of the rapid ventricular rates that usually accompany it, although loss of the atrial contribution to ventricular filling may contribute to the deterioration in patients with poor left ventricular function. Management of the patient with atrial flutter is aimed at terminating the arrhythmia or slowing the ventricular response by administration of medications that slow AV nodal conduction and by withdrawal of medications that enhance it. The exact management program chosen depends on the hemo-

dynamic state of the patient at the time, the patient's underlying cardiovascular state, and the medication that the patient has taken up to that point. Atrial flutter can generally be terminated by direct current cardioversion with electrical discharges of 10 to 100 watt-seconds. In the patient with 1:1 AV conduction, the patient who has a rapid ventricular rate and is tolerating it poorly, and the patient who has no other cardiac disease and in whom converting the arrhythmia in advance of medication administration seems to carry little risk, electrical conversion is advisable.

The ventricular response to atrial flutter may be slowed with digitalis preparations, beta-blocking agents, and verapamil, but the latter two are best avoided in patients with poor left ventricular function, for they may precipitate or worsen congestive heart failure. Digitalis, beta-blocking agents, and verapamil* may be given intravenously or orally; the route of administration is chosen on the basis of the speed with which slowing of the ventricular rate is desired. The dosage of propranolol required to slow the ventricular rate is in the range of 5 to 10 mg orally three times daily, much lower than that needed for treatment of angina pectoris or hypertension. Patients who have no problem from atrial flutter with 2:1 AV conduction may be given oral digitalis or propranolol and sent home from the emergency department to return for follow-up, while sicker patients might best be managed by monitoring their cardiac rhythm in a holding area of the emergency department or in the hospital.

As digitalis or propranolol is administered to the patient in atrial flutter, the AV conduction ratio generally changes from 2:1 to a bigeminal rhythm in which the average AV conduction ratio is 3:1 (Fig. 50–19). During this bigeminal rhythm, the shorter R-R intervals are slightly longer than the R-R intervals during 2:1 AV conduction, and the longer intervals are slightly shorter than twice the R-R intervals during 2:1 AV conduction. Further digitalis and/or propranolol administration results in predominantly 4:1 AV conduction and a perfectly regular ventricular response at a rate of about 70 to 80 beats/minute. When the average AV conduction ratio is 3:1 or 4:1, quinidine or procainamide may be administered in the usual therapeutic doses for 24 to 48 hours. These medications may convert the atrial flutter to sinus rhythm, and they seem to aid in the maintenance of sinus rhythm once it is achieved. However, both quinidine and procainamide often slow the flutter rate slightly before they convert the rhythm. If they are given to patients whose flutter rates are initially relatively slow (less than about 260/minute), they may slow the atrial rate to a rate at which the normal AV node can conduct every impulse, resulting in 1:1 AV conduction with a dangerously rapid ventricular rate. Thus, before quinidine or procainamide is administered to patients with relatively slow flutter rates, it is advisable to depress AV nodal conduction, as evidenced by an average AV conduction ratio of 3:1 or 4:1, with digitalis and/or beta-blocking medications, and/or verapamil. Occasionally, during the administration of digitalis, beta-blocking agents, quinidine, or procainamide, or following a low-energy (less than about 75 watt-second) electrical discharge, atrial flutter may convert to atrial fibrillation; in this case, management of that specific arrhythmia must be undertaken.

---

*At the time of this writing verapamil is available only for IV use.

Paroxysmal Supraventricular Tachycardia

The term *paroxysmal supraventricular tachycardia* (PSVT) refers to a rapid regular rhythm that, in the overwhelming majority of patients, is due to reentry within the AV node. On occasion, however, it may be caused by reentry within the sinus node or atrial tissue. In patients with accessory AV conduction pathways, the mechanism of PSVT usually entails conduction from atrium to ventricle via one of the two pathways, and from ventricle to atrium via the other pathway.

PSVT is recognized in the surface ECG by the regular occurrence of QRS complexes at rates in the range of 140 to 220 per minute, usually between 160 and 170 per minute (Fig. 50–20). The QRS complexes are usually identical to sinus-stimulated QRS complexes in that same patient, although they may be different on occasion because of aberrant intraventricular conduction of the supraventricular impulses. When PSVT occurs in patients with accessory AV conduction pathways, the supraventricular impulse usually enters ventricular tissue via the normal AV node-His-Purkinje system pathway and returns via the accessory pathway to the atrium, from which it reenters the AV node; thus, the QRS complexes are usually normal. Rarely, the directions of conduction in the two pathways are reversed; in this instance, the QRS complexes may be very wide and bizarre, because ventricular activation is initiated via the accessory pathway in an area well away from those areas in which the His-Purkinje system normally initiates ventricular activation. When the rate of PSVT is above 200 beats/minute, it is likely that an accessory pathway is involved in the reentry circuit.

In AV nodal reentrant PSVT, the AV node behaves as if it has two pathways that are isolated from each other in the mid-portion of the node, but are joined together in the upper portion of the node, near the atrium, and in the lower portion of the node, near the His bundle (Fig. 50–21). During PSVT, one AV nodal conduction pathway transmits impulses from the upper portion of the node to the lower portion of the node; from that point it may enter both the His bundle, from which it can activate the ventricles, and the lower portion of the other AV nodal pathway in which it travels retrogradely to the upper portion of the AV node; at this point it can both enter the atrium to stimulate a P wave and *reenter* the upper portion of the other AV nodal pathway to begin another cycle.

In PSVT due to AV nodal reentry or to accessory pathway reentry, both atrial and ventricular rhythms are dependent on maintenance of the reentry circuit; thus, there is *always* a 1:1 relationship of P waves to QRS complexes. When sinus node or atrial reentry is the mechanism of PSVT, however, the ventricular rhythm depends on the atrial rate and on the conduction prop-

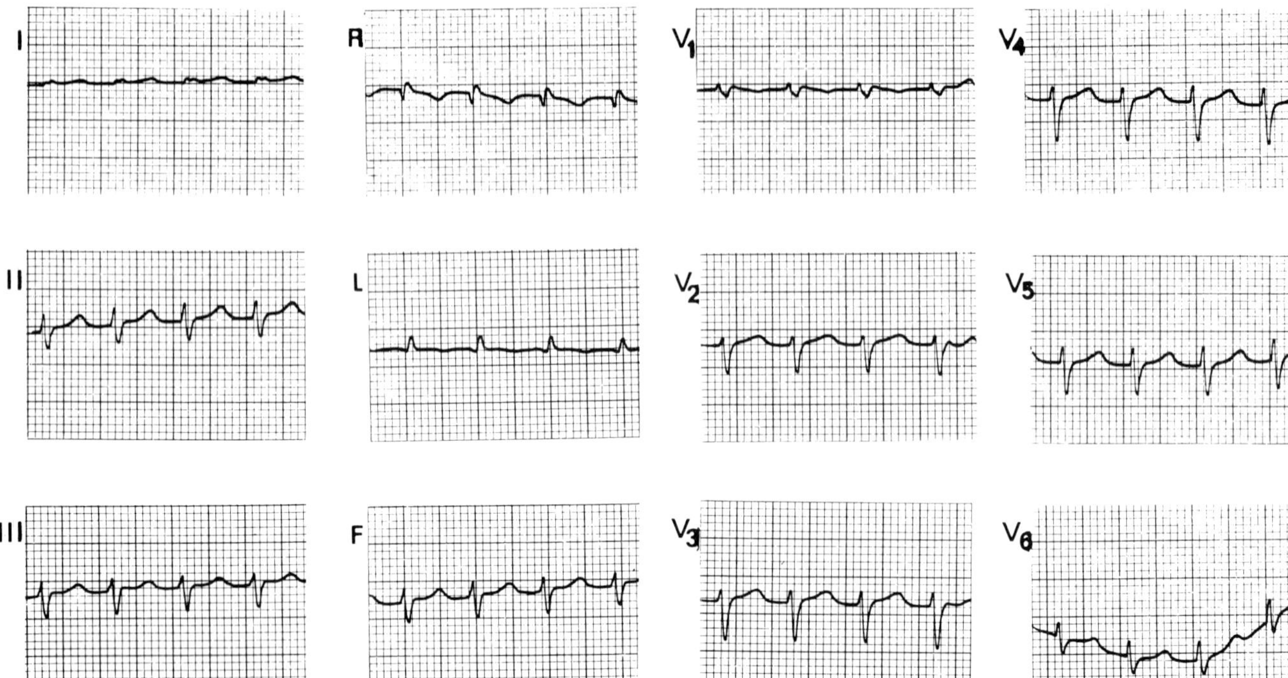

Figure 50–20   ECG Showing AV Nodal Reentrant PSVT. *Note:* This 12-lead ECG was recorded from a patient during an episode of AV nodal reentrant PSVT. P waves are not clearly identifiable, because they fall within the QRS complexes.

---

erties of the AV node. At times of 1:1 AV conduction, there is a 1:1 relationship between P waves and QRS complexes, but at other times, when AV conduction is depressed the ventricular rate is less than the atrial rate.

In AV nodal reentrant PSVT, the P waves usually fall within or close to the QRS complexes and are ob-

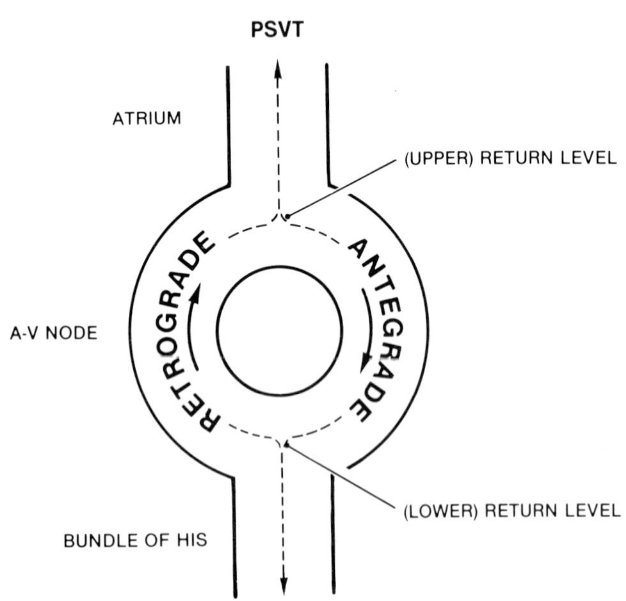

Figure 50–21   Movement of Electrical Impulses during AV Nodal Reentrant PSVT.

scured by them (Fig. 50–20). In accessory pathway reentry PSVT, the P waves usually occur outside of (later than) the QRS complexes and are thus somewhat easier to identify (Fig. 50–22). In sinus node or atrial reentry PSVT, the P waves precede the QRS complexes.

Patients with PSVT generally complain of rapid heart action. The occurrence of other symptoms depends on the hemodynamic effects of the tachycardia and the underlying cardiovascular status of the patient. In most patients, the deleterious hemodynamic effects result from the rapid heart rate; in some patients, they result from the loss of the normal atrial and ventricular contraction sequences because of the simultaneous activation of atria and ventricles. It is not unusual at the onset of PSVT for the patient—even a healthy one—to have presyncope or syncope if the rate of the tachycardia is very rapid and the ability of the cardiovascular system to adjust to sudden decreases in stroke volume and blood pressure is depressed.

The rate of PSVT is determined by the conduction velocities of the tissues that comprise the reentrant circuit; the arrhythmia persists only when the impulses travel in the reentrant pathways at specific velocities. Alterations of the conduction velocities and refractory periods of the reentrant pathways may interrupt the circus movement and, thus, terminate PSVT. In fact, PSVT is generally terminated by administering medications or by inducing changes in autonomic nervous system traffic that alter conduction velocities or refrac-

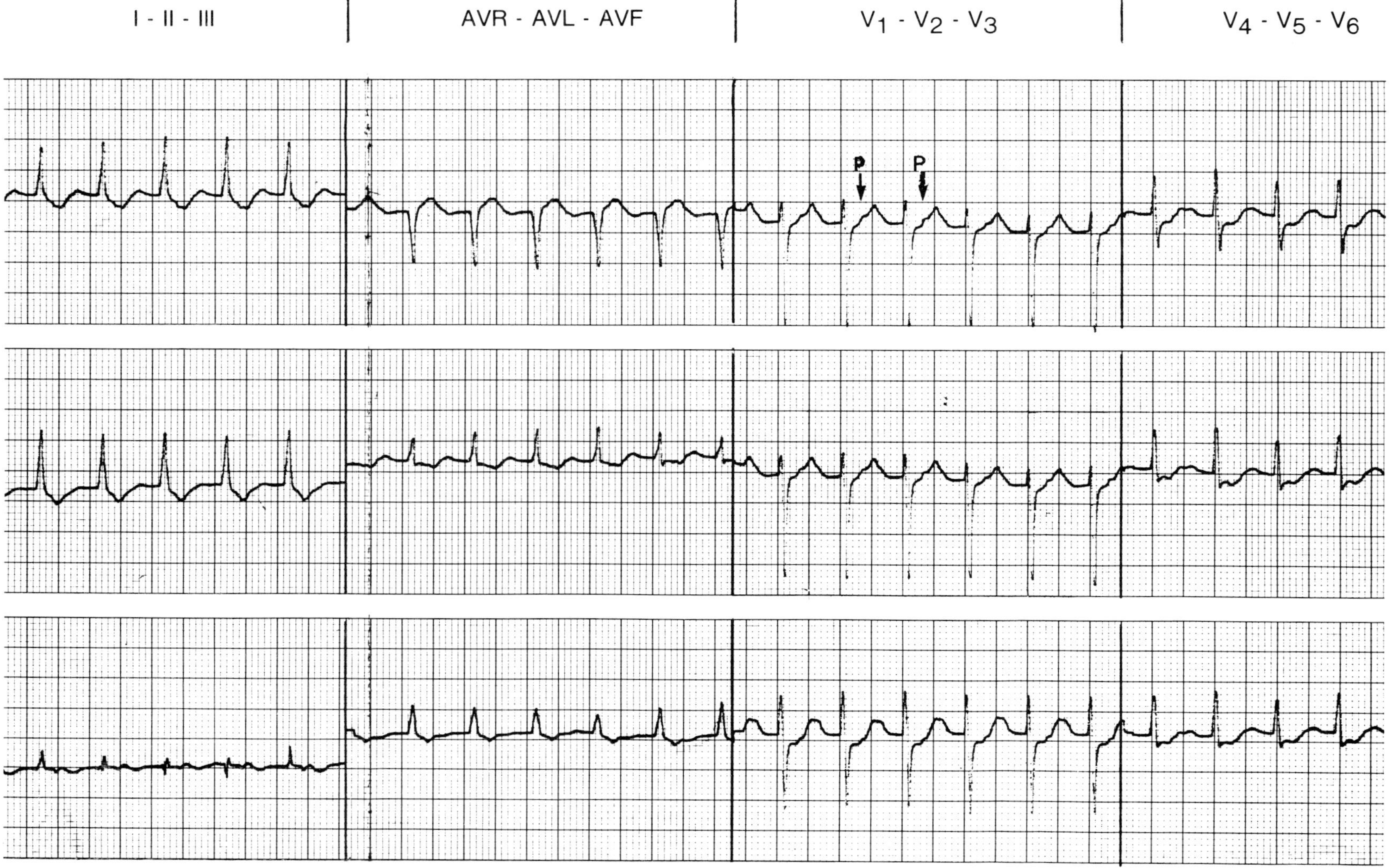

Figure 50–22   ECGs Showing PSVT Due to Accessory Pathway Reentry. *Note:* This 12-lead ECG was recorded during PSVT in a patient with an accessory AV conduction pathway and Wolff-Parkinson-White syndrome. The P waves fall well after the QRS complexes, whereas in AV nodal reentrant PSVT (Fig. 50–20) the P waves fall within the QRS complexes. The QRS complexes in this tracing are normal because the ventricles are activated normally via the His-Purkinje system.

tory periods of the reentrant pathways. The following medications and maneuvers are commonly used in attempts to terminate PSVT:

- vagal stimulation: carotid sinus massage, Valsalva's maneuver
- alpha-adrenergic stimulating agents: Vasoxyl, Aramine, Neo-Synephrine
- parasympathetic stimulating agents: Tensilon
- calcium blocking agents: verapamil
- beta-adrenergic blocking agents: Inderal, Lopressor
- digitalis preparations
- procainamide
- quinidine preparations
- Norpace
- lidocaine
- direct current cardioversion

Carotid sinus massage, Valsalva's maneuver, and elevation of the blood pressure with sympathomimetic amines such as methoxamine hydrochloride (Vasoxyl), metaraminol (Aramine), or phenylephrine hydrochloride (Neo-Synephrine), result in sympathetic withdrawal from and increased parasympathetic traffic into the AV nodal reentrant pathways; such changes may slow conduction or effect a block of one or both pathways, thus interrupting the circus movement and terminating the arrhythmia. Tensilon, a rapidly acting but short-lived cholinesterase inhibitor, allows the sudden buildup of large quantities of acetylcholine within the AV node, transiently blocking impulse conduction in one or both pathways and terminating the circus movement. Verapamil, a calcium-blocking agent, acts by directly slowing conduction in AV nodal pathways. Digitalis preparations probably act both by stimulating increased parasympathetic traffic into and by directly depressing conduction through the AV node. Beta-blocking agents, such as propranolol hydrochloride (Inderal) and metoprolol tartrate (Lopressor), act by slowing conduction in AV nodal pathways by virtue of their ability to block the effects of catecholamines. Quinidine, procainamide, and disopyramide (Norpace) are capable of slowing conduction in AV nodal pathways and in accessory AV conduction pathways; thus, they may be extremely effective in terminating PSVT that is due either to AV nodal reentry or to accessory pathway reentry. Lidocaine may be effective in terminating PSVT due to accessory pathway reentry, for it is capable of suppressing conduction in some accessory pathways.

The specific treatment selected for an individual depends on the potential effectiveness, the potential risk, and the simplicity of administering the therapy. For example, carotid sinus massage may quickly and effec-

tively terminate PSVT in a young, healthy adult, but it may result in a CVA in an older individual with extracranial cerebrovascular disease. Carotid sinus massage, Valsalva's maneuver, and Tensilon may be ineffective when the arterial blood pressure is low (i.e., less than 110 mm Hg systolic), but each may rapidly terminate PSVT when the blood pressure is normal, or has been increased to 140 to 180 mm Hg systolic. Such an elevation in blood pressure may be achieved by the administration of sympathomimetic amines, preferably at a slow rate but also at a rapid rate. The blood pressure must be measured frequently during the administration of such medications to avoid an excessive elevation, especially in patients with coronary artery disease, cerebrovascular disease, or severe left ventricular dysfunction. Occasionally, elevation of the blood pressure itself terminates PSVT, and there is no need for a vagal maneuver. Tensilon is best avoided in the asthmatic, in whom it may initiate bronchospasm, and in the patient with acute or chronic gastrointestinal disease, in whom it may induce nausea, vomiting, abdominal cramping, or evacuation of the bowels. Verapamil and beta-blocking medications are best avoided in patients with sick sinus syndrome in whom it may dramatically prolong the period of standstill that follows termination of PSVT, and in patients with poor ventricular function. Digoxin and verapamil are best avoided in the patient with Wolff-Parkinson-White syndrome *if* the patient has a history of atrial fibrillation and rapid ventricular rates because of rapid accessory pathway conduction, for these medications may enhance AV conduction if atrial fibrillation occurs. Lidocaine is likely to be effective only when a limb of the reentrant circuit is an accessory pathway, but its IV administration in a dosage of 50 to 150 mg is generally quite safe. Procainamide is extremely effective in terminating PSVT due to AV nodal reentry, as it blocks retrograde conduction in the conducting AV nodal pathway; however, when administered intravenously too rapidly, it may result in profound hypotension. Direct current cardioversion can be safely used to terminate PSVT regardless of the underlying mechanism, but it requires anesthesia. Occasionally, attempts at electrical conversion of PSVT result in atrial fibrillation rather than sinus rhythm, in which case the atrial fibrillation must be managed.

As PSVT tends to be recurrent and is initiated by APCs and PVCs, it is important to consider prescribing chronic antiarrhythmic therapy for suppression of ectopic beats in patients who have frequent or poorly tolerated episodes of the arrhythmia. Furthermore, before they are sent home from the emergency department, such patients might be taught how to perform carotid sinus massage, Valsalva's maneuver, and other vagal stimulatory maneuvers. They may also be advised to take specific medications in specific dosage schedules in an attempt to terminate the arrhythmia shortly after its onset and thus avoid a trip to the hospital. If an accessory AV conduction pathway is clearly involved in the PSVT, cardiologic evaluation seems appropriate.

Nonparoxysmal Junctional Tachycardia

A rarely encountered arrhythmia, nonparoxysmal junctional tachycardia is due to acceleration of the automatic rate of an AV junctional pacemaker (Fig. 50–16). In order for this accelerated pacemaker to emerge during sinus rhythm, it must have a more rapid rate of discharge than the sinus node at the time; usually, the junctional rate is just slightly in excess of the sinus rate. In the presence of atrial fibrillation or flutter, or ectopic atrial tachycardia, the junctional rhythm emerges only when there is such a high-grade AV block that the interval between consecutive atrial impulses traversing the AV node and reaching the AV junctional (His bundle) pacemaker exceeds the escape interval of the junctional pacemaker. This arrhythmia is generally seen only in the presence of digitalis excess and in very ill patients in the early hours after cardiac surgery.

Nonparoxysmal junctional tachycardia can be recognized by the regular occurrence of QRS complexes that are normal, i.e., usual for the patient (Fig. 50–23). Typically, there is a retrograde conduction block of these junctional impulses, so retrograde atrial activation does not occur (Fig. 50–16). However, antegrade conduction of sinus or atrial impulses through the AV node is usually unimpaired, although it may be depressed. If antegrade AV conduction is normal, atrial impulses reaching the AV junctional pacemaker before it is set to discharge are conducted through the AV junction and into the ventricles to stimulate a QRS complex that will occur prematurely. The premature QRS complex may have a contour identical to that of the usual QRS complexes if intraventricular conduction of this impulse is normal, but a different contour if intraventricular conduction is aberrant (Fig. 50–23).

Nonparoxysmal junctional tachycardia per se causes only mild to moderate hemodynamic deterioration, attributable to the intermittent loss of the atrial contribution to ventricular filling due to the AV dissociation resulting from the junctional automatic rate exceeding the sinus rate. As digitalis excess is the cause of this arrhythmia in most patients seen in the emergency department, management of the patient involves withdrawing digitalis. Continued digitalis administration to patients with nonparoxysmal junctional tachycardia may result in an increase in the rate of the arrhythmia and may be followed by ventricular tachycardia and ventricular fibrillation. It may be prudent to hospitalize

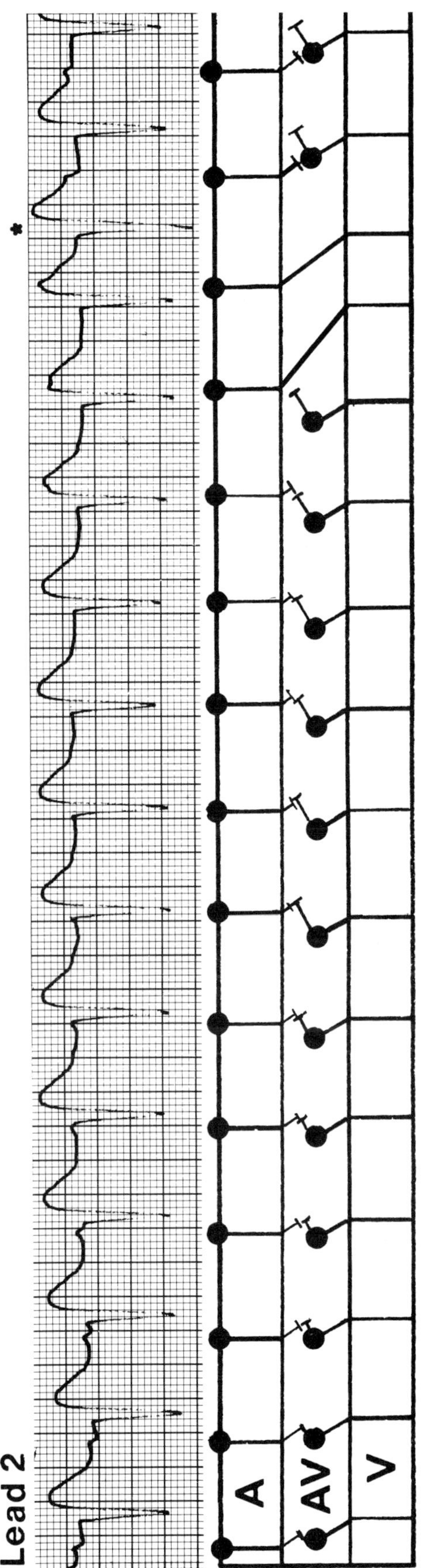

Figure 50–23 ECG Showing Nonparoxysmal Junctional Tachycardia in a Patient with Digoxin Excess. *Note:* The independent atrial rhythm is able to capture the ventricles only when the P wave falls shortly after the QRS complex. The wider QRS complex near the end of the strip (*asterisk*) is an aberrantly conducted sinus beat. The closed circles (●) in the latter diagram represent impulse formation in the sinus node (*top line*) and AV junction (*middle panel*). The vertical lines represent impulse conduction through the atria (A) and ventricles (V), while the slanted lines represent conduction through the AV node and His bundle (AV).

these patients for cardiac rhythm monitoring until the arrhythmia disappears.

Ventricular Tachyarrhythmias

Accelerated Ventricular Rhythm

Accelerated ventricular rhythm (AVR) is recognized by the emergence, during slowing of the sinus rate or during the slow phase of sinus arrhythmia, of wide and abnormal but generally not very bizarre QRS complexes that occur with regularity and are dissociated from the atrial rhythm (P waves) (Fig. 50–24). Fusion QRS complexes, which reflect activation of the ventricles by both the sinus impulse and the ectopic ventricular impulse, typically occur at the times of emergence and disappearance of the abnormally wide QRS complexes. Generally, accelerated ventricular rhythm will disappear when the sinus rate increases to the point that it consistently exceeds the rate of the accelerated ventricular rhythm.

Accelerated ventricular rhythm occurs exclusively in acute myocardial infarction, usually during the initial hours or days of the event. It is felt to reflect enhanced automaticity within the ischemic myocardium that bridges infarcted and normal tissue. AVR does *not* degenerate into ventricular fibrillation and does *not* cause hemodynamic deterioration because of its rate which is very close to the prevailing sinus rate at the time of its appearance. However, in patients with significant left ventricular dysfunction it may result in a mild to profound fall in blood pressure resulting from the loss of the atrial contribution to ventricular filling that occurs during transient AV dissociation. If the fall in blood pressure is felt to be clinically disadvantageous, the accelerated ventricular rhythm can generally be suppressed by increasing the sinus rate with intravenously administered atropine (0.5 to 1 mg), a phenomenon termed *overdrive suppression*. Generally, accelerated ventricular rhythm is most clinically significant because it indicates that acute myocardial necrosis has occurred within hours to days of its appearance.

Ventricular Tachycardia

Ventricular tachycardia (VT) is defined as the occurrence of at least three PVCs in a row at a rate in excess of 100 beats/minute. Ventricular tachycardia is initiated by PVCs; it may be sustained, i.e., lasting minutes to days, or nonsustained, lasting several seconds to a minute or so and terminating spontaneously (Figs. 50–4, A, and 50–25). The QRS complexes during ventricular tachycardia may vary in contour from mildly abnormal to very bizarre; the more bizarre complexes usually occur at more rapid rates, in specific clinical

settings, and in enlarged hearts. In sustained ventricular tachycardia, the QRS rhythm is generally perfectly regular; in nonsustained ventricular tachycardia, especially if rapid, the QRS complexes usually occur at variable intervals that are often very difficult to accurately measure.

The majority of patients with ventricular tachycardia have an awareness of abnormal cardiac action. Although most patients with ventricular tachycardia are symptomatic, some are totally asymptomatic and the tachycardia is unexpectedly detected on routine physical or electrocardiographic examination. In some, the rapid ventricular rate and the absence of the normal atrial and ventricular contraction sequence may result in such dramatic falls in cardiac output and blood pressure that the patient experiences profound weakness, presyncope, syncope, shortness of breath, and chest discomfort that suggests myocardial infarction. Recognition of ventricular tachycardia is of critical importance because it may degenerate into ventricular fibrillation and thus lead to circulatory arrest.

Ventricular tachycardia occurs most commonly in patients with cardiac disease, particularly coronary artery disease. It may occur in the initial seconds to days following acute myocardial infarction, or weeks to years afterwards as a manifestation of recurrent ischemia or infarction, or aneurysm. In a patient with coronary artery disease, runs of abnormally wide QRS complexes must be considered ventricular tachycardia until proved otherwise; however, they must be differentiated from accelerated ventricular rhythm and from supraventricular impulses with aberrant intraventricular conduction. In some patients, ventricular tachycardia may be a manifestation of digitalis excess.

Management of the patient with sustained ventricular tachycardia involves termination of the tachycardia and prevention of its recurrence.* If the patient is on the verge of or has already suffered cardiovascular collapse, direct current countershock, preferably synchronized, is the therapy most likely to restore sinus rhythm (Fig. 50–26, A). The energies needed to terminate ventricular tachycardia may be as low as about 10 watt-seconds, although much higher energy levels are sometimes required. For the patient with cardiovascular collapse, an initial high-energy (200 to 400 watt-second) discharge is advisable. Closed chest cardiac massage may be used to support the circulation until the electrical discharge can be administered. Many patients with hemodynamically significant ventricular tachycardia may be hypoxemic or acidemic, and correction of these abnormalities may improve the chances for successful

---

* For a detailed discussion of the pharmacologic treatment of ventricular arrhythmias associated with acute myocardial infarction, see Chapter 49.

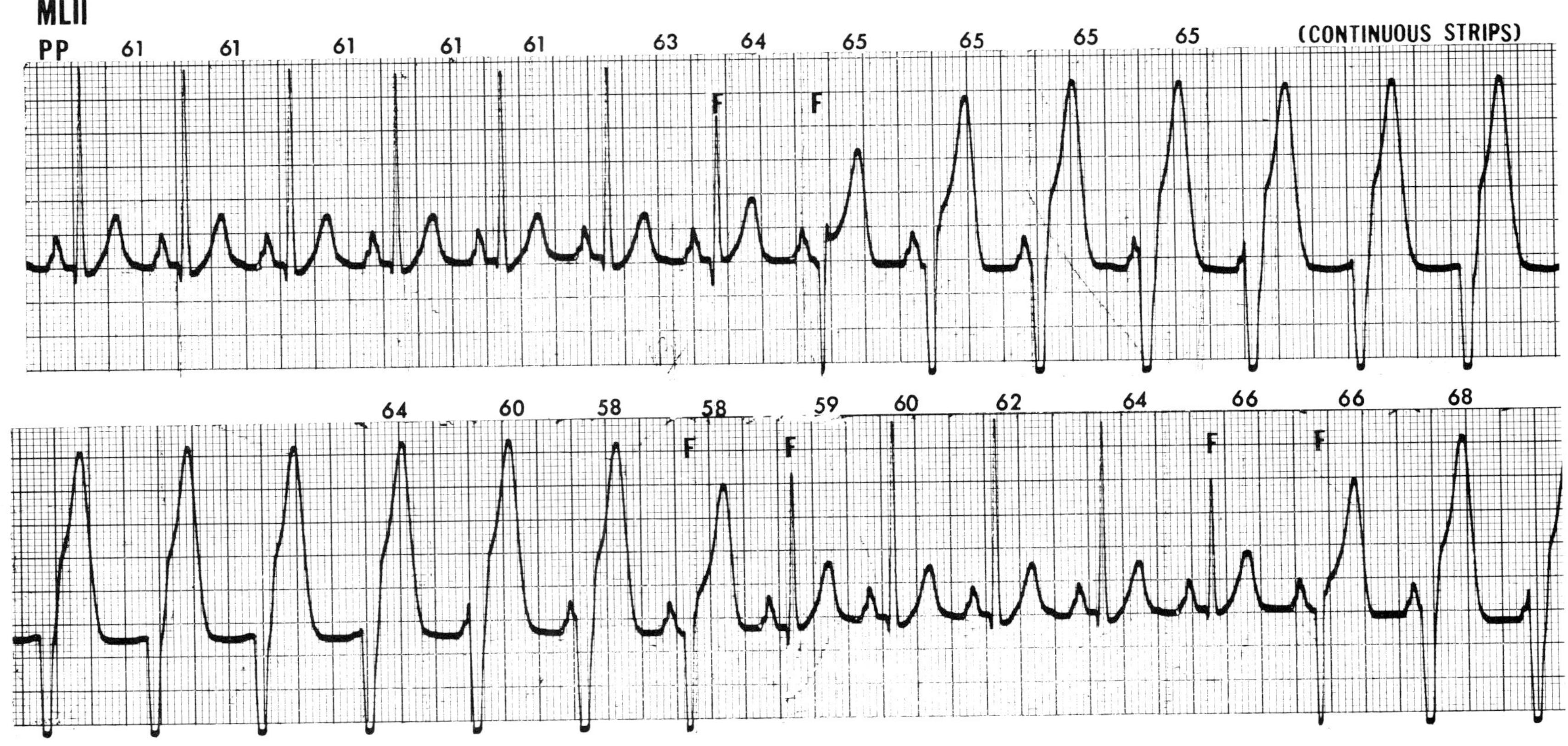

Figure 50–24   ECGs Showing Accelerated Ventricular Rhythm. *Note:* These strips, showing accelerated ventricular rhythm, were recorded from a patient with acute anterior wall myocardial infarction. The intervals between sinus P waves (PP) are in hundredths of a second. In the top strip, as the sinus rate slows, i.e., PP intervals lengthen, there appears a wide but reasonably organized and regularly occurring ventricular rhythm at a rate close to the sinus rate. Near the end of the top strip, the P waves disappear within the QRS complexes. In the bottom strip, the P waves reappear as the sinus rate accelerates; for a few seconds, they stimulate QRS complexes. When the sinus rate again slows, however, the wide, regular ventricular rhythm reappears. At the time of transition from one rhythm to another, the ventricles are activated by both sinus and ventricular impulses, resulting in fusion beats (F).

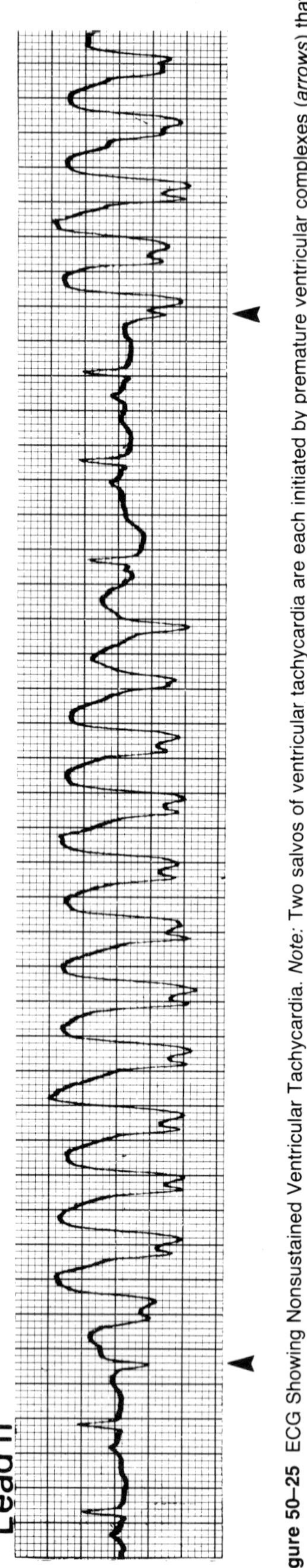

Figure 50–25 ECG Showing Nonsustained Ventricular Tachycardia. *Note:* Two salvos of ventricular tachycardia are each initiated by premature ventricular complexes (*arrows*) that fall in the T waves of sinus-stimulated QRS complexes. (*Source:* Reprinted with permission from Jacobson LB, Goldschlager N: *Arrhythmias: Case Studies.* Garden City, NY, Medical Examination Publishing, © 1978.)

termination of ventricular tachycardia and prevention of its recurrence.

In the less seriously ill patient with ventricular tachycardia, the IV administration of lidocaine (50 to 150 mg over 30 seconds to 5 minutes) or procainamide (50 mg/minute up to a dose of about 1,000 mg) may terminate the arrhythmia (Fig. 50–26, B). In the patient with recurrent ventricular tachycardia that is neither suppressed nor terminated by lidocaine or procainamide, bretylium tosylate (Bretylol) may be administered (see Chapter 49). Once sinus rhythm has been restored, medication aimed at suppressing PVCs, such as lidocaine, procainamide, quinidine, or disopyramide may be started, the specific medication and route of administration to be based on the patient's clinical condition, the likelihood that ventricular tachycardia will recur, and the hemodynamic effects of the tachycardia in the individual patient.

Paroxysms of self-terminating ventricular tachycardia may occur in patients whose ECGs show long QTU intervals (Fig. 50–27). In some of these patients, the long QTU interval is congenital and may be associated with deafness; in others, it may be acquired, or it may result from hypokalemia, coronary artery disease, or the administration of tricyclic antidepressants, phenothiazines, and antiarrhythmic medications (i.e., quinidine preparations, procainamide, and disopyramide). The runs of QRS complexes comprising ventricular tachycardia in association with long QTU intervals have a characteristic morphology termed *torsade de pointes.* This term describes the gradual and cyclic transition in the directions of the QRS complexes from upright to biphasic to inverted and vice versa (Fig. 50–28). It is critical to identify torsade de pointes and self-terminating paroxysms of ventricular fibrillation related to the long QTU interval, for the administration of quinidine, procainamide, or disopyramide to these patients may prolong the QTU interval even more, facilitating the appearance of ventricular tachycardia and increasing its severity. These patients must be managed by withdrawal of medications that may be contributing to the long QTU interval; by correction of hypokalemia, if present; and by the administration of lidocaine, diphenylhydantoin, or propranolol, in that order of preference. Occasionally, repeated electrical terminations of the arrhythmia may be required while the reversible abnormalities are being corrected. Atrial, but not ventricular, overdrive pacing may be helpful in shortening the QTU interval. If the heart rate is very slow both atrial and ventricular overdrive pacing may decrease the predisposition to the PVCs that initiate torsade de pointes.

When ventricular tachycardia is due to digitalis excess, termination of the arrhythmia by direct current cardioversion is often followed by more serious ven-

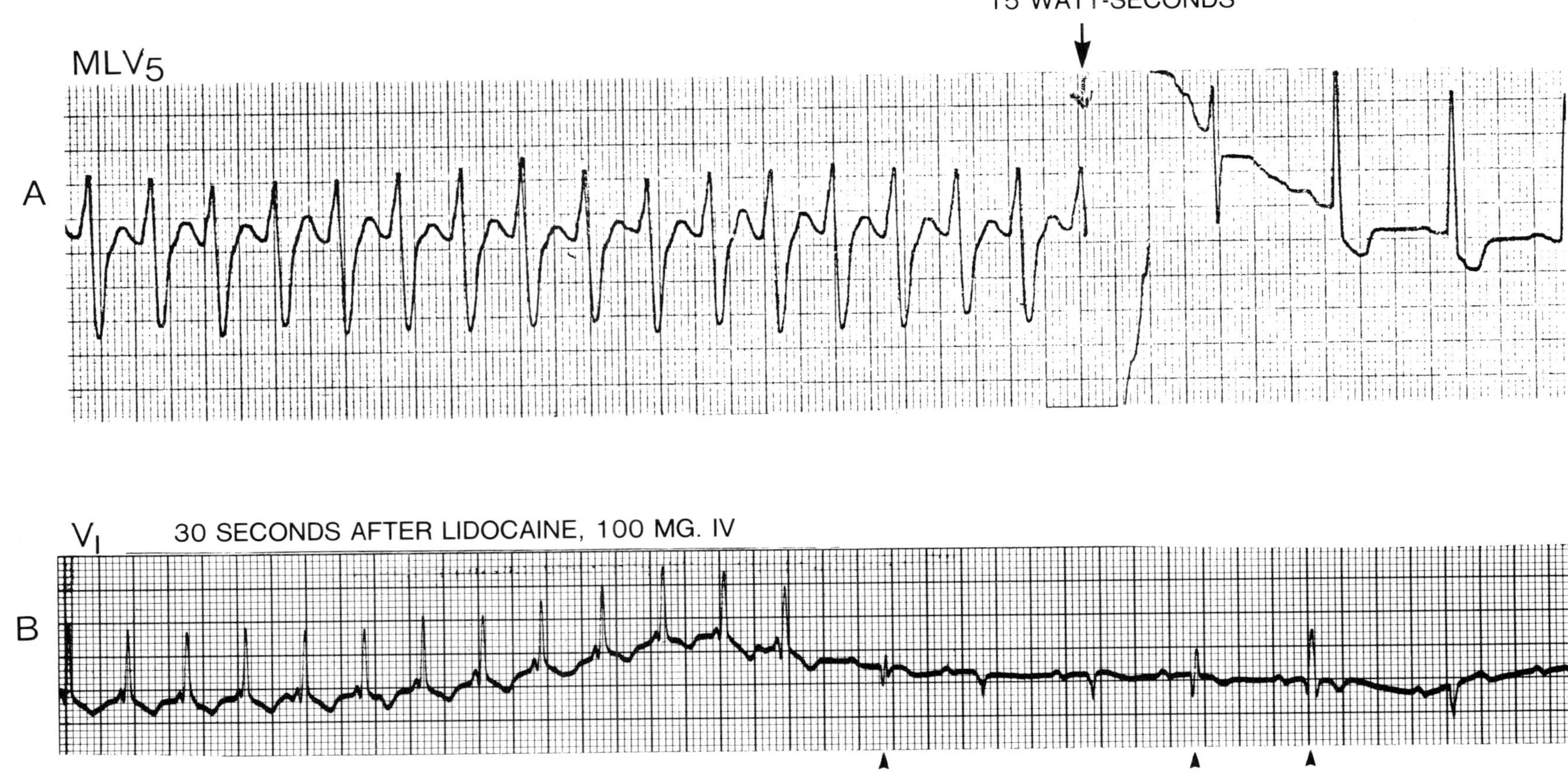

Figure 50–26   ECGs Showing Terminations of Sustained Ventricular Tachycardias. *Note: A* Sustained ventricular tachycardia at a rate of about 167 beats/minute is converted to sinus rhythm at a rate of about 90 beats/minute by a 15 watt-second synchronized direct current electrical discharge. *B.* Sustained ventricular tachycardia at a rate of about 170 beats/minute is terminated by the IV administration of lidocaine. Following termination of the ventricular tachycardia, the underlying atrial rhythm stimulates the QRS complexes. Some PVCs occur in the first few seconds after termination, and as they fall in late diastole result in fusion complexes (*arrows*).

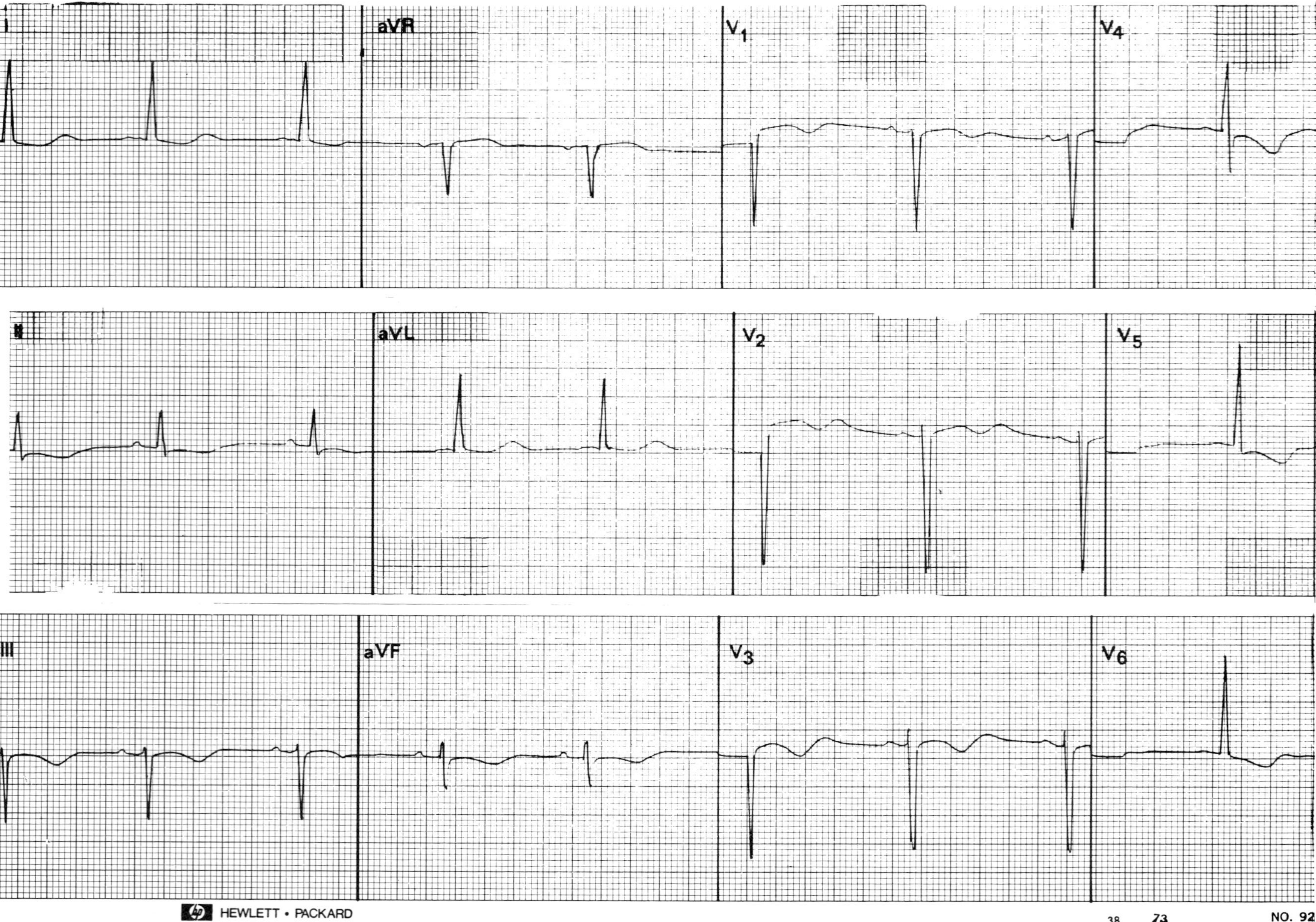

Figure 50–27   ECG Showing Prolongation of QTU Intervals. *Note:* This 12-lead ECG was recorded from a patient with tricyclic antidepressant-related prolongation of the QTU interval. This patient had paroxysms of ventricular tachycardia and ventricular fibrillation, as shown in Figure 50–28.

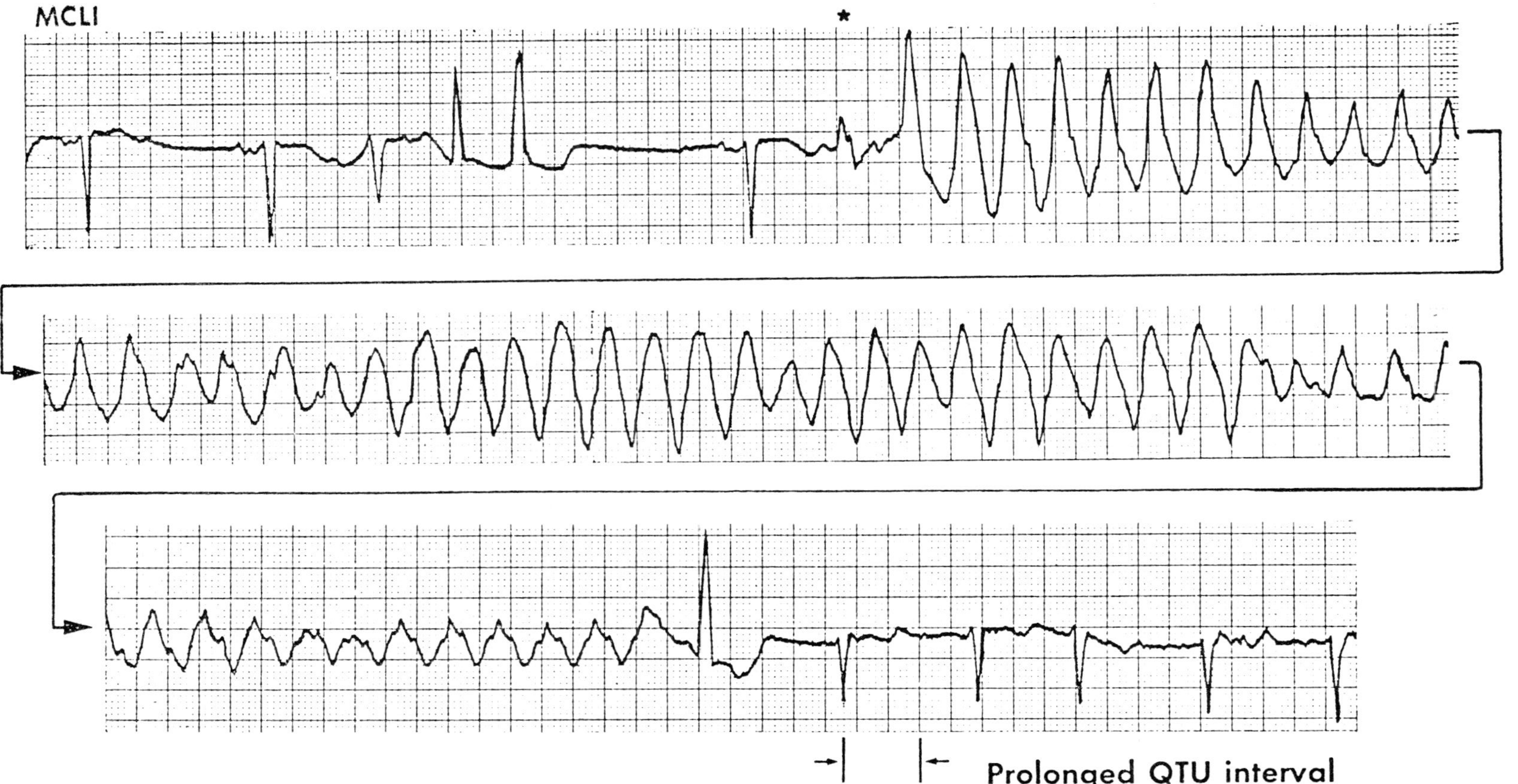

Figure 50–28   ECG Showing Torsade de Pointes. *Note:* These strips were recorded from the same patient whose 12-lead ECG appears in Figure 50–27. Beginning in the top strip, two sinus beats are followed by three PVCs. There then appears a sinus beat, in the U wave of which falls a PVC (*asterisk*), which initiates a 17-second run of bizarre ventricular tachycardia at a rate of about 200 beats/minute. This tachycardia terminates spontaneously, and sinus rhythm resumes. During tachycardia, the QRS complexes are initially upright, then equiphasic, and then inverted. This alternation in direction then repeats itself.

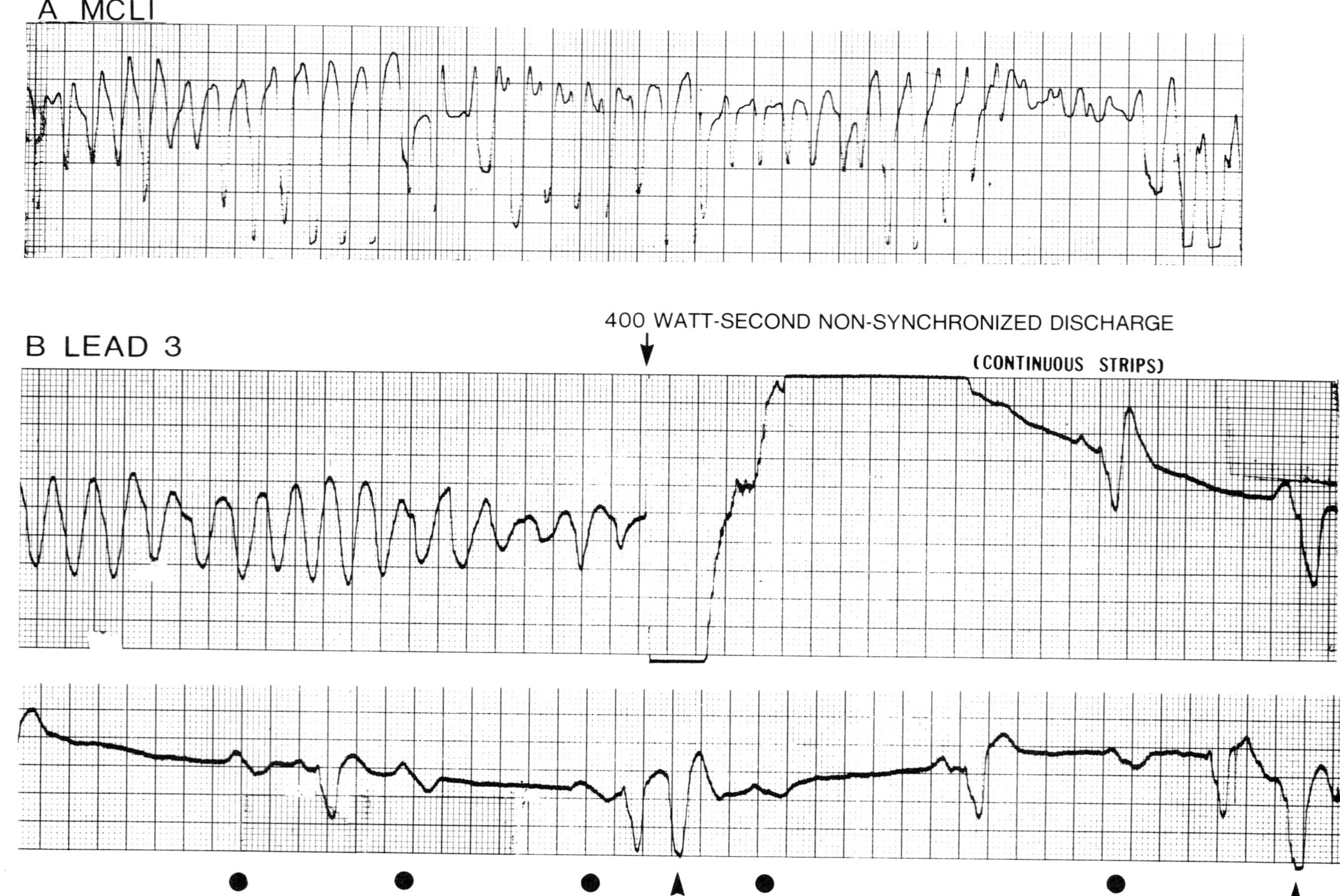

Figure 50–29   ECGs Showing Ventricular Fibrillation. *Note: A* This ECG shows coarse, rapid, irregular electrical activity representing ventricular fibrillation in a patient with acute inferior wall myocardial infarction. *B* These two continuous strips show the termination of ventricular fibrillation by a 400 watt-second nonsynchronized electrical discharge. Following termination of ventricular fibrillation, slow sinus rhythm with premature ventricular beats (*arrows*) appears. The unusual electrical deflections identified by the closed circles (●) are attributable to the closed chest compression that is being performed at the time.

tricular arrhythmias and even ventricular fibrillation. Thus, it is preferable to attempt to terminate ventricular tachycardia with IV lidocaine or procainamide in this setting. Furthermore, as hypokalemia is often present in such patients, management might include correction of hypokalemia by the cautious administration of KCl.

Ventricular Fibrillation

Ventricular fibrillation (VF), the most common cause of sudden death from acute myocardial ischemia and infarction, is recognized in the surface ECG by the absence of identifiable QRST complexes and by the presence of irregular oscillating electrical activity that may be fine or coarse (Figs. 50–4, B, and 50–29). Ventricular fibrillation may be induced during electrical conversion of ventricular tachycardia, even when there has been appropriate synchronization of the electrical discharge to the QRS complex; it may occur in the setting of long QTU intervals. As ventricular fibrillation is a mechanically useless rhythm that results in circulatory arrest, it must be terminated if the patient is to survive. Defibrillation is best achieved using nonsynchronized direct current countershock at high (approximately 400 watt-second) energy levels (Fig. 50–29, B). If defibrillation does not occur after two or three maximum energy direct current discharges, it may reflect the presence of hypoxemia, acidemia, or hyperkalemia, and closed chest cardiac massage should be performed while attempts are made to correct the abnormalities. More recently, bretylium tosylate has become available for rapid IV injection in an attempt to achieve a chemical defibrillation. When electrical defibrillation has failed despite correction of metabolic abnormalities, this medication may terminate the ventricular fibrillation and allow restoration of an effective cardiac rhythm. (See Chapter 49.)

Regular, Wide QRS Tachycardias

The regular, rapid occurrence of abnormally wide QRS complexes could reflect PSVT with aberrant intraventricular conduction of the supraventricular impulses or sustained ventricular tachycardia. As these cardiac rhythm disturbances may have dramatically different clinical significances and respond to very different therapies, differential diagnosis is crucial, though often difficult. As shown in Table 50–3, the rate of the QRS complexes during tachycardia is not generally helpful in determining whether or not the rhythm is supraventricular or ventricular in origin. The wider and more bizarre the QRS complexes, and the more superior and rightward the mean frontal plane axis of the

TABLE 50–3 Differential Diagnosis of Regular Wide QRS Tachycardia

	Ventricular Tachycardia	PSVT
Rate	130–180 (100–200)	140–180 (120–220)
QRS contours	Often bizarre	Rarely bizarre
QRS axis	Superior, rightward	Usually normal
P:QRS relationships	1:1, 1:2, dissociated	1:1 almost exclusively

complexes, the more likely the rhythm is to be ventricular tachycardia. The identification of atrial and ventricular relationships during tachycardia is extremely helpful in the differential diagnosis; although there are 1:1 atrial and ventricular relationships in virtually all episodes of PSVT and in many episodes of ventricular tachycardia, the finding of AV dissociation excludes the diagnosis of PSVT and establishes the diagnosis of ventricular tachycardia. Examination of ECGs taken prior to the tachycardia may assist in differential diagnosis. If the contours of sinus-stimulated QRS complexes are *identical* to the wide, bizarre QRS complexes that occur during tachycardia, the diagnosis of PSVT is established. The clinical history may also be helpful; if a patient with regular tachycardia at a rate of about 160 to 170 beats/minute has had similar episodes over a period of years, the arrhythmia is almost certainly PSVT. Figures 50–30 and 50–31 display 12-lead ECGs during PSVT with aberrant intraventricular conduction and during ventricular tachycardia, respectively.

Faced with a patient who has a rapid, regular, wide QRS tachycardia with 1:1 atrial and ventricular relationships, the emergency department physician may perform a number of maneuvers that might have both diagnostic and therapeutic effects. Carotid sinus massage and the IV administration of Tensilon or verapamil may terminate PSVT but would not be likely to terminate ventricular tachycardia. Lidocaine may terminate ventricular tachycardia and, occasionally, PSVT when one of the reentry pathways is an accessory pathway that has properties like those of bundle branch and Purkinje fibers. Elevation of the blood pressure with sympathomimetic amines may terminate both PSVT and ventricular tachycardia and is therefore of little diagnostic help, but it would be useful if it terminated the arrhythmia. So, the emergency department physician faced with a patient whose wide QRS tachycardia could be either supraventricular or ventricular in origin may find it valuable to apply carotid sinus massage or to inject Tensilon or verapamil, or lidocaine intravenously to see the effect on the rhythm.

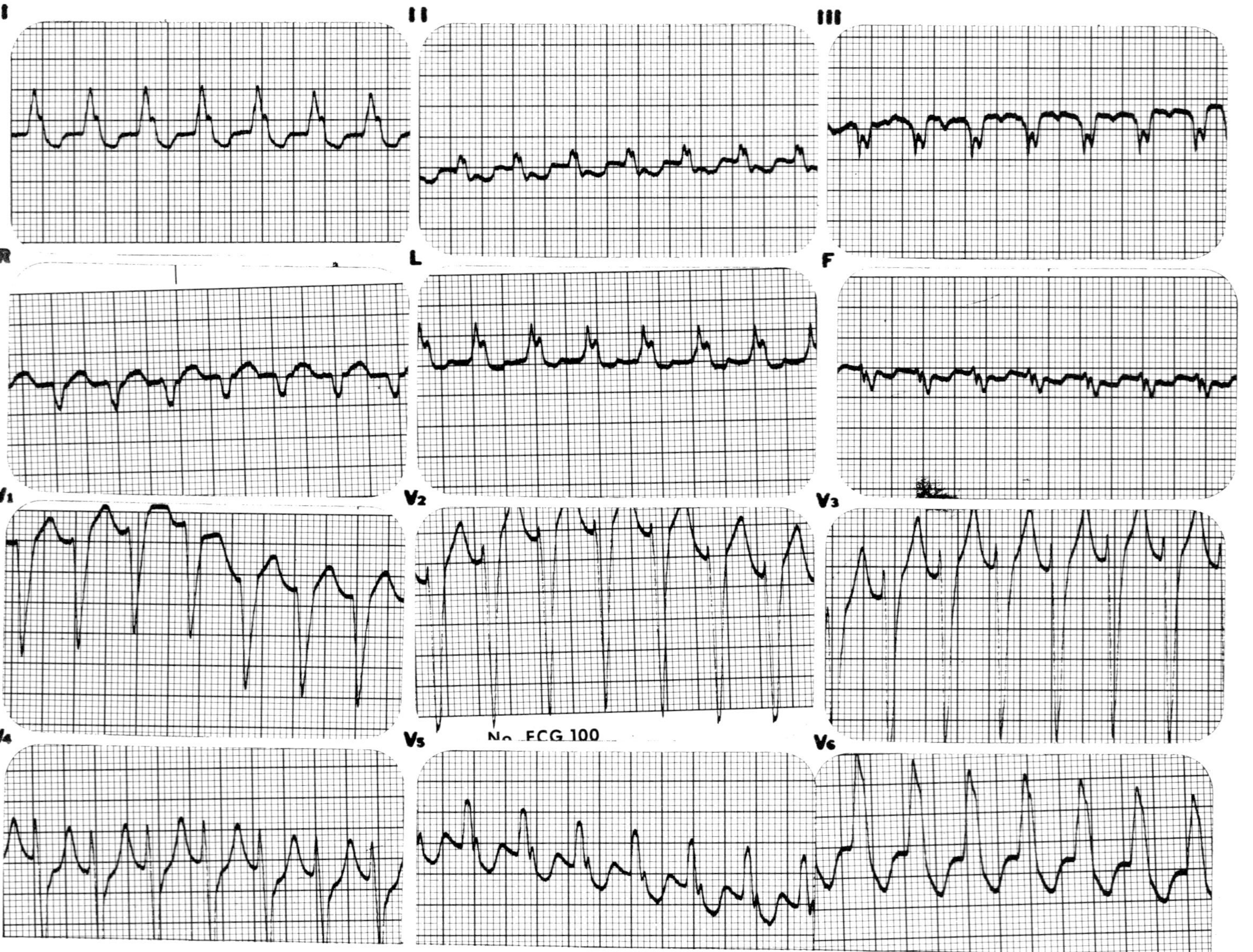

Figure 50–30   ECG Showing PSVT with Aberrant Intraventricular Conduction. *Note:* This 12-lead ECG shows PSVT at a rate of 167 beats/minute. The wide QRS complexes have a rather "pure" left bundle branch block type pattern and a normal mean frontal plane axis. (*Source:* Reprinted with permission from Jacobson LB, Goldschlager N: *Arrhythmias: Case Studies.* Garden City, NY, Medical Examination Publishing, © 1978.)

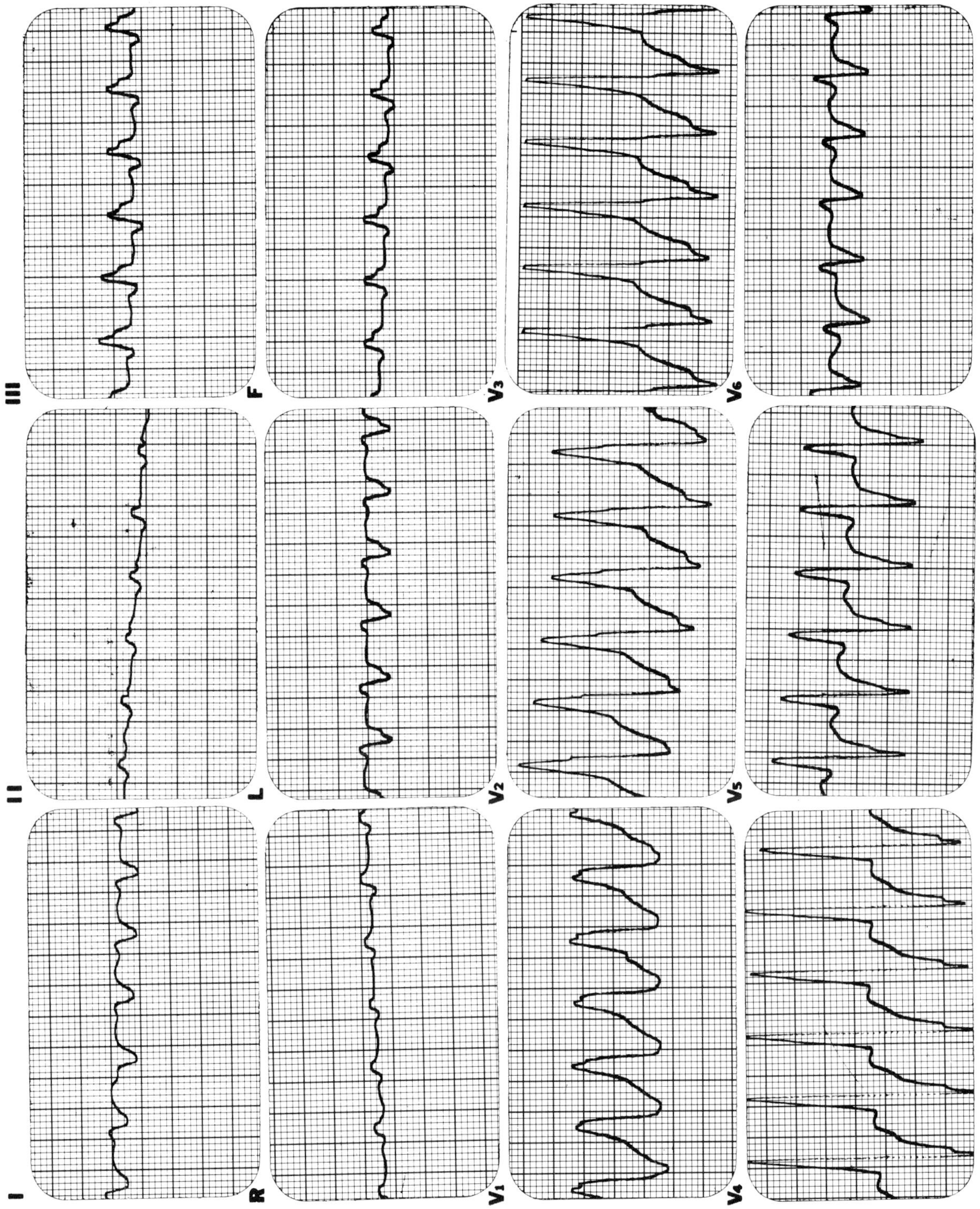

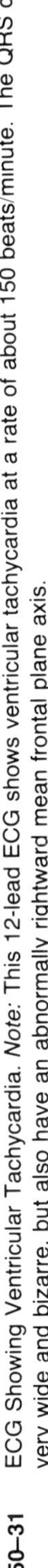

Figure 50–31 ECG Showing Ventricular Tachycardia. *Note:* This 12-lead ECG shows ventricular tachycardia at a rate of about 150 beats/minute. The QRS complexes not only are very wide and bizarre, but also have an abnormally rightward mean frontal plane axis.

THE WOLFF-PARKINSON-WHITE SYNDROME

Some patients have, in addition to the normal AV node-His-Purkinje system pathway connecting atria to ventricles, another AV conduction pathway. Such accessory AV conduction pathways usually enter ventricular tissue well away from the areas in which ventricular activation is normally initiated and are capable of conducting impulses more rapidly than is the AV node. Thus, QRS complexes stimulated by supraventricular impulses entering the ventricles via an accessory AV conduction pathway are grossly abnormal, typically showing a slow initial deflection (the delta wave) and an abnormally long duration, typically greater than 0.12 seconds. The PR interval in these patients is often shorter than normal and typically less than 0.12 seconds, presumably because the impulse can travel from atrium to ventricle more rapidly via the accessory pathway than via the AV node-His-Purkinje system. Figure 50–32 shows a 12-lead ECG recorded from a patient with an accessory AV conduction pathway during accessory pathway conduction. Patients with accessory AV conduction pathways and supraventricular tachyarrhythmias are said to have the Wolff-Parkinson-White syndrome. In addition to PSVT, these patients may experience atrial flutter and fibrillation.

As accessory AV conduction pathways exhibit electrophysiologic properties like those of bundle branches and Purkinje fibers, they have conduction velocities, refractory periods, and responses to antiarrhythmic medications that usually differ dramatically from those of the normal AV conduction system, which contains the relatively slowly conducting AV node. Specifically, accessory pathways may have such rapid conduction velocities and such short refractory periods that they are capable of conducting impulses from atrium to ventricle at rates in excess of 300/minute. While quinidine, procainamide, and disopyramide generally lengthen refractory periods of, and slow conduction velocities in, accessory pathways, beta-blocking agents, digoxin, and verapamil generally do not. In fact, digoxin commonly effects a slight shortening of the refractory period of an accessory pathway which has a very brief refractory period to begin with. When atrial fibrillation and flutter occur with accessory pathway conduction that results in ventricular rates above 240 beats/minute, digoxin and beta-blocking drugs usually do not slow the ventricular rate; on occasion, digoxin may even increase the already dangerously rapid rate. Quinidine, procainamide, and disopyramide, however, generally do slow the ventricular rate. Thus, in the presence of atrial flutter and fibrillation with rapid ventricular rates attributable to accessory pathway conduction, the IV administration of procainamide may help to slow the ventricular rate.

However, if the patient is experiencing or is on the verge of experiencing cardiovascular collapse, direct current cardioversion at the energy levels usually used for atrial flutter and fibrillation is a more appropriate therapy; it is probably less risky than the IV administration of quinidine preparations or of disopyramide to such critically ill patients.

Accessory pathway conduction during atrial fibrillation is recognized by the occurrence of wide, very bizarre QRS complexes at irregularly irregular intervals (Fig. 50–33). Accessory pathway conduction in atrial flutter with 1:1 AV conduction can be recognized by the regular occurrence of wide and very bizarre but essentially identical QRS complexes at rates of about 300/minute, well in excess of the rates of most sustained ventricular tachycardias. Atrial flutter with 1:1 AV conduction via an accessory pathway is more likely than ventricular tachycardia if the patient is a young adult, has no other symptoms of heart disease, and has a history of recurrent episodes of tachycardia, such as PSVT.

In most patients with Wolff-Parkinson-White syndrome, the mechanism of PSVT usually, but not always, involves a reentrant impulse traveling from atrium to ventricle via the normal AV node-His-Purkinje system pathway and from ventricle to atrium via the accessory pathway. Thus, during PSVT, the QRS complexes usually have normal contours (Fig. 50–22). PSVT may be terminated by maneuvers or medications that slow conduction through the normal and/or the accessory AV conduction pathways. Carotid sinus massage, Tensilon, verapamil, Valsalva's maneuver, beta-adrenergic blocking agents, and sympathomimetic amines that increase arterial blood pressure may terminate PSVT by slowing conduction through the AV node and may be used in doses similar to those used in PSVT in patients without accessory pathways. Lidocaine, procainamide, quinidine, and disopyramide may terminate PSVT by slowing conduction in the accessory pathway. As lidocaine is the safest, most rapidly acting, and simplest to administer, a 50- to 125-mg bolus of this medication might be the first therapeutic maneuver. While digoxin may terminate PSVT by slowing conduction in the AV node, some authorities feel it should not be used in the presence of antegradely conducting accessory pathways because it may enhance accessory pathway conduction and thus increase the ventricular rate if the rhythm changes from PSVT to atrial fibrillation or flutter, which not uncommonly occurs.

PERMANENT CARDIAC PACING SYSTEMS

Most patients with permanent artificial cardiac pacing systems have had the system implanted for prevention

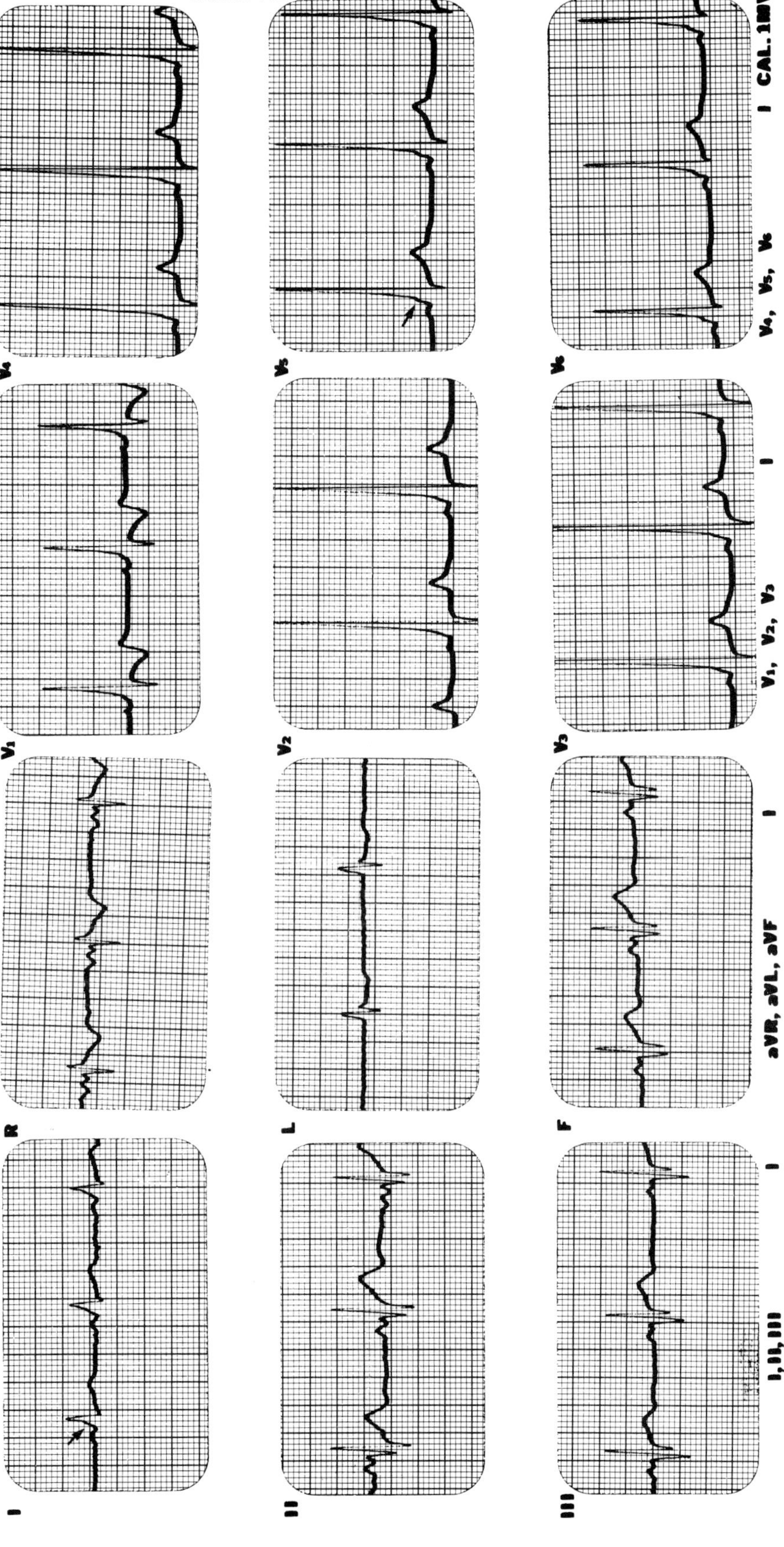

Figure 50–32   ECG from Patient with Wolff-Parkinson-White Syndrome. *Note:* This 12-lead ECG recorded from a patient with Wolff-Parkinson-White syndrome shows the short PR interval, the wide QRS complexes, and the delta waves, two of which are indicated by the arrows (Leads I and V_5). (ECG is at 81% of original.)

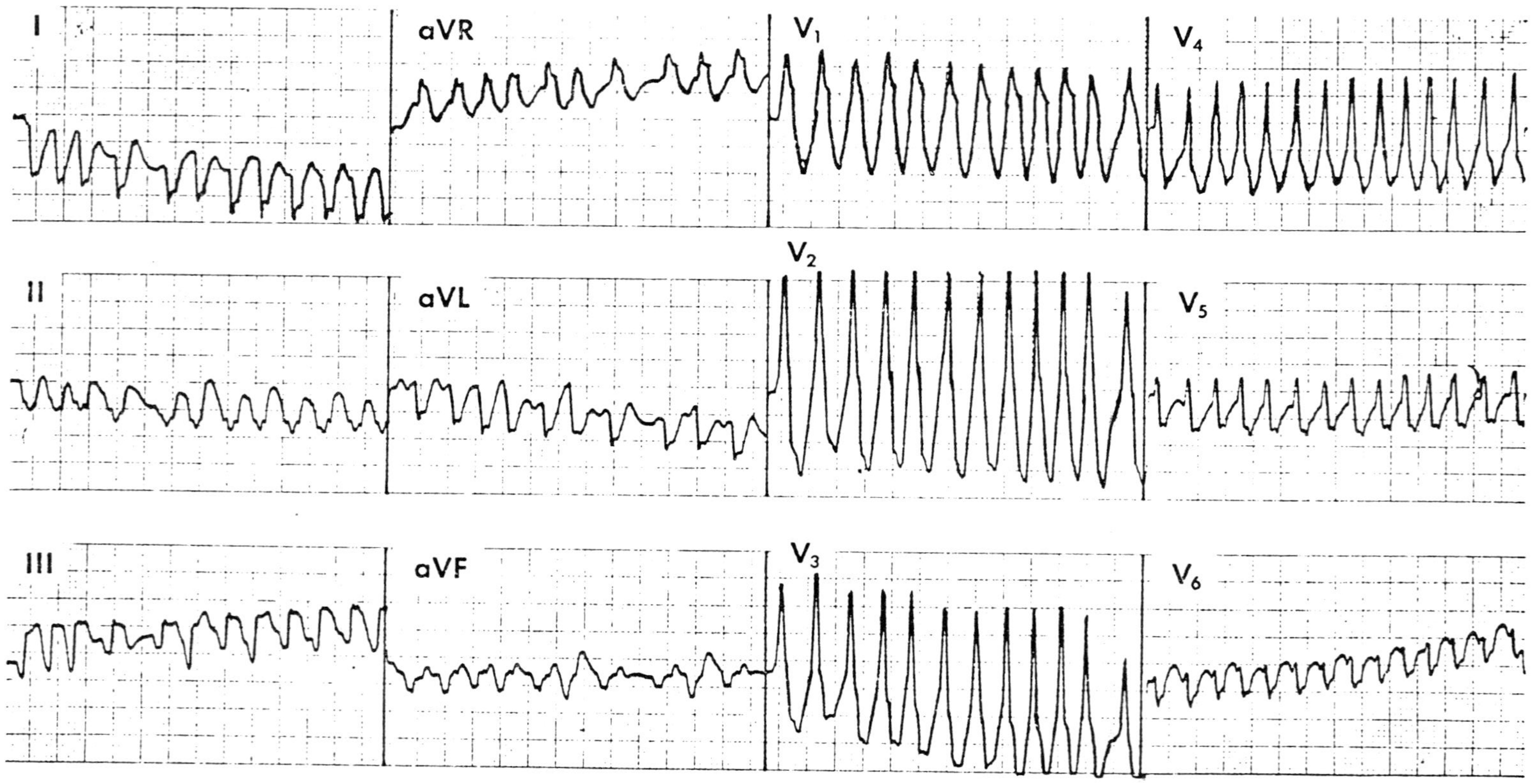

Figure 50–33   ECG Showing Atrial Fibrillation in a Patient with Wolff-Parkinson-White Syndrome. *Note:* This 12-lead ECG was recorded from a patient with Wolff-Parkinson-White syndrome during atrial fibrillation. The very wide bizarre QRS complexes that occur at irregular intervals at an average rate of about 280/minute reflect ventricular activation via the accessory AV conduction pathway, which obviously has a very short refractory period.

or treatment of bradycardias. Because bradycardias are the functional manifestations of disease processes that are usually progressive, the abnormality in cardiac rhythm present after months to years of pacing may be more profound than that present before pacing was instituted. Thus, failure of a permanent cardiac pacing system may result in profound bradycardia with catastrophic consequences. The appearance or recurrence of symptoms suggesting bradycardia in a patient with a permanent cardiac pacing system raises the strong possibility that the pacing system has malfunctioned or failed.

Cardiac pacing systems consist of two parts, a pacemaker generator and a lead system (Fig. 50-34). The pacemaker generator contains the energy source of the system and the electronic components necessary to generate the electrical impulses (pacing stimuli) that depolarize the heart and to sense spontaneous cardiac electrical activity. The lead system, which carries electrical impulses from the pacemaker generator to the heart and spontaneous cardiac electrical activity from

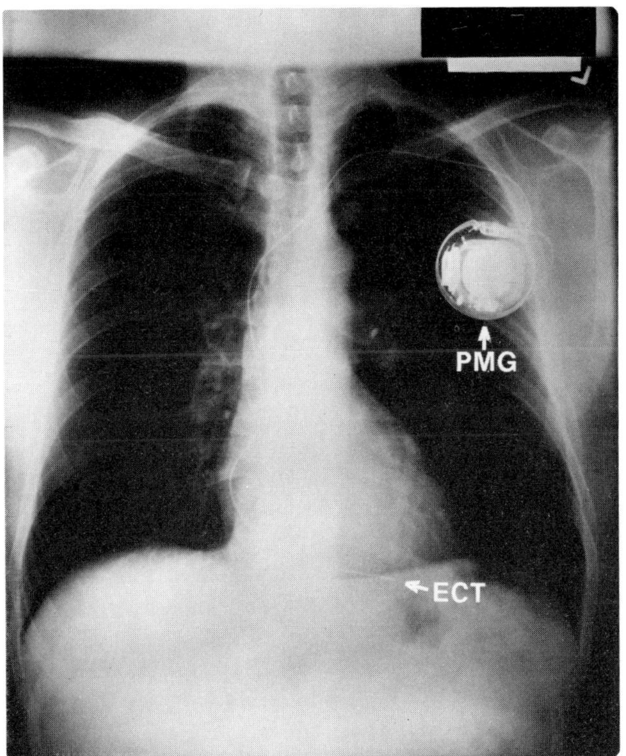

Figure 50–34 Roentgenogram Showing Permanent Transvenous Ventricular Pacing System. *Note:* This posteroanterior chest roentgenogram of a patient with a permanent transvenous ventricular pacing system shows that the lead, an electrode catheter, has been introduced into the left cephalic vein. The electrode catheter tip (*ECT*) lies in the apex of the right ventricle, and the pacemaker generator (*PMG*) lies in the left infraclavicular area.

the heart to the sensing circuit within the pacemaker generator, consists of an insulated wire. At one end of this wire is a metallic pin that inserts into the pacemaker generator; at the other end is a bare metallic surface (the electrode) that makes contact with cardiac muscle.

The emission of a pacing stimulus into body tissues is recorded on the surface ECG as a sharp deflection of very brief duration, termed a *pacing artifact* (Fig. 50–35). When pacing artifacts initiate ventricular activation, they are seen at the onset of the QRS complex. The interval at which pacing stimuli are emitted from a pacemaker generator is termed the *pacing,* or *automatic, interval* of the device; the corresponding rate is termed the *pacing,* or *automatic rate* (Fig. 50–35). The rate of many pacemaker generators may be changed noninvasively by application of a small "programmer" onto the skin overlying the generator.

Pacing systems may fail to function properly because of energy source depletion, electronic component failure, fracture or insulation break within the lead system, a change in the interface between the electrode portion of the lead system and the myocardium with which it makes contact, and interaction between the pacing system and high-energy radiation fields. As a discussion of all types of permanent cardiac pacing systems is beyond the scope of this chapter, an evaluation of only demand ventricular pacing systems—those most widely implanted—is presented. A technique for the insertion of a pacemaker is reviewed in Chapter 71.

Permanent Demand Ventricular Pacing Systems

Demand ventricular pacing systems are designed to emit pacing stimuli only when spontaneous cardiac electrical activity is not sensed within a specific time interval, termed the *escape interval* (Figs. 50–35 and 50–36). Pacing stimuli are not emitted if spontaneous QRS complexes are sensed at intervals shorter than the escape interval. However, in order to keep it from sensing a portion of a paced QRST complex or the later portion of a spontaneous QRST complex, the initial portion of which has already been sensed, the sensing circuit of a demand pacemaker generator is designed not to process incoming signals for a specific time interval after the emission of a pacing stimulus or after the sensing of spontaneous cardiac electrical activity. The duration of this *sensing refractory period* is generally in the range of 300 ± 75 milliseconds, but it varies among pacemaker generators.

Figure 50–35, A illustrates the sensing refractory period. In this strip, the first two QRS complexes are stimulated by the P waves that precede them; the last two QRS complexes are paced. The first QRS complex

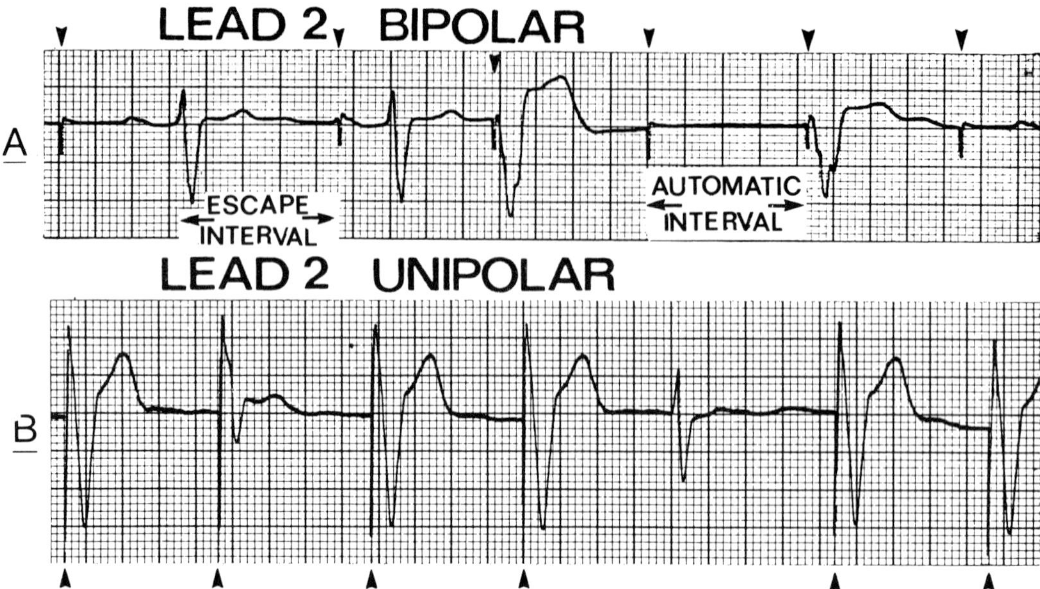

Figure 50–35 ECGs Showing Pacing Artifacts. *Note:* These lead 2 rhythm strips from two different patients display pacing artifacts (*arrows*). The bipolar pacing artifacts (*A*) are small relative to the QRS complexes that they stimulate, while the unipolar pacing artifacts (*B*) are larger and distort the onsets of the QRS complexes that they stimulate. In *A*, the first, second, fourth, and sixth pacing artifacts do not stimulate QRS complexes because the energy output of the pacing system in this patient was intermittently too low to activate the ventricles. The second QRS complex is not sensed, but does not reflect "faulty sensing," for this complex falls within the sensing refractory period of this pacemaker generator.

must have been sensed, for a pacing artifact follows its onset at an interval of about 0.88 seconds, slightly longer than the pacemaker generator escape interval of about 0.84 seconds. However, the second QRS complex must *not* have been sensed, for a pacing artifact follows its onset at an inteval much shorter than the escape interval (0.58 seconds versus 0.84 seconds). This second QRS complex was not sensed because it fell about 0.26 seconds after emission of the second pacing stimulus, within the 0.32 ± 0.05 second sensing refractory period of this pacemaker generator. The first QRS complex was sensed because it has its onset about 0.64 seconds after the first pacing artifact, well after the sensing refractory period of 0.32 ± 0.05 seconds had elapsed.

In order to permit an evaluation of pacing function when the rate of the spontaneous QRS rhythm exceeds the demand pacing rate of the pacemaker generator, all demand ventricular pacemaker generators are designed to emit pacing stimuli at regular intervals without regard for the underlying rhythm, i.e., to function in an asynchronous or fixed rate mode when a specifically designed magnet is placed on the skin overlying the pacemaker generator (Fig. 50-36). The rate at which pacing stimuli are emitted when a magnet overlies the pacemaker generator is called the magnetic rate. The magnetic rate may be similar to, identical to, or faster than the pacing (automatic) rate during demand function, depending on the design specifications of the pace-

maker generator. The pacemaker generator is usually designed such that the magnetic rate either decreases linearly with energy source depletion or shows a quantum decrement when energy source depletion is extreme. Thus, accurate assessment of pacing system function requires a thorough knowledge of the design specifications of the particular pacemaker generator being evaluated.

In the evaluation of pacing system function, the occurrence of specific ECG phenomena generally allows an accurate diagnosis of the mechanism of the abnormality. For example, the failure of pacing artifacts to be recorded in the ECG at a time when the spontaneous ventricular rate is lower than the expected demand pacing rate indicates abnormal pacing system function (Fig. 50–37, A). There may be no pacing artifacts because (a) the pacemaker generator energy source is depleted to the point where the demand pacing rate has fallen below the spontaneous ventricular rate at that time; (b) the energy source is depleted to the point where not enough is left to emit a pacing stimulus; (c) electronic circuitry malfunction is prohibiting the generation or emission of stimuli from the pacemaker generator; (d) complete fracture of the lead system is preventing the emitted stimuli from reaching body fluids, which they must do if pacing artifacts are to be detected in the surface ECG; (e) the pacemaker generator is sensing, and being recycled by, signals other than spontaneous

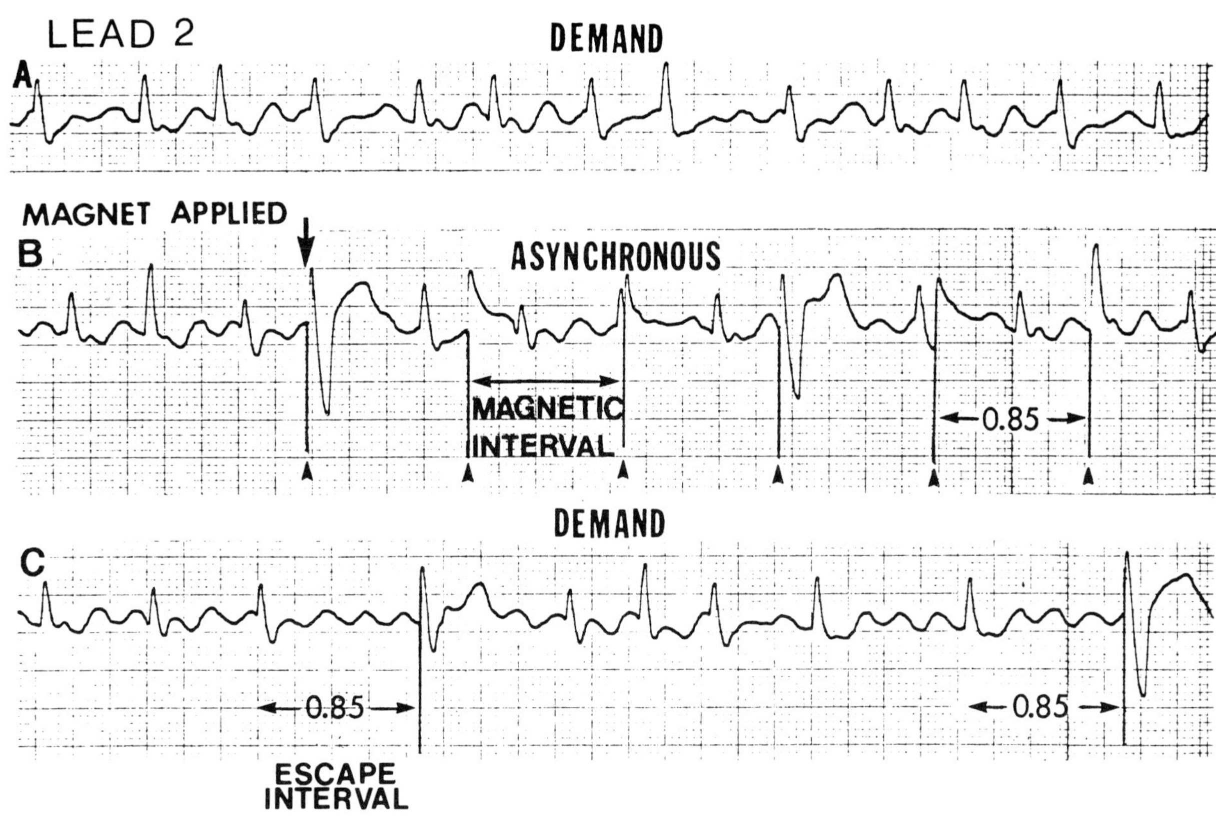

Figure 50–36 ECGs Showing Normal Function of a Permanent Demand Ventricular Pacing System. *Note:* These three lead 2 rhythm strips were recorded from a patient with a permanent demand ventricular pacing system. The atrial rhythm is fibrillation in all three strips. *A* Pacing artifacts are not seen, as the intervals between spontaneous QRS complexes never exceed the escape interval (0.85 seconds) of the pacemaker generator. *B* Application of the magnet onto the skin overlying the pacemaker generator results in the emission of pacing stimuli at regular intervals of 0.85 seconds. The first, fourth, and sixth pacing artifacts initiate or contribute to ventricular activation, but the others do not because they fall within the refractory period of ventricular tissue. *C* Recorded at a later time, pacing artifacts appear when the intervals between spontaneously occurring QRS complexes exceed the pacemaker generator escape interval.

QRS complexes, so-called spurious signals. Application of the magnet over the pacemaker generator would result in the appearance of pacing artifacts only if explanations (a) and (e) were correct. If (a) were correct, the pacing artifacts would appear at a rate slower than the usual magnetic rate of the pacemaker generator; if (e) were correct, the pacing artifacts would occur at the expected magnetic rate. Explanation (d) may be evaluated by the technique of radioauscultation, which involves placing the antenna of a portable FM radio over the pacemaker generator, tuning the dial between stations, and placing the amplitude at maximum level. Because a pacing stimulus that originates within the pacemaker generator emits a radio frequency signal even if the pacing stimulus does not exit from the pacemaker generator or the lead system, a "click" can be heard on the radio speaker every time a pacing stimulus is generated. Thus, when a pacemaker generator is emitting impulses appropriately but pacing artifacts are not

seen on the surface ECG, radioauscultation may allow the diagnosis of lead fracture to be established.

If pacing artifacts are being emitted at a rate faster than that expected on the basis of the pacemaker generator design specifications, a phenomenon termed *runaway,* electronic component or circuitry failure is the mechanism of the abnormal function.

If pacing artifacts follow spontaneous QRS complexes at intervals shorter than the escape interval of the pacing system, the QRS complexes in question are not being sensed appropriately (Fig. 50–37, B). Such a failure is usually due to suboptimal location of the electrodes within the heart; the amplitude of spontaneous ventricular electrical activity, i.e., the QRS complexes, that is reaching the pacemaker generator sensing circuit is too small to be detected by it. This problem usually occurs because the tip of an electrode catheter changes position within the heart. Rarely, it occurs as a transient phenomenon in patients with acute myocardial infarc-

REFERENCES

1. Devereux RB, Perloff JK, Reichek N, Josephson ME: Mitral valve prolapse. *Circulation* 54:3–14, 1976.
2. Leahey EB Jr, Bigger JT Jr, Butler VP Jr, Reiffel JA, O'Connell GC, Scaffidi LE, Rottman JN: Quinidine-digoxin interaction: Time course and pharmacokinetics. *Amer J Cardiol* 48:1141–1146, 1981.
3. Jacobson LB: Spontaneous ventricular parasystole initiating ventricular tachycardia. *J Electrocardiol* 6:63–70, 1973.

51. Congestive Heart Failure

RICHARD G. FRIEDMAN, M.D.

The dyspneic patient presents a diagnostic and therapeutic challenge to the emergency physician. The correct diagnosis and therapy can rapidly change an anxious, frightened, critically ill patient into a calm, asymptomatic one. Incorrect or inadequate therapy can just as easily make the patient profoundly worse. Since congestive heart failure (CHF) is the most common etiology of dyspnea in emergency department patients with infiltrates on their chest roentgenograms,[1] it is important for the physician to be thoroughly familiar with its diagnosis and management. A physician must quickly decide the most pressing problems and determine whether the patient is safe or in immediate danger. This approach is similar for any medical emergency. While examining the patient and obtaining a history and laboratory data base, the physician or paramedic in the field should already be deciding the most likely etiology of the dyspnea. Is it cardiac, pulmonary, psychogenic, or caused by a less commonly diagnosed disorder? Conservative therapy should be initiated as soon as possible, and definitive therapy should be started once the diagnosis is established. An approach to the diagnosis and management of the patient with CHF will be presented here, along with a brief review of the pathophysiology that leads to the common signs and symptoms of CHF.

DEFINITION

Heart failure refers to any condition in which an alteration in myocardial function results in the heart's inability to circulate enough oxygenated blood to meet the body's metabolic needs during rest or exercise.[2,3] Congestion is found in the organs that are in the anatomic circuit located behind the failing ventricle. In right-sided CHF, the liver is engorged with fluid; while in predominant left-sided CHF, the lungs may be engorged.

CHF may be an acute or chronic condition. Either form involves some element of elevated ventricular filling pressures, but the rate of rise and the ability for compensatory mechanisms to increase cardiac output will determine the level of symptoms that the patient will experience. Compensatory mechanisms involved in regulating cardiac output are outlined below:[3,4]

  I. Cardiac
    A. Ventricular hypertrophy
    B. Ventricular dilatation (Frank-Starling mechanism)
    C. Sympathetic nervous system
      1. Heart rate
      2. Contractility
  II. Peripheral Circulation
    A. Venous constriction
    B. Arteriolar constriction
 III. Renal
    A. Increased sodium retention (increases preload)
    B. Inappropriate secretion of antidiuretic hormone

The functional class of the patient with CHF is based on the relationship of symptoms of CHF to the activity level of the individual. According to the New York Heart Association classification the functional classes of CHF include:[4]

- *Class I:* normal basal output in the absence of circulatory congestion. Lesser degrees of myocardial dysfunction such as hypertrophy without failure may be seen. No symptoms are noted at rest or with activity.
- *Class II:* moderate elevations of systemic and pulmonary venous pressures. Symptoms may occur with greater than normal activity.
- *Class III:* compensated CHF. The resting cardiac output is normal with excessive elevation of pulmonary venous pressure. Symptoms may occur with normal levels of activity.
- *Class IV:* decompensated CHF. Inability of the heart to maintain basal cardiac output. Symptoms occur at rest.

In chronic compensated CHF, the left ventricular end-diastolic pressure (LVEDP) and end-diastolic volume may be elevated, which causes the heart to operate at a different point on the Frank-Starling curve.[5] The increased diastolic myocardial stretch developed as a result of the increased LVEDP causes an increase in forward stroke volume as the diastolic reserve is tapped, but this is at the expense of increased filling pressures, which may result in symptoms of dyspnea and congestion with any increased demands.[5] Similarly, flow to the central nervous system and heart may be maintained through sympathetic nervous system mediated arteriolar and venous vasoconstriction and tachycardia at the expense of decreased peripheral blood flow to the skin, splanchnic, and renal beds.[4,5] All the compensatory mechanisms listed previously can lead to the classic symptoms of CHF, which include dyspnea, tachycardia, diaphoresis, paroxysmal nocturnal dyspnea, orthopnea, vasoconstriction, and edema if increased metabolic demands are made on the compensated ventricle.[6] In acute CHF, either the insult occurs so rapidly that the compensatory mechanisms cannot handle the situation or the mechanisms were already being utilized chronically and no reserve capacity remained. Patients seeking aid in the emergency department will usually have some element of decompensated CHF. Patients with class I or II CHF will most often be asymptomatic and are managed as outpatients without emergency care. If, however, there is increased metabolic demand, CHF can decompensate and symptoms are apparent. In decompensated left-sided CHF, forward flow can no longer be maintained adequately even at rest, and any increased demand on the circulatory system may cause

fluid to move from the edematous pulmonary interstitium and into the alveolar sacs, resulting in pulmonary edema.[7] In the most severe form of heart failure, cardiogenic shock, the heart fails to perfuse the tissues and all compensatory mechanisms are inadequate or have failed.

This chapter will focus on those forms of heart failure that result from a defect in the myocardium and will not deal at length with CHF caused by acute volume overload or with high output failure that results from increased peripheral demands.

PATHOPHYSIOLOGY

Cardiac function is predominantly determined by the following interrelated parameters:[6,8,9]

- afterload, defined as the resistance to forward flow from the ventricle or the intraventricular systolic tension developed during ejection
- preload, the Frank-Starling mechanism or the diastolic stretch of myocardial fibers
- heart rate
- contractility, defined as the inotropic state of the heart
- normal temporal sequence of segmental contraction of the ventricle.

Any condition that significantly alters any of these parameters or their interrelationship may result in decreased forward blood flow consistent with CHF. Various pathologic mechanisms that can give rise to CHF and conditions that are associated with them are listed in Table 51–1.

Ideally, the therapy for CHF is linked to its etiology. If the problem is increased afterload from systemic hypertension, then afterload reducing agents would be a logical measure. If increased preload is present, then diuresis or peripheral venous pooling would be helpful. If the CHF is caused by decreased contractility, then inotropic agents are useful. However, if the problem is cardiac tamponade or hypovolemia, the use of diuretics would be potentially harmful. In a patient with a high output heart failure with a diminished afterload, further afterload reduction might be injurious.

Availability of the flow-directed pulmonary artery catheter allows the clinician to determine the precise pathophysiology at the patient's bedside. Since treatment varies with the etiology of the CHF, it is often useful to pass a Swan-Ganz catheter. Direct pressure measurements can be made in the right atrium, right ventricle, and pulmonary artery. The pulmonary artery wedge pressure approximates the left atrial pressure, which approximates the LVEDP, which represents pre-

TABLE 51–1   Pathophysiologic Mechanisms Causing CHF

Mechanism	Associated Conditions
Global decrease in contractility	Cardiomyopathy Hypothermia Infiltrative disorders Ischemia Metabolic disorders Toxins
Regional decrease in contractility	Ischemia Trauma
Decreased quantity of myocardium	Infarction
Increased afterload	Aortic stenosis Hypertension Idiopathic hypertrophic subvalvular aortic stenosis Pulmonary stenosis Tricuspid stenosis
Increased forward flow with volume overload	Aortic regurgitation Mitral regurgitation Tricuspid regurgitation Ventricular septal defect
Dyssynergy of contraction	Aneurysm Atrioventricular dissociation
Inadequate heart rate	Disorders of rhythm and conduction
Decreased return of blood to heart	Cardiac rupture Constriction Hypovolemia Mitral stenosis Restriction Tamponade Vena cava obstruction
High output failure with increased peripheral demand	Arteriovenous communication Beri-beri Hyperthermia Hyperthyroidism Sepsis
Abnormal anatomy	Congenital heart disease
Inability to handle volume	Iatrogenic volume overload

TABLE 51–2   Pulmonary Artery Flow-Directed Catheter Findings in Conditions Causing CHF

Condition	Finding
Constriction or restriction	Equalization within 5 mm Hg of the diastolic right and left ventricle pressures with RA mean and PAW
Right ventricular infarction	↑ RA, ↑ RV, normal or ↓ PAW, normal or ↓ PA
Pulmonary hypertension	↑ PA, normal PAW
Left ventricular infarction	↑ PAW, ↑ RA
Hypovolemia	↓ RA, ↓ PAW
Mitral regurgitation	V wave in PAW tracing
Tricuspid regurgitation	↑ V wave in RA tracing
Noncardiac pulmonary edema	All pressures normal or decreased

Note: ↑ = increased; ↓ = decreased; PA = pulmonary artery pressure; PAW = pulmonary artery wedge pressure; RA = right atrial pressure.

load. Clinical conditions causing CHF that have typical findings with a Swan-Ganz catheter are listed in Table 51–2. In general, interstitial edema is present in the lungs with a pulmonary artery wedge pressure of 13 to 20 mm Hg, symptoms of CHF develops at a pressure of 20 to 24 mm Hg, and pulmonary edema occurs with a pressure greater than 725 mm Hg.[7] In chronic situations, higher levels of the pulmonary artery wedge pressure may be compensatory and may not be associated with symptoms at rest.

The Swan-Ganz catheter can also be used to measure cardiac output by thermal dilution, and the cardiac index can be calculated. Serial saturation samples can be obtained to determine whether an intracardiac shunt may be present. Simultaneous pulmonary artery and arterial saturation samples and a hemoglobin value may be used to determine the arteriovenous oxygen (AVO_2) difference. The AVO_2 difference is the amount of oxygen extracted from the blood as it passes through the tissues and is important in validating the cardiac output measurements. Tissue perfusion will not correlate with cardiac output in all cases. If cardiac output is normal or elevated but the red blood cells hold onto oxygen more avidly than usual, the AVO_2 difference would be narrow, reflecting a lack of perfusion independent of the cardiac output. Conditions that may cause increased avidity for oxygen by the red blood cell include hypophosphatemia, hypothermia, alkalosis, carbon monoxide poisoning, methemoglobinemia, sepsis, and some hemoglobinopathies.

Other valuable measurements that may be calculated with the use of a Swan-Ganz catheter and an arterial line include the systemic vascular resistance, which reflects afterload, and pulmonary vascular resistance. Swan-Ganz fiberoptic catheters provide continuous determinants of oxygen saturation and allow cardiac output determination by green dye as well as by thermal dilution. (See Chapter 57 for a technique used in inserting the Swan-Ganz catheter.)

DIAGNOSIS

Accurate and rapid diagnosis is crucial to ensure the comfort and safety of the dyspneic patient. As the patient is evaluated, any prehospital treatment that may alter the physical findings must be considered.[10] When first entering the patient's room, the patient should be watched carefully and the following observations made:

- Is the patient sitting or lying? If lying, is the patient either less dyspneic or so hypoxic that he or she may be semistuporous and unable to sit up?
- What does the cardiac monitor show?
- What is the respiratory rate, and are the accessory muscles of respiration being used?
- Is the patient cyanotic?
- Is there evidence of diaphoresis or peripheral edema?
- When questioned, is the patient gasping for breath or able to speak freely?

If the history is inadequate, the physician should consult friends, relatives, the old hospital chart, and the private physician as soon as possible.

While examining the patient, emergency care personnel must look for findings that may suggest an etiology for the patient's dyspnea:

- What are the vital signs?
- Is there evidence of a paradoxical pulse that may suggest chronic obstructive pulmonary disease (COPD), tamponade, pericardial effusion, constriction, or restriction?
- Is there a mechanical alternating pulse suggestive of tamponade?
- Are there postural blood pressure changes suggestive of hypovolemia?
- On auscultatory examination, is there an S_3 gallop rhythm? If so, is it right- or left-sided in origin?
- Are there murmurs, suggestive of aortic stenosis, idiopathic hypertrophic subvalvular aortic stenosis, pulmonic stenosis, tricuspid stenosis, or mitral stenosis, or of regurgitation with increased volume overload such as mitral, tricuspid, aortic, or pulmonary regurgitation?
- Is there any evidence of congenital heart disease or a murmur suggestive of a ventricular septal defect or other intracardiac shunt?
- Are there any unusual findings such as a pericardial knock suggestive of constrictive disease?
- Are the heart sounds faint, suggestive of pericardial effusion, or do the peripheral pulses decrease with inspiration when inspecting the neck?
- Is there jugular venous distention or a positive hepatojugular reflex?
- Is there a large V wave or cannon wave suggestive of tricuspid regurgitation or atrioventricular dissociation?
- Is Kussmaul's sign, found in COPD, cor pulmonale, right ventricular infarction, or constriction, present?

- On auscultation of the lungs, are there rales or wheezes?
- Is there evidence of pleural effusion?
- Is there any suggestion of a pneumothorax or of foreign body aspirations that might cause dyspnea?
- Are there physical findings of hyperthyroidism, arteriovenous fistulas, dialysis shunts, sepsis, or any other systemic disorders that can lead to CHF?

Observation of the patient and completion of the examination outlined above should take only a few moments, and the examiner should quickly be able to determine whether a primary cardiac problem is involved or whether the CHF is secondary to a problem in another oxygen system. While the patient is being examined, routine measures should be performed simultaneously if not already done en route to the hospital. These include establishing an intravenous line and an airway, administering supplemental low flow oxygen (see Chapter 57), starting cardiac monitoring, and administering diuretics, morphine sulfate, and lidocaine if indicated. An ECG, chest roentgenogram, arterial blood gas values, and baseline laboratory data (including sodium, potassium, carbon dioxide, chloride, creatinine, creatine phosphokinase, lactic dehydrogenase, magnesium, phosphorus, and a urinalysis) should be obtained as soon as possible. Conservative therapy should be started immediately and should be directed by new data as they become available.

TREATMENT

Treatment of CHF can be divided into five phases: (1) conservative measures to ensure oxygenation and make the patient comfortable; (2) elimination of the underlying etiology; (3) classic therapy including digitalis and diuretics; (4) optimizing preload, afterload, and inotropic states (Table 51–3)[6,11–14] and (5) unusual techniques, including intra-aortic balloon pumping, phlebotomy, and artificial pacing.

When confronted with a dyspneic patient, it is important to eliminate any reversible causes of CHF or dyspnea. A careful, rapid physical examination may reveal any evidence of tamponade or cardiac arrhythmias or may point to noncardiac causes of dyspnea, including pneumothorax or airway obstruction. (See Section XI.) The laboratory data may show electrolyte abnormalities that may depress myocardial function. Arterial blood gas values may suggest a pulmonary embolus, and the roentgenogram may reveal pulmonary infarction. An attempt should be made to reverse any underlying cause of CHF or conditions that mimic it while temporary therapy is continued.

TABLE 51–3   Drugs Used in Congestive Heart Failure

Drug	Route	Dose	Effects
Aminophylline	IV	2.75 mg/kg IV	Decreased bronchospasm Mild inotropic effect
Captopril	Oral	25– to 150–mg initial dose	Arterial and venous dilatation
Digoxin	IV or oral	0.5–mg loading dose	Increased contractility Increased cardiac output Reflex decrease in peripheral vasoconstriction
Dobutamine	IV	2.5–15μg/kg/min	Increased contractility Increased cardiac output
Dopamine	IV	2–5μg/kg/min; up to 30 mg/kg/min	Increased contractility Increased cardiac output Vasodilatation of renal vascular bed
Ethacrynic acid	IV or oral	50 mg	Diuresis
Furosemide	IV or oral	10–100 mg	Diuresis Increased peripheral venous capacitance
Hydralazine	IV Oral	20–50 mg 25–200 mg	Arterial dilatation Reflex tachycardia not found when treating CHF
Isoproterenol	IV	Starting at 1–3μg/min	Increased contractility Increased heart rate β-mediated vasodilatation
Metolazone	Oral	2.5–10 mg/day	Potentiates effect of loop diuretics
Morphine	IV	2– to 3–mg increments	Decreased anxiety Decreased preload
Nitroglycerin	IV	5–100μg/min and titrate to effect	Venodilatation Slight arterial dilatation
	Sublingual Topical Oral	1/150 grain 1/2–1 inch 10–40 mg	
Nitroprusside	IV	20–300μg/min	Arterial and venous dilatation
Prazosin	Oral	1–10 mg	Arterial and venous dilatation

Conservative initial measures that may be started in the field include establishment of an airway and administration of supplemental oxygen. If there is any history or suspicion of chronic lung disease, then low flow oxygen at 1 to 2 liters/minute should be used until the patient is in a fully monitored setting where endotracheal intubation equipment is available. An intravenous line should be established and maintained at a keep-open rate. All medications preferably should be given intravenously. Intramuscular injections may cause an elevation in creatine phosphokinase, which may confuse the early diagnosis of a myocardial infarction. Vasoconstriction to the skin may decrease absorption of intramuscular injections. Oral medications may be erratically absorbed secondary to bowel edema or decreased splanchnic blood flow. Morphine sulfate may be given intravenously in doses of 2 to 3 mg to decrease anxiety and reduce preload. An initial intravenous dose of a diuretic such as furosemide, 20 to 40 mg, may be given.

Furosemide increases venous capacitance peripherally and reduces preload even before diuresis begins. If there does not appear to be an acute myocardial infarction and the patient is not already on digitalis, then digoxin, 0.5 mg, may be given intravenously. If wheezing is present, aminophylline may be given intravenously with a loading dose of 2.75 mg/kg over 20 to 30 minutes. Lidocaine may be given as a 75- to 100-mg intravenous bolus for ventricular ectopy and may be repeated if necessary. (See Chapter 49.) If available, rotating tourniquets may be used to reduce preload. While therapy is continuing, the patient should be in a comfortable position (usually sitting up) and all laboratory specimens should be obtained, the rest of the history should be taken, and the physical examination should be completed. If there is an inadequate response to the diuretic, the dose may be repeated or increased.

In recent years, treatment of CHF has been expanded to include manipulation of contractility, preload, and

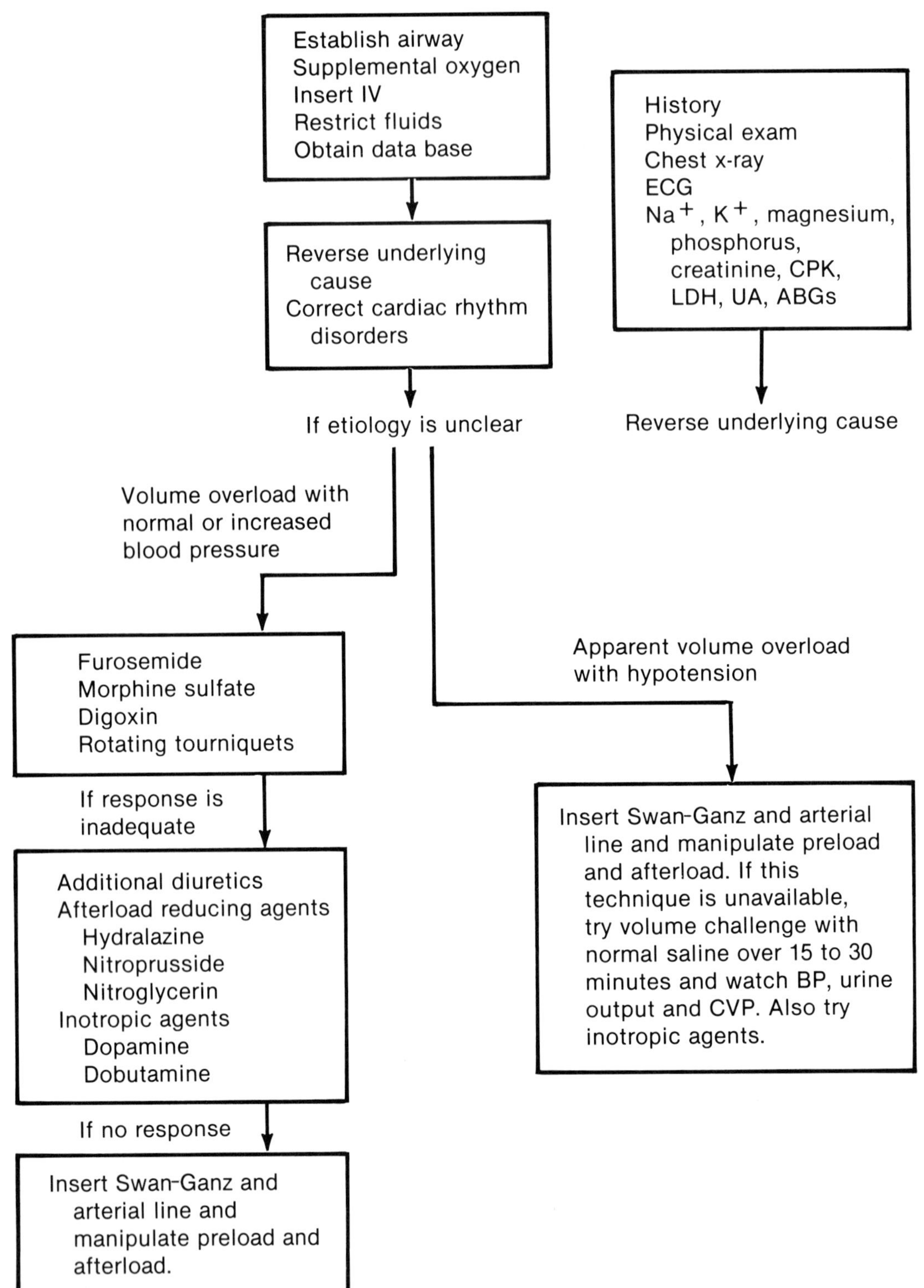

Figure 51–1   Emergency Treatment of Congestive Heart Failure.

afterload. If forward flow is restricted by increased afterload, arteriolar vasodilators including nitroprusside, hydralazine, prazosin, and captopril may be useful. While hydralazine is a pure arteriolar vasodilator, nitroprusside and prazosin predominantly dilate the arterial bed but also dilate the venous beds. Nitroglycerin and isosorbide dinitrate predominantly dilate the venous beds and decrease preload. The inotropic agents dopamine and dobutamine may decrease preload and afterload indirectly by increasing cardiac output and decreasing reflex vasoconstriction and directly by β-mediated vasodilatation.[12] If hypovolemia is clinically suspected, a volume challenge of 250 ml of normal saline given intravenously over 20 to 30 minutes may be used, while urine output, blood pressure, and central venous pressure are monitored.

The rational use of potent vasodilators or inotropic agents and volume administration is best managed by hemodynamic measurements obtained by pulmonary artery catheter and an arterial line. A simple central venous pressure line may give erroneous information regarding filling pressures. The doses of most commonly used agents in congestive heart failure are listed in Table 51–3.

SUMMARY

CHF refers to any condition that results in failure of the myocardium to pump enough oxygenated blood to maintain tissue perfusion. The body has several mechanisms that are invoked to maintain cardiac output, and the signs and symptoms of CHF may be a part of these reflex mechanisms. The patient who presents in the emergency department with congestive heart failure should have a careful history and physical examination, and an adequate data base should be obtained while conservative therapy is being administered. Definitive therapy is based on the underlying etiology. Current therapy of CHF based on decreased contractility consists of fluid and salt restriction, oxygen, diuretics, and digitalis. Vasodilators, inotropic agents, and mechanical support may be useful in certain situations. Early

use of a Swan-Ganz catheter may help in the differential diagnosis and may direct therapy so that the CHF may be treated effectively with minimal risk to the patient. A decision algorithm for guidance in the treatment of congestive heart failure is found in Figure 51–1.

REFERENCES

1. Gerard S: Shortness of breath in emergency room patients. *Radiol Clin North Am* 16:113–121, 1978.
2. Mantle J, et al: Advances in the treatment of heart failure. *Cardiovasc Clin* 2:49–64, 1981.
3. Mason DT: The failing heart. *DM*, January 1977.
4. Mason DT, et al: Alternations of hemodynamics and myocardial mechanics in patients with congestive heart failure: Pathophysiologic mechanisms and assessment of cardiac function and ventricular contractility. *Prog Cardiovasc Dis* 12:507–557, 1970.
5. Weber KT, Janick JS: The heart as a muscle-pump system and the concept of heart failure. *Am Heart J* 98:371–384, 1979.
6. Zelis R, et al: Circulatory dynamics in the normal and failing heart. *Ann Rev Physiol* 43:455–476, 1981.
7. Smulyan H, et al: Pulmonary effects of heart failure. *Surg Clin North Am* 54:1077–1087, 1974.
8. Kaplan S: New aspects of management of congestive heart failure. *Cardiovasc Clin* 22:293–299, 1981.
9. Cohn, JN: Vasodilator therapy of congestive heart failure. *Adv Intern Med* 26:293–315, 1980.
10. McManus WF, et al: Prehospital advanced emergency care: A potential pitfall. *J Trauma* 18:305–307, 1978.
11. Atkinson AB: Captopril in the treatment of clinical hypertension and cardiac failure. *Lancet* 2:836–839, 1979.
12. Goldberg L, et al: Newer catecholamines for treatment of heart failure and shock: An update on dopamine and a first look at dobutamine. *Prog Cardiovasc Dis* 14:327–340, 1977.
13. Chatterjee K, Parmley W: The role of vasodilation therapy on heart failure. *Prog Cardiovasc Dis* 14:301–325, 1977.
14. Mason DT: Afterload reduction and cardiac performance. *Am J Med* 65:106–125, 1978.

52. Hypertensive Emergencies

JEFFREY A. SANDLER, M.D.

Emergencies associated with elevations in blood pressure are fortunately quite rare, despite the large number of patients known to have chronic hypertension. Not only the emergencies themselves, but also their overtreatment can be life-threatening. It is estimated that less than 1 percent of patients with hypertension will experience a hypertensive crisis, and this low figure is probably due to better and more effective treatments of hypertension.

DEFINITION[1]

The terms *accelerated* and *malignant* hypertension are frequently used interchangeably; however, a fine line may be drawn between the two. Accelerated hypertension indicates a rapid rise in blood pressure, usually in the face of previously known hypertension. Malignant hypertension generally implies a more severe form. Both accelerated and malignant hypertension have an extremely poor prognosis without treatment.

The signs and symptoms of accelerated hypertension include central nervous system symptoms, such as headache, nausea, vomiting, and visual disturbances. Over time, the illness may progress to seizures and coma. Physical examination reveals an elevated blood pressure with diastolic pressures as high as 130 to 140 mm Hg. However, lower diastolic readings can be seen in patients with hypertension of shorter duration, and relatively asymptomatic patients who do not fulfill the criteria for accelerated or malignant hypertension can have

these values. Other physical findings include funduscopic changes such as hemorrhages, exudates, and, in the case of malignant hypertension, papilledema. There may be signs of left ventricular enlargement and cardiac failure. (See Chapter 51.) A brief laboratory evaluation reveals mild to moderate azotemia with elevation of both the blood urea nitrogen (BUN) and creatinine; urinalysis shows proteinuria, red cells, and red cell and white cell casts. Examination of the peripheral smear may demonstrate evidence of microangiopathic hemolytic anemia with fragmented red blood cells and thrombocytopenia. The electrocardiogram may show left ventricular hypertrophy and strain, and the chest roentgenogram may confirm the left ventricular enlargement, as well as the presence of heart failure.

ETIOLOGY

The most frequent cause of a hypertensive crisis is underlying essential hypertension. Rarely, emergencies are seen in patients with the more unusual secondary forms of hypertension, such as primary hyperaldosteronism, Cushing's syndrome, or renovascular disease. Hypertension can also occur in the face of a central nervous system catastrophe, such as an intracerebral or subarachnoid hemorrhage; a dissecting or leaking aortic aneurysm; acute left ventricular failure; or coronary ischemia. Toxemia of pregnancy with convulsions, edema, and proteinuria is also associated with an elevation in blood pressure. A rare cause of accelerated hypertension can be the catecholamine crisis seen in a patient with an undiagnosed pheochromocytoma or an individual who is taking monoamine oxidase inhibitors and has ingested foods containing tyramine.

The pathology seen in patients with accelerated hypertension consists mainly of a necrotizing arteriolitis. Spasm of the arterioles can be visualized in the fundi; this usually represents generalized arteriolar spasm. The vascular injury leads to fibrin deposition with intraluminal thrombosis and subsequent organ damage in the kidney, brain, and other organs of the body.

PATHOPHYSIOLOGY

The cause of accelerated and malignant hypertension is not completely understood. It has been postulated that the reninangiotensin system participates and that further fluid retention and vasospasm occur secondarily.[2] The inciting events are not, however, well delineated. In addition, the pathophysiology of hypertensive encephalopathy is not yet clear. Recognizing that there is an autoregulation of cerebral blood flow over a wide range of mean arterial pressures from 60 to 160 mm Hg, some investigators have suggested that an overregulation of cerebral blood flow leads to decreased perfusion; others that a failure of the autoregulatory mechanism leads to higher central nervous system perfusion pressures.[2] The end result is the same—hemorrhages, edema, and infarction of the brain.

The major hemodynamic aspect of accelerated hypertension is increased peripheral vascular resistance. Clinically, this is manifested as encephalopathy that may lead to stupor and coma in 12 to 48 hours, renal damage, and congestive heart failure with left ventricular enlargement and pulmonary congestion on examination.

DIAGNOSIS

The diagnosis is provided through the history and physical examination. Laboratory evaluation plays a minor role in the emergency approach to the hypertensive crisis: complete blood count (CBC), BUN and creatinine determinations, and urinalysis should be performed but the results may be normal. Chest and abdominal roentgenograms should be obtained to demonstrate the presence of left ventricular enlargement and cardiac failure, and to evaluate the kidney size. Small kidneys usually imply chronic underlying renal disease; normal-sized kidneys bespeak an acute process. A lumbar puncture may be performed if the patient's neurologic status is changing. Generally, this reveals an increase in pressure and protein. If there is xanthochromia or fresh red blood cells, then an intracerebral or subarachnoid hemorrhage has occurred.

DIFFERENTIAL DIAGNOSIS

In the clinical setting of a patient with an elevated blood pressure and a changing neurologic status, the physician must determine whether the central nervous system deficit is primary or secondary to malignant hypertension. Frequently, only treatment of the blood pressure can elucidate the problem. If the patient's condition improves as the blood pressure is lowered, then the problem was primarily hypertensive. If further neurologic deterioration ensues, then a primary neurologic etiology must be sought.

Unusual causes of accelerated hypertension need to be considered. If the patient has a history of palpitations, pallor, and sweats, the diagnosis of a pheochromocytoma must be entertained; however, the patient may be taking monoamine oxidase inhibitors and recently have ingested tyramine-containing foods, such as red wine, cheese, or chicken liver.

TREATMENT

A good clinical rule to follow in hypertensive emergencies is to treat first and investigate later, since the entities considered here are life-threatening and frequently fatal unless therapy is begun promptly. Little can be done in the prehospital setting, except to treat concomitant congestive heart failure. In that case, the patient should be sitting up, and oxygen should be administered. Future studies will be required to determine whether the administration of a loop diuretic (furosemide or ethacrynic acid) IV in the field by trained paramedical personnel will improve survival rates in patients with hypertensive crises.

On arrival at the hospital, the patient is examined immediately; if a hypertensive crisis is suspected, an intravenous line is begun and loop diuretic administered. Because many of the antihypertensive medications used require continuous blood pressure monitoring, the patient should be placed in an intensive care unit that is equipped for such monitoring, preferably by the intra-arterial technique. Routine orders include salt restriction, careful monitoring of intake and output, and daily weights. The mainstay of management remains pharmacologic. Treatment may be initiated with a diuretic, preferably furosemide, 40 to 80 mg, or ethacrynic acid, 50 to 100 mg, given IV by bolus. Within 30 minutes, the diuretic effect occurs. Peripheral venodilation provides a "tourniquet" effect, an extra advantage in the face of left ventricular failure. Importantly, these drugs do not reduce renal blood flow.

The major antihypertensive medications may temporarily impair renal function, but it is hoped that their use will preserve long-term function. It is important in the treatment of hypertensive crises to attempt to switch to oral medications as soon as possible so that the use of more potent and risky parenteral antihypertensive medications can be ended.

ANTIHYPERTENSIVE MEDICATIONS

Sodium nitroprusside (Nipride), the most potent and predictable antihypertensive medication, is the drug of choice for the treatment of uncomplicated accelerated or malignant hypertension. Its mechanism of action is by direct peripheral vasodilation (Table 52–1), both arterial and venous. Consequently, there may be either a decrease in cardiac output or an actual increase, owing to afterload reduction. Its effect is seen within seconds and is dose-dependent. When administration is stopped, the patient's blood pressure usually returns to pretreatment levels within one to ten minutes. The use of the medication is limited by its toxicity; its metabolic products include cyanide and thiocyanate. There are now some experimental approaches to reduce the problem of cyanide intoxication; at the present time, however, it is recommended that, if the drug is to be used for more than 72 hours, thiocyanate levels should be monitored and the toxic range avoided. The drug is quite light-sensitive and needs to be shielded. It is diluted in 5 percent dextrose and water to a final concentration of 50 mg/500 ml or 100 μg/ml. The infusion rate is begun at 0.5 μg/kg/minute and may be increased slowly to as high as 8 μg/kg/minute.

Diazoxide (Hyperstat) is the second most commonly used parenteral antihypertensive medication. It is structurally related to the thiazide diuretics, but has a different mechanism of action. It directly relaxes arteriolar smooth muscle, causing an increase in cardiac output with reflex tachycardia (which may be blocked by concomitant administration of propranolol). The advantage of diazoxide is that once blood pressure is controlled, it returns to pretreatment levels only gradually, i.e., over four to ten hours. Thus, it requires less frequent monitoring. The maximum response occurs within 10 to 30 minutes after a rapid intravenous bolus of 75 to 300 mg. The injection must be rapid to prevent the diazoxide from binding to plasma proteins. The disadvantage of this medication is that the fixed dose may produce hypotension requiring treatment with sympathomimetic amines. Because of reflex cardiac stimulation, diazoxide is not recommended for treatment of aortic dissection or leakage. It is also not recommended for patients with ischemic heart disease because reflex tachycardia may exacerbate angina. Other side-effects include hyperglycemia due to inhibition of insulin release, hyperuricemia, and sodium retention. The drug crosses the placenta and may lead to fetal hyperbilirubinemia and abnormal carbohydrate metabolism. An alternative dose regimen to the 300-mg intravenous bolus is a 50- to 75-mg bolus every ten minutes; this approach is currently under investigation.

Trimethaphan (Arfonad) is a ganglionic blocking agent that is especially useful in the treatment of dissecting aneurysm. Since it decreases cardiac output and cardiac

---

TABLE 52–1 Drug Treatment of Hypertensive Emergencies

Drug	Mode of Action	Effect on Cardiac Output	Dosage	Time Course Onset	Time Course Duration	Adverse Effects
Nitroprusside (Nipride)	Vasodilator	Decrease or increase	0.5–8 μg/kg/min	1–2 min	1–5 min	Cyanide and thiocyanate toxicity
Diazoxide (Hyperstat)	Vasodilator	Increase	75–300 mg IV bolus	1–2 min	30 min–18 hours	Hyperglycemia, hyperuricemia, sodium retention, nausea
Trimethaphan (Arfonad)	Ganglionic blockade	Decrease	0.25–15 mg/min	1–2 min	10 min	Hypotension
Hydralazine	Vasodilator	Increase	10–50 mg IM or IV	10–20 min	3–8 hours	Tachycardia
α-Methyldopa	Decreased sympathetic stimulation		250–500 mg IV every 4–8 hours	2–3 hours	6–12 hours	Central nervous system depression
Reserpine	Decreased sympathetic stimulation		0.25–5 mg IM every 4–6 hours	1–2 hours	6–24 hours	Central nervous system depression
Propranolol	β Blockade "central"	Decrease	1–3 mg IV, or 40–120 mg orally 4 times/day	1–2 min 1–1½ hours	T ½ = 3½–6 hours	Left ventricular failure, bronchospasm, bradycardia

contractility, less ejection pressure is exerted at the site of the leak or tear. Trimethaphan decreases systemic vascular resistance by arteriolar dilation. To achieve maximal effect with this medication, the head of the patient's bed should be elevated. Its main advantages are (1) it is potent, (2) it acts immediately, and (3) it is rapidly reversed by discontinuing administration and placing the patient in the Trendelenburg position. The drug also promotes venous pooling, which has a "tourniquet effect" on patients with acute left ventricular heart failure. It is prepared in a solution of 500 mg/liter dextrose and water, and given at a dose of 0.25 mg/minute; the dosage may be increased to as high as 15 mg/minute, depending on blood pressure response. This difficulty in determining the appropriate dosage is one disadvantage; another is that it may cause hypotension.

Hydralazine affects hypotension by decreasing peripheral resistance. It maintains renal blood flow and thus can be used in the presence of acute glomerulonephritis or toxemia of pregnancy. It is unpredictable, however, and it rarely controls severe hypertension. It is also accompanied by a reflex tachycardia and an increase in cardiac output; therefore, it should not be used in patients with unstable ischemic heart disease. The dosage ranges between 10 and 50 mg IM or by slow intravenous injection (over 10 to 15 min.) every three to six hours. It usually begins to act within 10 to 20 minutes, and its effect lasts three to eight hours.

α-Methyldopa is a second-line drug that decreases sympathetic stimulation either centrally or peripherally. It is given in a dose of 250 to 500 mg (some recommend a dose as high as 1,000 mg)[2,3] IV every four to eight hours. Its onset of action occurs within two to three hours, and its effect lasts six to twelve hours. Its major adverse effect is central nervous system depression. α-Methyldopa is frequently used orally as a transition drug when the intravenous medications are being tapered off and stopped.

Parenteral reserpine is rarely used, although it was one of the first drugs available for the treatment of hypertensive crises. It is given intramuscularly (IM) in a dose ranging from 0.25 to 5 mg every four to six hours; it produces marked central nervous system depression, however.

Another drug to be considered is propranolol. This has not been a primary drug in the treatment of malignant hypertension, but it has been used in conjunction with other medications. It is a β blocker that may also have a central hypotensive effect. It decreases cardiac output and can be given in a dosage of 1 to 3 mg IV or 40 to 120 mg orally, four times a day. Adverse effects include a decrease in left ventricular function, precipitation of congestive heart failure, and bronchospasm in patients with underlying obstructive lung disease. It should be avoided in any patients with suspected congestive heart failure. It is also relatively contraindicated in patients with known or suspected pheochromocytoma, since β blockade may lead to protracted and unopposed α stimulation, worsening the hypertension.

SPECIAL THERAPEUTIC PROBLEMS

Hypertensive Encephalopathy

If neurologic symptoms in a patient with hypertension worsen with treatment, then hypertensive encephalopathy is unlikely and underlying central nervous system disease, such as intracerebral or subarachnoid hemorrhage, must be considered. Lumbar puncture and other diagnostic studies, including a computerized axial tomography (CT) scan must be undertaken. In patients who do have hypertensive encephalopathy, hypertension should be rapidly but not excessively lowered. A diastolic pressure of 100 mg Hg should be the goal. This level is adequate, since most patients with hypertensive encephalopathy have underlying chronic hypertension and the autoregulatory mechanisms function quite well at this level.

Pheochromocytoma

A very rare and unusual form of accelerated hypertension, pheochromocytoma can be diagnosed with phentolamine (Regitine). A test dose of 0.5 to 1 mg is given IV; if no precipitous drop in blood pressure occurs, 5 mg may be given. A fall in blood pressure of 35 mm Hg/25 mm Hg lasting longer than four minutes is suggestive of a pheochromocytoma with 75 percent accuracy. Many false-positive Regitine tests occur in patients under stress, however. If the hypertension is indeed significant, even in the presence of a pheochromocytoma, nitroprusside can be used safely with good results (Table 52–2).

Acute Dissecting Aneurysm

Many factors are involved in the evaluation of an acute dissecting aneurysm: the site of the leak, the age and condition of the patient, and the availability of a cardiac surgery team. Vasodilating drugs such as hydralazine, diazoxide, or nitroprusside may actually worsen the problem because of reflex cardiac stimulation. The drug of choice in the treatment of acute dissecting or leaking aortic aneurysm is trimethaphan because it decreases myocardial contractility.

Acute Left Ventricular Heart Failure

Hypertension is treated with intravenous diuretics and trimethaphan or nitroprusside. These drugs promote

Table 52–2   Selection of Parenteral Drug Regimen for Specific Hypertensive Crises*

Emergency	Preferred	Secondary	Drugs to Avoid
Accelerated or malignant hypertension	Nitroprusside, trimethaphan, diazoxide	Hydralazine, α-Methyldopa, reserpine	
Hypertension in the presence of			
Intracerebral or subarachnoid hemorrhage	Nitroprusside, trimethaphan	α-Methyldopa	Reserpine
Dissecting or leaking aortic aneurysm	Trimethaphan		Diazoxide, hydralazine, nitroprusside
Acute left ventricular failure	Nitroprusside, trimethaphan		Propranolol, hydralazine
Coronary ischemia	Nitroprusside		Hydralazine
Toxemia of pregnancy	Magnesium sulfate	Diazoxide hydralazine	Trimethaphan
Pheochromocytoma	Phentolamine	Nitroprusside	α-Methyldopa, reserpine

* A loop diuretic (furosemide or ethacrynic acid), given intravenously, should accompany all drug treatment regimens.

venous pooling and decrease blood return to the heart. Digitalization may be required. (See Chapter 51.)

Acute Cerebrovascular Accident

Hypertension in the face of an acute cerebrovascular accident is a "tightrope situation." (See Chapter 46.) If the blood pressure is too high, there is a risk of direct vascular damage to the peri-infarction area. If the blood pressure is lowered too far, there is a risk of hypoperfusion, ischemia, and extension of the injury. Some authors recommend that the mean arterial pressure be maintained at approximately 120 mm Hg (the diastolic pressure plus one-third the pulse pressure),[2] or the systolic between 160–180, the diastolic 100–120.[4] Vasodilating drugs have a theoretical disadvantage in that blood may be diverted from the peri-infarction area. Trimethaphan may be the drug of choice under these circumstances. In the face of a subarachnoid hemorrhage, aggressive hypotensive therapy, including trimethaphan and tilting of the bed, has been recommended by some.[3] α-Methyldopa may reduce the pressure more gently.

Toxemia of Pregnancy

Magnesium sulfate lowers the blood pressure and decreases the neuromuscular irritability associated with toxemia of pregnancy. It is administered IV in a dosage of 4 gm of a 50 percent solution (over 30 min.), then 1 gm every hour. Diuretics, hydralazine, and diazoxide are also used. However, there is some placental transfer of diazoxide and side-effects can be seen in the fetus. For specifics of hypertension in pregnancy, see Chapter 64, Obstetric and Gynecologic Emergencies.

Acute Ischemic Heart Disease

Hypertension in the face of acute ischemic heart disease is best treated with nitroprusside, which lowers the blood pressure and maintains coronary blood flow. Propranolol, in the absence of left ventricular heart failure, may also be used. Of course, nitroglycerin, 0.4 mg given sublingually as needed, and its long-acting derivatives may be effective in treating refractory angina in the face of hypertension.

CONCLUSION

Follow-up of patients who have experienced a hypertensive crisis includes gentle weaning from parenteral treatment to an oral program as soon as possible. Under most circumstances, a multiple drug regimen, i.e., a diuretic plus a variety of drugs currently available for the management of chronic hypertension, is recommended. In the days following the treatment of the hypertensive crisis, it is important to measure blood pressure in both the supine and standing position, since dramatic changes in intravascular volume and vasomotor tone have taken place during the hospitalization.

REFERENCES

1. Moser M: When hypertension is an emergency. *Drug Therapy*, March 1976, pp 6–20.
2. Becker CE, Benowitz NL: Hypertensive emergencies. *Med Clin North Am* 63:127–140, 1977.
3. Koch-Weser J: Hypertensive emergencies. *N Engl J Med* 290:211–214, 1974.
4. AMA Committee on Hypertension: The treatment of malignant hypertension and hypertensive emergencies. *JAMA* 228:1673–1679, 1974.

53. Vascular Injuries

LUKE K. LI CALZI, M.D.
MORRIS D. KERSTEIN, M.D.

The effective management of vascular trauma depends on early diagnosis. This, in turn, requires a high degree of clinical suspicion in both penetrating and blunt trauma and recognition of the *patterns* of injury. For example, blood vessel trauma is often associated with certain bone fractures, and awareness of this allows prompt diagnosis and early therapy. Vascular injuries occur in a wide variety of settings and are becoming increasingly frequent in a motorized, mechanized, and militaristic society.[1-5] Most often, they occur in combination with injuries to other organs and contribute significantly to the morbidity and mortality of the traumatized patient.

The initial approach to the patient with a suspected vascular injury depends on a number of factors. Blood loss from penetrating injuries of the extremities can usually be controlled with compressive bandages, allowing an orderly but rapid assessment of the patient's condition. However, penetrating injuries of the visceral or intrathoracic vessels can easily cause exsanguinating hemorrhage and often necessitate immediate surgery. Injuries due to blunt trauma and fractures are often insidious. They are manifested by the signs of arterial insufficiency, i.e., absence of pulses, pallor, paresthesias, pain, and paralysis. It should be remembered that complete arterial disruption can occur without the immediate loss of peripheral pulses and that the late sequelae of thrombosis include ischemia or arteriovenous fistulas. The close anatomical association of nerves and vessels should increase the index of suspicion of vascular injury when nerve injury is evident.

The early management of the critically injured patient includes the establishment of several large-bore intravenous cannulas for rapid fluid administration. Fluid resuscitation is accomplished initially with isotonic salt solution (Ringer's lactate) and then with typed whole blood when available. The patient's general condition then determines whether further diagnostic procedures may be done in the emergency department. Vascular injuries require the 24-hour availability of angiography. Persistent hypotension, other than that caused by cardiac tamponade or major long bone fractures, is due to intra-abdominal or intrathoracic blood loss and is best treated by early laparotomy or thoracotomy in the operating room. Time is the limiting factor, however, and it does not always permit the treatment of tamponade in the operating room.

The condition of the stable patient may be evaluated further by angiography to delineate the site of arterial injury.[6] This is especially helpful in the presence of multiple penetrating wounds of the extremities when the exact site of injury cannot readily be determined. Angiography is of paramount importance in the stable patient with suspected visceral (*e.g.*, liver or superior mesenteric artery) or thoracic arterial injury. It is not necessary, however, to perform angiography when the trajectory of penetrating arterial injury is obvious.[7]

It is difficult to generalize because of the complex variations and combinations of major trauma; however, several axioms may be stated:

- Vascular injuries must be suspected in certain modes and sites of injury.

- Initial resuscitation and stabilization of the patient is essential.
- Acute peripheral vascular occlusion must be treated within six hours to prevent tissue necrosis.
- Complete arterial disruption can occur even though the distal pulses remain intact.
- Absent pulses in the traumatized patient should never be attributed to "spasm."
- Tourniquets should be avoided and direct compression used to control hemorrhage.
- Tense hematomas and active bleeding indicate significant vascular injury.
- Arteriographic facilities and a vascular surgical team are essential.
- The ability to recognize patterns of associated injuries allows early diagnosis and treatment of vascular trauma.
- It must be determined whether there is a history of any bleeding disorder or any ingestion of drugs that may interfere with coagulation.

PATTERNS OF INJURY

Arterial Trauma Associated with Fractures and Dislocations

Perhaps the most frequently overlooked vascular injuries are those associated with fractures and dislocations. Although significant soft tissue damage may occur in the extremities, the high amputation rate is due in part to delay in diagnosis and treatment of vascular injuries.[8] The peripheral blood vessels should be carefully assessed in all cases of orthopedic trauma, especially the following:

1. knee, elbow, and ankle dislocations
2. sternoclavicular dislocations and fractures
3. supracondylar fractures of humerus and femur
4. first and second rib fractures
5. pelvic fractures
6. femoral and humeral shaft fractures

The failure of the peripheral circulation to return to normal following reduction of dislocations is an indication for urgent arteriography. Dislocations of the ankle, elbow, and, especially, the knee should be reduced by an orthopedic surgeon without delay. (See Chapter 8.) Both anterior and posterior knee dislocations are associated with popliteal artery compromise in over 50 percent of cases, and an arterial injury should be confirmed or excluded by arteriography in all instances.[9,10] Popliteal vein injuries also frequently occur with knee dislocations.

Dislocations and fractures associated with vascular trauma should be reduced prior to arterial repair; stabilization should be maintained postoperatively by external fixation. The importance of adequate splinting of fractures and dislocations during patient transport should be emphasized. Occasionally, satisfactory results can be obtained with internal fixation; but, in most cases, the degree of soft tissue damage and the prolonged operative time required for internal fixation jeopardize the survival of the limb. A delayed approach to ligament and definitive bone repair is most satisfactory.

Supracondylar fractures of the humerus and femur are associated with disruption of the brachial and superficial femoral arteries, respectively. This occurs less commonly with humeral and femoral shaft fractures.[11]

Sternoclavicular dislocations, clavicular fractures, and, rarely, anterior shoulder dislocations have caused laceration of the innominate and subclavian arteries. Signs of hypovolemia and shock, together with pulse and blood pressure differentials between the two arms, should alert the examiner to the diagnosis. The unstable patient requires immediate exploratory surgery, while the stable patient should undergo arteriography to delineate the lesion. The thoracic outlet syndrome is sometimes a late sequela of clavicular fractures, especially with malunion, but it is uncommon to see an acute thoracic outlet syndrome. However, fractures of the clavicle or of the first and second ribs may result in permanent neurologic damage secondary to ischemic neuritis and unrecognized vascular injury.

First and second rib fractures, although not directly responsible for vascular injuries, often signal severe intrathoracic trauma.[12,13] The aortic arch, subclavian artery, and vertebral artery may be disrupted, and cardiac and pulmonary contusions may occur. These rib fractures are often associated with other major intra-abdominal, neurologic, and orthopedic injuries; and the inhospital mortality of these patients approaches 30 percent.

Pelvic fractures can cause significant retroperitoneal hemorrhage and are often associated with other major injuries.[14] (See Chapter 62.) These two factors result in a 12 percent mortality rate among these patients. Major vessel disruption (iliac or femoral arteries) occurs rarely (one percent), but often in open pelvic fractures (including rectal or perineal laceration) and in those with a double break in the pelvic ring.[14–16] These patients are in profound shock when they are first seen and require emergency resuscitation and subsequent surgical exploration. The mortality rate approaches 75 percent currently. Venous bleeding can often be controlled with packing and compression in the emergency department. The stable patient with continued blood loss or expanding hematoma should undergo arteriography for localization of the bleeding point and possible Gelfoam embolization.[17] Nonexpanding retroperitoneal hematomas should be left undisturbed.

Deceleration Injuries

Injuries caused by deceleration, as occur in a fall or a high-speed auto accident, often involve disruptions of the thoracic aorta and, occasionally, the aortic arch branches.[18,19] In most cases, such injuries are fatal. In the 10 to 20 percent of patients surviving the initial injury, roentgenographic findings often include first and second rib fracture, pleural capping, widened mediastinum, deviation of the trachea to the right, or deviation of the normal straight course of a nasogastric tube. Aortography confirms the diagnosis, with intimal dissection occurring usually just distal to the left subclavian artery. The high hospital mortality rate is due to free rupture into the pleural space prior to exploration and the frequent association of a deceleration injury with other severe injuries. Occasionally, patients survive with these injuries unrecognized until they develop the late sequelae of false aneurysms in the thoracic aorta and pseudocoarctation syndrome. (See Chapter 54.)

Intimal disruptions can occur in any of the aortic arch branches in deceleration injuries. They are manifested by neurologic defects, which may be transient or permanent; variable arterial pulses; and the presence of bruits. Again, aortography is essential in delineating the injury.

Thoracotomy in the emergency department has no role in the salvage of these patients.

Blunt Trauma

The greatest challenge to the emergency physician and surgeon is posed by blunt trauma. The detection of significant organ and vessel injury is most difficult and necessitates meticulous examination of the patient and judicious use of highly sensitive diagnostic tests, such as abdominal paracentesis and lavage. Most often, significant hemorrhage is caused by organ injuries (e.g., to the liver or spleen), but specific and isolated vascular injuries do occur.

Blunt trauma to the carotid and vertebral arteries is rare in comparison with penetrating injuries.[20] These vessels can become completely or partially occluded from fracture and disruption of the intima, however. The injury may result from either a direct blow or a forcible hyperextension-flexion of the neck; it occurs usually at the carotid bifurcation. (See Chapter 43.) Cervical hematoma or bruit may be present, and the patient may have either an initial or delayed hemiplegia. Such an injury commonly has neurologic effects, such as Horner's syndrome. The newer noninvasive vascular tests (oculoplethysmography or directional Doppler) and a CT scan of the head may be helpful in differentiating the cause of the neurologic deficit in craniocervical trauma, but the diagnosis of carotid artery trauma is confirmed by arteriography. Surgical repair is successful only if the diagnosis is made early.

Blunt thoracic trauma can cause a host of life-threatening cardiovascular injuries. (See Chapter 61.) Pericardial tamponade; cardiac contusion; atrial, ventricular, and septal perforations; and rupture of the valves, chordae, and papillary muscle can all occur.[21,22]

Abdominal aortic injuries due to blunt trauma are much rarer than penetrating injuries and have only recently been recognized. Although they are most often related to steering wheel or seat belt injuries, they may occur after any blunt abdominal injury.[23] Commonly, the arterial intima is disrupted, resulting in thrombosis of the aorta. Femoral and distal pulses may be absent. If only partial occlusion occurs, the diagnosis may be missed. Several patients have been reported with manifestations of aortic occlusion several months after the initial injury.

Blunt trauma to the major visceral vessels occurs less frequently than that to the visceral organs (e.g., spleen, liver, kidney, pancreas, bowel), but it is associated with much greater mortality. Renal pedicle injuries are associated with gross or microscopic hematuria and usually with serious injuries.[24] A "one-shot" intravenous pyelogram (IVP) should be obtained either in the emergency department or on the operating table in the unstable patient with multiple injuries. If the patient is stable following the initial evaluation and resuscitation, a complete sequence IVP should be obtained. Arteriography is then done if nonfunction, significant distortion, or extravasation is shown. Blunt renal artery and vein laceration or thrombosis has been less successfully managed than penetrating injuries. The renal vein may be ligated, especially when divided close to the vena cava, without loss of the kidney; however, there is a high nephrectomy rate in these injuries.

Vena caval injuries are often lethal, especially if they occur at the level of the intrahepatic cava. Major hepatic vein lacerations also occur with blunt trauma. These patients are in shock and show signs of massive intraabdominal bleeding. Salvage requires emergency laparotomy. Control of the bleeding at operation may be exceedingly difficult; exposure is facilitated by either a combined thoracoabdominal incision or a median sternotomy. Several techniques for vascular isolation of the inferior vena cava have been developed for use during surgery.[25] Despite all measures, the mortality rate remains high.

Penetrating Trauma

The majority of vascular injuries seen today are penetrating injuries, and they can occur to any of the major vessels. Stab wounds can completely transect an artery without loss of the distal pulse. The proximity of the wound to a major vessel should direct further investigation. As mentioned earlier, when a stab wound has caused obvious vascular injury, preoperative arteriography is usually not necessary.[7] It is useful, however, in verifying the diagnosis and in investigating gunshot wounds with indirect trajectories and multiple pellet injuries.

With gunshot wounds, the velocity and mass of the missile are important factors. The fact that the kinetic energy dissipated by the bullet is proportional to the square of the velocity is the most important consideration. High-velocity (2,500 feet/second) and high-caliber bullets cause a great deal of secondary tissue destruction due to "shock waves." Intimal and medial arterial wall damage can occur over long distances. Failure to recognize the full extent of the injury can lead to early failure of arterial reconstruction. Gunshot wounds frequently require arteriography unless the patient is unstable.

Penetrating neck wounds can involve the carotid, vertebral, subclavian, or innominate arteries, as well as the veins, esophagus, and trachea. Injuries deep to the platysma muscle with continued hemorrhage, expanding or pulsatile hematomas, neurologic deficits, or airway obstruction require emergency exploration. The condition of the stable patient without obvious vascular, neurologic, or airway sequelae of neck wounds should be evaluated with angiography and endoscopy (bronchoscopy and esophagoscopy) to identify possible sites of injuries.[26–28] In most large series, about 50 percent of patients may be managed conservatively, i.e., exploration can be avoided, when the results of these examinations are normal.

Carotid artery injuries with active bleeding require emergency surgery; when there is no bleeding, arteriography is valuable in defining the site and extent of injury. With the advances in vascular surgical technique, the outcome in these patients following repair seems to depend mostly on their preoperative neurologic status. Patients with preoperative neurologic deficits or coma have a very high incidence of postoperative cerebrovascular accident and death, probably resulting in part from inadequate collateral circulation via the circle of Willis and the branches of the external carotid artery.[29] There is general agreement that dense hemiplegia and/or coma should preclude attempts at arterial repair in carotid injury.

Injuries to the vertebral artery occur less frequently and are usually not recognized initially. The classic delayed presentation is a vertebral arteriovenous fistula with symptoms of vertebrobasilar insufficiency and a cervical bruit that is often audible to the patient. Ligation of the fistula is safe and effective therapy.[30]

Patients with innominate and subclavian artery injuries have often experienced massive blood loss by the time they are first seen and require emergency exploration. Preoperative angiography in the stable patient allows precise operative planning. All patients should be examined carefully for the status of pulses, the presence of thrills or bruits, and neurologic deficits. The risk of exsanguinating hemorrhage is very high in these patients.[31,32]

Penetrating abdominal injuries to the aorta, iliac arteries and veins, splanchnic arteries (celiac, superior mesenteric, and inferior mesenteric), visceral arteries and veins (hepatic and renal), and inferior vena cava and portal vein are life-threatening and are most often associated with multiple intra-abdominal injuries.[33–36] Prompt and effective resuscitation of the patient and emergency exploration are required. Because of the extent of injury, seldom is arteriography indicated. A one-shot IVP is helpful in establishing the extent of renal function bilaterally. Vascular repair may consist of any combination of ligation, lateral suture, or graft interposition.

Peripheral arterial injuries are managed according to the same general principles. Obvious injuries with ischemic extremities, absent pulses, massive hemorrhage, and direct missile trajectories should be explored. Preoperative arteriography is useful when the site of multiple pellet or variable projectory injuries must be determined or when there is only a clinical suspicion of injury. Vascular repair can salvage the limb in a great percentage of cases; occasionally, however, primary amputation must be done because the extent of soft tissue or bone injury precludes a viable, useful extremity. Popliteal artery injuries are especially serious, with amputation rates of about 50 percent.[37–39]

Recent advances in microvascular surgery make repair of vessels distal to the brachial and popliteal artery bifurcations a feasible alternative to ligation.[40]

Intra-arterial Injection of Drugs

A severely ischemic hand or digit may result from intra-arterial injections of drugs of either medical use or abuse. (See Chapter 35.) Numerous pharmacologic agents have been implicated. This condition is being observed with increasing frequency in addicts seeking additional routes for drug administration.[41] Initial treatment involves chemical sympathectomy by stellate ganglion block; intra-arterial vasodilators, such as reserpine or papaverine; and rheologic agents, such as dextran.[42] Arteriography should be performed to delineate the level of injury. Occasionally, injury to the brachial, radial, or ulnar arteries that is amenable to surgical repair is discovered. Occlusion usually occurs at the level of digital arteries, however, and therapy is limited to surgical dorsal sympathectomy. A good response to chemical dorsal sympathectomy, as shown by improvement in digital plethysmography or skin temperature, is fairly predictive of a good response to surgical sympathectomy.

Another vascular injury seen in the emergency department, also due to repeated intra-arterial drug injection, is the infected (mycotic) false aneurysm of a peripheral artery. Such an aneurysm may appear to be a simple abscess, but the history of injection and location of the mass should alert the physician to the diagnosis. Puncture should be avoided until vascular control is obtained in the operating room. Direct compression is the best method to control hemorrhage from peripheral mycotic aneurysm in the prehospital setting or in the emergency department. If this should fail, tourniquet control should be obtained during transit to the operating room.

Late Complications of Vascular Injuries

Arteriovenous fistulas and false aneurysms occur most frequently in penetrating injuries to the extremities and less frequently in injuries to the neck, thorax, and abdomen. They are common with multiple small fragment injuries, although most lesions are single.[43] Late complications include high output cardiac failure, infection, and rupture of false aneurysms.

The intravascular migration of bullets is a fascinating phenomenon.[44,45] Bullet wounds to the pulmonary veins, left heart, or the thoracic or abdominal aorta may migrate to the distal arterial tree and should be suspected when there is no exit wound and the bullet is not visible on a roentgenogram. Following repair of the initial injury, it is advisable to remove the bullet to prevent arterial occlusion and ischemia. Missiles that have entered the major veins or vena cava may likewise migrate to the right heart or pulmonary arteries and should be removed to prevent endocarditis. Peripheral small-caliber missiles or fragments thereof in the pulmonary artery as emboli need not be removed. Paradoxical movement of bullets through a patent foramen ovale has been reported.

Acute arterial occlusion for any reason can cause an ischemic myopathy with rhabdomyolysis, myoglobinuria, hyperkalemia, and acute renal failure.[46] (See Chapter 63.) Treatment includes early restoration of circulation via bypass, arterial repair or embolectomy, and correction of fluid deficits, hyperkalemia, and metabolic acidosis. Alkalinization of the urine with osmotic diuresis is essential to avoid precipitation of myoglobin in the renal tubules.

Compartment syndromes occur in the forearm and leg in response to crush type trauma, arterial injury, and venous hypertension.[47] They are seen frequently in unconscious drug addicts with compression of a limb.[48] Arterial occlusion leads to muscle and nerve death and finally to the myopathic-renal failure syndrome. Treatment consists of fasciotomy to relieve the compartmental pressure.

In young children, peripheral arterial injuries leading to stenosis or occlusion result in limb growth disparities of 2 to 4 cm. Careful evaluation and repair of vascular injuries (especially in the legs) in these patients will prevent future deformity.[49]

Upper extremity post-traumatic ischemia can occur as a direct result of arterial injury or as a late manifestation of the thoracic outlet syndrome.[50] Volkmann's contracture following supracondylar fractures is a good example of a compartment syndrome due to arterial compression and trauma. Failure of orthopedic reduction to restore circulation is an indication for angiography. In addition, patients with or without concomitant nerve damage may exhibit post-traumatic causalgia. These cold, paretic, painful, vasospastic hands are best treated by dorsal sympathectomy.[51]

REFERENCES

1. Hardy JD, Raju S, Neely WA, et al: Aortic and other arterial injuries. *Ann Surg* 181:640–653, 1975.
2. Bole PV, Purdy RT, Munda RT, et al: Civilian arterial injuries. *Ann Surg* 183:13–23, 1976.
3. Perry MD, Thal ER, Shires GT: Management of arterial injuries. *Ann Surg* 173:403–408, 1971.
4. Drapanas T, Hewett RL, Weichert RF, et al: Civilian vascular injuries: A critical appraisal of three decades of management. *Ann Surg* 172:351–360, 1970.
5. Rich NM, Spencer FC: *Vascular Trauma.* Philadelphia, WB Saunders Co, 1978.
6. Burnett HF, Parnell CL, Williams GD, et al: Peripheral arterial injuries: A reassessment. *Ann Surg* 183:701–709, 1976.
7. Turcotte JK, Towne JB, Bernard VM: Is arteriography necessary in the management of vascular trauma of the extremities? *Surgery* 84:557–562, 1978.
8. Sher MH: Principles in the management of arterial injuries associated with fracture/dislocations. *Ann Surg* 182:630–634, 1975.
9. Dart CH, Braitman HE: Popliteal artery injury following fracture or dislocation at the knee. *Arch Surg* 112:969–973, 1977.
10. Jones RE, Smith EC, Bone GE: Vascular and orthopedic complications of knee dislocation. *Surg Gynecol Obstet* 149:554–558, 1970.
11. Kodstra G, Schipper JJ, Boontje AH, et al: Femoral shaft fracture with injury of the superficial femoral artery in civilian accidents. *Surg Gynecol Obstet* 142:399–403, 1976.
12. Richardson JD, McElvein RB, Trinkle JK: First rib fracture: A hallmark of severe trauma. *Ann Surg* 181:251–254, 1975.

13. Wilson JM, Thomas AN, Goodman PC, et al: Severe chest trauma: Morbidity implication of first and second rib fracture in 120 patients. *Arch Surg* 113:846–849, 1978.

14. Rothenberger DA, Fischer RP, Strate RG, et al: The mortality associated with pelvic fractures. *Surgery* 84:356–361, 1978

15. Rothenberger DA, Fischer RP, Perry JF: Major vascular injuries secondary to pelvic fractures: An unsolved clinical problem. *Am J Surg* 136:660–662, 1978.

16. Raffa J, Christensen NM: Compound fractures of the pelvis. *Am J Surg* 132:282–286, 1976.

17. Urk HV, Perlberger RR, Muller H: Selective arterial embolization for control of traumatic pelvic hemorrhage. *Surgery* 83:133–137, 1978.

18. Plume S, Deweese JA: Traumatic rupture of the thoracic aorta. *Arch Surg* 114:240–243, 1979.

19. Hoffman TH, Richardson JD, Flint LM: Intimal disruption of major cerebral vasculation following blunt trauma. *Surgery* 87:441–444, 1980.

20. Krajeuski LP, Hertzer NR: Blunt carotid artery trauma: Report of two cases and review of the literature. *Ann Surg* 191:341–346, 1980.

21. Jones JW, Hewitt RL, Drapanas T: Cardiac contusion: A capricious syndrome. *Ann Surg* 181:567–574, 1975.

22. Saunders CR, Doty DB: Myocardial contusion. *Surg Gynecol Obstet* 144:595–603, 1977.

23. Dajee H, Richardson IW, Iype MD: Seat belt aorta: Acute dissection and thrombosis of the abdominal aorta. *Surgery* 85:263–267, 1979.

24. Sturm JT, Perry JF, Cass AS: Renal artery and vein injury following blunt trauma. *Ann Surg* 182:696–698, 1975.

25. Schrock T, Blaisdell FW, Mathewson C: Management of blunt trauma to the liver and hepatic veins. *Arch Surg* 96:698–702, 1968.

26. Lundy LJ, Mandal AK, Lou MA, et al: Experience in selective operations in the management of penetrating wounds of the neck. *Surg Gynecol Obstet* 147:845–848, 1978.

27. O'Donnel VA, Atik M, Pick RA: Evaluation and management of penetrating wounds of the neck: The role of emergency angiography. *Am J Surg* 138:309–313, 1979.

28. Meinke AH, Bivins BA, Sachatello CR: Selective management of gunshot wounds to the neck. *Am J Surg* 138:314–319, 1979.

29. Ledgerwood AM, Mullins RJ, Lucas CE: Primary repair vs. ligation for carotid artery injuries. *Arch Surg* 115:488–493, 1980.

30. Beesinger DE, Thal ER, May RO, et al: Vertebral arteriovenous fistula associated with an anomalous arterial vessel. *Surgery* 85:230–234, 1979.

31. Sehalf HV, Brawley RK: Operative management of penetrating vascular injuries of the thoracic outlet. *Surgery* 82:182–191, 1977.

32. Lim LT, Saletta JD, Flanigan OP: Subclavian and innominate artery trauma. *Surgery* 86:850–897, 1979.

33. Nance FC, Wennar MA, Johnson LW, et al: Surgical judgment in the management of penetrating wounds of the abdomen: Experience with 2212 patients. *Ann Surg* 179:639–646, 1974.

34. Myles RA, Yellin AE: Traumatic injuries of the abdominal aorta. *Am J Surg* 138:273–277, 1979.

35. Mattox KL, Rea J, Emmy CL, et al: Penetration injuries to the iliac arteries. *Am J Surg* 136:663–667, 1978.

36. Graham JM, Mattox KL, Beall AC, et al: Injuries to the visceral arteries. *Surgery* 84:835–839, 1978.

37. Conkle DM, Richie RE, Sawyers JL, et al: Surgical treatment of popliteal artery injuries. *Arch Surg* 110:1351–1354, 1975.

38. Snyder WH, Watkins WL, Whiddon LL, et al: Civilian popliteal artery trauma: An eleven year experience with 83 injuries. *Surgery* 85:101–108, 1979.

39. Daugherty ME, Sachatello CR, Ernst CB: Improved treatment of popliteal arterial injuries. *Arch Surg* 113:1317–1321, 1978.

40. Kelley G, Eiseman B: Management of small arterial injuries: Clinical and experimental studies. *J Trauma* 16:681–686, 1976.

41. Wright CB, Lamoy RE, Hobson RW: Hemodynamic effects of intra-arterial injection of drugs of abuse. *Surgery* 79:425–431, 1976.

42. Wright CB, Geelhoed GW, Hobson RW: Acute vascular insufficiency due to drugs of abuse, in Rutherford RB (ed): *Vascular Surgery*. Philadelphia, WB Saunders Co, 1977, pp 451–460.

43. Rich NM, Hobson RW, Collins GJ: Traumatic arteriovenous fistulas and false aneurysms: A review of 558 lesions. *Surgery* 78:817–828, 1975.

44. Mattox KL, Beall EC, Ennix CL, et al: Intravascular migratory bullets. *Am J Surg* 137:192–195, 1979.

45. Ledgerwood AM: The wandering bullet. *Surg Clin North Am* 57:97–109, 1977.

46. Haimovici H: Muscular, renal and metabolic complications of acute arterial occlusions: Myonephropathic-metabolic syndrome. *Surgery* 85:461–468, 1979.

47. Matsen FA, Krugmire RB: Compartmental syndromes. *Surg Gynecol Obstet* 147:943–949, 1978.

48. Owen CA, Mubarak SJ, Hargens AR, et al: Intramuscular pressures with limb compression: Classification of the pathogenesis of the drug-induced muscle-compartment syndrome. *N Engl J Med* 300:1169–1172, 1979.

49. Whitehouse WM, Coran AG, Stanley JC, et al: Pediatric vascular trauma. *Arch Surg* 111:1269–1275, 1976.

50. Roos DB: Thoracic outlet and carpal tunnel syndromes, in Rutherford RB (ed): *Vascular Surgery*. Philadelphia, WB Saunders Co, 1977, pp 605–621.

51. Barker WF: *Peripheral Arterial Disease*, ed 2. Philadelphia, WB Saunders Co, 1975, pp 370–386.

54. Heart and Great Vessel Emergencies

NEAL W. SALOMON, M.D.

Most emergencies of the heart and great vessels develop in a dramatic manner and require both immediate diagnosis and therapy; a smaller proportion is associated with more subtle signs and symptoms and requires careful and deliberate diagnosis to elucidate the problem. In all cases, effective management depends on a high index of clinical suspicion for certain injuries, as well as on a firm knowledge of basic cardiovascular physiology and anatomy. Traumatic emergencies involving the heart and aorta may be seen as isolated cardiac problems, particularly when related to penetrating injuries, but they are often associated with multiple injuries, particularly when the mechanism of injury is massive blunt (nonpenetrating) trauma. (See Chapter 7.)

PATTERNS OF PRESENTATION

There are four major patterns of presentation of traumatic or nontraumatic emergencies of the heart and great vessels. The first and most obvious is hemorrhage, which may result from either laceration or rupture of the heart or any of the great vessels secondary to either blunt or penetrating trauma. The second major presentation is cardiac tamponade, which may be caused by either blunt or penetrating cardiac trauma or rupture of an ascending aortic dissection into the pericardium. Other nontraumatic causes of acute pericardial tamponade include severe hemorrhage in a patient medicated with anticoagulants or tamponade secondary to malignant or uremic pericardial effusions. The third pattern is primary cardiac injury (contusion) secondary to blunt concussive forces. The final major pattern of presentation is acute pain, with or without hemodynamic decompensation, such as that associated with acute aortic dissection in either the ascending or the descending thoracic aorta.

GENERAL PRINCIPLES

After general resuscitative measures have been carried out, standard therapy for treatment of hypovolemic shock must be instituted if this condition is present. This presupposes a sufficient number of both central and peripheral intravenous (IV) lines, most probably an endotracheal tube if indicated (see Chapter 56) and, if at all possible, either a radial or femoral arterial line for continuous measurement of blood pressure and immediate access to the bloodstream for arterial blood gas analysis. Blood specimens should be sent for blood type and cross-match, and electrolytes and hematocrit levels should be determined.

It is critical for the physician to have a high index of suspicion for acute cardiac tamponade. The diagnosis should be considered in any patient with poor peripheral perfusion and hypotension that seems out of proportion to the severity of blood loss, and in any patient with hypotension and elevated venous pressure (high central venous pressure or elevated neck veins). If acute pericardial tamponade is suspected, immediate pericardiocentesis should be performed with a 14- or 16-gauge catheter inserted from the subxiphoid approach. (See Chapters 7 and 70.) Ideally, this should be done with electrocardiographic monitoring (V lead clipped to exploring needle) to detect epicardial surface contact.[1] It is important to recognize that an unsuccessful attempt at pericardial aspiration of blood does not necessarily rule out the diagnosis. A significant amount of blood may be located posteriorly and may be inaccessible to the exploring catheter. If the clinical situation warrants further attempts at pericardial decompression, a subxiphoid incision or left anterior thoracotomy can be used to enter the pericardium. This can be done either in the emergency department or in the operating room.

OPEN CHEST RESUSCITATION

One of the basic tenets of vigorous resuscitation in an emergency department is that any case of cardiocirculatory arrest secondary to trauma that does not respond to the usual resuscitative efforts should be treated by open cardiac massage. The immediate reason for the cardiac arrest may not be initially evident. Possible causes include ventricular fibrillation, asystole, pericardial tamponade, hypovolemia, or myocardial contusion. (See Chapters 49 and 50.)

The diagnosis of cardiocirculatory arrest must be made rapidly on clinical grounds alone. The absence of any palpable peripheral pulses or blood pressure is the most important indication of arrest. The extremities may be cool, cyanotic, and mottled; the patient may exhibit apnea or agonal respiratory efforts. If peripheral circulation is ineffective following trauma, there should be no delay in instituting open cardiac resuscitation. It is most critical to establish adequate circulation of oxygenated blood to the brain, heart, and other vital organs with the minimal possible delay. The patient must be intubated and placed on manual or mechanical ventilatory support while—simultaneously—the chest and pericardium are opened through a left thoracotomy and cardiac massage is instituted. Open cardiac massage permits the immediate decompression of any element of pericardial tamponade. In addition, once the pericardium is open, cardiac hemorrhage, if present, can be controlled. Hypovolemia and metabolic acidosis must also be corrected.

The technique for open cardiac massage and resuscitation is similar for virtually all cases of traumatic cardiac arrest, particularly those involving injury to the heart and great vessels. The most expedient technique is to perform an anterior left thoracotomy with an incision extending from the left sternal border in the fourth or fifth intercostal space laterally to the left anterior or midaxillary line (Fig. 54–1). Minimal time should be spent preparing and draping the patient. Once the pericardium is visible and the left pleural space is entered, a rib retractor should be inserted and the incision opened (Fig. 54–1, A). The pericardium should then be opened with a vertical incision, with care to avoid injury to the left phrenic nerve (Fig. 54–1, B). The heart is inspected and an attempt can be made to control any cardiac hemorrhage under direct vision. Immediate control can be accomplished by digital pressure or insertion of a Foley catheter into the wound, followed by partial inflation of the balloon. When the catheter is retracted, the balloon seals the wound.

If the patient is intubated and adequately oxygenated, the red arterial blood should be easily distinguishable from the unoxygenated blood on the right side of the circulation, allowing the physician to locate the source of bleeding. Simultaneously, lactated Ringer's solution must be infused to correct hypovolemia. The obligatory metabolic acidosis must be corrected as well, with rapid IV administration of at least two ampuls (50 mEq each) of sodium bicarbonate. During this time, manual compression of the heart should be carried out at a rate of approximately 70 to 80 compressions/minute, and it should be possible to judge the adequacy of the patient's circulating volume by palpation of the heart. Care must be observed in performing manual cardiac compression. Using either a one- or two-handed technique, the operator must be wary to provide rhythmic compression lasting approximately one second, followed by rapid relaxation. An arrested heart must be handled gently, as the soft myocardium can easily be punctured and disrupted.

Once adequate circulating volume has been restored, further attention should be paid to the cardiac rhythm. In the presence of ventricular fibrillation, 100 mg intracardiac lidocaine should be given and attempts at direct epicardial defibrillation with sterile paddles should be made starting at 60 to 100 watt-seconds direct current. Several repetitions may be required. The longer the period of arrest, the more difficult the defibrillation. If the heart is asystolic, intracardiac calcium chloride (1 gm) and epinephrine (3 to 5 ml 1:10,000 solution) should be used to attempt to convert the rhythm to ventricular fibrillation.[1] Extreme care must be taken to maintain rhythmic cardiac compressions and thus prevent distention of the heart. Even a short period of left ventricular distention can result in a heart that is refractory to any further resuscitative effort.

One additional maneuver that may temporarily provide more effective circulation to the heart and brain

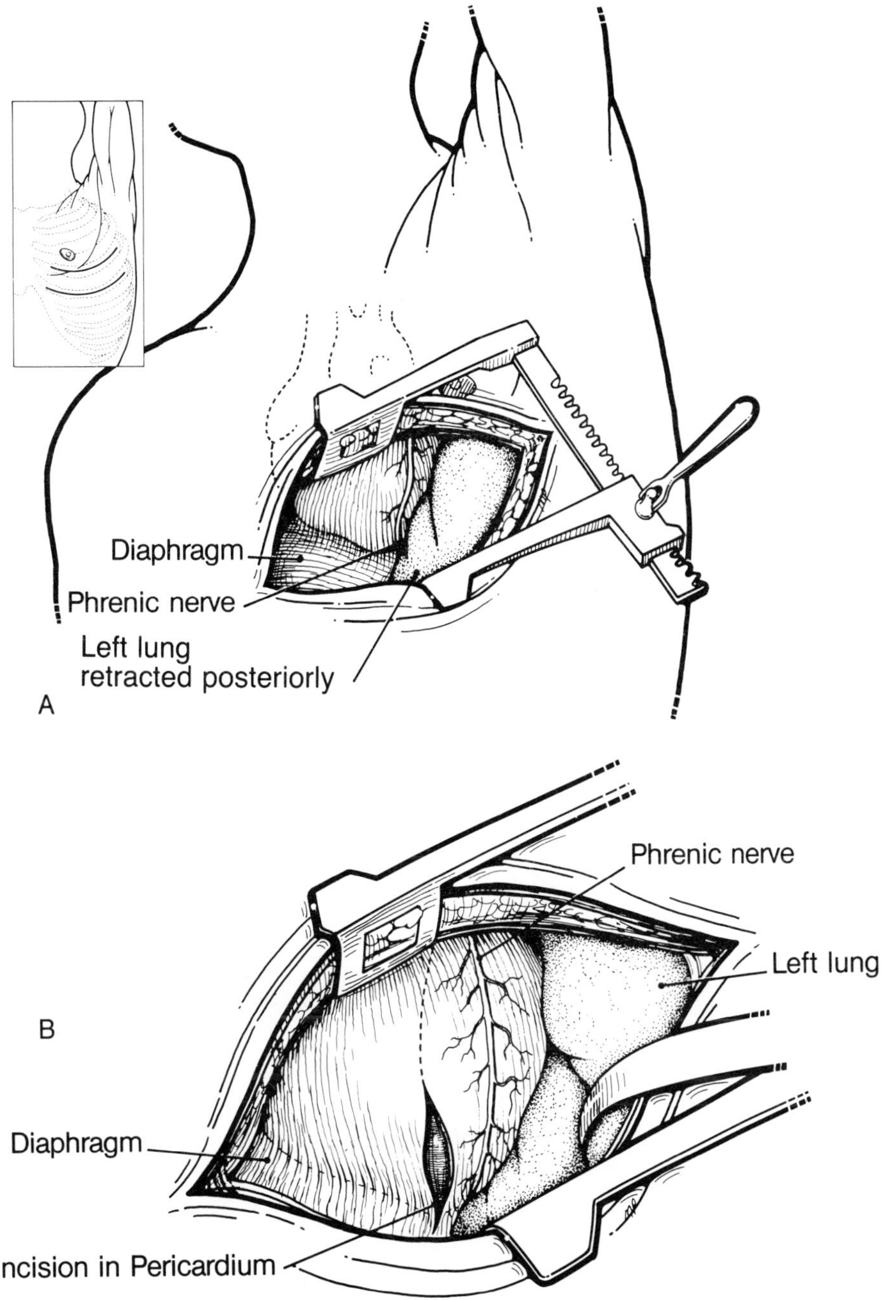

Figure 54–1   *A.* Position and Anatomic Landmarks for Emergency Left Thoracotomy. *B.* Appropriate Placement of Pericardial Incision through a Left Thoracotomy. Note: This provides pericardial decompression and wide exposure of the heart.

involves intermittent occlusion of the descending thoracic aorta. This maneuver is most readily accomplished by manual compression or occlusion of the descending aorta with the left lung retracted anteromedially.

In a situation of marked hypovolemia with a flaccid, nonpulsatile aorta that is difficult to recognize, the vertebral bodies are the best palpable landmark; the descending thoracic aorta lies immediately adjacent and lateral to the bony vertebral column. The aorta may be isolated by blunt digital dissection. A vascular clamp can be placed across the aorta once it is encircled with the operator's left index finger. Coupled with manual cardiac massage, cross-clamping the descending thoracic aorta permits selective perfusion of the coronary and cerebral circulation until the circulating volume is adequate.

If the initial emergency department cardiac resuscitation is successful and effective circulating volume is restored, the patient should be taken to the operating room for thorough irrigation, debridement, and sterile closure of the thoracotomy incision. Definitive operative repair of any cardiac lacerations should be performed at this time. The pericardiotomy should be loosely approximated to prevent cardiac herniation through the pericardium into the left hemithorax. This portion of the patient's care should be performed by an experienced cardiothoracic surgeon.

SPECIFIC CARDIAC INJURIES

Myocardial Contusion

It is said that myocardial contusion is the most underdiagnosed injury sustained by patients subjected to multiple blunt trauma. The injury can easily be missed unless the clinician's index of suspicion is high. (See Chapter 61.) In otherwise healthy patients, the sequelae of the injury are generally well tolerated, and the usual clinical criteria may not be evident on physical examination. Direct myocardial contusion is most commonly secondary to sternal or anterior thoracic compression.[2] The injury can be thought of as a localized myocardial infarction in terms of its pathologic appearance and pathophysiologic sequelae. (See Chapter 49.) The actual tissue damage can be confined to a partial thickness, e.g., subepicardial or subendocardial, or it may be transmural in extent.[3]

Clinical Correlates

The most common clinical sequela of a myocardial contusion is a supraventricular or ventricular arrhythmia, depending on the area of the heart injured. Just as it is in a myocardial infarction, the tendency toward cardiac arrhythmia in a myocardial contusion is exacerbated by concomitant hypoxia, hypercapnia, acidosis, or electrolyte imbalance. The next most common early clinical consequence of myocardial contusion is primary pump failure, which may or may not be associated with concomitant arrhythmias; the degree of failure depends on the amount of tissue damage. Reduced cardiac output has been shown to be a common physiologic consequence of myocardial contusion, although the reduction in overall cardiac function is most often subclinical.[4]

In a multiply injured patient, the clinical picture of myocardial contusion may be obscured. Its associated signs, symptoms, and sequelae—both immediate and long-term—parallel those of a myocardial infarction secondary to ischemia. Symptoms may include precordial pain, which may be immediate in onset or may be delayed until several hours or days following the injury. The patient may experience palpitations, and the entire symptom complex may be exacerbated by the pain of the direct external injury itself. There may be fracture of the sternum or anterior ribs; external bruising may or may not be evident. The patient usually exhibits tachycardia, but it is uncommon for the patient to have an early pericardial friction rub.[5]

Diagnosis

As in a myocardial infarction, the electrocardiogram (ECG) is perhaps the most specific, although not the most sensitive, way of establishing the diagnosis of myocardial contusion. The actual incidence of electrocardiographic alterations following direct myocardial injury is variable. ECG changes may develop immediately, or they may take several days to develop. They are almost always reversible. The most common alterations observed while the patient is in the emergency department are ST-T wave elevations or depressions. Less common changes are QRS widening, which is indicative of intraventricular conduction defects, or even acute pathologic Q waves, which is indicative of transmural injury. Cardiac arrhythmias, both ventricular and supraventricular, are another common ECG manifestation of myocardial contusion. The origin of the arrhythmia may be helpful in determining the particular site of injury.[1] (See Chapter 50.)

Probably the most sensitive index of myocardial damage presently available is the determination of creatine phosphokinase (CPK) enzyme levels. That portion of CPK specifically indicative of myocardial damage is the MB fraction. When the diagnosis is suspected, blood should be drawn for measurement of total CPK and MB fraction levels. Serial samples should be drawn for approximately four days following the injury.

Therapy

The primary therapy for myocardial contusion involves expectant treatment of the possible complications, namely, life-threatening arrhythmias and/or myocardial pump failure. Continuous ECG monitoring is essential. Any evidence of ventricular arrhythmias should prompt the use of a 100-mg IV lidocaine bolus. The patient should then be started on a continuous lidocaine infusion at 2 to 4 mg/minute. Supraventricular arrhythmias, i.e., rapid atrial fibrillation or paroxysmal supraventricular tachycardia, should be treated with digitalis, even when there is no evidence of hemodynamic compromise secondary to tachyarrhythmia. All patients should have at least one central venous pressure monitoring line. If there is evidence of inadequate peripheral perfusion, it is advisable to have a Swan-Ganz pulmonary artery catheter in place for pressure measurements, as well as for serial cardiac output determinations. Rarely, bradyarrhythmias develop, and any evidence of hemodynamic compromise secondary to slow heart rate should prompt the use of a temporary transvenous endocardial pacemaker when indicated. (See Chapter 50.)

In the absence of any other significant injuries, the patient should be transferred from the emergency department to the intensive care unit for electrocardiographic and hemodynamic monitoring until all evidence of arrhythmias and low cardiac output has disappeared. If, on the other hand, the patient requires immediate surgery, the risk of general anesthesia is superimposed on the hemodynamic instability associated with the acute myocardial contusion. Electrocardiographic and hemodynamic monitoring with an arterial line and a Swan-Ganz pulmonary artery catheter and maintenance of optimal filling pressures are very important adjuncts to successful surgery. Elective procedures should be delayed until the patient's condition is stable, which may take from several days to several weeks.

Pericardial Rupture

Rupture of the pericardium is an uncommon injury and one that is difficult to diagnose. It can occur secondary to blunt abdominal or thoracic trauma and may involve either pleural cavity, although rupture into the left cavity is more common. The pericardium can also rupture through the diaphragmatic pericardial reflection into the peritoneal cavity. Traumatic defects of the pericardium may follow either blunt or penetrating injuries and may be present despite an intact sternum or rib cage. Not infrequently, this compressive trauma of the chest causes pulmonary parenchymal rupture as well, resulting in a pneumothorax and pneumopericardium. If the pericardial tear is of sufficient size, there is a risk of herniation of the heart through the pericardial defect, which reduces venous return and, consequently, cardiac output. The diagnosis is difficult to make both on physical examination and on chest roentgenogram; the only hints are abnormal displacement of the heart to the left and prominence of the left heart border.[6]

If the diaphragmatic portion of the pericardium is ruptured and the heart displaced into the peritoneal cavity, there is less likelihood of hemodynamic compromise and a greater potential for cephalad displacement of bowel and stomach into the pericardial and/or pleural cavities. The major risk associated with this injury is incarceration or strangulation of the abdominal contents at the diaphragmatic pericardial reflection.

Most often, pericardial rupture is part of a multiple trauma constellation and, thus, is commonly missed. In the emergency department, the standard guidelines for open cardiac resuscitation should be followed. If the patient demonstrates markedly low cardiac output following blunt or penetrating trauma, the chest should be opened as discussed previously. This direct exploration permits immediate diagnosis of pericardial rupture.

The treatment of this purely mechanical problem is straightforward. The heart is replaced in an anatomical position, and the pericardial defect is repaired with heavy nonabsorbable suture material to prevent subsequent herniation through it. It is virtually always possible to repair an acute pericardial tear without the use of patch material. This repair should take place in the operating room if at all possible.

Cardiac Lacerations and Hemopericardium

Either blunt or penetrating injuries to the heart may present as hypovolemic shock or as pericardial tamponade. The clinical picture of hypovolemic shock is the most obvious; it results from massive, uncompensated blood loss from the heart or great vessels through a pericardial defect, either externally or into one or both pleural cavities. Often, however, concomitant injuries add to the blood loss. Pericardial tamponade results from the accumulation of blood in the pericardial sac after a cardiac laceration. Because the intact pericardium is an inelastic fibrous membrane, the intrapericardial collection of only 150 to 250 ml blood can markedly reduce cardiac diastolic filling (Fig. 54–2). Rising intrapericardial pressures obstruct venous return, resulting in elevated central venous filling pressures. Inadequate diastolic ventricular filling diminishes ventricular stroke volume and decreases cardiac output despite compensatory tachycardia and peripheral vasoconstriction. Volume infusion and inotropic stimulation is only temporarily effective in supporting cardiac output. The primary problem of hemopericardium must be resolved.

Characteristically, patients with either blunt or penetrating cardiac wounds have rapid, feeble pulses; hypotension; pale, cool extremities; and rapid, panting respiratory efforts. The neck veins may or may not be distended, depending on the circulating blood volume and the presence of cardiac tamponade. The patients may be combative and restless from cerebral hypoxia, or they may be moribund as a result of hypoxia, ethanol intoxication, or associated head trauma. Restlessness and agitation are often mistaken for signs of well-being, when actually they indicate that the patient may be in extremis. The heart sounds may be faint, and there may be auscultatory evidence of a left-to-right shunt, particularly following penetrating trauma. Not uncommonly, associated injuries include hemothorax and/or pneumothorax, which may or may not be under tension.

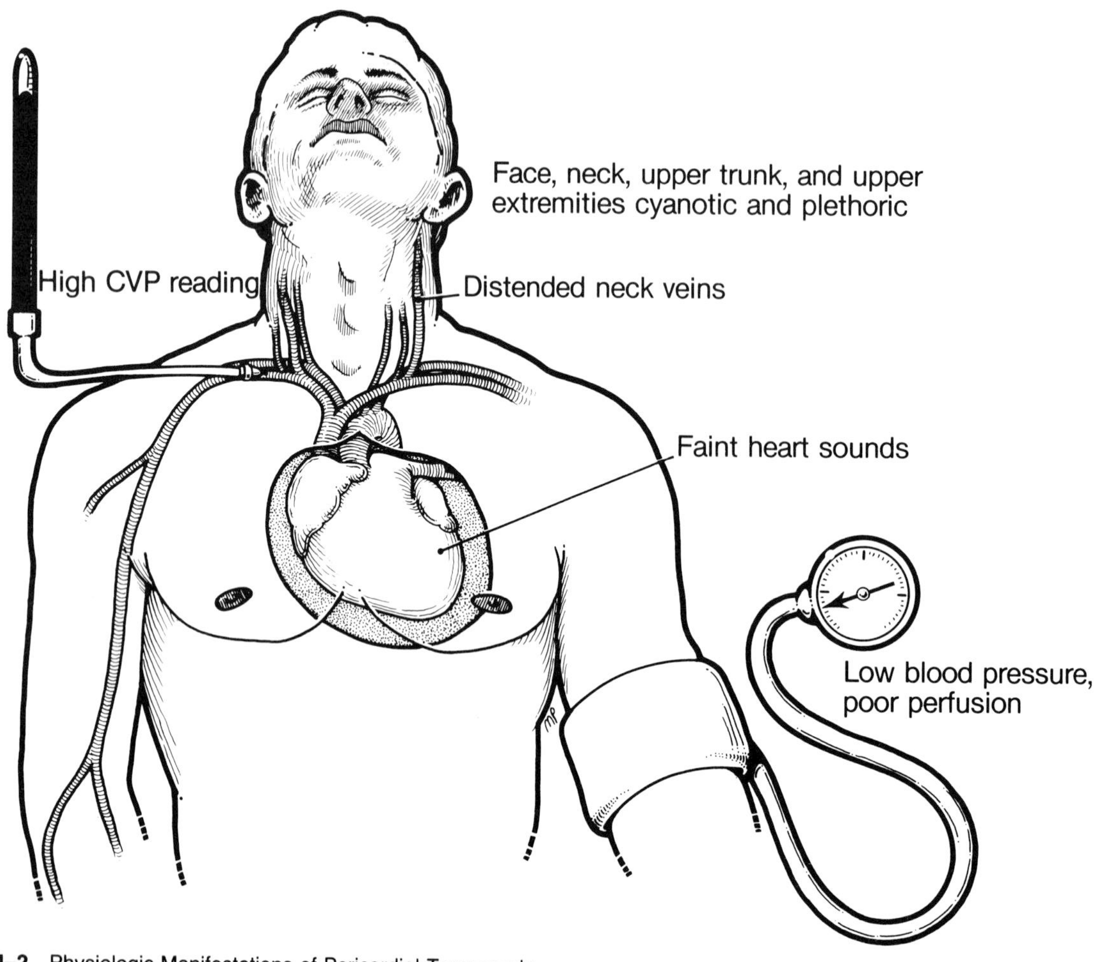

Figure 54–2   Physiologic Manifestations of Pericardial Tamponade.

Pericardial Tamponade

Even when the clinical picture is complete, the diagnosis of acute cardiac tamponade requires a high index of suspicion. If the condition is suspected, immediate pericardiocentesis should be performed via the subxiphoid approach, with the patient either supine or at a 45° angle elevation. A 14-gauge needle through which a 16-gauge catheter can be passed should be introduced at the angle of the xiphoid process just to the left of the midline. The needle should be directed toward the left shoulder. If possible, an indifferent lead of the ECG should be attached to the aspirating needle. S-T segment elevation indicates contact with the heart. Once blood has been withdrawn, the catheter should be passed through the needle, the needle removed, and as much blood as possible aspirated through the catheter. (See Chapter 70.)

Blood in the pericardium is often defibrinated and will not clot. Even if this is true of the aspirated blood, it is not an absolute indication of pericardial blood. In fact, it may be difficult to determine whether or not the needle has penetrated the heart. Several techniques have been used to localize the position of the needle or catheter tip. For example, the intrapericardial pressure can be measured with a water manometer connected to the end of the needle or catheter. If this pressure is less than the central venous pressure, there is probably no significant pericardial tamponade, and the needle is probably not within the heart. If the patient's clinical condition permits and the facilities are available, a small amount (10 ml half-diluted Renograffin 60) of radiopaque contrast material can be injected through the catheter and a chest radiograph taken at the end of the injection.[1] Persistence of the contrast material indicates an intrapericardial location of the catheter. Any contrast material injected into a cardiac chamber will be rapidly cleared and diluted; thus, it will not be apparent on the radiograph.

Successful decompression of a hemodynamically significant tamponade should result in dramatic improvement of the patient's condition. The catheter should be left in place, however, for reaccumulation and clinical deterioration may quickly recur. If this occurs, operative decompression is clearly indicated. If time permits, this should be performed in the operating room, but it can be done by means of a small subxiphoid incision or left anterior thoracotomy in the emergency department.

Penetrating Wounds of the Heart

The relative incidence of penetrating injury to each chamber of the heart roughly corresponds to the proportion of the heart's surface that each chamber comprises, as seen from an anterior plane. As the right ventricle takes up the majority of the surface area in this projection, penetrating injuries of the right ventricle account for approximately two-thirds of the total. Wounds of the right atrium account for approximately 10 to 20 percent; wounds of the left ventricle and left atrium account for approximately 10 percent.

Treatment of penetrating cardiac wounds requires an awareness of several techniques for attaining hemostasis, depending on the specific site of injury. Ventricular wounds of the heart should be controlled initially by thoracotomy and digital pressure on the spurting area, followed by repair with interrupted nonabsorbable horizontal mattress sutures (2-0 or 3-0) as the finger is gradually moved off the laceration (Fig. 54–3). Bleeding from wounds of the atrial chambers is most conveniently controlled by means of a partially occluding curved vascular clamp. Atrial lacerations can be sutured with either interrupted or running sutures. Another convenient technique that can be used to control bleeding in any chamber is the insertion of a sterile Foley catheter into the laceration, subsequent inflation of the balloon, and slight outward traction on the catheter.[1] Suturing is then performed as previously described. If the area of injury is adjacent to a major coronary vessel, care must be taken to place the sutures so that they pass under the vessel so as not to occlude it when the sutures are secured.

It is important to minimize the risk of infection by limiting the use of any prosthetic material in the emergency repair of these injuries. Consequently, patches or bolster materials are avoided unless they are essential for hemostasis. Any clots within the pericardium or pleural cavity must be evacuated, and the cavity must be thoroughly irrigated with sterile saline to allow adequate visualization and full exploration. Care must be taken in the handling of this delicate and friable tissue, as unnecessary force in the performance of these maneuvers exacerbates the injury.

In cases of massive hemorrhage, several autotransfusion devices are available, and experience has shown

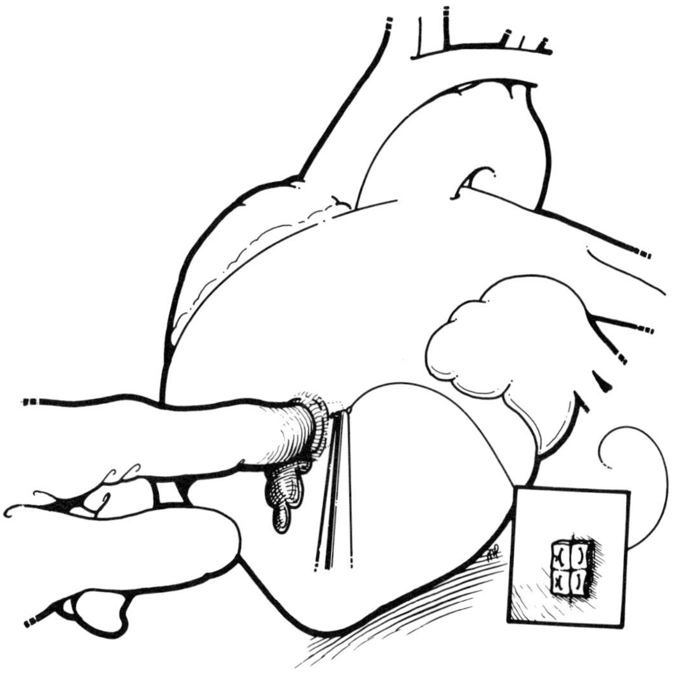

Figure 54–3 Primary Suture Repair of Cardiac Laceration.

them to be of value in selected situations. In general, the simplest systems have proved to be the most efficacious. Nearly all patients with signs of hemodynamic collapse after a blunt or penetrating injury to the heart and great vessels benefit from open cardiac resuscitation and a full attempt at repair of the significant injuries. After hemostasis has been attained and the heart resuscitated both electrically and mechanically, the patient should be transferred to a formal operating room for definitive repair of the wound and sterile closure of the incision.

Long-Term Sequelae

Wound infections are surprisingly uncommon in emergency thoracotomy and cardiac exploration. However, care must be taken during the wound closure to perform thorough irrigation and sterile closure. Any devitalized tissue should be debrided. One common postoperative finding is pericarditis, as manifested by a pericardial friction rub, serial ECG changes, and symptomatic precordial pain. Penetrating cardiac injuries can result in a wide variety of intracardiac injuries, such as ventricular septal defects, papillary muscle damage, valvular injuries, and bullet emboli. These intracardiac injuries are not often diagnosed accurately during the initial examination in the emergency department. These intracardiac injuries are usually discovered at a later date, following successful initial therapy. Subsequent surgical correction, if necessary, is performed on an elective basis.[7]

AORTIC INJURIES

Pathophysiology

Traumatic rupture of the aorta has been recognized as an increasingly common injury within the last two decades. It is clearly associated with the increase in the number of high-speed automotive deceleration injuries, since it has been estimated that 10 to 15 percent of patients who die from motor vehicle accidents sustain aortic rupture. The injury itself is very often associated with other potentially lethal conditions, such as ruptured abdominal viscus, closed head injury, pelvic or extremity fractures, or other fatal cardiopulmonary injuries.[8]

Although several mechanisms of injury have been proposed, horizontal acute deceleration that creates sheer stress between the relatively immobile attachments of the aortic arch and the more mobile descending thoracic aorta seems to be the mechanical explanation that corresponds best with the observed anatomical locations of aortic ruptures. The most common site of injury is at the ligamentum arteriosum, which is the point of maximum aortic fixation to the posterior mediastinum. Other mechanisms of injury to the thoracic aorta include severe thoracic compression and vertical deceleration.[1]

The majority of patients who survive to reach the emergency department have an aortic laceration just distal to the left subclavian artery in the area of the ligamentum arteriosum. These patients actually represent a selected population, however, because patients with aortic ruptures commonly have other, fatal injuries as well and do not survive long enough to reach the emergency department. Pathologically, the injury is usually a linear transverse (Fig. 54–4) or spiral laceration extending either partially or circumferentially around the thoracic aorta. The laceration usually extends through the intima and media of the aortic wall so that only the adventitia, parietal pleura, and surrounding mediastinal tissues remain intact to contain the aortic blood pressure. Once this thin outer layer ruptures, the patient immediately exsanguinates. Preexisting aortic pathology, such as atheroma formation, does not predispose the aorta to this injury.[9,10] In fact, the greatest incidence is among those who are 20 to 30 years old, and the injury occurs much more commonly in men than in women (approximately 10:1).

In a classic study by Parmley et al.,[11] of patients with isolated aortic rupture, approximately 20 percent survived to reach an emergency department. Those patients who sustained a traumatic aortic rupture but were fortunate enough to have the thin-walled adventitia remain intact then formed a false aneurysm. The subsequent natural history of this thin-walled and tenuous aneurysm overlying the aortic rupture was somewhat unpredictable. Of the initial 20 percent of patients who survived at least 1 hour, 30 percent died within 6 hours of injury, 40 percent died within 24 hours, and a total of 72 percent of the original surviving 20 percent died within eight days.

Because up to one-half of the patients sustaining aortic rupture have no external evidence of thoracic injury, the cornerstone of successful therapy with this injury is a high index of suspicion. For this reason, one of the keys to successful diagnosis is the evaluation of the nature of the traumatic event. If an acceleration-deceleration mechanism can be implicated in the injury, careful consideration must be given to the diagnosis even in the absence of any signs or symptoms. Depending on associated injuries, the patients may complain of substernal or interscapular pain, dyspnea, hoarseness, or dysphagia.[8] (See also Chapter 61.)

Diagnosis

Although a variety of clinical signs have been ascribed to aortic injury, taken either individually or together, they remain both insensitive and nonspecific. Upper extremity hypertension may be found in 30 to 40 percent of patients and may be due to partial compression of the aortic lumen by periaortic hematoma or by a partial one-way valve flap mechanism that can result in distal propagation of a periaortic dissection (quite rare).

A bloody left pleural effusion, if a consequence of an aortic laceration, is an ominous sign of impending rupture. Hematoma or ecchymosis at the base of the neck can have many causes, including extension of hematoma from an aortic tear.

The chest roentgenogram should be used as an important adjunct in the evaluation of this lesion. Classically, the most common findings associated with aortic injury are a widened superior mediastinum, obscuration of the aortic knob, and a left pleural cap above the left lung (Fig. 54–5). Among the other roentgenographic signs that may be seen are a left pleural effusion, left first rib fracture, deviation of the trachea to the right, and depression of the left main stem bronchus.[1] Although suggestive, none of these roentgenographic findings are truly diagnostic; they may be due to mediastinal bleeding from other causes or may not be associated with mediastinal hemorrhage at all. Supine anteroposterior portable chest roentgenograms are

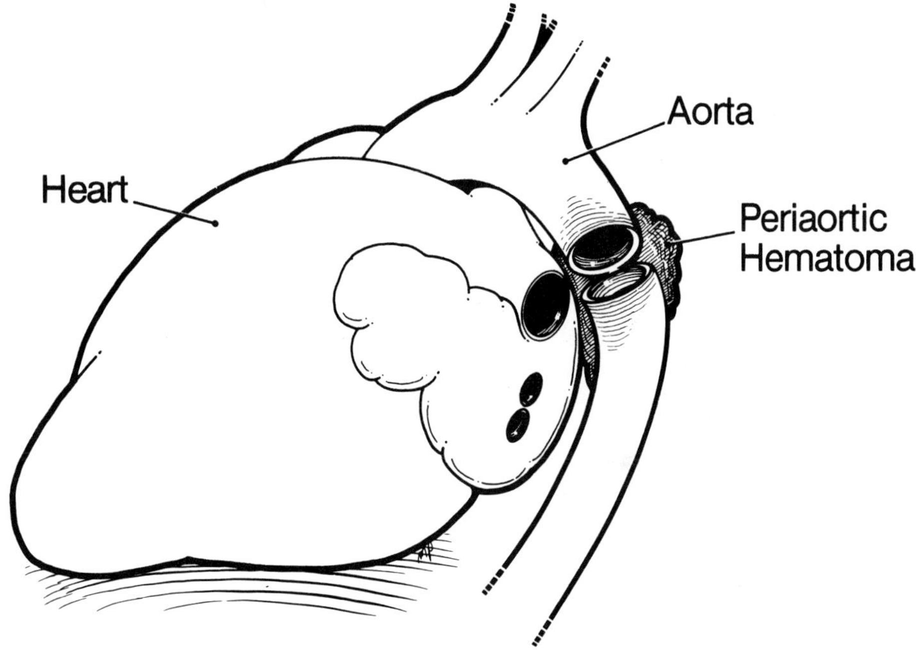

Figure 54–4   Schematic Representation of Location and Appearance of Traumatic Aortic Laceration.

notorious for accentuating the mediastinal silhouette; if the patient's condition permits, a standard, erect posteroanterior and lateral roentgenogram should be obtained. However, traumatic aortic rupture has been found in patients with normal chest roentgenograms. At this point, the emergency department physician must critically consider the nature of the accident and the possibility of traumatic aortic injury.

Aortography

The definitive diagnostic test with regard to aortic trauma is aortography, although computerize axial tomography is becoming an important diagnostic tool. The indications for aortography are consequently very liberal. It should generally be performed on any patient who has sustained a significant acceleration-deceleration injury, even when there are no external clinical signs or definitive radiologic evidence of mediastinal hematoma. Aortography carries a very low risk, and it can be done through either a transaxillary or a transfemoral approach. The general purpose is to rule out a suspected aortic rupture. The physician should be prepared to continue even after many study results have been negative rather than risk omitting a study that would be helpful. Accurate diagnosis and anatomical localization of the site of injury is of importance in the surgical approach. The vast majority of injuries involve either a partial or complete separation of the intima and media of the descending thoracic aorta that occurs within several centimeters of the origin of the left sub-

clavian artery. The intimal flap can often be identified, as can the false aneurysm and periaortic hematoma in the region of the laceration. There may or may not be demonstrable extravasation of contrast material (Fig. 54–6).

The presence of this injury is an indication for immediate left thoracotomy and surgical repair. Although traumatic rupture of the aorta is often an isolated event, consideration must be given to the order of priorities when it is associated with other life-threatening situations. Most commonly, decompression of closed head injuries, stabilization of cervical spine or thoracic spine fractures, the consideration of intra-abdominal bleeding, and care of fractures of the pelvis or long bones take precedence.

Treatment

Surgical repair of aortic injury entails performing a left posterior lateral thoracotomy, attaining proximal and distal aortic control, and opening the mediastinal hematoma after proximal and distal cross-clamping. The injury can often be repaired primarily by debriding the edges of the aorta and performing an end-to-end anastomosis. Occasionally, because of the wide separation of the proximal and distal ends of the transected aorta, it is necessary to insert a tubular length of dacron graft material.

Perhaps the most important technical point of this procedure is how best to protect the distal aortic per-

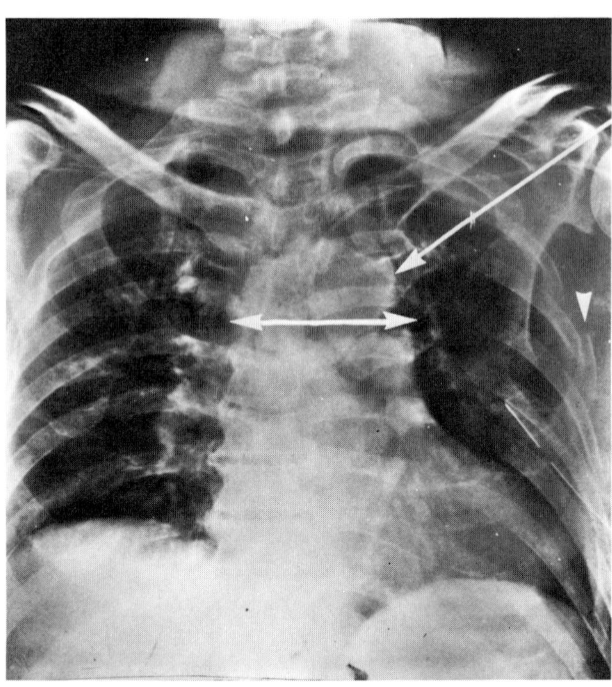

Figure 54–5 Chest Radiograph of Patient with an Aortic Transection. *Note:* Shows a widened mediastinum, obscuration of the aortic knob, and fractured ribs.

fusion while the aorta is cross-clamped. The cardiothoracic surgeon has several options, including the simple method of clamping and repairing without providing any adjuvant protection. One option is to use a partial femoral arterial bypass to allow perfusion of the body distal to the cross-clamp while the heart perfuses the

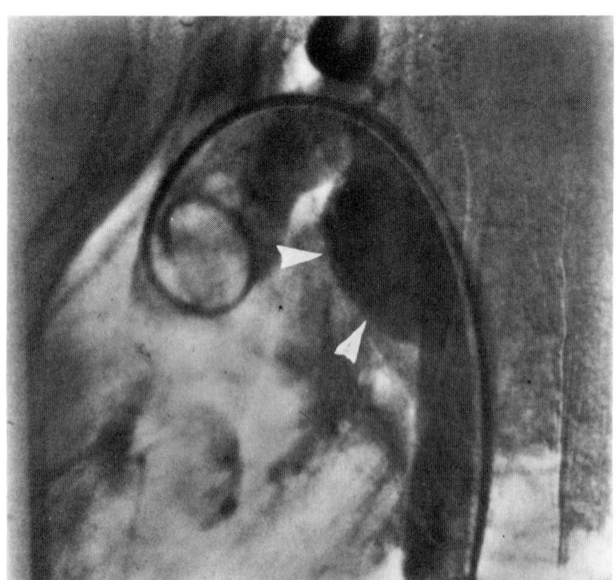

Figure 54–6 Lateral View of Thoracic Aortogram. *Note:* Illustrates the extraluminal periaortic hematoma.

upper body. Another possibility is to insert an external bypass shunt, which is most conveniently placed in the ascending aorta proximally and in either the descending thoracic aorta distal to the area of repair or in the left femoral artery.

The most significant complication following this surgery is postoperative paraplegia. Because of the vagaries of origin of the aortic contribution to the anterior spinal artery and our inability to detect the critical connections accurately, we are unable to determine which level is the critical one in a given patient for spinal arterial perfusion. There is considerable debate among cardiovascular surgeons as to which method minimizes distal ischemia.[12,13]

ACUTE AORTIC DISSECTIONS

Pathophysiology

Acute aortic dissections are one of the most common, as well as the most lethal, nontraumatic disorders involving the heart or great vessels. Although the exact pathogenesis of aortic dissections is not completely known, the basic underlying pathophysiology is an intimal tear with propagation of a dissecting hematoma for variable lengths along the aorta. The lesion is not rare; it has been estimated that the incidence is 10 to 20 cases per million population per year in the United States.[14] The intimal tear may arise anywhere along the thoracic aorta. Perhaps the most rational classification defines basically two types of aortic dissections. If the ascending aorta is involved, despite the site of primary intimal tear, the dissection is termed type A. If the descending thoracic aorta is involved to the exclusion of the ascending aorta, this is classified as type B. Type B dissections usually start in the proximal descending thoracic aorta just beyond the origin of the left subclavian artery.

To a large extent, the clinical picture and subsequent sequelae of the dissection are predicated upon the site of origin and the extent of distal propagation. When the ascending aorta is involved, the primary morbidity and mortality is caused by rupture of the dissection into the pericardium, resulting in tamponade, free rupture into the pleural cavities or mediastinum, extension of the dissection into the coronary arteries (causing occlusion), or severe aortic regurgitation. In addition, cerebral and upper extremity ischemia may result from occlusion of the arch vessels. When the descending thoracic aorta is involved, any of the branches of the descending thoracic or abdominal aorta may be occluded by the dissecting hematoma, which could result in mesenteric or bowel infarction, paraplegia, renal infarction, or free rupture.[15]

Diagnosis and Treatment

The signs and symptoms of aortic dissections are extremely variable,[16] and are usually accompanied by an excruciating, sharp, tearing pain that may be localized to either the precordium or the posterior chest and back, with extension of the pain into the abdomen, lower back, legs, or neck. The pain is almost always of sudden onset and is described as severe. The usual differential diagnosis includes myocardial infarction, pulmonary embolism, arterial occlusion, or an acute abdomen. Subsequent signs and symptoms are dependent on the specific branch vessels affected. The patients often have a history of hypertension and may well be hypertensive at the time of their initial examination. It is essential to maintain a high index of suspicion; the combination of the acute onset of severe back or chest pain in a hypertensive patient with any suggestion of pulse deficit or pressure differential in either the upper or lower extremities heralds the diagnosis of an acute aortic dissection until proved otherwise.

Control of the patient's blood pressure is of critical importance. (See Chapter 52.) A continuous IV drip of sodium nitroprusside 50 mg/250 ml D_5W is one choice of therapy. Patients should have several IV lines in place, including a central venous pressure monitoring line as well as a radial arterial line, for continuous monitoring. IV propranolol (Inderal) in 1-mg increments should also be administered as necessary to maintain a mean arterial pressure of approximately 80 mm Hg.

Aortography should be performed as soon as possible if the diagnosis of aortic dissection is being considered. Aortography is currently the best means to determine the site of intimal tear and the extent of propagation of the dissection. Once the site and extent of the aortic dissection has been demonstrated, the subsequent management can be planned. Patients with type A dissections are virtually always candidates for emergency surgical repair. However, patients with type B dissections, although usually considered for emergency surgery, may best be treated medically, e.g., with antihypertensive therapy, depending on the specific patient variables.

REFERENCES

1. Kirsh MM, Sloan H: *Blunt Chest Trauma: General Principles of Management*, ed. 1. Boston, Little, Brown & Co, 1977, pp 143–212.
2. Liedke AJ, Demuth W: Nonpenetrating cardiac injuries: A collective review. *Am Heart J* 86:687–697, 1973.
3. Jones J, Hewitt R, Drapanas T: Cardiac contusion: A capricious syndrome. *Ann Surg* 181:567–574, 1975.
4. Pomerantz M, Delgado F, Eisman B: Unsuspected depressed cardiac output following blunt thoracic and abdominal trauma. *Surgery* 70:865–870, 1971.
5. Levitsky S: New insights in cardiac trauma. *Surg Clin North Am* 55:43–55, 1975.
6. Mattila S, Silvola H, Ketonen P: Traumatic rupture of the pericardium with luxation of the heart, case report and review of the literature. *J Thorac Cardiovasc Surg* 70:495–498, 1975.
7. Symbas P, DiOrio D, Tyras D, et al: Penetrating cardiac wounds: Significant residual and delayed sequelae. *J Thorac Cardiovasc Surg* 66:526–532, 1973.
8. Borrie J: *Management of Thoracic Emergencies*, ed 3. New York, Appleton-Century Crofts, 1980, pp 456–476.
9. Reul GJ, Rubio PA, Beall AC: The surgical management of acute injury to the thoracic aorta. *J Thorac Cardiovasc Surg* 67:272–281, 1974.
10. Turney S, Attar S, Ayalla R, et al: Traumatic rupture of the aorta: A five-year experience. *J Thorac Cardiovasc Surg* 72:727–734, 1976.
11. Parmley L, Mattingly TW, Manion WC, et al: Nonpenetrating traumatic injury of the aorta. *Circulation* 17:1086–1091, 1958.
12. Applebaum A, Karp R, Kirklin J: Surgical treatment for closed thoracic aortic injuries. *J Thorac Cardiovasc Surg* 71:458–460, 1976.
13. Crawford E, Rubio P: Reappraisal of adjuncts to avoid ischemia in the treatment of aneurysms of the descending thoracic aorta. *J Thorac Cardiovasc Surg* 66:693–704, 1973.
14. Pate JW, Richardson RL, Eastridge CE: Acute aortic dissections. *Am Surg* 42:395–404, 1976.
15. Daily PO, Trueblood HW, Stinson EB, et al: Management of acute aortic dissections. *Ann Thorac Surg* 10:237–247, 1970.
16. Slater EE, DeSanctis RW: The clinical recognition of dissecting aortic aneurysm. *Am J Med* 60:625–633, 1976.

55. Cardiopulmonary Resuscitation

THOMAS CLARKE KRAVIS, M.D.

In 1983, approximately 1.5 million people will sustain a myocardial infarction. A large percentage of these patients will die, and half will succumb precipitously within two hours after the onset of symptoms before they can receive care in a hospital. Widespread standardized cardiopulmonary resuscitation (CPR) techniques and sophisticated paramedic treatment and transport systems have been developed with the purpose of preventing these prehospital deaths.

A number of factors alter the possibility of survival of patients following out-of-hospital cardiopulmonary arrest:[1,2]

- the underlying state of the myocardium
- recognition of the early signs of myocardial ischemia
- response time of prehospital care personnel
- the interval from cardiovascular collapse to initiation of CPR and definitive intervention (defibrillation, intubation, medication)
- the level of training of the prehospital care personnel
- initiation of CPR by a lay bystander
- patient age
- type of cardiac rhythms responsible for arrest
- blood pressure at the time of collapse
- the level of sophistication of in-hospital cardiac care

Cardiopulmonary arrest is defined as the sudden collapse of an individual with circulatory arrest and apnea. Sudden death usually refers to those patients who die within one hour of the onset of symptoms. Basic life support is that phase of emergency cardiac care in which the circulation and respirations of a victim of cardiopulmonary arrest are externally supported through CPR. Although CPR is not definitive therapy, it increases the amount of time the body can tolerate a lethal arrhythmia without suffering irreversible organ damage before advanced life support is available.[3] Some have expanded CPR to include cardiopulmonary-cerebral resuscitation (CPCR) because maximum cerebral blood flow is one of the major objectives of CPR, and arrest periods longer than four minutes are associated with postarrest encephalopathy and low survival rate.[1,4] Successful CPR should return a victim of cardiac arrest to a status similar to that preceding the arrest.[5] The technique of CPR may be modified according to the age of the patient, the mechanism of the arrest, whether it was witnessed or unwitnessed, and the number of rescuers.

Advanced cardiac life support includes basic life support plus the use of adjunct techniques and equipment, such as intravenous lines, pharmacologic agents, electrocardiogram (ECG) monitoring, and electrical defibrillation.

Other therapeutic tools available to resuscitate a patient include artificial airway maintenance and ventilation, the application of MAST trousers, pericardiocentesis, placement of central venous pressure lines, pacemaker insertion, open chest cardiac massage, and intra-aortic balloon-pump assistance.[6]

The author is indebted to Regina Atcheson, M.D., for her assistance with the development of this chapter.

STEPS OF CPR

When an individual suffers a cardiopulmonary arrest, the following six steps should be started immediately:

1. Establish unresponsiveness.
2. Obtain assistance if available, and activate the emergency medical service (EMS) system.
3. Place the patient in the proper position.
4. Establish an airway.
   a. Open the airway.
   b. Establish breathlessness (look, listen, feel).
5. Provide positive pressure mouth-to-mouth breathing (rule out foreign body airway obstruction).
6. Ensure circulation.
   a. Establish presence or absence of pulse.
   b. Begin chest compression if the patient has no pulse.

The only exception to this basic procedure occurs when a monitored patient develops ventricular fibrillation. For this patient, electrical countershock defibrillation (followed by other advanced life support measures if available) is the immediate first treatment of choice.[6]

1.   Establish Unresponsiveness.

The first step to be taken when a person has suddenly collapsed or is found unconscious is to determine whether in fact the patient has had a cardiopulmonary arrest. Other causes of apparent unresponsiveness include upper airway obstruction, trauma to the head and neck, poisonings and drug overdose, drowning, respiratory failure, sepsis, and hypovolemia. Any of these processes may subsequently *result* in cardiopulmonary arrest and each should be borne in mind when examining the unresponsive patient, since the management of such patients may require special treatment in addition to CPR. For example, in patients with cardiopulmonary arrest in association with head and neck injuries, airway management must be instituted with great care, since injury to the spinal cord and subsequent paralysis may be caused by manipulation of the neck. Cardiopulmonary arrest as a consequence of opiate overdose may require CPR, but intravenous antagonists, e.g., naloxone hydrochloride (Narcan), are required to treat the reversible underlying process. Finally, some causes of upper airway obstruction can be treated immediately; for example, a foreign body can be removed.

In the out-of-hospital setting, the first step in managing a patient who is unresponsive is to firmly but gently shake and shout at the patient. In order to determine the adequacy of respiratory motion, the rescuer should remove any clothing over the patient's chest, and place a cheek close to the patient's nose and mouth to feel the patient's exhalations, if present. Retraction of soft tissues in the suprasternal notch or intercostal spaces suggests airway obstruction. If the patient is unresponsive, then an airway should be immediately established, since complete obstruction of the airway for longer than four to six minutes will usually cause death.

2.   Obtain Assistance If Available.

If two rescuers are present, one person should be sent to activate the EMS system. The shorter the time between collapse and initiation of CPR and advanced cardiac life support, the more likely is the survival of the cardiac arrest victim.

3.   Place the Patient in the Proper Position.

CPR should usually be performed at the site where the victim was found, with the victim placed in a supine position. In the emergency department or hospital bed, a firm support that extends from the shoulder to the waist should be provided underneath the patient's back. Spine boards utilized by prehospital care personnel are sufficient. Elevation of the lower extremities may promote venous return and augment artificial maintenance of circulation.[6]

4.   Establish an Airway.

The tongue commonly causes airway obstruction in the unconscious victim. It may also act as an obstructing valve during inspiration. In the presence of normal muscle tone, tilting the head back often adequately opens the airway. In the absence of sufficient muscle tone, it is necessary to move the jaw forward as well, which lifts the tongue away from the posterior aspect of the throat.

Once the airway has been established, the rescuer can watch the chest and abdomen while placing an ear near the victim's nose and mouth to *look* for spontaneous rise or fall of the chest wall, *listen* for escape of air during exhalation, and *feel* the flow of air on the cheek.

Head Tilt

The first step in opening the airway is the head tilt, which can be augmented by either the chin lift or neck lift. One of the rescuer's hands is placed underneath the victim's neck; the other hand is placed on the patient's forehead (Fig. 55–1). The neck is lifted with one hand while the other hand tilts the head gently back-

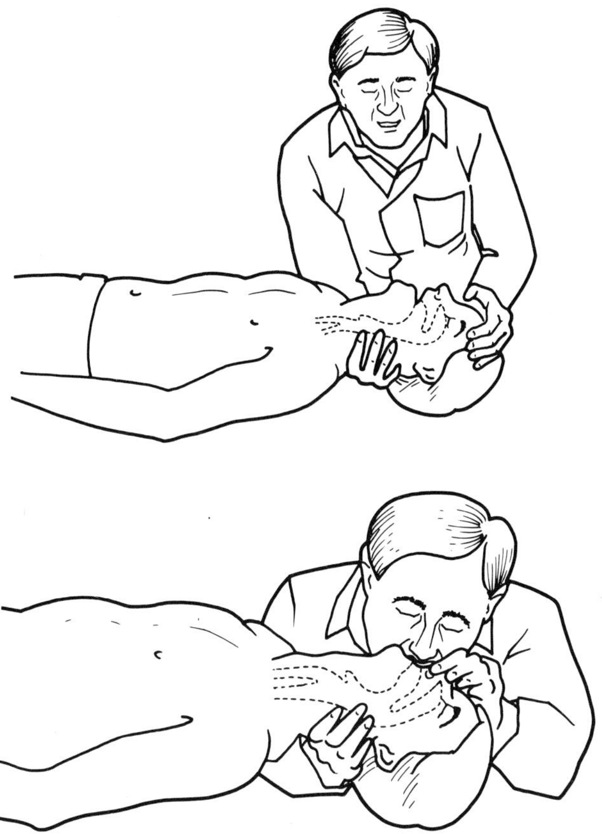

Figure 55–1 Cardiopulmonary Resuscitation Method 1, Head Tilt-Neck Lift.

---

ward with slight pressure on the forehead. Elevating the patient's shoulders may help in tilting the head. These maneuvers may open the patient's mouth so that spontaneous ventilations are observed. If not, positive airway pressure by mouth to mouth (or stoma) may be accomplished. In some patients, however, additional manipulations to displace the mandible forward are required.[6]

Head Tilt-Neck Lift

The rescuer tilts the head by placing one hand on the victim's forehead and applying firm, gentle, backward pressure. This tips the victim's head backward naturally. The rescuer places the other hand beneath the neck, supporting the neck and moving it upward. The hand lifting the neck should be positioned close to the back of the head in order to minimize cervical spine extension and the risk of spinal cord injury in patients with head or neck trauma. If this maneuver does not open the patient's mouth so that adequate spontaneous ventilation is achieved, then positive airway pressure by mouth to mouth may be accomplished from this position. In some patients, however, it is also necessary to displace the mandible forward by chin lift.

Head Tilt-Chin Lift

In combination with head tilt, the chin lift is a highly effective maneuver in opening the airway. It may be effective in some persons in whom the head tilt-neck lift has not been successful (Fig. 55–2). In this maneuver, the rescuer lifts the victim's chin by taking the hand that had been used to lift the neck and placing the tips of the fingers of that hand under the lower jaw, or the bony part of the chin, and lifting the chin forward while supporting the jaw. The fingers should not compress the soft tissues under the chin. The rescuer's other hand continues to press firmly on the victim's forehead in order to tilt the head back. The chin is lifted so that the teeth are merely brought together, but the mouth is not closed completely. Rarely, the rescuer's thumb is required to depress the lower lip slightly in order to keep the mouth open.

Jaw Thrust with Head Tilt

If further displacement of the jaw forward is required, the jaw thrust with head tilt can be accomplished. The rescuer places the hands at the side of the victim's head, grasping the angles of the victim's lower jaw and lifting

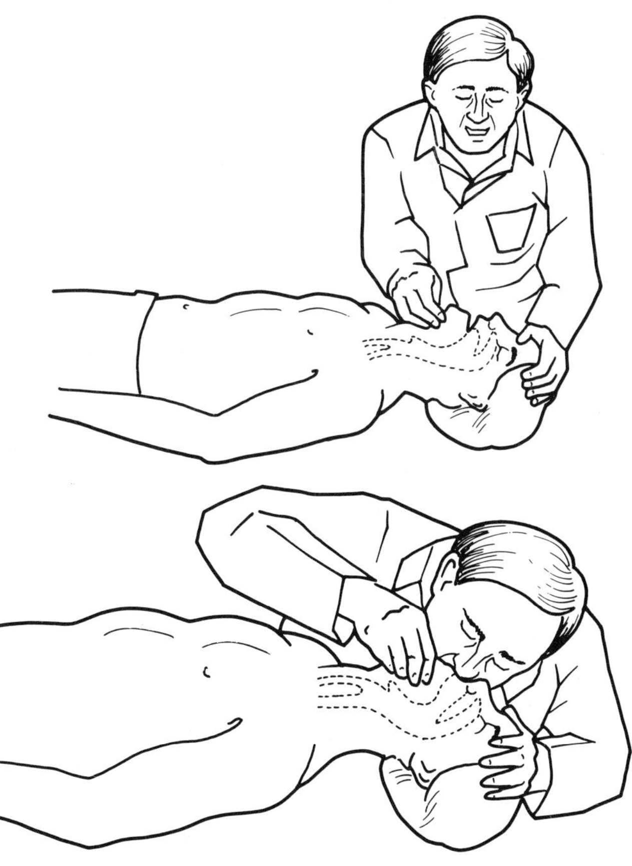

Figure 55–2 Cardiopulmonary Resuscitation Method 2, Head Tilt-Chin Lift.

with both hands, displacing the mandible forward by tilting the head backward. The rescuer's elbows rest on the surface on which the victim is lying. The lower lip can be retracted with the rescuer's thumb.

Modified Jaw Thrust without Head Tilt

In patients with a suspected neck injury, a modified jaw thrust without head tilt should be utilized. The rescuer places one hand on each side of the victim's head, maintaining the head in a neutral position (no backward tilt). The rescuer's fingers are placed behind the angles of the jaw to displace the mandible forward. The rescuer's thumb may be utilized if necessary to retract the lower lip. The head is then carefully supported. The rescuer's index fingers are used to displace the mandible forward without tilting the head back or turning it to one side.

These maneuvers should be successful in lifting the tongue off of the posterior pharynx, where it may cause obstruction in cases where there is a loss of pharyngeal muscle tone and control of the tongue.

5. Provide Positive Pressure Breathing.

Once the victim's mouth has been opened, the airway established, and the head tilted back, the rescuer gently pinches the patient's nostrils with the thumb and index fingers, making an airtight seal (Fig. 55–1 and Fig. 55–2). After taking a deep breath, the rescuer places an open mouth widely around the outside of the victim's mouth to make a seal and forcibly exhales the air into the patient's mouth. The volume exhaled should be approximately twice the normal resting adult tidal volume (1,000 to 1,500 ml). Four ventilations are delivered in rapid succession without allowing passive exhalation from the victim's lungs. The rescuer *looks* at the victim's chest to determine if it falls during exhalation, *feels* the resistance to flow in the victim's lungs as they inflate, and *listens* to the sound of air escaping from the victim's airways with lung deflation.

In instances of severe maxillofacial trauma, mouth-to-nose ventilation may be more effective. The rescuer keeps the victim's head tilted back with one hand; with the other hand, the rescuer lifts the victim's lower jaw and closes the mouth. The same steps of "look, feel, and listen" are followed, although it may be necessary to open the victim's mouth to allow the air to escape during exhalation because of nasopharyngeal obstruction caused by a soft palate. Finally, mouth-to-stoma ventilation may be indicated in patients with a laryngectomy. The rescuer's hand or a tightly fitting mask (placed around the stoma) may be required for patients with a temporary tracheostomy tube in the airway.

If the chest does *not* fall, upper airway obstruction should be suspected and appropriate management initiated. (See Chapter 57.) If the chest does fall during exhalation, then cycles of positive pressure ventilation should be initiated. Two quick full breaths (without allowing time for lung deflation between breaths) are delivered after each cycle of five chest compressions for a single rescuer CPR. Mouth-to-nose, stoma, or tracheostomy tube ventilation follows these same principles. Oxygen enrichment and other adjuncts to airway management are instituted as soon as possible.[6]

6. Ensure Circulation.

In addition to airway maintenance and positive pressure ventilation, forward flow of blood and tissue perfusion by oxygenated blood is required for effective resuscitation. If the chest rises and falls in response to positive pressure ventilation, the rescuer then seeks a pulse in the unresponsive patient by gently palpating with two fingers the carotid (or femoral) pulse on the same side as the rescuer. Although the palpation of a pulse is not a reliable method of assessing blood flow or mean blood pressure,[7] the absence of a pulse suggests cardiac arrest.

It is theoretically possible to generate forward blood flow during CPR by two distinct mechanisms: the cardiac pump mechanism and the thoracic pump mechanism.[8] The predominant mechanism of flow in a given victim probably depends on a number of factors, e.g., the ventral/dorsal chest diameter, the presence of cardiomegaly, the compliance of the chest wall and lung, whether ventilations are applied simultaneously or intermittently with chest compressions, and at what lung volume and pressures the ventilations are applied.

External Chest Compression

Cardiac Pump Mechanism. Forward blood flow simulating artificial systole can be accomplished from external compression of the chest either manually or mechanically. A traditional view is that, during CPR, the compression of the victim's heart between the sternum and the vertebral spine causes a pressure gradient that forces blood from the heart to the peripheral circulation. This cardiac pump mechanism theory of forward flow suggests that cardiac compression generates a higher pressure in the ventricle than elsewhere in the thorax. With chest compression, the mitral and tricuspid valves close while the aortic and pulmonic valves open, blood is ejected into the great arteries, and a positive arterial-venous pressure difference is generated in the thorax. Upon release of pressure on the sternum, intracardiac pressure falls, the mitral and tricuspid valves open, and the heart fills from the systemic and pulmonary venous reservoirs. The airways vent the thorax during chest compression, and a small inflow of air occurs when compression is released. The tidal volume generated, however, is insufficient for adequate alveolar gas exchange, so positive pressure ventilation must be provided. Mechanisms that limit filling or emptying of the cardiac pump may limit blood flow. One such factor is hypovolemia, because filling of the pump during diastole is dependent on the pressure difference between the systemic veins and the right ventricle.[8,9]

Thoracic Pump Mechanism. Another hypothesis is that the compression of the chest increases intrathoracic pressure on the pulmonary vascular bed as well as the heart.[10] In this thoracic pump mechanism theory of forward blood flow, the displacement of the sternum and direct cardiac compression are not relevant. The heart serves not as a pump, but rather as a conduit for blood from the lungs. Thus, flow into the extrathoracic vessels depends on whether they remain open or collapse. Forward flow may result from a pressure gradient between the carotid artery and the more compressible jugular vein. During artificial systole, thoracic compression (or cough) generates increased intrathoracic pressure that is vented by arterial outflow to peripheral tissues. Release of intrathoracic pressure permits artificial diastolic filling. The site at which the force is applied is not important.[8,11]

If the patient is awake, forward blood flow can be accomplished with coughing. Intrathoracic pressure is increased by the contraction of the diaphragm, as well as intercostal and abdominal muscles, against a closed glottis. This so-called cough CPR maintains cerebral blood flow. The technique has several advantages: it is patient-initiated, it is not hazardous, it increases venous return to the heart, and each cough is preceded by a small negative pressure inspiration.[11,12]

CPR TECHNIQUES

Rescuer's Position for Providing Chest Compressions

The rescuer should be close to the side of the victim's chest, the knees just touching the patient's side, and the rescuer's legs slightly spread apart.[6] The rescuer's middle and index fingers locate the inferior margin of the rib cage at the point where the ribs make an angle with the sternum. After placing one finger in this notch, the rescuer places the other finger adjacent to the first finger on the lower end of the sternum. The heel of the rescuer's hand is placed on the lower half of the sternum. The heel of the other hand is placed *above* the xiphoid, over the lower one-half of the sternum (next to the finger of the first hand that located the notch) and

on top of the other hand. The fingers are always kept off the chest wall and interlocked. The heels of both hands are parallel to each other, and the fingers are directed straight away from the rescuer (Fig. 55–3).

The rescuer's elbows are straight and locked with the shoulders parallel to the patient's sternum so that the thrust is straight down. In an adult with cardiopulmonary arrest, the rescuer should apply sufficient compression to depress the sternum 1.5 to 2 inches (3.8 to 5 cm) at a rate of 60 cycles/minute. The duration of compression or "duty cycle" is an important determinant in producing forward blood flow and a ratio of *at least* 50 to 60 percent compression should be delivered.[13,14]

One-Rescuer CPR

With one rescuer, the chest compressions must be interrupted to provide the ventilation. Therefore, the chest compression rate must be increased to 80 cycles/minute. The compression/ventilation ratio should be 15:2, i.e., 15 chest compressions to 2 ventilations. The

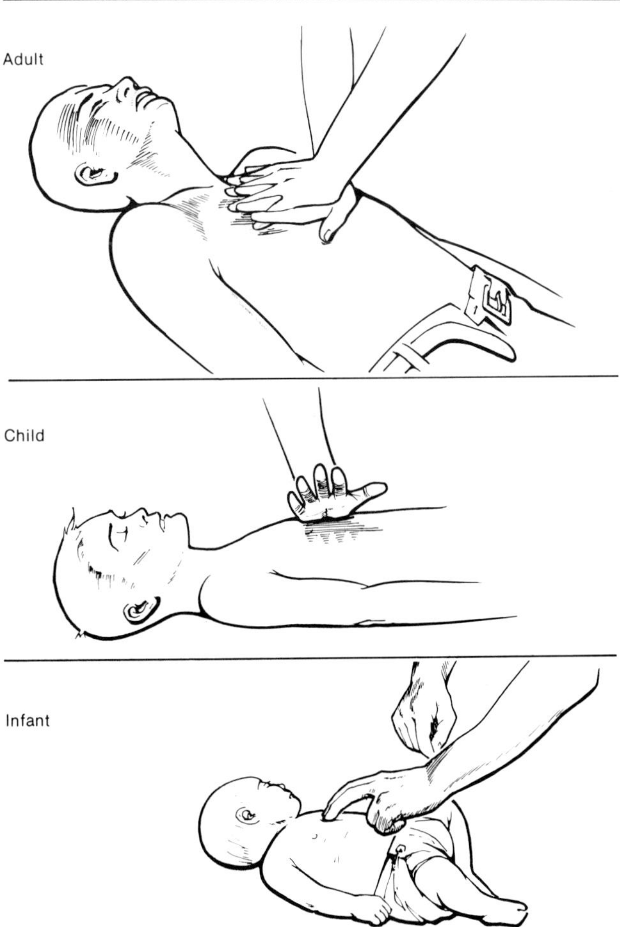

Figure 55–3 Cardiopulmonary Resuscitation Variations.

ventilations are provided in a volume approximately twice the normal adult resting tidal volume, i.e., 1,000 to 1,500 ml quickly (in a period of five to six seconds) without allowing the victim to have full exhalations between the first and second breaths.[6]

External chest compression and mouth-to-mouth ventilation should proceed until definitive care, such as endotracheal intubation, defibrillation, or drug therapy, are provided.

A second rescuer can verify that the pulse is absent by palpating the carotid pulse during the five-second interval when chest compression is discontinued.

Two-Rescuer CPR

The advantage of two-rescuer CPR is that one rescuer on one side of the patient can maintain artificial circulation by external chest compressions, while the second rescuer, at the patient's head, establishes the airway and provides artificial positive pressure ventilation. During two-rescuer CPR, the compression rate is 60 cycles/minute and the compressions are smooth, regular, and uninterrupted. The second rescuer provides cycles of one lung inflation interposed during the upstroke of the fifth chest compression. This ratio (five compressions to one ventilation) is maintained until the rescuers choose to change position, at which time the rescuer who is managing the airway replaces the rescuer at the victim's side immediately after a lung inflation and the rescuer who has been performing the cardiac compressions now provides the mouth-to-mouth ventilation. The carotid pulse of the victim is rechecked at the time the rescuers change roles.[6]

ARRHYTHMIAS ASSOCIATED WITH CARDIOPULMONARY ARREST

Ventricular fibrillation is the arrhythmia most commonly associated with cardiac arrest, but ventricular tachycardia, ventricular asystole, electromechanical dissociation, a variety of bradyarrhythmias, and other arrhythmias can also occur. (See Chapter 50.)

Ventricular Fibrillation

The Monitored Patient

Inadequate cardiac output in cardiopulmonary arrest is usually caused by ineffective myocardial contraction due to arrhythmias: ventricular fibrillation is the most common arrhythmia in this setting. If ventricular fibrillation is observed on an ECG monitor, or if it is known that the patient has been in cardiac arrest for less than two minutes, then electrical defibrillation should be accomplished immediately. When the time period from collapse is unknown and ventricular fibrillation is recognized, it has been recommended that basic life support be performed for two minutes before defibrillation is attempted.[6,15] Monitored ventricular fibrillation may also be treated by a "precordial thump," which consists of a sharp, quick, single blow to the victim's midsternum with the fleshy portion of a closed fist. This technique is not recommended in pediatric patients, however. If this maneuver does not succeed in terminating the arrhythmia, electrical defibrillation should be attempted immediately.

Defibrillation

A number of factors determine whether or not a human heart in ventricular defibrillation can be successfully defibrillated electrically. The longer a heart is in ventricular fibrillation, the less likely electrical defibrillation will be successful. Basic and advanced cardiac life support extend the time during which subsequent defibrillation is likely. Since a critical mass of myocardium must be depolarized in close temporal sequence in order to defibrillate successfully, the larger the size of the heart, the greater the energy required. The underlying cardiac pathology, as well as the metabolic milieu (e.g., the presence of arterial or tissue hypoxemia, acidosis, hypothermia, electrolyte abnormalities, or drug toxicity), determines the success of the defibrillation. Finally, previous electrical countershocks affect subsequent defibrillation, since the transthoracic resistance decreases with repeated electrical shock.

In defibrillation across the chest, the largest amount of energy distributed is a vector, the direction of which is determined by paddle placement and the path of current through the myocardium. Paddles should be placed on the chest in a position that maximizes current flow through the myocardium. In the usual situation, one paddle at least 10 to 13 cm in size is placed just to the right of the upper sternum below the right clavicle; the second paddle, just to the left of the left nipple in the anterior axillary line. Each paddle should be pressed at a pressure equal to 10 kg.[6,15] (See Chapter 71.) With an *anterior-posterior* paddle placement, the paddles face each other, spreading the current flow between them. With this placement the electrical current may be more effectively directed through the heart, ensuring more even depolarization. However, additional studies are required to determine the usefulness of this approach.

Using a sufficient amount of electrolyte gel and applying pressure to both paddles facilitates defibrillation, since firm contact with the skin is important to provide a low resistance to electrical current flow. Resistance can be decreased with the use of a low-impedance medium, such as moist saline pads, between the paddles and the skin. The optimum amount of electrical energy required has not been firmly established; however, 200 to 300 joules is usually adequate. At times 400 joules is required for successful defibrillation.

The Unmonitored Patient

If a patient develops cardiopulmonary arrest when the cardiac rhythm is not being monitored, then CPR should be immediately begun. The cardiac monitor-defibrillator should be utilized, and the paddles should be quickly placed in the appropriate anatomical position, allowing a "paddle check" or "quick look" at the cardiac rhythm. In the presence of ventricular fibrillation, CPR should be momentarily disrupted and defibrillation accomplished at 200 to 300 joules.[6,15]

If the first attempt at electrical defibrillation is unsuccessful, then a second countershock at the same energy level should be administered. CPR should be continued throughout these events, except when electrical cardioversion is attempted immediately. If a second electrical cardiac countershock does not restore an effective cardiac rhythm, basic life support should be continued for two minutes and/or additional advanced cardiac life support measures initiated, e.g., mask valve, esophageal airway, or endotracheal intubation. In addition, an intravenous line should be established. If these are ineffective, a third defibrillation attempt should be made, but usually at no more than 360 joules. In patients weighing less than 50 kg, a dose of 6 watt-seconds/kg has been recommended.[14]

Pharmacologic Agents

Epinephrine

Various pharmacologic agents have been found to be useful in advanced cardiac life support. The level of these agents in the circulation of patients during CPR depends on the dose, rate and route of administration, and the effectiveness of CPR. It has been suggested that CPR be performed for at least one minute after drug administration because it takes at least that long to achieve the desired pharmacologic effect.[16] Epinephrine is an adrenergic catecholamine that increases heart rate by increasing automaticity of cardiac pacemakers, increasing the force of myocardial contraction. Epinephrine also increases systemic vascular resistance, and therefore blood pressure, aortic diastolic pressure, and coronary perfusion during diastole, and increases myocardial oxygen demands. Often, it facilitates electrical cardioversion of ventricular fibrillation. This agent is indicated in the advanced life support of patients with asystole, electromechanical dissociation, and ventricu-

lar fibrillation. Epinephrine may convert fine ventricular fibrillation to coarse fibrillation.[17]

A dose of 0.5 to 1 ml 1:10,000 solution is given intravenously. If an intravenous line has not been established, 10 ml of this solution can be instilled directly into the trachea via the endotracheal tube. Epinephrine administered by this route achieves a maximum blood concentration in 15 seconds, but its concentration is only one-tenth that of epinephrine administered intravenously. However, it remains metabolically active in the circulation longer than epinephrine administered intravenously, probably because of continued slow absorption.[17,18]

Injection of epinephrine into the ventricle itself from a subxiphoid approach may be attempted, but this procedure may be associated with complications because of intramyocardial injection of the material and hemopericardium.

Sodium Bicarbonate

Patients in cardiopulmonary arrest may require sodium bicarbonate. When the peripheral tissues do not receive an adequate supply of oxygen, metabolic (lactic) acidosis may result. In addition, the associated alveolar hypoventilation (or apnea) can cause carbon dioxide retention and respiratory acidosis. Acidosis and hypercapnia each have profound effects upon cardiac performance. Respiratory acidosis secondary to alveolar hypoventilation should be treated by airway maintenance, ventilation, and, if necessary, hyperventilation.

Sodium bicarbonate is used to treat the metabolic acidosis. One mEq/kg (usually one ampul of an 8.4 solution of 50 mEq solution) should be administered as the initial dose to an adult of normal size. Repeat intravenous administration of bicarbonate may be required in one-half of this dose every 10 to 15 minutes, but such therapy should be guided by determinations of arterial blood gas levels, pH, and base deficit. Administration of excessive sodium bicarbonate may not only result in metabolic alkalosis, hypernatremia, or hyperosmolality, but may also be responsible for "postarrest cerebral dysfunction." Attempts should be made to obtain an arterial pH near the normal value of 7.38, and a PCO_2 near the normal value of 38 to 40 mm Hg.[15]

Lidocaine

Other pharmacologic agents may be required in the treatment of ventricular fibrillation if the previously mentioned steps are not successful. Lidocaine is useful in suppressing ventricular arrhythmias and may terminate ventricular tachycardia, but it cannot itself terminate ventricular fibrillation. However, following the termination of ventricular fibrillation, it may prevent the recurrence of ventricular tachyarrhythmias. Lidocaine is usually administered IV in a dose of 1 mg/kg as a bolus (50 to 100 mg), followed by a constant infusion of 1 to 4 mg/minute (15 to 60 mg/kg/minute) in order to maintain the serum concentration in the range of 1.5 to 4 mg/liter.[19,20]

Bretylium Tosylate (Bretylol)

If therapeutic maneuvers such as precordial thump, electrical defibrillation, and the administration of epinephrine, sodium bicarbonate, or lidocaine have failed to control ventricular fibrillation, bretylium tosylate may be utilized. Bretylium tosylate, a quaternary ammonium compound which is an adrenergic blocker, is a potent antidysrhythmic medication with a positive ionotropic effect. The antidysrhythmic mechanism of action of bretylium is not clear, but it elevates the ventricular fibrillation threshold and increases the action potential duration; it may prevent reentry from ischemic cardiac zones by prolonging the refractory period. Its unique feature is the ability to terminate ventricular fibrillation.

The dose of bretylium tosylate is 5 to 10 mg/kg IV diluted one part bretylium tosylate with four parts of dextrose injection USP or sodium chloride in a bolus. If ventricular fibrillation does not terminate in ten minutes, electrical conversion may be attempted. If defibrillation still can not be achieved, a 10 mg/kg IV bolus may be administered and repeated up to five times at intervals of 15 to 30 minutes to a maximum dose of 30 mg/kg while CPR continues.[15]

Arrhythmias Following Defibrillation

Ventricular fibrillation, premature ventricular contractions, ventricular tachycardia, asystole, sinus bradycardia, supraventricular tachyarrhythmia with rapid ventricular response, junctional or ventricular escape rhythm, or virtually any arrhythmia may follow defibrillation. (See Chapter 50.) While the mechanisms responsible for these postdefibrillation arrhythmias remains unclear they probably reflect the underlying process responsible for the initial episode of ventricular fibrillation and the metabolic electrolyte changes that occurred during the arrest. However, the electrical discharge itself may contribute, for high electrical current concentrations across the heart can cause "prolonged depolarization" that may induce morphological changes and damage the neuroelectrical system of the heart, thus producing potentially lethal arrhythmias.[19] Arrhythmias may be dependent on the amplitude of the electrical shock.[20] Regardless of the mechanism, pa-

tients with postdefibrillation arrhythmias require not only specific treatment of the arrhythmia, but also treatment of the underlying metabolic factors that may significantly alter therapy, such as alveolar ventilation, acid-base balance, and electrolyte abnormalities.

Other Arrhythmias in CPR

Ventricular Tachycardia

In some patients ventricular tachycardia may be responsible for cardiopulmonary arrest. After the paddles have been placed in the appropriate position and a rapid evaluation of the cardiac rhythm has been obtained, ventricular tachycardia is treated with a synchronized electrical discharge of 20 to 200 joules. If the lidocaine at the above dosage schedule is ineffective or ventricular tachycardia is refractory or recurrent, a 500 mg dose of bretylium tosylate (5 to 10 mg/kg) in 50 ml dextrose 5% and water is injected intravenously over 8 to 10 minutes. Following the loading dose of bretylium tosylate, administration may continue IV at a rate of 1 to 2 mg/min if required.

Ventricular Asystole

In approximately one-quarter of all patients found in cardiac arrest, the rhythm is ventricular asystole (cardiac standstill). In these patients, CPR should be immediately begun, an airway established, and an intravenous line established. Epinephrine (0.5 to 1 mg 1:10,000 solution) is given intravenously, then sodium bicarbonate (1 ampul 50 ml of an 890 mEq/liter solution) intravenously if clinically indicated. If a spontaneous rhythm does not appear, atropine (1 to 2 mg) by intravenous push is given. If this fails to elicit a spontaneous rhythm, calcium chloride (5 ml 10% solution) is given IV. This medication, which has the ability to increase myocardial contractile force, is most useful when there is electromechanical dissociation, i.e., spontaneous cardiac electrical activity but no corresponding cardiac mechanical activity.

Calcium chloride in this amount can elevate serum calcium to dangerous levels (12.9 to 18.2 mg/dl) within 5 minutes of administration, but serum calcium returns to a normal level in 15 minutes. In addition to its positive ionotropic effects, calcium may suppress sinus impulse formation, enhance ventricular excitability, and may cause ventricular ectopy.[21] If ventricular asystole persists despite the treatment discussed, epinephrine 0.5 to 1 mg of a 1:10,000 solution is administered IV every 5 minutes and calcium chloride 5 ml 10% solution may be given intravenously at 10 minute intervals. If this fails, isoproterenol (1 to 4 μg/minute) by constant IV infusion may be given. A temporary transvenous or transthoracic pacing electrode may be tried if isoproterenol is not successful.

Electromechanical Dissociation

Patients with cardiopulmonary arrest may exhibit electromechanical dissociation, i.e., organized electrical activity on an ECG monitor without evidence of cardiac mechanical contraction or peripheral perfusion. The mechanism of this occurrence is not clear; it may result from a failure of calcium transport, since this ion is required for the coupling of electrical with mechanical events. Clinically, electromechanical dissociation is similar to and therefore must be distinguished from pericardial tamponade and myocardial rupture. CPR should be initiated, followed by the intravenous administration of epinephrine. If this is ineffective, calcium chloride should be given at the dosage described earlier. Arterial blood gas levels should be measured to determine pH, base deficit, and the need for sodium bicarbonate. In the field, sodium bicarbonate may be given empirically at 10-minute intervals during electromechanical dissociation. Isoproterenol or epinephrine may be given, antishock trousers applied (or an intra-aortic balloon pump may be helpful) to improve the hemodynamic state during electromechanical dissociation.

ADJUNCTS TO CPR

After establishment of an airway, oxygen enrichment should be provided to the patient with cardiopulmonary arrest. In patients with cardiopulmonary arrest as a consequence of trauma and acute blood loss, volume expansion is also required. A peripheral intravenous infusion with dextrose 5 percent in water should be started immediately by advanced life support personnel for the purpose of introducing therapeutic agents, when indicated. Often, central (internal jugular, subclavian, femoral) venous catheters are required.

Complications of CPR

As with any therapeutic intervention, complications may occur with CPR. Laceration of the liver or other internal injury may result if the xiphoid is depressed. Other complications that can occur include pulmonary edema, rib fractures, splenic injury, myocardial injury (including rupture), fracture of the sternum, costochondral separation, pneumothorax, hepatic injury, aortic rupture, hemothorax, aspiration pneumonia, lung contusion, and fat and bone marrow emboli.[22] Gastric distention should not be managed by continuous pressure on the abdomen, since this may rarely cause gastric laceration, pulmonary aspiration or trapping, and laceration of the liver.[14,23] The stomach should be decompressed by means of a nasogastric tube if severe gastric distention limits ventilation.

Open Chest Cardiac Resuscitation

Some patients with cardiac arrest require open chest cardiac massage. The surgical approach for this technique is discussed in Chapter 54. The clinical indications for opening the chest and manually compressing the heart include the following list of absolute and relative indications:

- vertebral abnormalities, such as marked scoliosis, lordosis, or kyphosis
- severe sternal malformations, such as pectus excavatum and pectus carinatum, that make it impossible to compress the heart against the vertebrae
- cardiac arrest secondary to penetrating wounds of the myocardium and thorax
- major mediastinal shifts as a consequence of tension pneumothorax or pleural effusion
- cardiac tamponade
- extracardiac intrathoracic hemorrhage
- flail chest
- massive air embolism, requiring needle aspiration by direct visual approach and massage
- ruptured abdominal aortic aneurysm
- failure of the closed chest procedure, particularly in a young, apparently healthy individual
- ventricular aneurysm in association with cardiac arrest
- severe hypothermic cardiac arrest
- cardiac arrest occurring in the operating room in the patient whose chest is already opened
- third trimester of pregnancy
- crushed chest injury when the chest cannot be stabilized laterally.[1]

Pneumatic Antishock Trousers

As an adjunct to cardiopulmonary resuscitation, particularly when a patient is hypovolemic, pneumatic antishock trousers (MAST trousers) may be useful. These trousers allow emergency care personnel to deliver an immediate "autotransfusion" to the critically ill or injured patient. The antishock trousers have three independently controlled compartments: the abdominal compartment extends from the abdomen to the pubis; two lower compartments extend from the ankles to the upper thighs. Placement of the trousers compresses the venous and capillary systems beneath the compartments and shunts blood away from the legs and the abdomen. The external pressure also increases local arterial blood pressure by increasing the peripheral resistance. Theoretically then, the trousers increase the central blood volume, increase the venous return of blood to the chest, decrease the perfusion of the lower body, and increase perfusion of the brain. They also increase central venous pressure, pulmonary capillary wedge pressure, stroke volume, supradiaphragmatic arterial blood flow, and the lung blood volume. Inflation of the trousers reflexly decreases the heart rate and decreases infradiaphragmatic arterial blood flow and vital capacity.

During cardiopulmonary resuscitation, inflation of the antishock trousers may increase systolic blood pressure, as well as carotid and coronary artery blood flow. The mechanisms are unclear, but they may be related to a reduction in the size of the vascular compartment and preferential distribution of the cardiac output to the heart-lung-brain circulation; an increase in the intrathoracic pressure; and increased pressure within the abdominal aorta, which elevates diastolic blood pressure and thereby improves coronary artery blood flow.[24]

The antishock suit should not be used in acute myocardial infarction and cardiogenic shock associated with high pulmonary venous and systemic pressures, because it may aggravate left ventricular heart failure. (See Chapter 6.)

Intra-aortic Balloon Counterpulsation in Cardiac Arrest

An intra-aortic balloon may theoretically be useful in some patients with cardiogenic shock in cardiopulmonary arrest, particularly in a patient who is unresponsive to volume expansion or advanced cardiac life support measures. A deflated single-chamber balloon is inserted percutaneously into a disease-free femoral artery. The balloon is positioned under fluoroscopy into the descending thoracic aorta. It is inflated during diastole, just after aortic valve closure, and is deflated at the time of ventricular systole as sensed by the R wave of a surface ECG. Theoretically, the inflation of the balloon displaces blood into the coronary arteries during diastole, while in systole the sudden deflation decreases left ventricular work.[15]

Chest Compressors during Cardiopulmonary Arrest

Chest compressors can compress the chest at an optimal rate and depth. A manual chest compressor is a simple hand-operated compressor that may deliver an adjustable stroke volume at 1.5 to 2 inches (3.8 to 5 cm) of sternal compression, but the adequacy of compression and appropriate position must be monitored continuously. An automatic chest compressor may have an adjustable depth of compression and a mechanism for automatically ventilating the lungs, and the relationship between compression and ventilation can be programmed. These devices may have a role in protracted CPR and during transport, but they may cause sternal fracture and require constant monitoring for proper position and depth of ventilations and compressions.

Central Venous Lines

It has been suggested that central venous lines be established in patients requiring advanced life support to facilitate the rapid delivery of medications to the central arterial circulation.[25] The size and configuration should be chosen so that an artificial pacemaker, if required, can be inserted. (See Chapter 71.)

Artificial Pacemakers in CPR

Often, effective cardiac rhythm cannot be established by medication and external emergency cardiac pacing is indicated at that point. The pacing electrode catheter or wire can be passed to the heart either through a central vein or through the chest wall. In either event, once contact is established with the ventricular myocardium, the electrode should be connected to a pacemaker generator. The generator should be set in an asynchronous (fixed rate) mode, and its output turned to maximal in order to establish capture. Once the situation has stabilized, optimal pacemaker generator setup and electrode placement can be determined.

BASIC CPR IN INFANTS AND CHILDREN

Cardiopulmonary arrest in infants and children is rarely the result of cardiac disease; it is usually caused by a primary respiratory event, such as foreign body obstruction, near-drowning, trauma, drug overdose, smoke inhalation, or sudden infant death syndrome. Two additional processes that may present as an acute respiratory event are epiglottitis and laryngotracheobronchitis. (See Chapter 57.)

CPR in infants and children differs from that in adults, but the principles of basic life support and advanced cardiac life support are the same: establish unresponsiveness or respiratory difficulty; call for help if available; position the victim properly; establish an airway; provide positive pressure breathing; and ensure circulation.

The difference in providing CPR to a child or infant is in the priorities chosen and the modification required in the resuscitative techniques to account for the differences of the anatomy and physiology of the younger patient. For example, in the infant and small child, the larynx is located more anteriorly and cephalad; the epiglottis is shorter and U-shaped, rather than flat; the angle formed by the epiglottis and vocal cords is more acute; the gums are soft, vascular, and easily indented; the deciduous teeth are poorly anchored and easily dislodged; the heart is situated higher in the chest; and the lungs are of a smaller volume. Furthermore, the cartilaginous structures in the airways are pliable in infants under two years of age.[15,26]

Unresponsiveness

A child or infant who is found apparently unresponsive should be tapped and shaken to determine if there is subsequent movement, respirations, or a cry. If there is evidence of airway obstruction, suctioning and sweeping for foreign bodies should be considered since upper airway obstruction is a more common cause of cardiopulmonary arrest in the younger patient than in the adult.[6] If acute epiglottitis is suspected, however, the airway should not be manipulated unless a physician highly skilled in airway maintenance is immediately available.

Position

Trauma is a common cause of death and injury in the younger age group, and great care must be taken in manipulating an infant or child with cardiopulmonary arrest associated with trauma. The patient should be rolled to the back without movement of the neck so as to avoid possible cervical spine injury. An infant less than one year old or a small child should be placed in the sniffing position, i.e., with the occiput of the head lifted slightly off of the flat surface of the bed or ground and supported with a rolled towel or the rescuer's hand.

Airway

If the child is apneic or cyanotic, or if the child is struggling to breathe, the airway should be opened. The head tilt-neck lift as previously described usually moves the tongue forward and relieves obstruction. In infants less than two years of age, the cartilaginous structures in the airways are soft, pliable, and easily collapsible. Thus, extension of the neck should not be exaggerated, since this maneuver may in itself cause obstruction.

After these maneuvers have been performed, the patient is examined for breathlessness. The rescuer *looks* for movement of the chest; *listens* with the ear over the victim's mouth for exhaled breaths; and *feels* the movement of exhaled air on the cheek. If the airway has been successfully opened and respirations are spontaneous (and a pulse is present), the patient should be immediately transported to an emergency department. However, if there are no spontaneous respirations, positive pressure ventilation should be delivered.

Breathing

In infants and small children who are not breathing, the rescuer can provide positive pressure ventilation by placing the entire mouth over the mouth and nose of the victim. The rescuer delivers four breaths in rapid succession without permitting the victim's lungs to deflate until after the fourth breath. Since the lungs and airways are smaller than those of an adult, the volume required to inflate the lungs is smaller (approximately 8 ml/kg), but the resistance is greater. In the infant, small puffs of air may be sufficient. The volume delivered should be that required for the chest to rise and subsequently fall. The rate of ventilation increases inversely according to the patient's age. In the neonate, the frequency is 24/minute; in infants, 20/minute; in a child, 15/minute. If air cannot enter or the chest does not collapse during exhalation, the possibility of foreign body obstruction of the upper airway should be considered. If air freely enters and leaves the victim's lungs, the rescuer checks for a pulse.[6]

Circulation

After the airway has been opened and four quick breaths have been successfully delivered, the rescuer should check for the presence of a pulse. Using the finger tips, the rescuer palpates the brachial artery in an infant or the carotid in a child. Precordial activity may not be a reliable sign of a peripheral pulse that is adequately perfusing vital organs. If there is a pulse but there are no respirations, only positive pressure ventilation is required. If there is no pulse, compression of the chest, in addition to artificial ventilation, is indicated.[26]

The site of external cardiac compression differs in the child, not only because the position of the heart is higher in the thorax than that of the adult, but also because the left lobe of the liver of the child is under the sternum and xiphoid. In the child, the lower one-half of the sternum is utilized; in the infant, the midsternum is the site of external compression (Fig. 55–3). The standard technique of locating the notch in the center of the chest with the middle finger is utilized, as in the adult. In the child, the heel of the hand is placed over the lower one-half of the sternum. The fingers are kept off the chest, and the sternum is displaced 1 to 1.5 inches (2.6 to 4 cm) at a rate of 80/minute. In the infant, two fingers are used to compress an area over the midsternum between the two nipples 0.5 to 1 inch (1.3 to 2.6 cm) at a rate of 100/minute. In the neonate, the rate of compression is 124/minute. In each of these situations, the ratio of compressions to ventilations is the same, i.e., 5:1.

Drugs in Resuscitation of Infants and Children

Oxygen enrichment is required for the treatment of underlying hypoxemia at an FIO_2 of 0.5 to 1.

Epinephrine at a dose of 0.1 ml/kg at a dilution of 1:10,000 administered either intravenously or via the endotracheal tube is given for indications as described for CPR in the adult.[26]

Adequate alveolar ventilation is the proper treatment for respiratory acidosis, and sodium bicarbonate may be required for metabolic acidosis. The initial dose introduced empirically is 2 mEq/kg. After blood gas levels and pH measurements have been determined, an additional dose can be calculated according to the following formula: mEq sodium bicarbonate = 0.3 × weight (kg) × base deficit (mEq/liter). In the prehospital care setting, when blood gas and pH measurements are not available, 1 mEq/kg may be given intravenously every ten minutes after the initial dose.

Calcium is indicated for electromechanical dissociation and, in some instances, ventricular asystole. Calcium chloride 10 percent is administered slowly at a dose of 0.3 ml/kg (8 mEq/kg) or 5 to 10 mg/kg. Calcium may precipitate if administered intravenously with bicarbonate and should be used with great caution in the patient who has taken a digitalis preparation.

Atropine may be administered for symptomatic bradyarrhythmias. It is given intravenously at a dose of 0.01 to 0.03 mg/kg to a maximum of 0.5 to 1 mg.

Lidocaine may be administered intravenously or via the endotracheal tube at a dose of 0.5 to 1 mg/kg for ventricular fibrillation or ventricular tachycardia.

Bretylium may be given at a dose of 5 mg/kg for refractory ventricular fibrillation or ventricular tachycardia; the maximum dosage is 30 mg/kg.

Airway Adjuncts

Basic principles of airway maintenance are the same for infants and children as they are for adults. Oxygen enrichment and an oral, pharyngeal, and nasopharyngeal airway should be used, but the use of an esophageal obturator airway in the infant and child is not yet recommended.

When endotracheal intubation is indicated, the size of the endotracheal tube that is required can be calculated according to the following formula: the size in millimeters of the internal diameter of the tube is equal to 16 plus the age of the patient in years, divided by 4. Two additional tubes, one 0.5 mm larger and one 0.5 mm smaller than the first, should also be available. If the patient is under the age of eight years, an uncuffed tube is used. (See Chapter 71 for a discussion of the curved blade technique of intubation of a child or infant.)

Defibrillation

While ventricular fibrillation is the most common arrhythmia associated with cardiac arrest in the adult, children and infants with cardiopulmonary arrest experience bradyarrhythmias and heart block more frequently. Thus, defibrillation is indicated only in the monitored patient, not in the patient with an unwitnessed, unmonitored arrest. The technique for defibrillation is the same as that for adults, but the size of the electropaddles is reduced to 4.5 cm for infants and 8 cm for older children. The optimum amount of electrical energy required to defibrillate has not been clearly established, but an initial dose of 2 to 3 joules/kg discharge is usually sufficient. If this is unsuccessful, then the energy dose is doubled.[26]

Intravenous Therapy

A peripheral or central intravenous line is required for advanced cardiac life support in the infant or child. The anatomical site and location chosen is determined by the clinical condition of the patient, ease of access, and the skill of the rescuer.[25] In the prehospital care setting, peripheral intravenous lines can be introduced in a scalp vein (frontal superficial, temporal, posteriooricular, supraorbital, occipital and posterior facial). The scalp is prepared with povidone-iodine solution, a rubber band tourniquet is placed around the head, and a 23 to 25 gauge butterfly needle with the bevel up is advanced until there is free flow of venous blood. Then the tourniquet is released.[15]

Upper Extremity

The veins of the dorsum of the hand (cephalic, basilic, and the dorsal venous arch) are accessible with a 23 to 25 gauge butterfly needle or plastic intracath. The cephalic, median, basilic, and median antecubital veins may also be utilized.

Lower Extremity

Veins in the lower extremity (saphenous, median, marginal, dorsal arch, and femoral) are accessible. The extremity is immobilized in a position that stretches the veins. The puncture site is prepared with povidone-iodine and the needle or cannula introduced with the bevel down. The needle is advanced with gentle aspiration until free flow of venous blood is observed.

Central Venous Catheters

The technique for introducing a central venous line via the internal jugular vein is described in Chapter 71. The subclavian vein approach is not recommended because of the associated complications. The external jugular and femoral veins are also possible sites of cannulation.[15,25]

Because the external jugular vein is distended and easily identified in the crying infant, it is often the site of entry chosen by prehospital care personnel in the critically ill or injured infant or child. The child is placed in 20° Trendelenburg position, and the head is turned to the contralateral side at 45°. The skin is prepared with povidone-iodine, anesthetized with 0.5 to 1 percent lidocaine, and the needle or intracath is introduced into the vein until free venous flow is observed.

In the femoral vein technique, the leg is externally rotated and immobilized. The anatomical site is one fingerbreadth inferior to the inguinal ligament, just medial to the femoral artery. After aseptic preparation, the needle or intracath is advanced at a 45° angle in the skin until free venous flow of blood is observed. A guide wire is introduced and advanced, and the plastic catheter is advanced to the desired position.

REFERENCES

1. Babbs CF, Winslow EBJ: Knowledge gaps in C.P.R.: Synopsis of a panel discussion. *Crit Care Med* 3:181, 1980.
2. Bergner L, Eisenberg M, Hallstrom A, et al: Evaluation of Paramedic Services for Cardiac Arrest. National Center for Health Services Research, Research Report Series, December 1981.
3. Lilja GP, et al: Clinical assessment of patients undergoing C.P.R. in the emergency department. *JACEP* 2:81, 1979.
4. Lund I, Skulberg A: Cardiopulmonary resuscitation by lay people. *Lancet* 2:702, 1976.
5. Safar P: *Cardiopulmonary Resuscitation*. New York, Springer Verlag, 1977, p 195.
6. Standards and guidelines for cardiopulmonary resuscitation (CPR) and emergency cardiac care (ECC): Parts I-VII—Adult basic life support. *JAMA* 5:453–509, 1980.
7. Vaagenes P, et al: On the technique of external cardiac compression. *Crit Care Med* 3:176, 1976.
8. Rudikoff MJ, et al: Mechanisms of blood flow during cardiopulmonary resuscitation. *Circulation* 2:345, 1980.
9. Chandra N, et al: Simultaneous chest compression and ventilation at high airway pressure during cardiopulmonary resuscitation. *Lancet* 1:175, 1980.
10. Werner JA, et al: Two-dimensional echocardiography during C.P.R. in man: Implications regarding the mechanism of blood flow. *Crit Care Med* 5:375, May 1981.
11. Criley JM, et al: The heart is a conduit in C.P.R. *Crit Care Med* 5:373, 1981.
12. Niemann JT, et al: Cough C.P.R. *Crit Care Med* 3:141, 1980.
13. Luce JM, et al: New developments in cardiopulmonary resuscitation. *JAMA* 12:1366, 1980.
14. Redding JS: Cardiopulmonary resuscitation: An algorithm and some common pitfalls. *Am Heart J* 6:788, 1979.
15. McIntyre KM, Lewis AJ (eds): *Textbook of Advanced Cardiac Life Support*. American Heart Association, 1981.
16. Barsan WG, et al: Lidocaine levels during C.P.R. *Ann Emerg Med* 2:73, 1981.
17. Roberts JR, et al: Blood levels following intravenous and endotracheal epinephrine administration. *J Amer Coll Emerg Phys* 8(2):53, February 1979.
18. Roberts JR, et al: Endotracheal epinephrine in cardiorespiratory collapse. *JACEP* 12:515, 1979.
19. Ewy G: Defibrillation. Current Problems in Cardiology, Vol. 2, No. 11, 1978, Year Book Medicine Publication.
20. Jones JL, Jones RE: Post shock arrhythmias—A possible cause of unsuccessful defibrillation. *Crit Care Med* 8:167–171, 1980.
21. Dembo DH: Calcium in advanced life support. *Crit Care Med* 5:358, 1981.
22. Bodily K, et al: Aortic rupture and right ventricular rupture induced by closed chest cardiac massage. *Minn Med* 62(4):255, April 1979.
23. Nagal EL, et al: Complications of C.P.R. *Crit Care Med* 5:424, 1981.
24. Lilja GP, Long RS, Ruiz E: Augmentation of systolic blood pressure during external cardiac compression by use of the MAST suit. *Ann Emerg Med* 10:182, 1981.
25. Kuhn GJ: Peripheral vs. central circulation times during C.P.R.: A pilot study. *Ann Emerg Med* 8:417, 1981.
26. Orlowski, JP: Cardiopulmonary resuscitation in children. *Ped Clin N Amer* 3:495, 1980.

Alterations of Respiratory System Functions

The author of "Airway Management" (Chapter 56) offers a state-of-the-art review on the advanced technology and manipulative techniques of emergency airway maintenance that have developed over the past 30 years. Various methods and specific indication techniques for oxygen administration, and partial and full artificial airways, are reviewed. The iatrogenic problems that may result from these maneuvers and their prevention and treatment are summarized.

Emergency patients with conditions that alter the respiratory system may have a variety of symptoms, such as cough, dyspnea, hemoptysis, chest pain, or sudden respiratory collapse. In evaluating patients with apnea, hypoventilation, dyspnea, or wheezing, "Alterations of Central Nervous System Functions" (Section IX), "Poisoning and Drug Overdose" (Chapter 24), "Alcohol Abuse" (Chapter 36), and "Cardiopulmonary Resuscitation" (Chapter 55) should be consulted. "Alterations of Circulatory System Functions" (Section X) should be reviewed in evaluating the condition of patients with signs and symptoms that are not primarily of pulmonary origin, but result from either traumatic or nontraumatic events involving the heart or great vessels. Inflammatory diseases of the upper respiratory tract that are usually not life-threatening, such as acute pharyngitis, sinusitis, and abscess, are discussed in "Infectious Disease Emergencies" (Chapter 20).

"Obstructive Lung Diseases" (Chapter 57) first addresses emergencies involving the upper airway, such as acute epiglottis, croup, and foreign body obstruction; then, the reversible obstructive lower airway conditions commonly associated with cough and shortness of breath (e.g., acute exacerbation of bronchitis, emphysema, and asthma) are considered. A common therapeutic approach for the emergency treatment of these patients and their continued ambulatory outpatient care, if required, is presented.

In Chapter 58 the common clinical manifestations, diagnostic tests, and therapy of pulmonary embolism and its usual source (deep venous thrombosis) are described in detail and summarized in a succinct algorithm.

"Respiratory Failure" (Chapter 59) deals with conditions that may be associated with respiratory failure, such as unconsciousness due to central nervous system changes, obstruction, cardiorespiratory failure, or trauma. The clinical signs of respiratory failure are presented in a form which will be of interest to the prehospital and emergency department personnel. A review of pertinent pulmonary physiology and a method for simply but accurately interpreting arterial blood gas changes, analyzing the efficiency of the lung as an O_2 exchanger for patients on supplemental O_2, and determining the alveolar-arterial O_2 difference is reviewed. Other pulmonary emergencies are included in "Miscellaneous Respiratory Emergencies" (Chapter 60). Finally, "Chest Trauma" (Chapter 61) presents a concise outline of traumatic chest injuries that the reader may wish to consider in conjunction with "Heart and Great Vessel Emergencies" (Chapter 54).

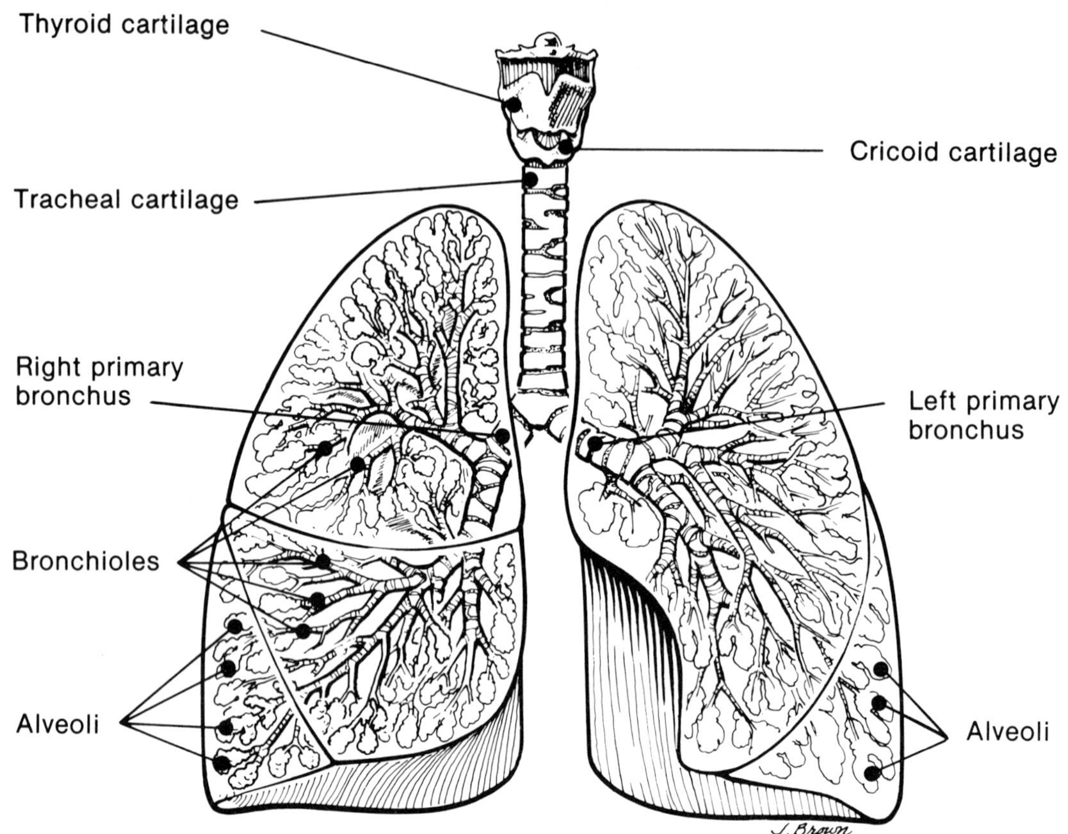

Normal Anatomy of the Respiratory Tract

56. Airway Management

STUART J. MENN, M.D.

There is no area of technologic understanding that has contributed more to improvement in emergency respiratory care during the past 30 years than airway management. Control of the airway permitted a major advance in the intensive care unit—it allowed the application of positive-pressure ventilation to critically ill patients for extended periods of time. Additionally, artificial airway care is an integral part of surgery and postoperative care. The emergency department and its extension—the paramedical mobile unit—use airway management as a vital component of resuscitation. Finally, long-term airway management has been applied to such neurologic conditions as slowly progressive demyelinating disease, chronic spinal cord injury, as well as the obstructive sleep apnea syndrome.

Unfortunately, the initial use of artificial airways produced several iatrogenic complications. Some were minor and in view of the condition being treated, these complications could be considered insignificant. However, others caused serious setbacks and even death. Improvement in equipment and a better understanding of airway function has led to a sharp reduction in serious complications. All medical personnel involved in airway care must be mindful of the potentially lethal results that can arise in advanced emergency care.

AIRWAY CARE *WITHOUT* AN ARTIFICIAL AIRWAY

Oxygen Enrichment

Although not commonly thought of as a part of airway management, a brief discussion of oxygen administration is appropriate since this gas must be applied to and pass through the airway on the way to the alveolus. There are four major methods of oxygen administration, each with specific patient indications. The most common and principal method of long-term oxygen administration is through a nasal catheter or prongs. The range of oxygen flow rate in this method is 1 to 4 liters/minute. Flow rates above this level often irritate the nasal mucosa. The limit of oxygen enrichment by this method is approximately 35 percent.

For oxygen levels of 30 to 60 percent, an open oxygen mask is used. Flow rates should be at least 4 liters/minute to provide adequate venting of expired CO_2. Rates as high as 10 to 15 liters/minute can provide 50 percent O_2. Patients with hypoxemia and hypercapnia require a method of oxygen administration that tightly controls the oxygen mix reaching the trachea. This can be provided by the high air flow with oxygen enrichment (HAFOE) technique of the Venturi mask introduced by Campbell in the 1960s. This mask has special application for the patient with chronic obstructive pulmonary disease (COPD) in the ambulance, emergency department, or intensive care unit. Its safety feature is the prevention of severe CO_2 retention due to poorly controlled oxygen administration. The Venturi mask provides low levels of oxygen enrichment between 22 and 40 percent.

When the fractions of the inspired oxygen (FIO_2) go beyond 50 to 70 percent, oxygen can be provided on a short-term basis by the non-rebreathing oxygen mask with a reservoir bag set at 15 liters/minute. While this mask is comfortable to wear, its limitation is that oxygen administration is interrupted during coughing and suctioning.

The most recent technique, which allows very high oxygen administration (greater than 80 percent FIO_2) in a patient who will not permit or tolerate an artificial airway, is a soft plastic positive-pressure mask (Hudson Corporation, Ohio, CA). This mask uses a phalange design that creates a tight seal around the face and allows the application of positive end-expiratory pressure (PEEP) levels of up to 15 cm H_2O. One elderly woman with acute myocardial infarction, papillary muscle rupture, and severe congestive heart failure used such a mask for 17 hours. PEEP levels of 10 to 15 cm H_2O have been used successfully by others. The limitations of this method include the discomfort of a tightly applied mask, interruption during routine suctioning, and air swallowing causing gastric distention. Vomiting represents a serious complication, and this mask should always be used with a nasogastric tube.

Oxygen Toxicity

Oxygen toxicity is rarely associated with patients receiving oxygen by mask or cannula. Since FIO_2 seldom exceeds 50 to 60 percent in these patients and the ill effects of oxygen have been described in people receiving over 80 percent for over 36 continuous hours, clinical toxicity would be very rare.[1] One report, however, does show that even modest levels of oxygen of 40 to 60 percent can diminish mucociliary function, but the clinical significance of such data is not certain. Finally, it is essential that dry oxygen directly from a cylinder is not given directly to patients. Otherwise, all of the tracheobronchitic symptoms that mimic acute oxygen toxicity will be produced. A nonproductive cough and irritation on deep inspiration is caused by the damage to the mucociliary lining of the upper airway by lack of proper humidification.

Humidification

It is essential to maintain the water balance of the lower airway mucosa. When air or oxygen has insufficient water vapor pressure, the nasal and oral mucosa must add moisture to bring the water content up to 100 percent saturation at 37°C (46 cm H_2O/ml gas). This causes a drying of the mucosa, a thickening of the mucus produced by the glands lining the airway, and a dysfunction of the cilia. Dry gas that bypasses the normal upper airway (e.g., by tracheostomy) will cause major irritation to the lower airways of the bronchi and a serious cough with secretion problems.

Humidifiers serve to raise the water content of gas and must be heated to allow for full saturation at core temperature. Cold bubble humidifiers used with gas tanks are only adequate for nasal administration. A device such as the heated cascade humidifier is required for adequate treatment of gas bypassing the nose or mouth.

Nebulization

The technique of producing droplets of fluid in a gas medium is called mist, aerosol, or nebulization therapy. It is a different process than humidification and should be used during special situations. Nebulization allows for supersaturation of the water vapor, allowing for a positive fluid balance. This method is used when a patient has a negative airway water balance and has very dried secretions. Nebulization therapy also is used to deposit droplets of medication such as β_2-sympathomimetic drugs and corticosteroids to different levels of the airway. (See Chapter 57.) This technique is widely used in the treatment of asthma and less frequently used for acute epiglottitis and postextubation problems. Since bacteria can "ride on the back" of these aerosol particles, sterility of the nebulization fluid must be ensured. Heated nebulization is particularly dangerous and should be avoided to lower the risk of bacterial contamination of the airway.

Suctioning

Many emergency and intensive care patients will not be capable of coughing effectively. In order to mobilize secretions from the upper airways, suctioning through the nose is required. (See Chapter 71.) All patients without a spontaneous cough need suctioning. This is particularly true of obtunded patients even though they may not appear to have secretions. Waiting until patients sound "junky" is not good practice in airway care. Clear plastic catheters with a low friction coefficient and adequate side holes with ring tips designed to diminish airway mucosal tearing by the vacuum should be used. Suction pressure should be limited to -60 to -80 mm Hg. If secretions cannot be removed at this level of vacuum, a larger bore catheter and more attention to "liquefication" of secretions are required. The immediate complication seen with improper suctioning techniques is hypoxemia, arrhythmias, hypotension, and atelectasis (HAHA). These dangers can be sharply reduced by preoxygenation of the hypoxemic patient before suctioning, by inserting the catheter without vacuum, by limiting the suctioning time to 10 seconds or less, and by hyperinflating lung units with a voluntary deep breath or a resuscitation bag following suctioning.

Most serious complications of suctioning occur in critically ill patients receiving mechanical ventilation through endotracheal or tracheostomy tubes. For the past 5 years, these complications have been avoided by requiring all suctioning through a disposable bronchoscopy adaptor (Instrumentation Industries, Inc., Pittsburgh, Pa.) attached to the artificial airway. Utilizing this approach, the patient is not disconnected from the ventilator and can receive oxygen supplementation and assisted ventilation during suctioning.

A delayed complication of suctioning is infection. The procedure employing disposable catheters and semisterile techniques has reduced but not completely eliminated this problem.

A common error in suctioning techniques is the improper placement of the catheter in the airway. In order to extract secretions from the trachea, the catheter tip must be below the vocal cords. Medical personnel all too frequently mistake secretions from the pharyngeal region as being from the trachea and believe their suctioning technique has been adequate. When suctioning through an endotracheal tube, the catheter should extend out beyond the tip of the artificial airway. Although much has been written about directing catheter tips into the right and left main-stem bronchi while using conventional catheters, the standard manuevers have not proved satisfactory. Patients requiring specific suctioning of the main-stem bronchi, especially the left bronchus, require fiberoptic bronchoscopy.

Resuscitation Mask Devices

The final airway technique that does not employ an artificial airway is the self-inflation bag or positive-pressure demand valve. Both of those techniques use a face mask, which is often the Achilles heel of the system. The bag or demand valve is used during cardiorespiratory arrests, during the postoperative period, or after suctioning. The two most common errors in this system are (1) underinflation due to poor mask fit with leaks and (2) overinflation due to overenthusiastic but poor technique. The author has witnessed a tension pneumothorax produced by excessive squeezing of a resuscitation bag. It must be remembered that the total volume of the bag of 1.5 to 2.0 liters need not be emptied into the airway rapidly. This will only serve to subject the lungs to extremely high airway pressures. Demand valve resuscitation systems (Hare-Elder Lightweight Portable Demand Valve Resuscitator, Dynamed Co., Carlsbad, Calif.) can be powered by a 50-psi tank of compressed air or, more likely, oxygen. This is an excellent portable emergency technique since the valve can also be triggered without patient demand and therefore function as a miniventilator. These devices are gaining popularity in hazardous industrial cases such as in mines and at firefighting locations.

In the comatose patient, the triple airway maneuver is necessary to ensure upper airway patency.[2] The triple airway maneuver includes (1) tilt head backward, (2) displace mandible forward, and (3) open mouth. Oropharyngeal and nasopharyngeal tubes substitute for the last two components of the triple maneuver (jaw thrust and opening of the mouth). Even with these partial artificial airways in place, head tilt backward is required to guarantee an open airway.

PARTIAL ARTIFICIAL AIRWAYS

Oropharyngeal Device

The oropharyngeal airway has limited use as an emergency tool in the comatose patient. As consciousness returns, this airway may produce gagging, vomiting, and laryngospasm. The most important use of this device is to prevent the tongue from falling back against the upper palate. A secondary use is to prevent teeth from sealing off the mouth so that oral secretions could not be suctioned. The oropharyngeal airway should only be left in place until one of the more permanent solutions to upper airway obstruction can be employed.

Nasopharyngeal Airway

The nasopharyngeal airway (affectionately called "the trumpet") is an excellent temporary technique to manage upper airway problems. It is hollow, made of a latex rubber, and shaped to follow the posterior wall curvature of the nasopharynx. The tip is beveled, and with lubrication and topical anesthesia of the nose the airway is easily placed in position. The sharp side of the airway is inserted along the medial aspect of the nose, which is devoid of the rich blood vessel supply of the lateral mucosa. An α-sympathomimetic such as phenylephrine will prepare the nose adequately. The tip of the catheter helps separate the tongue from the posterior pharyngeal wall. In addition to its use in preventing upper airway obstruction, the nasopharyngeal tube facilitates nasal suctioning with a small ($-12F$) catheter. This technique can avoid the repeated trauma of placing a catheter down the naris during each attempt. A nasopharyngeal tube should be repositioned in the opposite naris every 4 days to avoid pressure necrosis.

FULL ARTIFICIAL AIRWAYS: ENDOTRACHEAL TUBES

Indications for Use

There are five accepted indications for placing an endotracheal tube in a patient (Table 56–1): (1) non-

TABLE 56–1   Indications for Endotracheal Intubation

Indication	Clinical Example
Maintain patent airway	Stroke
Protect against aspiration	Drug overdose
Tracheobronchial suctioning	Acute asthma
Positive-pressure mechanical ventilation	Guillain-Barré syndrome
High-level oxygen administration	Viral pneumonia

patency of the upper airway, (2) protection of the airway from aspiration, (3) tracheobronchial suctioning, (4) mechanical ventilation, and (5) severe hypoxemia without hypercapnia.

Nonpatency of the Upper Airway

Upper airway obstruction is frequently encountered as part of a larger medical emergency. It accompanies the unconsciousness of a cardiopulmonary arrest and the coma following severe cerebrovascular accident and drug overdose. In these cases, obstruction is due to a loss of pharyngeal muscle tone and control of the tongue. A recently discovered episodic loss of tone of the pharyngeal muscles during sleep is the basis of obstructive sleep apnea.

A second source of upper airway obstruction results from medical conditions such as allergic anaphylaxis, direct laryngeal trauma, inhalation burns, subglottic edema, and bleeding. In these cases, the soft tissues surrounding the airway swell and obstruct the air channel. The third mechanism is due to a foreign body or particular aspiration. A clue to the presence of partial obstruction is a low-pitched snoring or high-pitched stridor sound during inspiration. The latter should not be mistaken for asthma, which is usually worse during expiration. When complete obstruction occurs, there will be no sound made by the patient; marked inspiratory efforts without air flow are observed. A patient will often clutch the throat with one hand, and this has become an almost universal emergency sign of complete upper airway obstruction.

The first step in the emergency care of airway obstruction is to position the patient (if unconscious) in the lateral decubitus position, extend the neck, and clear the mouth of the tongue and vomitus. In a conscious patient, the Heimlich or an equivalent maneuver may be employed to increase intrathoracic pressure and to expel the foreign body. Oropharyngeal or nasopharyngeal airways can be quickly inserted. Ventilation by face mask should be carried out. If these measures do not ensure a clear upper airway, an endotracheal tube should be inserted. Massive soft tissue swelling from

irritation or trauma are two of the rare situations that require a cricothyroidotomy or emergency tracheostomy. These techniques will be discussed in greater detail later in the chapter. Attempts to introduce an endotracheal tube down such an airway could lead to tragic results with complete obstruction and death.

Protection of Airway

Even more common than the loss of pharyngeal muscle tone during the obtunded state of consciousness is the loss of the airway's protective reflexes. The "gag and swallowing reflex" via the glossopharyngeal nerve is the first one to be diminished. The vagus nerve mediates the laryngeal reflex protecting the epiglottis and, more distantly, the cough reflex of the upper trachea and carina. As these protective mechanisms are lost in descending order, the airway becomes vulnerable to both massive aspiration from vomiting and more subtle, continuous aspiration of gastric and pharyngeal contents. The patient who is comatose secondary to drug overdose has the additional risk of iatrogenic aspiration during gastric lavage. All airways that are unprotected for more than a brief time require a cuffed artificial airway to prevent aspiration. In some situations, such as recovery from anesthesia or after the lavage attempt, this airway can be rapidly removed, if consciousness is restored.

A particularly difficult problem is the patient with neurologic deficit from degenerative or demyelinating disease or cerebral vascular disease who has intermittent incompetency in airway protection. In this case, major problems originate from aspiration of pharyngeal content rather than gastric vomitus. Cuffed tracheostomy tubes are used in these patients. The length of time these airways are utilized is usually determined by the progression of the primary neurologic disease. With better equipment and the education of both the patient and society, a trend toward permanent tracheostomy has taken place. With a permanent artificial airway, the patient can avoid those problems resulting from poor coughing ability particularly during periods of upper airway infection. With proper airway care, the incidence of infection due to the tracheostomy has been reduced to a minimum.

Long-term use of a tracheostomy tube to prevent aspiration is not effective. A cuffed tube cannot be inflated indefinitely, and without such protection the airway is vulnerable to aspirated oral secretions. There is some evidence that placement of a tracheostomy tube without an inflated cuff can even promote aspiration, especially during eating and sleeping. A feeding esophagoscopy is a more permanent solution for a neurologically disabled patient who can not protect the airway.

Tracheobronchial Suctioning

An artificial tube should rarely be utilized solely for the purpose of improving bronchial toilet. In most clinical situations, coaching and encouragement by nursing or respiratory therapy personnel will produce an adequate cough effort by the patient. This can be further aided with postural drainage, additional chest physical therapy, and appropriate nasal suctioning techniques. Patients who are not helped by these conservative measures because of extreme weakness or an altered state of consciousness are also in danger of airway obstruction.

Occasionally, the patient with COPD who is quite alert develops severe dehydration, very thick mucus plugs in the airway, and a severely impaired cough due to fatigue. In these cases, an orotracheal or nasotracheal tube is placed to carry out limited lavage through a fiberoptic bronchoscope and repeated short-term suctioning.

A rare candidate for short-term intubation is the patient with lobar atelectasis in whom a trial of incentive spirometry or spontaneous sighing has not been successful. The use of a hyperinflation resuscitation bag (e.g., Ambu) and positioning is a valuable adjunct in these patients.

Mechanical Ventilation

The use of positive-pressure ventilators is the major indication for intubation. Except for the pediatric age-group, all endotracheal tubes have balloon cuffs that permit sealing of the airway so that pressure produced by an external device can be applied directly to the lungs. The seal also prevents gastric distention and aspiration. The selection of the type of endotracheal tube or tracheostomy tube is not based on the specific positive-pressure ventilator. A universal 15-mm connector permits the attachment of any ventilator to most tubes. Consideration of such factors as the estimated duration of ventilatory support or the level of peak airway pressure will determine the choice of artificial airway.

Ultrashort-term support during the intraoperative or the immediate postoperative period would favor the use of the orotracheal tube. Longer ventilatory support for several days may be expected in patients with acute CO_2 retention secondary to COPD. These cases may be best managed with nasotracheal tubes. However, some physicians continue to prefer oral over nasal tubes in all cases.

The tracheostomy tube is usually reserved for patients who require ventilatory support for weeks to months. In patients with neurologic respiratory failure secondary to Guillain-Barré syndrome or tetanus, an endotracheal tube should be replaced by a tracheostomy early in the treatment period.

Another consideration about tube selection relates to the level of peak airway pressure. The Kamen-Wilkenson Fome cuff tube with a self-inflating cuff will often not permit application of positive airway pressures exceeding 70 cm H_2O. In all other cases, this tube seems to be very satisfactory. One advantage of the self-inflating cuff tube is that it requires no addition of air by nursing personnel. This feature minimizes problems with leaks and overdistention.

Severe Hypoxemia without Hypercapnia

Endotracheal tubes are occasionally placed in patients who do not require mechanical ventilation but who will benefit from PEEP. This can be achieved in a variety of ways in the spontaneously breathing patient; the most common way is to apply continuous positive airway pressure (CPAP) through a cuffed endotracheal tube. Patients who benefit from such pressure are grouped into the adult respiratory distress syndrome (ARDS). Management with an endotracheal tube and PEEP without mechanical ventilation is becoming a popular ventilation modality in such patients.

Rarely, an endotracheal tube is placed solely to permit the patient to breathe the highest supplemental oxygen possible. Levels of oxygen very close to 100 percent with good humidification can be given to the patient over an extended period. Without intubation, the highest level of oxygen that can be consistently administered by mask approaches 70 to 80 percent.

Selection of Orifice: Orotracheal versus Nasotracheal Tube

There are two choices in placing an endotracheal tube into the patient: (1) the oral and (2) the nasal route (Table 56–2). The advantages of orotracheal intubation are speed of placing the tube through the cords and establishing airway control and tube size. In a resuscitation situation, the oral route is the only choice since it provides the quickest entrance into the trachea. This

TABLE 56–2   Indications for Orotracheal and Nasotracheal Tubes

Criterion	Orotracheal	Nasotracheal
Rapid intubation	x	
Better stabilization		x
Mandibular-cervical problems		x
Larger diameter airway	x	
Bleeding diathesis	x	
Sinus infection	x	
Long-term intubation		x

also applies to many emergency department situations in which seconds rather than minutes count. The oral route also allows placement of a tube 0.5 to 1.0 mm larger in internal diameter than a nasal tube. This is sometimes critical in allowing bronchoscopic procedures through the tube.

Disadvantages of an oral tube are more discomfort for the patient, inability to sip fluids, and poor stabilization of the tube, leading to accidental extubation or main-stem bronchial intubation.

Nasotracheal intubation affords increased patient comfort and better stability of the tube in the awake patient requiring intubation. In addition, there are situations in which access to the airway via the oral route cannot be gained. Temporomandibular dislocation, masseter spasm, tetanus, oral cavity pathology and cervical vertebral pathology are examples of situations where nasotracheal intubation must be used.

A final advantage of the nasal tube is the use of the blind nasotracheal intubation technique. The patient who does not require emergency intubation within seconds can have a tube placed through the nose into the trachea without the use of a laryngoscope. In skilled hands, this is a simple procedure very well accepted by the patient.

The contraindications to nasal intubation are increased bleeding tendencies or acute sinusitis and central nervous system infection secondary to fracture of facial or skull bones. Patients on anticoagulant therapy or with severe thrombocytopenia should not be subjected to the chance of a posterior nasopharyngeal bleed following placement of a nasal tube. Acute epiglottitis is a contraindication to nasotracheal intubation that is performed blindly.

Selection of Tubes

Large Volume Cuff

Major advances in technology over the past 10 years provide the emergency physician with a wide selection of satisfactory endotracheal tubes. Problems related to toxic materials utilized in the manufacture of tubes have been eliminated through the use of inert synthetic polyvinyl chloride or Silastic material. Construction of the cuff allows for a large volume with little pressure exerted to the surrounding tracheal wall. The high-volume/low-pressure principle of the modern cuff only works if the cuff is not overinflated to achieve a seal. Proper size selection of the endotracheal tube will eliminate leaks around a cuff that is too small for the airway. Frequently, a seal cannot be achieved at certain areas of the trachea due to preexisting tracheomalacia. Even a large volume cuff does not guarantee definite prevention of aspiration, since secretions can drain down

the folds of a not fully inflated cuff.[3] Specially designed tubes, such as the directional tip-control tubes (Endotrol), may be particularly useful for blind nasotracheal intubation.

Radiopaque Marker

One feature of the modern endotracheal tube is a radiopaque line running down the length of the tube all the way to the tip. This line is very useful in the radiologic determination of tube placement. Endotracheal tubes can be used for oral or nasal intubation. Tubes are maufactured 6 to 10 cm longer than necessary for oral use, and this extra length should be removed after an orotracheal tube is placed in a patient.

Lumen Size

Selection of the size of a tube is very important. Unfortunately, there is no uniform system to designate tubes made by different manufacturers. Endotracheal tubes are usually designated according to the internal diameter (ID). The range of tubes for adults goes from 5.0 to 10.0 mm ID (20 to 40 French gauge). Most of the time, selection will be from 6.0 to 8.5 mm for women and 7.0 to 9.5 mm for men. Tracheostomy tubes, on the other hand, are labeled with outer diameter (OD) sizes and range from 8 to 12 mm OD (24 to 42 French gauge). With experience, one can select the proper tube for a patient based on overall body size. The correct choice is the largest tube that can get through the vocal cords and cricoid cartilage area without difficulty. It is best to avoid a tube so large that it must be forced through the vocal cords. Tubes that are too large are associated with increased tracheal damage.

Endotracheal tubes that are too small may not provide an adequate cuff seal, are difficult to suction through, and will not allow a fiberoptic bronchoscope to be placed down the lumen. When switching from an oral tube to a nasal tube, it is necessary to use a tube with a 0.5 to 1.0 mm smaller ID.

Methods of Intubation

The positioning of the patient's head and neck, the identification of proper anatomical landmarks, the preparation of the endotracheal tube, and the premedication of the pharynx for direct oral intubation have been adequately described in several textbooks,[4] and there is no substitute for "hands-on" execution of these steps under skilled supervision. Each patient presents unique challenges, and only through this experience can one feel secure about intubation skills. (See Chapter 71.)

There are a few principles that will aid in providing a safety factor for the patient. There are two vital considerations every time a patient is intubated: oxygenation and suctioning. The first step in treating a severely hypoxemic patient in respiratory distress is *not* to place a laryngoscope blade into the mouth and search for the vocal cords. Cardiac arrest can result from attempting to intubate the hypoxemic patient. Instead, a face mask attached to a resuscitation bag with 100 percent oxygen should be applied to the patient. Several seconds of oxygen delivery will raise the arterial oxygen tension and permit a safe and controlled intubation. In some borderline patients, pretreatment with 0.5 mg IV atropine is recommended to avoid excessive vagal tone leading to severe bradycardia or laryngospasm. A resuscitation bag attached to a properly sized mask should be available at the bedside.

A second important factor is to have available adequate suctioning. This entails a device capable of extracting a large volume of material from the oral cavity (such as a Yankawer tip) and a suction capability of at least -115 mm Hg wall pressure. Concern about gastric content aspiration during intubation is so great that some physicians have recommended prior treatment with antacids.[5]

Orotracheal intubation is frequently aided by a stylet inserted into the tube, resulting in a favorable shape to the tube. This will increase the chances of a tracheal rather than an esophageal intubation. Care must be taken to lubricate the stylet so that it can be easily removed once the tube enters the trachea. Assurance that the tip of the stylet does not extend beyond the endotracheal tube will prevent mucosal damage. Muscle relaxants are occasionally needed to open the clenched jaw and get adequate visualization of the cords. One should only use these drugs after a thorough understanding of their pharmacology and with confidence that the tube can be placed into the trachea.

The keys to blind nasal intubation are the preparation of the nose and posterior pharynx, the positioning of the head in the forward flexed position, and the advancement of the tube simultaneous with a deep inspiration.

The nasal orifice with the largest lumen should be chosen. A topical anesthetic and a vasoconstrictor should be applied to the nasal channel. This combination is ideally served using topical cocaine 4% sprayed down the nose. Following this medication a lubricated nasopharyngeal tube is placed in the nose and then removed. This alerts one to possible obstruction of the passage and also dilates the area for easier insertion of the nasotracheal tube. The tube is lubricated and slowly passed through the naris using firm but controlled pressure. The tube should not be forced through a very tight obstruction. Great resistance means that the tip of the tube must be redirected or replaced with a smaller lumen tube. Once the narrow nasal passage is entered,

the tube will easily advance toward the vocal cords. By monitoring the air flow through the tube looking for clear breath sounds and water vapor that alternately condenses during inspiration and evaporates during expiration, the tube can be blindly thrust forward during the next inspiration. If this technique does not succeed after three or four tries with repositioning of the head, then the visual approach using a McGill forceps and a laryngoscope should be attempted. This is a two person technique. One person visualizes the tip of the tube and the vocal cords with one hand and guides the tube in the direction of the cords with the McGill forceps in the other hand. Care must be taken not to damage the cuff with the forceps. A second person pushes the distal end of the tube through the nose upon demand. The endotracheal tube is aligned with the larynx by appropriate flexion and extension of the head. Translaryngeal anesthesia using a 22-gauge 1″ needle and 2.0 ml of 4% lidocaine injected midline into the cricothyroid membrane has been recommended by some to facilitate blind nasotracheal intubation, avoid laryngospasm and prevent excess reflex sympathetic discharge. Adequate oxygenation during this procedure can be maintained by administering 10 liter/min oxygen flow through a nasal catheter passed down the opposing nare. The use of the bronchoscope provides a new method of intubation in difficult cases. The tube is placed through the nose to the back of the pharynx. The flexible fiberoptic bronchoscope is placed through the tube and directed through the vocal cords into the midtrachea. Then the endotracheal tube is placed over the bronchoscope through the cords. The smallest lumen tube that allows easy movement of the bronchoscope is 7.5 mm. An 8.0–9.0 mm ID tube is preferred.

A checklist for endotracheal intubation is presented below:

- Check tube and cuff prior to intubation.
- Preoxygenate patient.
- Have adequate suction equipment available.
- Check position of tube tip after intubation by radiology or bronchoscopy.
- Stabilize the tube to prevent movement.
- Monitor cuff volume and pressure.
- Use humidification and catheter suction to maintain tube patency.

Care and Troubleshooting

Tube Placement

Attention to simple but significant detail is the key to good endotracheal care. Immediately on placement of the tube, the cuff should be inflated (unless a passive cuff is being used) to 5 to 8 ml or until an obvious leak is sealed while gently ventilating the patient with a self-inflating bag. Breath sounds should be checked in the axillary region and these should be symmetrical on both sides. For oral intubation, observation of the centimeter scale along the length of the tube is helpful. The 22 to 24 cm mark opposite the teeth generally indicates good placement. Initially, intubation of the right main bronchus occurs in up to 10 percent of the cases. Radiographic or bronchoscopic confirmation of proper tube placement is helpful.[6] The tip of the tube should be 4 to 6 cm above the carina with the patient's head in a neutral position. Flexion of the neck can cause a 2 cm descent of the tube. Temporary overinflation of the cuff with palpation of the neck to feel the trachea rise is an additional technique to check for inadvertent endobronchial intubation.

Overinflation of Cuff

The introduction of the Kamen-Wilkenson Fome self-inflating cuff, the Shiley tube with the pressure relief valve, and the Lanz tube with the external pilot balloon reservoir are all attempts to prevent overdistention of the cuff, leading to tracheal damage. Only the amount of air needed to seal the airway, and *no* more, should be used. Many physicians recommend a "minimal leak" be present as long as tidal volume during mechanical ventilation is not lost.

The volume of air in the cuff and the intercuff pressure should be measured using the gauge of a blood pressure cuff. These pressures can be recorded on a piece of tape applied to the cuff inflation site. This allows the medical staff to monitor the pressure two to three times a day. Intracuff pressure in a proper-sized tube with a large volume cuff should be under 20 mm Hg. The chest roentgenogram provides an additional clue to cuff size for the air shadow of the cuff can be seen surrounding the tube.[7] Stabilization of the tube is vital to prevent accidental movement into the right mainstem bronchus and extubation. After proper placement of the tip of the tube is confirmed, the tube should be taped to the face using the area above the upper lip and below the lower lip on the chin. If an oral tube is used, it should be anchored at the corner of the mouth. An oropharyngeal airway is also placed in the mouth to prevent biting of the tube and to facilitate oral suctioning. Stabilizing nasal tubes is easier. Commercial tube holders are available and helpful in long-term intubation. Frequently in orotracheal intubation, several centimeters of the distal portion of the tube can be cut off.

Tube Obstruction

Problems with lumen obstruction due to mucous crusting or herniation of the cuff have been largely eliminated by suctioning techniques, humidification, and proper tube construction. Occasionally a suction catheter will not completely pass through the length of the tube. This will signal either mid-tube compression, especially in nasointubation, or placement of the tip of the tube too close to the carina. Repositioning the head will usually relieve the obstruction due to compression while slight withdrawal of the tube will prevent carinal contact.

Cuff Leak

Cuff leak is perhaps the most common problem associated with an endotracheal tube. It is usually detected by observation of air passing out of the oral cavity instead of through the tube. In situations in which large amounts of positive pressure are being used, small air leaks are expected. As long as there is no significant loss of tidal volume, this so-called minimal leak is not objectionable and may even be a good protection against excessive cuff pressure. Differentiation between a cuff that has lost volume due to a temporary leak and a defective cuff that cannot hold air volume must be made. If a cuff is structurally damaged, large volumes of air can be injected into the cuff but the amount cannot be recovered when attempts are made to evacuate the air. A defective cuff requires a tube change while a temporary leak only needs the addition of the lost volume and/or repositioning of the tube. Sometimes the defect is not with the cuff itself, but with the cuff injection device. In this case, a temporary adaptor can be used and the endotracheal tube can be salvaged. It should be noted that persisting leak may be due to the cuff being situated at the level of the cords. Repositioning is required. A common mistake made by medical and nursing personnel is to routinely deflate the cuff every few hours to reduce the possibilities of pressure necrosis. There is no evidence or justification for this practice. In addition, aspiration can result if secretions that accumulate in the larynx above the cuff are not removed each time. There is no need to routinely change well-functioning endotracheal tubes. Experience has shown that maintenance of the same tube for several weeks is possible without major morbidity.[8,9] Some physicians suggest that a nasotracheal tube should be repositioned into the opposite naris every week in prolonged nasointubation, but this is not an established view.

Postextubation Problems

Patients must be carefully watched immediately following extubation. After short-term intubation, there is a risk of upper airway obstruction due to laryngospasm or subglottic edema. Extubation following long-term use of an endotracheal tube can lead to airway obstruction due to granuloma. Inspiratory stridor is a common sign of these events. Occasionally, upper airway obstruction will appear several weeks to months following extubation. In this case, obstruction is due to tracheomalacia and circumferential stenosis is due to scarring at the site where the inflated cuff had been positioned.

Rare complications of prolonged endotracheal intubation include tracheoesophageal fistula and vocal cord paralysis. The combination of a large-bore nasogastric tube with an endotracheal or tracheostomy tube seems to aid in the development of these fistulas. Some physicians recommend immediate nebulization of a vasoconstrictor and corticosteroid therapy for several hours following extubation to prevent or treat subglottic edema.

CRICOTHYROIDOTOMY AND TRACHEOSTOMY

The major indication for a tracheostomy tube is to maintain an artificial airway for periods of weeks and more. Tracheostomy as the immediate emergency measure without prior endotracheal intubation is performed only in the rarest situations. Maxillary-mandibular trauma and trauma to the larynx with inhalation burn injury are examples of these uncommon situations. The use of immediate emergency tracheostomy in acute epiglottis in children is still being debated.[10] (See Chapter 57.)

Cricothyroidotomy

Experience has shown that tracheostomy when done as an emergency procedure outside the operating room is associated with high morbidity and occasional mortality.[11] The complication rate in emergency tracheostomy is five times higher than in elective tracheostomies. In cases in which quick entrance to the lower airway must be gained, a cricothyroidotomy should be attempted. After quickly infiltrating the area with a topical anesthetic and injecting some through the cricoid membrane, a sharp scapel blade is used to penetrate the membrane. A 4 to 5 mm ID tracheostomy tube can be placed through the triangular membrane located above the cricoid cartilage. Only minor bleeding should occur. In extreme emergencies, a 14-gauge needle passed through the cricothyroid membrane will suffice until a more satisfactory airway can be obtained.

The cricothyroidotomy technique can be carried out successfully in 30 to 45 seconds and should be the special procedure used in the emergency department when approach to the lower airway from the mouth or nose is impossible. Cricothyroidotomies should be converted to a standard tracheostomy once the patient has been stabilized if an artificial airway is still required. (See Chapter 71.)

Emergency Tracheostomy

In only the rarest conditions such as direct laryngeal trauma to the hyoid bone, the thyroid cartilage, and the cricoid cartilage or subglottic stenosis will a cricothyroidotomy not be effective. A rapid tracheostomy using a deep vertical incision from the cricoid cartilage to the sternal notch is employed. The cervical trachea will not be visible but can be palpated following this incision. Several rings are rapidly cut vertically, and an airway is placed.

Only after airway patency is ensured can attention be paid to the brisk bleeding that accompanies all emergency tracheostomies. This total procedure can take 60 to 90 seconds.

The materials and cuff construction of a tracheostomy tube are very similar to an endotracheal tube produced by the same manufacturer. Therefore, airway care related to the cuff is identical. Some tracheostomy tubes (e.g., Shiley) have an inner cannula that must be routinely removed and cleaned. Immediately following a tracheostomy, the site around the incision requires special attention to avoid serious wound infection. Tracheostomy wound care is discussed in several standard surgical texts. (See Chapter 71.)

Tracheostomy Complications

An uncommon but grave complication occurring in about 0.4 percent of tracheostomies is innominate artery erosion.[12] While this is usually associated with cancer of the trachea, it can also occur in any tracheostomy owing to anterior erosion at the tracheostomy site or with low placement of the tracheostomy below the third cartilaginous ring. The emergency care in this case is to remove the tracheostomy tube, place an endotracheal tube distal to the erosion, and inflate the cuff to prevent aspiration of blood. This may require intubating the right main-stem bronchus. A second endotracheal tube should be placed into the tracheostomy site with the balloon inflated to tamponade the bleeding point. Direct finger pressure through the tracheostomy can also be applied.

Although changing tracheostomy tubes is usually a routine procedure in a healed tracheostomy site, problems can occur with changing new tubes. Misplacement of the tube in the paratracheal soft tissue can occur, and if not quickly detected this catastrophe can lead to cardiac arrest. Displacement of the tube resulted in a 25 percent mortality in one series.[11] It takes 5 to 7 days before a clear tract is formed between skin and the entrance into the trachea. Frequently there will be great difficulty in placing the new tube back into the trachea. Therefore, it is recommended that the tube not be removed for the first few days. If an emergency occurs, such as a defect in the cuff, then a suction catheter should be placed through the old tube into the trachea and left in place as the tube is removed over the catheter. The new tracheostomy tube is then inserted back over the suction catheter, which serves as a guide wire. Whenever a tracheostomy tube is being replaced, a mask and a resuscitation bag connected to oxygen should be available. The patient should be placed in the identical position in which the tracheostomy was originally done. This will help to line up the skin site with the entrance into the trachea.

Two complications particularly associated with tracheostomy are mediastinitis from extension of local infection at the tracheostomy site and subcutaneous and mediastinal emphysema from too tight a wound closure.

ESOPHAGEAL AIRWAYS

A recent addition to emergency airway care has been the esophageal obturator airway (EOA). This technique was especially introduced in 1973 to aid paramedics not skilled in the use of a laryngoscope. The EOA consists of a 33 cm curved cuffed tube that is not open at the distal end. It is designed to enter the esophagus, a procedure that is generally easy to accomplish. The cuff is inflated to 35 ml of air. Above the cuff, which seals off the esophagus from the trachea, are 16 holes. Through these passages air can be directed throughout the posterior pharynx. Since it cannot enter the esophagus it is forced into the trachea. A sealed mask fits around the nose and mouth that prevents air from exiting above. This technique has only had limited popularity and is adequate for short-term ventilation only. Contraindications to the use of the EOA are in (1) pediatric population, (2) conscious patients, (3) patients known to have ingested caustic substances, and (4) patients with known esophageal disease.

The major complications with using the EOA are (1) inadvertent tracheal intubation, (2) esophageal perfo-

ration, and (3) gastric fluid aspiration at the time of removal. Midesophagus perforations have been reported in 0.1 to 2 percent of a series of survivors.[13] It has been suggested that the cuff inflation be limited to 20 ml of air to reduce the incidence of perforation.

Since the tube is not placed through the vocal cords, airway patency is not assured with an esophageal airway. There is still need to maintain backward tilt of the head. This technique, therefore, should be considered only better than a simple mask and self-inflating bag during resuscitation. Its use ends when endotracheal intubation can be accomplished.

REFERENCES

1. Menn SJ, Tisi M: Oxygen as a drug: Chemical properties, benefits and hazards of administration, in Burton G (ed): *Respiratory Care*. Philadelphia, JB Lippincott Co, 1977, pp 386–398.
2. Safar P: *Cardiopulmonary Cerebral Resuscitation*. Stavenger, Norway, Asmund S. Laerdal, 1981, pp 21–24.
3. Pavlin EG, Van Nimwegan D, Hornbein TF: Failure of a high-compliance, low-pressure cuff to prevent aspiration. *Anesthesiology* 42:216–219, 1975.
4. Rattenborg C: *Clinical Use of Mechanical Ventilation*. Chicago, Year Book Medical, 1981, pp 186–195.
5. Roberts RB, Shirley MA: Reducing the risk of acid aspiration during caesarean section. *Anesth Analg* 53:859–868, 1974.
6. Goodman LR, Conrardy PA, Lange F, et al: Radiographic evaluation of endotracheal tube position. *Am J Roentgenol* 127:433, 1976.
7. Khan F, Reddy N, Khan A: Cuff trachea ratio as an indicator of tracheal damage. *Chest* 70:431, 1976.
8. Taylor H, Mhoon E, Matz G: *Complications due to Tracheostomy and Endotracheal Tubes*. Chicago, Year Book Medical, 1981, chap 25.
9. Freeman GR: A comparative analysis of endotracheal intubation in neonates, children and adults: Complications, prevention and treatment. *Laryngoscope* 82:1385, 1972.
10. Schuller DE, Birck HG: The safety of intubation in croup and epiglottitis: An eight year follow-up. *Laryngoscope* 85:33, 1975.
11. Chew J, Cantrell RW: Tracheostomy complications and their management. *Arch Otolaryngol* 96:538, 1972.
12. Cooper JD: Tracheo-innominate artery fistula: Successful management in three consecutive cases. *Ann Thorac Surg* 24:439, 1977.
13. Kassels S, Robinson W, O'Bara K: Esophageal perforation associated with esophageal obturator airway. *Crit Care Med* 8:386, 1980.

57. Obstructive Lung Diseases

THOMAS CLARKE KRAVIS, M.D.

This chapter addresses the prehospital treatment and emergency care of patients with obstructive respiratory emergencies (see Fig. 57–1). In the first section the common causes of acute upper airway disease are reviewed. Supraglottitis (epiglottitis), a common disease of children and increasingly recognized in adults, is distinguished from croup. A discussion of foreign body obstruction of the upper airway is followed by a review of anaphylaxis, since this process may involve upper airway obstruction and is mechanistically similar to allergic asthma.

The discussion on obstructive diseases of the lower airways concentrates on the potentially reversible components of asthma, emphysema, and bronchitis. A common therapeutic approach for the acute treatment of patients with lower airways diseases is presented.

UPPER AIRWAY DISEASES

Acute Supraglottitis or Epiglottitis

Definition

Acute supraglottitis is the rapid development of inflammation of the mucous membranes involving the supraglottic portion of the larynx above the true vocal cords including the epiglottis, aryepiglottic folds, ventricular bands, pharynx, and arytenoid cartilage. This process may lead to acute upper airway obstruction.

Etiology

Acute supraglottitis commonly occurs in children aged 2 to 7, but is being increasingly recognized in the adult patient.[1] Cultures taken from the epiglottis and blood have suggested *Hemophilus influenzae* (group B) as the most common etiologic agent in children.[2] *Streptococcus* group A, *Streptococcus pneumoniae*, and *Staphylococcus pyogenes* have been implicated particularly in adult patients.[3] Parainfluenza virus, adenovirus, *Streptococcus viridans*, nonpathogenic *Neisseria*, and respiratory syncytial virus have each been associated with the process. No seasonal predilection is noted.

Pathology

The infectious agents induce an acute inflammatory response, with the histological appearance of polymorphonuclear leukocytes, edema, erythema, and submucosal abscess of the structures in the most cephalad portion of the larynx.

Pathophysiology and Clinical Correlates

The development of acute epiglottitis may rapidly lead to acute and total airway obstruction. A number of different mechanisms have been postulated that may be responsible for the development of airway obstruction. Obstruction may be related to the rate at which the inflammatory response occurs and the size of the airway opening. For example, the process is frequently observed in children where the tracheal diameter is small,

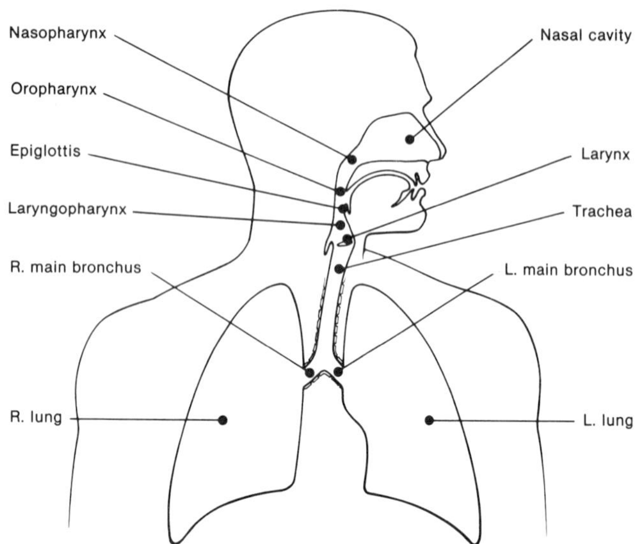

Figure 57–1 Anatomy of the Respiratory Tract.

and the course often fulminant, whereas in the adult patient the disease is not so common and may have a longer prodromal state.

Chronic inflammatory changes usually do not cause obstruction. It is possible that the loosely attached structures become edematous and fold back over the glottic opening thereby producing obstruction. Aspiration of pooled secretions into a partially compromised glottic opening may also contribute. The tongue, floor of the mouth, and the supraglottic structures are hypersensitive to stimulation, and this may cause reflex laryngospasm. Irritation of the vocal cords in the setting of hypoxemia and hypercapnia may also cause laryngospasm. Finally, respiratory failure as a result of increased work of breathing in an exhausted, fatigued patient may lead to respiratory arrest. (See Chapter 59.)

History

The history usually commences with difficulty breathing, fever to 104°F (40°C), and stridor. The abrupt onset may be associated with sore throat, dysphagia, painful swallowing, and cough. A muffled voice (not a brassy croup-like cough or hoarseness) may result from the inflamed mucosa tightly adhering to the mucosal covering of the vocal cords. These symptoms characteristically progress rapidly.

The signs and symptoms are often out of proportion to the objective clinical physical findings. The patient may sit erect with the mouth open and tongue protruding, and appear apprehensive and fearful. Severe dysphagia results in the accumulation of saliva and secretions causing drooling. There may be inspiratory dyspnea and findings of inspiratory-expiratory stridor

with retraction. The appearance of cyanosis, exhaustion, prominent retraction, and tachycardia suggests severe hypoxemia and hypercapnia, imminent respiratory failure, and the requirement for immediate intervention.

Physical Examination

The patient with suspected acute supraglottitis should be examined by a physician skilled and experienced in the technique of airway maintenance. The physical exam should follow a lateral roentgenographic examination (portable equipment) of the neck unless the patient is in extremis. The patient should be sitting with the head extended and the mouth open, but in infants and small children this probably can be safely done in the supine position. The epiglottis may be visualized directly or with an illuminated mirror attachment. A tongue blade may be inserted into the oropharynx, and moved gently and laterally against the buccal mucosa. This may reveal the characteristic swollen, cherry-red epiglottis. The cephalad position of the epiglottis makes visualization easier in the child than in the adult.

If the epiglottis is not visualized, then the patient should be placed on O_2 in the supine head-tilt position, and examined with a laryngoscope. If the characteristic findings of epiglottitis are visualized, then endotracheal intubation at the time of the procedure can be accomplished, and the patient reintubated with a nasotracheal tube subsequently, if desired. Alternatively, the patient may be ventilated with a mask and bag and humidified O_2 until airway establishment can be accomplished under controlled settings in an operating room.

Laboratory Diagnosis

When the diagnosis of supraglottitis is not obvious a lateral roentgenogram of the soft tissues of the neck should be obtained in the presence of a physician who can intubate the patient or perform a cricothyreotomy if necessary. The roentgenogram of the neck should be done with the patient sitting and the neck in extension. In a normal lateral neck roentgenogram the epiglottis resembles an adult's little finger on lateral projection; a wide rounded configuration of an inflamed epiglottis resembles an adult's thumb (Fig. 57–2 A).

Several diagnostic pitfalls must be appreciated when interpreting the lateral neck roentgenogram.[4] For example, the roentgenogram may appear normal early in the clinical course of acute epiglottitis. On expiration the posterior pharynx may bulge into the pharynx simulating a space-occupying retropharyngeal mass. The roentgenologic finding suggestive of an enlarged epiglottis is not always indicative of acute epiglottitis: supraglottitis may also be observed in foreign body re-

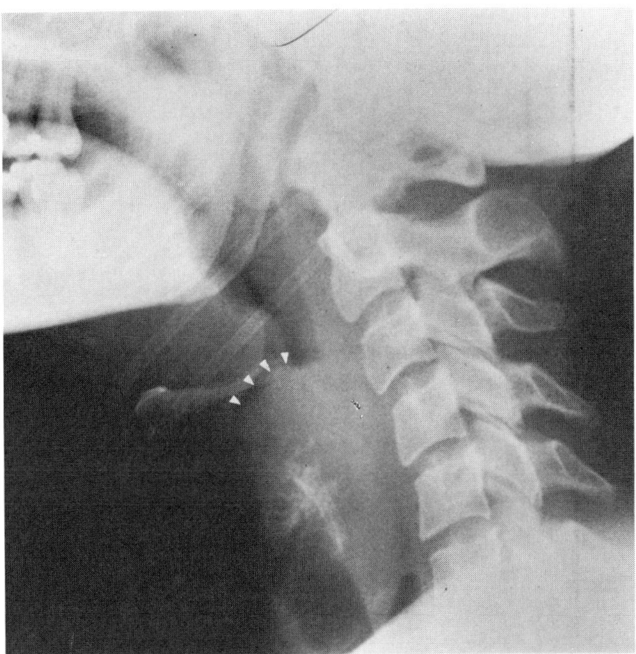

Figure 57–2 A Lateral Roentgenogram of the Structures in the Neck Demonstrating Enlargement of the Epiglottis and Arytenoids.

action, angioneurotic edema, chronic epiglottitis, and mucous membrane injury secondary to steam inhalation or swallowing hot liquids. Anteroposterior (AP) roentgenologic exams may reveal subglottic narrowing indistinguishable from croup (Fig. 57–2 B). The peripheral WBC count is elevated and the arterial blood gases abnormal, but neither is diagnostic.

Differential Diagnosis

In making the diagnosis of acute epiglottitis, a number of other processes should be considered: angioneurotic edema, aspiration of foreign bodies, blunt and penetrating traumatic injuries of the vocal cords, tumors, laryngismus, congenital lesions, acute spasmodic laryngitis, thermal and chemical burns, and reflex laryngospasm.[5] One should also consider Ludwig's angina, irritant fumes, near-drowning, laryngomalacia, and papillomas. Other infectious processes that may clinically mimic supraglottitis include diphtheria; pertussis; peritonsillar, peripharyngeal, and retropharyngeal abscesses; allergic drug reactions; and croup.

Treatment

Patients with suspected acute supraglottitis should be kept calm without unnecessary disturbances or manipulation of the upper airway.[6] The patient should never be left alone and medical personnel skilled in removing

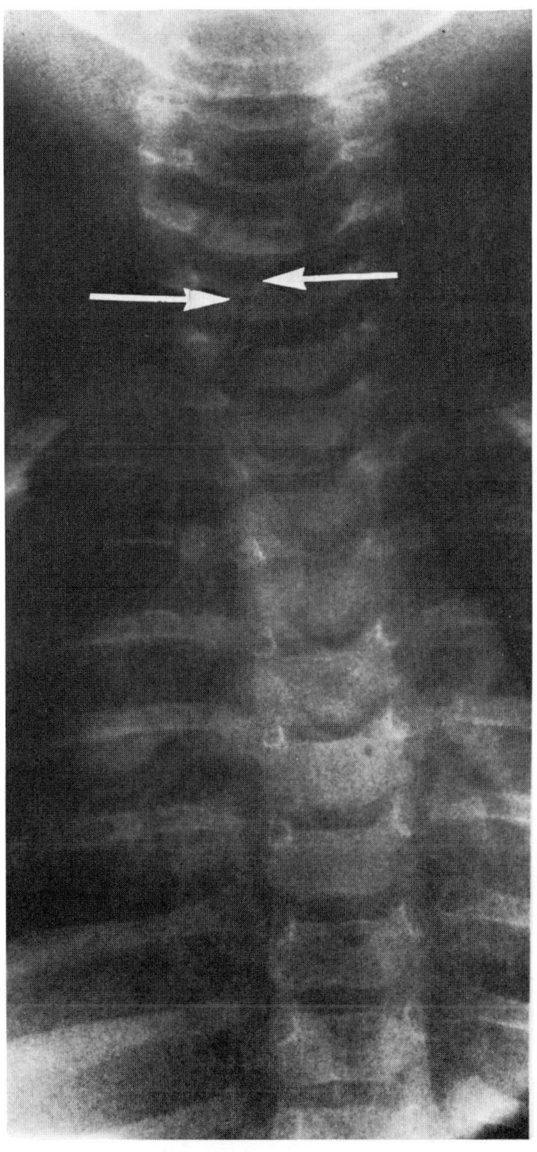

Figure 57–2 B AP Roentgenogram of the Neck Showing Subglottic Edema in a Patient with Croup.

or bypassing upper airway obstruction should always be present. Thus, the prehospital care of a patient with supraglottitis includes rapid transport in an emergency vehicle in the erect position.

When the diagnosis of acute supraglottitis is suspected, the aim of treatment is to be in a position to secure the airway at the time the epiglottis is visualized. At the time of examination, nasotracheal or endotracheal intubation may be required in the emergency department. The patient should be kept in the sitting position and an intravenous (IV) solution of 5 percent dextrose and water (D_5W) begun in a peripheral vein along with Valium for sedation if required. If the endotracheal tube cannot be introduced, then an endotracheal tube of one size smaller should be tried.

After intubation the patient should be placed in the supine position. Initial endotracheal intubation for 24 to 36 hours may be sufficient, and may avoid some of the major complications of nasotracheal tubes or tracheostomy. If stridor increases, hypercarbia or severe hypoxemia develops, or vital signs deteriorate, then immediate cricothyreotomy may be required in the rare patient who cannot be ventilated or intubated. Alternatively, the patient can sometimes be maintained on an air bag and mask on humidified O_2 while being brought to the operating room for elective intubation.[7]

Whether or not epinephrine and other β-adrenergic agonists used in other forms of acute airway disease are helpful in acute supraglottitis is controversial. Certainly the initiation of pharmacologic agents that may alleviate reversible airway obstruction regardless of the etiology should be considered once mechanical obstruction by foreign body has been ruled out. These can be administered in the field by prehospital care personnel, during transport, and in the emergency department. Stridor and airway spasm may be partially resolved with nebulized racemic epinephrine (2.25 percent Vaponephrine) with humidified O_2, and may be administered by mask or mouth piece. Anti-inflammatory agents such as steroids may be effective for inflammatory edema, but whether these pharmacologic agents are more effective than simple artificial airway management and antibiotics remains controversial.[8]

After appropriate cultures of blood and epiglottis have been obtained, the patient should be placed on ampicillin, 100 to 200 mg/kg/day every four hours IV. Because of the emergence of ampicillin-resistant *Hemophilus influenzae,* chloramphenicol at 50 mg/kg/day every six hours should also be given IV.

Complications of supraglottitis include up to a 5 percent mortality, respiratory failure, *Hemophilus influenzae* meningitis or pneumonia, and pulmonary edema.

Croup

Laryngotracheitis or laryngotracheal bronchitis is a subglottic inflammatory process involving structures below the true vocal cords including the larynx, bronchial tree, and trachea. Edema of these subglottic tissues may produce airway obstruction. The process commonly is a disease of children between the ages of 3 months and 3 years, and is usually associated with parainfluenza virus type 1, 2, and 3, coxsackievirus, echovirus, adenovirus, influenza virus type A and B, and respiratory syncytial virus.[9] In a large number of cases no organism is recovered. There is seasonal variation, with 80 percent of the cases occurring during the months of October through April.

Pathophysiology, History, and Clinical Correlates

The infectious agent proliferates in the upper respiratory tract, and the ensuing inflammatory changes, including edema and mucous exudation, decrease the size of the laryngotracheobronchial tree.

The clinical course includes the onset of upper respiratory tract-type symptoms, including brassy, barking, cough and fever. Although the clinical course may be milder than epiglottitis, except for fever, these signs and symptoms do not distinguish croup from epiglottitis. There may be hoarseness, inspiratory stridor, and expiratory wheezing with or without retraction, and the symptoms are often worse at night. Drooling is not prominent, and stridor is not aggravated by the patient's being in the supine position. A total of 2.5 percent of patients require an artificial airway.[10] Hypercapnia and hypoxemia secondary to alveolar hypoventilation and ventilation-perfusion abnormalities may develop.

The diagnostic approach for croup is similar to that for epiglottitis. The patient should be kept calm, a lateral roentgenogram of the neck should be obtained with portable equipment. The presence of a physician skilled in intubation or performing emergency cricothyreotomy-tracheostomy is mandatory. The lateral roentgenogram of the neck does not show an enlarged (inflamed) epiglottis. The AP view may show a convex inward subglottic narrowing at the level of the false cords (Fig. 57–2 B).

Differential Diagnosis

Croup must be distinguished from acute supraglottitis and the other processes that may mimic supraglottitis.

Treatment

Prehospital care of the patient with suspected croup includes rapid transport in the erect position while keeping the patient calm. Humidified O_2 and nebulized Vaponephrine (racemic epinephrine) 2.25 percent, 1 percent L-epinephrine, or terbutaline may be effective for symptomatic relief and may also help to avoid the subsequent need for intubation. These patients should be admitted and observed since the pharmacologic relief of the airway obstruction may be only temporary. Mild cases can be treated at home using a cool mist vaporizer and 40 percent O_2. Oral fluids should be encouraged and the respiratory rate monitored. If the patient is admitted, IV hydration may be required if the patient is unable to take liquids orally. Antibiotics are not required, and use of steroids is controversial. Complications of croup are respiratory failure, requiring intubation, and pulmonary edema.

Foreign Body Obstruction

Definition

Any material other than air saturated with water vapor is considered a foreign body in the tracheobronchial tree.

Etiology, Pathophysiology, and Clinical Correlates

Obstruction of the upper airway occurs commonly because of redundancy of the tongue in the patient with coma from drug overdose, central nervous system (CNS) depression, and cardiopulmonary arrest. Simple maneuvers such as the head tilt, jaw thrust and jaw lift, or the insertion of an oropharyngeal or nasopharyngeal airway may relieve the obstruction. Mucus, saliva, food, blood, and gastric contents may obstruct the airway, and in these instances prevention of aspiration is most important. In a patient with CNS depression, endotracheal intubation may be required in order to protect the airway from aspiration.

Aspirate may originate from above or below the epiglottis. Foreign materials from below the epiglottis usually originate from the vomiting of gastric contents. This may occur following a seizure, during cardiopulmonary resuscitation, at the time an esophageal obturator airway is removed, and in conditions where the CNS is depressed. Inhalation of as little as 0.3 ml/kg of gastric fluids may result in aspiration pneumonitis. This is a function not only of a low pH (usually a pH below 2.2) but also of factors such as the tonicity of the gastric material and the presence of food particles.[11]

In the older age-group the so-called cafe coronary may be seen in patients with dentures. It is caused by the combination of eating, drinking alcohol, and talking, during which time a large food particle such as meat may be caught in the upper airway. Aspiration of a foreign body is the leading cause of in-home accidental death among children under the age of 6. The foreign body is commonly food or food derivatives—particularly peanuts, nuts, and seeds—that may penetrate deeply into the tracheobronchial tree.[12] With the cough reflex the foreign body may be expelled, or alternatively, a startled response may force inspiration and concomitant dilatation of the airway, permitting the foreign material to penetrate deeper into the tracheobronchial tree. A foreign body may be trapped in the upper airway or lower airway and the subsequent obstruction may be complete or partial. Lower airways obstructions caused by foreign bodies in the bronchi may be divided into four types:[13]

1. A check-valve mechanism in which air is inhaled but cannot be exhaled causing air-trapping and unilateral hyperinflation on the affected side.
2. A stop-valve mechanism caused by a large foreign body (or the inflammatory changes secondary to a small foreign body) with subsequent atelectasis distal to the lesion.
3. A ball-valve mechanism which involves partial expulsion and reimpaction of the foreign body during inspiration and expiration with subsequent atelectasis on the affected side.
4. A bypass valve mechanism caused by partial airway obstruction with subsequent decreased ventilation and an opacity visualized on the affected side.

Subsequent inflammatory changes in the lower airways because of foreign bodies include atelectasis, abscess, or bronchiectasis.

A history of aspiration or a choking episode accompanied by a paroxysm of coughing is the most common presenting complaint.[14] This episode may be followed by a relatively asymptomatic interval. The inhalation of a foreign body may be asymptomatic or produce the symptom of pain, a sticking sensation in the larynx, laryngeal spasm, inspiratory dyspnea, cough, or a change in the quality of the voice. The patient may clutch the throat. If the foreign body is loose in the larynx and there is movement of air, a wheeze or other sounds produced by air transmitted across the foreign body may be auscultated. In complete airway obstruction there may be aphonia, cyanosis, and no wheezing.

The patient appears restless, with a rapid respiratory rate, decreased tidal volume, stridor, retraction, and cyanosis. Anxiety and agitation may be followed by stupor and coma. If the foreign body penetrates beyond the bifurcation of the trachea, the material may enter the lower airways into either the right or left main-stem bronchus with equal frequency.[14] In such cases there may be no clinical signs, unilateral wheezing, decreased breath sounds, asymmetry, and hyperresonance secondary to air-trapping on the affected side. Fever may be present in the patient with an inflammatory response in the area of the foreign body.

Diagnosis

The inability to provide positive pressure ventilation to an unresponsive patient suggests airway obstruction. Direct visualization with a laryngoscope or flashlight and tongue blade may be diagnostic. Routine chest roentgenograms may be normal in approximately one-third of the cases, since most foreign bodies are not radiopaque.[15] Unilateral emphysema may be demonstrated and is exaggerated during inspiration and expiration. The technique of assisted expiration may eliminate the problem of patient movement and poor radiograph exposure timing: a lead-gloved hand exerts pressure to the epigastrium during expiration at the time of exposure. Signs of lower airway obstruction secondary to a foreign body include atelectasis and air-trapping which may be manifested by a mediastinal shift to the opposite side during exhalation and hyperlucency of the involved side. Inspiratory and expiratory films may show a paradoxical decrease in the heart size during expiration. Fluoroscopy is used only as a supplemental technique since 50 percent of fluoroscopic exams are normal. If routine roentgenograms fail to identify a foreign body and clinical suspicion is high, fluoroscopy is followed by a lung ventilation-perfusion scan or CT scan. If these are negative, bronchoscopy is indicated.

Treatment

Before treatment the patient with suspected foreign body obstruction of the airway should be assessed to distinguish this condition from other processes that cause sudden respiratory arrest, such as myocardial infarction, drug overdose, and processes that cause central nervous depression. An evaluation should be made to determine whether there are contraindications to movement, such as fracture of the cervical spine. In the absence of trauma, a *comatose* patient with a partial soft tissue upper airway obstruction should be placed in the head down anterior recumbent position.[16] This permits the tongue to fall anteriorly from the posterior wall of the pharynx and permits regurgitated gastric contents to drain from the mouth rather than into the airway. The *conscious* patient should be in the erect position, flexed forward from the hips with the head in a sniffing position.[16] This allows the tongue to fall anteriorly away from the posterior wall of the pharynx and maximizes the musculoskeletal portion of the tongue. Manual or mechanical methods of opening the airway are reviewed in Chapter 56.

Foreign bodies may cause partial or complete obstruction of the upper or lower airways. If the victim with a partial airway obstruction is capable of good air exchange and is able to cough forcefully, prehospital and emergency care personnel should not interfere with these attempts to expel a foreign body. With adequate respiration the normal cough can exert pressures greater than those achieved by back blows or the manual thrust. However, the patient with partial obstruction may deteriorate clinically as air exchange becomes ineffective, and the work of breathing increases. At this point the patient is managed as though there were a complete airway obstruction.

The sequence recommended by the American Heart Association for the choking patient with airway obstruction is as follows:

The *conscious* choking patient *without trauma*

- Determine if the patient has a complete airway obstruction by asking the victim if he is able to speak
- Four back blows in rapid succession
- Four manual thrusts

Repeat above sequence until the obstruction is cleared or the victim becomes unconscious.

The *unconscious* choking patient *without trauma*

The unconscious patient is approached in the manner described in Chapter 55. The rescuer follows the sequence of calling for help, opening the airway, and providing positive pressure airway ventilation. If the rescuer *looks, feels,* and *listens* to the victim and determines that there is a foreign body obstructing air flow, then the following steps are performed.

- Obtain help, if possible, and activate the EMS system
- Four back blows in rapid sequence
- Four manual thrusts
- Finger sweep
- Reopen the airway, reposition the head, and provide positive pressure ventilation

The above sequence should be repeated until the obstruction is cleared.

There are three basic maneuvers that are useful in the prehospital care setting for the emergency relief of foreign body airway obstruction: back blows, manual thrusts, and finger sweep.

Back Blows. A "back blow" consists of a series of four sharp, rapid blows with the heel of the hand over the victim's thoracic vertebrae in an area between the scapulae. This maneuver is to be accomplished in rapid sequence with the patient erect or supine. If a conscious victim is erect, the rescuer takes a position at the side and slightly behind the patient. While delivering the blows over the victim's thoracic vertebrae, the other hand can be placed over the mid-sternum acting as support for the victim. The victim's head can be placed in such a position that it is lower than the chest so as to allow the effect of gravity to assist in removal of the foreign body. The unconscious patient is rolled to the side facing the rescuer with the patient's chest against the rescuer's thigh. The blows are delivered to the back as described above.

Manual Thrust. A "manual thrust" consists of a series of four lower chest or upper abdominal thrusts that have the effect of forcing air out of the lungs so that the foreign body is expelled from the upper airway. The *chest thrust* is the procedure of choice for the pregnant or obese patient who is conscious. In this maneuver the rescuer's arms are placed under the patient's armpits around the patient's chest from behind. The thumb side of the fist is placed on the midsternum avoiding the xiphoid process. The rescuer grasps the fist with the other hand and exerts four rapid backward thrusts. The unconscious patient may be supine with the rescuer kneeling close to the side.

In the *abdominal thrust* the rescuer stands behind the conscious patient, and encircles the arms around the patient's waist from behind. The rescuer grasps one fist with the other hand and places the thumb of the fist against the patient's abdomen between the waist and rib cage. The rescuer's fist is then pressed into the patient's abdomen with a quick upward inward thrust.[17]

With the unconscious patient lying supine the rescuer straddles the hips or one thigh of the victim. The rescuer's hand is placed against the victim's abdomen between the waist and rib cage. The second hand is then placed on top of the first. With the rescuer's shoulders directly over the victim's abdomen, an upward and inward thrust is applied to the victim, without turning the victim's head to the side.

If these sequences are ineffective then a *finger probe* of the mouth and oral pharynx should follow. However, light finger pressure can convert a partial to a complete obstruction. In relieving upper airway foreign body obstruction there is a 50 percent success rate with back blows, 85 percent using manual thrusts, and 55 percent using finger probe. Since all the procedures probably contribute to success, they should all be employed to maximize the possibility of relieving obstruction.

In the event that the therapeutic maneuvers discussed above are ineffective, other devices sometimes available to prehospital care personnel and readily available in the emergency department may be utilized to remove a foreign body. Suctioning may be an effective way to remove mucus, saliva or aspirated particles. During these maneuvers, supplemental oxygen should be provided when possible to treat hypoxia. Visualization of the upper airway with a laryngoscope should be accomplished, and foreign materials can be suctioned or removed with McGill forceps. If a foreign body is not observed, but is suspected below the glottis (or not visualized), then roentgenologic examinations or other diagnostic tests including perfusion lung or CT scans may be useful. Bronchoscopy remains the ultimate treatment of choice if the therapeutic maneuvers are unsuccessful or the clinical index of suspicion is high even in the absence of confirming diagnostic tests.

Cricothyroid membrane puncture with a 14 gauge needle may be effective in establishing an airway when obstructing foreign materials that have not been impacted past the vocal cords cannot be removed by these procedures.

Anaphylaxis

Definition

Anaphylaxis is a complex potentially life-threatening event that occurs soon after an individual previously sensitized to an antigen has been exposed to that antigen. The mechanisms involved are similar to those of IgE-mediated (allergic) asthma (described below). In allergic asthma the specific antigen is introduced via the respiratory tract, and the subsequent reaction is manifested primarily in the lungs, the target organ. In systemic anaphylaxis the reaction occurs in response to a specific antigen within seconds or minutes after the antigen has been introduced, usually by injection, or less commonly by ingestion. Anaphylaxis involves the integumentary, respiratory, cardiovascular, and digestive systems, either singly or in combination. A variety of materials are capable of producing the reaction, and include antibiotics (particularly penicillin), antisera, hormones, venoms, pollen, blood, vaccines, and foods including seafood, fish, berries, nuts, eggs, chocolate, pork, and milk.

Diagnosis

After exposure to the offending specific antigen, the patient may develop shortness of breath, wheezing, chest tightness, cyanosis, hypotension, and ultimately unconsciousness. Laryngoedema may produce a feeling of fullness in the throat, hoarseness, and stridor. A characteristic pruritic, erythematous rash may occur locally or coalesce to form giant hives. Death may occur by airway obstruction via the upper airway, or shock without pulmonary symptoms or findings. In other patients there may be only mild symptoms including gastrointestinal (GI) complaints, lightheadedness, dizziness, apprehension, or itching of the nose and mouth.

Anaphylaxis should be distinguished from other processes that cause urticaria, and from those that cause symptoms suggestive of upper airway obstruction. For example, in hereditary angioedema (HA), edema of the mucosa of the respiratory and GI tracts occurs but it is accompanied by a family history of HA, abdominal pain (frequently mimicking a surgical abdomen), angioedema without urticaria, and C1 esterase inhibitor deficiency noted in the patient's serum.

Treatment

An IV should be introduced into a peripheral vein if a patient is suspected of having systemic anaphylaxis, since the reaction may progress rapidly. Oxygen should be provided for patients with respiratory complaints. Mild symptoms such as pruritic urticaria can be treated simply by administering Benadryl, 50 mg intramuscularly (IM), and/or epinephrine, 0.2 to 0.5 ml subcutaneously of a 1:1,000 solution. If the anaphylactic reaction is caused by the injection of the antigen into an extremity, proximal tourniquets, local application of ice packs, and injection of epinephrine into the entry site may reduce absorption of the antigen into the blood stream.

In the patient with bronchospasm, in the absence of hypotension, aminophylline, 5 to 6 mg/kg IV over 20 minutes, may be useful. In the presence of hypotension, 0.5 to 1 mg of a 1:10,000 solution of epinephrine IV push may be required. If epinephrine fails to control the hypotension, then volume expanders and IV dopamine may be life-saving. (See Chapter 6.) Corticosteroids such as Solu-Cortef, 250 mg IV, are not required in the initial management of anaphylaxis, but are useful in controlling or preventing the subsequent development of persistent bronchospasm and hypotension.

LOWER OBSTRUCTIVE LUNG DISEASES

Lower obstructive lung diseases include a number of respiratory conditions that are distinct entities, each characterized by airway obstruction in different parts of the lung. These conditions include emphysema, in which air flow is obstructed in the peripheral airways; bronchitis, where central airway narrowing occurs; and asthma, in which airway narrowing occurs both in central and peripheral airways. The obstruction in these processes may be acute, chronic, reversible, or irreversible. This section deals primarily with the acute processes involved in the conditions that are potentially reversible.

Asthma

Asthma is a disease process of the lungs characterized by widespread reversible narrowing of the peripheral airways, an increased reactivity or sensitivity to a variety of stimuli, and often signs or laboratory findings of an allergic disorder. Asthma, a common respiratory disorder, affects approximately 2.5 percent of the population, with more than half of these patients between the ages of 5 and 15 years. Asthma causes 2,000 to 5,000 deaths per year. The etiology of asthma is not clear, but current understanding of the process includes allergic and nonallergic asthma.

Allergic Asthma

Allergic or intrinsic asthma is associated with a positive family history of asthma, and an increased level in serum IgE antibody.

A common associated finding is immediate hypersensitivity reaction manifested by a wheal-and-flare reaction when the skin is tested with specific antigens. IgE antibody specifically directed against the antigen is increased in the patient's serum. Bronchospasm may be produced by aerosol challenge with the offending antigen. Approximately 5 percent of patients with asthma have IgE-mediated asthma, and an understanding of the mechanisms of asthma has been developed using human and animal models of IgE-mediated asthma.

IgE is the antibody class that mediates type I or immediate hypersensitivity. Specific IgE antibody is generated in response to exposure to antigens via the oral, parenteral, or aerosol route. IgE attaches to basophils in the blood as well as mast cells in perivascular and peribronchial tissue, thereby sensitizing them to specific antigens. Reexposure to the antigen permits the formation of an antigen-IgE-antibody complex that forms a bridge on the surface of the mast cell or basophil. This biochemical event effects a complex change in both the cell membrane and the intracellular contents, such that a variety of pharmacologic agents are released or secreted. These chemical agents, when released, may have an effect on the other cells, nervous tissue, airways, blood vessels, and ultimately the ventilation and perfusion of the lungs. (Figure 57–3 demonstrates the structures associated with the basic ventilation-perfusion unit of the lung.)

The bronchiolar muscle tone of the airway is influenced by a complex interaction of nerve transmission and intracellular chemical events that regulate airway size and the response to injury. The sympathetic nerv-

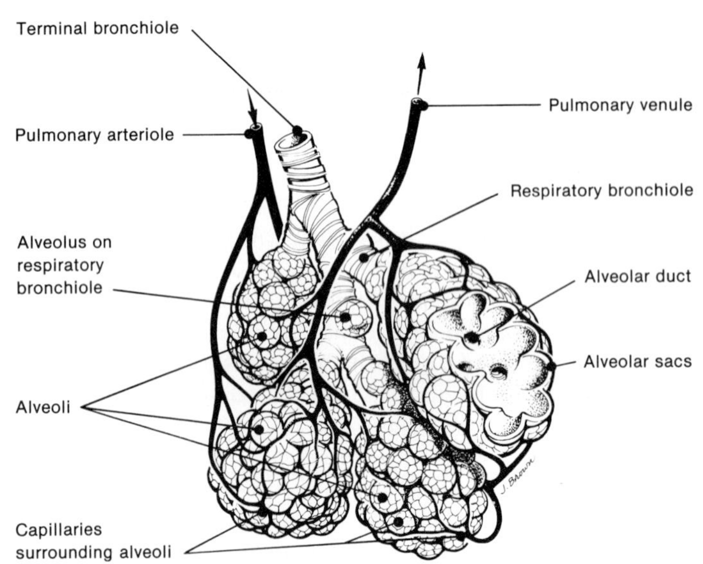

Figure 57–3 Structures of the Lower Airway.

ous system relaxes bronchiolar smooth muscle; the parasympathetic system increases smooth muscle tone via stimulation through the vagus nerve. The vagal reflex may be triggered by stimuli to the J receptors in the epithelium of the airways.

A patient with asthma and hyperirritable airways may experience bronchoconstriction as a result of contact with allergens, as well as nonallergic stimuli such as dust, smoke, sulfur dioxide, hypoxemia, ammonia, cold air, and emotion. Intracellular levels of cyclic adenosine monophosphate (AMP) modulate the release of potentially injurious mediators from mast cells located in the airway epithelium, perivascular lung tissue, and basophils. An increase in intracellular cyclic AMP inhibits mediator release, and decreases muscle tone thereby causing airway dilatation. Decreased concentration of intracellular cyclic AMP effects the reverse. Other cyclic nucleotides such as guanosine monophosphate, as well as cations such as calcium, are also involved in the control of these complicated cellular events.

Chemical Mediators of Asthma. A variety of chemicals have been identified in association with IgE-mediated reactions. A partial list of these mediators of inflammation includes:

- Histamine, a low molecular weight amine that causes constriction of smooth muscle and edema of bronchiole mucosa thereby increasing permeability;
- Slow-reacting substance (SRS-A), a lipid that causes constriction of bronchiole smooth muscle;
- Platelet activating factor (PAF), a material released from basophils (PAF-B) or lung (PAF-L),[18] which causes the release of serotonin and histamine from platelets;
- Eosinophilic chemotactic factor (ECF-A), which causes eosinophils to migrate into the affected area and is associated with the increased number of eosinophils in the peripheral blood;
- Prostaglandins, some of which have been associated with allergic lung inflammation.

The first three materials alter permeability and constrict the airways. Other putative agents of inflammation have been identified in vitro and in vivo, and therapeutic agents designed to inhibit the release or modify the pharmacologic action or physiologic effects of these mediators provide a rationale for the drug therapy of acute asthma.

Pathophysiology and Clinical Correlates. The inciting or injurious event, whether it is allergic (IgE-related) or nonallergic, has similar pathologic and physiologic consequences. The release of chemical mediators causes the histological appearance of edema in bronchial mucosa and excessive production of mucus by the bronchial glands. There is hypertrophy of smooth muscles, thickened basement membrane, an eosinophilic infiltrate, mucus plugging, and impaired ciliary clearance.

Bronchoconstriction and mucus plugging increase airway resistance, decrease expiratory flow rates, and increase work of breathing. This leads to air-trapping and hyperinflation. There are underlying changes in elastic recoil and a heterogeneous mismatch of ventilation and perfusion (V/Q mismatch). The degree of V/Q mismatch is detected by arterial blood gas measurements. Initially there is alveolar hyperventilation, the $PaCO_2$, is reduced, and there is respiratory alkalosis. The worsening V/Q abnormalities cause a reduction in the PaO_2 (hypoxemia). As the V/Q disturbance worsens along with fatigue from the work of breathing, the $PaCO_2$ may become normal, while the PAO_2 remains low. In extreme cases there is severe hypoxemia, acute CO_2 retention, and respiratory acidosis. (See Chapter 59.)

Nonallergic Asthma

Nonallergic, idiosyncratic, or extrinsic asthma is a respiratory disease experienced by a heterogeneous population of patients who develop recurrent reversible bronchospasm in response to a variety of stimuli. For example, in these patients exercise, inhalation of cold air, emotion, combustion fumes, grains, metals, proteolytic enzymes, hypoxemia, and detergents may precipitate bronchospasm. The patient may be hypersensitive to aspirin (or other analgesics), which in some patients is associated with nasal polyps. The physiologic, clinical, and pathologic findings are similar to those found in IgE-mediated asthma except that usually there is no family history of asthma nor is there a peripheral blood eosinophilia, an elevated serum IgE level, or a positive response to inhalation or to skin challenges with various antigens.

Clinical Correlates. The acute asthma patient may be sitting forward in a leaning position and frequently has a disturbing cough. Breathing may be rapid or labored with the use of accessory muscles of respiration, decreased diaphragmatic excursion, and hyperresonance to percussion. Wheezing is heard when obstruction is mild or moderate, but may be absent when bronchoconstriction is severe enough to impede the movement of air required to produce a wheezing noise. Hyperinflation and pulsus paradoxus may be additional findings.

There are helpful guidelines for assessing acute asthma and determining the requirement for hospital admission for further care.[19-21] The amount of expiratory dyspnea, pulse rate, respiratory rate, pulsus paradoxus, expiratory flow rate, wheezing, accessory-muscle use, and arterial blood gases can assist in predicting the relapse rate and need for hospitalization in many cases. Dyspnea is an important complaint, but a subjective sensation that can occasionally correlate poorly with the degree of airway obstruction. Usually the alert patient can estimate the severity of airway obstruction better than the examining physician.[22,23] Wheezing is one of the less discriminating factors. Sustained tachycardia (120) may be associated with an increased incidence of complications, and such patients are usually admitted.

Although a variety of pulmonary and nonpulmonary conditions can cause pulsus paradoxus in acute asthma, a decrease of greater than 10 mm Hg indicates severe airway obstruction. Some 90 percent of patients with prebronchodilator FEV_1 of less than .6 liters or post-treatment FEV_1 of less than 1.6 liters/minute will require hospitalization (and/or will deteriorate within 48 hours).[21] However arterial blood gases do not always correlate with the severity of airway obstruction, and a normal or increased $PaCO_2$ can be an ominous sign of incipient respiratory failure.

The complications of asthma that can be demonstrated roentgenographically include pneumothorax, atelectasis, pneumonia, and pneumomediastinum,[24] and such patients require hospital admission.

Status asthmaticus deserves special consideration since it is a complication of 5 to 10 percent of patients with asthma. Status asthmaticus is defined as a severe asthmatic attack unresponsive to all inhaled or injected sympathomimetic amines, including: the patient's own maintenance regimen; injectable beta agonists such as subcutaneous epinephrine or specific beta-2 agonists; and IV methylxanthines in appropriate doses.

Clinical signs include the findings of unremitting acute airway obstruction, severe respiratory distress, changes in the level of consciousness, and cyanosis despite oxygen therapy. Retinal vein distention or papilledema are late signs. Severe narrowing of the airways increases the work of breathing, which increases O_2 consumption and CO_2 production. Hypoxemia and ultimately respiratory acidosis result from V/Q mismatch. Such patients are in respiratory failure and require IV therapy and corticosteroids. Intubation and mechanical ventilation may be necessary. (See Chapter 59.)

Differential Diagnosis of Lower Obstructive Airway Disease

Apnea

If the patient is apneic or hypoventilating, CNS depression as a consequence of trauma, cerebrovascular accident, or drugs must be ruled out. For example, the prehospital treatment of the apneic patient should include consideration of the use of IV Narcan if the pupils are constricted.

Dyspnea, Wheezing, and Fatigue

A common presentation of patients with obstructive lung disease is dyspnea, wheezing, and fatigue. This may be a manifestation of a number of different lung disease processes. In asthma the obstructive process is acute and potentially reversible. In other diseases, such as bronchitis and emphysema, the obstructive process is chronic. Understanding the amount of potentially reversible obstruction and the degree of chronic irreversible obstruction of chronic obstructive airway disease makes expectations of treatment more reasonable.

Upper Airway Obstruction

Foreign body aspiration may cause symptoms that are confused with asthma. The upper airway should be examined when these processes are suspected, except in the prehospital setting when epiglottitis is suspected.

Congestive Heart Failure ("Cardiac Asthma")

Pulmonary edema may commonly present with dyspnea and wheezing. The characteristic history and physical findings in cardiac and noncardiac pulmonary cases are reviewed in Chapters 48 and 51.

Drugs and Other Causes

Certain pharmacologic agents such as Inderal and other beta-blocking agents cause or enhance bronchospasm. Other conditions to be distinguished from asthma include systemic vasculitis, pulmonary emboli, carcinoid syndrome, and allergic alveolitis. Infections including bronchitis, pneumonia, bronchiolitis, anaphylactic reactions, and worm infestation may present with a clinical picture of airway obstruction.

Treatment of Lower Airways Obstruction

Reversibility of airways obstruction is the sine qua non of asthma. Patients with chronic airways obstruction due to emphysema and bronchitis have airway abnormalities that are not immediately amenable to acute treatment. All chronic obstructive airways diseases (asthma, emphysema, and bronchitis) may have potentially reversible components such as bronchospasm, excessive secretions, mucous membrane swelling, and dynamic compression of airways. These reversible components have similar pathophysiologic consequences resulting in V/Q mismatch, a widening of the alveolar-arterial oxygen gradient, and a potential to develop hypoxemia and hypercarbia. Thus, the prehospital and emergency department treatment of patients with lower airways obstruction may be managed with many common therapeutic modalities.

Oxygen Therapy

The terms high- and low-flow oxygen are often used incorrectly. A high-flow system is one in which the gas flow of the apparatus is sufficient to meet all inspiratory requirements, and the patient breathes only the gas that is supplied by the device. A low-flow system is one in which the gas flow is insufficient to meet the patient's inspiratory requirement and room air is used to provide part of the inspired gas.

High-flow systems usually utilize a Venturi device, which uses the Bernoulli principle to entrain room air in a fixed proportion to oxygen. This system provides a constant flow regardless of the patient's breathing pattern. Low-flow systems provide a FIO_2 that is dependent on the tidal volume and respiratory rate of the patient. As tidal volume or respiratory rate increases the FIO_2 decreases.

Oxygen delivered to a patient with chronic obstructive pulmonary disease (COPD) in an emergency department should be of the high-flow variety to ensure a stable flow. When low-flow oxygen is delivered to an oxygen sensitive patient with chronic lung disease the chance of producing oxygen-induced apnea is increased. If the patient hypoventilates the FIO_2 will increase and produce more hypoventilation; a deadly cycle.

Pending arterial blood gas measurement, nasal prongs delivering 2 liters of oxygen per minute or a 28 percent ventimask should be instituted for patients suspected of having COPD and potential O_2 sensitivity and CO_2 retention. In the acute setting it is not possible to accurately predict whether a patient with chronic obstructive airway disease will be O_2 sensitive. A previous history of O_2 sensitivity, the setting of an acute exacerbation, and the findings of arterial hypoxemia and respiratory acidosis are warnings for potential development of CO_2 narcosis in response to O_2 therapy. Arterial blood gases are mandatory to guide acute O_2 therapy to reverse life-threatening hypoxemia while avoiding the potential serious complication of O_2 sensitivity. (See Chapters 56 and 59.)

IV Fluids

An IV solution of 5 percent dextrose and water or one-half normal saline at a rate of 100 to 125 ml/hour should be established in the field in a peripheral vein in patients with lower airways obstruction. This provides a route for the introduction of medications and treating dehydration if present. There is no compelling evidence that fluids decrease the viscosity and loosen airway secretions in the normally hydrated patient, and indeed such fluids may cause extravasation of fluid into the interstitial space and aggravate airway narrowing.[25]

Adrenergic Sympathomimetic Agents

Sympathomimetic agents remain a potent pharmacologic tool in the treatment of patients with lower airways obstruction with reversible components. These pharmacologic agents may induce a rapid and effective bronchodilation in a few minutes, and produce a beneficial effect that may last from one to eight hours. These agents are usually delivered subcutaneously or by aerosol.

Sympathomimetic agents alter the response to lung injury by a variety of mechanisms. It has been postulated that on the surface of target cells a number of different receptors or effector cells discriminate or recognize structural components of various drugs. Stimulation of these receptors is accomplished through a complex mechanism involving the recognition, binding, and activation of these specific receptors by these drugs. The adrenergic receptors have been designated alpha or beta, depending on the anatomic site and location in the various tissues. (For example, alpha receptors are located mainly in the blood vessels and their stimulation mediates vasoconstriction.) Beta receptors comprise two subpopulations: beta-1 receptors increase heart rate and the force of cardiac contraction; and beta-2 relax the airways.

Beta-receptor stimulation is postulated to lead to the activation of the enzyme adenylate cyclase, located in the intracellular membrane of the bronchiole smooth muscle, which increases the intracellular synthesis and therefore the concentration of cyclic AMP. This increase in the intracellular cyclic AMP level facilitates the transport of calcium out of the cell; the consequent fall of intracellular calcium relaxes the contractile proteins and smooth muscle, subsequently dilating the airways. The beta agonist also inhibits the liberation of mast cell- and basophil-derived mediators of inflammation via this cyclic AMP mechanism. Thus, the inflammatory lung reaction can be controlled or modulated through therapeutic beta agonists by two mechanisms: dilatation of the airways by relaxing smooth muscle, or inhibition of the liberation of chemical mediators that cause airway constriction.

The side-effects of these pharmacologic agents may also be ascribed to their relative alpha or beta activity. The vasoconstrictor effect of these agents increases the systemic blood pressure via the stimulation of alpha receptors located in the smooth muscle of blood vessels. The activation of beta-1 receptors of the heart may be responsible for the development of cardiac arrhythmias such as ventricular fibrillation.

Since there is a difference in the relative amount of alpha and beta activity of the various pharmacologic agents that might have an effect on the inflammatory lung reaction, an agent may be chosen that produces the desired therapeutic effect, but introduces few unwanted side-effects. Epinephrine has alpha, beta-1, and beta-2 activity, and not only dilates the airways and inhibits mediator release, but also may induce tachycardia and vasoconstriction. Some of the newer agonists have specific beta-2 activity, and therefore limited extrapulmonary effects.

In vitro evidence suggests synergism between the phosphodiesterase inhibitors (methylxanthines), which increase intracellular cyclic AMP by inhibiting cyclic AMP phosphodiesterase, and the beta agonists, but whether or not this occurs clinically remains controversial.[26–28]

Aerosolization of Adrenergic Sympathomimetic Agents. Beta agonists are used to relieve airway obstruction, and aerosolization is an effective means of delivery. The pharmacologic agent should be diluted in sterile normal saline. Nebulization should be achieved with compressed air or oxygen. Approximately 10 percent of the inhaled aerosol dose reaches the airways, much of the material is trapped in the nasopharynx, and some may be absorbed into the circulation through the mucous membranes. The dose of the pharmacologic agents delivered locally to the lungs depends on the size of aerosol droplet, the concentration of the pharmacologic agent, and the respiratory rate and tidal volume of the patient. Aerosols offer a theoretical advantage in that a smaller total dose of the pharmacologic agent can be delivered to the patient with a concentrated amount delivered directly to the affected organ, the lungs. Thus, the possibility of extrapulmonary side-effects is minimized.

The technique of delivery of the aerosol is important. There is greater pulmonary deposition of droplets with slow inspiratory rates and larger tidal volumes. With a pressurized aerosol the valve is activated shortly after the patient begins a slow inhalation. The actuator may be placed just outside the patient's open mouth and directed toward the hypopharynx.[29] The breath-holding phase should be maintained at least ten seconds. A face mask or mouth piece offers no significant advantage for the delivery of nebulized bronchodilators, and it has been suggested that patients be allowed to choose their preferred method of delivery.[30] Intermittent positive pressure offers no advantage in the delivery of pharmacologic agents in patients with airways obstruction, and indeed, may be contraindicated since it may increase airway obstruction, decrease cardiac output, and cause a pneumothorax.[31]

Epinephrine. Epinephrine is an adrenergic sympathomimetic agent with alpha, beta-1, and beta-2 activity.

The beta effect dilates the airways and inhibits the release of chemical mediators of inflammation. The main alpha activity of epinephrine is constriction of the peripheral blood vessels, which often induces a temporary increase in the arterial blood pressure. Larger doses stimulate the myocardium and increase cardiac output, heart rate, AV conduction, and also irritability. Complications of epinephrine administration include fever, tremors, nervousness, and cardiac arrhythmias. Severe reactions include intracerebral hemorrhage and pulmonary edema. Epinephrine should be used only with extreme caution in patients with heart disease, tachycardia, cardiac arrhythmias, hypertension, diabetes, pregnancy, or hyperthyroidism. Epinephrine is useful in the treatment of the younger patient with acute asthma, but is not as effective and may be harmful to the older patient because of the above side-effects.

In the treatment of patients with asthma epinephrine may be given subcutaneously in a 1:1,000 aqueous solution at intervals of 20 to 30 minutes for three doses. In children the dose is 0.01 ml/kg subcutaneously to a maximum dose of 0.5 ml. In adults the usual dose is 0.2 to 0.5 mg of a 1:1,000 solution, and 0.5 mg is the optimal dosage.[32] Onset of action occurs in five minutes and the duration is approximately 90 minutes.

Susphrine. Susphrine is a long-acting preparation of an epinephrine base in aqueous suspension at a dilution of 1:200. Thus, it has all the alpha and beta actions of epinephrine as well as the side-effects and potential complications. Susphrine is commonly used in the child with asthma following the initial successful therapy with epinephrine. Susphrine is given subcutaneously at 0.005 ml/kg to children of less than 30 kg. The maximum dose is 0.15 ml. The material has an onset action in 15 minutes and lasts up to eight hours. The rapid action is due to the 20 percent of epinephrine in the solution, while the sustained activity is due to the crystalline epinephrine base in suspension. The material is usually not given any more frequently than every six hours, and never IV.

Terbutaline Sulfate (Bricanyl, Brethine). This synthetic sympathomimetic amine exerts a preferential effect on beta-2 adrenergic receptors such as those located in bronchial smooth muscle. Terbutaline relieves bronchospasm in asthma as well as bronchospasm in association with bronchitis and emphysema. Terbutaline can be given subcutaneously, orally, or, in some countries, by nebulization. Whether terbutaline has a clear advantage over epinephrine in relieving acute reversible airways obstruction remains controversial. Evidence suggests that terbutaline has fewer extrapulmonary side-effects.[33]

Terbutaline tablets have an onset of action in 10 to 30 minutes, the maximum effect usually occurs between 20 and 180 minutes, and the pharmacologic effect lasts from four to eight hours. The usual adult dosage is 2.5 to 5 mg every six to eight hours; and for children 2.5 mg three times daily, not to exceed 7.5 mg in a 24-hour period.

Terbutaline may also be given subcutaneously, which produces a measurable change in air flow rates within five minutes, a maximum effect at 30 to 60 minutes, and action that may persist from four to six hours.

The duration of clinically significant improvement is comparable to that found with equal doses of epinephrine. The side-effects of terbutaline are similar to those of epinephrine and include tachycardia, nervousness, palpitations, dizziness, headache, nausea, vomiting, and anxiety. Although the agent has not been available for children under the age of 12, one study suggests that in children terbutaline has no advantage over epinephrine.[33]

The usual subcutaneous dose of terbutaline is 0.25 mg. If clinical improvement is not apparent in 15 to 30 minutes, a second dose of 0.25 mg may be administered with a total dose not over 0.5 mg within a four-hour period. If the patient does not respond to a total dose of 0.5 mg, then other therapeutic measures should be considered. In some countries, terbutaline sulfate is available in a pressurized air-filled form that delivers a dosage of 0.25 mg per puff; or nebulized in a dose of 0.25 to 0.50 mg in 1.5 to 3 ml of normal saline every four to six hours.

Isotherine (Bronkosol). Bronkosol is an adrenergic sympathomimetic amine with preferential affinity for beta-2 receptor sites and a lower affinity for beta-1 receptors. It is useful as a bronchodilator for asthma and for the reversible bronchospasm that may occur in association with bronchitis and emphysema. Bronkosol may be administered by hand nebulizer, two to seven inhalations every three to four hours, or aerosol on room air or with oxygen. When administered with oxygen the flow rate is 2 liters/minute (or up to 6 liters if the patient is hypoxic and not oxygen sensitive) over a period of 10 to 20 minutes. The usual dose is 0.5 ml of Bronkosol in a dilution of 1:3 to 1:5 with sterile normal saline or other diluent for 10 to 20 minutes depending on the therapeutic response desired.

The onset of action is 1 to 2 minutes, bronchodilation persists up to one to three hours, and there is little tachycardia. Repeated, frequent administration may produce chemical bronchorrhea, increased myocardial irritability, or paradoxical bronchospasm. The bronchodilating effects may act synergistically with theophylline. The side-effects include palpitations, nervousness, nausea, headache, tremor, and cardiac arrhythmias.

Isoproterenol (Isuprel). Isoproterenol is a sympathomimetic amine which acts almost exclusively on beta-1 and beta-2 receptors. Isoproterenol relaxes smooth muscle of both large and small components of the airway, but also has cardiac effects, and for this reason is not the drug of choice in the older patient or the patient with coronary artery disease.

Isuprel may be used to treat bronchospasm in association with acute asthma or reversible lower airways obstruction in association with chronic bronchitis or emphysema. Isoproterenol may be administered by aerosol, nebulized with oxygen or room air, or in a mist.

For adults and children a 1:200 solution may be administered by hand-bulb nebulization in a dose of 5 to 15 deep inhalations. In adults the 1:100 solution may be used if the stronger solution seems to be indicated. The usual dose is two to seven deep inhalations.

Isuprel may be delivered in a more dilute form over a long period of time. For example, 0.5 ml of a 1:200 solution can be diluted to 2 to 2.5 ml with normal saline to achieve a concentration of 1:800 to 1:1,000. This can be administered with oxygen or with compressed air. The material is usually nebulized over a period of 10 to 20 minutes. Side-effects include tachycardia, palpitation, nervousness, nausea, headache, dizziness, sweating, and angina-type pain. Isoproterenol is occasionally given IV in children with status asthmaticus.

Salbutamol or Albuterol (Proventil). By virtue of its relatively select action of beta-2 adrenoceptors, salbutamol relaxes smooth muscle of the bronchi, uterus, and the vascular supply to skeletal muscles, and may have less cardiac stimulant than does isoproterenol. Salbutamol is long acting by any route of administration in most patients because it is not a substrate for cellular uptake process for catecholamines nor for catechol-o-methyltransferase. The material is gradually absorbed from the bronchi, and systemic levels are low after inhalation of recommended doses. Maximum plasma concentrations occur 2 to 4 hours after aerosol administration. The usual aerosol dose is 2 inhalations every 4 to 6 hours, and the onset of improvement in pulmonary function is 15 minutes with clinical improvement up to 4 hours. In countries where the material is available in oral form, the syrup can be provided to children at a dose of 2 to 4 mg t.i.d. or 0.05 to 0.15 mg/kg. In the adult a dose of 4 to 8 mg t.i.d. (0.15 mg/kg) causes improvement in 20 to 30 minutes with persistence of pharmacologic activity to 3 hours.

Metaproterenol Sulfate (Metaprel). Metaproterenol is a sympathomimetic agent with primarily beta-2 activity that is available in liquid or tablet and in the metered-dose inhaler. When the material is administered orally in tablet or liquid form, decreased bronchospasm can last up to four hours. The usual oral dose is 2 mg/kg divided into doses over 24 hours. When administered by metered-dose inhalation, relief of bronchospasm persists from one to five hours. The usual single dose is two to three inhalations which should not be repeated more often than every three hours, and a total dosage should not exceed 12 inhalations.

Theophylline (Aminophylline). Methylxanthines may provide prophylaxis for the development of lower airway obstruction and are also useful in the treatment of the acute episode. Aminophylline is available in IV or oral form in a regular or in a sustained-release capsule. Serum theophylline levels in the therapeutic range correlate highly with effective bronchodilatation.

However, the dosage of theophylline is critical, and careful attention must be paid to the various factors affecting the rate of elimination of the agent and the serum concentration since the range between therapeutic efficacy and toxicity is narrow.

It is well known that aminophylline is beneficial in the management of obstruction to airway flow, and it is thought that this occurs through a number of mechanisms. The methylxanthines increase the concentration of intracellular cyclic AMP by inhibiting the enzyme phosphodiesterase. The subsequent increase of cyclic AMP inhibits the release of potentially injurious mediators of inflammation. The same cyclic AMP mechanism is involved in the relaxation of smooth muscles in the airway. The methylxanthines may also improve diaphragmatic contractility particularly in fatigued muscles. The methylxanthines offer additional beneficial extrapulmonary pharmacologic properties in that they increase cardiac output and the glomerular filtration rate. Aminophylline thus remains an important therapeutic tool in treating patients with bronchospasm, particularly in the prehospital care of patients when the etiology of the bronchospasm is unclear.

Theophylline is not without side-effects, and for this reason a careful history of previous theophylline ingestion as well as the presence of heart or liver disease is important. Theophylline may cause insomnia, irritability, and headaches, and the CNS and cardiac effects may occur prior to GI changes of nausea and vomiting. Seizures may be induced, and are associated with a high mortality rate. Thus, it is important to carefully monitor patients with an ECG during administration and obtain sequential serum theophylline levels.

Prophylaxis of bronchospasm with theophylline may be commenced orally with a dose of 16 mg/kg/day or 400 mg/day (whichever is less) in divided doses. If side-effects are not observed, then the amount can be increased biweekly, until the age-related mean dose required to produce the therapeutic level or the serum therapeutic level is reached. The therapeutic serum concentration ranges from 10 to 20 μg/ml. The final dosage requirement is based on peak serum concentrations, which occur approximately two hours after administering oral liquid or uncoated tablet, or four hours after administering sustained-release material.

Theophylline elimination rates vary greatly among individuals: the pharmacokinetics is determined by a number of factors including individual variability in normal people and the patient's age, weight, and history of cigarette smoking, and the presence of heart or liver disease. Since theophylline clearance per kilogram decreases with increasing age, infants generally have the highest clearance values per weight. Thus, small children may require higher or more frequent doses if therapeutic levels of theophylline are to be maintained.

Aminophylline is the form of theophylline that may be introduced IV and is usually given over 20 to 40 minutes. The usual adult IV loading dose in patients not previously treated with aminophylline is 5.5 to 6 mg/kg; the average effective dose in adults is 13 mg/kg/day; the average effective dose in children is 24 mg/kg/day; the usual maintenance IV therapy dosage is 0.9 mg/kg/hour.

In patients who have been previously treated with aminophylline preparations or who have conditions that would reduce the dosage required, the following guidelines apply:

- A 1 mg/kg loading dose for each 2 μg/ml increase desired in the measured level of theophylline with the target level being 10 μg/ml of serum.
- Infusion rates for neonates is 0.15 mg/kg/hour; 0.2 to 0.8 mg/kg/hour in infants less than 1 year; 0.5 to 1 mg/kg/hour in children aged 1 to 9; 0.65 to 1 mg/kg/hour in children over 9 years of age and healthy adult smokers; 0.4 to 0.7 mg/kg/hour in healthy nonsmokers.
- Infusion rates in patients with congestive heart failure, liver dysfunction, hypoalbuminemia, or age over 55 is 0.2 mg/kg/hour.

Aminophylline is available in tablet, rectal suppository, or IV solution. Under 6 years of age it is given 10 mg/kg/24 hours. Over 6 years of age it is given 20 mg/kg/24 hours divided into six-, eight-, or twelve-hour doses depending on the clinical response and therapeutic blood levels. Theophylline is available in tablet or capsule form. Given in the above dosages, theophylline (anhydrous, Slo-Phyllin) is available in capsules and given every eight hours; theophylline (anhydrous) sustained-action (Theo-Dur) is available in tablets of eight- or twelve-hour doses; and oxtriphyllin (Choledyl) is available in tablet form and given on a six- to eight-hour schedule. (See also Chapter 24.)

Corticosteroids. Corticosteroids may be useful in the treatment of patients with obstructive airway disease and acute exacerbation because of their anti-inflammatory effect, which may decrease airway edema. Corticosteroids may also improve the bronchodilating effect of adrenergic sympathomimetic amines by improving the beta-receptor function, which may be impaired in patients with allergic airway diseases. There remains controversy on the indications for corticosteroids in acute reversible lower airways obstruction, but two factors should be considered if these agents are chosen. Corticosteroid therapy does not replace bronchodilator therapy such as that achieved with theophylline and the beta agonists; and if corticosteroids are chosen, initial IV dosage should be high and then rapidly tapered until the desired therapeutic effect has been achieved.

Hydrocortisone methylsuccinate (Solu-Cortef) may be given in doses of 250 to 1,000 mg IV and may be required in similar quantities every four to six hours IV. Intravenous methylprednisolone (Solu-Medrol) may be as effective. Patients recovering from acute episodes requiring corticosteroids may require maintenance, oral methylxanthines or beta agonists, and a tapering of the corticosteroid to a dose that produces the desired clinical effect or one that suppresses the total peripheral eosinophil count below 50/cu mm.

Beclomethasone Aerosol (Becotide, Vanceril). Inhalation therapy with this steroid preparation may avert some of the systemic side-effects often observed with long-term oral or parenteral use of steroids. The favorable effects of Beclomethasone do not begin until after several days of treatment, and therefore it is not indicated in the acute treatment of the asthmatic. The daily aerosol dose of 0.4 mg is equal to 7.5 mg of prednisone. After 0.8 mg are given, systemic side-effects can be demonstrated by measuring a depression in adrenocorticoid function. Local side-effects include oral thrush and candidiasis.

Cromolyn. Cromolyn is not a bronchodilator and is not to be used during an acute attack of bronchospasm. This agent prevents allergic, exercise-, or cold-induced bronchospasm particularly in children. An inhaler delivers the medication by aerosol, and is provided when the patient is free of symptoms.

Steps in the Treatment of Asthma

Patients Not Previously Treated

In addition to oxygen, patients with acute asthma who are not taking medications for this condition can be treated initially with epinephrine subcutaneously. Epinephrine is administered subcutaneously in a dilution of 1:1,000, and may be repeated every 20 to 30 minutes for two to three doses. In children the dose is 0.01 mg/ kg to a maximum of 0.5 ml. In adults, the dose is 0.2 ml to 0.5 ml, which may be repeated every 20 to 30 minutes for a maximum of three doses.

An alternative to epinephrine is terbutaline, 0.25 to 0.5 mg subcutaneously and repeated in four to six hours, if required. A third alternative in the treatment of patients with acute asthma who have not received previous therapy is aerosolization of an adrenergic sympathomimetic agent with relative beta-2 activity, such as isotherine (or terbutaline, in countries where it is approved).

If the patient responds favorably to any of these treatments, then maintenance bronchodilator therapy should be prescribed (see below).

Patients Unresponsive to Beta-Adrenergic Agents or Oral Theophylline

A patient with an acute episode of asthma who is unresponsive to the above treatment or who currently has been using inhaled beta-adrenergic agents or oral theophylline unsuccessfully requires an IV line and the commencement of aminophylline therapy. If the patient has not previously been treated with aminophylline, then an adult may be given 5.5 to 6 mg/kg IV over 20 minutes followed by maintenance therapy. Indications for reduced dosage and side-effects are discussed above. Patients at this stage may not benefit from repeated subcutaneous administration of epinephrine or terbutaline. Nebulization of a specific beta-2 agent may be effective.

Patients Unresponsive to Beta-Adrenergic Agents and IV Theophylline

Patients who have not responded to beta-adrenergic agents (subcutaneously or by aerosol) in combination with IV theophylline should be considered for hospital admission. In these patients IV corticosteroids and inpatient care may be required. Hydrocortisone methylsuccinate may be started at a dose of 200 to 1,000 mg IV and repeated every four to six hours until the desired therapeutic effect is achieved.

Respiratory acidosis is an ominous sign during an acute asthma attack and heralds the development of impending respiratory decompensation. The early response to airway constriction is hyperventilation and respiratory alkalosis. Respiratory acidosis may develop later in the course of the attack from a combination of worsening ventilation-perfusion mismatch, increasing air-trapping, and respiratory muscle fatigue.

When CO_2 retention occurs acutely despite optimal pharmacologic management then intubation and mechanical ventilation must be considered. If severe metabolic acidosis coexists with CO_2 retention a cautious trial of bicarbonate therapy IV may be tried. This treatment is not without hazard because bicarbonate is converted to CO_2 as it exerts its buffering effect on hydrogen ion and may accentuate the CO_2 retention by presenting an increased load of carbon dioxide to an already overburdened respiratory system. The potential theoretical advantage of treating the metabolic acidosis is to enhance the effect of beta-adrenergic agonists which are not optimally effective in the presence of acidosis. An alternative approach is to increase the dose of beta agonists, titrating the dose until either a therapeutic response or an undesired side-effect occurs.

Antibiotics

Infection is a common precipitating event in patients with acute asthma, but in most instances, pathogenic bacteria cannot be cultured from the respiratory tract. Antibiotic therapy should be reserved for patients with clinical evidence of bacterial infection.

Intubation and Mechanical Ventilation

Patients with acute asthma may develop respiratory failure or arrest, in which case intubation and artificial airway maintenance may be required. (See Chapter 56.) In instances when respiratory failure is evident, the patient should be intubated and placed on mechanical ventilation. (See Chapter 59.)

Maintenance Therapy of Patients with Asthma

The most important measure in maintenance therapy of patients with asthma is to prevent the initiating event. Thus, in patients with cold air-, exercise-, or allergen-induced bronchospasm, these must be avoided. The emergency care of patients with acute asthma should always be followed by pharmacologic maintenance therapy whether a patient is admitted or discharged. The methylxanthine preparations alone or with a beta-sympathomimetic agent orally or by aerosol may be effective. The average theophylline maintenance dose is 2 to 4 mg/kg every six hours, or 900 mg/day (whichever is less). This can be achieved with theophylline or a sustained-release theophylline preparation. Oral terbutaline at an average dose of 2.5 to 5 mg every six to eight hours may be effective because of its beta-2 activity.

A severe asthma attack, or repeated attacks within a short time period, is a potentially life-threatening event that must be treated aggressively. The longer the attack persists the more likely it is to progress to status asthmaticus. A patient who has continued bronchospasm for more than 24 hours and does not respond with two hours of aggressive treatment in the emergency department should be admitted to the hospital for further observation and treatment. If the initial attack is aborted with intravenous aminophylline only to recur within hours it is because the underlying basic process has not been adequately controlled. The patient should be treated with intravenous corticosteroids and admitted to the hospital.

Patients who have received corticosteroids in the emergency department will require a tapering of the dose. For example, prednisone, 1 mg/kg/24 hours divided into doses, or beclomethasone, 100 μg inhalation four times a day, may be given until appropriate maintenance therapy can be determined by the patient's own pulmonary specialist.

Emphysema

Emphysema is a respiratory disease process involving the small components of the lungs that is characterized by abnormal, permanent enlargement of the air spaces distal to the terminal bronchioles, accompanied by destruction of the alveolar wall. Pulmonary capillaries in the walls of alveoli are lost with varying degrees of inflammatory changes, including fibrosis of the interstitium.

The etiology of emphysema remains unclear, although the association with cigarette smoking has been strong. Clinical and in vitro evidence suggest that potentially injurious proteolytic enzymes are released from cellular elements such as leukocytes sequestered in the lung and alveolar macrophages. These enzymes (elastase and collagenase) digest elastin and collagen, the main supporting structural elements of the walls of the alveoli. Lung destruction may be a consequence of excess proteolytic enzymatic activity in relation to the concentration or activity of naturally occurring serum inhibitors such as alpha-1-antitrypsin.

The destruction of elastin and collagen and the enlargement of the acinus is associated with a change in the lung's elasticity, the loss of elastic recoil, and the subsequent collapse of the airways during expiration, thereby obstructing airflow. With an increase in airway resistance in the affected parts of the lung, ventilation of alveolar units decreases in comparison with perfusion. These areas of low V/Q result in abnormal oxygen exchange, which may lead to arterial hypoxemia and an increase in arterial carbon dioxide.

Patients with pure emphysema have been referred to as pink puffers. The patient characteristically is thin with a barrel-shaped chest, is acyanotic, and has minimal productive cough and shortness of breath. Their work of breathing is such that the arterial PAO_2 and $PACO_2$ remain relatively normal. The patients maintain a high minute ventilatory rate and volume that initially compensates for the hypoxemia and CO_2 retention. With progression of the disease or exacerbation by coexisting diseases, the patient's work of breathing may increase with ultimate retention of CO_2 and hypoxemia late in the disease. There is minimal evidence of a right-to-left shunt (PaO_2 greater than 500 mm Hg with the patient on 100 percent oxygen for 20 minutes).

The chest examination reveals increased intercostal interspaces, hyperresonance to percussion, limited diaphragmatic excursion, and prolonged expiration. The patient may also exhibit use of accessory muscles for respiration, abdominal breathing, and the characteristic pursed lips. Wheezing is usually heard on auscultation, but in the presence of severe obstruction or hypoventilation, movement of air through the airway may be insufficient to produce the air turbulence manifested as wheezing. The liver may be palpable as a consequence of right ventricular heart failure, which may appear late in the disease. Clubbing of the nails and peripheral edema may be present.

Patients with emphysema commonly seek emergency care because of cough, wheezing and shortness of breath, or the emergence of acute bronchitis or other injurious events. A bulla or bleb may not only compress normal lung tissue, but may also spontaneously burst, producing a pneumothorax. The sudden deterioration of patients with obstructive disease should also alert the clinician to consider the development of GI bleeding secondary to peptic ulcer disease, pulmonary emboli, cardiac failure, or arrhythmias.

Laboratory Diagnosis

Roentgenograms of the chest in patients with emphysema suggest air-trapping, which is manifested by hyperinflation, low, flat diaphragms, wide interspaces, and the appearance of a small heart. Static lung volumes suggest hyperinflation with an increase in the ratio of residual volume to total lung capacity, a normal vital capacity, and an increase in the residual volume. Dynamic flow rates show a decreased ratio of FEV_1 to forced vital capacity, suggesting expiratory flow obstruction; normal airway resistance, indicating peripheral airway disease; and an increase in compliance, consistent with the loss of elastic recoil. There is little or no reversibility of air flow with bronchodilators. The diffusion capacity is reduced, indicating a loss of functioning lung tissue. The ECG may reveal right ventricular hypertrophy.

Treatment

Emergency care personnel must identify and treat the process that causes acute exacerbation of the patient's emphysema. Thus, the patient with a pneumothorax may require a chest tube, and the patient with acute infection, antibiotics. The prehospital treatment and emergency care is directed at the pathologic consequences of these injurious events.

Hypoxemia. Since obstruction to airflow may result in alveolar hypoventilation, V/Q mismatch, and hypoxemia, the prehospital care of patients with emphysema with acute exacerbation should include treatment with oxygen. Oxygen in the appropriate concentration will relieve irritability and somnolence, assist in correcting underlying metabolic lactic acidosis, and alleviate hypoxemia and its possible sequelae (including cardiac arrhythmias, pulmonary hypertension, cor pulmonale, and respiratory failure).

There is a risk involved in giving oxygen to patients disposed to carbon dioxide retention. Such patients depend upon hypoxia as an important stimulus for respiration and the elimination of hypoxia with oxygen may lead to increasing alveolar hypoventilation, respiratory acidosis, CO_2 narcosis, and ultimately apnea. Oxygen may be administered conveniently via nasal prongs, but a Venturi mask-type apparatus will provide more accurate delivery of the various concentrations of oxygen. Oxygen therapy in the emergency department should be accomplished with careful attention to the clinical appearance of the patient and arterial blood gas determinations.

Bronchospasm. A second potentially reversible and thus a treatable component associated with acute exacerbation of emphysema is bronchospasm. Intravenous theophylline preparations remain a potent pharmacologic tool in the prehospital treatment and emergency care of patients with bronchospasm in association with emphysema. This agent is approved for use by prehospital care personnel in many areas of the country, is effective in treating bronchospasm resulting from a variety of different mechanisms, and may be life-saving (as well as relatively safe) even though the etiologic cause of the bronchospasm is not clear. Thus, in the patient with emphysema who is not currently taking aminophylline, a loading dose of 5 to 6 mg/kg in D_5W may be given IV over 20 minutes. Patients who do not respond to IV aminophylline therapy may require concomitant treatment with sympathomimetic agents. Maintenance therapy is indicated for patients admitted for further inpatient care, as well as those who clinically improve and are discharged from the emergency department.

Beta-sympathomimetic agents are effective in treating bronchospasm in patients with emphysema. These agents may be delivered by aerosol or subcutaneously either alone or concurrently with the IV administration of aminophylline. Beta-2 sympathomimetic agents such as Bronkosol, 0.5 cc of 1:100 in 5 cc normal saline, may be aerosolized for 10 to 20 minutes. Alternatively, 2.5 to 5 mg of terbutaline sulfate can be given subcutaneously and repeated at four to six hours if required. The rationale for using agents with these mechanisms of action and side-effects is discussed elsewhere in this chapter.

Infection. In the emergency care setting, infection is a common coexisting or precipitating event in the patient with emphysema. In such patients common bacterial flora cultured from the respiratory tract include *Hemophilus influenzae* or *Streptococcus pneumoniae*. When there is evidence of bacterial respiratory infection, antimicrobial agents, such as ampicillin (500 mg four times a day) or amoxicillin (500 mg three times a day) or tetracycline (500 mg three times a day) each for ten days may be useful. Appropriate cultures should be taken before initiation of therapy.

In patients with acute severe exacerbation of emphysema, corticosteroids may be effective. Solu-Medrol can be administered (200 to 1,000 mg IV followed by tapering of the dose). Digoxin should be used in emphysema only when left ventricular heart failure is evident and then with caution since the incidence of arrhythmias increases in the presence of hypoxemia and hypokalemia (conditions often associated with emphysema). Diuretics may be helpful when there is left or right ventricular failure. Pharmacologic agents directed at sedation are to be avoided since they cause CNS depression of respiration. Antihistamines are contraindicated since they dry the secretions.

Finally, there is controversy regarding whether or not expectorants are useful in patients with emphysema. Fluids in the form of water orally or delivered by aerosol may help liquefy secretions.

Chronic Bronchitis

Bronchitis is a respiratory disease characterized by inflammation of the bronchiole tree with the subsequent secretion of excessive mucus. Chronic bronchitis, a disease of the central airway, is characterized by cough and the production of mucus sufficient to expectorate on most days for at least three months of each year for more than two successive years. The excessive mucus production is associated with hypertrophy of the submucosal glands, decreased size of the airway lumens, edema of the walls, muscle hypertrophy, inflammatory cells, enlargement of goblet cells, and possibly interstitial fibrosis.

Cigarette smoke is a major contributing factor in the development of bronchitis and frequent smoking is associated with increase in the size of the mucous glands. Tobacco smoke may not only inhibit ciliary mobility, and thus clearance of bacteria and secretions, but may also increase airway resistance by reflex bronchoconstriction. Environmental pollution and bacterial, viral,

and microplasma infections are associated with acute exacerbations in patients with bronchitis; the most common organisms are *Hemophilus influenzae* and *Streptococcus pneumoniae*. These recurrent episodes of inflammation may be related to injury of the small components of the airway, which may not be manifested as breathlessness until late in the progressive course of the disease. Thus, by the time a patient presents with moderate dyspnea, pulmonary function is already significantly impaired.

Patients with bronchitis exhibit obstructed air flow, overinflation, and maldistribution of ventilation compared with perfusion. The static lung volumes reveal hyperinflation with an increase in the ratio of residual volume to total lung capacity and a reduction in the vital capacity. Dynamic flow rates suggest expiratory obstruction as demonstrated by a decrease in the ratio of FEV_1 to forced vital capacity, and an increase in airway resistance consistent with central airway narrowing. Bronchodilator therapy improves the static lung volumes and improves expiratory flow rates. The diffusion capacity and compliance are decreased. Arterial blood gases usually reveal moderate arterial hypoxemia, arterial hypercapnia consistent with alveolar hypoventilation, and a chronic compensated respiratory acidosis (until late in the disease or during acute exacerbation).

The response to 100 percent oxygen may suggest right-to-left shunting. The chest roentgenogram reveals a typical obstructive pattern of hyperinflation with the addition of increased markings and "tram lines." Right ventricular heart failure occurs earlier than in pure emphysema, and the ECG may suggest pulmonary hypertension.

Patients with chronic bronchitis are sometimes referred to as blue bloaters because hypoxemia and carbon dioxide retention tend to occur relatively early, as compared with emphysema, and produce cyanosis and edema. The patient appears dyspneic at rest, is stocky in build, and has a relatively normal thoracic configuration. Cyanosis can be present with accompanying productive cough, pulmonary hypertension, and right ventricular heart failure. Pulmonary wedge pressure may be elevated during exercise, and left ventricular compliance may be decreased. Secondary polycythemia may develop from chronic hypoxia, reducing capillary wall contact of O_2-carrying RBCs.

Treatment

The treatment of the potentially reversible components of lung injury associated with bronchitis is similar to those associated with emphysema, and includes the treatment of hypoxemia with O_2, beta-2 bronchodilators for bronchospasm, the empirical use of antibiotics for bacterial infection, and liquefaction of sputum. Mechanical ventilation may be required for respiratory failure. (See Chapter 56.)

REFERENCES

1. Procino ND: Acute epiglottitis in adults. *J Ear Nose Throat* 57:30–34, 1978.
2. Hannallah R, Rosales JK: Acute epiglottitis: Current management and review. *J Can Anesth Soc* 25(2):84–91, 1978.
3. Lindquist JR, Franzen RE, Ossoff RH: Acute infectious supraglottitis in adults. *Ann Emerg Med* 9(5):256–259, 1980.
4. Mills JL, Spackman TJ, Bornes P, et al: The usefulness of lateral neck roentgenograms in laryngotracheobronchitis. *Am J Dis Child* 133(4):1140–1148, 1979.
5. Maze A, Block E: Stridor in pediatric patients. *Anesthesiology* 50(2):132–135, 1979.
6. Jordon WS: Nonsurgical treatment of epiglottitis and laryngotracheobronchitis. *Otolaryngology* 86:508–512, 1978.
7. Glicklich M, Cohen RD, Jona J: Steroids and bag and mask ventilation in the treatment of acute epiglottitis. *J Pediatr Surg* 14(3):247–257, 1979.
8. Tunnessen WW, Feinstein AR: The steroid-croup controversy: An analytic review of methodological problems. *J Pediatr* 96(4):751–756, 1980.
9. Lazarus GM: The child with croup. *J Am Med Wom Assoc* 32(11):406–408, 1977.
10. Mitchell DP, Thomas RL: Secondary airway support in the management of croup. *J Otolaryngol* 9(5):419–422, 1980.
11. Little JW: Pulmonary aspiration. *West J Med* 13(2):122–129, 1979.
12. Cohen SR, Herbert WI, Lewis GB Jr, et al: Foreign bodies in the airway: Five-year retrospective study with special reference to management. *Ann Otol Rhinolaryngol* 89:437–442, 1980.
13. Chatterji S, Chatterji P: The management of foreign bodies in air passages. *Anesthesia* 27:390–395, 1972.
14. Rothmann BF, Boeckman CR: Foreign bodies in the larynx and tracheobronchial tree in children: A review of 225 cases. *Ann Otol Rhinolaryngol* 89:434–436, 1980.
15. Aytac A, Yurdakul Y, Ikizler C: Inhalation of foreign bodies in children: report of 500 cases. *J Thorac Cardiovasc Surg* 74(1):145–151, 1977.
16. Linscott MS, Horton WC: Management of upper airway obstruction. *Otolaryngol Clin North Am* 12(2):351–373, 1979.
17. Heimlich HJ, Hoffman KA, Canestri FR: Food-choking and drowning deaths prevented by external subdiaphragmatic compression. *Ann Thorac Surg* 20(2):188–195, 1975.
18. Kravis TC, Henson PM: IgE-induced release of platelet activating factor from lung. *J Immunol* 115(6):1677–1681, 1975.
19. Brandstetter RD, Silver RT, Verina TK: Identifying the acutely ill patient with asthma. *South Med J* 74(6):713–715, 1981.
20. Bilgi C, Jores RL, Sproule BJ: Relation between pulsus paradoxus and pulmonary function in patients with chronic airway obstruction. *J Can Med Assoc* 117(12):1389–1392, 1977.
21. Nowak RM, Gordon KR, Wroblewski DA, et al: Spirometric evaluation of acute bronchial asthma. *JACEP* 8(1):9–12, 1979.
22. Shim CH, Williams HM Jr: Evaluation of the severity of asthma: Patients versus physicians. *Am J Med* 68(1):11, 1980.
23. Shim CH, Williams HM Jr: Pulsus paradoxus in asthma. *Lancet* 8063(1):530–531, 1978.
24. Petheram IA, Kerr IH, Collins JV: Value of chest radiographs in severe acute asthma. *Clin Radiol* 32(3):281–282, 1981.
25. Stalcup AS, Mellins RB: Mechanical forces producing pulmonary edema in acute asthma. *N Engl J Med* 297(11):592–596, 1977.
26. Smith JA, Weber RW, Nelson HS: Theophylline and aerosolized terbutaline in the treatment of bronchial asthma: double-blind comparison of optimal doses. *Chest* 78(6):816–818, 1980.
27. Josephson GW, MacKenzie EJ, Lietman PS, et al: Emergency treatment of asthma: A comparison of two treatment regimens. *JAMA* 242(7):639–643, 1979.
28. Josephson GW, Kennedy HL, MacKenzie EJ, et al: Cardiac dysrhythmias during the treatment of acute asthma. *Chest* 78(3):429–435, 1980.
29. Harper TB, Strunk RC: Techniques of administration of metered-dose aerosolized drugs in asthmatic children. *Am J Dis Child* 135(3):218–221, 1981.
30. Steventon RD, Wilson RS: Facemask or mouthpiece for delivery of nebulized bronchodilator aerosols? *Br J Dis Chest* 75(1):88–90, 1981.
31. McCombs RP, Lowell FC, Ohman JL Jr: Myths, morbidity and mortality in asthma. *JAMA* 242(14):1521–1524, 1979.
32. Brandstetter RD, Gotz VP, Mar DD: Optimal dosing of epinephrine in acute asthma. *Am J Hosp Pharm* 37(10):1326–1329, 1980.
33. Simons FE, Gillies JD: Dose response of subcutaneous terbutaline and epinephrine in children with acute asthma. *Am J Dis Child* 135(3):214–217, 1981.

58. Pulmonary Embolism

MARK ALLEN ROSEN, M.D.
BARRY E. BRENNER, M.D., Ph.D.
ROBERT R. SIMON, M.D.

INCIDENCE

Pulmonary embolism is a potentially lethal syndrome, commonly seen by the emergency medical clinician. Yet the incidence, pathophysiology, diagnosis, treatment, and prevention remain controversial. While some authors contend that pulmonary embolism is greatly over-diagnosed and overtreated,[1] many feel the opposite is true, particularly when the pulmonary vasculature is examined closely.[2]

Most studies estimate that approximately 50,000 deaths per year in the United States are directly due to pulmonary embolism.[3] In this country, it is estimated that 500,000 to 600,000 people experience a pulmonary embolism each year, since less than 10 percent are fatal.[3,4] Varying with the techniques used in postmortem examinations, the incidence of pulmonary embolism is reported to be between 10 and 64 percent. If a careful search for embolic traces such as a healed residua and fibrous bands and webs is undertaken, one or more embolic episodes may be shown in 64 percent of lungs at autopsy.[2] Without searching for these subtle signs of pulmonary embolism, only 29 percent of these patients would have had their conditions diagnosed.

The frequency of all pulmonary embolism found at routine autopsy (12.3 percent) and of major pulmonary embolism (7.1 percent) has remained essentially unchanged from that detected 20 years previously (13.6 percent and 8.6 percent, respectively).[5] Of the patients studied, the rate of diagnosis was only 9.3 percent and has been essentially unimproved during the past decade.

ETIOLOGY

Pulmonary emboli arise from a venous thrombosis of the lower extremity in 80 to 90 percent of the cases.[3] Of these, it is the large thrombi located in the veins above the knee that are more likely to embolize. Likewise, although the pelvic veins can thrombose, these veins are usually small, so the thrombi, and therefore the emboli, tend to be smaller.[3] Superficial veins usually totally occlude when inflamed and carry less of an embolic risk.[3] However, if the thrombus extends into the deeper veins, the risk is markedly elevated.

The incidence of pulmonary embolism rises dramatically with the patient's age. About 90 percent of fatal pulmonary emboli occur after age 50.[6] Jones and Sabiston note, however, that in children under 16 years of age, nearly 1 percent of 10,000 necropsies had documented pulmonary emboli.[7] In children, the nidus was found frequently in larger vessels. Thus, the emboli were often of larger size than those commonly seen in adults. Involvement was noted in the intracranial sinuses, intra-abdominal vessels, superior vena cava, right side of the heart, and pulmonary artery.

Pulmonary embolism is three and one-half times more frequent in patients with heart disease, the most frequent predisposing factor. Atrial fibrillation or congestive heart failure are both additional predisposing factors. In these conditions, the enlarged right atrium and slow circulation may result in the formation of a mural thrombus in the right atrium that serves as the source of the embolus.

Following trauma to the leg, there is an 800 percent increase in the risk for pulmonary embolism.[8] Even minor trauma increases the risk. Patients with fractures of the pelvis and lower extremity are particularly predisposed to pulmonary embolism. Neoplasms, especially those originating from the gastrointestinal tract, lung, or genitourinary system, significantly increase the chances of thromboembolism.[9,10] Emboli associated with malignancies tend to be resistant to conventional therapy.

Stasis from bed rest, prolonged standing, or excessive sitting can cause thromboembolism. Immobility after surgery should be avoided as much as possible. Deep vein thrombosis varies from 5 percent or less after surgical hernia repairs or cholecystectomy to 44.4 percent after prostatectomies.[11] Cardiac, biliary, and gastric surgery also are associated with a high risk of deep vein thrombosis.

Obesity, particularly in young people, predisposes the patient to thromboembolism.[12] The risk is doubled in extreme obesity.[13]

There is a sevenfold increase in pulmonary embolism in age-matched women during pregnancy and the early postpartum period.[14] Young women increase their risk by threefold if they are being treated with estrogens.

Blood disorders such as sickle cell anemia or trait, polycythemia vera, and leukemia with leukostasis predispose to thromboembolism owing to the stasis of venous return.[6]

THROMBOGENESIS

Virchow was the first to describe the triad of stasis, intimal damage, and increased coagulability of the blood as causative factors in thrombogenesis. There is a delayed clearance of activated clotting factors during stasis secondary to such common entities as congestive heart failure or bed rest. If the coagulation cascade is allowed to continue unopposed, thrombosis may occur. Even with minor trauma to the lower extremities, there are transient elevations in the end products of the coagulation cascade. However, most investigators feel that stasis alone will not cause venous thrombosis.[15] Additional factors, such as increased platelet adhesiveness, have been postulated. With the use of electron microscopy, thromboemboli in rabbits were shown to contain a thin eosinophilic rim consisting of platelets that had undergone some degree of metamorphosis.[16] In ad-

dition, these platelet aggregates were prevented in heparinized animals.

When a thrombus detaches, it migrates in a matter of seconds through the venous system to reach the lungs. Hemodynamic changes will occur instantaneously as the clot lodges in the pulmonary vasculature. Over the course of several days, the clot will contract and then endothelialize. Pulmonary vasculature obstruction and resultant hemodynamic abnormalities may persist for weeks.[17]

Following an embolic event, three mechanisms are involved in the restoration of normal vasculature: (1) mechanical changes, (2) fibrinolysis, and (3) organization. Subtle movement of an embolus due to dislodgement or fragmentation can markedly alter pulmonary blood flow.[4] Movement or fragmentation of an embolus can cause sudden clinical improvement in patients in shock or cardiac arrest. Sometimes the exact moment of dislodgement of the embolus can be noted by seeing a red flush due to increased blood flow pass over the patient's face.[18] The major mechanism that leads to resolution of pulmonary vascular occlusions is fibrinolysis.[4] If the thrombus has aged or become organized before embolization, it will be less sensitive to organization.[19] Organization takes days or weeks for completion. The smaller the amount of fibrinolysis, the more remains for organization and the more likely there is to be significant pulmonary arterial obstruction.[3] Vascular patency usually is restored, even with massive emboli, in less than 4 weeks.

PATHOPHYSIOLOGY

Patients may exhibit wheezing secondary to massive bronchoconstriction.[20–26] Some of this is due to thrombin-facilitated serotonin release from platelet aggregates. Bronchoconstriction probably is not, however, the primary etiologic factor in the dyspnea of pulmonary embolism, since the increase in large airway resistance experimentally is not enough to cause the sensation of breathlessness.[27]

Immediately after the embolus lodges, the pulmonary vascular resistance increases and pulmonary hypertension ensues. In the absence of previous cardiopulmonary disease, the mean pulmonary arterial pressure is usually not greater than 40 mm Hg, even with massive obstruction, probably because the normal nonhypertrophied heart cannot attain this high pressure.[28] In the patient with a mean pulmonary artery pressure greater than 40 mm Hg, with no previous cardiopulmonary disease, embolization is probably recurrent. In patients free of preembolic cardiopulmonary disease, the hemodynamic response to pulmonary embolism is most closely related to the extent of embolization.[29] The cardiac index is usually normal or increased, unless there is a massive embolization, in which case the cardiac index is often decreased. Patients with prior heart or lung disease tend to have pulmonary hypertension out of proportion to the magnitude of the embolic obstruction of the pulmonary vasculature.[29] It is believed that the rapid and often transient increase in pulmonary artery pressure is under humoral control. Experimentally, vagotomy, sympathectomy, and parasympathetic or sympathetic drugs do not significantly alter these hemodynamic changes. Therefore, the neural reflex, once postulated as responsible for the pulmonary hypertension of pulmonary embolism, has not gained widespread acceptance.[29] Seemingly insignificant emboli have been observed to cause major changes in pulmonary vascular resistance. Therefore, pure mechanical obstruction does not explain completely the etiology of pulmonary hypertension with pulmonary embolism.

Alveolar duct constriction and a decrease in production of alveolar surfactant probably account for much of the atelectasis seen with pulmonary embolization. After impaction, the affected alveoli receive no carbon dioxide from venous return, thus diluting the alveolar carbon dioxide content. This induces a compensatory reflex bronchiolar and alveolar duct constriction that tends to decrease the ventilation-perfusion mismatch. In addition, distal to the occluded vessel, there is a decreased concentration of surfactant,[16] probably secondary to hypoxia of the bronchiolar and alveolar cells that produce the surfactant.[27] Atelectasis may occur owing to constriction of the smaller airway in combination with parenchymal instability from lack of functioning surfactant.

Pulmonary infarction, actual necrosis of lung tissue, occurs in less than 10 percent of pulmonary emboli owing to the dual vascular supply of the lungs. An increase in the blood flow through bronchial and pulmonary artery anastomosis at the precapillary level probably begins within 2 hours following embolization.[27] These vessels enlarge rapidly, begin to resemble muscular arterioles, and may eventually provide the lung tissue distal to the embolus with greater flow than before the embolization.[27]

After a lobar or segmental branch of the pulmonary vasculature has been obstructed, the alveoli become transiently filled with red blood cells. If necrosis of lung parenchyma occurs, a pulmonary infarction has taken place. If not, this event is known as transient infarction, pulmonary hemorrhage, or incomplete infarction. Half of true infarctions will heal with residual fibrotic changes persistent on roentgenograms in 3 to 12 months despite the age of the patient.[17] Transient infarction will not, however, produce long-term roentgenographic abnormalities.

DIAGNOSIS

Signs and Symptoms

A high index of suspicion is required for diagnosis of acute pulmonary embolism. It is uncommon for a patient to present with dyspnea, pleuritic chest pain, hemoptysis, and pleural friction rub. Dyspnea is the only subjective finding present in most patients (Table 58–1).[30,31] Classically, the patient will exhibit a shallow tachypnea, with respiratory rates up to 50 breaths per minute. The exact etiology of chest pain associated with pulmonary embolism is controversial. The pain may be due to stimulation of the pain fibers located in the parietal pleura, if pulmonary infarction has occurred. Alternatively, pain secondary to pulmonary vasculature stretch has been postulated. When present, the pain may be pleuritic or a dull, substernal pressing sensation simulating angina. Indeed, hypoxia may be so severe as to produce angina. Dizziness or syncope due to cardiac arrhythmias from hypoxia or due to a marked reduction in cerebral blood flow may occur, particularly if the embolus is massive. Hemoptysis, secondary to congestive atelectasis or infarction, occurs in only one-third of patients.

Tachypnea and tachycardia are the only consistent signs of pulmonary embolism. However, since they are both transient phenomena, absence of their findings on arrival to a medical facility does not exclude pulmonary

TABLE 58–1   Manifestations of Pulmonary Embolism

Clinical Feature	*% Patients (Duke Study)**	*% Patients (UK Pulmonary Embolism Study)†*
Dyspnea	77	81
Pleuritic pain	63	72
Hemoptysis	26	34
Cough		54
Pulse >100	59	43
Tachypnea	38	88
Pleural rub	81	
Fever	43	42
Thrombophlebitis	23	34
Increased pulmonic sound	11	54
Rales	42	54

* Data from Wolfe WG, Sabiston DC: *Pulmonary Embolism.* Philadelphia, WB Saunders Co, 1980.

† Data from Urokinase-Streptokinase Pulmonary Embolism Trial Group: A national cooperative study. *JAMA* 236:1477, 1976. © 1976, American Medical Association.

Note: Dyspnea is seen in most patients but may not be present by the time the patient seeks medical attention. Other "classic" signs and symptoms such as hemoptysis and clinical evidence of thrombophlebitis are notoriously infrequent.

embolism. Wheezing from bronchoconstriction, due to loss of surfactant, may occur.[3] If pulmonary infarction is present, a pleural friction rub, pleural effusion, or fever may be present. Pleural rubs are heard most commonly over the lower lobes, where emboli occur most often. Fever, most commonly from 100°F to 101°F (37.8°C to 38.3°C), may peak at 104°F (40.0°C) and can persist as a low-grade, sustained, or spiking fever for more than 1 week.[32]

In patients with previous cardiopulmonary disease or recurrent embolization, cor pulmonale may develop with an S_3 gallop rhythm, right-sided ventricular heave, loud pulmonic sound, jugular venous distention, large A wave, cyanosis, and/or shock. Fixed splitting of the second heart sound is an ominous finding because it develops only in patients with marked ventricular compromise. The two factors contributing to its development are (1) early closure of the aortic valve as the left ventricle rapidly empties the reduced blood volume received from the lungs and (2) a delay in pulmonic closure due to the failure of the right ventricle to pump against an elevated pulmonary artery resistance.[33] A new systolic or diastolic murmur heard over the second left intercostal space or an interscapular bruit may be auscultated owing to a partial obstruction of the pulmonary vasculature by a large embolism.[18]

If present, signs and symptoms of deep vein thrombosis are helpful but they are only present in about one-third of patients.[31] Warmth, tenderness, and an increase in the diameter of the extremity may be noted. Homans' sign (discomfort behind the knee on forced dorsiflexion of the foot) is often inaccurate.[30,34] Inflating a blood pressure cuff to the point of pain (using the normal extremity first) has been advocated by some as a bedside test of thrombophlebitis,[35] but results of this test are inaccurate.[34,36,37]

In 2 years at Peter Bent Brigham Hospital, five cases of paradoxical embolism were diagnosed.[38] Thirty-five percent of the population had a patent foramen ovale wide enough to pass a dissecting probe; yet paradoxical embolism occurred only in a minority, owing to the left-to-right shunt across the foramen. The most common mechanism causing a reversal of this shunt and the potential for paradoxical embolism has been pulmonary embolism producing pulmonary hypertension, right ventricular failure, and subsequent right atrial hypertension.[38] In addition, Swan showed that in many atrial left-to-right shunts, there often exists a small right-to-left shunt, owing to streaming of venous blood from the inferior vena cava toward the region of the fossa ovalis and across the septal defect.[39] Whenever an arterial embolism, myocardial infarction, or cerebrovascular accident occurs in patients without obvious etiology, paradoxical embolism should be considered, especially in patients with pulmonary hypertension.

Patients with hemoglobin S-C disease are predisposed to develop pulmonary emboli. Bashour and Lindsay caution that the occurrence of an acute febrile episode with chest pain and pulmonary infiltrates in a black patient should alert the physician to search for pulmonary embolism subsequent to hemoglobin S-C disease since these patients often are not diagnosed as having sickle trait until past the second decade.[40]

In short, pulmonary embolism can occur in a wide variety of clinical settings. Yet only dyspnea, tachypnea, and tachycardia are reliable clinical features. Thus, clinical suspicion is crucial in the diagnosis of this entity.

Laboratory Findings

In pulmonary embolism, the white blood cell count rarely is greater than 15,000/cu mm and in many instances is less than 10,000/cu mm.[29] Leukocytosis in excess of 20,000/cu mm with a marked left shift favors another diagnosis, such as pneumonia. However, it must be remembered that pneumonia can be a late complication of pulmonary embolism. A triad of elevated levels of serum lactic dehydrogenase (LDH), normal levels of glutamic oxaloacetic transaminase, and elevated levels of bilirubin has been proposed as suggestive of embolism, but it is nonspecific and usually not present.[41] Patients with pulmonary emboli have a higher mean LDH_3 level than patients with congestive heart failure or pneumonia, but the pattern is not sufficiently characteristic to be of clinical use in the differential diagnosis of patients suspected of having pulmonary embolism.[42]

In almost all patients with pulmonary embolism, there is systemic arterial hypoxemia. Virtually all patients will have a PO_2 less than 90 mm Hg.[29] A diffuse and non-uniform bronchoconstriction secondary to serotonin release from thrombin-mediated platelet aggregates may account for the hypoxemia.[43] Occlusion of the pulmonary vasculature by emboli causes the remaining fraction of the vascular bed to accept a higher blood flow in order to sustain the normal cardiac output.[44] This right-to-left shunting has also been implicated as a main cause of hypoxemia.[44] Perfusion-ventilation mismatch and venous admixture causes an increased A-a gradient. Respiratory alkalosis may be present from hyperventilation.

Electrocardiographic Findings

Serial electrocardiograms in 135 patients with angiographic evidence of pulmonary embolism led to the following observations by Stein and associates.[45] In massive and submassive pulmonary embolism, the electrocardiogram was normal in 6 percent and 24 percent, respectively. The most common abnormality was

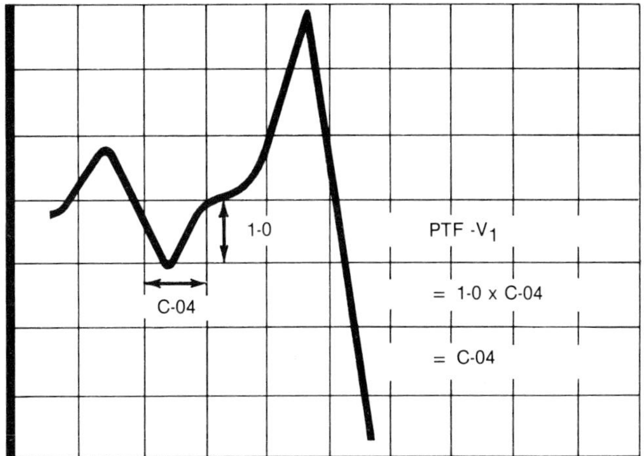

Figure 58–1 Method of Calculating PTF-V$_1$. *Source:* Abraham A: P-wave analysis in myocardial infarction, pulmonary edema and embolism. *Am Heart J* 89:301, 1975. Reproduced with permission.

nonspecific ST-T wave changes, seen in 42 percent. Only 26 percent of patients had the classic signs of acute cor pulmonale (i.e., $S_1 Q_3 T_3$, right bundle branch block, P pulmonale, or right-axis deviation). Surprisingly, left-axis deviation occurred as frequently as right-axis deviation (7 percent). An important finding was transient low voltage seen in the frontal plane in 6 percent of the patients. It was noted that the patients with electrocardiographic abnormalities had larger defects on lung scan and arteriogram and more significant elevation in the mean pulmonary arterial pressure and right ventricular diastolic pressure.[45] The PO_2 did not differ significantly between the groups of patients with or without electrocardiographic changes. Stein and associates concluded that acute ventricular dilation is a probable causative factor for the electrocardiographic changes in acute massive and submassive pulmonary embolism.[45]

When the patient presents acutely in the emergency department, it is often difficult to distinguish chest pain and dyspnea due to acute pulmonary edema, acute myocardial infarction, or acute pulmonary embolism. Abraham proposed that the algebraic product of the duration in seconds and the amplitude in millimeters of the terminal half of the P wave in lead V_1, (PTF-V_1) may be useful in these cases (Fig. 58–1).[46] He found that none of his 35 patients with acute pulmonary embolism had PTF-V_1 values more negative than -0.03. Yet 34 of 35 patients with acute pulmonary edema and 31 of 35 patients with acute myocardial infarction had values more negative than -0.03. Thus, PTF-V_1, a seldom-noted finding, may be of use clinically in separating patients with acute pulmonary embolism from those with acute or impending pulmonary edema.

Pulmonary Perfusion Scanning

Pulmonary blood flow can be assessed by use of radioisotopes such as iodine 131, technetium 99m, or chromium 51 tagged to albumin. With the patient in the supine position after intravenous injection of these macroaggregated particles, the pulmonary blood flow can be delineated. The six views obtained are anterior, posterior, right and left lateral, and right and left anterior oblique (Fig. 58–2, A). The particles become lodged in a small portion of the pulmonary alveolar and capillary beds without causing detectable hemodynamic alterations. Areas of defect in flow can be seen if pulmonary emboli are present. However, regional blood flow can be altered by a variety of cardiopulmonary diseases other than pulmonary embolism. Consequently, a positive perfusion lung scan is not specific for diagnosing pulmonary emboli. However, this technique has a high degree of sensitivity; a normal lung scan virtually excludes the diagnosis of embolization.[47] Cheely and co-workers point out the difficulty in analyzing the data comparing lung scanning, a noninvasive study, to angiography, an invasive test considered to be the "gold standard" for diagnosis.[48] They state that many studies are subject to criticism because the lung scans were performed with anterior, posterior, and lateral views with a rectilinear scanner, whereas a multiview gamma camera with oblique views in conjunction with a ventilation scan is currently considered the standard of practice. Commonly, despite adequate treatment, serial lung scans may demonstrate increased perfusion in some areas and decreased perfusion in others. This change in blood flow is due to the dynamic state of the pulmonary vasculature during resolution of emboli, whereby there is a redistribution of blood from areas of good perfusion to areas of previously poor perfusion, as the emboli resolve.

Ventilation-Perfusion Scanning

Aerosolized xenon 133 or indium 113m tagged to albumin may be administered to the patient after the perfusion scan to enhance the specificity of the lung scan. Theoretically, since pulmonary embolism is a vascular disease, there should be normal ventilation in abnormally perfused areas, creating a ventilation-perfusion mismatch (Fig. 58–2, A, B, and C). Likewise, if the perfusion defect is due to previous pulmonary disease, there should be a matching ventilatory defect. However, these generalizations are often not entirely accurate, since emboli to the pulmonary vasculature can cause ventilatory defects by bronchoconstriction and "transient" pulmonary infarction as well as "true" pulmonary infarction. Cheely and coworkers noted that two perfusion-ventilation patterns had an excellent correlation with subsequent pulmonary angiography.[48] There was a greater than 90 percent probability of pulmonary embolism if the lung scan showed multiple segmental and lobar perfusion defects with a normal ventilation. In none of their patients was there an angiographically proved pulmonary embolism if subsegmental or non-segmental matching defects existed. They concluded that if a patient is not in this high or low probability group (27 percent of their patients were in one of these groups), then pulmonary angiography is required, since its risks are less than that of long-term anticoagulation. Lung scanning may not be sensitive enough to diagnose a large intravascular embolus if there is a generalized reduction in pulmonary arterial blood flow.[33] A normal lung scan is usually interpreted as incompatible with the diagnosis of pulmonary embolism.[34] Rarely, a normal scan may, in fact, be produced if more blood enters the lung with the less obstructed circulation, so that sufficient pulmonary-capillary perfusion is produced. Small areas of decreased perfusion in the diaphagmatic area may be difficult to detect with ventilation-perfusion scans.[49]

The accuracy of a ventilation-perfusion scan is improved considerably when the scan is compared with the chest radiograph with regard to number and sizes of the perfusion defects (Table 58–2). In a retrospective analysis of 146 patients with suspected pulmonary embolism, Biello and associates note that when the ventilation-perfusion study demonstrated at least two moderate-sized mismatches (between 25 and 75 percent

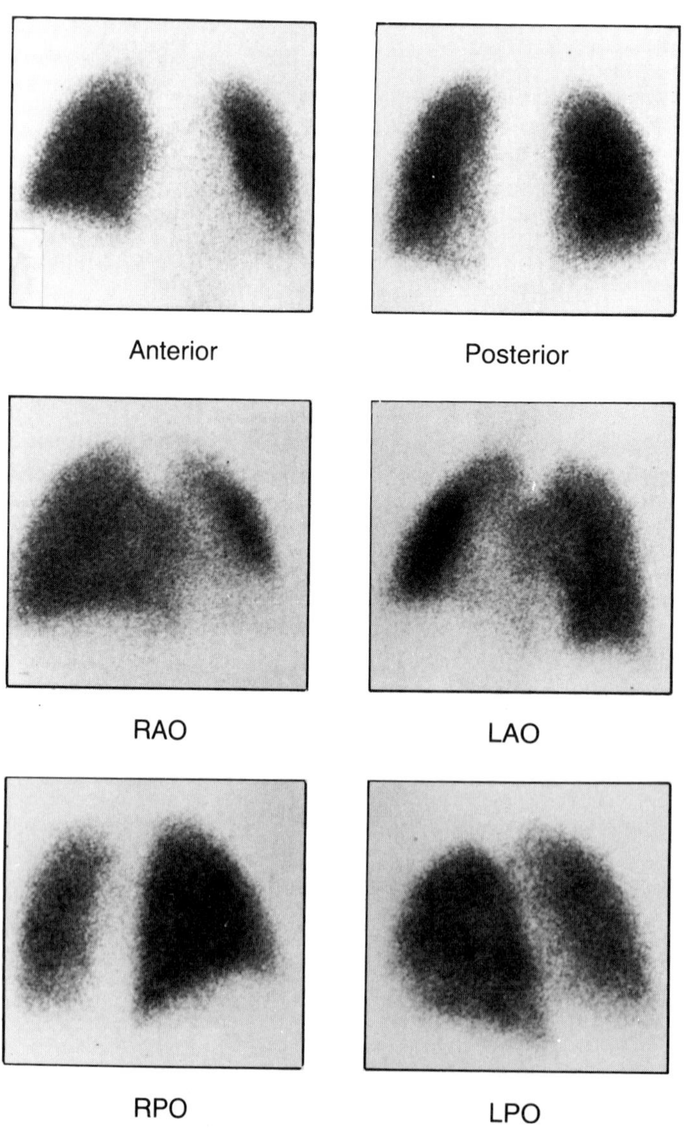

Figure 58–2 *A*   Six Views of A Normal Perfusion Lung Scan.

of segmental volume) or one large area of mismatch (greater than 75 percent of a segment), there was a 92 percent probability of pulmonary embolism.[47] Patients with either single or multiple small subsegmental perfusion defects did not have angiographically proved emboli. The single moderate-sized mismatch remained a diagnostic problem. There was only a 7.7 percent chance of pulmonary embolism, when the perfusion defect was substantially smaller than the corresponding abnormality of the chest roentgenogram. When the perfusion defect was larger than the defect on the chest roentgenogram, there was an 87 percent incidence of pulmonary embolism.

Some groups propose that due to the inherent risks of anticoagulation, pulmonary angiography is essential and should be performed on all patients suspected of pulmonary embolism. Menzoian and Williams at Boston University Medical Center performed a retrospective review of the accuracy of diagnosis of pulmonary embolism, based on clinical impression, arterial blood gas determination, and lung scanning. Although it is unclear what criteria were used in their ventilation-perfusion scan interpretation, there were 14 false-positives and 7 false-negatives of the 70 patients studied.[50] Many other studies favor lung scanning,[51-56] especially if the interpretation is enhanced by methods previously discussed.[47] In addition, lung scanning is relatively safe, is noninvasive, and can be used to follow the progress of the patient. Therefore, lung scanning should be used as a rapid screening procedure for all

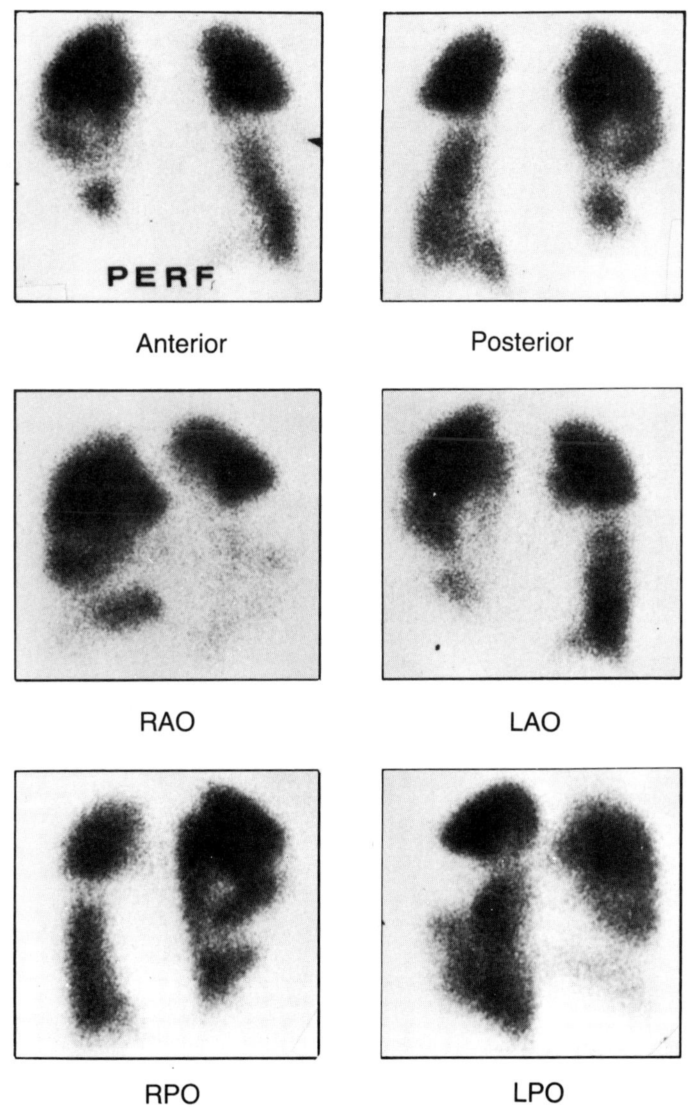

Figure 58–2*B*   Perfusion Lung Scan of a Patient with Pulmonary Embolism.

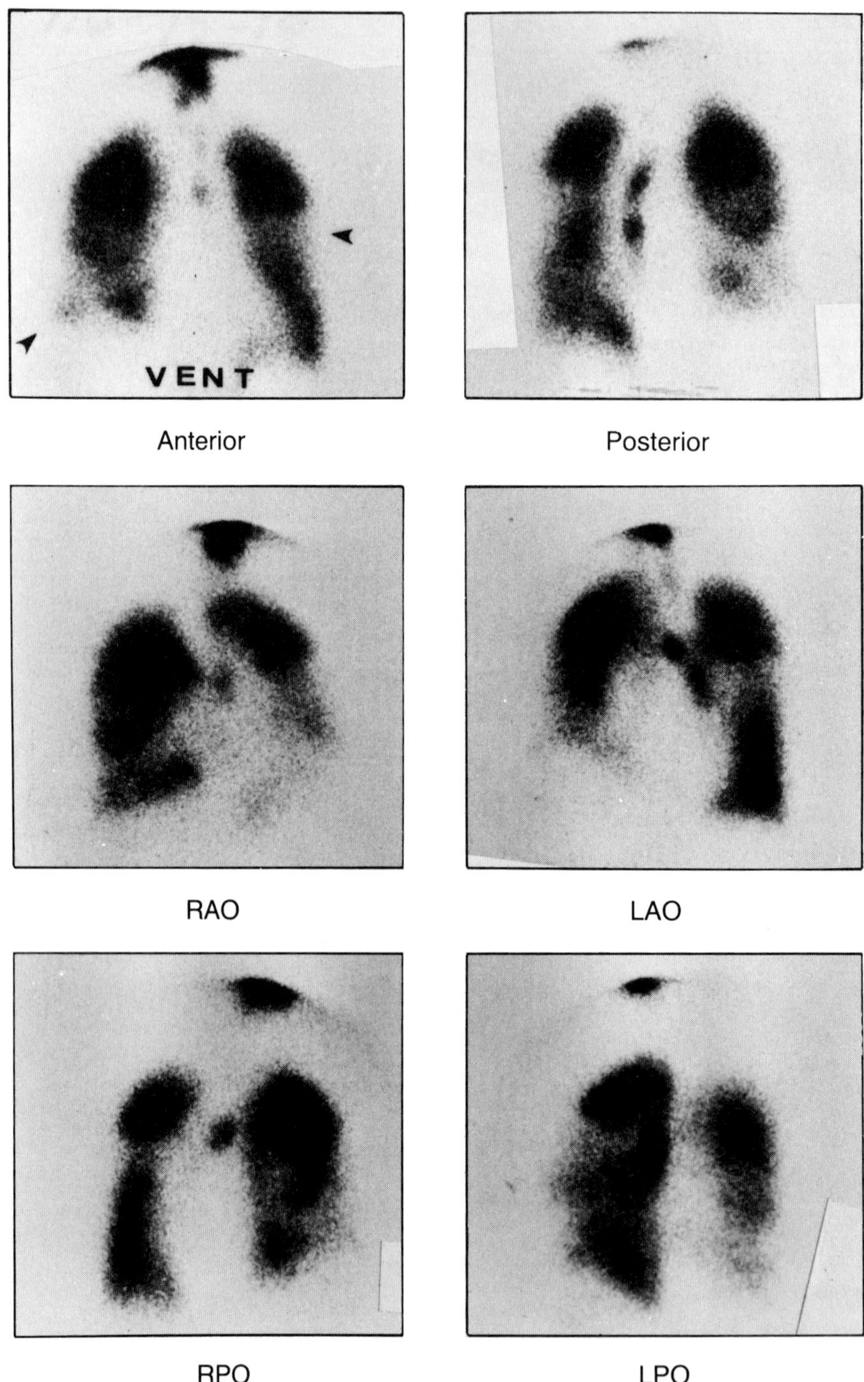

Figure 58–2 *C*   Ventilation Lung Scan of a Patient with Pulmonary Embolism.

patients suspected of pulmonary embolism, whenever possible. If the results of the lung scan are completely normal, a positive diagnosis is doubtful so angiography is not required. Otherwise, angiography should be performed, since the risks of anticoagulation exceed those of angiography.

Angiography

Although angiography is uniformly accepted as the most definitive procedure for the diagnosis of pulmonary embolism, it too has its limitations. Small emboli may go unnoticed since angiography cannot give clear

TABLE 58–2   Scheme for Interpretation of Ventilation-Perfusion Lung Scan

Interpretation	Pattern	Frequency Pulmonary Embolism (%)
Normal	Normal perfusion	0
Probability of pulmonary embolism:		
Low	Small V-Q mismatches	0
	Focal V-Q matches with no corresponding radiographic abnormalities	4.8
	Perfusion defects substantially smaller than radiographic abnormalities	7.7
Intermediate	Diffuse, severe airway obstruction	20
	Matched perfusion defects and radiographic abnormalities	27
	Single moderate V-Q mismatch without corresponding radiographic abnormality	33
High	Perfusion defects substantially larger than radiographic abnormalities	87
	1 or more large, or 2 or more moderate-sized, V-Q mismatches with no corresponding radiographic abnormalities	92

Source: Biello D, et al: Ventilation-perfusion studies in suspected pulmonary embolism. *Am J Roentgenol* 133:1033, 1979. © 1979.

whereby the catheter is advanced further, under fluoroscopy, and contrast material is injected into the pulmonary arteries or one of their subdivisions. The dye will exhibit less dilutional effect and a clearer, more definitive study will be obtained. With the use of this technique with magnification filming, pulmonary emboli or vessel cut-offs as small as 0.5 mm in diameter can be demonstrated (Fig. 58–3, A, B).[57,59] However, even with this technique, minimal changes such as fibrous webs and strands, detectable at autopsy, will go unnoticed.

The incidence of complications due to pulmonary angiography is approximately 4 percent (Table 58–3).[60,61] Mortality averages 0.2 percent and usually occurs in a patient with a right ventricular end diastolic pressure greater than 20 mm Hg.[61] Hypertonic contrast agents transiently increase pulmonary artery and right ventricular pressure, which is poorly tolerated in a patient with a severely compromised right ventricle.[61]

resolution of vessels 2 mm or less in caliber. However, emboli smaller than 2 mm do not appear to affect mortality and morbidity and need not be treated.[57] In addition, larger emboli can be missed if the physician looks only for a sharp "cut-off" of blood flow. A sharp "cut-off" is not seen as commonly as a "filling defect," which is created as contrast medium streams around a partially occluded thrombus.[3] The examination is reliable only if performed within 48 hours of the clinical episode.[30] After that time, significant fragmentation and resolution of the embolus may have begun, resulting in a negative study.[30] However, complete resolution may take 7 to 19 days[3,58] or more.[4]

If there is prior cardiopulmonary disease and the angiogram shows nonspecific abnormalities such as absence of smaller branches (i.e., "pruning"), retarded flow, or abnormal tapering of vessels, it is difficult to determine whether these findings are due to the underlying disease or to embolization. It is in these cases that selective or subselective angiography can be performed,

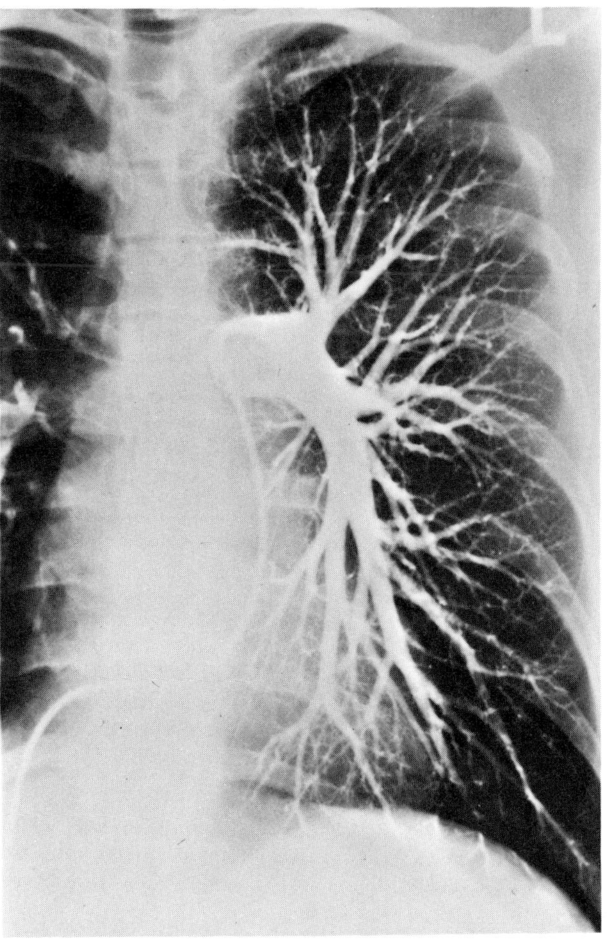

Figure 58–3 *A* Normal Pulmonary Angiogram of the Left Lung.

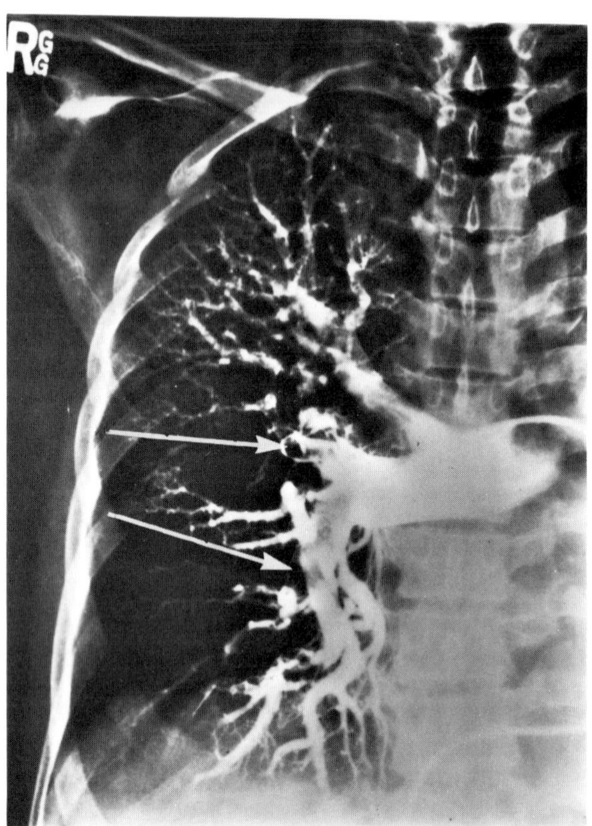

Figure 58–3 *B*   Pulmonary Angiogram of the Right Lung of a Patient with Pulmonary Embolism. *Note:* The upper arrow denotes a large embolus in the lateral segmental artery to the right middle lobe. The lower arrow indicates a second embolus obstructing the anterior basal and lateral basal segmental arteries to the right lower lobe.

TABLE 58–3   Complications of Pulmonary Angiography in a Study of 1,350 Patients

Complication	No. of Patients
Death (all patients had pulmonary hypertension)	3
Cardiac perforation	14
Endocardial or myocardial injury	6
Major cardiac arrhythmia	11
Cardiac arrest	5
Contrast material reactions	11
Miscellaneous	11
Total	61

Source: Mills S, et al: The incidence, etiologies and avoidance of complications of pulmonary angiography in a large series. *Radiology* 136:295, 1980.

MEDICAL THERAPY

Anticoagulation

Treatment of pulmonary embolism is aimed at preventing further embolization and controlling hemodynamic embarrassment while endogenous mechanisms attempt to restore the pulmonary vasculature (see algorithm in Figure 58–4). If pulmonary embolism is suspected, treatment should be initiated in the emergency department while further diagnostic studies are being pursued. Heparin, by preventing activation of factors IX and XI and by potentiating antithrombin III, is the mainstay in therapy for halting the thrombotic process.[3] The half-life of heparin is shorter in experimental pulmonary embolism than in venous thrombosis (12.0 minutes and 18.2 minutes, respectively).[62] Although the mechanism for increased heparin clearance in pulmonary embolism is uncertain, larger initial doses of heparin prevent this reduction in its half-life.[62] No oral form of heparin is available, since it is not absorbed from the gastrointestinal tract. Treatment is similar to treating deep venous thrombosis. Heparin is infused intravenously at 1,500 units/hour or 25 U/kg/hour.[63] Continuous infusion appears to have a lower incidence of bleeding.[29,63–66] However, if continuous infusion is not practical, a bolus of 5,000 units can be given intravenously every 4 hours. If venous access is a problem, 5,000 units of heparin can be administered every 4 hours or 10,000 units every 8 hours by the subcutaneous route. The partial thromboplastin time should be maintained at two to two and one-half times normal.[63] For a witnessed acute pulmonary embolism, the first dose of heparin should be 15,000 to 20,000 units.[3,62,67] Data suggest that vasoactive amines, released from platelets coating the embolus, may exaggerate the acute cardiopulmonary consequences of the embolism.[3] Heparin, in large doses, inhibits the release of these amines.

If the patient is no longer at risk of deep vein thrombosis or pulmonary thromboembolism, anticoagulation should be maintained for at least 7 to 10 days to allow the venous thrombus to become adherent to the wall of the vein and commence resolution and organization.[68] If risk still exists, 6 to 12 months of therapy is arbitrarily chosen by many physicians, although data documenting optimal length of anticoagulation are lacking. Prolonged therapy can be maintained with "minidose" heparin, in which case hematologic monitoring is not required, or with sodium warfarin (Coumadin). Sodium warfarin inhibits production of factors VII, IX, and X and prothrombin in the liver. Since sodium warfarin does not produce an anticoagulant effect for at least 48 hours, it can not be utilized as initial therapy for pulmonary embolism. This oral anticoagulant may be administered a few days before cessation of heparin

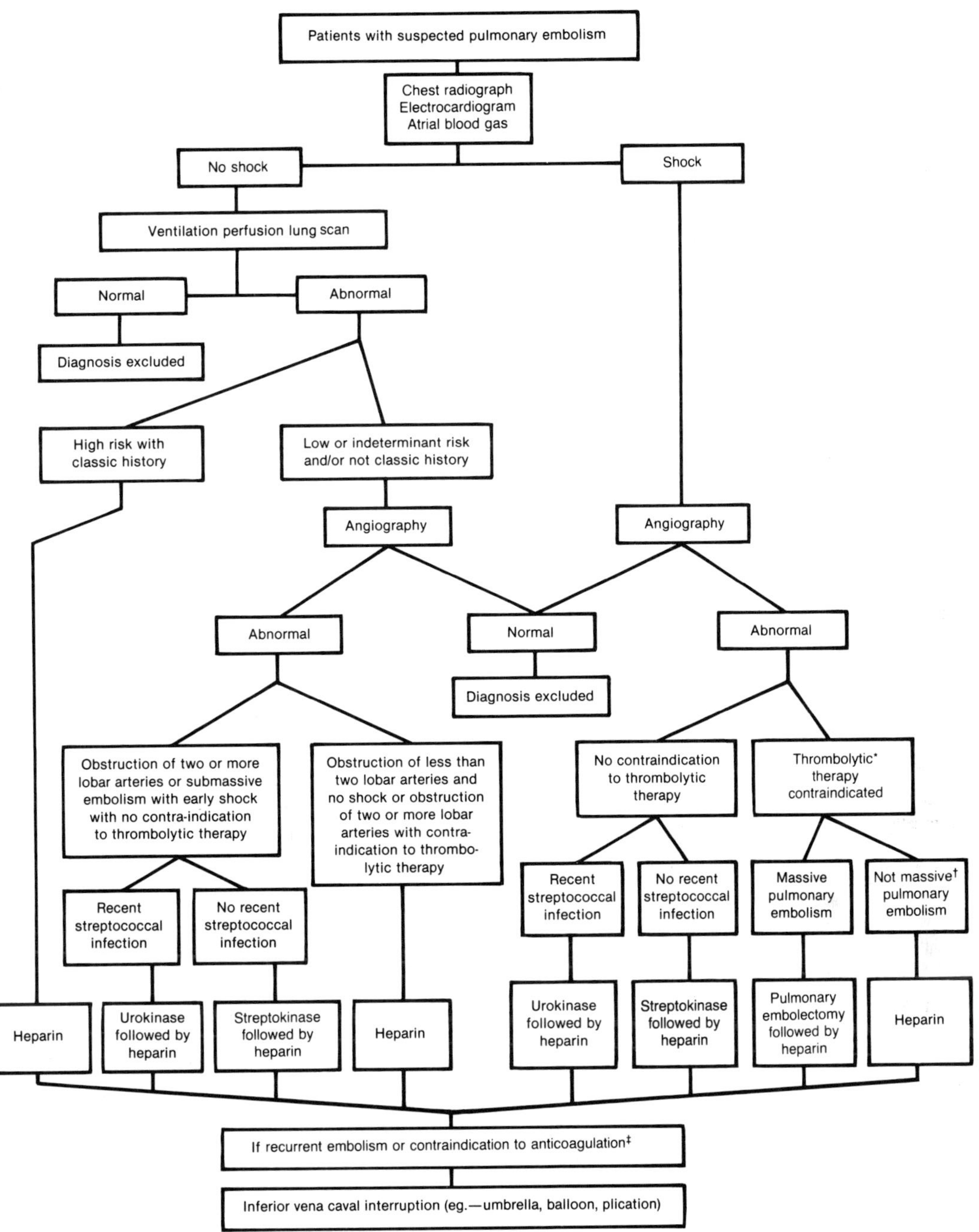

Figure 58–4 An Approach to Diagnosis and Therapy for Pulmonary Embolism. *Note:* * Contraindication to thrombolytic therapy: recent surgical procedure, bleeding diathesis, intracranial lesion, diastolic blood pressure greater than 120 mm Hg, allergy. † Shock due to another etiology. ‡ Contraindications to heparin therapy: uncontrollable active bleeding, allergy.

therapy to permit the prothrombin time to prolong. Doses of 5 to 10 mg are usually required to prolong the prothrombin time to two to two and one-half times normal.

It is crucial to discontinue all other intramuscularly administered medicines to minimize the risks of bleeding in patients treated with heparin. Oxygen and, if necessary, vasopressors should be administered to maintain a normal blood pressure.

Thrombolytic Therapy

In recent years, drugs known to activate plasminogen, and thus form the nonspecific proteolytic enzyme plasmin to bring about clot dissolution, have been studied for their potential use in the therapy of embolism. There are presently two prototypes: streptokinase and urokinase. Streptokinase is a nonenzymatic protein excreted by group C, β-hemolytic streptococci that can be used unless the patient presents with a high titer of antistreptococcal antibody.[69] If the patient has a recently documented streptococcal pharyngitis, urokinase should be used instead of streptokinase. Urokinase is a more expensive, enzymatic protein produced by human renal parenchymal cells.[69] In a study of the effect of thrombolytic therapy on pulmonary capillary blood volume in patients with pulmonary emboli, it was shown that thrombolytic agents allowed a more complete resolution of emboli than did heparin.[14] When evaluated at 2 weeks and subsequently at 1 year, capillary perfusion and diffusion were consistently improved in the group receiving thrombolytic agents, whereas in the group treated with heparin, the values remained more impaired.

Elliot and associates showed 80 to 100 percent lysis of clots in two-thirds of patients with streptokinase and no lysis in any of acute proximal venous thrombosis with heparinized patients.[70] In addition, 10 of 26 streptokinase-treated patients had a completely normal deep venous system at 3 months, as compared with none of the heparinized patients.

The Food and Drug Administration's indications for the use of thrombolytic agents include massive pulmonary emboli with obstruction equivalent to two or more lobar arteries and submassive emboli accompanied by shock or impending shock.[69] Streptokinase also has been approved for deep vein thrombosis with extension into the inferior or superior vena cava and arteriovenous cannula occlusion.[69]

The degree of thrombolysis is decreased if lesions are older than 7 days, if lesions are located in vessels with poor blood flow (small or totally occluded vessels), or if there is massive thromboemboli, hyperthermia, or hypothermia.[70]

In a national cooperative study, the National Heart and Lung Institute evaluated the efficacy of urokinase.[71] Although there was significant resolution of pulmonary emboli after 24 hours, there was no significant decrease in the recurrence of embolization or in the 2-week mortality as compared with the heparin group. Bleeding complicated treatment in 45 percent of patients in the urokinase group as compared with 27 percent in the heparin group.

During therapy with these agents, the thrombin time should be prolonged between two to five times the control. An initial loading dose of streptokinase, 250,000 IU, diluted in saline or dextrose administered over 30 minutes should precede the maintenance dose of 100,000 IU/hour for 24 to 72 hours. If urokinase is used, 4,400 IU/kg is given over 10 minutes followed by 4,400 IU/kg/hour for 12 hours.

Thrombolytic agents are used acutely to induce thrombus dissolution and improve the altered cardiopulmonary hemodynamics. They should not replace conventional anticoagulants. Once thrombolytic therapy is discontinued and the thrombin time falls to less than twice normal values (usually in 2 to 4 hours), a continuous heparin infusion should be instituted.[69]

Therapy with streptokinase or urokinase is contraindicated owing to the risk of hemorrhage if any surgical procedure has been performed in the past 10 days or if there is bleeding diathesis, any disease that can potentiate bleeding from a central nervous system embolism such as cerebrovascular accident in the past 2 months, bacterial endocarditis or mitral valve disease with atrial fibrillation, recent trauma, intracranial neoplasm, diastolic blood pressure greater than 125 mm Hg, active and progressive cavitating pulmonary disease, acute or chronic renal or hepatic disease, or history of allergic reaction to these drugs.[71,72]

Except for bleeding, which occurs in up to 45 percent of patients, other common side-effects such as fever or mild allergic reaction can be treated symptomatically. If bleeding is life threatening, ε-aminocaproic acid in doses of 5 gm initially followed by 1 gm/hour for 2 to 4 hours intravenously or orally can be used to reverse the effects of the thrombolytic agents.[69]

Dextran

Plasma expanders have been used on an experimental basis in treatment of massive pulmonary embolism.[73] Dextran has been utilized to redistribute blood flow into areas of lung previously underperfused because of pulmonary artery vasoconstriction and small vessel closure. This treatment can cause a dramatic increase in PO_2 and the cardiac index with a decreased pulmonary venous admixture. Dextran may be chosen as the plasma expander of choice because it has a known antithrombotic effect, reduces platelet activity, and facilitates lysis of fibrin clots.

SURGICAL THERAPY

In approximately 6 percent of patients, a surgical procedure is necessary to prevent recurrent embolization.[74] Common indications for surgery include recurrent embolization despite adequate anticoagulation, contraindication to anticoagulation, and septic pelvic emboli. If the location of the thrombi permit, bilateral femoral vein ligation is usually performed since long-term edema and stasis are infrequently encountered.[33] If this procedure is unsuccessful or contraindicated owing to thrombi located proximal to the groin, surgery on the inferior vena cava should be performed. Possible surgical procedures include caval ligation, caval plication, insertion of intraluminal devices such as an umbrella or sieve, or placement of mattress sutures in the vena cava to create a grid. There is a 30 to 35 percent incidence of postligation sequelae, including recurrent phlebitis, pain, and edema.[75] There is at least a 20 percent incidence of recurrent pulmonary embolization due to collateral flow after caval ligation or placement of an intraluminal umbrella. Intraluminal devices may be improperly inserted into the iliac or renal vein. In addition, migration into the right atrium, right ventricle, or pulmonary artery may occur. Greenfield designed an intraluminal device with hooks designed to grasp the wall of the inferior vena cava without penetration to prevent proximal migration of the thrombus.[76] Plication of the vena cava allows small multiple emboli to pass. In two-thirds of the patients, recurrent thrombosis with extension at the site of plication is so severe that complete caval obstruction occurs.[77] The use of a mattress suture to form a grid also seems to cause the same problem.

Pulmonary embolectomy is rarely performed in recent years. It is reserved for patients with massive pulmonary embolism with shock, those unresponsive to alternative forms of therapy, and those who probably would not survive without immediate embolectomy. Depending on the population studied and the expertise of the surgical team, mortality varies from 10 to 100 percent, averaging usually between 35 to 40 percent. Heinbacher and associates reported their success with embolectomy in 11 patients in shock, including 4 patients who had suffered cardiac arrest.[78] Pulmonary angiograms were performed on all patients before surgery, at times with partial cardiopulmonary bypass from femoral vein to artery through a portable pump oxygenator. Closed compression cardiac massage tended to fragment and propel proximal emboli distally, thus improving circulation. Only 1 of the 11 reported patients died.

Sabiston and coworkers suggest pulmonary embolectomy as the treatment of choice for a small but definite group of patients with chronic emboli that do not resolve and may cause a state of cor pulmonale.[79] In these patients, the emboli become fibrotic and adherent to the arterial wall instead of resolving. These investigators postulate inadequately functioning endogenous thrombolysins or emboli arising from an older than usual and fibrotic thrombus as the possible etiology of this syndrome. Patency of the pulmonary artery distal to the obstruction seems to be the main determinant of success. In five of six patients with chronic pulmonary emboli, status post embolectomy, there was an improvement of dyspnea and cyanosis with an increase in the PO_2 and a decrease in the mean pulmonary artery pressure. This uncommon illness could be detected earlier if follow-up lung scans are done several months after embolization to document return of normal or near-normal pulmonary perfusion.

MORTALITY

Mortality of untreated pulmonary embolism averages 30 percent.[4] Two-thirds of patients who die of pulmonary embolism do so within the first 2 hours, usually before hospitalization. Mortality appears to be related more closely to the underlying cardiopulmonary status of the patient than to the magnitude of the embolus. In addition, patients with associated heart disease have a slower rate of recovery.[80] In patients who survive long enough to have the diagnosis established and appropriate prophylactic therapy begun, the morbidity of patients with massive pulmonary embolism without shock (6 percent) is essentially the same as that of patients with submassive embolism (5 percent).[81] Only 8 percent of patients with documented pulmonary embolization die of this entity.[81] Mortality is closely related to the hypotension secondary to acute right ventricular failure, which seems to correlate with the patients' previous cardiovascular status. In a study of late prognosis of acute pulmonary embolism, 36 of 42 patients without prior left ventricular failure survived for follow-up at 1 to 7 years later, as compared with only 3 of 16 with prior heart failure.[82]

REFERENCES

1. Robin E: Overdiagnosis of pulmonary embolism: The emperor may have no clothes. *Ann Intern Med* 87:775, 1977.
2. Freidman D, Suyemoto J, Wessler S: Frequency of thromboembolism in man. *N Engl J Med* 272:1278, 1965.
3. Moses K: Pulmonary Embolism. *Am Rev Respir Dis* 115:829, 1977.
4. Dalen J, Alpert J: Natural history of pulmonary embolism. *Prog Cardiovasc Dis* 17:259, 1975.
5. Coon W: The spectrum of pulmonary embolism. *Arch Surg* 111:398, 1976.
6. Parker BN, Smith JR: Pulmonary embolism and infarction. *Am J Med* 24:402, 1958.
7. Jones RH, Sabiston DC: Pulmonary embolism in childhood. *Surg Sci* 3:35, 1966.
8. Bauer G: Thrombosis following leg injuries. *Acta Chir Scand* 90:229, 1944.
9. Byrd RB, Divertie MD, Spittell JA, Jr: Bronchogenic carcinoma of thromboembolic disease. *JAMA* 202:1019, 1967.
10. Amundsen MA, Spittel JA, Jr, Thompson JH, Jr: Hypercoagulability associated with malignant disease. *Ann Intern Med* 58:608, 1963.
11. Hartsuck J, Greenfield L: Post-operative thromboembolism. *Arch Surg* 107:733, 1973.
12. Kent DC, Reid D: Pulmonary embolism in active duty servicemen. *Arch Environ Health* 12:509, 1966.

13. Coon W, Willis P: Deep vein thrombosis and pulmonary embolism. *Am J Cardiol* 4:611, 1959.
14. Sharma GV RK, Burleson V, Sasahara A: Effect of thrombolytic therapy on pulmonary-capillary blood volume in patients with pulmonary embolism. *N Engl J Med* 303:842, 1980.
15. Virchow R: Postoperative pulmonary embolism. *Am J Cardiol* 12:451, 1963.
16. Thomas D, Gurewich V, Ashford T: Platelet adherence to thromboemboli in the relation to the pathogenesis and treatment of pulmonary embolism. *N Engl J Med* 274:953, 1966.
17. Dalen J, Banas J, Brooks H, et al: Resolution rate of acute pulmonary embolus in man. *N Engl J Med* 280:1194, 1969.
18. Gorham LW: A study of pulmonary embolism. *Arch Intern Med* 108:76, 1961.
19. Freiman DG, Wessler S, Lertsman M, et al: Experimental pulmonary embolism with serum-induced thrombi aged in vivo. *Am J Pathol* 39:95, 1961.
20. Boyer NH, Curry JJ: Bronchospasm associated with pulmonary embolism: Respiratory failure. *Arch Intern Med* 73:403, 1944.
21. Gurewich V, Thomas D, Stein M, et al: Bronchoconstriction in the presence of pulmonary embolism. *Circulation* 27:339, 1963.
22. Jewett JF: Asthma emboli and cardiac arrest. *N Engl J Med* 288:265, 1973.
23. Olazabel F, Jr, Roman-Irizarry LA, Oms JD: Pulmonary emboli masquerading as asthma. *N Engl J Med* 278:999, 1968.
24. Rebhun J: Pulmonary embolism in asthmatics. *Ann Allergy* 28:586, 1970.
25. Webster JR, Jr, Saadeh GB, Eggun PR, et al: Wheezing due to pulmonary embolism: Treatment with heparin. *N Engl J Med* 274:931, 1966.
26. Windebank WJ, Boyd G, Moran F: Pulmonary thromboembolism presenting as asthma. *Br Med J* 1:90, 1973.
27. Soloff LA, Rodman T: Acute pulmonary embolism: I. Review. *Am Heart J* 74:710, 1967.
28. Scully R, Galdabini JJ, McNeely B: Case records of Massachusetts General Hospital. *N Engl J Med* 296:33, 1977.
29. Sharma GV RK, Sasahara A, McIntyre K: Pulmonary embolism: The great imitator. *DM* 72:4, 1976.
30. Wolfe WG, Sabiston DC: *Pulmonary Embolism.* Philadelphia, WB Saunders Co, 1980.
31. Urokinase-Streptokinase Pulmonary Embolism Trial Group: A national cooperative study. *JAMA* 236:1477, 1974.
32. Murray H, Ellis G, Blumenthal D, et al: Fever and pulmonary thromboembolism. *Am J Med* 67:232, 1979.
33. Soloff L, Rodman T: Acute pulmonary embolism: II. Clinical. *Am J Med* 74:829, 1979.
34. Ortiz-Ramirez T, Serna-Ramirez R: New early diagnostic sign of phlebitis of the lower extremities. *Am Heart J* 50:366, 1955.
35. Lowenberg R: Early diagnosis of phlebothrombosis with aid of a new test. *JAMA* 155:1566, 1954.
36. DeWeese J, Rogoff S: Phlebographic patterns of acute deep venous thrombosis of the leg. *Surgery* 53:99, 1963.
37. Barner H, DeWeese J: An evaluation of the sphygmomanometer cuff pain test in venous thrombosis. *Surgery* 48:915, 1960.
38. Dalen JE: Cardiovascular responses to experimental pulmonary embolism. *Am J Cardiol* 20:3, 1967.
39. Meister SG, Grossman W, Dexter L, et al: Paradoxical embolism: Diagnosis during life. *Am J Med* 53:292, 1972.
40. Boshour T, Lindsay J: Hemoglobin S-C disease presenting as acute pneumonitis with pulmonary angiographic findings in two patients. *Am J Med* 58:559, 1975.
41. Wacker WE, Rosenthal M, Snodgrass P, et al: Diagnosis of pulmonary embolism and infarction. *JAMA* 178:8, 1961.
42. Light R, Bell W: LDH and fibrinogen—fibrin degradation products in pulmonary embolism. *Arch Intern Med* 133:372, 1974.
43. Levy S, Simmons D: Mechanism of arterial hypoxemia following pulmonary thromboembolism in dogs. *J Appl Physiol* 39:41, 1975.
44. Wilson JE III, Pierce AK, Johnson RL, Jr, et al: Hypoxemia in pulmonary embolism: A clinical study. *J Clin Invest* 50:481, 1971.
45. Stein P, Dalen JE, McIntyre KM, et al: The electrocardiogram in acute pulmonary embolism. *Prog Cardiovasc Dis* 17:247, 1975.
46. Abraham A: P-wave analysis in myocardial infarction, pulmonary edema and embolism. *Am Heart J* 89:301, 1975.
47. Biello D, Mattar AG, McKnight RC, et al: Ventilation-perfusion studies in suspected pulmonary embolism. *Am J Roentgenol* 133:1033, 1979.
48. Cheely R, McCarthey WH, Perry JR, et al: The role of non-invasive tests versus pulmonary angiography in the diagnosis of pulmonary embolism. *Am J Med* 70:17, 1981.
49. Fred H, Burdine JA, Jr, Gonzalez DA, et al: Arteriographic assessment in the diagnosis of pulmonary thromboembolism. *N Engl J Med* 275:1025, 1966.
50. Menzoian J, Williams L: Is pulmonary angiography essential for the diagnosis of acute pulmonary embolism? *Am J Surg* 137:543, 1979.
51. Isawa T, Hayes M, Taplin G: Radioaerosol inhalation lung scanning: Its role in suspected pulmonary embolism. *J Nucl Med* 12:606, 1971.
52. DeNardo GL, Goodwin DA, Ravasini R, et al: The ventilatory lung scan in the diagnosis of pulmonary embolism. *N Engl J Med* 282:1334, 1976.
53. McNeil BJ, Ventilation-perfusion studies and the diagnosis of pulmonary embolism: Concise communication. *J Nucl Med* 21:319, 1980.
54. McNeil BJ, Holman BL, Adelstein SJ: The scintigraphic definition of pulmonary embolism. *JAMA* 227:753, 1974.
55. McNeil BJ: A diagnostic strategy using ventilation-perfusion studies in patients suspected for pulmonary embolism. *J Nucl Med* 17:613, 1976.
56. Taplin GV, Chopra SK: Lung perfusion-inhalation scintigraphy in obstructive airway disease and pulmonary embolism. *Radiol Clin North Am* 16:491, 1978.
57. Novelline R, Baltarouch O, Christos A, et al: The clinical course of patients with suspected pulmonary embolism and a negative pulmonary arteriogram. *Radiology* 126:561, 1978.
58. Fred HL, Axelrod MA, Lewis JM, et al: Rapid resolution of pulmonary thromboemboli in man: An angiographic study. *JAMA* 196:1137, 1966.
59. Bookstein JJ: Segmental arteriography in pulmonary embolism. *Radiology* 93:1007, 1969.
60. Dalen J, Brooks H: Pulmonary angiography in acute pulmonary embolism: Indications, techniques and results in 367 patients. *Am Heart J* 81:175, 1971.
61. Mills S, Jackson D, Older R, et al: The incidence, etiologies and avoidance of complications of pulmonary angiography in a large series. *Radiology* 136:295, 1980.
62. Chiu H, VanAken W, Hirsh J, et al: Increased heparin clearance in experimental pulmonary embolism. *J Lab Clin Med* 90:204, 1977.
63. Simon TL, Hyers TM, Gaston JP, et al: Heparin pharmacokinetics: Increased requirements in pulmonary embolism. *Br J Haematol* 39:111, 1978.
64. Lundblad R, Brown W, Mann K, et al: *Chemistry and Biology of Heparin.* New York, Elsevier-North Holland, 1981.
65. Salzman EW, Deykin D, Shapiro R, et al: Management of heparin therapy. *N Engl J Med* 292:1046, 1975.
66. Glazier RL, Crowell EB: Randomized prospective trial of continuous vs. intermittent heparin therapy. *JAMA* 236:1365, 1976.
67. Thomas D: Therapeutic role of heparin in acute pulmonary embolism. *Curr Ther Res* 18:21, 1975.

68. Taylor HE, Sheperd WE, Robertson CE: An immunohistochemical examination of granulation tissue with glomerular and lung antiserums. *Am J Pathol* 38:39, 1961.

69. Bell W, Meek A: Guidelines for the use of thrombolytic agents. *N Engl J Med* 301:1266, 1979.

70. Elliot MS, Immelman EJ, Jeffery P, et al: A comparative randomized trial of heparin versus streptokinase in the treatment of acute proximal venous thrombosis: An interim report of a prospective trial. *Br J Surg* 66:838, 1979.

71. Urokinase Pulmonary Embolism Trial Study Group: Urokinase pulmonary embolism trial phase I results. *JAMA* 214:2163, 1970.

72. American Hospital Formulary Service: *Streptokinase and Urokinase.* Washington, DC, American Society of Hospital Pharmacists, 1979.

73. Hauser C, Shoemaker W: Volume loading in massive acute pulmonary embolus. *Crit Care Med* 7:304, 1979.

74. Thomas DP: Treatment of pulmonary embolic disease. *N Engl J Med* 273:885, 1965.

75. Schwartz SI, Lillehei RC, Shires GT, et al: *Principles of Surgery.* New York, McGraw-Hill Book Co, 1974.

76. Greenfield LJ: A new intracaval filter permitting continued flow and resolution of emboli. *Surgery* 73:599, 1973.

77. Bergan J: Prevention of pulmonary embolism. *Arch Surg* 92:605, 1966.

78. Heimbecker RO, Keon WJ, Richards KU: Massive pulmonary embolism: A new look at surgical management. *Arch Surg* 107:740, 1973.

79. Sabiston DC, Jr, Wolfe WG, Oldham HW, Jr, et al: Surgical management of chronic pulmonary embolism. *Ann Surg* 185:699, 1976.

80. Tow D, Wagner H, Jr: Recovery of pulmonary arterial blood flow in patients with pulmonary embolism. *N Engl J Med* 276:1053, 1967.

81. Alpert J, Smith R, Carlson J: Mortality in patients treated for pulmonary embolism. *JAMA* 236:1477, 1976.

82. Parakos JA, Adelstein SJ, Smith RE, et al: Late prognosis of acute pulmonary embolism. *N Engl J Med* 289:55, 1973.

59. Respiratory Failure

DAVID ROSE, M.D.

Ventilation serves two basic purposes: maintenance of the arterial pH and oxygenation of the arterial blood. Respiratory failure then, by definition, is the inability to defend the arterial pH against either respiratory or metabolic acidosis or the inability to adequately oxygenate the arterial blood. Acute respiratory failure may arise *de novo* or may be superimposed on underlying chronic lung disease. This discussion will center on the physiology of breathing and the relationship of the mechanics of breathing to the etiology of respiratory failure. The pathophysiology of respiratory failure will be viewed from two perspectives: clinical assessment of ventilation and arterial blood gas interpretation.

Ventilation moves fresh gas into the alveoli (alveolar ventilation) and removes CO_2 from the body. Gas moves into the lungs because a pressure gradient is developed between the airway and the alveoli. This pressure difference may be initiated in either of two ways. Spontaneous ventilation creates a pressure in the lungs that is below ambient pressure by dropping the diaphragm and expanding the chest wall. Air moves into the lungs because pleural pressure and hence alveolar pressure is less than atmospheric pressure. Mechanical ventilation produces a pressure at the airway that is greater than atmospheric pressure and forces air into the lungs under positive pressure. Air moves along a gradient from an area of higher pressure, the airway, to one of lower pressure, the lungs, until the pressure differential between these two areas equalizes.

The work of breathing is normally expended during inhalation; exhalation is passive. Some of the work done during the inspiratory cycle to expand the thorax and move the diaphragm is stored as potential elastic energy and released during the expiratory phase. The recoil of the rib cage and the elastic recoil of the lung normally serve to move air out of the lung as a passive event. Only when flow is obstructed or when the respiratory rate is high is there an active component to assist exhalation.

CONTROL OF VENTILATION

The two major areas responsible for the control of ventilation are a central and a peripheral chemoreceptor area. The brain stem, the central area, is responsible for about 85 percent of the respiratory drive. The central chemoreceptor cells are stimulated primarily by the pH of the cerebrospinal fluid (CSF) which bathes the brain stem.

Carbon dioxide diffuses freely between the blood and the CSF and regulates the ventilatory drive through an effect on hydrogen ion concentration (pH). A fall in pH (rise in hydrogen ion concentration) of the CSF stimulates the brain stem chemoreceptors and increases the output from both the inspiratory and vasomotor centers. The ventilatory cycle is normally controlled by the arterial PCO_2 through its effect on the CSF pH. The normal response from an increase in arterial CO_2

(fall in arterial pH) is an increase in the depth of respiration followed shortly by an increase in respiratory rate. The change in arterial pH, through its effect on CSF pH, stimulates the vasomotor center to increase both cardiac output and peripheral vascular resistance. It is the central mechanism that is responsible for the respiratory depression seen with narcotics. Morphine and other opiates shift the CO_2 response curve down and to the right.

The peripheral chemoreceptors reside primarily in the aortic and carotid bodies found at the bifurcation of the carotid artery and on the aortic arch. They are stimulated primarily by a decrease in oxygen supply from such causes as a low arterial oxygen tension, decreased blood flow, anemia, and changes in arterial pH. Stimulation of these bodies causes an increase in tidal volume and ventilatory rate, tachycardia, hypertension, increase in pulmonary vascular resistance, and an outpouring of catecholamines from the adrenal gland.

The central receptors will respond to changes in arterial PCO_2 of 1 mm Hg while the peripheral chemoreceptors will not respond unless the CO_2 tension changes by more than 10 mm Hg. The central chemoreceptors do not respond to hypoxemia while the peripheral receptors are activated only when the arterial PO_2 falls below 60 mm Hg. Excessively high levels of CO_2 will eventually depress rather than stimulate the central chemoreceptors.

Chronic Obstructive Pulmonary Disease (COPD)

High levels of O_2 in the arterial blood may depress ventilation in patients with COPD. Most patients with COPD and acute respiratory failure respond to an increase in inspired O_2 with an increase in arterial O_2 tension and an improvement in clinical status. Some patients however, experience progressive hypercapnia and acidosis with resultant stupor or coma and may require mechanical ventilation.

The typical COPD patient is chronically ill, always hypoxemic, may retain CO_2, has poor exercise tolerance, and depends on cardiac reserve to maintain homeostasis. The low arterial PO_2 is the "hypoxic drive" which maintains ventilation. The poor distribution of ventilation and the high degree of venous admixture seen with this disease state will produce large changes in alveolar O_2 tension with small increases in the inspired O_2 concentration. A patient with COPD, when given supplemental O_2, will primarily decrease cardiac and pulmonary work and not change arterial PO_2, because the primary determinant of ventilatory effort in COPD is tissue oxygenation. The increase in alveolar O_2 will allow the patient to decrease cardiopulmonary work and still maintain arterial PO_2 at an acceptable, albeit low, level.

This disease, by producing high airway resistance, increased dead space, and a large intrapulmonary shunt has led to an increase in the work, and the O_2 cost of breathing. Work of breathing is held to the minimal acceptable level by settling for a low arterial PO_2 and an inadequate alveolar ventilation. The drive to breathe with COPD comes primarily from the peripheral chemoreceptors (hypoxemia) and the work of breathing is kept at the minimal level that will supply the tissue O_2 needs. The adaptive result is that the work of breathing will decrease and a low arterial PO_2 will be maintained rather than the work of breathing being maintained at a high level and arterial PO_2 rising. The decrease in alveolar ventilation results in an increase in arterial CO_2 and a respiratory acidosis.

The use of a high inspired O_2 concentration has produced acute ventilatory failure superimposed on chronic respiratory insufficiency. The obvious treatment for this type of ventilatory failure is to lower or discontinue the O_2 therapy. The primary goal of O_2 therapy in patients with chronic ventilatory failure is to minimize the work of breathing and not to increase the arterial PO_2. The judicious use of O_2 will serve to support the patient's cardiopulmonary system by improving the ventilatory status while other measures are instituted to reverse the course of the acute ventilatory failure. Oxygen therapy is never curative and only buys time until other definitive measures can be undertaken.

AIRWAY SUPPORT

Five major situations may require airway support for respiratory failure:

- Unconsciousness
  a) Drugs
  b) CNS (central nervous system)
- Obstruction
- Cardiorespiratory failure
- Neurologic dysfunction
- Trauma

Unconsciousness

The most obvious of these is unconsciousness. Any patient in an obtunded state must have an airway evaluation to assess two functions: (1) Are the patient's reflexes intact enough to protect the airway? and (2) Is ventilation adequate? The clinician must be able to answer strongly in the affirmative to both of these questions or must intervene.

The lung must be protected from aspiration of oropharyngeal and gastric contents by either an orotracheal or nasotracheal tube if the patient is unable to protect the airway. The use of an endotracheal tube is vastly preferred to an emergency tracheostomy. An adequate tidal volume must also be assured by whatever method is most suitable. If the tidal volume is not deemed adequate or there are signs of upper airway obstruction, the head should be extended, unless contraindicated by neck injury, and the jaw lifted upward to move the tongue from the posterior pharynx. (See Chapter 56.)

The airway may be obstructed by secretions, foreign bodies, soft tissue swelling, or malposition of the head in an obtunded patient. The signs of obstruction may be subtle if there is minimal ventilatory effort. Partial obstruction is indicated by stridor or a snoring sound and may be accompanied by retractions and the use of accessory muscles. Severe obstruction will often be accompanied by cyanosis and, in the conscious patient, agitation. A person found unconscious may appear to be sleeping but may be truly apneic. The examiner must look at the chest, listen for breath sounds, and feel for the movement of air from the mouth or nose. If ventilation is inadequate then immediate steps must be taken to ensure adequate alveolar ventilation.

Obstruction

Obstruction may be caused by bleeding, masses, croup, epiglottitis, or foreign bodies. Removal of the offending object is the obvious treatment when possible. Dorsiflexion of the head and forced elevation of the jaw will open the hypopharynx blocked by a retrolapsed tongue. Care should be taken when inserting instruments into the mouth if the cause of the obstruction is unknown. Patients with vascular or necrotic tumors, retropharyngeal abscess, or epiglottitis may be harmed by blunt probing with suction catheters or oral airways. Nasotracheal intubation can be done when the jaw cannot be opened because of fractures, trismus, or facial trauma. (See Chapter 57.)

Cardiorespiratory Failure

Cardiorespiratory failure may also require airway support. Patients with asthma, pulmonary edema, cardiac arrest, or chronic lung disease may need intubation and ventilation if they are unable to do the work of breathing adequately.

Neurologic Dysfunction

Neurologic problems such as poliomyelitis, myasthenia gravis, and the effects of neurotoxic drugs may prevent the patient from protecting the airway or from adequately moving the diaphragm. Especially when mental state is altered it is necessary to assess ventilation and intervene if needed.

Trauma

Trauma, especially of the chest, should alert the clinician of the need for airway assistance. Paradoxical respiration in the presence of an unstable chest wall may lead to an inadequate tidal volume. Cord lesions will also cause paradoxical breathing because of intercostal muscle paralysis.

CLINICAL SIGNS

Respiratory distress is the objective sign of a patient with cardiorespiratory failure; dyspnea is the subjective symptom. Dyspnea describes any state in which the patient becomes conscious of difficulty or effort in breathing or the need for greater respiratory efforts to satisfy air hunger. Dyspnea may be predominately inspiratory or expiratory. Inspiratory dyspnea occurs primarily with obstruction from such causes as tumor, foreign body, upper airway infection, or extrinsic compression of the trachea that impedes the free flow of air during inspiration. There is often retraction of the intercostal spaces and a low-pitched crowing sound called stridor. Expiratory dyspnea is associated with obstruction to the smaller airways as in asthma, bronchitis, and obstructive emphysema. Expiration is prolonged, expiratory wheezes may be audible, and often the intercostal spaces bulge outward.

The signs to alert the clinician to the possibility of respiratory failure are many and varied, but often the only clue to elevation in arterial CO_2 is the presence of hypertension and tachycardia or headache and flushing. Hypoxemia may be heralded by an altered mental state without a sensation of distress. If any question exists regarding the adequacy of ventilation an arterial blood gas must be drawn to confirm the diagnosis.

The key to the evaluation, diagnosis, and treatment of respiratory failure is clinical assessment and arterial blood gases. A normal blood gas does not necessarily mean the patient is doing well if the clinical evaluation reveals a respiratory rate of 40 breaths per minute with marked retractions and the use of accessory muscles. On the other hand a patient may appear quiet, comfortable, and breathing easily because the arterial CO_2 is 120 mm Hg and the mental state depressed.

Respiratory Evaluation

The clinical respiratory evaluation must begin with observation, preferably with the patient disrobed. Ensuring an airway and adequate tidal volume take precedence over all other maneuvers. Once assured that the patient's ventilatory status is stable enough so that no acute intervention is required the clinical exam should begin.

The same guidelines are followed as in the evaluation of the airway: look, listen, and feel. Observation begins at the patient's head looking for the use of accessory muscles. Patients with marked distress use the temporalis muscle, wiggle the ears, raise the eyebrows on inspiration, flare the nostrils, and breathe through an open mouth. The nose is the source of 75 percent of the upper airway resistance to breathing. Open-mouth breathing and nasal flaring are mechanisms to decrease resistance to inspiration. Patients, such as asthmatics, with expiratory resistance do not flare the nostrils because inspiratory resistance is not a major obstacle for them.

The neck is observed for the use of the sternocleidomastoid muscle which is an accessory muscle of inspiration. This is best evaluated by gently pushing on the belly of the muscle to feel a contraction during inspiration. The trachea and suprasternal notch are observed for the presence of "tracheal tug" which is the exaggerated inward movement of this area during inspiration. It is a sign of increased intrapleural pressure and is seen with upper airway obstruction primarily, but also when the lungs are stiff (decreased lung compliance).

The chest is observed for symmetry of expansion and the presence of intercostal retractions. Retractions are caused by increases in pleural pressure above that generated by normal inspiration. As the chest wall forcefully expands, the soft tissue between the ribs is sucked inward. This is a normal occurrence with rapid respiratory rates, but is also seen when a decrease in lung compliance prevents the lung from expanding easily during inspiration so that a large pleural pressure gradient is created.

Abdominal muscles are accessory muscles of exhalation and are used to force air out of the lungs. They come into play when exhalation is obstructed such as during an asthma attack or other intrathoracic airway obstruction. The abdominal muscles may also be used during rapid breathing to shorten the expiratory time and allow more time for inhalation. A hand is gently placed on the abdomen to feel the contraction of the abdominal muscles during exhalation. Exhalation is normally passive and no muscles are used.

Auscultation

Auscultation is the best technique to compare the state of bronchial patency of various lung areas and to detect abnormal respiratory sounds arising from dis-

eased areas although the patient with respiratory distress may not be able to fully cooperate with the exam. The chest roentgenogram has done so much to elucidate pulmonary pathology that the art of auscultation is being lost. Its greatest value lies in the acute situation while awaiting the chest roentgenogram when it is necessary to rule out pneumothorax, tension pneumothorax, and other potentially life-threatening problems.

Chest Percussion

Percussion of the chest is of less utility in the acute situation than in the evaluation of chronic disease, but important information may be gained by laying hands on the chest. Careful examination should include palpation of the thorax for areas of crepitation, tenderness, masses, and pulsations. Differences in expansion of one hemithorax in comparison with the other can be more easily appreciated by palpation than by visual examination. The hands are placed over the lower anterolateral aspect to the chest with the thumbs along the costal margin each pointing toward the xyphoid. Expansion may be limited by pleurisy, fractured ribs, or other trauma to the chest.

Ventilation in Disease

The ventilatory pattern seen in a diseased state is determined by the work of breathing. A patient will choose a ventilatory pattern to minimize energy expenditure rather than to maximize efficient physiologic ventilation. This important concept allows the clinician to deduce important information about airway resistance and lung compliance from the rate and depth of breathing. The work necessary to overcome elastic recoil (lung compliance) is increased when breathing is deep and slow, just as a stiff balloon is harder to inflate with a single deep breath than with a series of smaller breaths.

On the other hand, the work necessary to overcome airway resistance is increased when breathing is rapid and shallow. There is a ventilatory frequency at which the total work of breathing is minimal for any given lung compliance and airway resistance. When compliance falls (stiff lungs), ventilatory frequency will increase and tidal volume will decrease. When airway resistance increases, the respiratory rate decreases and tidal volume increases. Figure 59–1 shows the plot of elastic work (lung compliance), resistance work (airways), and total work as a function of ventilatory frequency.

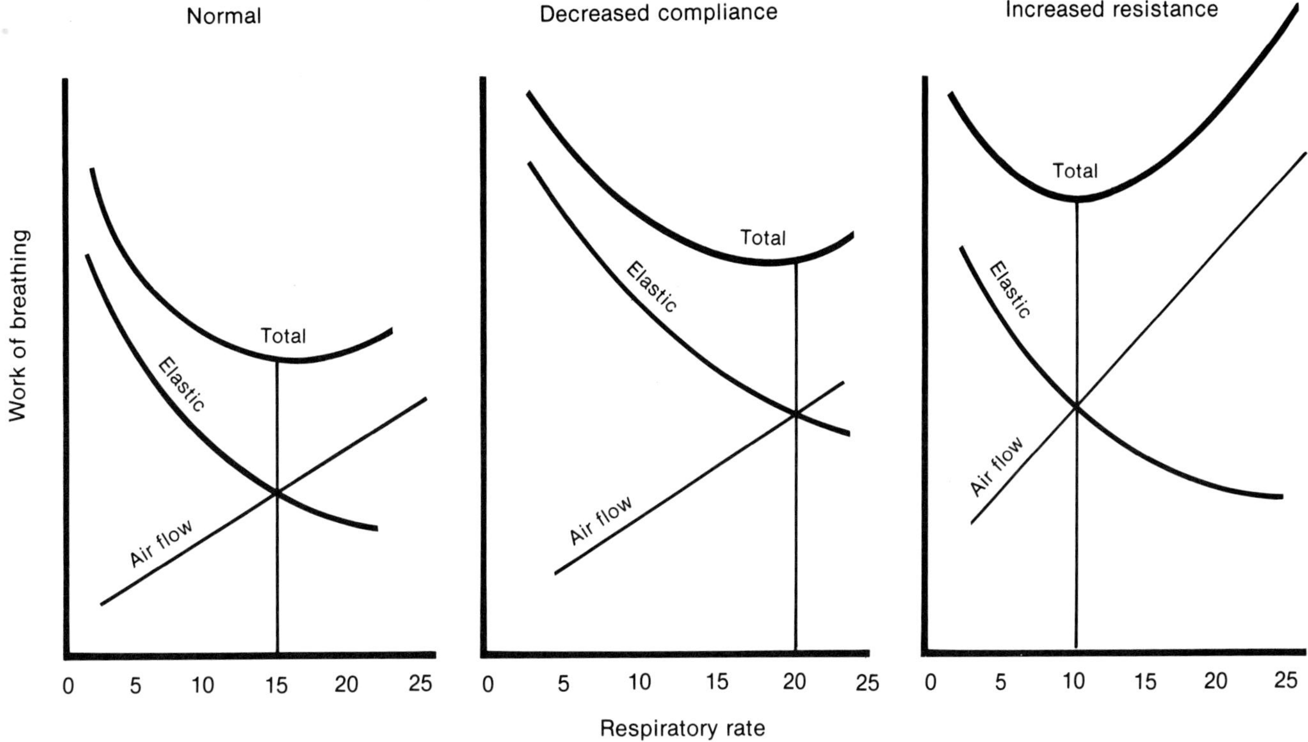

Figure 59–1   The Work of Breathing at Different Ventilatory Frequencies. The frequency at which total work is minimum depends on elastic resistance and airways resistance.

ARTERIAL BLOOD GASES

Clinical assessment is the first and most important aspect of acute care, and laboratory tests are all of secondary importance. A patient with respiratory failure is best evaluated and followed with serial arterial blood gas monitoring and with repeat clinical evaluations. The increased availability of arterial blood gas monitoring in the emergency department has made it imperative that the physician have the expertise to rapidly analyze these samples. Decisions regarding the adequacy of ventilation, oxygenation, and acid-base status can be readily assessed and closely regulated by such arterial samples.

The term arterial blood gases really refers to two gases, O_2 and CO_2 and to two serum measurements which are not gases, pH and bicarbonate. The gases and the pH are usually measured directly using appropriate specific electrodes while the bicarbonate is calculated from the pH and $PaCO_2$ according to the Henderson-Hasselbach equation.

Partial Pressure

The layer of gas that surrounds the earth is most dense at the surface and thins out at altitude. This gas has weight and exerts a pressure termed the atmospheric pressure. This pressure may be expressed in units of weight such as pounds per square inch or millimeters of mercury (mm Hg) or in a unit of pressure such as torr which is not related to weight or gravity. The atmospheric pressure decreases with increasing altitude because the number of gas molecules per unit volume decreases relative to that at sea level. Most discussions use sea level as the reference for barometric pressure, which is 760 mm Hg or 760 torr (1 torr = 1 mm Hg at 1 g of gravity).

The sum of the pressures of each gas in a mixture must add up to ambient pressure. Each gas exerts a partial pressure in the mixture, which is proportional to the fractional concentration of that gas in the mixture. Each gas exerts its pressure independent of the other gases and dependent only on its concentration. Oxygen makes up 21% of the atmosphere so it exerts a partial pressure of 21% of 760 mm Hg or 160 mm Hg. Nitrogen makes up 79% of the atmosphere and exerts a partial pressure of 79% of 760 mm Hg or 600 mm Hg.

The concentration of the various gases in our atmosphere remains relatively constant with increases in altitude even though the barometric pressure falls. At 18,000 ft barometric pressure is approximately half that at sea level, but O_2 still makes up 21% of the molecules and contributes 21% of the pressure, while N, which makes up about 79% of the atmosphere, contributes 79% of the pressure. The partial pressures of O_2 and N at ½ atm (380 mm Hg) equal 80 mm Hg and 300 mm Hg, respectively.

Carbon Dioxide

The $PaCO_2$ is solely determined by two factors, CO_2 production (V_{CO_2}) and CO_2 elimination, the alveolar ventilation (V_A). The partial pressure of CO_2 in the arterial blood is directly proportional to the amount of CO_2 produced and inversely proportional to the alveolar ventilation.

$$PaCO_2 \, \alpha \, \frac{V_{CO2}}{V_A}$$

Production of CO_2 may be increased acutely by such states as shivering, fever, sepsis, seizures, hyperalimentation, and will lead to an increase in $PaCO_2$ if alveolar ventilation remains constant. Alveolar ventilation serves to bring fresh gas into the alveoli and remove CO_2 from the body. The partial pressure of CO_2 in the arterial blood is inversely proportional to the alveolar ventilation when CO_2 production is constant. The term alveolar hypoventilation is applied when the $PaCO_2$ is greater than 40 torr and alveolar hyperventilation when the $PaCO_2$ is less than 40 torr. Alveolar ventilation is defined as the tidal volume (V_T) minus the dead space (V_D).

$$V_A = V_T - V_D$$

A patient with a constant CO_2 production and minute ventilation and a sudden increase in $PaCO_2$ (alveolar hypoventilation) must have either a decrease in tidal volume or an increase in dead space. Dead space is wasted ventilation, which is defined as ventilation in excess of perfusion. Hemodynamic factors that affect pulmonary blood flow may cause an increase in $PaCO_2$ without an absolute decrease in ventilation.

An acute rise in $PaCO_2$ causes an immediate rise in serum bicarbonate because CO_2 is directly converted into bicarbonate through the action of carbonic anhydrase.

$$CO_2 + H_2O \underset{\text{anhydrase}}{\overset{\text{carbonic}}{\rightleftharpoons}} H_2CO_3 \rightleftharpoons H^+ + HCO_3^-$$

A chronic elevation in $PaCO_2$ will lead to a greater increase in bicarbonate than will acute changes because of renal compensatory mechanisms. Patients with persistently elevated arterial levels of CO_2 will increase

their renal reabsorption of bicarbonate in an attempt to return the pH toward normal.

The following rules allow the clinician to quantify and evaluate changes in pH, $PaCO_2$, and bicarbonate. These rules help to determine if changes in $PaCO_2$ are acute or chronic by the extent of the deviation in bicarbonate from normal. These rules also allow for rapid interpretation of disorders of pH when used in conjunction with the premise that the body does not overcompensate for acid-base disorders. Assume that the normal $PaCO_2$ is 40 torr and the normal bicarbonate is 24 mEq/liter.

Rule 1. For every *acute* 10-torr rise in $PaCO_2$ the bicarbonate will rise by 1 mEq/liter.
Rule 2. For every *chronic* 10-torr rise in $PaCO_2$ the bicarbonate will rise by 4 mEq/liter.
Rule 3. For every 10-torr *fall* in $PaCO_2$ the bicarbonate will fall by 2 mEq/liter.
Rule 4. For every *acute* 10-torr change in $PaCO_2$ the pH will change in the same direction by 0.1 unit.

Acid-Base Status

Serum bicarbonate level is affected by changes in $PaCO_2$ because CO_2 is converted into bicarbonate through the action of carbonic anhydrase. An elevation in $PaCO_2$ will cause an increase in serum bicarbonate and a decrease in $PaCO_2$ will cause a decrease in serum bicarbonate. The bicarbonate level in the blood may reflect metabolic as well as respiratory alterations because a metabolic acidosis will convert bicarbonate and hydrogen ions to CO_2 and water. The term base excess is used to quantify the changes in serum bicarbonate due to metabolic causes.

Base excess is defined as the deviation in bicarbonate from that predicted by a change in $PaCO_2$. It is the change in bicarbonate due to metabolic causes. In effect, respiratory alterations are accounted for using rules 1, 2, and 3; any deviation in the measured bicarbonate from this predicted level must be due to metabolic causes. Base excess is a way to quantify metabolic acid-base changes and to differentiate metabolic from respiratory changes in pH. Base excess is the difference between the patient's measured bicarbonate concentration and the predicted bicarbonate according to the patient's $PaCO_2$ using rules 1, 2, and 3.

A patient with an acute rise in $PaCO_2$ from 40 to 50 torr and a measured bicarbonate of 25 mEq/liter has a base excess of 0 because according to rule 1, for every acute 10-torr rise in $PaCO_2$ bicarbonate will rise by 1 mEq/liter above the normal level of 24 mEq/liter. A base excess of 0 implies that there is no metabolic component to the acid-base derangement; it is purely respiratory. If the above rise in $PaCO_2$ were chronic then the base excess would be -3 mEq/liter because according to rule 2, for every chronic 10-torr rise in $PaCO_2$ bicarbonate will rise by 4 mEq/liter. The difference between the predicted 28 mEq/liter and the measured 25 mEq/liter is -3 mEq/liter. This would indicate that in addition to a chronic respiratory acidosis ($PaCO_2 = 50$) there is also a metabolic acidosis (-3 mEq/liter). Base excess is calculated by predicting what the bicarbonate should be for the measured $PaCO_2$ and then concluding that any deviation from this prediction is due to metabolic causes. The normal range for base excess is -2 to $+2$ mEq/liter.

Efficiency of Oxygenation

Hypoxemia is defined as an arterial O_2 tension below normal. In practice the utility of this definition hinges on what is considered normal. The generally accepted "normal value" for PaO_2 on an F_1O_2 of 0.21 (room air) is 90 to 100 torr, but this is based on the theoretical alveolar PO_2 of 100 torr and does not reflect the age-related decrease in oxygenation that is seen clinically. A more useful estimation is obtained by the following formula:

$$PaO_2 = 105 - (\tfrac{1}{2}\ patient's\ age)$$

The analysis of the partial pressure of O_2 in the blood is facilitated by an understanding of the major physiologic causes of hypoxemia. Arterial hypoxemia is due to either decreased alveolar oxygen tension or right-to-left intrapulmonary shunting of blood.

Decreased alveolar O_2 tension can result from alveolar hypoventilation, a decrease in venous hemoglobin saturation, or venous admixture.

Decreased Alveolar Oxygen Tension

Alveolar Hypoventilation. Alveolar hypoventilation while breathing room air is the most obvious cause of a low alveolar PO_2. Alveolar ventilation brings fresh gas into the alveoli and removes CO_2. The partial pressure of O_2 in the alveolus and hence the blood must decrease as CO_2 builds up from hypoventilation. When breathing room air the sum of the partial pressures of CO_2 plus O_2 must remain constant; as the pressure of CO_2 in the alveolus (P_ACO_2) builds up the pressure of O_2 in the alveolus (P_AO_2) must decrease. The alveolar air equation (Fig. 59–2) is the formula which describes the relationship between O_2 and CO_2 in the alveolus. The graphic solution for the alveolar air equation is also shown in Figure 59–2 for room air.

Nitrogen is a relatively insoluble gas that exerts the same pressure in the alveoli as in the atmosphere. The

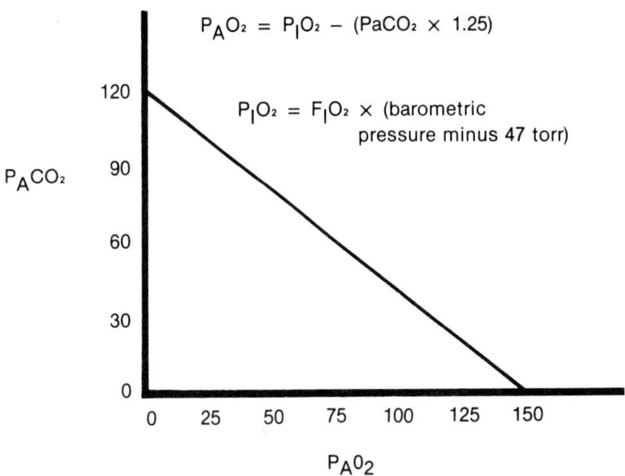

Figure 59–2 The Aveolar Air Equation. *Note:* While breathing room air, as $PaCO_2$ increases P_AO_2 falls. When $PaCO_2$ increases above 60 torr PaO_2 may fall to a dangerous level.

pressure of O_2 in the alveoli will be decreased below that in the trachea by an amount directly proportional to the partial pressure of CO_2 added to the lung from the venous blood. Normally, CO_2 is produced and O_2 consumed in a constant ratio, the respiratory exchange ratio (respiratory quotient). This is the ratio of the volume of CO_2 produced by the body to the volume of O_2 consumed. Oxygen is consumed and CO_2 produced in a ratio of 10 to 8 (respiratory quotient = 0.8). Carbon dioxide is exchanged for O_2 in the alveoli so that the partial pressure of O_2 falls as the partial pressure of CO_2 rises (Fig. 59–2). This relationship, a decrease in P_AO_2 for a rise in P_ACO_2 and vice versa, is extremely important.

Venous Hemoglobin. A decrease in venous hemoglobin saturation will lower alveolar O_2 tension. The oxyhemoglobin dissociation curve dictates that the less saturated the hemoglobin, the greater the volume of O_2 necessary to achieve a predicted increase in O_2 tension. A decrease in mixed venous hemoglobin saturation may be seen when the peripheral tissue demand for O_2 is greater than the supply. This may be seen clinically with a low cardiac output state, anemia, seizures, shivering, and other conditions of O_2 supply-demand imbalance.

The removal of O_2 from the alveolus in a volume greater than that supplied by the alveolar ventilation will produce a lower P_AO_2 than the maximum predicted by the alveolar air equation. Arterial hypoxemia may ensue because arterial PO_2 is always less than alveolar PO_2.

Venous Admixture. Venous admixture is alveolar underventilation in relation to perfusion. It is the most common clinical phenomenon responsible for hypoxemia that is responsive to O_2 administration.

The volume of fresh gas delivered to the alveolus (alveolar ventilation) must contain a quantity of O_2 adequate to fully saturate the amount of hemoglobin in the blood perfusing that alveolus. The delivery of an inadequate amount of O_2 will lead to a fall in P_AO_2 as O_2 moves into the blood. The hypoxemia caused by venous admixture is correctable with a high inspired concentration of O_2 because this will lead to an increased volume of O_2 being delivered to the alveolus.

The alveolar ventilation may be adequate to remove the volume of CO_2 produced even though it may be inadequate to supply the O_2 needs of the blood perfusing the lung. The ultimate example of this phenomenon is ventilation with an anoxic gas such as pure N. The arterial CO_2 will not rise as long as alveolar ventilation is adequate, but hypoxemia will rapidly ensue, because an adequate volume of O_2 is not being delivered to the alveolus. Alveolar PO_2 and hence arterial PO_2 will fall as the blood perfusing the lung removes O_2 from the alveolus at a faster rate than it is replaced by the fresh gas of alveolar ventilation. A similar situation may develop while breathing room air, but is easily correctable with the administration of O_2.

Physiologic Shunt

Intrapulmonary shunting of blood, physiologic shunt, is defined as that portion of the cardiac output that does not exchange with alveolar gas. It is the sum total of the anatomic shunt, the capillary shunt, and the venous admixture. A physiologic shunt causes hypoxemia, because, in effect, desaturated blood from the right heart enters the left heart without coming into contact with ventilated alveoli. This "shunted" venous blood, in effect, is added to normally oxygenated blood and a decreased arterial O_2 content results. The degree to which a shunt will cause arterial hypoxemia is dependent not only on the magnitude of the shunt, but on mixed venous hemoglobin saturation.

Arterial to Alveolar Ratio

The standard method of analyzing the efficiency of the lung as an O_2 exchanger for patients on supplemental O_2 has been the alveolar-arterial O_2 difference or gradient (the A-a difference or A-a gradient). This is determined by calculating the alveolar PO_2 using the alveolar air equation (Fig. 59–2).

$$P_AO_2 = P_IO_2 - (PaCO_2 \times 1.25)$$

The measured arterial value for O_2 is subtracted from the calculated alveolar value to determine the A-a difference.

One of the difficulties with the use of the A-a difference is that the normal range changes with varying concentrations of inspired O_2. A more useful calculation is the arterial to alveolar ratio (a/A ratio) based on the same measurement and calculation as the A-a difference, except that the values are divided to form a ratio rather than subtracted to form a difference. The a/A ratio is more useful because it remains relatively constant at any F_IO_2. It may be used to predict what the PaO_2 will be when a change is made in F_IO_2 because the ratio of arterial PO_2 to alveolar PO_2 will remain constant.

Example:

The lower limit of normal for PaO_2 is 75 torr while breathing room air. Alveolar PO_2 while breathing room air is approximately 100 torr. What is the lower limit of normal for the a/A ratio?

Answer:

$$\text{a/A ratio} = \frac{\text{arterial } PO_2}{\text{alveolar } PO_2} = \frac{75}{100} = 0.75$$

The lower limit of normal for the a/A ratio is 0.75. The a/A ratio should be greater than 0.75 regardless of the inspired O_2 concentration. Whenever the PaO_2 is less than 75% of the P_AO_2 the lung is not working well as an O_2 exchanger.

Example:

A patient has a $P_aCO_2 = 40$ torr and a $PaO_2 = 82$ torr, $F_IO_2 = 0.3$. What is the a/A ratio?

Answer:

$$P_AO_2 = F_IO_2 \times (760 - 47) - (PCO_2 \times 1.25)$$
$$= (0.3 \times 713) - 50$$
$$= 164 \text{ torr}$$
$$\text{a/A ratio} = 82/64 = 0.5$$

The a/A ratio of 0.5 implies that 50% of whatever partial pressure of O_2 is in this patient's alveolus will be transported into the arterial blood. This patient's arterial PO_2 will equal to 50% of the alveolar PO_2 regardless of the fraction of O_2 being inspired.

Example:

A patient in the emergency department has a $PaCO_2 = 40$ torr and $PaO_2 = 240$ torr, $F_IO_2 = 0.5$. What is the a/A ratio?

Answer:

$$P_AO_2 = (0.5 \times 713) - (40 \times 1.25)$$
$$= 300 \text{ torr}$$

This patient's lungs are working well as an O_2 exchanger because 80% of the partial pressure of O_2 in this alveoli is transmitted to the arterial blood.

Example:

The patient in the above example is ready for transfer to the ward from the emergency department. Will this patient need supplemental O_2 on transfer? What is the expected PaO_2 while breathing room air?

Answer:

$$P_AO_2 = (.21 \times 713) - (40 \times 1.25)$$
$$= 100$$
$$\text{arterial } PO_2/100 = 80$$
$$\text{arterial } PO_2 = 80$$

This patient could be expected to have a $PaO_2 = 80$ torr on an $F_1O_2 = 0.21$.

The alveolar PO_2 is approximately 100 torr while breathing room air. This convenient number allows the a/A ratio to be used to predict the expected PaO_2 on room air regardless of the F_1O_2 used to calculate the a/A ratio. The a/A ratio multiplied by 100 will predict the PaO_2 expected while breathing room air.

Example:

A patient has a $PaO_2 = 188$ torr, $PaCO_2 = 40$ torr, $F_1O_2 = 0.4$. The a/A ratio = 0.8. What is the predicted PaO_2 while breathing room air?

Answer:

The a/A ratio = 0.8 means that 80% of the alveolar PO_2 is transmitted into the arterial blood regardless of the F_1O_2. On room air alveolar $PO_2 = 100$ torr. a/A ratio $\times$ 100 = predicted PaO_2; $0.8 \times 100 = 80$ torr.

Example:

A patient has a $PaO_2 = 100$ torr; $PaCO_2 = 40$ torr, $F_1O_2 = 0.4$. How well are the lungs working as an O_2 exchanger?

Answer:

$$P_AO_2 = (0.4 \times 713) - (40 \times 1.25)$$
$$= 235 \text{ torr}$$
$$\text{a/A ratio} = 100/235$$
$$= 0.42$$

This patient could be expected to have a $PaO_2 = 42$ torr while breathing room air. It is easier to understand the amount of pulmonary disability involved to produce a $PaO_2 = 42$ torr while breathing room air than it is to appreciate the extent of lung dysfunction signified by a $PaO_2 = 100$ torr while breathing an $F_1O_2 = 0.4$.

BIBLIOGRAPHY

Comroe J: *Physiology of Respiration.* Chicago, Year Book Medical Publishers Inc, 1974.
Hedley-Whyte J, Burgess G, Feeley T, Miller M: *Applied Physiology of Respiratory Care.* Boston, Little Brown & Co, 1976.
Shapiro B, Harrison R, Trout C: *Clinical Application of Respiratory Care.* Chicago, Year Book Medical Publishers Inc, 1975.

60. Miscellaneous Respiratory Emergencies

TODD D. BAILEY, JR., M.D.
BARRY E. BRENNER, M.D., Ph.D.
ROBERT R. SIMON, M.D.

PLEURAL EFFUSION

Normally there are 5 to 10 ml of clear, alkaline fluid (pH approximately 7.6) in the pleural space between the parietal and visceral pleura. Pulmonary disease, as well as pathologic processes in other organs and systems, can lead to increased production of pleural fluid. Evaluation of the liquid can be of great diagnostic and therapeutic benefit to the clinician. (Figure 60–1 illustrates a pleural effusion of the right side.) Most of the visceral pleura is supplied by branches of the pulmonary artery, and venous drainage is into the pulmonary veins. The parietal pleura is supplied by branches of the intercostal arteries and drains into the azygous, hemiazygous, and internal mammary veins. The passage of fluid from these vessels into the pleural space is a function of the hydrostatic and colloid osmotic pressures. There is a net pressure difference of 9 cm H_2O favoring movement of fluid from the parietal pleura into the pleural space. Because the capillaries of the visceral pleura are at the same pressures as the pulmonary circulation, the hydrostatic pressure in these capillaries is much lower, and there is a net pressure of 10 cm H_2O "driving" fluid from the pleural space into the visceral pleura. Thus, fluid normally flows from the systemic capillaries in the parietal pleura to the pleural space and then to the pulmonary capillaries in the visceral pleura. Lymphatics in both the visceral pleura and the parietal pleura drain protein, particulate matter, erythrocytes, leukocytes, and fluid from the pleural space.

Several mechanisms can cause the abnormal accumulation of pleural fluid: increased capillary permeability as occurs in any inflammatory process, increased hydrostatic pressure as occurs in congestive heart failure, decreased osmotic pressure as occurs in hypoalbuminemia, increased intrapleural pressure as occurs in atelectasis, and impaired lymphatic drainage, often because of obstruction of lymphatic vessels.

Pleural effusions have classically been divided into transudates and exudates. Transudates result from an increase in hydrostatic pressure or a decrease in plasma colloid osmotic pressure; exudates result from inflammation and changes of the pleural surface leading to increased capillary permeability or lymphatic obstruction. The following characteristics have been shown to be most helpful in distinguishing transudative from exudative effusions:

1. pleural fluid protein concentration divided by serum protein concentration greater than 0.5
2. pleural fluid lactic acid dehydrogenase (LDH) divided by serum LDH greater than 0.6
3. pleural fluid LDH greater than two-thirds of the upper limit of normal for serum LDH

Other criteria have been used in the past to differentiate transudates from exudates. For example, effusions with

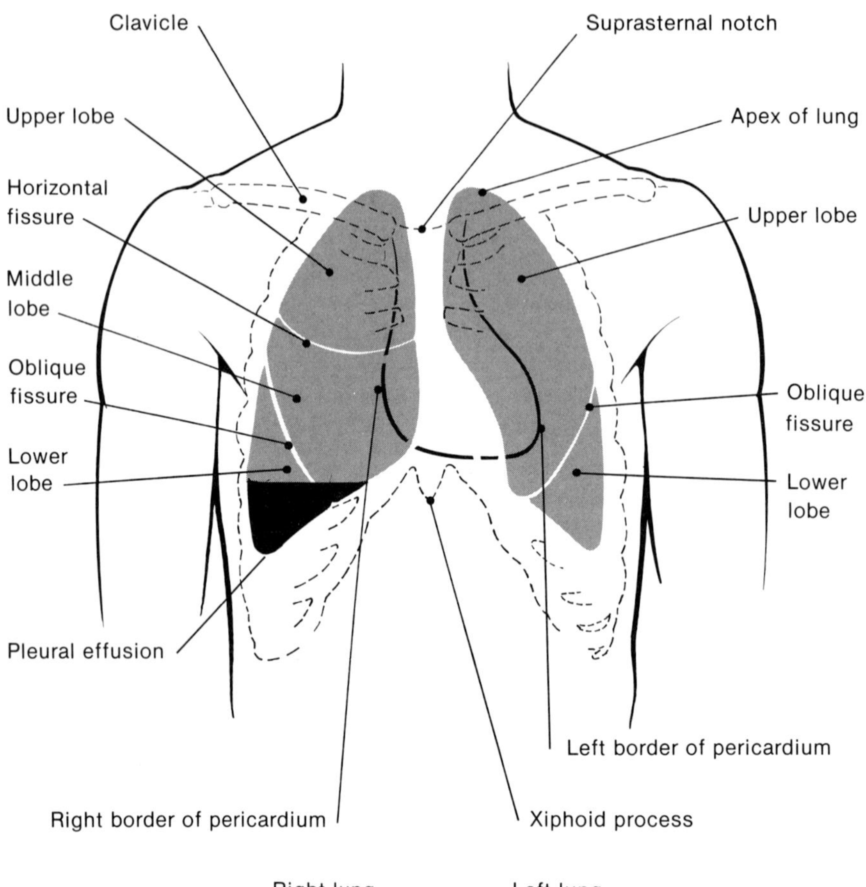

Figure 60–1 Anatomy of Chest and Lungs Showing Pleural Effusion in Right Lung.

a white cell count less than 1,000/ml, specific gravity less than 1.016, and a protein level less than 3 percent were once considered transudates. Unfortunately, use of either of the last two criteria results in an incorrect classification of over 10 percent of pleural effusions.

The signs and symptoms of pleural effusions are usually those of the underlying disease. Sometimes, the patients are asymptomatic, and the effusion is found routinely on chest roentgenogram. In the presence of greater than 300 ml fluid, the physical findings are likely to include decreased lung expansion on the side of the effusion, dullness to percussion, decreased breath sounds, and egobronchophony.

When diagnostic thoracocentesis is indicated, the procedure should be done high in the pleural space to avoid hepatic or splenic puncture and as close to the location of the fluid as possible to avoid pneumothorax. An uncomplicated case of congestive heart failure does not require thoracocentesis. A bleeding diathesis and advanced chronic obstructive pulmonary disease are relative contraindications to a thoracocentesis; in the latter case, a complicating pneumothorax might lead to demise.

The differential diagnosis of pleural effusions is long, especially for exudative effusions:[1,2]

Transudative Pleural Effusion
  Congestive heart failure
  Cirrhosis
  Nephrotic syndrome
  Acute glomerulonephritis
  Myxedema
  Peritoneal dialysis
  Hypoproteinemia
  Meigs' syndrome
  Sarcoidosis
Exudative Pleural Effusion
  Infectious diseases
    Tuberculosis
    Bacterial infections
    Viral infections
    Fungal infections
    Parasitic infections
  Neoplastic diseases
    Mesothelioma
    Metastatic disease

Collagen vascular disease
  Systemic lupus erythematosus
  Rheumatoid pleuritis
Pulmonary infarction—embolization
Gastrointestinal diseases
  Pancreatitis
  Esophageal rupture
  Subphrenic abscess
  Hepatic abscess
  Whipple's disease
  Diaphragmatic hernia
Trauma
  Hemothorax
  Chylothorax
Drug hypersensitivity
  Nitrofurantoin
  Methysergide
Miscellaneous diseases
  Asbestos exposure
  Uremia
  Post–myocardial infarction syndrome
  Trapped lung
  Post–radiation therapy

Pleural fluid should be analyzed, and the analysis should include a differential cell count; measurement of protein, LDH, and glucose concentrations; determination of pH, specific gravity, and amylase level; Gram stain; culture and sensitivity tests; and, if indicated, cytology and hyaluronic acid and complement level measurements.

Grossly purulent, exudative effusions containing large numbers of polymorphonuclear leukocytes with cytoplasm that shows toxic granulation are typical of empyema. A low pH (less than 7.20) suggests that the empyema will not resolve without a chest tube.[2] The pleural glucose level may be low with an empyema. Pleural effusion is infrequently seen (10 to 15 percent) with viral or mycoplasmal pneumonia, and these do not lead to a frank empyema.[3] Pleural effusion is seen in 50 percent of patients with bacterial pneumonia.[3] A clear or bloody fluid that is quite viscous suggests a malignant mesothelioma, in which case hyaluronic acid levels in the fluid are elevated.[4]

Patients with rheumatoid disease or systemic lupus erythematosus (SLE) have low levels of pleural complement and glucose. Pleural fluid in patients with SLE usually shows LE cells. Lymphoid predominance and a paucity of mesothelial cells is typical of tuberculosis. Grossly bloody fluid (erythrocyte count greater than 100,000/ml) should alert the physician to carcinoma, trauma, or pulmonary embolus. Chylothorax due to a tear or obstruction of the thoracic duct is characterized by white milky fluid. Pleural effusion complicates pancreatitis in approximately 6 to 10 percent of cases.[1,2]

The pleural amylase level is high in pancreatitis as well as in esophageal rupture. In the latter, the amylase is salivary in origin. Esophageal rupture and pancreatic pseudocyst are also associated with a pleural fluid pH of as low as 6 to 7.[3]

INHALATION INJURIES

Structural fires, industrial accidents, and transportation mishaps are the most common causes of inhalation injuries. Aside from carbon monoxide and chlorine, no single gas causes a significant number of chemical inhalation injuries; however, a relatively large number of gases may cause bronchopulmonary injury.[5]

Smoke is a suspension of solid or liquid particles in a gas medium; therefore, by definition, it can have many different components. The most common form of smoke inhalation injury is a chemical tracheobronchitis caused by the inhalation of numerous toxic substances in smoke,[6] although pulmonary alveolar disease occurs as well. Chemical irritation of the upper respiratory tract is due to the inhalation of smoke alone because it is frequently found in the absence of cutaneous burns.[7] Factors that prolong exposure to smoke, such as confinement in a closed area, history of drug or ethanol ingestion, head injury, or significant organic brain syndrome, all contribute to the shortness of breath, cough, and burning sensation in the throat and chest seen in association with smoke inhalation. Bronchospasm, conjunctivitis, and carbonaceous sputum also accompany severe upper respiratory tract inhalation injuries.[7] (See Chapter 21.)

Injuries to the respiratory tract can be divided into thermal and chemical injuries. Direct thermal injury to the tracheobronchial tree is rarely seen clinically unless steam has been inhaled.[8] Certain criteria are helpful in predicting whether a respiratory burn has occurred:[6]

1. flame burns about the face
2. singed areas about the lips, face, and pharynx
3. skin burns inflicted during exposure to smoke in a closed area

The presence of facial burns in smoke inhalation patients is frequently associated with the later development of pneumonia, and the pneumonia contributes significantly to the high mortality rate.[7]

The definitive diagnosis of significant upper airway inhalation injury is made by bronchoscopy as soon as the patient's condition is stable. The characteristic findings are edema and erythema above the level of the true vocal cords. PaO_2 may be decreased, and there may be carboxyhemoglobinemia. The chest roentgenogram is usually normal. Treatment of upper airway obstructive disease is empiric, involving humidified oxygen and bronchodilators. Antibiotics should not be used prophylactically, as they may lead to the emergence of resistant bacterial strains. Most recent studies suggest that steroids are contraindicated in patients with inhalation injuries.[7,9,10] In most patients with upper airway disease from smoke inhalation, symptoms resolve completely, although chronic severe pulmonary disease, including bronchiectasis, has been reported.[7]

A second syndrome associated with smoke inhalation involves the smaller airways and alveoli and may lead to the adult respiratory distress syndrome (ARDS). This disease, however, is probably due to complicating factors such as sepsis, fat embolization, aspiration, oxygen toxicity, or massive central nervous system injury. It is characterized by

1. hypoxemia despite elevation of the inspired oxygen concentration
2. a progressive decrease in pulmonary compliance
3. roentgenogram indications of interstitial edema that progresses to widespread areas of consolidation[7]

The increased use of plastics and synthetic fabrics for decorative and structural purposes exposes victims of fires to new types of inhalation hazards. Hydrochloric acid is the principal offending agent in polyvinyl chloride combustion and chloride gas inhalation. When heated, polyvinyl chloride may release (besides carbon monoxide) up to 58 percent of its weight in hydrochloric acid. The released hydrochloric acid is not visible, and those firefighters who take off their masks may inhale toxic amounts of hydrochloric acid up to one hour after the fire has been extinguished.[11] Another toxic manifestation of polyvinyl chloride smoke inhalation is the development of cardiac extrasystoles. These may be found in approximately 20 percent of patients for up to two hours after exposure. In two-thirds of these patients, the extrasystoles are premature ventricular contractions.[11]

Exposure to chlorine gas most often results from storage tank leakage, but it may result from prolonged exposure at home to bleaches containing sodium hydrochloride. People expect cleaning agents to be harsh and, not recognizing the risk, may voluntarily prolong exposure. The extent of injury depends on the concentration of the gas, the duration of exposure, and the water content of the tissue exposed. The injury to the lungs, gastrointestinal tract, eyes, and skin caused by chlorine gas is due partially to the interaction of hydrochloric acid with sulfhydryl groups and disulfide bonds on protein.[12]

Minor burns and conjunctivitis can be treated symptomatically. High concentrations of chlorine gas in contact with the skin can produce extensive deep partial and total thickness burns. The primary site of major injury is the respiratory system, with disease ranging from tracheobronchitis to pulmonary edema. Treatment of minor injury is outlined in Exhibit 60–1.

Polyurethane is an explosive, flammable plastic that produces carbon monoxide, toluene, 2,4-diisocyanate, and hydrocyanic acid when it burns. Burning nylon also releases hydrocyanic acid and can produce cyanide poisoning. Cyanide acts by interrupting cellular electron transport so that cells cannot utilize oxygen. Oxyhemoglobin remains saturated, however; the patient is not cyanotic. Cyanide also binds the ferric ion in the cellular cytochrome enzymes.

Treatment of cyanide poisoning is begun with amyl nitrite pearls followed by 10 ml 3 percent sodium nitrite given slowly intravenously over two to four minutes. This treatment oxidizes ferrous hemoglobin, producing methemoglobin that binds the cyanide ion and forms cyanomethemoglobin. Fifty ml 25 percent solution of sodium thiosulfate converts the cyanomethemoglobin to nontoxic thiocyanate.

Acrylics are another large group of plastics that may cause inhalation injuries because they produce acrolein, an aldehyde, when they burn. Burning wood is a common source of acrolein. Aldehydes fix or denature proteins by bonding to sulfhydryl groups. Exposure to 0.25 ppm causes mucosal irritation, and prolonged exposure to 21 ppm causes pulmonary edema.

Anhydrous ammonia is used as a fertilizer and yields a pH of 11.6 when hydrolyzed. It destroys tissue by alkaline hydrolysis, producing liquefaction necrosis.

Exhibit 60–1 Treatment of Minor Injuries due to Chlorine Gas

I. Tracheobronchitis
  A. Humidification with cold steam (40% FIO_2, if needed)
  B. Bronchodilation
    1. Epinephrine (1:1,000 strength): in adults, 0.3 ml subcutaneously every 20 minutes three times, if required; in children, 0.01 ml/kg subcutaneously every 20 minutes three times, if required; or
    2. Aminophylline, 6 mg/kg in 150 ml D_5W over 20 minutes intravenously, then 0.7 mg/kg/hr maintenance; or
    3. Intermittent positive pressure breathing with 0.3 ml metaproterenol in 2.5 saline every 60 minutes two times, if required.
II. Conjunctivitis and Corneal Defects
  A. Irrigation of eyes with 1 liter saline after topical anesthesia.
  B. Fluorescein stain; antibiotic ointment, patch, and ophthalmology referral for corneal defect.
  C. If no corneal defect, one drop ophthalmic solution every one to two hours.
III. Cutaneous Burns
  A. Cleansing with saline.
  B. Tetanus prophylaxis.
  C. Topical burn cream (e.g., silver sulfadiazine) and bandage.

Unlike acid substances, alkaline substances are not neutralized by tissue fluids and continue to react with tissue until they are removed or neutralized. Anhydrous ammonia can cause blindness, as well as laryngeal and pulmonary edema and death.

Metal fume fever is an acute illness of short duration that occurs when fumes from metals heated above their melting point are inhaled. Zinc, copper, and magnesium are the most common offending agents. Symptoms of thirst and a metallic taste in the mouth usually begin within 4 to 8 hours after exposure. The patient may develop fever, rigors, weakness, and muscle aches. Some metals, especially cadmium, can cause severe chemical pneumonias and death. Usually, however, the disease resolves spontaneously in 24 to 48 hours. Treatment is symptomatic in most patients, but high-dose steroids may be life-saving in patients with severe chemical pneumonitis.[13]

HEMOPTYSIS

There are few symptoms as worrisome to both patients and physicians as hemoptysis. Whether the patient is first seen with massive hemoptysis or simply blood-streaked sputum, the emergency physician should be prepared to manage rapid bleeding from the airway and then to embark on the appropriate diagnostic workup.

For many years, hemoptysis was almost synonymous with tuberculosis, as noted in Hippocrates' aphorism, "the spitting of pus follows the spitting of blood, consumption follows the spitting of this, and death follows consumption."[14] The differential diagnosis of hemoptysis is long. More than 100 etiologies have been reported,[15,16] including

- inflammatory causes
  tuberculosis
  bronchiectasis
  lung abscess
  pneumonia (particularly that caused by *Klebsiella*)
  bronchitis
- neoplastic causes
  bronchogenic carcinoma
  bronchial adenoma
- vascular causes
  left ventricular failure
  mitral stenosis
  pulmonary thromboembolism
  primary pulmonary hypertension
  arteriovenous malformations
  Eisenmenger's syndrome
  pulmonary vasculitis: Wegener's granulomatosis and Goodpasture's syndrome
  idiopathic pulmonary hemosiderosis
  amyloidosis of the respiratory tract
- traumatic causes
  foreign body
  lung contusion
- hemorrhagic causes
  hemorrhagic diathesis
  anticoagulant therapy

The most common causes of hemoptysis are bronchitis and bronchiectasis, lung cancer, and tuberculosis, depending on the patient population of a given study. The incidence of hemoptysis in various diseases is shown in Table 60–1. It should be remembered that hemoptysis is relatively infrequent in metastatic carcinoma to the lung.[15] Also, hemoptysis that occurs in association with viral or bacterial pneumonia is usually scanty, and its occurrence in such cases should always raise the suspicion of some other underlying process.[15] In 5 to 15 percent of cases, the etiology of hemoptysis may not be discovered.[15–17]

One of the first considerations when evaluating the condition of a patient with hemoptysis is to determine that the blood is actually coming from the lung and not from the nasopharynx or gastrointestinal tract. A careful history and physical examination should make that distinction clear and provide further clues to the etiology of the hemoptysis. A male smoker over 40 years old with a greater than one-week history of hemoptysis is a likely candidate for carcinoma.[15,17] Chronic hemoptysis over months or years in an otherwise healthy young female suggests bronchial adenoma.[15] Chronic hemoptysis with sputum production of more than 30 ml/day and air bronchograms and cysts seen on chest

Table 60–1   Incidence of Hemoptysis in Various Diseases: Study of 1,316 Patients with Chest Disease

Disease	Patients with Hemoptysis (%)
Bronchogenic carcinoma	56.0
Lung abscess	49.0
Pulmonary infarct	44.0
Bronchiectasis	43.5
Tuberculosis	36.5
Congenital cyst	25.8
Empyema	24.5
Metastatic carcinoma	24.0
Mediastinal tumor	20.0
Cardiac disease	17.5
Esophageal obstruction	9.0

Source: Reprinted with permission from American Thoracic Society: The management of hemoptysis. *Am Rev Respir Dis* 93:471–474, 1966.

roentgenograms strongly suggests bronchiectasis, while putrid sputum suggests lung abscess.[15] If the patient complains of pleuritic chest pain, has a pleural friction rub, and develops hemoptysis, a pleural lesion should be suspected, e.g., pulmonary infarct, lung abscess, coccidioidomycosis cavity, or vasculitis.[15] A low-pitched rumbling diastolic murmur in a patient with pulmonary hypertension and a history of rheumatic fever suggests mitral stenosis. A murmur over the lung fields and a sharp coin lesion on chest roentgenogram should make the clinician think of Osler-Weber-Rendu disease with pulmonary arteriovenous malformation.

Most clinicians believe that all patients with hemoptysis should undergo bronchoscopy; only a few patients are excepted, notably those with malignant cells or acid-fast bacilli in their sputum before bronchoscopy.[18] Furthermore, the bronchoscopy can be performed during the bleeding episode.[17]

Massive hemoptysis is a life-threatening event. The results of the bleeding assume greater importance than the cause, since the patient is at risk of dying of suffocation, not blood loss. Massive hemoptysis has been variably defined as expectoration of greater than 600 ml blood in a 16- to 48-hour period.[17,18] The rapidity of the bleeding is more important than the total volume lost, however, and brisk bleeding over a short time can cause serious respiratory difficulty. Massive hemoptysis is frequently caused by chronic infection, usually tuberculosis,[17] but it may also be caused by lung abscess, bronchiectasis, and aspergillosis.[15]

Over 87 percent of patients with massive hemoptysis have had previous bleeding.[18] Emergency thoracotomy and pulmonary resection are considered by many to be the treatments of choice for massive hemoptysis. Crocco and associates reported an 81 percent survival rate among 32 patients with massive hemoptysis who were treated surgically, as compared with a 21 percent survival rate for 9 patients who were treated nonsurgically.[18] The thoracic surgeon should be called as soon as massive hemoptysis is diagnosed. Patients with massive hemoptysis should undergo bronchoscopy immediately, preferably rigid bronchoscopy. If bleeding subsides, the flexible fiberoptic bronchoscope can be used.[18,19]

In the emergency management of massive hemoptysis, the patient should be placed in the Trendelenburg position with the site of bleeding dependent. Blood volume should be replaced and clotting abnormalities corrected. Endobronchial balloon tamponade has been successfully employed in some patients who need emergency airway management or who could not tolerate or refused resection of the lung.[20] Contraindications to pulmonary resection might be terminal carcinoma, von Willebrand's disease, Goodpasture's syndrome, or poor pulmonary reserve; it might also be contraindicated when

the bleeding site has been localized.[21] Pulmonary hemorrhage secondary to mitral stenosis is best controlled by emergency cardiac surgery rather than pulmonary resection.[21]

CARBON MONOXIDE POISONING

An odorless, colorless, tasteless, and nonirritating gas, carbon monoxide causes nonspecific symptoms of headache, nausea, and confusion. It is produced both from the normal catabolism of hemoglobin and from many environmental sources. Prompt recognition and treatment of carbon monoxide poisoning can avoid the neurologic deficits seen after hypoxic insults of any etiology.

Space heaters in poorly ventilated apartments and automobile exhaust fumes are two notorious causes of carbon monoxide poisoning. Also, smoke from sterno stoves, hibachis, charcoal briquette fires, as well as from cigars, pipes, or cigarettes, can elevate carbon monoxide levels. Methylene chloride, a hydrocarbon solvent used in strippers and other aerosols can be converted in vivo to carbon monoxide.

Carbon monoxide is endogenously produced from the α-methane carbon atom of the protoporphyrin ring during the natural degradation of hemoglobin. This leads to carboxyhemoglobin levels of approximately 0.5 percent in normal individuals and as high as 5 to 6 percent in persons with hemolytic anemia. Although most carbon monoxide is combined with hemoglobin, approximately 15 percent is present in extravascular tissues, probably in combination with myoglobin and other iron-containing hemoprotein.

The major effect of carbon monoxide poisoning results from its tendency to combine with hemoglobin to form carboxyhemoglobin (COHb), according to Haldane's law:

$$\frac{\text{Concentration of COHb}}{\text{Concentration of O}_2\text{Hb}} = M \times \frac{\text{Partial pressure of CO}_2}{\text{Partial pressure of O}_2}$$

The ratio of carboxyhemoglobin to oxyhemoglobin is dependent, therefore, on the partial pressure of carbon dioxide and oxygen in the environment. M is the affinity constant, which refers to the relative ability of a gas to bind to hemoglobin, compared with that of oxygen.

The affinity of carbon monoxide for hemoglobin is 240 times greater than that of oxygen; while carbon monoxide combines with hemoglobin at only one-tenth the rate that oxygen combines, it dissociates from hemoglobin 2,400 times as slowly as oxygen. By comparison, the affinity constant of carbon monoxide for myoglobin is only 40, and myoglobin may facilitate oxygen delivery to the tissues when there is a large amount of carbon monoxide in the blood.

Carbon monoxide, by competing with oxygen for binding sites on hemoglobin, reduces oxyhemoglobin saturation in direct proportion to the concentration of carboxyhemoglobin. Also, carbon monoxide shifts the oxyhemoglobin dissociation curve to the left, requiring a far greater decrease in tissue oxygen tension to produce dissociation and release of oxygen from hemoglobin (Fig. 60–2). There is then a lower tissue oxygen partial pressure than is found with a similar oxyhemoglobin saturation caused by hypoxia or anemia alone. Carbon monoxide also may inhibit the actions of the cytochrome system by binding to iron-containing proteins, especially cytochrome A3 and P450.[22,23]

The amount of tissue hypoxia and the subsequent development of symptoms from carbon monoxide poisoning depend on many factors, including the metabolic activity during exposure. Animals with high metabolic rates, such as the parakeet, are more susceptible to the effect of carbon monoxide and may even die before symptoms are observed in humans. Other important factors are total carboxyhemoglobin concentration, length of exposure, and underlying disease. Because the cardiovascular and central nervous systems have high metabolic rates, they account for a majority of the toxic manifestations in carbon monoxide poisoning.

The electrocardiogram (ECG) may show ischemia, infarction patterns, or conduction defects. Cerebral edema with increased intracranial pressure, pulmonary edema, hyperglycemia, and proteinuria may occur. Decreases in visual and auditory function may be measured. The characteristic cherry red complexion due to the color of carboxyhemoglobin is not always present, and it should be remembered that cyanohemoglobin can produce the same bright red color as blood.

At carboxyhemoglobin levels of 5 to 9 percent, patients with underlying coronary artery disease show a lowered threshold for exercise-induced angina. Levels of 20 percent may cause a healthy person to complain of nausea, vomiting, headache, and loss of manual dexterity. At levels of 50 percent, normal persons may become comatose with convulsions. Levels of 60 to 70 percent are potentially lethal.[23]

Diagnosis is made most reliably by spectrophotometric documentation of the actual percentage of carboxyhemoglobin in the blood. Estimates based on expired carbon monoxide are less accurate. The arterial PO_2 is usually normal in carbon monoxide poisoning, reflecting dissolved oxygen in the blood and not the actual hemoglobin saturation.

Treatment begins immediately by removing the victim from the contaminated environment and administering oxygen in high concentrations. The half-life of carboxyhemoglobin is five to six hours and is decreased to one to two hours by breathing 100 percent oxygen through a tight-fitting mask.[23] Hyperbaric oxygen at 3 atm reduces the half-life to 30 minutes, although transportation to a hyperbaric chamber should never delay initial treatment.[23] Therapy should begin before the carboxyhemoglobin level has been determined by the laboratory and should continue until the carboxyhemoglobin level is less than 10 percent.[24]

Some clinicians believe that a patient with a carboxyhemoglobin level of 25 percent or greater should be treated in a hyperbaric chamber because the patient will thus be spared the headache and nausea that often follow carbon monoxide poisoning.[24] Kindwall recommends that a patient who has a carboxyhemoglobin level of 40 percent or more and is in a hospital without hyperbaric facilities should be transported to a hyperbaric chamber. If the level is 39 percent or less, the patient with mild symptoms only may be treated with oxygen at the original hospital. However, if there are any neurologic signs, mental impairment, or S-T segment depression on the ECG, the patient should be referred for hyperbaric treatment. Complications of hyperbaric oxygen therapy are discomfort, seizures, and pulmonary oxygen toxicity.[24]

Patients who have carboxyhemoglobin levels of 25 percent or more, as well as those with impaired mentation or histories of cardiac decompensation and levels of 15 percent or more, should be hospitalized.[23] There may be a latent period of four to nine days between apparent recovery and onset of later sequelae, such as psychosis, incontinence, deafness, dysphasia, visual impairment, and temporospatial disorientation. Recovery may not be complete for up to two years.[24,25]

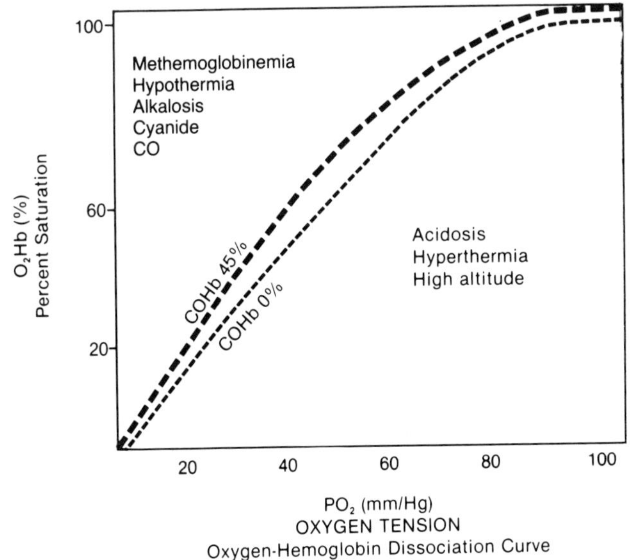

Figure 60–2 Oxygen-hemoglobin Dissociation Curve.

FAT EMBOLISM

When fat droplets large enough to occlude capillaries and arteries appear in the circulation, fat embolism occurs. It is characterized by confusion, hypoxia, and petechiae, and it is most frequently associated with skeletal trauma. The actual source of the fat globules is still debated, but there is agreement on the pathophysiology of fat embolism and the treatment of the resulting respiratory failure.

Multiple fractures of the long bones, ribs, and pelvis are most commonly associated with fat embolism, and the number and severity of fractures correlates directly with patient mortality.[26] Fat embolism has been suspected following total hip replacement, especially during insertion of the femoral component,[27] and has been seen in patients with decompression sickness, diabetes mellitus, sickle cell disease, chronic alcoholism, and acute hemorrhagic pancreatitis.[26]

Several major theories have been advanced to explain the presence of the fat in the circulation. The first is the marrow globular theory. According to those who espouse this theory, fat cells from the bone marrow of fractured bones enter the venous system at the time of trauma and travel to the lungs, where they are filtered and trapped. This theory requires an increase in marrow pressure to a level above systemic venous pressure, at least transiently, which has been verified experimentally.[27]

A second theory is that the loss of the stability of the chylomicron emulsion, which occurs in severe trauma, causes fat emboli.[27] Chylomicrons, normally approximately 1 μm in size, coalesce to form fat microglobules of 10 to 20 μm, which are then large enough to block pulmonary capillaries. In addition, large amounts of catecholamines and adrenal steroids are released during stress. Lipolysis of mobilized neutral fat releases free fatty acids, which produce a delayed chemical inflammatory process in the circulation, lungs, and brain on the second and third day post-trauma. Free fatty acids are normally bound to albumin with less than 1 percent unbound. Because of catabolic conditions in severe trauma, albumin levels fall and, thus, the levels of unbound free fatty acid rise. Free fatty acids that are unbound are potent cellular toxins.[28]

When fat globules of significant size are trapped in the lung, right atrial and pulmonary artery pressures rise, leading to signs and symptoms of acute cor pulmonale. Hypoperfusion of the pulmonary capillary bed leads to improper function of Type III pneumocytes and decreased surfactant production. Pulmonary vascular endothelial injury, edema, hemorrhage, and atelectasis occur, leading to hypoxia.

Thrombocytopenia to as low as 75,000 platelets can occur because the fat droplets become coated with a thin layer of platelets, decreasing the actual number of circulating platelets. The release of amines, serotonin, and 5-hydroxytryptamine by platelets may cause bronchospasm and vasospasm.

Several clinical signs have been rather consistently described in association with fat embolism, e.g., pyrexia, tachycardia, tachypnea, and mental status abnormalities due in part to acute hypoxemia. Head injury, electrolyte imbalance, drug ingestion, and other causes of change in mental status must be considered, however. Petechiae may be present, owing to thrombocytopenia. Fat globules may be seen in the blood, urine, and/or sputum. Chest roentgenogram may show patchy infiltrates, and the ECG manifests signs of right heart strain. Serum lipase levels are elevated because the presence of neutral fat emboli in the lungs stimulates the formation of lipase by lung parenchyma.[26]

The most important laboratory test is the blood gas determination and a PO_2 of 50 to 60 mm Hg in the presence of the other findings mentioned is sufficient for a diagnosis of fat embolism syndrome. The signs and symptoms of fat embolism can appear within the first 12 to 48 hours after injury. There is no "latent period."[26,27]

Prevention and treatment of fat embolism begin in the prehospital phase of care for the trauma patient. A cervical collar and backboard should be used, and fractures must be splinted. Support of respiration is the most important aspect of treating fat embolism syndrome.[27] Heparin and low-molecular-weight dextran are not used.[27]

Steroids are given in large doses (methylprednisolone, 13 mg/kg/day) to decrease cerebral edema and platelet adhesiveness, to stabilize lysosomal membranes, and to reduce the inflammatory effect of free fatty acids on the alveolocapillary membranes.[27]

AIR EMBOLISM

There are two types of air embolism: venous and arterial. Air may enter a systemic vein, obstructing the right ventricular outflow tract (venous air embolism), or it may enter the pulmonary veins, ultimately obstructing systemic arteries, especially those of the heart and central nervous system. Both types of air embolism can be catastrophic, but they differ in many respects. Initial therapy should be instituted in the prehospital setting and may be life-saving.

Venous air embolism can occur whenever air is forced into the body, as during a radiographic contrast study. Blood transfusion under pressure, as well as blood or fluid infusion by gravity alone, can lead to air embolism if proper precautions are not taken. The urogenital tract is very susceptible to air embolism, especially in pregnant women. Air frequently enters the venous sinuses of the uterus, either during insufflation of the vagina for therapeutic reasons, oral-genital sex, or abortion attempts.[29] Stab or gunshot wounds to the chest or neck can cause air embolism, as can rapid decompression in diving or flying.

Death in humans from air embolism following subclavian venipuncture has been reported. It has been shown that there is a pressure drop in the central venous system in patients with hypovolemia and negative inspiratory, intrapleural pressure, permitting volumes of air as high as 100 ml/second to enter the central veins.[30]

Venous air embolism probably produces death through the following sequence of events. A bubble of air flows from the systemic veins into the right atrium, right ventricle, and the pulmonary artery, preventing most or all pulmonary blood flow. Pulmonary arterial pressure rises and systemic arterial pressure falls, leading to shock and cardiorespiratory arrest. Sometimes, the air proceeds to the lungs, where acute pulmonary hypertension may lead to pulmonary edema. The patient may complain of chest pain or cough; severe cyanosis is often present. The classic diagnostic sign of venous air embolism is the "millwheel murmur," which is a loud, churning sound heard over the entire precordium and probably represents blood flow against the air bubbles in the right heart or outflow tract. The ECG may show evidence of ventricular ischemia or injury.

Venous air embolism can produce deaths in dogs if the amount of air is only 7 to 8 ml/kg injected rapidly over five seconds. If less than 1 ml/kg is given to dogs at a slow rate of less than 1 ml/minute, however, tremendously large quantities can be given before death ensues.[31] The cross-sectional area of the right outflow tract at its most superior point also is probably important in determining the amount of air necessary to cause death. There are no reliable data for lethal doses in humans, but any amount greater than 300 ml is probably dangerous. Air causes ischemia in the coronary arteries in dogs, both by vascular spasm secondary to direct irritation from the gas and by arterial obstruction. The ischemia is demonstrated grossly by ECG changes, with the most superior areas of myocardium being affected.

Arterial air embolism can occur when less than 1 ml air enters the pulmonary veins and may follow chest trauma, surgery, pneumothorax, or thoracocentesis. The air travels to the left ventricle, aorta, and those branches of the aorta that are most superiorly oriented, given the patient's body position at the time of the insult. It may pass to the coronary arteries, causing ischemia; to the cerebral arteries, causing neurologic deficit; or to the kidneys, liver, and other organs. Venous air also can pass from the right heart through pulmonary arteriovenous shunts or a patent foramen ovale to cause arterial air embolism, especially in patients with pulmonary hypertension.[31]

The signs and symptoms of arterial air embolism may be immediate or delayed. The patient may complain of feeling "dizzy or faint." Cyanosis is noted frequently, as is chest pain if the coronary arteries are involved. Patients with cerebral artery embolism may experience loss of consciousness, convulsions, hemiplegia, hemiparesis, nystagmus, strabismus, or cortical blindness. Shock soon develops. The murmur associated with venous air embolism is not present. The presence of air streaming through retinal vessels is considered diagnostic for arterial air embolism. A sharply defined area of pallor of the tongue (Liebermeister's sign) has been described, as well as marbling of the skin due to embolism in skin vessels.[31] An incision into the skin may produce blood with air, so-called air bleeding.

Because venous and arterial air embolism are relatively rare, the disease may easily be overlooked; however, recognition is the key. Immediate management of *venous air embolism* includes placing the patient in the head-down, left lateral decubitus position (Durant's maneuver), which permits the air bubble to rise away from the right ventricular outflow tract and proceed into the right ventricle where large emboli are "crushed" into smaller ones.[29,32] The patient with *arterial air embolism* should also be placed head down to permit the air bubble to move proximally away from the cerebral and coronary circulation.[31] A volume respirator at 100 percent oxygen should be applied to effect an exchange of the inert air. Some clinicians give heparin to patients with arterial or venous air embolism to reduce the possibility of thromboembolic phenomena occurring behind the air bubble. Also, a high incidence of fat emboli and platelet aggregation is associated with air embolism. Finally, some authors have recommended hyperbaric oxygen at 3 atm until symptoms resolve or until there is no further improvement.[33]

FOREIGN BODIES

A discussion of aspiration of foreign bodies will be found in Chapter 57.

ASPIRATION

A frequent problem for all providers of emergency care is aspiration of stomach contents. A high index of suspicion, especially in certain patient populations, is required to recognize the condition and manage it properly in the prehospital setting.

Aspiration is defined as any nongaseous material in the tracheobronchial tree. Of the multiple predisposing settings for aspiration, one of the most common is drug overdose. Many patients who have ingested toxic amounts of one or more drugs, especially sedative or hypnotic agents, aspirate before the arrival of paramedics. These patients are at further risk of aspiration during gastric lavage or endotracheal intubation. Aspiration often occurs during resuscitation from a cardiac arrest. Trauma victims frequently aspirate blood, stomach contents, or teeth. Aged and debilitated patients, as well as those with esophageal abnormalities (e.g., reflux, hiatal hernia, achalasia, esophageal diverticula, and tracheo-esophageal fistula), are at high risk for aspiration. Other particularly dangerous situations are small bowel obstruction and diabetic ketoacidosis with change in mental status or gastroparesis due to electrolyte abnormalities.

The term *Mendelsohn's syndrome*, or *toxic aspiration pneumonitis*, has become synonymous with aspiration of stomach contents with a pH of less than 2.5. Mendelsohn was the first to conclude that acid was the main determinant of pulmonary injury after aspiration.[34] Morbidity and mortality depend on the volume, nature, and distribution of the aspirated material as well.[35] Studies have shown that most people aspirate pharyngeal secretions during their sleep,[36] and that injury or infection occur only when normal pulmonary defense mechanisms are either overwhelmed or in some way impaired in their ability to clear the material.

The immediate danger of aspiration is that of mechanical obstruction of the tracheobronchial tree. After aspiration of acid with a pH less than 2.5, hypoxia can occur within minutes, owing to reflex airway closure. This airway narrowing is exacerbated by a decreased surfactant activity caused by the acid pH. Finally, there is an outpouring of fluid and protein into damaged tissue, causing interstitial and alveolar edema and hemorrhage. The alveolar-arterial oxygen difference increases as pulmonary shunting occurs. Pulmonary vascular resistance is increased, probably because of hypoxic vasoconstriction of pulmonary arterioles, and pulmonary artery pressure falls secondary to a decreased cardiac output from loss of intravascular volume.[37] Aspiration of less acidic material (pH greater than 2.5) can cause transient or sustained damage, depending on the volume, toxicity, and size of the particles. Many of the same changes occur as with Mendelsohn's syndrome, but to a lesser degree.

Under most circumstances, true bacterial infection does not occur for three to four days after the initial aspiration. Anaerobes are the most frequently implicated organisms in both adults and children,[38] although gram-positive and gram-negative aerobes can be found.[39]

Dyspnea, bronchospasm, frothy sputum, cyanosis, tachycardia, and hypotension or shock may accompany severe aspiration. In Mendelsohn's syndrome, the chest roentgenogram is usually abnormal, showing a patchy peribronchial infiltrate that may progress to ARDS.[40] Arterial blood samples usually show a low PO_2. A leukocytosis is present, reflecting demargination during stress.

Priorities in prehospital care management are securing the airway and placing the patient in a head-down, left lateral decubitus position. Suctioning and cardiovascular stabilization procedures should be instituted.

In the emergency department, nasogastric intubation should be followed by cimetidine or antacid administration. The patient must be treated in the same way that any patient with ARDS is treated. This includes positive end-expiratory pressure (PEEP) when adequate oxygenation cannot be maintained otherwise. The pulmonary edema associated with aspiration is not due to increased left ventricular pressures and should not be treated as such. Proper fluid management frequently requires the use of measurements obtained by means of a Swan-Ganz catheter. Aminophylline may be helpful in reversing bronchospasm. Immediate bronchoscopy is necessary to remove large particulate matter, especially if chemical or radiographic signs of lung volume loss are present. Pulmonary lavage of any kind should not be performed.[41]

Most authors currently recommend that neither steroids nor antibiotics be given initially.[42] About 25 to 45 percent of patients with aspiration develop pneumonia,[43] and the signs and symptoms of infection are generally obvious. Prophylactic administration of penicillin has not been shown to reduce morbidity and mortality, but it has resulted in a higher incidence of gram-negative pneumonias.

In patients with severe aspiration and shock, the mortality rate is reported as high as 60 to 90 percent.[35,40–42] Most patients who recover, however, do so almost completely; only radiologic evidence of pulmonary fibrosis, scarring, and/or mild changes in pulmonary function tests remains.

NEAR-DROWNING

Approximately 8,000 people die each year as a result of drowning, and 40 percent of these are children.[44] These figures do not take into account those who survive but are left with irreversible neurologic deficits. As more swimming pools are built, these statistics will continue to increase. The expertise of the emergency care physician is vital in directing prehospital care of drowning victims, as well as in managing them in the emergency department. Chapter 32, "Drowning and Near-Drowning," provides a comprehensive review of this respiratory emergency.

REFERENCES

1. Light RW: Pleural effusions. *Med Clin North Am* 61:1339–1351.

2. Black L: The pleural space and pleural fluid. *Mayo Clin Proc* 47:493–505.

3. Sahn SA: Pleural manifestations of pulmonary disease. *Hosp Pract*: 73–89, 1981.

4. Rasmussen L, Faber V: Hyaluronic acid in 247 pleural fluids. *Scand J Respir Dis* 48:366–371.

5. Done AK: The toxic emergency: It's a gas. *Emerg Med* 8:305–314.

6. Wroblewski DA, Bower GC: The significance of facial burns in acute smoke inhalation. *Crit Care Med* 7:335–338.

7. Horvitz JH: Pulmonary complication in the burn patient. *Cutis* 22:489–496.

8. Divincenti FC, Pruit BA, Reckler JM: Inhalation injuries. *J Trauma* 11:109–117.

9. Moylen JA, Chan C: Inhalation injury—An increasing problem. *Ann Surg* 138:34–37.

10. Dressler DP, Skornik WA, Kupersmith S: Corticosteroid treatment of experimental smoke inhalation. *Ann Surg* 183:46–52.

11. Dyer RF, Esch VH: Polyvinyl chloride toxicity in fires. *JAMA* 235:393–397.

12. Hedges JR, Morrissey WL; Acute chlorine gas exposure. *JACEP* 8:59–63.

13. Dula DJ: Metal fume fever. *JACEP* 7:448–450.

14. Pursel SE, Lindskog GE: Hemoptysis. *Am Rev Respir Dis* 84:329–336.

15. Tisi GM, Braunwald E: Cough and hemoptysis, in Harrison TR, Thorn GW, et al (eds): *Principles of Internal Medicine*, ed 8. New York, McGraw-Hill, 1977, pp 164–166.

16. American Thoracic Society: The management of hemoptysis. *Am Rev Respir Dis* 93:471–474.

17. Selecky PA: Evaluation of hemoptysis through the bronchoscope. *Chest* 73:741–745.

18. Crocco JA, Rooney JJ, Fankushen DJ, et al: Massive hemoptysis. *Arch Intern Med* 121:495–498.

19. Landa JF: Indications for bronchoscopy. *Chest* 73:686–690.

20. Saw EC, Gottlieb LS, Yokoyama T, et al: Flexible fiberoptic bronchoscopy and endobronchial tamponade in the management of massive hemoptysis. *Chest* 70:589–591.

21. McCollum WB, Mattox KL, Guin GA, et al: Immediate operative treatment for massive hemoptysis. *Chest* 67:152–155.

22. Jackson D, Menges H: Accidental carbon monoxide poisoning. *JAMA* 243:772–774.

23. Myers RA, Linberg SE, Cowley RA: Review of carbon monoxide poisoning: The injury and its treatment. *JACEP* 8:479–484.

24. Kindwall E: Carbon monoxide poisoning, in Dairs JC, Hung TK (eds): *Hyperbaric Oxygen Therapy*. Undersea Medical Society, Inc, 1977, pp 177–190.

25. Winter PM, Miller JN: Carbon monoxide poisoning. *JAMA* 236:1502–1504.

26. Peltier L: Fat embolism. *Orthop Clin North Am* 1:13–19.

27. Oh W, Mital M: Fat embolism: Current concepts of pathogenesis, diagnosis and treatment. *Orthop Clin North Am* 9:769–779.

28. Moylan JA, Birnbau M, Katz A: Fat emboli syndrome. *J Trauma* 16:341–347.

29. Gottlieb JD, Ericsson JA, Sweet RB: Venous air embolism: A review. *Anesth Analg* 44:773–779.

30. Flanagan JP, Gradisar IA, Gross RJ: Air embolus: A lethal complication of subclavian venipuncture. *N Engl J Med* 281:488–489.

31. Durant TM, Oppenheimer MJ, Webster MR: Arterial air embolism. *Am Heart J* 38:489–500.

32. Durant TM, Long J, Oppenheimer MJ: Pulmonary (venous) air embolism. *Am Heart J* 33:269–281.

33. Hart GB: Treatment of decompression illness and air embolism with hyperbaric oxygen. *Aerospace Medicine* 45:1190–1193.

34. Mendelsohn CL: The aspiration of stomach contents into the lungs during obstructive anesthesia. *Am J Obstet Gynecol* 52:191–205.

35. Cameron JL, Mitchell WH, Zuidema GD: Aspiration pneumonia. *Arch Surg* 106:49–52.

36. Huxley E: Pharyngeal aspiration in normal adults and patients with depressed consciousness. *Am J Med* 64:564–568.

37. Rebaudo CA, Grace WJ: Pulmonary aspiration. *Am J Med* 50:510–519.

38. Brook I, Finegold SM: Bacteriology of aspiration pneumonia in children. *Pediatrics* 65:1115–1119.

39. Lorber B, Swenson RM: Bacteriology of aspiration pneumonia. *Ann Intern Med* 81:329–331.

40. McCormick PW. Immediate care after aspiration of vomit. *Anaesthesia* 30:658–665.

41. Wynne JW, Modell JH: Respiratory aspiration of stomach contents. *Ann Intern Med* 87:466–474.

42. Bynum LJ, Pierce AK: Pulmonary aspiration of gastric contents. *Am Rev Respir Dis* 114:1129–1136.

43. Murray HW: Antimicrobial therapy in pulmonary aspiration. *Am J Med* 66:138–190.

44. Hoff BH: Multisystem failures: A review with special reference to drowning. *Crit Care Med* 7:310–320.

61. Chest Trauma

THEODORE L. JACKSON, M.D., F.A.C.S.

Most of the examination and some of the treatment of a patient with a chest injury must be carried out simultaneously if valuable time is not to be lost and the patient is to survive. The orderly progression of the medical procedures to be done on the patient is best described by the use of algorithms. These algorithms are extremely helpful and facilitate the learning process for the care of these injuries. For this reason an algorithm is presented in Figure 61–1 to enable the reader to better understand the treatment as each event is described.

If the patient with chest trauma is in or goes into cardiopulmonary arrest while being examined, the chest must be opened quickly and the major catastrophe corrected.[1] It is rare, if ever, that a patient with a chest injury in cardiopulmonary arrest can be resuscitated without performing a thoracotomy except in cases such as bilateral pneumothorax. A large bore intravenous line must be inserted, and the patient should be intubated immediately. There are other occasions when the chest must be opened, but cardiopulmonary arrest with chest trauma is the most urgent occasion and should be remembered by all emergency department physicians.[2]

PNEUMOTHORAX

Pneumothorax is the presence of free air in the chest cavity. In a patient with respiratory distress the chest cavity must be decompressed of free blood and air, which occupy volume and restrict lung expansion, caus-ing dyspnea. The dyspnea progresses to respiratory distress, which, if severe, causes tachycardia, tachypnea, cyanosis, hypotension, and death.

Pneumothorax can be spontaneous or traumatic. The traumatic type is usually more severe because it may involve other insults as well as be complicated by hemorrhage. The most frequent cause of pneumothorax is iatrogenic, often being the result of subclavian punctures or cardiac massage, for example.

Spontaneous pneumothorax is usually caused by the rupture of a bleb and is seen in infectious conditions such as tuberculomas. These air pockets may be small, medium, or total and unilateral or bilateral. Unless tension is present they are not dangerous unless they are bilateral or emphysematous, in which case mediastinal shift and/or tension may develop. Ruptured emphysematous blebs start out as unilateral disease but often progress to bilateral ruptures.

The signs of tension pneumothorax are tracheal deviation, distended neck veins, cyanosis, and hypotension. If a tension pneumothorax is suggested, the physician should needle the second interspace on the affected side and if the plunger of the syringe blows outward, a tension pneumothorax can be diagnosed without a roentgenogram. A chest tube should be inserted immediately. Tension pneumothorax results in both increased intrathoracic pressure and anatomic obstruction of the superior vena cava (SVC). This results in a decrease of blood pressure as well as increasing markedly the work required for adequate ventilation. Treatment

"

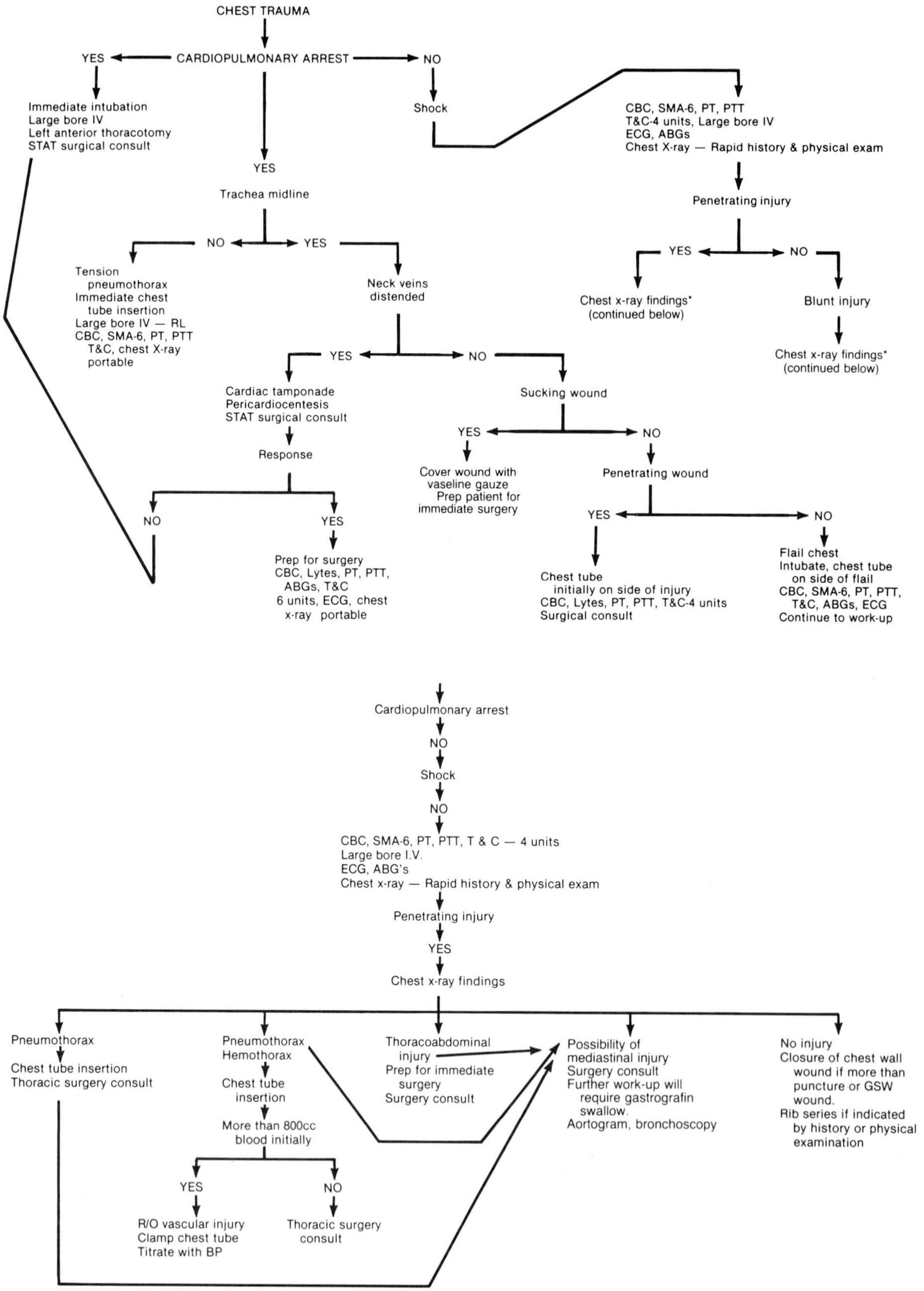

Figure 61–1 Algorithm for Chest Trauma. *Note*: CBC, complete blood cell count; SMA, Sequential Multiple Analyzer; PT, prothrombin time; PTT, partial thromboplastin time; T&C, type and cross match; ABGs, arterial blood gases; CVP, central venous pressure; COPD, chronic obstructive pulmonary disease; CVD, collagen vascular disease.

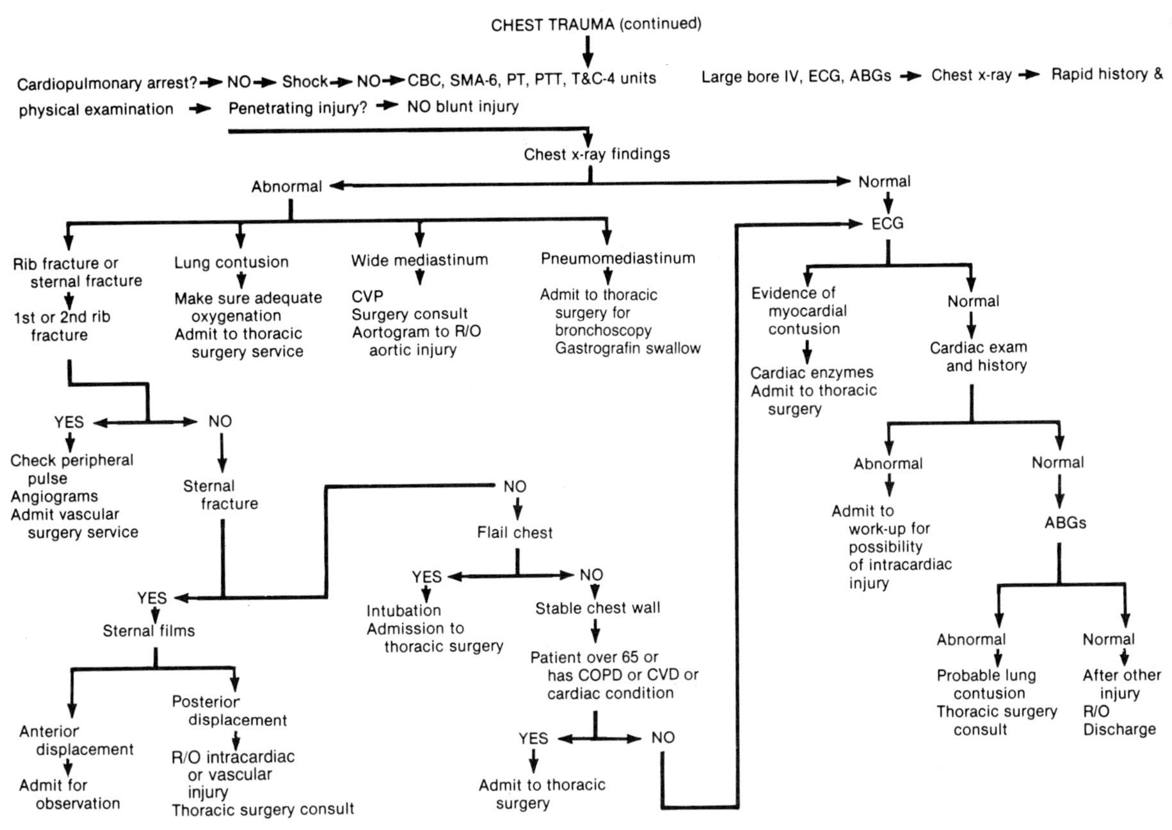

Figure 61–1 continued

should never be delayed to confirm or document the presence of the pneumothorax by chest roentgenogram or arterial blood gas determinations.

Spontaneous pneumothorax (Fig. 61–2) is classified according to size in order to determine appropriate treatment. Accordingly, a pneumothorax less than 10 percent can be observed with follow-up roentgenograms; one from 10 to 20 percent is probably best treated by placing a chest tube in the patient. The tube can be removed in 48 hours if the roentgenogram shows expansion of the lung. It is best to use a chest tube thoracotomy because of the infrequency of complications and the ease of monitoring the patient.

Traumatic pneumothorax can be either blunt or penetrating. Blunt pneumothorax results from trauma to the chest that causes rupture of the lung tissue and leaking of air into the pleural space (Fig. 61–3). Penetrating pneumothorax is caused by broken ribs and knife and bullet wounds and is usually more serious. It frequently results in chest hemorrhage and bleeding from intercostal vessels. The penetrating type also is more frequently of the tension variety and is especially severe when associated with emphysema; hypovolemia frequently is associated. Decompression is mandatory for even a small traumatic pneumothorax. These pa-

tients often are treated with assisted respiration and anesthesia for operative procedures, both of which make them more susceptible to developing tension. They should be decompressed by insertion of a posterior chest tube in the eighth intercostal space. (See Chapter 71.)

FRACTURED RIBS

Even a single fractured rib can lead to serious consequences if treated too casually. This is particularly true in older patients whose ribs are more brittle and rigid. If atelectasis or pneumonitis supervenes, patients with poor cardiac reserves do poorly.

Rib fractures are infrequent until adult life and even then require considerable force. They are usually associated with intrathoracic injuries that frequently are undetected unless the physician has a high index of suspicion. The force of the trauma and the manner in which it was inflicted must be considered. The number, position, and type of rib fractures enters into the determination of concomitant injury.

Fractures above the fourth rib imply excessive trauma because these ribs are usually protected by heavy musculature, the clavicle, and the arms. These fractures are frequently associated with other intrathoracic injuries,

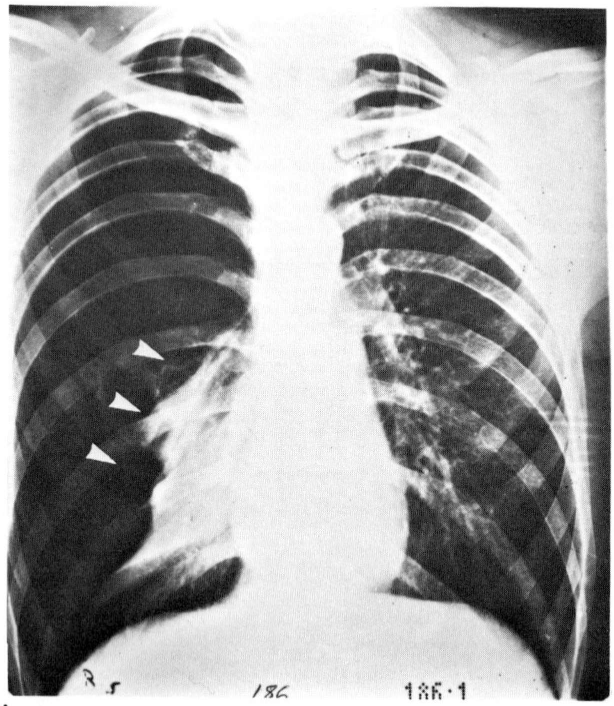

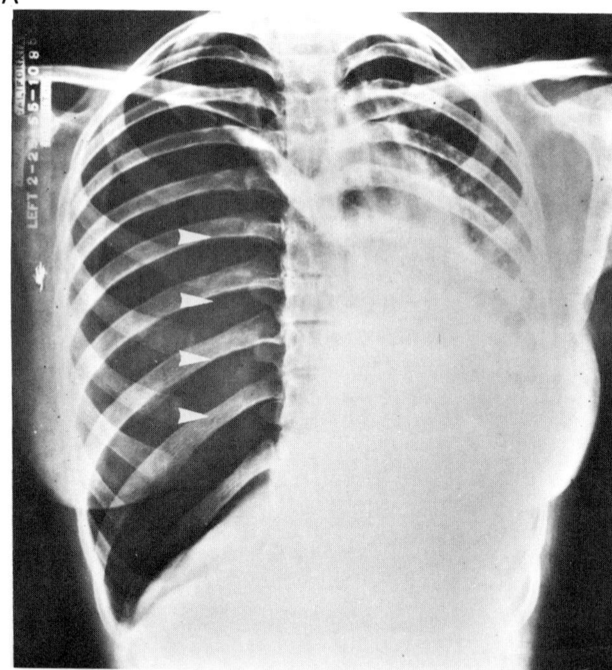

Figure 61–2 *A* Chest Roentgenogram Demonstrating a Right Spontaneous Pneumothorax without Evidence of a Mediastinal Shift. *B* Chest Roentgenogram Demonstrating a Right Spontaneous Pneumothorax with Tension. *Note:* There has been a marked shift of the mediastinal contents to the left.

a major vascular injury was found. The presence of pulses does not rule out vascular injuries. Angiography must be performed on all these patients if their other injuries do not mandate immediate exploration.

Posterior fractures of the lower ribs may occur from direct force and are frequently associated with injury to the spleen and kidneys. The fifth through the ninth ribs are most frequently broken because they are the site of most blunt trauma.

The "spring fracture" usually results from antero-posterior compression of the thorax and causes little or no lung damage. A direct blow tends to drive the rib into the lung and causes more damage. A hemothorax or pneumothorax usually accompanies this type of injury.

Diffusely applied trauma will result in numerous fractures on both sides of the impact. "Flail chest" may result from this condition.

Pain at the fracture site with point tenderness and crepitus is usually present in rib fractures. Pain is accentuated by coughing, deep breathing, and changes in position. Splinting on respiration is frequently the only early sign of fractured ribs. Anteroposterior pressure will elicit pain at the fracture site, which is often the only symptom present.

Radiographic examination is not always specific but is especially helpful in injuries to the heavily muscled areas of the chest. These roentgenograms aid in detecting air, fluid, and associated injuries, as well as in confirming the position and displacement of the rib.

The treatment of rib fractures depends on the following factors:

- advanced age
- underlying cardiopulmonary disease
- significant associated disease
- difficulty of the patient to cooperate
- jagged rib fragments with inward displacement
- bleeding dyscrasias or anticoagulant therapy
- multiple fractures
- lack of control of pain.

Multiple fractures usually can be treated with analgesics, with care being taken to see that the patient can breathe adequately after being given the drug. Patients should be rechecked in 24 to 48 hours with chest roentgenograms. They should be encouraged to cough and breathe deeply. Intercostal nerve block is excellent treatment in patients with discrete fractures.

The use of adhesive strapping is debatable, but it can be used in simple discrete fractures. The physician must be sure that it does not limit expansion of the chest and predispose to atelectasis. A wide expanse of tape might interfere with examination and should be avoided. The strapping may cause blistering and is often no more

such as rupture of the aorta or the tracheobronchial tree (see Fig. 61–4). Posterior first rib fractures are seen frequently in deceleration accidents. In 70 to 85 percent of patients studied after first and second rib fractures,

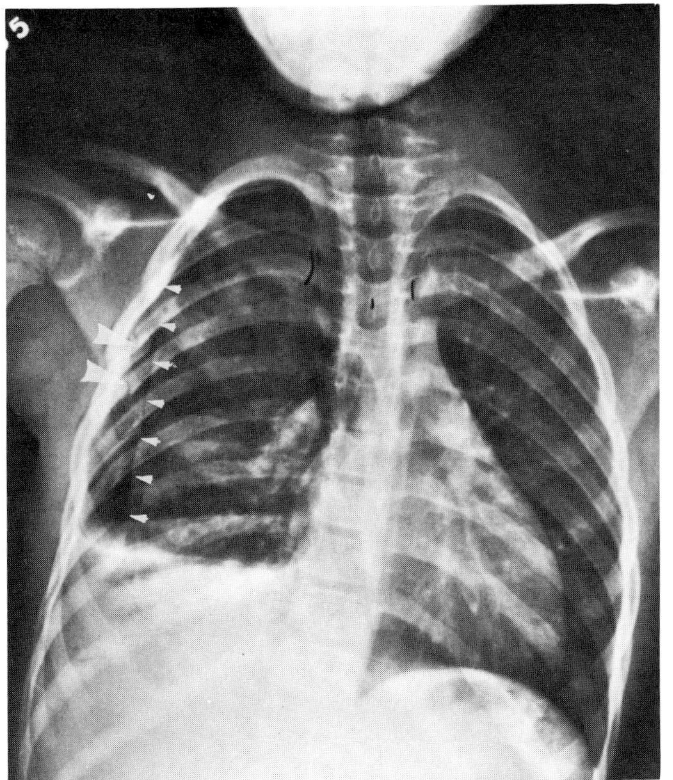

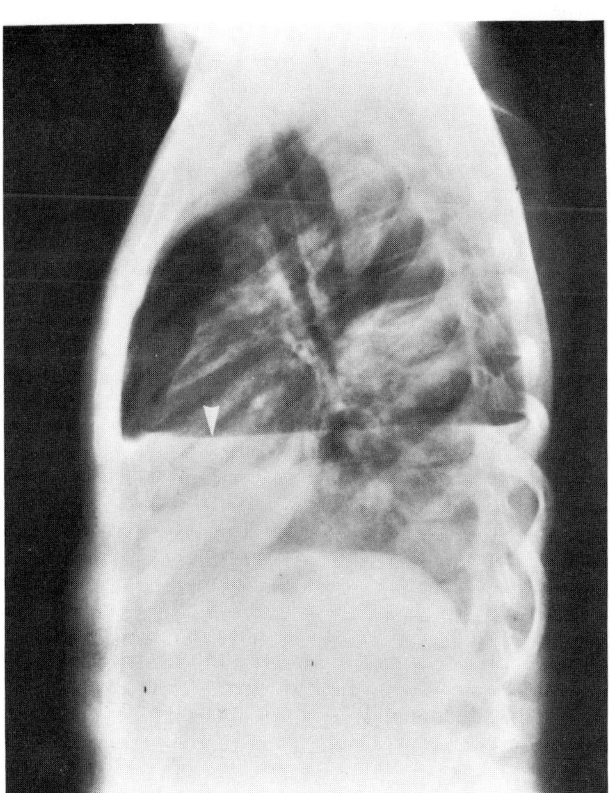

Figure 61–3 *A* Chest Roentgenogram Indicating by the Large Arrows Two Fractured Ribs; the Smaller Arrows Indicating a Right Pneumothorax. *Note:* The air fluid line at the base of the right lung indicates a hemopneumothorax. *B* Lateral Chest Roentgenogram Demonstrating a Hemopneumothorax. *Note:* The air fluid line can be seen, but the fractured rib is not visualized in this view.

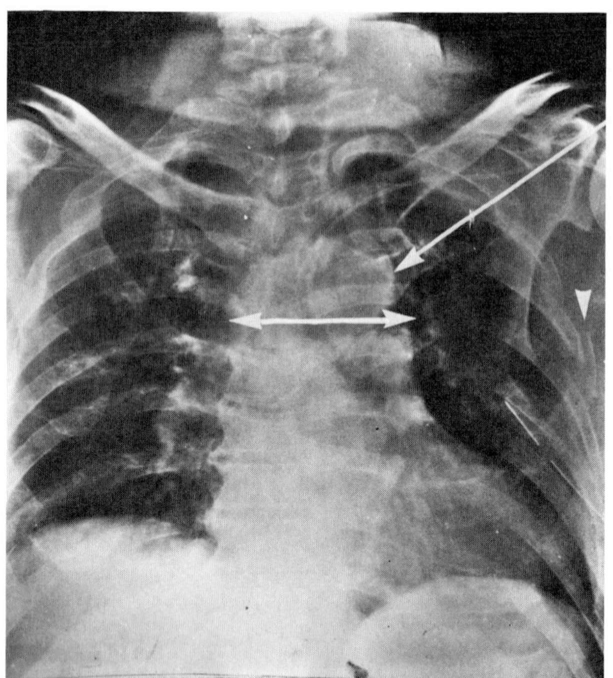

Figure 61–4 Chest Roentgenogram Revealing a Widened Mediastinum, a Prominent Aortic Knob, and Fractured Ribs.

effective than analgesics, although it is more effective in lower rib fractures.

FLAIL CHEST

The paradoxical movement of the chest wall, inward on inspiration and outward on expiration, is known as flail chest. Flail chest occurs when two or more contiguous ribs are broken in more than one place. (See Figure 61–5.) These fractures result in an unstable portion of the chest wall, which permits the paradoxical motion. This rarely occurs when the fractures are under the scapula or any large muscle mass that tends to splint the area. Flail chests are usually accompanied by severe chest injuries: chest wall contusion, hemopneumothorax, interruption of intercostal vessels, and/or injury to the cardiovascular system. Respiratory distress is usually proportional to the size of the area of instability of the chest wall and the degree of the injury to the underlying lung.

Flail chest has been noted in several series to be the most frequently missed diagnosis in patients with chest injuries that result in mortality and morbidity. The physiologic abnormalities seen with flail chest usually become more serious in the first 48 hours after injury.

Flail chest is diagnosed by observation, or it may be asymptomatic, in which case arterial blood gases should be evaluated. If respiratory distress occurs, respiration should be assisted. Progressive hypovolemia and hypercapnia should be placated by the use of ventilators. Intubation or tracheostomy may be required in the severely dyspneic patient. The decision as to the amount of oxygen to be given is made by the result of blood gas evaluations, which are also used to determine total volume and to maintain the normal range of the gases. The patient should be gradually weaned from the respirator on or about the third day. If the levels of the blood gases return to normal, the tracheostomy tube can be discontinued and assisted respiration stopped.

SUBCUTANEOUS EMPHYSEMA

Subcutaneous emphysema may be caused by fractured ribs, but it also may occur from penetrating wounds of the chest. Delayed pneumothorax must be watched for if a previous infection or injury has caused synthesis of the parietal and visceral pleura.

Subcutaneous emphysema of the *neck only* may be the earliest sign of undetected major intrathoracic injury to the esophagus or major airways. Diagnosis is made by observation, palpation, and/or chest roentgenograms. When the emphysema is very extensive, incisions into the area are used to relieve the symptoms.

TRAUMATIC ASPHYXIA

Compression injuries to the chest account for most cases of traumatic asphyxia. The injury usually compresses the right atrium and forces blood backward into the veins of the upper chest, neck, and head. Stasis and hemorrhages in the veins of the skin result in bluish mottling of the skin. Traumatic asphyxia is usually self-limiting and clears in a few weeks.

SUCKING WOUNDS OF THE CHEST

Disruption in the continuity of the chest wall will result in sucking wounds. (See Figure 61–6.) When the size of the rupture is smaller than the trachea, sucking wounds can be tolerated fairly well, but a large hole, larger than the trachea, will result in the preferential ingress and egress of air through the larger leak, resulting in respiratory embarrassment.[3] Petrolatum gauze should be used to cover the hole, and a tracheostomy tube should be placed before the hole is closed. This will prevent the conversion of a sucking wound into a tension pneumothorax from closing the hole before placing the thoracotomy tube.

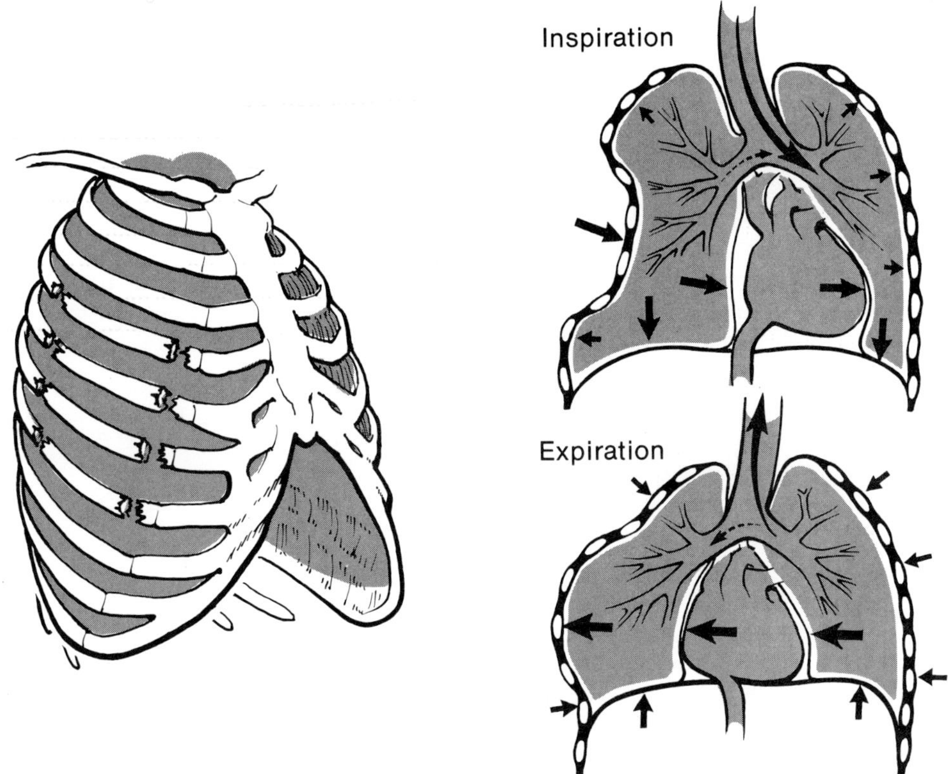

Figure 61–5 Flail Chest.

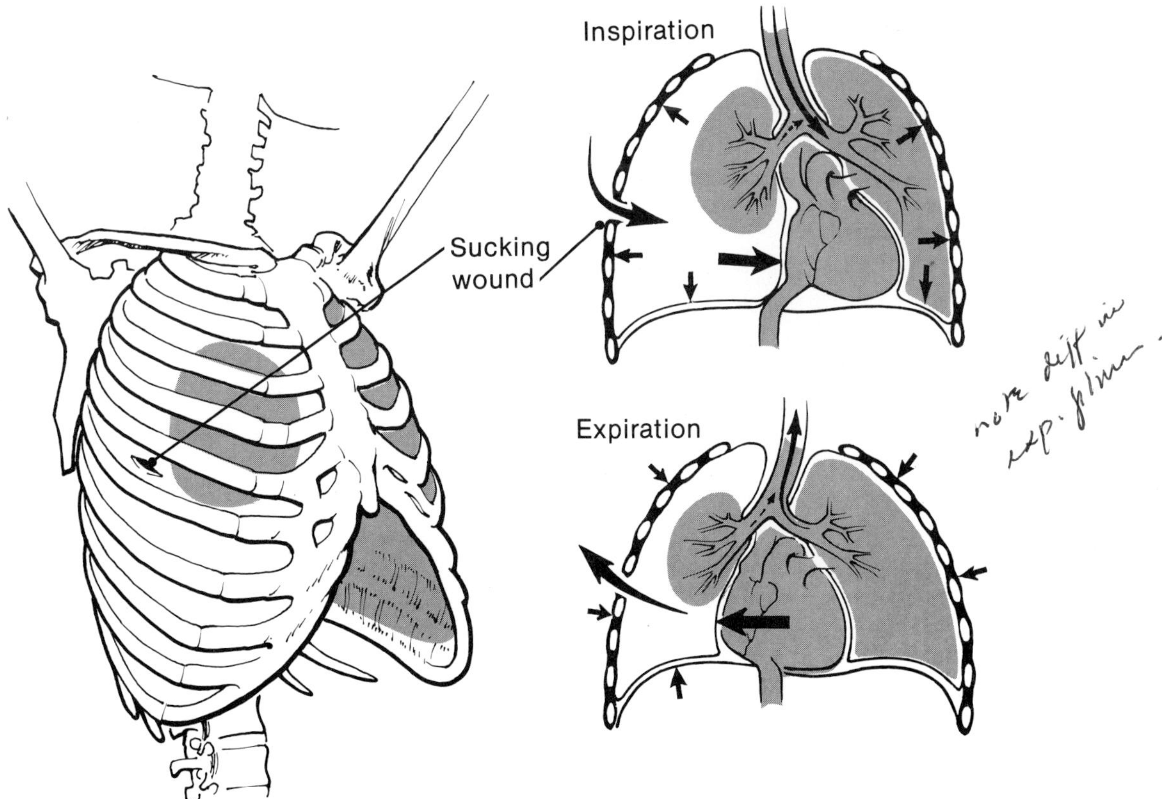

Figure 61–6 Sucking Wound of Chest.

PENETRATING OR BLUNT INJURY OF MAJOR AIRWAYS

Penetrating wounds of the lower neck or upper chest may involve the trachea or major bronchi (Fig. 61–7). Complete tear of the trachea or major bronchi may result from severe blunt trauma to the chest.[4]

The severity of the airway injury depends on the size of the wound in the tracheobronchial tree, the level of the injury, the magnitude of the injury to the other lung, or whether the flow of air from the tracheobronchial lumen to the pleural space is bidirectional, unidirectional, or stopped because of obliteration of the traumatic defect by surrounding tissues. Patients with unilateral air flow are more likely to be severely symptomatic with dyspnea and hypertension because of the frequent development of tension pneumothorax.[2] Symptoms of bidirectional air flow are directly related to the size of the hole in the tracheobronchial tree.

Patients with a defect sealed by adjacent tissues are relatively asymptomatic unless an unstable area causes the trachea to collapse, particularly during expiration. This is especially true in those patients in whom the placing of one or two chest tubes does not result in improvement. Penetrating wounds of the lower neck or upper chest should always be watched, especially when accompanied by hemoptysis or subcutaneous emphysema.

If the patient is in shock and a penetrating chest wound is the only injury, the differential diagnosis is vascular injury with massive bleeding or bilateral pneumothorax. If while the patient is in the emergency department, the chest tube drains more than 300 cc/hr exploratory thoractomy should be done. If there is no evidence of major vascular injury, the patient should be admitted to the thoracic surgery service after placement of bilateral chest tubes.

TRAUMATIC PERFORATION OF THE ESOPHAGUS

Traumatic perforation of the esophagus is usually caused by instrumentation, caustic ingestion, or missile and knife wounds and, less frequently, by blunt abdominal trauma.[2,4] Pain is dependent on the site of perforation, and it is the most prevalent symptom. Fever, hoarseness, dysphasia, and respiratory distress may be present. Cervical esophageal perforation usually results in local tenderness, subcutaneous emphysema, and resistance of the neck on passive motion. Intrathoracic esophageal perforation causes mediastinal emphysema,

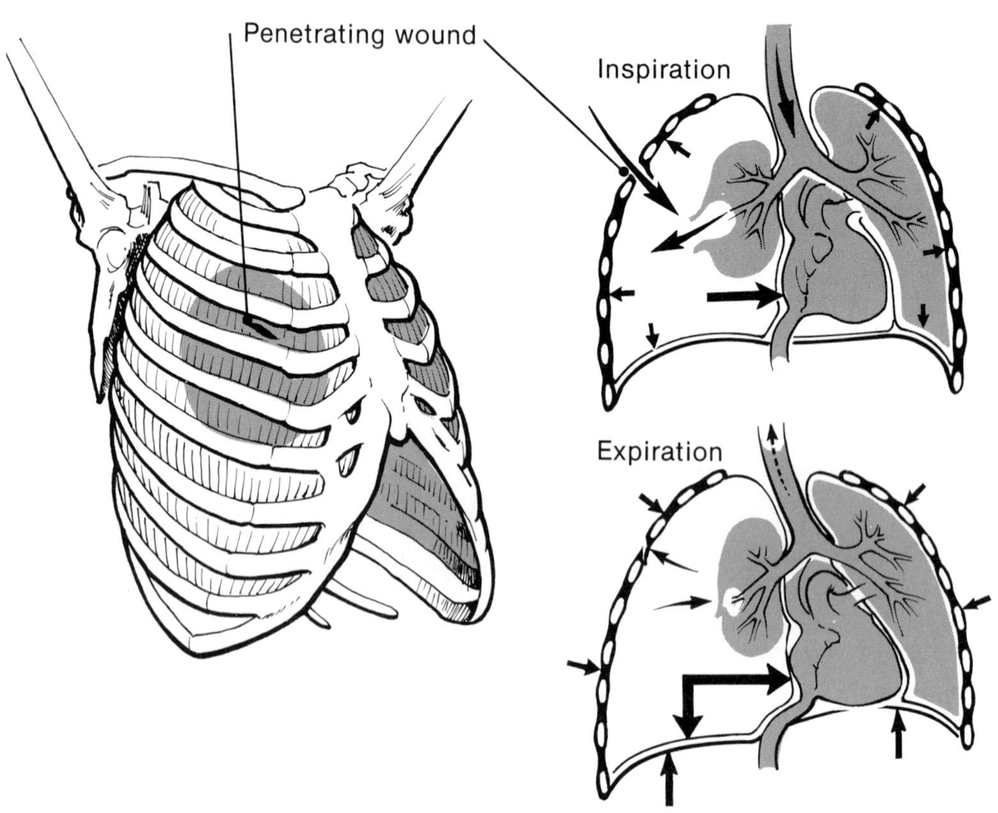

Figure 61–7   Penetrating Wound

mediastinitis, subcutaneous emphysema in the neck, mediastinal crunch, splinting of the chest wall, respiratory distress, and shock. Intra-abdominal perforation causes abdominal tenderness and rigidity, which may also occur from rupture of the lower thoracic segment.

Patients with cervical perforation should have chest and neck roentgenograms, which may show widening of the mediastinum in its upper portion, subcutaneous emphysema in the neck, and an increase in the prevertebral shadow. Thoracic perforation reveals an increase in the entire mediastinal shadow, mediastinitis or subcutaneous emphysema in the neck, and hydrothorax or pneumothorax. Since one or all of these findings may be present, perforation must be confirmed by esophagography with meglucamine diatrizoate (Gastrografin), especially when penetrating wounds are near the esophagus or the wounds traverse the mediastinum, such as those caused by bullets. The contrast media may be either absorbable or nonabsorbable, and roentgenograms must be frontal and lateral, both during and after swallowing. Treatment is emergent, with suspension of oral alimentation, constant gastric suction, antibiotics, and volume expanders as needed. Surgery should follow immediately. Esophageal perforation has a high mortality and morbidity rate.

DIAPHRAGMATIC INJURIES

The widespread use of the knife and gun has made injury to the diaphragm one of the most frequently encountered traumatic injuries.[2] The symptoms and signs that result are related to the organs that are injured and are frequently accompanied by hemothorax, pneumothorax, peritonitis, or signs relating to the intrathoracic or intraperitoneal structures involved in the penetrating injury. Penetrating injuries can be suspected radiographically and confirmed at laparotomy or thoracotomy.

Injury to the diaphragm frequently is caused by severe blunt injury to the upper abdomen and lower chest. It usually involves the membranous portion in the left chest because the right diaphragm is protected by the liver.

Rupture of the left half of the diaphragm results in a diaphragmatic hernia; the intraperitoneal contents herniate into the left chest and the mediastinum shifts toward the left.[4] (See Fig. 61–8.) Because of these anatomic changes, cardiac and respiratory embarrassment occur, the bowel increases in size, and the blood supply of the herniated material is compromised, causing obstruction, visceral ischemia, and gangrene.

Symptoms may occur immediately or days, months, and years later. When a diagnosis is suggested, the physician should listen to the chest to determine if bowel

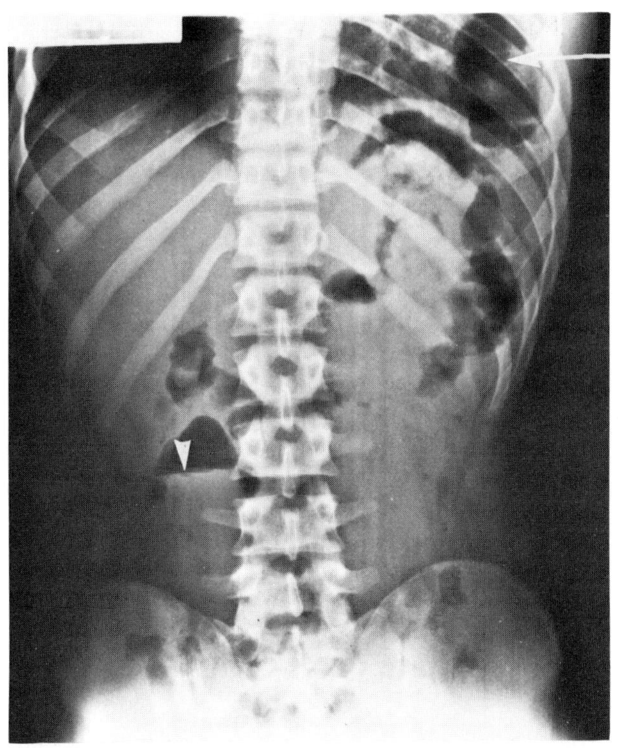

A

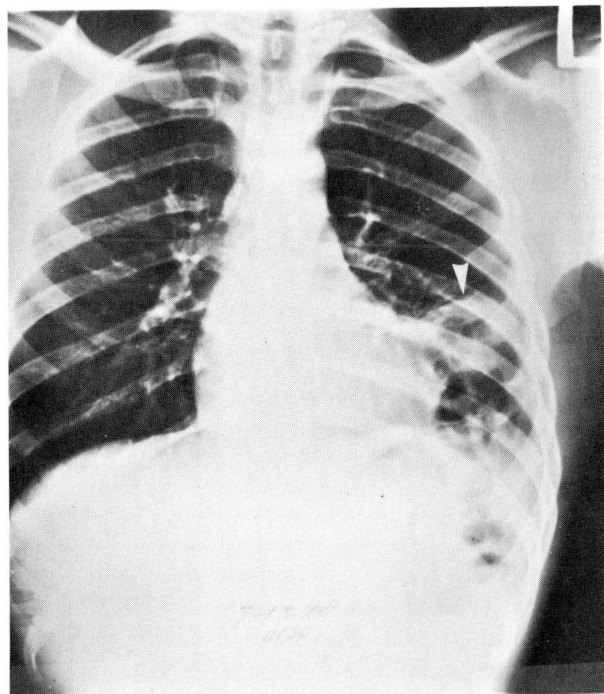

B

Figure 61–8   *A* Abdomen Roentgenogram with the Patient in the Erect Position Demonstrating Air Fluid Levels and Dilated Loops of the Bowel, Suggestive of Obstruction or Ileus. *Note:* The left hemidiaphragm is not visualized. *B* Chest Roentgenogram of the Same Patient Demonstrating a Ruptured Left Hemidiaphragm with the Appearance of Bowel in the Left Chest.

sounds are present. A Levine tube is inserted, and roentgenograms are taken. The physician can also order a Gastrografin upper gastrointestinal series. If the results of any of these tests are positive, surgery should be done as soon as possible.

PENETRATING WOUNDS OF GREAT VESSELS

Penetrating wounds of the great vessels usually involve the chest, abdomen, and neck and are caused by missiles and stab wounds. These wounds are accompanied by massive hemothorax, shock, cardiac tamponade, absent or weak subclavian or carotid pulse, or enlarging hematomas. Hematomas may cause compression of any structure, such as the vena cava, trachea, esophagus, great vessels, and heart. Arteriovenous fistulas are common. Arteriography is helpful in making the diagnosis, but at times the diagnosis is not confirmed until surgery is performed. Treatment of penetrating wounds of the great vessels usually involves restoring the blood volume, relief of tamponade, and provision of unobstructed respiration or artificial ventilation. Autotransfusion is very helpful in hypovolemic patients.

One of the simplest methods of autotransfusion described is to recover the blood by thoracostomy in a water-sealed chest bottle containing 0.9 percent normal saline.[5] Regulated suction of 10 mm Hg is applied. Another bottle is substituted when the first is filled or used for transfusion through a micropore filter. Some physicians add anticoagulant to the bottle.

More recently a satisfactory unit has been devised that collects blood in an autoclaved plastic bag that is in a rigid nonsterile plastic cannister using 10 mm Hg vacuum. This bag is fitted with a separate inlet valve to mix citrate brought in by a suction tip. The entire element is suspended from an IV pole after the anticoagulant inlet is connected by sterile tubing to citrate-phosphate-dextrose (CPD) anticoagulant. CPD is mixed with blood in a ratio of 1:7 regulated by the height of the reservoir bottle above the patient. The CPD flows only when the suction tip vent is occluded. Blood is aspirated only from below the surface to pervent hemolysis. The blood in the filled bag is infused through a micropore filter and blood set.

The complications of autotransfusion are not as numerous as one would expect. When more than 4,000 ml blood is used, coagulopathies occur that must be countered with platelet concentrates and fresh-frozen plasma. Excessive hemolysis may occur from prolonged exposure of the blood to the pleura; therefore, blood more than 6 hours old should not be used. Sepsis is not a problem nor is embolism since the routine use of the micropore filter. The usual cause of death is air embolism as a result of faulty technique.

AORTIC RUPTURE

Aortic rupture should be suspected in any victim of a high-speed deceleration accident regardless of absent physical findings or negative roentgenographic findings. (See Figure 61–9.) Ten percent of all automobile injury deaths are due to aortic rupture, and 20 percent of victims have multiple trauma, which should alert the physician to the possibility of aortic rupture. Many associated conditions should suggest possible aortic rupture, such as rib and sternal fractures, head injuries, extremity hypertension, differences in pulses, and blood in the carotid sheath.

Every trauma surgeon is familiar with widening of the mediastinum on an upright chest roentgenogram in aortic rupture, but the less obvious signs should come to one's attention, such as heart contusions, right deviation of the trachea, depressed left main-stem bronchus, and left pleural effusion. The diagnosis of aortic rupture can only be confused with patent ductus by aortography and that is because most ruptures take place at the site of the ligamentum arteriosum.

If patients with aortic rupture are diagnosed in the emergency department at once and operated on immediately, most will survive even in the presence of other injuries. If other injuries are present, the ruptured aorta is always repaired first. Primary repair is the treatment of choice. The use of a graft with a bypass shunt is next. The literature refers to a frequently seen triad in aortic rupture of (1) increased pulse amplitude and blood pressure of the upper extremities, (2) decreased pulse amplitude and blood pressure of the lower extremities, and (3) roentgenographic evidence of widening of the mediastinum.

PENETRATING WOUNDS OF THE HEART

Penetrating wounds of the heart are usually caused by stab or bullet wounds (Fig. 61–10) and are immediately fatal in 50 percent of patients.[6,7] If these wounds are diagnosed and operated on quickly, some patients will survive. The signs and symptoms depend on whether the blood flows freely through the pericardium. Signs of hemorrhage are present when the pericardium remains patent, but cardiac tamponade results when clot or blood is trapped in the pericardial sac.[8]

The patient with tamponade may show signs of shock and may be cyanotic.[2] The neck veins may be distended,

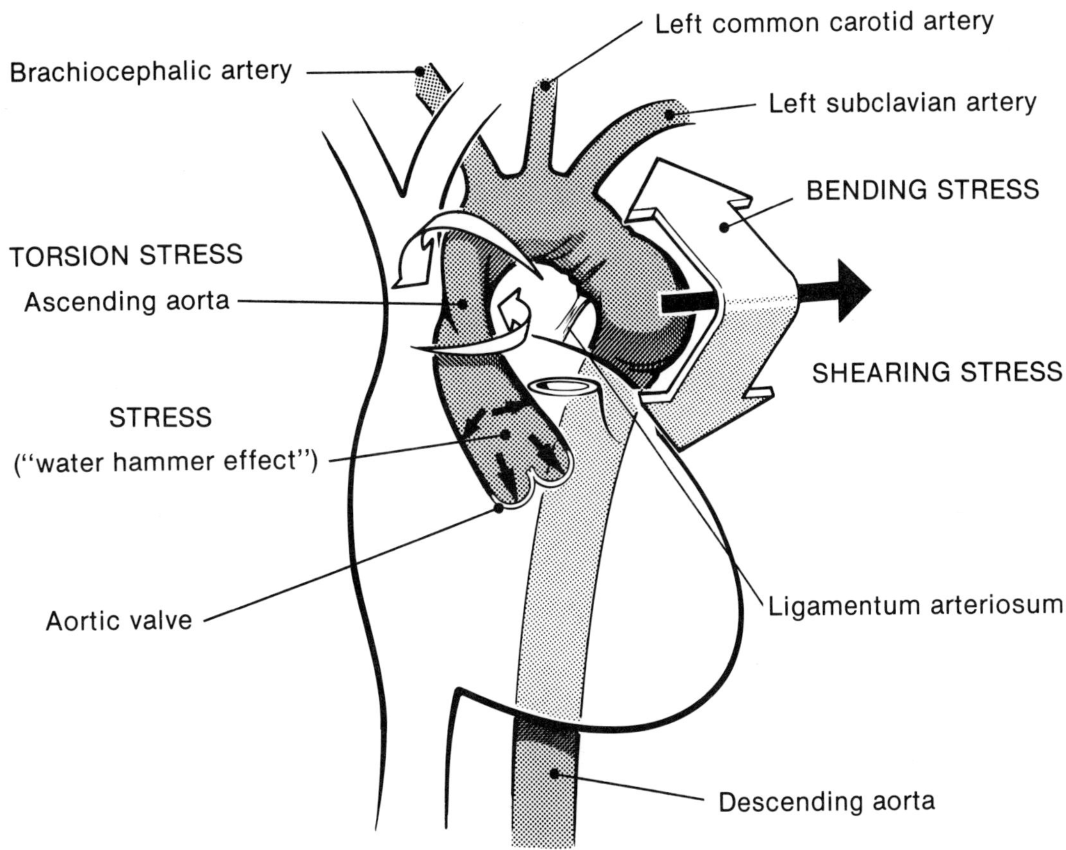

Figure 61–9   Aortic Rupture.

and there may be Kussmaul's sign (i.e., paradoxical filling of neck veins during inspiration). The physician may have difficulty hearing normal heart sounds and distended neck veins depend on a near normal intravascular volume; therefore, the signs of pericardial tamponade may only become apparent as the patient's intravascular volume is expanded during the resuscitation. The pulse is rapid and hypodynamic, and the pulse pressure is narrow. If a central venous pressure line is in place, the pressure will be elevated and will return toward normal after pericardiocentesis. When tamponade is suggested, the pericardium should be drained immediately and if possible electrocardiographic monitoring should be utilized to detect possible penetration of the myocardium. The subxiphoid approach should be used, and a 14- to 16-gauge needle is attached to the V lead of the electrocardiogram machine.

If the patient with signs of pericardial tamponade fails to respond after pericardiocentesis, then immediate left anterior thoracotomy should be performed and the pericardium opened vertically to remove clotted blood from the pericardial sac. The patient's vital signs should be monitored constantly during transfer to the operating room for repair of the cardiac wound. Declining blood pressure and an increase in central venous pressure in-

dicate the need for repeat pericardiocentesis, leaving a catheter in the pericardial space.

When hemothorax is the presenting sign of a penetrating wound, without evidence of tamponade, closed chest tube drainage is indicated. If the hemothorax is massive and the patient is hypovolemic, autotransfusion is indicated.

In general, all patients with penetrating wounds of the heart should have immediate surgery. Coronary lacerations should be repaired, and if necessary saphenous vein grafts should be done. The patient should be followed closely postoperatively for shunts, valvular lesions, aneurysms, or retained foreign bodies. These lesions can be repaired electively.

BLUNT INJURY TO THE HEART

Blunt trauma to the heart most often is caused by "steering wheel" injury in automobile accidents. This type of injury results from acceleration and deceleration pressure of the heart against the thorax, from compression of the heart between the sternum and vertebral column, or from sudden changes in the intrathoracic pressure. Myocardial contusion or rupture of the wall, interventricular septum, or any of the valves may occur.

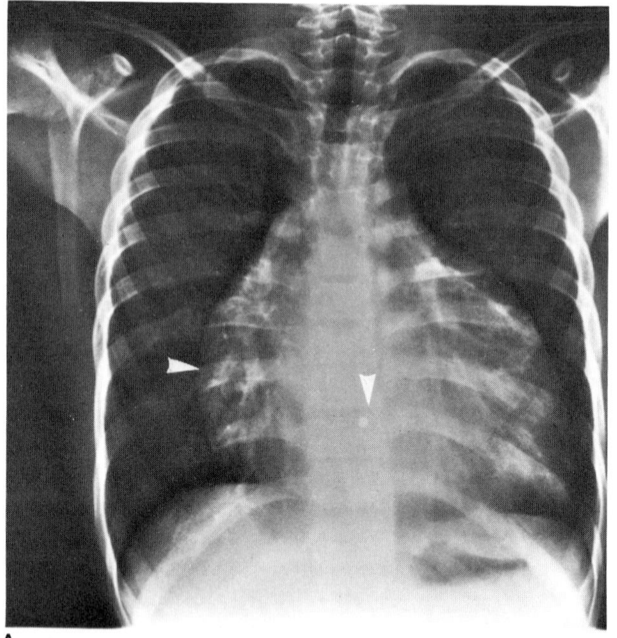

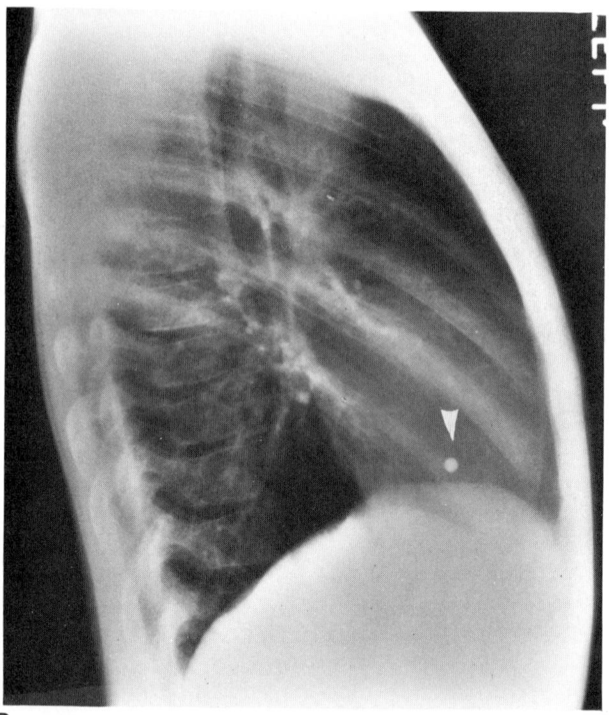

Figure 61–10 *A* Chest Roentgenogram Demonstrating a Buckshot Wound in the Heart with the Pericardium Filled with Blood. *B* Lateral Chest Roentgenogram in the Same Patient Demonstrating the Location of the Missile in the Heart.

CONTUSION OF THE HEART

The patient who enters the hospital with pain identical to that of myocardial infarction and a history of chest trauma not relieved by coronary dilating drugs must be suspected of having myocardial contusion.[6] There may be palpitation, tachycardia, and dyspnea, and the patient may be hypotensive. Premature atrial or ventricular contractions are the most common irregularities, but all kinds of irregularities have been reported. Pericarditis or pericardial tamponade may be associated.

The 12-lead electrocardiogram should be obtained in all patients with blunt injury to the heart, especially of the precordium. Serial electrocardiograms should be done because the changes may be late in developing. These changes may be transient or long lasting—from focal damage to pericarditis. Enzyme determinations are not reliable except for isoenzymes of creatine phosphokinase. The treatment is the same as that for myocardial infarction.

RUPTURE OF THE HEART

Rupture of the heart may be associated with immediate trauma or may be delayed 2 to 3 weeks as a result of a weakened myocardium from trauma. The heart can be compressed between the chest wall and vertebrae or from penetration by a rib, missile, or sternal bone. The rupture may involve any part of the heart, septum, or valves. The patient usually gives a history of trauma and presents with either cardiac tamponade or congestive heart failure. Pericardiocentesis should be followed by immediate surgery.

The diagnosis of rupture of the cardiac valves or intraventricular septum should be suspected in any patient who develops congestive heart failure immediately after trauma.[6] Decompensation may be immediate or late. Cardiac valve and ventricular septal rupture should be suspected in patients with valvular regurgitant murmur or murmur of ventricular septal defect following severe trauma.

Treatment is supportive. Cardiac catheterization should be performed if the patient fails to respond to treatment. Surgery should be considered depending on the findings.

TUBE THORACOSTOMY

The tube thoracostomy is one of the best methods of treatment open to the chest physician.[9] The placement of a chest tube is often life-saving, but when poorly placed the tube can be the source of increased morbidity and mortality. All physicians have seen chest tubes placed in the subcutaneous tissues and vital structures.

The primary use of the tube is to obliterate space between the parietal and visceral pleura usually caused by air or blood.[9] This creates the so-called pleural space and, depending on the size of this space, can cause tension pneumothorax or open pneumothorax with shift in the mediastinum, causing embarrassment to the contralateral hemothorax. Normally there is no such thing as intrapleural pressure, because there is no true intrapleural space.

It is essential to perform a tube thoracotomy to drain air or fluid from the thorax, maintain negative intrathoracic pressure, and monitor fluid or air loss from the intrapleural space. This reestablishes intrathoracic pressure equivalents. Once the tube is inserted it can be effective by simple drainage or by use of suction. This is determined by the need for a source of negative pressure or the need to evacuate persistent accumulation of fluid. Simple drainage can be used for well walled off accumulation. The evacuation from the chest of air and fluid is usually done by the use of Pleurovacs. These commercial systems allow for adequate evacuation of the chest. In addition they prevent aspirated fluid from being sucked back into the chest by means of valves placed in the system.

Tube thoracostomy is the treatment of choice in hemothorax and pneumothorax.[9] Indeed, some patients do well with aspiration or simple observation. Chest tubes are inserted preoperatively in patients with injury to the chest who may develop a hemothorax or pneumothorax during surgery. These tubes should be inserted and radiographs taken for location before anesthesia is given.

As is known, when supine, a patient will collect fluid posteroinferiorly and air superiorly. It would seem natural to place tubes accordingly. In trauma patients, however, a pure pneumothorax, which does not eventually include an accumulation of blood or fluid is seldom seen and a low-placed tube in a supine patient will eliminate most instances of pneumothorax.

The trauma tube is ideally placed in the fifth interspace in the mid axillary line. They are usually 34 or 35 French gauge. The skin must be *surgically* prepped and draped. The intercostal area is infiltrated with local anesthesia, and a 2- to 3-cm horizontal incision is made. The area is dissected with a clamp, moving the neurovascular bundle and staying close to the superior margin of the lower rib. The pleura is entered, and a gushing noise ensues along with air and fluid. The finger is inserted to ensure free access to the pleural space, and the tube is inserted posteriorly and superiorly with a large clamp. All the holes in the tube must enter the space. The area is closed with interrupted black silk sutures, with the tube included in a tie of one suture. Dressings should be applied. Roentgenograms should always be taken to determine the position of the tube and if there has been reexpansion of the lung. Extreme care must be used in transporting the patient with a chest tube. Too often a patient with a satisfactorily placed chest tube will have difficulty while being taken to radiology due to improper handling.

A physician or well-trained technician should accompany the patient to radiology. This individual can be prepared for sudden changes in the respiratory dynamics of the patient and be sure that the bottles are kept below the level of the patient and are not clamped or kinked. Portable radiographs can be used as indicated.

For a simple procedure, the placement of a chest tube is accompanied by myriads of complications. Malposition may occur, which has initiated the rule of not placing the tube below the fifth interspace (to avoid puncture of the liver or diaphragm) nor above the second interspace. The lung can be penetrated, but this can be prevented by putting a finger in the hole before the tube is inserted.

Infiltrations and location of compartmentalized fluid should be checked with a radiologist for identification and location. Problems with chest bottle connections, especially associated with transfer of patients, occur frequently. When massive bleeding occurs, the tube should be clamped and the patient prepared for surgery. When a massive air leak occurs, suction should be diminished.

Tube thoracostomy when properly applied is truly life-saving, but all tubes should be placed by a qualified physician. Some indications for bilateral chest tube placement include bilateral pneumothoraces, especially if spontaneous; lung contusions (put tube in worse side, other side if necessary, and both sides if patient is going to surgery); and subcutaneous emphysema in absence of pneumothorax, especially if patient is going to surgery.

EMERGENCY THORACOTOMY

At Denver General Hospital, between May 1974 and September 1978, 146 thoracotomies were performed in the emergency department on patients who arrived in cardiac arrest and did not respond in 2 to 3 minutes of resuscitative efforts. For those patients whose blood pressure did not rise above 60 mm Hg systolic in 5 to 10 minutes, the aorta was cross clamped. Those patients who arrived with suspected cardiac injuries with any signs of life were taken immediately to the operating room. Forty-eight of these patients had blunt injury to the chest, and none survived despite signs of life in the field or arriving at the emergency department. In penetrating abdominal injuries if signs of life were present at the scene 19 percent survived; if still alive in the emergency department 36 percent survived. There were no survivals in patients with no signs of life who were taken directly to the operating room.

In two subsequent large studies the patients with the highest survival rate were those with mediastinal injuries with cardiac tamponade, who presented with signs of life. Some of those series reported a mortality rate of as low as 11 percent. In addition to the indication for early (immediate to 72 hours) thoracotomy discussed above, Mandel and associates list the following:[10-12]

- penetrating wounds of the heart and great vessels
- cardiac arrest in the emergency department
- persistent bleeding through the chest tube that averages 150 to 200 ml/hour
- esophageal injuries
- intracardiac or intravascular missile fragments
- massive chest wall defects
- tracheobronchial injuries or ruptures
- pericardial tamponade
- ruptured diaphragm.

REFERENCES

1. Moore EE, et al: Post injury thoracotomy in the emergency department: A critical evaluation. *Surgery* 86:590–597, 1979.
2. Pellegrim RV, Layton TR, et al: Multiple cardiac lesions from blunt trauma. *J Trauma,* 1980.
3. Graham JM, Mattox K, et al: Air embolism following penetrating thoracic trauma. *Curr Concepts Trauma Care,* Fall 1979, pp 7–9.
4. Feliciano DV, Mattox, KL, et al: Hazards and pitfalls of thoracic inlet injury. *Curr Concepts Trauma Care,* Fall 1979, pp 5–7.
5. Davidson SJ: Autotransfusion from hemothorax. *Curr Concepts Trauma Care,* Fall 1979, pp 2–4.
6. Symbas PN: Chest and heart injuries. In *Principles and Practice of Emergency Medicine,* pp 653–673.
7. Trinkle JK, et al: Affairs of the wounded heart: Penetrating cardiac wounds. *J Trauma* 19:467–470, 1979.
8. Boeaut EP, et al: Cardiac tamponade following penetrating mediastinal injuries: Improved survival with early pericardiocentesis. *J Trauma* 19:461–466, 1979.
9. Bricker DL, Mattox KL: About chest tubes. *Curr Concepts Trauma Care,* Fall 1979, pp 16–19.
10. Mandel AK, Oparah SS: Penetrating stab wounds of the chest (Experience with 200 consecutive cases). *J Trauma* 16:336–339, 1976.
11. Mandel AK, Oparah SS: Penetrating gunshot wounds of the chest (Experience with 250 consecutive cases). *Br J Surg* 65: 1:45–48.
12. Peters RM: Chest trauma. In Warner CG (ed): *Emergency Care Assessment and Intervention,* ed 2. St. Louis, CV Mosby Co, 1978.

Alterations of Urinary and Reproductive System Functions

In "Genitourinary Emergencies" (Chapter 62), the author considers blunt and penetrating injuries of the kidney, the ureter, urinary bladder, and external genitalia, and provides the clinical and diagnostic approaches to treatment. The discussion of acute flank and intrascrotal pain is followed by a review of acute urinary retention. Infections of the genitourinary tract are discussed in "Infectious Disease Emergencies" (Chapter 20).

As discussed in "Renal Failure" (Chapter 63), evaluation of renal failure should be quickly and efficiently accomplished because the process is potentially reversible and its many causes are treatable. The author discusses renal failure, its identification and its etiology, including extrarenal causes, and management. Emergency conditions that may be a consequence of renal failure are discussed in "Disturbances in Cardiac Rhythm" (Chapter 50), "Congestive Heart Failure" (Chapter 51), and Metabolic and Endocrine Emergencies (Section III).

In "Obstetric and Gynecologic Emergencies" (Chapter 64), the authors review conditions that are responsible for a tremendous amount of morbidity and mortality among young women, and focus on lower abdominal pain with or without vaginal bleeding, ectopic pregnancy, and pelvic inflammatory disease.

Finally, in "Rape and Sexual Assault" (Chapter 65), the author addresses the physical and emotional injuries of patients who are the victims of rape and sexual assault. A rationale for medical, physiologic, and legal diagnostic tests is presented. Male and geriatric patients are also considered.

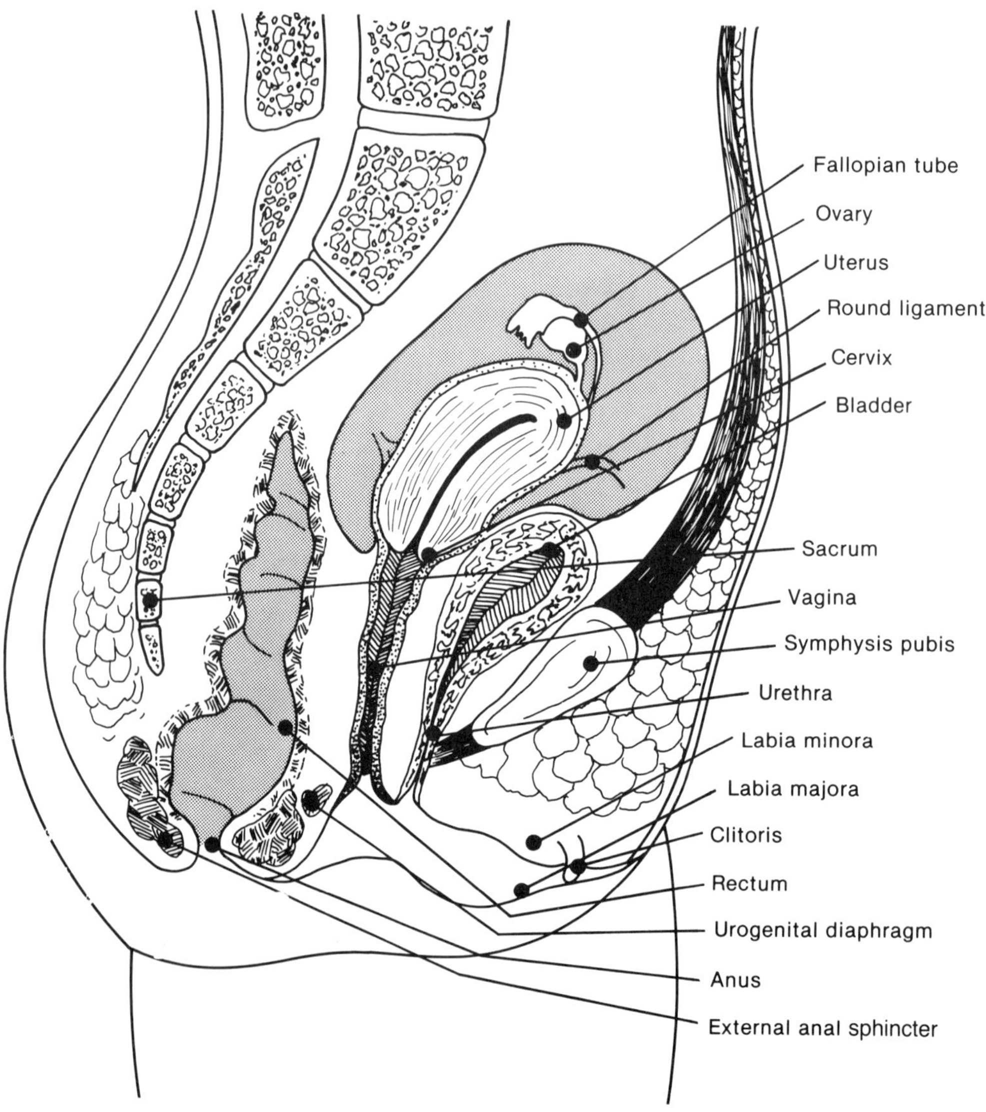

Female Urinary and Reproductive Structures

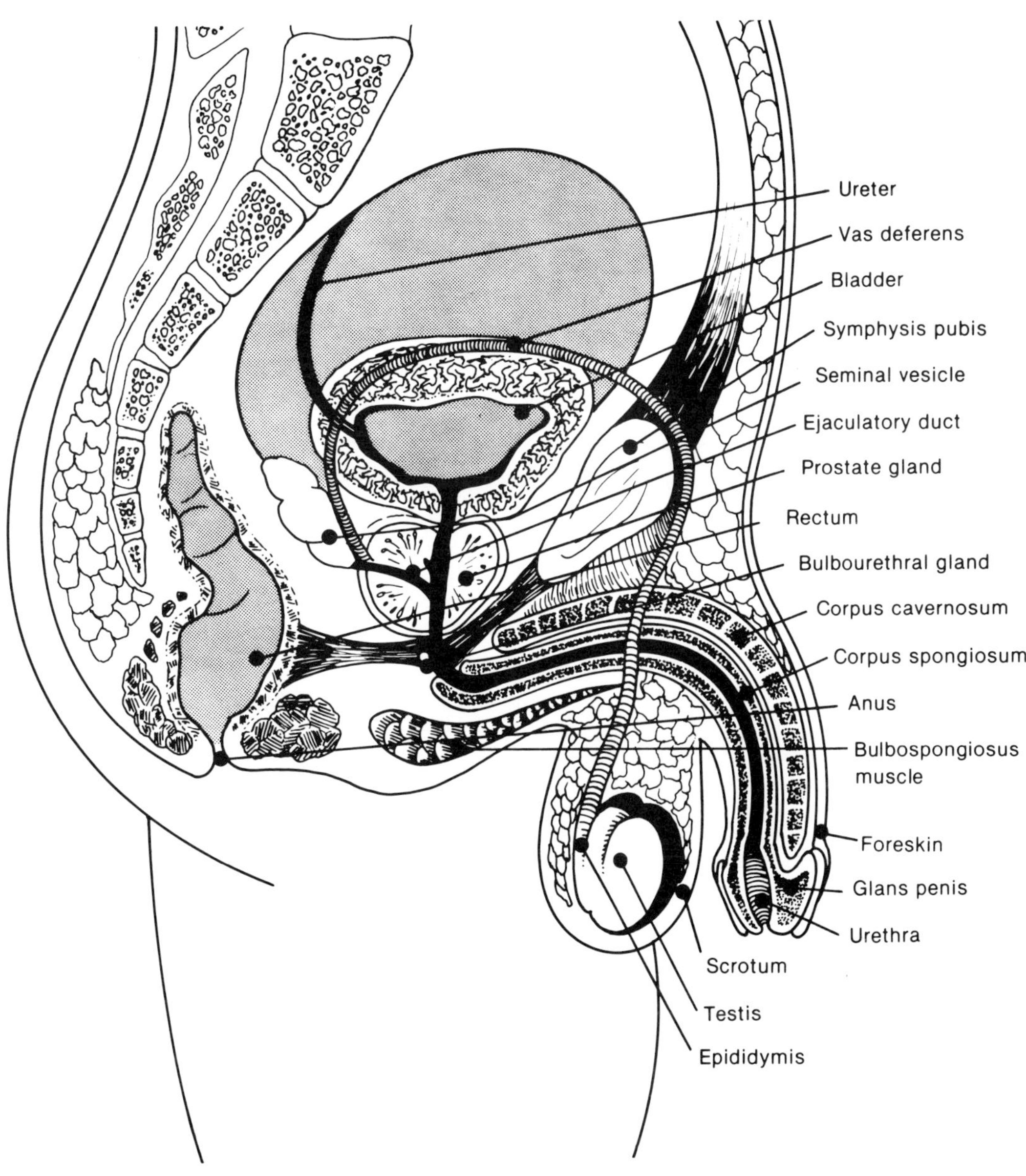

Male Urinary and Reproductive Structures

62. Common Genitourinary Emergencies

ALEXANDER D. VARGAS, M.D., F.A.C.S.

INJURIES TO THE KIDNEY

Although the kidneys are well protected in the retroperitoneum by the lower ribs, lumbar muscles, and the spine, traumatic injuries are seen frequently in an emergency environment. The etiology as well as the pathologic classification according to the extent of renal damage are important factors in determining the modality of treatment.

According to the etiology, renal injuries are classified into blunt and penetrating injuries. Blunt injuries most commonly are associated with sudden deceleration of the body. This mechanism usually occurs as a result of an automobile accident or a fall from a height. Direct blows to the abdomen or back may also involve the kidney directly. Penetrating injuries are seen as a result of external violence and usually are caused by gunshot wounds or stab wounds with the point of entrance through the abdomen, flank, or back.

According to the extent of damage, renal injuries may be classified pathologically as follows (Fig. 62–1): In contusions the renal capsule remains intact and the kidney shows ecchymosis and bruising. Occasionally, a subcapsular hematoma develops. Lacerations occur when the renal capsule is torn. The parenchymal defect may be superficial or, on occasion, deep and may involve the calyceal system, resulting in urinary extravasation. Lacerations may be multiple and severe with involvement of the entire kidney. In these cases, the pathologic event is called a shattered kidney. In pedicle injuries the renal artery or vein could be involved as a result of

direct injury or, as it happens in blunt renal injuries, in the form of an arterial intimal tear, with subsequent formation of a thrombus. Intimal tears occur as a result of sudden deceleration and stretching of the renal artery.

Following a renal injury, varying degrees of intrarenal or extrarenal bleeding may occur. Intrarenal bleeding presents as a subcapsular hematoma or as hematuria. Extrarenal bleeding results in a perirenal hematoma that usually is limited by Gerota's fascia. If the calyceal system is involved, extravasation of urine occurs, resulting in the formation of a urinoma. On rare occasions, a penetrating injury may present as a urinary cutaneous fistula.

Blunt Renal Injuries

Blunt renal injuries are most often sustained in automobile accidents, followed by falls, fighting, football, and crushing and swinging accidents.[1] A review of 252 cases of blunt renal injuries at the Los Angeles County–USC Medical Center revealed that associated injuries were found in 44 percent of the patients. The viscera that most commonly were injured were the spleen, liver, and lung.

Clinical Manifestations

Hematuria usually alerts the physician to suspect a renal injury. This sign is found in more than 95 percent of patients.[1,2] At the Los Angeles County–USC Medical

"

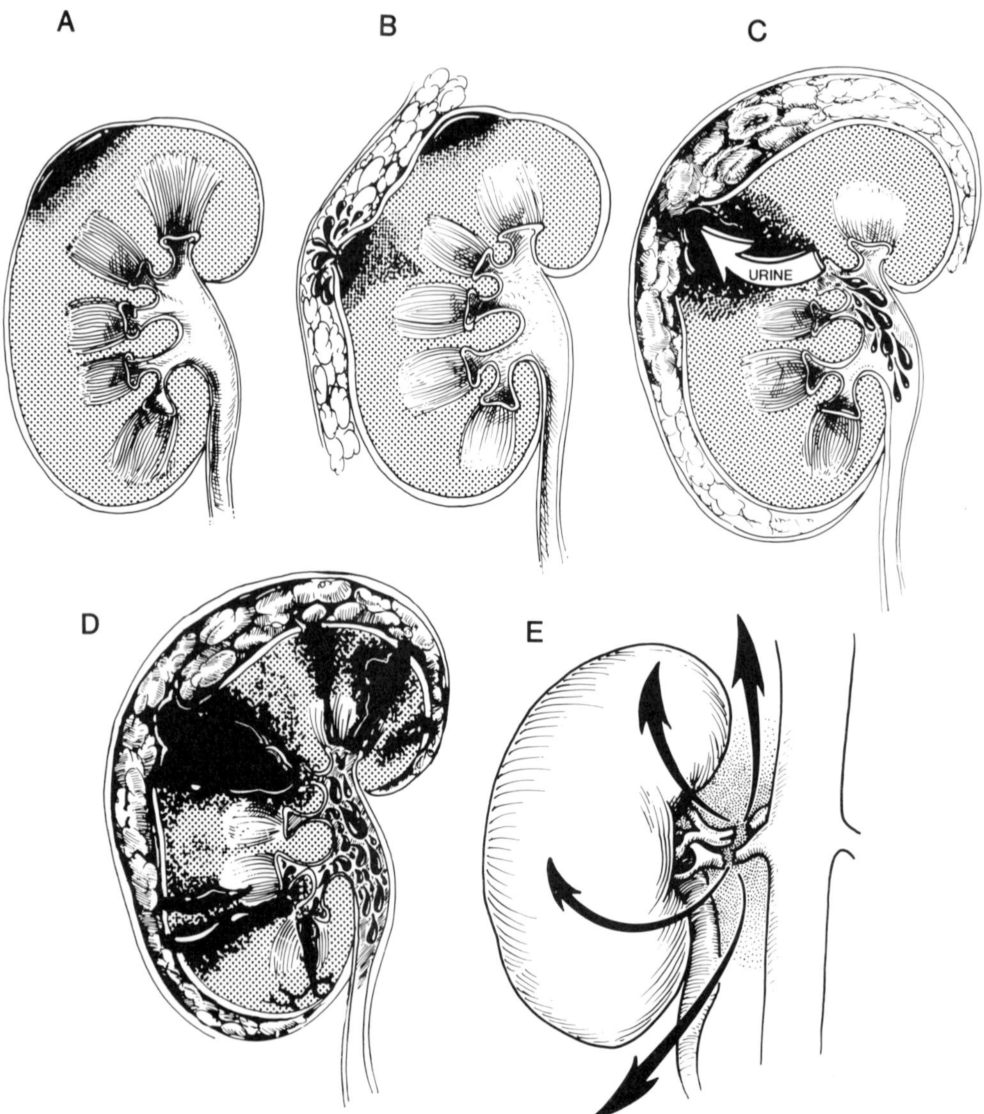

Figure 62–1   Classification of Renal Injuries. Note: *A*, contusion; *B*, superficial laceration; *C*, deep laceration; *D*, shattered kidney; *E*, pedicle injury.

Center 67 percent of patients presented with gross hematuria and 32 percent with a microscopic hematuria.

The history surrounding the circumstances of the accident should be thoroughly assessed, taking into consideration the magnitude and characteristics of the accident. The vast majority of patients present with symptoms of flank pain, abdominal pain, or a palpable mass (Table 62–1).

The physical examination most commonly reveals flank or costovertebral pain. Ecchymosis of the flank area or the clinical evidence of a rib fracture may be found. Since abnormal kidneys are more susceptible to renal injuries, assessment of preexisting renal lesions is important, particularly in the presence of minor trauma with disproportionate renal symptomatology. The Los Angeles County–USC Medical Center series indicates an incidence of preexisting lesions in 3 percent of the patients.

Radiographic Studies

After clinical stabilization, appropriate radiographic examinations are indicated in the search for associated injuries, particularly of the skull, chest, spine, ribs, and pelvis. If a renal injury is suspected, an excretory urogram should be performed.

Excretory Urography. The excretory urography should be performed by infusion technique or double-dose injection of contrast media. The urogram is abnormal in over 40 percent of the patients (Fig. 62–2). The most common findings are delayed visualization, extravasation of dye, and renal nonfunction (Table 62–2).

TABLE 62–1   Clinical Manifestations in 252 Patients with Blunt Renal Injuries

	No. Patients	Percent
Flank pain	160	63
Abdominal pain	88	35
Palpable mass	7	3
Gross hematuria	168	67
Microhematuria	80	32
Asymptomatic	4	2

TABLE 62–2   Results of Excretory Urography in 235 Patients with Blunt Renal Injuries

	No. Patients	Percent
Normal	125	53
Delayed excretion	35	15
Extravasation	27	11
Major	9	
Minor	18	
Nonvisualization	10	4
Preexisting abnormal	8	3
Equivocal	30	13

Renal Scan. A renal scan complements the excretory urogram and provides information about renal flow, renal function, and the existence of parenchymal defects. It is a noninvasive test that unfortunately lacks the detail obtained with renal angiography. It is the test of choice when the excretory urogram is normal or equivocal.

Aortography and Renal Angiography. Aortography and renal angiography is without doubt the most accurate test to disclose renal architecture (Fig 62–3).[3] Since this method is relatively invasive, it is best indicated when the excretory urogram reveals a nonvisualizing kidney, extravasation, or delayed excretion or when there is severe bleeding.

Ultrasonography. Ultrasonography is simple, noninvasive, and of value when the urogram shows a nonvisualizing kidney to assess the presence of a kidney. It may also be extremely helpful to evaluate the extent and course of a retroperitoneal collection.

Retrograde Urography. Retrograde urography is seldom indicated unless a ureteral injury is strongly suspected.

Computerized Axial Tomography. Utilizing high resolution techniques, computerized axial tomography may reveal lesions not identified by the previously discussed diagnostic tests.

Management

Based on the clinical and radiographic findings, blunt renal injuries may present as a contusion, laceration, shattered kidney, or pedicle injury (Table 62–3). The accurate anatomical definition of the injury dictates the most appropriate modality of treatment.

The vast majority of blunt renal injuries are amenable to conservative treatment. In fact, 88 percent of the 252

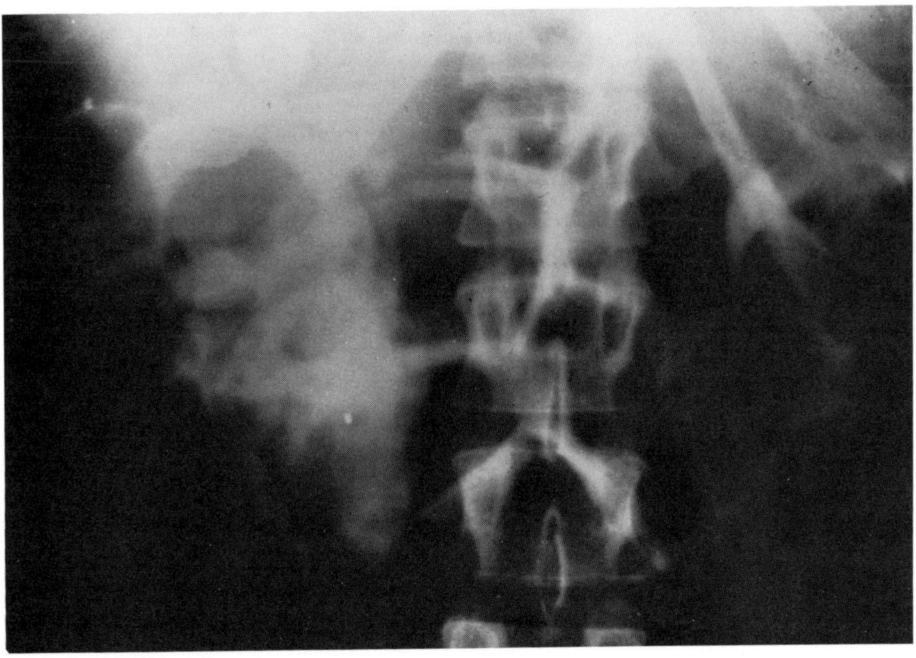

Figure 62–2   Intravenous Urogram. *Note:* Extravasation of urine is present on right kidney following blunt trauma.

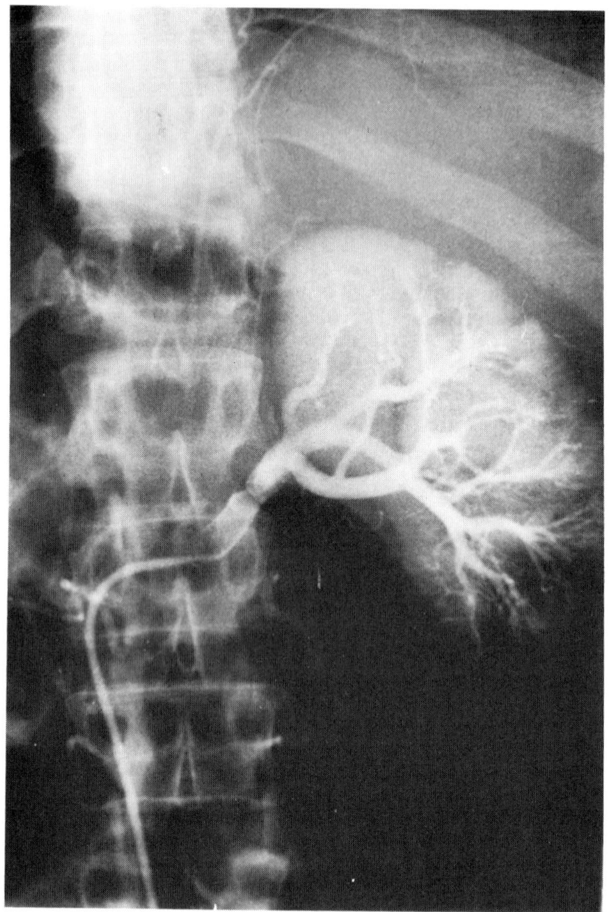

Figure 62–3   Selective Angiogram of Kidney. *Note:* Arterial injury in the form of an intimal tear of main renal artery is evident. Intravenous urogram revealed delayed function of the kidney.

blunt renal injuries reviewed at the Los Angeles County–USC Medical Center were treated conservatively. The management will depend on the radiographic evaluation and the clinical conditions of the patient.

Medical treatment is based on observation, bed rest until gross hematuria has resolved, and analgesia. Renal exploration is indicated by and large in the following

TABLE 62–3   Types of Renal Injury in 252 Patients with Blunt Trauma

Injury	No. Patients	Percent
Contusions	197	78
Major lacerations	23	9
Minor lacerations	13	5
Shattered kidneys	10	4
Pedicle injuries	9	3

situations: pedicle injuries, extensive parenchymal damage (shattered kidney), severe recurrent hematuria and/or progressive perirenal hemorrhage, severe urinary extravasation, and if an expanding hematoma is found at the time of laparotomy for associated visceral injuries. If surgical exploration is indicated, mobilization of the kidney should be performed only after the renal pedicle is secured with vascular clamps in order to prevent renal bleeding that could lead to an unnecessary nephrectomy.[4] After discharge, periodic follow-up is necessary for several months.

Penetrating Renal Injuries

Penetrating renal injuries are usually caused by gunshot or stab wounds. Injuries to the kidney are found in 8 percent of patients with gunshot wounds and in 6 percent of patients with stab wounds to the abdomen in large series.[5]

Associated injuries are seen with higher incidence as compared with blunt renal injuries. At the Los Angeles County–USC Medical Center, 94 percent of 148 patients with penetrating renal injuries had an associated visceral injury.

The injuries caused by gunshot wounds are in direct proportion to the velocity of the missile and also are related to the position and distance of the assailant.[6] On occasion, the bullet is deflected after hitting a bony structure.

Clinical Manifestations

Usually in penetrating renal injuries, the symptoms are related to associated intra-abdominal injuries and in the vast majority of patients there is abdominal or flank pain. It is important to assess the characteristics surrounding the trauma, the relative position of the assailant, and the type of weapon used.

Hematuria may be present and is suggestive of renal or ureteral injury. However, in a significant number of cases urinalysis is normal. According to our experience with 148 cases of penetrating renal injuries, hematuria was absent in 14 percent of the patients. Other investigators have encountered even a higher incidence of false-negative results of urinalysis.[4] The physician should keep a high index of suspicion when a patient has a penetrating abdominal injury, and if clinically advisable, an excretory urogram should be obtained in all cases of suggested renal injuries.

Initial physical examination will reveal a small entrance wound (and sometimes, a larger exit wound). Generalized abdominal tenderness with or without peritoneal signs is usually present.

TABLE 62–4 Results of Excretory Urography in 101 Patients with Penetrating Renal Injuries

	No. Patients	Percent
Normal	29	29
Delayed excretion	9	9
Extravasation	14	14
Nonvisualization	6	6
Equivocal	43	42

Radiographic Studies

After a thorough general evaluation of the patient and after stabilizing the clinical conditions, pertinent radiographic studies are needed.

Excretory Urography. Excretory urography in penetrating renal injuries has a limited accuracy. At the Los Angeles County–USC Medical Center, a false-negative excretory urogram occurs in 40 percent of patients. Therefore, a normal urogram occasionally may

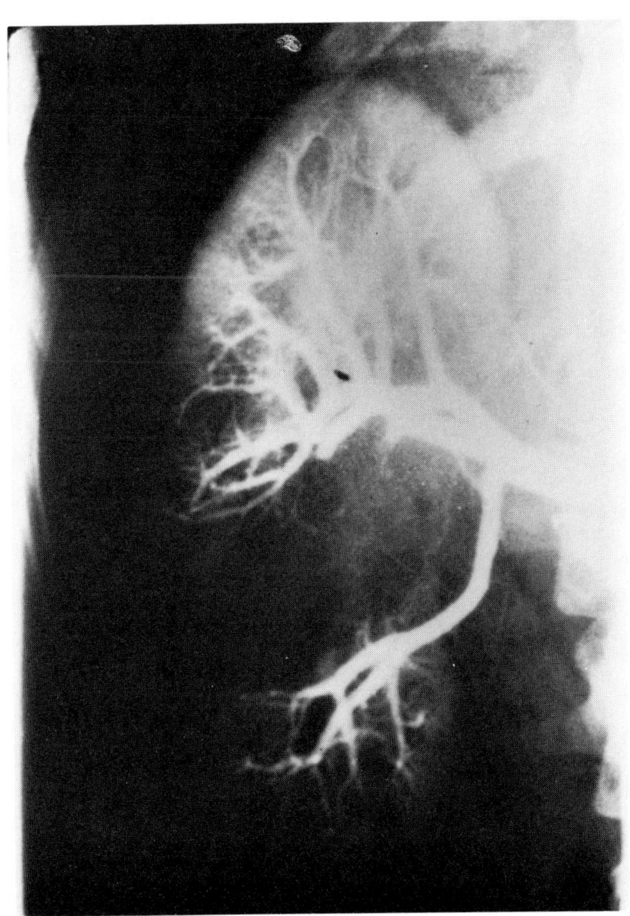

Figure 62–4 Selective Angiogram of Kidney. *Note:* Deep laceration of the kidney was caused by a gunshot wound.

give a false sense of security to the surgeon. The excretory urogram findings in this study are seen in Table 62–4. As in cases with blunt renal injuries, an infusion technique or a double-dose injection of contrast media should be utilized.

Aortography and Renal Angiography. In these cases, as in blunt renal injuries, aortography and renal angiography will demonstrate the renal anatomy with accuracy. In fact, it is the best diagnostic tool available for a thorough assessment in penetrating renal injuries. Unfortunately, since the procedure is relatively invasive and many of these patients are in critical condition, it is not unusual that a surgical exploration to control serious bleeding cannot be delayed and time is not available to perform angiography (Fig. 62–4).

Renal Scan. Renal scanning is noninvasive and may be useful in cases when the excretory urogram is normal or equivocal.

Retrograde Urography. Retrograde urography is only indicated when a ureteral injury is suspected.

Computerized Axial Tomography. CT scanning may identify small lesions.

Management

The management of penetrating renal injuries remains controversial. Some investigators advocate surgical exploration in all cases,[4] and others claim that conservatism may lead to the same or even better long-term results.[7,8]

Unquestionably, renal exploration is indicated in serious lacerations, shattered kidneys, or when there is pedicle involvement in an attempt to prevent immediate complications and to preserve renal parenchyma. An important consideration in the planning of management of penetrating renal injuries is the accurate definition of the extent and nature of the renal injury, which can be obtained by renal angiography. In general, stab wounds are more suitable for thorough radiographic evaluation and, in studies at the Los Angeles County–USC Medical Center, 59 percent of the angiograms were performed in these cases. The pathoanatomical findings in 148 cases treated at the Los Angeles County–USC Medical Center are shown in Table 62–5.

Superficial and moderately deep renal lacerations are successfully treated by conservative measures, provided that the clinical conditions of the patient are stable, angiography indicates no serious vascular derangement, significant urinary extravasation is absent, and on surgical exploration (in a search for unrelated intra-abdominal lesions), the perinephric hematoma is not expanding.

As in blunt renal injuries, renal exploration should be performed after complete control of the renal pedicle

TABLE 62–5   Types of Renal Injury According to Etiology in 148 Patients with Penetrating Trauma

| | Gunshot Wound | | Stab Wound | |
	No. Patients	Percent	No. Patients	Percent
Contusions	4	5		
Lacerations	45	52	60	97
Shattered kidneys	21	24		
Pedicle injuries	16	19	2	3

to avoid unnecessary bleeding. Periodic follow-up is needed for several months.

INJURIES TO THE URETER

By virtue of its size, anatomical position, and relative mobility, the ureter is rarely damaged. When injuries do occur they may be classified as either traumatic or iatrogenic. Early diagnosis is the single most important parameter affecting the success of repair.

Traumatic Ureteral Injuries

The vast majority of traumatic ureteral injuries result from penetrating wounds to the abdomen or the flank. As seen in Table 62–6, results of a study at the Los Angeles County–USC Medical Center indicate that gunshot wounds are responsible for 90 percent of the cases; stab wounds, 7 percent; and blunt trauma, 3 percent. Published figures indicate that 3 to 17 percent of penetrating abdominal wounds result in ureteral injuries.[9] These injuries predominate in males and are frequently seen in young active individuals. The proximal or mid ureter is involved more often in penetrating injuries. However, the distal ureter may be involved in lower abdominal gunshot wounds. Ureteral injuries that result from blunt trauma (fall from heights) occur at the ureteropelvic junction and are usually seen in children. In gunshot wounds the ureteral damage is in direct proportion to the velocity of the missile (blast effect).[6] According to this study, in gunshot wounds, associated visceral intra-abdominal injuries are found in over 90 percent of the patients. The organs usually involved are the large or small intestine, followed by the liver, large vessels, and pancreas. Stab wounds have a lower incidence of associated injuries, particularly if the entrance is through the flank (50 percent).

Iatrogenic Ureteral Injuries

The ureter may be injured during an abdominal or a retroperitoneal surgical procedure. However, the ma-

jority of injuries occur during pelvic procedures. Occasionally, the injury may be sustained during an endoscopic procedure (e.g., catheterization, stone manipulation) (Table 62–6).

The incidence of ureteral injuries in benign gynecologic operations has been reported to be between 0.4 and 2.5 percent,[10,11] however, for radical pelvic operation it has been described with an incidence as high as 30 percent.[12] The lower third of the ureter is by far the most predominant portion involved in pelvic operations.

Diagnosis

According to the time at which the ureteral injury is recognized, the diagnosis may be described as occurring in an immediate or delayed period. It is of utmost importance to recognize a ureteral injury at the time of presentation in case of trauma, or at the time of the surgical accident in iatrogenic injuries.

A high level of suspicion by the physician should be maintained in the presence of a gunshot wound or a stab wound to the abdomen or the back. In these cases, specific clinical manifestations are usually not identified in the immediate post-traumatic period since they are often obscured by the signs and symptoms of other associated visceral injuries. Hematuria may be present and is helpful in making the diagnosis. However, in the author's experience hematuria was absent in 46 percent of the patients; therefore, a normal urinalysis may be misleading (Table 62–7).

A high-dosage excretory urogram is the single most valuable diagnostic study, with an accuracy as high as 90 percent.[5] Unfortunately, a significant number of these cases remain undiagnosed since an excretory urogram is not obtained before laparotomy (indicated for associated injuries). The surgeon should then make certain

TABLE 62–6   Etiology of 111 Ureteral Injuries

Etiology	No. Patients	Percent
Traumatic		
Gunshot wounds	53	90
Stab wounds	4	7
Blunt trauma	2	3
Total	59	100
Iatrogenic		
Ob-gyn procedures	35	67
Urologic procedures	12	23
Endoscopic	5	10
Open	7	13
General Surgical Procedures	5	10
Total	52	100

TABLE 62–7   Hematuria in 48 Immediately Recognized Penetrating Ureteral Injuries

Type	No. Patients	Percent
Gross hematuria	11	23
Microhematuria	15	31
None	22	46

that a ureteral injury has not been sustained by directly visualizing the ureters at the operative field (Fig. 62–5). On occasion, a urine collection may be encountered, suggesting a ureteral compromise. If doubt exists, the intravenous injection of indigo carmine dye is a helpful maneuver to define urinary extravasation.

During a surgical procedure close to the retroperitoneum the ureter may be totally or partially transected, crushed, devascularized, or litigated. Since the ureter is mobile, small, and usually adherent to the posterior peritoneum, the surgeon must always keep a high index of suspicion, particularly when performing a difficult pelvic or abdominal operation. Preventive measures should be taken if a difficult surgical procedure is anticipated. The placement of ureteral catheters preoperatively may be helpful to prevent a ureteral injury. Undoubtedly, the identification of the ureter as it crosses the operative field is the most optimal preventive surgical maneuver.

The recognition of a significant number of ureteral injuries is delayed. For example, at the Los Angeles County–USC Medical Center the recognition of 19 percent of the traumatic injuries and 63 percent of the iatrogenic injuries is delayed (Table 62–8).

As opposed to immediate recognized injuries, the clinical manifestations are more specific in this group of patients, owing to hydronephrosis, tissue inflammation, infection, urinary extravasation, or fistula formation. The most prominent clinical manifestations are pain, fever, hematuria, and/or a palpable mass. A ureterocutaneous or ureterovaginal fistula occurs in a significant number of cases, the majority resulting from iatrogenic injuries (Table 62–9). The excretory urogram followed by a retrograde urogram usually confirms the diagnosis of ureteral injury in these cases.

Management

Once the ureteral injury is recognized, the surgical treatment depends on the location, extent, and type of injury. A meticulous surgical technique must be fol-

TABLE 62–8   Immediate and Delayed Recognition of 111 Ureteral Injuries

Diagnosis	Traumatic		Iatrogenic	
	No. Patients	Percent	No. Patients	Percent
Immediate	48	81	19	37
Delayed	11	19	33	63

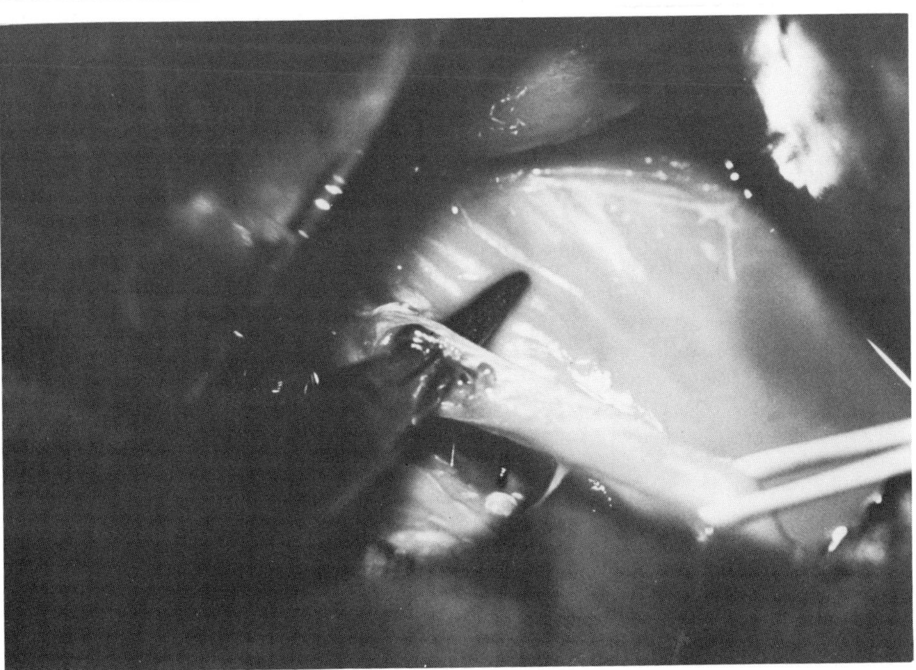

Figure 62–5   Ureteral Injury Due to Gunshot Wound.

TABLE 62–9   Delayed Recognition of 44 Ureteral Injuries

Clinical Finding	No. Patients	Percent
Pain and fever	23	52
Ureterocutaneous fistula	8	18
Ureterovaginal fistula	7	16
Palpable mass	2	4.5
Hematuria	2	4.5
Hypertension	1	2
Asymptomatic	5	11

lowed, with adequate debridement of damaged tissue and care to preserve the ureteral vascular supply. Simple maneuvers such as deligation or catheter placement may be adequate in certain cases. However, a careful assessment of the vascular ureteral supply should be made.

The preferred method of repair of lower third ureteral injuries is ureteroneocystostomy (Fig. 62–6). After adequate mobilization of the proximal ureter to gain sufficient ureteral length, an antireflux subcutaneous tunnel should be obtained. If an adequate length cannot be obtained, a psoas hitch may be performed.[13] On occasion, a simple end-to-side anastomosis can be safely performed. A Boari flap is an alternative that may successfully bridge a long lower ureteral defect (Fig. 62–7).[14]

An end-to-end ureteral anastomosis is the preferred method to treat injuries to the upper or mid third of the ureter. Adequate debridement, tension-free watertight anastomosis, and adequate drainage of surrounding tissues are basic principles to be followed. A generous spatulation of the ureteral ends should be performed, and a stent is left indwelling for alignment and drainage (Fig. 62–8).

If a long segment of ureter is resected and an end-to-end anastomosis is not feasible, a transureteroureteral anastomosis, autotransplantation, a posterior vesical flap, or an ileal ureter may be utilized.[13,15] Occasionally, a nephrectomy is the best alternative, particularly if the patient's clinical condition is less than optimal.

Excellent results are obtained after immediate repair of traumatic or iatrogenic injuries. In injuries in which recognition is delayed, the incidence of failure may be high after repair. At the Los Angeles County–USC Medical Center a failure rate of 20 percent in this group of patients (9 of 44 cases) has been noted.

INJURIES TO THE BLADDER

Injuries to the bladder are relatively infrequent, since the organ is well protected in the pelvic area. The diagnosis of bladder injury is easily made by radiographic methods; however, a high index of suspicion should be maintained by the physician who initially evaluates the patient. The bladder may be injured during a surgical procedure or by external trauma.

Iatrogenic Injuries

The bladder may be injured during pelvic surgery or urinary instrumentation. Surgical injuries occur more

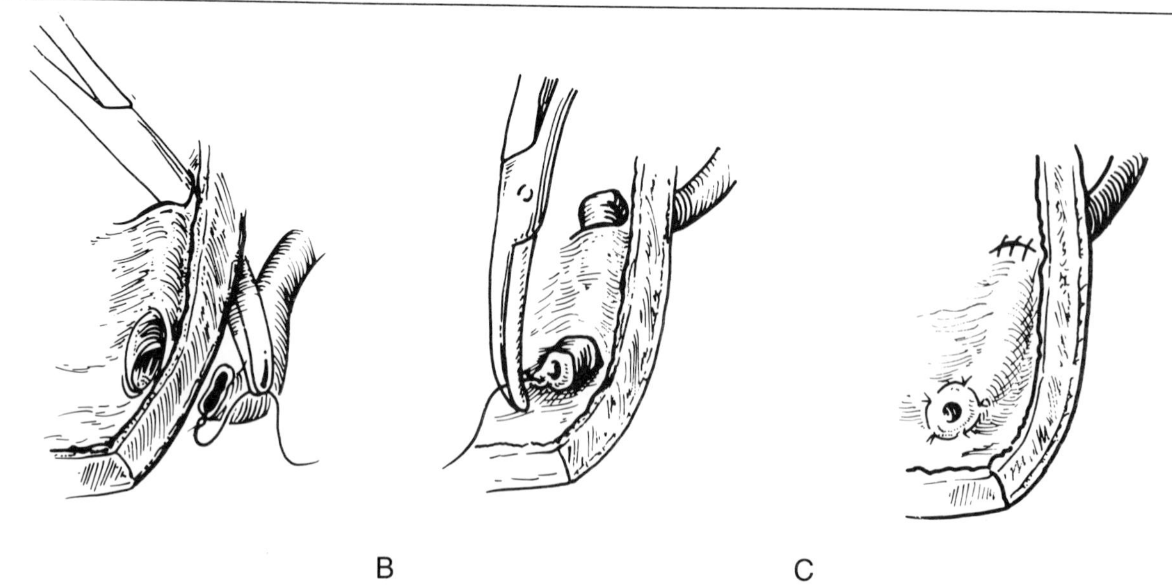

A   B   C

Figure 62–6   Ureteroneocystostomy.

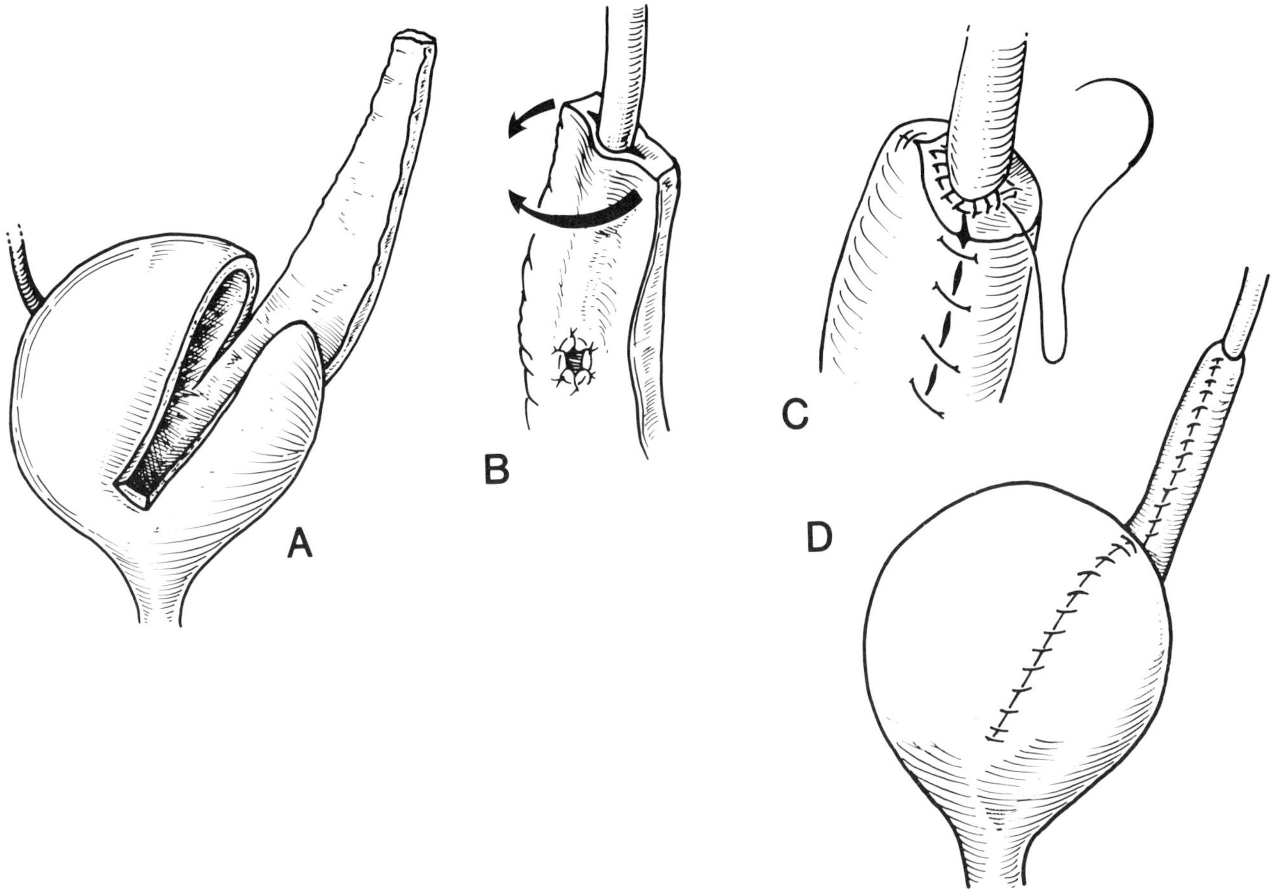

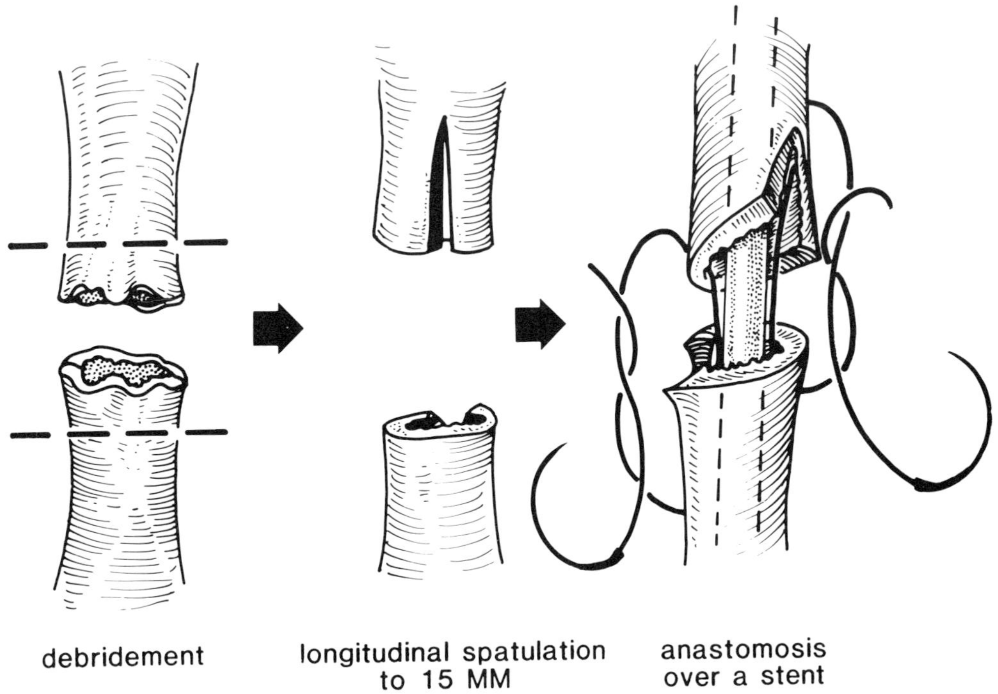

Figure 62–7   Use of Boari Flap to Repair Ureteral Injuries.

Figure 62–8   End-to-End Ureteral Anastomosis.

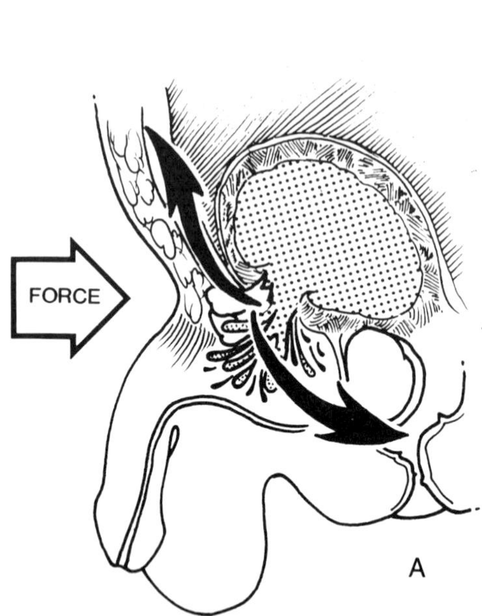

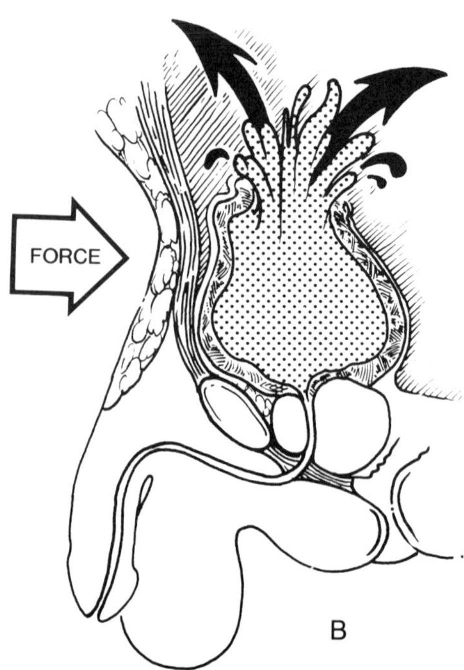

Figure 62–9   Rupture of the Bladder. *Note: A*, extraperitoneal rupture; *B*, intraperitoneal rupture.

frequently during a difficult operation, particularly when the anatomy is distorted as a result of an inflammatory process, neoplasms, or previous surgery.

Traumatic Injuries

According to the extent of damage, these injuries may be classified into contusions, extraperitoneal rupture, or intraperitoneal rupture. Extraperitoneal rupture usually results from bony fragments penetrating into the vesical wall. Most commonly, this occurs as a result of a pelvic fracture (Fig. 62–9, A). Intraperitoneal rupture is seen in patients sustaining a lower abdominal trauma while the bladder is distended with urine. Usually, the rupture occurs at the dome of the bladder and the urine flows freely into the abdominal cavity (Fig. 62–9, B).

The most common causes of penetrating injuries to the bladder are gunshot wounds and stab wounds to the lower abdomen. The vast majority of these patients will present with associated intra-abdominal injuries. Small intestinal, rectal, or pelvic vascular structures are most often involved.

Clinical Manifestations

A history of a lower abdominal injury followed by lower abdominal pain and hematuria is usually suggestive of a urinary bladder injury. Hematuria is seen in the vast majority of patients, with an incidence as high as 94 percent.[16] A fractured pelvis is commonly associated with a bladder injury. If there has been a delay in diagnosis, peritoneal signs may be present.

The majority of patients will not be able to urinate because of pain, neurologic disorders, or urinary extravasation. Physical examination may reveal tenderness in the suprapubic area. Ecchymosis of the adjacent skin may be found, and, on occasion, a suprapubic mass develops as a result of extravasation and bleeding.

Diagnosis

A plain roentgenogram may reveal fractures of the pelvic bones. Five to 10 percent of patients with a pelvic fracture will present with a ruptured bladder.[16,17]

A cystogram is the most reliable test to diagnose a bladder rupture. An anteroposterior and oblique view should be performed followed by a drainage film (Figs. 62–10 and 62–11).

When the pelvis is fractured, it is important to obtain a retrograde urethrogram before attempting urethral catheterization in order to rule out a urethral injury. In these cases, the passage of a catheter may convert a partial urethral laceration into a complete laceration.

Management

After adequate debridement of damaged tissue, immediate repair by anatomical layers with the use of

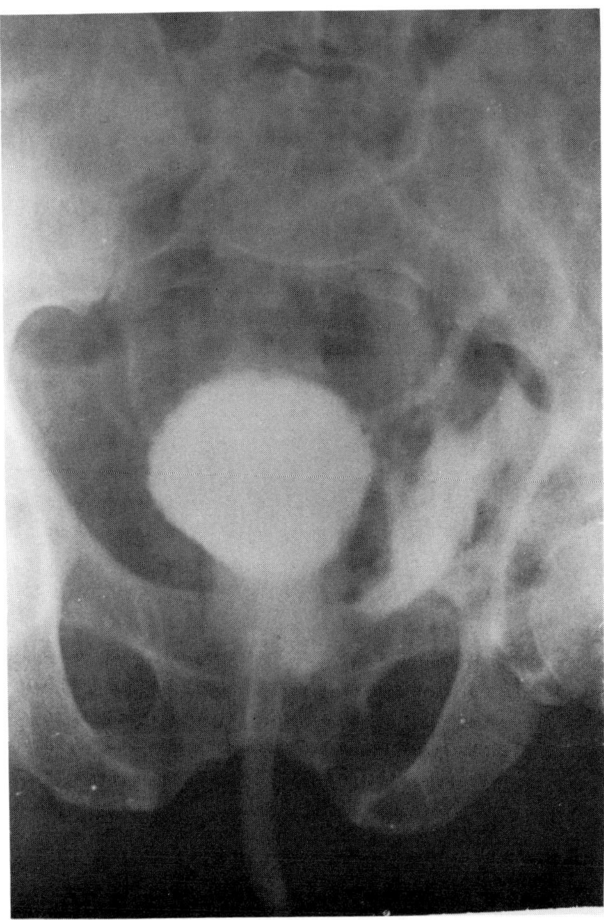

Figure 62–10   Cystogram Showing Extraperitoneal Bladder Rupture.

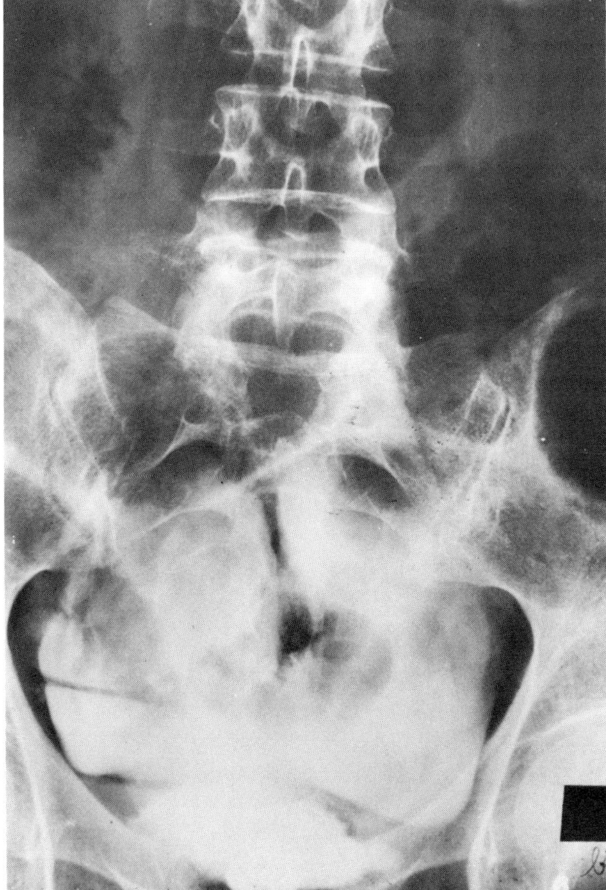

Figure 62–11   Cystogram Showing Intraperitoneal Bladder Rupture.

absorbable sutures is the most widely accepted repair in bladder injuries. Bladder rest for 7 to 14 days is preferred by most surgeons, together with appropriate drainage of the perivesical space.

If associated injuries are suspected, it is advisable to explore the abdominal cavity thoroughly. A suprapubic cystostomy or a urethral catheter is used for vesical drainage. The former is best indicated in the presence of large lacerations and in male patients.

In selective cases, particularly in the presence of an extraperitoneal bladder rupture, the simple placement of a urethral catheter, without surgical exploration, may be utilized with good results.[18,19] At the Los Angeles County–USC Medical Center this approach is used only in small extraperitoneal tears with appropriate antibiotic coverage and judicious observation.

With prompt diagnosis and treatment the prognosis of these injuries is excellent, with minimal morbidity and mortality. However, if the treatment is delayed, a significant incidence of complication and mortality is expected.

INJURIES TO THE URETHRA

Injuries to the urethra are relatively rare. Prompt diagnosis and adequate initial treatment is essential to prevent severe sequelae. In a male patient the clinical implications and management varies with the site of the injury. For this purpose, a separate description of injuries occurring at the membranous urethra, bulbous urethra, and pendulous urethra will follow.

Injuries to the Membranous Urethra

This type of injury usually presents in the form of a prostatomembranous disruption that is commonly associated with a pelvic fracture. The prostate is separated from its attachments to the genitourinary diaphragm. The laceration may be complete or incomplete. When a complete disruption occurs, the bladder and prostate are displaced upward and the defect is filled with blood clots and urine. Bony fragments may penetrate into the posterior urethra or bladder (Fig. 62–12). Injuries to the posterior urethra also may result from instrumentation, penetrating injuries (gunshot wounds or stab wounds), or iatrogenically during the course of an abdominoperineal rectal resection.

Clinical Manifestations

A history of a severe injury, usually the result of an automobile accident, is always obtained. There may be pain in the lower abdomen and in the perineum. Associated injuries are usually present, and the amount of hemorrhage at the level of the pelvis may be considerable. Urethral bleeding may be present and should alert the physician to the possibility of a urethral injury. The patient commonly is unable to urinate.

The physical examination usually reveals signs of urethral bleeding. There may be tenderness and/or a mass palpable in the suprapubic area due to extravasation, hematoma, or urinary retention. Rectal examination may reveal that the prostate is displaced upward, suggesting a complete prostatomembranous disruption.

Diagnosis

A pelvic fracture may be evident on a plain roentgenogram. If a urethral disruption is suspected, a retrograde urethrogram should be performed to confirm such diagnosis. Ten to 15 cc of diluted contrast medium is injected per urethra and usually shows extravasation (Fig. 62–13). The excretory urogram may show a teardrop vesical deformity with upward displacement of the bladder in patients with complete disruption.

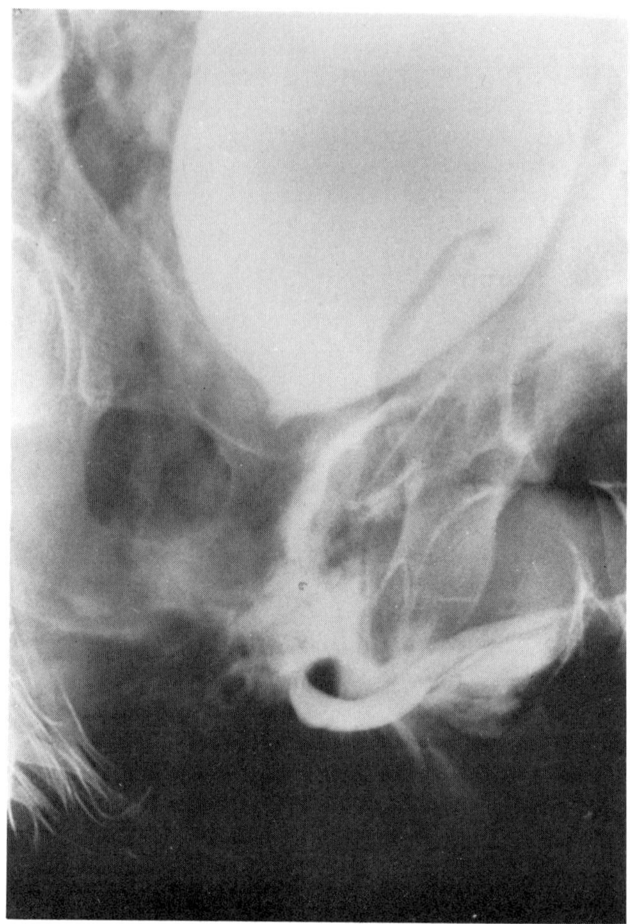

Figure 62–13   Retrograde Urethrogram of Membranous Urethral Injury. *Note:* Extensive extravasation of dye at the membranous urethra is shown in a patient with complete urethral disruption secondary to a pelvic procedure.

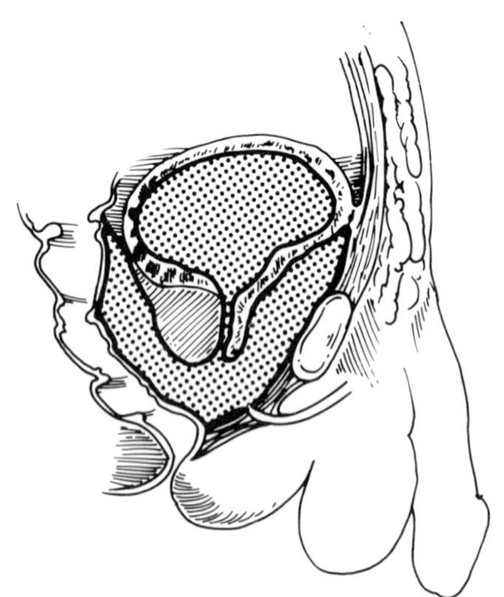

Figure 62–12   Membranous Urethral Disruption. *Note:* Hemorrhage is confined to the pelvis, above the genitourinary diaphragm.

A note of caution is in order regarding urethral catheterization. A forceful catheter insertion may convert a partially lacerated urethra into a completely lacerated one. In these cases, if catheterization is advisable, it should be performed by a urologic surgeon under strict sterile conditions. If a catheter is passed to the bladder, it should be left indwelling and its position confirmed radiographically.

Management

If a urethral catheter of adequate size can be passed to the bladder, it usually indicates a minor partial laceration and should be left indwelling for 10 to 14 days. Frequently, a more serious laceration occurs and surgical intervention is necessary. Some investigators advocate suprapubic cystostomy for urinary diversion initially, with urethral reconstruction, if needed, performed at a later date.[20] Others advocate early urethral realignment with a perineal traction of the prostate.[21]

At the Los Angeles County–USC Medical Center, these injuries have been managed by the initial placement of a suprapubic cystostomy without attempting to enter the pelvic area. Only in the presence of minimal pelvic hematuria has urethral realignment been attempted 7 days after the injury. The most significant complication is urethral stricture, which may require periodic dilatations or surgical correction.

Injuries to the Bulbous Urethra

Most commonly, bulbous urethral injuries result from perineal contusion by falling astride an object. The urethral laceration may be incomplete or complete, with the formation of a perineal hematoma and urinary extravasation. If Buck's fascia is disrupted, the extravasation will be limited only by Colles' fascia with spread to penis, scrotum, and abdominal wall (Fig. 62–14). Injuries to the bulbous urethra may also be caused by instrumentation or penetrating injuries and usually consist of partial tears.

Clinical Manifestations

The history of perineal trauma or instrumentation is usually present. Local pain and urethral bleeding are seen in the majority of patients. Most commonly, the patient is unable to urinate.

Physical examination reveals tenderness in the perineal region. Edema and extravasation may be palpable in the perineal, penile, scrotal, or even the lower abdominal wall. If seen late, signs of inflammation or infection may appear.

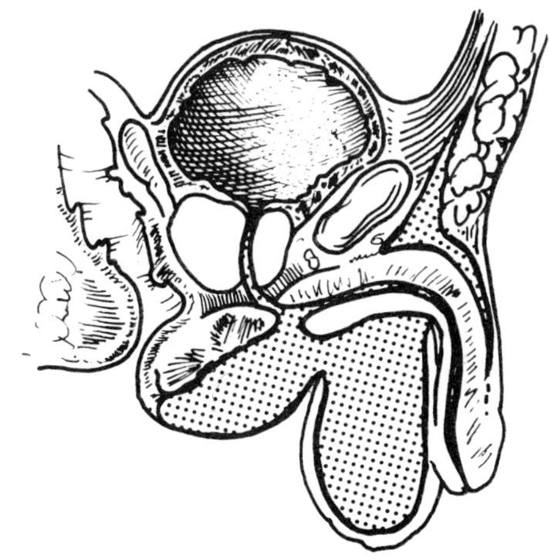

Figure 62–14 Bulbous Urethral Injury. *Note:* Hemorrhage is below genitourinary diaphragm and limited by Colles' fascia.

Diagnosis

As opposed to membranous urethral injuries, in bulbous urethral lacerations, the hemorrhage and urinary extravasation is below the genitourinary diaphragm. The retrograde urethrogram will ascertain the diagnosis with accuracy, showing extravasation at the site of injury (Fig. 62–15).

Management

The initial management of bulbous urethral laceration depends on the extent of the injury. Caution should be used in the passage of a urethral catheter since a partial injury may be converted into a complete tear. If a catheter is passed, this is left indwelling for 10 to 14 days to allow healing of the laceration. In cases of complete laceration, an end-to-end reanastomosis can be performed; however, the placement of a suprapubic cystostomy has been advocated by the majority of clinical investigators with successful results.[16,22] Subsequently, if a stricture develops, urethral reconstruction is planned several months later. If extensive extravasation is present, drainage of the periurethral area is indicated. This latter approach with the initial placement of a suprapubic cystostomy and urethral reconstruction at a later date if a stricture develops is favored.

Urethral stricture is the most serious complication. Antibiotic coverage may prevent a periurethral infection.

Injuries to the Pendulous Urethra

Most commonly, the pendulous urethra is injured by forceful traumatic instrumentation. Usually, this type of injury is sustained while passing a catheter or a sound in the presence of a stricture.

Penetrating wounds to the penile urethra are rare owing to the extreme mobility of the penis. On occasion, foreign bodies inserted into the urethra, usually for the purpose of masturbation, may injure the penile urethra. As a result, periurethral bleeding and urinary extravasation may occur.

Clinical Manifestations

Urethral bleeding is present in the majority of patients. Varying degrees of penile or scrotal swelling may be seen as a result of extravasation, and the patient may present with urinary retention.

Diagnosis

The diagnosis of an injury to the pendulous urethra is confirmed by a retrograde urethrogram.

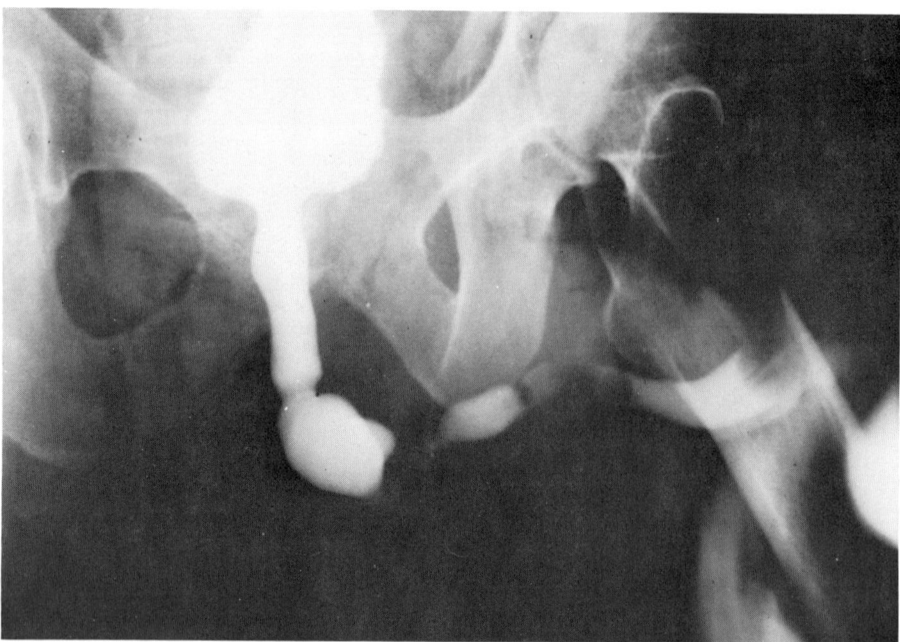

Figure 62–15 Retrograde Urethrogram of Bulbous Urethral Injury. *Note:* Bulbous urethra is completely blocked secondary to a straddle injury.

Management

Minor mucosal lacerations may be managed conservatively without the passage of a urethral catheter if voiding is normal. A partial laceration may be treated with the passage of a urethral catheter. If significant extravasation occurs, it is advisable to drain the periurethral area. In the presence of a complete urethral rupture, immediate surgical repair with end-to-end anastomosis should be attempted. However, if the clinical conditions are critical, a suprapubic cystostomy should be placed, followed by a urethral reconstruction at a later date.

INJURIES TO THE EXTERNAL GENITALIA

Penile Injuries

Penile injuries are unusual due to the anatomical position and mobility of the penis. As a result, the skin, urethra, or the erectile bodies may be injured.

The penis may be injured by blunt trauma, penetrating trauma, or strangulation. Blunt trauma may be sustained when the penis is flaccid and results in varying degrees of contusion. The most significant blunt injury occurs when the penis is erect and rupture of the corpora cavernosum or the urethra occurs.

Penetrating injuries to the penis may be superficial, with involvement of the skin and subcutaneous tissue, or deep, resulting in a laceration of the corpora cavernosum and/or the urethra. Extensive damage may occur when the genitalia is caught by large industrial machines.

Strangulation occurs as a result of ischemia caused by condoms, catheters, strings, or metal bands around the penis.

Clinical Manifestations

When the corpora cavernosum is fractured, a significant hematoma with associated local deformity is usually present. Occasionally, the urethra is lacerated, resulting in urinary extravasation. The skin commonly shows ecchymosis. On rare occasions, priapism may develop as a result of external trauma.

The extent of laceration will depend on the type of injury and the weapon involved. The urethra, corpora, and skin may be compromised. On rare occasions, the penis may be totally amputated, an event that is usually self-inflicted by mentally ill patients (Figs. 62–16 and 62–17).

Ischemia and necrosis are the complications that result from strangulation of the penis. A metal ring or a string, if found, should be removed immediately.

Management

Simple contusions are successfully treated by conservative measures. Rupture of the corpora cavernosum should be surgically repaired to prevent damage of the erectile function or a penile deformity.

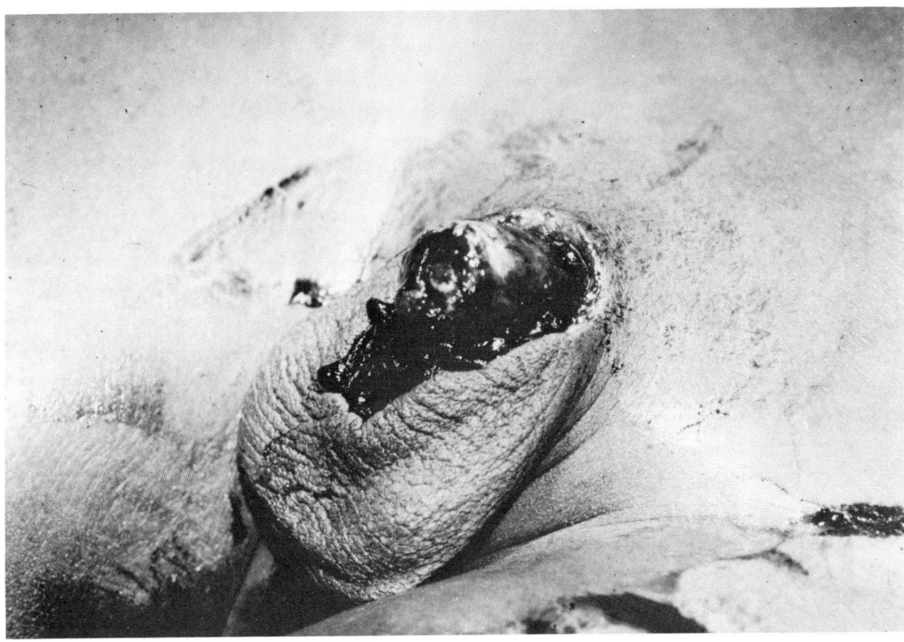

Figure 62–16   Traumatic Amputation of the Penis in a Child.

In penetrating injuries, it is important to assess fully the extent of the injury. Each structure should be repaired individually, achieving complete hemostasis.

Avulsion of the penile skin may be treated with a split-thickness skin graft when the lesion is extensive. Small lacerations are simply closed with absorbable suture material. If the urethra is compromised, repair should be attempted immediately and a catheter left indwelling for 7 to 10 days.[23]

Complete amputation of the penis should be repaired by reanastomosis with the aid of microsurgical techniques. Successful reanastomosis has been achieved even after several hours of penile amputation.

In patients presenting with penile strangulation, the

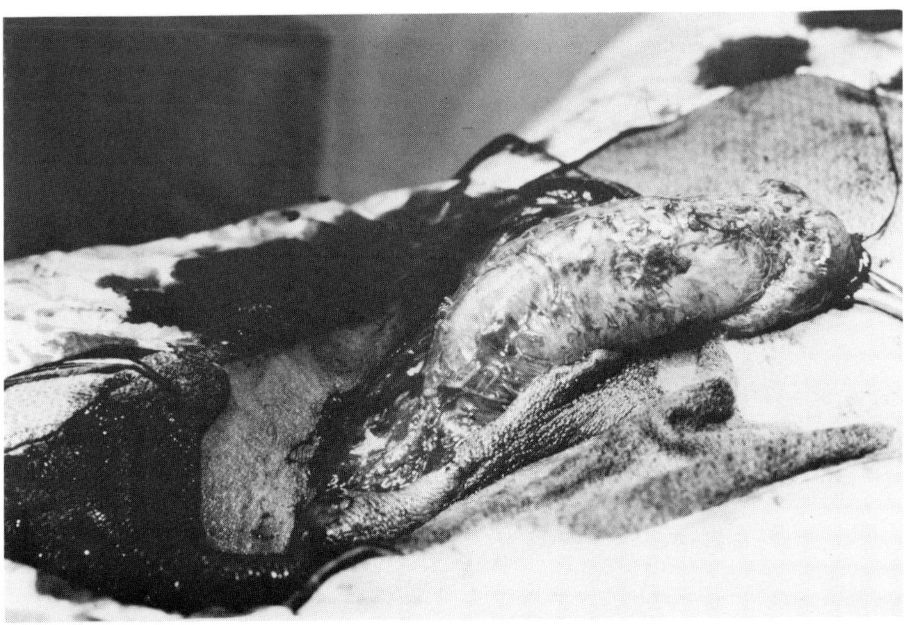

Figure 62–17   Self-Inflicted Lacerations of Penile Skin by a Mentally Ill Patient.

foreign body around the penis should be removed immediately. A metal band is best removed in the operating room with the patient under anesthesia.

Injuries to the Scrotum and Testicle

Injuries to the scrotum or testicle may be caused by penetrating injuries or blunt trauma. These injuries are uncommon, owing to the mobility and the anatomical position of the scrotum.

Clinical Manifestations

In penetrating injuries it is essential to determine the extent and deepness of the scrotal laceration. A scrotal hematoma is usually present, and if the tunica vaginalis is compromised a hematocele is formed. If the tunica albuginea of the testicle is compromised, seminiferous tubules may be seen extruding from the wound. Local pain associated with nausea and vomiting is common.

In blunt injuries severe pain associated with nausea and vomiting is usually present. The physical examination usually reveals swelling, localized pain, and a scrotal hematoma. The local inflammation and the hematoma formation usually depends on the severity of the injury. If the testicle is ruptured, a hematocele occurs (Fig. 62–18). If the clinical manifestations are disproportionate to the severity of the trauma, the physician should keep in mind the differential diagnosis of epididymitis or testicular torsion.

Management

In penetrating injuries, superficial lacerations are treated by simple skin closure. However, if the laceration is deep, with compromise of the dartos fascia and/or the tunica vaginalis, a thorough debridement, repair, and layered closure is necessary. If the testicle is ruptured, after thorough debridement, it should be repaired by closing the tunica albuginea.

In blunt injuries, prompt surgical exploration is necessary in most cases except if only minimal swelling and tenderness are present. Conservative treatment is based on scrotal elevation, ice packs, and rest for a few days. Scrotal exploration, however, prevents the chance of testicular loss and decreases the mobility to the patient. Extensive avulsions of the scrotal skin should be treated by transposition of the testis into a subcutaneous pouch in the thigh.[24]

ACUTE FLANK PAIN

The emergency department physician often sees patients with acute flank pain. In the majority of cases, flank pain is caused by a urinary problem. The pain is

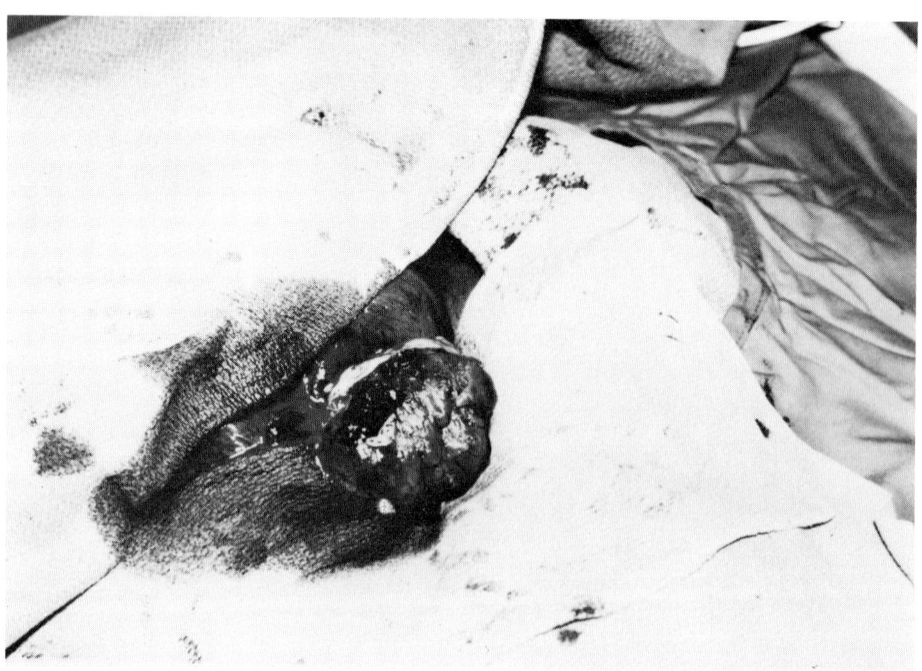

Figure 62–18 Testicular Rupture Secondary to Blunt Trauma. *Note:* Seminiferous tubules are seen protruding through the tunica albuginea of the testicle.

usually caused by renal disease or a ureteral obstruction. Renal pain is caused by sudden distention of the capsule that results from hydronephrosis, inflammation, or edema. Ureteral pain occurs as a result of capsular distention combined with periodic smooth muscle spasms.

Ureteral colic is the most common form of flank pain and results from a sudden ureteral obstruction with subsequent hyperperistalsis and smooth muscle spasms.[25] This form of colic is usually due to obstruction caused by a calculus. Ureteral colic may also be caused by hematuria with clots or papillary necrosis. Acute renal pain is caused by acute pyelonephritis, renal rupture, acute hydronephrosis, or an acute vascular disorder.

Clinical Manifestations and Differential Diagnosis

In ureteral colic the pain is usually severe and starts in the flank area, radiating to the lower abdominal quadrant following the course of the ureter. The pain is colicky with periods of relief. Nausea and vomiting may be present. On occasion, the physician may be able to ascertain the location of the obstruction by the characteristics of the pain. If the obstruction occurs in the upper ureter, the pain may radiate to the testicle in men or labia in women since the sensory nerve supply of the upper ureter follows a similar pathway (T11–12). If a stone is close to the bladder, vesical irritability may occur as a result of inflammation at the ureteral orifice.

Physical examination usually reveals pain localized to the costovertebral angle of the side involved. When calculi are present, the urinalysis may show microscopic hematuria and/or crystalluria. When infection occurs, pyuria is usually present. Gross hematuria is present when the etiology is the passage of clots. A flank mass may be palpable in patients with hydronephrosis or tumors. Papillary necrosis is caused by ischemic necrosis of the renal papilla. This disease may be caused by prolonged ingestion of analgesics, diabetes, sickle cell trait, or severe infections.

Patients with acute renal pain usually have constant and less sharp pain than the patient with typical ureteral colic. This pain often radiates along the subcostal area toward the umbilicus and occasionally to the lower abdomen. Sometimes it resembles ureteral colic, making the clinical diagnosis difficult.

Acute pyelonephritis is characterized by sudden flank pain associated with chills and fever. A history of urinary tract infection or ureterovesical reflux may be present. Infundibular obstruction may mimic ureteral colic inasmuch as a similar mechanism occurs with hyperperistalsis and muscle spasms. Intermittent hydronephrosis is usually the result of a congenital malformation

causing obstruction at the level of the ureteral pelvic junction; it is usually caused by rapid diuresis. A perinephric abscess frequently originates from a preexisting renal infection; the history of calculi or obstruction is usually present. On rare occasions a perinephric abscess occurs as a result of hematogenous spread. Spontaneous renal rupture occurs in the presence of preexisting renal disease and usually is noted in association with hydronephrosis or renal cysts; a history of minor trauma is obtained frequently. Acute renal artery occlusion occurs usually in patients with a history of rheumatic heart disease, atrial fibrillation, or myocardial infarction or after cardiac catheterization. It results from embolic occlusion of the main artery or its branches. Acute renal vein thrombosis is a rare clinical entity that is seen in infants or adults. The most important causes are amyloidosis, perirenal disease, thrombophlebitis, and trauma.

Diagnosis

In the presence of obstruction an excretory urogram will show delayed excretion with a prominent nephrogram effect. A calcified calculus may be seen along the ureteral area; however, when the calculus is radiolucent, the diagnosis will mainly depend on the excretory or retrograde urogram (Fig. 62–19). If the kidney is nonfunctioning, a vascular lesion should be suspected; in these cases a retrograde urogram will show normal upper tracts. A vascular lesion can be confirmed by angiography or venography.

Retrograde urethrography is useful to better define the renal architecture, particularly when the excretory urogram is nondiagnostic.

Management

Potent analgesics are usually needed to treat ureteral colic. Because of the magnitude of pain, meperidine (Demerol) or morphine sulfate are the preferred drugs. Proper hydration is important, particularly in patients with calculous disease.

Specific measures depend on the cause of the acute flank pain. A superimposed infection in the presence of obstruction is a particularly alarming situation that necessitates prompt treatment with broad-spectrum antibiotics and urinary drainage.

ACUTE INTRASCROTAL PAIN

Pain within the scrotum is seen frequently in medical practice. Inasmuch as a correct diagnosis will determine the best treatment to follow, the different causes for scrotal pain should be in the mind of the physician who initially evaluates the patient. The most common causes

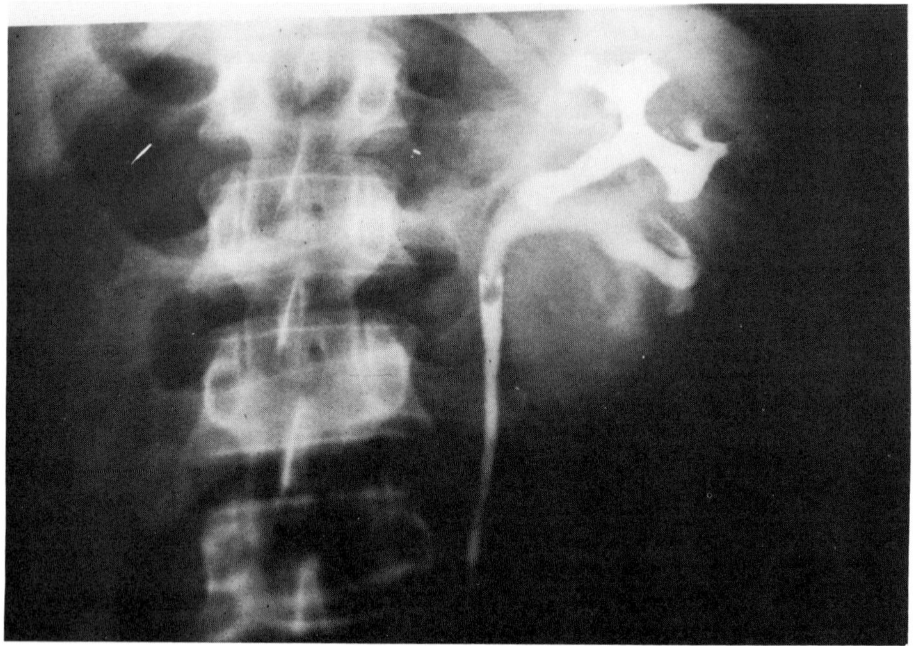

Figure 62–19 Retrograde Urogram Shows Radiolucent Calculus in Proximal Ureter.

for scrotal pain include acute epididymitis, testicular torsion, acute orchitis, trauma, incarcerated hernia, and torsion of testicular appendages.

Acute Epididymitis

Acute epididymitis implies an acute inflammatory process located within the epididymis. It is rarely seen in childhood and the majority of cases occur in the young adult. Organisms invade the epididymis mainly through the vas deferens and only rarely through a hematogenous or lymphatic route.[26]

Clinical Manifestations

The history of severe physical strain or urethral manipulation may be obtained. Pain is usually severe and develops rapidly. Fever is usually present. On physical examination the scrotum is enlarged and the skin is hyperemic. The epididymis is very tender and indurated. The epididymal induration may be localized in the tail, or it may involve the entire epididymis or even the testicle (orchioepididymitis). The urine may be infected or there may be evidence of urethral discharge.

Specific Epididymitis. Although several types of specific bacteria and fungus may invade the epididymis and cause various diseases (meningococcosis, blastomycosis, brucellosis, syphilis), two disorders deserve special comment: tuberculosis and gonorrhea.

Tuberculous epididymitis usually follows a prostatic or seminovesicle lesion. The epididymis may contain multiple nodules and "cold abscesses." The vas deferens may appear indurated and beaded. Usually, tuberculous epididymitis follows a subacute or chronic course and an epididymocutaneous fistula may occur.

Gonorrheal epididymitis was a common complication of gonococcal urethritis in the past. It is rarely seen now because of the availability of antibiotics. The epididymis usually appears extremely tender and inflamed. Chills and fever as well as prostration may be present. Symptoms of acute urethritis are usually noted, and there may be a history of urethral discharge.

Nonspecific Epididymitis. Nonspecific epididymitis is usually a purulent type of inflammation caused by common pyogenic bacteria. It often is associated with urinary tract infection, but occasionally the route of contamination is hematogenous. These infections are more apt to suppurate and an abscess may form. A history of trauma may be obtained; however, it is not clear whether this event precipitates epididymal infection.

Differential Diagnosis

On occasion there may be difficulties in differentiating acute epididymitis from torsion of the testicle, testicular tumors, torsion of the testicular appendages, trauma, and mumps orchitis.

Management

Important local measures that provide comfort to the patient include elevation of the scrotum, bed rest, ice packs, analgesics, and anti-inflammatory agents. The antibiotic of choice will depend on the etiology. The bacteria may be isolated by culturing the urine or urethral secretions when present. In nonspecific epididymitis a broad-spectrum antibiotic is recommended for 10 days.

Excellent prognosis is expected after appropriate therapy. Occasionally, an epididymal blockage develops, a situation that may lead to infertility when there is bilateral involvement.

Acute Orchitis

Many infectious diseases may involve the testicle through a hematogenous route. The most common form of orchitis is caused by mumps and occurs only after puberty. It usually involves one testicle, but bilateral involvement can be seen.

Clinical Manifestations

Usually, there is a sudden onset of pain and swelling of the testis. The scrotum becomes edematous and hyperemic. Associated fever is seen in most patients and prostration is marked. Usually, there is clinical evidence of an infectious disease. The testis is usually enlarged and severely tender. The epididymis in most cases cannot be separated from the testis itself, and an acute hydrocele may develop.

Differential Diagnosis

On occasion, it is difficult to differentiate this clinical entity from acute epididymitis or even testicular torsion. The findings of leukocytosis, normal urinalysis, and the clinical evidence of an infectious disease may help in defining the diagnosis.

Management

Bed rest is necessary. The use of scrotal elevation is helpful to relieve the edema and pain. Antibiotics are only indicated when the etiologic agent is a bacterium. Atrophic changes occur in one-third to one-fourth of the patients and may jeopardize fertility when there is bilateral involvement.[27]

Testicular Torsion

Testicular torsion is a condition in which the testicular circulation is compromised as a result of twisting of the spermatic cord. Two forms may be defined: intravaginal torsion and extravaginal torsion.

Intravaginal Torsion

Intravaginal torsion is the most common intrascrotal disorder in children[28] and results as a consequence of an anomalous suspension of the testicle caused by an overdevelopment of the tunica vaginalis. This type of torsion may occur at any age but is found more often around puberty (Fig. 62–20).

Intrascrotal pain usually is the initial presenting complaint. The pain may develop suddenly; however, on occasion it may be insidious. It may occur during activity or develop during sleep. Testicular torsion may resolve spontaneously and recur later. A past history of a similar episode may be obtained in a significant number of cases.

Physical examination reveals shortening of the spermatic cord, and the testicle often lies higher in the scrotum. The epididymis may be located anteriorly with normal characteristics. Later, both testes and epididymis become involved. The presence of nausea and vomiting together with radiation of the pain into the lower abdomen may be noted.

Testicular torsion may mimic acute epididymitis, torsion of testicular appendages, acute orchitis, incarcerated hernia, or acute hydrocele. Epididymitis occurs in an older age-group and is usually accompanied by fever. There may be a history of urinary tract infection. Torsion of the appendix testicle may be impossible to differentiate from testicular torsion. However, occasionally, a tender nodule may be felt at the upper pole of the testicle. Mumps orchitis is usually associated with parotitis. In patients with incarcerated hernia the cord appears thickened and a wide inguinal ring may be felt.

Although occasionally a testicle could be saved after ischemia for as long as 18 hours,[29] most of the surviving testicles had been operated on within 7 hours. The tes-

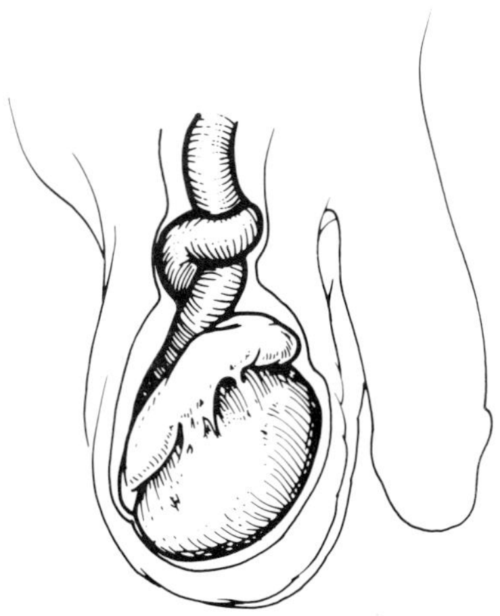

Figure 62–20 Intravaginal Form of Testicular Torsion.

ticle is approached through the scrotum and is untwisted. Warm saline is useful to restore circulation. If the testicle remains ischemic after a period of observation, an orchiectomy should be performed. In all cases an orchiopexy of the contralateral testicle should be performed.

Extravaginal Torsion

Extravaginal torsion is a rare condition that accounts for less than 6 percent of all testicular torsions.[30] It is seen usually in newborns and, in most instances, the event occurs in utero.

This form of torsion presents as a smooth, firm painless mass that produces thickness and discoloration of the scrotal wall. Usually, diagnosis is simple since testicular tumors are virtually nonexistent in the neonatal period. In most instances at operation the testicle is found to be necrotic, with the torsion at the level of the external inguinal ring. Infarction of the testicle is the rule.

Scrotal exploration with the aim of removing the infarcted testicle is indicated in most cases. Exploration of the opposite side does not appear to be necessary.

ACUTE URINARY RETENTION

Acute urinary retention is the sudden inability to urinate. Except in some cases of neurogenic bladder, it is usually associated with severe lower abdominal discomfort and urgency. This clinical entity is seen frequently in an emergency department environment.

The cause that precipitates urinary retention may be at the level of the urethra or the bladder itself. It may be of acquired or congenital nature. Urethral causes include prostatic obstruction, stricture, urethral valves, trauma, foreign bodies, and extraurethral obstruction. Bladder causes include calculi, tumors, neurogenic dysfunction, ureteroceles, blood clots, and bladder neck contraction.

Pathogenesis

The vast majority of cases presenting as acute urinary retention are due to obstruction at the level of the bladder outlet or the urethra. At times, however, urinary retention is the result of a neurogenic impairment or detrusor imbalance.

In the presence of obstruction, in order to overcome the urethral resistance, the vesical musculature hypertrophies. Soon the bladder will appear grossly trabeculated and the mucosa protrudes through the muscular bundles, forming diverticuli. During this event, two stages may be clearly identified: (1) the stage of compensation, when the bladder is able to empty, and (2) the stage of decompensation that results in increasing amounts of residual urine culminating in urinary retention.[31]

Clinical Manifestations

A thorough clinical history should be obtained in an effort to identify the underlying etiology. In patients with prostatic enlargement, a history of prostatism may be present. A history of urethritis suggests a possible urethral stricture. A neurologic disorder may be present in a patient with a neurogenic bladder.

The patient is usually in acute distress, except in some cases of neurogenic bladder with sensorial impairment. The pain is located in the lower abdomen and often is associated with severe urgency.

On physical examination the bladder is palpated and percussed above the pubis and close to the umbilical

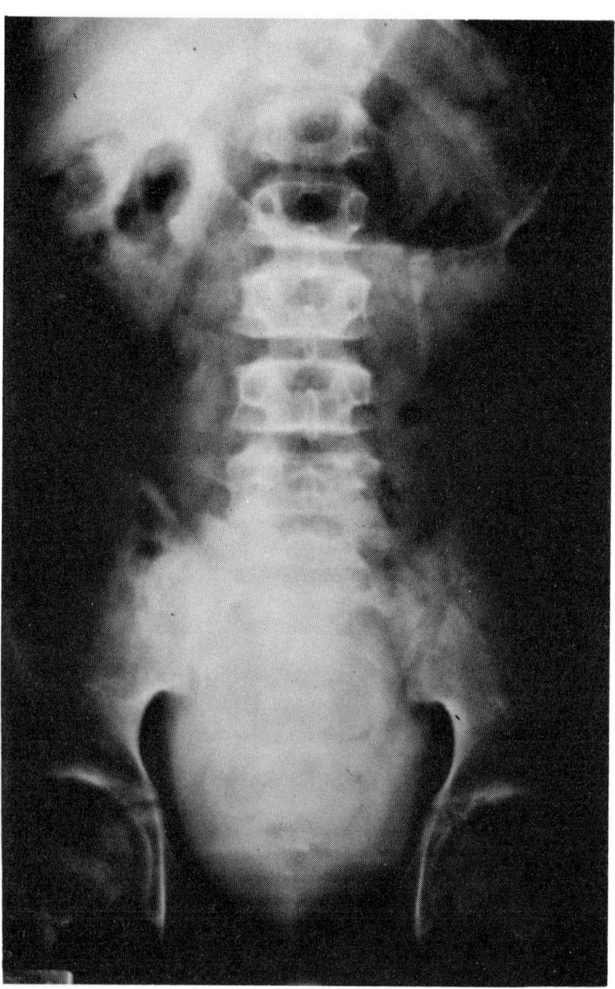

Figure 62–21 Intravenous Urogram of Child with Neurogenic Bladder. *Note:* The upper urinary tracts reveal mild ureterectasis and caliectasis.

line. Palpation of the urethra may reveal an induration suggestive of a stricture or a calculus. A careful neurologic examination should be performed to rule out a neurogenic component. Rectal examination may reveal an abnormal anal sphincter tonus suggestive of a neurogenic etiology. At the same time, rectal examination may reveal the presence of a pelvic mass or prostatic enlargement.

Laboratory Findings

Gross hematuria with formation of clots may result in urinary retention. The bleeding may occur at a renal, vesical, or prostatic level. A plain abdominal roentgenogram will reveal an enlarged bladder, and spinal deformities (spina bifida) are strongly suggestive of a neurogenic component.

The intravenous urogram is usually diagnostic, revealing a distended bladder and the anatomical conditions of the upper tracts (Fig. 62–21). A retrograde urethrogram is useful when a urethral obstruction is suspected. Finally, instrumental examination with the passage of a catheter is in most cases diagnostic. Cystourethroscopy will accurately assess the anatomy of the lower urinary tract.

Management

The establishment of bladder drainage is the immediate goal. The insertion of a catheter under sterile conditions is usually diagnostic and therapeutic. A small 16F catheter is usually of adequate size except in cases due to clot retention in which a large caliber catheter is preferred with the purpose of thoroughly irrigating the bladder. Catheterization is more difficult to perform in male patients owing to anatomical factors. In the presence of a urethral stricture, care should be taken not to injure the urethral mucosa or cause a false passage that may make further attempts to pass a catheter impossible. An adequate diagnosis is necessary and in the presence of a urethral stricture, the passage of filiforms and followers is a relatively simple measure that will adequately establish bladder drainage (Fig. 62–22). If drainage cannot be obtained through urethral catheterization, a cystostomy tube (trocar) should be inserted under local anesthesia (Fig. 62–23).[32]

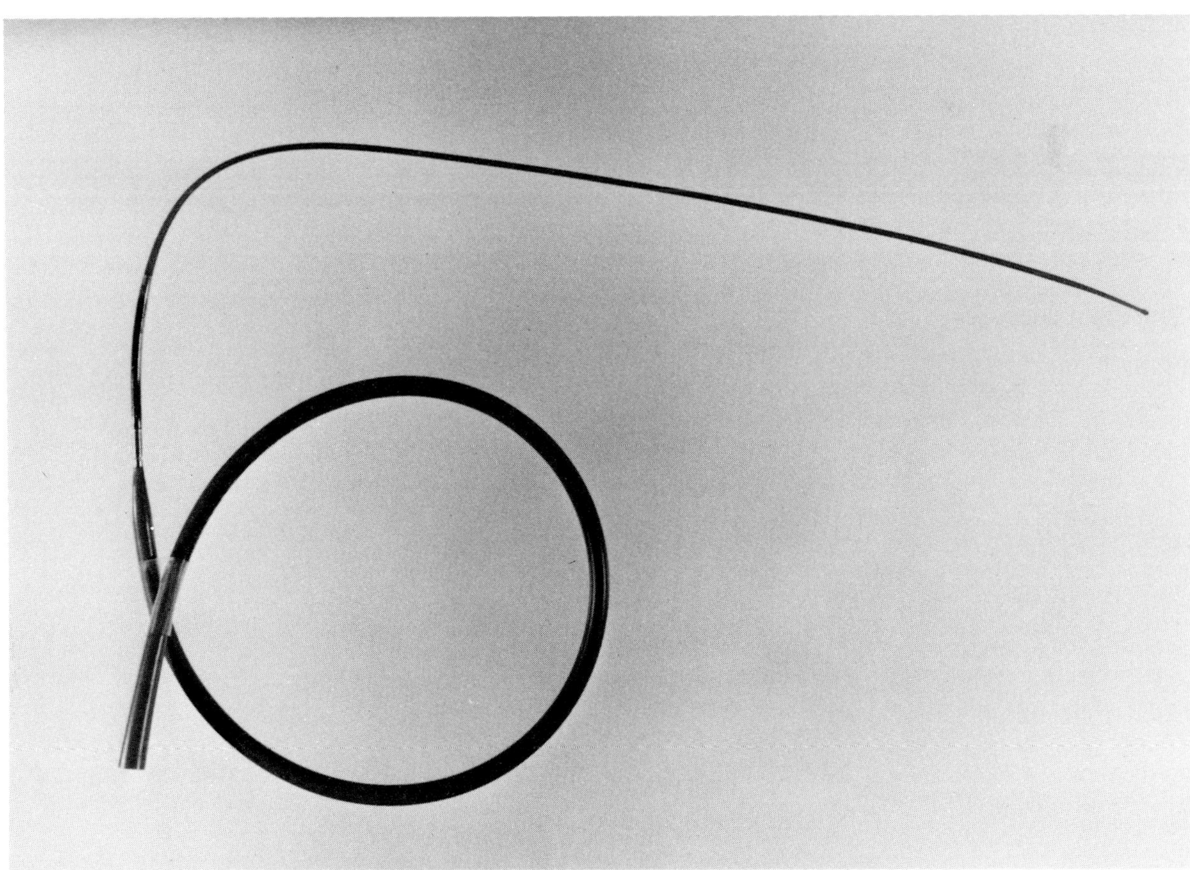

Figure 62–22 Filliform and Follower.

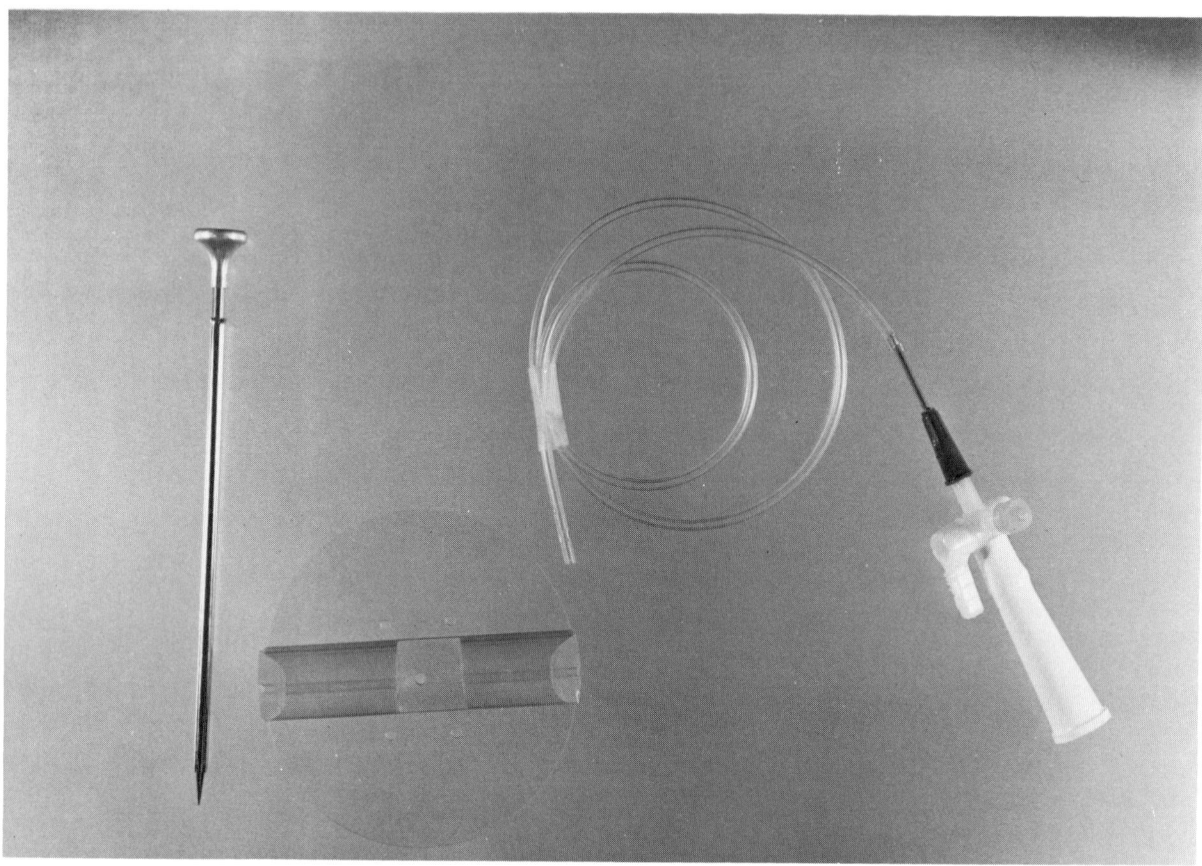

Figure 62–23 Suprapubic Cystostomy Tube.

If left untreated, urinary retention will lead to urinary tract infection that may spread throughout the entire urinary system. Bilateral hydronephrosis occurs as a consequence of chronic urinary retention and may result in renal insufficiency.

REFERENCES

1. Peters PC, Bright TC: Blunt renal injuries. *Urol Clin North Am* 4:17, 1977.
2. Glenn JF, Harvard BM: The injured kidney. *JAMA* 173:93, 1960.
3. Elkin M, Chien-Hsing M, de Paredes RG: Roentgenologic evaluation of renal trauma with emphasis on renal angiography. *Am J Roentgenol* 98:1, 1966.
4. Carlton CE, Scott R, Goldman M: The management of penetrating injuries of the kidney. *J Trauma* 8:1071, 1968.
5. Carlton CE: Injuries of the kidney and ureter, in Campbell MF, Harrison JH (eds): *Urology*, ed 4. Philadelphia, WB Saunders Co, 1978, p 881.
6. Stutzman RE: Ballistic and the management of ureteral injuries from high velocity missile. *J Urol* 118:947, 1977.
7. Tynberg PLH, Koch WH, Persky LP, Zellinger RH: The management of renal injuries coincident with penetrating wounds of the abdomen. *J Trauma* 13:502, 1973.
8. Peterson WE, Kirakole LU: Renal trauma: When to operate. *Urology* 3:537, 1974.
9. Holden S, Hicks CC, O'Brien DP, Harlan HS, Walker JA, Walton KN: Gunshot wounds of the ureter: A 15-year review of 63 consecutive cases. *J Urol* 116:562, 1976.
10. Newel QU: Injuries to the ureters during pelvic operations. *Ann Surg* 109:981, 1939.
11. Bright TC, Peters PC: Ureteral injuries secondary to operative procedure: Report of 24 cases. *Urology* 9:22, 1977.
12. St. Martin EC: Ureteral injury in gynecologic surgery. *J Urol* 70:51, 1953.
13. Persky L, Hoch WH, Kursch ED: Surgical management of the ureter, in Campbell MF, Harrison JH (eds): *Urology*, ed 4. Philadelphia, WB Saunders Co, 1978, p 188.
14. Thompson IM: Bladder flap repair of ureteral injuries. *Urol Clin North Am* 4:51, 1977.
15. Vargas AD, Silva E: Mobilization of the ureter by a posterior vesical flap in dogs: Preliminary report of a new technique. *Urology* 107:742, 1972.
16. Bright TC III, Peters PC: Injuries to the bladder and urethra, in Campbell MF, Harrison JH (eds): *Urology*, ed 4. Philadelphia, WB Saunders Co, 1978, p 906.
17. Montie J: Bladder injuries. *Urol Clin North Am* 4:59, 1977.
18. Richardson JR, Jr, Leadbetter GS, Jr: Nonoperative treatment of ruptured bladder. *J Urol* 114:213, 1975.
19. Mulkey AP, Witherington R: Conservative management of vesical rupture. *Urology* 4:426, 1974.

20. Morehouse DD, McKinnon JK: Posterior urethral injury: Etiology, diagnosis, initial management. *Urol Clin North Am* 4:69, 1977.
21. Turner-Warwick R: A personal view of the immediate management of pelvic fracture urethral injuries. *Urol Clin North Am* 4:81, 1977.
22. Roberts M: Injuries to the lower urinary tract, in Blandy J (ed): *Urology*. London, Blackwell Scientific, 1976, p 954.
23. Culp DA: Genital injuries: Etiology and initial management. *Urol Clin North Am* 4:143, 1977.
24. Bright TC, Peters PC: Injuries of the external genitalia, in Campbell MF, Harrison JH (eds): *Urology*, ed 4. Philadelphia, WB Saunders Co, 1978, p 931.
25. Smith DR: Symptoms of disorder of the genitourinary tract, in Smith DR (ed): *General Urology*, ed 9. Los Altos, Calif, Lange Medical Publications, 1975, p 25.
26. Nickel WR: Other infections and inflammations of the external genitalia, in Campbell MF, Harrison JH (eds): *Urology*, ed 4. Philadelphia, WB Saunders Co, 1978, p 640.
27. Whitaker RH: Benign disorders of the testicle, in Blandy J (ed): *Urology*. London, Blackwell Scientific, 1976, p 1182.
28. Allen TD: Disorders of the male external genitalia, in Kelalis PP, King LR (eds): *Clinical Pediatric Urology*. Philadelphia, WB Saunders Co, 1976, p 636.
29. Parker RM, Robison JR: Anatomy and diagnosis of torsion of the testicle. *J Urol* 106:243, 1971.
30. James T: Torsion of the spermatic cord in the first year of life. *Br J Urol* 25:56, 1953.
31. Smith DR: Urinary obstruction and stasis, in Smith DR (ed): *General Urology*, ed 8. Los Altos, Calif, Lange Medical Publications, 1975, p 112.
32. Leadbetter GW: Diagnostic urologic instrumentation, in Campbell MF, Harrison JH (eds): *Urology*, ed 4. Philadelphia, WB Saunders Co, 1978, p 358.

63. Renal Failure

JOHN A. MITAS II, M.D., F.A.C.P.

The presentation of renal failure may be as varied as the patients who enter the emergency department or who seek care for a seemingly unrelated symptom. For example, renal failure may be diagnosed in the 58-year-old diabetic who recently underwent a diagnostic radiographic procedure; the young expectant mother who arrives with altered mentation, edema, and hypertension; the child with a recent onset of dark urine; the victim of a hit-and-run driver; or the 75th person presenting with weakness after severe vomiting during a viral epidemic or during the hottest week on record. Because of the multiple functions of the kidney (Table 63–1) renal dysfunction must be considered in each of these patients because of different signs or symptoms. Renal failure no longer equates with oliguria[1] but must now be defined as a decrease in renal function, specifically glomerular filtration rate (GFR), with or without oliguria. Current series report that 30 to 60 percent of patients are nonoliguric.[2] The hallmarks of renal failure are azotemia and the biochemical consequences of decreased GFR, which may include abnormal volume regulation; hyperkalemia, hyperphosphatemia, and hypocalcemia; occasional hyponatremia; metabolic acidosis when the GFR is below 15 ml/minute; and abnormal handling of drugs and metabolites (physiologic and pharmacologic). Although renal failure is not always a true emergency when discovered, it does demand urgent evaluation because it is potentially reversible, many etiologies *are* treatable, and it is associated with a high mortality.

TABLE 63–1   Functions of the Kidney

Systems Regulated	Examples
Volume regulation	Diuresis or antidiuresis
Acid-base control	H^+ excretion, HCO_3^- reclamation and regeneration
Electrolyte conservation or excretion	Na^+, K^+, Cl^-, Ca^{++}, Mg^{++}, PO_4
Blood pressure regulation	Na^+, volume control; renin-angiotensin-aldosterone; vasodilator systems (prostaglandins, kallikrein-bradykinin)
Excretion of metabolites and waste products	Physiologic and pharmacologic substances
Maintenance of hematocrit	Erythropoietin production or formation
Metabolic	Insulin metabolism, amino acid conservation

This chapter will present a workable approach to renal failure, its identification, etiology, and management. Management of the functional abnormalities will be considered individually.

ETIOLOGY

Although the recognized causes of renal failure are numerous,[2] they may conveniently be consolidated in the time-honored classification of prerenal, parenchymal, and postrenal causes. Such a classification under-scores the concept that many causes are potentially reversible and many are treatable.

The suspicion of renal failure is confirmed by the findings of elevated blood urea nitrogen (BUN) and serum creatinine. The normal values for BUN are 10 to 20 mg/dl and for creatinine up to 1.5 mg/dl (depending on the individual's size and muscle mass). Because a number of factors may influence the concentration of BUN (e.g., diet, medications, gastrointestinal hemorrhage, hydration), it is best to consider the creatinine value. Values of 1.6 to 3 or 3.5 mg/dl may be considered representative of "renal insufficiency" (unless there is continued elevation), while values exceeding 3 to 3.5 mg/dl indicate "renal failure." Any of the three classes may cause a markedly elevated serum creatinine, although values of greater than 6 mg/dl are less commonly found in prerenal states and should lead to the consideration of other causes.

Prerenal causes have the common feature of decreased effective arterial volume—whether true or merely perceived. Although there has been a report of "non-oliguric prerenal failure,"[3] the majority of these patients will manifest oliguria because of an intact renal concentrating mechanism. Oliguria is defined by most nephrologists as a volume insufficient to excrete a maximally concentrated urine (of approximately 1,200 mOsm), which contains the waste products, obligate electrolytes, and osmoles that must be excreted daily. Such a volume would be at least 400 ml/day. The entities are multiple but may be roughly divided into cardiovascular, vascular, and hypovolemic states. The former include myocardial infarction, congestive heart failure, and arrhythmias—all of which lower the cardiac output (or cardiac index)—and mechanical factors such as cardiac tamponade, which reduces filling and cardiac output. Vascular factors such as arterial or venous obstruction may be perceived as low volume states, as may vascular pooling, which is associated with decreased vascular resistance in states of sepsis or the extreme of acidosis. True hypovolemic causes may be due to renal losses, extrarenal losses, or sequestration. Renal-mediated volume losses may be the result of prior diuretic use or excess, osmotic diuresis associated with uncontrolled diabetes mellitus, or diabetes insipidus. Extrarenal volume losses may occur via the skin (e.g., burns or excessive sweating, gastrointestinal tract (e.g., nausea, vomiting, diarrhea, hemorrhage), or hemorrhage. Sequestration without true loss occurs in burns, ascites, peritonitis, and occasionally with marked peripheral edema. The importance of these situations is that many are treatable and *if* successfully treated may prevent ischemic renal parenchymal damage from occurring. The major problem in identifying these pre-

renal states from established parenchymal damage will be discussed in a later section.

The parenchymal causes of renal failure may be subdivided according to the sites of involvement. These sites are vascular, glomerular, and tubular or tubulo-intestinal. Only the last of these represents true acute tubular necrosis (ATN), although the term is frequently used (inappropriately) for all forms of parenchymal renal failure. Vasculitis encompasses disorders such as systemic lupus erythematosus, Henoch-Schönlein purpura, large vessel polyarteritis, and small vessel polyarteritis (hypersensitivity angiitis). Scleroderma, Wegener's granulomatosis, and malignant hypertension may present as renal failure owing to their vascular involvement. The glomerulonephritides may be immunologically mediated in bacterial endocarditis,[4] gram-negative abscess,[5] occasional poststreptococcal glomerulonephritis, or rapidly progressive glomerulonephritis (RPGN). RPGN is a clinical syndrome of rapidly decreasing renal function with or without significant proteinuria but accompanied by hematuria and hypertension. Occasionally this is representative of Goodpasture's syndrome, in association with antiglomerular basement membrane antibodies in the serum. The tubular disorders occur as a result of hypercalcemia; hyperuricemia; tubular precipitation of myeloma protein (light chains), uric acid, and sulfonamides; oxalate nephropathy (ethylene glycol ingestion, methoxyflurane, Crohn's disease); and ATN due to ischemia or toxins such as drugs and diagnostic agents. Pregnancy-related renal failure may occur in toxemia or the postpartum state after a normal pregnancy.[6,7] The pathogenesis of pregnancy-related renal failure seems to be a combination of vascular, coagulation, and possible toxin-induced changes to tubules that do not fit neatly into a single category. The hepatorenal syndrome does not fit into any of these categories but consists of a *functional* derangement of unknown etiology without histologic changes.[8,9] (These kidneys could be transplanted and function normally.)

True ATN includes the ischemic damage resulting from untreated or inappropriately treated prerenal states and direct nephrotoxic damage. Ischemic injury is still the most common etiology of renal failure (and ATN) in adults.[1,2] In contrast, the pediatric patient is much more likely to have glomerulonephritis or the hemolytic-uremic syndrome.[2]

Nephrotoxins are classically considered to be the aminoglycosides, but numerous antibiotics have been recognized to cause ATN, including sulfonamides, cephaloridine, colistin, polymixin, neomycin, vancomycin, and amphotericin B.[10] These agents do not require prior sensitization, and injury is not strictly dose dependent. In some instances immunologic mechanisms are involved with the use of drugs. The best delineated association has been methicillin where there is evidence of antibodies directed against dimethoxypenicilloyl moiety, but other penicillin derivatives have been implicated.[11] Many diagnostic and therapeutic agents other than antibiotics have been identified,[12-14] but are too numerous to list.

Endogenous nephrotoxins may be found in compounds such as myoglobin and hemoglobin, but the "precipitation" of this disorder is not solely nephrotoxic because some other factors such as dehydration and acidosis may be necessary along with tubular obstruction and tubular cell anoxia.[15] Mismatched blood, transfusion reactions, and hemolysis from other causes should be considered. Myoglobinuria commonly follows trauma but perhaps is even more frequent following severe exercise (such as in joggers or unconditioned individuals), heat stroke, prolonged seizures, prolonged coma, and viral myositis.[15,16] The last of these should be considered in older individuals especially.[17,18]

Rhabdomyolysis with myoglobinuria should also be considered in patients with drug abuse—especially those using amphetamines and PCP (phencyclidine).[19,20] One report even indicates that total parenteral nutrition leading to hypokalemia can induce rhabdomyolysis and severe renal failure.[21]

Contrast materials for radiographic studies deserve special mention. These iodinated agents are commonly in use for a variety of procedures. The agents most frequently involved in nephrotoxicity are employed for excretory urography and angiography, intravenous cholangiography, oral cholecystography, and computed tomography with contrast.[22,23] The agents implicated are sodium diatrizoate, meglumine diatrizoate, meglumine iodipamide, iopanoic acid, and sodium ipodate. Special risk factors for developing dye-induced ATN include increased age, underlying renal disease, insulin-dependent diabetes (especially with onset before age 30 and/or creatinine exceeding 4 mg/dl), dehydration, proteinuria, liver disease, hyperuricemia, and radiographic study with contrast in the preceding 3 days. It is not definitely preventable by drip infusion techniques or by prior rehydration.[24]

Obstructive phenomena occur as a result of intrinsic or extrinsic obstruction. In order to cause azotemia the obstruction need not be complete but must be at the bladder outlet or bilateral to involve both ureters. If both ureters or collecting systems are not involved, the unobstructed kidney is capable of compensating for the unilateral loss of function. This is an important fact to remember when the diagnostic evaluation is undertaken.

PATHOLOGY

The pathologic features of renal failure vary according to the etiology. In prerenal conditions the renal blood vessels, glomeruli, and tubules are normal. Also, in occasional instances of well-defined clinical ATN, the histology may be totally normal. This emphasizes the point that in ATN there is poor correlation between histologic findings and functional impairment.[25] Focal and minimal tubular damage may be present in patients with severe functional changes. (Conversely, patients without renal failure may have autopsy findings similar to those in patients with ATN.)

The most common histologic findings in ATN depend on whether the damage is ischemic or toxin induced. In the former, tubular necrosis is patchy, with only short segments being affected. The pars recta of the proximal tubule seems to be most vulnerable. The basement membrane may be disrupted at sites of necrosis, and cell rupture may be present. In toxic damage, confluent areas of necrosis are noted in the convoluted and straight portions of the proximal tubule. However, the basement membranes remain intact. Necrotic lesions occur in all nephrons after toxic insult, whereas ischemic injury is patchy. Tubular casts are present in either type and form in the distal tubule. Casts consist of Tamm-Horsfall protein secreted by the thick portion of the ascending limb of the loop of Henle. In this matrix, cellular debris is deposited, forming the characteristic pigmented casts that are finely or coarsely granular and that must be distinguished from red blood cell casts. This can be done by focusing up and down through the cast while viewing through the high-power objective. Granular casts will appear as such, while red blood cell casts are identifiable by the presence of red blood cells at all depths of the matrix, distinguishing them from casts with red blood cells adherent to the exterior. For the histology associated with the various forms of glomerulonephritis or vasculitis, the interested reader is referred elsewhere to more detailed texts.

In obstructive disorders, hydroureter and hydronephrosis ensue. Depending on the duration and completeness, the dilation of the ureter and renal pelvis may be mild to severe. Because glomerular filtration and urine production continue, the dilation is progressive. Patients with the more severe cases may develop dilated collecting ducts, collecting tubules, and even Bowman's spaces with glomerular compression. When the disorder is prolonged there may be significant loss of renal parenchyma.

PATHOGENESIS AND CLINICAL FEATURES

The prerenal states will result in reduced renal perfusion. This may be due to either real or perceived reductions in circulating volume. As renal blood flow (RBF) and renal plasma flow (RPF) decrease, the GFR falls from a normal of 180 liters/day to much lower levels. The duration as well as degree of reduced perfusion may vary considerably between patients without parenchymal damage. During this reduced perfusion the BUN and creatinine concentrations rise. In conditions with diminished total body water, part of this rise is due to hemoconcentration (and can be substantiated by a rise in hematocrit, total protein, and albumen concentrations). Accompanying decreased effective arterial volume there may be reduced clearance of urea, creatinine, and metabolic wastes, leading to retention. As mentioned earlier, the rise in serum creatinine is to values of 6 mg/dl or less in most instances, although there are individual case reports of values of 9 to 10 mg/dl. In states in which the blood pressure is reduced several factors may play a role, including decreased RPF, reduced perfusion pressure, and reduced filtration. If appropriately treated with volume expansion, increased cardiac filling pressure, or relief of mechanical factors, the BUN and creatinine will return to normal or baseline values.

In glomerulonephritis or vasculitis, inflammation of the capillaries and/or preglomerular vessels alter the hemodynamics, as well as potentially alter the glomerular surface area and filtration.[26]

In one review of the literature of acute renal failure the results of eight large series (2,500 cases) were compiled. Of these cases, 43 percent were related to surgery and 9 percent to trauma; 26 percent occurred in a medical setting and 13 percent were pregnancy related.[25] Only 9 percent were caused by nephrotoxins. Of all causes of renal failure, ATN may be the underlying disorder in approximately three-fourths. The ischemic causes are those associated with untreated or inadequately treated prerenal disorders with resultant tubular damage. Occasionally, ischemic damage results from very brief periods of hypoperfusion, such as during operative procedures. Decreased perfusion pressure is normally accompanied by autoregulatory changes (i.e., decreased afferent arteriolar resistance as the mean arterial pressure [MAP, diastolic + one-third pulse pressure] falls to 80 mm Hg). Total RBF may remain the same but with redistribution to the juxtamedullary cortex, as demonstrated by studies using inert gas washout and microsphere methods. In other studies, RBF may be decreased with a uniform distribution in the cortex, using the same microsphere technique. As the MAP falls still lower (50 to 70 mm Hg) the RBF, GFR, and single nephron GFR fall to one-half to two-thirds of control values and alter the Starling forces. Below 40 to 45 mm Hg MAP, single nephron GFR stops completely in the superficial and deep nephrons.

Significant renal ischemia may occur in the absence of recognized hypotension and with only a modest decrease in cardiac output. This has been demonstrated by experiments using tilt tables or leg tourniquets to decrease the effective blood volume.[25] Although blood pressure may not change, the RPF may fall by more than one-third and be accompanied by a fall in GFR and urine flow.

ATN resulting from toxin exposure may occur from any of a number of agents identified.[10,12–14] However, the factors that establish and maintain renal failure in one patient but not another after similar exposure are multiple. Several experimental models have been devised in an attempt to identify the predominant factor responsible for a decreased GFR. The results vary between agents and among species. It is sufficient to say that vascular and tubular effects are interrelated and play roles of varying importance in each patient. The mechanisms leading to a reduced GFR include diminished RPF, altered glomerular capillary ultrafiltration coefficient (implying altered permeability and/or effective filtering surface area), tubular obstruction, and backleak.[25,27] The no-reflow phenomenon (i.e., cellular swelling preventing normal blood flow) does not appear to have experimental support. In established ATN, iodinated contrast material often yields a dense immediate nephrogram. This material is excreted by glomerular filtration not by tubular secretion, thus, glomerular filtration continues, although at a lower level. The role of the renin-angiotensin system remains in doubt. No protection has been noted in attempts to immunize with renin, to utilize angiotensin II blockade, or vasodilators. Owing to the proximity of the renin-containing macula densa to the glomerulus, a local role for this system in ischemic and toxin-induced ATN cannot be excluded.

Obstructive uropathy results when intrarenal or extrarenal obstruction alters the normal fall in pressure from kidney to bladder. Common etiologies in adult males are prostatic hypertrophy or carcinoma, calculi, and urethral strictures. In women, pregnancy, calculi, or malignancy are the most common etiologies. In children, congenital anomalies should be considered. Continued GFR and urine production lead to increased volume and pressure proximal to the obstruction, whether it is mechanical or functional. RBF and GFR are eventually diminished owing to increased tubular pressure opposing filtration. Additionally, blood flow is redistributed to the inner cortex while flow to the outer cortex and the inner medulla is reduced.[28]

Intrinsic obstruction should be considered in patients with a history of hematology-oncology disorders. In multiple myeloma, Bence Jones proteinuria seems to be the major determinant of renal failure and results from intratubular precipitation.[29] Patients with leukemia or lymphoma undergoing chemotherapy or irradiation may develop hyperuricemic nephropathy with obstruction, when serum uric acid exceeds 20 to 21 mg/

dl, urinary uric acid/creatinine exceeds 1.0, and tubular precipitation occurs.[30,31] Obstruction resulting from precipitation of uric acid in the ureters as well as in the tubules is now less common.[31]

DIAGNOSIS

A diagnosis of renal failure must be considered in the appropriate setting if it is to be made. Patients will not readily recognize that they have renal failure and may complain only of pain or generalized malaise. A fairly common presentation is the older adult who simply feels more fatigued or who has unexplained weakness or the younger patient who notes decreased exercise tolerance (with a creatinine of 10 mg/dl). Thus, the symptoms may not point immediately to the kidneys. In the trauma victim, dehydrated patient, or postoperative patient, renal failure comes to mind more readily. Symptoms that should raise the possibility of renal disease include edema of recent onset, scant or dark urine, or the new onset of hypertension. Altered mental status of short duration—confusion, somnolence, sleep disorders, short attention span—should instigate an investigation of renal function. The tests to request initially include BUN and serum creatinine, as well as serum electrolytes (Na^+, K^+, Cl^-, HCO_3^-). If the BUN and creatinine are elevated, the differential considerations must be entertained. The volume status and urine production must be discerned.

How high a BUN or creatinine should be accepted as normal? The BUN value should not exceed 20 mg/dl and the creatinine value should be less than 1.5 mg/dl. Women and men with small frames have somewhat lower values. In pregnancy, values that otherwise would be considered within the normal range are elevated if the BUN value exceeds 13 mg/dl and the creatinine value is greater than 0.8 mg/dl.[32] This is due to the normally increased RBF and GFR that accompanies the gravid state. In renal failure, the BUN value rises by 10 to 20 mg/dl each day as the creatinine value increases daily by 0.5 to 1.5 mg/dl. In trauma or severe rhabdomyolysis, these values may increase at a more rapid rate (doubled), with the creatinine value elevated out of proportion to that of the BUN.

Hyperkalemia becomes a risk factor when the GFR is less than 10 ml/minute. A rise of 0.5 mEq/liter/day or less is expected, but a rise of 1 to 2 mEq/liter in a matter of hours is possible in trauma patients.

Acidosis generally occurs as a result of the inability to excrete the acid load of 50 to 100 mEq generated per day. As the GFR falls and tubular function declines, the body is incapable of reclaiming HCO_3^- in the proximal tubule or of regenerating HCO_3^- at the distal tubule. Thus, the serum HCO_3^- concentration falls by 1 to 2 mEq/liter each day in patients with uncomplicated conditions, and by a more rapid rate if the patient is hypercatabolic. To compensate for the reduced HCO_3^- concentration, CO_2 must be exhaled. However, unmeasured anions begin to accumulate.

A number of secondary problems ensue that will be considered individually in the treatment section. Renal failure may involve other organ systems with resultant cardiac arrhythmias, heart failure, or pericarditis; altered mental status, electroencephalographic changes, and asterixis; nausea and vomiting, increased incidence of ulcers, and hemorrhage; respiratory problems related to volume excess; anemia, white blood cell dysfunction, and altered hemostasis; and altered thermoregulation and endocrine function.

Mortality remains high after the onset of renal failure despite the use of hemodialysis, owing to the severity of the underlying illness and current spectrum of disease.[2] The major determinants of mortality are infection and the primary illness that precipitated the disorder. Patients who are at increased risk include older patients, burn victims, those with a large number of complications, and possibly patients with a second episode of ATN.[2,25] Nonoliguric ATN is not a benign disorder as claimed in some studies but does have a mortality of 21 to 26 percent. Even the recovery or diuretic phase of oliguric ATN is the setting for approximately one-fourth of the deaths.

DIFFERENTIAL DIAGNOSIS

Because of the possibility of reversible conditions, it is important to establish as early as possible the category of renal failure in a given patient. Thus, a quick assessment of hydration (effective and total volume status), including cardiac function, and search for an obstructive component must be performed. Historical features such as flank pain or alternating anuria and urine production suggest obstruction. Has there been a history of nausea and vomiting, diarrhea, limited access to fluids, orthostatic symptoms, dyspnea, angina, orthopnea, arrhythmias, hemorrhage, or documented hypotension during surgery?

Prerenal azotemia is supported by dry skin, dry mucous membranes, low volume, and oliguria. Skin over the forehead or sternum is less susceptible to changes associated with aging and may be used to assess skin turgor. If dependent edema is noted in the legs or presacral area, the patient is not volume deficient. Additionally, "sheet lines" may be assessed over the back—if imprints are made in the skin of a supine patient, it is unusual for total body water to be significantly reduced. For patients in the cardiac care unit, intensive care unit, or trauma unit, the pulmonary capillary wedge

(PCW) pressure, cardiac output, and cardiac index can identify cardiac performance and adequacy of filling pressure. When a more rapid assessment is needed (and realizing that the central venous pressure [CVP] does not perfectly correlate with pulmonary artery diastolic or PCW pressures) the CVP can be used to assess the volume status. If there is *any* consideration of using furosemide or mannitol, it must *first* be established that a patient has an adequate volume. When the CVP is low, a volume challenge should be administered with normal saline, 500 ml over 15 to 20 minutes, with a recheck of the CVP at the completion of the infusion and 15 minutes later. Since the intravascular volume is normally one-fourth of the extracellular fluid and thus one-twelfth of the total body water,[33] a solution must be chosen that will not rapidly diffuse throughout the body space as dextrose 5 percent and water (D_5W) or hypotonic solutions may. Establishing that the hemodynamic parameters are normal should suggest other etiologies. However, it is not always possible to easily distinguish prerenal causes from parenchymal damage, so a variety of indexes and ratios have been devised that may identify the correct diagnosis.[34,35] These indexes are of greatest use in an oliguric patient who does not have underlying renal insufficiency. It is preferable to assess these indexes without the prior use of diuretics or other agents if possible. The application of these tests will be discussed after the assessment of renal obstruction has been discussed.

This order is appropriate in the usual diagnostic scheme because obstructive uropathy may be the most commonly overlooked diagnosis. Patients with a history of renal calculi, hematuria, diabetes (with or without neurogenic bladder), lymphoma, or malignancy should be considered, but the potential causes are too numerous to list.[28] Precipitation of substances in the ureters such as uric acid should be considered in patients with leukemia or lymphoma who have recently been treated with chemotherapy or radiation.

Evaluation for obstruction may be quickly carried out. Percussion and palpation for bladder enlargement and prostatic examination are simple measures. If enlargement is noted, a catheter may be placed for sterile drainage and sequential determination of urine volumes. A urine sample should be used to evaluate electrolytes, uric acid, and urinary creatinine as well as the sediment for crystals (uric acid, sulfa, oxalate) and blood. If there is very little urine in the bladder, the upper tracts must be assessed. Ultrasound can accurately determine renal size and degree of dilation of the ureters and renal pelvis. This procedure will not miss patients with obstructions but may yield a false-positive result in equivocal cases.

If ultrasound is not available, it may be necessary to catheterize one ureter. One ureter is sufficient because a single patent orifice and ureter rules out obstruction as an etiology (since one functioning kidney would be capable of compensating for obstruction of the contralateral side). This approach also avoids the risk of bilateral orifice edema. If an obstruction is found, a catheter can be placed to relieve the obstruction. Percutaneous nephrostomy is a reasonable alternative to alleviate the obstruction while other therapy is rendered. A catheter or nephrostomy may be temporary if hemodialysis can relieve uric acid or myeloma protein precipitation.[31,36]

As parenchymal causes, glomerulonephritis and vasculitis should be suspected when hematuria (especially red blood cell casts) is present and associated with proteinuria. Although these casts may be seen in patients with acute interstitial nephritis and occasional ATN, significant proteinuria (nephrotic range) is more common with glomerulonephritis. Oliguria and hypertension are additional important clues to glomerulonephritis. Acute interstitial nephritis should be considered if there is a history of recent medication use, rash, fever, peripheral eosinophilia, or eosinophils noted in the urine along with hematuria.[37,38] The kidneys may appear large on ultrasound or on an abdominal roentgenogram. For further information the reader should refer to a major nephrology text.

On occasion it is not possible to distinguish which patient has prerenal azotemia or ATN. In this situation, urinary indexes become quite important.[34,35] ATN requires support of the numerous functional deficiencies while the tubules repair themselves (usually over 5 to 10 days), while prerenal causes are potentially reversible. The various ratios and parameters are listed in Table 63–2. Because there is so much overlap using urinary osmolality, ratio of urine to plasma osmolality, and ratio of urine to plasma urea, these indexes are not particularly helpful. Osmolality of the urine depends to a large extent on urea handling, but urea is affected by states of hydration, medications (corticosteroids are catabolic; tetracyclines are antianabolic), gastrointestinal hemorrhage, hepatic function, and diet. Urinary sodium (U_{Na^+}) is usually less than 10 mEq/liter in prerenal states and greater than 25 mEq/liter in 81 percent of oliguric ATN patients (and 32 percent of nonoliguric ATN patients). This also is an imperfect test because values of 10 to 25 mEq/liter and less than 10 mEq/liter were reported in 13 percent and 6 percent of one series of oliguric patients, respectively.[25] Using urinary to plasma creatinine ratios, values of greater than or equal to 40:1 are seen in prerenal conditions and less than 10:1 in ATN. This leaves a large potential gray zone, which can be resolved by using a "break point" of 20:1, with the realization that this is usually correct but not always accurate. Improved diagnostic accuracy comes

TABLE 63–2   Useful Urinary and Plasma Parameters in Renal Failure

Test	Prerenal	ATN	Comments
Microscopic evaluation of urine	Normal; occasional hyaline or granular casts	Pigmented casts; epithelial cells	Red blood cell casts suggest glomerulonephritis or acute interstitial nephritis
Concentrating ability			
Specific gravity	> 1.015	$1.010-1.025$	Indistinguishable
Urinary osmolality (mOsm/liter)	> 500	< 350	Considerable overlap
$\dfrac{\text{Urine osmolality}}{\text{Plasma osmolality}}$	$\dfrac{2-3}{1}$	< 1.1 in oliguric patients < 1.2 in nonoliguric patients	Not always reliable
$\dfrac{\text{Urinary creatinine}}{\text{Plasma creatinine}}$	$> 40{:}1$	$< 10{:}1$	Because of large gray zone 20:1 may be more practical division
Urinary sodium (mEq/liter)	< 10	> 25 $10-25$ < 10	In 81% oliguric; 32% nonoliguric In 13% oliguric; 56% nonoliguric In 6% oliguric; 12% nonoliguric
Renal failure index $\dfrac{(U_{Na+})}{(U_{Creat}/P_{Creat})}$	< 1.0	> 1.0	Specific volume not needed Most useful in oliguric patients
Fractional excretion of sodium $\dfrac{(U_{Na+}\,P_{Na+})}{(U_{Creat}/P_{Creat})} \times 100$	$< 1\%$	$> 1\%$	Specific volume not needed Most useful in oliguric patients

from use of the renal failure index RFI $= (U_{Na+})/(U_{Creat}/P_{Creat})$ which yields values less than 1.0 for prerenal states and greater than 1.0 for ATN. Further refinement considers plasma sodium to determine the fractional excretion of sodium $FE_{Na} = 100$ $(U_{Na+}/P_{Na+})/(U_{Creat}/P_{Creat})$ which is $U_{Na}/P_{Na}/U_{Creat}/P_{Creat} \times 100$. Values less than 1 percent indicate avid sodium reabsorption while values greater than 1 percent indicate abnormal tubular handling of sodium. These indexes are useful in mixed disorders in which prerenal causes have been corrected or in which obstruction has been alleviated and yet the clinical state does not improve.

TREATMENT

The functional abnormalities common to most forms of renal failure will be discussed after mention of specific items.

The treatment of obstruction when it is found is the relief of that obstruction via catheter, suprapubic catheter, or percutaneous nephrostomy. After complete or bilateral obstruction is relieved, a marked fluid diuresis may occur. It will be necessary to monitor intake and output closely so that dehydration or vascular collapse does not follow. Special attention should be paid to repletion of K^+, HCO_3^-, and Mg^{++} losses, which may occur with a brisk diuresis. This replacement should prevent severe weakness from hypokalemia, acidosis

from HCO_3^- loss, or tetany or cardiac problems secondary to a low Mg^{++} causing hypocalcemia.

"Prerenal" patients should have their volume status normalized if it is truly depleted, and optimized if due to cardiac dysfunction. This may involve treatment of arrhythmias with appropriate medications, use of cardiac pacemakers, digitalization (with levels closely followed due to impaired renal excretion), and hemodynamic monitoring.

Glomerulonephritis may require corticosteroids, immunosuppressive agents, and even plasmapheresis if it is progressive and unrelenting.[39]

Acute interstitial nephritis accompanied by rash, fever, eosinophilia, or eosinophils in the urine may respond to high-dose corticosteroids (1 to 1.5 mg/kg/day prednisone). Occasionally these patients will require hemodialysis support.

The following recommendations for treatment apply predominantly to the renal parenchymal diseases.

Volume Regulation

Once adequate volume is assured but renal failure persists, it is important not to overload the patient. Furosemide or mannitol occasionally cosmetically improve urine production but do not improve the quality of the urine or attendant functions. There is the risk of causing ototoxicity from increasing doses of furosemide as well as hyperosmolality if the mannitol is not excreted. Mannitol is contraindicated when anuria, pulmonary congestion, marked dehydration, or heart failure exists. Either agent may prevent ATN if given prophylactically, but neither will reverse established ATN.

The importance of volume regulation is that too much volume is as bad as too little. Each individual generates 400 ml water daily from endogenous catabolism of proteins and lipids. The administration of 300 to 500 ml more than daily output (plus an additional 100 ml/day for each degree C fever) prevents volume excess. Ideally the patient should lose 0.5 kg/day. Patients with renal failure may replace body mass (muscle and adipose tissue) with water weight, and this can be significant over long periods. Excessive fluid administration may cause pulmonary edema and difficulty in weaning patients from the ventilator owing to requirements for increased constant positive airway pressure to permit better oxygenation. Data from studies of military personnel in Southeast Asia indicate that pulmonary edema frequently may develop even in patients who have nonoliguric ATN (9 of 14 cases).[40] Patients in precarious hemodynamic status can develop congestive heart failure and will then require medications or dialysis to correct the iatrogenic problem. In other individuals, excess volume may induce hypertension. Ascites may develop and cause wound dehiscence following abdominal surgery. Theoretically, marked peripheral edema could cause an increased fluid phase, slowing mass transfer into and out of cells. Thus, relative restriction of volume can reduce many iatrogenic complications. When possible, fluids should be administered orally for patient comfort and to remove a potential source of infection. Foley catheters should not be used if a patient can void spontaneously or if there is negligible urine output. Despite the best efforts at good catheter care, catheters invite possible infection that may result in death. When the patient enters the polyuric phase, the volume administered should be increased, but one should be cautious not to "chase one's tail." If the volume administered exceeds 2 to 3 liters, it is possible that sufficient function has been recovered and the physician is now "driving" the polyuria by the volumes administered. Therefore, after a few days of polyuria, begin decreasing the volume given to 500 ml less than the output.

Acid-Base Disorders

Renal failure is a well-recognized cause of metabolic acidosis. This occurs as a result of the inability of the patient to excrete the daily generated acid load as well as the inability to regenerate HCO_3^-. The accumulation of sulfate and phosphate, for example, leads to an increased anion gap (normal 12 ± 2 mEq/liter) usually exceeding 15 mEq/liter.[41] When the HCO_3^- falls, some of the decrement is replaced by chloride. However, when HCO_3^- is less than 16 mEq/liter, it is advisable to treat the patient with HCO_3^- or bicarbonate equivalent (lactate, acetate, or bicitrate—Shohl's solution), depending on the severity of the acidosis and hepatic function. In extremes of acidosis, the liver and other organs have an intracellular acidosis with impaired conversion of these anions to bicarbonate. In such patients the optimal replacement is with $NaHCO_3$, either orally or intravenously, to maintain the HCO_3^- concentration above 18 mEq/liter. The rationale of this therapy is to benefit enzyme systems, improve bone metabolism, and aid white blood cell function. An important point to consider is that there should be a compensatory respiratory alkalosis. Because compensatory acid-base adjustments *never* overcorrect, an alkalosis out of proportion to that expected should be considered an early clue to infection or sepsis and should initiate blood cultures and possible antibiotic coverage. Guidelines to follow in assessing mixed acid-base disorders and correction may be found elsewhere.[41,42] (See Chapter 18.)

Electrolyte Imbalance

Phosphate retention will cause a corresponding decrease in calcium. This fall in calcium induces the release of parathyroid hormone. It is rare that the hypocalcemia is clinically significant. However, when the calcium-phosphate product exceeds 70, metastatic calcification may occur in blood vessels, skin, lung, heart, and other sites. When hypocalcemia occurs in states of severe rhabdomyolysis, a rebound *hypercalcemia* should be expected as these deposits mobilize in the recovery phase. Hyperphosphatemia may be controlled by dietary restriction or phosphate-binding antacids if the patient has an oral intake. (If parenteral alimentation is used, these methods will not be successful.) Since phosphate and potassium accompany each gram of protein at approximately 1 mg and 1 mEq, respectively, the diet may be limited to 40 to 60 gm protein to control urea production, hyperphosphatemia, and hyperkalemia. Aluminum hydroxide phosphate binders may be given at the end of each meal to lessen absorption of phosphate from the gastrointestinal tract. The initial doses are Amphojel or Basaljel, 30 ml orally with each meal, or ALternaGEL, 15 ml orally with each meal. The dose may be raised if needed or lessened if the patient becomes hypophosphatemic (less than 2.5 to 3.0 mg/dl) to lessen the risk of severe hypophosphatemia (less than 1.0 mg/dl) and the complications of pulmonary, cardiac, or neurologic dysfunction.[43] Magnesium-containing antacids are contraindicated as phosphate binding agents, because of the risks of hypermagnesemia, which include death.

Sodium should not be given to excess. One gram of sodium equals 43 mEq, and a 4-gm Na^+ diet is equivalent to a 10-gm salt diet. Less than this quantity is usually required on a daily basis and will avoid increased thirst and volume overload. The dietary needs can be assessed by determining the total urinary losses and the intravenous saline administered and by following serum sodium concentrations for the development of hyponatremia or hypernatremia. Hyponatremia is more common, occurring partly as a consequence of obligate urinary sodium loss but more frequently from excessive volume administration.

Serum potassium elevations occur mainly from *dietary* intake, as well as medications, transfusion of old blood, hematoma resorption, and tissue injury. Potassium administration should be avoided during the oliguric phase or corrected cautiously if large extrarenal losses are evident. (During periods of polyuria, a marked kaliuresis may occur requiring supplementation.) When hyperkalemia greater than 7.0 mEq/liter occurs and electrocardiographic changes are evident, the first treatment should be intravenous 10% calcium gluconate (up to three ampuls at a rate of 3 to 5 minutes to administer each with constant electrocardiographic monitoring) in order to counteract the cardiac effects. This may then be followed by two or three ampuls of $NaHCO_3$ (50 mEq each), which induces the cellular uptake of potassium within minutes and may last for hours. This treatment may be followed by regular insulin, 1 unit/10 kg body weight by intravenous push, followed by a continuous insulin infusion. To prevent hypoglycemia, 2 to 3 gm glucose should be given per unit of insulin infused. These measures only temporize and shift potassium to an intracellular location. Therefore, they must be continued until potassium can be removed from the body. This may be accomplished by the use of sodium polystyrene sulfonate (Kayexalate), 15 to 20 gm three or four times a day in 20 ml of 70% sorbitol for oral use or 50 gm in 50 ml of 70% sorbitol plus 100 ml tap water as a retention enema. The obvious risk of this therapy is significant sodium loading. The ultimate means of potassium removal is via hemodialysis with a potassium-free dialysate. In some trauma cases, dialysis may be required twice daily in addition to other measures (e.g., peritoneal dialysis) to control hyperkalemia.

Hypertension

Hypertension in renal failure is often related to hypervolemia. However, it also may be mediated by a variety of factors, including increased cardiac output, increased activity of the renin-angiotensin system, increased peripheral vascular resistance, autonomic nervous system dysfunction, or a vasodilator deficiency.[44] Control of volume should obviate the need for medications to lower the blood pressure or improve cardiac performance. However, if hypertension is a problem in a previously normotensive individual or if there is a significant risk for a stroke or myocardial infarction, it is imperative to lower the blood pressure. Medications that are used should be titrated to the blood pressure and not to the level of renal function.[44] In renal failure, diuretics usually are not effective; therefore, other agents must be employed such as methyldopa, clonidine, propranolol, hydralazine, and prazosin. With either intravenous or oral methyldopa the maximal effect is evident at 4 to 6 hours. Hydralazine may be given intravenously or intramuscularly (at 15 to 25 mg) for rapid effect. Clonidine has the advantages of prompt onset, early maximal effect, and usefulness in moderate and severe hypertension but must be given orally. Because its half-life is prolonged in renal failure, clonidine should be given in the minimal effective dose. Minoxidil and nitroprusside can be used in malignant hypertension even when hemodialysis is necessary to support the patient. If the hypertension is clearly volume-mediated, this may be an indication for early hemodialysis. (See Chapter 52.)

Metabolic Disorders

Diet is important in renal failure because patients are frequently catabolic but unable to excrete the metabolic wastes. If the patient can eat, a diet of 20 to 40 gm/day of high biologic-value protein may be given. This may be liberalized to 60 gm/day as renal function improves or dialysis is initiated. This diet will not give excessive potassium or phosphate as noted earlier. If the patient is unable to eat, 100 gm glucose should be given daily to slow protein catabolism. Essential amino acid replacement has been shown to be of benefit in treating renal failure by lowering of the BUN through utilization of urea and possibly enhancing recovery.[45] These amino acids may be given intravenously as Nephramine or orally as Amin-Aid. The daily dose should be gradually increased while glucose, osmolality, and electrolytes are monitored on a daily basis.

Medications may require adjustment of dosage in renal failure as a result of an impaired excretory capacity. Most notably, digitalis compounds and antibiotics should be considered for alteration based on the half-life and route of excretion. Drugs such as gentamicin and carbenicillin used for serious infections may inactivate each other unless the times of administration are altered.[46] An extremely valuable reference is the updated dosing guidelines for adults by Bennett and coworkers.[47] Certain medications should be avoided if possible until resolution has occurred, namely K^+ and Mg^{++} containing drugs, salicylates, and anticoagulants, because of the increased incidence of gastrointestinal hemorrhage in uremia, sulfonamides, and nitrofurantoin. Sedatives and hypnotics should be used with extra caution because of prolonged half-lives and altered protein-binding and volumes of distribution in uremia. Drugs that may be needed include oral phosphate binders, water-soluble vitamins, and folic acid, 1 mg/day, if hemodialysis is employed.

Hematologic Disorders

Anemia is to be expected in patients with renal failure because of decreased production and shortened red blood cell survival. The hematocrit stabilizes at 20% to 25% and rises slowly after recovery. There is usually no need to routinely transfuse these patients. Notable exceptions occur if there is active hemorrhaging or if angina is precipitated. If angina develops, particularly in an older patient, it may be necesssary to maintain a hematocrit of 30%. If pulmonary edema or volume overload is present, it may be advantageous to give packed red blood cells during hemodialysis.

White blood cell function is impaired as azotemia worsens; thus attempts should be made to minimize sources of infection, such as unneeded intravenous lines and urinary catheters. It is best to *expect* infection (especially in the surgical, obstetric, or trauma patient) and be aggressive in treatment. Hyperosmolality also impairs white blood cell function, and this should be considered when amino acid solutions are employed. Dialysis to improve the uremia and hyperosmolality may be crucial to recovery.

Platelet function and hemostasis become progressively impaired as uremia deepens. Platelets are decreased in number through reduced production as well as utilization; qualitative defects appear as the BUN and creatinine near 100 mg/dl and 10 mg/dl, respectively; coagulation factors may decline and the bleeding time increases. As the risk of hemorrhage increases, dialysis is often initiated. If possible, medications that inhibit platelet aggregation should be avoided.

Endocrine Disorders

The values for hormone levels frequently appear abnormal in the uremic state owing to altered production, altered metabolism, abnormal protein binding, and alterations in the individual hormonal axis.[48] Thus, an assessment of endocrine function may be misleading unless these factors are taken into account. It is beyond the scope of this discussion to attempt to identify those changes—with one exception: insulin with a molecular weight of 6,000 is normally freely filtered at the glomerulus and taken up by the proximal convoluted tubule for catabolism. In uremia, despite what appears to be peripheral resistance to insulin and elevated lipids, insulin catabolism is decreased. Therefore, exogenous insulin may have more of an effect and attention should be given to decreasing the dose, if necessary, to prevent hypoglycemia.

Indications for Dialysis

Dialytic intervention is indicated in the patient with renal failure when any of the following are noted:

- central nervous system alterations such as altered mentation
- neurologic deficits with a sensory or motor neuropathy
- pericardial friction rub
- hyperkalemia, especially if accompanied by electrocardiographic changes
- BUN value greater than or equal to 100 mg/dl or creatinine value greater than or equal to 10 mg/dl
- massive volume excess
- severe acid-base disorders.

Factors that favor earlier initiation of dialysis include sepsis (with increased catabolism and the need for normal white blood cell function); trauma; diabetes, because of the associated risks; and the need for, or recent completion of, surgery in order to enhance wound healing, to prevent coagulopathies and hemorrhage, and to minimize the problems of infection and extracellular volume control.

Patients presenting with acute renal failure should be hospitalized until renal function has been recovered, a protracted recovery is evident, or the patients are considered to be chronic hemodialysis or peritoneal dialysis patients. Since some of these patients may require hemodialysis, it is beneficial to the patient to have one arm spared from phlebotomies and intravenous infusions. This will facilitate surgery for an arteriovenous fistula, polytetrafluoroethylene (PTFE) graft, or Quinton-Scribner shunt placement. Vessel damage, thrombosis, and phlebitis will also be minimized. Because the number of potential vascular access sites is strictly limited, blood pressures should not be determined in the extremity in which one of these types of access has been placed, owing to the additional risk of stasis leading to thrombosis and loss of the access. The viability of an access can be confirmed by a palpable thrill and audible bruit in the case of arteriovenous fistulas and PTFE grafts. For shunts, an uninterrupted column of blood is visible in all portions of the tubing. (The high flow through these devices may give a high venous return and transmit a bruit to the thorax, simulating a new murmur.) A thrombosed access requires prompt attention from a vascular surgeon.

Hemodialysis offers advantages over peritoneal dialysis: rapid access via femoral catheters, subclavian dialysis catheters, or extremity access as noted above; more rapid clearance of potassium and metabolic wastes; avoidance of respiratory depression and potential volume overload resulting from fluid in the peritoneum; and rapid correction of acid-base disorders. Peritoneal dialysis is preferred in patients in whom hemodynamic instability or hypotension (unsupportable with pressor agents) will not permit safe hemodialysis, in those with severe thrombocytopenia, in patients with a recent myocardial infarction, and in small children.

The morbidity and mortality remain high in renal failure owing to infection and underlying disorders,[2,25,40] but close attention to detail and anticipation of problems with volume overload, infection, and bleeding will improve the chance of survival. Patients with prolonged renal failure (i.e., greater than 4 to 6 weeks) have diminished chances of recovery but can be managed by chronic hemodialysis, peritoneal dialysis, or later renal transplantation.

REFERENCES

1. Anderson RJ, Linas SL, Berns AS, Henrich WL, Miller TR, Gabow PA, Schrier RW: Nonoliguric acute renal failure. *N Engl J Med* 296:1134–1138, 1977.
2. Anderson RJ, Schrier RW: Clinical spectrum of oliguric and non-oliguric acute renal failure, in Brenner BM, Stein JH (eds): *Acute Renal Failure*. New York, Churchill Livingstone, 1980, pp 1–16.
3. Miller PD, Krebs RA, Neal BJ, McIntyre DO: Polyuric prerenal failure. *Arch Intern Med* 140:907–909, 1980.
4. Gutman RA, Striker GF, Gilliland BC, Cutler RE: The immune complex glomerulonephritis of bacterial endocarditis. *Medicine* 51:1–25, 1972.
5. Beaufils M, Morel-Maroger L, Sraer J, Kanfer A, Kourilsky O, Richet G: Acute renal failure of glomerular origin during visceral abscesses. *N Engl J Med* 295:185–189, 1976.
6. Kelleher SP, Berl T: Acute renal failure in pregnancy. *Semin Nephrol* 1:61–68, 1981.
7. Grunfeld JP, Ganeval D, Bournerias F: Acute renal failure in pregnancy. *Kidney Int* 18:179–191, 1980.
8. Conn HO: A rational approach to the hepatorenal syndrome. *Gastroenterology* 65:321–340, 1973.
9. Gordon JA, Anderson RJ: Hepatorenal syndrome. *Semin Nephrol* 1:37–42, 1981.
10. Appel GB, Neu HC: The nephrotoxicity of antimicrobial agents. *N Engl J Med* 206:663–670, 722–728, 784–787, 1977.
11. Ditlove J, Weidmann P, Bernstein M, Massry SG: Methicillin nephritis. *Medicine* 56:483–491, 1977.
12. Cogan MG: Tubulo-interstitial nephropathies: A pathophysiologic approach. *West J Med* 132:134–140, 1980.
13. Porter GA, Bennett WM: Nephrotoxin-induced acute renal failure, in Brenner BM, Stein JH (eds): *Acute Renal Failure*. New York, Churchill Livingstone, 1980, pp 123–162.
14. Roxe DM: Toxic nephropathy from diagnostic and therapeutic agents: Review and commentary. *Am J Med* 69:759–766, 1980.
15. Knochel JP: Rhabdomyolysis and myoglobinuria. *Semin Nephrol* 1:75–86, 1981.
16. Koffler A, Friedler RM, Massry SG: Acute renal failure due to nontraumatic rhabdomyolysis. *Ann Intern Med* 85:23–28, 1976.
17. Grossman RA, Hamilton RW, Morse BM, Penn AS, Goldberg M: Nontraumatic rhabdomyolysis and acute renal failure. *N Engl J Med* 291:807–811, 1974.
18. Cunningham E, Kohli R, Venuto RC: Influenza-associated myoglobinuric renal failure. *JAMA* 242:2428–2429, 1979.
19. Kendrick WC, Hull AR, Knochel JP: Rhabdomyolysis and shock after intravenous amphetamine administration. *Ann Intern Med* 86:381–387, 1977.
20. Cogen FC, Rigg G, Simmons JL, Domino EF: Phencyclidine-associated acute rhabdomyolysis. *Ann Intern Med* 88:210–212, 1978.
21. Nadel SM, Jackson JW, Ploth DW: Hypokalemic rhabdomyolysis and acute renal failure: Occurrence following total parenteral nutrition. *JAMA* 241:2294–2296, 1979.
22. Swartz RD, Rubin JE, Leeming BW, Silva P: Renal failure following major angiography. *Am J Med* 65:31–37, 1978.
23. Byrd L, Sherman RL: Radiocontrast-induced acute renal failure: A clinical and pathophysiologic review. *Medicine* 58:270–279, 1979.
24. Carvallo A, Rakowski TA, Argy WP, Schreiner GE: Acute renal failure following drip infusion pyelography. *Am J Med* 65:38–45, 1978.
25. Levinsky NG, Alexander EA, Venkatichalam MA: Acute renal failure, in Brenner BM, Rector FC (eds): *The Kidney*, ed 2. Philadelphia, WB Saunders, 1981, vol 1, pp 1181–1236.
26. Blantz RC, Hostetter TH, Brenner BM: Functional adaptations of the kidney to immunological injury, in Wilson CB, Brenner BM, Stein JH (eds): *Immunologic Mechanisms of Renal Disease*. New York, Churchill Livingstone, 1979, pp 122–143.
27. Patak RV, Lifschitz MD, Stein JH: Acute renal failure: Clinical aspects and pathophysiology. *Cardiovasc Med* 4:19–38, 1979.
28. Wright FS, Howard SS: Obstructive injury, in Brenner BM, Rector FC (eds): *The Kidney*, ed 2. Philadelphia, WB Saunders, 1981, vol 2, pp 2008–2044.
29. DeFronzo RA, Cooke CR, Wright JR, Humphrey RL: Renal function in patients with multiple myeloma. *Medicine* 57:151–166, 1978.
30. Kelton J, Kelley WN, Holmes EW: A rapid method for the diagnosis of acute uric acid nephropathy. *Arch Intern Med* 138:612–615, 1978.
31. Kjellstrand CM, Campbell DC, von Hartitzsch B, Buselmeier TJ: Hyperuricemic acute renal failure. *Arch Intern Med* 133:349–359, 1974.
32. Lindheimer MD, Katz AI: Renal disease and pregnancy, in Suki WN, Eknoyan G (eds): *The Kidney in Systemic Disease*. New York, Wiley & Sons, 1976, pp 237–254.
33. Feig PU, McCurdy DK: The hypertonic state. *N Engl J Med* 297:1444–1454, 1977.
34. Espinel CH: The FE_{Na} test: Use in the differential diagnosis of acute renal failure. *JAMA* 236:579–581, 1976.
35. Miller TR, Anderson RJ, Linas SL, Henrich WL, Berns AS, Gabow PA, Schrier RW: Urinary diagnostic indices in acute renal failure: A prospective study. *Ann Intern Med* 89:47–50, 1978.
36. Brown WW, Hebert LA, Piering WF, Pisciotta AV, Lemann J, Garancis JC: Reversal of chronic end stage renal failure due to myeloma kidney. *Ann Intern Med* 90:793–794, 1979.
37. Lyons H, Pinn VW, Cortell S, Cohen JJ, Harrington JT: Allergic interstitial nephritis causing reversible renal failure in four patients with idiopathic nephrotic syndrome. *N Engl J Med* 288:124–128, 1973.
38. Linton AL, Clark WF, Driedger AA, Turnbull DI, Lindsay RM: Acute interstitial nephritis due to drugs: Review of the literature with a report of nine cases. *Ann Intern Med* 93:735–741, 1980.
39. Warren SE, Mitas JA, Golbus SM, Swerdlin AR, Cohen IM, Cronin RE: Recovery from rapidly progressive glomerulone-

phritis: Improvement after plasmapheresis and immunosuppression. *Arch Intern Med* 141:175–180, 1981.

40. Lordon RE, Burton JR: Post-traumatic renal failure in military personnel in Southeast Asia: Experience at Clark USAF Hospital, Republic of the Philippines. *Am J Med* 53:137–147, 1972.

41. Narins RG, Emmett M: Simple and mixed acid-base disorders: A practical approach. *Medicine* 59:161–187, 1980.

42. Bear RA, Grimbek M: Assessing acid-base imbalances through laboratory parameters. *Hosp Pract*, November 1974, pp 157–165.

43. Knochel JP: The pathophysiology and clinical characteristics of severe hypophosphatemia. *Arch Intern Med* 137:203–220, 1977.

44. Mitas JA, O'Connor DT, Stone RA: Hypertension in renal insufficiency: A major therapeutic problem. *Postgrad Med* 64:113–118, 1978.

45. Abel RM, Beck CH, Abbott WM, Ryan JA, Barnett GO, Fischer JE: Improved survival from acute renal failure after treatment with intravenous essential I-Amino acids and glucose: Results of a prospective double-blind study. *N Engl J Med* 288:695–699, 1973.

46. Weibert R, Keane W, Shapiro F: Carbenicillin inactivation of aminoglycosides in patients with severe renal failure. *Trans Am Soc Artif Int Organs* 22:439–443, 1976.

47. Bennett WM, Muther RS, Parker RA, Feig P, Morrison G, Golper TA, Singer I: Drug therapy in renal failure: Dosing guidelines for adults. *Ann Intern Med* 93:62–89, 286–325, 1980.

48. Emmanouel DS, Lindheimer MD, Katz AI: Endocrine abnormalities in chronic renal failure: Pathogenetic principles and clinical implications. *Semin Nephrol* 1:151–175, 1981.

64. Obstetric and Gynecologic Emergencies

CARL DAVID CUCCO, M.D.
ATEF H. MOAWAD, M.D.

Emergency care personnel are frequently called on to assess complaints and care for problems related to female sexual and reproductive function. In order to care for women on an emergent basis, an understanding of menstrual and reproductive physiology is essential. In addition, it is important to have a thorough knowledge of the differential diagnoses of the pathologic conditions of the female genitalia (Fig. 64–1).

The most frequently encountered complaints of women who do not have an intrauterine pregnancy are those of lower abdominal pain with or without associated vaginal bleeding. A large proportion of women with these complaints will be found to have either pelvic inflammatory disease or an ectopic pregnancy. Because these conditions are responsible for a tremendous amount of morbidity and mortality among young women, each will be discussed in some detail.

PELVIC INFLAMMATORY DISEASE

Pelvic inflammatory disease (PID) is a major health problem in the United States. It is estimated that between 3 and 4 million new cases of gonorrhea are occurring each year. Because in up to 85 percent of women and 15 percent of men gonorrheal infections are asymptomatic, diagnosis is often difficult. Yet if left untreated, 10 to 20 percent of female gonorrheal infections will progress to involve the internal genitalia. From 1973 to 1977, acute PID accounted for approximately 8 million patient visits to physicians' offices.[1]

Gonorrhea is caused by the gram-negative diplococcus *Neisseria gonorrhoeae*, discovered by Neisser in 1879. Acquired through sexual contact, the organism finds its main refuge in the cervical glands, the Skene and Bartholin glands, the periurethral glands, and the rectal mucosal crypts. Although an infected woman may complain of dysuria, frequency, a purulent vaginal discharge, and vulvar pruritus, typically the infection is asymptomatic. When present, the above features are unimpressive, and a culture is essential for accurate diagnosis. A Gram-stained smear revealing the classic paired, coffee-bean–shaped, intracellular gram-negative diplococci is recovered in only 50 to 75 percent of the patients. Thus, specimens from all women should be cultured from the urethra, cervix, and anus on Thayer Martin or Transgrow media. Once taken, the cultures should be stored in a concentrated CO_2 atmosphere by use of a candle jar.

Once a positive culture is obtained or a patient has symptoms and a reliable history of exposure, treatment consists of probenecid, 1 gm po, followed in 30 minutes by aqueous procaine penicillin, 2.4 million units, administered intramuscularly in each buttock. The probenecid blocks the tubular reabsorption of penicillin, prolonging elevated blood levels. This regimen will cure 98 percent of gonorrhea and virtually all incubating syphilis. A VDRL test should be done at the time of treatment and repeated in 3 months. If the patient is allergic to penicillin, she should be treated with spectinomycin, 2 gm IM, or tetracycline, 500 mg orally every

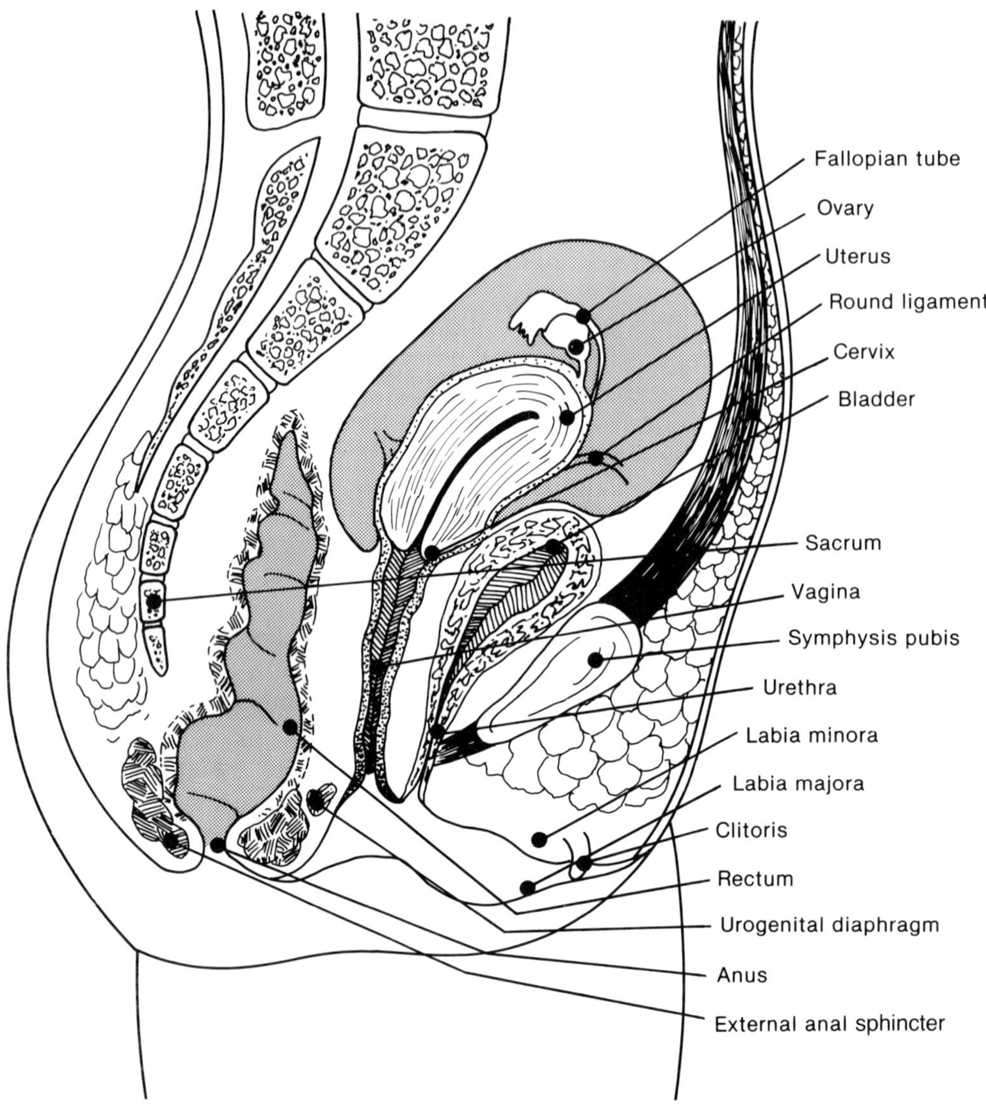

Figure 64–1 Normal Anatomy: Female.

6 hours for 5 days. She must refrain from intercourse until all of her contacts have been treated and another culture has been taken. This should be done 14 days after initial therapy. If the repeat culture remains positive, the patient should receive spectinomycin, 2 gm, intramuscularly.

The gonococci enter the uterus at the time of menstruation by spreading along the mucosal surface. Because of menstrual shedding, successful culturing of gonococci from the endometrium is rare. The fallopian tubes are morbidly affected, becoming edematous, erythematous, and purulent. Pus leaks from the fimbriated end of the tube into the cul-de-sac, causing a pelvic peritonitis. In time, the fimbriated end of the tube becomes clubbed, forming a pyosalpinx. In other cases,

a pelvic abscess will form. If the abscess involves the ovary and infundibulopelvic ligament, it is termed a tubo-ovarian abscess. In more severe cases purulent exudate may reach the liver surface via the right gutter, inciting a perihepatitis with adhesion formation between the capsule of the liver and undersurface of the diaphragm. This condition is known as the Fitz-Hugh–Curtis syndrome.

Once treated, the acute infection subsides to a chronic state that is characterized by scarring and adhesion formation. The pyosalpinx becomes a sterile hydrosalpinx, and the tubes become thickened and immobile. The patient experiences chronic, dull, aching lower abdominal pain, which is usually worse at menses. This chronic course is punctuated by acute reinfection with symptomatic flare-ups. Unlike the initial infection, gonococci are less often responsible for the reinfections. Once the tubal mucosal surface has been damaged, it is highly susceptible to infection by any of the common vaginal or gastrointestinal flora. Thus, the organisms responsible for acute flare-ups of chronic PID are usually anaerobic and gram-negative species, especially *Bacteroides, Escherichia coli*, and anaerobic streptococci.

Patients with PID present with lower abdominal pain and fever. Most often the pain begins as a suprapubic dull ache. With spreading peritonitis, the pain becomes generalized and exacerbated by movement. Patients with chronic PID complain of low back pain and lower abdominal pain, which worsens around menses. Dyspareunia, typically during deep penetration, is common, as is tenesmus and rectal pain during defecation. It is essential to remember that any patient with known or suspected chronic PID presenting with lower abdominal pain may have an ectopic pregnancy. The fact that patients with chronic PID frequently have dysfunctional uterine bleeding secondary to ovarian damage compounds the difficulty in making the correct diagnosis. The fever and chills associated with PID may be slight or marked, depending on the severity of the disease. Tachycardia, dehydration, and leukocytosis with a shift to the left are common. Anorexia, nausea, and vomiting may also play a role in the dehydration. Frequently, an associated anemia of chronic illness is discovered.

Physical examination reveals a febrile toxic patient in acute distress. She is typically lying on her side in the "fetal position," clutching her lower abdomen. There is abdominal distention with decreased or absent bowel sounds. Suprapubic and bilateral lower quadrant tenderness to palpation is a hallmark of PID. Classic signs of peritoneal irritation (i.e., rebound, referred pain, and involuntary muscle guarding) are apparent, especially in the lower quadrants. Upper abdominal signs suggest disseminated intraperitoneal infection and possible Fitz-Hugh–Curtis syndrome. On pelvic examination the vagina is quite warm and a purulent discharge may be seen coming from the cervical os. The cervix is exquisitely tender to motion, with pain referred bilaterally to the lower abdomen. It is commonly impossible to evaluate the uterus and adnexae secondary to severe pain and guarding, but when feasible the uterus is usually found to be small and firm. Chronic infection with scarring and adhesion formation produces a fundus that is immobile, commonly retroverted, and slightly tender. A cystic sausage-shaped adnexal mass is a hydrosalpinx, pyosalpinx, or tubo-ovarian abscess. Fluctuant bulging of the cul-de-sac also heralds the presence of a pelvic abscess.

After a thorough history and physical examination have been completed, intravenous lines are established and correction of dehydration and acidosis is begun.

Blood is obtained for a complete blood cell count (CBC), differential, electrolytes, culture, erythrocyte sedimentation rate, and quantitative C-reactive protein (CRP). The latter two studies are useful in following the course of infectious diseases. A CRPQ value of less than 2 indicates eradication of the acute infectious process. Urine specimens are obtained for urinalysis and a 2-minute immunologic pregnancy test. If the latter is positive, a rethinking of the diagnosis of PID is mandatory, because salpingitis is rarely, if ever, seen concomitant with an intact intrauterine pregnancy since protection of the internal genitalia is afforded by the thick cervical mucous plug. Also, ectopic pregnancy must always be ruled out in any patient having lower abdominal pain and a positive pregnancy test. During the pelvic examination, cervical, urethral, and anal cultures are taken.

If an intrauterine device (IUD) is in place, it is removed as soon as adequate serum levels of antibiotics are established in an attempt to prevent significant bacteremia. If pelvic examination rules out an abscess, it is suggested by some that a culdocentesis be performed in order to Gram-stain and culture the fluid obtained. It is questionable whether this is of value in helping to choose an antibiotic regimen for a particular patient. Finally, a nasogastric tube is placed when an adynamic ileus has resulted in severe abdominal distention and vomiting.

Criteria for hospitalization include a white blood cell count greater or equal to 16,000/cu mm; severe anorexia, nausea, vomiting, dehydration, and metabolic derangement; generalized abdominal peritonitis; and pelvic abscess. Often, however, the disease is of a milder nature and the patient can be released after being treated with the probenecid and intramuscular penicillin regimen described above. This should be followed with several days of oral ampicillin or amoxicillin. Specific instructions for follow-up care must be given.

When hospitalization is deemed necessary, the patient is given nothing by mouth and placed on bed rest in semi-Fowler's position so that the infected pelvis remains the most dependent area. Rehydration is continued, and analgesics and antipyretics are used as indicated. The initial acute attack of PID usually responds adequately to intravenous aqueous penicillin, 2 to 4 million units "piggy back" every 4 hours. Acute exacerbation of chronic PID requires coverage for gram-negative and anaerobic species, especially *Bacteroides fragilis*. This can be accomplished by adding an aminoglycoside, such as gentamicin, 3 to 5 mg/kg/day, IVPB in three divided doses with clindamycin, 600 mg administered in the same manner every 6 hours. Alternatively, chloramphenicol, 1 gm IVPB every 5 hours may be used. The response should be dramatic. If not, the patient must be thoroughly reevaluated and an intraperitoneal abscess must be ruled out. Should an abscess be discovered, surgical drainage is the treatment of choice. A ruptured tubo-ovarian abscess is a true surgical emergency, which formerly carried a mortality rate of 80 to 90 percent. With appropriate surgical and antibiotic management, mortality is markedly reduced.

With resolution of both fever and peritoneal signs, the pelvic examination is repeated. The patient will be more cooperative, and a hydrosalpinx or chronic tubo-ovarian abscess missed at the time of initial examination is easily palpated. Removal of the pelvic organs may at times be necessary to control recurrences of chronic PID and its attendant manifestations.

ECTOPIC PREGNANCY

An ectopic gestation is the implantation and growth of a fertilized ovum in a location other than the endometrium of the uterine fundus (Fig. 64–2). The incidence of ectopic pregnancy is increasing, with approximately 25,000 cases occurring annually in the United States. This is a frequency of one in 100 to 200 pregnancies, with the highest incidence in young, nonwhite, economically deprived urban women. Because ectopic pregnancy is responsible for 5 to 10 percent of the maternal deaths in the United States each year (second only to eclampsia) it is essential when any woman presents at the emergency department with lower abdominal pain or in shock that ectopic pregnancy be ruled out.

The most common predisposing factors to ectopic gestation are inflammatory or mechanical conditions that lead to a degree of occlusion or kinking of the fallopian tubes. Physiologic or hormonal dysfunction may also interfere with normal ovum transport.

Forty to sixty percent of ectopic pregnancies are associated with PID and the resulting chronic salpingitis and peritubular adhesions. Aggressive hospital management of acute PID is purported to preserve subsequent fertility. However, although these high-dose, broad-spectrum antibiotic regimens cure the infection, they have little effect on tubal patency. In fact, by preventing total occlusion of the tubal lumen in the face of a damaged epithelial lining, aggressive antibiotic management of acute PID may actually increase the risk of future ectopic pregnancy.

The presence of adhesions secondary to prior abdominal surgery, especially for ruptured abscess or manipulation of the fallopian tubes (i.e., tuboplasty, tubal ligation, or tubal reanastomosis) is another important etiologic factor for ectopic pregnancy. Previous elective abortion may produce a subclinical endometritis and perisalpingitis, which may also place the patient at increased risk. The IUD, which is excellent in preventing

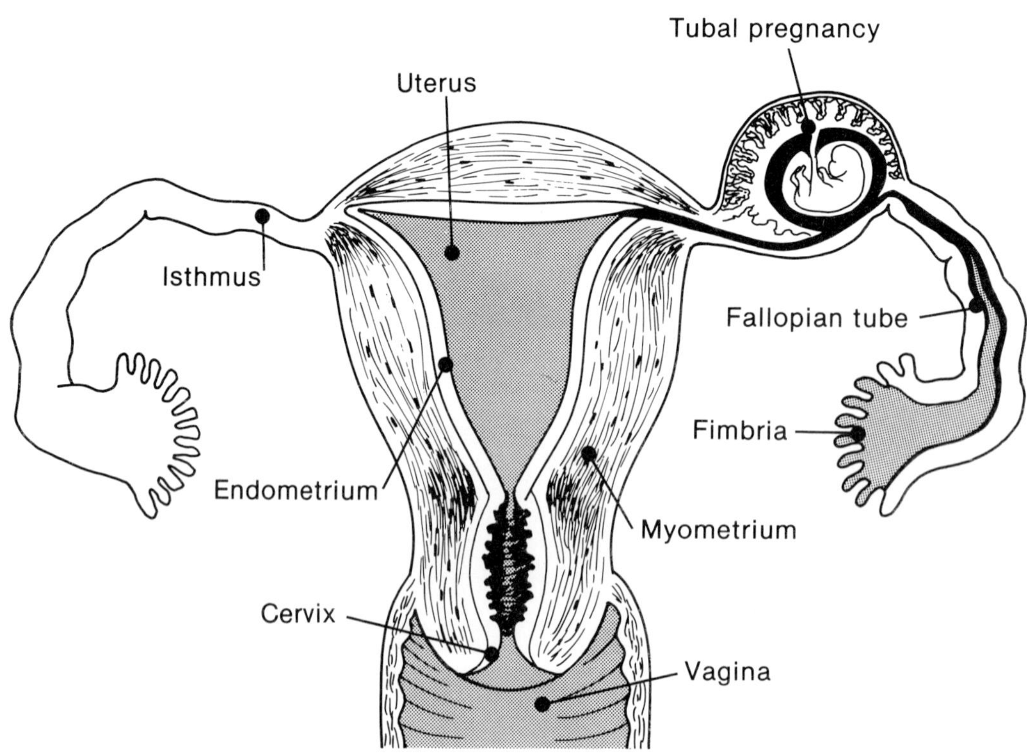

Figure 64–2 Ectopic Pregnancy.

intrauterine pregnancy, becomes progressively less effective in preventing pregnancy at a site farther from the endometrial cavity. Thus, while the incidence of intrauterine and tubal pregnancies is markedly reduced, the incidence of ovarian pregnancy is not reduced at all. Interestingly, virtually all reported cases of ovarian pregnancy associated with an IUD have been on the right side. Finally, once a woman has had an ectopic pregnancy, she is at a much higher risk for having another. In fact, 10 to 30 percent of these women will have future ectopic pregnancies while only one-third will ever deliver a term infant.

Still, despite all of the above, some 50 percent of fallopian tubes removed at salpingectomy for ectopic pregnancy are grossly and histologically normal as far as infection is concerned. This finding has led to theories of accessory ostia, congenital diverticula, tubal spasm, and impaired tubal transport of the ovum secondary to a deranged hormonal milieu as important, although unproved, etiologies for ectopic pregnancy.

The overwhelming majority of ectopic pregnancies (greater than 90 percent) occur in the fallopian tube, with over 50 percent of these in the ampullary portion. Cornual, ovarian, cervical, and abdominal pregnancies occur much less frequently. Often, the exact location is not diagnosed until the time of surgery.

There are no pathognomonic signs or symptoms of ectopic pregnancy; yet a specific constellation of complaints and findings is highly suggestive of the diagnosis. Since the key to successful treatment is dependent on early, accurate diagnosis, any woman complaining of lower abdominal pain with or without associated menstrual irregularities must be considered to have an ectopic pregnancy until proved otherwise.

The clinical triad in the diagnosis of ectopic pregnancy includes vaginal bleeding, lower abdominal pain, and a palpable adnexal mass. Unfortunately, this classic presentation is rarely the case, and often the signs and symptoms will be surprisingly minimal. For this reason a high degree of suspicion is always necessary if early unruptured ectopic pregnancies are not to be missed.

At the outset, the patient should be questioned regarding subjective signs of pregnancy. She may admit to breast changes, fatigue, and morning sickness. Since most women with ectopic pregnancies have been delivered of a child in the past, it is not rare for the patient to state that she "feels pregnant" once again.

Just about one-half of the patients will describe some irregularity of her own normal menstrual cycle, most complaining of 6 to 8 weeks of amenorrhea followed by spotting. Although the remaining patients will have had no amenorrhea, often the last period will have been abnormal in duration or amount of flow. Thus, a specific detailed questioning of the patient regarding the character of her menses is essential. At the time of admission

to the emergency department, most patients will report a variable amount of vaginal bleeding. This bleeding is often a scanty "spotting" of dark blood, unlike the bright red and, at times, profuse bleeding associated with incomplete abortion. The bleeding is due to involution of the uterine decidua secondary to fluctuating levels of hormonal support. Rarely is the ruptured ectopic pregnancy itself responsible for external vaginal bleeding. Occasionally, the decreasing levels of human chorionic gonadotropin (HCG) will cause sloughing of the entire endometrium in the form of a decidual cast. One must always keep in mind, however, that vaginal bleeding occurs in up to 20 percent of early intrauterine pregnancies so that a positive pregnancy test, coupled with a slightly enlarged uterus and vaginal bleeding, does not always mean ectopic pregnancy.

The pain associated with ectopic gestation may vary from vague and crampy to sharp, well localized, and intense. It is in response to irritation of the bowels and bladder from leaking blood and from stretching of the tubal peritoneum. For similar reasons, anorexia, nausea, and vomiting are frequent complaints. Sudden cessation of pain, especially after straining or pelvic examination is not to be taken lightly, since it may signal rupture of a tubal pregnancy. Abdominal examination reveals distention, decreased bowel sounds, and, at times, a doughy consistency to palpation secondary to hemoperitoneum. In very rare cases with massive hemoperitoneum a bluish discoloration of the skin around the umbilicus (Cullen's sign) may be noted. Tenderness to palpation, guarding, rebound, and referred pain to one or both lower quadrants is the rule.

A mass is palpated on pelvic examination in only 25 to 50 percent of patients with ectopic pregnancies. If felt, it is lateral to the uterus, ill defined, and tender and usually described as vague or doughy. The uterus is softened and enlarged, at times up to 12 weeks' gestational size. Unless the pregnancy is cornual in location, the fundus is not particularly tender. The cervix remains fairly firm in consistency with a closed os. A markedly softened cervix with an open os suggests threatened or incomplete abortion. The cervix may be slightly cyanotic (Chadwick's sign), and a slight movement usually results in exquisite pain.

Shoulder pain is an ominous complaint, since it signals massive intraperitoneal hemorrhage. The patient previously may have experienced agitation, dizziness, or fainting. Often she will state that she first noted these symptoms during or after exertion, sexual relations, or straining at defecation. A fairly typical picture is presented of an upset, pale woman with cold, clammy skin, a thready pulse, a narrowed pulse pressure, and orthostasis. When hemorrhage is severe the patient may present in shock. If traumatic hemorrhage can be ruled out, ectopic pregnancy must be considered. The distended abdomen and decreased bowel sounds secondary to hemoperitoneum have been mentioned. A boggy bulging of the cul-de-sac is found in pelvic examination, and the patient will complain of rectal pressure and tenesmus.

Culdocentesis may be used in the diagnosis of intraperitoneal hemorrhage in the absence of obvious clinical signs. The procedure is performed by inserting an 18-gauge spinal needle attached to a glass syringe between the uterosacral ligaments and into the cul-de-sac (Fig. 64–3, see also Chapter 71). If a plastic syringe is used, any blood obtained should be quickly transferred to a glass tube. The test is described as positive if non-clotting blood is obtained and negative if straw-colored peritoneal fluid is obtained. It is designated failed with no interpretation possible when blood that clots or no fluid at all is obtained. Inadvertent needle puncture of the bowel causes no significant sequelae.

It is essential to remember that a negative result of culdocentesis does not rule out an unruptured ectopic pregnancy. This fact coupled with a moderate rate of both false-positive and false-negative punctures has prompted the employment of culdocentesis in the following manner. Based on the history, physical examination, and laboratory evidence, the physician must first conclude whether the patient has a high probability of harboring an ectopic pregnancy. If so, a culdocentesis is performed as indicated. If the result is negative, the patient must still undergo laparoscopy to rule out an unruptured ectopic pregnancy or a false-negative culdocentesis. If the culdocentesis is positive, however, the laparoscopy may be omitted and immediate exploratory laparotomy performed. A patient never should be sent home on the basis of a negative or failed culdocentesis if, before the procedure, the examining physician had a high degree of suspicion of an ectopic pregnancy.

Emergency laboratory investigation as an aid in diagnosing ectopic pregnancy is relatively straightforward. A spun hematocrit is performed, and blood is obtained for an immediate CBC and differential. A 2-minute urine immunologic pregnancy test is obtained. Only 50 percent of ectopic pregnancies will be associated with a positive test. Thus, when negative the result must be disregarded. A serum test for the β-subunit of HCG is very sensitive and specific and allows the diagnosis of conception 8 days post ovulation.

Because the signs and symptoms of ectopic pregnancy are not always classic and because several other conditions may mimic the disease, the patient's history and a high index of suspicion are vital for correct diagnosis.

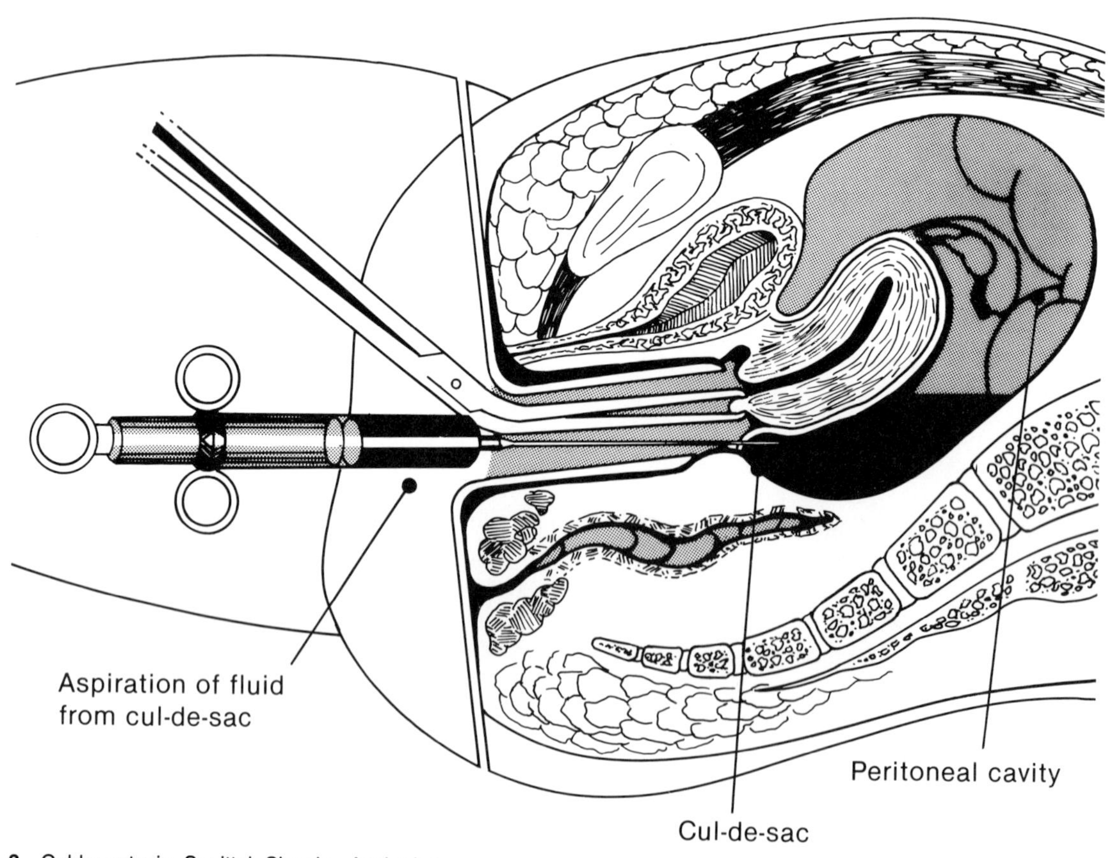

Figure 64–3   Culdocentesis: Sagittal, Showing Aspiration.

Threatened abortion, early intrauterine pregnancy, hemorrhagic corpus luteum, and PID are most frequently confused with ectopic pregnancy.

In threatened or complete abortion, the uterus is usually larger and softer than seen with ectopic pregnancy and the pain is comparable to severe menstrual cramps. The bleeding is likely to be profuse and bright red. The cervix is usually softer and there may be tissue (i.e., products of conception) protruding from an open os. On the other hand, PID is associated with fever, a marked leukocytosis, and a systemically toxic appearance. There is likely to be a history of previous pelvic infections, and subjective signs of pregnancy and orthostasis are not found. In addition, the uterus is small and firm. Early intrauterine pregnancy with a coexistent (hemorrhagic) corpus luteum may be quite difficult or impossible to differentiate from ectopic pregnancy prior to direct visualization of the pelvis. Halban's disease consists of a persistent corpus luteum leading to the palpation of an adnexal mass and spotting after a variable period of amenorrhea. Appendicitis begins with periumbilical pain, more numerous gastrointestinal complaints, leukocytosis, and fever. Rarely is it associated with cervical tenderness to motion or a change in the character of menses. Torsion of the adnexa presents with sudden excruciating unilateral lower abdominal pain, with radiation to the anterior and medial thigh. The patient is prostrate, and a large tender adnexal mass is palpated.

In the treatment of ectopic pregnancy, especially if ruptured, speed is of the utmost importance. Once the diagnosis is seriously entertained the patient should be hospitalized. There is no place for outpatient management of a patient who may have an ectopic pregnancy.

Once the diagnosis is made, two or more large-dose intravenous lines are immediately established. For the patient who is severely orthostatic or in shock, a central venous pressure (CVP) catheter is also secured. Correction of intravascular volume loss must be prompt, utilizing Ringer's lactate solution and blood, albumin, and low molecular weight dextran if necessary. When indicated because of severe hypertension and shock, type-specific blood should be immediately transfused. The patient is placed in Trendelenburg's position, and oxygen by mask is begun.

When starting the intravenous line, blood is obtained for an immediate CBC and differential, VDRL, and blood type and crossmatch. A hematocrit is spun, keeping in mind that despite massive intraperitoneal hemorrhage the value obtained may be normal or only slightly depressed until fluid replacement is begun. A 2-minute urine pregnancy test is performed. The role of culdocentesis has been discussed previously.

After appropriate work-up and stabilization of the patient has been completed, rapid consultation is obtained to facilitate transfer to the operating room. The only method of unequivocally ruling out an ectopic pregnancy is by direct visualization of the fallopian tubes. Besides being much less costly than laparotomy, laparoscopy is a timesaving procedure of low morbidity. Following a negative laparoscopy the patient can usually be discharged the next day. As a general rule, the surgeon should be willing to accept a 15 to 20 percent incidence of negative laparoscopy findings. If an ectopic pregnancy is found every time laparoscopy is performed, it is likely that many patients with early unruptured ectopic pregnancies are being sent away from emergency departments.

When laparotomy is indicated, salpingectomy with or without uterine cornual wedge resection is usually performed. The ipsilateral ovary may be bound to the fallopian tube and infundibulopelvic ligament in a mass of clot, necessitating a salpingo-oophorectomy. Conservative surgery, partial salpingectomy with later reanastomosis, salpingostomy, and milking the ectopic gestation from the ampullary portion of the tube have been advocated with the intention of better preserving subsequent fertility. The condition of the opposite tube, along with the age, parity, and desires of the patient must be considered before a decision of this type is made.

HYPERTENSION IN PREGNANCY

Normotensive women may become hypertensive during pregnancy. During any stage of gestation, a diastolic blood pressure of 90 mm Hg or above is abnormal. Likewise, a 30 mm Hg rise in the systolic blood pressure or a 15 mm Hg rise in the diastolic blood pressure over previously recorded values is significant. Thus, a patient with a blood pressure of 110/60 at 12 weeks' gestation is considered hypertensive should her blood pressure reach 140/80 at a later date. Whenever a gravida is admitted to the emergency department with an elevated blood pressure, an attempt must be made to differentiate chronic hypertension from pre-eclampsia (formerly referred to as toxemia). Although each of these conditions is hazardous to the mother and the fetus, the treatment varies according to the ultimate diagnosis.

Chronic hypertension can usually be diagnosed if the patient gives a reliable history of past hypertension. This is especially true if she has been treated with antihypertensive medication prior to pregnancy. Chronic hypertension is also diagnosed if the patient becomes hypertensive before the 20th week of gestation. Pre-eclampsia, on the other hand, is a syndrome consisting not only of hypertension but also of proteinuria of at least 0.3 gm/day (or a +1 reading by standard urine dipstick) and peripheral pitting edema. Uncontrolled, pre-eclampsia progresses to eclampsia, which is characterized by grand mal seizures.

Pre-eclampsia may vary from mild to severe. Severe pre-eclampsia is diagnosed when the diastolic blood pressure is equal to or greater than 110 mm Hg or when the dipstick urine protein is +3 or +4 (which correlates to greater than 5 gm/day). Epigastric pain, headaches, and visual complaints imply imminent seizure. Oliguria, with urine output of less than 30 ml/hour, is an equally ominous finding.

The precise cause of pre-eclampsia is not known. Generalized vasoconstriction causes an increase in peripheral vascular resistance and leads to an increase in blood pressure. During a normal pregnancy, owing to a physiologic increase in plasma volume, the glomerular filtration rate and renal plasma flow are increased. In pre-eclampsia, these are reduced, along with the 24-hour urine creatinine clearance rate.

The lesion responsible for the decrease in renal function is a swelling of the endothelial cells known as glomerular capillary endotheliosis. This lesion is wholly reversible, and renal biopsies become normal post partum. In addition to the kidney, the liver may also be affected, exhibiting a periportal necrosis and subcapsular hemorrhage. On very rare occasions the subcapsular hematoma ruptures into the abdominal cavity.

During a normal pregnancy, there is a 40 percent increase in plasma volume. This physiologic hypervolemia does not occur in pre-eclamptic patients. Rather, a hemoconcentration occurs concomitant with an increase in extracellular fluid. In severe pre-eclampsia anasarca may result.

All pregnant women with hypertension should be suspected of having pre-eclampsia until proved otherwise. Diabetic gravidas and those carrying multiple fetuses are at special risk, as are young mothers from socially deprived environments. Patients with chronic hypertension often develop a "superimposed" pre-eclampsia and need to be carefully monitored.

The diagnosis of pre-eclampsia is based on the finding of hypertension associated with proteinuria and edema. The level of hypertension may be in a range that is commonly thought to be borderline; yet it must again be emphasized that diastolic blood pressures of 90 mm Hg are distinctly abnormal at any time during pregnancy and when associated with edema and proteinuria, treatment for pre-eclampsia is required. The edema is of a peripheral pitting nature, with swollen ankles, hands, and a classic puffy "pre-eclamptic facies." The patient often gives a history of sudden weight gain. This is the result of edema and often precedes hypertension. The amount of proteinuria is variable from patient to patient and even at different times within the same patient. The urine to be tested should be obtained by catheterization, since contamination with vaginal discharge, amniotic fluid, or blood renders the dipstick result unreliable. Hyper-reflexia reflects irritation of the central nervous system, and severe hyper-reflexia associated with clonus warns that convulsions are imminent. Another warning of imminent convulsions is epigastric pain. This is also thought to be secondary to generalized central nervous system irritation, perhaps coupled with stretching of the liver capsule. At times, patients complain of visual changes, especially blurred vision and photophobia. Retinal vasospasm leading to edema has been implicated as the cause. Rarely, pre-eclampsia may present as a sudden loss of vision secondary to retinal detachment.

Laboratory findings reflect the hemoconcentration, along with hepatic and renal changes. The hematocrit is relatively high and falls precipitously post partum. The uric acid level is usually increased secondary to decreased renal clearance. It has been stated that the increase in uric acid does not occur in chronic hypertension and may be a way to distinguish the latter from pre-eclampsia. Blood urea nitrogen (BUN), creatinine, and liver transaminase values are increased in patients with severe pre-eclampsia. Also, in severe pre-eclampsia, the fibrinogen level is decreased from normal pregnancy levels of 0.4 to 0.8 gm/100 ml.

In-hospital management of pre-eclampsia is essential if excellent maternal and fetal outcomes are to be achieved. The blood pressures of these patients are quite labile, and a mild pre-eclamptic may progress to convulsions within minutes.

At the outset of treatment, careful assessment of the mother and fetus is mandatory. The gestational age, estimated fetal weight, presentation, and character of the fetal heart tones must be known if intelligent management decisions are to be made. Two intravenous lines are quickly established and blood is obtained for an immediate CBC and differential, platelet count, prothrombin time, partial thromboplastin time, liver enzymes, BUN, creatinine, fibrinogen, magnesium, uric acid, and blood type and crossmatch. It must be appreciated that the generalized vasospasm causes a contracted vascular space, rendering these patients exquisitely sensitive to intravascular fluid fluctuations. Iatrogenic congestive heart failure is surprisingly easy to precipitate. Thus, oliguria should be treated with a very carefully managed fluid challenge. Diuretics have no place in the treatment of oliguria unless it is associated with definite clinical evidence of congestive heart failure. A Foley catheter is essential to monitor urine output as well as proteinuria.

Once the diagnosis of pre-eclampsia is established, the patient should be protected from seizures by the administration of magnesium sulfate. Before the administration of this potentially dangerous drug, a Foley catheter must be placed and peripheral reflexes checked.

Toxic levels of magnesium sulfate cause respiratory and cardiac arrest. Before this, however, peripheral reflexes are lost. Thus, the patellar reflex is used to titrate the dose. Since magnesium sulfate is excreted in the urine, it is necessary to be cognizant of changes in urine output. With increasing oliguria the serum level of magnesium sulfate rises, the patellar reflexes become depressed or unobtainable, and the doses must be decreased. Generally, 4 gm magnesium sulfate over 10 minutes is given as an initial loading dose in a slow intravenous push. A continuous intravenous drip of 1 to 2 gm/hour is then begun. The magnesium sulfate is given for the sole purpose of preventing eclamptic seizures, not for the control of hypertension, although a transient decrease in blood pressure may follow the initial loading dose.

A consistently reproducible diastolic blood pressure of 110 mm Hg or greater should be treated with Apresoline. A continuous intravenous drip is established, and the diastolic blood pressure is titrated to a level that remains stable between 90 and 100 mm Hg. Intravenously or intramuscularly administered boluses of Apresoline are contraindicated in hypertensive pregnancies for fear of acutely depressing the blood pressure to levels that jeopardize uteroplacental blood flow and lead to fetal hypoxia, acidosis, and possibly death. For the same reason, when titrating the intravenous apresoline drip, the diastolic blood pressure should never be allowed to fall below 90 mm Hg.

As soon as feasible the patient should be transferred to the labor room for further evaluation, treatment, and a disposition regarding the timing and method of delivery. In general, once the pre-eclamptic mother's condition has been stabilized by the magnesium sulfate and Apresoline, induction is begun and vaginal delivery is attempted. Cesarean section is usually performed for obstetric indications only.

If the patient is diagnosed as having chronic hypertension rather than pre-eclampsia, she should still be admitted to the hospital if her diastolic blood pressure is 90 mm Hg or above. These patients do not require treatment with magnesium sulfate, unless, of course, they develop signs of pre-eclampsia (i.e., superimposed on their chronic hypertension). The mother and fetus remain at increased risk, and in-hospital evaluation of fetal parameters (i.e., estriol levels, fetal heart rate testing, ultrasound, fetal maturity studies) and maternal kidney function is justified. Treatment is begun with oral methyldopa (Aldomet) and Apresoline, and the pregnancy is prolonged as long as maternal and fetal conditions remain stable.

BLEEDING IN PREGNANCY

Vaginal bleeding during pregnancy is commonly discussed according to the stage of gestation during which it occurs. Spontaneous abortion is the most important cause of bleeding in early pregnancy, whereas later in pregnancy the serious causes of vaginal bleeding include abruptio placentae (placental abruption) and placenta previa.

Bleeding in Early Pregnancy

An abortion is traditionally defined as the birth of a fetus weighing less than 500 gm. Alternatively, the passage of a fetus of less than 20 weeks' gestation is an appropriate definition. Abortions are either spontaneous or induced. The incidence of spontaneous abortion has been estimated to be 10 to 20 percent of all pregnancies, however the true incidence is impossible to determine accurately because many early miscarriages are masked as part of a slightly irregular menstrual cycle.

Both fetal and maternal factors play a role in pregnancy wastage. Abnormal development of the fetus or placenta is the most common cause of early pregnancy loss. These spontaneous abortions, usually occurring in the first trimester, are associated with a high incidence of genetic defects and congenital anomalies that are incompatible with life. Maternal factors, including viral infections, endocrinologic disorders, and uterine malformations such as incompetent cervix and intrauterine septa, are more apt to be associated with second-trimester abortions. By and large, these infants are genetically normal.

By the time a patient in the first trimester of pregnancy presents with significant bleeding, the fetus has usually succumbed. The bleeding begins in the decidua basalis, and as it increases the expanding hematoma causes a dissection of the placenta from its myometrial attachment. The resulting irritation of the uterine musculature initiates contractions that eventually dilate the cervix and culminate in the passage of the products of conception into the vagina. Occasionally, the bleeding will be contained and no contractions will take place. This is referred to as a missed abortion.

Spontaneous abortions are classified as threatened, inevitable, incomplete, and complete. A threatened abortion is diagnosed when the patient complains of vaginal bleeding and mild cramps, yet has a cervical os that is closed. An inevitable abortion is one associated with definite uterine contractions and a dilated cervical os but with no passage of tissue into the vagina. Once any portion of the products of conception is seen at the external cervical os or in the vagina, an incomplete abortion has occurred. A complete abortion refers to the total passage of the fetus, membranes, and intact placenta from the womb.

When a patient complaining of vaginal bleeding is admitted to the emergency department, it should first be determined whether or not she is pregnant. Ectopic pregnancy must always be considered. Often the patient will know that she is in her first trimester. However, it is not infrequent that the pregnancy will be diagnosed for the first time by the emergency department physician. Once the pregnancy has been diagnosed, a detailed history of the patient's recent menstrual pattern, the character of her vaginal bleeding, and the quality of her pain, if any, should be elicited. Specific questioning regarding attempts at intrauterine manipulation is mandatory. Other common causes of vaginal bleeding (e.g., cervical erosion, polyps, vaginitis, trauma, and carcinoma) should be ruled out. The bleeding secondary to threatened abortion commonly begins as the spotting of dark thick blood and may remain as such for many days. A spun hematocrit affords a general idea of the amount of actual bleeding. As contractions become stronger, the passage of clots is common. Once tissue is passed (i.e., fetal parts, fetal membranes, or placenta), the bleeding increases and is bright red. The pain typically begins as suprapubic cramps and may involve the lower back. It is similar to severe dysmenorrhea and is not truly exacerbated by motion. Also, unlike ectopic pregnancy or PID, the abdominal examination is generally benign with normal bowel sounds and without the peritoneal signs of rebound tenderness, guarding, or rigidity. Fetal heart tones may be auscultated using a Doppler stethoscope.

Pelvic examination reveals a softened uterus enlarged to more or less the appropriate size for the period of amenorrhea. The fundus may be slightly tender. During the first trimester a corpus luteum may be palpated in one of the adnexa. Great care is necessary to distinguish an early threatened abortion with a palpable corpus luteum from an ectopic pregnancy. The cervix is cyanotic and softened, and may or may not be dilated. Fetal or placental tissue in the cervical os and vagina leaves little doubt as to the correct diagnosis.

Not all women with vaginal bleeding in early pregnancy progress to abortion. It is held that 20 percent of all women will bleed during early pregnancy, and only 5 percent of these will progress to spontaneous abortion. Therefore, if the patient is stable, the treatment for threatened abortion is conservative and expectant. There is no adequate evidence that treating these patients with either tocolytic (ritodrine, terbutaline, or isoxsuprine) or progestational agents improves fetal salvage. A majority of these pregnancies are genetically defective. With minimal bleeding and a stable hematocrit, the patient can be sent home on bed rest and vaginal rest. She should be instructed to return for reevaluation should fever, increasing abdominal pain, or vaginal bleeding or passage of tissue occur.

The treatment of inevitable, incomplete, and complete abortion is identical. An intravenous line using Ringer's lactate solution with 40 units of oxytocin (Pi-

tocin) per liter is established. The oxytocin increases uterine tone, facilitating the passage of remaining tissue and decreasing the amount of vaginal bleeding, thereby rendering uterine curettage safer and easier. A hematocrit is spun, and blood is obtained for an immediate CBC with differential and type and crossmatch. The patient is then admitted for dilatation and curettage. Even when a spontaneous abortion appears complete by clinical inspection, placental tissue and necrotic decidua may remain in the uterus and if not removed may incite a subclinical or overt endometritis with formation of intrauterine synechiae. Thus, all spontaneous abortions should be followed with a uterine curettage. The use of prophylactic antibiotics for noninfected spontaneous abortion is controversial. A hematocrit and blood type should be checked before hospital discharge. When the mother is Rh negative and unsensitized, she should receive 300 μg RhoGAM intramuscularly. In order to keep the uterus well contracted, it is a wise precaution to treat the patient with methylergonovine, 0.2 mg, orally every 8 hours for several days.

A patient who presents with fever and uterine tenderness has an infected abortion. As the infection spreads lower, abdominal peritoneal signs will be noted. It must be determined whether instrumentation has taken place. If so, cervical trauma and uterine perforation should be suspected. This is especially true if shock seems out of proportion to the amount of external hemorrhage. Shock coupled with hypothermia suggests gram-negative endotoxin as the etiologic factor. (See Chapter 7.)

Patients with septic abortion have virtually constant lower abdominal pain. The abdomen is distended, and palpation yields obvious peritoneal signs. Pelvic examination reveals a boggy and markedly tender uterus and parametrium. Cervical movement also causes exquisite pain, and a foul purulent discharge will be coming from the os. Should the patient be icteric and oliguric, clostridial infection must be ruled out.

Treatment of septic abortion must be aggressive. Intravenous lines and a CVP catheter should be placed. A hematocrit is spun, and a smear of peripheral blood is examined. Anemia associated with spherocytosis and evidence of intravascular hemolysis heralds clostridial infection. Blood is transfused as necessary. A Foley catheter is inserted, and a urinalysis is performed. Strict recording of intake and output is begun. As soon as possible an upright chest roentgenogram and flat plate of the abdomen are obtained in order to rule out free air under the diaphragm, intraperitoneal abscess formation, foreign bodies, or gas patterns consistent with clostridial infection.

The key treatment of septic abortion is the removal of all infected material from the uterus. Concurrent adequate antibiotic coverage is essential for optimal results. Broad-spectrum bactericidal antibiotics that cover β-streptococci, gram-negative species, and anaerobes should be chosen. Popular combinations include ampicillin with an aminoglycoside and clindamycin or very high doses of penicillin with chloramphenicol. In patients allergic to penicillin, erythromycin is the drug of choice for clostridial infection. Usually, a thorough uterine curettage will adequately remove the source of infection, allowing the antibiotics to take effect. However, hysterectomy may be necessary for clostridial infection, uterine perforation, or pelvic abscess formation.

Finally, a missed abortion is one in which no products of conception have been expelled from the uterus despite fetal demise. Diagnosis is based on the loss of fetal heart tones and a disappearance of the signs and symptoms of pregnancy. The patient reports loss of fetal movement, and the fundus is often smaller than anticipated. A brownish discharge may be coming from the cervix. The 2-minute immunologic urine pregnancy test may or may not remain positive. Real-time ultrasonographic screening for fetal heart motion has become an important adjuvant in the diagnosis of intrauterine fetal death and helps to differentiate this condition from molar pregnancy.

The greatest danger associated with missed abortion is a coagulation defect caused by the release of thromboplastins secondary to fetal autolysis. The defect is rarely seen within 6 weeks of fetal death. The patient should be thoroughly examined and an immediate platelet count and prothrombin time, partial thromboplastin time, and fibrinogen determinations obtained. She should be thoroughly questioned regarding any bleeding diathesis or new tendencies to bleed easily when bruised or brushing teeth, for example. If this history is positive or if the fibrinogen value is found to be less than 0.15 gm/100 ml, the patient should be admitted for evacuation of the uterine contents by means of suction curettage, intravaginal prostaglandin E_2 suppositories, or intravenous oxytocin, depending on the age of gestation and the state of the cervix. Fibrinogen replacement using cryoprecipitate may be necessary.

Bleeding in Late Pregnancy

The most serious causes of vaginal bleeding in late pregnancy are placental abruption and placenta previa. Other common causes of vaginal bleeding, such as polyps, bloody show, severe vaginitis, carcinoma, and cervical trauma secondary to intercourse or recent pelvic examination must be ruled out. It is crucial to understand that when a woman presents with vaginal bleeding in late pregnancy, a vaginal or rectal examination of the cervix is distinctly contraindicated and is indefensible in a setting in which provisions for immediate operative delivery are unavailable.

Placenta previa, which occurs once in every 200 pregnancies, is a condition in which placental tissue precedes the fetal presenting part. A total placenta previa is one in which the entire cervical os is covered by placental tissue. In a partial placenta previa a portion of the cervical os is covered. A marginal placenta previa occurs when the edge of the placenta is encroaching on the edge of the cervical os. Finally, a low-lying placenta is one that has implanted abnormally in the lower uterine segment. All of these conditions are more frequently encountered in multiparous patients and in patients who have previous incisions of the lower uterine segment.

The hallmark of placenta previa is painless vaginal bleeding after 20 weeks' gestation. As a pregnant woman approaches term, the previously irregular Braxton-Hicks contractions become increasingly more organized and cause a thinning of the cervix and lower uterine segment. This stretching causes the margins of a low-lying placenta to tear away from the uterine wall, resulting in maternal bleeding. The blood is free flowing and bright red. Commonly, the patient states that she was awakened by a sensation of wetness to find herself in a pool of blood. Although quite disconcerting, the first episode of bleeding is rarely fatal and usually stops spontaneously.

On physical examination, the uterus is soft and of normal tonus between contractions. The fundus is neither tender nor irritable. If labor is occurring, it is not hyperactive. An oblique or transverse lie of the fetus is usually discovered (via ultrasound or abdominal examination), and this is more common when the placenta occupies space in the lower uterine segment. Fetal heart tones are within normal limits (120 to 160 beats per minute) unless hemorrhage is severe. Under no condition is a vaginal examination permissible in the emergency department in order to "rule out" a placenta previa. Even the most gentle and carefully conducted cervical examination can result in torrential hemorrhage and exsanguination should a placenta previa exist.

Of all women presenting with third-trimester bleeding, fewer than one-half actually have placenta previa or abruption. Yet, the diagnosis of placenta previa must be initially based on history alone, and the pregnant woman near term complaining of vaginal bleeding must be admitted to the hospital until the definite diagnosis is established. If the maternal condition is stable, expectant management coupled with ultrasonographic localization of the placenta has proved safe and reliable in skilled hands. However, if the patient is in labor or bleeding profusely, a "double set-up" cervical examination is indicated. This procedure consists of surgical preparation and draping the patient on the operating room table for both a vaginal delivery and cesarean section. With the anesthesiologist and pediatrician present and the surgical team scrubbed and gowned, a careful cervical examination is performed. If placental tissue is palpated, the infant is delivered by immediate cesarean section.

The other main diagnosis that must be considered when a woman complains of third-trimester vaginal bleeding is placental abruption, or premature separation of a normally implanted placenta. This condition is encountered in approximately 1 percent of all pregnancies. Like placenta previa, abruption is more common in multiparous women and in gravidas over 35 years of age. A distinct correlation exists between placental abruption and hypertension during pregnancy.

Initially, retroplacental bleeding sheers the placenta away from the uterine wall. Usually, this expanding clot dissects between the membranes and the myometrium, resulting in external vaginal bleeding. This is not always the case, however, and an "occult" abruption is not uncommon. The clot eventually ruptures into the amniotic cavity, staining the amniotic fluid a "port wine" color. The bleeding also dissects into the uterine musculature, itself, separating the myometrial cells. This results in a uterus that is characteristically tender, irritable, and hyperactive. The resulting hyperactive contractility is associated with an increased uterine tonus between contractions. The patient complains of continuous, repeated contractions without relief. This is detrimental to the fetus, secondary to the lack of intravillous blood flow during periods of increased intrauterine pressure.

The expanding retroplacental clot and damaged myometrium result in the release of large quantities of thromboplastin into the maternal circulation. Disseminated intravascular coagulation may result. In addition, the expanding clot consumes maternal fibrinogen faster than it can be manufactured by the liver. The resulting "consumptive coagulopathy" coupled with disseminated intravascular coagulation renders severe placental abruption one of the most hazardous situations in obstetrics. Total renal shutdown may follow, resulting in either acute tubular necrosis or irreversible acute cortical necrosis. (See Chapter 63.) Fetal outcome is directly related to the amount of placental separation and the time from abruption to delivery.

Placental abruption is associated with mild to severe abdominal pain. Initially tearing in nature, the pain becomes continuous and severe. The uterus is quite tender and is boardlike and unyielding to palpation. It is irritable, and palpation alone stimulates hypertonic contractions and exacerbation of pain. Contractions appear to come right after each other, with no return to normal uterine tonus between them. Vaginal bleeding may vary in character and amount yet is usually less profuse than seen with placenta previa. The passage of

large clots is common. When the abruption is mild, the major concern is differentiating it from placenta previa. This can usually be accomplished after admission to the birth rooms via the double set-up examination described above. In the emergency department intravenous lines and a CVP catheter should be established. Blood is obtained for an immediate CBC and differential, a platelet count, and prothrombin time, partial thromboplastin time, and fibrinogen determinations. Fetal heart tones should be frequently auscultated. The fundus height is marked on the mother's abdomen, and the level is followed as an indication of intrauterine hemorrhage.

In the case of an obvious severe abruption, the fetal membranes should be immediately ruptured. The resulting reduction in uterine size serves to decrease bleeding and allows more efficient progress of labor. Cryoprecipitation is indicated for hypofibrinogenemia, and the loss of the other clotting factors is corrected with fresh-frozen plasma. Blood is transfused as indicated. Delivery should be by the most expeditious route, with most patients requiring immediate cesarean section. Vaginal delivery is preferred in patients with life-threatening coagulopathy and in cases associated with fetal death. In these latter circumstances, cesarean section is reserved for severe deterioration of maternal condition, usually associated with uncontrollable hemorrhage.

Postpartum Vaginal Bleeding

Vaginal bleeding in the postpartum period can be divided into immediate or chronic. Immediately post partum, vaginal bleeding is most often secondary to uterine atony, trauma of the birth canal, or retained products of conception. In the days and weeks following delivery, vaginal bleeding may persist or recur. This chronic postpartum bleeding is usually due to retained placental fragments or uterine subinvolution with some degree of infection.

Uterine atony should be suspected immediately as the cause of profuse vaginal bleeding shortly after the delivery of an infant at home or in the emergency department. Bimanual examination reveals a large boggy uterus filled with blood clots. A large-bore intravenous line should be immediately established, and Ringer's lactate solution with 40 to 80 units of oxytocin per liter should be infused at a brisk rate. In addition, bimanual uterine massage should be performed. Usually these methods are successful in stopping the hemorrhage and effecting strong uterine contractions. Ergonovine (Ergotrate), 0.2 mg, may be given intramuscularly. Rarely, if ever, is intravenous ergonovine indicated.

Once the uterus is firmly contracted the birth canal should be meticulously inspected for vulvar, vaginal, or cervical lacerations. Good lighting and adequate exposure are mandatory for optimal examinations. Large, deep vaginal and cervical lacerations are best treated by tight vaginal packing and immediate transfer to the operating room where conditions are more suitable for vaginal surgery.

Retained placental fragments may cause both immediate and chronic postpartum vaginal bleeding. A delivery taking place outside the hospital, manual removal of the placenta, and delivery of multiple fetuses are among the common situations in which portions of the placenta may remain in the uterus. Patients with retained secundines may have infection, in addition to bleeding, which may be characterized by a soft tender uterus, purulent vaginal discharge, and fever. As a preparation for definitive therapy in the operating room the patient should be given antibiotics intravenously. Broad-spectrum antibiotics that provide good gram-negative and anaerobic coverage are begun in the emergency department, and the patient is admitted for a uterine curettage.

Subinvolution refers to the lack of normal regression of uterine muscular hypertrophy that is expected during the first 4 to 6 weeks post partum. This condition is sometimes hard to differentiate from that discussed previously. The patient complains of passing blood clots from her vagina but is otherwise feeling fine. A large fleshy uterus is felt, which is only minimally tender. The condition is self-limiting and treatment consists of correction of blood loss, ferrous sulfate tablets, and oral oxytocics.

URINARY TRACT INFECTION/ PYELONEPHRITIS IN PREGNANCY

Among the most important changes during pregnancy are those affecting the urinary tract. A physiologic hydroureter develops early in pregnancy and continues until term. This is caused by the smooth muscle–relaxing properties of progesterone in combination with the weight of the gravid uterus impinging on the ureters. The tone of the bladder also decreases so that its total volume may double in pregnancy without causing discomfort or urgency.

In addition to these physiologic changes, asymptomatic bacteriuria is found in 4 to 8 percent of women in early pregnancy. If this condition is left untreated, 20 to 40 percent of these women will develop acute pyelonephritis.[2]

Thus, it is not uncommon for the pregnant patient to present with complaints and findings of cystitis and pyelonephritis. The pyelonephritis in pregnancy has a predilection for the right kidney. Diagnosis and management is only a little different than that of a nonpregnant patient, and only several key points require emphasis. (See Chapter 62.)

A clean catch urine specimen should be examined microscopically and a portion sent for culture and sensitivity. Catheterization is not justified because each manipulation carries with it a 4 to 6 percent incidence of subsequent cystitis. Treatment of uncomplicated urinary infection consists of a 7- to 10-day regimen of an oral sulfonamide or ampicillin. Over 90 percent of the usual urinary pathogens are sensitive to one of these two drugs. Follow-up cultures are mandatory. Sulfa-containing antibiotics should not be used during the last 4 to 6 weeks of pregnancy because they cross the placenta and compete with bilirubin binding sites, worsening neonatal hyperbilirubinemia. Pyelonephritis requires hospitalization, hydration, and treatment with intravenous antibiotics. Ampicillin and cephalothin (Keflin) are the usual drugs of choice. Premature labor has been associated with urinary tract infections, and labor should always be ruled out in these patients.

VENOUS THROMBOSIS

Pregnancy is associated with a hypercoagulable state characterized by an increase in serum levels of fibrinogen, the vitamin K–dependent clotting factors. Coupled with this is a generalized increase in venous distensibility, especially of the lower extremities. This is due both to hormonal changes and to the uterine enlargement of advancing gestation interfering with venous return. It is not hard to see why the most common vascular disease related to pregnancy is venous thrombophlebitis. If thrombophlebitis is undiagnosed, pulmonary embolism, an important cause of maternal mortality, may result. (See Chapter 58.)

In the nonpregnant patient, symptomatology is a poor reflection of the severity of thromboembolic disease and relates little to diagnosis of impending pulmonary embolism. In pregnancy, the diagnosis is even more difficult. Superficial venous distention of the lower extremities, leg pain, and edema are common in the gravid female and may obscure the diagnosis of early thrombophlebitis. In order to make the correct diagnosis, a high index of suspicion is necessary.

Despite the above, the initial clues in the diagnosis of thromboembolic disease are found in the history and early physical findings. Since symmetric involvement of the lower extremities is rare, any asymmetry in physical findings should arouse suspicion. The circumference at the ankles, midcalves, and midthighs should be compared.

The superficial veins, especially about the knee, may be dilated, and the leg may be erythematous and slightly warm. An indurated "cord" may be palpated. The Homans sign (leg pain or dorsiflexion of the foot) is of little diagnostic value, and the finding of calf tenderness is only slightly better. Doppler flow studies, performed in the emergency department, are becoming increasingly more important in the diagnosis and are highly reliable. If there is still doubt, the patient should be hospitalized for further diagnostic procedures, such as ascending phlebography.

Anticoagulation in pregnancy causes very real risks both to the mother and the fetus. Therefore, the diagnosis must be established with certainty before embarking on months of anticoagulant therapy. Whether or not the patient needs treatment will also affect her life style post partum, especially concerning breastfeeding and choice of contraception.

Immediate hospitalization with aggressive anticoagulation has been shown to decrease the maternal mortality from 12.8 to 0.7 percent.[3] Continuous intravenous infusion of heparin is the treatment of choice after initial diagnosis. This effectively prevents extension of the venous thrombus and recurrent pulmonary emboli. The main advantage of heparin is that it does not cross the placenta as do oral anticoagulants. Antibiotics are also indicated in most cases. Bed rest, leg elevation, warm moist heat, and elastic stockings are also beneficial.

HERPES GENITALIS

Herpes genitalis is a disease that commonly brings women to the emergency department with complaints of perineal pain. The disease caused by this DNA virus is divided into types I and II on the basis of differences in antigenic structure. Herpesvirus type I is usually contacted early in childhood and is responsible for over 90 percent of nongenital herpes lesions. Herpesvirus type II, on the other hand, is thought to be transmitted via sexual contact and causes well over 90 percent of genital herpetic lesions. (See Chapter 20.)

Some 80 percent of women become infected after having sexual contact with an infected partner. However, slightly more than three-fourths of these women will remain asymptomatic, making diagnosis difficult. The emergency department physician, having discovered a patient with genital herpes must answer two important questions: Is the patient pregnant? Is this the primary attack or a recurrent episode? The initial attack of herpes genitalis is usually of much greater severity than the recurrent episodes. It is characterized by vulvar, vaginal, and cervical vesicles or ulcers appearing 2 to 8 days following exposure. The most common initial symptom is a profuse watery vaginal discharge, leading to intense pruritus and pain on friction. Dyspareunia and dysuria are universal complaints. The dysuria, due to herpetic trigonitis and irritation with urine of the vulvar lesions, may be so intense that it results in acute urinary retention.

The vesicles usually rupture spontaneously, especially those around the vaginal orifice and labia minora where moisture is present. The vulva is typically erythematous, edematous, and tender. The ulcers are shallow and less than 5 mm in diameter. The edges are flat and not indurated. The crater is usually covered with a dirty yellow-white exudate that may become secondarily infected. Tender regional lymphadenopathy is present. Especially characteristic of the initial infection are the constitutional features that usually accompany the genital lesions. These include fever, headache, neuralgias, malaise, and myalgia.

The entire illness lasts from 7 to 10 days and is self-limiting. Exceptions to this are the pregnant patient and those with secondarily infected lesions in whom the illness may linger 4 to 6 weeks. It should be emphasized that not every patient with a primary herpes genitalis infection presents with all of these classic findings. The reason for this is thought to be that previous exposure to herpesvirus type I lessens the severity of subsequent type II infections.

Recurrent episodes of herpes genitalis are much less dramatic than the primary infection, probably owing to the development of antibodies. The area of perineal involvement is much less, lymphadenopathy is rare, and the constitutional symptoms are lacking. Still the patient is frequently miserable owing to vaginal discharge, dyspareunia, and dysuria.

The diagnosis of herpes is based on identifying the classic eosinophilic intranuclear inclusion bodies in material obtained from Papanicolaou smear or tissue scraping or by growing the actual virus in tissue culture. The Papanicolaou smear is easily performed and is highly diagnostic in the hands of an experienced cytopathologist. In addition to the Papanicolaou smear, the ulcer craters should be swabbed and scraped and any unruptured vesicles should be aspirated. Tissue biopsy may be helpful in ruling out other ulcerative lesions of the vulva. Serologic analysis is most helpful in differentiating primary from recurrent infection. Serum should be obtained for specific herpesvirus antibody titer at the time of initial diagnosis and 10 days afterward. An increase in the titer is seen with recurrent infection.

Treatment is symptomatic because no cure for herpes genitalis exists. Hot sitz baths and compresses are beneficial. A topical antibiotic and a local anesthetic, such as 1 percent oxytetracycline (Terramycin) cream, are indicated in infected cases. *Candida albicans* frequently coexists with herpes and should be treated with antifungal creams. The use of topical corticosteroids is distinctly contraindicated. A gonorrheal culture and a syphilis serologic test should be obtained with follow-up treatment, if indicated.

Hospital admission is advisable for patients with severe disease in whom urinary retention is common. A Foley catheter is inserted and urine is obtained for herpes culture. Phenazopyridine (Pyridium), two 100 mg tablets t.i.d., is useful in relieving dysuria. Formerly, painting the lesions with 0.1% neutral red dye followed by exposure to fluorescent light was used because of the dramatic symptomatic relief and decreased recurrence rate. Recently, however, investigation has suggested that there is oncogenic transformation of cells in tissue culture treated with photodeactivation, making this a form of treatment that is dangerous and inadvisable.

Herpes Genitalis in Pregnancy

Because herpes infection has a neonatal mortality of up to 75 percent, the diagnosis of herpes genitalis in a pregnant woman is vital. The usual route of neonatal infections is via passage through the birth canal. Thus, if there is good evidence of herpesvirus infection and intact membranes a prophylactic cesarean section is recommended. Several studies suggest that abdominal delivery is indicated when the membranes have been ruptured for less than 4 hours. Therefore, it is unwise to perform a vaginal examination on a woman with recently ruptured membranes and known herpesvirus infection for fear of carrying the organisms to the amniotic cavity.

LABOR/PREMATURE RUPTURE OF MEMBRANES

It is common for a pregnant patient, especially one with poor prenatal care, to present to the emergency department when she suspects that her membranes have ruptured or that she is in labor. Labor is characterized by uterine contractions that cause progressive effacement and dilatation of the cervix. The Braxton Hicks contractions in late pregnancy lead into a period of prelabor during which irregular uterine contractions of varying intensities occur. These uncoordinated contractions do not effect much cervical effacement or dilatation. Active labor, on the other hand, is diagnosed when regular strong contractions with intervals of 3 to 5 minutes produce cervical dilatation and effacement. At times the diagnosis of active labor may be difficult. The simplest method for establishing the diagnosis is to reassess the results of the cervical examination after several hours of observation in the emergency department or other appropriate setting.

Accurate diagnosis of ruptured membranes is always important, but it is especially critical in those patients presenting at 36 weeks' gestation or less. Most of the time the maternal history of an uncontrollable gush of clear fluid from the vagina and the finding of clear fluid with flecks of vernix coming from the cervical os make the diagnosis obvious. Frequently, however, the history is vague and the findings are equivocal. This is especially true near term when the increasing vaginal discharge leads many women to seek medical attention.

A correct approach to the diagnosis of ruptured membranes in patients 36 weeks pregnant or less is crucial to neonatal outcome. The preterm patient, or the patient with unsure dates, should never receive a digital vaginal or rectal examination in the emergency department when rupture of membranes is suggested. Of course, before the sterile vaginal examination is made one has to ascertain the well-being of the infant by hearing the fetal heart tones. This is especially important in alerting the physician to the possibility of a prolapsed cord. A speculum examination should be performed after the patient is thoroughly prepared (not vaginally) and draped under meticulously sterile conditions. The cervical os is visualized, and the presence of fetal small parts or prolapsed cord is ruled out. Any fluid coming from the os in the posterior fornix is tested in a sterile manner with nitrazine paper. This test is based on the fact that normally the vaginal pH is acidic, but amniotic fluid is alkaline. Thus, the latter turns the nitrazine paper a dark blue. However, blood and discharge due to severe vaginitis may also be alkaline and render the test unreliable. Therefore, every effort must be made to visualize fluid coming from the cervical os. When in doubt, one may ambulate the patient for several hours and repeat the test. In any case, once the diagnosis of ruptured membranes is confirmed, no digital examination of the cervix is performed for fear of carrying vaginal pathogens to the amniotic cavity and risking the development of premature labor or chorioamnionitis. Instead, the patient is hospitalized and her temperature, white blood cell count, and erythrocyte sedimentation rate are followed. She is treated expectantly until the fetus is mature, unless labor or signs of infection make intervention mandatory.

TRAUMA DURING PREGNANCY

Traumatic injury to the pregnant woman should be carefully evaluated with several considerations in mind.

- It must be remembered that the physiologic changes of pregnancy offer some protective measure to the mother. The increased blood volume (an increment of 50 percent by the 30th week of gestation) permits her to tolerate more blood loss than the nonpregnant patient. It is worth mentioning in this regard that the central venous pressure falls to one-third its usual level.

- Changes in the cellular components of the blood (e.g., the relative decrease in the hematocrit as well as the physiologic leukocytosis [as much as 50 percent]), should be acknowledged during the initial evaluation of these parameters.

- Changes in the urinary tract, hypertrophy of the kidneys, and dilatation of the calyces and the ureters should be considered when the urograms are interpreted.

- During the third trimester, in some patients when lying in the supine position the weight of the gravid uterus on the inferior vena cava hampers the venous return, leading eventually to decreased cardiac output and supine hypotensive syndrome, which has deleterious effects on both mother and fetus.

- Infections within the uterus are very serious and cannot be treated safely by antibiotics. Termination of pregnancy is necessary regardless of the stage of gestation.

- Fetal considerations should be adhered to if one is to protect its well-being. Maternal hypoxia as well as hypotension may cause very serious fetal deterioration, and one has to maintain an effective uterine blood flow as well as reasonable blood gases at all times. This would be of prime importance when one is correcting blood loss or during administration of anesthetics.

Fetal survival should be ascertained promptly in the emergency department and if there is any question one should freely consult the obstetric department. With modern tools, such as the use of Doppler and real-time ultrasonography to visualize fetal heart motion, this question can be resolved very quickly. In this regard, a proper evaluation of the fetal status is of prime importance in deciding further management. Electronic fetal heart rate monitoring could offer early assessment of its well-being. Analgesics can cause fetal depression; however, one cannot withhold necessary maternal treatment, especially if the delivery is not imminent. Aggressive management of fever is necessary since it is poorly tolerated by the fetus.

The gravid human uterus is by nature very vulnerable to irritation by physical stimuli. Therefore, injury to the abdomen may initiate active labor. Initially as well as periodically one has to evaluate the uterine activity to make an early diagnosis of this condition.

Ultrasonography has added immeasurably to the prenatal diagnosis for both fetal as well as placental status.

The presence of hematomas and retroplacental clots can be diagnosed. Proper consultation with competent personnel cannot be overemphasized.

Pelvic findings are crucial in deciding management. If the uterine cervix is open and delivery is imminent, prior arrangements with obstetricians and neonatologists can improve the survival of a premature infant. Statistics from today's intensive care nurseries are very encouraging, and one should not deny an infant this privilege at the time of delivery even if it is not within the delivery room of an institution.

Finally, combating infection with the proper antibiotics is essential, since in the gravid as well as the postpartum patient serious pelvic infections and septic shock are life threatening.

TABLE 64–1   Common Side-Effects of Drugs Used in Pregnancy

Drug	Side-Effects
Progestogens with or without estrogens and androgens	Masculinization of female fetus; vertebral, cardiac, limb defects
Diethylstilbestrol (DES)	Adenosis; clear cell cancer of cervix and vagina
Folic acid antagonists	Abortifacient; variety of degrees of congenital malformation
Alcohol	Fetal alcohol syndrome; intrauterine growth retardation
Salicylates	Achondroplasia; hydrocephalus; joint defects; cardiac lesion
Dextroamphetamines	Congenital heart disease; urogenital defects; limb deformities; cleft palate
Antiepileptic drugs Phenytoin Barbiturates	Hypoplasia of distal phalanges; diaphragmatic hernia; microcephaly; cleft lip
Narcotics	Fetal respiratory depression; addiction withdrawal syndrome
Diazepam (Valium)	If taken shortly before delivery may cause hypoactivity, hypotonicity, and hypothermia of fetus
Tetracycline, chlortetracycline, oxytetracycline	Stunting of bone growth; staining of deciduous teeth (greenish yellow-orange)
Streptomycin and aminoglycosides	Hearing impairment
Ampicillin	Decrease in maternal estriol levels in plasma and urine
Antithyroid drugs	Hypothyroidism of infant; neonatal goiter
Thiazide diuretics	Thrombocytopenia
Heavy cigarette smoking	Intrauterine growth retardation

DRUGS DURING PREGNANCY

Every drug given to the pregnant woman will potentially exert its effect on both the mother and the fetus (Table 64–1). Most drugs cross the placenta in varying degrees. Whether a drug should be administered to a pregnant woman depends more or less on its possible risks to the fetus and its value or necessity for treatment of the mother.

IRRADIATION DURING PREGNANCY

There is no safe level of x-irradiation to the fetus. Therefore, one must use sensitive pregnancy tests prior to ordering any diagnostic radiography for a woman who may be pregnant. One also should use ultrasonography to replace radiography as a diagnostic tool whenever possible.

An absorbed dose of 10 rads to the fetus at any time during gestation can be considered as a threshold for producing fetal pathology. Abdominal radiography can cause an exposure of 50 to 300 mrad/exposure. Fluoroscopy exposure results in 1 to 3 rads/minute.

REFERENCES

1. Pelvic Inflammatory Disease: United States. *Morbidity Mortality Weekly Rep* 28(51):606, 1980.
2. Kunin CM: *Detection, Prevention, and Management of UTI*, ed 2. Philadelphia, Lea & Febiger, 1972.
3. Villasanta U: Thromboembolic disease in pregnancy. *Am J Obstet Gynecol* 93:142–160, 1965.

BIBLIOGRAPHY

Breen JL: A 21 year survey of 654 ectopic pregnancies. *Am J Obstet Gynecol* 106:1004, 1970.
Clark DO: Gonorrhea: Changing concepts in diagnosis and management. *Clin Obstet Gynecol* 16:3, 1974.
Martin JD, Jr: *Trauma to the Thorax and Abdomen.* Springfield, Ill, Charles C Thomas Publisher, 1969.
Pritchard JA, MacDonald PC: *Williams Obstetrics*, ed 16. New York, Appleton-Century-Crofts, 1980.
Queenan JT: *Management of High Risk Pregnancy.* Oradell, NJ, Medical Economics Co, 1980.
Schroeter AL, Lucas JB: Gonorrhea: Diagnosis and treatment. *Obstet Gynecol* 39:274, 1972.
Swan KG: *Gunshot Wounds.* Littleton, Mass, PSG Publishing Co, 1980.

65. Rape and Sexual Assault

CARMEN GERMAINE WARNER, R.N., M.S.N., F.A.A.N.

Despite the achievements of emergency care throughout the past decade, patients of social and domestic violence continue to struggle alone. Adult men and women who are victims of rape represent a very special and unique emergency patient for several reasons:

First, their physical injuries may require careful and thorough assessment. Because of the probability of internal trauma, which is frequently unknown to the patient, it is imperative that a thorough evaluation be completed. The patient may not recall being injured and may even be unaware of pain.

Second, the patient is experiencing intense emotional injuries, all of which are very complex, and very real. Inappropriate responses are commonly noted and must be evaluated in concert with the total patient assessment. This presents a sensitive and frequently difficult situation as a result of a third factor—the personal feelings and reactions of emergency care personnel.

The intimacy and sensitivity of the rape situation, laced with evidence of considerable anger, fear, and hostility, produce a very emotional, potentially volatile environment. The need for empathic, thorough, gentle assessment is a challenge unlike that posed by any other patient.

MAGNITUDE OF THE PROBLEM

Statistical data on the incidence of rape reflect only those individuals who choose to report the crime. These data, known as the "crime rate," are the number of crimes per 100,000 vulnerable people. In essence, this rate may be classified as a "victim" risk rate. Unfortunately, this rate is primarily identified in terms of the risk for a woman and does not include potential male patients.

Several factors must be kept in mind when reviewing the following statistical data:[1,2]

- Reported forcible rape is rising faster than any other violent crime.
- Reported rape was up 166 percent over the past 15 years compared with an increase of 142 percent in assault and 19 percent in homicide.
- Forcible rape is one of the most underrated of all crimes.
- The "victim" risk rate that a woman may be raped in her lifetime is as high as 1 in 3.
- A rape is reported every 3 minutes.
- Approximately 560,000 rapes go unreported each year.
- In 1977 only half of all *reported* rapes resulted in arrest compared to two-thirds for assault and three-fourths for homicide.
- Of all adults arrested for forcible rape in 1977, 65 percent were prosecuted, 40 percent were dismissed or acquitted, 13 percent were found guilty of lesser offenses such as simple assault, and only 2 percent were found guilty of rape.

DEFINITIONS OF RAPE

Emergency care personnel, confronted with the possibility of testifying in court, are conscious of the various legal definitions of rape. These definitions vary from state to state and represent the profile of legislators along with the influence of patient advocates within each state. There are numerous working definitions of rape that may be identified. Some of these include the following:

- *Aggravated assault.* The perpetrator causes or attempts to cause serious physical and/or emotional injury to an individual, recognizing the seriousness of the act. This may be classified as a second-degree felony or a first-degree misdemeanor.
- *Attempted rape.* Actions taken by the perpetrator toward completion of an act of rape. The perpetrator must have been exposed and attempted to subdue and penetrate the victim, either male or female, but was unable to complete the act.
- *Indecent assault.* Touching the private parts of the body of a male or female, when the perpetrator recognizes this action may cause alarm. It includes contact with the genital area, breasts, or buttocks. This is a second-degree misdemeanor.
- *Involuntary sexual intercourse.* Forcible oral or anal intercourse with a male or female without consent, using threat of force, or when the individual is unconscious, mentally deranged, or under the age of 14. This is a first-degree felony.
- *Sexual abuse.* Sexual intercourse, marriage, or cohabitation with a blood relative without regard to the legitimacy of such acts. This is a first-degree misdemeanor.
- *Simple assault.* The perpetrator attempts to cause bodily harm or injury to a male or female. This is a third-degree misdemeanor.
- *Statutory rape.* Sexual intercourse between an individual 18 years of age or older with a male or female under 14 years of age. This is a second-degree felony.

Specific laws have addressed the various circumstances surrounding rape. Notation of legislative changes occurring throughout the United States are recorded in Table 65–1. These must be recognized, understood, and used in the testimony of patients who have become "victims" of such action. Rape is an extremely sensitive issue, and emergency care personnel must familiarize themselves with existing state interpretations.

Professionals may encounter situations they feel have not been specifically defined. These may refer to a situation resulting from a social relationship between two parties. It is most critical that under such circumstances emergency care personnel address *only* the presenting physical and emotional trauma and completely refrain from individual interpretation.

Factors involving a male or female who has been raped should be assessed with the same attitude as a patient experiencing chest pain. Emergency care personnel do not question whether the patient with chest pain really wanted this pain or whether they put themselves in this situation deliberately. Likewise, patients who have been raped rely on the support and guidance of personnel to assist them through this period of assessment and intervention. Only the patient and the perpetrator have the right to interpret and judge the situation, since they were the only ones present during the assault.

In today's society, it is common practice for unmarried individuals to enjoy sexual communication. This act constitutes an expression of giving and sharing, one of pleasure and fulfillment, not one of hostility, aggression, and violence. This is the critical difference that must be remembered. The pain, the fear, the humiliation, the terror, and the degradation of rape are feelings resulting from violence. Personnel must attempt to provide sensitivity, gentleness, and support in a manner that will restore the patient's belief and trust.

REDEFINING RAPE

In the past, rape has been defined emphasizing three separate factors: (1) carnal knowledge of a woman, (2) lack of consent to this carnal knowledge, and (3) use of force to accomplish the act. These factors were interpreted quite narrowly, with carnal knowledge being construed as penetration of the vagina by the man's penis; lack of consent construed as forcible resistance; and use of force considered to be physical violence or use of a weapon.[3]

Professionals recognized that these definitions were limiting and excluded many types of sexual assault. In an attempt to correct this, individual states have either broadened their definition of rape or eliminated certain traditional factors of rape. Examples of some of these changes include the following.

Form of Contact

Genital contact was previously noted as the only type of contact. Now states are recognizing contact between the genitals and the mouth or anus. *Penetration* has been expanded to include fingers, tongue, mechanical devices, and foreign objects. *Ejaculation* has almost completely disappeared in the definition of rape.

TABLE 65–1   Summary of Legislative Issues (1973 to 1976)

| Jurisdiction | New Legislation | Redefinition of the Crime | | | | | Revision of Proof Requirements | | | | Other Issues | | |
	Passed/ Proposed	Sex Neutral	Oral/ Anal	Degrees	Sexual Contact	Husband/ Wife Exclus.	Chastity Evid. Stand.	Chastity Evid. Proc.	Corrob- oration	Caution- ary Inst.	Victim* Com- pensation	C.J.S. Training	Privacy
Alabama	(X)	(X)	(X)	(X)	(X)		(X)	(X)	(X)				(X)
Alaska	X		X		X		X	X		(X)	X	X	
Arizona	(X)	(X)	(X)	(X)	(X)	(X)	(X)	(X)					
Arkansas	X	X	X		X			(X)			(X)		
California	X						X	X		X	X		(X)
Colorado	X	X	X	X	X		X	X		X	(X)		
Connecticut	X	X	X	X	X	X	(X)	(X)	X				
Delaware	X					X		X	X			X	
District of Columbia								X					
Florida	X	X	X				X	X		X	(X)		X
Georgia	X			(X)	(X)	(X)	X	X	(X)				X†
Hawaii	X			X	X			X			X		
Idaho	(X)		(X)	(X)			(X)	(X)	(X)				
Illinois	(X)			(X)			(X)	(X)			X	(X)	
Indiana	X	X	X	X			X	X					
Iowa	X	X	X	X		X	X	X	X	X	X		
Kansas	X	(X)				(X)	X	X			(X)		
Kentucky	X	X	X	X	X		X	X			X		
Louisiana	X		X	X			X						
Maine	X	X	X	X	X	X			X				
Maryland	X			X			X	X			X		
Massachusetts	X	X	X				(X)	(X)				X	(X)
Michigan	X	X	X	X	X	(X)	X	X	X				X
Minnesota	X	X	X	X	X	X	X	X	X	X	X	X	
Mississippi	(X)						(X)	(X)					
Missouri													
Montana	X	X			X	X	X	X					
Nebraska	X	X	X	X	X	X	X	X			(X)		
Nevada	X	(X)	(X)	(X)	(X)	X	X	X		X	X		
New Hampshire	X	X	X	X	X	X	X		X				
New Jersey	X			(X)			(X)	(X)	(X)		X	(X)	(X)
New Mexico	X	X	X	X	X	X	X	X	X				
New York	X					X‡	X		X		X		
North Carolina	(X)	(X)	(X)	(X)			(X)					(X)	X
North Dakota	X	X	X	X	X		X	X			X		
Ohio	X	X	X	X	X	X	X	X	X		X	X§	X
Oklahoma	X						X		X				
Oregon	X				X		X						
Pennsylvania	X	X				X	X	X	X	X		(X)	
Rhode Island	(X)	(X)	(X)	(X)	(X)		X‖	X‖					(X)

TABLE 65–1   Summary of Legislative Issues (1973 to 1976)—Continued

Jurisdiction	New Legislation	Redefinition of the Crime					Revision of Proof Requirements				Other Issues		
	Passed/ Proposed	Sex Neutral	Oral/ Anal	Degrees	Sexual Contact	Husband/ Wife Exclus.	Chastity Evid. Stand.	Chastity Evid. Proc.	Corrob- oration	Caution- ary Inst.	Victim* Com- pensation	C.J.S. Training	Privacy
South Carolina	(X)	(X)	(X)	(X)	(X)	(X)	(X)	(X)			(X)		X
South Dakota	X	X	X		X		X						X
Tennessee	(X)	(X)	(X)	(X)	(X)	(X)	X	X	(X)				
Texas	X	X	X	X			X	X	X		X		X
Utah	(X)					(X)	(X)	(X)			(X)		
Vermont	(X)	(X)	(X)	(X)	(X)	(X)	(X)	(X)	(X)				(X)
Virginia	(X)						(X)						X
Washington	X	X	X	X			X	X	X		X		
West Virginia	X	X	X	X	X		X						
Wisconsin	X	X	X	X	X	X	X	X			X		
Wyoming	(X)	(X)	(X)	(X)	(X)	(X)	(X)	(X)	(X)	(X)	(X)		(X)

(X) = Legislation proposed; X = legislation passed.

* This category encompasses victim payments under traditional victim compensation statutes as well as special medical services provided through local facilities.

† The Georgia privacy statute was declared unconstitutional.

‡ Rape charges between spouses in New York are referred to family court.

§ Ohio statute requires standard hospital protocol for evidence gathering.

‖ Restrictions promulgated by Rhode Island Supreme Court in 1975.

Source: Forcible Rape: An Analysis of Legal Issues. US Department of Justice, Law Enforcement Assistance Administration, National Institute of Law Enforcement and Criminal Justice, 1978.

Lack of Consent/Use of Force

This area has proved to be quite controversial since it is difficult to assess and interpret one's state of mind. There is minimal distinction between the resistance necessary to negate consent and the actions that may increase violence.

Certain changes reflect the recognition of circumstances that may be extremely dangerous, and the act is identified as a crime exclusive of the victim's state of mind. These include[4]:

- use of a dangerous weapon
- serious physical injury to the victim
- attempting the act during the commission of a felony, such as kidnapping or breaking and entering
- involuntary administration of drugs or alcohol to the victim, resulting in incapacitation
- reliance on the vulnerability of the victim, such as youth or special relationship
- use of threats of serious injury or death to the victim or a third person.

Degrees of Rape

Rape may include a plethora of criminal sexual activities, each of which may vary considerably. It is important to ensure proper punishment for the appropriate crime and to design a mechanism by which the reality of the crime is accurately reflected.

Several states have initiated such actions, identifying several degrees of rape and drafting rape laws allowing the less serious offense to be included within the most serious degrees of rape. This allows the flexibility of juries and prosecutors to make the appropriate decisions.

Penalties

Concomitant with the restructuring of degrees of rape is the need to examine the penalties prescribed. If legislature mandates a penalty that is too harsh, juries will return fewer convictions, hence the argument against statutes prescribing a life sentence for rape.

THE REALITY OF RAPE

The ugliness and devastating effects of rape can only be a reality to the patient and associated friends and family. Unless emergency care professionals have had the horror of rape invade their lives, it continues to remain "something that happens to the other person." Consequently, myths concerning rape continue to exist in the minds and practice of many individuals. Some of these myths include:

- The rapist is a sexually unfulfilled man carried away suddenly with an uncontrollable urge.
- Rapists are pathologically sick and perverted.
- Rapists are usually strangers to the victim.
- Rapes occur in dark alleys. So long as a person stays home, he or she will be safe.
- Raped individuals are at fault and probably provoked the attack.
- Rape is impossible without consent from the victim.
- Only people in lower socioeconomic classes get raped.
- Women report rape that is unfounded in order to seek attention.
- Every woman has rape fantasies.
- A woman cannot be raped by her husband.
- A hitchhiking man or woman encourages rape.
- Only young, beautiful women or promiscuous women are raped.
- Rape occurs primarily in large cities.
- Rapes are interracial.
- It is easy to prosecute rapists.
- Rape is a minor crime only affecting a few men and women.
- Rape is primarily a warm weather evening crime.

Fortunately, there are a number of factors attempting to dispel these myths. The media have made great commitments toward the investigation and presentation of factual data. Human service programs, universities and hospitals, and professional organizations have designed seminars to educate personnel concerning the realities of rape and the appropriate assessment and intervention. Upgraded reporting and management protocols, concomitant with utilization of sensitive listening personnel, encourage more rape patients to report the crime. Many of these patients include men, married women, and the elderly.

The bottom line reality is that *every man, woman, and child is a potential "victim" of rape.* Recognizing this, there is no way categories of "types of rape" patients could be identified other than being human.

EMERGENCY CARE MANAGEMENT

"The woman who is raped is doubly victimized . . . first by the attacker and again by the attitudes of society."[5] This is true with all stages of postrape intervention, but nowhere is potential invasion of self and dignity more immediate than in an emergency department. It is here that men and women reiterate the events of the rape incident; face the fact that his or her story may be doubted; feel subject to public scrutiny; wait for hours, frequently uninformed and alone; and are subjected to an embarrassing and potentially traumatizing physical examination.

Fortunately there are many emergency care personnel actively working to improve the assessment and intervention process for rape patients. This commitment has identified the health profession and its interaction with patients as a vital link in the overall community response to rape.

Medical-Legal Interaction

It is essential that emergency care personnel coordinate with the criminal justice system in order to encourage patients through gentle, supportive management to continue their coordination efforts throughout the follow-up and prosecutory process and ensure that proper evidence is collected and maintained.

Experience has proved that the evidence collected following a rape incident is frequently crucial in the successful identification and prosecution of the perpetrator. This medical examination—the initial contact the patient experiences with the system—has a profound effect on the response and cooperation displayed by the patient throughout the entire process.

As a means of assuring the completion of this integral first step, emergency care personnel must appreciate the value of protocol design along with personnel education and development.

Protocol Design

Recognizing the environment of a busy emergency department, the volume of emergencies handled, the rotation of personnel, and the sensitive issue of the rape itself, it is imperative that a standardized rape protocol be designed, developed, and implemented. Each facility, in respect of its potential diversification, should recognize and apply the following elements:

- Identify the facility's philosophy concerning management of rape patients.
- Outline specific goals and objectives of the proposed protocol.

- Clarify personnel responsibilities.
- Identify details of personnel communications and interactions.
- Establish a standard of excellence concerning assessment and intervention.
- Describe the structural parameters required for service delivery.
- Clarify the essential provisions to ensure proper emotional and physical management.
- Develop specific procedures required to ensure a complete and accurate medical record, proper collection of evidence, and maintenance of the chain of evidence.
- Outline ongoing requirements for continuing education.
- Incorporate an evaluation component for service delivery.

Personnel Education and Development

Concomitant with the design and implementation of a protocol is the need to standardize and upgrade the assessment and intervention of patients, along with the collection of evidence. This linkage is valuable for the following reasons: to identify the most appropriate and expeditious intervention for rape patients, to coordinate the specific protocol recommendations with actual levels of performance, and to establish a means through classroom performance to evaluate the protocol design.

The credibility of the course and its value to the participants is only as effective as its original planning, design, and implementation. In ensuring this credibility, there is a checklist of questions to be reviewed and answered. Some of these questions are noted in Exhibit 65–1.

Prehospital Care

The personnel who are the first to respond to the call of the rape patient establish the foundation for the continued ease of intervention. If the first responder is supportive, comforting, and expresses a willingness to listen, the rape patient will find it easier to develop an element of trust and will cooperate more fully with other medical and law enforcement personnel.

It is important to note that the initial reactions of the patient may vary greatly. Responses of both total hysteria and complete tranquillity have been recorded as reactions to the rape incident. Personnel should refrain from interpreting the patient's response, since each individual will react differently.

There are several key points to be remembered by the first responder:

- Attempt to comfort the patient.
- Secure the needed facts concerning the incident to enable appropriate support.

Exhibit 65–1 Rape Protocol Course Checklist

	Yes	No
1. Did the course design include input and participation from medical, law enforcement, and legal agencies, rape crisis centers, and social and mental health agencies?	______	______
2. Is the course designed to reinforce previous learning or provide new information?	______	______
3. Does the course material coincide with the level of expertise of the proposed participants?	______	______
4. Have you assessed the needs and attitudes of each potential student?	______	______
5. Has the program design included a philosophy, goals and objectives, conceptual framework, course curriculum, learning resources, facilities and equipment, pre-tests and post-tests, an evaluation component, and an up-to-date reading list?	______	______
6. Were participants involved in establishing the appropriate course hours, frequency, and scheduling?	______	______
7. Are participants in agreement with the arrangement for time off, CEUs, cost of materials, faculty remuneration, and employee compensation?	______	______
8. Are the instructors qualified to conduct the course?	______	______
9. Were key administrators or board members invited to comment on the program?	______	______
10. Has the course been opened to personnel from other facilities?	______	______
11. Has the course been designed to specifically link to the protocol?	______	______
12. Has an official education course been written to ensure the availability of repeated material?	______	______
13. Has a time schedule been designed for additional and ongoing courses?	______	______

- Relate the importance of reporting the incident to law enforcement officials, if they have not already been contacted.
- Inform law enforcement officials if need be.
- Activate all efforts to preserve the evidence. Therefore, make certain that the patient does not change clothing, eat, drink, take any medications (e.g., a tranquilizer), gargle, brush teeth, urinate, defecate, shower, or delay getting to the emergency department. (If the patient is informed of the value of this request, but insists he/she must clean up, this request should be respected.)
- Assess physical injuries and perform essential intervention.
- Assist the patient in contacting family or friends if desired.
- Initiate first-stage crisis intervention.
- Establish communication with the nearest emergency department or contract facility for rape patients.
- Accompany the patient to the medical facility.
- Check with admitting.
- Establish rapport with the emergency department nurse who will be coordinating ongoing care.

The first responder may choose to remain with the patient for a short period of time. This is recommended whenever possible as a means of facilitating a positive and comfortable transition, relating appropriate information concerning the patient and his or her condition, and ensuring that the patient will not be left alone in the examining room.

Emergency Department Response

Rape is a serious crime of assault on the body but more grievously on the psyche of the patient.[6] Despite the fact that the rape incident may not be physically life threatening, the psychological and sociological implications may indeed be life threatening as far as emotional stability is concerned. The initial interaction with emergency care personnel is equally important as that with the first responder. Specific guidelines of an adopted protocol are to be respected as just that—"guidelines." The needs and fears of each patient may vary. If adamant opposition to certain procedures arises, they must be thoroughly explained regarding eventual patient-perpetrator outcome. Should the patient maintain a continued stand against the procedure, the right of the patient must be respected.

A specific example might relate to the consent forms. Emergency departments must obtain written permission in order to conduct a physical examination and to collect physical evidence. Recognizing the trauma of rape, patients may refuse a pelvic examination for fear of pain or recollection of the event. They may agree only to attention to physical emergencies. If this occurs, personnel should attempt to clarify the value and purpose of physical evidence; yet the patient must never be forced or made to feel guilty.

The emergency visit, although difficult for the patient, family, and personnel, can be made easier for everyone if protocol guidelines are followed and if the patient is explained everything in complete detail prior to initiation of the procedure.

Management Philosophy

The emergency department philosophy should be designed to enable personnel to provide assessment and intervention to the rape patient as a total person, assign rape patients priority over all admissions except urgent and life-threatening emergencies, and collect physical evidence to substantiate a possible charge of rape/sexual assault in court.[7] It should be noted that all evidence collected in a criminal case is automatically the responsibility of the local law enforcement agency. Under normal circumstances, when law enforcement officials are present, emergency care personnel are to turn all evidence over to the responding agency. Should law enforcement officials be absent, emergency department personnel must properly preserve the evidence until officials arrive. It is also important to instruct and explain to the patient about each procedure, its purpose, steps, and anticipated results.

Special Patient Considerations

Despite the fact that continuity of care will be administered by one nurse, one physician, and one social worker, it is important for all emergency care personnel to administer the following considerations as the opportunity arises:

- Ensure immediate attention to every rape patient, guiding them to a private examining room. Even in the presence of life-threatening emergencies, someone should ensure that the patient is comfortable and relate the reason for any possible delay.
- Make arrangements for family and/or friends to be with the patient if desired.
- Identify the patient by proper name or a preassigned code name to protect him or her from further humiliation.
- Notify the physician and triage nurse of the patient's arrival.
- Recognize the chart as legal evidence and record accurately all statements, procedures, and actions.
- Inquire if the patient has pain or bleeding that might require immediate attention.

- Provide maximum emotional support and reduce any potentially traumatizing actions or statements.
- Advise the patient that a rape crisis advocate is available should contact be desired.
- Supply the patient with informational material concerning follow-up instructions, a list of community resources, and a voluntary evaluation form. The patient is not to be expected to read this material in the emergency department, but encouraged to look at it later in a comfortable setting.
- Notify the hospital social service department of the patient's arrival.

Responsibilities of Emergency Care Personnel

Emergency department rape protocols may vary depending on the design of each facility, while keeping in mind the ultimate privacy, safety, and support of each patient. Some of the functions to be addressed in a protocol include:

- Admit the patient in the privacy of a specially designed rape examination room.
- Explain the entire assessment and intervention procedure, allowing ample time for questions and answers.
- Recommend that the patient remain dressed in his or her own clothes until the examination begins.
- Serve as a liaison between family, friends, and the patient.
- If the patient desires the presence of a friend or family member during the examination, aid them

in the decision of whom to request. (Someone who is visibly disturbed may upset the patient.)
- Inquire whether the patient (if female) has children and, if so, how they are being cared for. If these children need attention, secure assistance from social service, law enforcement personnel, or family members.
- Assess if sedation or counseling is appropriate for those accompanying the patient.
- Secure the evidence collection kit and the examination set, placing them in the examining room, out of view, until the examination begins.
- Maintain the presence of a nurse throughout the assessment and intervention process.
- Carefully explain all procedures.
- Complete all labels, the examining reports, evidence envelope labels, and envelopes with patient information.
- Inquire as to patient's familiarity with pelvic and/or rectal examinations.
- Assess the patient's ability to tolerate these examinations physically and psychologically.
- Observe, collect, and preserve the patient's clothing as noted in Exhibit 65–2.[8]
- Collect urine samples for possible alcohol or drug use, even if not suspected.
- Assist with any photographs that are needed.

History

Obtaining an accurate verbal history of the rape is essential, not only for the strengthening of a legal case but also for the protection of the patient's well-being and integrity. Unfortunately, recollection is similar to

---

Exhibit 65–2 Care of Rape Victim's Clothing

1. Note clothing and record observations on chart.
2. Examine all clothing for soilage, tears, or presence of blood or semen.
3. Arrange for fresh clothing to be brought to the emergency department, should the patient's clothes need to be collected.
4. Collect patient's underwear. *Do not crumple*—place loosely in ample-sized paper container.
5. Attempt to air dry wet evidence. *Do not fan dry or use heat.*
6. Circle wet marks with laundry marker to circumscribe the evidence.
7. Place clean paper over stain and place in clean container. Do not allow stained areas to contact clean areas.
8. If female patient is menstruating, collect the tampon or sanitary napkin.
9. Place appropriate clothing in separate individual bags, seal properly, and mark with collector's initials and date.
10. Record on chart who collected the clothing and who it was turned over to.
11. All clothing used as evidence should be forwarded to appropriate scientific laboratory by law enforcement personnel.

Source: Warner CG, Koerper MJ, Spaulding D, et al: San Diego County protocol for the treatment of rape and sexual assault victims. City of San Diego, California, Fall 1978, p. 14.

reliving the entire event, and the patient may be reluctant to participate in the interview.

There are several alternatives that may assist the patient through this process. First, the rationale and value of the history should be slowly and clearly outlined. Frequently, a gentle hand and a supportive nature will gain the cooperation required. Second, the medical history, physical assessment, and collection of evidence may be conducted by the physician, with the history of the rape incident being recorded when the patient has become more stable. Finally, the rape history, usually recited once each for law enforcement, medical, and social service personnel, could be combined, with the essential information being tabulated by one person and disseminated appropriately. The historical data to be obtained is outlined in Table 65–2.

Physical Examination

Concern has been raised related to the gender of the examining physician. Some professionals feel the need for a woman rather than a man, thus minimizing potential fear. It has been proved that the sex of the examining physician is irrelevant; it is the personal attentiveness and interaction that are critical. In fact, it is valuable for the female patient to experience the immediate interaction with a supportive, understanding man. This greatly aids in diminishing the "fear of men" these patients often develop. All portions of the physical examination should be performed with special attention to the avoidance of pain, trauma, and further humiliation.

Each phase of the examination should be initiated with a step-by-step explanation. This is essential for the ultimate emotional well-being of the patient. In addition, the patient should not be requested to undress or be placed in stirrups until just prior to the examination. Considerations for a physical examination are noted in Table 65–3.

Medical, Physiologic, and Legal Laboratory Tests (Evidence Collection)

This portion of the examination is vital. The potential for legal pursuit is enhanced or destroyed as a result of proper, careful, and accurate collection and documentation of the results of medical tests and the collection and preservation of evidence.

There are numerous medical tests that need to be

TABLE 65–2   Rape and General History

Health History	Personal History: Female	Personal History: Male and Female	Rape History	Postrape History
Current immunizations (primarily tetanus)	Reactions to estrogens	Present venereal disease	Time, day, and date	Recall of:
Recent illness, injury, or surface or internal trauma (past month)	Current practice of birth control	Past venereal disease	Physical surroundings (e.g., sand, grass, leaves, flowers, water)	Gargling
Prescribed medications	Previous or current sterilization	Present or past rectal bleeding or discharge	Physical forms of violence	Brushing teeth
History of sickle cell anemia	Early signs of pregnancy	Present or past lacerations or sores in the mouth	Weapon(s) used	Vomiting
Any medication, topical, or food allergies	Most recent consensual intercourse or sexual activity		Restraint(s) used	Douching (if female)
	Past pregnancies		Verbal forms of violence	Urinating
	Viable children		Threats of violence	Defecating
	Recent gynecologic injury or surgery		Blindfolds used	Taking an enema
	Last menstrual period		Number of perpetrators	Bathing
	Wishes regarding hormonal pregnancy prevention, abortion, or menstrual extraction		Forced use of alcohol and/ or drugs	Changing clothes
	Present or recent vaginal infection		Loss of consciousness	Washing hair
			Fondling	Eating
			Vaginal entry or approach	Drinking
			Oral entry or approach	Taking medication
			Anal entry or approach	
			Forced to perform lewd acts	
			Ejaculation, urination, or defecation on body (be specific)	
			Use of condom or lubricant	
			Did perpetrator claim to be sterile?	

TABLE 65–3　Considerations of Physical Examination

General	Female Genitalia	Male Genitalia	Rectal
Note patient's general demeanor and emotional state.	Carefully examine the vulva, noting signs of trauma or foreign matter, semen, dirt, grass, or pus.	Examine penis for signs of trauma, foreign material, or infection.	Examine area for signs of trauma.
Record vital signs.		Examine scrotum for signs of trauma or foreign material.	Assess presence of lubricant, blood, semen, pus, or any foreign matter.
Assess physical appearance.	Gently examine introitus and hymen for signs of trauma.		Gently examine the rectum for possible trauma, placement of foreign objects, and internal lacerations and bleeding.
Examine skin (collect and label any foreign material such as seminal stains, botanical material, grass, plastic, paper, or blood).	Very carefully assess vaginal area for trauma, signs of foreign objects, or internal lacerations and bleeding.*		
Assess upper trunk, noting breast trauma and sexual maturity.	Gently inspect cervix for evidence of parity, signs of pregnancy, presence of menstruation, evidence of trauma, and signs of infection.		
Examine lower trunk for signs of trauma, noting sexual maturity.	Perform general pelvic assessment.		
Note extremities for bruises, fractures and sprains, and scratches.	Palpate uterus rectally.		
Record head and neck trauma including mouth, ears, and scalp. Collectible evidence may be secured from mouth, hair, or other orifices.	Utilizing a Wood's light (ultraviolet),[†] note signs of semen around the perineal area.		

* It is critical that water be used to lubricate the speculum rather than a lubricant to prevent altering the results of the acid phosphatase test.
[†] Obtain photographs as necessary.

run in both the assessment and the intervention stages of the patient examination. These tests include:

- gonorrheal cultures (Papanicolaou smear, oral and rectal specimens)
- syphilis test (blood test)
- evidence of sperm/semen
- follow-up test for syphilis
- follow-up test for gonorrhea (Papanicolaou smear, oral and rectal specimens)
- radiography for any physical injuries
- "morning after" medication to prevent pregnancy
- follow-up test for pregnancy
- follow-up test for injuries
- other unspecified tests (e.g., to assess internal injuries).

The collection of physiologic samples should be a routine part of the evidence collection procedure. Both blood and urine samples are to be collected according to proper hospital procedure. Special considerations given to the collection of blood and urine include blood grouping, medication and alcohol assessment, VDRL, serum test for pregnancy (β-human chorionic gonadotropin [β-HCG]), and collection of urine for medication assessment and pregnancy testing.

All evidence collected in a case of rape is automatically the responsibility of local law enforcement officials, despite the fact that it is collected by emergency care personnel. Under normal circumstances, all evidence is turned over to law enforcement personnel. If law enforcement officials are not present, the evidence

should be properly preserved until law enforcement officials arrive. This preservation should not exceed 6 hours. In all rape cases, the information noted in Exhibit 65–3 will be collected by the responding emergency physician.

Evidence collection kits may vary from facility to facility, but the important consideration is that the kit remain standardized. It should maintain all the essentials required for proper collection of evidence and should be prepared and readily available at all times. A sample of an evidence collection kit is noted in Table 65–4.

The chain of evidence is referred to as the custody of evidence.[10] Evidence collected by emergency care personnel in the previously mentioned medical, physiologic, and legal tests is essential for assessment and management of the rape patient, in addition to establishing a basis for legal prosecution. Despite the value of this evidence, it becomes invalid unless the following steps are activated:

- Record each step of the collection process.
- Maintain continuity of evidence transmission, ensuring that the proper samples are delivered and received.
- Label each piece of evidence with the patient's name; hospital number; day, date, and time of collection; specific material collected and from where; the collector's name; and to whom the evidence was delivered.
- Recognize that some tests, such as a Papanicolaou smear, pregnancy test, and tests for syphilis and gonorrhea, are medical procedures and must be

Exhibit 65–3 Legal Tests (Properly Identified)

Foreign materials on body and hair
Foreign matter such as seminal stains, blood, and other organic or synthetic materials located on the skin and hair should be collected, packaged, and properly labeled.

Head hair
Hair must be plucked or trimmed according to protocol.

Saliva (for blood group antigens)
In collecting saliva samples, obtain the specimen on the paper disk or swabs provided.

Oral swab (for sperm in cases of oral copulation)
This evidence will provide the most valuable results if collected from the upper and lower teeth along the gumline.

Nail scrapings (for foreign material)
Although this is not a mandatory procedure and may not always prove useful, skin tissues or other identifiable materials may be obtained from under the patient's fingernails.

Perineal area (for foreign material)
Foreign material, blood, or lubricant should be collected and properly packaged and labeled.

Pubic hair combings (for foreign material)
A towel should be placed beneath the patient, allowing him or her to comb the area, collecting any loose hairs.

Pubic hair trimmings or pluckings
Each protocol may vary with respect to the number of hairs required. Also controversy exists with the need to retraumatize the patient by plucking pubic hairs in the emergency department or to secure them later if specific proof is required.

Vaginal swabs (see Figure 65–1)
Using two swabs, collect evidence from the vaginal orifice, placing it in the proper container. Use two additional swabs for obtaining evidence from liquid poolings deep within the vaginal vault. Use these swabs in making slides for sperm motility. Add saline to prevent evidence from drying out and examine immediately under a high-powered microscope.

Specific considerations should be taken to test for:
- sperm motility and morphology
- acid phosphatase
- blood group antigens

Vaginal aspirants (see Figure 65–1)
This represents collection of evidence from the deepest possible source. Clear plastic tubing and a 10-cc syringe are used to collect the fluid directly.

Vaginal washings
Normal saline (10 cc) may be used to wash the vaginal vault if sufficient material is not available through other means.

Anal swabs
This is a critical part of the evidence collecting process. Since many patients are uncomfortable admitting sodomy has occurred, inquire whether or not there has been anal penetration.

Penile shaft swabs (for suspect only) (see Figure 65–2)[9]
In male suspects when appropriate, examine for vaginal epithelium or fecal stains.

Penile urethral swabs (for suspect only) (see Figure 65–2)[9]
In male suspects when appropriate, secure a Gram stain and culture for gonorrhea.

Clothing handling and preparation
Assessment should be made for foreign matter, semen, blood, or other secretions. Refer to Exhibit 65–2 for specific handling.

Photography
Signs of physical trauma can be permanently recorded. This is not required by all protocols.

processed in the hospital, while all others are transferred to law enforcement officials.[10]
- Be familiar with crime laboratory proceedings and their requirements.

This cooperative effort displayed by emergency care personnel will not only aid personnel but also directly benefit the patient and the patient's family.

Emergency Department Intervention

In essence, this phase of the response may begin at any stage of the examination when issues concerning

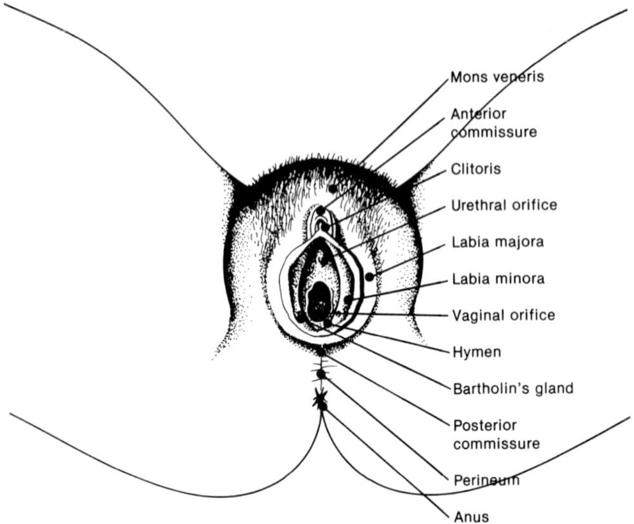

Figure 65–1 Female External Anatomy. (*Source:* Warner CG, Koerper MJ, Spaulding D, et al: San Diego County Protocol for the Treatment of Rape and Sexual Assault Victims. City of San Diego, Calif, Fall 1978, p 28.)

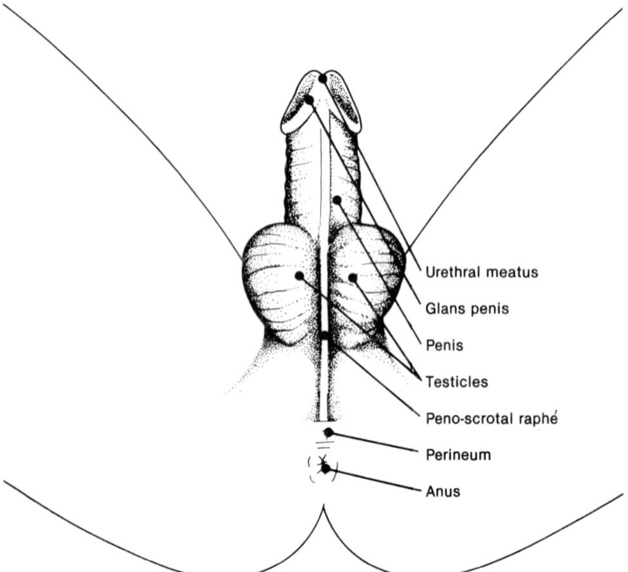

Figure 65–2 Male External Anatomy. (*Source:* Warner CG, Koerper MJ, Spaulding D, et al: San Diego County Protocol for the Treatment of Rape and Sexual Assault Victims. City of San Diego, Calif, Fall 1978, p 50.)

physical injuries, venereal disease, possible pregnancy, or psychologic difficulties arise. It is imperative that all emergency care personnel share responsibilities, affording the best possible care to the patient throughout his or her stay. Specific notation should be made to initiate the following measures prior to specific intervention.

TABLE 65–4   Evidence Collection Kit and Related Materials

Test	Equipment
Record of rape and personal history	Appropriate forms
Collection of clothing	Paper bags
	Butcher paper
	Labels
Physical examination	Appropriate forms
Urine for pregnancy test and drug test	Two containers
	Labels
Fingernail scrapings	Fingernail file
	Envelope
	Label
Saliva sample	Paper disk or swabs
	Envelope
	Label
Blood samples	Tourniquet
	Gauze pad (nonalcohol)
	Syringe (20-cc)
	Needle (21-gauge)
	Gray, red, and lavender top tubes
	Labels
Pubic hair combings	Plastic comb
	Towel
	Envelope
	Label
Pelvic exam (Papanicolaou smear)	Gloves
	Lubricant
	Speculum
	Cervical scraper (Ayre stick)
	Two slides
	Fixative
Vaginal swabs	Four cotton swabs
	Two plastic containers
	Saline
	Two glass slides
	Labels
	Pencil
Vaginal washing	Normal saline, 10 cc
	Aspiration pipette and bulb
Microscopic examination for sperm motility	Microscope
	Slides
	Slide covers
	Vaginal swabs
	Normal saline
Photography (optional)	Camera
	Film
	Flash cube

- Explain the concept of venereal disease and the importance of its treatment.
- Outline the value of pregnancy testing when applicable.
- Identify every phase of the examination procedure prior to initiating it.
- Explain each step of the examination as initiated.
- Assess the presence and severity of wounds, contusions, lacerations, abrasions, internal injuries, and the extent, degree, and location of pain.
- Identify acute anxiety reactions.

Venereal Disease Prophylaxis. The patient must be fully informed about the possibility of having contracted a venereal disease and the possible modes of treatment. It is essential to explain that there is evidence that 1 to 3 percent of all "victims" of sexual assault will contract venereal disease as a result of the assault and that up to 3 percent will prove to have unrecognized, established venereal disease.[8] The patient should be reassured with information regarding proved treatment and agencies available for follow-up care. The patient must be reminded that venereal disease can be transmitted through all mucous membranes (oral, genital, and anal) and that sexual relations are not safe until it has been determined whether or not a venereal disease was contracted or that prescribed treatment has been successful.

If the patient chooses to be treated for venereal disease or if personnel choose to provide care as a precautionary measure, it should be noted that in females, antibiotic therapy may disrupt the normal balance of bacterial organisms in the vagina, resulting in a yeast infection. One must also consider that the rape may have produced genital tissue irritation or the perpetrator may have transmitted something other than gonorrhea or syphilis (e.g., trichomoniasis, genital herpes, venereal warts, or crabs).

The patient must be informed that urinary tract infections can result from irritation or injury and that intercourse may become painful. Encouragement to seek medical attention should these problems develop is important.

Specific treatment for venereal disease is noted in Table 65–5.

TABLE 65–5   Gonorrhea and Syphilis Prophylactic Treatment

Gonorrhea	*Syphilis*
Probenecid, 1.0 gm orally, followed in 30 minutes with aqueous procaine penicillin G, 4.8 million units intramuscularly	(Prophylactic treatment not recommended) Benzathine penicillin G, 2.4 million units intramuscularly
Ampicillin, 3.5 gm orally, with probenecid, 1.0 gm orally	If allergic to penicillin: Tetracycline hydrochloride, 500 mg orally four times a day for 15 days or Erythromycin 500 mg, orally four times a day for 15 days
If patient is allergic to penicillin: Tetracycline hydrochloride, 1.5 gm orally stat and 500 mg orally four times a day for 4 days	
Spectinomycin hydrochloride, 2.0 gm intramuscularly	*Note:* Advise patient to have a repeat VDRL in 4 to 6 weeks.
Note: Advise patient to have a repeat examination in 7 to 10 days.	

Pregnancy. There is a 1 percent chance that a woman may become pregnant as a result of the attack.[10] Specific considerations must be taken by emergency care personnel concerning these patients.

The patient's capacity to become pregnant must be established by obtaining the following information:

- Is she sterile?
- Has she had a tubal ligation or hysterectomy?
- Has she reached the age of menarche or passed menopause?

If pregnancy is possible, determine:

- On what day of her cycle did the rape occur?
- What is the length of her regular cycle?
- What present methods of contraception, if any, are being used?

If she is currently pregnant (2 to 3 percent of women who are raped will prove to already be pregnant at the time of the attack[8]), this needs to be clarified through a pregnancy test in the emergency department. Pregnancy can be determined through a urine sample (accurate only after 4 weeks of pregnancy) or through a newer serum test (β-HCG) that detects pregnancy following 1 week of pregnancy.[10]

If the patient becomes pregnant, there are four alternatives:

1. β-HCG administered on the day of the physical examination. The results of this test will not return for 2 weeks, which is when the patient is to return for her checkup. If, on return, the test is positive, it signifies that the woman was already pregnant at the time of the rape. If the test results are negative, repeat the β-HCG test. Should the results after the second test be positive, it indicates that the patient probably became pregnant as a result of the rape and a suction curettage may be offered to the patient as an alternative.
2. Intravenous conjugated estrogens (Premarin), 25 mg, repeated once after 12 hours. There has been some associated nausea and vomiting, although considerably more compliance than diethylstilbestrol (DES).
3. The morning-after pill (DES). This alternative has very little compliance since 60 percent of the patients discontinue taking the medication following 2 to 3 days of nausea and vomiting.
4. Abortions or a menstrual extraction. (This is discussed in the follow-up care section later in this chapter.)

Psychological Reactions. It is vital that all people assisting or questioning a victim immediately after a sexual assault recognize that the patient is undergoing *legitimate* psychological reactions. Characteristics of the reactions may differ from person to person. However, psychological trauma is almost always present and must be treated along with medical and evidentiary examinations.

Approaching the patient in a caring manner, providing a safe, supportive environment, and legitimizing his or her experience will facilitate the process to follow and aid in restoring balance and mental health.

Rape creates an immediate and unanticipated crisis in the life of the patient. Mental disorganization that helps a patient psychologically survive the ordeal usually occurs. This may be manifested by inconsistencies in the patient's story, incoherence in speech, confusion of numbers, and loss of sense of time sequence. Shock and disbelief, which are similar to that suffered by victims of automobile accidents and natural disasters, may be characterized by one of two different styles of reactions:

1. The *expressed* style in which the patient is showing outward signs of fear, anger, and anxiety. Behavior may include sobbing, crying, restlessness, and tenseness.
2. The *controlled* style in which feelings are masked with a seemingly calm, composed or subdued affect. For instance, the patient may answer questions in a matter-of-fact manner or smile or laugh inappropriately.

In cases that were documented by Burgess and Holstrom,[11] about half the victims reacted with the expressed style and about half with the controlled style. It is important to keep this in mind since emergency and law enforcement personnel may mistake the patient with a controlled reaction as not telling the truth because he or she does not appear to be upset. Also, nervous laughter may lead some personnel to the assumption that the patient is not to be taken seriously.

Both law enforcement and emergency personnel must be able to recognize these shock reactions as normal and reassure the patient. People who first come in contact with the patient after a rape play an important role in the patient's eventual resolution of the rape trauma syndrome. A negative interchange may delay mental reorganization, whereas a positive, supportive interchange will facilitate not only moving through the process at hand (i.e., examination and investigation), but also the patient's future ability to deal with the rape.

All too often, when confronted with a difficult emotional situation, personnel react in one of the following ways:

- appearing extremely busy—running in and out of the room without communicating verbally with the victim
- leaving the patient completely alone—finding it easier to deal with rape by avoiding it
- relating to the patient on a very unemotional level—avoiding any possibility for touching, holding, or caring.

These are common avoidance reactions of personnel to patients. Refraining from the use of certain modes of communication will prove valuable, save time, and prevent misunderstandings. A few common communication barriers are:

- making premature comments and evaluations
- making statements that are too general
- interrupting the patient or family
- talking instead of actively listening
- talking down to patient and family
- asking loaded questions
- placing the blame
- arguing
- displaying irritating listening habits
- repeatedly telling the patient and family what to do.

It is important to establish good communication and let the patient know that attending personnel are caring and supportive. The following are some suggestions for personnel to keep in mind during the initial contact with the patient.

- Help the patient get in touch with his or her feelings. The patient may feel angry, depressed, guilty, dazed, or numb—these are all legitimate reactions. The expression of feelings at this time may be a healthy way for the patient to deal with rape.
- Help the patient accept his or her own feelings.
- Be sensitive to nonverbal signals (e.g., body posture, fidgeting, shakiness, incoherence in speech).
- Be the receiver. Listen to what the patient is saying *without judging*.
- Hear the patient's story and take it seriously—help legitimize the experience. (Our society often blames the patient: the victim brought it on; the victim did not resist; the victim wanted to be raped—these are common myths.)
- Communicate your own sense of stability by remaining calm and empathic.
- Establish a common language and "tune in" to the patient's terminology.

A patient who is anxious and fearful will naturally react in a fashion that may seem uncooperative, hostile, or emotional. This may be due to any one or a combination of the following factors: the nature of the rape/sexual assault, the meaning of the rape to the patient, the patient's ability to cope, the attitudes and response from others significant to the patient, the attitudes and responses of attending personnel, and the physical setting of the exam itself.

In order for personnel to intervene appropriately and reduce anxiety, they must:

- Know and understand the nature of rape/sexual assault.
- Assess how the patient perceives the assault.
- Identify and reinforce the patient's coping abilities.
- Assist "significant others."
- Coordinate care, be an interpreter and advocate if the victim needs assistance, and mobilize community resources.

Additionally, an important method of reducing the patient's anxiety is to explain procedures before initiating them. This includes: why the procedure is being done, the specific steps to be followed, how the patient's cooperation will aid in prosecuting the criminal and in his or her own recovery, and what may be done to assist in the procedure. Providing the patient with information and eliciting cooperation will also restore the patient's ability to control his or her own life and to make decisions after having been rendered helpless and out-of-control by the unanticipated assault.

SPECIAL CONSIDERATIONS OF MALE PATIENTS

Rape incidents involving men are extremely traumatic, and it is of the utmost importance that emergency care personnel interact in a sensitive and supportive manner.

The male patient experiences many of the same physical and emotional injuries as the female patient, and it is essential that he *not* be viewed any differently. In fact, the commonalities of all rape patients should be stressed rather than the differences.

Unfortunately, recognizing that the willingness of male patients to report rape is at the stage female rape patients were a decade ago, it is essential for all law enforcement and medical personnel to encourage male victims to report the crime through their support, sensitivity, and understanding.

A few factors to be noted concerning male patients include:

- It is a myth that rapes occur only to male prisoners or homosexuals.

- Male rapes are usually forceful and quite violent.
- The medical history, physical examination, and treatment should be the same as for a female patient, with special attention placed on rectal trauma, bleeding, or discharge; penile trauma, bleeding, or discharge; soreness, infection, or trauma to the mouth or pharynx; and internal injuries, soreness, or pain throughout the body.
- If the patient's anus is swollen and tender, assessment can be made through a rectal aspirate. This is performed by inserting 10-cc normal saline into the rectum and aspirating the fluid after 5 to 10 minutes. This sample can be saved for acid phosphatase and/or sperm analysis.[10]

SPECIAL CONSIDERATIONS FOR GERIATRIC PATIENTS

Geriatric patients generally are quite vulnerable to victimization, thus making the attack even more appalling. Factors contributing to this vulnerability include:

- age
- diminished sensory capacities
- bone and muscle changes
- impaired ability for mobility and self-control
- increased sensitivity of genitourinary organs
- living alone
- established daily routines, obvious to the observer
- lack of transportation.

Valid statistics are unavailable concerning rape incidents of the elderly, primarily because of embarassment, fear of reprisal, doubt about whether their complaint will be believed, and feeling overwhelmed by the system.

One analysis of those rape patients (over 50 years of age) who did report the crime affords a profile of these sexual assaults (Table 65–6). Older rape patients experienced a high degree of severe physical injury, particularly to the genital area. Aggression rather than any sexually exotic behavior presented the greatest difficulties. The resulting loss of control over their lives has a permanent impact. It has also been found that intense feelings of fear result in increased isolation.

SOCIAL SERVICE INTERVENTION

The role of the social worker is most valuable because it affords continuity of care for the patient and establishes the necessary linkages between medical manage-

TABLE 65–6   Profile of 78 Raped Patients Over Age 50

Criteria	Percent
Victim lived alone	97
Physical force was used	97
Victim raped in the home	73
Victim raped by a total stranger	68
Rape was associated with theft	65
Victim was actually beaten	50
Victim allowed perpetrator into the home as a repairman, official, or acquaintance	43
Perpetrator gained entrance through window or unlocked door	36
Perpetrator used forcible entry	21

Source: Adapted from information in Davis LJ: Rape and Older Women. In Warner CG (ed): *Rape and Sexual Assault: Management and Intervention.* Rockville, Md: Aspen Systems Corp, 1980, pp 93–119.

ment, follow-up psychological intervention, and return medical follow-up care. It is imperative that the social service department be notified immediately on admission of a rape patient. If emergency care personnel are busy with life-threatening emergencies, it prevents the patient from having to wait in the examining room unattended.

Special considerations to be followed by social service department personnel include:

- See the patient as quickly as possible.
- Communicate with friends, family, or law enforcement personnel to determine the nature of the assault and the condition of the patient.
- Orient patient to anticipated proceedings if emergency care personnel have not already done so.
- Assist the patient in contacting family or friends if he or she is alone.
- Explain the consent forms, their purpose, and value.
- Encourage the patient to relate his or her feelings, discuss the attack, and vent any anger, fear, guilt, or hostility.
- Listen.
- If the history of the attack has been obtained by the social worker, provide this information to emergency care personnel so the questioning process need not be repeated.
- Explain follow-up care and provide material to assist in this procedure.
- Assist in arranging follow-up appointments.
- Arrange for someone to accompany the patient home or to another place of comfort.
- Place a follow-up telephone call to the patient in a few days to assess his or her condition.

FOLLOW-UP CARE

The effectiveness of recovery is only ensured if a follow-up care plan is developed, activated, and assessed. Patients will not recall anything presented to them while in the emergency department, but an informational brochure placed in a pocket, purse, or wallet will be examined once the patient is home. The following information represents a sample of a follow-up guide proved to be of value and support to many patients.

Follow-Up Medical Care

Following the initial examination in the emergency department for collection of evidence and emergency medical treatment of sexual assault, the patient may still need basic medical care for general bodily injury, prevention of pregnancy, prevention of venereal disease, and psychologic reactions.[12]

This section is designed to relate medical problems encountered by other victims of sexual assault, to describe methods of care, and to provide resources for ongoing care at various levels of cost, from low-cost clinics to private care.

General Bodily Injury

Injuries sustained as a result of the sexual assault may require radiographs, laboratory work, dressing changes, minor surgical care, and/or medications. The patient should be informed as to how these injuries are to be cared for at home and when to return to the hospital or other community resource for follow-up care. The patient should be given an appointment card and written instructions before he or she leaves the hospital.

Prevention of Pregnancy

There may be a chance that a female patient may have become pregnant as a result of the sexual assault. *Emergency care personnel should discuss the probability of pregnancy with the patient.* Two alternatives are available to avoid pregnancy if it is determined that the patient is at risk: (1) the morning-after pill (DES) and (2) abortion or menstrual extraction, which is early abortion.

The morning-after pill (DES) involves a large dose of synthetic estrogen, which prevents implantation of the fertilized egg in the wall of the uterus. A full course of 25 mg taken two times a day for 5 days must be taken beginning within 24 hours of the sexual assault if it is to be effective. Compliance with this regimen is quite poor, since 60 percent of all patients discontinue the medication following the second or third day of nausea and vomiting, which are the usual side-effects of DES. However, DES is known to be linked with a rare form of vaginal cancer in *daughters* of women who took DES from 1945 to 1970 as an antimiscarriage drug during their pregnancy with those daughters. (Should the patient become aware that she is a DES daughter, she should seek medical advice for thorough testing.) The choice to take DES is the patient's, and she should be made aware of the following facts before signing the consent form.

Possible side-effects of DES include danger to the fetus if the patient is already pregnant at the time of the assault but was unaware of it and danger to the fetus if the patient remains pregnant as a result of the rape. (Counseling regarding abortion is recommended in the above two cases.) Nausea and vomiting, possible vaginal spotting, breast tenderness, insomnia, and/or rash during treatment may also be noted.

A pregnancy test done at the time of the sexual assault will show if the patient is already pregnant. If the patient should miss her menstrual period following the sexual assault, a second pregnancy test is advised approximately 6 weeks after the first day of her last period. Legal abortions and menstrual extractions are available in physicians' offices, clinics, and hospitals. Health facilities where pregnancy tests are done provide referrals for abortions.

Prevention of Venereal Disease

It is recommended that a gonorrhea culture be taken immediately and 7 to 10 days after the sexual assault and/or treatment. If oral or rectal penetration has occurred, swabs should be taken from those areas as well as the vaginal swab. Gonorrhea is more difficult to detect in the female than the male regardless of the testing used, and active cases can go unrecognized and untreated. It is, therefore, strongly recommended that preventive antibiotic therapy be undertaken. A blood test for syphillis (VDRL) should be taken immediately and repeated 4 to 6 weeks after the sexual assault.

Preventive antibiotic treatment may be given at the time of the sexual assault to prevent possible infection from the attacker. If the cost is prohibitive, there are many clinics where treatment and testing for venereal disease are available at low cost. If the patient chooses to be treated, he or she may not know for sure whether venereal disease has been contracted, but it is imperative that the patient have follow-up checks to ensure that the treatment has been effective.

If the patient chooses to be treated for venereal disease at the time of the sexual assault (and is female), such antibiotic therapy may disrupt the normal balance of bacterial organisms in the vagina. A yeast infection may develop but is readily treatable. In addition, the assault itself may also have an irritating effect on the genital tissues, or the attacker may have transmitted another kind of infection to the patient. These factors may lead to a female patient developing other venereal vaginal infections, such as trichomoniasis, genital herpes, venereal warts, or crabs.

Urinary tract infections can result from irritation or injury, and intercourse may become painful. If the patient experiences an unusual or heavy discharge from the vagina, sores, burning on urination, vaginal itching, or painful intercourse, she should seek medical attention promptly. Again, low-cost care at clinics is available if the cost of private care is prohibitive.

Follow-up Psychological Care

In most crisis situations, people can become upset and may be faced with unexpected changes in their lives. Since sexual assault may present a serious threat to the patient's safety and well-being, it is understandable that he or she may experience mental or emotional stress as an aftereffect of such an assault. In addition, the patient's family and friends may also be affected by what has happened. The patient needs to be around people who can be supportive and sympathetic. Some women's antirape groups offer woman-to-woman support throughout the procedures following a sexual assault. They are available to assist the patient. The patient may also wish to seek short- or long-term counseling. Members of the patient's immediate family may also benefit from counseling assistance. Sexual problems arising as a result of sexual assault are also treatable. The patient should be aware that many victims experience nightmares, phobias, fear of going out alone, fear of the dark, and a general suspicion of men. All these symptoms can be alleviated with proper care and support from friends, family members, and/or counselors.

EVALUATION OF RAPE INTERVENTION

The assessment, planning, design, development, and implementation of a rape management program is incomplete without the addition of an evaluation component. Professionals may have designed a program felt to be ideal for rape patients, which may not be meeting the needs of these patients at all. Consequently, each facility should develop and integrate an evaluation and feedback network used to strengthen and reinforce the original goals and objectives of the program.

One area of controversy involves the use of appropriate personnel, their role, and their function. Each facility should examine its particular protocols and determine the blueprint of personnel appropriate for their system. Identification of personnel and their strengths and weaknesses is shown in Table 65–7.[3]

In addition to personnel assessment, feedback from patients receiving care should be elicited. This type of evaluation should *not* be pursued prior to a 6-week follow-up visit. If social service personnel maintain contact with these patients, the evaluation process would be easily implemented with their assistance. An ex- ample of a patient evaluation form is noted in Exhibit 65–4.[13]

Other means of evaluation should be integrated based on program design. Quality assurance personnel in each facility will be able to provide specific and appropriate direction in the design and implementation of a desired standard of excellence for the care of all rape patients.

TABLE 65–7   Personnel Available to Perform Rape Examinations

Personnel	Possible Advantages	Possible Disadvantages
Emergency department physician	Experienced in dealing with emergency cases; expertise in handling patient trauma; may have more experience in dealing with criminal justice system.	May be somewhat inured to the problems of the rape patient; possibility of "burnout"; possible conflicts with other, more serious emergency cases.
Gynecologist	May be best able to recognize and treat injuries associated with rape; may be most experienced in requirements of evidence collection; may have extensive experience in dealing with women's concerns and fears during a pelvic examination.	May tend to treat rape patient as own ob-gyn patient rather than a patient in crisis; may present difficulties in availability for 24-hour service; may be inexperienced in crisis; may be unable to attend male patients.
Specially designated physician experienced in sexual assault examinations	Experienced in handling both the medical and emotional aspects of sexual assault cases; may develop rapport with criminal justice officials.	Possibility of "burnout"; may have problems in maintaining 24-hour availability; difficulty in "recruiting" physicians for this position due to legal involvement in case.
Private physician	May have a previously established rapport with patient; may ease burden on emergency department staff and physicians; may result in cost savings to the hospital and patient.	May be inexperienced in handling the medical, emotional, and legal aspects of rape; possible problems in maintaining 24-hour availability; possible reluctance to treat sexual assault patients.
Nurse-practitioner	May be able to establish good rapport with patient; may ease burden on emergency department personnel; may result in cost savings to hospital and patient; may develop extensive experience in handling rape cases.	Limited availability in many locations; expertise may be more open to question; may not have sufficient experience to recognize subtle signs of evidence; may require special training in rape investigation.
Coroner or medical examiner	Experienced in providing testimony on medical evidence; fewer problems in establishing 24-hour availability; possibility of developing substantial expertise in rape examinations.	May lack expertise in dealing with patients on a day-to-day basis; may be inexperienced in handling the medical and emotional aspects of rape; patient may have negative associations concerning the coroner or medical examiner.
Hospital intern	Readily available in most emergency department facilities; may be willing to adopt new procedures and/or methods of dealing with rape patients.	May be inexperienced in handling the medical, legal, and emotional aspects of rape; may not have sufficient expertise to recognize subtle signs of evidence; may not be available for medical testimony; expertise may be challenged if called to testify.
Hospital resident	Readily available in most emergency department facilities; may be willing to adopt new procedures and/or methods of dealing with rape patients; may have developed more medical expertise than interns.	May be inexperienced in handling the medical, legal, and emotional aspects of rape; may be unavailable for testimony; many residents are foreign-born and may experience language difficulties.

Source: Carrow DM: *Rape: Guidelines for a Community Response.* US Department of Justice, Law Enforcement Assistance Administration, National Institute of Law Enforcement and Criminal Justice, January 1980, p 130.

Exhibit 65–4 Evaluation Form for Hospital Examination, Laboratory Testing, and Counseling

Our concern is that the best possible care be provided to you and other patients of sexual assault. In order to evaluate and improve this program, your suggestions are needed. Please take a few moments to answer these questions and return the form at your convenience. Thank you for your cooperation.

1. Which hospital were you taken to?
   (List available hospitals)

2. Date of hospital exam ____________________
   Time of hospital exam ____________________
   Date this application was filled out

   ____

3. Were you left alone at the hospital? __________ If so, for how long? _______________________
   Did this bother you? __________ Was an explanation provided? _______________________

4. Please check any of the following areas that were explained to you prior to the procedure.

	Yes	No		Yes	No
• Reason for physical exam	___	___	• Reasons for asking personal questions	___	___
• Collection of evidence process	___	___	• Reasons for lab test(s)	___	___
• Steps in physical exam	___	___	• Possible treatment for venereal disease/pregnancy	___	___
• Other: ____________________	___	___			

5. Were the following counseling services satisfactory?

	Yes	No	Not given
• Advice on birth control measures	___	___	___
• Advice on the prevention of venereal disease	___	___	___
• Counseling on pregnancy prevention measures	___	___	___
• Other: ____________________________	___	___	___

6. What type of social service counseling did you receive?
   ________ Were you counseled by the hospital social worker?
   ________ Were you referred to outside community resources?
   ________ Were family and friends involved in the counseling?
   Was the counseling satisfactory?   Yes ________   No ________

COMMENTS

7. What type of follow-up recommendations were made?
   ________ Medical follow-up care was recommended
   ________ Signs and symptoms to watch for in case of complications were described
   ________ Psychological follow-up care was recommended

8. Did you receive a follow-up call from the hospital? ________ If yes, what did they recommend? ____________
   ____
   ____

9. Were you pleased with your care and treatment? ________ If not, what did you dislike? _____________
   ____
   ____

10. What improvements would you suggest for the care of future patients of sexual assault? ____________
    ____
    ____

11. How did you feel about your interview with the police officer? ______________________________
    ____

    The plain clothes officer? ____
    ____

12. Other comments: ____
    ____
    ____

If you feel comfortable signing your name, it would be most helpful, but please recognize that this is not required.

____

REFERENCES

1. *FBI Uniform Crime Reports,* 1977. US Department of Justice, 1978.
2. Keller E, Remus S: Statistics on sexual assault. In Keller E (ed): *Training Manual.* St Paul, Minnesota Program for Victims of Sexual Assault, 1979.
3. Carrow DM: *Rape: Guidelines for a Community Response.* US Department of Justice, Law Enforcement Assistance Administration. National Institute of Law Enforcement and Criminal Justice, January 1980, pp 130, 170, and 253–255.
4. *Forcible Rape: An Analysis of Legal Issues.* US Department of Justice, Law Enforcement Assistance Administration, National Institute of Law Enforcement and Criminal Justice, 1978, pp 8, 16, 17, and 20.
5. Caplan GM: *Rape and Its Victims: A Report for Citizens, Health Facilities, and Criminal Justice Agencies.* US Department of Justice, Law Enforcement Assistance Administration, 1975.
6. Report of the task force to study treatment of the victims of sexual assault, Prince Georges County, Maryland, March 1973.
7. Bay Area Hospital Conference on Sexual Assault: *Medical Protocol for Victims of Sexual Assault.* Queen's Bench Foundation, 1976, p 4.
8. Warner CG, Koerper MJ, Spaulding D, et al: San Diego County protocol for the treatment of rape and sexual assault victims. City of San Diego, California, Fall 1978, pp 14, 19, and 20.
9. Braen GR: Sexual assault examination protocol for medical personnel. (unpublished) August 1980.
10. Braen GR: Physical assessment and emergency medical management for adult victims of sexual assault. In Warner CG (ed): *Rape and Sexual Assault: Management and Intervention.* Rockville, Md, Aspen Systems Corporation, 1980, pp 57, 60, and 69.
11. Burgess AW, Holmstrom LL: *Rape: Victims of Crisis.* Bowie, Md, Robert J. Brady Co, 1974.
12. Subcommittee on Sexual Assault and Intrafamily Violence of the Advisory Board on Women: *Taking Care of Yourself, a Self-Help Guide.* City of San Diego, California, 1979–1980.
13. Subcommittee on Sexual Assault and Intrafamily Violence of the Advisory Board on Women: Evaluation form for hospital examination, lab testing and counseling. City of San Diego, California, 1980.

BIBLIOGRAPHY

Abarbanel G: Helping victims of rape. *Social Work* 21:478–482, 1976.
Bohmer C, Blumberg A: Twice traumatized: The rape victim and the court. *Judicature* 58:391–399 (March) 1975.
Brodyaga L, Gates M, Singer S, et al: *A Prescriptive Package: Rape and Its Victims: A Report for Citizens, Health Facilities and Criminal Justice Agencies,* Publication no. 1976–0–211–063/560. US Department of Justice, Law Enforcement Assistance Administration, National Institute of Law Enforcement and Criminal Justice, 1975.
Brownmiller S: *Against Our Will: Men, Women and Rape.* New York, Simon & Schuster, 1975.
Burgess AW, Holmstrom LL: Coping behavior of the rape victim. *Am J Psychiatry* 133:413–418 (April) 1976.
Burgess AW, Holmstrom LL: *Rape: Crisis and Recovery.* Bowie, Md, Robert J. Brady Co, 1979.
Burgess AW, Holmstrom LL: Rape trauma syndrome. *Am J Psychiatry* 131:931–986, 1974.
Burgess AW, Holmstrom LL: *Rape: Victims of Crisis.* Bowie, Md, Robert J. Brady Co., 1974.
Chappel D, Geis R, Geis G (eds): *Forcible Rape: The Crime, the Victim, and the Offender.* New York, Columbia University Press, 1977.
Fox S, Scherl D: Crisis intervention with victims of rape. *Social Work* 17:37–42, 1972.
Gager N, Schurr C: *Sexual Assault: Confronting Rape in America.* New York, Grosset & Dunlap, 1976.
Klingbeil KS, Anderson SC, Vontver L: Multidisciplinary care for sexual assault victims. *Nurse Practitioner* 1(6):21–25 (July-August) 1976.
Medea A, Thompson K: *Against Rape.* New York, Farrar, Straus & Giroux, 1974.
Metzger D: It is always the woman who is raped. *Am J Psychiatry* 133:405–408 (April) 1976.
National Center for the Prevention and Control of Rape, *Regional Directory: Rape Prevention and Treatment Resources.* US Department of Health, Education and Welfare, National Institute of Mental Health.
Russell DEH: *The Politics of Rape: The Victim's Perspective.* New York, Stein & Day, 1974.
Schultz LG (ed): *Rape Victimology.* Springfield, Ill, Charles C Thomas, 1975.
Simpson K, et al: *A Doctor's Guide to Court Handbook on Medical Evidence.* London, Butterworth, 1967, p 197.
Symonds M: The rape victim: Psychological patterns of response. *Am J Psychoanal* 36:27–34 (Spring) 1976.
Talbert S, White S, Bowen J, et al: Improving emergency department care of the sexual assault victim. *Ann Emergency Med* 9:293–297 (June) 1980.
Viano EC: Rape and the law in the United States: An historical and sociologic analysis. *Int J Crime Penology* 2:317–328 (November) 1974.
Walker MJ, Brodsky SL (eds): *Sexual Assault.* Lexington, Mass, Lexington Books, 1976.

APPENDIX 65–A

Glossary of Terms

ABO: Classification of blood; blood grouping in determinations in criminology. One blood grouping system. This blood grouping system can be found in blood, semen, saliva, perspiration, and vaginal discharge.

Acid phosphatase: A test that checks samples of fluid to see if semen is present.

Advocate: One who speaks in favor of, defends, recommends; an intercessor.

Alleged rapist: See *Defendant.*

Anal sex: See *Sodomy.*

Carnal knowledge: The act of a man having sexual intercourse with a woman. The male genitalia entering the vulva or labia is sufficient, and it is not necessary that the vagina be entered or the hymen ruptured.

Coitus: Sexual intercourse.

Cunnilingus: An act committed with the female sexual organ and the mouth.

Defendant: A person who is charged with a crime.

DES: Diethylstilbestrol, the morning-after pill used immediately after unprotected intercourse to prevent pregnancy; a controversial drug.

Fellatio: To put one's mouth on the male sex parts.

Forensic: Belonging to or suitable to courts of judicature, argumentative, i.e., forensic medicine or forensic science. Legal medicine or legal jurisprudence.

Gonorrhea: Contagious inflammation of the genital mucous membrane.

Gram stain: Method of staining bacteria or tissues. Those retaining stain are gram-positive; those losing stain are gram-negative. A test for gonorrhea.

Herpes: Groups of watery blisters on mucous membranes.

Incest: Sexual intercourse between persons closely related by blood.

Introitus: Entrance of the vagina.

Labia majora: Hairy fold of skin on each side of vulva.

Menstrual extraction: Procedure of emptying contents of uterus.

Modus Operandi: Method of operation.

Mons veneris: Pubic eminence.

Perineum: Area between anus and genital organs.

Perpetrator: The person who commits the assault/crime.

Perversion: Indulgence in unnatural sexual acts.

Prophylaxis: Preventive treatment.

Rape: In criminal law, the unlawful carnal knowledge of a woman by a man, not her husband, forcibly against her will and with penetration, however slight, of the male genitalia into those of the female.

Rape crisis line: A telephone number to call where someone is trained to help a victim talk about the rape and to answer questions.

Semen: Liquid portion of ejaculate, containing sperm.

Sexual assault: Any type of sexual act when committed without the consent to the act of one of the parties.

Sexual molestation (carnal abuse): An act performed by one person on another amounting to noncoital sexual contact without consent. May involve rape or forcible oral and anal sex acts, but most commonly fondling of a child's genitals.

Sodomy: Anal copulation.

Spermatozoa: Mature male germ cell (specific output of the testes).

Syphilis: Contagious venereal disease.

Unlawful sexual intercourse: The crime of having sexual intercourse with a female, under statutory age (18 years old) with or without the female's consent.

Vagina: The opening in the female that leads to the reproductive system.

VDRL: Serologic test for syphilis.

Venue: Place where a crime is committed. Change of, change of place of trial.

Victim compensation agency: A public office that gives money to victims of violent crimes.

981

Head and Neck Emergencies

The author of "Ocular Emergencies" (Chapter 66) presents a practical and comprehensive approach to emergencies involving the eye, reviewing the eye's anatomy as examined with the slit lamp, inflammatory changes of the eye that may result from injury or infection, and ocular events that may reflect systemic disease. The author then discusses the judicious use of pharmacologic agents in ocular emergencies.

In "Ear, Nose, and Throat Emergencies" (Chapter 67) and "Laryngeal Emergencies" (Chapter 68), commonly encountered problems are discussed, e.g., epistaxis, its complications and treatment; perforations of the tympanic membrane; foreign bodies; and blunt trauma to the larynx. Infectious processes of the ear are also discussed in "Infectious Disease Emergencies" (Chapter 20). Foreign bodies in the airway are also reviewed in "Obstructive Lung Diseases" (Chapter 57).

"Maxillofacial Injuries" (Chapter 69) includes the pathophysiology and clinical correlates of trauma, prehospital care, emergency department stabilization and evaluation, and treatment of injuries to the soft tissues, lips, mouth, tongue, eyebrow, and nose, and fractures of the mandible, zygoma, orbit, and maxilla.

In "Dental Emergencies" (Chapter 70), the author discusses some of the most prevalent diseases in the United States and their potential serious consequences: common decay, pulpitis, pulpal necrosis, alveolar abscess, dental alveolar trauma, fractured teeth, temporal mandibular joint dislocation, postextraction bleeding, and mucosal ulcerations and infections.

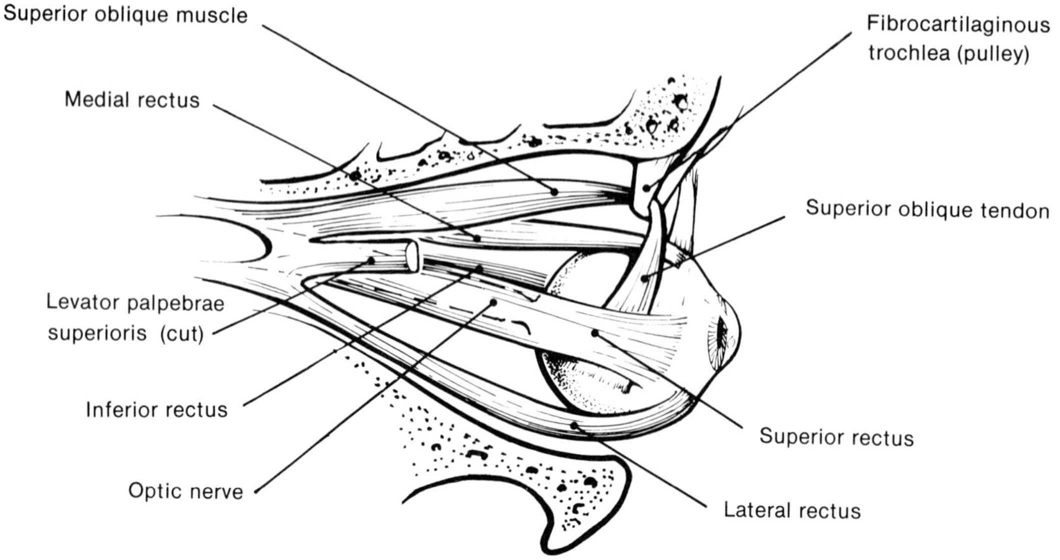

Superior view

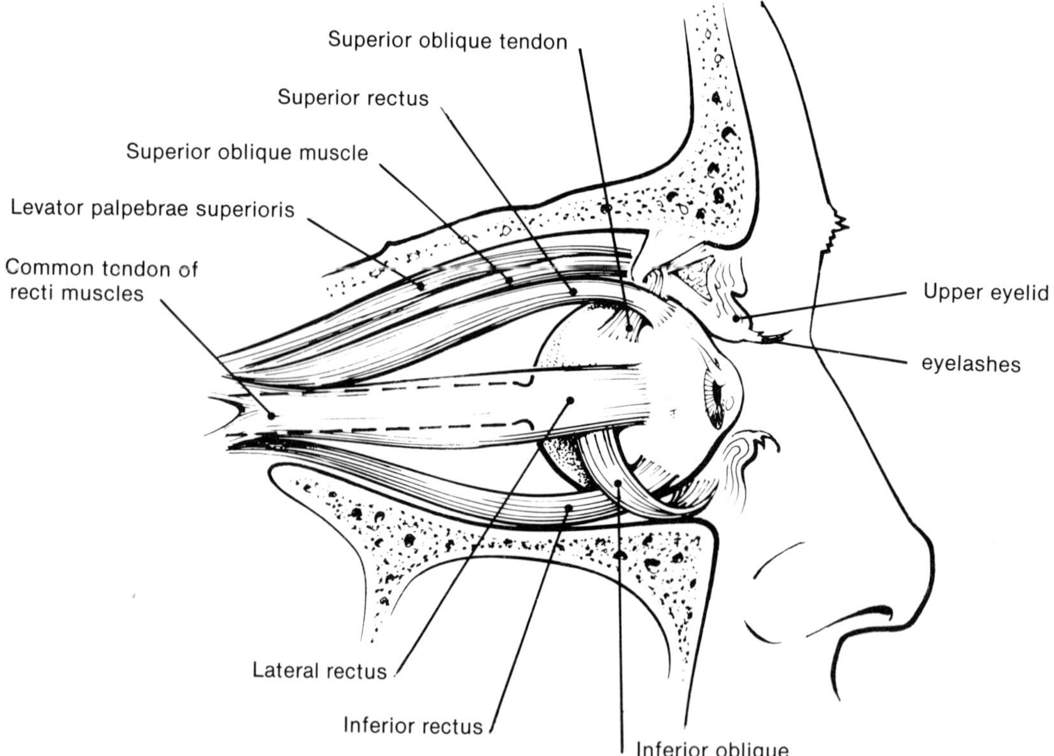

Lateral view

Ocular Muscles and Related Structures

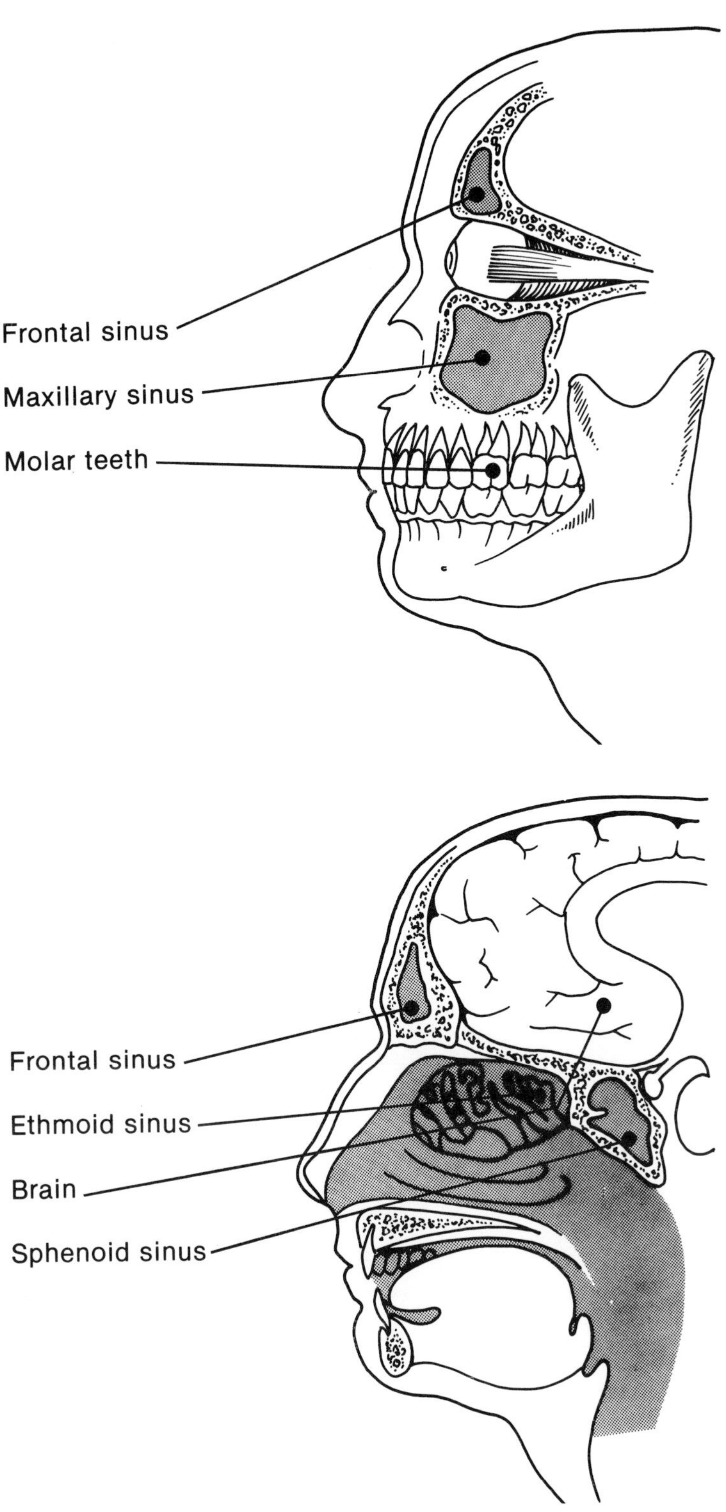

Paranasal Sinuses

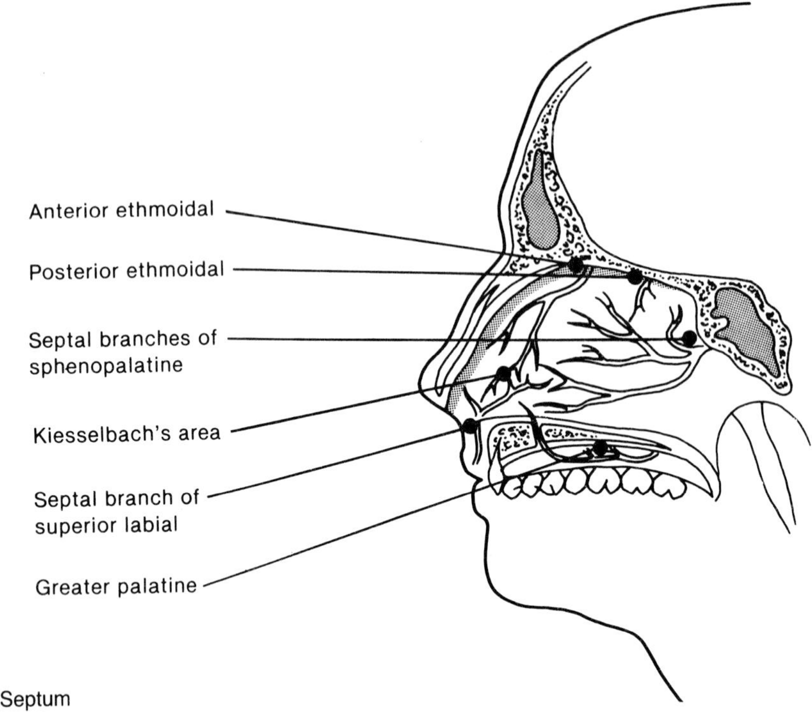

Blood Supply to the Nasal Septum

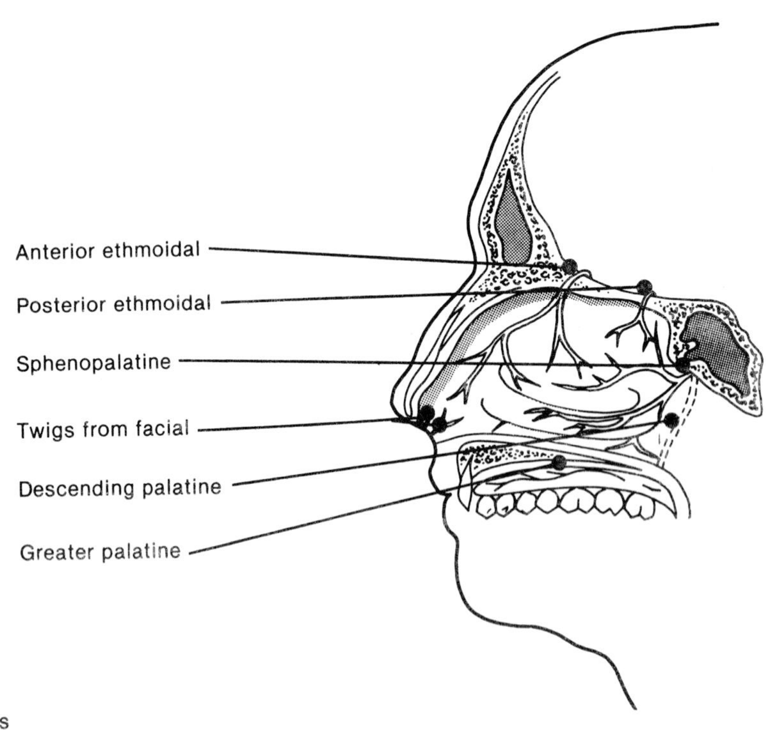

Blood Supply to the Turbinates

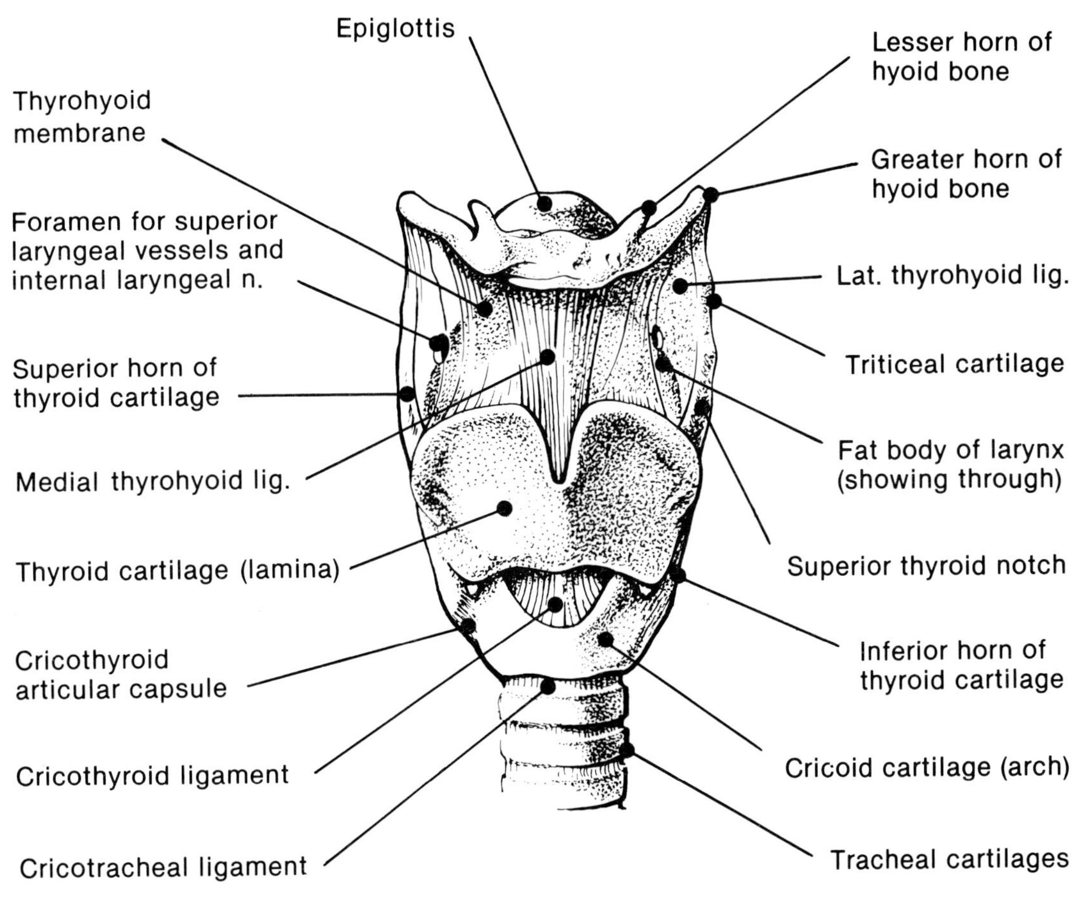

Cartilagenous Framework of the Larynx

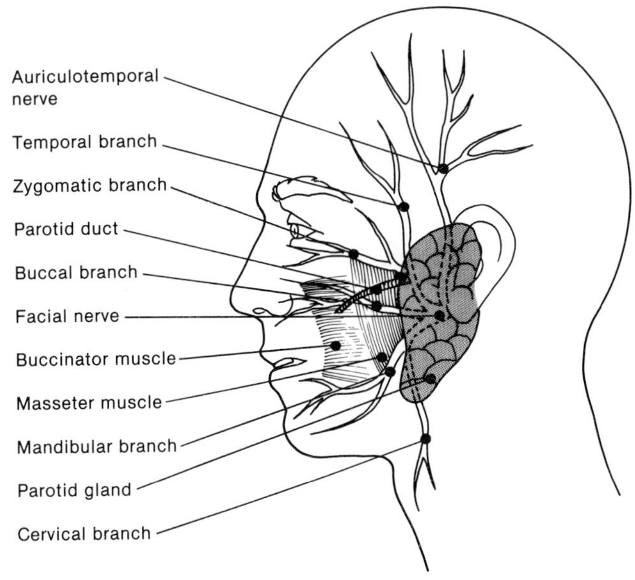

Muscles, Nerves, and Glands of the Head

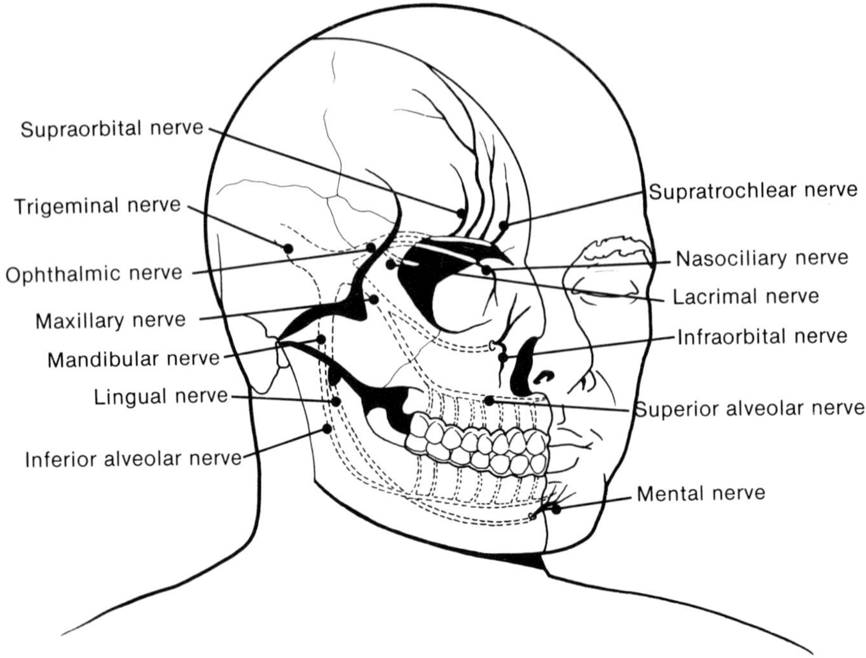

Trigeminal Nerves

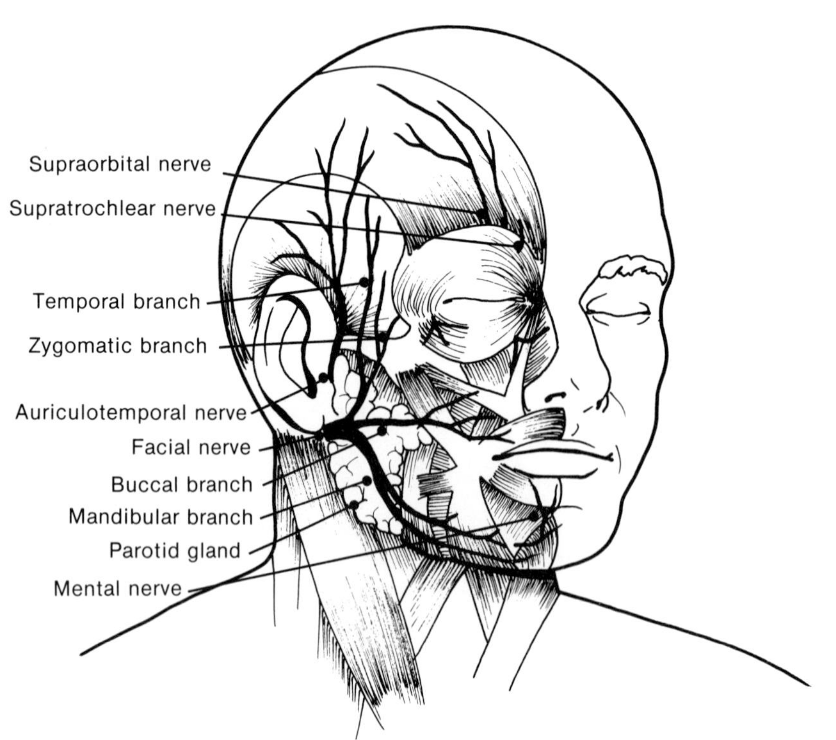

Facial Nerves

66. Ocular Emergencies

JAMES CABRAL, M.D.

Within the general medical community, the emergency physician should be considered second only to the ophthalmologist in ability to manage ocular problems. People living in isolated communities remote from major medical centers may actually look to the emergency department physician as the person most competent to manage ocular emergencies. Consequently, the emergency department physician must have a thorough understanding of the following factors:

- the eye's gross anatomy as well as the anterior and posterior anatomy as viewed with both a direct ophthalmoscope and a biomicroscope (the slit lamp),[1,2] including the eye muscles and related structures. (See Figure 66–1.)
- the range of ocular tissue response to exogenous infection, to chemical and physical trauma, and to endogenous agents[2–4]
- the types of ocular manifestations and responses to systemic disease[2,5,6]
- the mechanisms and routes of invasion of the ocular tissues by infectious agents[2,5,7,8]
- the bony anatomy of the skull and facial bones examined radiographically and accurately by palpation[1,2]
- the pharmacology and clinical applications of a limited number of ocular drugs.[2,5,9]

Certain skills also are essential, including the ability to

- recognize, and to a reasonable extent appraise, ocular inflammatory response in the different regions of the eye and adnexa[5–7]
- obtain an exceptionally well-documented history of ocular trauma, including the circumstances and mechanisms of trauma, as well as the sequence of ocular symptoms that develop during ocular medical disorders[2–5]
- perform a relatively thorough and accurate ocular examination[2,5,6]
- determine a patient's approximate visual status that may have existed prior to ocular trauma or disease and measure in a reproducible manner visual acuity and at least gross visual fields in the emergency department prior to both instilling ocular medications and manipulating the eye[2]
- communicate ocular history and clinical findings in the jargon of the ophthalmologist (Appendix 66–A)[5,10]
- obtain useful and reliable bacterial specimens for culture and ensure timely and proper inoculation in correct media[8,11–14]
- use commonly available emergency department instruments for both the examination and the treatment of the eye
- gain confidence and skill in a limited number of emergency ocular surgical procedures[3,4]
- prepare an ocular trauma patient for safe transport to another facility[3,4]
- develop a high index of suspicion, a fair degree of confidence, and a reasonable degree of caution.

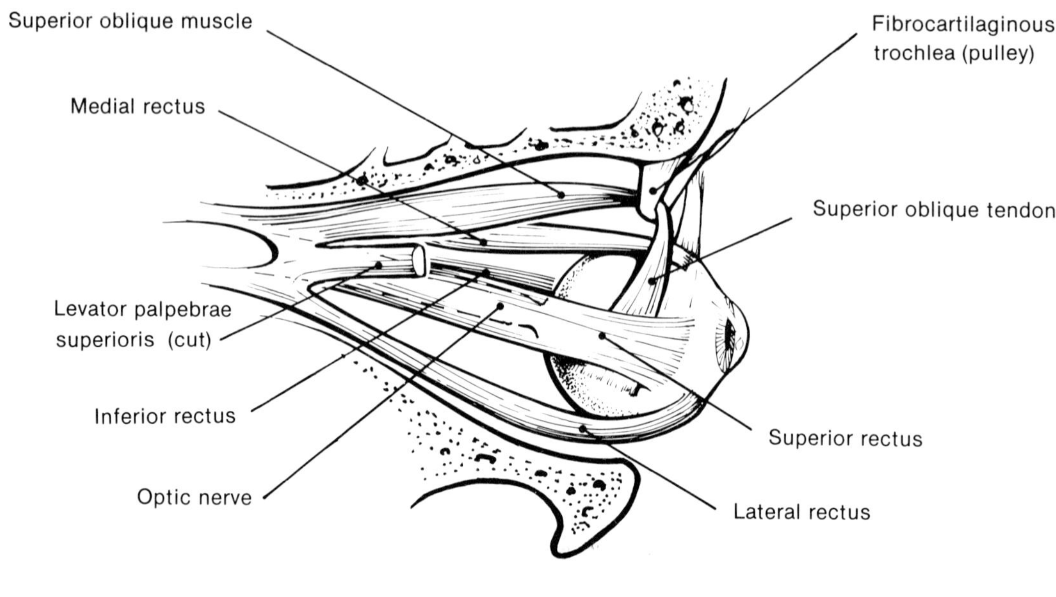

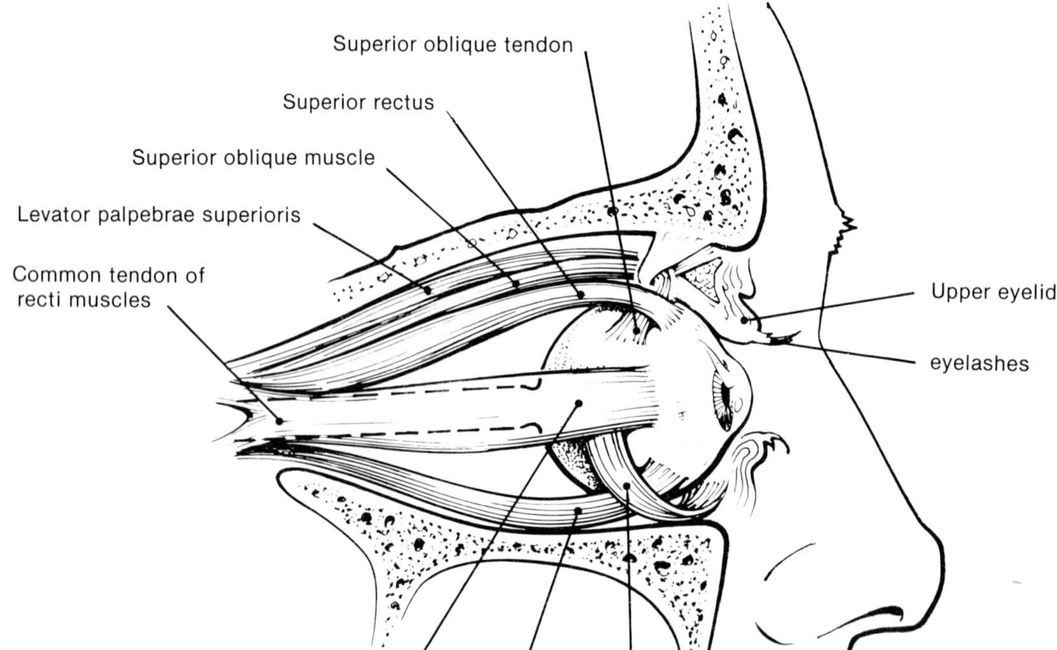

Figure 66–1 Superior and Lateral Views of Right Eye Showing Muscles and Related Structures.

THE OCULAR HISTORY

Since no two ocular problems are identical, and since many minor ocular problems are potentially devastating, prehospital care personnel and the emergency department physician should approach the ocular emergency with the same openmindedness and concern with which fever of unknown etiology, chest pain, or acute abdomen is evaluated. Ocular symptoms are frequently precipitated by a systemic disease or by a disorder remote from the eye. Prior to conducting the ocular examination, it is safer, and ultimately more efficient, to approach the patient with the objective of first obtaining, in an orderly manner, a classic history, which should include the following:

- chief complaint
- present illness
- past history of ocular disorders:
  - previous eye diseases
  - surgery, intraocular lens implant
  - infections and inflammations
  - trauma
  - previous use of eyeglasses and approximate age of current eyeglass prescription
  - status of previous visual acuity, noting particularly any history of visual deficit or asymmetry
- list of drug allergies and sensitivities
- list of currently employed drugs, vitamins, and mood-altering substances
- habits of smoking and drinking
- review of systems
- occupation and hazardous exposures, including sports, industry, and hobbies
- time of last oral intake, including nature of food and fluids ingested
- past medical history
- family history of ocular disorders, including specific questions in reference to cataracts, glaucoma, severe refractive errors, retina detachment, diabetic retinopathy, eye tumors, and severe visual loss.

A careful review of Freeman's trauma history checklist (Exhibit 66–1) will give the emergency department physician insight to the extent to which the ophthalmologist may pursue the history of ocular trauma in order to understand the mechanisms of injury, to conduct examinations and special studies, to plan treatment and aftercare, and, if necessary, to prepare for the medical-legal consequences of trauma.[3]

After cardiopulmonary resuscitation and the control of shock, the immediate care of chemical burns of the eye by freshwater irrigation takes priority over all other

Exhibit 66–1 Trauma History Checklist

 I. Details of Accident
   A. Date
   B. Time
   C. Location
   D. Accidental?
   E. Intentional?
   F. Self-inflicted?
   G. While at work?
   H. Goggles worn?
   I. Glasses worn?
   J. Damage to glasses or goggles or frames?
   K. Names and addresses of witnesses

 II. Object Producing Injury
   A. Blunt injury
     1. Description of object
     2. Distance traveled to eye
     3. Direction traveled to eye
   B. Foreign body cases
     1. Suspected composition of foreign body
     2. Single or multiple
     3. Possible contamination
     4. Pathway of foreign body to eye
       a. Distance traveled
       b. Direction traveled
       c. Position of patient's head at impact
       d. Direction of gaze at impact
     5. Tool or machinery involved in producing foreign body
       a. Description of tool or machinery
       b. Composition of tool or machinery
       c. Composition of grinding surface
       d. Possible contamination of surface

 III. Events Before Examination
   A. Name and address of other professional personnel examining patient
   B. Previous treatment?
     1. Ocular
     2. Systemic
     3. Antitetanus
   C. Transported
     1. Lying
     2. Sitting
   D. Change in vision
     1. Sudden
     2. Gradual
   E. Time fluid or food last taken by mouth

 IV. Visual Status Before Accident
   A. Injured eye
   B. Uninjured eye
   C. Preexisting ocular disease or amblyopia?
   D. Previous ocular surgery?
   E. Family history of ocular disease?

 V. Animal Bites
   A. Animal provoked?
   B. Probable location of animal for follow-up

Source: Freeman HM, McDonald PR, Scheie HG: Evaluation and examination of the traumatized eye. In Freeman HM (ed): *Ocular Trauma.* New York, Appleton-Century-Crofts, 1979.

emergency department procedures and protocols.[15] It is important to remember, however, that preoccupation with an ocular disaster must not cause the physician to overlook a less apparent life-threatening injury or disorder. Treat first the patient, then the eye.

VISUAL ACUITY TESTING

Because in ocular trauma, claims of loss of vision may be associated with future compensation, it is crucial to establish a probable visual status of both of the patient's eyes prior to an accident. The most reliable information is probably obtainable when the patient is distracted during the initial examination in the emergency department rather than later when compensatory reimbursement may influence the patient's recall.

Visual acuity ideally should be measured prior to both the instillation of eye drops and any manipulation of the eyes. Severe ocular discomfort and secondary blepharospasm may necessitate the use of topical anesthetic drops prior to acquiring a reliable visual acuity, which should be obtained in both eyes and preferably with and without eyeglasses. If the patient's eyeglasses are not available, the pinhole visual acuity may also be recorded. If treatment is initiated prior to testing vision, visual loss may be attributed to the therapy itself.

The examining physician must exercise extreme caution in guaranteeing that while testing the vision of one eye, the fellow eye is well covered. Not uncommonly, a patient will innocently perform visual acuity tests while viewing with the "covered" eye and inadvertently deceive the unwary examiner. Reliability of vision testing is further enhanced by testing first the eye with the least visual acuity, thus denying the patient the opportunity to inadvertently memorize a visual acuity chart or to identify test objects.

The successive levels of decreasing distance visual acuity are identified by the terms expressed in Table 66–1. If visual acuity is less than 20/400, the patient should be moved toward the distant visual acuity chart or vice versa until the 20/400 figure is identified. Visual acuity is then recorded as a fraction, the numerator of which is the distance in feet from the chart and the denominator is 400. Thus, if the 20/400 letter is first seen at 10 feet, acuity is recorded as 10/400.

If the patient is confined to a stretcher, it may prove convenient simply to hand-carry the distance visual acuity chart to a point 20 feet distant from the patient, who may turn his or her head to the side to view the chart, which is then rotated 90 degrees in order that the figures may be viewed in a normal manner relative to the patient's immediate posture. For this type of patient, every emergency department must be equipped simply to test near visual acuity with a standard type near visual acuity

TABLE 66–1   Distance Visual Acuity

Feet	Metric	Decimal
20/15	6/4.5	1.33
20/20	6/6	1.0
20/25	6/7.5	0.8
20/30	6/9	0.66
20/40	6/12	0.5
20/50	6/15	0.4
20/60	6/18	0.33
20/70	6/21	0.3
20/80	6/24	0.25
20/100	6/30	0.2
20/200	6/60	0.1
20/300	6/90	0.07
20/400	6/120	0.05

C.F. = Counting fingers at ______feet/meters
H.M. = Hand motion at ______feet/meters
L.P.& P. = Light perception and projection (identifies direction of light source)
L.P. = Light perception without projection
N.L.P. = No light perception

card as illustrated in Figure 66–2. If standard test charts are not available, one must improvise with a test that is reproducible, such as various sizes of newsprint, telephone directory print, or commonly known small objects held at recorded distances. Confrontation visual fields may be obtained even while the patient remains in either the prone or supine posture and may provide the first indication of an intracranial injury or a retinal detachment.

The uncooperative child or adult who is suspected of having a severe ocular injury may require ocular examination under anesthesia. Common sense may dictate that the examiner not persist in any attempts to perform the classic ocular examination but should pass this responsibility on to the ophthalmologist as soon as possible and record reasons for failing to acquire the visual acuity during the initial phases of management.

EXAMINATION OF THE GLOBE AND CONJUNCTIVAL FORNIX

Exposure of the globe

Displacing the eyelids to permit direct examination of the globe can be accomplished by lid retraction, eversion, and double eversion. If the examiner suspects a perforated or lacerated globe, pressure on the globe must be avoided at all costs. Prior to manipulation of the injured globe, the globe of the uninjured eye should be gently ballotted through the uninjured lid to acquire

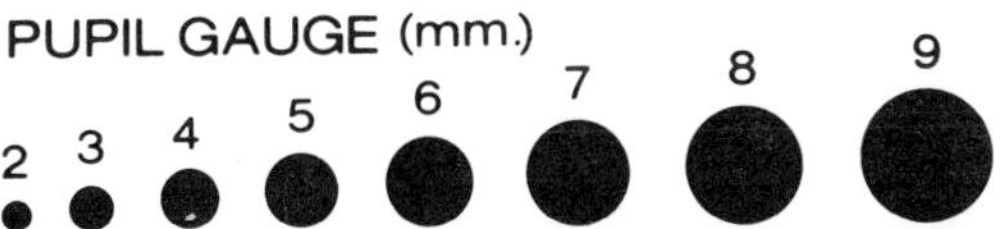

Figure 66–2 Standard Type Near Vision Acuity Card. *Source:* J.G. Rosenbaum. Reproduced with permission.

a feel for the normal tension of the globe and the normal resilience of the orbit. If necessary, the same trial examination could be performed on a cooperative emergency assistant. If very gentle ballottement of the injured eye with a delicate finger suggests the presence of hypotony, the examiner must assume the presence of a perforated or ruptured globe and proceed to examine the eye with greater caution.

Retraction of the Upper and Lower Lids

Simultaneous retraction of both the upper and lower lids is accomplished by applying the thumbs to the pa-tient's brow just above the superior orbital rim and to the malar eminence just below the inferior orbital rim, respectively, and *gently* applying pressure away from the globe. Even in a very healthy patient, these bony prominences can be tender. The maneuver can be accomplished, however, very successfully with a minimum amount of pressure.

Eversion of the Upper Lid

Since eversion of the upper lid is usually performed for purposes of removing a superficial foreign body, the physician should be prepared to remove the foreign body immediately on everting the lid. Thus, the patient probably should have received a topical anesthetic. A good source of oblique illumination should be available, preferably held by an assistant. The physician should be wearing a loupe or have an alternate source of magnification available, such as a simple magnifying glass. Immediately at hand should be an instrument such as a moistened cotton-tipped applicator or a jewelers forceps for removing extremely fine foreign bodies such as tiny splinters of glass or the delicate spines of a cactus. The patient should be comfortably seated at a slit lamp or placed in the supine position and be sufficiently informed to be both confident and helpful to the physician.

Eversion of the upper lid is initiated with the patient gazing downward. The lid is grasped by the central eyelashes and pulled downward with one hand while the physician's second hand applies the cotton-tipped applicator centrally to the upper margin of the tarsus and then gently flips the upper lid into eversion over the applicator tip, which is removed from behind the everted lid and reapplied to stabilize the upper lid margin. The key to success at this point is the patient's cooperation in avoiding blepharospasm and in maintaining a steady downward gaze. Return of the lid to normal position is accomplished by gently pulling the lid outward as the patient assumes an upward gaze.

Double Eversion of the Upper Lid

Double eversion of the upper lid becomes essential in exploring the upper fornix of the conjunctival sac in a search for multiple foreign bodies and the elusive single foreign body. This is accomplished by first simply everting the upper lid and then inserting the blade of a Desmarres retractor behind the already everted lid and then elevating the lid gently away from the globe with rotation of the retractor arm away from the globe and toward the forehead in order to open up the upper fornix. The hand grasping the retractor handle should be resting on the patient's forehead in order to maintain

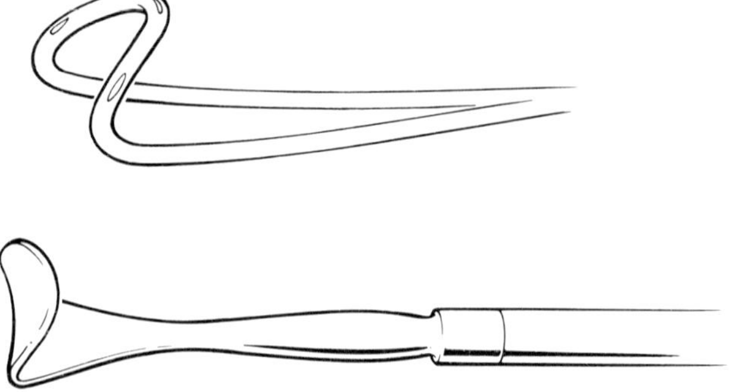

Figure 66–3 Desmarres Retractor Fashioned from a Medium-Sized Paper Clip.

a sustained and gentle traction. The patient must maintain a steady downward gaze. The examiner's second hand can then apply the tip of a moistened cotton-tipped applicator to the upper fornix and very gently retract inferiorly the folds of conjunctiva, thus opening the crevices to expose any small residual foreign bodies and wounds. A readily available substitute for the Desmarres retractor can be fashioned from a medium-sized or large paper clip (Fig. 66–3).

HERPETIC OCULAR DISEASE

Ocular herpetic disease may present solely in one of the following acute clinical forms:

- "itchy eye"
- "corneal abrasion"
- "corneal foreign body"
- "pink eye"
- primary keratoconjunctivitis (usually in children)
- vesicular ulcerative blepharitis
- blepharoconjunctivitis
- acute follicular conjunctivitis
- coarse epithelial keratitis
- dendritic keratitis
- geographic keratitis
- acute or recurrent iridocyclitis
- panuveitis
- nodular episcleritis
- interstitial keratitis

Although acute ocular herpes usually presents as a combination of these clinical forms, this list serves to emphasize the danger of using topical corticosteroids to treat what may appear to be a less dangerous problem. These clinical forms may present before the appearance of keratitis, or keratitis may never actually appear. It is advisable to examine carefully with magnification any

lesions of the lid, lid margins, and conjunctiva in order to detect small or sparse herpetic vesicles.

The signs and symptoms of dendritic keratitis include the following:

- gradual onset of symptoms
- watery ocular discharge
- ocular discomfort varying from a very mild itching sensation to an intense foreign body sensation or irritation
- photophobia of varying degrees
- conspicuous absence of a sudden onset of symptoms from an accurately detailed history in considering a diagnosis of corneal abrasion or a corneal foreign body
- single or clustered, large or small vesicles appearing on the skin, lid margin, or conjunctiva
- punctate keratitis developing into dendritic keratitis within 1 week
- ciliary and/or conjunctival injection
- conjunctival smears demonstrating lymphocytes, mononuclear cells, and a few polymorphonuclear leukocytes
- markedly reduced corneal sensitivity to light touch when tested with a wisp of cotton (a valuable diagnostic sign that may persist long after the initial dendritic lesion has healed).

The unfavorable manner in which corticosteroids influence herpetic ocular disease is best considered at this point. Topical and systemic corticosteroids do not increase the recurrence of ocular herpes but do increase the severity of spontaneously recurring herpetic infections by enhancing viral replication, enhancing viral penetration of deep corneal tissues by increasing the permeability of stromal ground substance, and inhibiting lymphoid immune response.[14,16] Corticosteroids are therefore contraindicated in the treatment of simple dendritic keratitis and are inadvisable in treating the acute phase of most forms of acute follicular conjunctivitis. Caution should be exercised in applying corticosteroids to eyes that possess corneal scars suggestive of a previous herpetic keratitis.

Prophylactic Therapy

If acute herpetic dermatitis is in close proximity to an otherwise unaffected eye, the patient should instill antiviral ointment or eye drops into the conjunctival sac six times per day until the rash begins to resolve and then twice daily until the skin rash has completely healed. Acceptable antiviral medications might include: trifluorothymidine, also known as trifluridine (Viroptic ophthalmic solution); adenine arabinoside, also known as Ara A (Vidarabine ophthalmic ointment); and idoxuridine, also known as IDU (Stoxil ophthalmic solution and ointment).

If the patient is being treated with systemic corticosteroids concurrent with herpetic keratitis in one eye, it is prudent to administer antiviral drops prophylactically to the uninvolved eye.

When the physician is uncertain but suspects an acute or chronic herpetic process, it is probably safest to document the clinical observations carefully, initiate antiviral therapy, and refer the patient to an ophthalmologist as soon as possible.

Treatment of Active Herpetic Keratitis

Since the first physician treating this vision-threatening disorder has the best chance of effecting a permanent cure, the emergency department physician should be relatively aggressive and precise in selecting the initial therapeutic regimen and in arranging adequate follow-up care.[12,16] The complications of herpetic ocular disease can be very difficult to manage. The unfavorable effects on vision tend to be cumulative. The therapeutic objectives include the following:

- to quickly eliminate the virus from the epithelium
- to reduce the risk of corneal stromal keratitis and scarring
- to avoid uveitis and glaucoma
- to avoid side-effects of treatment.

Removal of virus-replicating epithelium is probably safely accomplished only by the physician who is skilled at performing procedures on the cornea with the use of slit lamp magnification. A topical anesthetic solution is applied to the cornea. It may be advantageous to instill a few drops of an antiviral ophthalmic solution just prior to and just after debridement. It must be emphasized that the objective is to debride gently the infected corneal epithelium, the dendrite, without spreading the infection to adjacent healthy epithelium, and more importantly without damaging the underlying Bowman's membrane. This deeper damage could lead to viral invasion of the stroma and eventually to increased corneal scarring.

Although it is frequently recommended, it may be safer to avoid both wiping the dendrite with a cotton-tipped applicator and scraping with a sharp instrument. A safer instrument might be a semi-sharp, chisel-ended wooden stick, the tip of which has been moistened with a 10% phenol solution.[16]

With the aid of slit lamp magnification, the physician may identify the infected epithelium by means of fluorescein staining. The involved area may then be gently outlined by scoring the epithelium with the semi-sharp tip of the wooden stick, which is then used to elevate the involved epithelium away from the underlying Bowman's membrane.

The major contraindication to debridement and patching is the coexistence of a nearby herpesvirus reservoir (e.g., the vesicles of herpes blepharoconjunctivitis) that can reinfect open corneal wounds.

Until the corneal lesion has healed, antiviral eye drops should be instilled hourly during the day. Antiviral ointments may be employed every 2 hours at night and may be applied to involved areas of the conjunctiva, eyelid, and skin immediately adjacent to the eye. When the corneal lesions have healed, the regimen may be progressively decreased over a 2 to 3-week period.

In general, the eye should not be patched unless debridement has been performed, there is an irregular and uncomfortable corneal wound, and the area to be patched is free of any virus reservoir. Topical antibiotics should be administered in the presence of corneal ulceration, particularly after debridement. The routine prophylactic use of topical antibiotics in the presence of only a dendritic keratitis and in the absence of concurrent corticosteroid therapy should be discouraged. Antibiotic therapy should be specific and when possible based on sensitivity testing.

Cycloplegia for the relief of photophobia, ciliary spasm, and uveitis may be accomplished with one of the following ophthalmic solutions: cyclopentolate hydrochloride 2%, one drop four times daily; scopolamine hydrobromide 0.25%, one drop twice daily or homatropine 5%, one drop four times daily. Secondary glaucoma may best be controlled with acetazolamide (Diamox), 125 mg to 250 mg, orally four times a day and with one drop timolol maleate (Timoptic) 0.5% twice daily. Very high initial intraocular pressures may require the use of systemic osmotic agents such as 75 to 100 ml citrus-flavored 50% glycerin served over cracked ice and sipped via a straw, or mannitol, 12 to 25 gm, administered as a 20% intravenous solution over a 30-minute period.

The use of corticosteroids in the treatment of ocular herpes is generally dangerous and contraindicated in the clinical setting of the emergency department, unless the patient is already on a regimen of topical or systemic corticosteroids. In general, the physician should attempt to attain an acute reduction in the dose schedule of corticosteroid therapy, while avoiding the complications associated with a sudden total cessation of corticosteroid therapy. Corticosteroid therapy for the complications of ocular herpes requires considerable judgment and can be safely and effectively administered only under close observation in reliable patients and at times only during hospitalization. This therapy must be conducted by an ophthalmologist.

Oral analgesics, including codeine-containing compounds or synthetic narcotics, may be required for ocular discomfort. Young children may require hand restraint and the application of a shield to both protect the eye and avoid further contamination and spread of infection. Sunglasses and a large-brimmed hat may help to reduce photophobia due to iritis.

The principles of hygiene must be emphasized. The patient should avoid spreading the infection to any personal contacts and should particularly avoid patients who may be immunosuppressed. The physician should be cautious to avoid self-inoculation or inoculation of other patients through contamination of digits or ophthalmic instruments.

The emergency department physician should ensure follow-up by an ophthalmologist within 72 hours. This need should be reinforced by instructing the patient both on the complications of the immediate disease and of the possibility of developing recurrences within the same eye.

CORNEAL ABRASIONS AND FOREIGN BODIES

Corneal epithelial defects due to corneal abrasions and foreign bodies frequently extend into Bowman's membrane and occasionally into the corneal stroma. Both foreign bodies driven with force and high-speed projectiles may penetrate to the deepest corneal layers and occasionally penetrate to attain the deepest spaces of the globe and orbit.[3,4] This possibility must be suspected when there is a history of high speed, violent force, or explosion and when only one corneal foreign body is identified in the presence of multiple corneal defects. On these occasions, the patient's pupils must be dilated and the eyes examined with indirect ophthalmoscopy and gonioscopy. The emergency department physician should obtain radiologic studies when the possibility of an intraocular foreign body exists and should consult a radiologist and ophthalmologist immediately. Moderate to deep corneal wounds are usually associated with some degree of iritis or iridocyclitis. When there is a delay of at least 24 hours between injury and presentation at the emergency department, the wound may have progressed to a bacterial corneal ulcer if the offending agent was contaminated or if the patient had a concurrent infection.

Because the patient usually experiences a sudden intense sharp pain and foreign body sensation, the exact time of injury can usually be identified. When the patient is vague and uncertain of the exact time of injury, a differential diagnosis should be developed to include viral keratitis, especially herpes simplex keratitis; ultraviolet radiation keratitis; and infections or disorders involving the lid margins. The foreign body sensation is typically experienced with any corneal epithelial defect and does not require the presence of a true foreign body. The burden of proof remains with the physician who may have to doubly evert the upper lid and carefully examine the upper fornix to rule out a foreign body that may be hidden in the upper folds of the conjunctival sac. Very uncomfortable photophobia and blepharospasm may be induced by a corneal wound, by a foreign body, and by an iritis.

Although a corneal epithelial defect or foreign body may be grossly visible, the full extent of injury, inflammation, and complications can only be appreciated by examination with magnification and fluorescein stain and topical anesthesia. The emergency department physician must be careful to develop the habit of everting both the upper or lower eyelids and examining also the fornices to rule out the possibility of a second foreign body that may become masked by topical anesthetic and to not become distracted by the first readily visible corneal foreign body.

The irrigation method of removing superficial particulate or plaquelike foreign bodies requires the use of a syringe or intravenous-type tubing to direct a steady stream of normal saline or balanced salt solution against the edge of the foreign body in order to float the object away from the cornea. This method may be particularly useful when the cornea and conjunctiva are covered by numerous small particulate foreign bodies that are not imbedded. Subsequent examination of the eye may then reveal the presence of a few residual imbedded foreign bodies that must be removed by a different method.

The moistened cotton-tipped applicator is useful for removing individual very superficial or only slightly imbedded foreign bodies. The vigorous use of a cotton-tipped applicator may prove more destructive to normal corneal epithelium than the gentle use of a sharper instrument when trying to remove a foreign body that is firmly adherent and more deeply imbedded. In this circumstance, it is less traumatic to directly manipulate the foreign body with a sterile spud or with a modified 21- or 25-gauge hypodermic needle mounted either on a cotton-tipped applicator or on a hypodermic syringe (Fig. 66–4). The tip of the disposable hypodermic needle is modified by forcefully dragging the tip of the needle against the inner sterile surface of the plastic cylinder in which the needle itself is delivered. Under magnification one can bend the scalpel-like tip of the needle 45 to 90 degrees in order to effect the desirable microscopic instrument, which more efficiently permits surgical dissection immediately around the edge of the foreign body and also provides a surgical blade for excising necrotic tissue and rust. The physician's hand holding such an instrument should be resting on the patient's brow or cheek, while the patient is stabilized against the examining chair or slit lamp. The instrument itself is advanced tangentially to the anterior surface of the cornea in order that the cornea not be perforated

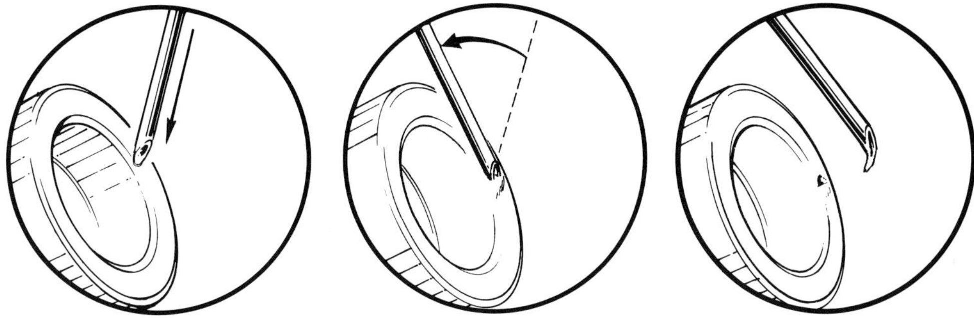

Figure 66–4 Modification of a 21 or 25 Gauge Needle Used to Manipulate a Foreign Body.

in the event that the patient lunges forward during manipulation.

All reasonable attempts should be made to remove a rust ring by sharp and precise dissection during the initial therapy. The ophthalmologist should be consulted immediately if after a reasonable and cautious effort the foreign body or rust cannot be satisfactorily removed from the visual axis in the center of the cornea. If, however, the rust is distant from the visual axis, the foreign material may be removed more easily within 24 hours, as it is sloughed toward the surface by the inflammatory reaction and by softening of the adjacent corneal tissue. In general, there will be a greater deal of corneal scarring at the site of such a wound.

Because of the frequency with which the emergency physician is called on to treat corneal abrasions and foreign bodies, and because of the possibility of very serious complications that may arise even from an apparently simple corneal abrasion, the physician must strive to be consistently successful and efficient in managing this problem. If the physician's management is cavalier or incomplete, the patient may leave the emergency department feeling briefly relieved and comfortable but may soon experience considerable inconvenience and suffering. The management of corneal abrasions and foreign bodies must span the following objectives:

- relief of acute pain, including foreign body sensation, photophobia, blepharospasm, and ciliary spasm
- acquisition of a sufficiently accurate history and examination to rule out small occult wounds and intraocular foreign bodies
- detection and safe, efficient removal of anterior segment foreign bodies
- restoration of corneal epithelial integrity
- prevention of infection due to the primary offending agent or that which may arise at the levels of primary care and aftercare
- reduction of ocular inflammatory responses including conjunctivitis, keratitis, and iritis
- reduction of corneal surface abrasion by limiting ocular and lid motility and by reducing friction and adhesion between the lids and globe
- assurance of rapid corneal healing and reduction in ocular inflammation through effective relief of ocular discomfort by local eye care and proper selection of oral medications and effective patient instruction regarding the proper use of medications and the necessity of sound rest and sleep to the healing process
- prevention of severe complication by ensuring timely and appropriate aftercare
- return of the patient to full normal activity as soon as possible.

The steps in management of corneal abrasions and foreign bodies are listed below:

1. Obtain a careful ocular history as described earlier.
2. Check and record the visual acuity.
3. Relieve ocular pain and blepharospasm with topical anesthesia.
4. Reevaluate the visual acuity after the patient is comfortable if the loss of visual acuity seems out of proportion to the apparent injury.
5. Complete the gross, microscopic, and direct fundus examination of both eyes. Be certain to examine the discs and maculas for signs of other ocular disease. *Always examine carefully both fundi of all diabetic patients:* the physician may be the first physician to diagnose diabetic retinopathy and save the patient from total blindness by timely referral to an ophthalmologist.
6. Initiate bacteriologic studies of the corneal wound and foreign bodies if indicated by history and examination.
7. Initiate cycloplegia and mydriasis if history and physical examination suggest the possibility of an

Exhibit 66–2 Preparation of Fortified Antibiotic Eye Drops

Penicillin G
1. Remove 5 ml "tears" from a 15-ml tear substitute squeeze bottle.
2. Add 5 ml "tears" to 1 vial penicillin G (5 million units).
3. Replace 5 ml reconstituted penicillin into tear squeeze bottle (10 ml + 5 ml = 15 ml).
4. Final concentration of penicillin = 333,000 U/ml.

Oxacillin
1. Remove 7 ml "tears" from a 15-ml tear substitute squeeze bottle.
2. Add 7 ml "tears" to 1 ampul oxacillin (1 gm).
3. Replace 7.2 ml reconstituted oxacillin into tear squeeze bottle (8 ml + 7.2 ml = 15.2 ml).
4. Final concentration of oxacillin = 66 mg/ml.

Carbenicillin
1. Reconstitute 1 vial carbenicillin (1 gm) with 9.5 ml sterile water.
2. Add 1.0 ml reconstituted carbenicillin into 15-ml tear substitute squeeze bottle (15 ml + 1 ml = 16 ml).
3. Final concentration of carbenicillin = 6.2 mg/ml.

Ticarcillin
1. Reconstitute 1 vial ticarcillin (1 gm) with 10 ml sterile water.
2. Add 1.0 ml reconstituted ticarcillin into 15-ml tear substitute squeeze bottle.
3. Final concentration of ticarcillin = 6.3 mg/ml.

Cephaloridine
1. Remove 2 ml "tears" from a 15-ml tear substitute squeeze bottle and discard.
2. Add 2 ml sterile saline to 1 ampul cephaloridine (500 mg).
3. Replace 2.4 ml reconstituted cephaloridine into tear squeeze bottle (13 ml + 2.4 ml = ml).
4. Final concentration of cephaloridine = 32 mg/ml.

Cefazolin
1. Remove 2 ml "tears" from a 15-ml tear substitute squeeze bottle and discard.
2. Add 2 ml sterile saline to 1 ampul cefazolin (500 mg).
3. Replace 2.2 ml reconstituted cefazolin into tear squeeze bottle (13 ml + 2.2 ml = 15.2 ml).
4. Final concentration of cefazolin = 33 mg/ml.

Vancomycin
1. Remove 9 ml "tears" from a 15-ml tear substitute squeeze bottle and discard.
2. Add 10 ml sterile water to 1 vial vancomycin (500 mg).
3. Replace 10.2 ml of reconstituted vancomycin into tear substitute squeeze bottle.
4. Final concentration of vancomycin = 31 mg/ml.

Gentamicin
1. Add 2 ml parenteral gentamicin to the 5-ml dropper bottle of commercial ophthalmic gentamicin.
2. Final concentration of gentamicin = 14 mg/ml.

Tobramycin
1. Remove 2 ml "tears" from a 15-ml tear substitute squeeze bottle and discard.
2. Add 2 ml parenteral tobramycin (80 mg) to tear substitute squeeze bottle (13 ml + 2 ml = 15 ml).
3. Final concentration of tobramycin = 5 mg/ml.

Amikacin
1. Remove 2 ml "tears" from a 15-ml tear substitute squeeze bottle and discard.
2. Add 2 ml parenteral amikacin (100 mg) to tear substitute squeeze bottle (13 ml + 2 ml = 15 ml).
3. Final concentration of amikacin = 6.7 mg/ml.

Bacitracin
1. Remove 9 ml "tears" from a 15-ml tear substitute squeeze bottle.
2. Add 3 ml "tears" to each of three commercial vials of bacitracin (50,000 U each).
3. Replace 9.6 ml reconstituted bacitracin into tear squeeze bottle (9.6 ml + 6 ml = 15.6 ml).
4. Final concentration of bacitracin = 9,600 U/ml.

Neomycin
1. Remove 2 ml "tears" from a 15-ml tear substitute squeeze bottle.
2. Add 2 ml "tears" to 1 vial neomycin (500 mg).
3. Replace 2 ml reconstituted neomycin into tear squeeze bottle (13 ml + 2 ml = 15 ml).
4. Final concentration of neomycin = 33 mg/ml.

Source: Baum JL: Antibiotic use in ophthalmology. In Duane TD (ed): *Clinical Ophthalmology.* Hagerstown, Md, Harper & Row, 1980, vol 4, chap 26.

intraocular foreign body or other intraocular disorders.

8. Remove foreign bodies of the cornea and conjunctiva by the least traumatic method under the given circumstances.

9. Instill broad-spectrum antibiotic eye drops (Exhibit 66–2 and Table 66–2).

10. Perform the dilated eye examination of the fundus by direct and/or indirect ophthalmoscopy as indicated.

11. Instill antibiotic eye drops and apply a light gauze dressing prior to transferring the patient for radiographic studies to rule out foreign bodies and/or bony injury.

12. Review radiographs, preferably with the radiologist, and determine the need for ophthalmologic consultation and/or specialized radiographic studies such as computerized axial tomography.

13. If there is no need for further consultation or special studies, prior to discharge the patient should receive the following local eye care:

    a. Repeat the instillation of topical anesthetic eye drops, such as Proparacaine 0.5%.

    b. If homatropine 5% eye drops are used to rest the eye and relieve spasms, advise the patient to anticipate blurred vision for the first 24 to 48 hours after instillation.

    c. Use a broad-spectrum antibiotic eye drop such as gentamicin, chloramphenicol, or a combination such as Neosporin.

    d. Instill into the conjunctival sac a broad-spectrum antibiotic ointment to lubricate opposing surfaces (Table 66–3).

    e. Ask the patient to close the eyelids until completion of the dressing and to avoid attempts to open the eyelids beneath the dressing in order to avoid inverting the eyelids and causing further abrasion by the eyelashes.

    f. Apply two gauze dressings to the injured eye. The patient may assist by gently holding the dressings in place.

    g. The skin area to which the adhesive tape shall be applied may be cleansed with either acetone or alcohol sponges. If necessary, apply tincture of benzoin to ensure a secure dressing.

    h. Prepare three strips of 1-inch paper tape, long enough to extend from the center of the forehead diagonally across the eye to just below the malar bone. Apply the first strip of tape by anchoring it to the forehead. Extend the tape diagonally downward across the eyepatch. With the second hand, draw the skin of the cheek up toward the eye and simulta-

TABLE 66–2　Commercially Available Antibiotic Eye Drops

Antibiotic	Trade Name	Concentration	Preservative
Tetracycline	Achromycin	1%	—
Gentamicin	Garamycin	3 mg/ml	Benzalkonium chloride, 1:10,000
Colistin	Coly-Mycin S ophthalmic	1.2 mg/ml	Thimerosal, 0.002%
Sulfacetamide	Belph 10	10%	Thimerosal, 0.005%
	Belph 30	30%	Thimerosal, 0.005%
	Sodium Sulamyd 10%	10%	Methylparaben, 0.5 mg/ml
	Sodium Sulamyd 30%	30%	Propylparaben, 0.1 mg/ml
	Sodium sulfacetamide 10%	10%	Disodium edetate, 0.1%
	Sodium sulfacetamide 30%	30%	Benzalkonium chloride, 0.005%
	Sulfacef–15	15%	Methylparaben, 0.05%
			Propylparaben, 0.01%
Sulfisoxazole	Gantrisin	4%	Phenylmercuric nitrate, 1:100,000
Chloramphenicol	Chloroptic	0.5%	Chlorobutanol, 0.5%
	Antibiopto	0.5%	—
	Ophthochlor	0.5%	—
	Econochlor	0.5%	Thimerosal, 0.01%
Polymixin B-neomycin-gramicidin	Neosporin	Polymixin B, 5000 U/ml	Thimerosal, 0.001%
		Neomycin sulfate, 2.5 mg/ml	—
		Gramicidin, 0.025 mg/ml	—
Polymixin B-neomycin	Polyspectrin	Polymixin B, 5000 U/ml	Thimerosal, 1:100,000
		Neomycin sulfate, 5 mg/ml	—
Polymixin B-neomycin	Statrol	Polymixin B, 16,250 U/ml	Benzalkonium chloride, 0.004%
		Neomycin sulfate, 3.5 mg/ml	—

Source: Baum JL: Antibiotic use in ophthalmology. In Duane TD (ed): *Clinical Ophthalmology.* Hagerstown, Md, Harper & Row, 1980, vol 4, chap 26.

TABLE 66–3 Commercially Available Antibiotic Ointments

Antibiotic	Trade Name	Concentration	Preservative
Tetracycline	Achromycin	1%	—
Chlortetracycline	Aureomycin	1%	—
Gentamicin	Garamycin	3 mg/gm	Methylparaben, 0.5 mg/gm
			Propylparaben, 0.1 mg/gm
Sulfacetamide	Cetamide	10%	Methylparaben, 0.05%
			Propylparaben, 0.01%
	Sodium Sulamyd	10%	Methylparaben, 0.5 mg/gm
			Propylparaben, 0.1 mg/gm
			Benzalkonium chloride, 0.25 mg/gm
Sulfisoxazole	Gantrisin	4%	Phenylmercuric nitrate, 1:50,000
Chloramphenicol	Chloroptic S.O.P.	1%	Chlorobutanol, 0.5%
	Antibiopto	1%	—
	Chloromycetin	1%	—
	Econochlor	1%	—
Polymixin B-bacitracin-neomycin	Neosporin	Polymixin B sulfate, 5,000 U/gm	—
		Zinc bacitracin, 400 U/gm	—
		Neomycin sulfate, 5 mg/gm	—
Polymixin B-bacitracin	Polysporin	Polymixin B sulfate, 10,000 U/gm	—
		Zinc bacitracin, 500 U/gm	—
Polymixin B-bacitracin-neomycin	Polyspectrin S.O.P.	Polymixin B sulfate, 5,000 U/gm	Chlorobutanol, 0.5%
		Zinc bacitracin, 400 U/gm	—
		Neomycin sulfate, 5 mg/gm	—
Polymixin B-neomycin	Statrol	Polymixin B sulfate, 6,000 U/gm	Methylparaben, 0.05%
		Neomycin sulfate, 3.5 mg/gm	Propylparaben, 0.01%

Source: Baum JL: Antibiotic use in ophthalmology. In Duane TD (ed): *Clinical Ophthalmology.* Hagerstown, Md, Harper & Row, 1980, vol 4, chap 26.

neously secure the free end of the tape to the cheek. Apply the second and third strips above and below and parallel to the first strip. Tell the patient that the dressing is deliberately applied with tension in order to provide a firm splint to the eye. *Advise the patient that the dressing is to be removed within 24 hours, preferably by an ophthalmologist but definitely by the patient if no physician is seen.*

14. Prescribe oral analgesics equivalent to the efficacy of 5 grains of aspirin combined with 30 mg codeine to be administered every 4 to 6 hours for the first 24 hours only.

15. *Under no circumstances should the physician prescribe any form of topical anesthetic.* The sustained use of a topical anesthetic is damaging to the cornea, may mask a corneal ulceration, and may of itself result in corneal opacification, degeneration, and ulceration.

16. Instruct the patient what to do if symptoms develop in the first 18 to 24 hours after discharge from the emergency department.

17. Insist that the patient restrict activities, rest, and preferably obtain as much sleep as possible in the ensuing 24 to 48 hours to facilitate reepithelialization of the cornea and relief of the iritis. To ensure the quality of rest and comfort, the patient should be encouraged to use the analgesics as prescribed.

18. Strongly urge the patient to have follow-up care within 24 hours.

19. Prescribe an antimicrobial eye solution such as sulfacetamide 10% eye drops, gentamicin, or chloramphenicol (Exhibit 66–2 and Table 66–2).

20. Instruct the patient on the need for caution since the patient is leaving the emergency department as a one-eyed person and will experience unexpected hazards in driving and using machinery.

LABORATORY AIDS IN THE DIAGNOSIS OF OCULAR INFECTIONS

In the majority of ocular infections, simple culture of the proper specimen and cytologic examination of tissue scrapings or aspirates together with clinical findings are sufficient to obtain a specific or presumptive diagnosis.[8,11] Though laboratory studies are not routinely indicated in obvious situations, laboratory studies

TABLE 66–4   Culture Media in Ocular Microbiology

Suspected Infection	Blood Agar	Chocolate Agar	Thayer-Martin Medium	Lowenstein-Jensen Medium	Cystine-Glucose-Blood Agar	Sabouraud's Agar	Fluid Thioglycolate Medium
Acute bacterial conjunctivitis	+	+ (southern US)					
Blepharitis	+	+				+	
Chronic conjunctivitis	+	+				+	
Hyperacute conjunctivitis (purulent)		+					
Neonatal conjunctivitis		+	+				
Oculoglandular conjunctivitis		+		+	+	+	+
Canaliculitis	+	+				+	+
Dacryocystitis	+	+				+	+
Corneal ulcer	+	+		+*		+	+
Endophthalmitis	+	+		+*		+	+
Orbital cellulitis	+	+		+*		+	+

* If cytology suggests a mycobacterium infection.

Source: Wilson LA, Sexton RR: Laboratory aids in diagnosis. In Duane TD (ed): *Clinical Ophthalmology.* Hagerstown, Md, Harper & Row, 1980, vol 4, chap 1.

should be performed when the diagnosis is in question and are mandatory in the following clinical situations:

- neonatal conjunctivitis (ophthalmia neonatorum)[17]
- corneal ulcers (non-herpetic)[12–14]
- membranous conjunctivitis[2,8]
- hyperacute (very severe) conjunctivitis[2,8]
- post-traumatic/postoperative infection[2]
- unresponsive ocular inflammation or infection
- preseptal and orbital cellulitis[7]
- dacryocystitis[18]
- infections in immunosuppressed patients
- ocular wounds associated with either highly contaminated foreign objects or with concurrent infections[3]
- endophthalmitis.[18]

The emergency department physician must have a reasonable facility in selecting proper solid and liquid bacteria culture media as well as the most useful stains for cytologic examination of corneal ulcers and conjunctival scrapings.[8,11] Without becoming a bacteriologist, the physician must develop and maintain skills in obtaining reliable specimens for culture, smear, and stain.

The solid culture media are relatively inexpensive and convenient (Table 66–4). The bacterial specimen is easily streaked on a medium's surface with the inoculating swab or spatula (Figs. 66–5 and 66–6). Bacterial growth within the streak is considered positive while growth off the streak is assumed to be a contaminant. Simultaneous cultures from the uninvolved eye permit the

physician to roughly quantitate isolated bacteria by comparing the numbers of colony-forming units (cfu) and the confluency of growth between the cfu from different regions of the same eye and by comparing cfu growth with that of the uninvolved eye.[11]

Although blood agar is readily available and inexpensive, chocolate agar is enriched to support the growth of more fastidious pathogens such as *Hemophilus*, gonococcus, and meningococcus. All bacteria that can be cultured on blood agar may also be cultured on chocolate agar but not vice versa—a culture difference that could be very significant in dealing with acute ocular infections in children. Thayer-Martin medium is an enriched chocolate agar containing antibiotics and anti-

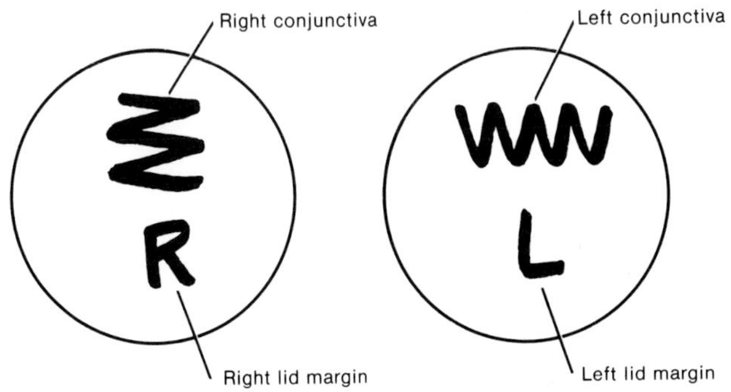

Figure 66–5   Pattern of Inoculating Streaks on Solid Media for Routine Culture of the Right and Left Eyes. (*Source:* Wilson LA, Sexton RR: Laboratory aids in diagnosis. In Duane TD (ed): *Clinical Ophthalmology.* Hagerstown, Md, Harper & Row, 1980, vol 4, chap 1.)

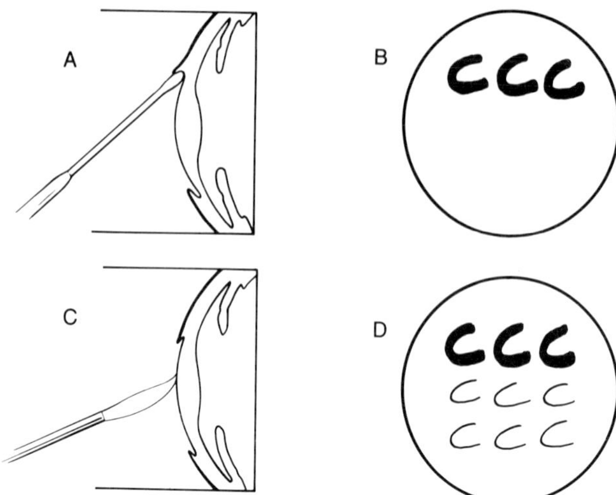

Figure 66–6 Method of Sampling of Corneal Ulcer and Inoculation of Media. Note: *A.* Initial sampling of a corneal ulcer with a sterile applicator stick. *B.* Inoculating first row of C streaks with applicator on solid media. *C.* The corneal ulcer is scraped centrally and at its advancing edges with a sterile, platinum spatula. *D.* The second and third rows of parallel C streaks are inoculated onto the same solid media as in *B.* (*Source:* Wilson LA, Sexton RR: Laboratory aids in diagnosis. In Duane TD (ed): *Clinical Ophthalmology.* Hagerstown, Md, Harper & Row, 1980. vol 4, chap 1.)

fungals that eliminate contaminants that may inhibit the growth of gonococcus, which is an important advantage in the diagnosis of neonatal and adult conjunctivitis and corneal ulceration.

Lowenstein-Jensen medium is used to isolate myco-bacteria, especially *M. tuberculosis,* as well as *Nocardia* organisms. Prior to obtaining the bacterial specimens, at least two tubes of Lowenstein-Jensen media should be prewarmed to room temperature. Immediately after obtaining the bacterial specimen, the culture media must be quickly inoculated and tightly sealed.

Fluid thioglycolate medium is suitable for cultivating strictly anaerobic, microaerophilic, and aerobic organisms that may be obtained from wounds and infections of the conjunctiva, corneal ulcers, lacrimal drainage system, aqueous, and vitreous. If an anaerobic organism is suspected, the specimen must be inoculated as quickly as possible after collection.

Cystine-glucose-blood agar selectively favors the growth of Pasteurella tularensis.

Most mycotic corneal ulcers are due to saprophytic fungi, which are inhibited by cycloheximide, a frequent component of fungal media. Cycloheximide must be avoided by selecting a fungal culture media such as Sabouraud's agar that has been fortified, preferably with a yeast extract to provide B-complex vitamins, essential

for most fungi, and with antibiotics such as chloramphenicol to suppress bacterial contamination.

A glucose-peptone-yeast extract broth inoculated with fungal specimen and incubated at 80.6°F (27°C) on a gyrotary shaker may demonstrate fungal growth as early as 36 hours after inoculation. Once fungal growth is observed, the fungus should be subcultured promptly to induce sporulation for further identification.

Swabs and scrapings for viral culture should be placed in a transport solution such as an antibiotic-treated Hanks' or Earle's balanced salt solution available through a viral laboratory and chilled in ice if it can be inoculated within 6 hours. If culture is to be delayed more than 6 hours, the specimen in the transport solution should be quick-frozen to $-4°F$ ($-20°C$) and kept frozen during transport to an appropriate laboratory facility.

Tissue scrapings and smears from any infection threatening the eye permit the physician to select the most useful staining techniques for cytologic study in order to determine the nature of the inflammatory response, the morphology of the offending organisms, or morphologic changes in the involved tissues such as the presence of inclusion bodies, multinucleation, and keratinization.

The Giemsa stain (Table 66–5) is the most useful in identifying the type of inflammatory cell response, the status of epithelial cells, the presence or absence of cytoplasmic inclusions, and the identification of hyphal fungal fragments and may therefore be more useful in determining whether a conjunctivitis is bacterial, viral, allergic, or fungal. Gram stain (Table 66–6) is useful to identify the morphologic features of bacteria and fungal hyphal fragments and as such to help determine the cause of conjunctivitis, but it is absolutely indispensable in determining the etiology of corneal ulcers.

Ideally, cytologic study should include both the Giemsa and Gram stain techniques. When the site of infection is too small to yield a sufficient specimen for multiple cultures and slides, the Gram and Giemsa stains are most likely to yield useful information regarding bacterial, viral, allergic, and fungal etiologies. When only one slide is prepared, however, the emergency department physician must exercise caution in selecting the single stain that will be most helpful in the given situation. In dealing with corneal ulcers, priority is always given to the Gram-stained slide.

Typical and atypical mycobacteria are selectively stained by both the older Ziehl-Neelsen acid-fast stain or by high-speed fluorochrome technique combined with fluorescent microscopy.

If sufficient infectious material is available, the physician may seek to identify fungal hyphal fragments by first placing a single drop of 10% or 20% potassium hydroxide on each of two precleaned glass slides. The

TABLE 66–5   Cytology of Conjunctival Scrapings in Acute and Chronic Conjunctivitis (Giemsa)

Cytology	Possible Diagnosis
Predominantly polymorphonuclear leukocyte (PMN) response	Fungal and bacterial conjunctivitis Canaliculitis, lacrimal conjunctivitis Neonatal inclusion conjunctivitis Any severe conjunctivitis with inflammatory membrane formation Erythema multiforme Reiter's syndrome Drugs (zinc sulfate, cocaine, silver nitrate) Early benign mucous membrane pemphigoid
Equal number of PMNs and lymphocytes	Presumed *Chlamydia* infection
Equal number of PMNs and lymphocytes plus fewer plasma cells, Leber cells, multinucleated cells with four or fewer nuclei	Trachoma, adult inclusion conjunctivitis
Predominantly mononuclear response (lymphocytes)	Epithelial keratoconjunctivitis Pharyngoconjunctival fever Herpes simplex conjunctivitis Newcastle disease conjunctivitis Toxic conjunctivitis (molluscum contagiosum, idoxuridine, miotics) Acute hemorrhagic conjunctivitis
Eosinophils and eosinophilic granules	Atopic keratoconjunctivitis Vernal conjunctivitis Hay fever conjunctivitis (ocular atopy) Erythema multiforme Benign mucous membrane pemphigoid

Epithelial cell changes
  Cytoplasmic inclusion
  Keratinization
  Increased goblet cells
	
	Definite *Chlamydia* infection
	Xerophthalmia, epithelial plaques, keratoconjunctivitis sicca (severe)
	Keratoconjunctivitis sicca, chronic conjunctivitis

Source: Wilson LA, Sexton RR: Laboratory aids in diagnosis. In Duane TD (ed): *Clinical Ophthalmology.* Hagerstown, Md, Harper & Row, 1980, vol 4, chap 1.

infected material, obtained with a platinum spatula, is immediately smeared and mixed with the potassium hydroxide on the glass slide and confined to a 1-cm surface area. A coverslip is immediately placed over this mixture and the borders are sealed with petroleum jelly (Vaseline) to prevent evaporation. The slide should be read immediately. If sufficient biologic material is available, two extra slides may be prepared with the assistance of the bacteriology technician and held in reserve for special fungal staining, including the use of periodic acid-Schiff (PAS) and Gormori methenamine silver (GMS) stains.

The ideal technique for obtaining culture specimens from the conjunctiva and lid margins employs sterile swabs, moistened with sterile saline or with bacteriologic broth prior to everting the eyelid and wiping the swab along the conjunctival fornix or cul-de-sac.[12] The upper and lower lid margins should be similarly swabbed. All swabs from a single eye are streaked on the same solid media culture plate in the manner described by

Wilson and Sexton (Fig. 66–5) to avoid confusion and to facilitate identifying the origins of the respective cultures.[11] Because the preservatives of topical anesthetic solutions markedly suppress bacterial growth, topical anesthetics should not be employed when obtaining these particular cultures.

Scraping epithelial surfaces for cytologic study requires both the instillation of a topical anesthetic into the conjunctival sac prior to everting the lids and the gentle scraping of the epithelial surface with a platinum spatula that has been flame sterilized and allowed to cool to room temperature. Scrapings are obtained from the sites of maximum infection and inflammatory response. Gentle scraping is mandatory to avoid conjunctival bleeding. The lid and conjunctival specimens from one eye may each be spread in a thin layer but on different identifiable sections of a single precleaned glass slide, and each should be confined to a 1-cm surface area to facilitate location and identification of organisms. The slide is then air dried for at least 5 minutes

TABLE 66–6   Gram Stain Cytology in Conjunctivitis and Corneal Ulcer

Staining Characteristics and Morphology	Most Probable Causative Organism	
	Conjunctivitis	Corneal Ulcer
Gram-positive		
Cocci; singly, in pairs, or in clusters	*Staphylococcus* sp.	*Staphylococcus* sp.
Cocci in chains	*Streptococcus* sp.	*Streptococcus* sp.
Lancet-shaped diplococci	Pneumococcus	Pneumococcus
Rods	Diphtheroids	*Bacillus* sp., atypical mycobacteria
Filaments	*Actinomyces* sp., fungus	Fungus
Gram-negative		
Diplococci	*Neisseria gonorrhoeae*	*N. gonorrhoeae*
	N. meningitidis	*N. meningitidis*
	N. catarrhalis	
Diplobacilli	*Moraxella* sp.	*Moraxella* sp.
Rods	*Hemophilus* sp.	*Pseudomonas aeruginosa* (until culture proves otherwise)
Filaments	Fungus	Fungus

Source: Wilson LA, Sexton RR: Laboratory aids in diagnosis. In Duane TD (ed): *Clinical Ophthalmology.* Hagerstown, Md, Harper & Row, 1980, vol 4, chap 1.

prior to immersion in a fixative of 95% methanol for 5 to 10 minutes and air dried a second time. Final staining may then be performed at the convenience of the physician or laboratory technician.

BACTERIAL CORNEAL ULCERS (BACTERIAL KERATITIS)

The bacterial corneal ulcer (bacterial keratitis) is an active invasion of the cornea by bacteria leading to stromal abscess formation associated with inflammatory findings of variable intensity. Since the cornea's resistance to bacterial invasion is attributable to the integrity of the outer epithelial layer, the cleansing mechanism and barrier protection of the normal eyelid, and the separate functions of the three layers of the precorneal tear film, defects in any one of these three defense mechanisms, whether from the slightest injury or from a chronic debilitating disease will dispose to bacterial corneal ulcers.

The clinical features of bacterial corneal ulcers may include the following:[8,12,13]

- preexisting infection such as a localized anterior segment ocular infection, an upper respiratory tract infection, a tracheostomy frequently in a comatose patient, contaminated surgical wounds, and contaminated eye medications and cosmetics
- predisposing disorders debilitating to the cornea specifically or to the patient in general
- epithelial injury and defect
- ulceration occurring within 72 hours of the initial inoculation
- sudden deterioration in visual acuity and in the clinical appearance of the cornea
- intense panconjunctival injection
- severe ocular pain usually, although the discomfort may be minimal or absent in the presence of a preexisting corneal anesthesia
- necrotic grayish stromal infiltrate at the base of an epithelial defect
- surrounding halo of white or gray epithelial and stromal edema
- radiating folds in the posterior cornea and Descemet's membrane
- abundant mucopurulent discharge clinging tenaciously to the ulcer
- central, paracentral, or peripheral localization on the corneal surface; centrally directed advancing ulcer border, undermined by replicating bacteria and overhung by a lip of necrotic stroma; and numerous microabscesses in the anterior corneal stroma
- anterior chamber reaction ranging from a mild flare and cell to an extensive sterile hypopyon and fibrin clot filling the entire anterior chamber and obscuring all iris detail and the fixation of a dense fibrin plaque to the endothelial surface behind the ulcer
- corneal melting (colliquative necrosis of the corneal stroma)
- extensive posterior synechia
- secondary cataract
- herniation of Descemet's membrane through an eroded corneal stromal defect manifest as a shiny black descemetocele
- corneal perforation within 3 to 7 days of injury or inoculation.

Because the clinical features of bacterial corneal ulcers are too variable and preclude etiologic diagnosis and a rationale for antimicrobial therapy, a laboratory workup for corneal ulcers is mandatory and must be approached methodically with considerable clinical discipline.[11–13]

The initial emergency and continued care of corneal ulcers is entirely the province of the ophthalmologist. Most patients with significant ulcers will be hospitalized because of the complex work-up, the intensity of nursing care required, the close monitoring of the clinical course, and the frequency of slit lamp examinations.

The realities of emergency medicine are such, however, that the emergency physician, particularly in a remote community or military outpost, may not have access to an ophthalmologist and adequate hospital facilities during the first 24 to 72 hours of this crisis. Because of the potential of the bacterial ulcer to involve the entire cornea, to impair vision severely, to perforate the cornea rapidly, and to lead eventually to loss of the globe, it is imperative that the physician be prepared to initiate swift and proper management. Subsequently, complete clinical and laboratory data must accompany the patient when the patient is transferred to the care of the ophthalmologist.

The one procedure most likely to renew and refresh the emergency physician's bacteriologic skills and train him to deal with a wide range of infectious problems is the work-up of a central corneal ulcer, the successful treatment of which is entirely dependent on meticulous technique and careful preparation in identifying the infecting orgnism and in initiating specific antimicrobial therapy.[8,11–13,18]

The therapeutic goals include the following:

- identifying the organism
- eliminating the organism
- minimizing the destructive effects of inflammation
- promoting rapid reepithelialization of the cornea.

To meet this challenge the physician's knowledge must span the following:

- the bacteria commonly known to cause corneal ulcers
- the Gram staining characteristics of these bacteria[8]
- the clinical signs suggestive of bacterial corneal ulcer
- a reliable technique for obtaining ulcer material for Gram stain cytology and culture[8,11,13,18]
- the antimicrobials used topically and subconjunctivally against organisms known commonly to cause bacterial corneal ulcers.[13,18]

Recognition of the corneal ulcer as bacterial is based on the Gram stain cytology of the smeared ulcer scraping. Probable specific etiology and selection of immediate antibiotic therapy are based on the physician's awareness of the common pathogens, the Gram stain characteristics and morphology, as well as their general antimicrobial sensitivity (Table 66–7). The physician should be quick to employ the services of a bacteriologist or bacteriology laboratory technician and prepare a checklist of desired smears, cultures, equipment, labels and charge slips, and instructions regarding early sensitivity testing.

The most common causes of corneal ulcers in the United States include the following:[11]

- *Pseudomonas aeruginosa:* gram-negative bacillus
- *Staphylococcus aureus:* gram-positive cocci
- *Streptococcus pneumoniae:* gram-positive diplococci
- *Moraxella lacunata:* gram-negative diplobacilli.

Less common causes of corneal ulcers include:

- *Staphylococcus epidermidis:* gram-positive cocci
- *Streptococcus viridans:* gram-positive cocci
- *Streptococcus pyogenes:* gram-positive cocci
- Enterobacteriaceae *(Escherichia coli, Proteus, Klebsiella pneumoniae, Serratia marcescens):* gram-negative bacilli
- *Neisseria gonorrhoeae:* gram-negative diplococci.

Rare causes of corneal ulcers are:

- anaerobic micrococci
- gram-positive baccilli
- nonhemolytic enterococcus *(Streptococcus faecalis).*

Smears and cultures should first be obtained from the conjunctiva, lid margins, and nasolacrimal sac reflux in the involved eye (Fig. 66–6). The cornea is then anesthetized with 0.5% proparacaine hydrochloride, which has less antiseptic than either cocaine or tetracaine. A sterile, dry Dacron or calcium alginate applicator is touched to the center of the corneal ulcer and is streaked first on bacterial and then on fungal culture plates, effecting an upper row of five C streaks in the **manner** described by Jones.[12] The applicator tip must not **touch** the lid margins or conjunctiva. Next, the **magnification** of the slit lamp or loupes is employed to obtain deeper ulcer scrapings with the platinum spatula applied first to the center of the corneal ulcer and then to the advancing edges (Fig. 66–6), yielding material that is **then** spread on a series of precleaned glass slides for Gram and Giemsa stains and lastly for special stains. In dealing with corneal ulcers priority is always given to the Gram stain slide.

In a similar manner, the corneal ulcer is scraped again deeper centrally and along the advancing ulcer edge. This material is used to inoculate the solid media, ef-

Table 66–7　Antibiotics of Choice

Organism	First Choice	Alternatives
Gram-positive cocci		
Staphylococcus aureus		
Non-penicillinase producing	Penicillin G	A cephalosporin, clindamycin, vancomycin
Penicillinase producing	Oxacillin, methicillin, nafcillin	A cephalosporin, clindamycin, vancomycin
Streptococcus pyogenes	Penicillin G	Erythromycin
Streptococcus, anaerobic	Penicillin G	Clindamycin, a tetracycline, erythromycin
Streptococcus pneumoniae	Penicillin G	A cephalosporin, erythromycin
Gram-negative cocci		
Neisseria gonorrhoeae	Penicillin G	Spectinomycin, tetracycline
Gram-positive bacilli		
Bacillus anthracis	Penicillin G	Erythromycin, a tetracycline
Clostridium perfringens (welchii)	Penicillin G	Erythromycin, a tetracycline
Corynebacterium diphtheriae	Erythromycin	Penicillin G
Listeria monocytogenes	Ampicillin with or without streptomycin	A tetracycline, erythromycin
Enteric Gram-negative bacilli		
Bacteroides		
Oropharyngeal strains	Penicillin G	Clindamycin, chloramphenicol, ampicillin, a tetracycline
Gastrointestinal strains	Clindamycin	Chloramphenicol, ampicillin, a tetracycline
Enterobacter	Gentamicin	Tobramycin, chloramphenicol, a tetracycline, carbenicillin
Escherichia coli		
Community acquired	Ampicillin	Gentamicin, a tetracycline, a cephalosporin
Hospital acquired	Gentamicin	Ampicillin, carbenicillin, a cephalosporin, tobramycin
Klebsiella pneumoniae	Gentamicin with or without cephalosporin	Tobramycin, a tetracycline, chloramphenicol
Proteus mirabilis	Ampicillin	Amoxicillin, a cephalosporin, gentamicin, tobramycin
Other *Proteus* species	Gentamicin	Tobramycin, carbenicillin, a tetracycline
Serratia	Gentamicin	Kanamycin, chloramphenicol, carbenicillin
Other Gram-negative bacilli		
Acinetobacter (Mima-Herellea)	Gentamicin	Tobramycin, chloramphenicol
Hemophilus influenzae	Chloramphenicol	Ampicillin
Pasteurella multocida	Penicillin G	A tetracycline
Pseudomonas aeruginosa	Carbenicillin or ticarcillin with tobramycin or gentamicin	
Actinomycetes		
Actinomyces israelii (actinomycosis)	Penicillin G	A tetracycline
Nocardia	A sulfonamide	Trimethoprim-sulfamethoxazole

Source: Baum JL: Antibiotic use in ophthalmology. In Duane TD (ed): *Clinical Ophthalmology.* Hagerstown, Md, Harper & Row, 1980, vol 4, chap 26, and modified from *The Medical Letter on Drugs and Therapeutics*, revised edition, 1976.

fecting the second and third parallel rows of five C inoculation streaks each. Attempts should be made to obtain scrapings from different depths and different regions of the corneal ulcer. The practice of effecting five C-streaked inoculations for each specimen tends to ensure effective inoculation and results in the highest success rate for culture (Fig. 66–7).[12]

Scrapings should be inoculated on a Lowenstein-Jensen slant to culture mycobacteria, which if cultured on blood agar could be misinterpreted as diphtheroids.

Lastly, scrapings obtained for a suspected viral corneal ulceration are placed in the transport media and prepared as described above.

Gram stained cytology of the corneal ulcer is the starting point in both diagnosis and treatment. The presence of organisms confers the infectious etiology. The staining characteristics and morphology permit classification of the organism. Based on this incomplete information on the infecting organism, initial therapy is selected according to the general effectiveness of the

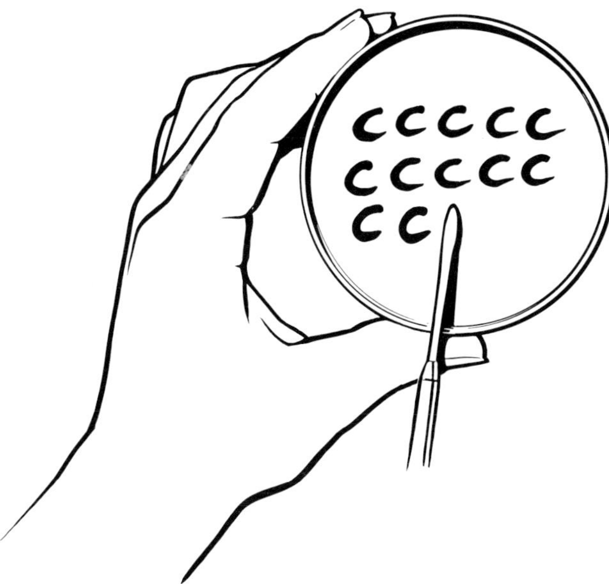

Figure 66–7 Direct Innoculation of an Agar Plate with Platinum Spatula. *Note:* Each row of C streaks represents a separate corneal scraping. (*Source:* Jones DB: Early diagnosis and therapy of bacterial corneal ulcers. *Int Ophthalmol Clin* 13(4):1, 1981.)

specific antibiotic agent against the group of bacteria in general. It must be assumed that the organisms identified by Gram stained cytology represent the most virulent and resistant within the group.[13] As subsequent laboratory data identify the specific organisms and the antimicrobial sensitivities, drug therapy may be altered to improve clinical response if indicated.[12,13,18]

An alternate regimen for the initial therapy of bacterial corneal ulcers is to employ multiple antibiotics known to be effective against the most virulent bacteria of both the gram-positive and gram-negative groups as outlined by Baum (Exhibit 66–3 and Table 66–8).

Within 18 to 24 hours, the preliminary identification of the isolated organisms may be possible by inspection of the culture plates, at which time antimicrobial sensitivity must be initiated even prior to final identification of the organism. The extent of visual impairment is ultimately determined by the severity of the inflammatory response elicited by the invading organism, the degree of pathogenicity of the organism, and the speed with which the organism is eliminated from the cornea. The 1- or 2-day advantage gained by determining the antimicrobial sensitivity early may be the deciding factor in determining the preservation of vision or indeed in preserving the eye.

UVEITIS

Although it is generally sufficient for the emergency physician to diagnose an ocular inflammatory process

Exhibit 66–3 Treatment of Bacterial Corneal Ulcers

Initial therapy for all suspected bacterial corneal ulcers
 1. Cefazolin, 100 mg (0.75 ml), and gentamicin, 40 mg (1.0 ml), subconjunctivally, daily for 4 to 5 days or until culture report and clinical condition suggest change
 2. Concentrated drops of cefazolin and gentamicin: 2 drops every 15 to 30 minutes around the clock for 48 hours or until culture report and clinical condition suggest change
 3. Cycloplegia
 4. Anticollagenase, especially if *Pseudomonas* suspected Acetylcysteine (Mucomyst) 20%, 2 drops every 1 to 2 hours
 5. Concentrated drops of cefazolin and gentamicin

Subsequent antibiotic therapy for specifically diagnosed bacterial corneal ulcers*
 Staphylococcus (penicillin-sensitive)
  Subconjunctival
   Penicillin G, 0.5–1.0 million units
   If patient is allergic to penicillin, gentamicin, 40 mg (1st choice), *or* cefazolin, 100 mg (if penicillin hypersensitivity unrelated to anaphylaxis or giant urticaria)
  Topical
   Bacitracin, 10,000 U/ml
 Staphylococcus (penicillin-resistant)
  Subconjunctival
   Cefazolin, 100 mg (1st choice), *or* oxacillin, 100 mg, *or* vancomycin, 25 mg
  Topical
   Bacitracin, 10,000 U/ml (1st choice), *or* vancomycin, 33 mg/ml
 Streptococcus (*S pyogenes, S viridans* or *S pneumoniae*)
  Subconjunctival
   Penicillin G, 0.5–1.0 million units
  Topical
   Bacitracin, 10,000 U/ml
 Enterococcus (*S fecalis*)
  Subconjunctival
   Penicillin G, 0.5–1.0 million units plus gentamicin or tobramycin, 40 mg (1.0 ml)
  Topical
   Vancomycin, 33 mg/ml
 Pseudomonas
  Subconjunctival
   Tobramycin, 40 mg (1.0 ml) *and* ticarcillin, 100 mg
  Topical
   Tobramycin, 15 mg/ml (1.5%)
   Ticarcillin, 6 mg/ml
 Proteus
  Subconjunctival
   Gentamicin, 40 mg (1st choice), *or* neomycin, 500 mg
  Topical
   Gentamicin, 14 mg/ml, *or* neomycin, 33 mg/ml
 Enterobacter, Escherichia coli, Klebsiella, Acinetobacter (*Mima-Herellea*)
  Subconjunctival
   Tobramycin, 40 mg (1.0 ml), *or* gentamicin, 40 mg (1.0 ml)
  Topical
   Gentamicin, 14 mg/ml

* Provided the organism is resistant to initial antibiotics, the ulcer continues to worsen, and the pathogen is sensitive to the suggested antibiotic.

Source: Baum JL: Antibiotic use in ophthalmology. In Duane TD (ed): *Clinical Ophthalmology.* Hagerstown, Md, Harper & Row, 1980, vol 4, chap 26.

TABLE 66–8   Parenteral and Subconjunctival/Retrobulbar Antibiotic Therapy in the Treatment of Bacterial Corneal Ulcers of Endophthalmitis

Generic	Trade Name	Subconjunctival or Retrobulbar	Parenteral
Penicillin G	Multiple	500,000–1 million units, 300–600 mg	2–6 million units every 3–4 hr*
Ampicillin	Multiple	100 mg	2.0 gm every 3–4 hr IV*
Methicillin	Staphcillin	75–100 mg	1.5 gm every 4 hr*
Oxacillin	Prostaphlin	75–100 mg	2.0–2.5 gm evey 4 hr*
Nafcillin	Nafcil-Unipen	†	1.5–2.0 gm every 4 hr IV*
Carbenicillin	Geopen	100 mg	2.0–4.0 gm every 3–4 hr IV*
Ticarcillin	Ticar	100–150 mg	3 gm every 4 hr IV*
Cephalothin	Keflin	‡	1.0–2.0 gm every 3–4 hr IV
Cephaloridine	Loridine	100 mg	1.0 gm every 3–4 hr IM§
Cefazolin	Kefzol, Ancef	100 mg	1.0 gm every 4 hr IV*
Cefamandole	Mandol	†	1.5–2.0 gm every 4 hr IV*
Cefoxitin	Mefoxin	†	1.5–2.0 gm every 4 hr IV*
Bacitracin	Bacitracin	10,000 units	Do not use, too toxic
Clindamycin	Cleocin	150 mg	0.5–1.0 gm every 8 hr IV
Gentamicin	Garamycin	20–40 mg	4 mg/kg every 24 hr
Tobramycin	Nebcin	20–40 mg	4 mg/kg every 24 hr
Amikacin	Amikin	†	5 mg/kg every 8 hr IM or IV
Neomycin	Mycifradin	250–500 mg	Do not use, too toxic
Vancomycin	Vancocin	25 mg	Do not use (nephrotoxic and ototoxic)
Chloramphenicol	Chloromycetin	50–100 mg	1 gm every 6 hr IV
Tetracycline	Multiple	2.5–5.0 gm	—
Doxycycline	Vibramycin	†	50–100 mg every 12 hr IV
Colistin	Coly-Mycin M	25 mg	5 mg/kg every 24 hr IM in 2–4 doses

* Use probenecid, 0.5 gm, orally four times a day.
† Undetermined.
‡ Very irritating, use cefazolin.
§ Maximum of 4 gm every 24 hours—nephrotoxic.
Source: Baum JL: Antibiotic use in ophthalmology. In Duane TD (ed): *Clinical Ophthalmology.* Hagerstown, Md, Harper & Row, 1980, vol 4, chap 26.

accurately as a form of uveitis (i.e., iritis, cyclitis, iridocyclitis, anterior uveitis, posterior uveitis, panuveitis), it is absolutely mandatory that all patients with any form of uveitis be referred to an ophthalmologist for definitive diagnosis, regardless of whether the uveitis was spontaneous in onset or secondary to an apparent traumatic event. For the welfare of the patient, it is safest for the physician to regard all forms of uveitis as symptomatic of a more serious latent underlying process.

The specific etiologic diagnosis of uveitis requires considerable diagnostic clinical acumen and the use of special diagnostic procedures, such as indirect ophthalmoscopy with scleral depression and contact lens biomicroscopy as well as the selection of laboratory tests.[6] Although many forms of acute uveitis respond without sequelae to a classic regimen, the physician should not accept the responsibility for diagnosing what is apparently an innocent and transient process. This applies particularly to the care of all children and to adults who experience the spontaneous onset of an iritis without apparent cause. Flare and cells, the hallmark of uveitis,

may actually be related to any one of the following entities:

- necrotic malignant intraocular tumor
- metastatic tumor
- leukemic infiltration
- transudation and cellular proliferation associated with a primary degenerative process or intraocular infection
- degenerative diseases involving the posterior eye
- retinal tear and retinal detachment
- retinal dystrophies.

The emergency physicians who accurately diagnose uveitis, initiate treatment, and make a reasonable effort to ensure proper aftercare have done their duty well. However, the physicians who are able to distinguish accurately between granulomatous and nongranulomatous uveitis in the different regions of the eye have greatly expanded their ophthalmologic skills, thus providing an increased level of competence in the general evaluation of all ocular disorders.

Signs and symptoms of uveitis include the following:[6,19]

- dull ipsilateral aching pain referred to any branch of the trigeminal nerve, but most commonly to the brow and the periorbital region
- spasmodic sharp pain associated with the pupillary light reflex and due to stimulation of trigeminal nerve pain fibers in the cornea, iris, or ciliary body
- epiphora—excessive tearing from trigeminal irritation
- blurred vision due to cloudiness of the media because of the inflammatory reaction in the aqueous and/or vitreous
- ciliary injection—a violaceous episcleral hyperemia involving the deep ciliary vessels radiating around the limbus and distinguished from conjunctival hyperemia by remaining fixed and not moving when the conjunctiva is manipulated with a cotton-tipped applicator
- altered iris color when compared with the iris color of the uninvolved eye
- smaller pupillary size when compared with the pupil diameter in the uninvolved eye
- flare—a milky homogenous relucency in the aqueous humor visible across the anterior chamber only when viewed with a narrowed beam of intense light against a dark background free of reflections and examined prior to any attempts at pupil dilation and applanation tonometry (Table 66–9). A flare is due to a transudate of protein across the inflamed uveal tissue and may be graded. "Plasmoid aqueous" signifies a low concentration of fibrin in the anterior chamber. "Plastic aqueous" designates such a high concentration of fibrin as to form a readily visible fibrin clot in the anterior chamber.

TABLE 66–9   Grading of Flare and Cells in the Anterior Chamber*

Grade	Flare		Cells	
½	Not visible	Normal	Rare cell	Normal
1	Very slight		Occasional cell	
1½	Mild		2–7	
2	Mild to moderate		8–15	
2½			16–30	
3	Moderate		Too many to count	
3½			Too many to count	
4	Severe		Largest number ever seen	

* Beam is 15 units wide, using the Haag-Streit 900 slit lamp; length is set at 2 units and is varied to optimum conditions.
Source: Schlaegel TF, Jr: Symptoms and signs of uveitis. In Duane TD (ed): *Clinical Ophthalmology.* Hagerstown, Md, Harper & Row, 1980, vol 4, chap 32.

- inflammatory cells in the aqueous humor and the retrolental and vitreous spaces (Fig. 66–8). The grading of cell concentration and media haziness in the separate regions of the eye (Tables 66–9 through 66–11) serve to indicate the major location of the inflammatory process and its severity. It should be emphasized that the evaluation of flare, cells, and media haziness is best determined in a darkened examining room by a dark-adapted examiner with intense illumination and both a narrowed and shortened slit beam of the slit lamp. The examiner must make a conscious effort to focus on the finest conceivable detail in the adjacent anatomy in order to properly focus the individual's eyes for the small detail within the media.
- keratic precipitates (KPs)—punctate aggregates of inflammatory cells deposited on the corneal en-

TABLE 66–10   Grading of Inflammation Behind the Lens*

Grade	Grade by Number of Cells	
	Retrolental Space	Anterior or Middle Vitreous
Mild		
½	Questionable	Questionable
1	1–7 cells	1–11 cells
Moderate		
1½	8–13 cells	12–19 cells
2	14–19 cells	20–34 cells
2½	20–25 cells	35–60 cells
Severe		
3	26–60 cells	61–120 cells
3½	Too many to count	
4	Too many to count	

* Long beam, 10 units wide, using the Haag-Streit 900 slit lamp.
Source: Schlaegel TF, Jr: Symptoms and signs of uveitis. In Duane TD (ed): *Clinical Ophthalmology.* Hagerstown, Md, Harper & Row, 1980, vol 4, chap 32.

TABLE 66–11   Vitreous Haze

Grade	Criteria
0	Crystal clear
1	Faint—must focus with direct ophthalmoscope
2	Mild haze
3	Moderate haze
4	Unable to see fundus with direct ophthalmoscope

Source: Kimura SJ, Thygeson P, Hogan MJ: Signs and symptoms of uveitis: II. Classification of the posterior manifestations of uveitis. Published with permission from The American Journal of Ophthalmology 47:171–176, 1959. Copyright by The Ophthalmic Publishing Company.

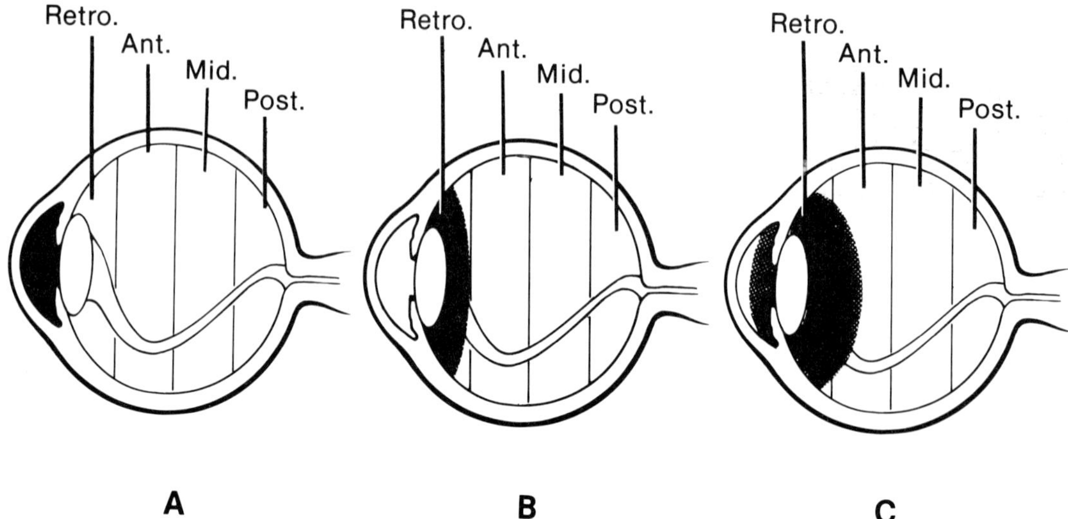

Figure 66–8 Location of Inflammatory Cells in the Diagnosis of Uveitis. *Note: A.* Iritis is diagnosed when all or almost all of the cells are found in front of the lens. *B.* Cyclitis is diagnosed when all or almost all of the cells are found behind the lens in the retrolental or anterior vitreous spaces. *C.* The most common diagnosis of anterior uveitis is that of iridocyclitis when a roughly equal number of cells is found in front of and behind the lens. (*Source:* Schlaegel TF, Jr: Symptoms and signs of uveitis. In Duane TD (ed): *Clinical Ophthalmology.* Hagerstown, Md. Harper & Row, 1980, vol 4, chap 32.)

TABLE 66–12 Differentiation of Granulomatous and Nongranulomatous Uveitis

Portion of Eye	Granulomatous	Nongranulomatous
Anterior segment	Insidious and mild; eye relatively white	Acute onset of severe inflammation (red eye)
	Nodules are superficial or deep in the iris	No nodules in the iris
	Floccules on the iris (evanescent)	No floccules on the iris
	Greasy exudates on the lens	May be heavy fibrinous exudate on lens
	Medium and large and often mutton-fat (greasy) keratic precipitates if patient is not on cortisone drops, which reduce the size of the keratic precipitate	Small, nongreasy keratic precipitates
Posterior segment	Common in choroid or retina	Rare in choroid or retina
	Heavy vitreous exudate or veils common	No or only fine punctate opacities in the vitreous
	Definite nodular lesion(s)	Diffuse—flat involvement characterized by edema and pigment changes

Source: Schlaegel TF, Jr: Symptoms and signs of uveitis. In Duane TD (ed): *Clinical Ophthalmology.* Hagerstown, Md, Harper & Row, 1980, vol 4, chap 32.

dothelial surface at or below the central cornea. KPs may be graded according to their distribution and composition and are described as being fibrinous, fine, medium, large, giant, hyalinized, "greasy" or "mutton-fat," discrete, coalescent, shrunken, pigmented, and shadow or ghost.

- nodules and precipitates—punctate cellular aggregates of the granulomatous "greasy or mutton-fat" variety detected on the iris surface, pupillary border, the trabecular meshwork, the anterior and posterior hyaloid (vitreous) faces, the anterior vitreous base, or the surface of the retina
- small pupillary size associated with a sluggish pupillary light response due to inflammation and edema of the uveal tissue
- intraocular pressure that tends to be normal or decreased depending on the extent to which the ciliary body is malfunctioning due to the inflammatory cyclitis. The physician must be constantly alert for the possibility of a secondary glaucoma due to obstruction of the trabecular meshwork in an eye that may have been already predisposed to glaucoma.

The prime reason for the physician's attempt to classify uveitis as granulomatous, nongranulomatous, or transitional (i.e., possessing features of the previous two forms of uveitis) (Table 66–12) is that the exercise trains the physician to observe, to record, and to report observations accurately in a disciplined manner. The secondary gains for the physician include greatly increased ophthalmologic skills and the opportunity to increase diagnostic acumen.

Since it is generally not the role of the emergency department physician to pursue the specific etiologic agents that may cause uveitis,[6,20] efforts should be directed at the nonspecific treatment of uveitis with the object of rapidly decreasing the inflammatory process in order to minimize or repair ocular damage and thereby minimize visual loss. Topical corticosteroid therapy remains the most effective method of eliminating the inflammatory process in the most frequent forms of uveitis. This route is more effective and is associated with less complications than systemic therapy. Once the physician is committed to the diagnosis of uveitis, topical corticosteroid therapy must be initiated without fear of inducing cataracts or glaucoma in the treated eye. These are problems that are consequent to long-term treatment and are the responsibility of the ophthalmologist attending to the patient's follow-up care. Once the physician is committed to using topical corticosteroids, the physician must be aggressive in prescribing a dose schedule that is sufficient to obtain the desired clinical response (Exhibit 66–4). By being too cautious and employing weaker corticosteroid solutions or a less aggressive dose schedule, the physician could do the patient a disservice. As topical corticosteroids eliminate the inflammatory process, the eye becomes more responsive to other medications and the late complications of uveitis are less likely to ensue.

Mydriatics and cycloplegics (Table 66–13) should be sufficient to provide patient comfort and yet be short acting enough to permit pupil mobility periodically through each day's cycle in order to avoid the complications of posterior synechia and a fixed immobile iris. The decision to employ such a long-acting mydriatic as atropine should be the responsibility of the ophthalmologist. The most useful mydriatic is homatropine 5% ophthalmic solution. The most useful topical corticosteroid is prednisolone 1% ophthalmic solution.

Oral analgesics containing a combination of ingredients such as aspirin and codeine might greatly relieve the periorbital pain. The prescription should be limited to cover a 36-hour period, however, to avoid masking a poor clinical response to the primary medications. The salicylate itself is a potent anti-inflammatory agent and will contribute to inhibiting prostaglandin synthetase within the eye.

Although uveitis is typically associated with a normal or decreased intraocular pressure, the emergency physician may unexpectedly be confronted with a secondary

Exhibit 66–4 Principles of Corticosteroid Therapy of the Eye

- Use enough, soon enough, often enough, and long enough to secure the desired results.
- Suppress inflammation until the pathogenic mechanism burns out. Determine the minimum necessary maintenance dose by a process of trial and error. Constantly attempt to decrease the dose by steplike decrements. Continue to reduce it if no relapse occurs. Increase the dose immediately if symptoms of inflammation reappear.
- In therapy that lasts longer than 2 weeks, never stop abruptly at a high dosage. If therapy must be discontinued, attempt to control the decrease with injections while tapering the systemic medication.
- Recognize that the contraindications to systemic corticosteroids apply less to the use of topical or periocular routes, although systemic absorption occurs.
- Realize that the reaction of a specific ocular entity may vary, depending on the route of administration.
- Never start with the assumption that a case is hopeless.
- Do not regard corticosteroids as 12th-hour therapy, but institute them immediately on indication.
- Start with high doses and decrease as the disease responds rather than starting with low doses and working up to the required amount.
- Do not decrease the dosage by some predetermined plan but according to the response of the patient.

Source: Gordon DM: Diseases of the uveal tract. In Gordon DM (ed): *Medical Management of Ocular Disease.* New York: Harper & Row, 1964.

glaucoma combined with uveitis. The physician should calmly evaluate the two entities separately. If the patient was known to have glaucoma prior to the onset of an apparent iritis, the inflammation is very likely due to uncontrolled glaucoma per se. Therapy should first be directed at controlling the glaucoma,[21] and the regimen for controlling the glaucoma may indeed include topical corticosteroids, which may enhance the eye's response to the antiglaucoma medications. If the patient has no antecedent history of glaucoma, if the fellow eye gives no suggestion of glaucoma, and if the affected eye does not show signs of an angle closure glaucoma,[21] it is probably safe to initiate the regimen for uveitis after first initiating control of the glaucoma with oral and/or intravenous hyperosmotic agents, topical timolol 0.5%

TABLE 66–13   Mydriatics and Cycloplegics

Parasympatholytic Drugs*

Atropine (0.5% to 2.0%): The most powerful cycloplegic available, producing mydriasis and cycloplegia lasting up to 2 weeks. It can be temporarily reversed by 1:100 intracameral acetylcholine.
Indication: Treatment of severe anterior uveitis
Oxyphenonium (Antrenyl) (1% and 5%): Produces a powerful mydriasis lasting up to 4 days and cycloplegia lasting up to 12 days.
Indication: Useful substitute for atropine in sensitive patients.
Hyoscine (Scopolamine) (0.25% and 0.5%): Produces a powerful mydriasis and cycloplegia lasting up to 5 days.
Indication: Treatment of severe anterior uveitis in atropine-sensitive patients
Homatropine (1% to 5%): Mydriasis lasts up to 2 days. It does not cause complete cycloplegia in children. It is augmented by cocaine and reversed by eserine.
Indication: Mild to moderate uveitis
Eucatropine (Euphthalmine) (5% and 10%): Effective mydriatic lasting only 4 hours, producing little cycloplegia.
Indication: Mild anterior uveitis
Cyclopentolate (Mydrilate, Cyclogyl) (0.5% to 2.0%): Short-acting cycloplegic.
Indications: Refraction, maximal cycloplegia occurs within 45 minutes; mild or moderate anterior uveitis. Particularly valuable in patients with heavily pigmented irises.
Tropicamide (Mydriacyl) (1% and 2%): Rapid-acting mydriatic and cycloplegic reaching its maximal activity in 20 minutes and lasting 6 hours. Good for bedtime use in patients with minimal flare and cells.
Indication: Mild anterior uveitis

Ocular side-effects:
blurring of vision and inability to accommodate due to cycloplegia;
precipitation of closed-angle glaucoma in patients with narrow angles;
Contact dermatitis of eyelids occurs in 5% of patients using atropine; less common in those using hyoscine.

Systemic side-effects:
Atropine, hyoscine, and (rarely) homatropine may cause dryness and flushing of the skin, thirst, and tachycardia, especially in infants. Delirium and confusion may also occur, particularly in the elderly. These effects are due to systemic absorption and can be prevented by pressing over the lacrimal sac or by tipping the head.

Sympathomimetic Drugs†

Phenylephrine (Neo-Synephrine) (10%): Produces mydriasis without cycloplegia within 20 minutes and lasts 3 hours. It is particularly effective when combined with a parasympatholytic mydriatic.
Indication: Breaking posterior synechias
Ephedrine (5%): Produces mydriasis within 30 minutes, lasting 3 hours.
Indication: Ophthalmoscopy
Hydroxyamphetamine (Paredrine) (1%): Produces mydriasis within 40 minutes.
Indication: Ophthalmoscopy
Epinephrine: Poor mydriatic when instilled into the normal eye, but a 1:1,000 solution dilates the pupil of a patient with Horner's syndrome.
Cocaine (2% to 4%): Produces mydriasis within 20 minutes which lasts 2 hours, together with a partial cycloplegia. It augments the action of homatropine and potentiates the action of Neo-Synephrine.
Indications: Breaking posterior synechias and as a local anesthetic

Ocular side-effects:
precipitation of closed-angle glaucoma in patients with narrow angles;
possible occurrence of transient corneal edema with phenylephrine;
melanin deposits in the conjunctiva and cornea with epinephrine;
macular edema with epinephrine (uncommon);
ocular pain and stinging;
desiccation of the corneal epithelium with cocaine;
shaking loose pigment floaters into the anterior chambers and the vitreous with phenylephrine.

Systemic side-effects:
The adrenergic drugs may produce tachycardia and palpitations; they should be used with caution in patients with hypertensive cardiovascular disease.
Cocaine may produce hyperreflexia, restlessness, delirium, tachycardia, irregular respiration, and chills and fever, all of which result from central nervous system stimulation, which may terminate in convulsions. These side-effects may be counteracted by a short-acting barbiturate.

* Parasympatholytics cause pupillary dilatation and paralysis of accommodation by rendering the sphincter pupillae and ciliary muscles insensitive to acetylcholine.

† Sympathomimetics imitate or potentiate the action of epinephrine and produce pupillary dilatation but no cycloplegia.

Note: These drugs potentiate the action of parasympatholytic drugs. Most mydriatics reach their maximal effect by 30 to 60 minutes, although in people with deeply pigmented irides this may take longer.

Source: Kanski JJ: Ophthalmological synopses: Mydriatics. *Br J Ophthalmol* 53:428, 1969.

eye drops, and oral or intravenous carbonic anhydrase inhibitors. When confronted with such a dilemma, the physician should seek the assistance of an ophthalmologist.

Topical antibiotic and antiviral (antiherpetic) eye drops should not be added to the regimen of topical medications, unless there is reasonable suspicion of infection of the external eye or if there is a remote concurrent infection that could inoculate the eye made vulnerable by corticosteroid therapy. Antiviral eye drops should be added to the regimen if the cornea of the affected eye shows the stigmata of old herpes keratitis or if the patient currently has any type of active herpetic infection.

Every reasonable effort should be made to improve the patient's sense of well-being by improving the patient's general health and by a genuine effort at obtaining both mental and physical rest. Through mechanisms yet to be defined, the patient's mental and physical health apart from any immediate ocular problems does seem to influence the clinical course of uveitis. Efforts should be made to control and eradicate concurrent infections or inflammatory disorders. Sunglasses and a large-brimmed hat (like a sombrero) may increase the patient's comfort by decreasing the spasmodic pain associated with the pupillary light reflex.

The patient must be advised of the urgency for follow-up care by an ophthalmologist in order to obtain the special diagnostic procedures essential to rule out a more serious underlying ocular disorder that may manifest itself as a uveitis. The therapeutic regimen usually requires modification throughout the 2 to 4 weeks of treatment during the acute phase. The clinical course of uveitis is unpredictable. Complications of uveitis can devastate the eye and lead to total blindness. The etiologic diagnostic work-up requires the skills and training of the ophthalmologist.

A summary of the nonspecific treatment of uveitis is presented in the following guidelines:

- prednisolone 1% ophthalmic solution, 1 drop every 1 to 2 hours during the waking hours and every 2 to 4 hours at night. To ensure that the patient receives the prescribed dose, the patient must vigorously shake the bottle of corticosteroid ophthalmic solution. To guarantee penetration of the eye by the medication after instilling the eye drops, the lids should be gently closed without squeezing and without blinking for at least 3 minutes. There should be a 3- to 5-minute interval between the instillation of separate eye medications. Ophthalmic solutions should be administered prior to the instillation of any ophthalmic ointments.
- homatropine 5% ophthalmic solution, 1 drop at bedtime only to as frequently as 1 drop every 4 hours according to the severity of the uveitis
- control of glaucoma, particularly pressures in excess of 30 mm Hg, with topical drugs specific for either angle closure or open angle glaucoma. When the clinical picture is confused by the presence of uveitis, the physician should consider the use of timolol 0.5% twice daily; intravenous acetazolamide, 500 mg (diluted in 5 ml sterile water), followed by 500-mg acetazolamide sequels (1 tablet orally every 12 hours); and hyperosmotic agents including oral glycerol and intravenous mannitol or intravenous urea.
- wearing of sunglasses and a broad-brimmed hat to relieve ocular pain due to the pupillary light reflex

- recommendation of complete and effective mental and physical rest
- use of appropriate topical antibiotic eye drops only in the presence of a concurrent infection of the external eye or one that may be transferred to the eye
- instillation of antiviral (antiherpetic) eye drops if the infected eye shows stigmata of old herpes keratitis or if the patient is currently exposed to any type of active herpetic infection
- appropriate patient referral for control and eradication of any other concurrent infection and inflammatory disorder
- mandatory referral to an ophthalmologist for completion of special diagnostic examinations and aftercare.

REFERENCES

1. Wolff E: *Anatomy of the Eye and Orbit.* London, HK Lewis & Co, 1968.
2. Duane TD (ed): *Clinical Ophthalmology.* Hagerstown, Md, Harper & Row, 1980.
3. Freeman HM, McDonald PR, Scheie HG: Evaluation and examination of the traumatized eye. In Freeman HM (ed): *Ocular Trauma.* New York, Appleton-Century-Crofts, 1979, pp 1–13.
4. Paton D, Goldberg MF: *Management of Ocular Injuries.* Philadelphia, WB Saunders Co, 1976.
5. Newell FW, Ernest JT: *Ophthalmology Principles and Concepts.* St. Louis, CV Mosby Co, 1974.
6. Schlaegel TF, Jr: *Essentials of Uveitis.* Boston, Little Brown Co, 1969.
7. Jones DB: Microbial preseptal and orbital cellulitis. In Duane TD (ed): *Clinical Ophthalmology.* Hagerstown, Md, Harper & Row, 1980, vol 4, chap 25.
8. Fedukowics HB: *External Infections of the Eye,* ed 2. New York, Appleton-Century-Crofts, 1977.
9. Havener WH: *Ocular Pharmacology.* St. Louis, CV Mosby Co, 1974.
10. Vaughan D, Asbury T: *General Ophthalmology.* Los Altos, Calif, Lange Medical Publications, 1974.
11. Wilson LA, Sexton RR: Laboratory aids in diagnosis. In Duane TD (ed): *Clinical Ophthalmology.* Hagerstown, Md, Harper & Row, 1980, vol 4, chap 1.
12. Jones DB: Early diagnosis and therapy of bacterial corneal ulcers. *Int Ophthalmol Clin* 13(4):1, 1981.
13. Wilson LA: Bacterial corneal ulcers. In Duane TD (ed): *Clinical Ophthalmology.* Hagerstown, Md, Harper & Row, 1980, vol 4, chap 18.
14. Pavan-Langston D: *Ocular Viral Disease.* Boston, Little Brown & Co, 1975, pp 19–35.
15. Ralph RA: Chemical burns of the eye. In Duane TD (ed): *Clinical Ophthalmology.* Hagerstown, Md, Harper & Row, 1980, vol 4, chap 28.
16. O'Day DM, Jones BR: Herpes simplex keratitis. In Duane TD (ed): *Clinical Ophthalmology.* Hagerstown, Md, Harper & Row, 1980, vol 4, chap 19.
17. Chandler JW, Rotkis WM: Ophthalmia neonatorum. In Duane TD (ed): *Clinical Ophthalmology.* Hagerstown, Md, Harper & Row, 1980, vol 4, chap 6.
18. Baum JL: Antibiotic use in ophthalmology. In Duane TD (ed):

Clinical Ophthalmology. Hagerstown, Md, Harper & Row, 1980, vol 4, chap 26.

19. Schlaegel TF, Jr: Symptoms and signs of uveitis. In Duane TD (ed): *Clinical Ophthalmology*. Hagerstown, Md, Harper & Row, 1980, vol 4, chap 32.

20. Schlaegel TF, Jr: Nonspecific treatment of uveitis. In Duane TD (ed): *Clinical Ophthalmology*. Hagerstown, Md, Harper & Row, 1980, vol 4, chap 23.

21. Kolker AE, Hetherington J, Jr: *Becker-Shaffer's Diagnosis and Therapy of the Glaucomas*. St. Louis, CV Mosby Co, 1976.

22. Moses RA (ed): *Adler's Physiology of the Eye: Clinical Application*. St. Louis, CV Mosby Co, 1981.

Appendix 66–A

The Terminology of Ocular Disorders

The list of ocular terms presented below is not very scientific and is not intended to suggest specific etiologies, but these terms are included in the jargon of the ophthalmologist, are very useful, and in a given clinical situation may permit the development of a differential diagnosis and a plan for management. This jargon accurately identifies and immediately communicates to the ophthalmologist the problem confronting the emergency department physician, who should strive to employ the terms accurately in order to maintain credibility as a clinician and to establish a strong rapport with ophthalmologic consultants.

All the disturbances of visual acuity listed below must at some time be evaluated with indirect ophthalmoscopy by an ophthalmologist. This particularly applies to such visual disturbances as visual field defects, photopsia or flashes of light, black spots or floaters, amaurosis fugax, sudden blurring of vision, morphopsia, and halos. The list of ocular signs and symptoms includes much of the phraseology employed by emergency department patients. The circumstances of emergency medical practice are such that the physician may become insensitive to vague, ill-defined, and apparently nonspecific symptoms. Most ocular symptoms are genuine and have as their basis real ophthalmologic disorders. Malingering and visual hysteria are relatively rare in the general ophthalmologic population, including that of the emergency department practice. Even our most intelligent and reliable patients with as devastating a disorder as retinal detachment or an intraocular tumor may only be able to describe their visual disturbances as a vague, ill-defined monocular or binocular visual disturbance. Because these visual signs and symptoms may reflect a medical disorder remote from the visual system itself, may be induced by medications, or may be related to a serious process within the brain or within the extracortical anatomy of the head, these signs and symptoms can be evaluated and treated appropriately only by an ophthalmologist.

amaurosis fugax—transient, brief, usually recurrent loss of vision in one or both eyes and described by the patient as a graying or darkening of visual images. The cause is usually vascular.

amblyopia—a lazy or weak eye

anisocoria—asymmetry of pupil size associated with either miosis or mydriasis that is congenital or acquired, permanent or transient

asthenopia—eye strain, visual discomfort

black eye

blepharoptosis—drooping upper eyelid

blepharospasm—persistent forcible eyelid closure

blindness (total)—no light perception

blurred vision

burning and itching

color blindness (partial or total)

dimness of vision

diplopia (monocular or binocular)

discharge from eye (serous, mucoid, purulent, fibrinous, bloody)

dry eyes

ectropion—outturning of lid margin

enophthalmos—sunken eye

entropion—inturning of lid margin

epiphora—excessive tearing

exophthalmos—bulging eyes

eyelid flutter (involuntary)—myokymia

floaters—black dots, threads, webs, smoke, crescents, and other silhouetted shapes observed as fixed or drifting across the visual field of one or both eyes periodically or constantly

foreign body sensation

hallucination (visual)—formed or ill-defined figures

hemorrhage or blood clot—ecchymosis of the lid, subconjunctival hematoma, hyphema

hyperopia—farsightedness

hysteria (visual)

iridescent vision (halos)

lack of depth perception

1015

lagophthalmos—eyelids do not cover the eyeball

leukocoria—a constant or transient appearance of a white image in the pupil of the eye (must be seen by an ophthalmologist)

loss of vision (gradual or sudden, isolated or recurrent, transient or sustained, partial or total)

morphopsia (micropsia, macropsia, or metamorphopsia)

myopia—nearsightedness

nyctalopia—night blindness

nystagmus—an involuntary repetitive movement or rotation of the eye

obscured vision (haziness or cloudiness of vision)

pain (palpebral, bulbar, retrobulbar, orbital or localized to specific regions of the face or head)

photophobia—abnormal or increased sensitivity to light

photopsia—a perception of illumination such as flashes of light, streaks, swirls, or bursts of light

presbyopia—holding newspapers and books at a progressively increasing distance for reading, occurring at the ages of 40 to 55 and associated with a decreased amplitude of accommodation

red or pink eye

strabismus (frequently manifest as "cross-eyed" or "wall-eyed")

swelling

trichiasis—eyelashes directed inward and scratching the globe

vertigo (objective or subjective)

visual field defect (total or partial, unilateral or bilateral, transient, recurrent, constant, positive or negative)

TABLE 66–A1   Distinguishing Features of Bacterial Preseptal Cellulitis, Orbital Cellulitis Secondary to Sinusitis, and Cavernous Sinus Thrombosis

Finding	Bacterial Preseptal Cellulitis	Orbital Cellulitis Secondary to Sinusitis	Cavernous Sinus Thrombosis
Lid edema	Moderate to marked	Marked	Marked
Color of lids	Red	Red	Blue-purple
Increased warmth of lids	Present	Present	Absent
Proptosis	Absent or slight	Marked	Marked
Chemosis	Moderate	Marked	Moderate
Sensation			
V-1	Normal	May be reduced	Reduced
V-2	Normal	Normal	Reduced
Vision	Normal	May be reduced	Generally reduced
Pupil	Normal	Normal	Dilated, sluggish reaction to light (III paresis)
Motility	Normal	Restricted in proportion to orbital edema	III, IV, VI paresis
Pain on motion	Absent	Present	Absent
Intraocular pressure	Normal	May be elevated	May be elevated
Ophthalmoscopy	Normal	May be normal	Venous congestion Disc edema
Temperature	Normal or slightly elevated	Elevated (102–104°F)	Elevated (102–104°F [38.9–40°C] or above)
White blood cell count	10,000–12,000/cu mm	15,000–20,000/cu mm	Above 15,000/cu mm
Other features	Evidence or trauma Purulent drainage	Radiographic changes of sinusitis Unilateral	Bilateral involvement Progressive loss of consciousness Intracranial complications

Source: Jones DB: Microbial preseptal and orbital cellulitis. In Duane TD (ed): *Clinical Ophthalmology.* Hagerstown, Md, Harper & Row, 1980, vol 4, chap 25.

Exhibit 66–A1 Routes of Infection in Orbital Cellulitis

Exogenous (direct inoculation)
  Post-traumatic
    Puncture wounds
    Retained foreign body
  Postsurgical
    Exploration for tumor
    Retinal reattachment procedure
    Strabismus surgery
Extension from adjacent structures
  Face and lids
    Posttraumatic cellulitis and abscess
    Erysipelas
  Paranasal sinuses
    Direct extension through the orbital wall
    Intravascular extension by venous
      communication
  Dental
    Anterior surface of the maxilla
    Maxillary sinus empyema
    Venous connection to the pterygoid plexus
  Intracranial
    Extradural abscess through the orbital roof
    Septic cavernous sinus thrombosis
Intraorbital
  Suppurative dacryoadenitis
  Panophthalmitis
Endogenous (metastatic)

Source: Jones DB: Microbial preseptal and orbital cellulitis. In Duane TD (ed): *Clinical Ophthalmology.* Hagerstown, Md, Harper & Row, 1980, vol 4, chap 25.

TABLE 66–A2 Selection of Initial Antibiotics in Posttraumatic Preseptal Cellulitis

Organisms in Gram Stain	Intravenous Antibiotics
Gram-positive cocci	Methicillin and penicillin G
Gram-positive rods	Penicillin G
Gram-negative rods	Gentamicin and penicillin G
None	Methicillin, penicillin G, and gentamicin

Source: Jones DB: Microbial preseptal and orbital cellulitis. In Duane TD (ed): *Clinical Ophthalmology.* Hagerstown, Md, Harper & Row, 1980, vol 4, chap 25.

Exhibit 66–A2 Standard Therapeutic Regimen for the Initial Treatment of Bacterial Endophthalmitis

Immediately following diagnosis of bacterial endophthalmitis and anterior chamber and vitreous aspiration for diagnostic purposes, commence therapy as follows:
Intravitreal injection
  Gentamicin, 0.1 mg (100 μg), in 0.1 to 0.2 ml. Following aspiration of fluid from the vitreous for diagnostic purposes, a 22-gauge needle remains in mid vitreous while a new tuberculin syringe containing antibiotic is exchanged and the material slowly injected into mid vitreous. In phakic eyes, both the diagnostic and therapeutic vitreal aspiration and injections are performed behind the lens through a tract made in the sclera 5.5 mm behind the corneal limbus.
Periocular injection
  Gentamicin, 40 mg (1 ml)
  Cefazolin, 100 mg (0.75 ml)
  Injections are made with a disposable tuberculin syringe, 25-gauge, ⅝-inch needle
Systemic
  Gentamicin, 4 mg/kg, IM daily in three divided doses
  Cefazolin, 1.0 gm, every 4 to 6 hr, IV
  Probenecid, 0.5 gm, orally, four times a day
Twelve hours after the above therapy, repeat the periocular injections of gentamicin and cefazolin and give:
Periocular injection
  Dexamethasone phosphate, 4 mg (1 ml), *or* prednisolone succinate, 25 mg (1 ml)
Prednisone, 60 mg, orally
The periocular injections are then given daily for 4 to 7 days, each drug in a separate syringe. Systemic antibiotic and corticosteroid therapy is continued for 10 to 14 days. Modify antibiotic therapy if necessary based on clinical condition and results of culture and sensitivity report of anterior chamber and vitreous tap.

Source: Baum JL: Antibiotic use in ophthalmology. In Duane TD (ed): *Clinical Ophthalmology.* Hagerstown, Md, Harper & Row, 1980, vol 4, chap 26.

TABLE 66–A3 Intraocular Pressures in Millimeters of Mercury for the Four Weights Supplied with Sklar-Schiotz Tonometer

Scale Reading	Plunger Load (In gms.)			
	5.5	7.5	10.0	15.0
0	41	59	82	127
.5	38	54	75	118
1.0	35	50	70	109
1.5	32	46	64	101
2.0	29	42	59	94
2.5	27	39	55	88
3.0	24	36	51	82
3.5	22	33	47	76
4.0	21	30	43	71
4.5	19	28	40	66
5.0	17	26	37	62
5.5	16	24	34	58
6.0	15	22	32	54
6.5	13	20	29	50
7.0	12	19	27	46
7.5	11	17	25	43
8.0	10	16	23	40
8.5	9	14	21	38
9.0	9	13	20	35
9.5	8	12	18	32
10.0	7	11	16	30
10.5	6	10	15	27
11.0	6	9	14	25
11.5	5	8	13	23
12.0		8	11	21
12.5		7	10	20
13.0		6	10	18
13.5		6	9	17
14.0		5	8	15
14.5			7	14
15.0			6	13
15.5			6	11
16.0			5	10
16.5				9
17.0				8
17.5				8
18.0				7

Note: This calibration scale includes the latest revisions of the scale adopted January 1955 by the Committee on Standardization of Tonometers of the American Academy of Ophthalmology and Otolaryngology

67. Ear, Nose, and Throat Emergencies

KEN KULIG, M.D.
GORDON GENTA, M.D.

A significant number of patients presenting to the emergency department have complaints referable to the ears, nose, or throat; yet most emergency physicians have had no formal, in-depth training in otolaryngology. This chapter is presented as an overview of some of the more common otolaryngologic problems seen in the emergency department.

ACUTE SINUSITIS

"Sinus problems" as understood by the lay public are responsible for a myriad of complaints, including nasal obstruction, headache, fatigue, nasal drainage, halitosis, and many others. True sinusitis refers to infection within one or more of the sinus cavities, usually bacterial in origin, but not infrequently viral or fungal. In general, acute sinusitis is a condition that has caused symptoms for hours to weeks and can usually be managed medically. Symptoms caused by chronic sinusitis have usually been present continually or intermittently for weeks to years. They are often refractory to medical treatment and patients may require a surgical procedure to establish adequate sinus drainage.

Anatomy and Development

The sinuses are irregular air cavities that lie within bones whose names they carry (Fig. 67–1). Although generally grouped into four pairs (frontal, ethmoidal, maxillary, and sphenoidal), there are about 12 sinuses on each side of the skull. The number is variable and frequently not the same on both sides.[1] Once the sinuses are fully developed (usually by adolescence), over half the circumference of the orbit is surrounded by sinus cavities and separated from them by only a thin plate of bone.[1,2]

The frontal sinus forms a portion of the roof of the orbit and extends posteriorly under the cranial cavity. The ethmoidal sinuses lie roughly between the orbits and the nasal cavities. The extremely thin bone separating the ethmoidal sinus from the orbit is appropriately termed the *lamina papyracea*.[3]

The maxillary sinus underlies the floor of the orbit, is the largest of the sinuses, and is the most frequently involved by an infectious process. The thickness of bone covering the apices of the teeth inferiorly is variable and occasionally absent. Odontogenic infection may be responsible for subsequent maxillary sinusitis in up to 10 percent of cases.

The sphenoidal sinus occupies the sphenoid bone and may extend into the wings of the sphenoid and even into the clinoid processes. The sphenoidal sinus is only very rarely infected.

The ethmoidal and maxillary sinuses are present at birth, although usually filled with amniotic fluid until several weeks of age. The frontal sinuses may be de-

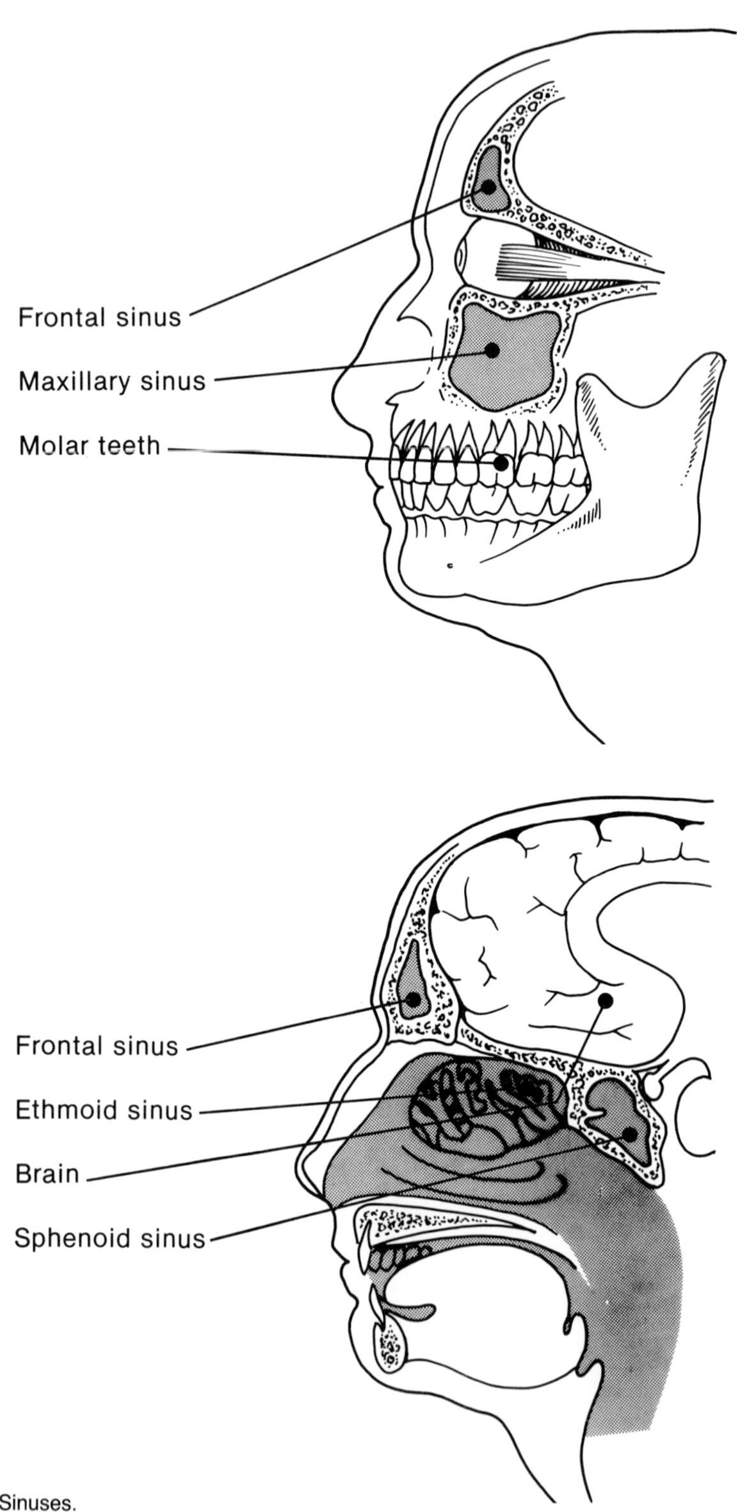

Figure 67–1 The Paranasal Sinuses.

tected radiographically after 5 or 6 years of age but are usually clinically significant only after 10 years of age.[4] Up to 20 percent of normal adults have absent frontal sinuses radiographically. The sphenoidal sinuses are the last to develop, reaching adult size in adolescence.

Of great importance is the venous drainage of the sinuses, from which infection may spread via valveless anastomosing veins to the orbit and also intracranially.[3] This will be further discussed in the section on complications.

The anterior sinuses (frontal, maxillary, and anterior ethmoidal) drain into the middle meatus beneath the middle turbinate. The posterior sinuses (sphenoidal and posterior ethmoidal) drain into the superior meatus and sphenoethmoidal recess. The close proximity of the ostia increases the likelihood of multiple sinus involvement.

Pathophysiology

The vast majority of cases of sinusitis are initiated by an obstruction of some type of the ostium draining that sinus (Table 67–1).[1,5] This most commonly occurs in the maxillary sinus, followed by the ethmoidal, frontal, and sphenoidal sinuses.[5,6] Because of the reasons cited above, it is more common to have sinusitis involving multiple cavities than an isolated process in one sinus.

The nature of the obstruction in the vast majority of cases is related to upper respiratory tract infections and/ or allergies, with resultant hyperemic and swollen mucosa surrounding the ostia. Subsequent interference with ciliary action along with mucus accumulation and in-

flammatory response provide the conditions for bacterial growth. Neoplasms, foreign bodies, and anomalies are other rare causes of obstruction.

Trauma may precipitate sinusitis by similarly interfering with normal mucus clearing and by introducing foreign material into the sinus cavity. Even relatively minor trauma may nevertheless cause a contusion of the sinus mucosa with similar results.[1]

Less common causes of acute sinusitis are also listed in Table 67–1. In many cases no etiology can ever be elucidated. The development of subacute or chronic sinusitis, however, should prompt a vigorous search for rare causes that may radically alter the therapy.

Clinical Manifestations

The most common symptoms seen in acute sinusitis are malaise (which may be pronounced), headache, and fever.[2] The fever is usually low grade unless a major complication of sinusitis has occurred. There may be a feeling of fullness and/or a dull throbbing pain over the involved area. Sudden movements frequently aggravate the pain, which may be referred to the teeth in the case of maxillary sinusitis.[6] The patient may complain of mucopurulent secretions coming from the nose, usually unilaterally. If the ethmoidal sinuses are involved, loss of vocal resonance may occur. The sense of smell may be lost, or there may be a persistent putrid odor.

Frontal sinusitis may cause the classic symptom of pain above the eyebrow, which is excruciating in the morning and lessens as the day progresses.[2,5] The patient is reluctant to allow anyone to touch the forehead over the involved area.

Ethmoidal sinusitis, particularly in children, frequently presents as orbital symptoms ranging from mild lid edema to orbital cellulitis or abscess.[3] It is prudent to evaluate every patient with nontraumatic periorbital swelling for sinusitis.

Physical signs found in cases of sinusitis are frequently nondiagnostic but may be pronounced when present. An accurate temperature should always be recorded. Tapping with the finger over the involved sinus may elicit excruciating pain in some individuals, but this sign is frequently absent. It is more likely to be found in cases of frontal sinusitis.

Ethmoiditis, as mentioned, often presents with orbital involvement. If this is absent, tenderness between the medial canthus and the bridge of the nose may be found. The ethmoidal sinuses, as is the case with the other sinuses, will rarely be involved by themselves, so that "pinpoint" tenderness is usually absent.

Unless the sinus ostia are completely obstructed, there will often be a mucopurulent discharge from the nose on the involved side, since purulent material under pres-

---

TABLE 67–1   Etiology of Acute Sinusitis

Obstruction
  Allergic (especially if polyps present)
  Infectious (viral upper respiratory infections most common)
  Anatomic (i.e., cleft palate, turbinate anomalies)
  Tumors (rare)
  Nasal foreign bodies
  Nasal packing for epistaxis control
  Adenoid hypertrophy

Trauma
  Fracture (i.e., orbital blowout)
  Penetrating wounds
  Contusion
  Barotrauma

Dental Infection
  Periodontitis
  Periapical abscess
  Sinus perforation (i.e., during tooth extraction)

Altered Immunity
  Hypogammaglobulinemia
  Chemotherapy-induced marrow depression
  Other immune deficiencies

Other
  Influenza
  Measles
  Cystic fibrosis
  Sepsis
  Pneumonia (particularly pneumococcal)
  Other pulmonary disease

sure is expelled from the sinus.[6] The absence of discharge, however, is often associated with more severe symptomatology.

Transillumination is often used but is generally not helpful in making the diagnosis.[1,2] Congenital absence of one or both frontal sinuses is common, and only the frontal and maxillary sinuses can be successfully transilluminated. With the advent of high-resolution sinus radiography, which is far more accurate diagnostically, transillumination has been employed less frequently.

Laboratory and Radiographic Studies

Since virtually all patients with sinusitis will eventually be placed on antibiotics, it is useful to obtain cultures beforehand if suitable material is available. The most valuable culture material is obtained from the sinus itself, but this necessitates a surgical procedure for retrieval.[7] If frank pus under the turbinates or in the posterior pharynx is present, this may be a good second choice as a site for obtaining cultures, but it is still likely to grow mixed flora.[1,2] It is important to use the smallest swab available to avoid contamination. Obtaining cultures of the anterior nasal secretions is useless and never recommended. The bacteriology of acute sinusitis is further discussed in the section on treatment and in Chapter 20.

In the case of a febrile toxic-appearing patient, a complete blood cell count and blood cultures should be obtained. In children with orbital involvement, a lumbar puncture is often recommended even in the absence of meningeal signs, particularly if the frontal sinus is involved, which is more likely to be associated with intracranial extension.[3,5] Whether or not to do a lumbar puncture is a difficult question with few guidelines available in the literature, and the decision should always be made in conjunction with the consulting services.

Radiographs are always necessary to make the diagnosis of acute sinusitis except in small children in whom they are extremely difficult to interpret. Even in adults the findings are frequently ambiguous and subject to a large degree of interpretation. Paranasal sinusitis is characterized radiographically by a decrease in the air content of the sinuses and by changes in the definition of the bony margins.[4] Initially the air space is reduced peripherally by edema and inflammation of the mucosal lining. The radiologic findings during this stage of sinusitis are virtually indistinguishable from those of chronic sinusitis or uncomplicated allergy.[1,4]

As the sinus fills with purulent material it becomes more opaque, and the radiographic diagnosis becomes more certain. It is essential to remember that differences in depth of the paired sinuses may give a cloudy appearance to the shallower air space even in the absence of disease and that overlying soft tissue swelling (i.e., cellulitis) may also cause the appearance of haziness of the sinus. Oblique radiographic projections in this setting may be helpful.[4]

Radiographs in infants and children are particularly difficult to interpret because the small, underdeveloped sinuses may be filled with normal redundant mucosa, leading to a "physiologic cloudiness."[4]

Air-fluid levels are the most valuable radiologic finding when present. These are most common in the large maxillary and frontal sinuses; supine horizontal radiographs may help define an air-fluid level in the sphenoidal and posterior ethmoidal sinuses.[1,6]

Rare radiographic findings secondary to complications of sinusitis include bony involvement characterized by local sclerosis of bony walls of the sinus, as seen in regional chronic osteitis, and bony destruction, as seen in osteomyelitis. The latter is more commonly seen in maxillary sinusitis in children.[3,5] Mucous cysts appear as peripheral thickening of the mucosa surrounding a well-rounded air space. Neoplasms in the paranasal sinuses cause opacity of the air space; secondary sinusitis is common. The use of tomography, radiopaque dyes, and other special techniques is occasionally useful in diagnosing neoplasms, cysts, or bony destruction.

Differential Diagnosis

Although there are many conditions that may mimic acute sinusitis in regard to pain, the diagnosis is generally not difficult to make based on a thorough history and physical examination, along with high-quality radiography. In the differential diagnosis the most common cause of confusion is pain of dental origin.[1] Dental caries, particularly when associated with infection and abscess, not only frequently mimics maxillary sinusitis but also frequently gives rise to it. (See Chapter 70.) The lining of the sinuses may appear thickened on the radiograph even in the absence of sinus infection per se. In difficult cases antral puncture may be required to rule out maxillary sinusitis.

Migraine headaches may mimic frontal sinusitis, but the character and onset of the headache are dissimilar from that seen in sinus headaches.

Trigeminal neuralgia is characterized by severe paroxysms of pain, commonly commencing after a "trigger" stimulus, that follow the distribution of the fifth cranial nerve.

Insect bites may produce local redness and swelling, and if the patient is unaware that such a bite occurred, there may be an initial confusion with sinusitis.

Neoplasms of the sinus usually present as facial pain and are commonly associated with acute sinusitis. Recurrent attacks or nonresolution of sinusitis, along with persistent radiographic abnormalities, suggest the diagnosis.

Foreign bodies in the nose may cause a persistent nasal discharge, and if any of the ostia are obstructed, may also result in sinusitis. A high index of suspicion and a thorough nasal examination will usually lead to the true diagnosis.

Complications

The incidence of complications of sinusitis has decreased greatly since the advent of the antibiotic era, but complications are still seen and are likely to present initially to the emergency department. The fact that the most serious complications are seen in otherwise healthy young people should prompt an aggressive approach.[3] The complications of sinusitis, in descending order of incidence, can be classified as orbital, intracranial, chronic sinusitis and mucocele formation, and osteomyelitis.[1,5]

Ethmoiditis is primarily responsible for the orbital complications seen in acute sinusitis, and this most frequently occurs in children. The degree of orbital involvement comprises a spectrum, beginning with eyelid edema and progressing to frank orbital cellulitis, that may be severe enough to result in limitation of gaze, proptosis, and interference with vision.[1,3,8,9] Sinusitis must always be considered when orbital cellulitis is present, regardless of the history given. Orbital abscess and cavernous sinus thrombosis are the endpoints of this process, the latter associated with an 80 percent mortality.

Intracranial extension of infection may result in epidural or subdural abscesses, intracranial thrombosis, or frank meningitis. The findings may initially be subtle and secondary to increased intracranial pressure. The presence of sinusitis should be considered in patients with meningitis caused by unusual organisms. (See Chapter 20.)

Chronic sinusitis results from chronic obstruction of the ostia and/or inadequate treatment of acute sinusitis. Once well established, chronic sinusitis usually necessitates a surgical drainage procedure for resolution.[2,6] Mucoceles may result from chronic sinusitis and also may need to be drained. They are generally innocuous but may enlarge and erode surrounding structures.

Osteomyelitis resulting from sinusitis is rare, although before the advent of antibiotics it was relatively common, particularly in children with maxillary sinusitis. Radiography may demonstrate bone erosion and loss of the intrasinus septa. Subperiosteal abscess may result in pain and marked swelling over the involved area (i.e., Pott's puffy tumor).

Treatment

Uncomplicated acute sinusitis can be treated on an outpatient basis if careful follow-up is available. Treatment consists of antibiotics, decongestants, and local heat.

An understanding of the bacteriology of sinusitis is essential in choosing antibiotic therapy; unfortunately the literature varies greatly as to the bacteria most commonly responsible for acute sinusitis. Although the percentages vary significantly, organisms most frequently recognized are pneumococcus, *Hemophilus influenzae, Streptococcus, Staphylococcus*, anaerobes, and *Klebsiella*.[1,6,7,10] Although rare, fungal infections are most commonly caused by mucormycosis, *Candida*, and *Aspergillus*. *Hemophilus influenzae* and pneumococcus combined are probably responsible for the majority of cases of acute sinusitis seen in otherwise healthy adults.[6,7] *Hemophilus* infections are more commonly seen in children. The significance of *Staphylococcus aureus* sinusitis is yet to be ascertained, but its existence is without question. For this reason, dicloxacillin or a cephalosporin is recommended for adults without complications.[1,6] A cephalosporin may be preferable to ensure gram-negative coverage in addition to *Staphylococcus*. Erythromycin may be substituted when the patient is penicillin and cephalosporin sensitive.

Because of the increased likelihood of *Hemophilus influenzae* in children, ampicillin is the drug of choice. The question of sinusitis caused by ampicillin-resistant *Hemophilus influenzae* has not been addressed in the literature.

In both adults and children with significant complications, intravenous oxacillin or nafcillin together with ampicillin is indicated.

Oral antibiotics in uncomplicated cases should be continued for 4 to 6 weeks. E.N.T. referral should be obtained immediately for complicated sinusitis, antibiotic unresponsiveness, or unusual organisms (i.e., fungi) on culture when identified.

Topical decongestants promote drainage by shrinking the nasal mucosa surrounding the ostia. Oxymetazoline is probably the most effective, with the least amount of rebound effect. Systemic decongestants and antihistamines are probably helpful, although not of proved benefit.

Local heat seems to be comforting to the patient and may promote sinus drainage. The patient should be advised to avoid swimming, smoking, flying, and physical exertion until the sinusitis has cleared. The possible complications of sinusitis should be explained to the patient so that a return visit can be scheduled should they occur.

The majority of cases of acute sinusitis will respond to the above measures. More difficult cases or those with complications should prompt referral to a specialist.

PERITONSILLAR ABSCESS (QUINSY)

Infection in the tonsil may occasionally extend through the capsule and form an abscess in the potential space between the capsule and the tonsil bed. The resulting "quinsy" is usually unilateral and located anterior and superior to the tonsil so that it is just behind the anterior tonsillar pillar.[11,12] For reasons not well understood, it is rare in children under 12 years of age. It may appear early or late in the course of tonsillitis.

Clinical Manifestations

The classic history is one of gradually increasing severe throat pain, resulting in dysphagia, drooling, and trismus. The pain is usually referred to the ear on the affected side. The patient is febrile, feels miserable, and appears "toxic"; the cervical lymph nodes are enlarged and tender.

Examination is difficult because of the patient's unwillingness to open the mouth. Examining the pharynx, however, confirms the diagnosis. The bright red peritonsillar swelling displaces the uvula to the opposite side, and the soft palate and uvula are edematous. The drooling and toxic appearance may simulate epiglottitis, but quinsy rarely causes stridor. (See Chapter 57.)

Bacteriology

In many instances the patient is already taking antibiotics so that cultures of the abscess contents are frequently negative. In one study of 68 patients, β-hemolytic *Streptococcus* was cultured from 16, α-hemolytic *Streptococcus* from 11, *Staphylococcus aureus* and *H. influenzae* from 1 each, and 39 cultures were negative. Anaerobes, although known to cause abscesses of the head and neck, were not cultured in this study.[13]

Complications

Although not common, peritonsillar abscess may result in airway compromise secondary to edema around the piriform sinus.[11,12] Rupture of the abscess may cause complete airway obstruction or pulmonary abscesses. Mediastinitis may occur via extension from the retropharyngeal space or carotid sheath.[13] Extension into the parapharyngeal space may erode the carotid artery or result in thrombophlebitis of the internal jugular vein with intracranial extension.[12] Rheumatic fever or glomerulonephritis may occur.

Treatment

Incision and drainage is always the treatment of choice, and referral to an E.N.T. specialist is mandatory. The procedure is done using local anesthesia, and the pus is allowed to drain freely out of the mouth. Classically, the tonsils are then removed 4 to 6 weeks later. However, many specialists are now advocating immediate tonsillectomy as a safe procedure that guarantees removal of the entire abscess, thus avoiding a second hospitalization.[13,14]

Once the problem is recognized in the emergency department, appropriate steps should be taken to admit the patient to the hospital with an E.N.T. referral. Active airway management is seldom necessary; however, if rupture should occur the patient should be sitting upright with the head down, and suction should be employed to remove the pus. (See Chapter 56.)

An intravenous loading dose of aqueous penicillin should be administered, even if the patient is already taking oral antibiotics. An adequate dose for the average adolescent or adult is 600,000 units.

EPISTAXIS

Epistaxis is an extremely common disorder affecting all age-groups. The peak incidence occurs in children/adolescents and the elderly and is much more common during the winter.

Anatomy

The blood supply of the superior septum and superior-lateral walls is derived from the internal carotid artery via the ethmoidal arteries, while the blood supply of the inferior portion of the septum and turbinates is derived from the external carotid artery via the palatine and sphenopalatine arteries (Figs. 67–2 and 67–3).[15] Kiesselbach's area, the anterior-inferior portion of the septum, receives an abundant blood supply from all arteries supplying the nose and is the most common site of epistaxis.[16] The three horizontally placed turbinates are located on the lateral walls of the nose and shield the sinus ostia. Most posterior epistaxis originates in branches of the sphenopalatine artery located posterior to the turbinates.

Pathophysiology

Most cases of epistaxis are anterior in location, so that the source can either be identified and cauterized or can be controlled by an anterior pack. The causes of anterior epistaxis are quite different from the causes of posterior epistaxis.

The mucosa in the anterior portion of the nose is extremely susceptible to drying, and particularly during the winter months when upper respiratory infections are epidemic, the atmospheric humidity is low, and nose-

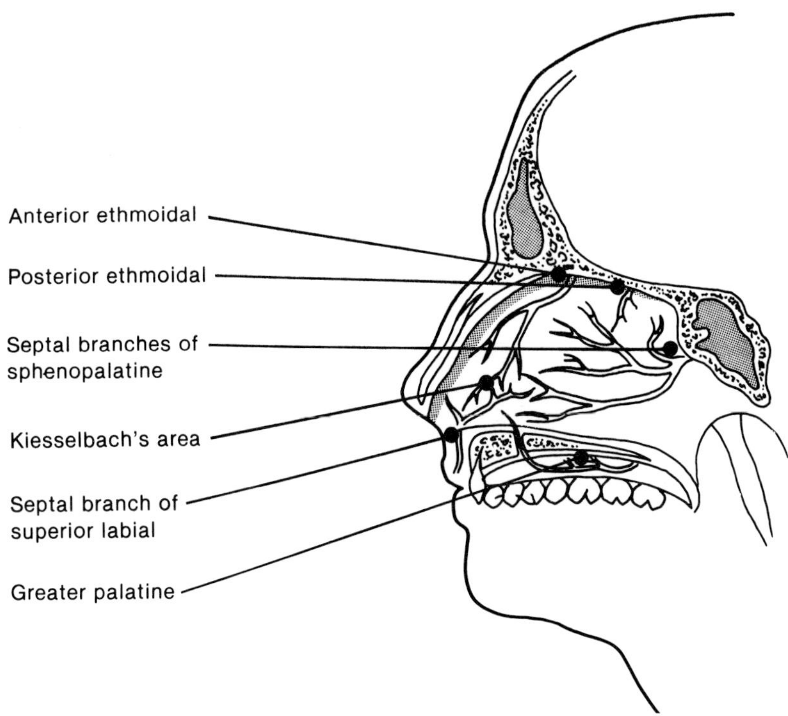

Figure 67–2   Blood Supply to the Nasal Septum.

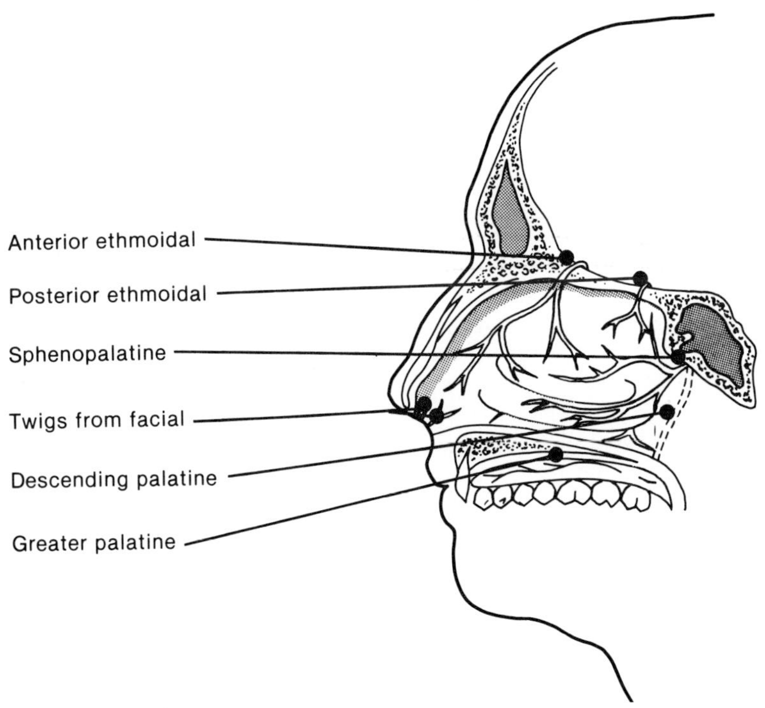

Figure 67–3   Blood Supply to the Turbinates.

picking is common, the extremely well-vascularized nasal mucosa is apt to break down and bleed. Allergies, environmental irritation, and overuse of local decongestants all result in a swollen, hyperemic mucosa, which,

especially when combined with the previously mentioned factors, is likely to cause epistaxis.

Nasal trauma and fracture frequently result in anterior epistaxis, probably from mucosal tears. The bleeding seen with trauma is often alarmingly profuse initially but self-limited and short in duration.[17]

A rare cause of anterior epistaxis is Rendu-Osler-Weber disease (hereditary hemorrhagic telangiectasia), in which cutaneous and mucosal telangiectasia appear in family members via an autosomal dominant transmission. Recurrent anterior epistaxis with a strong family history of the same is often the first clue to the diagnosis. Replacement of sections of nasal mucosa by skin grafting is sometimes necessary to prevent recurrence.[18,19]

Posterior epistaxis is usually seen in the elderly patient with a history of hypertension and/or atherosclerotic vascular disease.[15,20,21] The nasal arterioles are subject to the same changes seen in the retina,[22] with loss of the tunica media with age and narrowing with circumferential plaques. These vessels in the nose are susceptible to spontaneous rupture and because of loss of their ability to contract continue bleeding.

Coagulopathies only rarely cause epistaxis without evidence of bleeding elsewhere. Epistaxis secondary to a bleeding disorder is usually posterior in location and often resistant to tamponading attempts.[15,20] Fresh-frozen plasma may be required before hemostasis can be achieved.

Other rare causes of posterior epistaxis include pharyngeal and sinus neoplasms and rupture of internal carotid artery aneurysm. The history obtained in these disorders usually suggests the diagnosis.

History and Physical Examination

A brief history can usually be obtained while the equipment needed for a physical examination is being prepared. The most important questions to ask each patient are listed below:

- the duration of bleeding, frequency, and amount?
- with the head held horizontally, does blood run down the throat (posterior epistaxis) or out the front of the nose (anterior epistaxis)?
- past history of hypertension and treatment?
- thorough drug history: anticoagulants, aspirin?
- recent upper respiratory infections, allergies, nose-picking?
- possible foreign body; previous surgery or nasal packing that may have resulted in retained material in nose?
- family history of epistaxis or bleeding diathesis?
- history of liver disease or alcoholism?
- recent nasal trauma?
- general medical history: anemia; cardiac or pulmonary disease?

These questions are directed at finding an underlying condition responsible for the epistaxis. In most cases no such conditions are found. However, the history will often determine which laboratory studies may need to be ordered and even whether or not admission should be contemplated.

On physical examination, a comment on the overall condition of the patient should be made. Orthostatic vital signs should be obtained, and correction of volume loss begun if the pulse rate increases by more than 15 mm Hg or the systolic blood pressure decreases by more than 20 mm Hg upon standing.

The patient with epistaxis is frequently agitated, and sedation with meperidine (Demerol) or diazepam (Valium) often will facilitate the examination. The patient should be seated in front of the examiner with the head and neck in the classic "sniffing position." A bright head lamp or mirror with light source, point suction, bayonet forceps, nasal speculum, 4×4 gauze sponges, silver nitrate sticks, cotton with anesthetic/vasoconstrictor, and petrolatum gauze should be readily at hand. A quick look into the nose with adequate suctioning may instantly reveal the bleeding site; frequently, however, it is just necessary to anesthetize and vasoconstrict the nasal mucosa with 2% cocaine or a combination of epinephrine or 3% ephedrine and 1% tetracaine (Pontocaine) or 4% lidocaine (Xylocaine). Cotton can be shaped into the proper form by winding it around the bayonet forceps and, when soaked in the solution, is inserted into both sides of the nose. The patient is instructed to pinch the nose, or two tongue blades taped together on one end can be used in a pinching fashion.

Treatment

After a period of 15 minutes the cotton is removed and a thorough examination is conducted. Kiesselbach's area must always be thoroughly searched, since this is the site of the majority of epistaxis. Bleeding vessels here are usually easily cauterized using silver nitrate sticks, which should be gently touched to the septum for only several seconds at a time. Usually more than one stick is required, and all suspicious areas on the septum should be cauterized, because the vasoconstrictor may have temporarily stopped the bleeding from several sources or the actual bleeding source may now be masked.

If the epistaxis is not controlled by the above method, anterior nasal packing is now placed on the bleeding side if the epistaxis is unilateral. Petrolatum gauze inserted in a stairstep fashion with bayonet forceps should result in a nasal pack that will tamponade anterior bleeders. A broad-spectrum antibiotic such as ampicillin or a cephalosporin, and a decongestant, should be started to prevent bacterial sinusitis resulting from a now obstructed sinus ostia. The pack should remain in place for at least 48 hours.

If bleeding into the back of the throat continues, despite placement of what is felt to be an adequate anterior pack, posterior epistaxis can be assumed. Once this diagnosis is made, one must plan on hospital admission for the patient, E.N.T. referral, an intravenous line, and oxygen. Posterior nasal packing is an invasive procedure that should subsequently be managed only in a hospital setting.[15,16,20]

There are many methods used in placing a posterior pack, but probably the easiest and perhaps the safest is the one that employs the Foley catheter. A #14 French Foley is inserted into the bleeding side until its tip can be seen behind the uvula. The balloon is inflated with 10 ml water, and gentle traction is applied as both nostrils are packed with petrolatum gauze as described for anterior packing. It is imperative that the catheter not touch the skin of the nares as it emerges from the nose, since deforming pressure necrosis of the nose may result. The catheter should be securely taped to the skin of the face to ensure against slippage posteriorly. Antibiotics and a decongestant are indicated to prevent sinusitis.

Laboratory and Radiographic Studies

All patients who have had a history of prolonged epistaxis should at least have their hematocrit determined. This also applies to patients who demonstrate orthostatic changes in their blood pressure or to patients with a serious medical illness. Generally, all elderly patients with epistaxis should have a hematocrit, blood clotting studies and a platelet count. Information gained from the initial history will usually be the basis on which these studies are obtained. All patients who are admitted with a posterior pack in place should have blood clotting studies determined in addition to their routine admission laboratory tests and serial hematocrits.

Radiographs of the sinuses are indicated for recurrent epistaxis or for suspected sinusitis by history, particularly if there has been recent nasal packing done.

Complications

The majority of the complications of epistaxis are iatrogenic and are not rare. The septum may be perforated during the course of cauterization and subsequently require surgical repair. Nasal packing may force blood into the eustachian tube, the sinus ostia, or the nasolacrimal duct, with resultant pain and possibly infection. Patients with a posterior pack may have a febrile episode secondary to otitis or sinusitis. They may also become hypoxemic even with a patent airway.[23]

The most disastrous complication can occur if the packing material slips posteriorly, resulting in complete airway obstruction. Hypovolemic shock is only rarely seen with epistaxis, and if it is present a related event such as rupture of an aortic aneurysm should be sought. Anemia is more common and may be dangerous if it occurs in the presence of concurrent medical illness.

TYMPANIC MEMBRANE PERFORATIONS

Traumatic tympanic membrane perforation is frequently seen in the emergency department setting. Head and neck trauma or ear pain bring the patient to the physician, and routine examination may disclose a perforation. The cause is likely due to compression trauma seen in blows to the ear, overzealous use of cotton swabs and other foreign bodies, water skiing accidents, and instrumentation by a physician. Spontaneous rupture of the ear drum owing to acute or chronic infection generally presents as ear pain and drainage.

Evaluation

Initial evaluation includes pertinent history of the type of trauma and any associated symptoms, such as bloody or clear drainage, vertigo, abnormal taste, tinnitus, hearing loss, and prior ear diseases. Examination begins with careful inspection for other otolaryngologic or head and neck trauma, such as scalp lacerations, Battle's sign, maxillofacial fractures, facial nerve dysfunction, dental malocclusion, and any other obvious injury (including airway and vision). The examination is completed with careful otoscopic visualization of the tympanic membranes, ear canals, and auricle.

The hearing level must be documented prior to any treatment. If formal audiometrics are unavailable, a reasonable screening examination can be done by asking the patient to identify whispered words repeated at two to three feet from the ear or to distinguish a wristwatch held near the ear as a ticking or humming type. Standard Weber and Rinne tuning fork tests are also excellent screening tests. For medical-legal reasons the results of the audiologic tests should be documented on the patient's chart prior to treatment.

Management

Management begins with careful cleaning of the ear. This is most easily done with direct vision and suction. Local anesthesia may be required for adequate cleaning. If there is no middle ear damage, observation and good aural hygiene constitute conservative management. Water should be kept out of the ear by using ear plugs or cotton plugs covered with petrolatum. An antibiotic (balanced pH suspension) ear drop is used because of probable contamination of the middle ear. Oral antibiotics and decongestants are used only if there is a concurrent acute infection.

Immediate consultation by the otolaryngologist is necessary if there is severe vertigo, middle ear ossicular disruption, clear fluid drainage (perilymph or cerebrospinal fluid), facial nerve dysfunction, or more than scant bleeding. Eighty to 90 percent of traumatic perforations heal spontaneously with good auditory function. Surgical correction is indicated if the perforation has not healed within 3 to 4 months.[24–28]

FOREIGN BODIES

Foreign bodies of the ear, nose, and throat region are a common emergency department presentation. Problems range from the mild irritation from a foreign body in the ear to a life-threatening situation of respiratory distress caused by airway compromise following aspiration.

Ear

The ear can collect various objects such as beads, cotton tips, insects, beans, welding sparks, and any other conceivable small object. Symptoms include hearing loss, pain, tinnitus, and purulent drainage.

Evaluation begins with an assessment of hearing prior to manipulation. If audiography is unavailable, gross screening tests of whisper, watch tick, and tuning forks are recommended. Radiographs are rarely indicated.

Many patients with foreign bodies in their ear may have tried to remove them and the ear canal may be swollen and tender on presentation. An anxious child who will not cooperate makes extraction of the object difficult. In these cases, sedation or restraint may be necessary. Extraction is best accomplished under the operating microscope or the operating head of a hand-held otoscope. Simple irrigation and suction may accomplish removal, with care being taken not to use extremely hot or cold water. This may elicit the caloric vestibular response, causing the patient to become vertiginous and nauseated. Instruments that are useful are the cerumen curette, a blunt right angle ear hook, Hartman forceps, and Blake forceps. If the object cannot be grasped directly, the hook is introduced past the foreign body, rotated 90°, then withdrawn pulling the foreign body out (Fig. 67–4).

Certain organic foreign bodies (e.g., seeds, beans) may expand and require local anesthesia (four-quadrant block with lidocaine) (Fig. 67–5) for removal. After successful removal of the foreign body, the ear canal

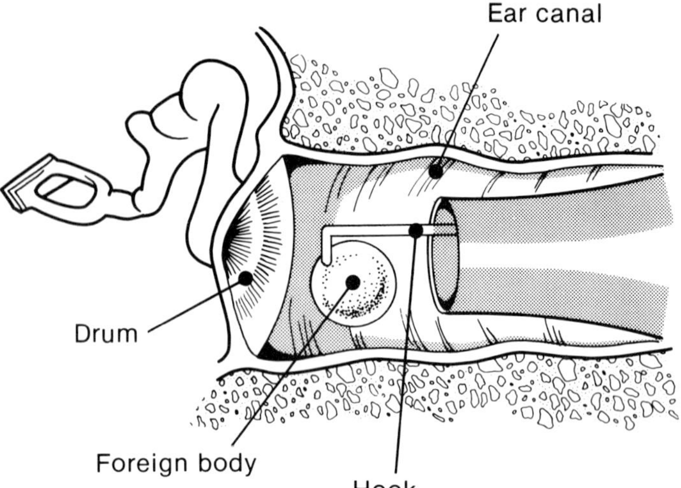

Figure 67–4   Foreign Body Removal Using Ear Hook.

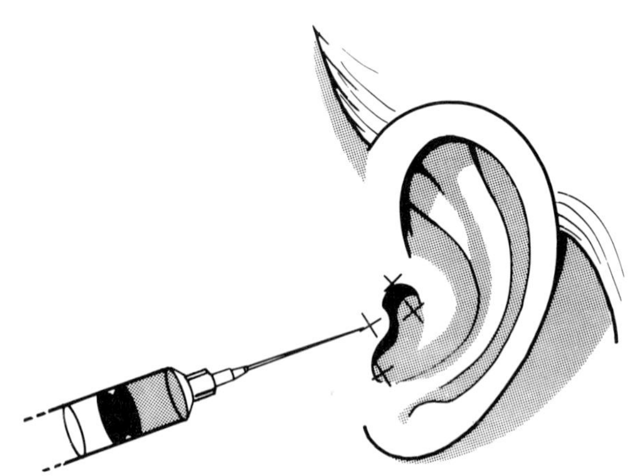
Figure 67–5   Four-quadrant Block of Ear Canal.

and tympanic membrane should be examined for injury. If there is a perforation, follow the guidelines described in the section on tympanic membrane perforation. Ear drops with antibiotics and corticosteroids should be used for several days if there is any bleeding, swelling, or signs of infection. If an insect is trapped in the ear, 70% alcohol or mineral oil is placed in the ear and then the insect is removed.

The otolaryngologist should be consulted if there is a perforation, moderate bleeding, or inexperience in removing foreign bodies of the ear.[29,30]

Nose

Foreign bodies in the nasal passages are more frequently seen in the pediatric age-group, usually children under 6 years of age. The classic presentation of a nasal foreign body is unilateral foul-smelling purulent discharge, unless the child is observed placing the foreign body in the nose. Nasal obstruction secondary to a foreign body may also present as general body odor. Paper, cloth, small toys, jewelry, and sponge remnants are common offenders.

Examination is facilitated by anesthetizing and shrinking the nasal mucosa with 10% cocaine or 2% lidocaine/phenylephrine mixture allowed to cover the nasal mucosa for several minutes. A good light source such as a head mirror is helpful for removal. Suction, right-angle hooks, or bayonet forceps are used to deliver the foreign body, being careful not to injure the nasal mucosa. Antibiotics and oral decongestants are useful for 5 to 6 days following removal to clear any obstructive sinusitis.[31,32]

Airway

A foreign body in the throat can be fatal and requires prompt diagnosis and management. Although treatment is usually directed by the otolaryngologist with assistance from the anesthesiologist and pediatrician, the diagnosis and initial care begin in the emergency department. Foreign bodies may lodge in the tracheobronchial tree or the esophagus. Rapid diagnosis is important because both may present with signs of airway distress.

Foreign bodies in the airway are commonly seen in children, in edentulous patients (denture aspiration), and following motor vehicle accidents. Dentures, coins, peanuts, or a large bolus of meat can be aspirated and lodged into any part of the tracheobronchial tree. The popular Heimlich maneuver has successfully saved many lives from sudden laryngeal obstruction. Immediate tracheostomy is occasionally necessary but is fraught with hazards even in the controlled setting. Several authors prefer emergency cricothyreotomy as an immediate airway opening measure, which can be converted to a more conventional tracheostomy in the operating room.

In less emergent situations of airway aspiration, the patient may present with a history of coughing, stridor, or wheezing or with a choking sensation after contact with small objects or following an automobile accident. Individuals at high risk include those with seizures, stroke patients, children running with food or other objects in their mouths, or someone who has recently eaten. Tracheobronchial foreign bodies may also present less acutely as a mild upper respiratory infection or more chronically with the signs and symptoms of pneumonia. Some studies have indicated that bronchial foreign bodies are more likely to be found in the right mainstem bronchus, owing to its more acute angle with the tracheal axis. Pulmonary foreign bodies may change position and cause a variety of clinical presentations.

Physical examination begins with observation of the patient in the emergency department. Coughing, stri-

dor, cyanosis, a rapid ventilatory rate, wheezing, and asymmetric chest movement with retractions of intercostal spaces may be observed separately or in combination.

When possible, the safest approach is to take anteroposterior and lateral soft tissue radiographs of the neck and chest. Then careful mirror exam of the larynx should be attempted. Many foreign bodies are not radiopaque and the radiograph may be normal. However, radiographs may show obvious foreign bodies, atelectasis, localized hyperinflation, or mediastinal shift.

The degree and location of the obstruction determines the urgency of treatment. As discussed above, sudden laryngeal obstruction requires removal of the foreign body using the Heimlich maneuver or establishing an artificial airway. Other tracheobronchial foreign bodies require rigid or flexible bronchoscopy as soon as available. More conservative therapy of distal foreign bodies includes chest percussion, dependent drainage, oxygen, and bronchodilator therapy. However, there is the risk of the foreign body dislodging into a more dangerous position in the trachea. As soon as available, there is no substitution for prompt endoscopic evaluation and removal of the foreign body.

Esophagus

Esophageal foreign bodies are frequently less emergent than airway obstructions but can develop into critical conditions if the esophagus is perforated. Small objects such as keys, coins, toys, fish or chicken bones, partial dentures, and a bolus of food make up the majority of esophageal foreign bodies.

History may reveal a motor vehicle accident, a child who suddenly "loses" a coin, or the patient who presents with "something stuck in my throat" after eating. Often there is gagging, choking, excessive salivation and drooling, odynaphagia, and dysphagia. There also may be the airway symptoms of dyspnea, wheezing, and cough if the esophageal foreign body pushes anteriorly against the trachea.

Diagnosis should include complete examination of the oral cavity, hypopharynx, and piriform fossae and a general neck examination. With any esophageal foreign body, there is a possibility of an esophageal perforation that can lead to severe mediastinitis and neck abscess. Symptoms include subcutaneous emphysema in the neck, fever, elevated white blood cell count, and decreased mobility of the thyroid cartilage on manipulation.

Radiographs are tne mainstay of diagnosis with anteroposterior and lateral neck and chest views. A radiopaque contrast medium (nonprecipitated) swallowed or string pledget soaked in the medium can give additional radiographic confirmation. Barium should not be used because it may obscure the object at endoscopy.

Conservative management, with consideration of the object, is to let the foreign body traverse the alimentary canal naturally. Liquids will usually not cause harm, but giving solid food to "push" the object into the stomach is contraindicated.

Endoscopic removal under direct vision is the safest and most reliable method of treatment. A newer method of removal for certain nonjagged esophageal obstructions in children is fluoroscopic removal by passing a Foley catheter beyond the object, inflating the catheter, and then pulling the foreign body out. This method is not entirely without hazard and requires a team experienced in the procedure. In esophageal foreign bodies as in airway foreign bodies, there is no substitution for removal of the object by an experienced endoscopist.[33–38]

ACUTE OTITIS MEDIA

Acute otitis media is one of the more common infectious diseases seen in the ambulatory patient. The highest incidence of infection occurs during the first 3 years of life.[39]

Clinical Manifestations

The individual with acute otitis often has a preceding upper respiratory infection. This is followed by earache, fever, malaise, loss of hearing, and otorrhea. Children may pull at the affected ear and may develop diarrhea and eat poorly. The objective signs of acute otitis include erythema, bulging of any portion of the tympanic membrane, loss of visualization of the bony landmarks, bullae formation, decreased mobility of the membrane on insufflation, and perforation with purulent drainage.

Etiology

The bacterial pathogens of acute otitis have been found to be *Streptococcus pneumoniae* and *Hemophilus influenzae* in 70 percent of cases cultured, with the latter predominating in children under 5 years of age. *Streptococcus pyogenes*, *Staphylococcus aureus* and *Neisseria catarrhalis* are also found. Less often, gram-negative bacteria, anaerobes, and *Mycoplasma* are associated with acute otitis. Although viral upper respiratory infections often precede acute ear infections, viral agents are rarely cultured from acute otitic infections.[40,41] The incidence of allergy in acute ear disease is unclear. Tympanocentesis has been the mainstay of diagnosis in the past but can be difficult, time consuming, and potentially dangerous, leading to damage of middle ear structures. Recent studies have shown a high correlation between middle ear and nasopharyngeal cultures.[42,43]

Treatment

The mainstay of therapy for acute otitis media is antibiotics. The choice of drug should include an antibiotic or combination that will eradicate the three primary pathogens. Ampicillin or amoxicillin is effective against pneumococci, most *H. influenzae*, and group A streptococci. The appropriate dose is administered orally with respect to weight and age of patient. The major side-effects are allergic reactions and diarrhea. (See Chapter 72.) Culturing of a purulent discharge obtained after the ear drum bursts or after the nasopharyngeal culture can be used to guide therapy.

In the older patient (over 6 years of age), penicillin is a good treatment of choice. The penicillin-allergic patient can be managed with erythromycin or sulfisoxazole.[44] Adjunctive measures in treatment, including nose drops and decongestants, have not consistently been shown to affect treatment or incidence of recurrences. These modalities may be of benefit in the relief of symptoms of the upper respiratory component of the illness.

Persistent and recurrent episodes of acute otitis media can be treated with a change from the original antibiotic to a combination drug such as trimethoprim-sulfamethoxazole. Once the infection has cleared, a regimen of chemoprophylaxis can be instituted. Studies have shown that chemoprophylaxis reduces the number of episodes of infection.[45] Unresolved and breakthrough episodes should be referred to the otolaryngologist for audiologic evaluation and possible surgical intervention. Published data now reveal a reduction in the number of infectious episodes when tympanostomy tubes are placed in the ear.[46] Otitis media with tympanostomy tubes in place is treated with medical regimens and antibiotic otic drops.

The major sequelae of acute otitis media are persistent serous otitis media (nonpurulent middle ear fluid with hearing loss) and chronic otitis media (perforation with or without cholesteatoma). These patients should be referred to the otolaryngologist for evaluation.

OTITIS EXTERNA

Anatomy

The external auditory canal in the adult is approximately 24 mm long and ends blindly at the tympanic membrane. The outer third of the canal is supported by cartilage that is continuous with the cartilage of the auricle. The skin lining the cartilaginous canal is thick and contains fine hairs, sebaceous glands, and glands that produce cerumen.[32] The auditory canal is oriented in an oblique direction inferiorly, medially, and anteriorly and also curves slightly superiorly, necessitating upward traction on the auricle for adequate visualization of the tympanic membrane.

The inner bony canal is lined with thin epithelium attached directly to bone. Directly anterior to the ear canal is the temporomandibular joint. Disease or dysfunction of this joint is often perceived as ear pain.

Pathophysiology

Infectious external otitis can be found in all age-groups, in all seasons, and in all climates. However the incidence increases dramatically during the summer when the disorder can be found frequently among swimmers. *Swimmer's ear* is the popular term for infectious external otitis. (See Chapter 20.)

Predisposing factors include anatomic considerations: narrow ear canal, excessive cerumen, mechanical blockage; traumatic origin: from placing foreign bodies in the canal; and environmental factors: heat, humidity, and conditions brought about by swimming.[47] Skin disease, particularly eczema, likewise predisposes to development of otitis externa.[48] Folliculitis and furuncles, which can develop in the thick skin of the cartilaginous canal, frequently set the stage for bacterial invasion.[49]

The normal ear canal may harbor *Staphylococcus albus* and diphtheroids but no pathogenic organisms.[50] The pathogenesis of infectious external otitis seems most likely to be the introduction of pathogenic organisms into a mechanically traumatized ear canal, which will then allow the growth of these organisms.

The bacteria most commonly cultured from patients with otitis externa are *Pseudomonas aeruginosa*, *Staphylococcus aureus*, *Proteus vulgaris*, and non-group-A *Streptococcus*.[47–51] *Aspergillus niger*, which produces a black growth, and *Candida* are infrequent causes of ear canal infection except in tropical climates. The true incidence of viral otitis externa is unknown but probably very low. There has been at least one case of documented gonococcal otitis externa,[52] a diagnosis suggested by the sexual history obtained and the presence of a urethral discharge.

Malignant otitis externa (also referred to as necrotizing otitis externa) is a particularly severe variant of the disease and is responsible for a high incidence of neurologic sequelae and a high mortality.[53–55] It most frequently occurs in diabetic, elderly adults and is usually caused by *Pseudomonas aeruginosa*. Several case reports describing this entity in children[56,57] with systemic disease testify to its invasive nature, with a very high incidence of neurologic sequelae, particularly peripheral facial nerve palsy.

Clinical Manifestations

In early or mild acute otitis externa, the patient will most commonly complain of ear pain that is aggravated by opening the mouth widely or by movement of the auricle. There is usually a yellow discharge from the ear, and low-grade fever may be present. Hearing loss or the feeling of a "blocked ear" may be present if the canal is obstructed.

In severe acute otitis externa, the ear pain will be intense, frequently involving the entire side of the face. Any manipulation of the ear will be excruciating to the patient. High fever may be present, and the purulent discharge may be profuse.

Lymphadenopathy is common in otitis externa, usually involving the preauricular and postauricular, posterior cervical, or occipital nodes. The nodes may be slightly tender.

The epithelium of the ear canal may be so edematous that the tympanic membrane cannot be visualized. A thick discharge, which is often foul smelling, should be obvious. If the tympanic membrane can be visualized, it may be inflamed like the ear canal,[47] but it is usually normal in appearance and mobility. The ear canal will usually appear pale and "soggy" and may be occluded by cerumen and desquamated epithelium. Irrigation of the ear will probably not allow better visualization and may be poorly tolerated by the patient because of the discomfort this procedure may induce.

Otitis externa is for all practical purposes a skin infection and may involve the skin of the auricle, which can become swollen and tender. Pustules and crusting may be present.

In chronic otitis externa, the ear canal is usually excoriated and itching rather than pain is the most common presenting symptom.[47] Patients will often attempt to relieve the itching by using a foreign body such as a pencil, often aggravating the condition by further damaging the epithelium.

Malignant external otitis will produce similar local symptoms but may also present as high fever, prostration, cranial nerve palsies, and osteomyelitis, progressing to seizures, coma, and death. The disease must be suspected early in patients with diabetes or other systemic disease and treated aggressively if significant sequelae are to be avoided.

Laboratory Findings

In all cases of otitis externa, cultures of the exudate should be obtained. Routine cultures should be adequate if the offending organism is *Pseudomonas*, *Staphylococcus*, *Streptococcus*, or *Proteus*. Fungal cultures may be useful if a monilial skin rash is present, if the growth on the canal is black (suggesting *Aspergillus niger*), or in cases not responding to antibacterial therapy.

If the local infection is particularly severe and spread outside the confines of the ear canal is suggested, radiographs of sinuses and mastoids are indicated. A complete blood cell count and blood cultures should be obtained if the patient appears to be septic, particularly if malignant external otitis is suggested.

Differential Diagnosis

Pain referred to the ear is common in the presence of dental infections, temporomandibular joint problems, and tumors or infections of the pharynx.[51] Otalgia without an evident cause mandates a thorough E.N.T. examination, particularly in the elderly, in whom a nasopharyngeal carcinoma may not be readily apparent.

Perhaps the most common confusion arises when otitis media is present with perforation of the tympanic membrane, in which purulent material fills the ear canal. A history of ear trauma, swimming, or prior episodes of otitis externa suggests infection limited to the ear canal. Hearing may be decreased in either otitis media or externa, but tragal palpation should elicit pain only if the ear canal is involved.[49,51] Fever, rhinitis, and sore throat suggest otitis media, while the presence of inflamed lymph nodes is more commonly found in association with otitis externa.

If the tympanic membrane can be visualized, otitis media should not be difficult to diagnose. Likewise, if enough debris can be removed to see the epithelial lining of the ear canal a normal appearance should be maintained in the presence of otitis media, even with perforation.

The results of bacterial cultures should likewise help make the correct diagnosis. *Pneumococcus* and *Hemophilus influenzae* are still the most common organisms causing otitis media and are not the cause of typical otitis externa. Confusion may result if *Staphylococcus aureus* is isolated, but the clinical examination is paramount.

Treatment

Treatment of all but the most severe forms of otitis externa consists of heat, analgesia, topical antibiotics (usually with cortisone), and use of an ear wick if the ear canal is swollen and occluded.

Heat seems to provide a good deal of comfort and may be provided by a heat lamp, hot wet compresses, or a heating pad.[50] Care should be taken not to accidentally burn the auricle. Analgesics should be prescribed according to the degree of pain present. Narcotics may be required in severe cases.

Most otolaryngologists have their own preference for the topical antibiotic of choice. Cortisporin otic solution or suspension, containing polymixin B, neomycin, and hydrocortisone, is widely used. The use of topical corticosteroids is recommended for their anti-inflammatory effect; the danger of worsening a fungal infection is remote except in tropical climates where fungal otitis externa is common.

The removal of significant amounts of debris from the ear canal employing a point suction is recommended if the ear canal is significantly occluded. The use of a microscope may be required for the procedure to be adequately performed. Irrigation is not generally recommended and is usually very painful for the patient.

Ear wicks consisting of cotton or gauze are useful when the ear canal is occluded; otherwise topical antibiotics cannot reach all of the involved area. The wick may be easily inserted using a bayonet forceps and should be kept moistened with the antibiotic at all times. As swelling subsides, the wick will usually fall out of the ear canal spontaneously. If it does not, it should be replaced in 2 to 3 days.

In severe cases of otitis externa, particularly in diabetic patients or in those with severe chronic disease, hospital admission and E.N.T. referral is recommended.

REFERENCES

1. Ballantyne J, Groves J (eds): *Scott-Brown's Diseases of the Ear, Nose, and Throat.* London, JB Lippincott, 1971, vol 3, pp 183–213.
2. Adams GL, Boies LR, Paparella MM (eds): *Boies Fundamentals of Otolaryngology,* ed 5. Philadelphia, WB Saunders, 1978.
3. Hawkins DB, Clark RW: Orbital involvement in acute sinusitis. *Clin Pediatr* 16:464–471, 1977.
4. Caffey J: *Pediatric X-Ray Diagnosis.* Chicago: Year Book Medical Publishers, vol 1, pp 104–111, 1973.
5. Sheffield RW, Cassisi NJ, Karlan MS: Complications of sinusitis. *Postgrad Med* 63:93–101, 1978.
6. Chapnik JS, Bach MC: Bacterial and fungal infections of the maxillary sinus. *Otol Clin North Am* 9:43–54, 1976.
7. Kinnman J, et al: Bacterial flora in chronic, purulent, maxillary sinusitis. *Acta Otolaryngol* 64:37–44, 1967.
8. Chandler Jr, Langenburnner DJ, Stevens ER: The pathogenesis of orbital complications in acute sinusitis. *Laryngoscope* 80:1414–1428, 1970.
9. Healy GB, Strong MS: Acute periorbital swelling. *Laryngoscope* 82:1491–1498, 1972.
10. Frederick J, Braude A: Anaerobic infection of the paranasal sinuses. *N Engl J Med* 290:135, 1974.
11. Ballantyne J, Groves J (eds): *Scott-Brown's Diseases of the Ear, Nose, and Throat.* London: JB Lippincott, 1971, vol 4, pp 113–118.
12. Levit GW: Cervical fascia and deep neck infections. *Laryngoscope* 80:409–435, 1970.
13. McCurdy JA: Peritonsillar abscess: A comparison of treatment by immediate tonsillectomy and internal tonsillectomy. *Arch Otolaryngol* 103:414–415, 1977.

14. Cantrell RW: Quinsy tonsillectomy. *Laryngoscope* 86:1714–1717, 1976.

15. Lingeman RE: Epistaxis. *Am Fam Physician* 14:79–83, 1976.

16. DeWeese DD, et al: Epistaxis: From A to Z in nosebleed control. *Patient Care* April 30, 1978, pp 66–83.

17. Moran WB: Nasal trauma in children. *Otolaryngological Clin North Am* 10:95–101, 1977.

18. Flessa HC, Glueck HI: Hereditary hemorrhagic telangiectasia (Osler-Weber-Rendu disease). *Arch Otolaryngol* 103:148–151, 1977.

19. McCaffrey TV, et al: Management of epistaxis in hereditary hemorrhagic telangiectasia: A review of 80 cases. *Arch Otolaryngol* 103:627–630, 1977.

20. Jaffe BF: Diseases and surgery of the nose. *Clin Symposia* 26:2–32, 1974.

21. Charles R, Corrigan E: Epistaxis and hypertension. *Postgrad Med* 53:260–261, 1977.

22. Ibrashi F, et al: Effect of atherosclerosis and hypertension on arterial epistaxis. *J Laryngol Otol* 92:877–881, 1978.

23. Lin YT, Orkin LR: Arterial hypoxemia in patients with anterior and posterior nasal packings. *Laryngoscope* 89:140–144, 1979.

24. Armstrong BW: Traumatic perforations of the tympanic membrane: Observe or repair. *Laryngoscope* 82:1822–1830, 1972.

25. Lee KG: *Essential Otolaryngology*. Garden City, NY, Examination Publishing Co, 1977.

26. Griffin WL: A retrospective study of traumatic tympanic membrane perforations in a clinic practice. *Laryngoscope* 89:261–283, 1979.

27. Juers AL: Traumatic tympanic perforations. *Trans Am Acad Otolaryngol* 78:261–283, 1974.

28. Pulec JL, Kinney SE: Diseases of the tympanic membrane, in Paparella MM, Shumrick DA (eds): *Otolaryngology*. Philadelphia, WB Saunders, vol 2, 1979.

29. Wood RP: *Handbook of Emergency ENT Care*. Denver, Colo, University of Colorado Medical Center Press, August 1973.

30. English GM: Trauma to the pinna and external auditory canal, in English GM (ed): *Otolaryngology, A Textbook*. Hagerstown, Md, Harper & Row, 1976.

31. Katz HP, et al: Unusual presentation of nasal foreign body in children. *JAMA* 241:1496, 1979.

32. Deweese DD, Saunders WH: *Textbook of Otolaryngology*, ed 5. St Louis, C V Mosby, 1977, p 234.

33. Heimlich HJ: Pop Goes the Cafe Coronary. *Emergency Med* 6:154–155, 1974.

34. Law U, Kosloske AM: Management of Tracheobronchial foreign bodies in children: A re-evaluation of postural drainage and bronchoscopy. *Pediatrics* 58:362–367, 1976.

35. Cantrell RW, et al: Foreign body and caustic ingestion: Management 1979. *Ann Otol Rhinol Laryngol* 88:872–879, 1979.

36. Ballentyne JJ: *Diseases of the Nose, Throat and Ear*, ed 12. Philadelphia, Lea & Febiger, 1977, chap 60.

37. Jackson C: Foreign bodies in the air and food passages, in English GM (ed): *Otolaryngology*. Hagerstown, Md, Harper & Row, 1979.

38. Wood RP, Northern JL: *Manual of Otolaryngology, A Symptom-Oriented Text*. Baltimore, Williams & Wilkins, 1979.

39. Howard JE, et al: Otitis Media of Infancy and Early Childhood. *Am J Dis Child* 130:965–970, 1976.

40. Brooke I: Otitis media in children: A prospective study of aerobic and anaerobic bacteriology. *Laryngoscope* 89:992–997, 1979.

41. Fairbanks DNF: Microbiology of ear, nose and throat infections. *Ear, Nose Throat J* 60:6–16, 1981.

42. Schwartz R, et al: The nasopharyngeal culture in acute otitis media: A reappraisal of its usefulness. *JAMA* 241:2170–2173, 1979.

43. Proctor B: Etiology of Otitis Media, in Wiet RJ, Coulthard SW (eds): Otitis Media: Proceedings of the Second National Conference on Otitis Media. Columbus, Ohio, Ross Laboratories, 1979, pp 21–25.

44. Paradise JL: Medical Treatment of Acute Otitis Media: A Critical Essay, in Wiet RJ, Coulthard SW (eds): Otitis Media: Proceedings of the Second National Conference on Otitis Media. Columbus, Ohio, Ross Laboratories, 1979, pp 79–84.

45. Shurin PA: Prevention of Otitis Media with Antimicrobial Drugs, in Wiet RJ, Coulthard SW (eds): Otitis Media: Proceedings of the Second National Conference on Otitis Media. Columbus, Ohio, Ross Laboratories, 1979, pp 67–69.

46. Gebhart DE: Tympanostomy tubes in the otitis media prone child. *Laryngoscope* 91:849–866, 1981.

47. Peterkin GA: Otitis externa. *J Laryngol Otol* 88:15, 1974.

48. Mawson SR: *Diseases of the Ear*. Baltimore, Williams & Wilkins, 1974, pp 233–241.

49. Farmer HS: A guide for the treatment of external otitis. *Am Fam Physician* 21:96, 1980.

50. DeWeese DD, Saunders WH: *Textbook of Otolaryngology*. St Louis, C V Mosby Co, 1978, pp 332–339.

51. Walike JW: Management of acute ear infections. *Otol Clin North Am* 12:439, 1979.

52. Pareek SS: Gonococcal otitis externa. *N Engl J Med* 300:1490, 1979.

53. Chandler JR: Malignant external otitis. *Laryngoscope* 78:1257, 1968.

54. Chandler JR: Pathogenesis and treatment of facial paralysis due to malignant external otitis. *Ann Otolaryngol* 81:648, 1972.

55. Schwarz G, Blumenkrantz M, Sundmaker W: Neurologic complications of malignant external otitis. *Neurology* 21:1077, 1971.

56. Sherman P, Black S, Grossman M: Malignant external otitis due to *Pseudomonas aeruginosa* in childhood. *Pediatrics* 66:782, 1980.

57. Rubinstein E, Ostfeld E, Ben-Zaray S, et al: Necrotizing external otitis. *Pediatrics* 66:618, 1980.

68. Laryngeal Emergencies

KEN KULIG, M.D.

Trauma to the larynx may be blunt or penetrating, iatrogenic (secondary to endoscopy or intubation) or autogenous (voice abuse), or result from thermal, chemical, or radiation burns (secondary to radiation therapy). In this section, emphasis will be placed on blunt laryngeal trauma and its diagnosis and management in the emergency department.

ETIOLOGY

Blunt trauma to the larynx is rare and is most frequently seen as a result of motor vehicle accidents in which severe multisystemic trauma is sustained. (See Chapter 7.) The mandible usually protects the larynx, with the head, neck, and face absorbing the major impact force.[1] However, in head-on automobile collisions the craniofacial complex is thrown forward and may strike the windshield, dashboard, or steering wheel. This movement extends the neck and exposes the larynx, which may strike the dashboard or steering wheel and be compressed against the cervical spine.[2] The most susceptible individual is the front seat passenger, followed by the driver.[3] The use of the lap belt without shoulder harness increases the risk of cervical and upper airway injury, since it causes the passenger to flex at the hips and thus extend the neck and chin.[4] One reason for the rarity of treated laryngeal fractures is that the patients often die from complete airway obstruction or related injuries before resuscitation can be instituted.[5]

Other causes of blunt laryngeal trauma include strangulation, fist blows, projectile rocks, and blows received during athletic events. Trailbike, snowmobile, and minibike riders encountering unexpected rope or cable barriers are presenting in increasing numbers with laryngeal trauma.[6]

Penetrating neck trauma has a low incidence of resulting laryngotracheal damage. In three separate series, the incidence of laryngeal or tracheal trauma associated with penetrating cervical wounds was 2 percent,[7] 9 percent,[8] and 8 percent.[9] In the majority of these cases the wounds are clean, do not involve major destruction of cartilaginous tissue, and are easily repaired at surgery.[7,8]

ANATOMY

The larynx consists of a cartilaginous framework interconnected by ligaments and membranes (Fig. 68–1). The three unpaired cartilages, the cricoid, thyroid, and epiglottis are the largest and form the foundation of the larynx. The three paired cartilages, the arytenoid, cuneiform, and corniculate, are important in phonation.

The true vocal cords are mucous membranes that cover the vocal ligaments and extend from the arytenoids to the interior, midportion of the thyroid cartilage. The fissure between the true cords is frequently termed the *glottis* (rima glottidis).

Easily palpable of the laryngeal structures are the thyroid cartilage (laryngeal prominence, or "Adam's

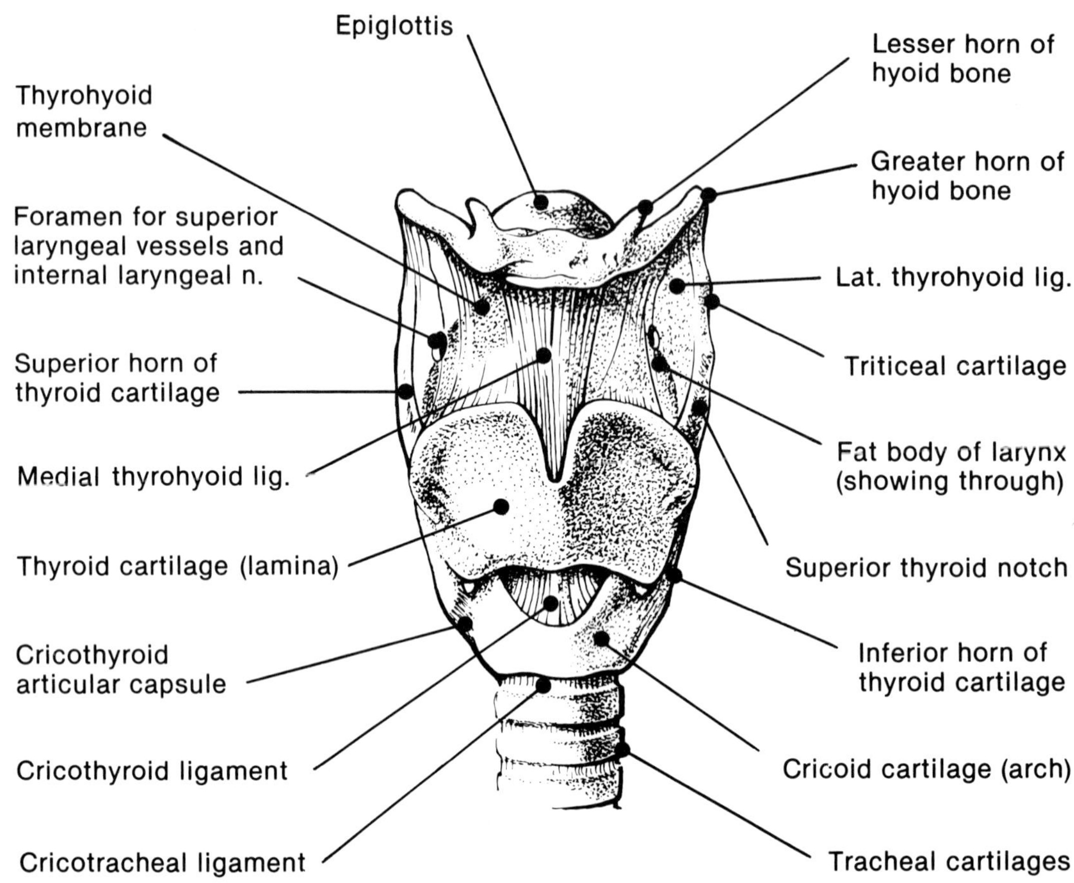

Figure 68–1   The Cartilaginous Framework of the Larynx Interconnected by Ligaments and Membranes.

apple"), the cricoid cartilage, and the first two tracheal rings. The hyoid bone, also easily palpable, is not formally considered to be part of the laryngeal complex. The cricothyroid ligament, an important access to the lower airway, is felt between the cricoid and thyroid cartilages.

Anatomically, laryngeal trauma may be limited to soft tissue edema and ecchymosis or may extend to mucosal laceration, vocal cord avulsion, linear fracture of the thyroid or cricoid cartilage, arytenoid joint subluxation, recurrent laryngeal nerve contusion or laceration, comminuted fracture of the cartilaginous structures, or complete laryngotracheal disruption.[10] Edema and hematoma formation in the loose supraglottic tissues is common to almost all laryngeal injuries and will resolve spontaneously and completely in the absence of any other injury.[11]

The most common laryngeal fracture is the vertical midline fracture of the thyroid cartilage (Fig. 68–2).[4,12] The fracture often extends from the thyroid notch to the cricothyroid membrane, and the anterior vocal cord attachments may be avulsed.

Supraglottic injuries include avulsion of the attachments of the epiglottis from the thyroid cartilage and fractures of the hyoid, which are painful but not dan-

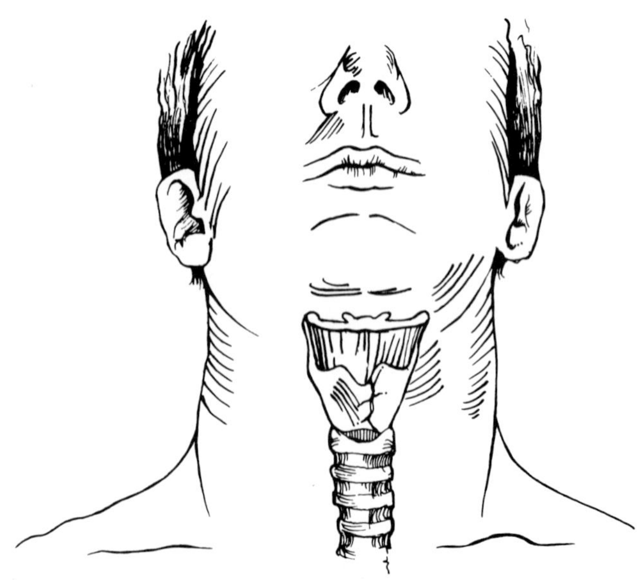

Figure 68–2   Vertical Midline Fracture of the Thyroid Cartilage.

gerous.[4,12] Infraglottis injuries involve fractures of the cricoid cartilage and possible separation from the upper tracheal rings, which may retract into the upper mediastinum. Associated thyroid cartilage fracture and recurrent laryngeal nerve damage are common.

ASSOCIATED INJURIES

The patient with laryngeal trauma usually also has severe multisystem trauma, including that to the extremities. However, once trauma to the larynx is suspected, several common associated injuries should be vigorously searched for.

Forces great enough to damage the flexible cartilaginous structures in the neck are great enough to damage any cervical structure, including the vertebrae. Fracture—dislocations of C2, C3, and C4 are the most common associated cervical spine injuries.[4] In one series 50 percent of patients with tracheal transection had associated cervical fractures.[13] The importance of the initial cross table cervical spine radiograph cannot be overemphasized in the patient with multiple trauma. (See Chapter 43.)

Aside from cervical spine fractures, the most common injuries associated with laryngeal trauma are chest trauma, pharyngeal or esophageal laceration, closed head injury, facial fractures, and recurrent laryngeal nerve injury.[13] Associated chest trauma (see Chapter 61) is common enough that, especially when it is obvious on physical examination, it is often mistakenly assumed to be the source of the subcutaneous emphysema actually caused by laryngeal disruption.[5,10,14]

Esophageal disruption from blunt cervical trauma has been reported and also should be considered when subcutaneous air is present.[15]

Vascular injuries secondary to blunt cervical trauma are rare and may present later as an aneurysm or an arteriovenous fistula.[14]

In general, blunt trauma to the larynx, esophagus, cervical vertebrae, and chest tends to occur concurrently and may be clinically subtle. For this reason, injuries to each structure must be diligently searched for in the presence of trauma to one of them. Associated head and facial trauma tends to be more obvious at the time of presentation to the emergency department.

CLINICAL MANIFESTATIONS

The presenting symptoms of the patient with laryngeal trauma are often minimal and may be attributed to some other cause.[4,5] When a good history is obtainable and not overshadowed by other major trauma, major complaints will be concerning problems with voice, swallowing, neck pain, and respiratory difficulties.

Dysphonia (change in the quality of voice, almost invariably hoarseness), or aphonia (total loss of voice) may be present in nearly one-half of patients. It is usually due to recurrent laryngeal nerve injury, thyroid cartilage fracture, anterior subluxation of the arytenoids, or hematoma in the area of the vocal cords.[4]

Dysphagia (difficulty in swallowing) and odynophagia (pain with swallowing) are both common in laryngeal fractures and can be attributed to distraction of fractured cartilage and/or disrupted tissue during the second stage of swallowing.[4,5] Either symptom can occur without esophageal injury.

The pain caused by neck motion, coughing, or speaking is common and due to distraction of fractured cartilage or damaged tissue.

Hemoptysis after laryngeal trauma is very common[13] but also very nonspecific in the patient with facial and cervical trauma who may swallow and/or aspirate blood from the upper airway. True hemoptysis (coughing up blood originating in the lower airway) secondary to trauma is rare.[16,17]

The most threatening symptoms of laryngotracheal damage are those of airway obstruction. (See Chapter 57.) The submucosal tissues of the supraglottic larynx permit rapid accumulation of fluid, and the resulting edema or hematoma formation may obstruct the airway and prevent intubation.[4] For this reason any subjective feelings of dyspnea or stridor on the part of the patient must be taken seriously and the patient monitored continuously.

The physical findings of laryngeal trauma vary with the extent of injury and injury to related structures. The most common findings are subcutaneous emphysema, changes in voice, loss of palpable landmarks, and airway obstruction (stridor or dyspnea as manifested by increased respiratory rate, use of accessory muscles, and agitation).[4,13]

Subcutaneous emphysema is almost universally present[13] but may vary from subtle to massive. It is often mistakenly attributed to a lower airway injury, and the larynx is overlooked.[5] Free air as seen on a soft tissue lateral roentgenogram of the neck may be the only sign of disruption of the upper airway.[4] The dissection of air from the larynx may spread into the mediastinum and pericardium without air leak elsewhere[10,12] and suggests contamination of deep cervical and thoracic structures by respiratory secretions and saliva.

Over 50 percent of patients will have some degree of airway obstruction, and although this may be minimal initially, complete obstruction may occur several hours after the injury.[4,13]

The loss of cartilaginous landmarks is common in laryngotracheal injury: the anterior neck may be flattened and the usual thyroid prominence may not be palpable.[11,12] Vigorous manipulation of the larynx during physical examination, however, is to be avoided, since this may aggravate existing injuries.[14]

The presence of a sucking wound in the neck, particularly after penetrating trauma, is almost always associated with upper airway perforation.[13]

Other less-specific signs include cervical swelling (which may represent large vessel injury), bony crepitus, and anterior neck tenderness. Changes in voice quality have already been mentioned.

It is important to realize that the external appearance of the neck may be quite misleading as far as the degree of laryngotracheal injury is concerned, since dangerous conditions may exist beneath nearly normal-appearing soft tissue.[14,18] A high index of suspicion, a meticulous physical examination, and continued observation are often necessary in assessing the true extent of injury.

RADIOGRAPHIC STUDIES

All patients who have sustained injuries to the neck serious enough to suggest a laryngeal injury should have a chest radiograph, cross table lateral view of the cervical spine, and soft tissue lateral view of the neck.[4,12,18] All three radiographs can be obtained as portables, keeping the unstable patient in the emergency department for observation. As an initial procedure in most patients, particularly if any degree of airway difficulty is present, a soft tissue lateral view of the neck with the cassette placed posteriorly to include the cervical spine should be done. This should demonstrate any subcutaneous emphysema if present (frequently this is unsuspected or obscured by a large hematoma), give a clear view of the laryngeal air column, and demonstrate any instability of the cervical spine that would contraindicate endotracheal intubation.[12,18] The information gained from this one portable radiograph is invaluable should it be necessary to actively support the patient's airway. At a later time a complete cervical spine series should be done in all patients with laryngeal trauma.

The chest radiograph is essential to rule out mediastinal emphysema and any associated injury such as hemothorax or pulmonary contusion. Mediastinal extension of cervical air implies contamination, and the patient should be started on antibiotics and taken to surgery.[12]

The cartilaginous structures in the neck are seen on routine radiographs only as indistinct shadows, and the diagnosis of a fracture of the larynx will require special studies including endoscopy to confirm the clinical impression. Clues to airway disruption observed on the soft tissue radiographs include emphysema, hyoid bone fracture, supraglottic or subglottic narrowing of the laryngeal air column, prevertebral soft tissue swelling, and flattening of the normal prominence of the thyroid notch.[18,19]

Further radiographic studies of the larynx may include xeroradiography, tomography, fluoroscopy, barium swallow, contrast laryngotracheography, and computerized axial tomographic scanning.[19] Each study offers a different perspective and depends on the skill of the radiologist for performance and interpretation.

MANAGEMENT IN THE EMERGENCY DEPARTMENT

Once laryngotracheal trauma has been recognized, the major decisions faced by the emergency department personnel are: When should active airway support be initiated, and should an attempt at endotracheal intubation be made or should tracheostomy be performed? Unfortunately the literature provides few guidelines for these very difficult questions. In most cases the true extent of injury is unknown, making any decision for intervention primarily one of clinical judgment and past experience. Attempts at laryngoscopy in the emergency department are controversial; in addition to usually being of questionable benefit, the manipulation required may be more than sufficient to totally obstruct the patient's airway.[4,5,12]

Several authors have used initial endotracheal intubation with success in laryngeal trauma patients with respiratory distress.[8,13,20] In one series of 23 patients with trauma to the larynx or trachea, 17 patients were successfully intubated; among these were 3 patients with complete laryngotracheal disruption.[13] The advantages of endotracheal intubation compared with tracheostomy are that it is faster, provides direct visualization of the area of damage, and allows immediate suctioning of the airway. Strong disadvantages include the necessity of neck manipulation when the status of the cervical spine may not be known, the possibility of dislodging the distal end of a complete laryngotracheal disruption, and the hazards of placing a tube through the area of trauma. Endotracheal intubation in these cases is always temporary. Tracheostomy in the operating room under more optimum conditions is performed as soon as possible.

The disadvantages of immediate tracheostomy in the emergency department are primarily those of technical difficulties in carrying out the procedure, particularly on a patient who may be awake and combative from hypoxemia or other reasons. However, some authors still recommend it as the initial procedure of choice.[4,5,10,12] The procedure has the obvious advantage of requiring minimal cervical manipulation and bypassing the area of trauma (usually).

Nasotracheal intubation in laryngeal trauma is to be condemned as too hazardous, as is cricothyroidotomy.

Perhaps the problem that presents the biggest management dilemma is the awake patient with known laryngeal trauma but with only mild (or even absent) respiratory distress. In closed injuries, it has been the experience of some authors that neither intubation nor tracheostomy were required in this type of case.[14,21] In one series of 22 closed injuries, 13 patients were managed in the hospital without tracheostomy or intubation and all recovered. The majority of these patients were symptomatic, with dysphonia, dysphagia, and emphysema. The management of the traumatized patient in this manner requires that an "attendant" be available constantly at the patient's bedside with an available tracheostomy set. Such practices are probably too risky to be considered adequate treatment for today's trauma patients.

REFERENCES

1. Nahum AM, Siegel AN: Biodynamics of injury to the larynx in automobile collisions. *Am Otolaryngol* 76:781–790, 1967.
2. Butler RM, Moser FH: The padded dash syndrome: Blunt trauma to the larynx and trachea. *Laryngoscope* 78:1172–1176, 1968.
3. Lambert GE, McMurray GT: Laryngotracheal trauma: Recognition and management, *J Am Coll Emergency Physicians* 5:883–886, 1976.
4. Zuidema GD, Rutherford RB, Ballinger WF (eds): *The Management of Trauma*, ed 3. Philadelphia, WB Saunders Co, 1979, pp. 347–352.
5. Whited RE: Laryngeal fracture on the multiple trauma patient. *Am J Surg* 136:354–355, 1978.
6. Alonso WA, Caruso VG, Roncace EA: Minibikes: A new factor in laryngotracheal trauma. *Am Otol Rhinol Laryngol* 82:800–804, 1973.
7. Blass DC, James EC, Reed RJ et al: Penetrating wounds of the neck and upper thorax. *J Trauma* 18:2–7, 1978.
8. Knightly JJ, Swaminathan AP, Rush BF: Management of penetrating wounds of the neck. *Am J Surg* 126:574–579, 1973.
9. Penn I: Penetrating injuries of the neck. *Surg Clin North Am*, 53:6, 1469–1478, 1973.
10. Larson DC, Cohn AM: Management of acute laryngeal injury: A critical review. *J Trauma* 16:858–862, 1976.
11. Ballenger JJ: *Diseases of the Nose, Throat, and Ear*, ed 11. Philadelphia, Lea & Febiger, 1969, pp 318–335.
12. Paparella MM, Shumrich DA (eds): *Otolaryngology*. Philadelphia, WB Saunders Co, 1973, vol 3, pp 609–615.
13. Lambert GE, McMurray GT: Laryngotracheal trauma: Recognition and management. *J Am Coll Emergency Physicians* 5:883–887, 1976.
14. Fitz-Hugh GS, Wallenborn WM, McGovern F: Injuries of the larynx and cervical trauma. *Am Otol Rhinol Laryngol* 80:419–442, 1971.
15. Spenler CW, Benfield JR: Esophageal disruption from blunt and penetrating external trauma. *Arch Surg* 111:663–667, 1976.
16. Lyons HA: Differential diagnosis of hemoptysis and its treatment, in Pierce AK (ed): *Basics of Respiratory Disease*. New York, American Lung Association, 1976, vol 5, p 2.
17. Wolfe JD, Simmons DH: Hemoptysis: Diagnosis and management. *West J Med* 127:383–390, 1977.
18. Greene R, Stark P: Trauma of the larynx and trachea. *Radiol Clin North Am* 15:309–320, 1978.
19. Momose KJ, Macmillan AS: Roentgenologic investigations of the larynx and trachea. *Radiol Clin North Am* 16:321–341, 1978.
20. Sheely CH, Mattox KL, Beall AC: Management of acute cervical tracheal trauma. *Am J Surg* 128:805–808, 1974.
21. Chadwick DC: Closed injuries of the larynx and pharynx. *J Laryngol Otol* 74:306–311, 1960.

69. Maxillofacial Injuries

STEPHEN V. CANTRILL, M.D.

Maxillofacial injuries are commonly encountered in the practice of emergency medicine and may run the gamut from a small lip laceration to a facial "crunch" associated with major trauma. The goal of this chapter is to provide guidance for the evaluation and treatment of this wide range of disorders.

There are many possible etiologies for maxillofacial injuries, including motor vehicle accidents, assaults, athletic injuries, home accidents, work-related injuries, animal and human bites, and nonaccidental childhood trauma (child abuse). More than 50 percent of these injuries, however, are sustained in motor vehicle accidents, and many of these (60 percent in some series) are associated with additional major trauma.

Maxillofacial injuries mandate special attention because of the importance of the face. The face contains the many important organs needed for seeing, hearing, smelling, breathing, eating, and talking, and the appearance of the structure has a major impact on daily life. Much of an individual's personality is embodied in the face, and any defect detracts from this. In working with facial injuries, care is required to avoid leaving any more of a defect than is absolutely necessary.

PATHOPHYSIOLOGY AND CLINICAL CORRELATES

Maxillofacial injuries may be inflicted by sharp or blunt instruments or both. Trauma from a sharp object is more likely to produce only a laceration, while blunt trauma may produce a contusion, avulsion, and/or bony disruption. Maxillofacial injuries resulting from vehicular trauma are usually deceleration injuries that might have been avoided if the patient had used the passenger restraint system available in the automobile. The kinetic energy present in a moving body is a function of the mass of the body times the square of its velocity; thus, it is the dispersion of this energy during deceleration that produces the force that causes the injury. It is easy to see why the magnitude of the injury can be greatly increased by only a moderate increase in speed.

Patients with massive facial trauma, hemorrhage, and airway obstruction may also present with severe, life-threatening injuries to other organ systems. These patients should have their maxillofacial trauma dealt with only to the degree of ensuring a patent airway and controlling the hemorrhage, and their other injuries must be evaluated and treated before attention is again given to the facial area. Facial injuries may appear grotesque, but except for airway and bleeding control they rarely present a true emergency. A further complicating factor is that vehicular accident patients are often under the influence of ethanol, thus making accurate evaluation of the patient more difficult. It should be remembered that shock is almost never due to maxillofacial trauma alone; an additional major cause must be sought elsewhere in the body.

DIAGNOSIS AND TREATMENT

Prehospital Care

The most important component of prehospital care in patients with maxillofacial trauma is the maintenance of a patent airway. The patient's airway can be compromised by bony or cartilagenous disruption or by obstruction of the airway by soft tissue, blood, or a foreign body. After the oropharynx is initially cleared of blood and debris, the method of airway management is a function of the patient's mentation and other suspected injuries. If a cervical spine injury is suspected, as it often is in vehicular trauma, the cervical spine must be immobilized, usually with the patient in a supine position. If the victim is obtunded but not bleeding into the airway, an oropharyngeal or nasopharyngeal airway may be adequate for maintenance of a patent airway. If the patient is comatose or bleeding into the oral cavity, nasotracheal intubation should be considered. It should be kept in mind that many paramedic programs do not permit endotracheal intubation or nasotracheal intubation in their accepted list of functions. In the case of respiratory arrest, orotracheal intubation may be necessary. In the rare case in which the patient has also sustained severe laryngeal trauma, a cricothyreotomy may be the only way of establishing an airway. If cervical spine injury is not suspected, the patient may be transported sitting, prone, or in a lateral decubitus position to avoid aspiration. Patients with isolated traumatic eye injuries should be transported in a sitting position.

Control of hemorrhage is second in importance, after ensuring an airway, in patients with maxillofacial trauma. Direct pressure, either by hand or pressure dressings, is almost always adequate in the field. (See Figures 69–1 and 69–2 for location of blood vessels.) Care must be taken not to further compromise the airway in applying the dressings to the head and face.

Impaled foreign bodies in the face and eye should be stabilized with gauze bandages prior to transport. Those involving *only* the cheek may be safely removed in the field, with finger pressure used to control hemorrhage. All other foreign bodies should be left in place until the patient is in the operating room.

Soft tissue injuries of the facial area should also be given prehospital attention. Large avulsion flaps should have any gross contamination removed by irrigation and then be replaced in their tissue bed. Completely avulsed tissues, especially ears, the nose, or teeth should be retrieved if possible, wrapped in gauze soaked in normal saline, and transported with the patient.

In cases where the eyes have been in contact with acid or alkali solutions, the eyes should be copiously irrigated on the scene. Any source of running water is adequate for this irrigation.

Emergency care personnel at the scene should also note the mechanism of injury and the position in which the patient was found. This information should be conveyed to those caring for the patient in the emergency department since it is frequently helpful in assessing the patient for other injuries. The patient's mental status both at the time of initial evaluation and during transport should be noted, because closed head trauma frequently accompanies maxillofacial injuries. Any change in mental status without evidence of shock should be assumed to be evidence of closed head trauma until proved otherwise. (See Chapter 7.)

Emergency Department Care

Initial Stabilization and Evaluation

On arrival in the emergency department, the patient may have been stabilized to varying degrees, based on the sophistication of the prehospital care system that was utilized. The initial care of the patient follows the same protocol as outlined above. A patent airway must be ensured, with intubation if necessary. A nasotracheal route is preferred if the patient is relatively stable or if there is concern about a possible cervical spine injury. In cases of massive facial and/or laryngeal trauma, a cricothyreotomy may be necessary as a life-saving measure. A true tracheostomy has no place in the emergency department in a "crash" situation, since it is often a very difficult and time-consuming procedure, even under the best of controlled circumstances.

If shock is present, it must be aggressively treated with fluid resuscitation, control of bleeding, and application of an antishock suit. As noted above, the presence of shock almost always indicates major trauma to areas other than the face. Head, chest, and abdominal etiologies for the hypotension must be ruled out. The presence of cervical spine trauma must be assumed until disproved in any person with altered mental status due to the trauma or other agents (e.g., ethanol). Any alert patient complaining of neck pain or paresthesia should also have the cervical spine immobilized until any injury can be discounted radiographically.

The patient should be completely evaluated for serious life-threatening injury before the maxillofacial trauma is evaluated. As noted, most facial hemorrhage can be controlled through direct pressure. Rarely, hemostats may be required to control an isolated bleeder. This should be done only under direct vision to avoid iatrogenic injury to important structures, such as the facial nerve and the parotid duct (Fig. 69–3). After evaluation, most clean facial lacerations may wait up to 24 hours for definitive care. If this is to be the case,

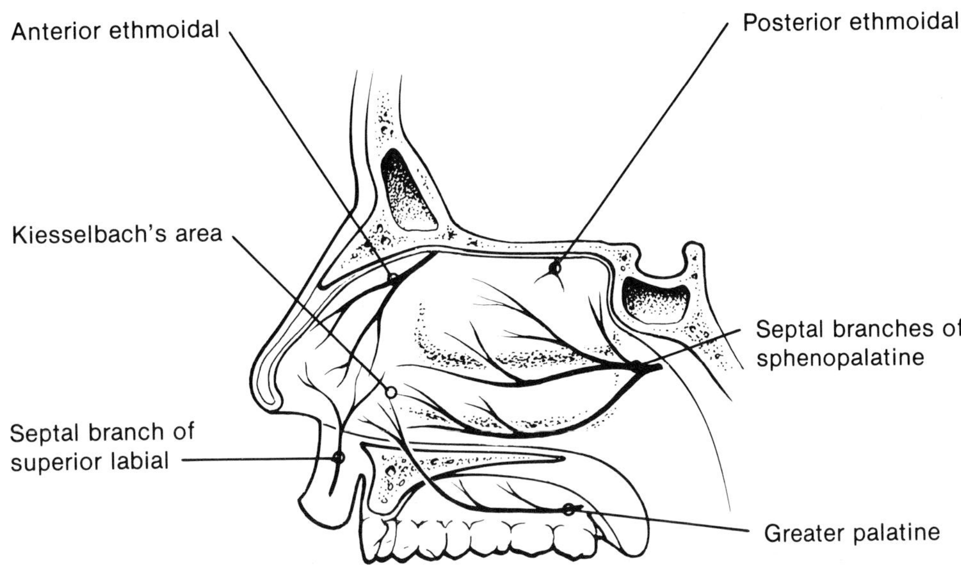

Figure 69–1   Blood Supply to the Nasal Septum.

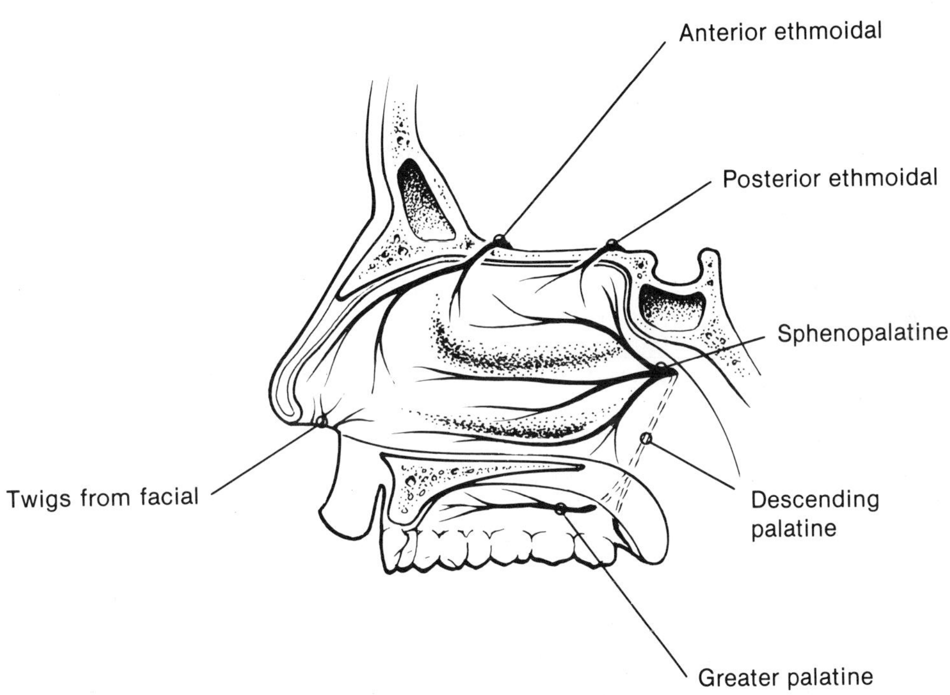

Figure 69–2   Blood Supply to the Turbinates.

the wound should be irrigated and the tissues placed in rough approximation. Grossly contaminated wounds, animal bites, human bites, and wounds with foreign body tattooing should be handled as soon as possible to provide maximum opportunity for a good result.

Evaluation of Maxillofacial Injuries

Much of facial trauma is obvious, but a surprising amount may elude the examining physician unless a thorough, systematic approach to evaluation is made.

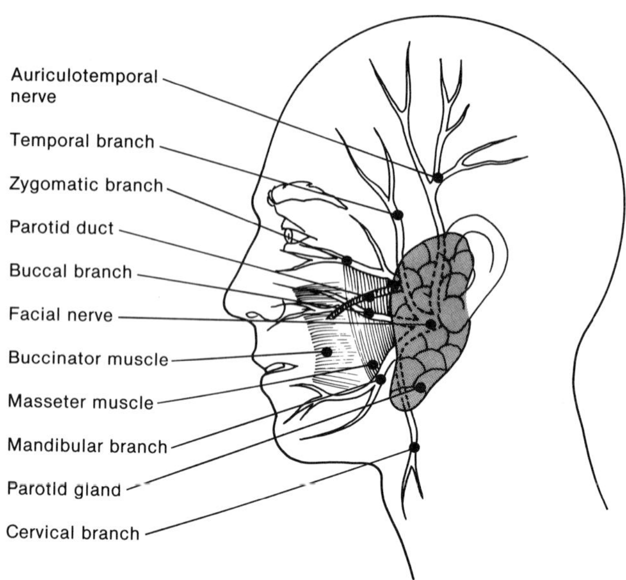

Figure 69–3   Muscles, Nerves, and Glands of the Head.

Since many maxillofacial injuries will be treated by a specialist, the main function of the emergency physician may only be to discover the injury. This is a crucial role. In many cases, if the injury is missed (e.g., a tripod fracture of the zygoma), the patient may end up with a healed injury that results in compromised function (e.g., diplopia) that may be extremely difficult to correct at a later date.

The evaluation of facial injuries begins with a history. This important source of data is often given short shrift, with unfortunate repercussions. It is important to understand the mechanism of injury to construct a differential diagnosis of what types of injury may have occurred and therefore must be ruled out. If alert, the patient can answer questions about sources of pain, but this may be unreliable since a greater pain (e.g., a femur fracture) may override the pain of other injuries. If mandibular trauma is a possibility, the patient should be asked if the dental occlusion feels normal. If it does not, the patient is assumed to have a mandibular fracture until proved otherwise.

Inspection of the facial area is performed, with deformity or asymmetry being sought as indicators of possible bony disruption. Enophthalmos (the sinking of the eye globe posteriorly in the orbit) and loss of consensual gaze should both be checked as indicators of possible disruption of the orbits. The bite should be inspected for malocclusion and the dentition should be inspected for evidence of a step deformity, both implying a mandibular fracture. If nasal trauma is suspected, the septum should be visually inspected for integrity and for existence of a septal hematoma. Excessive, watery rhinorrhea may be cerebrospinal fluid, indicating a frac-

ture of the cribriform plate. (Glucose determination of the rhinorrhea is not a valid method to differentiate cerebrospinal fluid from other fluids.) All soft tissue injuries must be thoroughly and carefully inspected. Often foreign material may be found deep in the wound, or a fracture may be directly visualized that is not seen on the radiograph. The integrity of the eye globes should be ensured by inspection. Tonometry may help in diagnosing penetrating violation by demonstrating an unusually low pressure. Fluorescein staining should be performed if nonpenetrating corneal injury is a possibility.

Documentation of what is observed is probably more important on the face than elsewhere. In one series it was noted that 24 percent of facial injuries resulted in personal litigation. This obviously requires the treating physician to be able to reconstruct carefully the nature of the initial injury. Photographs offer the best mechanism to do this. A camera with instantly developing film provides an easy mechanism for this, with the resultant picture stapled to the patient's record. Careful drawings with measurements should be supplied if photographs are unavailable.

The next step is evaluation of neuromuscular function. Motor function of the facial nerves may be easily evaluated by observing the face in repose and then by asking the patient to bare the teeth, smile, wrinkle the forehead, and close the eyes tightly. Sensory innervation of the three branches of the trigeminal nerve should be tested bilaterally (supraorbital, infraorbital, and mental branches). A fracture near the foramina of exit of any of these nerves will frequently present as anesthesia/hypoesthesia in the distribution of that nerve (Fig. 69–4). Extraocular movements should be completely tested as indicators of a possible orbital floor fracture. The patient should be asked about diplopia in each of the directions of movement. Visual acuity should be tested with a Snellen or similar chart if trauma to the eye is suspected. Palpation of the bony structure of the face, the next step, should be done in a systematic fashion (Fig. 69–5). Tenderness, step defects, crepitus, and false motion should all be searched for. Each is an indicator of potential facial fracture. The infraorbital area, the supraorbital ridge, the zygoma, the nasal bones, the lower maxilla, and the mandible should be carefully palpated. Stability of the teeth and the alveolar ridge should be tested by grasping the upper and lower incisors and attempting to move them.

Following the clinical evaluation and if the patient's condition allows, the physician should obtain radiographs, based on clinical suspicion as a result of the mechanism of injury and findings on physical examination. A multitude of radiographic views are possible. The workhorse of facial bone evaluation is the Waters projection (Fig. 69–6), which allows evaluation of the

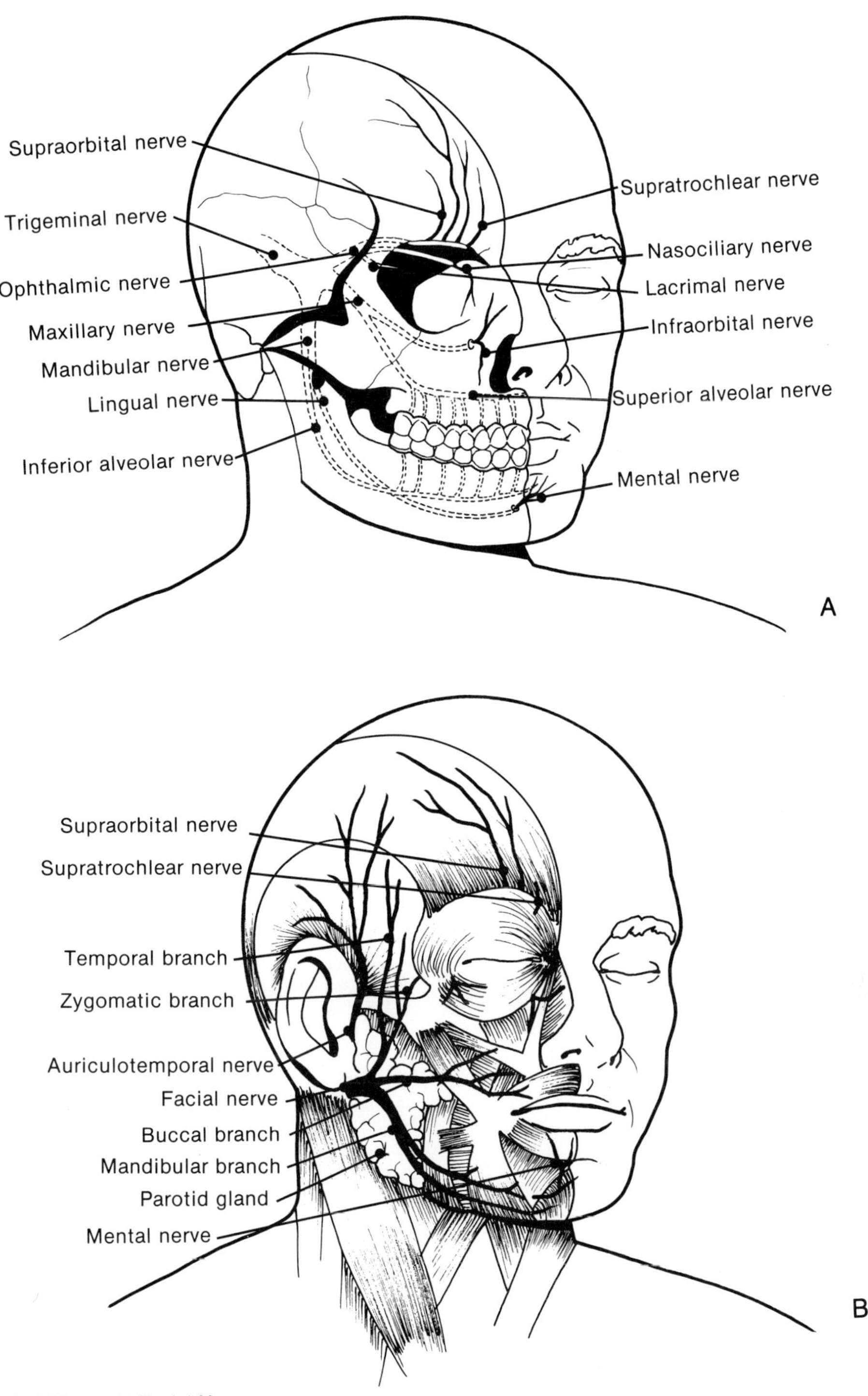

Figure 69–4 *A* Trigeminal Nerve. *B* Facial Nerves.

maxilla, maxillary sinuses, orbital floors, orbital inferior rims, and zygomas. This view is usually accompanied by posteroanterior and lateral facial bone views for routine screening. Other specific radiographs that may be indicated include those of the nasal bones, zygomatic arches, and lateral orbits. Mandible views may be ordered also, although Panorex views, if available, will show any mandibular fractures more clearly. Fractures,

fluid-filled sinuses, herniation of soft tissue into the sinuses, and subcutaneous air should all be searched for. All of these findings indicate probable skeletal disruption.

Use of Consultants

Decisions regarding consultants in maxillofacial trauma are sometimes difficult because of overlapping areas of

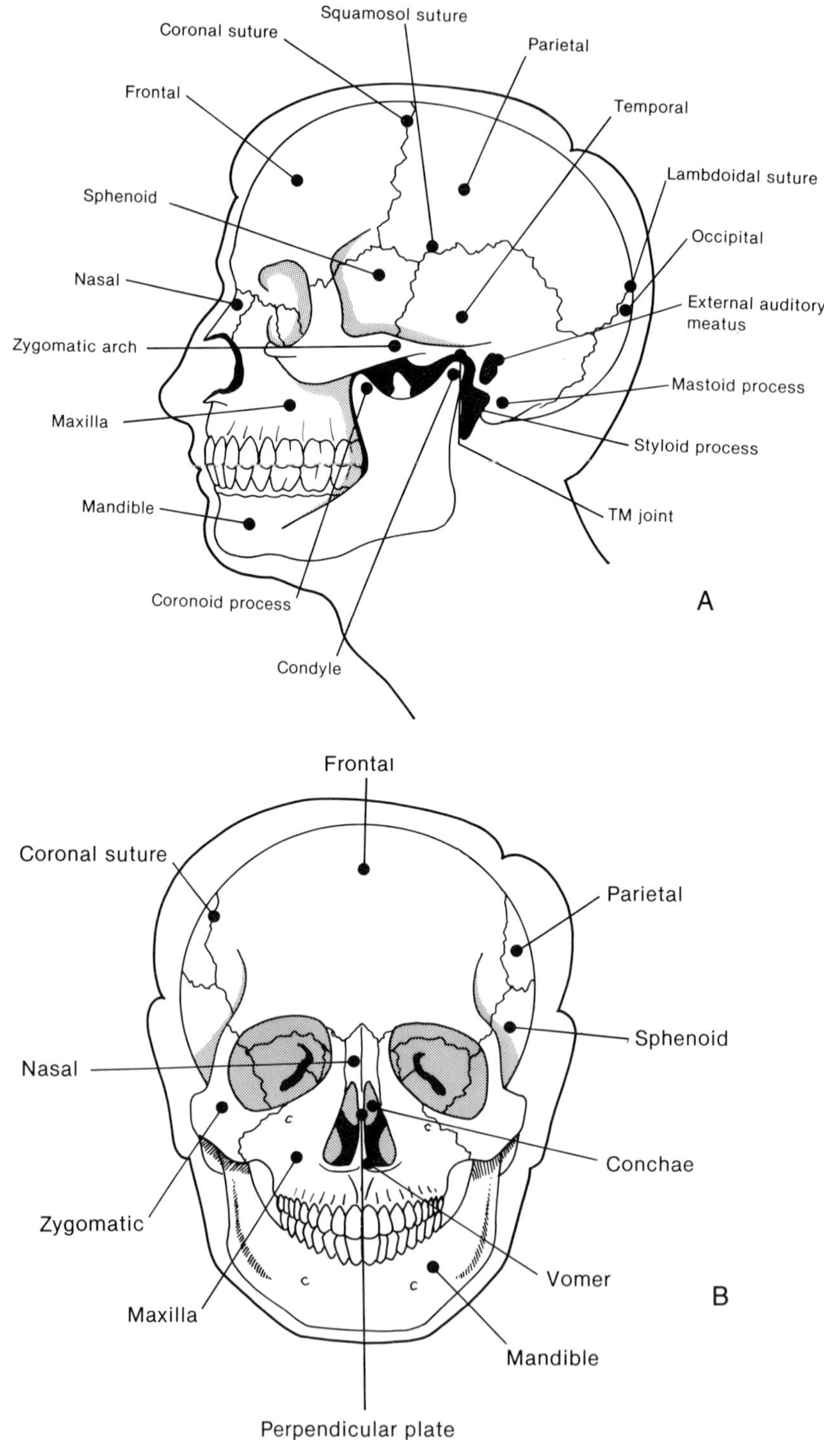

Figure 69–5 Normal Skull and Facial Bones. *Note: A. Sagittal view. B. Coronal View.*

clinical expertise. Different facial injuries may require consultation from plastic surgeons, otolaryngologists, ophthalmologists, and oral surgeons. Some specific recommendations are made in the sections that follow, but the best rule of thumb is for the emergency department physician to provide referral based on the interests and capabilities of the specialists immediately available. The decision for referral may at times be difficult, encompassing such facts as the emergency department physician's expertise in handling different injuries, the patient load in the emergency department at that time, and the complexity of the injury. Indicators for referral

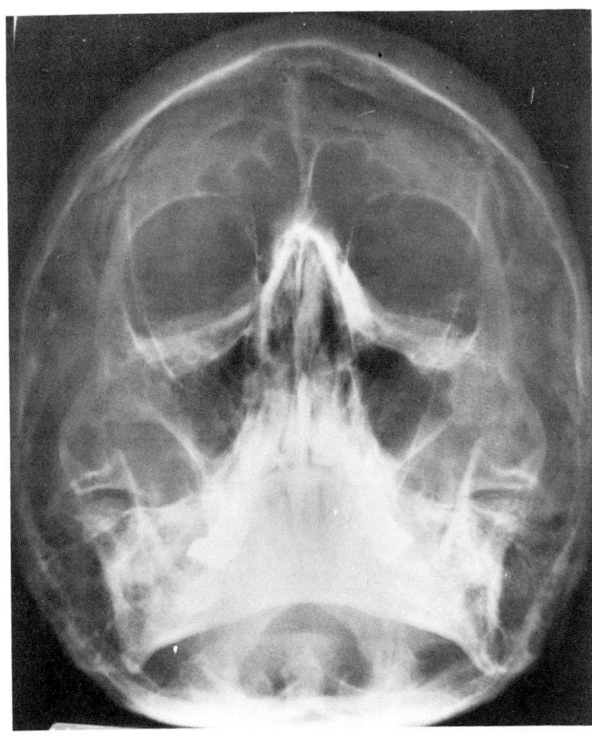

Figure 69–6 View of Facial Bones. Note: Head tilted back (Waters Projection).

include the necessity of general anesthesia for repair (such as in an uncooperative child), the possibility of nerve transection, the necessity of a delayed primary closure, the requirement that the patient be admitted due to severe injuries, the necessity of elaborate follow-up, the likelihood for successful repair being low, or the patient asking for a consultation or acting in a litigious manner.

Management of Soft Tissue Injuries

All soft tissue injuries regardless of location require consideration of tetanus prophylaxis. Patients with no history of prior tetanus immunization need treatment with tetanus hyperimmune globulin (Hypertet) as well as initiation of their tetanus immunization series. Patients with up-to-date immunization (within 5 years) but with grossly contaminated wounds probably should also have Hypertet. Normal wounds require only that the patient's last immunization be within the previous 5 to 10 years, with many institutions favoring the 5-year figure. Comatose patients with soft tissue injuries should receive a tetanus immunization.

The decision may be made not to close the soft tissue wound in the emergency department. This is indicated if the patient is unstable from other injuries. In this case, hemostasis should be achieved, the tissues of the wound loosely approximated, the wound covered with saline-soaked gauze, an occlusive dressing applied, and the patient started on antibiotics. Wound age may also be a consideration. Most wounds on the face can be closed up to 24 hours post injury. Older injuries should be referred for delayed primary closure. If the wound contains a foreign body or contamination that cannot be removed, it should not be closed. Severely contaminated wounds (e.g., bites, pavement injuries) should be closed only if they are less than 6 hours old. Any wound covering a fracture that will require later reduction should not be closed but rather dressed as noted above. All injuries that are not closed primarily should be carefully irrigated and dressed, and the patient should be given antibiotics.

Wound anesthesia is usually straightforward in maxillofacial injuries. Local infiltration of 1% lidocaine with 1:100,000 epinephrine will suffice in most cases, although epinephrine should not be used around the ear or the tarsal plate of the eye owing to the relative avascular nature of these structures. Plain lidocaine may also be preferable around large flaps that have tenuous circulation and about the nose. Up to 30 ml of 1% lidocaine may be used in adults and up to 60 ml of 0.5% lidocaine may be used. Infiltration is done with the smallest needle possible through the wound margins.

Additional anesthesia may be achieved, if necessary, through a regional block. Sensory innervation of the face is illustrated in Figure 69–4. One or 2 ml of 1% lidocaine instilled at the exit foramen of any of the major branches of the trigeminal nerve will produce anesthesia in the distribution of that branch. If both local and regional anesthesia are to be used, the regional block should be done first, with local augmentation supplied where necessary.

Children may require systemic analgesia to facilitate a facial repair. Meperidine (1 mg/kg) or a meperidine, promethazine, chlorpromazine combination may be administered intramuscularly. The disadvantages of this approach include the additional time required for the medication to take effect and the necessity of close monitoring of the patient's respiratory status, both during and after the repair. A "papoose board" is also advisable for restraint of small children. Care must be used to not overaggressively restrain young children, as this has resulted in respiratory arrest.

Wounds should be cleansed vigorously. Irrigation with a jet stream of normal saline (500 ml nominally) is preferred. Topical anesthesia of wounds requiring scrubbing (e.g., those with imbedded material) may be achieved through application of 4% lidocaine solution. To avoid a traumatic tattoo (which requires extensive treatment later for correction), all imbedded material should be removed. Any material not removed by scrubbing should be carefully picked out with a No. 11 scalpel blade or 16-gauge needle.

Following cleansing, the wound should be thoroughly explored in a search for any retained material, fractures of the bony skeleton, or injury to any specialized structures (e.g., lacrimal apparatus of the eye). Any devitalized tissue is then debrided, but conservatively so, limited if possible to 1 to 2 mm at the wound edge. Any excision of irreplaceable structures, such as the philtrum (Cupid's bow) of the lip, should be avoided. Clinical judgment is sometimes required to decide if closing a large defect might produce more scarring and deformity than allowing the wound to granulate in, with subsequent plastic revision if necessary. Any beveled wound edges should be revised so the edges of the wound are perpendicular to the surface, resulting in a smaller, smoother scar.

In all but the most superficial of wounds, a layered closure should be performed. The deep layers should be approximated with 4–0 or 5–0 absorbable sutures. The absorbable synthetics are probably superior because they last longer and cause less tissue reaction than chromic sutures. The skin layer is then closed with 5–0 or 6–0 monofilament synthetic nonabsorbable sutures. Landmarks, such as wrinkles, eyebrows, and the vermilion border of the lips should be approximated first to ensure continuity of these highly visible structures. The remainder of the wound may then be closed with interrupted simple or running sutures.

Dressings are usually not required over facial lacerations unless the patient is a child or a large forehead laceration has been repaired. A circumferential head dressing is advisable in the latter case to minimize hematoma formation. Adhesive bandages may be used in an attempt to avoid having a child pick at a wound. In all other cases, a thin layer of water-soluble antibiotic ointment is adequate.

Ongoing wound care consists of two basic principles: (1) keep the wound clean, removing any dried blood or serum with water or saline as needed, and (2) keep the wound soft and pliable, which is done by applying water-soluble antibiotic ointment several times per day. The patient should be informed of signs and symptoms of wound infection. Follow-up arrangements should be made for suture removal (normally in 4 to 6 days). Antibiotic usage during healing is probably only required in heavily contaminated wounds, such as animal or human bites.

Lip Injuries

The most important aspect of repair of lip injuries is the meticulous approximation of the vermilion border. Because infiltration of anesthetic may obliterate this border, the physician may wish to mark this structure on opposite sides of the wound with a small needle scratch prior to infiltration. A layered closure should be employed here if the injury violates the subcutaneous tissue. When placing the skin sutures, the first stitch should approximate the vermilion borders. The skin external to the lip may then be closed with synthetic nonabsorbable sutures. The vermilion section is then closed using fine silk for comfort with lip movement.

Mouth and Tongue Injuries

All but the most insignificant intraoral lacerations should be sutured. To not do so runs the risk of increased scar formation and subsequent functional impairment or a permanent soft tissue defect that may impair oral hygiene. Treatment of tongue lacerations follows the standard of a deep layer of absorbable suture if necessary, followed by a mucosal layer of silk or synthetic absorbable sutures. This exterior layer should have many knots placed to avoid having the tongue untie the suture material. Mucosal lacerations of the mouth are handled in a similar manner. Through-and-through lacerations (e.g., through the cheek into the oral cavity) require a three-layered closure. After irrigation, a watertight closure is made of the mucosal surface, using silk or synthetic absorbable sutures. The competency of this layer is tested by irrigating the wound from outside the mouth and checking for solution leaking into the mouth. The subcutaneous tissue and skin are then closed from outside in the standard manner. Patients with through-and-through lacerations and those with significant oral lacerations should have a course of antibiotics: 5 to 7 days of oral penicillin is probably adequate. Oral wound care consists of rinsing the mouth with a mild antiseptic three or four times per day.

The physician should be suspicious of all oral lacerations in the area of the parotid ducts or submandibular ducts. Patency of these structures should be demonstrated by milking the associated salivary gland and watching for flow of saliva from the duct. If there is a question of violation of these structures, the patient should be referred for careful exploration.

Ear Injuries

The major principle in treating ear injuries is the preservation of as much of the cartilagenous structure as possible. Small lacerations may be anesthetized by direct infiltration with lidocaine without epinephrine (due to the relative avascularity). Large defects are best anesthetized by raising a wheal around the base of the entire ear on the scalp. This will anesthetize all but the external canal and the concha, which may be directly infiltrated if necessary.

Injuries involving the cartilage require careful irrigation and closure of the perichondrium with fine absorbable sutures, followed by skin closure. If skin tissue loss does not allow the cartilage to be covered adequately, a consultant should be called in, since the cartilage may be saved in a subcutaneous pocket for later reconstruction. After repair, the ear should be splinted with wet cotton balls molded about the ear and held in place by a circumferential head bandage. Antibiotics are indicated if the perichondrium has been violated owing to the risk of a low-grade chondritis.

Injuries to the ear not violating the skin but causing swelling also require careful attention. The swelling is often a subperichondrial hematoma, which, if not treated, will calcify, forming a "cauliflower ear." This injury is treated by aseptically aspirating the blood and applying a compression dressing, as noted above, for 5 to 7 days.

Eye Injuries

Probably the most common eye injury is the corneal abrasion, an injury to the corneal epithelium due to direct trauma. These lesions are clearly seen with fluorescein stain under a Wood's light. Treatment is straightforward. The eye is anesthetized with topical ophthalmic solution, antibiotic ointment is placed in the eye, and the eye is patched. The patient is discharged with a prescription for oral pain medication and is told to consult an ophthalmologist in 24 hours for reevaluation. The patient should not drive with an eye patched because of the acute loss of binocular vision.

A related corneal injury is superficial keratitis or "flash burn" caused by ultraviolet radiation exposure. This uncomfortable entity is diagnosed by history and fluorescein stain. Treatment is identical for a corneal abrasion with the addition of instillation of a mydriatic (e.g., homatropine), before patching to help in decreasing the discomfort.

Foreign bodies on the surface of the eye require careful inspection after application of topical anesthetic. This evaluation is best done with a slit lamp, although magnifying glasses may be adequate. Careful attention is paid to the entire globe as well as to the conjunctival surfaces of the lids. The upper lid should be everted to allow careful inspection. Most foreign bodies may be removed by a moist cotton-tipped applicator, but some corneal foreign bodies may require sharp removal with an eye spud or a needle. After removal of the object, antibiotic ointment is instilled as above. The eye should be patched with ophthalmologic follow-up in 24 hours.

Chemical burns to the eye represent a true ocular emergency in that the action taken immediately following the injury is of extreme importance. The patient's eye should be copiously irrigated immediately after the accident. Specific antidotes should not be used since the heat produced by the chemical reaction could further damage the eye. Immediately after arrival in the emergency department the patient should have the affected eye locally anesthetized and gently irrigated with normal saline. If the chemical in question is alkali, the irrigation should continue for 1 hour since alkali is not inactivated by the tissues (as acid is) and therefore can continue to cause tissue destruction until physically removed. After irrigation, the injured eye should have a mydriatic and antibiotic ointment instilled and a patch applied. All ocular burns require ophthalmologic follow-up. The treatment of severe chemical burns, especially those caused by alkali, should be discussed with an ophthalmologist.

Corneal and scleral lacerations require immediate attention by an ophthalmologist. Nothing should be placed in the eye. It should be covered by a metal protective patch that gently covers the globe. The patient should be admitted to the hospital and kept fasting in the event that surgery is required.

Hyphemas, or gross blood in the anterior chamber due to direct blunt trauma, are not uncommonly seen in the emergency department. Patients with hyphemas should be admitted to the hospital and kept in a 30 degree-head-elevated position to allow the blood to layer out and clot. Bilateral eye patches may help to decrease eye motion.

Intraocular foreign bodies may be difficult to demonstrate if they are not radiodense. Posteroanterior and lateral orbital radiographs will help locate metallic foreign bodies. The localization of nonmetallic foreign bodies may require the assistance of an ophthalmologist. These patients should be admitted to the hospital.

Lacerations of the eyelids are not uncommon. Simple lacerations not involving the lid margin may be closed in the standard layered technique using 6–0 suture material, and the eye is patched. Lacerations involving the lid margin require meticulous technique and are best left for a plastic surgeon or ophthalmologist to repair. If necessary, artificial tears should be used to keep the cornea moist until the lid is repaired. Any laceration near the medial canthus requires that the integrity of the lacrimal apparatus be demonstrated by probing with a nylon or polypropylene suture and making sure it does not appear in the wound. Any violation of this structure requires repair by an ophthalmologist. (See Chapter 66.)

Eyebrow Injuries

The repair of soft tissue injuries of the eyebrow is straightforward. Debridement should be kept to a minimum. The eyebrow should not be shaved because it is a vital landmark in the repair. Any revision of the wound should be done parallel to the hair follicle roots (as opposed to perpendicular to the skin as is usually the case) to minimize any bald area in the resultant scar.

The first sutures should be placed to align the borders of the eyebrow to avoid any step defect.

Nasal Injuries

Nasal injuries include bony and soft tissue injuries. Nasal fractures may result in either lateral or posterior displacement of the bony fragments. Edema, tenderness, deformity, crepitus, and/or hypermobility are part of the clinical presentation. Radiographs are of limited usefulness except for documentation purposes. Gross lateral deformity can sometimes be corrected in the emergency department by lateral pressure. In all cases of documented or suspected fracture, follow-up 5 to 7 days postinjury is necessary to evaluate the nose after the swelling subsides. A high index of suspicion should be maintained for nasal fractures in children because the growth potential of the nose may be disrupted by an unrecognized fracture. In children, tenderness, swelling, and post-traumatic epistaxis are sufficient grounds to arrange follow-up.

In all cases of nasal trauma, the physician must be careful to check for a nasal septum hematoma. This presents as a big, bulging, purple grapelike structure on the septum. If such a lesion is missed, septal necrosis may ensue. Treatment involves a small vertical incision over the hematoma to drain it, an anterior nasal pack to guard against reaccumulation, oral antibiotics, and follow-up by an otolaryngologist or plastic surgeon.

Soft tissue injuries to the nose are best repaired with a combination of regional and local anesthesia. An infraorbital and supratrochlear block may be used. (The supratrochlear nerve is located 1.5 cm medial to the supraorbital foramen.) A layered closure should be used, with careful attention to covering any exposed cartilage and with careful irrigation after each layer. The nasal skin may be closed with a running subcuticular stitch of absorbable suture material to avoid the common problem of stitch abscesses in this area.

Abrasion/Avulsion Injuries

Facial abrasion/avulsion injuries are commonly seen when the patient's face impacts and skids along a roughened surface, such as highway pavement or a fractured windshield. The result is an area of abrasion with numerous small avulsions, some of which may contain foreign material (e.g., gravel, glass). These wounds require vigorous cleansing to avoid traumatic tattooing of the skin. All avulsion wounds require careful inspection and probing to ensure maximum removal of foreign material. It is not uncommon to find shards of glass deeply imbedded in the subcutaneous tissues from these injuries.

All full-thickness wound areas should be closed with nonabsorbable synthetic suture. Antibiotic gauze should then be applied to the entire area to help in the re-epithelization of the wound. Suture removal may be delayed to day 7 to allow for adequate healing and the gauze to loosen. The patient should be informed that the resultant healed wound may be uneven and "pebbly." This may be treated at a later date through dermabrasion.

Management of Fractures and Dislocations

Mandibular Fractures

Mandibular fractures are the third most common facial fracture, following nasal and zygomatic fractures. The cardinal sign of a mandibular fracture is dental malocclusion that is either observed or noted when the patient relates that his or her teeth do not fit right. These patients also have mandibular pain and tenderness. A step in dentition or an ecchymosis in the floor of the mouth are also indicators of fracture of the mandible. Any patient with these signs or symptoms following trauma must have a mandibular fracture ruled out. This is most elegantly done by a Panorex radiograph of the mandible. Failing that, standard anteroposterior and lateral views are obtained. Because the mandible is a ring-type structure, the traumatic impact may be transmitted about the ring, causing a fracture remote from the site of impact. This also explains the high (50 percent) incidence of multiple fractures of the mandible.

Almost all patients with mandibular fractures require admission to the hospital for occlusal fixation. If bony fragments are seen in the mouth or if periodontal bleeding is present near the site of the fracture, the fracture is considered an open fracture. These patients should be started on antibiotic therapy.

Temporomandibular Joint Dislocation

Dislocation of the temporomandibular joint (TMJ) may be seen following trauma or after opening the mouth excessively wide (e.g., with a yawn). Unilateral or bilateral dislocations may be present. In either case, the patient is unable to close the mouth and will have moderate TMJ discomfort, which will worsen with the passage of time owing to increased spasm of the muscles of mastication. If the dislocation is secondary to trauma, mandibular radiographs should be obtained prior to reduction to rule out a possible condylar fracture. TMJ dislocation occurs anteriorly and superiorly and is usually easily reduced by reversing this movement. This is accomplished by the physician placing gauze-wrapped thumbs (to avoid injury) on the patient's lower third molars with the fingers curled under the symphysis of the mandible. The mandibular condyles are then levered down with downward pressure on the molars and upward pressure on the symphysis of the mandible. The mandible is then slipped posteriorly for the completed reduction. If difficulty is encountered, diazepam may be administered intravenously to help overcome the muscle spasm. Postreduction roentgenograms are indicated if this is the initial TMJ dislocation for the patient. After reduction, if pain free, the patient may be discharged on a soft diet with instructions to avoid opening the mouth wide. However, if significant spasm or tenderness is present, admission for fixation of the mandible should be considered.

Maxillary Fractures

Maxillary fractures are usually seen as the result of massive facial trauma, frequently coexisting with other life-threatening injuries. These patients present with facial swelling, midface mobility to palpation, malocclusion, and/or cerebrospinal fluid rhinorrhea. Radiographic diagnosis is made by the Waters and lateral facial bone views. These fractures were classified, based on location, by LeFort. All combinations of these fractures may be seen.

Patients with maxillary fractures all require admission to the hospital. Emergency care consists of airway maintenance and ruling out other concomitant injuries. To protect the airway, intubation or, in severe cases, cricothyreotomy may be required. If cerebrospinal fluid rhinorrhea is present, the patient should be kept in a head-elevated position and started on antibiotic therapy.

Zygomatic Fractures

Zygomatic fractures are often caused by deceleration injuries. A common zygomatic fracture is the tripod fracture with fracture lines at the zygomaticotemporal suture, the zygomaticofrontal suture, and through the infraorbital foramen. These patients may present with a bony step defect, infraorbital hypoesthesia, flatness

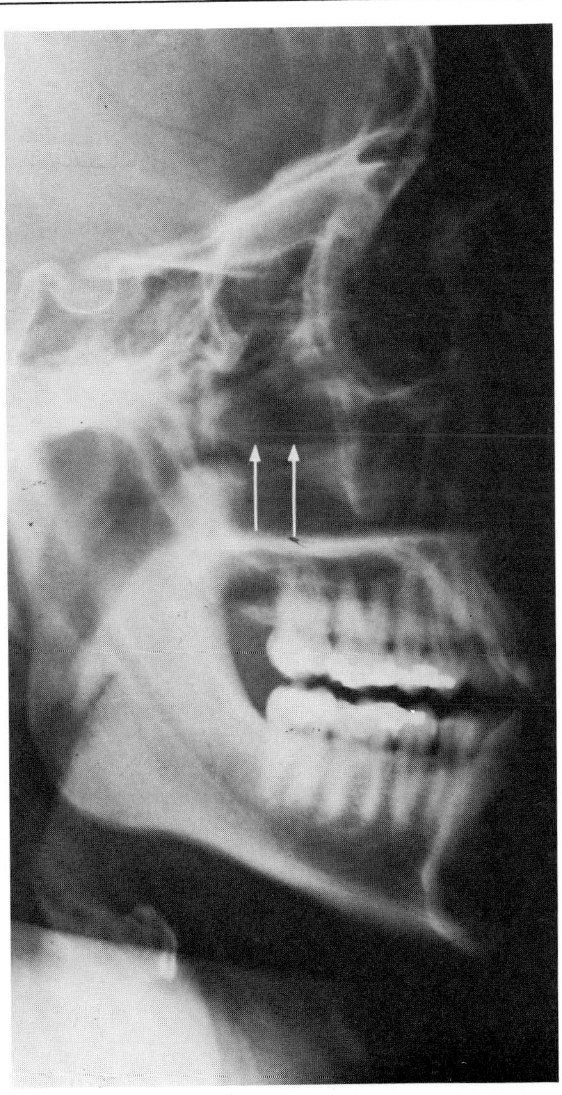

Figure 69–7 A   Lateral Roentgenogram of the Skull Demonstrating an Air Fluid Level in the Maxillary Sinus.

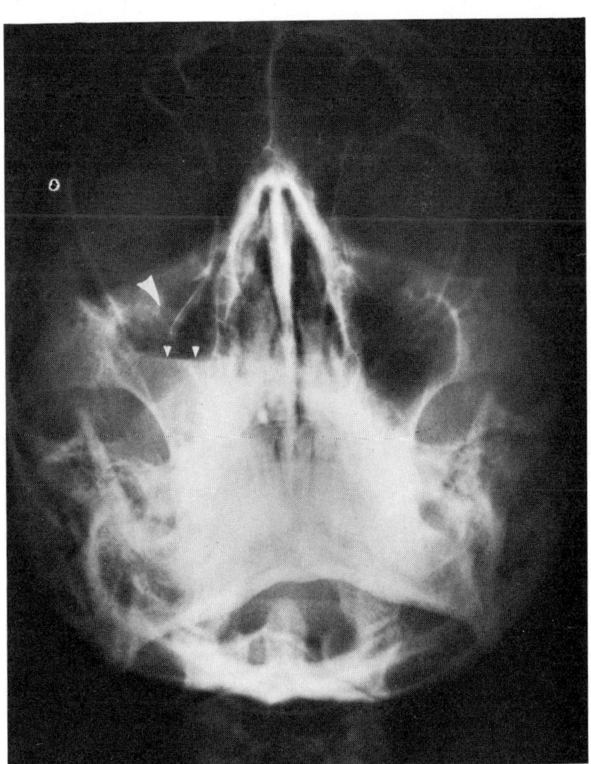

Figure 69–7 B   Waters View Roentgenogram of the Skull. *Note:* The small arrows demonstrate the air fluid level in the right maxillary sinus shown in *A*. The large arrow points to the herniated orbital contents. The findings suggest a "blowout" fracture of the right orbit.

of the malar eminence, diplopia, or change in consensual gaze. An isolated fracture of the zygomatic arch is often due to a roundhouse punch. These patients have tenderness over the arch and may have painful or limited mandibular movement due to encroachment by the arch on the mandible. Radiographs required to evaluate the zygoma include the Waters view and the submental-vertex view.

All patients with zygoma fractures require referral for possible elevation and fixation. If mandibular motion is not compromised and in the absence of other injuries, these patients may be followed as outpatients.

Orbital Floor Fractures

Fractures of the orbital floor are commonly seen following application of substantial force to the globe of the eye. This force is transmitted hydraulically to the interior orbit, fracturing the weakest portion, the inframedial area. Because of the architecture of the external orbit, the eye is well protected except from those objects less than 5 cm in radius (e.g., a knuckle or handball). As a result of the fracture, the inferior extraocular muscles may become entrapped or the fatty tissue surrounding the globe may herniate into the maxillary sinus. Muscle entrapment gives rise to diplopia and loss of full extraocular movements, especially upward gaze. Herniation of orbital contents may produce enophthalmos or the "hanging drop" sign on the ra-

diograph. The patient may also present with infraorbital hypoesthesia. However, the patient may have none of these findings and still a fracture may be seen on the radiograph. It should be stressed that clouding on a maxillary sinus without other explanation must be taken as indirect evidence of an orbital fracture until proved otherwise. These patients all require careful follow-up since operative intervention may be required to ensure proper binocular vision. Immediate admission is usually not indicated.

BIBLIOGRAPHY

Baker SP, Schultz RC: Recurrent problems in emergency room management of maxillofacial injuries. *Clin Plast Surg* 2:65–71, 1975.

Converse JM, et al: *Reconstructive Plastic Surgery*, vol II. Philadelphia, WB Saunders Co, 1977.

Curtis JW: Basic plastic surgical techniques in repair of facial lacerations. *Surg Clin North Am* 53:33–46, 1973.

Dingman RO, Natvig P: *Surgery of Facial Fractures*. Philadelphia, WB Saunders Co, 1969.

Dushoff IM: About face. *Emerg Med*, March 15, 1979.

Luce EA, Tubb TD, Moore AM: Review of 1000 major facial fractures and associated injuries. *Plast Reconstruct Surg* 63:26–30, 1979.

Paletta FX: Soft tissue injuries of face and scalp. *Clin Plast Surg* 4:479–490, 1977.

Schultz RC: *Facial Injuries*, 2nd ed. Chicago, Year Book Medical, 1977.

Schultz RC, Oldham RJ: An overview of facial injuries. *Surg Clin North Am* 57:987–1010, 1977.

Winspur I: Facial fractures and the ED physician. *Emerg Med Serv* May/June 1979, pp 31–36.

Zook EG, et al: *The Primary Case of Facial Injuries*. Littleton, Mass, PSG Publishing Co, 1980.

70. Dental Emergencies

JOHN P. KELLY, D.M.D., M.D.

Personnel in primary contact with patients seeking emergency care will frequently encounter complaints related to the oropharynx. The widespread prevalence of dental decay and the high incidence of pathology in and about the oral cavity will often result in acute symptoms for which the patients will seek emergency care. The nature of the patient's symptoms or the timing of their onset commonly brings the patient to the non-dental practitioner for whom the diseases of the oral cavity are unfamiliar.

With this review of the emergency conditions arising in the teeth, jaws, and oral soft tissues, the emergency care personnel with first contact with the patient will be more confident and capable of appropriate triage, emergency treatment, and definitive referral for continued care. Provision of adequate analgesia and initiation of antibiotic therapy where appropriate are the most critical components of initial emergency care.

ODONTOGENIC INFECTION

Pathology and Pathophysiology

Dental caries is the most prevalent disease in the United States. The action of oral microbes on the teeth in the presence of dietary carbohydrates and in the absence of adequate oral hygiene produces decalcification of enamel and subsequent decay of the underlying dentin. As decay progresses, recognizable patterns of pain will be described by the patient. The sensory receptors of the tooth are solely pain receptors; hence thermal or pressure stimuli are perceived only as painful stimuli by the dental pulp.

Incipient dental decay is only mildly symptomatic, producing mild pain when hot or cold liquids or sweet substances are ingested. The pain may be difficult to localize to an individual tooth, but the minimal and transient nature of the pain rarely brings such a patient to an emergency care facility.

As decay progresses deeper into the dentin and approaches the pulp chamber, the pulp becomes inflamed. The pain becomes considerably more debilitating; it may be stimulated by extremes of temperature, but it may also appear spontaneously and be unremitting, relieved only by therapeutic doses of narcotic analgesics. The same syndrome of pain can be experienced following restorative dental procedures when a filling is placed close to the pulp of the tooth. A fractured tooth can produce the same symptoms. In children, the pulpitis may be reversible; but in adults, the pulp usually becomes necrotic as a result of the inflammatory process.

When the necrotic pulp is infected, pain returns as the first evidence of a developing abscess. The pain in this instance is usually incited or aggravated by hot liquids and relieved by cold. Most often, the patient can localize the pain to a particular tooth with referral of pain from a mandibular tooth to the ear and from a maxillary tooth to the periorbital area. However, paradoxical referral of pain may make it difficult for the patient to determine whether the offending tooth is in the upper or lower jaw. Fever, swelling, and leukocytosis are not seen when the pain arises from a necrotic pulp.

Spread of infection from the necrotic pulp to the alveolar bone surrounding the root of the tooth gives a significant additional finding. The involved tooth is tender to the pressure of biting force; tenderness can be elicited by percussion of the tooth and the tooth may be mobile. Palpation of the soft tissues overlying the root may reveal fullness, frank swelling, or fluctuance as the abscess proceeds from the alveolus to the surrounding periosteum and adjacent soft tissue planes. The accompanying swelling usually spreads to the submandibular area from an infected mandibular tooth; abscessed maxillary teeth characteristically produce a cellulitis involving the cheek and periorbital tissues. The patient may present with malaise, fever, and leukocytosis.

An untreated alveolar abscess may progress to life-threatening infection if the process reaches the fascial spaces of the floor of the mouth (Ludwig's angina) or the vascular drainage system of the maxilla (cavernous sinus thrombosis). See Figure 70–1.

Painful infection associated with the soft tissues around partially erupted wisdom teeth is a frequently seen condition in the young adult population. In its mildest form, pericoronitis produces symptoms described as "teething." The more severe infections are accompanied by constant, throbbing pain, worsened by attempting to close the teeth together; the patient may be unable to open the mouth, the trismus resulting from spasm of the masticatory muscles adjacent to the mandibular third molars.

Diagnosis

A thorough history is required for evaluation of odontogenic pain and swelling. The various stages of dental infection have such historical characteristics that the diagnosis can often be made by addressing the specific questions of the pain's nature, onset, severity, duration, location, radiation, and aggravating and ameliorating factors (Table 70–1).

Initial examination requires comfortable positioning of the patient and a suitable lighting fixture for illuminating the mouth while leaving the examiner's hands free. Inspection of the mouth for fractured, decayed, or extensively restored teeth and inflammation or swelling of the soft tissues is easily accomplished. Palpation of the oral structures and percussion of the teeth with

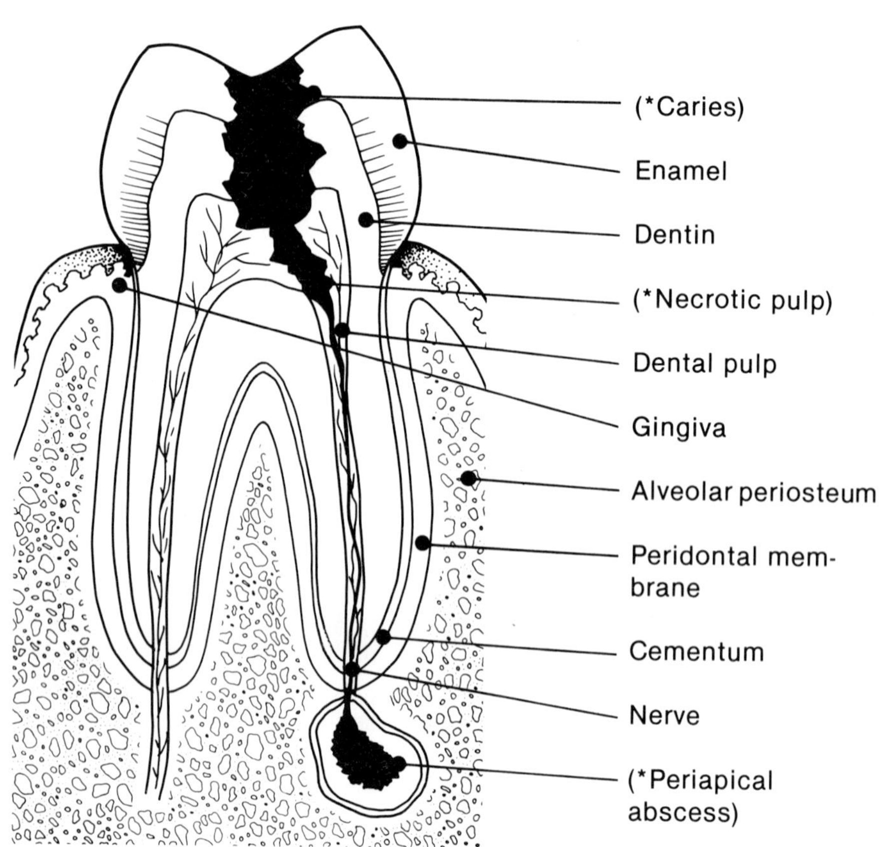

Figure 70–1   Abscessed Tooth and Gum. *Note:* * denotes abnormal conditions.

Table 70–1   Differential Diagnosis of Dental Pain

Disorder	Pain	Swelling	Emergency Treatment	Definitive Treatment
Decay	Dull; response to heat, cold, sweets	None	Analgesics	Dental restoration
Pulpitis	Sharp; response to heat, cold; may be spontaneous	None	Analgesics	Endodontic treatment or extraction
Pulpal necrosis	Throbbing; response to heat; relieved by cold	None	Analgesics	Endodontic treatment or extraction
Periapical abscess	Throbbing; tender to percussion or chewing	Usually none	Analgesics, antibiotics	Endodontic or surgical treatment
Alveolar abscess	Aching; tender to palpation	Present	Antibiotics, drainage	Surgical treatment

Source: Adapted from Kelly JP: Evaluation of facial pain and swelling, in Goroll AH, May LA, Mullae AG (eds): *Primary Care Medicine.* Philadelphia, JB Lippincott, 1981.

the handle of a dental mirror will aid in localization of the offending tooth; mobility and painful response to percussion are the significant findings, as are the nature and location of any swelling.

Unless dental radiography equipment is available in the emergency care location, radiographic studies are best deferred.

Laboratory studies are not indicated unless the odontogenic infection has produced systemic symptoms. In the latter case, white blood cell count and differential, blood sugar, and blood cultures may aid in subsequent management.

Differential Diagnosis

Differential diagnosis of odontogenic pain must include the various neuralgias (e.g., trigeminal, glossopharyngeal), maxillary sinusitis, salivary gland infection, masticatory muscle spasm, or temporomandibular joint afflictions. The nondental sources of pain often are more chronic in nature; acute exacerbation may lead the patient to seek emergency care, but definitive diagnosis and treatment is better deferred to the neurologist, oral and maxillofacial surgeon, or otorhinolaryngologist.

Treatment

Dental pain from caries, pulpitis, or pulpal necrosis requires referral to a dentist for definitive care; emergency treatment is confined to analgesic prescription. Codeine oxycodone or another of the synthetic narcotics in combination with aspirin or acetaminophen will usually be required. There is no evidence to suggest the use of antibiotics for these conditions. Emergency care by the dentist or endodontist may be appropriate.

When dental pain is accompanied by swelling or by the earlier signs of tooth mobility and sensitivity to percussion, initiation of antibiotic treatment is mandatory. The drug of choice is penicillin V, the usual dosage being 250 mg orally every 4 to 6 hours for 10 days. The alternative drug for patients allergic to penicillin is erythromycin in the same dosage. Tetracyclines, ampicillin, the cephalosporins, and other antibiotics have no place in the initial management of odontogenic infection, because the offending organisms are sensitive to penicillin in nearly all cases. A change in antibiotic is only mandated by subsequent sensitivity testing of cultured pathogens.

Treatment of acute pericoronitis associated with the erupting wisdom tooth is initiated with penicillin or erythromycin in the same dosage described above. Frequent mouth rinses with warm saline and the extraoral application of warm compresses will help to provide symptomatic relief.

Evaluation by an oral and maxillofacial surgeon is critical for the patient with facial cellulitis to determine the need for incision and drainage, tooth extraction, or other early management. Patients with toxic systemic symptoms or with massive swelling involving the airway may require hospital admission for parenteral antibiotic therapy and definitive care.

DENTOALVEOLAR TRAUMA

Fractured and Avulsed Teeth

The etiology of fractured teeth is similar to the causes of jaw fractures. (See Chapter 69.) They include injuries sustained in motor vehicle accidents, contact sports, and altercations. These minor injuries frequently may be accompanied by more severe problems, but, commonly, they are seen as isolated injuries or as trauma concomitant with such minor wounds as lip and chin lacerations. Hence, triage personnel must be familiar with the appropriate diagnosis and early management of such dental injuries.

Pathophysiology

The anterior teeth are most often those that are fractured or avulsed. The anatomic form of these teeth is a significant factor in their susceptibility, although their exposed location is obviously most important.

Whenever trauma to the anterior mouth is recognized, careful examination of the patient to rule out fractures of the mandibular condyles must be carried out. The condyles are most often fractured by a blow to the chin. Consequently, an innocent-appearing chin laceration or anterior chipped tooth may signify a much more serious injury, one that can become much more difficult to manage and treat successfully if it is not recognized at the earliest opportunity.

Diagnosis

Management of chipped teeth will depend on the amount of tooth structure that has been lost (Fig. 70–2). The simple enamel fracture is uncomfortable only to the extent that it presents a sharp or rough surface to the tongue and lip. Loss of enamel and dentin produces mild sensitivity to cold air and liquids. Exposure of the pulp of the tooth is exquisitely painful when the pulp is contacted by cold air or by the tongue or lip.

Teeth that have been loosened by trauma must be evaluated by dental radiographs to determine whether or not the mobility of the teeth is due to fractured roots or to partial avulsion of the tooth from the alveolar bone. Apparent mobility of the teeth is observed when an alveolar segment (teeth and their surrounding bone) is fractured. Complete avulsion of anterior teeth is also common; the preexisting status of the surrounding soft tissues and alveolar bone must be assessed in order to determine the feasibility of replanting the tooth.

Treatment

Minor fractures of enamel or dentin require no emergency treatment; routine dental restorative measures can be carried out to return the teeth to a comfortable and aesthetic condition.

A tooth fractured to the level of the pulp demands immediate attention in order to provide comfort to the patient. If the fracture is above the level of the alveolar bone, then immediate extirpation of the pulp and subsequent endodontic treatment can be carried out. However, if the fracture line extends below the level of the

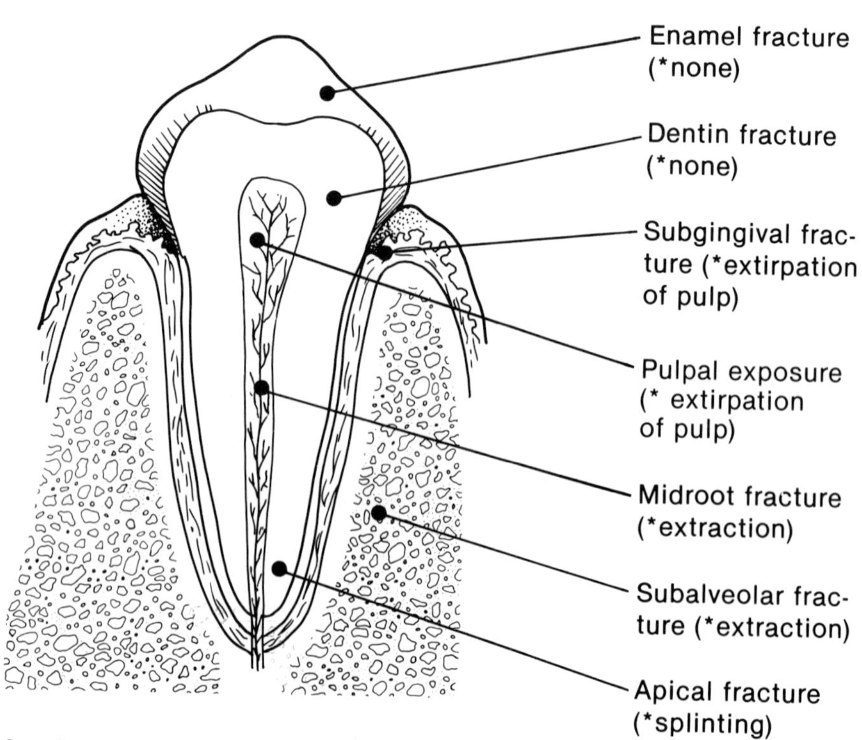

Figure 70–2   Tooth and Gum Anatomy. *Note:* * denotes recommended treatment.

alveolar bone, extraction of the tooth and its root is usually necessary.

Partially avulsed teeth may be repositioned with light finger pressure; local anesthesia may be necessary. Splinting of the teeth to adjacent teeth with wires, arch bars, or other suitable appliances should be carried out by the oral surgeon or dentist as an emergency procedure.

Replantation of completely avulsed teeth should always be attempted unless the condition of the surrounding bone and soft tissues or the patient's general condition makes such a procedure impossible. Prior to replantation, the tooth should be kept clean and moist. The best method of transport for the tooth is in the socket itself, if the patient can be instructed to do so prior to arrival in the emergency department. If the patient is unable to reposition the tooth, the tooth should be carried in the floor of the mouth; when the patient is uncooperative or otherwise unable to transport the tooth in this fashion, the tooth should be wrapped in clean, moistened gauze—it should neither be immersed nor allowed to dry. The oral surgeon should be consulted for definitive replanting and splinting of the tooth.

Fractured primary teeth can be treated in the same fashion described above for permanent teeth. Avulsed deciduous teeth are never replanted; when they are partially avulsed, they will usually require extraction.

Alveolar segment fractures are managed by wiring the teeth in the fractured segment to adjacent stable teeth.

TEMPOROMANDIBULAR JOINT (TMJ) DISLOCATION

Acute emergency conditions relating to the temporomandibular joint are confined to fractures, post-traumatic joint effusion, and dislocations. Fractures of the mandibular condyle have been previously discussed. Joint effusions in the absence of fracture are easily managed with warm compresses and analgesic and anti-inflammatory agents.

Pathophysiology of Dislocation

Dislocation of one or both temporomandibular joints is the result of displacement of the condylar process of the mandible anterior to the articular eminence of the temporal bone. The usual inciting event is a blow received while the mouth is open. Secondary muscle spasm prevents the mandible from returning to its normal position with the condyle in the glenoid fossa posterior to the articular eminence.

Diagnosis

The patient with a dislocated mandible presents with an open mouth that cannot be closed voluntarily; if the dislocation is unilateral, the jaw will be deviated to the opposite side. Because of the inability to close the mouth, the patient may be unable to swallow and, consequently, the common presentation will include drooling of saliva. Pain is a variable symptom with dislocation; in the presence of muscle spasm, pain and tenderness in the masseter muscle will be significant. The dislocated condyle can be palpated as a lateral prominence 1 or 2 cm anterior to the tragus of the ear.

Differential Diagnosis

Extrapyramidal reaction to a wide variety of drugs can produce symptoms similar to those of jaw dislocation. Phenothiazine tranquilizing agents, antihistamines, and antiemetic medications have all been implicated. The clinical signs of dislocation are absent in this instance. An intravenous dose of 50 mg diphenhydramine (Benadryl) produces dramatic resolution of the symptoms.

Acute episodes of the so-called TMJ syndrome are distinguished from dislocation by the inability of the patient to open the mouth in the former condition. Reassurance, analgesics, and referral to an oral surgeon are the only acute measures appropriate for the emergency management of the TMJ syndrome.

Treatment

Manual reduction of the dislocated mandible is most easily accomplished if it is attempted as soon as possible after the injury.

Relaxation of the patient is essential. In the presence of severe pain from muscle spasm, intramuscular administration of a narcotic (e.g., meperidine [Demerol], 50 mg) or diazepam (Valium) 10 mg, may be necessary to diminish the spasm and allow repositioning of the mandible. A good alternative to parenteral medication is the spraying of ethyl chloride on the skin over the masseter muscle; if the dislocation is not longstanding, this simple measure will often suffice.

The patient should be seated in a simple straight-backed chair placed against a wall so that the patient may brace the back of the head against the wall and so that the person doing the procedure can be directly in front of the patient. Reduction is accomplished by placing an index finger in the buccal sulcus just lateral to the posterior teeth on each side; the fingers should never be placed over the teeth themselves. At the same time, the thumbs are placed extraorally beneath the chin.

With the patient applying countertraction against the wall, steady, firm pressure in a downward and forward direction is applied with the thumbs and index fingers. Once sufficient pressure has been exerted to bring the condyle free of the articular eminence, muscular forces will provide the posterior motion necessary to return the condyle to the glenoid fossa. The patient must then be instructed to keep the teeth together while the muscular spasm subsides.

In instances of prolonged dislocation, attempts at simple reduction can only be accomplished with the use of general anesthesia and muscle relaxants.

Following reduction of the dislocation, the patient must limit jaw activity for several days; wide mouth opening and heavy chewing must be avoided. Aspirin or ibuprofen, 300 to 600 mg orally every 4 hours, are recommended for their analgesic and anti-inflammatory effects. Patients with chronic or habitual jaw dislocations should be referred to an oral and maxillofacial surgeon for further evaluation.

POSTEXTRACTION BLEEDING

Bleeding following the extraction of teeth is usually effectively managed by firm pressure with gauze sponges over the socket. However, rebleeding several hours after the procedure may bring the patient to the emergency department.

Pathophysiology

Postextraction bleeding may result either from local, surgical factors or from systemic coagulopathies. Following the removal of a tooth, the socket fills with blood and forms a clot by the familiar mechanisms; the adjacent soft tissues are compressed tightly against the alveolar bone and bleeding stops. Inadequacy of the clot or poor adaptation of the gingival tissues results in prolonged bleeding.

Diagnosis

A succinct history of prior bleeding episodes, concomitant medical problems or symptoms, current or recent drug usage, and familial bleeding problems should be obtained at the outset to determine the possibility of a nonsurgical cause of the bleeding. Hemorrhage occurring several days after extraction is more suggestive of a circulating factor deficiency than is bleeding several hours after the procedure.

Examination of the patient's mouth requires adequate lighting and suction apparatus. Excess clot must be rubbed or suctioned away so that the socket area can be visualized; in fact, exuberant clot may itself be the cause of prolonged, minor bleeding. A search should be made for any laceration or unsutured incision in the soft tissue adjacent to the socket since these are the most common causes of delayed bleeding; the effects of the vasoconstrictor used with the local anesthetic at the time of extraction may mask the potential for bleeding from minor mucosal interruptions until several hours have passed.

Treatment

When a systemic cause of bleeding is suspected, appropriate blood studies should be ordered to determine the number and function of platelets and the integrity of the coagulation cascade.

Removal of excessive coagulum and the application of firm pressure over the site of bleeding are the initial therapeutic steps to be taken. When mucosal apposition to the bone is inadequate or when lacerations can be identified, the placement of sutures (3-0 catgut or silk) will be necessary. The placement of gelatin sponge (Gelfoam) into the socket is occasionally useful in conjunction with suturing; topical thrombin powder, silver nitrate sticks, and other topical hemostatic agents are rarely of any value.

If medical causes of bleeding are diagnosed, subsequent care as an inpatient or on an ambulatory basis can be determined. When the bleeding has been controlled, patients should be instructed to bite firmly on gauze for 20 to 30 minutes, after which the socket is best left untouched. Any food or drink may be taken, but care should be exercised in order to protect the newly formed clot. For the same reason, mouth rinsing and gargling should be avoided for the following 24 hours. Analgesics containing aspirin should not be prescribed if there is any suggestion of a systemic etiology of the bleeding. Sutures are usually removed after 7 days.

MUCOSAL ULCERATIONS

Single or multiple erosive lesions of the oral mucosa are usually painful enough for the patient to seek emergency assistance. The more common acute ulcerative conditions of the mouth include aphthous ulcers, herpetic ulcers, Vincent's infection ("trench mouth"), and traumatic ulcerations beneath dental prostheses. Less commonly, erosive lesions of pemphigus, pemphigoid, lupus erythematosus, or lichen planus may be seen. The ulcers associated with oral syphilis or carcinoma are not usually painful; as a result, these diagnoses are rarely made in the emergency department.

Pathophysiology

Aphthous ulcers, which are acutely painful, shallow, well-demarcated lesions of the mucosa of the lip, cheek, or floor of the mouth, have no specifically proved cause. It is currently thought that the lesion results from an immune response to a streptococcal antigen. The condition frequently is associated with periods of emotional stress; young adults are most often afflicted.

Primary herpetic infection, common in the pediatric age-group, produces large clusters of ulcers throughout the mouth, in contrast to the solitary aphthous ulcers. Herpes zoster of the oral cavity results in ulcers along a sharply demarcated area that follows a division of the trigeminal nerve, just as the same infection in other parts of the body follows a dermatome distribution.

Vincent's infection is of bacterial origin and affects the gingival tissues. The gingival papillae between teeth are ulcerated and the adjacent gingiva is friable with a gray membranous coating; a foul smell accompanies the condition. Young adults are the usual victims.

Denture sores or traumatic ulcers associated with sharp or broken teeth can usually be identified by direct examination. Carcinoma must be included in the differential diagnosis of the apparently traumatic ulcer.

Treatment

No specific therapy can be offered for aphthous or herpetic ulcerations. Topical anesthetics in liquid or gel form can be used in order to allow the patient to have adequate nutrition. Orabase and Benzodent, which contain benzocaine, offer longer-lasting relief because of their mucosal-adhering properties and can be recommended for symptomatic relief. Creams and ointments containing corticosteroids offer few advantages and are contraindicated if herpetic infection is suspected.

Penicillin, 250 mg orally every 6 hours for 10 days, is the treatment of choice for acute Vincent's infection. Mouth rinses with dilute hydrogen peroxide often improve symptoms and are most effective in eliminating the accumulated gingival debris.

Removal of an irritating dental prosthesis is the only emergency treatment for the painful traumatic ulcer. Referral to a dentist or oral surgeon is required for correction of the inciting cause or for biopsy of the ulcer.

BIBLIOGRAPHY

Chow AW, Roser SM, Brady FA: Orofacial odontogenic infections. *Ann Intern Med* 88:392, 1978.

Guralnick WC, Donoff RB: Oral surgical disorders, in Wilkins EW (ed): *MGH Textbook of Emergency Medicine*. Baltimore, Williams & Wilkins, 1978, pp 550–558.

Kelly JP: Evaluation of facial pain and swelling, in Goroll AH, May LA, Mullae AG (eds): *Primary Care Medicine*. Philadelphia, JB Lippincott, 1981, pp 758–762.

Practical Applications of Emergency Care

The "Atlas of Common Emergency Department Procedures" (Chapter 71) was designed as a quick, clear, and accurate atlas of the procedures commonly performed by emergency care personnel. It contains a brief description of each procedure; the reader is referred to the previous chapters for a further description of the indications and alternative techniques. An extensive bibliography is provided following each procedure should more detailed discussions of the procedures be desired.

Equally useful is the "Emergency Drug Index" (Chapter 72) in which two registered pharmacists have succinctly summarized each of the pharmacologic agents and drugs mentioned throughout this text. For the reader's convenience, they are categorized according to their uses, but the reader is referred to the detailed explanations throughout the text for additional information on the clinical indications, complications, and alternative approaches to therapy.

71. Atlas of Emergency Procedures

THOMAS CLARKE KRAVIS, M.D.

1. SUBCLAVIAN VEIN CANNULATION

Indications

A. Determine and monitor central venous pressure.
B. Establish route for intravenous therapeutic agents, cardiac pacemaker, or Swan-Ganz catheter.
C. Determine the presence of pericardial tamponade, left ventricular heart failure, and shock.

Procedure

(Fig. 1.1) Place the patient in a supine, head-down 15° Trendelenburg position. Turn the head 90° to the opposite side of the procedure. Support the shoulders. Prepare and drape in usual sterile manner.

> *Note: In patients with penetrating wounds of the chest, the side of the injury should be used for the insertion of a central venous line.*

Identify the anatomical landmarks: the subclavian vein is anterior to the scalene muscle and courses over the first rib, anterior and inferior to the subclavian artery; it joins the internal jugular vein to form the innominate vein.

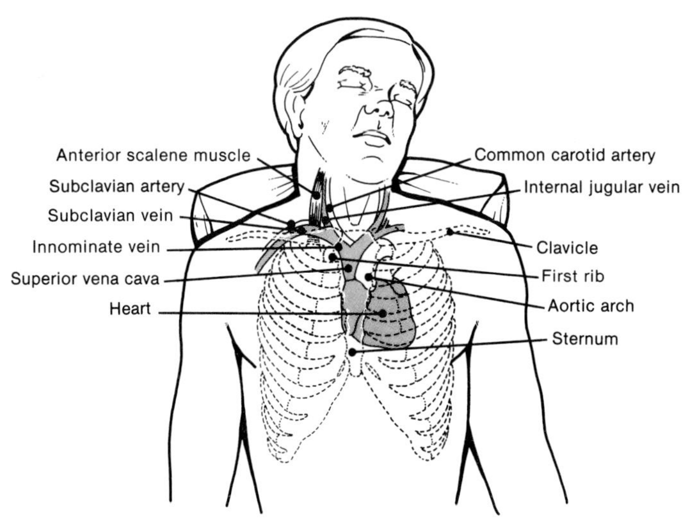

Figure 1.1 Anatomy.

(Fig. 1.2) Infiltrate 0.5 to 1 percent Xylocaine anesthetic one fingerbreadth (2 to 3 cm) below the inferior border of the midpoint of the clavicle. Allow the needle to pass underneath the clavicle.

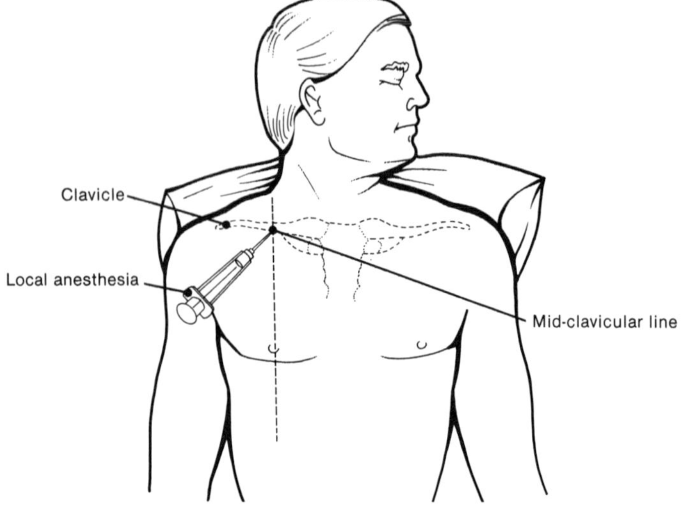

(Fig. 1.3) Attach a sterile 5- to 10-ml syringe filled with sterile saline to the angiocath or cannulation needle being introduced. Insert the needle into the anesthetized puncture site with the bevel of the needle upward; advance the needle toward the suprasternal notch parallel to the line of the lateral one-half of the clavicle, maintaining gentle negative pressure on the syringe. After the needle passes the first rib, gently aspirate.

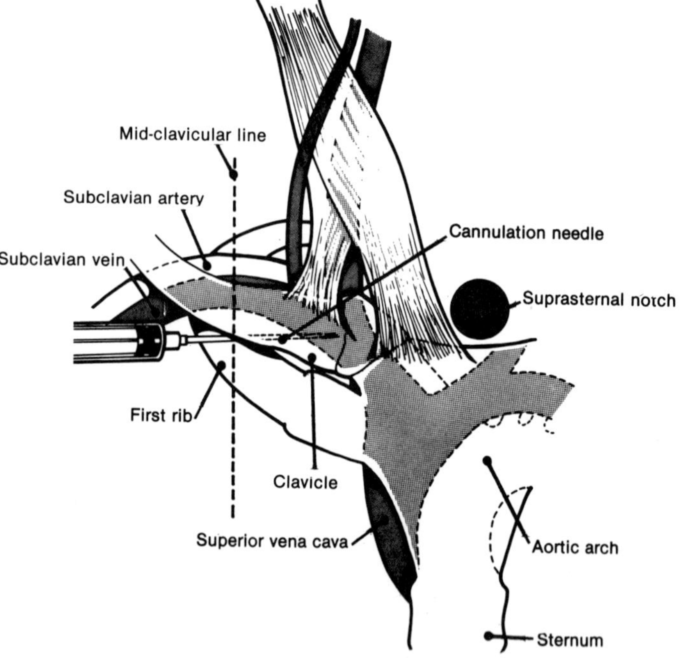

Figure 1.3   Cannulation needle entering subclavian vein.

(Fig. 1.4) After venous blood can be aspirated freely through the needle, rotate the bevel of the needle clockwise 90° and caudad; remove the syringe and slide the catheter through the needle into the subclavian vein. (If a plastic angiocath is being utilized, remove the needle, keeping the tip of the plastic catheter in the subclavian vein, introduce a flexible straight or J-tipped guide wire through the needle, and gently manipulate the guide wire into the subclavian vein. Advance the plastic catheter over the guide wire; remove the guide wire; reaspirate to confirm presence of free venous blood.)

Note: When the syringe is removed from the needle, instruct the patient to take and hold a deep breath; at the same time, cover the opening of the needle with a sterile-gloved finger to decrease the likelihood of air embolism. If the patient is on a mechanical ventilator, remove the syringe during inspiration. Raise the needle bevel in the anterior caudal position during cannulation. Rotate the patient's head to the ipsilateral side during cannulation, and rotate the needle 360°.

(Fig. 1.5) Aspirate free venous blood and flush the cannula with normal saline; attach the cannula to the intravenous line.

(Fig. 1.6) Secure the needle and tubing to the skin with a single suture—without compressing the catheter lumen—and apply a sterile dressing over the site, using povidone-iodine ointment at the puncture site. Tape the sterile dressing securely to the skin. Return the patient to a supine or head-up position, and obtain a chest roentgenogram to confirm that the tip of the cannula is located in the lower end of the superior vena cava, outside of the right atrium, and at the level of the interspace between the seventh and eighth thoracic vertebrae (i.e., 5 cm below the manubrial-sternal junction). Observe for the presence of complications of the procedure, e.g., hemothorax, pneumothorax, hematoma, hydrothorax, hydromediastinum, air embolism, subclavian vein thrombosis, catheter embolism, myocardial puncture, or cardiac tamponade.

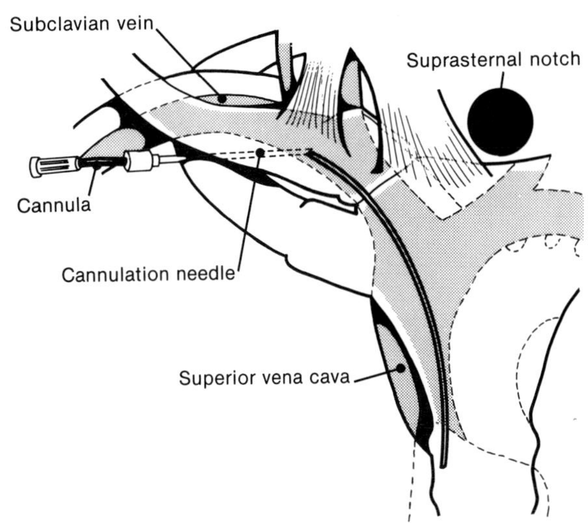

Figure 1.4   Cannula entering cannulation needle into subclavian vein.

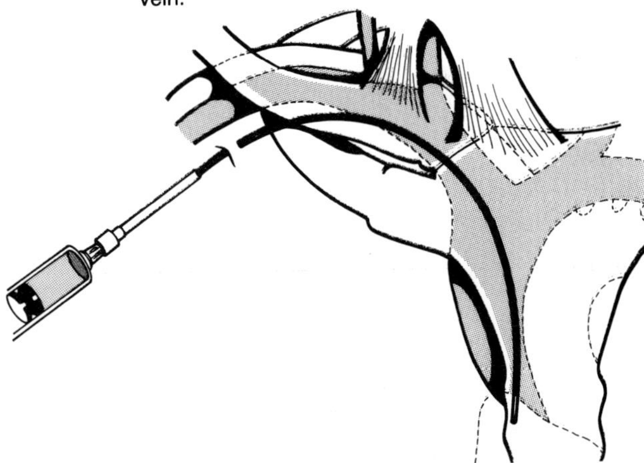

Figure 1.5   Flushing of cannula with saline.

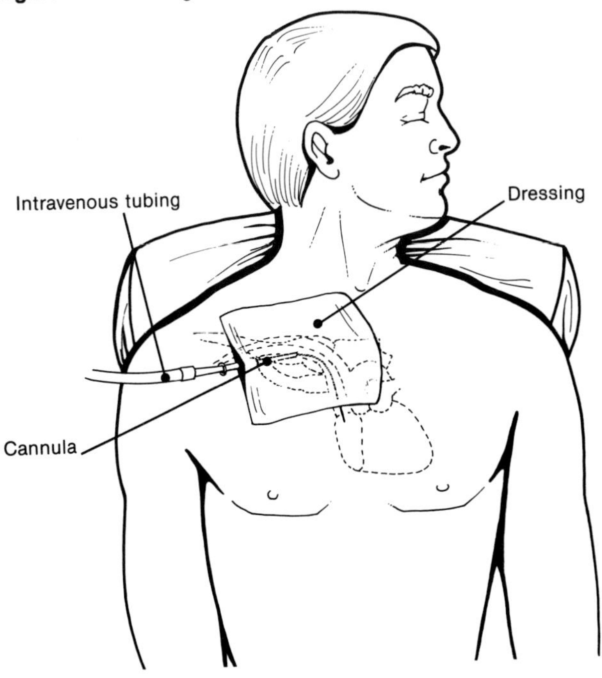

Figure 1.6   Dressing applied.

BIBLIOGRAPHY

Borja AR: Current status of infraclavicular subclavian vein catheterization. *Ann Thorac Surg* 13:615, 1972.

Borja AR, Hinshaw JR: A safe way to perform infraclavicular subclavian vein catheterization. *Surg Gynecol Obstet* 130:673, 1970.

Cosgriff JH: *An Atlas of Diagnostic and Therapeutic Procedures for Emergency Personnel*. Philadelphia, JB Lippincott Co, 1978.

Keeri-Szanto M: The subclavian vein, a constant and convenient intravenous injection site. *Arch Surg* 72:179, 1956.

McIntyre KM, Lewis AJ (eds): *Textbook of Advanced Cardiac Life Support*. Chicago, American Heart Association, 1981.

Vander Salm TJ, Cutler BS, Wheeler HB: *Atlas of Bedside Procedures*. Boston, Little Brown & Co, 1979.

Wilson JN, Grow JB, DeMong CV, et al: Central venous pressure in optimal blood volume to maintenance. *Arch Surg* 85:563, 1962.

2. INTERNAL JUGULAR VEIN CANNULATION

Indications

A. Determine and monitor central venous pressure.
B. Establish route for intravenous therapeutic agents, cardiac pacemaker, or Swan-Ganz catheter.
C. Determine the presence of pericardial tamponade, left ventricular heart failure, and shock.

Note: Cannulation of the internal jugular vein may be the method of choice to measure the central venous pressure because of the lower incidence of complications. If hematomas form, they are visible in the neck and compressible, and the procedure provides a direct route to the right atrium when a balloon-tipped flow-directed pulmonary catheter is inserted. The right internal jugular vein is usually chosen, since the right lung is lower than the left and this route does not endanger the thoracic duct. In penetrating wounds of the chest, the central venous catheter should be introduced on the same side as the penetrating injury. An alternative site may be indicated in suspected cervical spine injury.

Procedure

(Fig. 2.1) Place the patient in the supine, head-down 15° Trendelenburg position. Rotate the head 45° to the opposite side of the procedure.

Prepare and drape the patient in the usual sterile manner. Identify the anatomical landmarks: the internal jugular vein lies lateral to the carotid artery; the sternocleidomastoid muscle overlies the internal jugular vein in the lower half of the neck.

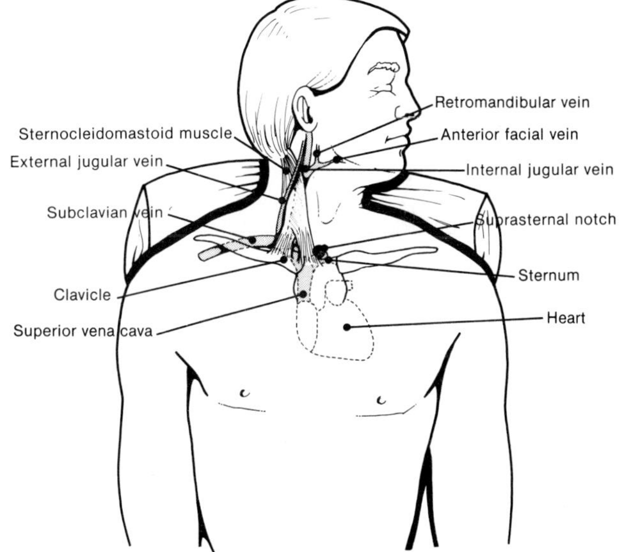

Figure 2.1 Anatomy.

(Fig. 2.2) Introduce 0.5 to 1 percent Xylocaine at a site under the posterior border of the sternocleidomastoid muscle 4 cm above the clavicle (i.e., two to three finger breadths), or just above the point at which the external jugular vein crosses the sternocleidomastoid muscle. Attach a 5- to 10-ml syringe filled with sterile saline to the angiocath or cannulation needle being introduced.

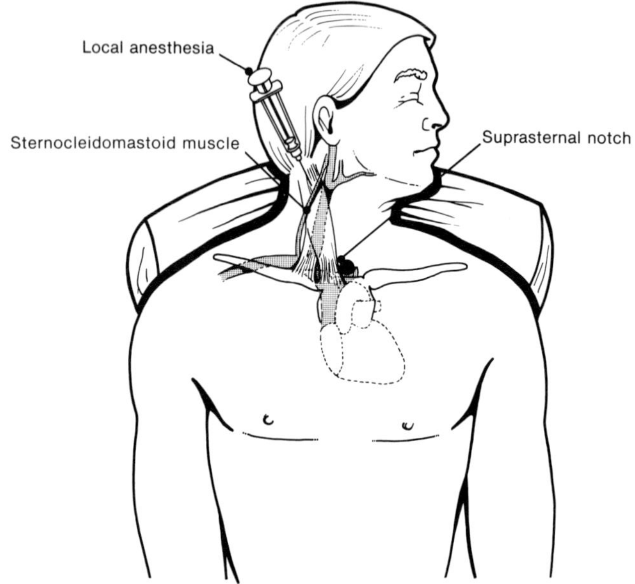

Figure 2.2 Local anesthesia.

(Fig. 2.3) Aim the needle caudally and ventrally toward the suprasternal notch underneath the sternocleidomastoid muscle at an angle that is 45° to the sagittal and horizontal planes and 15° forward in the frontal plane; advance and aspirate gently until there is free return of venous blood. Remove the syringe carefully. Have the patient take and hold a deep breath and at the same time cover the top of the needle with a gloved finger.

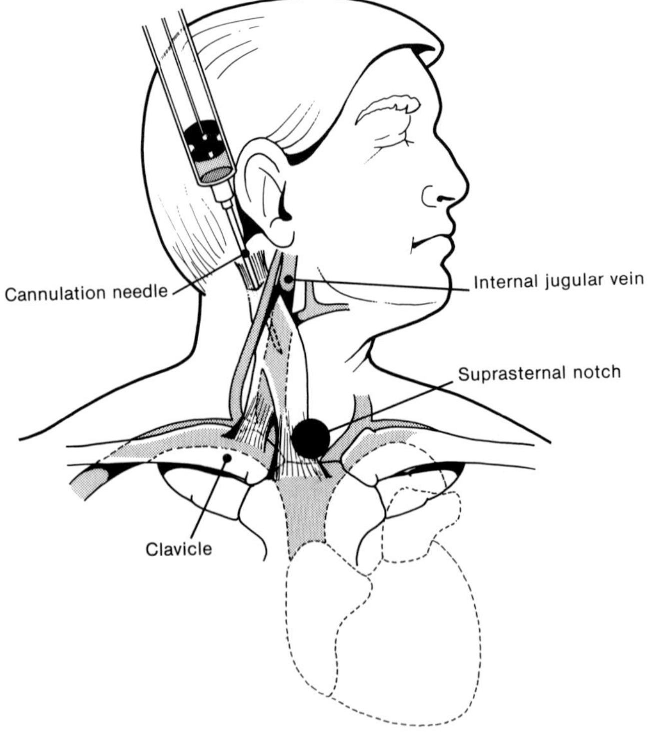

Figure 2.3 Cannulation needle entering internal jugular vein.

(Fig. 2.4) Then introduce the cannula into the needle. Insert the cannula through the needle into the internal jugular vein.

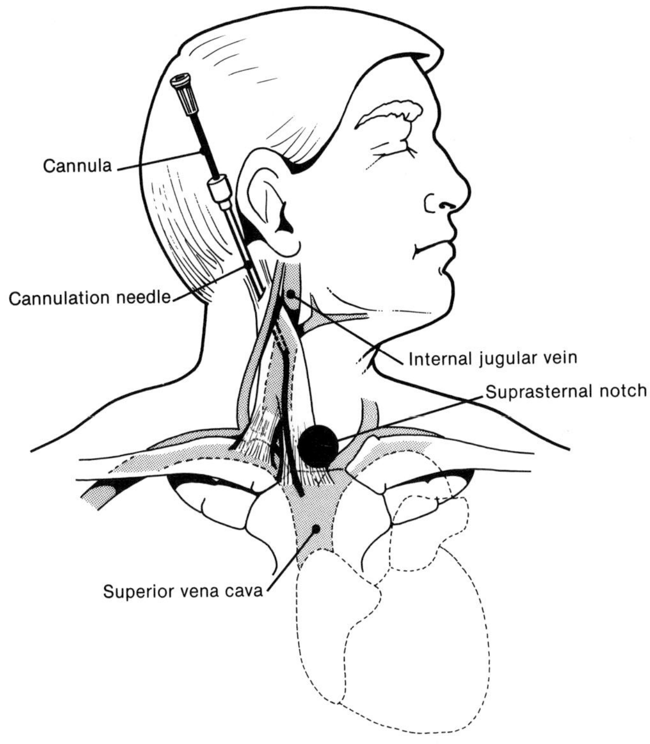

Figure 2.4 Cannula entering cannulation needle into internal jugular vein.

(Fig. 2.5) If a plastic angiocath is used, keep the tip of the catheter in the internal jugular vein and withdraw the needle.

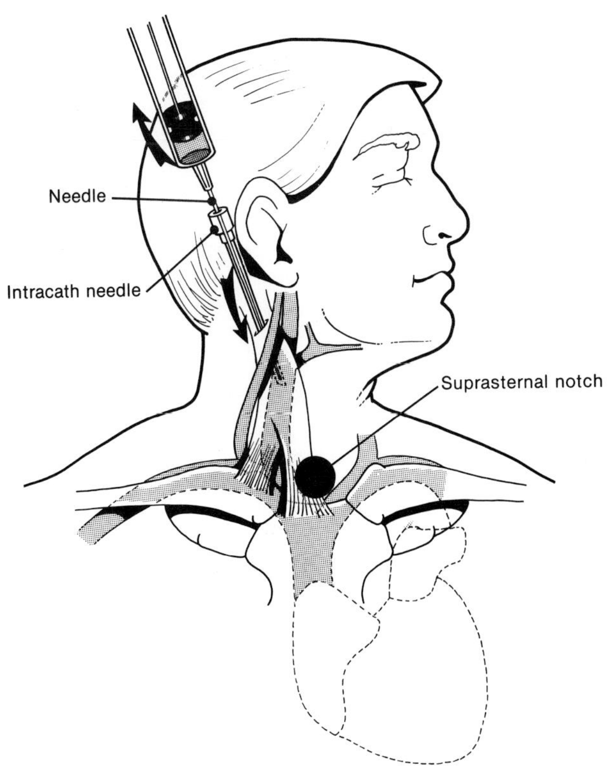

Figure 2.5 Alternate method.

(Fig. 2.6) Withdraw needle, aspirate to confirm flow of blood, and flush with saline; attach to intravenous line.

Suture, apply sterile dressing with povidone-iodine ointment, and secure with tape. Obtain chest roentgenogram to rule out complications and to establish position of the catheter in the superior vena cava (at the level of the seventh and eighth thoracic vertebrae).

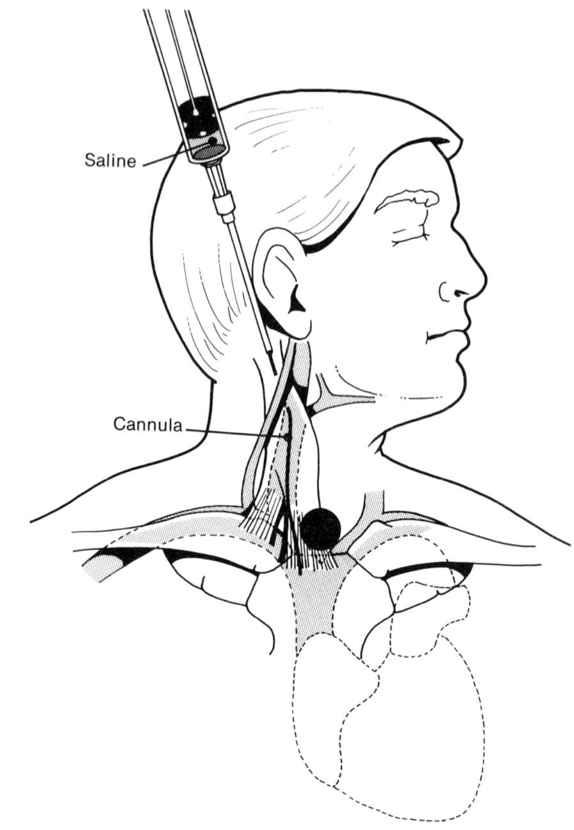

Figure 2.6 Flushing of cannula with saline.

(Fig. 2.7) *Note: In the supraclavicular or central technique of internal jugular vein cannulation, the needle is inserted in the apex of the triangle formed by the clavicle and the clavicular and sternal heads of the sternocleidomastoid muscle. The needle is advanced in a sagittal plane 30° posterior and caudad toward the ipsilateral nipple at a 50° angle with the frontal plane. Aspiration is performed until there is free return of venous blood.*

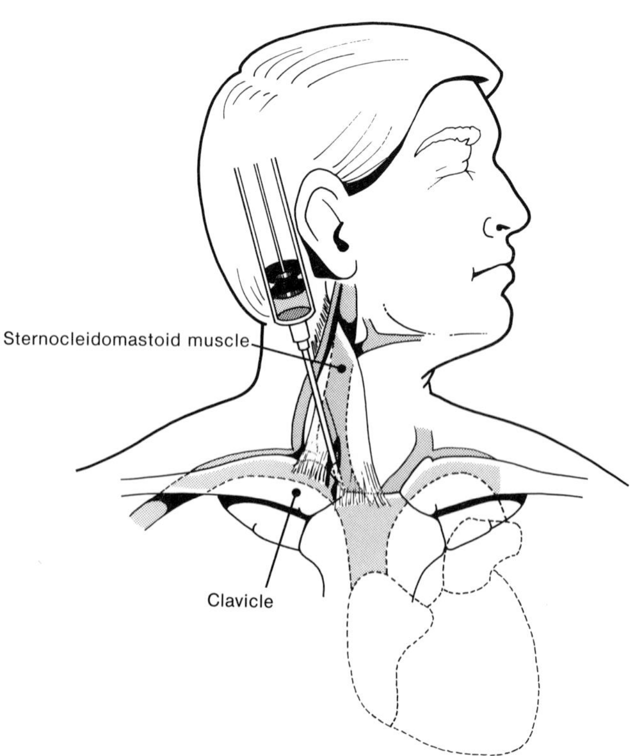

Figure 2.7 Supraclavicular technique.

BIBLIOGRAPHY

Civetta JM, Gabel JC, Gemer M: Internal jugular vein puncture with a margin of safety. *Anesthesiology* 36:622, 1972.

Cosgriff JH: *An Atlas of Diagnostic and Therapeutic Procedures for Emergency Personnel*. Philadelphia, JB Lippincott Co, 1978.

Daily PO, Griepp RB, Shumway NE: Percutaneous internal jugular vein cannulation. *Arch Surg* 101:534, 1970.

Jernigan WR, et al: Use of the internal jugular vein for placement of central venous catheter. *Surg Gynecol Obstet* 130:520, 1970.

McIntyre KM, Lewis AJ (eds): *Textbook of Advanced Cardiac Life Support*. Chicago, American Heart Association, 1981.

Vander Salm TJ, Cutler BS, Wheeler HB: *Atlas of Bedside Procedures*. Boston, Little Brown & Co, 1979.

3. PULMONARY ARTERY (SWAN-GANZ) CATHETERIZATION

Indications

A. Assess right and left ventricular function (hypovolemic, cardiogenic, and neurogenic shock; pericardial tamponade; pulmonary edema; and pulmonary embolism).
B. Measure pulmonary artery, pulmonary capillary wedge, right and left atrial pressures.
C. Measure cardiac output.
D. Sample right atrial and pulmonary arterial blood.

Procedure

(Fig. 3.1) Use a Swan-Ganz catheter with flotation balloon; a thermistor hub for measuring cardiac output; a proximal lumen hub to measure right atrial central venous pressure; a distal lumen hub to measure pulmonary artery wedge pressure; and rings indicating 10-cm intervals.

Place the patient in the supine 10° to 20° Trendelenburg position. Insert the catheter into the internal jugular vein, using a #16 angiocath (see 2. Internal Jugular Vein Cannulation), or the subclavian, femoral, or medial basilic vein.

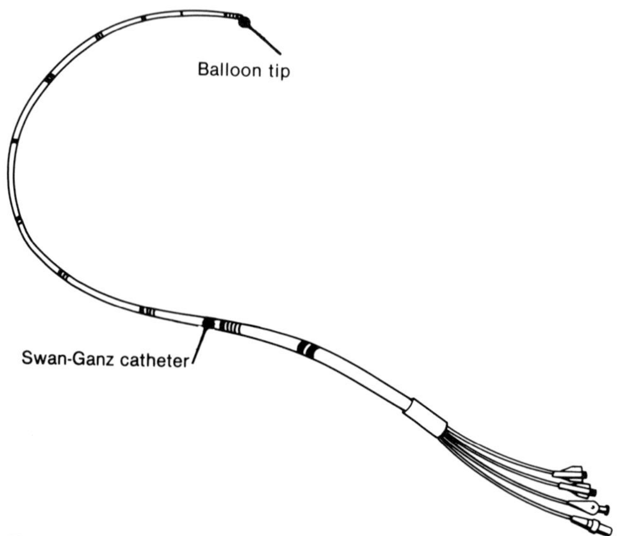

Figure 3.1   Swan-Ganz catheter.

(Fig. 3.2) Introduce a guide wire into the angiocath.

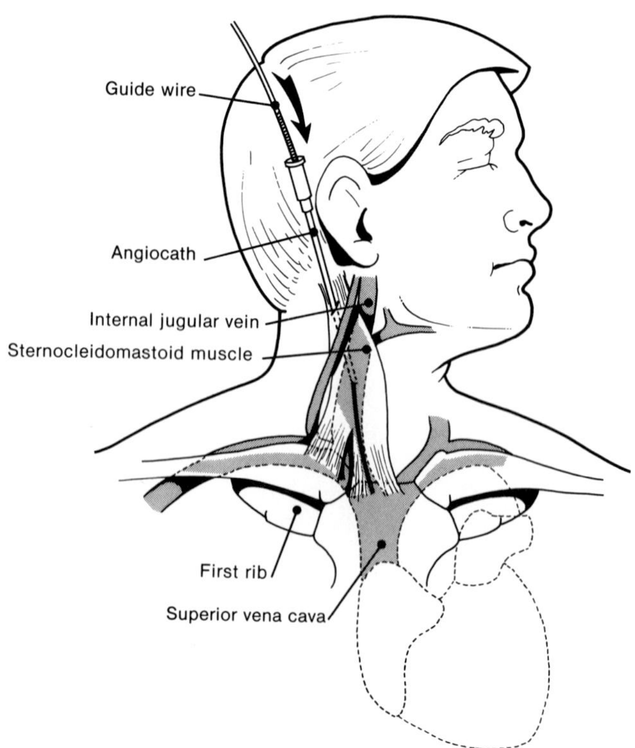

Figure 3.2   Guide wire slides through angiocath.

(Fig. 3.3, Fig. 3.4) Remove the angiocath and replace with an introducer and sleeve. Remove the guide wire. Remove the introducer and leave the sleeve in place. A sterile gloved thumb is placed over the end of the catheter to prevent air embolism and bleeding.

Slide the pulmonary artery catheter through the introducer sleeve.

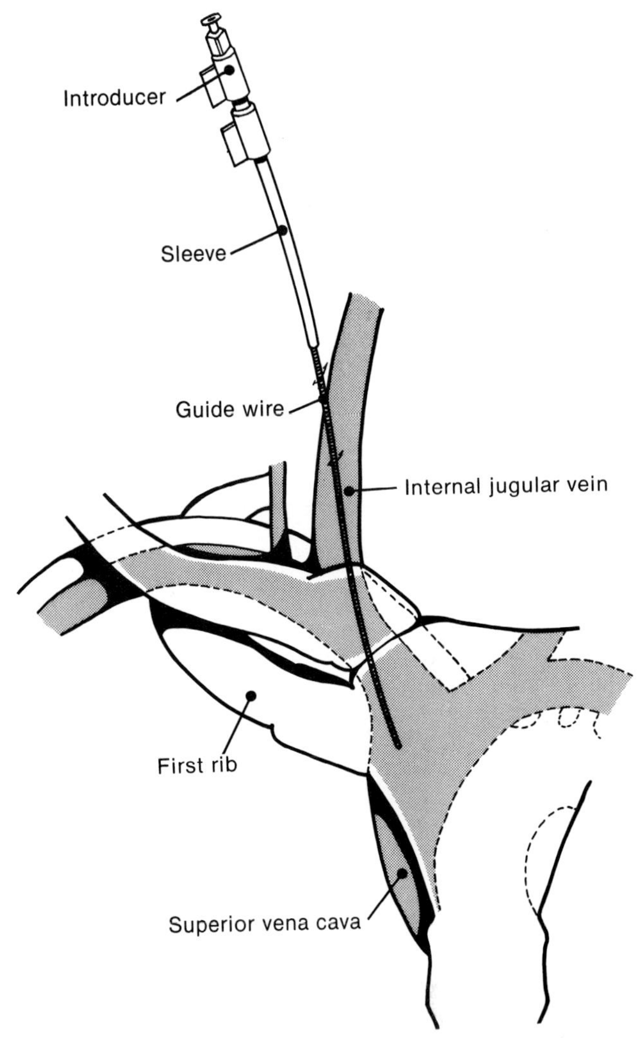

Figure 3.3 Introducer and sleeve replaces angiocath.

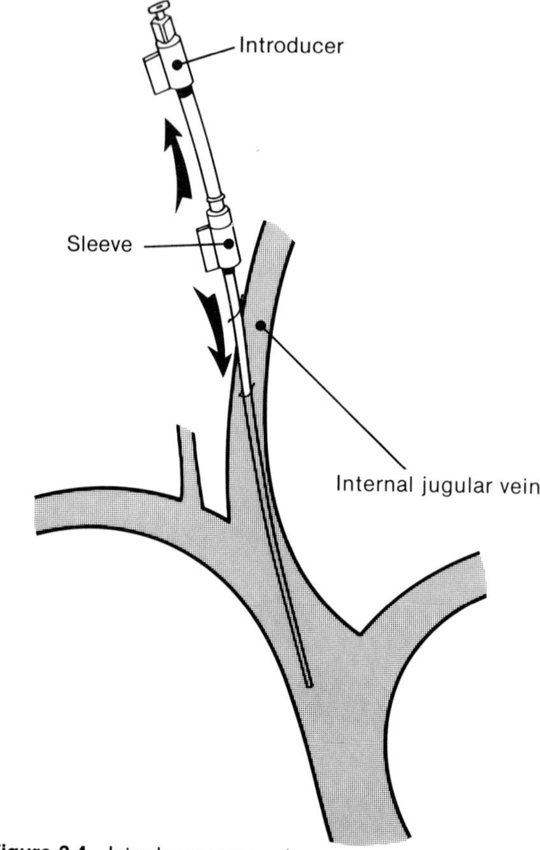

Figure 3.4   Introducer removed.

(Fig. 3.5) Advance the catheter centrally 10 to 15 cm into the right atrium. Advance the catheter into the right ventricle.

Attach a three-way stop-cock to the tube and flush it with heparinized saline. Note fluctuations on the monitor with the changes in respiration, which indicate the intrathoracic location of the catheter.

Inflate balloon to its full volume (1.25 to 1.50 ml). Observe the characteristic pressure changes. Advance the balloon into the pulmonary artery until the artery is occluded.

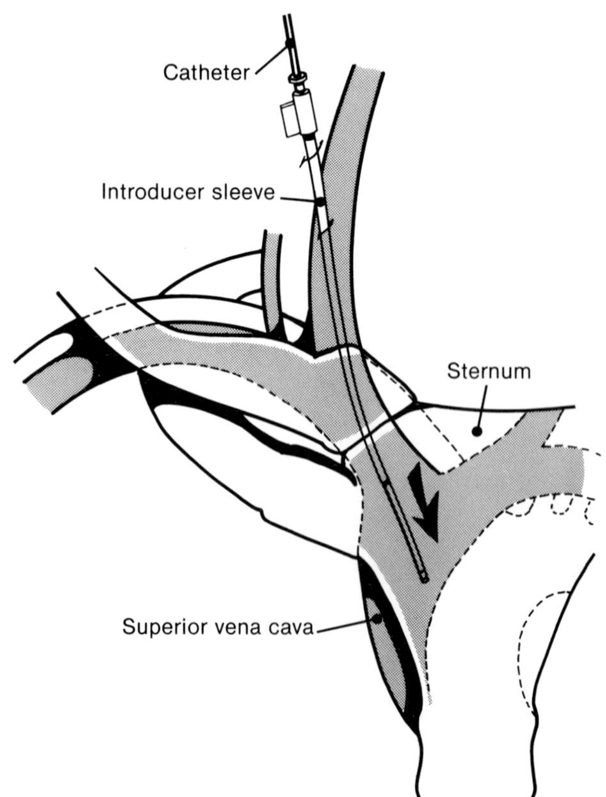

Figure 3.5   PA catheter slides through introducer sleeve.

(Fig. 3.6) Confirm that the tip of the catheter is in the pulmonary artery by the characteristic pressure wave on tracing and a chest roentgenogram. Secure catheter with suture. Commence heparin-saline flush. Apply dressing. Watch for complications of the procedure, such as pneumothorax, thrombosis of veins, pulmonary hemorrhage, cardiac dysrhythmias, endocarditis, fracture of the catheter, and balloon rupture.

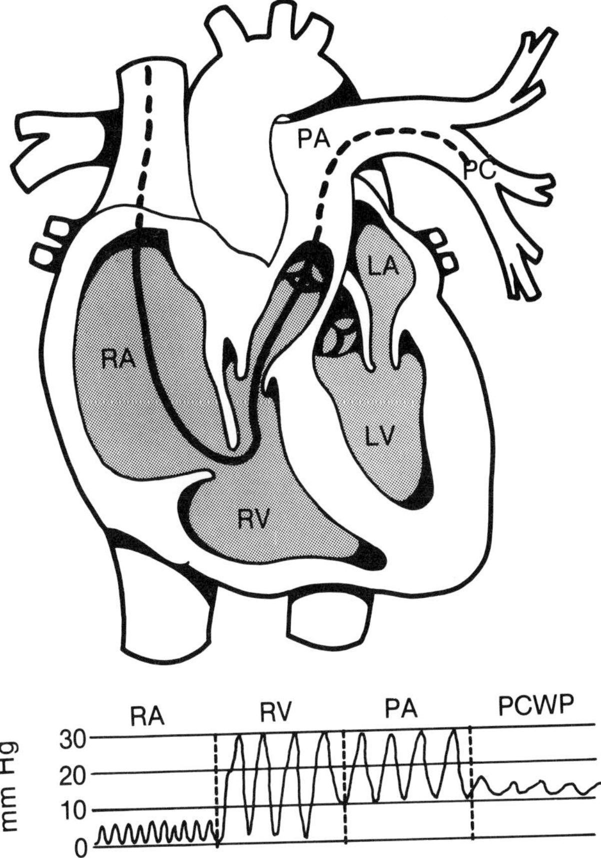

Figure 3.6   Catheter advanced to heart/sequential pressure tracings.

BIBLIOGRAPHY

Anderson WP, Dunegan JF, Knight DC, et al: Rapid estimation of pulmonary extravascular water with an instream catheter. *J Appl. Physiol* 39:843, 1975.

Fitzpatrick GF, Hampson LG, Burgess JH: Bedside determination of left atrial pressure. *Can Med Assoc J* 106:1293, 1972.

Foote GA, Schabel SI, Hodges M: Pulmonary complications of the flow-directed balloon-tipped catheter. *N Engl J Med* 290:927, 1974.

McIntyre KM, Lewis AJ (eds): *Textbook of Advanced Life Support.* Chicago, American Heart Association, 1981.

Swan HJC, Ganz W: Use of balloon flotation catheters in critically ill patients. *Surg Clin North Am* 55:501, 1975.

Swan HJC, Ganz W, Forrester J, et al: Catheterization of the heart in man with use of a flow-directed balloon-tipped catheter. *N Engl J Med* 283:447, 1970.

Vander Salm TJ, Cutler BS, Wheeler HB: *Atlas of Bedside Procedures.* Boston, Little Brown & Co, 1979.

4. TEMPORARY TRANSVENOUS PACEMAKER PLACEMENT

Indications

A. Identify hemodynamically compromising arrhythmias without adequate escape mechanism.
   1. Sinus node dysfunction
   2. Supraventricular bradycardia
   3. Disturbance of atrioventricular conduction
B. Prevent arrhythmias in association with acute myocardial infarction.
   1. Symptomatic bradycardia, sinoatrial block, and sick sinus syndrome
   2. Drug-resistant tachyarrhythmias
   3. Right bundle branch block with either left anterior fascicular block or left posterior fascicular block
   4. Acute onset of Mobitz II second-degree arterioventricular block with anterior myocardial infarction
   5. Alternating bundle branch block
C. Treat ventricular asystole.
D. Correct malfunction of implanted pacemaker.

Procedure

Fluoroscopic Control of Insertion

(Fig. 4.1) Use bipolar semifloating pacing catheter.

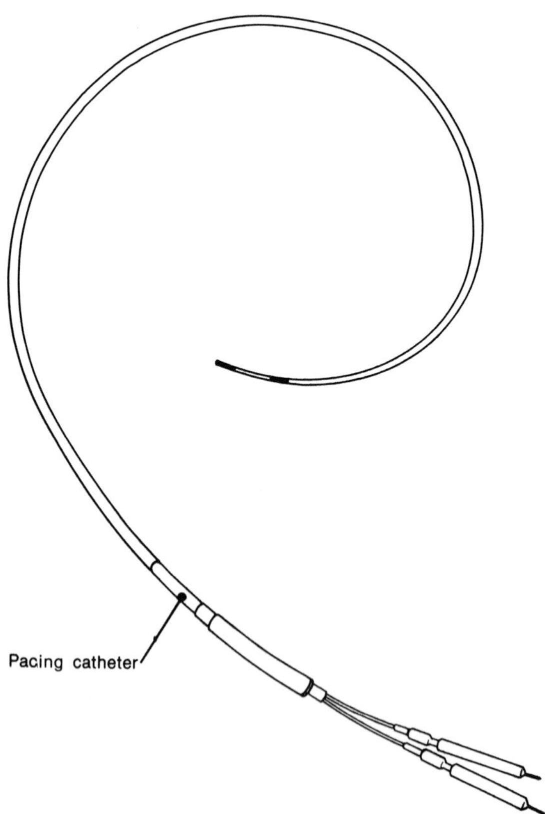

Figure 4.1 Pacing catheter.

(Fig. 4.2) Place the patient in the position for subclavian or internal jugular vein cannulation, and cannulate as previously described. Monitor electrocardiogram (ECG).

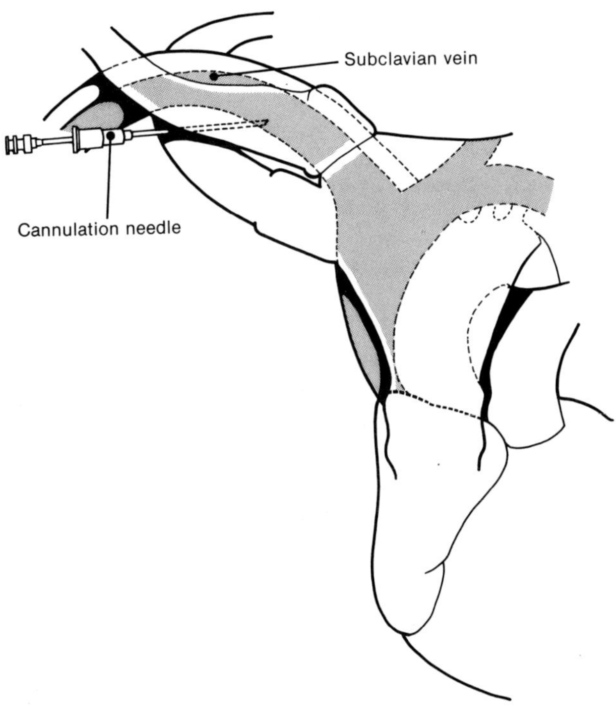

Figure 4.2   Cannulate superior vena cava.

(Fig. 4.3) Insert the catheter under fluoroscopic control. Introduce the catheter through the superior vena cava into the right atrium with the catheter tip against the lateral wall (Fig. 4.3, *A*). Advance the catheter across the tricuspid valve (Fig. 4.3, *B*). Float the catheter into the pulmonary artery, and withdraw to confirm its position in the right ventricle. Advance the catheter tip into the trabeculae of the right ventricle and confirm by fluoroscopy (Fig. 4.3, *C*).

ECG Control of Insertion

If the electrocatheter is to be introduced under ECG control, attach the pacing catheter to the V lead of a grounded ECG machine, and observe the P wave and QRS configuration during catheter introduction: when the catheter enters the right atrium, two large complexes are observed; as the catheter is advanced across the tricuspid valve into the right ventricle, the amplitude of the P wave decreases and a large amplitude QRS complex appears.

Blind Insertion

When fluoroscopic or ECG control is not possible, introduce a temporary transvenous pacemaker by the "blind" approach. Introduce the electrocatheter into the superior vena cava, attach it to the external pacemaker generator, and adjust it to a pacing rate of 70/minute at the highest output. Advance the catheter until ventricular pacing is observed.

Note: The electrical thresholds for pacing and sensing are determined immediately after the pacing catheter is positioned. For optimal temporary pacing, the threshold should be below one milliamp; for continuous maintenance pacing, the output should be 5 milliamps. Alternatively, the generator output can be increased until a pacing spike is immediately followed by a widened QRS complex. A 12-lead ECG with an operative pacemaker will display an ECG pattern suggestive of a left bundle branch block pattern.

Combined Pulmonary Artery Pressure Monitoring and Temporary Pacing

It is possible to combine pulmonary artery pressure monitoring and temporary pacing with a special Swan-Ganz catheter. After floating the catheter into the wedge position with the electrodes in the atrium and ventricle, choose the best threshold available. This technique allows AV sequential pacing.

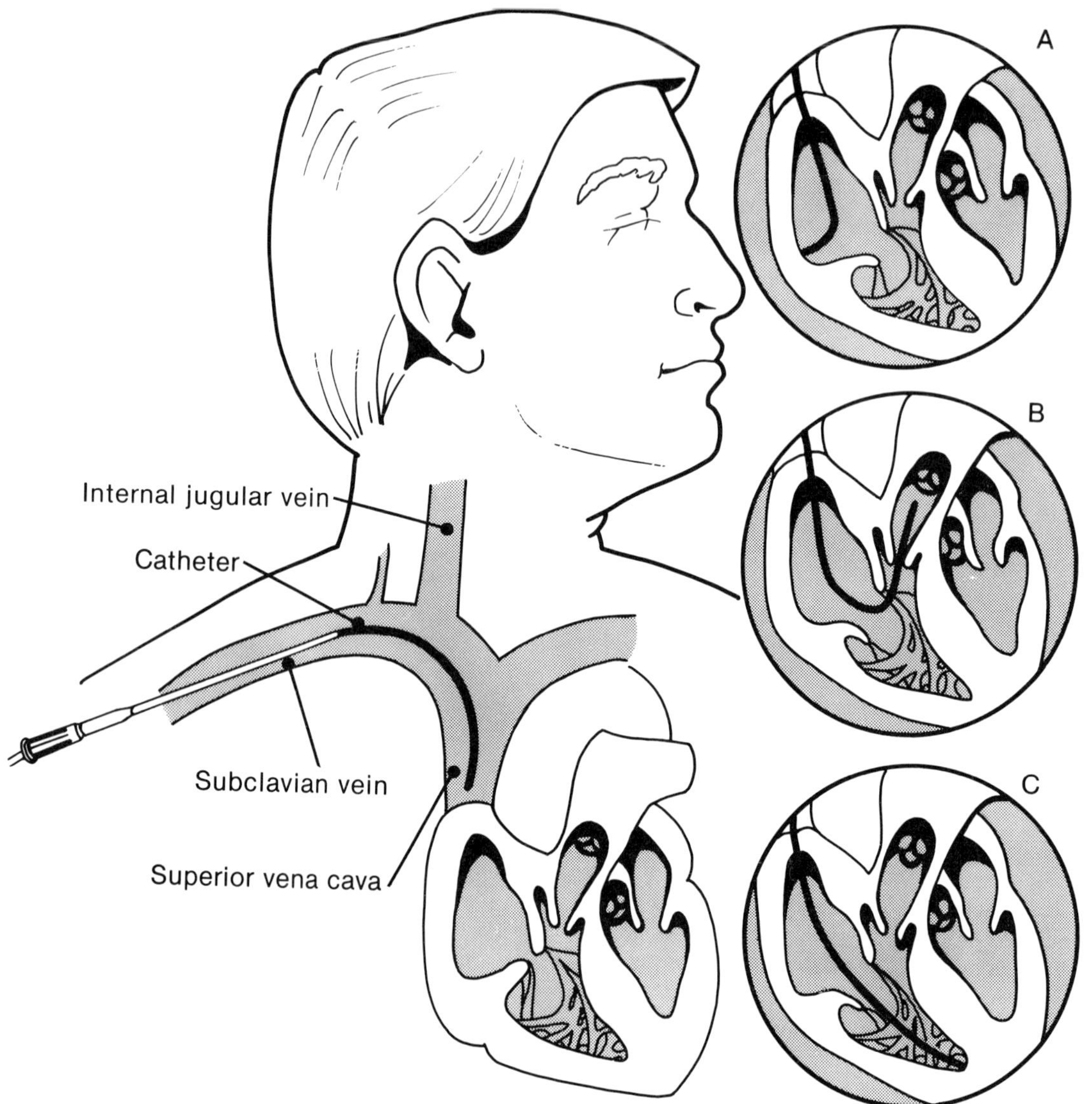

Figure 4.3 Insert electrode catheter.

BIBLIOGRAPHY

Atkins JM, Leshin SJ, Blomqvist G, et al: Ventricular conduction blocks and sudden death in acute myocardial infarction: Potential indications for pacing. *N Engl J Med* 288:281, 1973.

Castellanos A Jr, Zuckerman W, Berkovits BV: Cardiac pacemakers, in Harken DE (ed): *Cardiac Surgery* ed 2. Philadelphia, Davis, 1971.

Charduck WM: Cardiac pacemakers and heart block, in Sabiston DE, et al (eds): *Gibbon's Surgery of the Chest*, ed 3. Philadelphia, WB Saunders, 1976.

Cosgriff JH: *An Atlas of Diagnostic and Therapeutic Procedures for Emergency Personnel*. Philadelphia, JB Lippincott Co, 1978.

DeSantis RW: Short-term use of intravenous electrode in heart block. *JAMA* 184:544, 1963.

Furman S: Fundamentals of cardiac pacing. *Am Heart J* 73:261, 1967.

Furman S, Escher DJW: *Principles and Techniques of Cardiac Pacing*. New York, Harper & Row, 1970.

Furman S, Schwedel JB, Robinson G, Hurwit E: Use of an intracardiac pacemaker in the control of heart block. *Surgery* 49:98, 1961.

Lown B, Kosowsky BD: Artificial cardiac pacemakers I, II, III. *N Engl J Med* 283:907, 971, 1023, 1970.

McIntyre KM, Lewis AJ (eds): *Textbook of Advanced Cardiac Life Support*. Chicago, American Heart Association, 1981.

Parsonnet V, Zucker R, Gilbert L, Asa MM: An intracardiac bipolar electrode for interim treatment of complete heart block. *Am J Cardiol* 10:261, 1962.

Rubin I, Arbeit SR, Gross H: The electrocardiographic recognition of pacemaker function and failure. *Ann Intern Med* 71:603, 1969.

Schnedel JB, Escher DJW: Transvenous electrical stimulation of the heart. *Ann NY Acad Sci* 111:972, 1964.

Solomon N, Escher DJW: A rapid method for insertion of the pacemaker catheter electrode. *Am Heart J* 66:717, 1963.

Vander Salm TJ, Cutler BS, Wheeler HB: *Atlas of Bedside Procedures*. Boston, Little Brown & Co, 1979.

Weale FE: Cardiac resuscitation via jugular vein. *Lancet* 2:73, 1959

5. CULDOCENTESIS

Indication

Determine the presence of blood or inflammatory fluids in the cul-de-sac.

Procedure

Place the patient in the lithotomy position. Perform pelvic and rectovaginal examinations; insert the speculum; prepare the posterior vagina with povidone-iodine.

(Fig. 5.1) Gently grasp the posterior lip of the cervix with a tenaculum. Infiltrate 0.5 to 1 percent Xylocaine into the cervix in the midline posterior to the vaginal reflection.

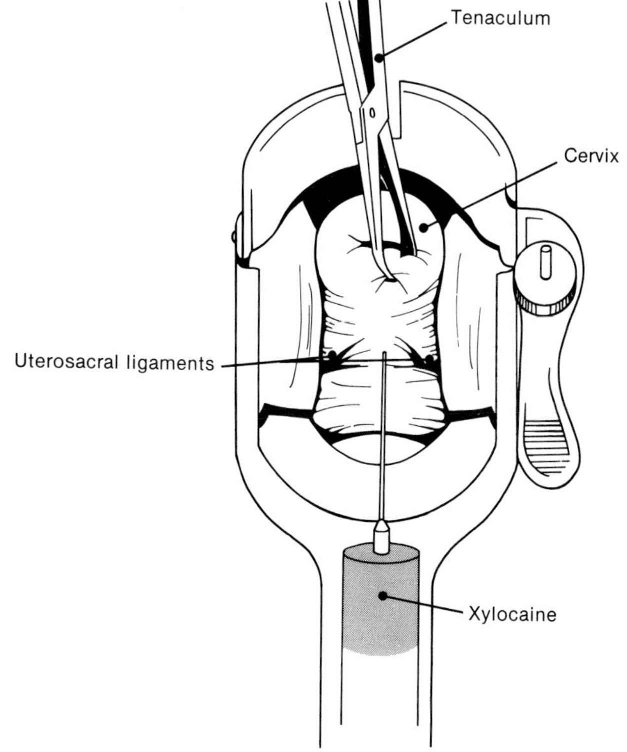

Figure 5.1 Culdocentesis needle inserted.

(Fig. 5.2) Insert an 18-gauge spinal needle attached to a glass syringe midline between the uterosacral ligaments and into the apex of the cul-de-sac. Keep the axis of the needle parallel to that of the uterus. Aspirate and place the contents into a glass tube. Examine the fluid: if nonclotting blood is obtained, the test is described as positive; if straw-colored peritoneal fluid is obtained, the test is described as negative. (If no fluid is obtained, the procedure may be repeated.)

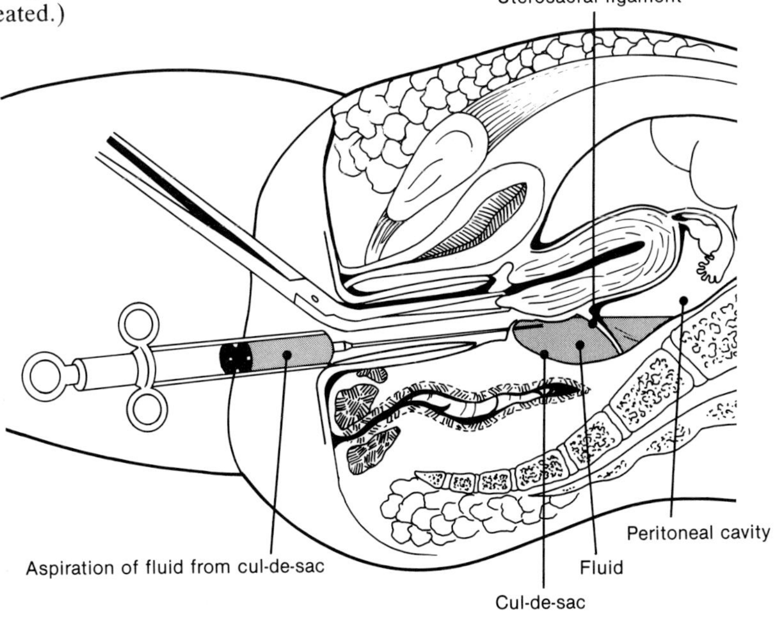

Figure 5.2 Aspirate cul-de-sac.

BIBLIOGRAPHY

Beacham DW, Beacham WD: Culdocentesis. *New Orleans Medical Surgical J* 103:283, 1951.

Cosgriff JH: *An Atlas of Diagnostic and Therapeutic Procedures for Emergency Personnel*. Philadelphia, JB Lippincott Co, 1978.

Decker A: *Culdoscopy*. Philadelphia, Davis, 1967.

Halpin TF: Ectopic pregnancy. *Am J Obstet Gynecol* 106:227, 1970.

Kelly HA: Treatment of ectopic pregnancy by vaginal puncture. *Johns Hopkins Hospital Bulletin* 7:209, 1896.

McGown L, Stein DB, Miller W: Cul-de-sac aspiration for diagnostic cytologic study. *Am J Obstet Gynecol* 96:413, 1966.

Vander Salm TJ, Cutler BS, Wheeler HB: *Atlas of Bedside Procedures*. Boston, Little Brown & Co, 1979.

6. PERITONEAL LAVAGE

Indication

Determine the presence of intraperitoneal bleeding or rupture of hollow viscus.

Procedure

(Fig. 6.1) After the patient has emptied the bladder, place the patient in the supine position. Prepare and drape the patient in the usual sterile manner. Infiltrate 0.5 to 1 percent Xylocaine with epinephrine 1:100,000 5 cm below the umbilicus in the midline from the skin to the peritoneum. Do not infiltrate into the peritoneum. Make a horizontal, 5-mm incision in the anesthetized area.

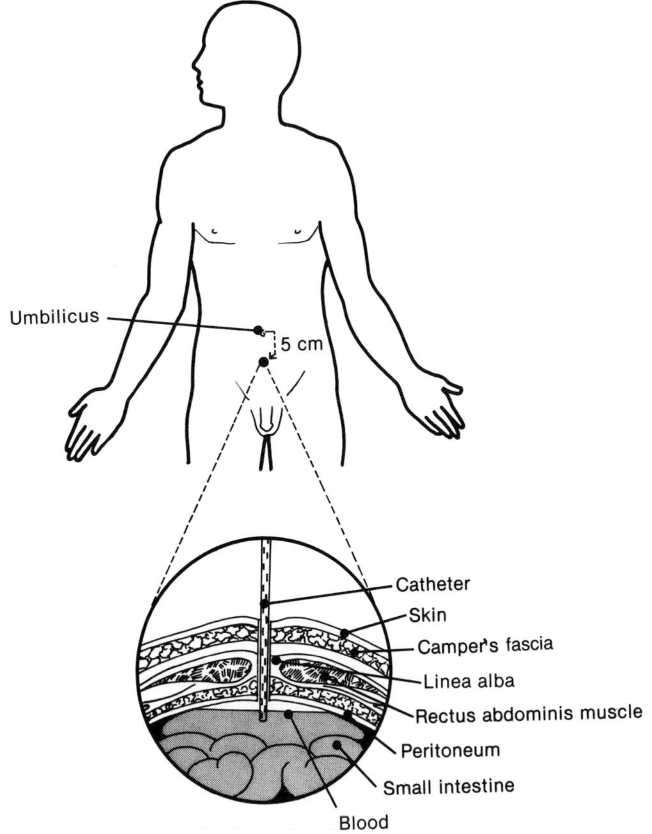

Figure 6.1   Insert catheter into peritoneal cavity.

(Fig. 6.2) Insert a trocar type peritoneal dialysis catheter, with the stylet protruding ⅛ inch (3 mm), through the incision site with the catheter in the midline, perpendicular to the abdominal wall. Have the patient lift the head to tense the abdominal wall. Advance the catheter with one hand while controlling excessive penetration with the other hand. Insert the catheter through the rectus muscle, and penetrate the linea alba through the peritoneum.

Gently advance the catheter retroperitoneally to the suspected site of injury. Remove stylet and immobilize the catheter with a clamp to the abdominal wall.

Aspirate with a syringe. If gross blood or bowel contents are aspirated, the test is definitive. Remove the catheter and apply a sterile dressing. In the absence of these findings, attach the peritoneal catheter to an intravenous line and infuse 10 ml/kg body weight (up to 1 liter) of Ringer's lactate into the peritoneal cavity. If possible, gently roll the patient in order to disperse the fluid.

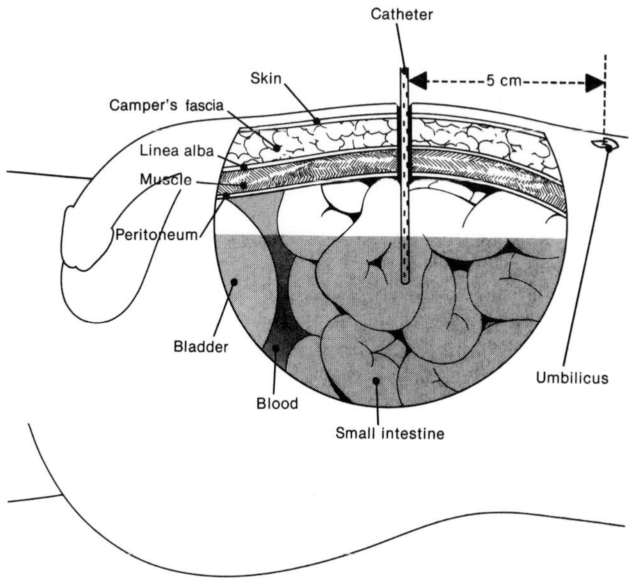

Figure 6.2   Advance catheter.

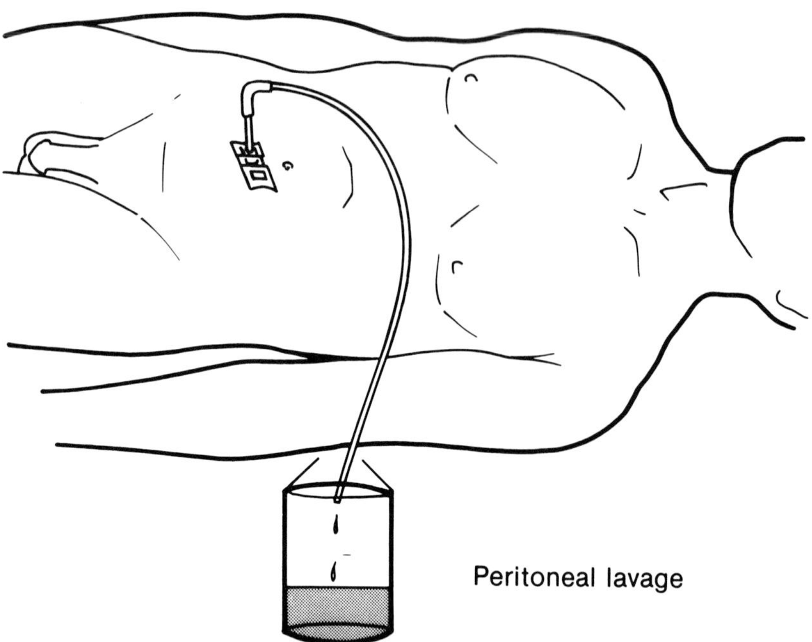

Figure 6.3   Peritoneal lavage.

(Fig. 6.3) After 5 to 10 minutes, reattach the intravenous tubing to the vent hole of the intravenous bottle and place the bottle below the level of the patient. Allow gravity to siphon the lavage fluid.

Interpret findings: if the intravenous tubing containing the lavage fluid is held over newspaper print, one of the following statements can be made:

1. No printing can be seen, indicating significant injury.
2. Printing can be seen, but not read, indicating a strong possibility of injury.
3. Fluid is bloody, but printing can be read, an equivocal test result.
4. Fluid is clear, a negative test result.

Alternatively, the test result may be positive if the hematocrit of the fluid obtained is greater than 2 percent; if the red blood cell count is greater than 100,000/cu mm; or the WBC count is greater than 500/cu mm (in unspun samples).

BIBLIOGRAPHY

Bivins BA, Jona JZ, Belin RP: Diagnostic peritoneal lavage in pediatric trauma. *J Trauma* 16:739, 1976.

Cosgriff JH: *An Atlas of Diagnostic and Therapeutic Procedures for Emergency Personnel*. Philadelphia, JB Lippincott Co, 1978.

Engrav LH, Benjamin CI, Strate RG, et al: Diagnostic peritoneal lavage in blunt abdominal trauma. *J Trauma* 15:854, 1975.

Jergens ME: Peritoneal lavage. *Am J Surg* 133:365, 1977.

Kazarian KK, Devanesan JD, Mersheimer WL: Diagnostic peritoneal lavage. *NY State J Med*, 75:2145, 1975.

Olsen WR, Redman HC, Hildreth DH: Quantitative peritoneal lavage in blunt abdominal trauma. *Arch Surg* 104:53, 1972.

Parvin TS, Smith DE, Asher WM, Virgilio RW: Effectiveness of peritoneal lavage in blunt abdominal trauma. *Ann Surg* 181:255, 1975.

Perry JF Jr, DeMueles JE, Root HD: Diagnostic peritoneal lavage in blunt abdominal trauma. *Surg Gynecol Obstet* 131:742, 1970.

Root HD, Hauser CW, McKin CR, LaFare JW: Diagnostic peritoneal lavage. *Surgery* 57:633, 1965.

Root HD, Keizer PJ, Perry JF Jr: The clinical and experimental aspects of peritoneal response to injury. *Arch Surg* 95:531, 1967.

Sachatello CR, Bivins B: Technic for peritoneal dialysis and diagnostic peritoneal lavage. *Am J Surg* 131:637, 1976.

Vander Salm TJ, Cutler BS, Wheeler HB: *Atlas of Bedside Procedures*. Boston, Little Brown & Co, 1979.

7. PERICARDIOCENTESIS (INDIRECT METHOD)

Indication

Identify acute pericardial effusion and tamponade.

Procedure

(Fig. 7.1) Position the patient at 60° elevation from the horizontal. Attach ECG leads to the patient. Prepare and drape the patient in the usual sterile manner. Identify the anatomical landmarks: the cardiac apex is 1 cm inside the left cardiac border (the angle between the left costal margin and the xiphoid). Infiltrate 0.5 to 1 percent Xylocaine just to the left of the xiphocostal angle, and infiltrate deeply to the costal arch.

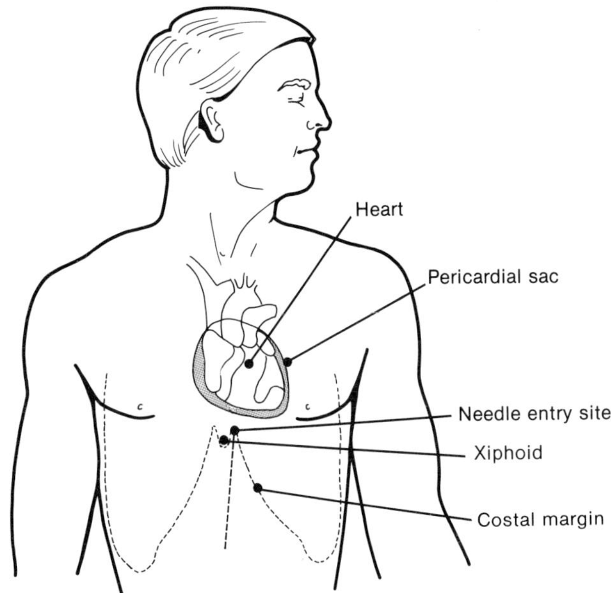

Figure 7.1   Anatomical location.

(Fig. 7.2) Connect the V lead to a sterile alligator clip, and place the sterile needle on a 10-ml syringe. Insert the needle into the anesthetized tract.

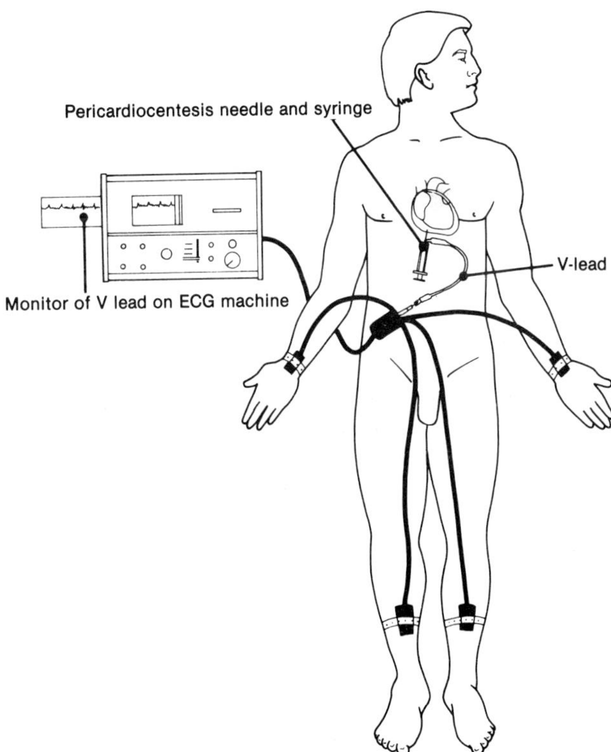

Figure 7.2   Monitor of V lead on ECG machine.

(Fig. 7.3) Advance the needle in the direction of the left shoulder while applying slight negative pressure to the attached syringe and continually monitoring the ECG. Advance the needle until the needle suddenly seems to "give," a sensation that signals pericardial penetration. If the ECG develops an "injury current" (ST segment elevation), which indicates contact with the epicardium, withdraw the needle slightly from the epicardium, simultaneously withdrawing pericardial fluid, if present. Examine the fluid: failure of the blood to clot in a glass tube establishes that the bloody fluid was not obtained from a cardiac chamber. Withdraw fluid until the patient's unstable hemodynamic state has been reversed or until fluid can no longer be aspirated.

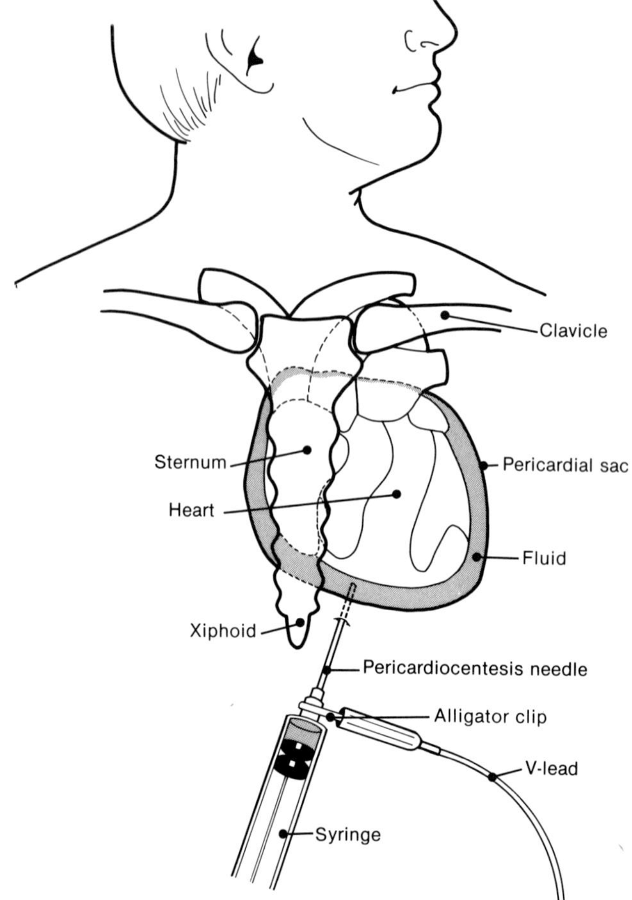

Figure 7.3   Insertion of pericardiocentesis needle.

(Fig. 7.4) Remove the syringe from the needle, and slide a plastic catheter through the needle into the pericardial space. Utilizing a three-way stop-cock, withdraw fluid from the pericardium. Leave the catheter in the pericardial sac for continued drainage if indicated. Alternatively, remove and apply sterile dressing and tape.

BIBLIOGRAPHY

Bains MS, Beattie EJ Jr: Cardiac tamponade. *Hosp Med* 12:47, 1976.

Bishop LH Jr, Estes EH Jr, McIntosh HDJ: The electrocardiogram as a safeguard in pericardiocentesis. *JAMA* 162:264, 1956.

Cosgriff JH: *An Atlas of Diagnostic and Therapeutic Procedures for Emergency Personnel*. Philadelphia, JB Lippincott Co, 1978.

Fredricksen RT, Cohen LS, Mullins CB: Periocardial windows or pericardiocentesis for pericardial effusions. *Am Heart J* 82:158, 1971.

Kilpatrick ZM, Chapman CB: On pericardiocentesis. *Am J Cardiol* 16:722, 1965.

McIntyre KM, Lewis AJ (eds): *Textbook of Advanced Cardiac Life Support*. Chicago, American Heart Association, 1981.

Neill JR, Hurst JW, Penfold ELJ: A pericardiocentesis electrode. *N Engl J Med* 264:711, 1961.

Schaffer AI: Pericardiocentesis with the aid of a plastic catheter and ECG monitor. *Am J Cardiol* 4:83, 1959.

Simpson JS: *Thoracic Injuries in Care of the Injured Child*. Baltimore, Williams & Wilkins, 1975, p 139.

Spodick DH: Acute cardiac tamponade: Pathologic physiology, diagnosis, and management. *Prog Cardiovasc Dis* 10:64, 1967.

Vander Salm TJ, Cutler BS, Wheeler HB: *Atlas of Bedside Procedures*. Boston, Little Brown & Co, 1979.

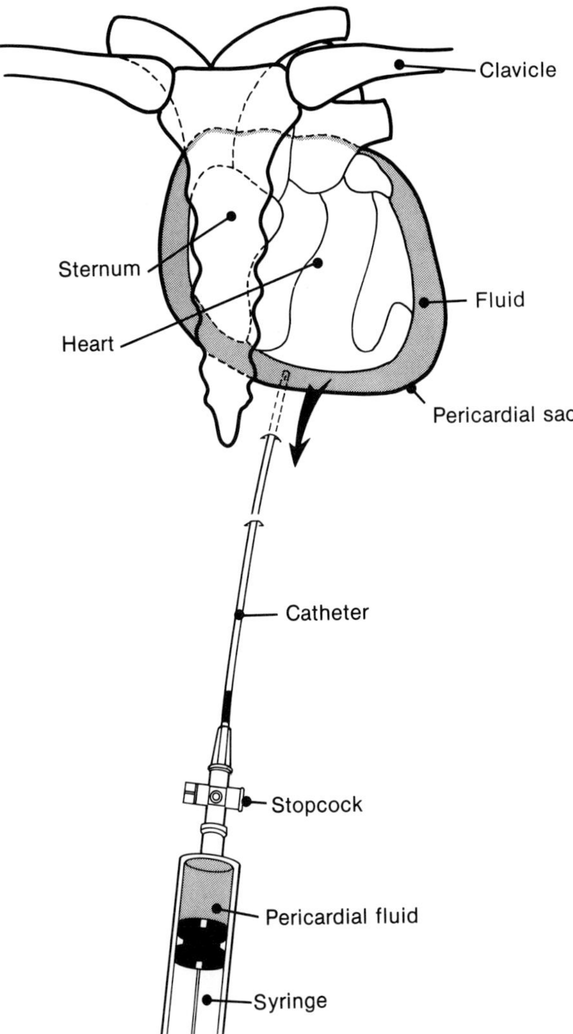

Figure 7.4   Catheter insertion.

8. DEFIBRILLATION AND ELECTRICAL CARDIOVERSION

Indication

Determine the presence of life-threatening ventricular or atrial arrhythmias causing hemodynamic compromise.

Procedure

Secure the direct current cardioversion apparatus, and select the appropriate mode and electrical charge required. (Fig. 8.1) Use electrode paste or saline pads to lower electrical impedance. Apply one paddle over the second right intercostal space, just below the right clavicle, and the second paddle over the fifth intercostal space, i.e., on the left mid-axillary line just lateral to the left nipple. If the patient is conscious and time permits, give diazepam (Valium), 5 to 10 mg, intravenously for sedation, and hyperventilate the patient with supplemental oxygen. Then apply the electrical shock.

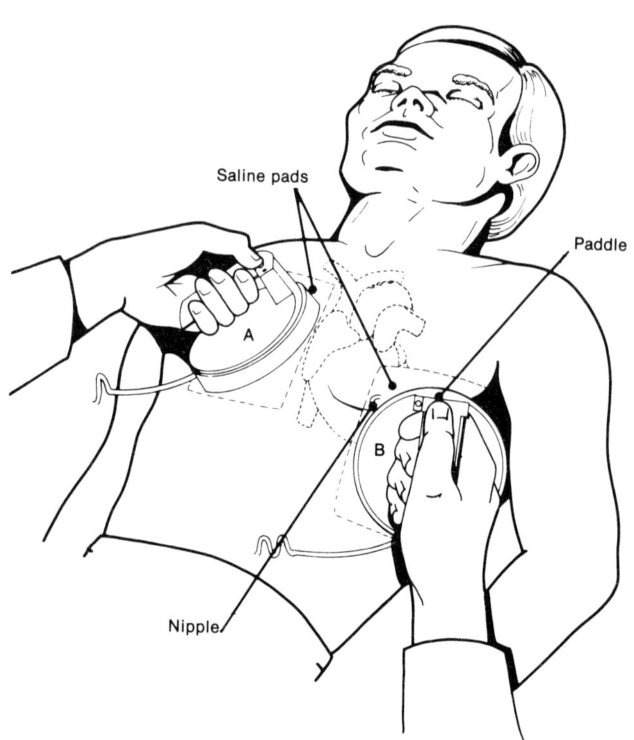

Figure 8.1   Apply paddles.

BIBLIOGRAPHY

Dorney ER: The use of cardioversion and pacemakers in the management of arrhythmias, in Hurst JW, et al (eds): *The Heart*, ed 3. New York, McGraw-Hill, 1974, pp 558–562.

Lown B, Neuman J, Amarasingham R, et al: Comparison of alternating current with direct current electroshock across the closed chest. *Am J Cardiol* 10:223, 1962.

McIntyre, KM, Lewis AJ (eds): *Textbook of Advanced Cardiac Life Support*. Chicago, American Heart Association, 1981.

Parker MR (ed): Defibrillation and synchronized cardioversion, in *Advanced Cardiac Life Support*. Chicago, American Heart Association, 1975.

Resnekov L: Theory and practice of electroversion of cardiac dysrhythmias. *Med Clin North Am* 60:325, 1976.

Vander Salm TJ, Cutler BS, Wheeler HB: *Atlas of Bedside Procedures*. Boston, Little Brown & Co, 1979.

9. NASOTRACHEAL SUCTIONING

Indication

Remove secretions or blood from the tracheobronchial tree.

Procedure

Position the patient in the sitting, semisitting, or supine position. Hyperventilate the patient with supplemental oxygen if the patient is in respiratory distress.

(Fig. 9.1) Select a sterile, clear, plastic, low-friction, coefficient #14 French suction catheter with adequate side holes. Lubricate the end of the catheter, and introduce it into the patient's nostril. Advance the catheter along the floor of the nose into the hypopharynx. Advance the catheter during inspiration.

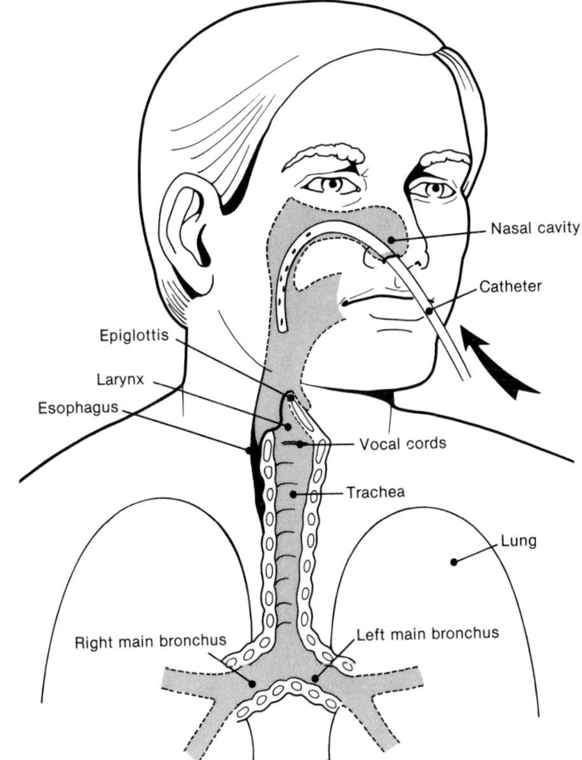

Figure 9.1 Catheter inserted into nose.

(Fig. 9.2) Alternatively, gently place light traction with a sterile-gloved hand and gauze on the tongue, pull it forward, and advance the catheter.

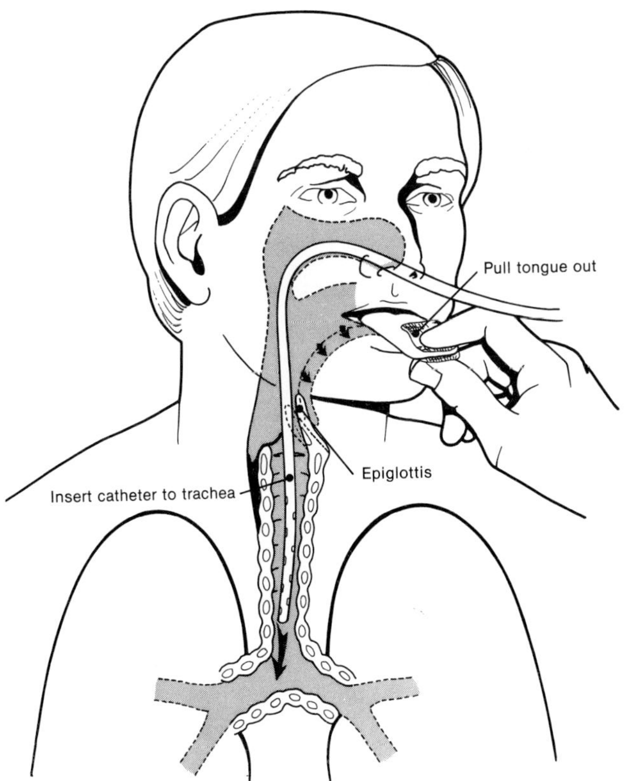

Figure 9.2 Advance catheter into trachea.

1088   EMERGENCY MEDICINE

(Fig. 9.3) Watch for patient coughing or changes in phonation, which suggest that the catheter tip has advanced into the trachea below the vocal cords. Apply suction via the vacuum tube for five to ten seconds at -60 to -80 mm Hg. Collect mucus in trap if indicated. Remove catheter.

BIBLIOGRAPHY

Haight C: Intratracheal suction in the management of postoperative pulmonary complications. *Ann Surg* 107:218, 1938.

Shim C, Fine N, Fernandez R, et al: Cardiac arrhythmias resulting from tracheal suctioning. *Ann Intern Med* 71:1149, 1969.

Vander Salm TJ, Cutler BS, Wheeler HB: *Atlas of Bedside Procedures*. Boston, Little Brown & Co, 1979.

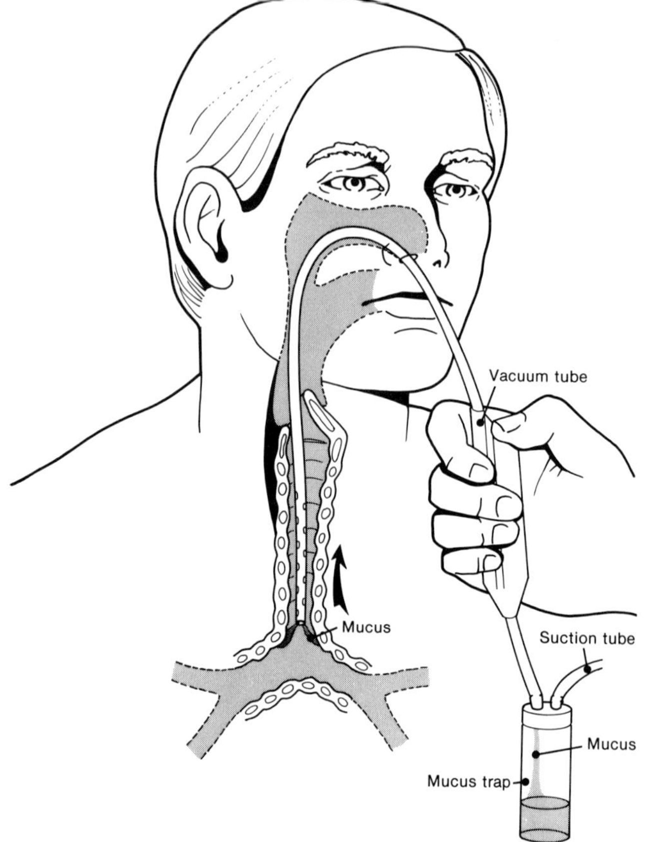

Figure 9.3   Apply suction vacuum.

10. NEEDLE CRICOTHYROID PUNCTURE

Indications

A. Provide an emergency airway when endotracheal intubation is not possible or indicated.
B. Provide an emergency airway when the upper airway is obstructed secondary to trauma or foreign body.

Procedure

Place the patient in the supine position with support under the shoulders.

(Fig. 10.1) Prepare and drape the patient in the usual sterile manner. Identify the anatomical landmarks: the cricothyroid membrane is located just below the thyroid cartilage and above the cricoid cartilage.

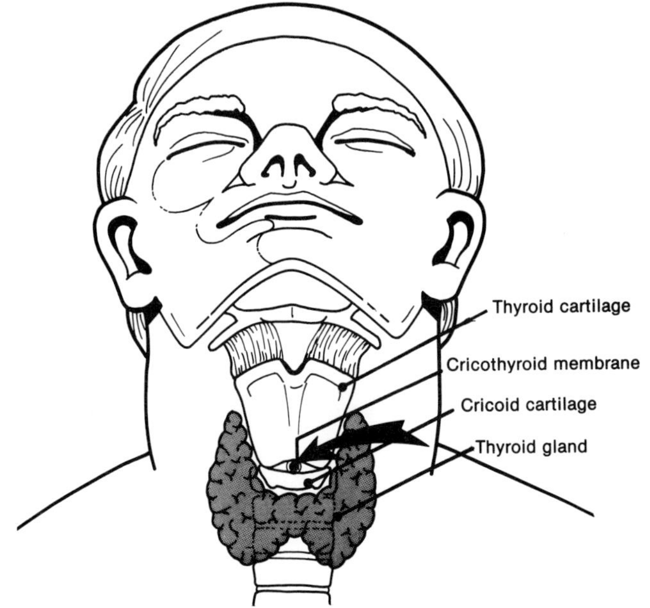

Figure 10.1 Anatomy.

(Fig. 10.2) Introduce 0.5 to 1 percent Xylocaine in the midline over the cricothyroid membrane.

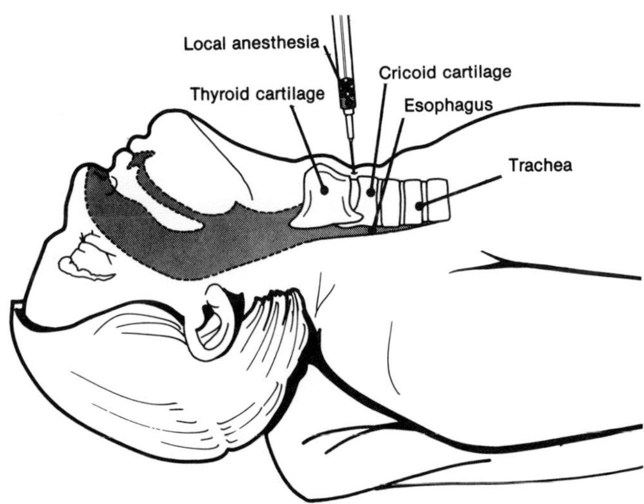

Figure 10.2 Local anesthesia.

(Fig. 10.3) Penetrate the cricothyroid membrane with a 14-gauge intracath needle on the end of an air-filled syringe. Keep the bevel of the needle up, and direct the point of the needle at an angle of 45° to the neck. Aspirate until the presence of air confirms the position of the needle in the trachea. Remove the syringe.

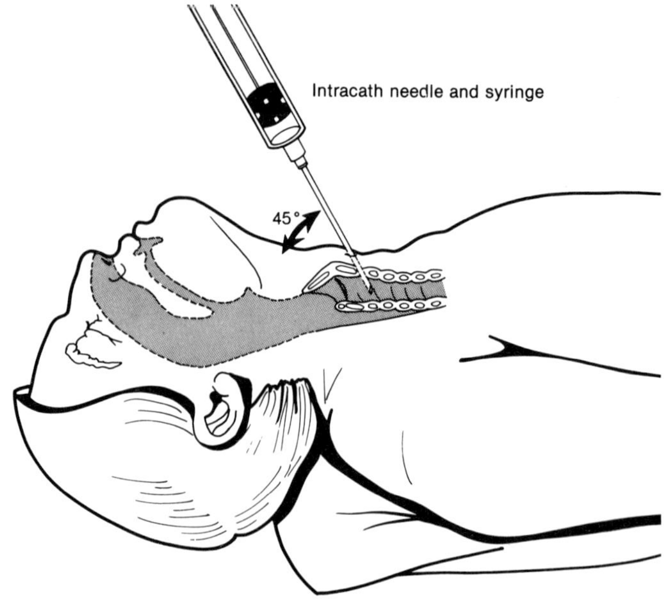

Figure 10.3   Intracath needle punctures cricothyroid membrane.

(Fig. 10.4) Thread the catheter through the needle into the trachea. Attach the catheter hub to a number 3.0 mm pediatric endotracheal tube adapter.

Apply supplemental oxygen apparatus, via a "Y"-connector at a high flow rate, to the opening of the catheter if the patient is ventilating. Attach to a mechanical ventilatory apparatus if the patient requires ventilatory assistance. A second catheter with a stopcock can be inserted adjacent to the first: with the stopcock closed during inspiration and opened during exhalation, CO_2 can be eliminated. Apply povidone-iodine to wound site and a sterile dressing. Visualize lung inflations and auscultate the chest for adequate ventilations.

BIBLIOGRAPHY

Bartlett JG, Rosenblatt JE, Feingold SM: Percutaneous transtracheal aspiration in the diagnosis of anaerobic pulmonary infection. *Ann Intern Med* 79:535, 1973.

Cosgriff JH: *An Atlas of Diagnostic and Therapeutic Procedures for Emergency Personnel.* Philadelphia, JB Lippincott Co, 1978.

Craig DB: Transtracheal ventilation. *JAMA* 235:2082, 1976.

Jacobs HB: Emergency percutaneous transtracheal catheter and ventilator. *J Trauma* 12:50–55, 1972.

Jacoby JJ, Hamelburg W, Ziegler CH, et al: Transtracheal resuscitation. *JAMA* 162:625–628, 1956.

Kalinske RW, Parker RH, Brandt D, et al: Diagnostic usefulness and safety of transtracheal aspiration. *N Engl J Med* 276:604, 1967.

Pecora DV: A method of securing uncontaminated tracheal secretions for bacterial examination. *J Thorac Cardiovasc Surg* 37:653, 1959.

Spencer CD, Beaty HN: Complications of transtracheal aspiration. *N Engl J Med* 286:304, 1972.

Vander Salm TJ, Cutler BS, Wheeler HB: *Atlas of Bedside Procedures.* Boston, Little Brown & Co, 1979.

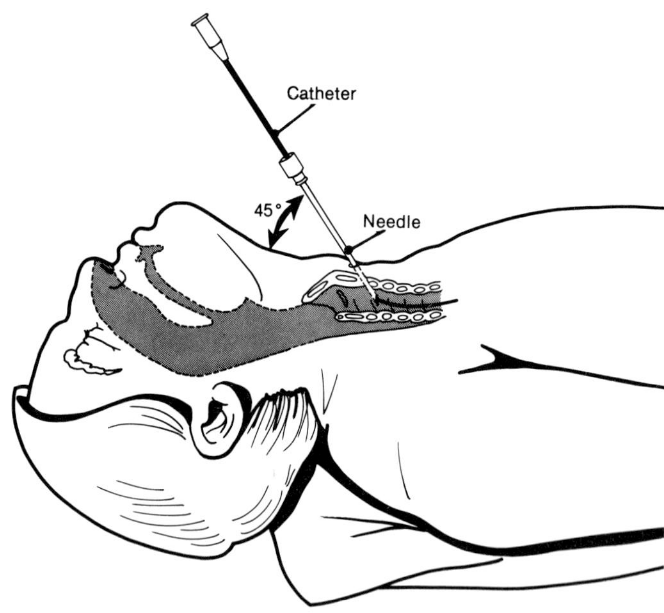

Figure 10.4   Catheter inserted into intracath needle.

11. ENDOTRACHEAL INTUBATION

Indications

A. Maintain an airway in a patient with respiratory or cardiac arrest.
B. Protect against aspiration.
C. Suction the tracheobronchial tree.
D. Provide positive pressure mechanical ventilation.
E. Administer high levels of oxygen.

Caution: Nasotracheal approach is indicated in suspected cervical spine injuries.

Procedure

Test the laryngoscope light and the balloon on the endotracheal tube. Provide supplemental oxygen and/or hyperventilate the patient with oxygen briefly before initiating the procedure.

(Fig. 11.1) Position the patient in the sniffing position (the neck flexed forward and the head extended backward). If necessary, place a support under the occiput to elevate the head a few centimeters above the horizontal.

Lubricate the tube and stylet, and introduce the metal stylet into the endotracheal tube with the desired tube configuration.

Straight Blade Technique

(Fig. 11.2) Insert the laryngoscope blade between the patient's teeth and open the patient's mouth with the right hand. Advance the blade to the right side of the mouth, displacing the tongue to the left, but observe the cords before advancing the tube. Utilizing the laryngoscope, visualize the glottic opening.

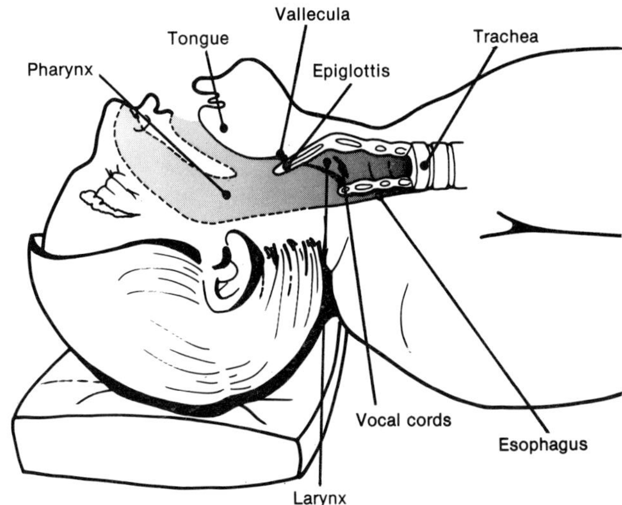

Figure 11.1   Anatomy.

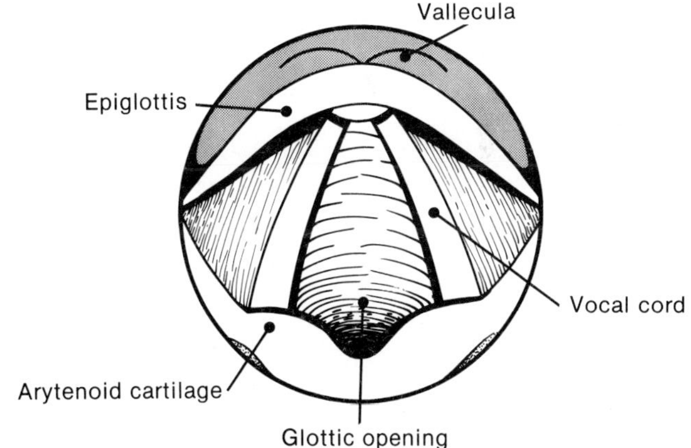

Figure 11.2   View through laryngoscope.

(Fig. 11.3) Advance the blade to just beyond the tip of the epiglottis. Aim it below the epiglottis.

Exert upward traction on the handle of the laryngoscope, displacing the base of the tongue and the epiglottis anteriorly to expose the glottic opening.

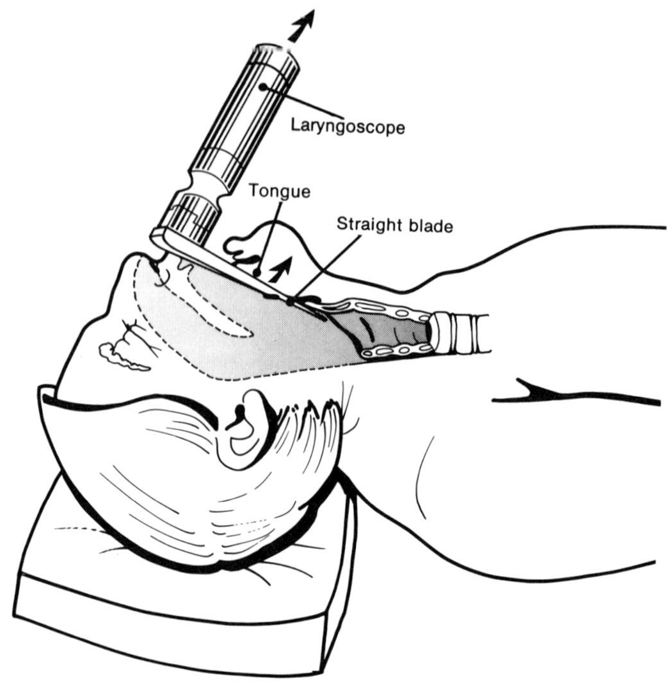

Figure 11.3　Straight blade technique.

Curved Blade Technique

(Fig. 11.4) Insert the tip of the blade into the vallecula. Displace the epiglottis anteriorly by upward traction with the tip of the blade. Gently lift the laryngoscope upward and forward at the base of the tongue and epiglottis.

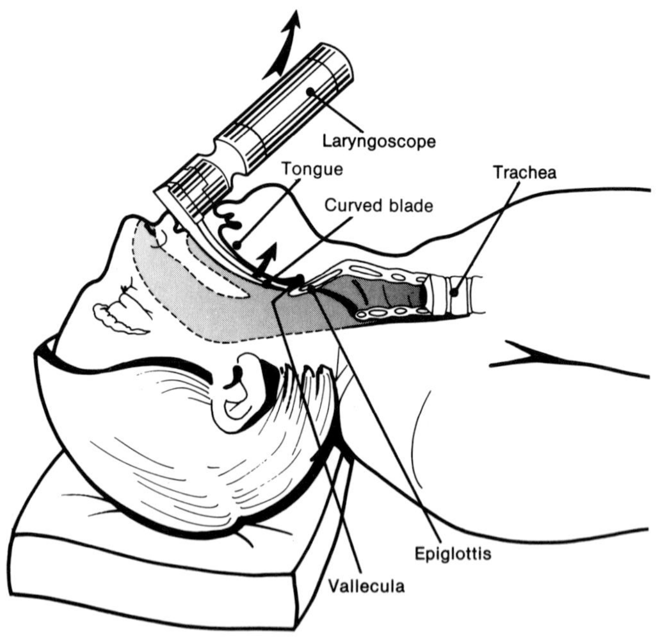

Figure 11.4　Curved blade technique.

(Fig. 11.5) As in the straight blade technique, observe the cords before advancing the tube. Advance the endotracheal tube between the vocal cords so that the balloon is just below the cords.

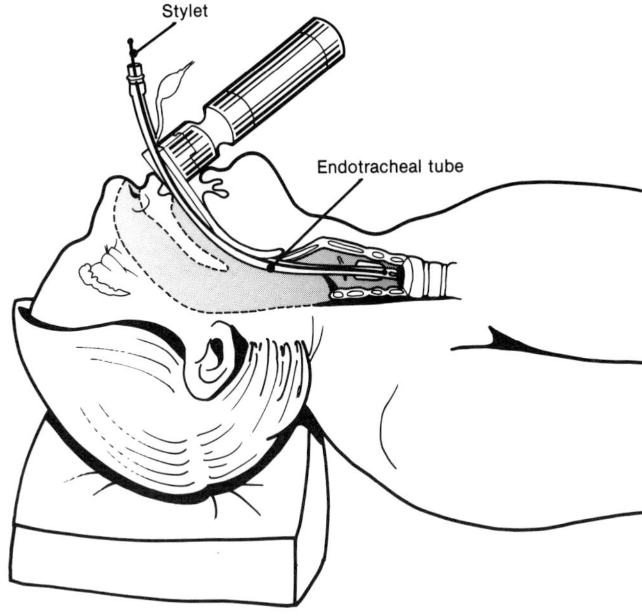

Figure 11.5 Endotracheal tube in place.

(Fig. 11.6) In a child or infant, utilizing the curved blade technique and applying pressure over the cricoid cartilage will occlude the upper end of the esophagus (Sellick maneuver) and may facilitate glottic visualization.

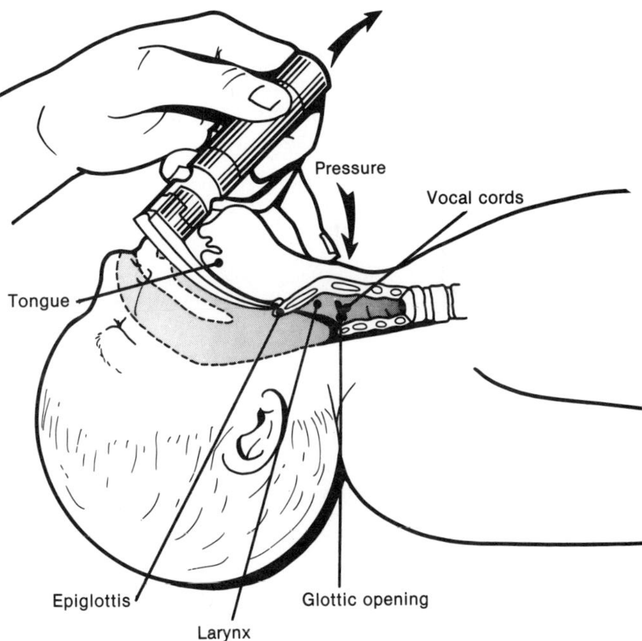

Figure 11.6 Intubation of infant.

(Fig. 11.7) Remove the stylet.

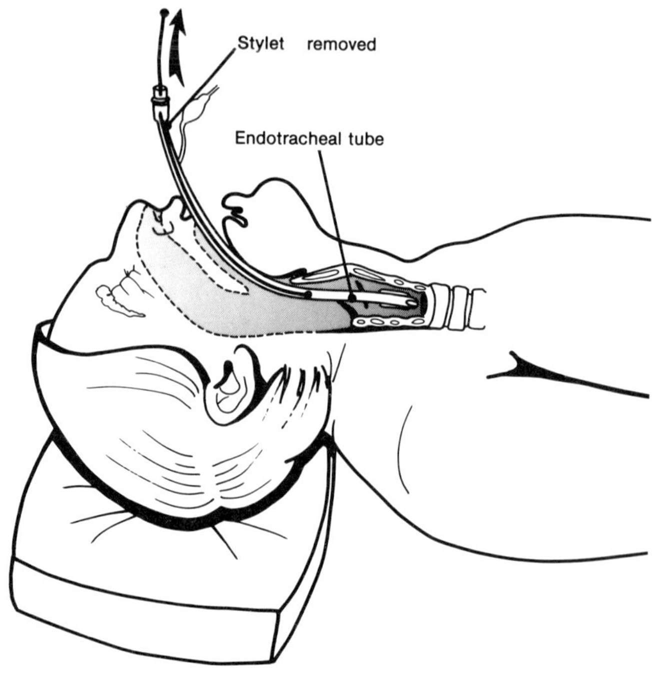

Figure 11.7   Stylet being removed.

(Fig. 11.8) Inflate the balloon. Confirm that no air is escaping around the tube by listening at the patient's mouth. Establish that both the right and left lungs are ventilated by auscultating the chest. Attach the tube to a bag valve device or mechanical respirator.

Tape the tube securely. Provide supplemental oxygen or mechanical ventilation as indicated. Obtain a chest roentgenogram to confirm the position of the endotracheal tube.

BIBLIOGRAPHY

Collins VJ: *Principles of Anesthesiology*, ed 2. Philadelphia, Lea & Febiger, 1976, p. 379.

Dripps R et al: Intubation of the trachea, in *Introduction to Anesthesia*, ed 4. Philadelphia, WB Saunders, 1972, pp 186–199.

Magill IV: Endotracheal anesthesia. *Am J Surg* 34:450, 1936.

McIntyre KM, Lewis AJ (eds):*Textbook of Advanced Cardiac Life Support*. Chicago, American Heart Association, 1981.

Vander Salm TJ, Cutler BS, Wheeler HB: *Atlas of Bedside Procedures*. Boston, Little Brown & Co, 1979.

Waters RM, Rovenstine EA, Guedel AE: Endotracheal anesthesia and its historical developments. *Anesth Analg* 12:196, 1933.

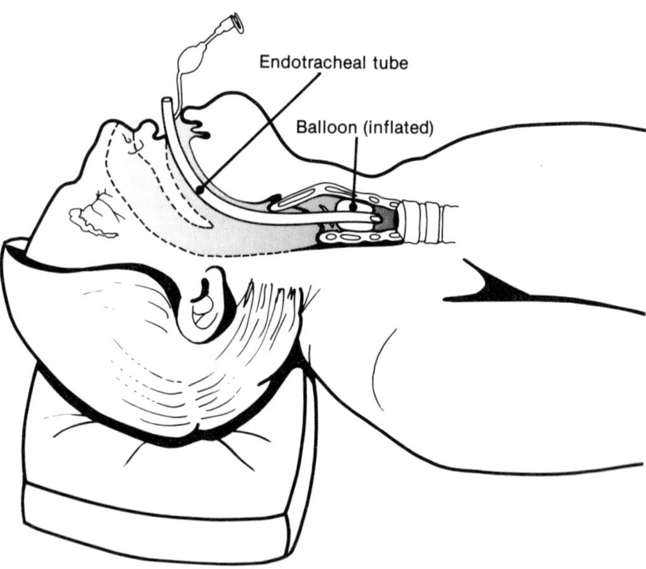

Figure 11.8   Inflate cuff.

12. CLOSED THORACOSTOMY

Indication

Remove fluid or air from the pleural space.

Procedure

For removal of air by the anterior apical approach, position the patient in the supine position, elevated 30°. Place the patient in the lateral decubitus position if the basilar or lateral apical tube approach is to be used. Prepare and drape the patient in the usual sterile manner.

(Fig. 12.1) Identify the anatomical landmarks: the second intercostal space on the midclavicular line or, alternatively, the midaxillary line at the caudal edge of the axillary line.

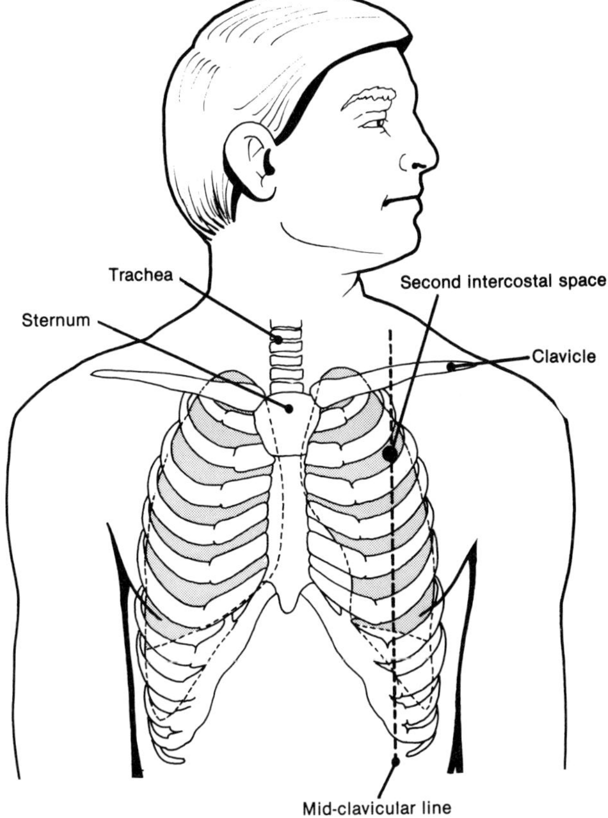

Figure 12.1   Anatomical position.

(Fig. 12.2) Introduce 0.5 to 1 percent Xylocaine into the skin muscle and fat to the parietal pleura above the superior border of the rib. Also infiltrate the skin over the next caudal interspace. Aspirate from the pleural space to confirm the presence of fluid or air.

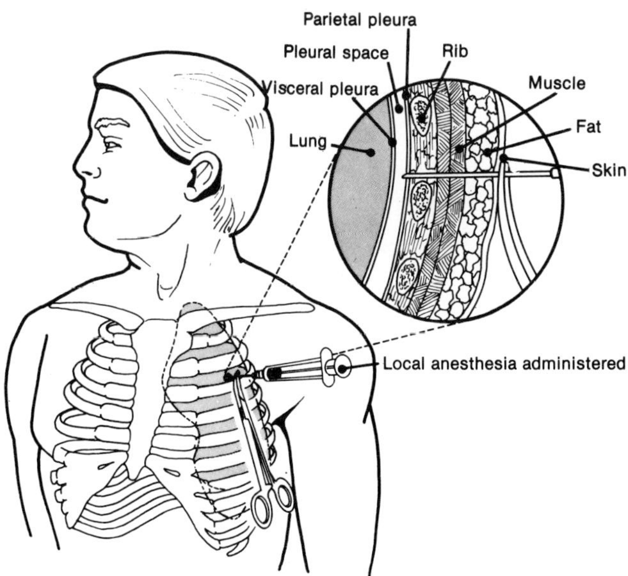

Figure 12.2   Local anesthesia.

(Fig. 12.3) With a #10 scalpel blade, make an incision in the area of the skin previously anesthetized. The space should be large enough to admit the small finger. Introduce a curved clamp into the incision site, and spread the fascia over the superior edge of the rib.

Perforate the pleura and enter the pleural space.

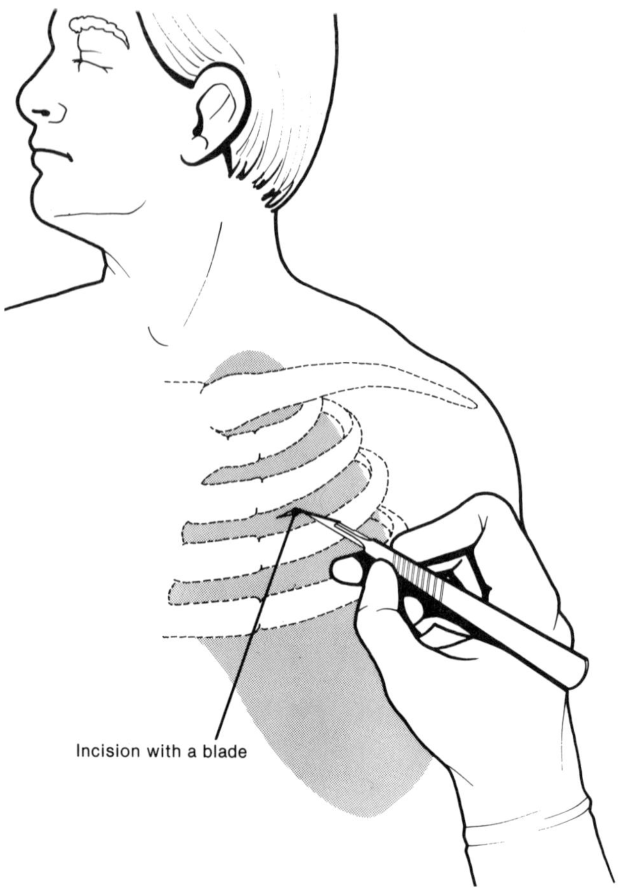

Figure 12.3   Incision of skin.

(Fig. 12.4) Introduce the fifth (small) finger into the pleural space to confirm the space and exclude the possibility that lung tissue is against the incision site.

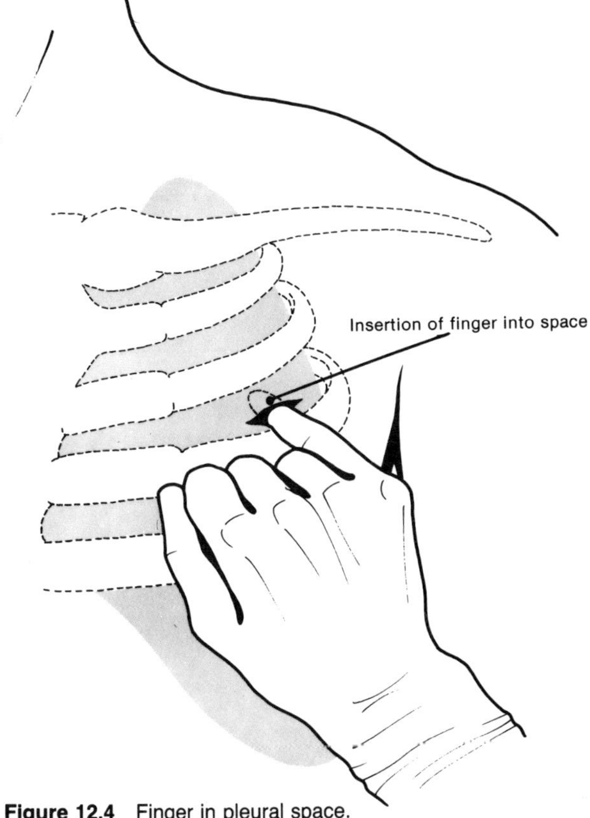

Figure 12.4 Finger in pleural space.

(Fig. 12.5) Insert the chest tube into the pleural space, advancing the tube toward the lung apex. Attach the chest tube to a water-sealed suction bottle apparatus. Suture the chest tube to the skin of the chest wall. Tape the tube to the chest wall and apply a sterile dressing. Obtain a chest roentgenogram to confirm the location of the chest tube and the success of therapy.

For treatment of hemothorax, utilize the sixth or seventh intercostal space on the midaxillary line. After the tube is advanced, position it posteriorly and basally.

BIBLIOGRAPHY

Bowditch HI: Paracentesis thoracis. *Am J Med Sci* 23:103, 1852.

Cosgriff JH: *An Atlas of Diagnostic and Therapeutic Procedures for Emergency Personnel*. Philadelphia, JB Lippincott Co, 1978.

Gott PH: A simplified method for thoracentesis and pleural fluid drainage. *Am Rev Respir Dis* 92:295, 1965.

Hoffmann L: A modified thoracentesis technique. *Am Rev Respir Dis* 89:106, 1964.

Neptune WB: Thoracentesis, in Nora PF (ed): *Operative Surgery*. Philadelphia, Lea & Febiger, 1972, pp 217–218.

Vander Salm TJ, Cutler BS, Wheeler HB: *Atlas of Bedside Procedures*. Boston, Little Brown & Co, 1979.

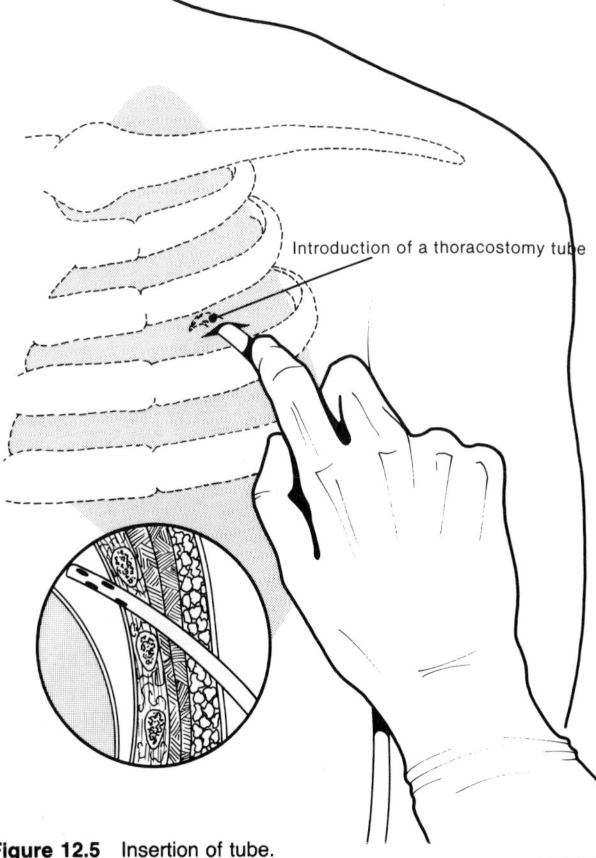

Figure 12.5 Insertion of tube.

13. ASPIRATION AND INJECTION OF JOINTS, BURSAE, AND TENDONS

Indications

A. Determine the presence of joint effusion.
B. Evacuate hemarthrosis or other effusion.
C. Instill therapeutic agents.

Procedure

Knee Joint

(Fig. 13.1, *A*) For the anterior approach, flex the knee to 90°. Insert the needle through the middle of the patellar tendon, directly to the intercondylar notch.

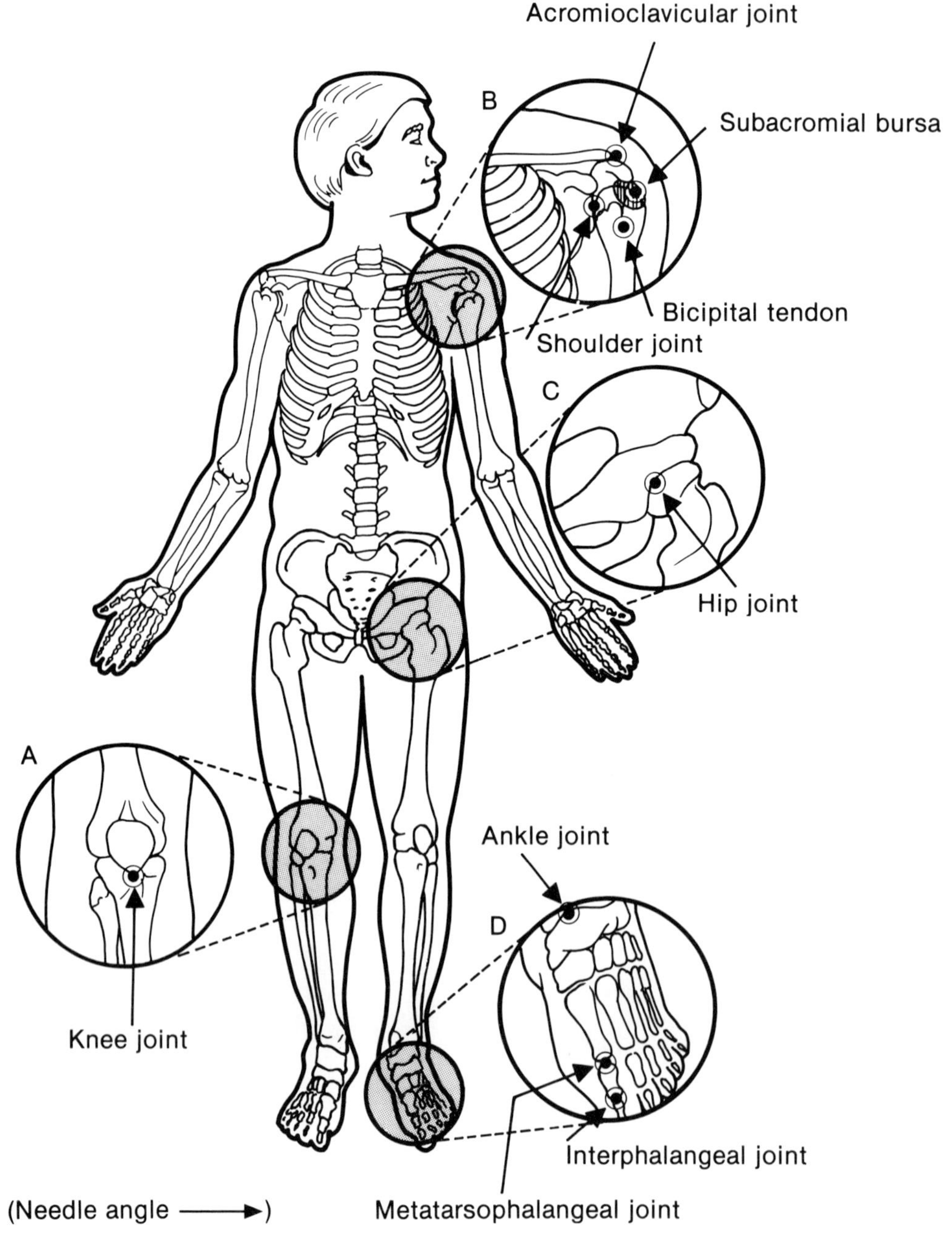

Figure 13.1 Anterior view.

Glenohumeral (Shoulder) Joint

(Fig. 13.1, *B*) Place the patient in a sitting position with the arm at the side and the hand across the abdomen. In the anterior technique, insert the needle lateral and inferior to the coracoid; direct it to the anterior rim of the glenoid.

Acromioclavicular Joint

Place patient in same position as for the glenohumeral joint, and palpate the joint. Insert the needle superiorly; direct it to the lateral end of the clavicle.

Subacromial Bursa

Place the patient in the same position, applying downward traction to the flexed elbow, and insert the needle laterally 1 cm below the tip of the acromion; direct it medially to the bursa.

Bicipital Tendon

With the patient in the same position, insert the needle anteriorly at the point of maximum tenderness; direct the needle to the bicipital groove.

Hip Joint: Anterior Approach

(Fig. 13.1, *C*) Place the patient in the supine position, hip straight and in neutral rotation. Insert the needle at the intersection of the parasagittal line through the anterior superior iliac spine and the transverse line through pubic symphysis.

Tibiotalar (Ankle) Joint

(Fig. 13.1, *D*) Place the foot in the plantar flexed position. Insert the needle medial to the anterior tibial tendon; direct it to the hollow at the anterior margin of the medial malleolus.

Metatarsophalangeal and Interphalangeal Joints

Flex toes to 15° to 20° and apply traction. Insert the needle dorsally, medial or lateral to extensor tendon.

Glenohumeral Joint: Posterior Technique

(Fig. 13.2, *A*) Insert the needle 2 cm inferior to posterior angle of acromion; direct it to posterior rim of glenoid.

Radiohumeral (Elbow) Joint

(Fig. 13.2, *B*) Place the patient in a sitting position, flexing the elbow 90°; pronate the forearm (palm down), and insert the needle between the lateral epicondyle and radial head; direct it medially.

Lateral Epicondyle

Place the patient in a sitting position with the elbow flexed 90°, pronate the forearm, and insert the needle at and directly to the point of maximum tenderness.

Olecranon Bursa

Flex the elbow to 90°, and insert the needle at the posterior tip of the olecranon; direct it along the shaft of the ulna.

Hip Joint: Lateral Approach

(Fig. 13.2, *C*) Place the patient in the supine position with the hip straight and internally rotated. Insert the needle anterior to the greater trochanter, directly beneath the midportion of Poupart's ligament.

Greater Trochanteric Bursa

Place patient in the same position as for a lateral approach to a hip joint, and insert the needle directly to the point of maximum tenderness.

Metacarpophalangeal and Interphalangeal Joints

(Fig. 13.2, *D*) Flex fingers to 15° to 20°, apply traction to finger, and insert the needle dorsally, medial or lateral to extensor tendon.

Carpometacarpal (Thumb) Joint

(Fig. 13.2, *E*) Oppose the thumb to little finger, applying traction to the thumb, and insert the needle proximal to prominence of base metacarpal on the palmar side of abductor pollicis tendon.

Radiocarpal (Wrist) Joint

(Fig. 13.2, *F*) Flex the wrist to 30°, apply traction to the hand, and insert the needle dorsally, distal to the dorsal tubercle, medial to extensor pollicus longus tendon, directly volarly to joint.

Knee Joint: Anteromedial Approach

(Fig. 13.2, *G*) Place the patient in a supine position with the knee extended. Insert the needle 1 cm medial to patella directly to intercondylar notch.

Anserine Bursa

Extend the knee, and insert the needle directly to the point of maximum tenderness.

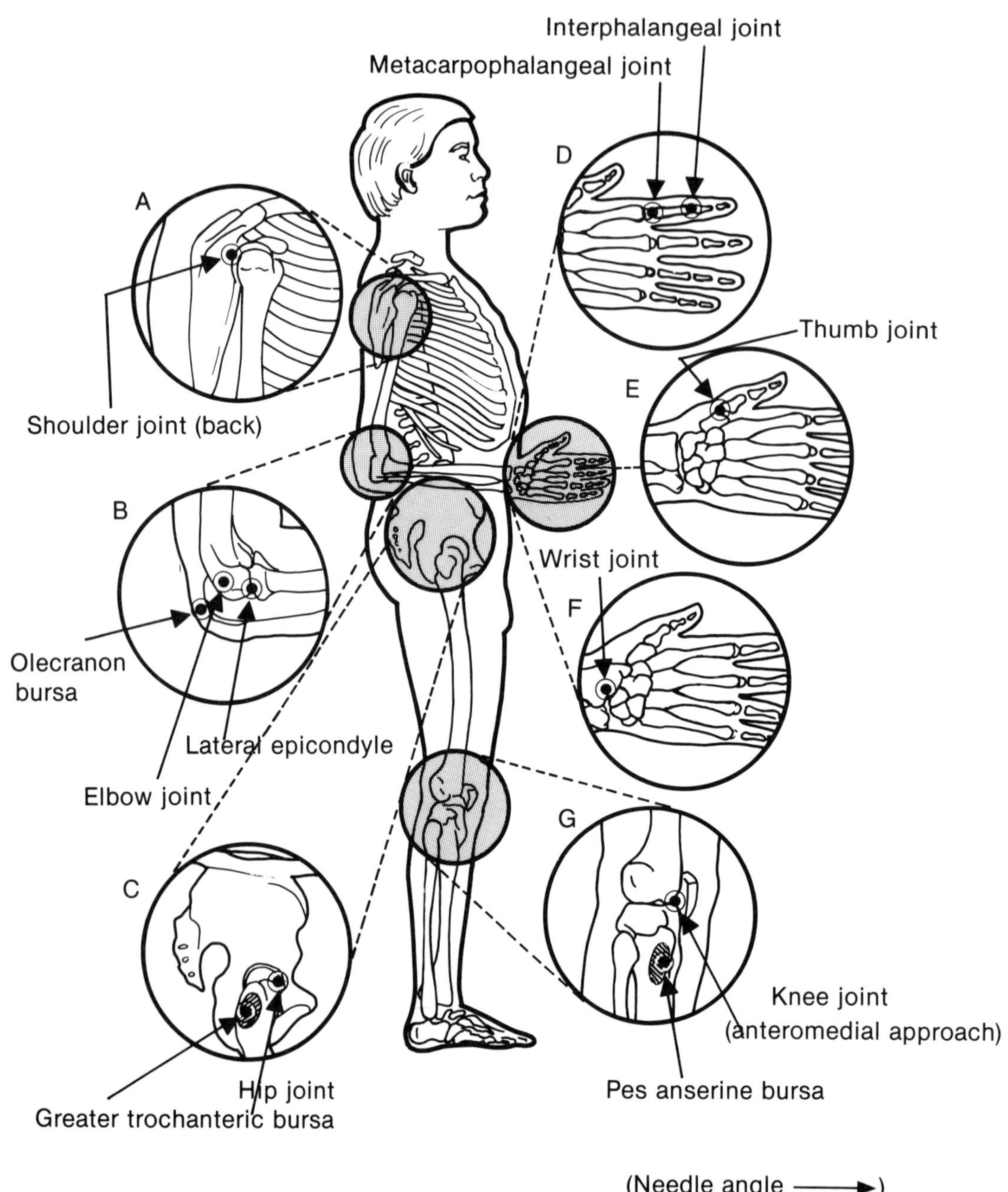

Figure 13.2 Lateral view.

BIBLIOGRAPHY

Calabro JJ: Rheumatoid arthritis. *Ciba Found Symp* 23:1, 1971.

Cosgriff JH: *An Atlas of Diagnostic and Therapeutic Procedures for Emergency Personnel*. Philadelphia, JB Lippincott Co, 1978.

Hollander JL: *Arthritis and Allied Conditions*. Philadelphia, Lea & Febiger, 1972, p 517.

Miller JA: Joint paracentesis from an anatomic point of view: I. Shoulder, elbow, wrist and hand. *Surgery* 40:993, 1956.

Miller JA: Joint paracentesis from an anatomic point of view: II. Hip, Ankle, and Foot. *Surgery* 41:999, 1957.

Pruce AM, Miller JA, Berger IR: Anatomic landmarks in joint paracentesis. *Ciba Found Symp* 16:19, 1964.

Steinbrocker OT, Neustadt DH: *Aspiration and Injection Therapy in Arthritis and Musculoskeletal Disorders*. Hagerstown, Md, Harper & Row, 1972.

Sweetnam R: Corticosteroid arthropathy and tendon rupture. *J Bone Joint Surg* 51B:397, 1969.

Vander Salm TJ, Cutler BS, Wheeler HB: *Atlas of Bedside Procedures*. Boston, Little Brown & Co, 1979.

72. Emergency Drug Index

CAROLYN M. STEWART, Pharm.D.
JAMES P. STEWART, Pharm.D.

CONTENTS

ANTIARRHYTHMICS, VASOPRESSORS, CARDIAC ARREST MEDICATIONS

Generic Name: ATROPINE (Parenteral)
Trade Name: Atropine
Dosage Form: Injection (IV), 1 mg/10 cc preloaded syringe or 0.4 mg, 0.5 mg, 0.6 mg/cc vials.
Uses: Anticholinergic, used for treatment of sinus bradycardia (pulse under 60) and improvement of atrioventricular conduction.
Adult Dosage (Parenteral): 0.5–1 mg IV push (range, 0.3–2 mg). Doses may be repeated q. 5 min. until pulse over 60 or 2 mg have been given. For improvement of atrioventricular conduction, 0.3–1.2 mg IV or subcutaneously q. 4 hours p.r.n. (maximum dosage of 4 mg/day).
Pediatric Dosage (Parenteral): 0.1–0.2 mg/10 kg IV (maximum dosage of 0.3–0.4 mg).
Precautions: Glaucoma, coronary artery disease (1 mg doses may produce ventricular arrhythmias).
Adverse Reactions: Dose-related. Keep IV rate at 1 mg/min or less. Adverse reactions that may occur include
- at 1 mg: tachycardia, dry mouth, pupil dilation
- at 2 mg: increase of symptoms that develop at 1 mg, blurred vision
- at 5 mg: aggravation of symptoms mentioned, speech disturbances, hot, dry skin
- at 10 mg: increased severity of all symptoms, atropine "flush," excitement, hallucinations, coma, arrest. (Antidote: physostigmine IV.)

Drug Interactions: Incompatible with sodium bicarbonate.

Generic Name: BRETYLIUM TOSYLATE
Trade Name: Bretylol
Dosage Forms: Injection (IV/IM), 500 mg/10 cc ampule (50 mg/cc).
Uses: Adrenergic-blocking and antiarrhythmic agent, used for treatment of life-threatening ventricular arrhythmias. Onset is rapid (within minutes), and duration is approximately 6–9 hours.
Adult Dosage (Parenteral): For emergency treatment, 5–10 mg/kg IV push (over 8 min.). May repeat with 2 doses of 10 mg/kg up to 15 to 30 min. apart. (Maximum total dosage of 30 mg/kg.) For prophylaxis, 5–10 mg/kg IV over 8 min., then either repeat bolus dose q. 6 hours or continuous IV infusion of 1–2 mg/min.

NOTE: Although the authors have been careful to provide general drug administration guidelines that are in agreement with current literature, we suggest that the reader refer to the text itself for specific indications and dosages. We also suggest that appropriate information sources be consulted when dealing with new and unfamiliar drugs. It remains the responsibility of every practitioner to evaluate the appropriateness of a particular opinion in the context of the actual clinical situation and with due consideration to any new developments in the field. A review of pharmacokinetics and drug overdose is found in Chapter 24.

Carolyn M. Stewart, Pharm.D.
James P. Stewart, Pharm.D.

Pediatric Dosage (Parenteral): 2–5 mg/kg IM (investigational).
Precautions: Short-term use only. Patient should be weaned over 3–5 days. Initial release of norepinephrine caused by bretylium may worsen digitalis-induced arrhythmias. No more than 5-cc IM dose in any one site. Repeated IM doses should be avoided.
Adverse Reactions: Nausea, vomiting, and hypotension after too rapid IV administration. Hypotension (incidence 50%–75%), to which tolerance usually develops, may be treated with dopamine or Levophed if supine diastolic blood pressure is less than 75 mm Hg. Bradycardia, substernal pressure, and angina have been reported.
Drug Interactions: Should not be mixed with any other medication.

Generic Name: CALCIUM CHLORIDE (IV, 10%)
Trade Name: Calcium Chloride
Dosage Form: Injection (IV/intracardiac), 10-cc (10% solution) preloaded syringe (13.6 mEq Ca^{++}).
Uses: Stimulation of myocardial contractility and treatment of severe hypocalcemia and tetany associated with hypermagnesemia. (Normal serum calcium level, 4.5–5.5 mEq/liter or 9–11 mg/dl.)
Adult Dosage (Parenteral): For CPR, 5–10 cc 10% solution slow IV or intracardiac.
Pediatric Dosage (Parenteral): For a child, 0.47 mEq/kg (0.35 cc/kg) IV. For an infant, 0.3 mEq/kg (0.22 cc/kg) intracardiac.
Contraindications: Relative contraindication in digitalized patients.
Precautions: Should not be given IM or subcutaneously because of risk of tissue necrosis. Rate of calcium ion infusion should not exceed 0.7–1.5 mEq/min. (less than 3 cc/min.). Caution must be used in digitalized patients.
Adverse Reactions: Most result from too rapid IV administration (toxic serum level of calcium, 15 mg/100 cc (7.5 mEq/liter) or more. Symptoms include tingling sensations, calcium taste, sense of heat waves, vasodilation, bradycardia, arrhythmias, ventricular fibrillation. Treatment of hypercalcemia includes hydration, IV furosemide, mithramycin, sodium sulfate solutions, or IV phosphates.
Drug Interactions: Incompatible with sodium bicarbonate, phosphates, cephalothin.

Generic Name: CALCIUM GLUCONATE (IV 10%)
Trade Name: Calcium Gluconate
Dosage Form: Injection (IV/intracardiac), 10 cc 10% solution (4.7 mEq Ca^{++}).
Uses: See calcium chloride.
Adult Dosage (Parenteral): For CPR, 10 cc of 10% solution IV or intracardiac. Dosage may be repeated q. 5–10 min. p.r.n. For tetany, 10–20 cc 10% solution slow IV over 5–10 min., then IV infusion of 15 mEq Ca^{2+}/kg in D$_5$W 1,000 cc over 4–12 hours.
Pediatric Dosage (Parenteral): IV, 0.47 mEq/kg (1 cc/kg); intracardiac, 0.3 mEq/kg (0.64 cc/kg). (Maximum dose for infants, 2 cc.)

Contraindications: See calcium chloride.
Precautions: See calcium chloride.
Adverse Reactions: See calcium chloride.
Drug Interactions: See calcium chloride.

Generic Name: CALCIUM SALTS (Oral)
Trade Names: Calcium Gluconate, Calcium Lactate
Dosage Forms: Tablets, Calcium Gluconate (300 mg, 500 mg, 600 mg, 1 gm) and Calcium Lactate (300 mg, 600 mg).
Uses: Treatment and prophylaxis of hypocalcemia.
Adult Dosage (Oral): Calcium Gluconate, 15 gm daily in divided doses; Calcium Lactate, 1.5–3 gm t.i.d with meals.
Pediatric Dosage (Oral): 500 mg/kg/day in divided doses.
Adverse Reactions: Constipation with oral use.

Generic Name: DIGOXIN
Trade Name: Lanoxin
Dosage Forms: Tablets, 0.125 mg, 0.25 mg, 0.5 mg; injection (IV/IM), 0.1 mg/cc (pediatric), 0.25 mg/cc; elixir, 0.05 mg/cc.
Uses: Digitalis glycoside for treatment of congestive heart failure, pulmonary edema, atrial and reentrant supraventricular arrhythmias.
Digoxin Dosage Parameters:
- therapeutic blood level: 0.8–2 ng/cc
- toxic blood level: 2–3 ng/cc
- half-life: approximately 36 hours (1.5 days)
- IV doses: 100% absorption (onset, 5–10 min.)
- oral doses: 80% absorption (onset, 1–2 hours)
- IM doses: approximately equal to oral doses but painful; no advantage unless other routes are contraindicated.

Adult Dosage (Oral): If patient has been on digitalis for past 2 weeks, one-half digitalizing dose. For digitalization, 0.5–0.75 mg by mouth initially, then 0.25–0.5 mg q. 6–8 hours until total loading dose is given (usually 1–1.5 mg/24 hours). For maintenance, 0.125–0.5 mg q.d.
Adult Dosage (Parenteral): For digitalization, 0.25–0.5 mg IV to start, then 0.25 mg q. 4–6 hours to full digitalizing dose (0.5–1 mg/24 hours). For maintenance, 0.125–0.5 mg IV q.d.
Pediatric Dosage (Oral): (*Note:* All maintenance doses are 20%–30% of digitalizing dose q.d.) For a child over 10 years, adult dosage; for a child 2–10 years, digitalizing dose of 40–60 μg/kg by mouth divided q.6 hours; for a child 2 weeks–2 years, digitalizing dose of 40–80 μg/kg by mouth divided q.6 hours.
Pediatric Dosage (Parenteral): For a child over 10 years, adult dosage; for a child 2–10 years, digitalizing dose of 25–40 μg/kg given IV and divided q. 6 hours; for a child 2 weeks–2 years, digitalizing dose of 35–50 μg/kg given IV and divided q. 6 hours.
Contraindications: Ventricular fibrillation, hypersensitivity to cardiac glycosides (rare).
Precautions: Hypokalemia, hypomagnesemia, and hypercalcemia may predispose or enhance toxicity. "Sick sinus" syndrome, incomplete atrioventricular block, or outflow obstruction in idiopathic hypertrophic subaortic stenosis may worsen. Atrial arrhythmias associated with hypermetabolic and febrile states are particularly resistant. Caution is needed

in the presence of renal impairment, premature infants, patients with severe types of cardiac and pulmonary disease. Digoxin toxicity may mimic many of the arrhythmias it is being used to treat.
Adverse Reactions: Gastric upset, e.g., anorexia, nausea, vomiting, diarrhea; visual disturbances, e.g., blurred, yellow vision, diplopia, halos; headache, weakness, drowsiness, paresthesias, cardiac arrhythmias, paroxysmal tachycardia with block and nodal rhythms common, as well as premature ventricular contractions.
Drug Interactions: With antacids, decrease in oral absorption of digitalis. With potassium-depleting diuretics and calcium salts, increase in digitalis toxicity. With sympathomimetics, may precipitate/exacerbate digitalis-induced arrhythmias. With β-blockers, may worsen atrioventricular block. With quinidine, may increase digoxin serum levels.

Generic Name: DIPHENYLHYDANTOIN (IV)
Trade Name: Dilantin
Dosage Forms: Injection, 50 mg/cc (IV use only recommended).
Uses: Antiarrhythmic agent used for premature ventricular contractions, ventricular tachycardia, and paroxysmal tachycardia, especially PAT with block secondary to digitalis toxicity.
Adult Dosage (Parenteral): 100–250 mg q. 5–15 min. slow IV up to toxicity or 750–1000 mg. (IV rate not to exceed 50 mg/min.)
Pediatric Dosage (Parenteral): 3–5 mg/kg slow IV.
Contraindications: Sinus bradycardia, sinoatrial block, second- and third-degree block, Stokes-Adams syndrome.
Precautions: Should be diluted in normal saline only. IV line should be flushed with normal saline after direct IV push to minimize venous irritation.
Adverse Reactions: Rapid IV injection may cause cardiovascular collapse. IM administration can cause tissue necrosis, and absorption is erratic.
Drug Interactions: Should not be mixed with any other medications.

Generic Name: DISOPYRAMIDE
Trade Name: Norpace
Dosage Forms: Capsules, 100 mg and 150 mg.
Uses: Antiarrhythmic, similar to quinidine and procainamide used for treatment of ventricular arrhythmias, particularly premature ventricular tachycardia and contractions.
Adult Dosage (Oral): 100–150 mg q. 6 hours. If loading dose is required, 200–300 mg (usual dosage range, 400–800 mg daily). Therapeutic serum level is 2–4 μg/cc (up to 7 μg/cc). For severe refractory ventricular tachycardia, up to 300–400 mg q. 6 hours with constant cardiac monitoring.
Pediatric Dosage (Oral): Not established.
Contraindications: Cardiogenic shock, preexisting second- or third-degree atrioventricular block (if no pacemaker present), torsade de pointes, hypersensitivity to disopyramide.
Precautions: Renal or hepatic insufficiency, pregnancy, lactation, diabetes. Effects are unpredictable in Wolff-Parkinson-White and "sick sinus" syndromes. Drug has negative inotropic effect. Caution must be used in congestive heart

failure and cardiomyopathies. Anticholinergic activity may be prominent, and may exacerbate myasthenia gravis, urinary retention, other conditions aggravated by anticholinergic activity.

Adverse Reactions: Toxic serum levels generally 9 μg/cc or more. Anticholinergic side-effects include dry mouth, blurred vision, urinary retention, and gastric upset. Drug may precipitate or worsen CHF and preexisting atrioventricular block; hypoglycemia, generalized malaise, hypotension, CNS derangements, hypersensitivity reactions, hepatic enzyme changes may occur.

Drug Interactions: Disopyramide may potentiate activity of other anticholinergic agents. With oral anticoagulants, possible potentiation of hypoprothrombinemic effects.

Generic Name: DOBUTAMINE
Trade Name: Dobutrex
Dosage Forms: Injection (IV), 250 mg.
Uses: Sympathomimetic for short-term inotropic support (direct β-adrenergic stimulation). It does not release endogenous catecholamines as does dopamine.
Adult Dosage (Parenteral): IV infusion of 2.5–10 μg/kg/min. (rates up to 40 μg/kg/min. have been used). Suggested dilution is 250 mg/500 cc normal saline or D_5W for a concentration of 500 μg/cc. (*Note:* Moderate doses decrease pre-load and have minimal chronotropic and blood pressure effects. The effects of high doses resemble those of isoproterenol, e.g., tachycardia and decreased peripheral resistance.)
Pediatric Dosage: Not established.
Contraindications: Idiopathic hypertrophic subaortic stenosis.
Precautions: May precipitate or exacerbate ventricular ectopic activity; increases atrioventricular conduction (digitalize p.r.n.). Exaggerated pressor response may be seen in the presence of preexisting hypertension. It may intensify and extend myocardial ischemia associated with acute myocardial infarction. It may be ineffective in patients who have recently received β-blocking agents.
Adverse Reactions: Dose-related effects seen with doses over 20 μg/kg/min. Ventricular ectopic beats, premature ventricular contractions, chest pain, palpitations, increased heart rate (5–15 beats/min.), increased blood pressure (10–20 mm Hg). Atrioventricular conduction is increased.
Drug Interactions: Incompatible with sodium bicarbonate and alkaline solutions, such as aminophylline and diphenylhydantoin. Dobutamine and nitroprusside together may result in higher cardiac output and lower pulmonary arterial wedge pressures than when either is used alone.

Generic Name: DOPAMINE
Trade Name: Intropin
Dosage Forms: Injection (IV), 200 mg/ampule, 400-mg vial, premixed solution of 400 mg/250 cc D_5W (1600 mg/cc).
Uses: Sympathomimetic for increasing cardiac output, blood pressure, and urine flow via direct, β-l receptor stimulation.
Adult Dosage (Parenteral): Suggested IV dilution is 400 mg/250 cc D_5W or 1600 μg/cc. IV infusion at 2–5 μg/kg/min. to start; may be increased by 5–10 μg/kg/min. up to 50 μg/

kg/min. Most patients require 20 μg/kg/min. or less, but rates of 50–100 μg/kg/min. have been used.
Pediatric Dosage (Parenteral): Safety and efficacy not established. IV doses of 9 μg/kg/min. have been used (range, 0.3–25 μg/kg/min.).
Contraindications: Pheochromocytoma, uncorrected tachyarrhythmias, or ventricular fibrillation.
Precautions: Hypovolemia should be corrected first. Hypoxia, hypercapnia, and acidosis all reduce dopamine effectiveness. Discolored solutions should not be used. Caution must be used with elderly patients, cardiovascular disease, hypertension, angina, hyperthyroidism.
Adverse Reactions: Dose-related. High doses cause vasoconstriction with resulting decrease in renal output, tachycardia, and ventricular arrhythmias. Low doses cause vasodilation with resulting hypotension. Occasionally, nausea, vomiting, and angina occur.
Drug Interactions: Incompatible with sodium bicarbonate and other alkaline solutions. Cyclopropane/halogenated hydrocarbon anesthetics sensitize myocardium to arrhythmias. Fatal ventricular arrhythmias have occurred. With MAO inhibitors, dopamine should be reduced to one-tenth the usual dose. Diphenylhydantoin produces additive bradycardia and hypotension.

Generic Name: EDROPHONIUM
Trade Name: Tensilon
Dosage Forms: Injection (IM/IV), 10 mg/cc.
Uses: Cholinesterase inhibitor with rapid onset (30–60 sec.) and brief duration (5–10 min.) It may be used for termination of paroxysmal supraventricular tachycardias not controlled by vagal maneuvers.
Adult Dosage (Parenteral): 5–10 mg by slow IV push over 30–60 sec. Dose may be repeated in 15–20 min. Failure to respond to two doses indicates alternate therapy should be tried.
Contraindications: Asthma
Precautions: May induce uterine contractions in pregnant women. Digitalis may sensitize myocardium to edrophonium.
Adverse Reactions: "Cholinergic crisis," with nausea, vomiting, diarrhea, blurred vision, increased salivations, bronchospasm, muscle cramps and fasciculations, paralysis, hypotension, bradycardia, cardiac arrest. (Antidote: atropine IV.)

Generic Name: EPINEPHRINE (Injection)
Trade Names: Epinephrine, Adrenalin, Sus-Phrine
Dosage Forms: Injection (subcutaneous) 5 mg/cc (1:200); (IM/subcutaneous IV) 1 mg/cc (1:1000) ampules; (IV/intracardiac) 1 mg/10 cc (1:10,000) preloaded syringe.
Uses: Sympathomimetic used in CPR to stimulate myocardial contractility and coarsen fine ventricular fibrillation before electrical defibrillation. Produces bronchodilation in anaphylactic shock and other hypersensitivity reactions.
Adult Dosage: For CPR, 0.5–1 mg (5–10 cc 1:10,000 solution) IV/intracardiac may be repeated q. 5–10 min. p.r.n. For bronchodilation, 0.2–0.5 cc 1:1000 solution subcutaneously. Dose may be repeated in 20 min. and again q 2 hours p.r.n.;

0.1–0.3 cc of 1:200 solution (Sus-Phrine) may be given subcutaneously and repeated in 4 hours if needed.

Pediatric Dosage: For CPR, 5–10 µg/kg (0.05–0.1cc/kg 1:10,000 solution) intracardiac; 10 µg/kg (0.1 cc of 1:10,000 solution) IV. For bronchodilation, 10 µg/kg (0.01 cc/kg 1:1000 solution) subcutaneously. Dose may be repeated every 4 hours or as often as every 20 min. p.r.n. to a maximum of three days; when utilizing Sus-Phrine at a 1:200 solution, 20–25 µg/kg (0.004–0.005 cc/kg) subcutaneously as a single dose.

Contraindications: (Excluding CPR use.) Narrow angle (congestive) glaucoma, organic brain damage, shock other than anaphylaxis, coronary insufficiency, labor, hypersensitivity to sympathomimetics.

Precautions: Elderly patients and those with hypertension, cardiovascular disease, hyperthyroidism, angina, diabetes, chronic emphysema with degenerative heart disease.

Adverse Reactions: Arrhythmias, palpitations, anginal pain, cerebral hemorrhage, pulmonary edema secondary to peripheral vasoconstriction, anxiety, tremor, local tissue necrosis at injection site.

Drug Interactions: Incompatible with calcium salts, sodium bicarbonate, aminophylline, and diphenylhydantoin. Simultaneous administration with isoproterenol may induce serious arrhythmias. Halogenated anesthetics/cyclopropane may sensitize myocardium to epinephrine-induced arrhythmias.

Generic Name: ISOPROTERENOL (Parenteral)

Trade Name: Isuprel

Dosage Forms: Injection (IM/IV/subcutaneous/intracardiac), 1:5000 ampules, or 1 mg/5 cc; 1:50,000 ampules, or 0.2 mg/10 cc.

Uses: Sympathomimetic for treatment of Stokes-Adams syndrome, cardiac arrest, heart block with ventricular arrhythmias. Primarily used to maintain heart rate in third-degree block.

Adult Dosage (Parenteral): As an IV push or intracardiac injection, 0.02–0.06 mg (1 cc 1:5000 solution diluted with 9 cc normal saline, 0.02 mg/cc). As an IV infusion, 1–5 µg/min. (Up to 40 µg/min. have been used.) Suggested IV dilution of 1 ampule 1:5000 in 250 cc D$_5$W for concentration of 4 µg/cc).

Pediatric Dosage (Parenteral): Usually one-half of adult dose (e.g., 0.01–0.03 mg IV push), then titrate with IV infusion.

Contraindications: Tachycardia due to digitalis toxicity.

Precautions: May worsen shock by systemic vasodilation. Volume deficits must be corrected first. Caution must be used in patients with coronary insufficiency, acute myocardial infarction, diabetes, hyperthyroidism, sensitivity to sympathomimetics. Infusion must be decreased or temporarily discontinued if heart rate rises above 110 beats/min. Light-sensitive; discolored solutions should not be used.

Adverse Reactions: Doses sufficient to increase heart rate to more than 130 beats/min. may induce ventricular arrhythmias. Other reactions include facial flushing, headache, nausea, vomiting, sweating, nervousness, mild tremor, anginal pain, tachycardia, palpitations.

Drug Interactions: Simultaneous administration with epinephrine may induce serious arrhythmias.

Generic Name: LIDOCAINE (Parenteral)

Trade Name: Xylocaine

Dosage Forms: Injection (IM/IV), 100 mg/5 cc preloaded syringe; 1 gm or 2 mg for IV infusions.

Uses: Antiarrhythmic for treatment of ventricular arrhythmias, especially premature extrasystoles and tachycardia.

Adult Dosage (Parenteral): Therapeutic serum levels of 2–6 µg/cc usually achieved by following regimen: IV bolus of 1–2 mg/kg (50–100 mg), followed by IV infusion of 1–5 µg/min. IV bolus may be repeated in 5 min. (maximum of 200–300 mg in 1 hour).

Pediatric Dosage (Parenteral): For a child, 0.5–1 mg/kg IV (not to exceed 100 mg/hour or total dose of 5 mg/kg); for an infant, 0.15–1 mg/kg IV every 20–60 min. p.r.n. (maintenance infusion of 10–50 µg/kg/min.).

Contraindications: Known hypersensitivity to local anesthetics of amide type. Stokes-Adams syndrome, severe degrees of sinoatrial, atrioventricular, or intraventricular heart block.

Precautions: Caution must be used in atrial flutter/fibrillation with preexisting rapid ventricular rate. Dosage adjustments may be necessary in cirrhosis, liver failure, cardiogenic shock, advanced heart failure.

Adverse Reactions: Appear to correlate with plasma levels of 5–9 µg/cc (or IV rates over 5 mg/min. or repeated IV boluses). CNS symptoms include drowsiness, dizziness, excitement, diplopia, tinnitus, muscle twitching, respiratory depression, convulsions. Cardiovascular side-effects include hypotension, bradycardia, prolongation of QRS and PR intervals. Hypersensitivity reactions of urticaria, rash, or edema may occur.

Generic Name: METARAMINOL BITARTRATE

Trade Name: Aramine

Dosage Forms: Injection (IV), 10 mg/cc (100 mg/10 cc in preloaded syringe).

Uses: Vasopressor (direct α- and β-adrenergic stimulation and norepinephrine release).

Adult Dosage (Parenteral): IV bolus of 1–5 mg (0.1–0.5 cc) over 10–30 sec., then IV infusion of 0.1–1 mg/min. (dilution, 100 mg/500 cc D$_5$W or normal saline).

Pediatric Dosage (Parenteral): Single IV dose of 10 µg/kg or IV infusion using dilution of 10 mg/250 cc.

Contraindications: Concomitant use of cyclopropane or halogenated anesthetics.

Precautions: Acidosis must be corrected first, since pressor responses are poor in presence of metabolic acidosis. Rapid IV rates can induce acute pulmonary edema and arrhythmias. Tachyphylaxis may occur. Rebound hypotension may occur after infusion stopped.

Adverse Reactions: See epinephrine.

Drug Interactions: See epinephrine.

Generic Name: METHOXAMINE

Trade Name: Vasoxyl

Dosage Forms: Injection (IM/IV), 10 mg/cc and 20 mg/cc.

Uses: Vasopressor (α-adrenergic vasoconstriction) that is also used to terminate paroxysmal supraventricular tachycardia.

Dosage (Parenteral): IM 10–15 mg; IV, 3–5 mg over 5 min., then 10–15 mg IM if indicated. For termination of PSVT, 5–15 mg IV slowly, or 10–20 mg IM (rarely used).

Contraindications: Shock due to myocardial infarction or peripheral mesenteric thrombosis.

Precautions: May exacerbate CHF or myocardial infarction. Caution is required with hyperthyroidism, hypertension, elderly patients. Volume deficits must be replaced.

Adverse Reactions: Excessive hypertension with severe reflex bradycardia, severe headache, precordial pain, nervousness, dizziness, vomiting, pilomotor response, severe peripheral and visceral vasoconstriction.

Drug Interactions: β-Blocking agents may increase vasoconstriction. Phenothiazines decrease pressor effect; anticholinergics increase pressor effect.

Generic Name: NOREPINEPHRINE (LEVARTERENOL)
Trade Name: Levophed
Dosage Forms: Injection (IV/intracardiac), 4 mg norepinephrine BASE/4 cc ampule (1 mg/cc).
Uses: Sympathomimetic vasopressor (predominantly direct α-stimulation) for restoration of blood pressure in cardiogenic shock.
Adult Dosage (Parenteral): Average initial infusion rate, 8–12 µg BASE/min., which is then adjusted to maintain systolic blood pressure about 80–100 mm Hg with an average maintenance infusion of 2–4 µg BASE/min. Dosage range up to 40–50 µg BASE/min. has been used. (*Note:* 4–8 mg BASE (1–2 ampules) should be diluted in 500 cc D$_5$W (not normal saline) to a final concentration of 8–16 µg/cc.)
Pediatric Dosage (Parenteral): For a child or infant: Initially 0.05 µg/kg/min. (usual IV rate, 2 µg/min.) Dilution is 0.5–1 mg BASE/500 cc D$_5$W to a final concentration of 1–2 µg/cc.
Contraindications: Hypotension secondary to uncorrected blood volume deficits, mesenteric or peripheral vascular thrombosis, pregnancy (causes fetal anoxia).
Precautions: Tissue necrosis may be caused by vasoconstriction or extravasation; treat with phentolamine infiltration of IV site or by IV infusion. Metabolic acidosis must be corrected first, because it inhibits cardiac response. Brownish colored solutions should not be used. Abrupt stopping of infusion may cause hypotensive relapse.
Adverse Reactions: Headache (first sign of overdose), severe hypertension, reflex bradycardia, decreased cardiac output, weakness, tremor, pallor, anxiety, insomnia.
Drug Interactions: Incompatible with diphenylhydantoin, sodium bicarbonate, aminophylline, metaraminol, ampicillin. Normal saline promotes oxidation of drug. With MAO inhibitors and tricyclic antidepressants, it causes severe hypertension. With some anesthetics, e.g., cyclopropane and halothane, may sensitize myocardium to arrhythmias.

Generic Name: POTASSIUM CHLORIDE
Trade Names: KCL, Klorvess, K-Lor, Slow-K, Klotrix
Dosage Forms: Tablets, 8 mEq slow release, 10 mEq slow release; capsules, 8 mEq; injection, 2 mEq/cc (IV only); oral elixirs/solutions, 10% (20 mEq/15 cc) and 20% (40 mEq/15 cc).
Uses: Potassium and chloride replacement in correction of hypokalemia.

Adult Dosage (Oral): 40–60 mEq/day in divided doses (adjust to patient's needs) up to 100–200 mEq/day.
Adult Dosage (Parenteral): Slow IV infusion up to 10 mEq/hour if serum potassium less than 2.5 mEq/liter. Up to 40 mEq/hour if serum potassium less than 2 mEq/liter (maximum recommended dose, 400 mEq/day). Constant cardiac monitoring is required with use of high concentrations. For treatment of digitalis toxicity, 10–15 mEq/hour for 2–4 hours with constant cardiac monitoring.
Pediatric Dosage (Oral/Parenteral): As needed.
Contraindications: Hyperkalemia, impaired renal function with oliguria or azotemia, Addison's disease.
Precautions: Concomitant use of potassium-sparing diuretics. With digitalis, it may induce atrioventricular conduction defects. It is extremely irritating to vein. *Never given IM.*
Adverse Reactions: With oral use, gastric upset, abdominal discomfort, bad taste. With parenteral use, local tissue necrosis. Hyperkalemia must be treated immediately if serum potassium greater than 6.5 mEq/liter:

- at 6–8 mEq/liter: weakness, fatigue, atrioventricular or intraventricular block, widened QRS complexes.
- at 8–9 mEq/liter: atrial arrest, neuromuscular paralysis
- over 9 mEq/liter: idioventricular rhythms, ventricular tachycardia, fibrillation, asystole

For treatment of hyperkalemia, discontinue all potassium chloride and obtain serum potassium level immediately. IV calcium (unless patient is on digitalis), glucose and insulin infusions, kayexalate enemas, dialysis may be given.

Generic Name: PROCAINAMIDE (IM/IV)
Trade Name: Pronestyl
Dosage Forms: Injection (IM/IV), 100 mg/cc; IV only, 500 mg/cc.
Uses: Treatment of ventricular tachycardia, especially that not controlled by lidocaine, or ventricular arrhythmias associated with digitalis toxicity.
Adult Dosage (Parenteral): 100–200 mg IV bolus (at 25–50 mg/min.), followed by 100 mg q. 5 min. p.r.n. (up to 1-gm loading dose). If control achieved, initiate IV drip at 1–5 mg/min. (2 mg/kg/hour).
Pediatric Dosage (Parenteral): 2 mg/kg IV slowly over 5–20 min. (range, 3–6 mg/kg), then IV infusion of 20–80 µg/kg/min.
Contraindications: See procainamide (oral). Infusion rates over 50 mg/min. are associated with increased toxicity. Keep infusion rate at less than or equal to 25–50 mg/min.
Adverse Reactions: See procainamide (oral).
Drug Interactions: See procainamide (oral).

Generic Name: PROCAINAMIDE (Oral)
Trade Names: Pronestyl and Procan
Dosage Forms: Capsules, 250 mg, 375 mg, 500 mg.
Uses: Antiarrhythmic agent similar in activity to lidocaine and quinidine for treatment of atrial and ventricular arrhythmias.
Adult Dosage (Oral): Initial therapy with regular, not sustained release, procainamide. For atrial fibrillation, 1–1.25 gm to start. Dose may be repeated in 1 hour with 750 mg, then 500 mg–1 gm q. 2 hours until arrhythmia stopped (maximum 4 gm/day); for maintenance, 500 mg–1 gm q. 4–

6 hours. For ventricular tachycardia and premature ventricular contraction, 1 gm to start, then 250–500 mg q. 3 hours.
Pediatric Dosage (Oral): 8–15 mg/kg q. 4–6 hours (maximum 1 gm/day) has been used.
Contraindications: Complete atrioventricular heart block, second- or third-degree atrioventricular block (unless pacemaker present), hypersensitivity to procainamide.
Precautions: Anticholinergic activity; therefore, caution is needed in myasthenia gravis, glaucoma, and other conditions aggravated by anticholinergic activity. "Vagolytic" effect can increase atrioventricular conduction. It may be necessary to digitalize patient to control ventricular rate during conversion of atrial flutter. Hepatic or renal disease, CHF, low output cardiac failure may require reduced dose. In hypokalemia, effectiveness is reduced.
Adverse Reactions: Symptoms of toxicity occur at plasma levels of 8–16 μg/cc. Cardiac effects include hypotension, widened QRS complexes, PR interval prolongation, heart block, ventricular tachycardia and fibrillation, asystole. Gastric upset, lupus-like syndrome (positive lupus erythematosus and antinuclear antibody test results, incidence about 50%), with or without symptoms, blood dyscrasias. CNS derangements, including mental depression, weakness, confusion, hallucinations.
Drug Interactions: See disopyramide. Neuromuscular blocking agents and aminoglycosides may be potentiated by procainamide.

Generic Name: PROCAINAMIDE (Sustained Release)
Trade Name: Procan SR
Dosage Forms: Tablets, 250 mg and 500 mg.
Uses: See procainamide. Sustained release tablets should be used for preventative maintenance only.
Adult Dosage (Oral): For a person who weighs 50 kg or less, 500 mg q. 6 hours; for 50–90 kg, 750 mg q. 6 hours; for over 90 kg, 1 gm q. 6 hours.

Generic Name: PROPRANOLOL
Trade Name: Inderal
Dosage Forms: Tablets, 10 mg, 20 mg, 40 mg, 80 mg; injection (IV), 1 mg/cc ampule.
Uses: β-Adrenergic blocker (both β-1 and β-2 receptors) for treatment of various atrial and digitalis-induced arrhythmias, angina, and hypertension.
Adult Dosage (Oral): Dosage must be titrated to response. For arrhythmias, 10–40 mg t.i.d. or q.i.d. For angina, 10 mg t.i.d to start; maintenance, 160–240 mg daily, divided doses. For hypertension, 20–40 mg t.i.d. (up to 480 mg daily).
Adult Dosage (Parenteral): 0.5–3 mg slow IV (1 mg/min. or less). Dose may be repeated in 2–5 min., but additional doses should be delayed at least 4 hours. Maximum dose is 10 mg in resistant ventricular fibrillation. Administration rates of more than 1 mg/min. may cause severe hypotension and asystole.
Pediatric Dosage (Oral): 1–2 mg/kg in three or four divided doses.
Pediatric Dosage (Parenteral): 10–20 μg/kg over 10 min. IV.

Contraindications: Congestive heart failure, right ventricular failure due to pulmonary hypertension, cardiogenic shock, sinus bradycardia, bronchial asthma, heart block greater than first degree, concurrent use of psychotropic agents such as MAO inhibitors, Raynaud's syndrome.
Precautions: May precipitate CHF, severe bradycardia in Wolff-Parkinson-White syndrome, bronchospasm, may mask symptoms of thyrotoxicosis and hypoglycemia (diabetes). Caution is required with hepatic and renal impairment.
Adverse Reactions: Bronchospasm, decreased respiratory function, hypotension, bradycardia, atrioventricular block. May precipitate or aggravate CHF. Hypoglycemia, fatigue, lethargy, vertigo, light-headedness, ataxia, mental derangements, paresthesias, gastric upset, ischemic colitis, mesenteric arterial thrombosis, and hypersensitivity reactions may occur.
Drug Interactions: Potentiates insulin and oral hypoglycemic agents; antagonizes bronchodilation of theophylline and other bronchodilators; worsens digitalis-induced bradycardia.

Generic Name: QUINIDINE GLUCONATE
Trade Name: Quinaglute
Dosage Forms: Tablets, 324 mg; injection (quinidine gluconate) (IM/IV), 80 mg/cc (50 mg BASE/cc).
Uses: Antiarrhythmic agent for atrial arrhythmias and premature ventricular contractions. Parenteral use for treatment of ventricular tachycardia. Long-acting oral forms used for preventive maintenance therapy.
Adult Dosage (Oral): 1–2 tablets (324–648 mg) q. 8–12 hours.
Adult Dosage (Parenteral): For ventricular tachycardia or premature ventricular contractions, 400–600 mg IM q. 2 hours as needed; IV, 16 mg/min. by infusion; 800 mg quinidine gluconate diluted in 50 cc D$_5$W and administered at 1 cc/min. Infusion should be stopped immediately if tachycardia controlled, toxicity appears, or significant hypotension and QRS prolongation (over 25%) occurs. (Caution: IV use is hazardous.)
Pediatric Dosage (Parenteral): IM, 5–10 mg/kg q. 6 hours; IV, 5 mg/kg over 10–15 min. (Extreme caution necessary.)
Contraindications: Digitalis toxicity (with atrioventricular conduction disturbances); hypersensitivity or idiosyncratic reaction to quinidine or quinine; heart block (second- or third-degree, complete); ectopic impulses and rhythms resulting from escape mechanisms.
Precautions: Toxic serum levels, 8–15 μg/cc. Significant hypotension, bradycardia, heart block, and idioventricular rhythms may occur (see also quinidine sulfate).
Adverse Reactions: Cinchonism, which includes nausea, vomiting, diarrhea, tinnitus, visual disturbances, dizziness. Cardiotoxicity, including bradycardia, hypotension, complete heart block with asystole, idioventricular rhythms. CNS effects of syncope, vertigo, confusion, delirium. Hypersensitivity reactions, hemolytic anemia, thrombocytopenic purpura, anaphylaxis.

Generic Name: QUINIDINE SULFATE (Oral)
Trade Names: Quinidine and others.
Dosage Forms: Tablets, 100 mg, 200 mg, 300 mg, (sustained release, 300 mg); capsules, 200 mg, 300 mg.

Uses: Antiarrhythmic agent for atrial arrhythmias (e.g., atrial premature contractions and paroxysmal tachycardia, atrial flutter and fibrillation, paroxysmal supraventricular tachycardia) and premature ventricular contractions.

Adult Dosage (Oral): Therapeutic blood levels, 2–8 µg/cc. For maintenance, 200–300 mg t.i.d or q.i.d. For premature atrial or ventricular contractions, 200–300 mg q.i.d. up to 200–400 mg q. 4–6 hours (maximum 3–4 gm/day). For PSVT, 400–600 mg q. 2–3 hours until paroxysm is terminated (maximum, 3–4 gm/day). For conversion of atrial fibrillation, 200 mg q. 2–3 hours for five to eight doses, then daily doses up to 3–4 gm/day until rhythm restored or toxicity seen.)

Pediatric Dosage (Oral): 10–30 mg/kg/day in divided doses.

Contraindications: See quinidine gluconate.

Precautions: Test dose of 200 mg orally or IM recommended before treatment. Renal or hepatic disease may require dosage adjustments. Hypokalemia may cause refractoriness or predispose to quinidine-induced arrhythmias. Caution in myasthenia gravis, bronchial asthma, hyperthyroidism, CHF, glucose-6-phosphate dihydrogenase (G6PD) deficiency.

Adverse Reactions: See quinidine gluconate.

Drug Interactions: May potentiate action of neuromuscular blocking agents and aminoglycosides.

Generic Name: SODIUM BICARBONATE (IV)

Trade Name: Sodium Bicarbonate

Dosage Forms: Injection (IV), 50 mEq/50 cc preloaded syringe (8.4%), 10 mEq/10 cc preloaded syringe (pediatric).

Uses: Treatment of metabolic acidosis.

Adult Dosage (Parenteral): 1 mEq/kg IV initially (approximately 1.5–2 ampules), then 1 ampule q. 5–10 min. p.r.n. Repeat doses should be governed by arterial blood gas and pH values. (*Note:* 2.5 ampules (150 cc) will raise serum pH approximately 0.05–0.1 unit.)

Pediatric Dosage (Parenteral): 1–2 mEq/kg (at rate less than 10 cc/min).

Precautions: In children under 2 years old, rapid injection rates (over 10 cc/min.) may cause hypernatremia, increased cerebrospinal fluid pressure, intracranial hemorrhage.

Drug Interactions: Direct IV admixture incompatible with calcium salts, sympathomimetics, dopamine, hydrocortisone, atropine, lidocaine.

Generic Name: VERAPAMIL (IV)

Trade Names: Calan, Isoptin

Dosage Forms: Injection (IV), 5 mg/cc (2 cc ampules).

Uses: Calcium slow-channel blocker used primarily for treatment of supraventricular tachyarrhythmias and control of ventricular rate in atrial flutter/fibrillation.

Adult Dosage: Initial dose of 5–10 mg (0.075–0.15 mg/kg) IV bolus over 2 min; repeated with 10-mg slow IV bolus in 30 min., if necessary. In older patients, dose given over 3 min.

Pediatric Dosage (Investigational): In patients 1–15 years old, 0.1–0.3 mg/kg single IV dose, which may be repeated in 30 min. In patients less than 1 year old, 0.1–0.2 mg/kg single IV dose, which may be repeated in 30 min.

Contraindications: As for oral verapamil. Concurrent administration of IV β-blocking agents.

Precautions: Slow IV over at least 2 min. Other precautions as for oral verapamil.

Adverse Reactions: Hypotension, bradycardia, severe tachycardia, dizziness, headache, CNS depression. (See also oral verapamil.)

Drug Interactions: See oral verapamil.

ANTIHYPERTENSIVES, ANTIANGINAL AGENTS

Generic Name: ALPHA-METHYLDOPA

Trade Name: Aldomet

Dosage Forms: Tablets, 125 mg, 250 mg, 500 mg; injection (IV only) 250 mg/5 cc.

Uses: Antihypertensive agent (depletes catecholamines).

Adult Dosage (Oral): 250 mg b.i.d. or t.i.d. (up to 3 gm/day in two to four divided doses).

Adult Dosage (Parenteral): 250–500 mg (diluted in 100 cc D_5W) given slowly IV over 30–60 min., repeated q. 6 hours p.r.n.

Pediatric Dosage (Oral): 10 mg/kg/day in two to four divided doses (up to 65 mg/kg/day or 3 gm/day).

Pediatric Dosage (Parenteral): 20–40 mg/kg/24 hours, slow IV in divided doses q. 6 hours p.r.n. Maximum dose is 65 mg/kg/day.

Contraindications: Hypersensitivity to methyldopa. Active hepatic disease, hepatitis, cirrhosis. Liver disorders associated with prior methyldopa therapy.

Precautions: Renal impairment. Paradoxical pressor response after parenteral doses.

Adverse Reactions: Transient sedation and drowsiness often occur initially. Occasional vertigo, lactation, dry mouth, nasal stuffiness, gastric upset, postural hypotension, edema, positive Coombs' test, liver damage, drug fever, depression, impotence may occur. Rarely, hemolytic anemia, thrombocytopenia, and systemic lupus erythematosus.

Generic Name: CLONIDINE

Trade Names: Catapres, Combi-pres (in combination with chlorthalidone)

Dosage Forms: Tablets, 0.1 mg, 0.2 mg.

Uses: Antihypertensive; acts centrally to decrease sympathetic outflow.

Adult Dosage (Oral): Initially, 0.1 mg b.i.d.; increased at weekly intervals by 0.1–0.2 mg to desired response. Maximum dose, 2.4 mg/day.

Precautions: Abrupt withdrawal may cause hypertensive crisis due to sudden catecholamine release; doses should be tapered slowly over 3–7 days. Concomitant administration of tricyclic antidepressants may lead to hypertension. Caution required in CHF, myocardial insufficiency, chronic renal failure, recent myocardial infarction.

Adverse Reactions: Dry mouth, sedation, drowsiness occur most frequently. Constipation, dizziness, orthostatic hypotension, impotence, and allergic manifestations occur occasionally. Edema, CNS depression and excitement, and increased alcohol sensitivity reported.

Drug Interactions: With tricyclic antidepressants, may lead to hypertension.

Generic Name: DIAZOXIDE (IV)

Trade Name: Hyperstat

Dosage Forms: Injection (IV), 300 mg/20 cc ampules.

Uses: Antihypertensive agent for emergency reduction of blood pressure in malignant hypertension.

Adult Dosage (Parenteral): Bolus of 150–300 mg (or 5 mg/kg) rapidly IV (10–30 sec.), which may be repeated in 30 min.; then at 4- to 24-hour intervals p.r.n.

Pediatric Dosage (Parenteral): 5–10 mg/kg rapidly by IV push.

Contraindications: Hypersensitivity to thiazides. Treatment of compensatory hypertension associated with aortic coarctation or arteriovenous shunt.

Precautions: Fall in blood pressure cannot be titrated. Tolerance may develop if edema not prevented by diuretic. Caution is required in diabetes, concomitant use of other vasodilator therapy, and impaired cardiac or cerebral circulation.

Adverse Reactions: Hyperglycemia, salt and water retention, edema, gastric distress, hyperuricemia, hypertrichosis, hypotension, pain at injection site, angina, vertigo, flushing.

Generic Name: GUANETHIDINE

Trade Name: Ismelin

Dosage Forms: Tablets, 10 mg, 25 mg.

Uses: Antihypertensive agent for treatment of moderate to severe essential hypertension.

Adult Dosage (Oral): 10 mg initially, increased by 10- to 25-mg increments at 5–7 day intervals, depending on response. Usual maintenance dose is 25–50 mg q.d.

Pediatric Dosage (Oral): 10–60 mg q.d.

Contraindications: Hypersensitivity to guanethidine. Use of MAO inhibitors. Pheochromocytoma. Frank congestive heart failure not due to hypertension.

Precautions: May significantly compromise renal blood flow, causing fluid retention. Caution in renal impairment, congestive heart failure, bronchial asthma, peptic ulcer, coronary insufficiency, cerebral vascular disease.

Adverse Reactions: Frequent dizziness, weakness, diarrhea, bradycardia, syncope, and orthostatic hypotension. Occasional inhibition of ejaculation, sodium and fluid retention, and blurred vision.

Drug Interactions: Decreased antihypertensive effect with concomitant use of tricyclic antidepressants, CNS stimulants, and phenothiazines. With MAO inhibitors, hypertensive crisis. With vasopressors, hypertension, risk of cardiac arrhythmias. With reserpine, excessive hypotension and mental depression.

Generic Name: HYDRALAZINE

Trade Name: Apresoline

Dosage Forms: Tablets, 10 mg, 25 mg, 50 mg, 100 mg; injection (IM/IV), 20 mg/cc ampules.

Uses: Antihypertensive for treatment of essential hypertension (direct arteriolar vasodilation).

Adult Dosage (Oral): 10 mg q.i.d. for first 2–4 days, increased slowly to 25–50 mg q.i.d. if necessary (maximum of 200–300 mg daily).

Adult Dosage (Parenteral): 20–40 mg IM or slow IV, repeated as needed (generally q. 4–6 hours).

Pediatric Dosage (Oral): 10–100 mg q.d., in divided doses.

Contraindications: Hypersensitivity to hydralazine. Coronary artery disease (may exacerbate angina). Rheumatic mitral valve disease (may precipitate congestive heart failure).

Precautions: Slow acetylators should not receive more than 200 mg q.d. Propranolol may be used to prevent tachycardia. Caution in patients with advanced congestive heart failure.

Adverse Reactions: Primarily dose/duration-dependent. Frequently headache, tachycardia, palpitation, flushing, anorexia, nausea, dizziness. Occasional sweating, drug fever, skin rash, peripheral neuropathy (treat with pyridoxine). Systemic lupus erythematosus may develop. This effect is primarily dose and duration dependent.

Generic Name: ISOSORBIDE DINITRATE

Trade Names: Isordil, Sorbitrate

Dosage Forms: Tablets (oral), 5 mg, 10 mg, 20 mg, 30 mg, 40 mg (sustained release); capsules, 40 mg (sustained release); sublingual tablets, 2.5 mg, 5 mg, 10 mg.

Uses: Antianginal vasodilator used sublingually for treatment of acute angina pectoris and orally for prophylaxis and long-term management.

Adult Dosage (Oral): 5–30 mg q.i.d. (regular tablets); 40 mg (sustained release) q. 6–12 hours; sublingual, 2.5–10 mg p.r.n. (q. 2–3 hours).

Contraindications: Severe postural hypotension. Severe anemia. Hypersensitivity to organic nitrates.

Precautions: See nitroglycerin.

Adverse Reactions: See nitroglycerin.

Drug Interactions: See nitroglycerin.

Generic Name: METOPROLOL

Trade Name: Lopressor

Dosage Forms: Tablets, 50 mg, 100 mg.

Uses: β-1 blocking agent for treatment of hypertension. Also used investigationally for treatment of paroxysmal supraventricular tachycardia.

Adult Dosage (Oral): 50–100 mg bi.d. or t.i.d. with meals (range, 100–450 mg daily). Should be withdrawn slowly over 1–2 weeks if discontinuation is necessary.

Contraindications: Sinus bradycardia, heart block greater than first degree, cardiogenic shock, overt congestive heart failure, right ventricular failure secondary to pulmonary hypertension.

Precautions: Asthma, congestive heart failure, atrioventricular conduction defects, Raynaud's defects, cardiomegaly, hyperthyroidism, labile diabetes (may mask symptoms of hypoglycemia), renal or hepatic impairment.

Adverse Reactions: Fatigue, dizziness, headaches, depression, bronchospasm, shortness of breath, diarrhea, gastric upset, mental disturbances, bradycardia, dry eyes and mucous membranes, rash, pruritus, reversible alopecia, decreased libido. Abrupt withdrawal may exacerbate angina or lead to myocardial infarction in ischemic patients.

Drug Interactions: With digitalis, additive bradycardia. With sympathomimetics, antagonistic effects. With catecholamine-depleting agents (e.g., reserpine), additive effects.

Generic Name: MINOXIDIL
Trade Name: Loniten
Dosage Forms: Tablets, 2.5 mg, 10 mg.
Uses: Antihypertensive. Nonadrenergic vasodilator for treatment of severe hypertension not manageable with maximal diuretic doses and other antihypertensive agents.
Adult Dosage (Oral): 5 mg q.d. to start, increased to 10, 20, then 40 mg q.d. in single or divided doses (up to 100 mg q.d.). Usual maintenance dose, 10–40 mg q.d.
Pediatric Dosage (Oral): For a child under 12 years old, 0.2 mg/kg/day to start (up to 50 mg q.d.). Usual maintenance dose, 0.25–1 mg/kg q.d. (*Note:* A diuretic, e.g., furosemide, should always be prescribed with minoxidil.)
Contraindications: Pheochromocytoma.
Precautions: Congestive heart failure, angina, recent myocardial infarction, renal impairment, patients on dialysis. Too rapid blood pressure control may precipitate cerebrovascular accident or myocardial infarction.
Adverse Reactions: Hypertrichosis (80% incidence), tachycardia, angina, (pretreatment with β-blockers or methyldopa required), edema, salt and water retention, rash, pericardial effusion and tamponade.
Drug Interactions: With CNS depressants, sedative-hypnotics, alcohol, and other antihypertensive agents, additive hypotension.

Generic Name: NADOLOL
Trade Name: Corgard
Dosage Forms: Tablets, 40 mg, 80 mg, 120 mg.
Uses: β-1 blocker for treatment of angina pectoris and mild to severe hypertension. Also used investigationally in treatment of atrial and ventricular arrhythmias.
Adult Dosage (Oral): 40 mg initially, increased p.r.n. every 3–7 days. Angina dosage range, 80–240 mg q.d.; hypertension dosage range, 80–320 mg q.d.
Contraindications: See metoprolol.
Precautions: See metoprolol.
Adverse Reactions: See metoprolol.
Drug Interactions: See metoprolol.

Generic Name: NIFEDIPINE
Trade Name: Procardia
Dosage Form: Capsules, 10 mg.
Uses: Calcium channel blocker used primarily for treatment of chronic angina and vasospastic (variant) angina.
Adult Dosage (Oral): 10 mg t.i.d. to start. Usual dose, 10–20 mg t.i.d. Coronary artery spasms may require 20–30 mg q.i.d. Maximum recommended daily dose, 120–180 mg.
Contraindications: Known hypersensitivity to nifedipine. Use in pregnancy not established.

Precautions: May precipitate angina in patients abruptly withdrawn from β-blocking agents. Decreased coronary perfusion, associated with decreased diastolic pressure and increased heart rate, may increase angina.
Adverse Reactions: (These are primarily a result of vasodilating effects and are dose-related.) Hypotension, dizziness, light-headedness, headache, flushing, weakness, peripheral edema. Also gastric upset, nasal and chest congestion with dyspnea, joint stiffness, muscle cramps, nervousness, blurred vision, dermatitis, fever, chills, sexual difficulties, increased angina.
Drug Interactions: With β-blocking agents, excessive hypotension and congestive heart failure symptoms.

Generic Name: NITROGLYCERIN
Trade Names: Nitrostat, Nitrol, Nitro-Bid, Transderm-Nitro, Nitro-Dur
Dosage Forms: Tablets (sublingual), 0.15 mg, 0.3 mg, 0.4 mg, 0.6 mg; ointment, 2%; transdermal disks, 5 mg, 10 mg; capsules (sustained release), 2.5 mg, 6.5 mg.
Uses: Venodilation and coronary artery vasodilation. Used intermittently to prevent or relieve acute attacks of angina pectoris. Sustained release forms available for prophylaxis.
Adult Dosage (Sublingual): 0.15–0.4 mg initially, which may be repeated at 5-min. intervals three times. Doses must be individualized; some patients require up to 0.6 mg.
Adult Dosage (Ointment): 1–2 inches applied q. 3–4 hours p.r.n. (up to 4–5 inches per application).
Adult Dosage (Transdermal Disk): One 5-mg or 10-mg disk applied to chest q. 24 hours.
Adult Dosage (Sustained Release): 2.5–6.5 mg p.o. q. 8–12 hours.
Contraindications: Hypersensitivity to nitroglycerin, increased intraocular pressure, severe anemia, increased intracranial pressure.
Precautions: Glaucoma, head trauma, cerebral hemorrhage. Concurrent use of drugs and/or conditions that may reduce myocardial oxygen supply or increase oxygen demand. Tablets should be kept in their original container and protected from heat to avoid potency loss.
Adverse Reactions: Headache, blurred vision, dry mouth, vertigo, weakness, postural hypotension, palpitations, syncope, rash, methemoglobinemia, iatrogenic organic nitrate dependence, and tolerance may develop.

Generic Name: NITROGLYCERIN (IV)
Trade Name: Tridil, Nitroglycerin
Dosage Forms: Injection (IV only), 25 mg/cc (must be diluted before use).
Uses: Venodilation to reduce cardiovascular preload and arteriolar dilation to reduce afterload. Used for blood pressure control in perioperative hypertension and during surgical procedures, treatment of congestive heart failure associated with acute myocardial infarction, and treatment of angina pectoris not responding to recommended doses of β-blockers and organic nitrates.
Adult Dosage: (Must be titrated to desired response.) Initially, 5 μg/min. Titrated with increments of 5 μg/min. q. 3–5 min. until response seen. If no response at 20 μg/min., titrated with increments of 10–20 μg/min. (suggested dilution of 25

mg/250 cc normal saline or D_5W, for a concentration of 100 µg/cc). Concentrations greater than 400 µg/cc should be avoided because propylene glycol in diluent may precipitate. (*Note:* Drug must be mixed in *glass* IV bottles only and administered through special non-PVC nitroglycerin infusion tubing; 40%–80% of dose may be absorbed by standard PVC IV tubing.)

Contraindications: Hypersensitivity to organic nitrates, uncorrected hypovolemia, increased intracranial pressure, constrictive pericarditis, pericardial tamponade.

Precautions: Renal and/or hepatic disease. Excessive hypotension may compromise effective coronary perfusion. Attendant risk of ischemia and thrombosis. Paradoxical bradycardia and increased angina pectoris may accompany nitroglycerin-induced hypotension.

Adverse Reactions: Primarily headache, then tachycardia, hypotension, nausea, vomiting, restlessness, apprehension, muscle twitching, retrosternal discomfort, palpitations, vertigo, abdominal pain.

Generic Name: PAPAVERINE

Trade Name: Pavabid, Papaverine

Dosage Forms: Tablets, 30 mg, 60 mg, 100 mg, 200 mg, 500 mg; capsules (sustained release), 150 mg; injection (IV), 30 mg/cc.

Uses: Spasmolytic and vasodilating agent for treatment of various obstructive and vasospastic diseases and cerebral vascular insufficiency. Questionable use in treatment of angina.

Adult Dosage (Oral): 150 mg q. 8–12 hours (sustained release form), up to 300 mg q. 12 hours.

Adult Dosage (Parenteral): 30–120 mg slow IV, which may be repeated q. 3 hours p.r.n. (with extreme caution to avoid arrhythmias).

Contraindications: Complete atrioventricular block.

Precautions: Glaucoma. Too rapid IV administration may produce arrhythmias, apnea.

Adverse Reactions: Nausea, gastric upset, abdominal discomfort, drowsiness, headache, flushing of face, hyperhidrosis, tachycardia, tachypnea, hepatic hypersensitivity reactions.

Generic Name: PRAZOSIN

Trade Name: Minipress

Dosage Forms: Capsules, 1 mg, 2 mg, 5 mg.

Uses: Antihypertensive agent. Produces direct arteriolar vasodilation and sympatholytic effect that blocks reflex tachycardia.

Adult Dosage (Oral): 1 mg b.i.d. or t.i.d. (up to 20 mg q.d.). Usual maintenance dose, 6–15 mg/day, divided q. 8–12 hours.

Precautions: When another antihypertensive agent is added, prazosin dose must be reduced to 1–2 mg t.i.d. and retitrated. Initial dose should be limited to 1 mg and increased slowly. Syncope, dizziness, light-headedness, loss of consciousness may occur within 30–90 min. of initial dose or with rapid dosage increases. Severe tachycardia, e.g., heart rate greater than 120–160 beats/min., may precede syncopal episode.

Adverse Reactions: See precautions. Also drowsiness, fatigue, gastric upset and disturbances, dry mouth, blurred vision,

diaphoresis, tinnitus, nasal congestion, urinary frequency, or incontinence.

Drug Interactions: With CNS depressants, sedative-hypnotics, alcohol, other antihypertensive agents—additive hypotension.

Generic Name: RESERPINE

Trade Name: Serpasil

Dosage Forms: Tablets, 0.1 mg, 0.25 mg, 1 mg; injection (IM), 2.5 mg/cc.

Uses: Antihypertensive agent for treatment of mild essential hypertension and hypertension emergencies.

Adult Dosage (Oral): 0.5 mg q.d. for 1–2 weeks, then 0.1–0.25 mg q.d.

Adult Dosage (Parenteral): For hypertensive emergency, 0.5–1 mg IM stat, then 2–4 mg q. 3 hours p.r.n.

Pediatric Dosage (Oral): 0.25–0.5 mg q.d.

Contraindications: Hypersensitivity to rauwolfia alkaloids. Mental and suicidal depression/electroshock therapy. Peptic ulcer, ulcerative colitis.

Precautions: Parenteral onset slow (1–3 hours). Severe withdrawal symptoms of depression after high doses. Severe hypotension with IM doses over 0.5 mg.

Adverse Reactions: Frequent CNS disturbances (depression, drowsiness, weakness, lethargy, vertigo, headache). Gastric upset, abdominal pain, diarrhea, hypotension, nasal congestion. Incidence of drug-induced depression seems to be dose-related.

Drug Interactions: With MAO inhibitors, may cause severe hypertension.

Generic Name: SODIUM NITROPRUSSIDE

Trade Name: Nipride

Dosage Forms: Injection (IV), 50 mg.

Uses: Antihypertensive vasodilator. Both arterial and venous pressures are lowered. IV onset is immediate and duration brief (1–10 min.).

Adult Dosage (Parenteral): IV infusion at 3 µg/kg/min. to start (range, 0.5–10 µg/kg/min.). Rate should not exceed 10 µg/kg/min. or 800 µg/min. Suggested dilution of 50 mg in 250 cc D_5W produces a 200 µg/cc concentration.

Pediatric Dosage (Parenteral): Same as adult dosage.

Contraindications: Arteriovenous shunt, coarctation of aorta.

Precautions: Solution must be protected from light and diluted in preservative-free D_5W only. Fresh solutions must be used and discarded after 4 hours. Infusion device should be used for administration. Metabolized to cyanide and thiocyanate in tissues/liver. Caution in renal and hepatic impairment, vitamin B_{12} deficiency, hypothyroidism. (Thiocyanate inhibits iodine uptake.)

Adverse Reactions: Thiocyanate toxicity with thiocyanate levels of 100 µg/cc. Tinnitus, blurred vision, fatigue, delirium, anorexia, skin rash, dyspnea, dilated pupils, pink skin color, coma. Also symptoms of rapid reduction in blood pressure, e.g., nausea, sweating, headache, palpitations, substernal distress.

Drug Interactions: With dopamine, higher cardiac output, lower pulmonary vascular resistance (synergistic). Should not be mixed with any other medications.

Generic Name: TRIMETHAPHAN CAMPHOR SULFO-
NATE

Trade Name: Arfonad

Dosage Forms: Injection (IV), 500 mg/10 cc (50/mg/cc).

Uses: Antihypertensive. Produces cholinergic and adrenergic
blockade.

Adult Dosage (Parenteral): Slow IV infusion (1 gm/500 cc
D_5W). Initially, 0.5–1 mg/min. (0.25–0.5 cc/min.); rate adjusted to response. In hypertensive emergency, may increase to 1–15 mg/min.

Contraindications: Hypovolemia, shock, uncorrected anemia,
asphyxia, uncorrected respiratory insufficiency.

Precautions: Use in children; pregnant women; elderly, debilitated patients; patients with hepatic, cardiac, or renal
disease; diabetes, degenerate CNS disease, allergic individuals (drug releases histamine).

Adverse Reactions: All side-effects of ganglionic blockade:
orthostatic hypotension, tachycardia, urinary retention,
constipation, parolytic ileus, angina, dry mouth, gastric upset, cycloplegia, mydriasis, weakness, xerostomia, urticaria, pruritus.

Drug Interactions: Incompatible with alkaline solutions.

Generic Name: VERAPAMIL (Oral)

Trade Name: Calan

Dosage Forms: Tablets, 80 mg, 120 mg.

Uses: Calcium slow channel blocker for treatment of angina
pectoris, including vasospastic (Prinzmetal's variant), unstable (crescendo), and chronic stable angina.

Adult Dosage (Oral): 80 mg t.i.d. to q.i.d. to start. Increased
at daily or weekly intervals until desired response obtained
(24–48 hours recommended between dosage increments).
Dosage range, 240–480 mg daily.

Contraindications: Severe left ventricular dysfunction, hypotension (systolic blood pressure under 90 mm Hg), cardiogenic shock, "sick sinus" syndrome (except with functioning pacemaker), second- or third-degree atrioventricular
block.

Precautions: Hepatic and/or renal impairment. Safe use during pregnancy/lactation not established.

Adverse Reactions: Hypotension, pulmonary/peripheral edema,
bradycardia, congestive heart failure, atrioventricular block
(third-degree), dizziness, headache, fatigue, gastric upset,
constipation, elevated liver enzymes. Occasional CNS
symptoms including blurred vision, paresthesias, equilibrium disorders, muscle cramps, syncope.

Drug Interactions: With β-blockers, additive negative ino-
tropic/chronotropic effects. May be therapeutically useful,
however. With digitalis, increases in serum digoxin levels
of 50%–75%; possible digitalis toxicity. With antihypertensive agents and quinidine, additive hypotensive effects.

ANTICONVULSANTS

Generic Name: CARBAMAZEPINE

Trade Name: Tegretol

Dosage Forms: Tablets, 200 mg.

Uses: Anticonvulsant for many types of seizures, including
psychomotor, grand mal, and mixed seizure patterns. Also
an analgesic agent for pain associated with trigeminal neuralgia.

Adult Dosage (Oral): For epilepsy, 200 mg b.i.d. initially,
increased by 200 mg/day p.r.n., up to 1600 mg daily. Usual
dose, 800–1200 mg q.d. in divided doses. For trigeminal
neuralgia, 100 mg b.i.d. to start, which may be increased
by 100 mg q. 12 hours (up to 1200 mg q.d. in divided doses).
Dose should be increased gradually over 7–10 days to minimize side-effects.

Pediatric Dosage (Oral): For epilepsy in a child 6–12 years
old, 400–800 mg q.d. in divided doses; for a child over 15
years old, 1000–1200 mg q.d. in divided doses.

Contraindications: Bone marrow depression, hypersensitivity
to carbamazepine or tricyclic compounds. Concurrent MAO
inhibitor therapy.

Precautions: Should not be used for petit mal seizures responsive to other agents. Pregnancy, MAO inhibitor cross-
allergenicity, hepatic impairment. Acute withdrawal of drug
may precipitate status epilepticus. Carbamazepine should
not be administered until at least 14 days after discontinuing
MAO inhibitors.

Adverse Reactions: Dizziness, gastric upset, diarrhea, ataxia,
headache are frequent. Also stomatitis, rashes, photosensitivity nystagmus and other visual disturbances, syncope,
congestive heart failure, pulmonary edema, thrombophlebitis, aggravation of hypertension and blood dyscrasias, including aplastic anemia, leukopenia, agranulocytosis have
been reported.

Drug Interactions: With MAO inhibitors, hyperpyrexia, excitability, seizures.

Generic Name: DIAZEPAM

Trade Name: Valium

Dosage Forms: Tablets, 2 mg, 5 mg, 10 mg; injection (IM/
IV) 10 mg/2 cc.

Uses: Benzodiazepin derivative for treatment of anxiety, skeletal muscle spasm, acute seizure episodes (including status
epilepticus).

Adult Dosage (Oral): 2–10 mg b.i.d. to q.i.d.

Adult Dosage (Parenteral): For muscle spasm, 10 mg IM, which
may be repeated in 3–4 hours with 5–10 mg. For seizures,
5–10 mg slow IV (no faster than 5 mg/min.), which may be
repeated in 10–20 min., up to 30 mg in 8 hours.

Pediatric Dosage (Oral): For a child over 6 months, 1–2.5 mg
t.i.d. to q.i.d. (muscle spasm or adjunctive anticonvulsant
therapy).

Pediatric Dosage (Parenteral): For seizures in a child 1 month
to 5 years, 0.2–0.5 mg slow IV, repeated q. 2–5 min. p.r.n.
to a maximum of 5 mg. For seizures in a child over 5 years,

1 mg slow IV repeated q. 2–5 min. p.r.n. to a maximum of 10 mg. May repeat seizure doses again in 2–4 hours.

Contraindications: Hypersensitivity to diazepam, neonates under 1 month old. Glaucoma (acute narrow angle and open angle). Psychosis, shock, coma, acute alcohol withdrawal seizures.

Precautions: IV administration may cause severe hypotension. Not recommended for seizure prophylaxis. Extravasation or intra-arterial administration should be avoided. Caution in elderly, debilitated, children, depression and/or suicidal tendencies. May be habit-forming and cause barbiturate-like withdrawal symptoms.

Adverse Reactions: From oral use: drowsiness, ataxia, fatigue, vertigo, dizziness, paradoxical hyperexcitation, hallucinations, nightmares (especially in elderly), rash, hepatic abnormalities, jaundice. From parenteral use: tissue necrosis, thrombophlebitis, hypotension, respiratory depression, premature ventricular contractions, laryngospasm, cardiovascular collapse.

Drug Interaction: See chlordiazepoxide.

Generic Name: DIPHENYLHYDANTOIN
Trade Name: Dilantin
Dosage Forms: Tablets, 50 mg (chewable); capsules, 30 mg, 100 mg; injection, 50 mg/cc (IV use only recommended); oral suspension, 30 mg/5 cc, 125 mg/5 cc.
Uses: Anticonvulsant for various types of seizures (e.g., grand mal and psychomotor seizures). Antiarrhythmic (see Diphenylhydantoin IV).
Adult Dosage (Oral): Loading dose of 1 gm in divided doses over 4 hours, then 300–400 mg q.d. This usually achieves therapeutic levels in 8–12 hours.
Adult Dosage (Parenteral): Loading dose of 750–1000 mg slow IV no faster than 50 mg/min. IM not recommended because of slow, erratic absorption.
Pediatric Dosage (Oral): Usual maintenance, 5–7 mg/kg/day divided q. 12–24 hours (up to 300 mg/day). Loading dose method: 500–600 mg divided doses to start, then usual maintenance dose q.d. (*Note:* Without a loading dose, steady state plasma levels are not achieved for 5–15 days. Therapeutic serum levels, 10–20 µg/cc.)
Contraindications: Hypersensitivity to hydantoins.
Precautions: Pregnancy, uremia (protein-binding displacement), liver disease, elderly and/or severely ill patients (variable clearance rates). Abrupt drug withdrawal may precipitate status epilepticus.
Adverse Reactions: Frequently dose-related (toxic serum level greater than 20 µg/cc):
- 20–30 µg/cc, nystagmus
- 30–40 µg/cc, ataxia, slurred speech
- over 40 µg/cc, mental confusion, somnolence, lethargy
- over 50 µg/cc, coma

Also gastric upset, gum hyperplasia, megaloblastic anemia, reversible lymph node hyperplasia ("pseudolymphoma"), rashes, blood dyscrasias, liver damage, toxic hepatitis, hirsutism.
Drug Interaction: Barbiturates may increase diphenylhydantoin metabolism, but effect varies and is unpredictable. Oral anticoagulants, disulfiram, phenylbutazone increase di-

phenylhydantoin toxicity. With chronic alcohol ingestion, anticonvulsant effect is decreased. High doses of tricyclic antidepressants and antipsychotics may increase seizure risk.

Generic Name: MAGNESIUM SULFATE (Parenteral)
Trade Name: Magnesium Sulfate
Dosage Forms: Injection (IM/IV), 1 gm/2 cc ampule (50%), 5 gm/10 cc ampule (50%) (4.06 mEq Mg^{++}/cc).
Uses: Anticonvulsant for treatment of seizures due to eclampsia and hypomagnesemia, and arrhythmias secondary to hypomagnesemia and digitalis toxicity.
Adult Dosage (Parenteral): For severe hypomagnesemia, 2–4 gm (16–32 mEq) daily IM or slow IV infusion in divided doses. Repeat daily until serum levels return to normal. For eclampsia, 1–2 mg IM initially then 1 gm q. 30 min. until relief obtained. (May also be given IV as 10% solution at rate no faster than 2–3 cc/min. Use Extreme Caution.) (Antiarrhythmic for paroxysmal tachycardia): 15–20 cc of 20% solution over 30–60 seconds (hazardous).
Pediatric Dosage (Parenteral): As an anticonvulsant, 20–40 mg/kg IM of 20% solution, 100–200 mg/kg IV as 1%–3% solution (severe cases only) over 1 hour.
Precautions: Renal impairment. Hypomagnesemia may predispose to digitalis toxicity. IV rate should not exceed 150 mg/min. (1.5 cc/min. of 10% solution).
Adverse Reactions: Disappearance of patellar reflex is useful sign of clinical toxicity. Normal serum level, 1.5–2.5 mEq/liter. Toxicities correlate well with serum levels:
- at over 4 mEq/liter, deep tendon reflexes decrease, hypotension, nausea
- at over 7 mEq/liter, CNS depression, muscular weakness, flushing, sweating
- at over 10 mEq/liter, loss of deep tendon reflexes, heart block, respiratory paralysis
- at over 12 mEq/liter, possibly fatal

Rapid IV administration may produce symptoms of flushing, intense heat in throat and radiating down body. (Antidote: 10–20 cc 10% calcium gluconate over 5–10 min. IV.)
Drug Interactions: Incompatible with calcium salts and sodium bicarbonate.

Generic Name: PARALDEHYDE
Trade Name: Paraldehyde
Dosage Forms: Injection (IM/IV) 2 cc, 5 cc, 10 cc amps.; oral solution 15 cc, 30 cc.
Adult Dosage (Oral): 5–10 cc p.o. q. 4–6 hours for 24 hours, then q. 6 hours (seizures)
Adult Dosage (Parenteral): (IM), 5–10 cc (avoid); (IV), 0.2–0.4 cc/kg diluted in NS (250–500 cc) by infusion.
Pediatric Dosage (Parenteral): approx. 0.15 cc/kg, slow IV (diluted in saline).
Contraindications: (Relative) Bronchopulmonary disease, hepatic insufficiency, gastroenteritis/ulceration.
Precautions: IM use causes sterile abscesses. Use *glass* syringes only. Solution oxidizes rapidly. Discard opened bottles after 24 hours.
Adverse Reactions: Gastric mucosal irritation with oral use. IM use causes sterile abscesses or permanent sciatic nerve injury. Pulmonary hemorrhage and edema, circulatory collapse, respiratory distress with IV use.

Generic Name: PHENOBARBITAL
Dosage Forms: Tablets, 8 mg, 16 mg, 30 mg, 32 mg, 60 mg, 65 mg, 100 mg; injection (IM/IV), 65 mg/cc, 130 mg/cc; drops, 16 mg/cc; oral elixir, 20 mg/5 cc.
Uses: Sedative-hypnotic. Also anticonvulsant orally for grand mal and partial seizures, and parenterally for status epilepticus.
Adult Dosage (Oral): For sedation, 15–30 mg b.i.d to q.i.d.; for hypnosis, 100–200 mg at bedtime; for epilepsy, 50–100 mg b.i.d. to t.i.d. or 100–200 mg at bedtime.
Adult Dosage (Parenteral): For sedation/hypnosis, IM injection as for oral dose; for status epilepticus, 260–390 mg (4–6 mg/kg) IM or slow IV, which may be repeated in 6 hours.
Pediatric Dosage (Oral): For sedation, 6 mg/kg/day divided q.i.d.; for epilepsy, 3–6 mg/kg/day in divided doses (may give entire dose at bedtime).
Pediatric Dosage (Parenteral): For hypnosis, 3–6 mg/kg IM; for status epilepticus, 3–6 mg/kg IM or slow IV (range, 100–400 mg).
Contraindications: IV infusion rate should not exceed 60 mg/min. See barbiturates.
Precautions: See barbiturates.
Adverse Reactions: See barbiturates.
Drug Interactions: See barbiturates.

Generic Name: THIAMINE
Trade Name: Vitamin B$_1$
Dosage Forms: Tablets, 5 mg, 10 mg, 25 mg, 50 mg, 100 mg, 200 mg, 500 mg; injection (IM/IV), 100 mg/cc, 200 mg/cc.
Uses: Prevention and treatment of thiamine deficiency (oral use). Used parenterally for treatment of severe deficiencies, such as Wernicke's encephalopathy, and high-output heart failure due to beriberi.
Adult Dosage (Parenteral): 100–200 mg IM or IV infusion (diluted in normal saline). Maintenance dose, 100 mg IM or p.o. q.d., then decreased to 5–10 mg t.i.d.
Pediatric Dosage (Oral): 10–50 mg daily in divided doses.
Pediatric Dosage (Parenteral): 10–25 mg IM or IV.
Contraindications: Hypersensitivity to thiamine.
Precautions: Glucose solutions may worsen symptoms in thiamine-deficient patients because carbohydrate metabolism uses up remaining thiamine.
Adverse Reactions: Primarily after large IV doses: feelings of warmth, tingling, pruritus, pain, sweating, nausea, tightness in throat, angioedema, respiratory distress, cyanosis, pulmonary edema, gastrointestinal bleeding, circulatory collapse.

ANTICOAGULANTS, ANTIFIBRINOLYTICS

Generic Name: ε-AMINOCAPROIC ACID
Trade Name: Amicar
Dosage Forms: Tablets, 500 mg; injection (IV), 250 mg/cc (5 gm/20 cc vial).
Uses: Antifibrinolytic agent for treatment of excessive bleeding resulting from systemic hyperfibrinolysis and urinary fibrinolysis.
Adult Dostage (Oral): Same as IV dosage.
Adult Dosage (Parenteral): IV infusion (diluted in normal saline or D$_5$W) of 4–5 gm for first hour, followed by 1 gm/hour for approximately 8 hours. More than 30 gm/24 hours not recommended.
Contraindications: Pregnancy (teratogenicity in animals). Evidence of active intravascular clotting process.
Precautions: Rapid IV administration should be avoided. Drug should not be administered without definite diagnosis and/or laboratory findings indicative of hyperfibrinolysis (hyperplasminemia).
Adverse Reactions: Rapid IV administration causes hypotension, bradycardia, arrhythmias. Thrombophlebitis with IV administration. Occasional nausea, cramps, diarrhea, hypotension, tinnitus, malaise, nasal and conjunctival congestion, rash, headache.

Generic Name: HEPARIN SODIUM
Trade Name: Heparin
Dosage Forms: Injection (IV/subcutaneous), 1,000, 5,000, 7,500, 10,000, 20,000, 40,000 units/ml.
Uses: Anticoagulant (see warfarin).

Adult Dosage (Parenteral): Must be titrated to prothrombin time responses. Therapeutic effect is 1.5–2.5 times control value using APTT or ACT. Half-life increases with increasing doses.
Adult Dosage (Intermittent IV): 100 U/kg IV q. 4 hours.
Adult Dosage (Continuous IV infusion): IV bolus of 35–70 U/kg followed by continuous infusion of 900–1,200 U/hour *or* 5,000 U IV bolus, followed by 1,000 U/hour IV infusion.
Adult Dosage (Subcutaneous): For prophylaxis, 5,000 U q. 8–12 hours.
Pediatric Dosage (Parenteral): As for adult, to yield clotting times of 20–30 min. or 2 to 3 times the control value.
Contraindications: See warfarin.
Precautions: IM injections should be avoided because of possible hematoma formation. Special risk patients include those with mild hepatic or renal disease, hypertension, in-dwelling catheters, women over 60 years old (see warfarin precautions).
Adverse Reactions: Hemorrhage, immune thrombocytopenia (reversible), hypersensitivity reactions including chills, fever, urticaria, anaphylaxis. Histaminelike reactions at injection site, delayed transient alopecia, osteoporosis (long-term use). Acute vasospastic reaction may develop 6–10 days after initiating therapy and includes pain, ischemia, cyanosis in affected limb, feeling of oppression, and headache (this reaction is unresponsive to protamine). For treatment of heparin overdose, 1–1.5 mg 1% protamine sulfate, slow IV, for every 100 units heparin to be neutralized (maximum, 50 mg in any 10-min. period).

Drug Interactions: Antiplatelet drugs that may increase risk of bleeding or hemorrhage include aspirin, dextran, dipyridamole, ibuprofen, indomethacin, oxyphenbutazone, phenylbutazone, glyceryl guaiacolate. Also coumarin anticoagulants, streptokinase, and urokinase potentiate heparin.

Generic Name: WARFARIN SODIUM
Trade Name: Coumadin
Dosage Forms: Tablets, 2 mg, 2.5 mg, 5 mg, 10 mg, 25 mg; injection (IM/IV), 50 mg.
Uses: Anticoagulant for prophylaxis therapy of venous thrombosis and pulmonary embolism, treatment of atrial fibrillation with embolization, and adjunctive therapy of coronary occlusion and cerebral transient ischemic attacks.
Adult Dosage (Oral): 10–15 mg/day for 2–3 days until desired prothrombin time is reached. Maintenance dosage range, 2–10 mg/day (based on prothrombin time determinations).
Adult Dosage (Parenteral): IM/IV as for oral dosage regimen.
Contraindications: Active bleeding or hemorrhagic tendencies, vitamin K deficiency. Pregnancy, severe hypertension, renal or hepatic disease, acute adrenal hemorrhage or insufficiency, open wounds, visceral carcinoma, gastrointestinal or genitourinary lesions, subacute bacterial endocarditis, recent eye, brain, or spinal cord surgery, retinopathy.
Precautions: Prothrombin time should be determined daily; stools and urine should be examined daily for blood. Altered anticoagulant activity may occur in congestive heart failure, vitamin C and vitamin K deficiencies, alcoholism, fever, diarrhea, severe diabetes and allergic disorders, hyperlipemia, hypothyroidism, edema, hereditary warfarin resistance, polycythemia vera.
Adverse Reactions: Bleeding, hemorrhage, "purple toes" syndrome, gastric upset, diarrhea, fever, dermatitis, alopecia, hemorrhagic infarction and skin necrosis, priapism, uterine bleeding, ovarian hemorrhage upon ovulation, hematuria. (Treat overdose with vitamin K [Phytonadione].)
Drug Interactions: Drugs that may potentiate response include anabolic steroids, chloral hydrate, chloramphenicol, clofibrate, cimetidine, dipyridamole, disulfiram, oxyphenbutazone, phenylbutazone, other nonsteroidal anti-inflammatory agents, thyroid drugs, tricyclic antidepressants, quinine, quinidine, salicylates, streptokinase, urokinase. Drugs that may decrease response include alcohol (chronic ingestion), barbiturates, corticosteroids, glutethimide, meprobamate, estrogens, vitamin K, vitamin C, griseofulvin, antacids.

ANTI-INFLAMMATORY/ANTIGOUT AGENTS

Generic Name: ALLOPURINOL
Trade Name: Zyloprim
Dosage Forms: Tablets, 100 mg, 300 mg.
Uses: Treatment of chronic gout, both primary and secondary, and treatment of primary or secondary uric acid nephropathy.
Adult Dosage (Oral): 100 mg daily to start, followed by weekly increases of 100 mg/day until serum uric acid falls to 6 mg/dl or less or until a maximum of 800 mg/day is reached. Average dose for mild gout is 200–300 mg/day; for moderately severe tophaceous gout, 400–600 mg/day. Doses over 300 mg should be divided.
Pediatric Dosage (Oral): For a child under 6 years, 150 mg/day, adjusted after 48 hours. For a child 6–10 years, 300 mg/day, adjusted after 48 hours.
Contraindications: Children (except for hyperuricemia secondary to malignancy) and location.
Precautions: Prophylactic doses of colchicine should be given with allopurinol for several months, owing to an initial increased risk of gouty attacks. Do not initiate during acute gouty episode. Fluid intake must be sufficient to keep urine output at least 2 liters/day. Renal impairment mandates reduced dosage. Caution in hepatic impairment. May be used with salicylates and uricosurics.
Adverse Reactions: Frequently, maculopapular skin rash occurs, but exfoliative, urticarial, purpuric, and erythema multiforme lesions also reported. Severe hypersensitivity reactions include vasculitis and epidermal necrolysis. Gastric upset, drowsiness, reversible hepatotoxicity reported. Rarely, alopecia, cataract formation, bone marrow depression.
Drug Interactions: With iron salts, increases hepatic iron concentration and toxicity.

Generic Name: BENOXAPROPHEN
Trade Name: Oraflex
Dosage Forms: Tablets, 400 mg, 600 mg.
Uses: Nonsteroidal anti-inflammatory analgesic for relief of signs and symptoms of rheumatoid arthritis and osteoarthritis.
Adult Dosage (Oral): 400–600 mg as a single daily dose, titrated to patient's needs (maximum daily dose, 1,000 mg).
Contraindications: Hypersensitivity to benoxaprophen or demonstrated hypersensitivity to aspirin or other nonsteroidal anti-inflammatory agents.
Precautions: Possible cross-sensitivity with aspirin or other nonsteroidal anti-inflammatory compounds. Renal impairment, peptic ulcer disease, compromised cardiac function or hypertension. Skin and nail phototoxicity with onycholysis. Skin toxicity usually reversible in 48 hours; onycholysis may take weeks to resolve. Use in pregnant or nursing mothers not recommended. Inhibits platelet function.
Adverse Reactions: More frequently gastric upset with dyspepsia, nausea, vomiting, abdominal pain, flatulence, diarrhea, constipation, rashes, pruritus, skin and nail phototoxicity reactions, dysuria, tinnitus, headache, vertigo, sleep disturbances, dry eyes and mucous membranes, peripheral edema, hypertension, aggravation of congestive heart fail-

ure. Occasional peptic ulcers, gastrointestinal bleeding, gastritis, palpitations, Stevens-Johnson syndrome, mental depression and confusion, paresthesia. Rarely, blood dyscrasias, thrombophlebitis, epistaxis, pancreatitis, cholecystitis, interstitial nephritis, and ocular toxicity, including diplopia, photophobia, toxic optic neuropathy.

Drug Interactions: Possible potentiation of oral anticoagulant and antiplatelet activity.

Generic Name: COLCHICINE
Trade Name: Colchicine
Dosage Forms: Tablets, 0.5 mg, 0.6 mg; injection (IV), 0.5 mg/cc (2 cc ampule)
Uses: Treatment of acute gouty attack and prophylaxis of chronic gout.
Adult Dosage (Oral): 0.6–1.2 mg initially, then 0.5–0.6 mg q. 1–3 hours until pain relieved or until gastrointestinal toxicity (up to maximum of 7–8 mg). A 3- to 4-day delay is required before repeating. Maintenance dose, 0.6–1.2 mg orally q.d. or q.o.d.
Adult Dosage (Parenteral): Slow IV (diluted in 10 cc normal saline), 1–2 mg initially, then 0.5 mg q. 3–6 hours (up to 4 mg/24 hours).
Contraindications: Anuria, pregnancy.
Precautions: Should be given slowly IV (diluted) with care to avoid extravasation. Drug should not be given IM or subcutaneously. Nausea, vomiting, diarrhea indicates full therapeutic dose has been attained. Caution in elderly, debilitated patients or those with renal, gastric, or cardiac disease.
Adverse Reactions: Primarily nausea, vomiting, diarrhea. Also hemorrhagic gastroenteritis, vascular damage, thrombophlebitis, nephrotoxicity, peripheral neuritis, paralysis. Prolonged use may cause bone marrow depression with agranulocytosis and aplastic anemia.

Generic Name: IBUPROFEN
Trade Name: Motrin
Dosage Forms: Tablets, 300 mg, 400 mg, 600 mg.
Uses: Nonsteroidal anti-inflammatory agent for treatment of rheumatoid arthritis and osteoarthritis. Mild-to-moderate analgesic action.
Adult Dosage (Oral): For analgesia, 400 mg q. 4–6 hours with food (up to 2,400 mg/day); for arthritis, 300–600 mg t.i.d. to q.i.d. with food (up to 2,400 mg/day).
Contraindications: See indomethacin.
Precautions: See indomethacin.
Adverse Reactions: See indomethacin.
Drug Interactions: See indomethacin.

Generic Name: INDOMETHACIN
Trade Name: Indocin
Dosage Forms: Capsules, 25 mg, 50 mg.
Uses: Nonsteroid anti-inflammatory agent for treatment of many forms of arthritis, including acute gouty arthritis.
Adult Dosage (Oral): 25 mg b.i.d. or t.i.d. with meals to start, increased by 25 mg at weekly intervals p.r.n. (maximum recommended dose, 150–200 mg/day). For acute gouty arthritis, 50 mg t.i.d. (maximum dose, 200 mg/day).
Contraindications: Children under 14 years. Pregnancy, lactation, history of gastrointestinal lesions (latent or active). Allergy to aspirin, indomethacin, and other nonsteroid anti-inflammatory agents if manifested by bronchospastic reactions.
Precautions: May aggravate psychiatric disorders, epilepsy, or Parkinsonism. Inhibits platelet aggregation (i.e., prolongs bleeding time). Caution in elderly (increased risk of ocular and CNS effects). Renal impairment. May mask clinical signs of infection.
Adverse Reactions: Frequent headache, dizziness, sedation, tinnitus, gastric upset, mental confusion. Hypersensitivity reactions include rash, urticaria, exacerbation of asthma, acute respiratory distress, angioedema. Also peripheral neuropathy, peptic ulcer with perforation, gastrointestinal inflammation, blood dyscrasias (with leukopenia, agranulocytosis), edema, hypertension, tachyarrhythmias, epistaxis, nasal polyps, hepatotoxicity.
Drug Interactions: Probenecid increases indomethacin serum levels. Aspirin exacerbates gastrointestinal upset/bleeding. With oral anticoagulants, possible potentiation of hypothrombinemia and increased risk of gastrointestinal bleeding.

Generic Name: NAPROXEN
Trade Name: Naprosyn
Dosage Forms: Tablets, 250 mg, 375 mg.
Uses: Nonsteroid anti-inflammatory agent for treatment of rheumatoid arthritis and osteoarthritis. Also used as analgesic in treatment of mild-to-moderate pain and dysmenorrhea.
Adult Dosage (Oral): 250–375 mg b.i.d. with meals. For analgesia, 500 mg to start, then 250 mg q. 6–8 hours p.r.n. (maximum daily dose, 1,250 mg).
Pediatric Dosage (Oral): Not established. Investigationally, 5 mg/kg/day in children under 50 kg has been used.
Contraindications: Hypersensitivity to naproxen or aspirin and other nonsteroidal anti-inflammatory agents when manifested by asthma, urticaria, bronchospasm.
Precautions: Renal impairment, peptic ulcer disease, or history of gastrointestinal bleeding.
Adverse Reactions: Gastric upset and CNS sedation and depression are frequent, but may be less severe than those due to indomethacin. Occasional tinnitus, allergic reactions, and edema. Visual disturbances, blood dyscrasias (rare).
Drug Interactions: Naproxen metabolite may cause false elevation in assay for urinary 17-ketogenic steroids. With oral anticoagulants, possible increased hypoprothrombinemic effect and gastrointestinal bleeding.

Generic Name: OXYPHENBUTAZONE
Trade Name: Tandearil
Dosage Form: Tablets, 100 mg.
Uses: See phenylbutazone.
Adult Dosage (Oral): See phenylbutazone.
Contraindications: See phenylbutazone.
Precautions: See phenylbutazone.

Adverse Reactions: See phenylbutazone.
Drug Interactions: See phenylbutazone.

Generic Name: PHENYLBUTAZONE
Trade Name: Butazolidin
Dosage Forms: Tablets, 100 mg; capsules, 100 mg with antacid added.
Uses: Anti-inflammatory agent beneficial in treatment of acute attacks of gouty arthritis.
Adult Dosage (Oral): 400 mg initially, then 100 mg q. 4 hours for 1 week. (Maintenance therapy for other anti-inflammatory indications, up to 400 mg/day.
Contraindications: Children under 12 years, senile patients. Phenylbutazone or oxyphenbutazone allergy. Severe renal, hepatic, or cardiac disease. Peptic ulcer/gastrointestinal inflammatory disease. Thyroid disease, hypertension. Concomitant use of oral anticoagulants. Parotitis, stomatitis, polymyalgia rheumatica, temporal arteritis, blood dyscrasias. Systemic edema.
Precautions: First trimester of pregnancy. Patients receiving antidiabetic or sulfonamide agents. Therapy in elderly must be restricted to 1 week, as the toxicity risk is greater after 40 years of age. Serious blood dyscrasias may occur many weeks after the drug has been withdrawn; therefore, blood count must be monitored every 2 weeks. Asthma and systemic lupus erythematosus may be exacerbated. Visual disturbances (blurred vision) may indicate toxicity. Therapy should be discontinued if leukopenia or granulocytopenia is significant.
Adverse Reactions: Nausea, vomiting, gastric distress, salt and water retention, edema, dizziness, exacerbation of peptic ulcer. Blood dyscrasias, including aplastic anemia and agranulocytosis; hepatotoxicity; nephritis; exfoliative dermatitis, including Stevens-Johnson syndrome.
Drug Interactions: Displaces many protein-bound drugs. With insulin/oral hypoglycemics, potentiation of hypoglycemic effects. Increases serum levels of diphenylhydantoin. With coumarin anticoagulants and heparin, potentiation of anticoagulant effects.

Generic Name: PROBENECID
Trade Name: Benemid
Dosage Forms: Tablets, 500 mg. Also in combination with colchicine as ColBENEMID.

Uses: Uricosuric agent for treatment of chronic gout and adjuvant to penicillin therapy.
Adult Dosage (Oral): 250 mg b.i.d. for 1 week, then 0.5 gm b.i.d. As an adjuvant to penicillin therapy, 2 gm/day in divided doses.
Pediatric Dosage (Oral): As an adjuvant to penicillin therapy in a child under 50 kg, 25 mg/kg/day to start, then 40 mg/kg/day in four divided doses. In a child over 50 kg, same as adult dosage.
Contraindications: Hypersensitivity to probenecid, uric acid kidney stones or blood dyscrasias, acute gouty attacks, salicylate therapy. Children under 2 years.
Precautions: If gout is exacerbated, colchicine should be added. Liberal fluid intake and urine alkalinization recommended. Renal impairment (probably ineffective if glomerular filtration rate is under 30 cc/min). Caution in peptic ulcer disease or G6PD deficiency. Hypersensitivity reactions necessitate discontinuance of drug.
Adverse Reactions: Gastric upset, hypersensitivity reactions (mild to severe) including rash, pruritus, fever, blood dyscrasias (hemolytic anemia, aplastic anemia [rare]). Genitourinary effects, including renal colic, hematuria, uric acid stones.
Drug Interactions: Increases plasma concentrations of penicillins, cephalothin, methotrexate, PAS, rifampin, indomethacin, sulfonamides, sulfinpyrazone. Salicylates inhibit uricosuric action of probenecid.

Generic Name: SULFINPYRAZONE
Trade Name: Anturane
Dosage Forms: Tablets, 100 mg; capsules, 200 mg.
Uses: Uricosuric agent for treatment of chronic or intermittent gouty arthritis.
Adult Dosage (Oral): 100–200 mg b.i.d. with meals. Increase over 1 week to 200 mg b.i.d. as necessary.
Contraindications: Hypersensitivity to sulfinpyrazone or phenylbutazone (and derivatives). Active peptic ulcer/gastrointestinal ulceration and inflammation. Blood dyscrasias (past or present).
Precautions: See probenecid. Sulfinpyrazone also inhibits platelet aggregation and may increase prothrombin time in patients on oral anticoagulants.
Adverse Reactions: See probenecid, although incidence of rashes may be lower.
Drug Interaction: See probenecid. With anticoagulants, additive hypoprothrombinemia.

ANTIDEPRESSANTS, ANTI-EMETICS, TRANQUILIZERS

Generic Name: AMITRIPTYLINE
Trade Names: Elavil, Endep
Dosage Forms: Tablets, 10 mg, 25 mg, 50 mg, 75 mg, 100 mg, 150 mg; injection (IM), 10 mg/cc.
Uses: Tricyclic antidepressant.
Adult Dosage (Oral): 75 mg/day, divided doses or single dose at bedtime to start. Dosage may be increased by 25- to 50-mg increments at bedtime to 150 mg/day.

Adult Dosage (Parenteral): 20–30 mg IM q.i.d. initially, replaced with oral therapy as soon as possible. (*Note:* Hospitalized patients may require 100 mg/day to start, followed by gradual increases up to 200–300 mg/day.)
Contraindications: Hypersensitivity to amitryptyline. Concomitant MAO inhibitor therapy. Myocardial infarction during acute recovery phase.
Precautions: Anticholinergic activity, so use with caution in

glaucoma (narrow angle), myocardial infarction, urinary retention, cardiovascular disease, hyperthyroidism. Psychotic, manic-depressive, or suicidal patients may worsen. Hepatic impairment may cause drug accumulation.

Adverse Reactions: Dry mouth, blurred vision, increased intraocular pressure (may precipitate acute attack in narrow angle glaucoma), hypotension, hypertension, tachycardia, palpitations, myocardial infarction, arrhythmias, heart block. Possible CNS disturbances include excitement, hallucinations, delusions, fatigue, sedation, peripheral neuropathy, ataxia, numbness, extrapyramidal symptoms. Gastric upset, black tongue, abnormal liver function tests, hepatitis, and allergic reactions (including rash and photosensitivity) may occur.

Drug Interactions: With MAO inhibitors, hyperpyrexia, convulsions, coma, death. With anticholinergics, increased anticholinergic effects. With sympathomimetics, severe hypertension, hyperpyrexia. With alcohol and other CNS depressants, additive CNS depression.

Generic Name: CHLORDIAZEPOXIDE
Trade Name: Librium
Dosage Forms: Capsules, 5 mg, 10 mg, 25 mg; injection (IM/IV), 100 mg.
Uses: Benzodiazepine derivative for treatment of moderate to severe anxiety, tension, and alcoholic withdrawal symptoms.
Adult Dosage (Oral): For anxiety, 5–10 mg t.i.d. or q.i.d. (up to 200 mg/day). For alcohol withdrawal, 50–100 mg repeated p.r.n. (up to 300 mg/day).
Adult Dosage (Parenteral): For anxiety, 50–100 mg IM initially, then 25–50 mg t.i.d. or q.i.d. p.r.n. For alcohol withdrawal, 50–100 mg IM q. 3–4 hours p.r.n. (up to 300 mg/day).
Pediatric Dosage (Oral): For a child over 6 years, 5–10 mg b.i.d. to t.i.d. p.r.n.
Contraindications: Hypersensitivity to chlordiazepoxide, shock, comatose states.
Precautions: For IV use, normal saline should be used as diluent; infusion should be slow, over 1 minute. Maximum parenteral dose recommended is 300 mg in any 6- to 24-hour period. Elderly or debilitated patients should be given one-half dose. Hepatic or renal impairment/concomitant psychotropic therapy. Barbiturate-like withdrawal symptoms may occur. Drug may be habit-forming.
Adverse Reactions: Drowsiness, vertigo, ataxia and oversedation (especially in elderly), gastric upset, paradoxical excitement, stimulation, acute rage (especially in psychiatric patients), allergic reactions with rash and drug fever, cholestatic jaundice. Parenteral use has caused syncope, hypotension, tachycardia, extrapyramidal symptoms, blurred vision, and respiratory depression.
Drug Interactions: Additive CNS depression with alcohol, tricyclic antidepressants, sedative-hypnotics, MAO inhibitors, and other CNS depressants.

Generic Name: CHLORPROMAZINE
Trade Name: Thorazine
Dosage Forms: Tablets, 10 mg, 25 mg, 50 mg, 100 mg, 200 mg; capsules (sustained release), 30–300 mg; injection (IM/IV), 25 mg/cc; suppositories, 25 mg, 100 mg; syrup 10 mg/5 cc; oral concentrate, 30 mg/cc, 100 mg/cc.
Uses: Phenothiazine antipsychotic tranquilizer and antiemetic.
Adult Dosage (Oral): As an anti-emetic, 10–25 mg q. 4–6 hours p.r.n. As an antipsychotic, 200–800 mg q.d., divided doses.
Adult Dosage (Parenteral): As an anti-emetic, 25 mg IM initially. If no hypotension, 25–50 mg IM q. 3–4 hours p.r.n. As an antipsychotic, 25 mg IM stat. MR in one hour with 25–50 mg.
Pediatric Dosage (Oral): As an anti-emetic, 0.55 mg/kg q. 4–6 hours p.r.n.
Pediatric Dosage (Parenteral): As an anti-emetic, 0.55 mg/kg IM q. 6–8 hours (up to 40 mg/day).
Contraindications: Hypersensitivity to phenothiazines. Circulatory collapse, severe hypotension. CNS depression, comatose states, presence of large amounts of CNS depressants. Bone marrow depression.
Precautions: Extrapyramidal symptoms, so use cautiously in children. Caution in hepatic and cardiovascular disease, chronic respiratory disorders, convulsive disorders, myasthenia gravis. Because the cough reflex is suppressed, patient may aspirate.
Adverse Reactions: CNS sedation and depression, thermoregulatory impairment (hyperpyrexia), seizures, cerebral edema, extrapyramidal effects (moderate for chlorpromazine), tardive dyskinesia, anticholinergic effects of tachycardia, dry mouth, blurred vision, urinary difficulty, constipation, orthostatic hypotension (due to α-adrenergic blockade), "quinidinelike" effect on heart, heart block, allergic reactions (including cholestatic jaundice), photosensitivity, blood dyscrasias.
Drug Interactions: Additive CNS depression with narcotics, sedative-hypnotics, alcohol, other tranquilizers.

Generic Name: HALOPERIDOL
Trade Name: Haldol
Dosage Forms: Tablets, 0.5 mg, 1 mg, 2 mg, 5 mg; injection (IM), 5 mg/cc; oral solution, 2 mg/cc.
Uses: Antipsychotic tranquilizer (butyrophenone derivative).
Adult Dosage (Oral): 0.5–2 mg b.i.d. or t.i.d. (up to 3–5 mg t.i.d. or more).
Adult Dosage (Parenteral): 2–5 mg IM q. 1–8 hours p.r.n.
Pediatric Dosage (Oral): 0.05–0.15 mg/kg/day (maximum 6 mg daily).
Contraindications: Hypersensitivity to haloperidol. Severe toxic CNS depression or comatose states. Parkinson's disease.
Precautions: Elderly and debilitated patients require reduced dosage. Convulsive disorders (lowered seizure threshold), severe cardiac disease.
Adverse Reactions: High incidence of extrapyramidal symptoms. Other side-effects similar to those of phenothiazines.
Drug Interactions: With lithium, encephalopathic syndrome characterized by weakness, lethargy, fever, tremulousness, confusion, extrapyramidal symptoms, blood dyscrasias, elevated serum enzymes, irreversible brain damage.

Generic Name: PROCHLORPERAZINE
Trade Name: Compazine
Dosage Forms: Tablets, 5 mg, 10 mg; capsules (sustained release), 10 mg, 15 mg, 30 mg, 75 mg; injection (IM/IV), 5 mg/cc; suppositories, 2.5 mg, 5 mg, 25 mg (adult); oral syrup and concentrate.
Uses: Phenothiazine anti-emetic.
Adult Dosage (Oral): 5–10 mg t.i.d. or q.i.d. or 25 mg b.i.d., rectally.
Adult Dosage (Parenteral): 5–10 mg IM q. 3–4 hours p.r.n. (maximum 40 mg/day).

Pediatric Dosage (Rectal): In a child over 2 years, 0.4 mg/kg/day (e.g., 2.5–5 mg b.i.d. or t.i.d.).
Pediatric Dosage (Parenteral); 1.32 mg/kg IM (usually one dose is sufficient).
Contraindications: Pediatric surgery (see chlorpromazine).
Precautions: Higher incidence of extrapyramidal side-effects than with chlorpromazine. Avoid use in children under 2 years or 20 lb weight.
Adverse Reactions: See chlorpromazine.
Drug Interactions: See chlorpromazine.

ANTIHISTAMINES/ANTIPRURITICS

Generic Name: CYPROHEPTADINE
Trade Name: Periactin
Dosage Forms: Tablets, 4 mg; oral syrup, 2 mg/5 cc.
Uses: Antihistamine, antipruritic agent.
Adult Dosage: 4 mg t.i.d. or q.i.d. (4–20 mg/day).
Pediatric Dosage: 0.25 mg/kg/day in three or four divided doses.
Contraindications: Hypersensitivity to drug, patients on MAO inhibitor therapy, elderly and debilitated patients, newborn and premature infants, conditions aggravated by anticholinergic action (e.g., glaucoma, stenosing peptic ulcer).
Precautions: See diphenhydramine. Also may cause increased appetite and weight gain in children. Antiserotonin activity may inhibit adrenocorticotropic hormone release in Cushing's disease.
Adverse Reactions: Frequent sedation, dizziness, disturbed coordination, dry mouth, thickening of bronchial secretions, epigastric distress. Also hypotension, headache, palpitations, tachycardia, CNS stimulation and depression, rashes, urticaria, blurred vision, urinary retention and frequency, photosensitivity.
Drug Interactions: With alcohol, other CNS depressants, additive CNS depression. With MAO inhibitors, increased anticholinergic side-effects.

Generic Name: DIPHENHYDRAMINE
Trade Name: Benadryl
Dosage Forms: Capsules, 25 mg, 50 mg; injection (IM/IV), 10 mg/cc, 50 mg/cc; elixir, 12.5 mg/5 cc.
Uses: Antihistamine for treatment of allergic reactions, adjunctive therapy of anaphylaxis, treatment of extrapyramidal drug reactions.
Adult Dosage (Oral): 25–50 mg t.i.d. or q.i.d. For hypnotic dose, 50–100 mg at bedtime.
Adult Dosage (Parenteral): 10–50 mg IM or IV (up to 400 mg/day).
Pediatric Dosage (Oral): In a child over 9 kg, 12.5–25 mg t.i.d.

or q.i.d., or 5 mg/kg/day in three or four divided doses (up to 300 mg/day).
Pediatric Dosage (Parenteral): Same as oral dosage.
Contraindications: Hypersensitivity to diphenhydramine or related compounds (dimenhydrinate). Newborn and premature infants, lactation, patients on MAO inhibitor therapy, conditions aggravated by anticholinergic action (e.g., glaucoma).
Precautions: Elderly over 60 years, bronchial asthma, glaucoma, hyperthyroidism, hypertension, cardiovascular disease, hypertension, stenosing peptic ulcer, prostatic hypertrophy.
Adverse Reactions: See cyproheptadine.
Drug Interactions: See cyproheptadine.

Generic Name: HYDROXYZINE
Trade Names: Vistaril, Atarax
Dosage Forms: Tablets (HCL), 10 mg, 25 mg, 50 mg, 100 mg; capsules (pamoate), 25 mg, 50 mg, 100 mg; injection (IM only), 25 mg, 50 mg, 100 mg; oral suspension, 25 mg/5 cc.
Uses: Antihistamine, antipruritic, antianxiety agent, and anti-emetic.
Adult Dosage (Oral): For anxiety, 50–100 mg q.i.d. For pruritus, 25–50 mg t.i.d. to q.i.d.
Adult Dosage (Parenteral): 25–100 mg IM q. 4–6 hours p.r.n.
Pediatric Dosage (Oral): For anxiety or pruritus in a child under 6 years, 50 mg q.i.d.; in a child over 6 years, 50–100 mg q.i.d.
Contraindications: Hypersensitivity to hydroxyzine.
Precautions: Should not be given IV or subcutaneously. Drowsiness may impair performance of potentially hazardous activities.
Adverse Reactions: Transient drowsiness, dry mouth, involuntary motor activity, including tremor and convulsions (rare).
Drug Interactions: Alcohol, tricyclic antidepressants, narcotic analgesics, sedative-hypnotics, and other CNS depressants cause increased CNS depression.

AMINOGLYCOSIDE ANTIBIOTICS

Generic Name: AMIKACIN
Trade Name: Amikin
Dosage Forms: Injection (IM/IV), 100 mg, 500 mg, 1 gm.
Uses: Aminoglycoside antibiotic useful in gentamicin- and kanamycin-resistant gram-negative organisms. Other indications as for gentamicin.
Adult Dosage (Parenteral): For uncomplicated infections, 250 mg IM b.i.d. For moderate to severe infections, 7.5 mg/kg q. 12 hours or 5 mg/kg q. 8 hours IM or slow IV (therapeutic serum levels, 15–30 μg/cc).
Pediatric Dosage (Parenteral): In the child and infant, same as adult. For sepsis in the newborn or neonate, 10 mg/kg IM or IV to start, then 7.5 mg/kg q. 12 hours.
Contraindications: Hypersensitivity to amikacin or other aminoglycosides.
Precautions: See gentamicin. If no definite clinical response in 3–5 days, recheck culture and sensitivity. Patient must be adequately hydrated to minimize renal irritation.
Adverse Reactions: Nephrotoxicity (mild to acute). Auditory damage with high doses (sometimes irreversible). CNS/neuromuscular effects, including dizziness, numbness, tingling, muscle twitching, neuromuscular blockade with apnea. Hypersensitivity reactions and superinfections may occur.
Drug Interactions: Increased nephrotoxicity with cephalosporins, vancomycin, other aminoglycosides, polymyxin. Increased ototoxicity with loop diuretics, other aminoglycosides. Increased neuromuscular blockade with anesthetics, curariform drugs, other aminoglycosides.

Generic Name: GENTAMICIN
Trade Name: Garamycin
Dosage Forms: Topical preparations; injection (IM/IV), 20 mg, 60 mg, 80 mg; intrathecal, 2 mg/cc (2 cc).
Uses: Aminoglycoside antibiotic for serious infections due to variety of gram-negative organisms, including *Pseudomonas* spp. Ineffective against anaerobes such as *Bacteroides* and *Streptococcus* spp.
Adult Dosage (Parenteral): Therapeutic levels, 2-10 μg/cc (usual, 4–8 μg/cc). Toxic levels, greater than 10–12 μg/cc. Dose varies with type and severity of infection. Usual dose, 3–5 mg/kg/day IM or IV in divided doses q. 8 hours (up to 6–8 mg/kg/day). Intrathecal dose, up to 5 mg q. 18–24 hours, in combination with systemic administration.
Pediatric Dosage (Parenteral): In a child, 2–2.5 mg/kg IM or IV q. 8 hours; in an infant, 2.5 mg/kg IM or IV q. 8 hours; in a newborn or neonate, 2.5 mg/kg IM or IV q. 12 hours. Intrathecal dose, 1–2 mg q.d. with or without systemic administration.
Contraindications: Hypersensitivity to gentamicin (absolute); hypersensitivity to other aminoglycosides (relative).
Precautions: IV doses should be diluted to less than or equal to 1-mg/cc concentration and given slowly over 30–60 min., depending on patient's renal function. Dosage adjustments required in renal insufficiency. Possible cross-allergenicity with other aminoglycosides. Monitor renal/auditory functioning periodically if treatment over 10 days duration.

Adverse Reactions: See amikacin.
Drug Interactions: See amikacin.

Generic Name: KANAMYCIN
Trade Name: Kantrex
Dosage Forms: Capsules, 500 mg; injection (IM/IV), 75 mg (pediatric), 500 mg, 1 gm.
Uses: Aminoglycoside antibiotic used orally for preoperative bowel sterilization and adjunctive treatment of hepatic encephalopathy. Parenterally for infections due to staphylococci and susceptible gram-negative organisms. *Pseudomonas* and anaerobes are resistant.
Adult Dosage (Oral): For hepatic encephalopathy, 6–12 gm orally or rectally as enema daily in divided doses. For bowel sterilization, 1 gm q. 1 hour for four doses, then 1 gm q. 4 hours for 24 hours.
Adult Dosage (Parenteral): 7.5 mg/kg q. 12 hours or up to 15 mg/kg/day IM or slow IV infusion in divided doses q. 8–12 hours (not to exceed 1.5 gm/day). Intraperitoneal irrigation should not exceed IM or IV dosage. (Therapeutic blood levels usually 15–20 μg/cc.)
Pediatric Dosage (Parenteral): In a child, same as adult. In an infant (2 kg or more), 15–20 mg/kg/day, divided q. 8–12 hours; in a newborn or neonate (under 2 kg), 7.5 mg/kg q. 12 hours.
Contraindications: See gentamicin.
Precautions: IV use should be avoided (unless IM use not feasible). Prolonged oral use may lead to malabsorption syndrome. Systemic absorption from oral, rectal, or irrigation use may occur in presence of renal impairment or denuded/ulcerated mucosa. For other precautions, see gentamicin.
Adverse Reactions: Primarily ototoxicity with cochlear, vestibular damage, especially with serum levels over 35 μg/cc or with prolonged therapy at lower doses. For other adverse reactions, see gentamicin.
Drug Interactions: See gentamicin.

Generic Name: NEOMYCIN
Trade Name: Mycifradin
Dosage Forms: Tablets, 500 mg; oral solution, 125 mg/5 cc; various topical preparations.
Uses: See kanamycin. Also used topically for a variety of skin and eye infections.
Adult Dosage (Oral): For hepatic encephalopathy, 6–8 gm (or rectally as enema) in four to six divided doses for 1–2 days, then decreased to 2–4 gm daily in divided doses. For bowel sterilization, 1 gm q. 1 hour for four doses, then 1 gm q. 4 hours for 24 hours.
Contraindications: Hypersensitivity to neomycin (absolute); hypersensitivity to other aminoglycosides (relative).
Precautions: See kanamycin.
Adverse Reactions: See kanamycin.
Drug Interactions: See kanamycin.

Generic Name: STREPTOMYCIN

Dosage Forms: Injection (IM only), 500 mg, 1 gm, 5 gm.

Uses: Aminoglycoside antibiotic for treatment of tuberculosis, bacterial endocarditis (adjunct), plague, tularemia.

Adult Dosage (Parenteral): For tuberculosis, 1 gm IM q.d. to start, then two to three doses weekly up to 1 year (given with other antituberculars). Usual dose for other infections, 1–2 gm IM daily divided q. 12 hours (maximum, 4 gm q.d.). For bacterial endocarditis, 1 gm IM b.i.d. for 1 week, then 0.5 gm b.i.d. IM for 1 week (with penicillin).

Pediatric Dosage (Parenteral): For a child, 20–40 mg/kg/day IM divided q. 6–12 hours (along with other anti-infectives). Not recommended for infants or newborns.

Contraindications: Hypersensitivity to streptomycin (absolute); hypersensitivity to other aminoglycosides (relative).

Precautions: Not for IV use. Caution in pregnancy, elderly, renal and auditory impairment, as well as in use with other ototoxic drugs. Therapeutic levels, 25–50 μg/cc. Toxic serum levels, greater than 50 μg/cc.

Adverse Reactions: Vestibular ototoxicity (frequent, sometimes irreversible). Nephrotoxicity, paresthesias, rash, fever, neuromuscular blockade, hepatic necrosis. See also gentamicin.

Drug Interactions: See gentamicin.

Generic Name: TOBRAMYCIN

Trade Name: Nebcin

Dosage Forms: Injection (IM/IV), 20 mg (pediatric), 60 mg, 80 mg.

Uses: As for gentamicin, except active against gentamicin-resistant strains of *Pseudomonas*.

Adult Dosage (Parenteral): 3.5 mg/kg/day IM or IV divided q. 8 hours, depending on severity of infection; should be decreased to 3 mg/kg/day as soon as possible.

Pediatric Dosage (Parenteral): Same as adult dose for child or infant. In the newborn or neonate (less than 1 week), up to 4 mg/kg/day IM or IV, divided q. 12 hours.

Contraindications: Hypersensitivity to tobramycin and/or other aminoglycosides.

Precautions: Culture and sensitivity testing necessary. Other precautions for gentamicin.

Adverse Reactions: Same adverse reactions as those for gentamicin, but less nephrotoxicity claimed.

Drug Interactions: See gentamicin.

CEPHALOSPORIN ANTIBIOTICS

Uses: Broad spectrum antibiotic class active against most gram-positive cocci, including penicillinase-producing staphylococci and many strains of gram-negative bacilli (e.g., *Escherichia coli, Proteus, Hemophilus influenzae,* and *Klebsiella* spp.). Second-generation cephalosporins (e.g., cefamandole) show increased activity against *Enterobacter* spp. and some anaerobes, while third-generation cephalosporins (e.g., cefoxitin, moxalactam, and cefotaxime) are more active still against *Bacteroides, Clostridium, Peptococcus,* and *Peptostreptococcus* spp. Moxalactam and cefotaxime also include in vitro activity against *Serratia, Providencia,* and some strains of *Pseudomonas aeruginosa.* Most strains of enterococci (e.g., *Streptococcus faecalis*) and methicillin-resistant staphylococci are resistant to cephalosporins, and the third generation compounds may have diminished gram-positive potency compared to the first- and second-generation agents. Cephalosporins are useful in treatment of urinary tract, lower respiratory tract, skin and soft tissue infections, as well as septicemia, and third-generation agents are especially useful for gynecological and intra-abdominal infections.

Contraindications: Hypersensitivity to cephalosporins.

Precautions: Possible cross-allergenicity with penicillin (7%–10% incidence). Renal impairment (dosage adjustments necessary when creatinine clearance is 50 ml/min. or less).

Adverse Reactions: Gastric upset, diarrhea, hypersensitivity reactions, serum sickness (especially with prolonged parenteral use), thrombophlebitis with IV use, eosinophilia and other transient blood dyscrasias, some renal impairment (including increased blood urea nitrogen and serum creatinine levels). Cephaloridine has the greatest nephrotoxic potential and should be avoided. Transient rises in liver enzymes may occur, as well as a positive direct Coombs' test, especially in azotemic patients. Superinfections with enterococci and yeasts may occur. (*Note:* Pseudomembranous colitis has occurred with moxalactam use. Also a disulfiram-like reaction to alcohol ingestion and a vitamin K-responsive hypoprothrombinemia with occasional bleeding tendencies has been associated with moxalactam and cefamandole.)

Drug Interactions: Probenecid increases serum levels of cephalosporins. Aminoglycosides, potent loop diuretics, increase nephrotoxicity.

PARENTERALLY ADMINISTERED CEPHALOSPORINS

Pediatric doses are for children greater than 3 months old.

Generic Name: CEPHALOTHIN

Trade Name: Keflin

Dosage Forms: Injection (IM/IV), 1 gm, 2 gm, 4 gm vials.

Adult Dosage: 500 mg–1 gm IV q. 4–6 hours (up to 12 gm daily).

Pediatric Dosage: 80–160 mg/kg/day, divided doses IV (IM use to be avoided as it is extremely painful).

Generic Name: CEPHAPIRIN

Trade Name: Cefadyl

Dosage Form: Injection (IM/IV)

Adult Dosage: 500 mg, 1 gm, 2 gm IV q. 4–6 hours (up to 12 gm/day).

Pediatric Dosage: 40–80 mg/kg/day IV, divided doses.

Generic Name: CEFAZOLIN
Trade Names: Ancef, Kefzol
Dosage Forms: Injection (IM/IV), 250 mg, 500 mg, 1 gm vials.
Adult Dosage: 250–500 mg IM q. 8 hours for mild infections; 500 mg–1 gm IV q. 6–8 hours (up to 12 gm/day) for severe infections.
Pediatric Dosage: 25–50 mg/kg/day IM or IV divided q. 6–8 hours (up to 100 mg/kg/day divided q. 6–8 hours for more serious infections). (*Note:* Significant biliary levels achieved with cefazolin.)

Generic Name: CEPHRADINE
Trade Name: Velosef
Dosage Forms: Injection (IM/IV), 250 mg, 500 mg, 1 gm, 2 gm, 4 gm.
Adult Dosage: 1–2 gm IM/IV q. 6 hours (up to 8 gm/day).
Pediatric Dosage: 50–100 mg/kg/day IM or IV, divided q. 6 hours.

Generic Name: CEFAMANDOLE
Trade Name: Mandol
Dosage Forms: Injection (IM/IV), 500 mg, 1 gm, 2 gm vials.
Adult Dosage: 500 mg–1 gm IV q. 4–8 hours (up to 12 gm/day); 500 mg–1 gm IM q. 8 hours for uncomplicated urinary tract infection.
Pediatric Dosage: 50–100 mg/kg/day IM/IV, divided q. 4–8 hours (maximum of 150 mg/kg/day for severe infections).

Generic Name: CEFOXITIN
Trade Name: Mefoxin
Dosage Forms: Injection (IM/IV), 1 gm, 2 gm vials.
Adult Dosage: 1 gm IM or IV q. 6–8 hours for uncomplicated infections; 1–2 gm IV q. 4–6 hours for moderate to severe infections (up to 12 gm/day).
Pediatric Dosage: 80–160 mg/kg/day IM or IV, divided q. 4–6 hours (up to 12 gm/day).

Generic Name: CEFOTAXIME
Trade Name: Claforan
Dosage Forms: Injection (IM/IV), 1 gm, 2 gm vials.
Adult Dosage: 1 gm IM or IV q. 12 hours for uncomplicated urinary tract infection or pneumonia; 1–2 gm IV or IM q. 6–8 hours for moderate to severe infections; 2 gm IV q. 4 hours for life-threatening infections (maximum, 12 gm/day).
Pediatric Dosage: Safety and effectiveness not yet established.

Generic Name: MOXALACTAM
Trade Name: Moxam
Dosage Forms: Injection (IM/IV), 1 gm, 2 gm vials (Oxa-beta lactam derivative).
Adult Dosage: 500 mg–2 gm IM or IV q. 8 hours for mild to moderate infections; 3–4 gm IV q. 8 hours for severe infections (maximum dose, 12 gm/day).
Pediatric Dosage: 50 mg/kg IM or IV q. 6–8 hours (up to 200 mg/kg/day). For neonates, 50 mg/kg IM or IV q. 8–12 hours (up to 200 mg/kg/day).

ORALLY ADMINISTERED CEPHALOSPORINS

Generic Name: CEFACLOR
Trade Name: Ceclor
Dosage Forms: Capsules, 250 mg, 500 mg; oral suspension, 125 mg/5 cc, 250 mg/5 cc.
Adult Dosage: 250 mg–500 mg p.o. q. 8 hours (up to 4 gm/day).
Pediatric Dosage: 20 mg/kg/day, divided q. 8 hours (up to 40 mg/kg/day for severe infections. (*Note:* Claimed especially useful for ampicillin-resistant *Hemophilus influenzae* in treatment of otitis media.)

Generic Name: CEFADROXIL
Trade Names: Duricef, Ultracef
Dosage Form: Capsules, 500 mg.
Adult Dosage: 1 gm p.o. q.d. to b.i.d., depending on severity of urinary tract infection; 1 gm/day single dose or divided b.i.d. for skin and soft tissue infections.

Generic Name: CEPHALEXIN
Trade Name: Keflex
Dosage Forms: Capsules, 250 mg, 500 mg; oral suspension, 125 mg/5 cc, 250 mg/5 cc.
Adult Dosage: 250–500 mg q. 6 hours (up to 4 gm/day).
Pediatric Dosage: 25–50 mg/kg/day, divided q. 6 hours (up to 75–100 mg/kg/day divided q. 6 hours for severe otitis media infections).

Generic Name: CEPHRADINE
Trade Names: Anspor, Velosef
Dosage Forms: Capsules, 250 mg; 500 mg; oral suspension, 125 mg/5 cc, 250 mg/5 cc.
Adult Dosage: 250 mg q. 6 hours or 500 mg q. 12 hours p.o. (up to 4 gm/day).
Pediatric Dosage: 75–100 mg/kg/day p.o. divided q. 6–12 hours (up to 4 gm/day).

PENICILLIN AND PENICILLIN DERIVATIVE ANTIBIOTICS

Generic Name: AMOXICILLIN
Trade Names: Amoxil, Larotid
Dosage Forms: Capsules, 250 mg, 500 mg; oral suspension, 125 mg/5 cc, 250 mg/5 cc; pediatric drops, 50 mg/cc.

Uses: See ampicillin. Higher blood levels than ampicillin, owing to oral absorption.
Adult Dosage (Oral): 250 mg q. 8 hours. For gonorrheal urethritis, 3 gm with 1 gm probenecid as an single dose.

Pediatric Dosage (Oral): Dependent on severity of infection. For a child weighing 20 kg or more, same as adult; for an infant weighing less than 20 kg, 20–40 mg/kg/day divided q. 8 hours. For an infant (6–8 kg), 50–100 mg q. 8 hours; for an infant less than 6 kg, 25–50 mg q. 8 hours.

Contraindications: Penicillin hypersensitivity.

Precautions: See ampicillin.

Adverse Reactions: See ampicillin, but may produce less diarrhea in children.

Drug Interactions: See penicillin.

Generic Name: AMPICILLIN

Trade Names: Polycillin, Amcill

Dosage Forms: Capsules, 250 mg, 500 mg; injection (IM/IV), 125 mg, 250 mg, 500 mg, 1 gm, 2 gm; oral suspension, 125 mg/5 cc, 250 mg/5 cc.

Uses: Penicillin-derivative antibiotic for various infections due to penicillin-G sensitive gram-positive and gram-negative cocci, *Hemophilus influenzae, Salmonella, Shigella, Escherichia coli, Proteus* spp. (penicillinase-producing staphylococciase resistant).

Adult Dosage (Oral): For mild to moderate infections, 250–500 mg (p.o. or IM) q. 6 hours. For gonococcal urethritis, 3.5 gm with 1 gm probenecid as a single dose.

Adult Dosage (Parenteral): For severe infections, 1–2 gm IV q. 4–6 hours (up to 8–14 gm daily in six to eight divided doses).

Pediatric Dosage (Oral): For a child weighing 20 kg or more, same as adult dosage; for a child weighing less than 20 kg, 50–100 mg/kg/day divided q. 8 hours.

Pediatric Dosage (Parenteral): IM or IV doses same as oral doses.

Contraindications: Penicillin hypersensitivity.

Precautions: Possible cross-allergenicity with cephalosporins (7%–10% incidence). β-hemolytic *Streptococcus* infections should be treated for at least 10 days. Not active against penicillinase-producing staphylococci. High incidence of rashes when used in patients with infectious mononucleosis.

Adverse Reactions: Gastric upset with oral use, diarrhea, pseudomembranous colitis, black hairy tongue. Hypersensitivity reactions, including "ampicillin rash" (erythematous, maculopapular). Superinfections, blood dyscrasias, neurotoxicity and convulsions with high doses especially in presence of renal impairment.

Drug Interactions: Probenecid increases ampicillin serum levels. With allopurinol, increased incidence of skin rashes.

Generic Name: CARBENICILLIN

Trade Names: Geopen, Geocillin, Pyopen

Dosage Forms: Tablets (Geocillin), 382 mg carbenicillin base; injection (IM/IV), 1 gm, 2 gm, 5 gm, 10 gm.

Uses: Broad spectrum semisynthetic penicillin active against variety of strains of gram-positive and gram-negative organisms, including *Pseudomonas*. (*Klebsiella* and penicillinase-staphylococci are resistant.)

Adult Dosage (Oral): For urinary tract infection, 1–2 tablets q.i.d.

Adult Dosage (Parenteral): 1–2 gm q. 6 hours IM for mild to moderate infections; 300–500 mg/kg/day IV in divided doses or continuous infusion (up to 30–40 gm/day).

Pediatric Dosage (Oral): For a child, 50–60 mg/kg/day, divided q. 6 hours (oral use not recommended, however).

Pediatric Dosage (Parenteral): For mild to moderate infection in a child, 50–200 mg/kg/day IM or IV divided q. 4–6 hours; for severe infections, 300–500 mg/kg/day IM or IV divided q. 6–8 hours. For a newborn or neonate, 75–100 mg/kg/day IM or IV divided q. 6–8 hours.

Contraindications: Penicillin hypersensitivity.

Precautions: High sodium content (4.7 mEq Na$^+$/gm). Renal or hepatic impairment. Must be well diluted for IV use to reduce incidence of thrombophlebitis. Gram-negative resistance may develop; culture and sensitivity must be checked frequently.

Adverse Reactions: See penicillin-G. Also, coagulation abnormalities, platelet dysfunction, bleeding have occurred, especially in the presence of renal impairment. Hypokalemic metabolic alkalosis, fluid overload, anicteric hepatitis may occur.

Drug Interactions: Synergism with gentamicin may permit a decrease in the dose of carbenicillin. They cannot be mixed together in same IV, however. Probenecid increases serum levels of carbenicillin.

Generic Name: CLOXACILLIN

Trade Name: Tegopen

Dosage Forms: Capsules, 250 mg, 500 mg.

Uses: Antistaphylococcal penicillin derivative.

Adult Dosage (Oral): 250–500 mg q. 6 hours, before meals; may be doubled in severe infection.

Pediatric Dosage (Oral): For a child weighing 20 kg or more, same as adult dosage. For a child weighing less than 20 kg, 50–100 mg/kg/day divided q. 6 hours (higher in severe infections).

Contraindications: Penicillin hypersensitivity.

Precautions: See methicillin. Methicillin-resistant staphylococci should be considered resistant to cloxacillin.

Adverse Reactions: See oxacillin.

Drug Interactions: See penicillin.

Generic Name: DICLOXACILLIN

Trade Name: Dynapen

Dosage Forms: Capsules, 125 mg, 500 mg, 250 mg; oral suspension, 62.5 mg/5 cc.

Uses: Antistaphylococcal penicillin with exceptionally good oral absorption.

Adult Dosage (Oral): 250–500 mg q. 6 hours, before meals; may be doubled in severe infections.

Pediatric Dosage (Oral): For a child weighing 40 kg or more, same as adult dosage; for a child weighing less than 40 kg, 25–50 mg/kg/day divided q. 6 hours; may be doubled in severe infections.

Contraindications: Penicillin hypersensitivity.

Precautions: Methicillin-resistant staphylococci should be considered resistant to dicloxacillin as well. (See also oxacillin.)

Adverse Reactions: See oxacillin and penicillin.

Drug Interactions: See oxacillin and penicillin.

Generic Name: METHICILLIN
Trade Name: Staphcillin
Dosage Forms: Injection (IM/IV), 1 gm, 4 gm, 6 gm.
Uses: Semisynthetic penicillin for infections due to penicillinase-producing staphylococci.
Adult Dosage (Parenteral): For mild to moderate infections, 1 gm q. 4–6 hours IM/IV. For severe infections, 1–2 gm q. 4–6 hours IV.
Pediatric Dosage (Parenteral): For a child, 100–200 mg/kg/day IM or IV divided q. 4–6 hours; for an infant, 100–200 mg/kg/day IM or IV divided q. 6–8 hours; for a newborn or neonate, 50–100 mg/kg/day IM or IV divided q. 12 hours.
Contraindications: Penicillin hypersensitivity.
Precautions: See penicillin-G. Also, methicillin is a potent inducer of penicillinase. Renal impairment may necessitate dosage adjustments. Newborns have a slower renal clearance of methicillin.
Adverse Reactions: See penicillin-G. Also, interstitial nephritis may occur (direct toxic effect). Thrombophlebitis with IV use. Blood dyscrasias and superinfections may occur.
Drug Interactions: See penicillin-G.

Generic Name: MEZLOCILLIN SODIUM
Trade Name: Mezlin
Dosage Forms: Injection (IM/IV), 1 gm, 2 gm, 3 gm, 4 gm.
Uses: Broad-spectrum penicillin active in vitro against a variety of gram-positive cocci (except penicillinase-producing strains) and gram-negative bacteria, including *Klebsiella, Enterobacter, Hemophilus, Escherichia, Serratia, Proteus, Bacteroides,* and *Pseudomonas* strains. High activity against enterococci.
Adult Dosage (Parenteral): For uncomplicated urinary tract infection, 1.5–2 gm IM or IV q. 6 hours. For severe infection, 3 gm IV q. 4–6 hours or 4 gm IV q. 6 hours. Maximum recommended dosage is 350 mg/kg/day or 24 gm/day.
Pediatric dosage (Parenteral): For a child over 1 month and under 12 years, 50 mg/kg IV q. 4 hours (300 mg/kg/day). For a neonate or newborn weighing less than 2 kg, 75 mg/kg q. 8–12 hours IV; weighing over 2 kg, 75 mg/kg q. 6–8 hours IV.
Contraindications: Hypersensitivity to penicillin.
Precautions: See penicillin. Sodium content, 1.85 mEq/gm. Inactive against penicillinase-producing organisms. In vitro sensitivities may not correlate with in vivo ones. Culture and sensitivity tests required in serious infections.
Adverse Reactions: Hypersensitivity reactions, including rashes, urticaria, drug fever, anaphylaxis. Gastric upset with nausea, vomiting, diarrhea reported. Blood dyscrasias and abnormalities in renal and hepatic function test may occur, as well as hypokalemia, convulsive seizures, and neuromuscular irritability with high doses. Thrombophlebitis with IV use and pain with IM administration.
Drug Interactions: See penicillin.

Generic Name: NAFCILLIN
Trade Names: Unipen, Nafcil
Dosage Forms: Tablets, 500 mg; capsules, 250 mg; injection (IM/IV), 500 mg, 1 gm, 2 gm, 4 gm; oral solution, 250 mg/5 cc.

Uses: Antistaphylococcal penicillin. (Significant biliary concentrations achieved).
Adult Dosage (Oral): 250 mg–1 gm q. 4–6 hours.
Adult Dosage (Parenteral): For mild infections, 500 mg IM q. 4–6 hours; for moderate to severe infections, 500 mg–2 gm IV q. 4–6 hours.
Pediatric Dosage (Oral): For a child, 50–100 mg/kg/day divided q. 6 hours.
Pediatric Dosage (Parenteral): For a child, 100–200 mg/kg/day IM or IV divided q. 4–6 hours; for an infant, 100–200 mg/kg/day IM or IV divided q. 6 hours; for a newborn or neonate, 50–100 mg/kg/day IM or IV divided q. 12 hours.
Contraindications: Penicillin hypersensitivity.
Precautions: See oxacillin. Caution in hepatic or renal impairment.
Adverse Reactions: See oxacillin.
Drug Interactions: See penicillin.

Generic Name: OXACILLIN
Trade Name: Prostaphlin
Dosage Forms: Capsules, 250 mg, 500 mg; injection IM/IV, 250 mg, 500 mg, 1 gm, 2 gm, 4 gm; oral solution, 250 mg/5 cc.
Uses: Antistaphylococcal penicillin (see methicillin).
Adult Dosage (Oral): 500 mg q. 4–6 hours, before meals for at least 5 days.
Adult Dosage (Parenteral): 250–500 mg IM or IV q. 4–6 hours for mild to moderate infection; 1–2 gm IV q. 4–6 hours for severe infection.
Pediatric Dosage (Oral): For a child over 40 kg, same as adult dosage; for a child weighing 40 kg or less, 50 mg/kg/day in divided doses q. 6 hours.
Pediatric Dosage (Parenteral): For a child over 40 kg, same as adult dosage; for a child weighing to 40 kg or less, 50–100 mg/kg/day IM or IV divided q. 4–6 hours. For a newborn or neonate, 25 mg/kg/day IM or IV divided q. 4–6 hours.
Contraindications: Penicillin hypersensitivity.
Precautions: See methicillin and penicillin. Methicillin-resistant strains of staphylococci should be considered resistant to oxacillin. Possible nephrotoxicity in newborns on high doses.
Adverse Reactions: See methicillin and penicillin. Also, nonspecific, cholestatic jaundice may occur.
Drug Interactions: See penicillin-G.

Generic Name: PENICILLIN-G
Trade Name: Pentids, Penicillin-G
Dosage Forms: Tablets, 125 mg, 250 mg (400,000 U), 500 mg (800,000 U); oral suspension, 125 mg/5 cc, 250 mg/5 cc; injection (IM/IV), 1, 5, 20 million units (potassium and sodium salts available); long-acting IM procaine PCN-G, 300,000 U/cc, 600,000 U/cc; benzathine PCN-G 300,000 U/cc, 600,000 U/cc.
Uses: Bactericidal antibiotic, for penicillin-G sensitive cocci, syphilis, *Neisseria gonorrhoeae, Clostridium* spp. (penicillinase-producing *Staphylococcus* are resistant).
Adult Dosage (Oral): 250–500 mg q. 6 hours, before meals.
Adult Dosage (Parenteral): Dependent on type and severity of infection. IV range, 1.2–24 million U q.d. divided q. 4–

6 hours. IM procaine PCN-G, 600,000 U–1.2 million U q. 12–24 hours.

Pediatric Dosage (Oral): For a child over 12 years, same as adult; for a child under 12 years, 25,000–100,000 U/kg/day in three to six divided doses (15–60 mg/kg/day).

Pediatric Dosage (Parenteral): For a child, 25,000–300,000 U/kg/day divided q. 8 hours; for an infant, 50,000–250,000 U/kg/day divided q. 8 hours; for a newborn/neonate, 50,000–100,000 U/kg/day divided q. 12 hours.

Contraindications: Penicillin hypersensitivity.

Precautions: Possible cross-allergenicity with cephalosporins. Potassium content of K salt, 1.7 mEq/million units; sodium content of Na salt, 1.7 mEq/million units. Caution in impaired cardiac or renal function, elderly patients, neonates, seizure disorders.

Adverse Reactions: Occasional gastric upset, hypersensitivity reactions, hyperkalemia and cardiac arrhythmias with large doses of potassium salts, CNS toxicity with seizures after massive IV doses or in presence of renal impairment. Pseudoanaphylactic reactions and cardiac arrest with inadvertent IV administration of procaine penicillin.

Drug Interactions: Probenecid increases serum levels of penicillins.

Generic Name: PENICILLIN-V
Trade Names: V-Cillin K, Pen-Vee K

Dosage Forms: Tablets, 125 mg, 250 mg, 500 mg; oral suspension, 125 mg/5 cc, 250 mg/5 cc.

Uses: See penicillin-G. Better oral absorption than penicillin-G.

Adult Dosage (Oral): See penicillin-G.

Pediatric Dosage (Oral): See penicillin-G.

Contraindications: See penicillin-G.

Precautions: See penicillin-G.

Adverse Reactions: See penicillin-G.

Generic Name: TICARCILLIN
Trade Name: Ticar
Dosage Forms: Injection (IM/IV), 1 gm, 3 gm, 6 gm.

Uses: See carbenicillin. Appears more active against *Pseudomonas* than carbenicillin.

Adult Dosage (Parenteral): IM, 1 gm q. 6 hours; IV, 200–300 mg/kg/day divided q. 3–6 hours.

Pediatric Dosage (Parenteral): In a child weighing less than 40 kg, 50–200 mg/kg/day divided q. 4–8 hours IV (depending on severity of infection). In a child weighing 40 kg or more, same as adult. In a newborn or neonate, 75–100 mg/kg/day IV divided q. 4 hours.

Contraindications: Penicillin hypersensitivity.

Precautions: See carbenicillin.

Adverse Reactions: See carbenicillin.

Drug Interactions: See carbenicillin.

SULFONAMIDES

Generic Name: SULFAMETHOXAZOLE/TRIMETHOPRIM (SMZ/TMP)
Trade Names: Bactrim, Septra
Dosage Forms: Tablets, 400 mg SMZ/80 mg TMP (single strength), 800 mg SMZ/160 mg TMP (double strength); injection (IV), 400 mg SMZ/80 mg TMP per 5-cc ampules; oral suspension, 200 mg SMZ/40 mg TMP per 5 cc.

Uses: Treatment of acute and chronic urinary tract infection, shigellosis, *Pneumocystis carinii* pneumonia.

Adult Dosage (Oral): For urinary tract infections, 1 double strength tablet q. 12 hours for 10–14 days. For shigellosis, same for 5 days; for *P. carinii* pneumonia, 15–20 mg/kg/day (TMP concentration) divided doses q. 6 hours for 14 days.

Adult Dosage (Parenteral): For urinary tract infection, 8–10 mg/kg/day IV (TMP concentration) divided q. 6 hours for 14 days; for *P. carinii* pneumonia, same as oral dosage but given slowly IV over 60–90 min. (Each 5 cc ampule should be diluted in at least 125 cc D_5W.)

Pediatric Dosage (Oral): For a child over 12 years, same as adult dosage; for an infant 2 months to 12 years, 1 cc suspension/kg/day divided q. 12 hours for 10–14 days. Not recommended for newborns and neonates.

Pediatric Dosage (Parenteral): For a child over 2 months same as adult dosage for *P. carinii* pneumonia. Not recommended for newborns and neonates.

Contraindications: See sulfisoxazole.

Precautions: See sulfisoxazole.

Adverse Reactions: See sulfisoxazole.

Drug Interactions: See sulfisoxazole.

Generic Name: SULFISOXAZOLE
Trade Name: Gantrisin
Dosage Forms: Tablets, 500 mg; injection (IV), 400 mg/5 cc ampule; oral suspension, 500 mg/5 cc; topical preparations.

Uses: Bacteriostatic antibiotic used primarily for acute and chronic urinary tract infections due to susceptible gram-negative organisms.

Adult Dosage (Oral): 2–4 gm initially, then 4–8 gm q.d. in divided doses q. 4–6 hours.

Adult Dosage (Parenteral): For meningitis, 50 mg/kg IV initially, then 100 mg/kg/day in divided doses q. 6 hours in a slow IV infusion over 60–90 min. well diluted.

Pediatric Dosage (Oral): For a child over 2 months, 75 mg/kg initially, then 150 mg/kg/day divided q. 6 hours (maximum, 6 gm/day). Not recommended for newborns or neonates.

Pediatric Dosage (Parenteral): For a child over two months, same as adult IV dosage.

Contraindications: Hypersensitivity to sulfonamides, pregnancy/lactation, severe renal or hepatic impairment.

Precautions: May exacerbate porphyria and G6PD deficiency. Caution in severely allergic or asthmatic patients because of high sensitivity risk. Topical preparations may be sensitizing.

Adverse Reactions: Gastric disturbances, stomatitis, hepatitis. Allergic reactions, e.g., rash, photosensitivity, drug fever, Stevens-Johnson syndrome. Renal/hepatic damage, kernicterus in newborns, blood dyscrasias, CNS toxicity, including headaches, peripheral neuropathy, mental derangements.

Drug Interactions: Can displace many drugs, such as oral anticoagulants, sulfonylureas, diphenylhydantoin from their protein-binding sites to potentiate their activity.

TETRACYCLINES

Generic Name: DOXYCYCLINE
Trade Names: Vibramycin, Vibratabs
Dosage Forms: Tablets, 100 mg; capsules, 100 mg; injection (IV only), 100 mg, 200 mg; oral suspension, 25 mg/5 cc.
Uses: See tetracycline. Also used for *Neisseria gonorrhoeae* infection in penicillin-allergic patients, and treatment of primary and secondary syphilis.
Adult Dosage (Oral): 100 mg q. 12 hours for 24 hours, then 100 mg q.d. (up to 100 mg q. 12 hours for severe infections); for syphilis, 300 mg q.d. for 10 days; for gonorrhea, 300 mg stat, then 100 mg b.i.d. for 3 days.
Adult Dosage (Parenteral): 200 mg IV initially, then 100–200 mg/day divided q. 12–24 hours. IV doses should be well diluted in at least 100 cc diluent.
Pediatric Dosage (Oral): For a child over 8 years, 4.4 mg/kg in two divided doses to start, then 2.2 mg/kg q.d. in single or divided doses; may be increased to 4.4 mg/kg in severe infections.
Pediatric Dosage (Parenteral): In a child over 8 years, 4.4 mg/kg IV in one or two divided doses at start, then 2.2–4.4 mg/kg daily in one or two divided infusions, depending on severity of infection.
Contraindications: Severe hepatic impairment.
Precautions: For patients with slower renal clearance, give dose q. 24 hours only. Drug should not be given IM since it causes severe tissue necrosis.
Adverse Reactions: See tetracycline. However, not significantly antianabolic as is tetracycline and will not further increase azotemia in renal failure.
Drug Interactions: See tetracycline.

Generic Name: TETRACYCLINE
Trade Names: Achromycin, Sumycin
Dosage Forms: Capsules, 250 mg, 500 mg; injection (IM), 100 mg, 250 mg (contains 2% procaine); injection (IV), 250 mg, 500 mg; oral syrup, 125 mg/5 cc; topical preparations.
Uses: Broad-spectrum antibiotic, useful in penicillin-sensitive patients, for infection due to susceptible gram-positive and negative cocci and bacilli, *Rickettsia*, *Chlamydia*, syphilis, amebiasis, gonorrhea.
Adult Dosage (Oral): 250 mg q. 6–12 hours on empty stomach.
Adult Dosage (Parenteral): 250 mg/day IM single or divided doses; 250–500 mg IV q. 6–12 hours, depending on infection severity. IV solutions for infusion should be well diluted in at least 100 cc of diluent.
Pediatric Dosage (Oral): For a child over 8 years, 25–50 mg/kg/day divided q. 12 hours.
Pediatric Dosage (Parenteral): For a child over 8 years, 10–20 mg/kg/day IV divided q. 12 hours; IM administration not recommended.
Contraindications: Renal impairment. Hypersensitivity to tetracycline.
Precautions: Not to be used in pregnancy, lactation, children less than 8 years old. Hepatic impairment. IM injections contain 2% procaine.
Adverse Reactions: Gastric upset, glossitis, enterocolitis, photosensitivity, hypersensitivity reactions, monilial superinfections, increased intracranial pressure, mottling and discoloration of fetal/children's teeth. Azotemia with renal insufficiency, fatty infiltration of liver with large IV doses (greater than 2 gm/day). Pain, thrombophlebitis with IV use.
Drug Interactions: Multivalent cations (Fe^{3+}, Mg^{2+}, Ca^{2+}) in food and antacids decrease oral absorption of tetracyclines.

MISCELLANEOUS ANTI-INFECTIVES

Generic Name: AMPHOTERICIN B
Trade Names: Fungizone
Dosage Forms: Injection, 50 mg (IV); topical preparations.
Uses: Antifungal agent for IV or intrathecal use for various fungal infections, including candidiasis and coccidioidomycosis.
Adult Dosage (Parenteral): 250 μ/kg/day initially as a single dose, slow IV infusion. May be increased by daily increments of 250 μg/kg/day up to total dose of 1.5 mg/kg/day (usual dose, 50 mg daily). For bladder irrigation, 15–50 mg/day (using up to 5 mg/10 cc concentration in sterile water). For intrathecal use, 300 μg/day or 500 μg two or three times weekly.
Pediatric Dosage (Parenteral): Same adult dosage in mg/kg.
Precautions: Impaired renal function, pregnancy (safe use not established). Should be diluted with D_5W only, not normal saline or electrolyte solutions. Recommended IV concentration, no more than 1 mg/10 cc. Dose should be infused over 2–6 hours.
Adverse Reactions: Fever, chills, nausea, headache, vomiting,

malaise, injection site pain are very common during infusing period. Cardiovascular collapse possible with rapid IV infusion. Renal tubular acidosis with hypokalemia and hypomagnesemia may occur in renal impairment (usually reversible). Intrathecal administration may cause peripheral neuritis, convulsions, chemical meningitis.

Generic Name: CHLORAMPHENICOL
Trade Name: Chloromycetin
Dosage Forms: Capsules, 250 mg; injection (IV), 1 gm; oral suspension, 150 mg/5 cc.
Uses: Broad-spectrum antibiotic (bacteriostatic), particularly useful for acute *Salmonella* infections and *Hemophilus influenzae* meningitis.
Adult Dosage (Oral): 50–100 mg/kg/day divided q. 6 hours to start, decreased to 50 mg/kg/day divided q. 6 hours as soon as possible.
Adult Dosage (Parenteral): 50 mg/kg/day IV divided q. 6 hours (average dose, 1 gm IV q. 6 hours).
Pediatric Dosage (Oral and Parenteral): For a child, same as adult dosage; for an infant (over 2 weeks), up to 50 mg/kg/day divided q. 6 hours IV or p.o. For a newborn or neonate (under 2 weeks), 25 mg/kg/day IV or p.o. divided q. 6 hours.
Contraindications: Hypersensitivity to chloramphenicol. Should not be used prophylactically.
Precautions: Should not be given IM because of erratic absorption. To be avoided in pregnancy at term/lactation. Renal and/or hepatic impairment require dosage adjustments. Blood studies recommended, at start of therapy and q. 2 days during therapy.
Adverse Reactions: Blood dyscrasias, bone marrow depression (reversible and irreversible), aplastic anemia (rare), hemolytic anemia in G6PD deficiency, "Gray syndrome" in neonates (cardiovascular collapse), gastric upset, allergic and febrile reactions. CNS injury, including optic neuritis and peripheral neuropathy.
Drug Interactions: With alcohol, Antabuse-like reaction. Increased anticoagulant effect with warfarin and dicumarol. Increased hypoglycemia with sulfonylureas. Chloramphenicol increases toxicity of diphenylhydantoin.

Generic Name: CLINDAMYCIN
Trade Name: Cleocin
Dosage Forms: Capsules, 75 mg, 150 mg; injection (IM/IV), 300 mg, 600 mg; oral suspension, 75 mg/5 cc.
Uses: Alternate antibiotic for penicillin-allergic patients for treatment of staphylococcal infections. Also used for anaerobic infections (outside CNS), particularly those due to *Bacteroides.*
Adult Dosage (Oral): 150–450 mg q. 6 hours.
Adult Dosage (Parenteral): 600–2700 mg/day IM or IV divided q. 6, 8, or 12 hours (usual dose, 300–600 mg IV q. 6 hours). Maximum dose, 4800 mg/day. IV infusion rate not to exceed 30 mg/min.
Pediatric Dosage (Oral): For serious infections, 8–16 mg/kg/day divided q. 6–8 hours; for more severe infections 16–20 mg/kg/day divided q. 6–8 hours. Not recommended for neonates and newborns.
Pediatric Dosage (Parenteral): In severe infections, not less

than 300 mg/day IV or IM. For a child over 1 month, 15–40 mg/kg/day IV or IM divided q. 6–8 hours. Not recommended for neonates and newborns.
Contraindications: Hypersensitivity to lincomycin and clindamycin, meningitis (no cerebrospinal fluid diffusion).
Precautions: Possible cross-resistance with lincomycin and erythromycin. Elderly patients and those with gastrointestinal disease, particularly colitis. Pregnancy and lactation, hepatic impairment.
Adverse Reactions: Gastric upset after oral administration, including nausea, vomiting, cramps, diarrhea, severe pseudomembranous colitis (rare with parenteral use and usually reversible on oral drug discontinuation). Also hypersensitivity reactions, rashes, jaundice, blood dyscrasias. Thrombophlebitis with IV use. Sterile abscesses with IM use.
Drug Interactions: General anesthetics, neuromuscular blocking agents may cause neuromuscular blockade and respiratory depression.

Generic Name: ERYTHROMYCIN
Trade Names: E.E.S., Ilosone, E-Mycin
Dosage Forms: Tablets, 125 mg, 200 mg, 250 mg, 400 mg, 500 mg; capsules, 125 mg, 200 mg, 250 mg, 400 mg, 500 mg; injection (IV only), 500 mg, 1 gm; topical preparations; oral suspension, 125 mg/5 cc, 200 mg/5 cc, 250 mg/5 cc, 400 mg/5 cc.
Uses: Alternative antibiotic for penicillin-allergic patients. Also effective against *Hemophilus influenzae, Mycoplasma pneumoniae,* and *Legionnaire's agent.*
Adult Dosage (Oral): 250 mg q.i.d. on empty stomach (up to 4 gm/day).
Adult Dosage (Parenteral): 15–20 mg/kg/day IV divided (usual dose, 500 mg q. 6–8 hours). Maximum dosage, 4 gm/day.
Pediatric Dosage (Oral): 30–50 mg/kg/day divided q. 6 hours; may be doubled in severe infection.
Pediatric Dosage (Parenteral): Same as adult dosage in mg/kg and dosage interval.
Contraindications: Hypersensitivity to erythromycin; hepatic impairment (estolate form only).
Precautions: Pregnancy, hepatic impairment.
Adverse Reactions: Gastric upset, cramping, hypersensitivity reactions with rash and urticaria, cholestatic jaundice (estolate form). Thrombophlebitis and pain frequent with IV use (doses must be diluted well). Rare ototoxicity with IV doses greater than 4 gm daily.
Drug Interactions: Erythromycin can cause elevated theophylline serum levels and toxicity.

Generic Name: KETOCONAZOLE
Trade Name: Nizoral
Dosage Form: Tablets, 200 mg.
Uses: Broad spectrum antifungal agent for treatment of candidiasis, coccidioidomycosis, histoplasmosis, chromomycosis, and paracoccidioidomycosis. (Should *not* be used for fungal meningitis owing to its poor penetration into cerebral spinal fluid.) Duration of therapy varies. Up to 12 months may be required for severe infections.
Adult Dosage (Oral): 200 mg as a single daily dose, initially.

Dose may be increased to 400 mg once daily for more severe infections.

Pediatric Dosage (Oral): For a child weighing 20 kg or less, 50 mg once daily; for a child 20 to 40 kg, 100 mg once daily; for a child weighing over 40 kg, 200 mg once daily.

Contraindications: Hypersensitivity to ketoconazole.

Precautions: Use should be avoided in nursing mothers. Teratogenic in rodents. Patients with achlorhydria should take tablets with meals or dissolve them in 4 cc 0.1–0.2 NHC1 and take through a straw to protect tooth enamel.

Adverse Reactions: Most frequently, nausea, vomiting, abdominal pain, and pruritus. Also reported are headache, dizziness, somnolence, fever, chills, photophobia, diarrhea, transient increases in liver enzymes.

Drug Interactions: Concomitant administration of antacids, anticholinergics, and H_2-blockers reduce absorption of ketoconazole. (These medications may be given at least 2 hours after ketoconazole.)

Generic Name: METRONIDAZOLE (IV)
Trade Name: Flagyl IV RTU
Dosage Form: Injection (IV only), 500 mg/100 cc.
Uses: Parenterally for serious infections caused by susceptible anaerobic bacteria, including *Bacteroides* and *Clostridia* spp. All aerobic organisms should be considered resistant.

Adult Dosage (Parenteral): 15 mg/kg over 1 hour by IV infusion, then 7.5 mg/kg q. 6 hours over 1 hour IV (maximum, 4 gm/24 hours). May be changed to oral therapy when conditions warrant, i.e., 7.5 mg/kg p.o. q. 6 hours.

Pediatric Dosage (Parenteral): Not recommended.

Contraindications: Hypersensitivity to metronidazole or other nitroimidazole derivatives. Should be avoided in pregnancy, especially in the first trimester.

Precautions: Hepatic disease (drug accumulation), pregnancy, lactation, patients with active CNS disease. Carcinogenic in rodents.

Adverse Reactions: Gastric upset, unpleasant metallic taste, *Candida* superinfections, hypersensitivity reactions, darkened urine, cystitis, leukopenia, thrombophlebitis (IV use only). CNS toxicity, including peripheral neuropathy, seizures, ataxia, vertigo, syncope.

Drug Interactions: Potentiates warfarin. Alcohol causes Antabuse-like reaction.

Generic Name: METRONIDAZOLE (Oral)
Trade Name: Flagyl
Dosage Form: Tablets, 250 mg.
Uses: Trichomonacide also used in treatment of enteritis due to *Giardia lamblia* or intestinal amebiasis.

Adult Dosage (Oral): For trichomoniasis, 2 gm single dose, or 250 mg t.i.d. for 7 days. For *Giardia lamblia* enteritis, 250 mg t.i.d. for 10 days. For intestinal amebiasis, 750 mg t.i.d. for 5–10 days.

Pediatric Dosage (Oral): For *Giardia lamblia* enteritis in a child, 15 mg/kg/day divided t.i.d for 10 days. For intestinal amebiasis, 30–50 mg/kg/day divided t.i.d for 7 days.

Contraindications: See metronidazole (IV).
Precautions: See metronidazole (IV).
Adverse Reactions: See metronidazole (IV).

Drug Interactions: Potentiates warfarin. Alcohol causes Antabuse-like reaction.

Generic Name: NITROFURANTOIN
Trade Name: Macrodantin
Dosage Forms: Capsules, 25 mg, 50 mg, 100 mg; oral suspension, 25 mg/5 cc.
Uses: Urinary tract infections.
Adult Dosage (Oral): 50–100 mg q.i.d. with food or milk.
Pediatric Dosage (Oral): 5–7 mg/kg/day divided q.i.d.
Contraindications: Significant renal impairment, pregnancy at term, infants under 1 month, hypersensitivity to nitrofurantoins.

Precautions: With long-term therapy, possible pulmonary fibrosis or interstitial pneumonitis. Hemolytic anemia in G6PD deficiency. Severe or irreversible peripheral neuropathy in high-risk patients (e.g., those with renal impairment, diabetes, debilitation).

Adverse Reactions: Frequent gastric upset, hypersensitivity reactions, blood dyscrasias, severe peripheral neuropathy, diffuse interstitial pneumonitis, pulmonary fibrosis, cholestatic jaundice, hepatitis, transient alopecia.

Drug Interactions: Probenecid and sulfinpyrazone increase serum level of nitrofurantoin.

Generic Name: NYSTATIN
Trade Names: Mycostatin, Nilstat
Dosage Forms: Tablets, 500,000 U; oral suspension, 100,000 units/cc; topical and vaginal preparations.
Uses: Treatment of candidiasis.

Adult Dosage (Oral): For oral candidiasis, 4–6 cc oral suspension q.i.d.; should be continued at least 48 hours after oral symptoms have cleared. For gastrointestinal candidiasis, 500,000–1 million units t.i.d. (tablets). For vaginal candidiasis, one vaginal tablet inserted b.i.d. for 2 weeks.

Pediatric Dosage (Oral): For a child or infant, 250,000 U q.i.d.; for a newborn or neonate, 100,000 U q.i.d.

Contraindications: Not for systemic use.

Precautions: Suspension should be retained in mouth as long as possible when treating oral candidiasis. Vaginal tablet should be retained in vagina as long as possible when treating vaginal candidiasis.

Adverse Reactions: Virtually nontoxic.

Generic Name: PHENAZOPYRIDINE
Trade Name: Pyridium
Dosage Forms: Tablets, 100 mg, 200 mg.
Uses: Urinary antiseptic and analgesic.
Adult Dosage (Oral): 100–200 mg t.i.d. after meals.
Contraindications: Renal insufficiency.

Precautions: May discolor feces and turn urine reddish orange. Hemolysis in G6PD deficiency. Yellow skin or sclera if drug accumulates (e.g., renal impairment).

Adverse Reactions: Gastric upset, methemoglobinemia, hemolytic anemia (especially with G6PD deficiency).

Generic Name: PYRIMETHAMINE
Trade Name: Daraprim
Dosage Form: Tablets, 25 mg.

Uses: Antimalarial agent also used for treatment of toxoplasmosis.

Adult Dosage (Oral): For toxoplasmosis, 50–75 mg q.d. with 1–4 gm of a sulfonamide for 1–3 weeks. Dosage of each drug then reduced by one-half and continued for 4–5 weeks more.

Pediatric Dosage (Oral): For a child, 1 mg/kg/day divided b.i.d. with pediatric dose of sulfonamide. After 2–4 days, dose reduced to one-half and continued for 1 month.

Contraindications: Large doses in first trimester of pregnancy.

Precautions: Blood counts should be done twice a week while patient is on initial high-dose therapy, every week when dose is reduced. (Pyrimethamine is a folic acid antagonist.)

Adverse Reactions: Gastric upset, anorexia, vomiting, megaloblastic anemia, bone marrow depression with leukopenia and thrombocytopenia. Blood dyscrasias may be treated with 3–9 mg folinic acid IM until blood cell count returns to normal.

Generic Name: QUINACRINE

Trade Name: Antabrine

Dosage Form: Tablets, 100 mg.

Uses: Anthelmintic, antimalarial, antiparasitic agent.

Adult Dosage (Oral): 100 mg t.i.d. for 5–7 days for *Giardia lamblia* enteritis.

Pediatric Dosage (Oral): For a child, 6–7 mg/kg/day divided t.i.d. for 5 days. (Maximum, 300 mg daily).

Precautions: Patients over 60 years old or those with history of psychosis. Pregnancy.

Adverse Reactions: Gastric upset, vomiting, dizziness, headache, toxic psychosis, hypersensitivity reactions, urticaria, blood dyscrasias, ocular disturbances, yellow staining of skin, blue and black nail pigmentation, acute hepatic necrosis.

Drug Interactions: Antabuse-like effect with alcohol. Primaquin has increased toxicity if given with quinacrine.

Generic Name: RIFAMPIN

Trade Names: Rifadin, Rimactane

Dosage Forms: Capsules, 300 mg.

Uses: Treatment of tuberculosis and prophylaxis of sulfonamide-resistant meningococcal meningitis.

Adult Dosage (Oral): For tuberculosis, 600 mg daily in combination with at least one other antitubercular drug. For meningococcal meningitis prophylaxis, 600 mg b.i.d. for 2 days.

Pediatric Dosage (Oral): For tuberculosis in a child over 5 years, 10–20 mg/kg/day as single dose (up to 600 mg/day) used in combination with at least one other antitubercular drug. For meningococcal meningitis prophylaxis in a child

1–12 years, 10 mg/kg b.i.d. for 2 days (up to 600 mg b.i.d.). For an infant under 1 year, 5 mg/kg b.i.d. for 2 days.

Contraindications: Previous rifampin-associated hepatitis.

Precautions: Pregnancy, lactation, hepatic disease. Caution in daily users of alcohol.

Adverse Reactions: More frequent and severe with intermittent high-dose therapy. Gastric disturbances, allergic reaction, subclinical hepatitis frequent (18%). Clinical hepatitis may occur, especially with preexisting liver disease. Flu-like syndrome, blood dyscrasias, and acute reversible renal failure with nephritis has occurred.

Drug Interactions: May decrease effect of oral anticoagulants and oral contraceptives.

Generic Name: SPECTINOMYCIN

Trade Name: Trobicin

Dosage Forms: Injection (IM), 2 gm, 4 gm.

Uses: Treatment of uncomplicated gonorrhea and an alternate for penicillin-sensitive patients. Not effective against syphilis.

Adult Dosage (Parenteral): 2 gm IM as single dose (4 gm if resistance is prevalent).

Pediatric Dosage (Parenteral): Not recommended.

Contraindications: Hypersensitivity to spectinomycin.

Precautions: Pregnancy, infants, children. May mask or delay symptoms of incubating syphilis (serologic tests should be done for syphilis).

Adverse Reactions: Pain at injection site, transient dizziness or nausea.

Generic Name: VANCOMYCIN

Trade Name: Vancocin

Dosage Forms: Injection (IV), 500 mg; oral solution 500 mg/6 cc (may use injection preparation orally).

Uses: Bactericidal antibiotic for serious infections due to gram-positive cocci resistant to less toxic agents.

Adult Dosage (Oral): 500 mg–1 gm q. 6 hours.

Adult Dosage (Parenteral): 2 gm/day IV divided q. 6–12 hours.

Pediatric Dosage (Oral): For a child, 20 mg/kg/day divided q. 6 hours. For an infant, 10 mg/kg/day divided q. 6 hours.

Pediatric Dosage (Parenteral): Same as oral dosage.

Contraindications: Renal/auditory impairment, hypersensitivity to vancomycin.

Precautions: Should not be given IM. Dosage adjustments necessary in renal impairment. Well diluted solutions and alternate injection sites may be required to reduce thrombophlebitis.

Adverse Reactions: Thrombophlebitis, ototoxicity, nephrotoxicity, hypersensitivity reactions, fevers, chills, peripheral neuropathy.

Drug Interactions: See gentamicin.

BRONCHODILATORS, ANTIASTHMATIC AGENTS

Generic Name: AMINOPHYLLINE (Oral)
Trade Name: Various generics available
Dosage Forms: Tablets, 100 mg, 200 mg; suppositories, 0.25 gm, 0.5 gm.
Uses: Bronchodilator.
Adult Dosage: For acute asthma symptoms in patients *not* currently receiving theophylline derivatives, loading dose of 7 mg/kg, followed by maintenance dose of 2.4–3.5 mg/kg q. 6–8 hours, depending on patient's status. For acute asthma symptoms in patients currently receiving theophylline derivatives, loading dose is deferred if serum theophylline level can be rapidly obtained. A loading dose of 2.5 mg/kg may be given if sufficient respiratory distress warrants a small risk. Maximum daily dosage, 15.2 mg/kg/day or 1100 mg/day (whichever is less).
Pediatric Dosage: For acute asthma symptoms in children (age 6 months to 9 years) *not* currently receiving theophylline derivatives, loading dose of 7 mg/kg, followed by maintenance dose of 4 mg/kg q. 6 hours. For children (9 to 16 years old), loading dose of 7 mg/kg, followed by maintenance dose of 3.5 mg/kg q. 6 hours. For acute asthma symptoms in children currently receiving theophylline derivatives, adult dosage guidelines for that patient type should be followed. Maximum daily dosage, 21.2–28.2 mg/kg/day or 1100 mg/day (whichever is less).
Contraindications: Hypersensitivity to aminophylline or theophylline. Active peptic ulcer disease.
Precautions: Severe cardiac or hepatic disease, hypertension, acute myocardial injury, hyperthyroidism. May exacerbate peptic ulcer. Rectal suppository absorption is slow and erratic.
Adverse Reactions: Gastric upset and irritation, including nausea, vomiting, anorexia, dyspepsia, bitter aftertaste. Dizziness, vertigo, headache, nervousness, agitation, insomnia. Palpitations, tachycardia, flushing, extrasystoles, tachypnea. (See also aminophyllin IV.)
Drug Interactions: See theophyllin.

Generic Name: AMINOPHYLLINE (Parenteral)
Trade Name: Aminophyllin
Dosage Form: Injection (IV), 25 mg/cc.
Uses: Bronchodilator for bronchial asthma, reversible bronchospasm in bronchitis, emphysema, pulmonary edema.
Dosage (Parenteral): (Therapeutic serum levels, 10–20 µg/cc.) Usual IV bolus of 5.6 mg/kg in D_5W 100 cc over 20-40 min., then maintenance infusion of 0.5–0.9 mg/kg/hour, depending on patient's status. (Note: Aminophylline contains 80% theophylline as the ethylenediamene salt.)

Maintenance Dose
(mg/kg/hour)

Adults	Next 12 Hours (mg)	Beyond 12 Hours (mg)
Young smokers	1.0	0.8
Healthy nonsmokers	0.7	0.5
Older patients	0.6	0.3
Patients with congestive heart failure or liver disease	0.5	0.2
Children		
6 months–9 years	1.2	1.0
9 years–16 years	1.0	0.8

Contraindications: Hypersensitivity to theophylline or aminophylline.
Precautions: Must be given slowly (25–40 mg/min.) or serious arrhythmias and/or convulsions can occur. IM administration to be avoided, as it is painful and absorption is incomplete.
Adverse Reactions: Most are related to toxic plasma levels over 20 µg/cc:
- over 20 µg/cc: nervousness, irritability, headache
- over 40 µg/cc: atrial tachycardia, ventricular arrhythmias
- over 60 µg/cc: seizures

Too rapid IV administration causes headache, flushing, dizziness, palpitation, hypotension, ventricular fibrillation, bradycardia, cardiac arrest.
Drug Interactions: Unstable at pH below 8. Incompatible with acidic drugs and pressor amines (e.g., dopamine, isoproterenol, epinephrine, levophed).

Generic Name: BECLOMETHASONE
Trade Names: Vanceril, Beclovent
Dosage Forms: Metered dose inhaler (42 µg/inhalation).
Uses: Adjunctive treatment of bronchial asthma requiring chronic corticosteroid therapy.
Adult Dosage: Two inhalations t.i.d. or q.i.d., or up to 20 inhalations/24 hours, if needed.
Pediatric Dosage: For a child 6–12 years old, one or two inhalations t.i.d. or q.i.d., or up to 10 inhalations/24 hours, if needed.
Contraindications: Hypersensitivity to beclomethasone or other components of inhaler. Primary treatment of status asthmaticus or acute asthmatic episodes requiring intensive measures.
Precautions: Fungal infections of mouth common (*Candida, Aspergillus*). Systemic steroid withdrawal symptoms may occur during transfer to inhaler.
Adverse Reactions: Pulmonary infiltrates with eosinophilia, bronchospasm (rare), hoarseness, dry mouth, suppression of hypothalamic-pituitary-adrenal function.

Generic Name: ISOPROTERENOL (Oral/Inhalation)
Trade Name: Isuprel
Dosage Forms: Tablets (sublingual), 10 mg, 15 mg; Isuprel Mistometer for oral inhalation (1:400); solution (1:200) for use in nebulizers.
Uses: Bronchodilator.
Adult Dosage (Oral): Sublingually, 10–15 mg t.i.d. to q.i.d. (maximum, 60 mg/day); By inhalation, one or two inhalations (with inhaler) q. 4 hours p.r.n.
Pediatric Dosage (Oral): 5–10 mg t.i.d. to q.i.d. (maximum, 30 mg daily).
Precautions: Inhalation route preferred because sublingual absorption is unpredictable.
Adverse Reactions: See parenteral isoproterenol.

Generic Name: METAPROTERENOL
Trade Names: Metaprel, Alupent
Dosage Forms: Tablets, 10 mg, 20 mg; solution for nebulization, 5%; oral syrup, 10 mg/5 cc; metered dose inhaler.
Uses: Bronchodilator (primarily β-2 receptor agonist).
Adult Dosage (Oral): 20 mg or 10 cc t.i.d. to q.i.d. For inhalation, two or three inhalations q. 3–4 hours (up to 12 inhalations/day).
Pediatric Dosage (Oral): For a child weighing less than 27 kg, 10 mg or 5 cc t.i.d. or q.i.d. For a child over 27 kg, adult dosage.
Contraindications: Cardiac arrhythmias associated with tachycardia.
Precautions: Excessive use of inhaler and other sympathomimetics may lead to paradoxical bronchoconstriction. Patients with hypertension, congestive heart failure, coronary artery disease, hyperthyroidism, diabetes, sensitivity to sympathomimetics.
Adverse Reactions: Tachycardia, hypertension, palpitations, nervousness, tremor, gastric upset, bad taste.
Drug Interactions: With sympathomimetic bronchodilators, additive adrenergic effects. Nonselective β-blockers antagonize bronchodilator effect.

Generic Name: N-ACETYLCYSTEINE
Trade Name: Mucomyst
Dosage Forms: Solution for nebulization, 10%, 20%.
Uses: Adjuvant therapy for patients with abnormal viscid or inspissated mucous secretions. Also used for treatment of acetaminophen overdose.
Adult Dosage: For nebulization, 6–10 cc 10% (or 3–5 cc 20%) t.i.d. or q.i.d. into facemask, mouthpiece, or tracheostomy; for direct instillation, 1–2 cc 10% or 20% q. 1 hour p.r.n. For treatment of acetaminophen overdose, 140/mg/kg 20% solution p.o. or via nasogastric tube to start. Then 70 mg/kg q. 4 hours for 16 doses (should be given within 12 hours after overdose).
Contraindications: Hypersensitivity to acetylcysteine.
Precautions: Because of increased bronchial secretions, suction may be required. In asthmatic patients, bronchospasm may occur.
Adverse Reactions: Stomatitis, nausea, rhinorrhea, reversible bronchospasm.

Generic Name: OXTRIPHYLLINE
Trade Name: Choledyl
Dosage Forms: Tablets, 100 mg, 200 mg; elixir, 100 mg/5 cc; pediatric syrup, 50 mg/5 cc (32 mg anhydrous theophylline/5 cc).
Uses: Bronchodilator.
Adult Dosage (Oral): 200 mg q.i.d. or 10 cc q.i.d. (elixir).
Pediatric Dosage (Oral): For a child 2–12 years old, 9.4 mg/kg.
Contraindications: None to the tablets or elixir (not theophylline). Pediatric syrup is a theophylline and, thus, is contraindicated in theophylline hypersensitivity.
Precautions: See aminophylline.
Adverse Reactions: See aminophylline.
Drug Interactions: See aminophylline.

Generic Name: TERBUTALINE
Trade Names: Bricanyl, Brethine
Dosage Forms: Tablets, 2.5 mg, 5 mg; injection (subcutaneous), 1 mg/cc ampules.
Uses: Bronchodilator (β-2 agonist). Oral terbutaline has longer duration of activity than metaproterenol.
Adult Dosage (Oral): 5 mg t.i.d. (at 6-hour intervals). Recommended maximum dose, 15 mg/day.
Adult Dosage (Parenteral): 0.25 mg subcutaneously in a single dose. MR in 15–30 min. (maximum 0.5 mg/4-hour period).
Pediatric Dosage (Oral): For a child over 12 years old, 2.5 mg t.i.d. (up to 7.5 mg/24 hours).
Pediatric Dosage (Parenteral): For a child over 12 years, 3.5–5 µg/kg subcutaneously, but safety not established.
Contraindications: Hypersensitivity to sympathomimetics.
Precautions: Diabetes mellitus, hypertension, hyperthyroidism, cardiac disease, pregnancy.
Adverse Reactions: (Dose-related, usually transient.) Increased heart rate, palpitations, headache, dizziness, nervousness, tremor, nausea, gastric upset, sweating, tinnitus.
Drug Interactions: Propranolol and β-blockers antagonize bronchodilator effects of terbutaline. With other sympathomimetics, additive cardiovascular effects.

Generic Name: THEOPHYLLINE (Sustained Release)
Trade Name: Theo-Dur
Dosage Forms: Tablets, 100 mg, 200 mg, 300 mg (sustained release).
Uses: Bronchodilator.
Adult Dosage (Oral): 300 mg q. 12 hours (up to 6.5 mg/kg q. 12 hours or maximum of 900 mg/day).
Pediatric Dosage (Oral): For a child under 9 years old, 100 mg q. 12 hours to start, then up to 24 mg/kg/day (maximum, 900 mg daily); for 9–12 years, 150 mg q. 12 hours to start, then up to 20 mg/kg/day (maximum, 900 mg daily); for 12–16 years, 200 mg q. 12 hours to start, then up to 18 mg/kg/day (maximum, 900 mg daily).
Contraindications: Hypersensitivity to theophylline; active peptic ulcer disease.
Precautions: See aminophylline. Also, cigarette smoking decreases serum half-life of theophylline.
Adverse Reactions: See aminophylline.
Drug Interactions: Ephedrine, other sympathomimetics, and other xanthine derivatives may cause increased theophylline levels and/or toxicity. Propranolol, β-blockers inhibit theophylline activity.

Generic Name: THEOPHYLLINE (Regular Action)
Trade Name: Slo-Phyllin, Theolair
Dosage Forms: Tablets, 100 mg, 200 mg (Slo-Phyllin); 125 mg, 250 mg (Theolair). Elixir, 80 mg/15 cc.
Uses: See aminophylline.
Adult Dosage: For acute asthma symptoms in patients *not* currently receiving theophylline derivatives, loading dose of 6 mg/kg followed by maintenance dose of 2–3 mg/kg q. 6–8 hours, depending on patient's status. For acute asthma symptoms in patients currently receiving theophylline derivatives, loading dose is deferred if serum theophylline level can be rapidly obtained. A loading dose of 2.5 mg/kg may be given if sufficient respiratory distress warrants a small risk. Maximum daily dosage, 13 mg/kg/day or 900 mg/day (whichever is less).
Pediatric Dosage: For acute asthma symptoms in children (age

6 months–9 years) and *not* currently receiving theophylline derivatives, loading dose of 6 mg/kg, followed by maintenance dose of 4 mg/kg q. 6 hours. For children (age 9–16 years), loading dose of 6 mg/kg, followed by maintenance dose of 3 mg/kg q. 6 hours. For acute asthma symptoms in children currently receiving theophylline derivatives, adult dosage guidelines for that patient type should be followed. Maximum daily dosage, 18–24 mg/kg/day or 900 mg/day (whichever is less).

Contraindications: See aminophylline.

Precautions: See aminophylline.

Adverse Reactions: See aminophylline.

CORTICOSTEROIDS

Uses: Corticosteroids are anti-inflammatory agents for the treatment of a variety of disorders, including endocrine, rheumatic, collagen, neoplastic, and respiratory diseases; dermatologic, allergic, and hematologic disorders; renal and gastrointestinal inflammatory disease. Parenterally, corticosteroids are primarily used as adjunctive treatment of shock (including septic), anaphylaxis, status asthmaticus, cerebral edema, and increased intracranial pressure.

Dosage Forms: Topical, parenteral, oral preparations.

Contraindications: Systemic fungal infections. Hypersensitivity to individual agents.

Precautions: Especially in long-term oral therapy—pregnancy, active or latent peptic ulcers, diabetes mellitus, osteoporosis, gastrointestinal perforations, tuberculosis, chronic or active infections, hypertension or other cardiovascular diseases, psychological conditions, myasthenia gravis.

Adverse Reactions: With prolonged therapy—acute toxic reactions, including peptic ulceration, gastrointestinal hemorrhage, impaired glucose tolerance, superinfections, impaired resistance to infection, psychosis, allergic reactions. Chronic toxic reactions include cushingoid syndrome, adrenal suppression, fluid and electrolyte imbalances (edema, hypokalemia, sodium retention, congestive heart failure), osteoporosis, easy bruising, poor wound healing, striae, muscle wasting, ocular cataracts, hyperglycemia, pseudotumor cerebri. Steroid withdrawal symptoms may occur after discontinuance of prolonged therapy.

Drug Interactions: With potassium-depleting diuretics, increased risk of hypokalemia; with oral hypoglycemics/insulin, hypoglycemic action antagonized.

Generic Name: DEXAMETHASONE

Trade Name: Decadron

Dosage Forms: Tablets, 0.25 mg, 0.5 mg, 0.75 mg, 1.5 mg, 4 mg; injection (IM/IV), 4 mg/cc, 10 mg/cc; long-acting suspension for IM use, 8 mg/cc (Decadron-LA).

Uses: For oral use, see corticosteroids. Parenterally for treatment of cerebral edema, shock, status asthmaticus.

Adult Dosage (Oral): 0.75–9 mg/day to start, then titrated dose to lowest clinically effective level.

Adult Dosage (Parenteral): 10–20 mg IV push (higher doses have been used), then 4 mg IM or IV q. 6 hours until symptoms subside. Response usually evident in 12–24 hours. Dosage may usually be reduced after 2–4 days. Change to oral dose when possible. For life-threatening shock, up to 1–6 mg/kg as a single IV injection or 40 mg IV q. 2–6 hours p.r.n.

Pediatric Dosage (Parenteral): 0.2 mg/kg IV.

Precautions: High-dose therapy should not be continued past 48–72 hours. Prophylactic antacid therapy may be indicated to prevent peptic or stress ulceration during high-dose therapy. Dexamethasone's effects may require 12–24 hours to become evident. Maximum neurologic benefits may require 3–4 days, and osmotic dehydration (e.g., mannitol) may also be needed.

Adverse Reactions: Short-term parenteral administration unlikely to produce harmful effects. Peptic ulcer, burning or tingling in perineal area, paresthesias, ataxia, convulsions, anaphylaxis have occurred.

Generic Name: FLUDROCORTISONE

Trade Name: Florinef

Dosage Form: Tablets, 0.1 mg.

Uses: Mineralocorticoid with moderate glucocorticoid effects. Useful for replacement therapy in chronic adrenocortical insufficiency (Addison's disease) and salt-losing forms of congenital adrenogenital syndromes.

Adult Dosage (Oral): 0.05–0.1 mg q.d. (up to 0.2 mg q.d.).

Adverse Reactions: Primarily fluid and electrolyte imbalances, e.g., edema, hypokalemia, sodium retention, hypertension, cardiac hypertrophy.

Generic Name: HYDROCORTISONE (Sodium Succinate)

Trade Name: Solu-Cortef

Dosage Forms: Injection (IM/IV), 100 mg, 250 mg, 500 mg, 1000 mg.

Uses: Severe shock. (See also dexamethasone.)

Adult Dosage (Parenteral): 0.5–2 gm IV slowly over one to several minutes, then q. 4–6 hours; or 50 mg/kg stat, slow IV, then repeat dose in 24 hours.

Precautions: See dexamethasone.

Adverse Reactions: See dexamethasone.

Generic Name: METHYLPREDNISOLONE (Sodium Succinate)

Trade Name: Solu-Medrol

Dosage Forms: Injection (IM/IV), 40 mg, 125 mg, 1000 mg.

Uses: See dexamethasone.

Adult Dosage (Parenteral): 30 mg/kg IV over 10–20 min.; may be repeated q. 4–6 hours for 48 hours. Large doses may be diluted in D_5W or normal saline for IV infusion.

Precautions: May cause peptic ulceration. Prophylactic antacid therapy every 2 hours may be necessary.

Adverse Reactions: Cardiac arrhythmias and circulatory collapse have been reported, primarily in renal transplant patients, with doses greater than 500 mg IV. Anaphylaxis, allergic reactions have been reported following parenteral corticosteroid therapy.

Generic Name: PREDNISONE
Trade Name: Deltasone
Dosage Forms: Tablets, 1 mg, 2.5 mg, 5 mg, 10 mg, 20 mg.
Uses: See corticosteroids.

Adult Dosage (Oral): Total daily dose is variable and depends on the clinical disorder. Oral range is 5–60 mg/day, followed by gradual reduction in dose to lowest level possible to maintain adequate clinical response. Every other day dosage regimen may be used for minimum pituitary-adrenal suppression. For acute asthma, allergy, bronchospasm, 30–60 mg q.d. (divided doses) tapered over 3–5 days.
Contraindications: See corticosteroids.
Precaution: See corticosteroids.
Adverse Reactions: See corticosteroids.
Drug Interactions: See corticosteroids.

DIURETICS

Generic Name: ACETAZOLAMIDE
Trade Name: Diamox
Dosage Forms: Tablets, 125 mg, 250 mg; capsules (sustained release), 500 mg; injection (IM/IV), 500 mg.
Uses: Carbonic anhydrase inhibitor for reduction of intraocular pressure (for long-term treatment of primary open angle glaucoma and other chronic glaucomas). Also an anticonvulsant and weak diuretic.
Adult Dosage (Oral): 250 mg q. 4–6 hours or 500 mg sustained release capsule q. 12 hours.
Adult Dosage (Parenteral): 500 mg IV or IM initially; may be repeated in 2–4 hours.
Pediatric Dosage (Oral): 10–15 mg/kg/day in divided doses.
Pediatric Dosage (Parenteral): 5–10 mg/kg q. 6 hours IV or IM.
Contraindications: Renal impairment, gout or chronic obstructive pulmonary disease, hypersensitivity to acetazolamide, long-term treatment of chronic noncongestive angle closure glaucoma.
Precautions: Should be avoided during pregnancy (teratogenic in rodents). Possible cross-allergenicity with sulfonamides.
Adverse Reactions: Frequent anorexia, gastric disturbances, malaise, lethargy, and depression. Also paresthesias, headache, dizziness, transient myopia, renal calculus formation and colic, sulfonamide-like nephropathy, hyperuricemia, blood dyscrasias, hypersensitivity reactions.

Generic Name: AMILORIDE
Trade Name: Midamor
Dosage Form: Tablets, 5 mg.
Uses: Potassium-sparing diuretic used as adjunctive treatment with thiazide in congestive heart failure and hypertension.
Adult Dosage (Oral): 5 mg q.d. with meals (up to 10–20 mg q.d.). Usually given with other kaliuretic diuretics or antihypertensive agents.
Contraindications: See triamterene.
Precautions: See triamterene.
Adverse Reactions: See triamterene.
Drug Interactions: Lithium excretion decreased. Predisposition to toxicity.

Generic Name: ETHACRYNIC ACID
Trade Name: Edecrin

Dosage Forms: Tablets, 25 mg, 50 mg; injection (IV), 50 mg.
Uses: Potent loop diuretic with activity and indications similar to those of furosemide.
Adult Dosage (Oral): 50–100 mg q.d. (titrated in 25- to 50-mg increments to desired response, up to 200 mg daily).
Adult Dosage (Parenteral): 50 mg or 0.5–1 mg/kg slow IV (over 2–3 min.), may be repeated once (maximum dose, 100 mg).
Pediatric Dosage (Oral): For a child, 25 mg q.d. to start, titrated by 25-mg increments. To be avoided in infants.
Pediatric Dosage (Parenteral): For a child, 0.5–1 mg/kg slow IV. To be avoided in infants.
Contraindications: Anuria (see furosemide).
Precautions: Should not be given IM or subcutaneously. Other precautions as for furosemide. Use should be discontinued in severe renal disease if oliguria, azotemia, electrolyte imbalances worsen.
Adverse Reactions: Similar to those of furosemide. However, hearing loss is *more frequent* and often permanent, especially in oliguric patients and those with preexisting auditory impairment. Oral tablets can cause gastric upset and bleeding. IV use frequently causes thrombophlebitis.
Drug Interactions: See thiazides. With aminoglycosides, additive ototoxicity.

Generic Name: FUROSEMIDE
Trade Name: Lasix
Dosage Forms: Tablets, 20 mg, 40 mg, 80 mg; injection (IM/IV), 10 mg/cc (20 mg, 40 mg, 100 mg ampules); oral solution, 10 mg/cc.
Uses: Potent loop diuretic for treatment of moderate to severe edema and hypertension. Also adjunctive treatment of hypercalcemia.
Adult Dosage (Oral): 20–80 mg q. morning (usual dose). If no response, may be increased by 20- to 40-mg increments q. 6–8 hours p.r.n. (up to 600 mg daily has been used).
Adult Dosage (Parenteral): 20–40 mg IM or IV push (over 1–2 min.) initially. May be increased by 20-mg increments q. 2 hours until desired response obtained. Doses up to 4–6 gm daily have been used in acute/chronic renal failure. (*Note:* IV administration rate should not exceed 4 mg/min. in elderly and renally impaired patients and 20 mg/min. in general.)

Pediatric Dosage (Oral): 2 mg/kg to start. May be increased by 1–2 mg/kg q. 6–8 hours, up to 6 mg/kg/day maximum.

Pediatric Dosage (Parenteral): 1 mg/kg IM or IV to start. May be increased by 1 mg/kg q. 2 hours until desired response. Maximum dosage, 6 mg/kg/day in divided doses.

Contraindications: Anuria. Hypersensitivity to furosemide. Pregnancy.

Precautions: Possible cross-allergenicity with sulfonamides. Caution in severe or progressive renal disease, liver disease, or cirrhosis (may precipitate hepatic encephalopathy), diabetes, gout, patients on digitalis glycosides, severe electrolyte imbalances.

Adverse Reactions: See hydrochlorothiazide. Also tinnitus and reversible or permanent hearing damage has occurred after rapid or large IV doses (generally occurs within 10–20 min. after administration).

Drug Interactions: See hydrochlorothiazide. Renal excretion of lithium and salicylates is decreased. Possible toxicity from resulting increased serum levels. With aminoglycosides, additive ototoxicity.

Generic Name: HYDROCHLOROTHIAZIDE (Representative Thiazide-type diuretic)

Trade Name: HydroDIURIL

Dosage Forms: Tablets, 25 mg, 50 mg, 100 mg.

Uses: Thiazide diuretic for treatment of mild to moderate hypertension and edema.

Adult Dosage (Oral): 50–100 mg q.d. or b.i.d. depending on response (up to 200 mg/day).

Pediatric Dosage (Oral): For a child 2–12 years old, 37.5–100 mg/day in two divided doses (2.2 mg/kg/day); for an infant under 2 years, 12.5–37.5 mg/day in two divided doses (2.2 mg/kg/day).

Contraindications: Anuria. Mild edema of pregnancy. Hypersensitivity to hydrochlorothiazide. Hypersensitivity to other sulfonamides (relative contraindication).

Precautions: Gout, diabetes mellitus, renal or hepatic impairment. Possible cross-allergenicity with sulfonamides.

Adverse Reactions: Fluid and electrolyte imbalances, e.g., dehydration, orthostatic hypotension, volume depletion, hyponatremia, hypokalemia, hypochloremic alkalosis, hyperuricemia, hyperglycemia, and decreased glucose tolerance. Also paresthesias, weakness, vertigo, muscle spasm, cramps, gastric upset, cholestatic jaundice, hypersensitivity reactions (including photosensitivity, urticaria, rash). Rarely, blood dyscrasias.

Drug Interactions: With antihypertensive agents, additive effects. With oral hypoglycemics/insulin, hypoglycemic effects antagonized. With steroids, increased risk of hypokalemia. With alcohol and CNS depressants, additive orthostatic hypotension. Thiazides decrease lithium excretion and predisposes to lithium toxicity.

Generic Name: MANNITOL

Trade Names: Mannitol, Osmitrol

Dosage Forms: Injection (IV), 5%, 10%, 20% (500-cc bottles), 25% (12.5 gm/50-cc vial, ampule).

Uses: Osmotic diuretic for treatment of cerebral edema and promotion of renal excretion of toxins.

Adult Dosage (Parenteral): For cerebral edema, 1–2 gm/kg slow IV over 30–60 min. (through in-line filter); for diuresis in toxin excretion, continuous IV infusion of 5%–20% solution to maintain urine output of 100–500 cc/ hour. (Maximum dose, 200 gm.)

Pediatric Dosage (Parenteral): For cerebral edema, 2 gm/kg over 30–60 min. IV (15%–20% solution); for diuresis in toxin excretion, 2 gm/kg as a 5%–10% IV solution to maintain high urine output.

Contraindications: Anuria or impaired renal function not responding to test dose of 200 mg/kg IV push. Severe pulmonary congestion or edema, congestive heart failure, dehydration. Active intracranial bleeding, edema associated with abnormal capillary fragility or membrane permeability.

Precautions: Pregnancy. Should not be administered with blood. Solutions more concentrated than 15% may crystallize.

Adverse Reactions: Fluid and electrolyte imbalances, particularly fluid overload with pulmonary edema, hypertension, water intoxication, congestive heart failure. Too rapid diuresis may lead to dehydration, hypovolemia. Tissue necrosis may occur if solution extravasates.

Generic Name: METOLAZONE

Trade Name: Zaroxolyn

Dosage Forms: Tablets, 2.5 mg, 5 mg, 10 mg.

Uses: Diuretic agent similar in activity to thiazides. Often given with furosemide for treatment of refractory edema.

Adult Dosage (Oral): For edema, 5–10 mg q.d. For hypertension, 2.5–5 mg q.d. (Maximum daily dose, 20 mg.)

Contraindications: Anuria, hepatic coma or precoma, hypersensitivity to metolazone.

Precautions: See hydrochlorothiazide.

Adverse Reactions: See hydrochlorothiazide.

Drug Interactions: See hydrochlorothiazide.

Generic Name: SPIRONOLACTONE

Trade Name: Aldactone

Dosage Forms: Tablets, 25 mg, 100 mg (also available with hydrochlorothiazide as Aldactazide).

Uses: Potassium-sparing diuretic for treatment of edema, essential hypertension, and primary aldosteronism.

Adult Dosage (Oral): For edema and hypertension, 50–100 mg q.d. divided doses (up to 200 mg); for primary aldosteronism, 100–400 mg q.d.

Pediatric Dosage (Oral): 3 mg/kg/day. Dosage should be adjusted after 5 days (up to 9 mg/kg/day), and duration of therapy should be limited to 1 month.

Contraindications: Significant renal impairment, anuria, acute renal insufficiency. Hyperkalemia.

Precautions: Excessive amounts of high potassium foods or salt substitutes should be avoided, as should prolonged use of aspirin or salicylates.

Adverse Reactions: Hyperkalemia, electrolyte imbalances, drowsiness, lethargy, dehydration, diarrhea, gynecomastia, gastric upset. (*Note:* Spironolactone produces no hyperuricemia or glucose intolerance.) Useful in patients with gout or diabetes.

Drug Interactions: Salicylates antagonize spironolactone activity.

Generic Name: TRIAMTERENE
Trade Name: Dyrenium
Dosage Forms: Capsules, 50 mg, 100 mg (available with hydrochlorothiazide as Dyazide).
Uses: Potassium-sparing diuretic.
Adult Dosage (Oral): 100 mg b.i.d. after meals (up to 300 mg/day).

Pediatric Dosage (Oral): For a child, 4 mg/kg/day initially. May be increased to 6 mg/kg/day in divided doses.
Contraindications: See spironolactone.
Precautions: See spironolactone.
Adverse Reactions: Similar to those with spironolactone, except hyperuricemia is possible. Diabetics are particularly prone to hyperkalemia. Gastric upset is frequent.

HYPOGLYCEMICS/ANTIHYPOGLYCEMICS

Generic Name: DEXTROSE (50%)
Trade Name: 50% Dextrose
Dosage Forms: Injection (IV), 25 gm/50 cc (50%) preloaded syringe.
Uses: Osmotic diuretic, treatment of hypoglycemia.
Adult Dosage (Parenteral): 25–50 cc (12.5–25 gm) slow IV push. Caloric content, 3.4 Kcal/gm.
Pediatric Dosage (Parenteral): 0.5–1 cc/kg at initial rate of 1 cc/min., then infused at 8–10 mg/kg/min.
Contraindications: Diabetic coma.
Precautions: Extremely hypertonic (2,526 mOsm/liter). Must not be given IM or subcutaneously. Should be given slowly (maximum infusion rate without causing glycosuria, 0.5 gm/kg/hour). Should be avoided in the presence of intracranial or intraspinal hemorrhage.
Adverse Reactions: Phlebitis, thrombosis, hyperglycemia.

Generic Name: GLUCAGON
Trade Name: Glucagon
Dosage Forms: Injection (IM/IV/subcutaneous), 1 mg, 10 mg.
Uses: Pancreatic hormone used in treatment of severe hypoglycemic reactions and insulin overdose.
Adult Dosage (Parenteral): For hypoglycemia, 1–2 mg IM or subcutaneously; may be repeated once, in 15 min. Maximum effects usually occur in 10–15 min.
Adverse Reactions: Mild hyperglycemia (with rebound hypoglycemia after glucagon stopped), hypokalemia, nausea, vomiting, hypocalcemia.

Generic Name: INSULIN
Trade Name: Iletin
Dosage Forms: Concentrations of 40, 80, 100 U/cc (pure beef, pure pork, and beef-pork mixtures available).

Insulin Type	Onset (hours)	Peak (hours)	Duration (hours)	Route
Rapid				
Regular (CZI)	0.5–1	2–4	5–7	IV/subcutaneous/IM
Semilente	1–2	4–6	12–16	IM/subcutaneous
Intermediate				
Globin Zinc	1–2 +	6–10	12–18	IM/subcutaneous
Isophane (NPH)	1–2	8–12	18–24 +	IM/subcutaneous
Lente	2–4	8–12	18–24 +	IM/subcutaneous
Prolonged				
Protamine Zinc (PZI)	4–8	16–20	36 +	IM/subcutaneous
Ultralente	4–8	16–20	36 +	IM/subcutaneous

Uses: Treatment of diabetes mellitus, diabetic ketoacidosis, and hyperglycemic nonketotic coma.
Dosage: For diabetic maintenance therapy, must be titrated to response. For diabetic ketoacidosis, 50 units regular insulin IM and 50 U IV stat, then 50–100 U IM q. 2 hours until blood sugar less than 250 mg/dl and plasma ketone reading no longer positive. With the microinfusion method for diabetic ketoacidosis, 4–8 U/hour as insulin drip (in normal saline) until blood sugar less than 250 mg/dl; once under control, patient may be switched to regular insulin administered subcutaneously (sliding scale) or an intermediate or long-acting insulin administered subcutaneously.
Contraindications: Hypersensitivity (although desensitization procedures may be warranted in some patients).
Precautions: Renal patients may be more sensitive to insulin's hypoglycemic effects. Patients becoming refractory to one animal source may be switched to another purified form.
Adverse Reactions: Hypoglycemia (symptoms include bradycardia with hypotension, diaphoresis, hypertension, tachycardia, lethargy, convulsions, coma, nausea, vomiting, diarrhea, hunger). Local reactions include urticaria, insulin allergy, lipodystrophy. Insulin insensitivity and resistance (immune or nonimmune mechanism) are sometimes treated with steroids or a switch to another animal source insulin.

GASTRIC ACID INHIBITOR

Generic Name: CIMETIDINE
Trade Name: Tagamet
Dosage Forms: Tablets, 200 mg, 300 mg, 400 mg; oral solution, 300 mg/5 cc; injection (IM/IV), 300 mg/2 cc.
Uses: Histamine H_2-receptor antagonist that inhibits gastric acid secretion. For prevention and treatment of active and recurrent duodenal ulcers. Also used in the treatment of pathological hypersecretory conditions.
Adult Dosage (Oral): For active duodenal ulcer, 300 mg q.i.d., with meals and at bedtime, continued for 6–8 weeks (unless healing demonstrated endoscopically); for prevention; 400 mg at bedtime. For hypersecretory condition, 300 mg q.i.d., with meals and at bedtime as long as clinically indicated (up to 2400 mg/day).
Adult Dosage (Parenteral): 300 mg IV (or IM) q. 6 hours.
May be given slow IV push over 1–2 min., but IV piggyback is preferred.
Pediatric Dosage: Not recommended for use in children under 16 years of age.
Precautions: With severe renal impairment, dosage interval should be adjusted to 12 hours. Elderly and/or severely ill patients may experience increased mental confusion, which is reversible within 48 hours of discontinuing drug.
Adverse Reactions: Dizziness, muscular pain, mild and transient diarrhea, neutropenia, and rash more frequent. Also mental confusion, dizziness, headache, blood dyscrasias, mild gynecomastia, hepatitis, pancreatitis, and interstitial nephritis have been reported. Rapid IV injection may cause cardiac arrhythmias and hypotension.
Drug Interactions: May potentiate hypoprothrombinemic effect of oral anticoagulants.

NARCOTIC AND NON-NARCOTIC ANALGESICS

Generic Name: ACETAMINOPHEN
Trade Names: Tylenol, Datril
Dosage Forms: Tablets, 325 mg, 500 mg, 80 mg (pediatric); capsules, 500 mg; elixir, 120 mg/5 cc (pediatric), 1 gm/30 cc (adult); drops, 60 mg/0.6 cc.
Uses: Analgesic and antipyretic agent.
Adult Dosage (Oral): 650 mg–1 gm q. 4–6 hours p.r.n. (up to 2.6 mg/day).
Pediatric Dosage (Oral): For a child 6–12 years old, one-half adult dosage; for a child 4–6 years old, 120–240 mg t.i.d. or q.i.d.; for a child 1–4 years old, 1 teaspoon elixir t.i.d. or q.i.d.; for an infant (under 1 year), 0.5 teaspoon elixir t.i.d. or q.i.d.
Adverse Reactions: Nontoxic in normal doses. Rare blood dyscrasias or hypersensitivity reactions. Toxic overdoses exhibit symptoms of nausea, vomiting, malaise, diaphoresis, hepatotoxicity, delirium, thirst, hypoglycemia, coma, convulsions. (Overdose treatment: acetcylcysteine 20% orally.)
Drug Interactions: With oral anticoagulants, slight increase in hypoprothrombinemic effect.

Generic Name: ASPIRIN
Trade Names: Various generics available
Dosage Forms: Tablet, 325 mg, 400 mg, 650 mg (with or without caffeine and antacids); timed release preparations, 486 mg (7½ gr), 650 mg (10 gr); suppositories, 65 mg, 100 mg, 325 mg, 650 mg; children's aspirin, 81 mg (1¼ gr).
Uses: Analgesic, antipyretic, anti-inflammatory agent. Also used as antiplatelet therapy.
Adult Dosage (Oral): For antipyretic/analgesic effect, 1–3 tablets (325–975 mg) q. 4 hours p.r.n. (up to 4 gm/day); for antiplatelet therapy; 325–650 q.d. (range, 325–1300 mg/day).
Pediatric Dosage (Oral): For a child 2–6 years old, 2.5–5 gr q. 4 hours (up to 5 doses q.d.); for a child 6–12 years old, 5–7.5 gr q. 4 hours (up to 5 doses q.d.).
Contraindications: Hypersensitivity to salicylates, hemophilia, hemorrhagic states, bleeding ulcer.
Precautions: Peptic ulcer disease, gastritis, coagulation abnormalities. Asthma, hay fever, nasal polyps may predispose to salicylate hypersensitivity.
Adverse Reactions: Gastric upset. "Salicylism," i.e., dose-related tinnitus at plasma level of 200–400 µg/cc. Severe or fatal toxicity at over 400 µg/cc. Symptoms include hearing impairment, tinnitus, visual disturbances, nausea, vomiting, hyperventilation, diaphoresis, vertigo, mental confusion, tachycardia, fever, hemorrhage, convulsions, vasomotor depressions, coma, respiratory failure and alkalosis, followed by metabolic and respiratory acidosis (especially in children).
Drug Interactions: With oral anticoagulants, potentiation of bleeding. With alcohol, corticosteroids, nonsteroidal anti-inflammatory agents, increased risk of gastrointestinal ulceration. With probenecid and sulfinpyrazone, decreased uricosuria.

Generic Name: BUTORPHANOL
Trade Name: Stadol
Dosage Forms: Injection (IM/IV) 1 mg/cc, 2 mg/cc.
Uses: Non-narcotic analgesic for moderate to severe pain. A 2 mg dose is approximately equal in potency to 10 mg morphine sulfate. Duration of analgesia is 3 to 4 hours. It also has narcotic-antagonist activity equivalent to 1/40 that of naloxone and 30 times that of pentazocine.
Adult Dosage (Parenteral): 2 mg IM q. 3–4 hours p.r.n. (range, 1–4 mg q. 3–4 hours); 1 mg IV q. 3–4 hours p.r.n. (range, 0.5–2 mg q. 3–4 hours).
Contraindications: Hypersensitivity to butorphanol. Not recommended for children under 18 years.
Precautions: Caution in respiratory decompensation, renal or hepatic impairment (severe), pregnancy, lactation, head injury and increased intracranial pressure, acute myocardial infarction, ventricular dysfunction, or coronary insufficiency. Possible addiction liability in emotionally unstable individuals or those with history of drug abuse. Because of its narcotic antagonist properties, butorphanol is not rec-

ommended for patients physically dependent on narcotics, and it may reduce the effectiveness of previously administered narcotics. Dosage of butorphanol should be reduced when administered concomitantly with phenothiazines and other tranquilizers.

Adverse Reactions: Most frequent include sedation, nausea, clamminess/sweating, headache, vertigo, dizziness, lethargy, and "floating" feeling. Also CNS excitation, including nervousness, unusual dreams, and hallucinations may occur, as well as palpitations, blood pressure changes, elevated cerebral spinal fluid pressure, flushing, cold intolerance, dry mouth, respiratory depression, rashes, hives, diplopia, or blurred vision. (Treatment of overdose: naloxone).

Drug Interactions: Narcotic withdrawal symptoms with methadone and other narcotics. Increased CNS depression with alcohol, tranquilizers, hypnotics, and other CNS depressants. With pancuronium, conjunctival changes may occur.

Generic Name: CODEINE
Trade Names: Various
Dosage Forms: Tablets, 15 mg, 30 mg, 60 mg; injection (IM/subcutaneous); in combination with other analgesics and antitussives (usually 10 mg codeine per 5 cc).
Uses: Narcotic analgesic and antitussive. Treatment of mild to moderate pain.
Adult Dosage (Oral): For analgesia, 15–60 mg q. 4 hours p.r.n.; for antitussive effect, 5–15 mg q. 4 hours p.r.n.
Adult Dosage (Parenteral): 15–60 mg IM or subcutaneous q. 4 hours p.r.n.
Pediatric Dosage (Oral): For analgesia, 3 mg/kg/day in six divided doses orally or subcutaneously; for antitussive effect, 1–1.5 mg/kg/day in divided doses.
Contraindications: Hypersensitivity to codeine.
Precautions: See morphine. May have lower addiction potential and lesser toxicity than other narcotics.
Adverse Reactions: Light-headedness, dizziness, sedation, gastric upset, constipation, respiratory depression, pruritus.
Drug Interactions: See morphine.

Generic Name: MEPERIDINE HCL
Trade Name: Demerol
Dosage Forms: Tablets, 50 mg, 100 mg; injection (IM/IV) 25 mg, 50 mg, 75 mg, 100 mg; elixir, 10 mg/cc.
Uses: Narcotic analgesic for severe pain; 80–100 mg meperidine approximately equal in potency to 10 mg morphine sulfate (duration, 2–4 hours).
Adult Dosage (Oral): 50–150 mg q. 3–4 hours p.r.n.
Adult Dosage (Parenteral): 50–150 mg IM q. 3–4 hours p.r.n.; or slow IV 50–100 mg diluted and titrated.
Pediatric Dosage (Oral): 1–2 mg/kg q. 3–4 hours (up to 100 mg per dose) p.r.n. (or 6 mg/kg/day in six divided doses).
Contraindications: See morphine. Administration of MAO inhibitors within last 14 days. Hypersensitivity to meperidine.
Precautions: Metabolite (nor-meperidine) has excitant properties that may precipitate seizures in epileptics. Subcutaneous route is to be avoided, as it causes pain and tissue necrosis.

Adverse Reactions: See morphine.
Drug Interactions: See morphine. With anticonvulsants, decrease in seizure threshold; increase in anticonvulsant dosage may be required.
Drug Interactions: Physically incompatible with all barbiturates, Librium, Valium, aminophylline, sodium bicarbonate, hydrocortisone. Additive CNS depression with other narcotics, sedative-hypnotics, tricyclic antidepressants, alcohol, antianxiety agents. With tricyclic antidepressants and anticholinergics, additive anticholinergic effects.

Generic Name: MORPHINE SULFATE
Trade Name: Morphine
Dosage Forms: Tablets, 10 mg, 15 mg, 30 mg; injection (IM/subcutaneous/IV), 2 mg, 4 mg, 6 mg, 8 mg, 10 mg, 15 mg.
Uses: Narcotic analgesic for severe pain. Duration of action, approximately 4–5 hours.
Adult Dosage (Oral): Serum levels usually not sufficient owing to rapid metabolism after oral absorption.
Adult Dosage (Parenteral): 5–20 mg IM or subcutaneously q. 4 hours p.r.n. For IV administration, 1–10 mg diluted and slowly injected; may repeat small doses q. 5–10 min., cautiously.
Pediatric Dosage (Parenteral): 100–200 µg/kg subcutaneously q. 4 hours p.r.n. (Maximum of 15 mg/dose.)
Contraindications: Hypersensitivity to morphine. Bronchial asthma or severe respiratory depression.
Precautions: Addicting. Dose must be decreased by one-half when other CNS depressants are used. Vagolytic action may increase ventricular rate (caution in paroxysmal supraventricular tachycardia). Caution in respiratory disorders, elderly or debilitated patients, myxedema, hepatic or renal impairment (severe), convulsive disorders, prostatic hypertrophy, head trauma with intracranial lesions or increased intracranial pressure.
Adverse Reactions: Primarily respiratory and circulatory depression. Also euphoria, dysphoria, hallucinations, urinary retention, gastric upset, constipation and biliary tract spasm (morphine sulfate more than meperidine). Also causes histamine release.
Drug Interactions: See meperidine.

Generic Name: PENTAZOCINE
Trade Name: Talwin
Dosage Forms: Injection (IM/IV/subcutaneous), 30 mg, 60 mg.
Uses: Non-narcotic analgesic for relief of moderate to severe pain.
Adult Dosage (Oral): 50–100 mg q. 3–4 hours p.r.n. (up to 600 mg/day).
Adult Dosage (Parenteral): 30–60 mg IM or subcutaneous, or 30 mg IV, q. 3–4 hours p.r.n. (up to 360 mg/day).
Contraindications: Hypersensitivity to pentazocine. Not recommended for children under 12 years old.
Precautions: See morphine. Addicting. Pentazocine is a mild narcotic antagonist that may reduce the effectiveness of a previously administered narcotic.
Adverse Reactions: Sedation, sweating, dizziness, nausea, euphoria, hallucinations are most frequent. Occasional anti-

cholinergic effects. After parenteral use, diaphoresis, respiratory depression, apnea.

Drug Interactions: See morphine.

Generic Name: PROPOXYPHENE
Trade Name: Darvon
Dosage Forms: Tablets, 50 mg, 100 mg with acetaminophen (Darvocet-N, Darvocet-N 100); capsules, 32 mg, 65 mg plain, 32 mg and 65 mg with APC (Darvon Compound-32 and Darvon Compound-65).
Uses: Non-narcotic analgesic for treatment of mild pain.
Adult Dosage (Oral): 65 mg q. 4–6 hours p.r.n., or 100 mg (Darvocet-N 100) q. 4–6 hours p.r.n.
Contraindications: Not recommended in children. Hypersensitivity to propoxyphene, pregnancy, suicidal or addiction-prone patients.
Precautions: Addicting. Mental impairment and reflex activity slowed.
Adverse Reactions: Dizziness, sedation, nausea, vomiting are most frequent. Constipation, euphoria, dysphoria, minor visual disturbances, and skin rashes also occur. Chronic ingestion of over 800 mg/day may cause toxic psychosis and convulsions. Acute overdoses cause CNS and respiratory depression, coma, convulsions, pulmonary edema, hypotension, arrhythmias. Toxic serum levels over 2 mg/100 cc alone or 1 mg/100 cc when combined with other CNS depressants can be fatal (lethal doses may be 0.5 gm or more). Naloxone is used to treat respiratory depression. Hemodialysis is of little value in treatment of overdose.
Drug Interactions: Other CNS depressants, tricyclic antidepressants, alcohol, and muscle relaxants potentiate CNS depression.

Generic Name: ZOMEPIRAC
Trade Name: Zomax
Dosage Form: Tablets, 100 mg.
Uses: Nonsteroidal anti-inflammatory, antipyretic, and analgesic agent for mild to moderate pain.
Adult Dosage (Oral): 100 mg q. 4–6 hours p.r.n.
Contraindications: Hypersensitivity to zomepirac or to aspirin or other nonsteroid anti-inflammatory agents manifested by bronchospastic reactions.
Precautions: Peptic ulcer disease and upper gastrointestinal inflammatory disease, renal impairment, hypertension, congestive heart failure, coagulation disorders.
Adverse Reactions: Frequent gastric upset, anorexia, dizziness, sedation, vertigo, tinnitus occurs. (See also indomethacin.) Also urinary tract infection and frequency, vaginitis, hematuria reported with prolonged use. Ocular changes have been reported in animals.

SEDATIVE-HYPNOTICS

BARBITURATES

Uses: Sedative-hypnotics also used in treatment of acute convulsive disorders and for preoperative sedation.
Dosage Forms: Various preparations are available for parenteral, oral, or rectal use. They may be rapid-acting (duration of minutes, as thiopental sodium IV) short- to intermediate-acting (duration of 5–8 hours, as pentobarbital), or long-acting (duration of 6–10 hours, as phenobarbital).
Contraindications: Hypersensitivity to barbiturates. Porphyria. Respiratory disease in which dyspnea or obstruction is present.
Precautions: Psychic and/or physical dependence with tolerance may develop. Severe hepatic or renal impairment (drug accumulation). Caution in pregnancy, severe cardiac disease, and elderly or debilitated patients. Respiratory depression, apnea, laryngospasm, and hypotension may occur with too rapid IV administration. Mental impairment and slowing of reflexes may prohibit the performance of potentially hazardous activities.
Adverse Reactions: Habit-forming, residual sedation ("hangover"), lethargy, paradoxical excitement or hyperactivity in children, hypersensitivity reactions, skin eruptions, serum sickness, CNS depression. IV use, especially, causes thrombophlebitis, severe respiratory depression, apnea, hypotension, coughing, hiccoughing, laryngospasm, bronchospasm, nausea, vomiting. For most barbiturates, toxic blood levels of 3.5 mg/100 cc (range, 1.5–3.5 mg/100 cc) are potentially lethal. Toxic symptoms usually appear at ten times the hypnotic dose, and include hypothermia, fever, sluggish or absent reflexes, respiratory depression, hypotension, circulatory collapse, pulmonary edema, miosis, or (in severe cases) mydriasis, oliguria, coma.
Drug Interactions: With alcohol, tranquilizers, and other CNS depressants, additive CNS and respiratory depression. With coumarin anticoagulants, decreased prothrombin time. Barbiturates stimulate hepatic microsomal enzymes, resulting in increased metabolism of many drugs metabolized in the liver (e.g., digitoxin, diphenylhydantoin, corticosteroids).

Generic Name: AMOBARBITAL (Barbiturate-derivative)
Trade Names: Amytal, Amytal Sodium
Dosage Forms: Tablets, 15 mg, 30 mg, 50 mg, 100 mg; elixir, 44 mg/5 cc.
Uses: Sedative-hypnotic used primarily as anticonvulsant for status epilepticus and acute agitation in psychotic and hysterical states.
Adult Dosage (Oral): See secobarbital.
Adult Dosage (Parenteral): 130–260 mg IM or slow IV (up to 500 mg slow IV). IV administration rate should not exceed 100 mg/min.
Adverse Reactions: See barbiturates.
Drug Interactions: See barbiturates.

Generic Name: ETHCHLORVYNOL
Trade Name: Placidyl

Dosage Forms: Capsules, 100 mg, 200 mg, 500 mg, 750 mg.
Uses: Sedative-hypnotic.
Adult Dosage (Oral): 500–750 mg at bedtime for 1 week only (maximum dose, 1 gm).
Contraindications: Hypersensitivity to ethchlorvynol. Porphyria.
Precautions: See barbiturates. Toxic levels are about 4 mg/100 cc.
Adverse Reactions: See barbiturates. Also, prolonged coma (days) with fluctuating levels of consciousness may occur with overdoses. Paradoxical excitement and seizures, hypothermia, and pancytopenia may occur. Lethal doses are not well defined (15 gm?). Chronic exposure may produce ataxia, incoordination, tremors, muscle weakness, peripheral neuropathy, slurred speech, confusion.
Drug Interactions: See barbiturates.

Generic Name: GLUTETHIMIDE
Trade Name: Doriden
Dosage Forms: Tablets, 0.25 gm, 0.5 gm; capsules, 0.5 gm.
Uses: Sedative-hypnotic.
Adult Dosage (Oral): 0.25–0.5 gm at bedtime p.r.n.
Contraindications: Hypersensitivity to glutethimide, porphyria.
Precautions: See barbiturates. Hemodialysis or peritoneal dialysis is of little value in overdose treatment. Toxic serum levels usually over 3 mg/100 cc.
Adverse Reactions: See barbiturates. Lethal adult dose probably 5–10 gm. Stupor or coma may alternate with alert, hyperactive behavior (owing to enterohepatic recirculation). Convulsions may occur.
Drug Interactions: See barbiturates.

Generic Name: METHAQUALONE
Trade Name: Mequin (formerly Quaalude)
Dosage Forms: Tablets, 150mg, 300mg.
Uses: Sedative-hypnotic.
Adult Dosage (Oral): 150–300 mg at bedtime p.r.n.
Contraindications: Hypersensitivity to methaqualone. Toxic serum level approximately 3 mg/100 cc.
Precautions: See barbiturates.
Adverse Reactions: See barbiturates. Convulsions and vomiting with aspiration pneumonitis and respiratory obstruction may occur. Toxic reactions usually follow acute ingestion of 2–4 gm. Dialysis may be helpful in treating overdoses.
Drug Interactions: See barbiturates.

Generic Name: PENTOBARBITAL (Barbiturate-derivative)
Trade Name: Nembutal
Dosage Forms: Capsules, 30 mg, 50 mg, 100 mg; injection (IM/IV), 50 mg/cc; suppositories, 30 mg to 200 mg.
Uses: See secobarbital.
Adult Dosage (Oral): See secobarbital.
Pediatric Dosage (Oral): See secobarbital.
Precautions: See secobarbital.

Generic Name: SECOBARBITAL (Barbiturate-derivative)
Trade Name: Seconal
Dosage Forms: Tablets, 50 mg, 100 mg; capsules, 30 mg, 50 mg, 100 mg; injection, (IM/IV), 50 mg/cc; suppositories, 30-200 mg; elixir 22 mg/5 cc.
Uses: Sedative-hypnotic.
Adult Dosage (Oral): For hypnosis, 100 mg at bedtime; for sedation; 20–40 mg b.i.d. to t.i.d.
Adult Dosage (Parenteral): For hypnosis, 100 mg IM at bedtime; for acute convulsions, 5–6 mg/kg IM or slow IV, repeated q. 3–4 hours p.r.n.
Pediatric Dosage (Oral): For sedation, 2 mg/kg/day divided doses (also rectally).
Pediatric Dosage (Parenteral): For acute convulsions; 3–5 mg/kg IM or slow IV, repeated q. 3–4 hours p.r.n.
Contraindications: Obstetric deliveries. (See also barbiturates.)
Precautions: See barbiturates.
Adverse Reactions: See barbiturates.
Drug Interactions: See barbiturates.

Generic Name: THIOPENTAL IV (Barbiturate-derivative)
Trade Name: Pentothal
Dosage Forms: Injection (IV only), 500 mg/20 cc.
Uses: Anesthesia for brief procedures, induction anesthesia, anticonvulsant. Also used for narcoanalysis in psychiatric disorders.
Adult Dosage (Parenteral): Dosage must be titrated to response.
Contraindications: Absence of suitable veins for IV administration. Hypersensitivity to barbiturates. Latent or manifest porphyria.
Precautions: Extravasation or intra-arterial injection should be avoided. Test dose of 25–75 mg recommended. Caution in advanced cardiac disease, increased intracranial pressure, asthma, myasthenia gravis, pregnancy.
Adverse Reactions: Repeated doses lead to prolonged anesthesia owing to drug accumulation in fatty tissues. IV reactions as for reactions to IV administration of barbiturates.

SKELETAL MUSCLE RELAXANTS

Generic Name: CARISOPRODOL
Trade Name: Soma
Dosage Forms: Tablets, 350 mg (also with codeine 16mg, phenacetin, caffeine).
Uses: Skeletal muscle relaxant.

Adult Dosage (Oral): 350 mg t.i.d. and at bedtime.
Contraindications: Acute intermittent porphyria. Hypersensitivity to carisoprodol or related compounds, such as meprobamate.
Precautions: Mental impairment and reflex slowing. Renal or

hepatic impairment. Mild withdrawal symptoms after large doses (100 mg/kg/day).

Adverse Reactions: See methocarbamol. Also idiosyncratic reactions after first dose have occurred and include CNS derangement, diplopia, temporary vision loss, ataxia, extreme weakness, confusion, disorientation.

Drug Interactions: Additive CNS depression with alcohol, tranquilizers, sedative-hypnotics.

Generic Name: METHOCARBAMOL
Trade Name: Robaxin
Dosage Forms: Tablets, 500 mg, 750 mg; injection (IM/IV), 100 mg/cc.
Uses: Skeletal muscle relaxant (centrally acting).
Adult Dosage (Oral): 1.5 gm q.i.d. for initial 48–72 hours, then 750 mg–1 gm q.i.d. (up to 4.5 gm daily).

Adult Dosage (Parenteral): 100–300 mg/day IM or IV for up to 3 days. May repeat after 48 hours; for tetany, 100-300 mg IV q. 6 hours until nasogastric tube can be inserted.
Pediatric Dosage (Parenteral): For tetany, 15 mg/kg or more, slow IV q. 6 hours (rate under 3 cc/min.).
Contraindications: Hypersensitivity to methocarbamol. Renal disease (contraindication with injectable form only).
Precautions: IV rate not to exceed 3 cc/min. Convulsive seizures have occurred after IV use.
Adverse Reactions: Oral administration may produce sedation, dizziness, lethargy, gastric upset, allergic reactions. Parenteral administration may produce nausea, vomiting, syncope, hypotension, tachycardia, blurred vision, facial flushing, respiratory depression, thrombophlebitis, anaphylaxis.
Drug Interactions: See carisoprodol.

PLASMA VOLUME EXPANDERS

Generic Name: ALBUMIN (Human)
Trade Name: Normal Serum Albumin, Albutein
Dosage Forms: Injection (IV), 250 mg/cc (12.5 gm/50 cc) 25%, 50 mg/cc (5%).
Uses: Plasma volume expander.
Adult Dosage (Parenteral): For hypovolemic shock, 25 gm (100 cc 25% solution) IV rapidly. May be repeated in 15–30 min. (up to 125 gm/day, maximum). As plasma volume returns to normal, IV infusion should be slowed to to 1 cc/min. or less to prevent circulatory overload.
Pediatric Dosage (Parenteral): For a child, 25 gm IV initially, then 25%–50% of adult dose, thereafter. For the newborn or neonate, 1 gm/kg IV.
Contraindications: Cardiac failure, severe anemia.
Precautions: Administration of albumin to dehydrated patients may be ineffective unless additional IV fluids are given. Rapid infusion rates, e.g., over 1 cc/min., may cause circulatory overload in patients whose plasma volume has almost returned to normal.
Adverse Reaction: See plasma protein fraction. However, since albumin is more highly purified than plasma protein fraction, it may be less likely to cause adverse allergic reactions and hypotension.

Generic Name: DEXTRAN 40, 70, 75
Trade Names: Rheomacrodex, Dextran 40, Dextran 70, Gentran-40, Gentran-75
Dosage Forms: Injection (IV), Dextran 40 in 500 cc normal saline or D_5W, Dextran 70 in 500 cc normal saline or D_5W, Dextran 75 in 500 cc normal saline or D_5W or 10% invert sugar.
Uses: Plasma volume expander. Dextran 70 and 75 are high-molecular-weight polymers, while Dextran 40 is a low-molecular-weight polymer.
Adult Dosage (Parenteral): For administration of Dextran 40 10–20 cc/kg slow IV (not to exceed 20/cc/kg/day); if therapy continued for more than 24 hours, total daily dose should not exceed 10/cc/kg/day. For administration of Dextran 70 or 75, 500–1,000 cc slow IV at 20–40 cc/min.; total dose should not exceed 20 cc/kg/day during first 24 hours.
Pediatric Dosage (Parenteral): Same as adult dosage.
Contraindications: Hypersensitivity to dextrans. Severe congestive heart failure, renal failure, hypervolemic states, bleeding disorders.
Precautions: Chronic liver disease, impaired renal function, or cardiovascular impairment. Antigenic potential (more with high-molecular-weight than with low-molecular-weight dextran). Antiplatelet action may increase clotting time.
Adverse Reactions: Hypersensitivity reactions include rash, urticaria, pruritus, nasal congestion, dyspnea, chest tightness, mild hypotension. Angioedema, bronchospasm, and anaphylaxis have occurred, as well as nausea, vomiting, and acute hypotension.

Generic Name: HETASTARCH (Hydroxyethyl starch)
Trade Names: Volex, Hespan
Dosage Forms: Injection (IV), 6% hetastarch in 500 cc normal saline.
Uses: Plasma volume expander.
Adult Dosage (Parenteral): 500–1,000 cc IV infusion (up to 1,500 cc/day or 20 cc/kg). For acute hemorrhagic shock, may be administered at 20 cc/kg/hour, for burns and septic shock, administered at less than 20 cc/kg/hour.
Contraindications: Severe bleeding disorders. Severe congestive cardiac and renal failure with oliguria or anuria.
Precautions: Circulatory overload; central venous pressure should be monitored. Hepatic disease. Large doses may prolong prothrombin and bleeding times.
Adverse Reactions: Minimal antigenic properties, but allergic reactions have been reported, including vomiting, mild fever, chills, itching, parotid gland enlargement, headaches, urticaria, peripheral and periorbital edema, and wheezing.

Generic Name: PLASMA PROTEIN FRACTION (Human)
Trade Name: Plasmanate
Dosage Forms: Injection (IV), 5% (250 cc, 500 cc).

Uses: Plasma volume expander.

Adult Dosage (Parenteral): For hypovolemic shock, 250–500 cc IV infusion at 10 cc/min. or less; as plasma volume approaches normal, rate should be slowed to 5–8 cc/min. For hypoproteinemia, 1,000–1,500 cc IV q.d.

Pediatric Dosage (Parenteral): 5–7cc/kg infused IV at rate of 10 cc/min. or less.

Contraindications: Cardiopulmonary bypass procedures. Severe anemia (possible contraindication).

Precautions: Does not provide coagulation factors. IV rate over 10 cc/min. may cause vascular overload with pulmonary edema and cardiac failure. Commercial preparations contain 130–160 mEq. Na^+/liter; must be used cautiously in patients with hepatic, renal, or cardiac failure.

Adverse Reactions: Infrequent, but include flushing, nausea, vomiting, chills, fever, headache, backpain, hypersalivation, erythema, urticaria.

THYROID/ANTITHYROID AGENTS

Generic Name: LEVOTHYROXINE

Trade Name: Synthroid

Dosage Forms: Tablets, 25 μg, 50 μg, 100 μg, 150 μg, 200 μg, 300 μg; injection (IV), 500 μg vial.

Uses: Thyroid preparation for treatment of hypothyroidism or absent thyroid function. Given parenterally for treatment of myxedema coma or stupor.

Adult Dosage (Oral): 25–50 μg/day initially, increased by 25–50 μg at monthly intervals until desired response is obtained (usual maintenance dose, 100–200 μg/day).

Adult Dosage (Parenteral): For myxedema coma without heart disease, 200–500 μg IV to start, repeated in 1–2 days with 100–300 μg.

Pediatric Dosage (Oral): For a child, 6 μg/kg/day; for an infant under 1 year, not less than 100 μg/day (therapy of cretinism).

Contraindications: Acute myocardial infarction, uncorrected adrenal insufficiency, thyrotoxicosis.

Precautions: Caution required in patients with cardiovascular disease or acute myocardial infarction. The status of other metabolic diseases, including diabetes, adrenal insufficiency, hyperadrenalism, hypopituitarism, may be affected by changes in thyroid status.

Adverse Reactions: Headache, nervousness, tremor, palpitations, tachycardia, angina, cardiac arrhythmias, diarrhea, abdominal cramps, heat intolerance, diaphoresis, and weight loss may occur. All are dose-related and may be avoided by slow dosage increases.

Drug Interactions: With oral anticoagulants, potentiation of hypoprothombinemic effect. With insulin and oral hypoglycemics, decreased hypoglycemic effect. With tricyclic antidepressants, potentiation of antidepressant effects. With diphenylhydantoin, possible increase in thyroxine blood level.

Generic Name: PROPYLTHIOURACIL

Trade Name: Propylthiouracil, PTU

Dosage Form: Tablet, 50 mg.

Uses: Treatment of hyperthyroidism and thyroid storm (antithyroid).

Adult Dosage (Oral): 100 mg q. 8 hours initially and continued for 6–8 weeks until patient is euthyroid. Then, dosage is reduced by one-third every 4–6 weeks to maintenance levels of 50–100 mg/day. Occasionally, resistant patients may require initial doses of 900–1,200 mg/day, divided q. 4–8 hours.

Pediatric Dosage (Oral): For a child 6–10 years old, 50–150 mg/day until euthyroid, then 50 mg b.i.d. For a child over 10 years, 150–300 mg/day until euthyroid, then 50 mg b.i.d.

Contraindications: Last few weeks of pregnancy/lactation.

Precautions: Pregnancy. Oral anticoagulants (hypoprothrombinemic effect), possible cross-sensitivity with methimazole (low incidence). Potentially serious agranulocytosis may develop.

Adverse Reactions: Skin rashes, urticaria (dose-related). Occasional gastrointestinal disturbances, headache, dizziness, paresthesias, arthralgia, hypoprothrombinemia, salivary gland and lymph node enlargement, loss of taste, visual disturbances, and edema may occur. Mild leukopenia (white blood cell count under 4,000/cu mm) occurs in about 10% of patients treated and is usually not an indication for discontinuation of the drug. However, severe leukopenia, thrombocytopenia, and agranulocytosis require discontinuance.

Drug Interactions: May potentiate action of oral anticoagulants.

ERGOT ALKALOIDS, OXYTOCICS, ESTROGENS

Generic Name: ERGOTAMINE TARTRATE

Trade Name: Ergomar, Gynergen

Dosage Forms: Tablets (sublingual), 2 mg; tablets (oral), 1 mg; injection (subcutaneous/IM), 0.5 mg/cc; inhalation, 9 mg/cc; also available as Cafergot tablets containing 1 mg ergotamine plus 100 mg caffeine, and Cafergot rectal suppositories containing 2 mg ergotamine plus 100 mg caffeine.

Uses: Ergot alkaloid for treatment of migraine headaches.

Adult Dosage (Oral): 2–3 mg initially (or 1–2 mg sublingually), then 1–2 mg q. 1 hour to a maximum of 6 mg/day or 10 mg/week. For inhalation therapy, one inhalation stat, then q. 5 min. p.r.n. (up to 6/day). Cafergot tablets are given as follows: 2 tablets at start of attack, then 1 tablet q. 30 min. p.r.n. (maximum of 6 tablets/attack or 10 tablets/week). In Cafergot suppository therapy, 1 suppository is given stat; may be repeated once (maximum of 2 suppositories/attack or 4 suppositories/week).

Adult Dosage (Parenteral): 0.25–0.5 mg IM or subcutaneously to start; repeated once in 2 hours (up to 1 mg/week).

Contraindications: Pregnancy, occlusive vascular disease, coronary heart disease, hypertension, hepatic or renal impairment, sepsis, severe pruritus, cellulitis.

Precautions: Overdosing or prolonged administration may lead to ergotism and eventual gangrene.

Adverse Reactions: Frequent nausea and vomiting, muscle weakness and pain in extremities, tingling in fingers and toes, occasional headaches. Also precordial distress, tachycardia, bradycardia, gangrene (rare).

Generic Name: METHYLERGONOVINE MALEATE
Trade Name: Methergine
Dosage Forms: Tablets, 0.2 mg; injection (IM/IV) 0.2 mg/cc.
Generic Name: ERGONOVINE MALEATE
Trade Name: Ergotrate
Dosage Forms: Tablets, 0.2 mg; injection (IM/IV) 0.2 mg/cc.
Uses: Used post partum after placental delivery to produce firm uterine contractions and decrease uterine bleeding.
Adult Dosage (Oral): 0.2 mg b.i.d. to q.i.d. for 2 days usually.
Adult Dosage (Parenteral): 0.2 mg q. 6 hours, repeated in 2–4 hours if bleeding is severe.
Contraindications: See ergotamine.
Precautions: See ergotamine.

Generic Name: METHYLSERGIDE MALEATE
Trade Name: Sansert
Dosage Forms: Tablets, 2 mg.
Uses: Serotonin antagonist for prevention and reduction in frequency of vascular headaches (severe and/or uncontrollable ones that necessitate prophylaxis).
Adult Dosage (Oral): 4–8 mg q.d. with meals (divided doses).
Contraindications: See ergotamine. Also pulmonary disease, collagen or fibrotic disease, valvular heart disease.
Precautions: With long-term uninterrupted treatment, retroperitoneal and pleuropulmonary fibrosis, fibrotic thickening of cardiac valves and murmurs may occur. Continuous administration should not exceed 6 months, with 3–4 weeks of no drug every 6 months.
Adverse Reactions: Cold, numb extremities, leg cramps, girdle and flank pain, urinary obstruction, nausea, vomiting, diarrhea, CNS changes, edema, and flushing.

Generic Name: OXYTOCIN
Trade Names: Pitocin, Syntocinon

Dosage Forms: Injection (IM/IV) 5 units (5,000 milliunits)/0.5 cc, 10 units (10,000 milliunits)/1 cc.
Uses: Oxytocic agent to induce or stimulate labor. Also used postpartum to prevent or control hemorrhage.
Adult Dosage (Parenteral): For labor induction, 10 units diluted in 1,000 cc D_5W and administered via infusion pump at 0.2–4 milliunits/min., until uterine response evaluated (optimum response, three or four good quality contractions in 10 min.). To prevent postpartum hemorrhage, 0.6–1.8 units (0.06–0.18 cc) diluted in 3–5 cc normal saline and injected slowly, IV; alternatively, 3–10 units (0.3–1 cc) administered IM.
Contraindications: Any contraindication to induction of labor.
Precautions: Hyperstimulation of uterus during labor may lead to uterine tetany (discontinue oxytocin stat). Concurrent administration of vasopressors may cause severe hypertension and cerebral hemorrhage.
Adverse Reactions: Severe water intoxication with convulsions and coma may occur with IV rates exceeding 20 milliunits/min. Hypertensive episodes, subarachnoid hemorrhage, rupture of uterus, anaphylactic reactions, and fetal arrhythmias may occur.
Drug Interaction: Vasopressors (such as vasoconstrictors in anesthetics used for caudal block) may produce severe hypertension.

Generic Name: CONJUGATED ESTROGENS
Trade Name: Premarin
Dosage Forms: Tablets, 0.3 mg, 0.625 mg, 1.25 mg, 2.5 mg; injection (IV), 25 mg.
Uses: Estrogen replacement therapy in menopause, dysfunctional uterine bleeding, prostatic carcinoma, estrogen deficiency, osteoporosis. Parenterally, used for emergency treatment of dysfunctional uterine bleeding.
Adult Dosage (Oral): In menopause, 0.3–1.25 mg q.d. or cyclicly.
Adult Dosage (Parenteral): For emergency uterine bleeding, 25 mg slow IV stat, then 25 mg q. 6–12 hours p.r.n. (given slowly to prevent flushing).
Contraindications: Known or suspected breast cancer if estrogen-dependent neoplasms suspected. Pregnancy. History of thrombophlebitic disorders or active thrombophlebitis. Undiagnosed abnormal vaginal bleeding.
Precautions: Renal or hepatic disease, metastatic bone cancer associated with hypercalcemia. Possible increased risk of gallbladder disease or malignant neoplasms. Hypertension, fluid retention, thromboembolism are all exacerbated.
Adverse Reactions: Nausea, vomiting, abdominal cramps, breakthrough bleeding, amenorrhea, breast enlargement, migraine headaches, cholestatic jaundice, edema, dermatologic changes, mental depression, steepening of corneal curvature, intolerance to contact lenses.
Drug Interactions: With oral anticoagulants, decreased anticoagulant effect. With tricyclic antidepressants, increased antidepressant side-effects.

HEMATINICS

Generic Name: FERROUS SULFATE
Dosage Forms: Tablets, 325 mg (containing 33 mg elemental iron, but other strengths available); elixir, 300 mg/5 cc (other strengths available).
Uses: Treatment of iron-deficient anemia.
Adult Dosage (Oral): 2–3 mg/kg/day elemental iron (usually 325 mg ferrous sulfate t.i.d.). After hemoglobin normalized, treatment continued for 3 months more.
Pediatric Dosage (Oral): For deficiency in a child, 4–6 mg/kg/day elemental iron in divided doses. For prophylaxis, 1 mg/kg/day elemental iron.
Contraindications: Hemochromatosis, hemosiderosis, hemolytic anemias, peptic ulcer, regional enteritis, ulcerative colitis.

Precautions: Liver disease. Gastric upset can be minimized by taking with small amounts of food. Both oral and parenteral effects slow to appear; (hemoglobin increase may take 2 weeks.) Severe, acute poisoning occurs frequently in children.
Adverse Reactions: Gastric irritation, black tarry stools, constipation, diarrhea, stained teeth (with liquid forms). Toxic dose for adult approximately 50 gm of ferrous sulfate. Toxic dose for children is 1 gm or more. Overdoses are treated with deferoxamine.
Drug Interactions: Vitamin C increases iron absorption. Food and antacids decrease absorption. Tetracycline chelated by iron and tetracycline absorption decreased. Allopurinol increases hepatic concentration of iron.

MISCELLANEOUS AGENTS FOR OVERDOSE TREATMENT

Generic Name: AMYL NITRITE
Trade Name: Amyl Nitrite
Dosage Forms: Vaporoles for inhalation (0.3 cc).
Uses: For inhalation. Used in preliminary treatment of cyanide and thiocyanate poisoning. Also used as antianginal agent.
Adult Dosage: One vaporole administered by inhalation for 15–30 sec. of every minute while sodium nitrite solution is being prepared for IV administration.

Generic Name: DEFEROXAMINE
Trade Name: Desferal
Dosage Forms: Injection (IM/IV), 500 mg.
Uses: Iron-chelating agent for treatment of iron intoxication.
Adult Dosage (Parenteral): 5–10 gm/50–100 cc normal saline via nasogastric tube or Ewald tube, followed by 1 gm IM or IV. Then, 500 mg IM or slow IV q. 4 hours for two doses. Depending on clinical response, subsequent doses of 500 mg may be given q. 4–12 hours. (Maximum dose, 6 gm/24 hours.)
Pediatric Dosage (Parenteral): 20 mg/kg IM or slow IV, then 10 mg/kg q. 4 hours for two doses (or q. 4–12 hours if needed).
Contraindications: Severe renal disease or anuria.
Precautions: Gastric aspiration should be done first, then a lavage with 1% sodium bicarbonate to form insoluble iron carbonates. Deferoxamine will turn urine red. Slow IV infusion not to exceed 15 mg/kg/hour.
Adverse Reactions: Too rapid IV infusion causes histamine release with erythema, urticaria, hypotension, shock. Also pain and induration at injection site.

Generic Name: NALOXONE HCl
Trade Name: Narcan
Dosage Forms: Injection (IM/IV/subcutaneous), 0.4 mg/cc, 0.02 mg/cc (neonatal).

Uses: Narcotic antagonist. Treatment of narcotic-induced respiratory depression. Also effective in respiratory depression due to pentazocine, propoxyphene, diphenoxylate, and possibly diazepam.
Adult Dosage (Parenteral): Usual 0.4 mg (1 cc) IV, IM, or subcutaneously. May be repeated at 2- to 3-min. intervals p.r.n.
Pediatric Dosage (Parenteral): 0.01 mg/kg IV, IM, or subcutaneously. May be repeated in 2–3 min. (until 0.1 mg/kg has been used).
Precautions: Ineffective in respiratory depression not due to narcotics (e.g., barbiturates, cocaine). If no improvement seen after 2–3 hours, another etiology must be suspected.
Adverse Reactions: In absence of narcotic, naloxone has no activity of its own. Rarely, nausea, vomiting, hypertension, tachycardia, pulmonary edema, ventricular arrhythmias have been reported in patients with coronary artery disease.

Generic Name: LACTULOSE
Trade Names: Chronolac, Cephulac
Dosage Forms: Oral syrup, 10 gm/15 cc.
Uses: Laxative. Also used for prevention and adjunctive treatment of portal-systemic encephalopathy, including hepatic coma and precoma.
Adult Dosage (Oral): For hepatic encephalopathy, 30–45 cc t.i.d. or q.i.d. (20–30 gm), dose adjusted q. 1–2 days p.r.n. to provide two or three soft stools daily. For acute portal-systemic encephalopathy, 30–45 cc q. 1–2 hours until laxative effect. As a laxative, 15–30 cc q.d. (up to 60 cc/day). (*Note:* May also be given as a retention enema of 300 cc lactulose and 700 cc water to be retained 1 hour.)
Contraindications: Low galactose diets (syrup contains galactose).
Precautions: Diabetics (syrup contains sugars).
Adverse Reactions: Flatulence, cramps, nausea, diarrhea.

Generic Name: PHYSOSTIGMINE
Trade Name: Antilirium
Dosage Forms: Injection (IV), 2 mg ampules.
Uses: Cholinesterase inhibitor. Treatment of anticholinergic overdoses.
Adult Dosage (Parenteral): Initially, 2 mg slow IV over 2 min. May be repeated with 1–2 mg until positive response or cholinergic signs develop.
Pediatric Dosage (Parenteral): Initially, 0.5 mg slow IV over 2 min. May be repeated with 0.5 mg IV q. 5 min. until positive response or cholinergic signs develop (maximum, 2 mg).
Precautions: Bronchial asthma. Repeated doses may be necessary if patients are experiencing seizures, arrhythmias, hypertension.
Adverse Reactions: Seizures, cholinergic crisis, severe bradycardia, arrhythmias if used with vasopressors. (Antidote: atropine in dose of 50% of injected amount of physostigmine.)

Generic Name: SODIUM NITRITE IV
Trade Name: Sodium Nitrite (contained in Cyanide Antidote Package)
Dosage Forms: Injection (IV), 300 mg/10 cc (3%), 2 vials/package.
Uses: Treatment of cyanide and thiocyanate poisoning.
Adult Dosage (Parenteral): To be given *before* the sodium thiosulfate solution: 10 cc (300 mg 3% solution) slow IV push over 2–4 min. Then, leaving needle in place, the sodium thiosulfate infusion is begun immediately.

Generic Name: SODIUM POLYSTYRENE SULFONATE
Trade Name: Kayexalate
Dosage Form: Powder, for oral or rectal use.
Uses: Ion exchange resin for treatment of hyperkalemia; exchanges approximately 1 mEq potassium/gm resin.
Adult Dosage: 15–40 gm q.i.d. suspended in sorbitol solution or as a rectal enema, 30–50 gm Kayexalate with equal amounts of sorbitol in 150–200 cc water. Should be retained for 45 min.–4 hours and may be repeated once or twice.
Precautions: Slow effect (hours). Should not be used alone in emergency situations. Is not selective for potassium; also binds calcium and magnesium. Caution in patients who cannot tolerate sodium load.
Adverse Reactions: Anorexia, nausea, vomiting, gastric irritation, and fecal impaction when given orally. Latter avoided by rectal use and addition of sorbitol to solutions.

Generic Name: SODIUM THIOSULFATE IV
Trade Name: Contained in Cyanide Antidote Package
Dosage Forms: Injection (IV), 12.5 gm/50 cc (25%), 2 vials/package.
Uses: Treatment of cyanide and thiocyanate poisoning.
Adult Dosage (Parenteral): 12.5 gm (50 cc of 25% solution) over 10 min., slow IV push. (To be given immediately *after* the sodium nitrite solution, with the same needle left in patient's arm). If symptoms recur, regimen may be repeated with half-doses of sodium nitrite and sodium thiosulfate.

BIBLIOGRAPHY

Eisenberg MS, and Copass MK (eds): *Manual of Emergency Medical Therapeutics.* Philadelphia, WB Saunders Co, 1978.

Geffner ES (ed): *The Hospital Pharmacy Compendium of Drug Therapy.* New York, Biomedical Information Corporation, 1981.

Hansten PD: *Drug Interactions,* ed 3. Philadelphia, Lea & Febiger, 1976.

Heinemann CJ: *Emergency Drug Reference.* Kettering, Ohio, Kettering Medical Center, 1981.

Knoben JE, Anderson PO, Watanabe AS: *Handbook of Clinical Drug Data,* ed 4. Hamilton, Ill, Drug Intelligence Publications, Inc, 1978.

Phillips RE, Feeney MK: *The Cardiac Rhythms: A Systematic Approach to Interpretation.* Philadelphia, WB Saunders Co, 1973.

Medical Letter on Drugs and Therapeutics. *Handbook of Antimicrobial Therapy,* Rev ed. New Rochelle, N Y , The Medical Letter, Inc, 1980.

Reilly MJ (ed): *The American Hospital Formulary Service.* Washington, D C , American Society of Hospital Pharmacists, 1981.

List of Pharmacologic/Therapeutic Drugs and Agents for Emergency Facilities*

Antihistamine Drugs
Diphenhydramine
(Benadryl®)
Antibiotics
Penicillins
Ampicillin
Benzathine Penicillin
Penicillin G Potassium
Penicillin G Procaine
Erythromycin
Oxacillin Sodium
Gentamicin Sulfate
Autonomic Drugs
Parasympathomimetic (Cho-
linergic) Agents
Edrophonium Chloride
(Tensilon®)
Neostigmine Methylsulfate
Physostigmine
Parasympatholytic (Cholin-
ergic Blocking) Agents
Atropine Sulfate
Sympathomimetic (Adrener-
gic) Agents
Dopamine
Epinephrine HCl
Isoproterenol HCl
Norepinephrine Bitartrate
*Blood Formation and
Coagulation*
Anticoagulants
Heparin Sodium
Anticoagulant Reversing
Agents
Protamine Sulfate
Aqueous Vitamin K
Cardiovascular Drugs
Cardiac Drugs
Sodium Bicarbonate

Calcium Chloride
Digoxin
Propranolol
Verapamil HCl
Bretylium HCl
Lidocaine
Procainamide HCl
Hypotensive Agents
Diazoxide (Hyperstat®)
Sodium Nitroprusside
(Nipride®)
Trimethaphan (Arfonad®)
Vasodilating Agents
Amyl Nitrite
Nitroglycerin

Central Nervous System Drugs
Analgesics and Antipyretics
Acetaminophen
Aspirin
Codeine
Meperidine HCl
(Demerol®)
Morphine Sulfate
Narcotic Antagonists
Naloxone (Narcan®)
Anticonvulsants
Diazepam (Valium®)
Phenobarbital
Phenytoin (Dilantin®)
Psychotherapeutic Agents
Chlorpromazine
(Thorazine®)
Diazepam
Haloperidol

Diagnostic Agents
Myasthenia Gravis
Edrophonium Chloride
Neostigmine Methylsulfate

Test tapes for urine bilirubin,
blood, sugar, ketones,
pH, urobilinogen, pro-
tein (Bili-Labstix®)
Stool Contents
Stool tests for occult blood
(Hemoccult®)
Blood Contents
Reagents for estimating
blood glucose
(Dextrostix®)
*Electrolytic, Caloric, and Water
Balance*
Replacement Solutions
Dextrose 5% with Water
Potassium Chloride
Ringer's injections,
lactated
Sodium Chloride
Diuretics
Furosemide (Lasix®)
Mannitol
Hypoglycemic Agents
Dextrose 50% in water
*Eye, Ear, Nose, and Throat
Preparations*
Local Anesthetics
Proparacaine
(Ophthaine®) ⎱
Tetracaine ⎰ either/or
(Pontocaine®)
Gastrointestinal Drugs
Adsorbents
Charcoal, activated
Emetics and Anti-Emetics
Ipecac Syrup
Prochlorperazine
(Compazine®)
Cathartics
Magnesium Salt
*Hormones and Synthetic
Substitutes*
Adrenals
Hydrocortisone (Solu-
Cortef®)

Methylprednisolone (Solu-
Medrol®)
Dexamethasone
(Decadron®)
Insulins and Antidiabetic
Agents
Glucagon HCl
Insulin, regular
Thyroid
Levothyroxine Sodium
Local Anesthetics
Lidocaine HCl
Serums, Toxoids, and Vaccines
Serums
Antivenin, Black Widow
Spider Bite, Equine Ori-
gin (geographic-area-
specific)
Antivenin, Snake-Bite,
Polyvalent, Equine
Origin (geographic-area-
specific)
Rabies Immune Globulin,
Human
Tetanus Immune Globulin
Toxoids
Diphtheria and Tetanus
Toxoids and Pertussis
Vaccine Adsorbed
Tetanus and Diphtheria
Toxoids Adsorbed, adult
and pediatric
Tetanus Toxoid Adsorbed

Spasmolytics
Parenteral
Aminophylline
Terbutaline Sulfate
Inhalation
Metaproterenol Sulfate

Vitamins
Vitamin B Complex
Thiamine HCl

Unclassified Agents
Cyanide Antidote Kit

* Common trade names have been selectively mentioned for purposes of clarification. This is not to be construed as any form of
endorsement.

* Reprinted from *Annals of Emergency Medicine* with permission,
© copyright 1982.

<h1>Index</h1>